Plain English Descriptions for
Procedures

2017

2017 Plain English Descriptions for Procedures

Published by DecisionHealth
9737 Washingtonian Blvd., Suite 502
Gaithersburg, MD 20878-7364
1-855-885-5341

Copyright © 2017 DecisionHealth
All rights reserved

Printed in the United States of America

ISBN: 978-1-58383-869-3

Item ID: MPB-PEDCPT-17

Acknowledgements

Tonya Nevin, *Vice-President, Medical Group Practice*
Lori Becks, RHIA, *Clinical Technical Editor*
Michelle L. Suitor, CPC, *Clinical Technical Editor*
Juli Folk, *Books Manager*
Bradley Clark, *Illustrator*
Jonus Croft, *Illustrator*
Marquia Parnell, *Desktop Publisher*

Contents

Introduction

The *Plain English Descriptions for Procedures* was created to provide the coder with an accurate clinical description of each CPT® code, written in plain English that can be understood by everyone. Billing accuracy can be greatly increased when the coder fully understands the medical relevance of assigned CPT codes for billing purposes, which can save both time and money.

Format

Plain English Descriptions for Procedures is presented in a two column format with sequential code descriptions presented for a single code standing alone or for a logical grouping of codes. The CPT code(s) is given, followed by the code description, and the Plain English Descriptions in plain English terms. Reading the entire lay description will help ensure the best possible code choice. Chapter headers and individual page ends identify the chapter and code ranges to provide a quick reference guide. The chapter divisions in the *Plain English Descriptions for Procedures* correspond to CPT chapters.

Plain English Descriptions for Procedures also contains a listing of prefixes and suffixes found in general medical terminology. A section of anatomy charts is also included.

Plain English Descriptions for Procedures will be most useful if used in conjunction with the official CPT code book and a comprehensive medical dictionary. Using all of these resources in tandem will enable the coder to make the most accurate code selection.

Illustrations have been included at the code level to enable the coder to more efficiently identify and locate body systems/parts.

Please note: In 2017, the codes that were previously included in Appendix G of the AMA's Current Procedural Terminology (CPT®) were revised with the removal of the moderate (conscious) sedation symbol. Those codes are not marked as revised in this publication unless additional revisions to the code or descriptions were indicated. For information/guidance on reporting moderate (conscious) sedation services, please refer to the official guidelines in your 2017 AMA CPT® code book.)

Prefixes and Suffixes

Prefixes and suffixes are elements used in medical terminology that consist of one or more syllables placed before or after root words to show various kinds of relationships. Prefixes come before the root word and suffixes come after the root word. They are never used independently but function to modify the meaning. Many prefixes and suffixes are added to other words with a hyphen, but medical dictionary publishers are opting to drop the hyphen on many of the more commonly prefixed medical words.

Examples:

Prefixes
micro = small
peri = surrounding

Suffixes
algia = pain
an = pertaining to

The following are lists of prefixes and suffixes typically seen in medical terminology.

Prefixes

a(d)-	towards
a(n)-	without
ab-	from
ab(s)-	away from
ad-	towards
allo-	other, another
ambi-	both
amphi-	on both sides, around
ana-	up to, back, again, movement from
aniso-	different, unequal
ante-	before, forwards
anti-	against, opposite
ap-, apo-	from, back, again
bi(s)-	twice, double
bio-	life
brachy-	short
cata-	down
circum-	around
con-	together
contra-	against
cyte-	cell
de-	from, away from, down from
deca-	ten
di(s)-	two
dia-	through, complete
di(a)s	separation
diplo-	double
dolicho-	long
dur-	hard, firm
dys-	bad, abnormal
e-, ec-	out, from out of
ecto-	outside, external
ek-	out
em-	in
en-	into
endo-	into
ent-	within
epi-	on, up, against, high
eso-	will carry
eu-	well, abundant, prosperous
eury-	broad, wide
ex-, exo-	out, from out of
extra-	outside, beyond, in addition
haplo-	single
hapto-	bind to
hemi-	half
hept-	seven
hetero-	different
hex-	six
homo-	same
hyper-	above, excessive
hypo-	below, deficient
im-, in-	not
in-	into, to
infra-	below, underneath
inter-	among, between
intra-	within, inside, during
intro-	inward, during
iso-	equal, same
juxta-	adjacent to
kata-	down, down from
macro-	large
magno-	large
medi-	middle
mega-	large
megalo-	very large
meso-	middle
meta-	beyond, between
micro-	small
neo-	new
non-	not
ob-	before, against
octa-	eight
octo-	eight
oligo-	few
pachy-	thick

pan-	all
para-	beside, to the side of, wrong
pent-	five
per-	by, through, throughout
peri-	around, round-about
pleo-	more than usual
poly	many
post-	behind, after
pre-	before, in front, very
pros-	besides
prox-	besides
pseudo-	false, fake
quar(r)-	four
re, red-	back, again
retro-	backwards, behind
semi-	half
sex-	six
sept-	seven
sub-	under, beneath
super-	above, in addition, over
supra-	above, on the upper side
syn-	together, with
sys-	together, with
tetra-	four
thio-	sulfur
trans-	across, beyond
tri-	three
uni-	one
ultra-	beyond, besides, over

Suffixes

-ase	fermenter
-ate	do
-cide	killer
-c(o)ele	cavity, hollow
-ectomy	removal of, cut out

-form	shaped like
-ia	got
-iasis	full of
-ile	little version
-illa	little version
-illus	little version
-in	stuff
-ism	theory, characteristic of
-itis	inflammation
-ity	makes a noun of quality
-ium	thing
-ize	do
-logy	study of, reasoning about
-megaly	large
-noid	mind, spirit
-oid	resembling, image of
-ogen	precursor
-ol(e)	alcohol
-ole	little version
-oma	tumor (usually)
-osis	full of
-ostomy	"mouth-cut"
-pathy	disease of, suffering
-penia	lack
-pexy	fix in place
-plasty	re-shaping
-philia	affection for
-rhage	burst out
-rhea	discharge, flowing out
-rhexis	shredding
-pagus	Siamese twins
-sis	idea (makes a noun, typically abstract)
-thrix	hair
-tomy	cut
-ule	little version
-um	thing (makes a noun, typically abstract)

Anatomy

The Right Eye
(Transverse Section)

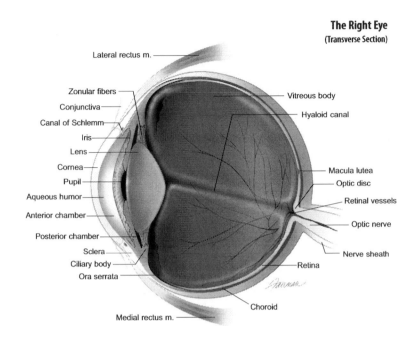

Lateral rectus m.
Zonular fibers
Conjunctiva
Canal of Schlemm
Iris
Lens
Cornea
Pupil
Aqueous humor
Anterior chamber
Posterior chamber
Sclera
Ciliary body
Ora serrata
Medial rectus m.

Vitreous body
Hyaloid canal
Macula lutea
Optic disc
Retinal vessels
Optic nerve
Nerve sheath
Retina
Choroid

The Right Ear

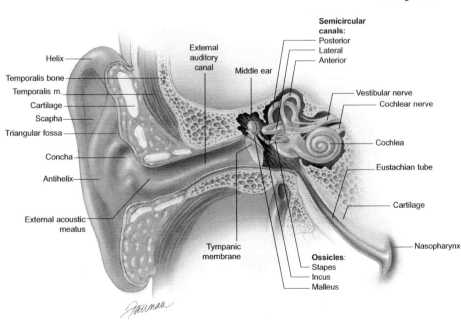

Helix
Temporalis bone
Temporalis m.
Cartilage
Scapha
Triangular fossa
Concha
Antihelix
External acoustic meatus

External auditory canal
Middle ear
Tympanic membrane

Semicircular canals:
Posterior
Lateral
Anterior

Vestibular nerve
Cochlear nerve
Cochlea
Eustachian tube
Cartilage
Nasopharynx

Ossicles:
Stapes
Incus
Malleus

Anatomy

Female Figure
(Anterior View)

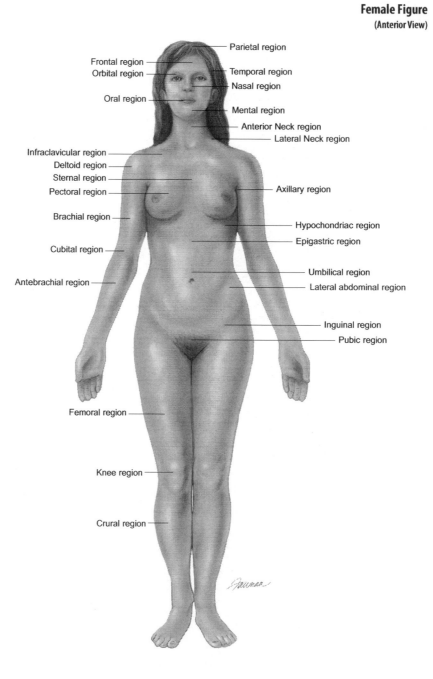

Parietal region
Frontal region
Orbital region
Temporal region
Nasal region
Oral region
Mental region
Anterior Neck region
Lateral Neck region
Infraclavicular region
Deltoid region
Sternal region
Pectoral region
Axillary region
Brachial region
Hypochondriac region
Epigastric region
Cubital region
Antebrachial region
Umbilical region
Lateral abdominal region
Inguinal region
Pubic region
Femoral region
Knee region
Crural region

© Fairman Studios, LLC, 2002. All Rights Reserved.

Female Breast

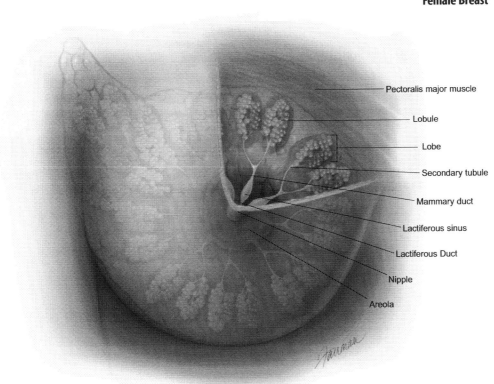

Pectoralis major muscle
Lobule
Lobe
Secondary tubule
Mammary duct
Lactiferous sinus
Lactiferous Duct
Nipple
Areola

Brain
(Inferior View)

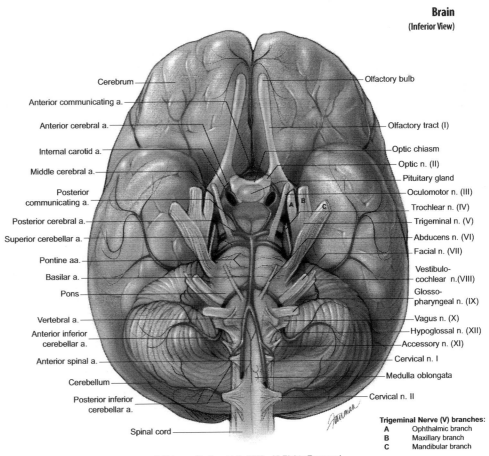

Cerebrum
Anterior communicating a.
Anterior cerebral a.
Internal carotid a.
Middle cerebral a.
Posterior communicating a.
Posterior cerebral a.
Superior cerebellar a.
Pontine aa.
Basilar a.
Pons
Vertebral a.
Anterior inferior cerebellar a.
Anterior spinal a.
Cerebellum
Posterior inferior cerebellar a.
Spinal cord

Olfactory bulb
Olfactory tract (I)
Optic chiasm
Optic n. (II)
Pituitary gland
Oculomotor n. (III)
Trochlear n. (IV)
Trigeminal n. (V)
Abducens n. (VI)
Facial n. (VII)
Vestibulo-cochlear n.(VIII)
Glosso-pharyngeal (IX)
Vagus n. (X)
Hypoglossal n. (XII)
Accessory n. (XI)
Cervical n. I
Medulla oblongata
Cervical n. II

Trigeminal Nerve (V) branches:
A Ophthalmic branch
B Maxillary branch
C Mandibular branch

Anatomy

Muscular System
(Anterior View)

Temporalis m.

Orbicularis oculi m.

Masseter m.

Buccinator m.

Sternocleidomastoid m.

Trapezius m.

Deltoid m.

Pectoralis major m.

Serratus anterior m.

Biceps brachii m.

Brachialis m.

External abdominal oblique m.

Brachioradialis m.

Extensor carpi radialis longus m.

Palmaris longus m.

Flexor carpi radialis m.

Superficial inguinal ring

Tensor fasciae latae m.

Sartorius m.

Adductor longus m.

Rectus femoris m.

Vastus lateralis m.

Iliotibial tract

Vastus medialis m.

Gracilis m.

Lateral patellar retinaculum

Tibialis anterior m.

Gastrocnemius m.

Peronius longus m.

Peronius brevis m.

Soleus m.

Extensor digitorum longus m.

Extensor hallucis longus m.

Extensor hallucis brevis m.

Frontalis m.

Zygomaticus minor m.

Zygomaticus major m.

Orbicularis oris m.

Depressor anguli oris m.

Levator scapulae m.

Pectoralis minor m.

Internal intercostal mm.

Coracobrachialis m.

Brachialis m.

Rectus sheath

Rectus abdominus m.

Linea alba

Internal abdominal oblique m.

Transversus abdominus m.

Palmaris longus m.

Flexor pollicis longus m.

Flexor digitorum superficialis m.

Abductor pollicis brevis m.

Flexor pollicis brevis m.

Abductor digiti minimi m.

Iliopsoas m.

Pectineus m.

Adductor brevis m.

Adductor magnus m.

Vastus lateralis m.

Vastus medialis m.

Patella

Patellar ligament

Medial patellar retinaculum

Tibia

Flexor digitorum longus m.

Abductor hallucis m.

Anatomy

Muscular System
(Posterior View)

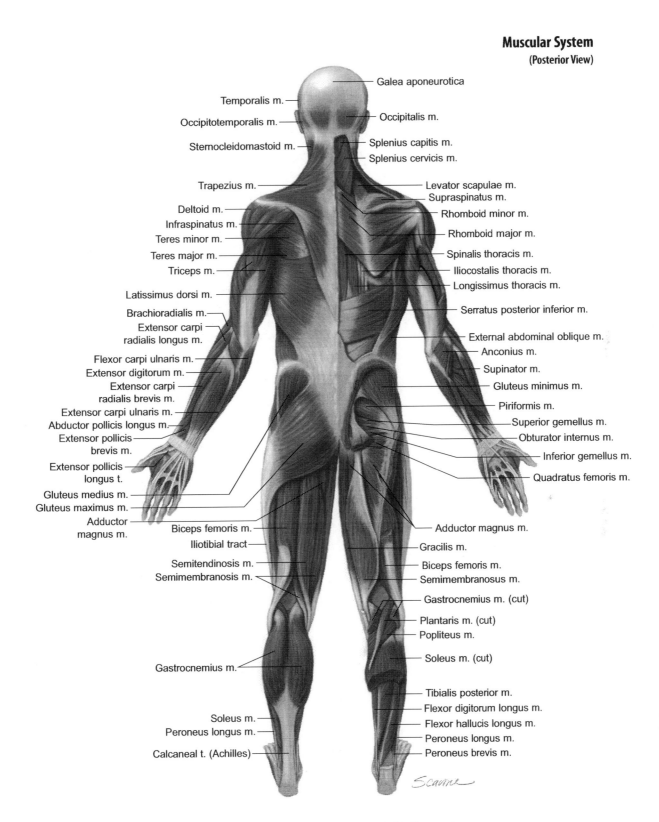

Galea aponeurotica

Temporalis m.

Occipitotemporalis m.

Occipitalis m.

Sternocleidomastoid m.

Splenius capitis m.

Splenius cervicis m.

Trapezius m.

Levator scapulae m.

Supraspinatus m.

Deltoid m.

Rhomboid minor m.

Infraspinatus m.

Teres minor m.

Rhomboid major m.

Teres major m.

Spinalis thoracis m.

Triceps m.

Iliocostalis thoracis m.

Longissimus thoracis m.

Latissimus dorsi m.

Serratus posterior inferior m.

Brachioradialis m.

Extensor carpi radialis longus m.

External abdominal oblique m.

Anconius m.

Flexor carpi ulnaris m.

Supinator m.

Extensor digitorum m.

Gluteus minimus m.

Extensor carpi radialis brevis m.

Piriformis m.

Extensor carpi ulnaris m.

Superior gemellus m.

Abductor pollicis longus m.

Obturator internus m.

Extensor pollicis brevis m.

Inferior gemellus m.

Extensor pollicis longus t.

Quadratus femoris m.

Gluteus medius m.

Gluteus maximus m.

Adductor magnus m.

Biceps femoris m.

Adductor magnus m.

Iliotibial tract

Gracilis m.

Semitendinosis m.

Biceps femoris m.

Semimembranosis m.

Semimembranosus m.

Gastrocnemius m. (cut)

Plantaris m. (cut)

Popliteus m.

Soleus m. (cut)

Gastrocnemius m.

Tibialis posterior m.

Flexor digitorum longus m.

Flexor hallucis longus m.

Soleus m.

Peroneus longus m.

Peroneus longus m.

Peroneus brevis m.

Calcaneal t. (Achilles)

Anatomy

Skeletal System
(Anterior View)

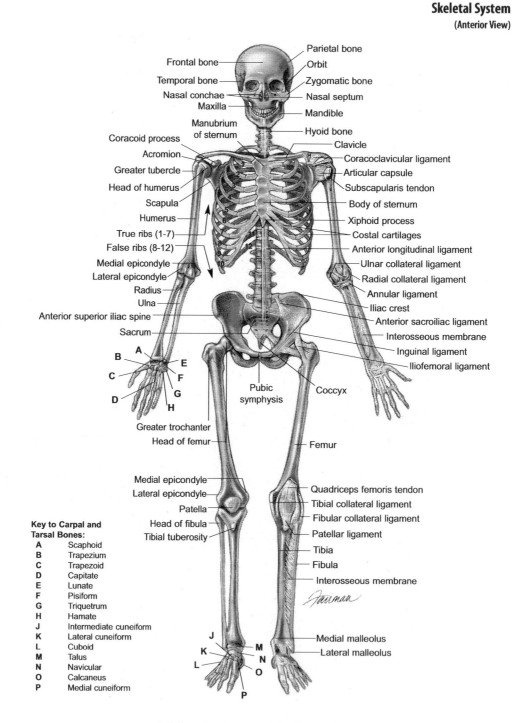

Parietal bone
Frontal bone
Orbit
Temporal bone
Zygomatic bone
Nasal conchae
Nasal septum
Maxilla
Mandible
Manubrium of sternum
Hyoid bone
Coracoid process
Clavicle
Acromion
Coracoclavicular ligament
Greater tubercle
Articular capsule
Head of humerus
Subscapularis tendon
Scapula
Body of sternum
Humerus
Xiphoid process
True ribs (1-7)
Costal cartilages
False ribs (8-12)
Anterior longitudinal ligament
Medial epicondyle
Ulnar collateral ligament
Lateral epicondyle
Radial collateral ligament
Radius
Annular ligament
Ulna
Iliac crest
Anterior superior iliac spine
Anterior sacroiliac ligament
Sacrum
Interosseous membrane
Inguinal ligament
Iliofemoral ligament
A
B
E
C
F
G
D
Pubic symphysis
Coccyx
H
Greater trochanter
Head of femur
Femur
Medial epicondyle
Quadriceps femoris tendon
Lateral epicondyle
Tibial collateral ligament
Patella
Fibular collateral ligament
Head of fibula
Patellar ligament
Tibial tuberosity
Tibia
Fibula
Interosseous membrane
Medial malleolus
Lateral malleolus
J
K
M
L
N
O
P

Key to Carpal and Tarsal Bones:

A	Scaphoid
B	Trapezium
C	Trapezoid
D	Capitate
E	Lunate
F	Pisiform
G	Triquetrum
H	Hamate
J	Intermediate cuneiform
K	Lateral cuneiform
L	Cuboid
M	Talus
N	Navicular
O	Calcaneus
P	Medial cuneiform

Anatomy

Skeletal System
(Posterior View)

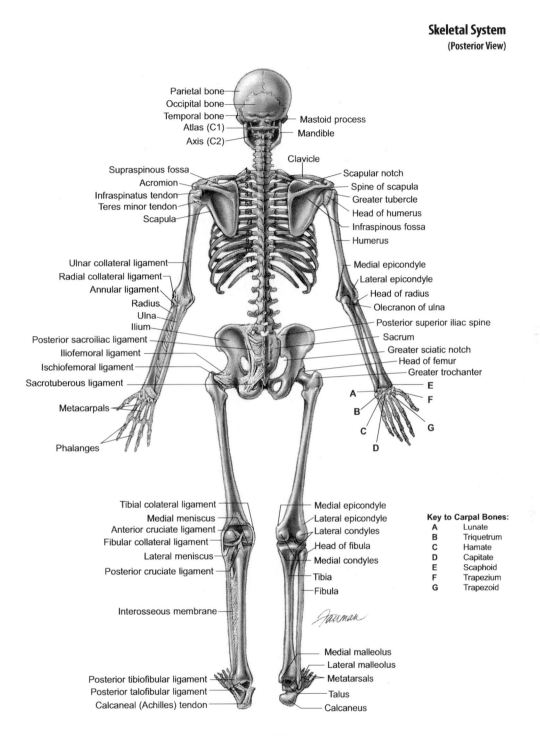

Parietal bone
Occipital bone
Temporal bone
Atlas (C1)
Axis (C2)
Mastoid process
Mandible
Clavicle
Supraspinous fossa
Acromion
Infraspinatus tendon
Teres minor tendon
Scapula
Scapular notch
Spine of scapula
Greater tubercle
Head of humerus
Infraspinous fossa
Humerus
Ulnar collateral ligament
Radial collateral ligament
Annular ligament
Radius
Ulna
Ilium
Posterior sacroiliac ligament
Iliofemoral ligament
Ischiofemoral ligament
Sacrotuberous ligament
Metacarpals
Phalanges
Medial epicondyle
Lateral epicondyle
Head of radius
Olecranon of ulna
Posterior superior iliac spine
Sacrum
Greater sciatic notch
Head of femur
Greater trochanter
E
F
A
B
C
G
D

Tibial colateral ligament
Medial meniscus
Anterior cruciate ligament
Fibular collateral ligament
Lateral meniscus
Posterior cruciate ligament
Medial epicondyle
Lateral epicondyle
Lateral condyles
Head of fibula
Medial condyles
Tibia
Fibula

Key to Carpal Bones:
A Lunate
B Triquetrum
C Hamate
D Capitate
E Scaphoid
F Trapezium
G Trapezoid

Interosseous membrane

Posterior tibiofibular ligament
Posterior talofibular ligament
Calcaneal (Achilles) tendon

Medial malleolus
Lateral malleolus
Metatarsals
Talus
Calcaneus

Anatomy

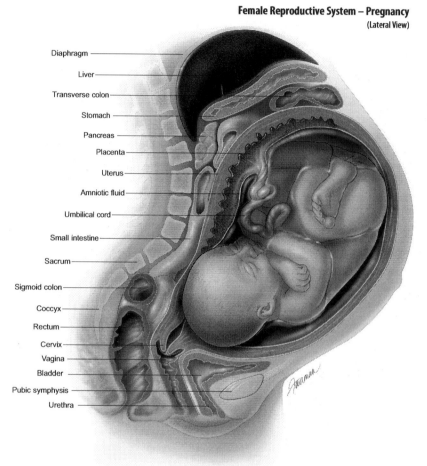

Female Reproductive System – Pregnancy
(Lateral View)

Diaphragm

Liver

Transverse colon

Stomach

Pancreas

Placenta

Uterus

Amniotic fluid

Umbilical cord

Small intestine

Sacrum

Sigmoid colon

Coccyx

Rectum

Cervix

Vagina

Bladder

Pubic symphysis

Urethra

Anatomy

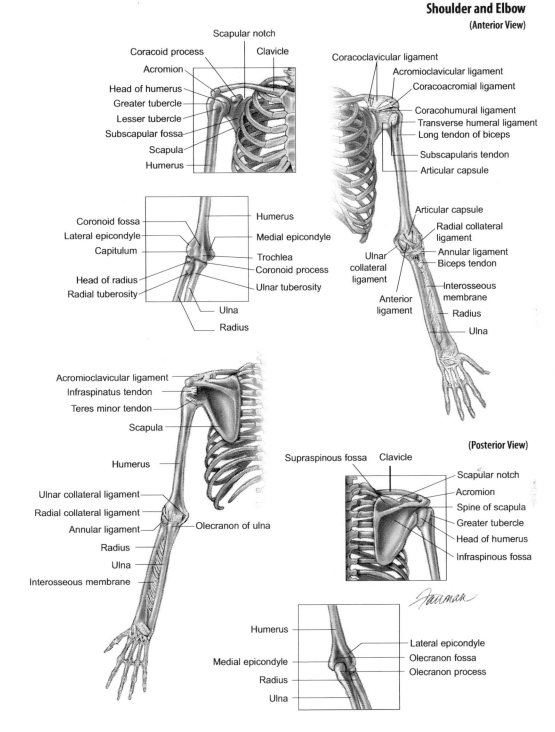

Shoulder and Elbow
(Anterior View)

Scapular notch
Coracoid process
Acromion
Head of humerus
Greater tubercle
Lesser tubercle
Subscapular fossa
Scapula
Humerus
Clavicle

Coracoclavicular ligament
Acromioclavicular ligament
Coracoacromial ligament
Coracohumural ligament
Transverse humeral ligament
Long tendon of biceps
Subscapularis tendon
Articular capsule

Coronoid fossa
Lateral epicondyle
Capitulum
Head of radius
Radial tuberosity
Humerus
Medial epicondyle
Trochlea
Coronoid process
Ulnar tuberosity
Ulna
Radius

Articular capsule
Radial collateral ligament
Annular ligament
Biceps tendon
Interosseous membrane
Radius
Ulna
Ulnar collateral ligament
Anterior ligament

Acromioclavicular ligament
Infraspinatus tendon
Teres minor tendon
Scapula
Humerus
Ulnar collateral ligament
Radial collateral ligament
Annular ligament
Radius
Ulna
Interosseous membrane
Olecranon of ulna

(Posterior View)

Supraspinous fossa
Clavicle
Scapular notch
Acromion
Spine of scapula
Greater tubercle
Head of humerus
Infraspinous fossa

Humerus
Medial epicondyle
Radius
Ulna
Lateral epicondyle
Olecranon fossa
Olecranon process

© Fairman Studios, LLC, 2002. All Rights Reserved.

Anatomy

Musculoskeletal System – Hand and Wrist
(Dorsal and Palmar Views)

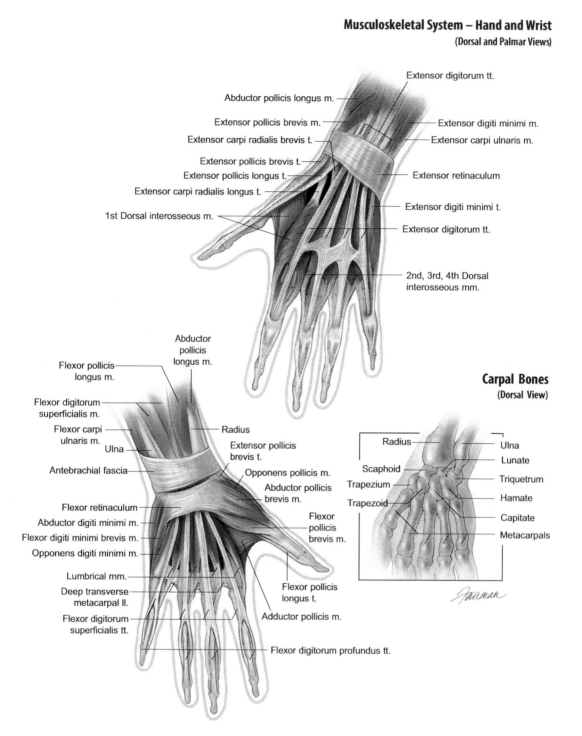

Extensor digitorum tt.

Abductor pollicis longus m.

Extensor pollicis brevis m.

Extensor carpi radialis brevis t.

Extensor digiti minimi m.

Extensor carpi ulnaris m.

Extensor pollicis brevis t.

Extensor pollicis longus t.

Extensor carpi radialis longus t.

Extensor retinaculum

1st Dorsal interosseous m.

Extensor digiti minimi t.

Extensor digitorum tt.

2nd, 3rd, 4th Dorsal interosseous mm.

Abductor pollicis longus m.

Flexor pollicis longus m.

Carpal Bones
(Dorsal View)

Flexor digitorum superficialis m.

Flexor carpi ulnaris m.

Radius

Ulna

Extensor pollicis brevis t.

Antebrachial fascia

Opponens pollicis m.

Abductor pollicis brevis m.

Flexor retinaculum

Abductor digiti minimi m.

Flexor digiti minimi brevis m.

Opponens digiti minimi m.

Flexor pollicis brevis m.

Lumbrical mm.

Deep transverse metacarpal ll.

Flexor digitorum superficialis tt.

Flexor pollicis longus t.

Adductor pollicis m.

Flexor digitorum profundus tt.

Radius

Ulna

Lunate

Scaphoid

Triquetrum

Trapezium

Hamate

Trapezoid

Capitate

Metacarpals

Musculoskeletal System – Hip and Knee
(Anterior and Posterior Views)

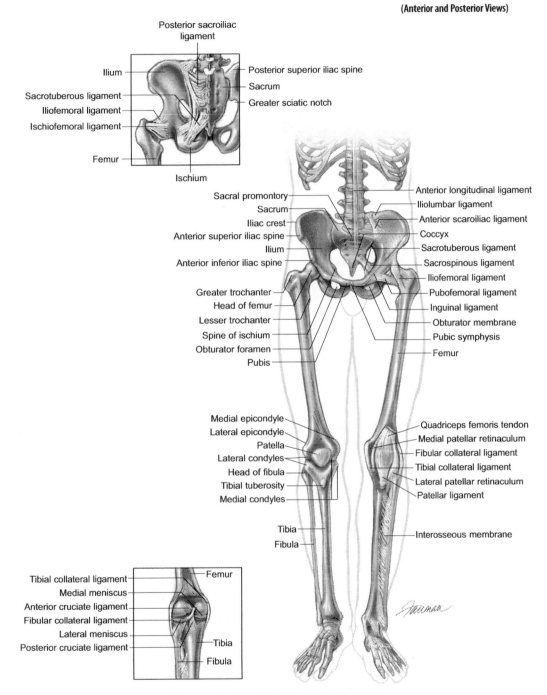

Posterior sacroiliac ligament
Ilium
Sacrotuberous ligament
Iliofemoral ligament
Ischiofemoral ligament
Femur
Ischium
Posterior superior iliac spine
Sacrum
Greater sciatic notch

Sacral promontory
Sacrum
Iliac crest
Anterior superior iliac spine
Ilium
Anterior inferior iliac spine
Greater trochanter
Head of femur
Lesser trochanter
Spine of ischium
Obturator foramen
Pubis

Anterior longitudinal ligament
Iliolumbar ligament
Anterior scaroiliac ligament
Coccyx
Sacrotuberous ligament
Sacrospinous ligament
Iliofemoral ligament
Pubofemoral ligament
Inguinal ligament
Obturator membrane
Pubic symphysis
Femur

Medial epicondyle
Lateral epicondyle
Patella
Lateral condyles
Head of fibula
Tibial tuberosity
Medial condyles
Tibia
Fibula

Quadriceps femoris tendon
Medial patellar retinaculum
Fibular collateral ligament
Tibial collateral ligament
Lateral patellar retinaculum
Patellar ligament
Interosseous membrane

Tibial collateral ligament
Medial meniscus
Anterior cruciate ligament
Fibular collateral ligament
Lateral meniscus
Posterior cruciate ligament
Femur
Tibia
Fibula

Anatomy

Musculoskeletal System – Foot and Ankle

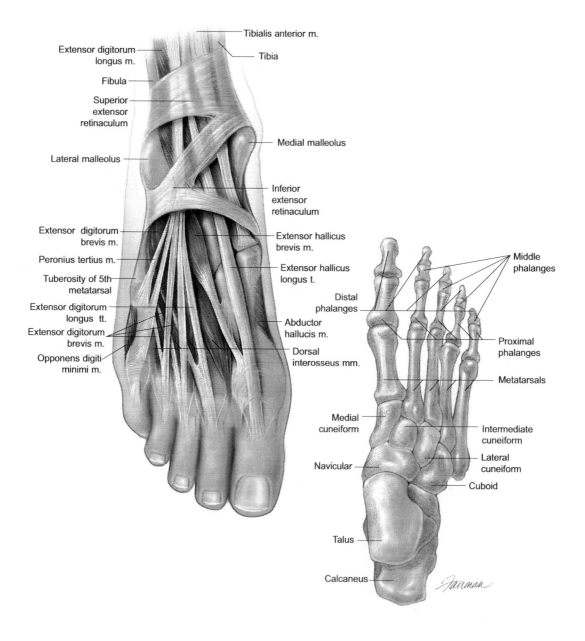

Tibialis anterior m.

Extensor digitorum longus m.

Tibia

Fibula

Superior extensor retinaculum

Medial malleolus

Lateral malleolus

Inferior extensor retinaculum

Extensor digitorum brevis m.

Extensor hallicus brevis m.

Peronius tertius m.

Extensor hallicus longus t.

Tuberosity of 5th metatarsal

Extensor digitorum longus tt.

Abductor hallucis m.

Extensor digitorum brevis m.

Dorsal interosseus mm.

Opponens digiti minimi m.

Middle phalanges

Distal phalanges

Proximal phalanges

Metatarsals

Medial cuneiform

Intermediate cuneiform

Navicular

Lateral cuneiform

Cuboid

Talus

Calcaneus

Vascular System

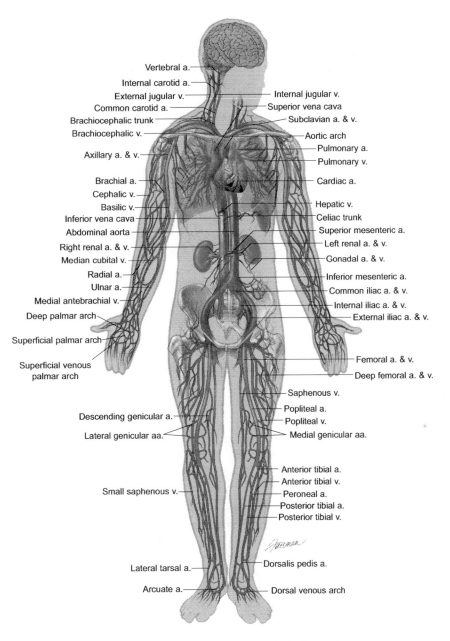

Vertebral a.
Internal carotid a.
External jugular v.
Common carotid a.
Brachiocephalic trunk
Brachiocephalic v.
Axillary a. & v.
Brachial a.
Cephalic v.
Basilic v.
Inferior vena cava
Abdominal aorta
Right renal a. & v.
Median cubital v.
Radial a.
Ulnar a.
Medial antebrachial v.
Deep palmar arch
Superficial palmar arch
Superficial venous palmar arch

Internal jugular v.
Superior vena cava
Subclavian a. & v.
Aortic arch
Pulmonary a.
Pulmonary v.
Cardiac a.
Hepatic v.
Celiac trunk
Superior mesenteric a.
Left renal a. & v.
Gonadal a. & v.
Inferior mesenteric a.
Common iliac a. & v.
Internal iliac a. & v.
External iliac a. & v.
Femoral a. & v.
Deep femoral a. & v.
Saphenous v.
Popliteal a.
Popliteal v.
Medial genicular aa.

Descending genicular a.
Lateral genicular aa.

Anterior tibial a.
Anterior tibial v.
Peroneal a.
Posterior tibial a.
Posterior tibial v.

Small saphenous v.

Lateral tarsal a.
Arcuate a.

Dorsalis pedis a.
Dorsal venous arch

© Fairman Studios, LLC, 2002. All Rights Reserved.

Anatomy

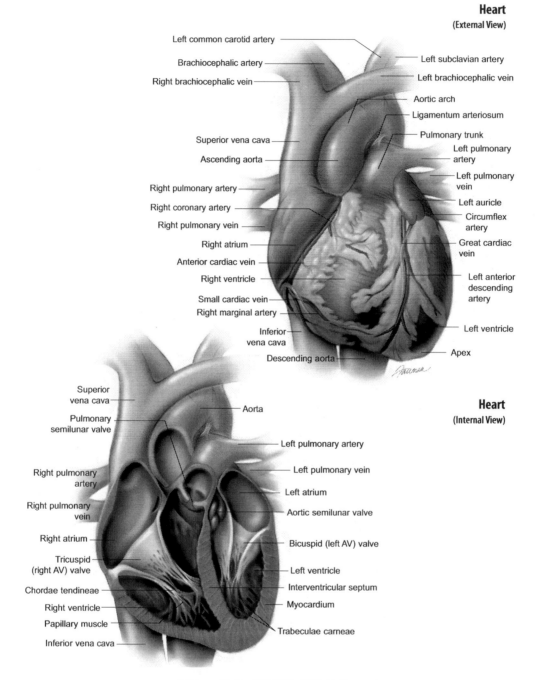

Heart
(External View)

Left common carotid artery

Brachiocephalic artery

Right brachiocephalic vein

Left subclavian artery

Left brachiocephalic vein

Aortic arch

Ligamentum arteriosum

Pulmonary trunk

Superior vena cava

Ascending aorta

Left pulmonary artery

Left pulmonary vein

Right pulmonary artery

Right coronary artery

Right pulmonary vein

Right atrium

Anterior cardiac vein

Right ventricle

Small cardiac vein

Right marginal artery

Inferior vena cava

Descending aorta

Left auricle

Circumflex artery

Great cardiac vein

Left anterior descending artery

Left ventricle

Apex

Heart
(Internal View)

Superior vena cava

Pulmonary semilunar valve

Aorta

Left pulmonary artery

Left pulmonary vein

Right pulmonary artery

Right pulmonary vein

Left atrium

Aortic semilunar valve

Right atrium

Tricuspid (right AV) valve

Bicuspid (left AV) valve

Chordae tendineae

Left ventricle

Right ventricle

Interventricular septum

Papillary muscle

Myocardium

Inferior vena cava

Trabeculae carneae

Respiratory System

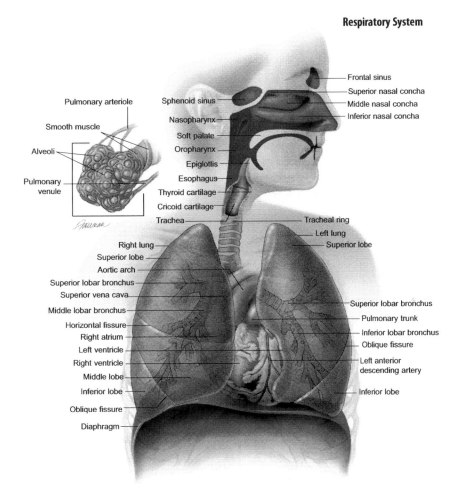

Pulmonary arteriole

Smooth muscle

Alveoli

Pulmonary venule

Frontal sinus

Superior nasal concha

Middle nasal concha

Inferior nasal concha

Sphenoid sinus

Nasopharynx

Soft palate

Oropharynx

Epiglottis

Esophagus

Thyroid cartilage

Cricoid cartilage

Trachea

Tracheal ring

Left lung

Superior lobe

Right lung

Superior lobe

Aortic arch

Superior lobar bronchus

Superior vena cava

Middle lobar bronchus

Horizontal fissure

Right atrium

Left ventricle

Right ventricle

Middle lobe

Inferior lobe

Oblique fissure

Diaphragm

Superior lobar bronchus

Pulmonary trunk

Inferior lobar bronchus

Oblique fissure

Left anterior descending artery

Inferior lobe

© Fairman Studios, LLC, 2002. All Rights Reserved.

Anatomy

Skeletal System
(Vertebral Column – Left Lateral View)

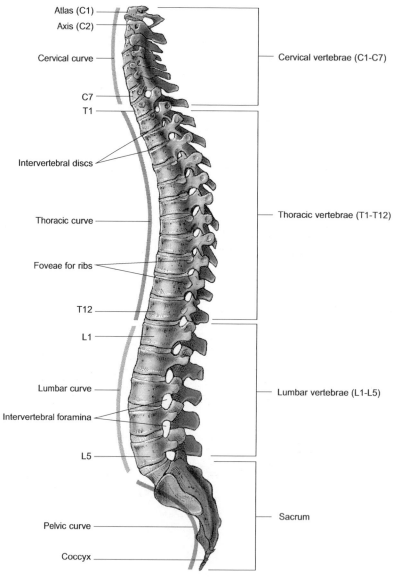

Atlas (C1)

Axis (C2)

Cervical curve

Cervical vertebrae (C1-C7)

C7

T1

Intervertebral discs

Thoracic curve

Thoracic vertebrae (T1-T12)

Foveae for ribs

T12

L1

Lumbar curve

Lumbar vertebrae (L1-L5)

Intervertebral foramina

L5

Sacrum

Pelvic curve

Coccyx

Anatomy

Digestive System

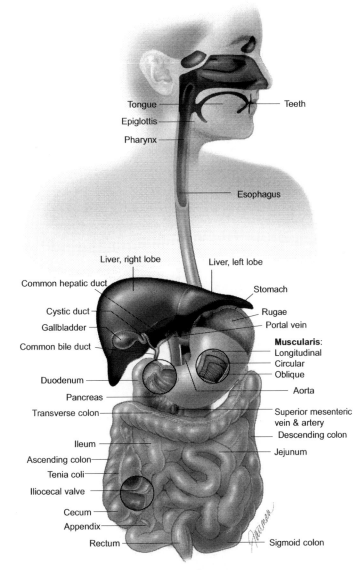

© Fairman Studios, LLC, 2002. All Rights Reserved.

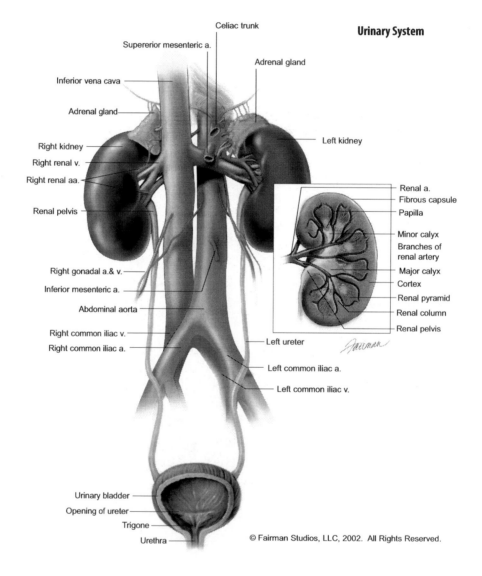

Urinary System

Celiac trunk

Supererior mesenteric a.

Adrenal gland

Inferior vena cava

Adrenal gland

Left kidney

Right kidney

Right renal v.

Right renal aa.

Renal pelvis

Renal a.

Fibrous capsule

Papilla

Minor calyx

Branches of renal artery

Major calyx

Cortex

Renal pyramid

Renal column

Renal pelvis

Right gonadal a.& v.

Inferior mesenteric a.

Abdominal aorta

Right common iliac v.

Right common iliac a.

Left ureter

Left common iliac a.

Left common iliac v.

Urinary bladder

Opening of ureter

Trigone

Urethra

© Fairman Studios, LLC, 2002. All Rights Reserved.

Anatomy

Male Genital System

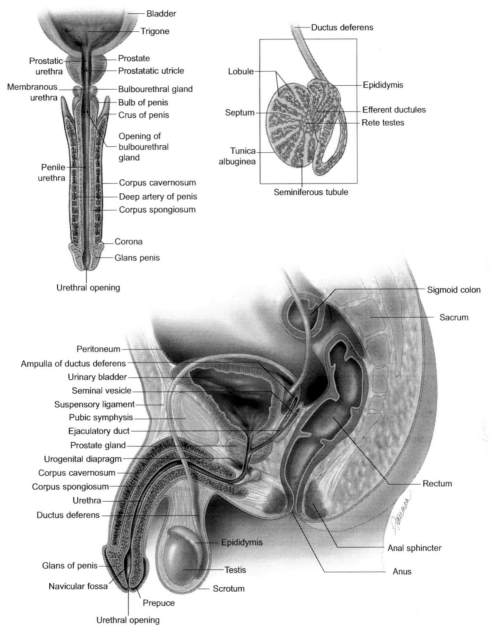

Bladder
Trigone
Prostatic urethra
Prostate
Prostatatic utricle
Membranous urethra
Bulbourethral gland
Bulb of penis
Crus of penis
Opening of bulbourethral gland
Penile urethra
Corpus cavernosum
Deep artery of penis
Corpus spongiosum
Corona
Glans penis
Urethral opening

Ductus deferens
Lobule
Epididymis
Septum
Efferent ductules
Rete testes
Tunica albuginea
Seminiferous tubule

Peritoneum
Ampulla of ductus deferens
Urinary bladder
Seminal vesicle
Suspensory ligament
Pubic symphysis
Ejaculatory duct
Prostate gland
Urogenital diapragm
Corpus cavernosum
Corpus spongiosum
Urethra
Ductus deferens
Glans of penis
Navicular fossa
Prepuce
Urethral opening
Epididymis
Testis
Scrotum

Sigmoid colon
Sacrum
Rectum
Anal sphincter
Anus

© Fairman Studios, LLC, 2002. All Rights Reserved.

Anatomy

Female Genital System

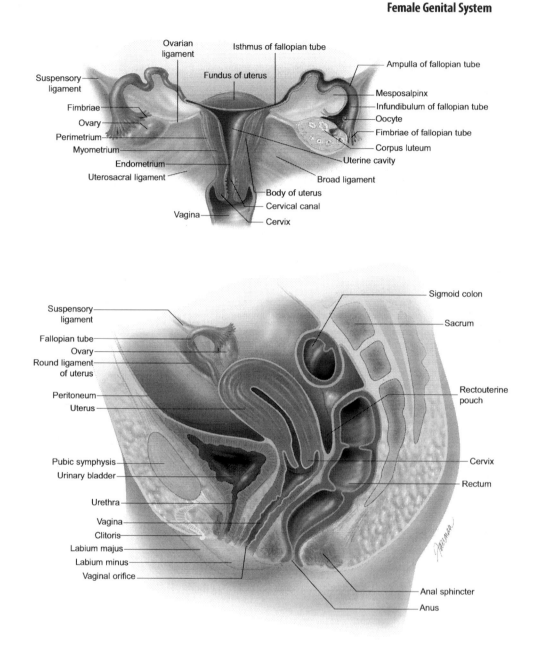

Ovarian ligament

Isthmus of fallopian tube

Fundus of uterus

Ampulla of fallopian tube

Suspensory ligament

Mesposalpinx

Fimbriae

Infundibulum of fallopian tube

Ovary

Oocyte

Perimetrium

Fimbriae of fallopian tube

Myometrium

Corpus luteum

Endometrium

Uterine cavity

Uterosacral ligament

Broad ligament

Body of uterus

Cervical canal

Vagina

Cervix

Suspensory ligament

Sigmoid colon

Fallopian tube

Sacrum

Ovary

Round ligament of uterus

Peritoneum

Rectouterine pouch

Uterus

Pubic symphysis

Cervix

Urinary bladder

Rectum

Urethra

Vagina

Clitoris

Labium majus

Labium minus

Vaginal orifice

Anal sphincter

Anus

10021-10022

10021 Fine needle aspiration; without imaging guidance
10022 Fine needle aspiration; with imaging guidance

A fine gauge needle (22 or 25 gauge) and syringe are used to percutaneously sample fluid from a cyst or remove clusters of cells from a solid mass. The fine needle aspiration (FNA) site is cleaned and the physician searches for the lump by palpation. If the lump is found and can be palpated, the physician guides the needle into the site. If the lump is found, but is non-palpable, imaging guidance is used to assist the FNA procedure. Fluoroscopic guidance or ultrasonographic guidance may be used. After the needle is placed into the breast in the lesion, a vacuum is created and multiple in and out needle motions are performed. Several needle insertions are usually required to ensure that an adequate tissue sample is taken. The samples are then smeared on a microscope slide and are: 1) allowed to dry in air, 2) are fixed by spraying, or 3) are immersed in a liquid. The fixed smears are then stained and examined by a pathologist under the microscope. FNA does not require stitches and is usually performed on an outpatient basis. A small bandage is placed over the site after the procedure. Many patients resume a normal routine the same day as the FNA procedure. Code 10021 if no imaging guidance is needed. Code 10022 when imaging guidance is used to localize the cyst.

10030

10030 Image-guided fluid collection drainage by catheter (eg, abscess, hematoma, seroma, lymphocele, cyst), soft tissue (eg, extremity, abdominal wall, neck), percutaneous

A soft tissue fluid collection such as an abscess, hematoma, seroma, lymphocele, or cyst is drained by percutaneous technique. Using fluoroscopy, ultrasound, or CT guidance, the fluid collection in the soft tissue is identified. The skin and soft tissue over the fluid collection is punctured and a catheter is placed. The fluid is drained. The soft tissue cavity may be flushed with sterile saline or antibiotic solution to clear all pus, blood, and other fluid from the site. The catheter may be removed or secured to the skin to provide continuous drainage.

10035-10036

10035 Placement of soft tissue localization device(s) (eg, clip, metallic pellet, wire/needle, radioactive seeds), percutaneous, including imaging guidance; first lesion
10036 Placement of soft tissue localization device(s) (eg, clip, metallic pellet, wire/needle, radioactive seeds), percutaneous, including imaging guidance; each additional lesion (List separately in addition to code for primary procedure)

Placement of a soft tissue localization device(s), such as a clip, metallic pellet, wire/needle, or radioactive seed is performed so that the physician can identify the exact site of the lesion prior to a biopsy or en bloc removal. The area of concern is marked on the skin and radiological images of the target tissue are obtained. Using these images, the needle is advanced into the lesion and additional images are taken to confirm placement of the needle within the mass. For wire localization, a hooked wire is inserted into the lesion at a perpendicular angle using a needle. The wire remains anchored within the mass when the needle is withdrawn, and a short length of wire extends out through the skin. Alternatively, a plastic stylette with a localization device such as a clip, metallic pellet, or radioactive seed at the end is inserted through the biopsy needle and advanced to the site of the lesion using radiographic guidance. The localization device is released into the soft tissue lesion and the stylette and needle are removed. Use 10035 for placement of the localization device in the first lesion and 10036 for each additional lesion.

10040

10040 Acne surgery (eg, marsupialization, opening or removal of multiple milia, comedones, cysts, pustules)

Acne surgery is performed using marsupialization or opening and removal of multiple milia, comedones, cysts, or pustules. Acne is characterized by several different types of lesions. Milia (whiteheads) and comedones (blackheads) are non-red, non-inflamed lesions. Cysts and pustules are red, inflamed lesions. Comedomes are removed mechanically using an extractor. Milia are opened and removed with a needle or fine blade. Cysts and pustules are incised and drained. Marsupialization is rarely used as it involves resecting the wall of the cystic lesion which can lead to scarring.

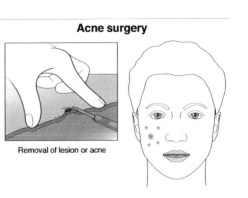

Acne surgery

Removal of lesion or acne

The physician creates a small incision over the acne site or lesion and removes the overlying skin. The lesion is either drained and cleansed to facilitate healing or removed outright.

10060-10061

10060 Incision and drainage of abscess (eg, carbuncle, suppurative hidradenitis, cutaneous or subcutaneous abscess, cyst, furuncle, or paronychia); simple or single
10061 Incision and drainage of abscess (eg, carbuncle, suppurative hidradenitis, cutaneous or subcutaneous abscess, cyst, furuncle, or paronychia); complicated or multiple

This skin is cleansed and local anesthetic injected as needed. A straight or elliptical incision is made spanning the entire area of fluctuance. Any pockets of pus are opened using blunt dissection. The abscess is drained and then irrigated with sterile solution. Use 10060 for incision and drainage of a simple or single abscess. Simple lesions are typically left open to drain and heal by secondary intention. Use 10061 for incision and drainage of a complicated or multiple abscesses. Complicated abscesses require placement of drain or packing.

10080-10081

10080 Incision and drainage of pilonidal cyst; simple
10081 Incision and drainage of pilonidal cyst; complicated

A pilonidal cyst is located just above the cleft of the buttocks and typically contains hair and skin debris. If the cyst becomes infected and an abscess forms, an incision and drainage is performed. The skin is cleansed and a local anesthetic injected. A straight or elliptical incision is made spanning the entire area of fluctuance. Any pockets of pus are opened using blunt dissection. The abscess is drained. Hair and debris are removed along with the epithelial lining which is removed by curettage. Use 10080 for a simple incision and drainage with local wound care to facilitate healing. Use 10081 for a complicated incision and drainage which includes placement of a drain or packing with gauze.

10120-10121

10120 Incision and removal of foreign body, subcutaneous tissues; simple
10121 Incision and removal of foreign body, subcutaneous tissues; complicated

Incision and removal of a foreign body embedded beneath the surface of the skin is performed. A straight or elliptical incision is made, the skin is separated, and the foreign body is identified. A hemostat or grasping forceps is then used to remove the foreign body. The incision may be closed or left open to heal by secondary intention. Use 10120 for a simple incision and removal. Use 10121 for a complicated incision and removal if the foreign body is deeply embedded and difficult to localize. The physician may need to dissect underlying tissues to remove the foreign body.

10140-10160

10140 Incision and drainage of hematoma, seroma or fluid collection
10160 Puncture aspiration of abscess, hematoma, bulla, or cyst

In 10140, an incision is made with a scalpel and fluid is drained. Any blood clots are removed with a hemostat. Gauze packing or a cannula may be utilized to facilitate further drainage if fluids continue to enter the site. A pressure dressing usually is applied over the site. The incision may be closed, or left open to heal secondarily. In 10160, the physician cleanses the skin above the subcutaneous fluid deposit. A large needle attached to a syringe is guided into the fluid deposit and aspirated with the syringe. A pressure dressing may be applied over the site of the procedure.

10180

10180   Incision and drainage, complex, postoperative wound infection

Incision and drainage is performed when infection occurs after an operation and the wound must be drained. The physician prepares the area by removing any sutures or staples or by creating additional incisions. Any necrotic (dead) tissue is removed after the wound has been drained. The wound is irrigated with saline and may be resutured or packed with gauze to allow additional drainage. Suction or latex drains may be used if the physician closes the wound. If the wound is left open, it may require future closure.

11000-11001

11000   Debridement of extensive eczematous or infected skin; up to 10% of body surface

11001   Debridement of extensive eczematous or infected skin; each additional 10% of the body surface, or part thereof (List separately in addition to code for primary procedure)

Foreign material and devitalized or contaminated tissue is removed from eczematous or infected skin until surrounding healthy tissue is exposed. After debridement, antibiotics or topical lubricants are applied to the skin. Code 11000 reports debridement of up to 10% of the body surface. Use code 11001 together with 11000 for each additional 10% of body surface area debrided or any additional percentage within that amount.

11004-11006

11004   Debridement of skin, subcutaneous tissue, muscle and fascia for necrotizing soft tissue infection; external genitalia and perineum

11005   Debridement of skin, subcutaneous tissue, muscle and fascia for necrotizing soft tissue infection; abdominal wall, with or without fascial closure

11006   Debridement of skin, subcutaneous tissue, muscle and fascia for necrotizing soft tissue infection; external genitalia, perineum and abdominal wall, with or without fascial closure

Skin, subcutaneous tissue, muscle, and fascia of the external genitalia and perineum are debrided due to necrotizing soft tissue infection (NSTI) in 11004. NSTI of the perineum is also referred to as Fournier's gangrene. The skin is incised. The area of NSTI is explored to determine the extent of tissue involvement. All apparent necrotic tissue is aggressively debrided, extending beyond the skin to subcutaneous tissues, fascia, and muscle, until the presence of arterial bleeding is noted and viable tissue is identified. All nonviable skin is resected, taking care to preserve as much viable skin and subcutaneous tissue as possible. Cultures are taken and sent to the lab for identification of infectious organisms and sensitivity testing. Use 11005 for debridement of skin, subcutaneous tissue, muscle, and fascia for NSTI of the abdominal wall, with or without closure of the fascia and 11006 for NSTI debridement of the external genitalia, perineum, and the abdominal wall, with or without closure of the fascia.

11008

11008   Removal of prosthetic material or mesh, abdominal wall for infection (eg, for chronic or recurrent mesh infection or necrotizing soft tissue infection) (List separately in addition to code for primary procedure)

Prosthetic material or mesh is removed from the abdominal wall due to infection that may be chronic or recurrent or due to necrotizing soft tissue infection (NSTI). An incision is made over the area of infection encompassing the previous surgical scar. The abdominal cavity is entered above or below the mesh or other prosthetic material. The medial borders of the rectus muscle are identified and blunt dissection is used to separate subcutaneous tissue, mesh, and the abdominal wall scar. The posterior abdominal wall is freed of all viscera. The infected mesh is removed and any mesh remnants are located and removed. Once all mesh or other prosthetic material is removed, separately reportable debridement, laparotomy, intestinal or fistula repair, and/or abdominal wall reconstruction is performed as needed.

11010-11012

11010   Debridement including removal of foreign material at the site of an open fracture and/or an open dislocation (eg, excisional debridement); skin and subcutaneous tissues

11011   Debridement including removal of foreign material at the site of an open fracture and/or an open dislocation (eg, excisional debridement); skin, subcutaneous tissue, muscle fascia, and muscle

11012   Debridement including removal of foreign material at the site of an open fracture and/or an open dislocation (eg, excisional debridement); skin, subcutaneous tissue, muscle fascia, muscle, and bone

Open fractures are those described as compound, infected, missile, puncture, or those with foreign bodies. In 11010, only skin and subcutaneous tissues at the site of the open fracture or open dislocation are debrided. The skin and subcutaneous tissues are copiously

irrigated with sterile saline. Devascularized skin and subcutaneous tissues are removed using sharp excision. Foreign material is also removed. In 11011, skin, subcutaneous tissue, muscle fascia, and muscle are debrided. The wound is irrigated and skin and subcutaneous tissue are removed as described above. Muscle tissue is inspected for viability by checking color, consistency, contraction, and circulation. The fascia is incised parallel to the muscle fibers. Nonviable muscle tissue is identified and excised. Any foreign material is removed. When all nonviable tissue has been removed as indicated by bleeding in the exposed surfaces, the physician may close the wound or leave it open to drain. In 11012, skin, subcutaneous tissue, muscle fascia, muscle, and bone are debrided. Skin, subcutaneous tissue, muscle fascia, and muscle are removed as described above. All devascularized bone is removed. Cortical bone fragments may also be removed or large cortical fragments may be removed and sterilized and then used in the fracture treatment to maintain integrity of the bone.

11042-11047

11042   Debridement, subcutaneous tissue (includes epidermis and dermis, if performed); first 20 sq cm or less

11043   Debridement, muscle and/or fascia (includes epidermis, dermis, and subcutaneous tissue, if performed); first 20 sq cm or less

11044   Debridement, bone (includes epidermis, dermis, subcutaneous tissue, muscle and/or fascia, if performed); first 20 sq cm or less

11045   Debridement, subcutaneous tissue (includes epidermis and dermis, if performed); each additional 20 sq cm, or part thereof (List separately in addition to code for primary procedure)

11046   Debridement, muscle and/or fascia (includes epidermis, dermis, and subcutaneous tissue, if performed); each additional 20 sq cm, or part thereof (List separately in addition to code for primary procedure)

11047   Debridement, bone (includes epidermis, dermis, subcutaneous tissue, muscle and/or fascia, if performed); each additional 20 sq cm, or part thereof (List separately in addition to code for primary procedure)

Debridement of skin, subcutaneous tissue, muscle, and/or bone is performed and foreign material is removed. In 11042 and 11045, subcutaneous tissue, including epidermis and dermis, is debrided. Devascularized, necrotic skin is removed. Using sharp excision, nonviable epidermis, dermis, and subcutaneous tissue is removed until viable tissue is encountered as evidenced by bleeding. Foreign material is also removed. The physician may close the wound or cover the wound with gauze. Use 11042 for the first 20 sq cm debrided and 11045 for each additional 20 sq cm or part thereof. In 11043 and 11046, skin, subcutaneous tissue, and muscle are debrided. The wound is irrigated and skin and subcutaneous tissue are removed as described above. Muscle tissue is inspected for viability by checking color, consistency, contraction, and circulation. The fascia is incised parallel to the muscle fibers. Nonviable muscle tissue is identified and excised. Any foreign material is removed. When all nonviable tissue has been removed as indicated by bleeding in the exposed surfaces, the wound may be closed or packed with gauze, or a drain placed. Use 11043 for the first 20 sq cm debrided and 11046 for each additional 20 sq cm or part thereof. In 11044 and 11047, skin, subcutaneous tissue, muscle, and bone are debrided. Nonviable skin, subcutaneous tissue, muscle fascia, and muscle are removed as described above. All devascularized bone is removed until viable bone is encountered as evidenced by bleeding. The physician may close the wound, place a drain, or pack the wound with gauze. Use 11044 for the first 20 sq cm debrided and 11047 for each additional 20 sq cm or part thereof.

11055-11057

11055   Paring or cutting of benign hyperkeratotic lesion (eg, corn or callus); single lesion

11056   Paring or cutting of benign hyperkeratotic lesion (eg, corn or callus); 2 to 4 lesions

11057   Paring or cutting of benign hyperkeratotic lesion (eg, corn or callus); more than 4 lesions

A benign hyperkeratotic lesion such as a corn or callus is removed by paring or cutting. A corn is a small area of thickened skin. A callus is a larger area of thickened skin. Corns or calluses that press on underlying tissues causing pain, such as corns that form on the toes or calluses that form on the bottom of the feet often require removal. The thickened area of skin is pared down or trimmed using a scalpel. Use 11055 for a single lesion, 11056 for two to four lesions, or 11057 for more than four lesions.

11100-11101

11100   Biopsy of skin, subcutaneous tissue and/or mucous membrane (including simple closure), unless otherwise listed; single lesion

11101   Biopsy of skin, subcutaneous tissue and/or mucous membrane (including simple closure), unless otherwise listed; each separate/additional lesion (List separately in addition to code for primary procedure)

The physician biopsies a skin, subcutaneous, or mucous membrane lesion and closes the biopsy site as needed. The lesion to be biopsied is cleansed and a local anesthetic injected. A scalpel is used to remove all or a portion of lesion. The tissue sample is then

Integumentary/Skin

sent to the laboratory for separately reportable histologic examination. The biopsy site may be closed in a single layer with sutures or left open to granulate. Use 11100 for biopsy of a single lesion and 11101 for each separate additional lesion.

11200-11201

11200 Removal of skin tags, multiple fibrocutaneous tags, any area; up to and including 15 lesions

11201 Removal of skin tags, multiple fibrocutaneous tags, any area; each additional 10 lesions, or part thereof (List separately in addition to code for primary procedure)

Skin tags are tiny projections of skin that may have a small, narrow stalk connecting to the skin surface. These can be found on any body region. Local anesthesia may or may not be used. A scalpel, ligature strangulation, or chemical/electrical cautery may be used to remove the tags. Code 11200 reports removal of up to or including 15 skin tags. Use code 11201 together with 11200 for each additional 10 lesions removed or any additional number of lesions within that amount.

11300-11303

11300 Shaving of epidermal or dermal lesion, single lesion, trunk, arms or legs; lesion diameter 0.5 cm or less

11301 Shaving of epidermal or dermal lesion, single lesion, trunk, arms or legs; lesion diameter 0.6 to 1.0 cm

11302 Shaving of epidermal or dermal lesion, single lesion, trunk, arms or legs; lesion diameter 1.1 to 2.0 cm

11303 Shaving of epidermal or dermal lesion, single lesion, trunk, arms or legs; lesion diameter over 2.0 cm

A single epidermal or dermal lesion of the trunk, arms or legs is removed by shaving. Pedunculated lesions, seborrheic keratoses, fibrous papules or other lesions with a minimal dermal component are commonly removed by shaving. Shaving extends no further than the middle dermis, leaving the subcutaneous layer intact. The area is cleansed and a local anesthetic administered. A blade is used to remove the lesion which is accomplished by transverse incision or by repetitive, horizontal slicing in the same direction. The physician inspects the surrounding tissue to ensure that the entire lesion has been removed. The edges of the wound are then smoothed and bleeding controlled using electrocautery or chemical cautery. The shaved specimen is sent to the laboratory for separately reportable histologic evaluation. Use 11300 for lesion diameter of 0.5 cm or less, 11301 for lesion diameter of 0.6-1.0 cm, 11302 for lesion diameter of 1.1-2.0 cm, and 11303 for lesion diameter over 2.0 cm.

11305-11308

11305 Shaving of epidermal or dermal lesion, single lesion, scalp, neck, hands, feet, genitalia; lesion diameter 0.5 cm or less

11306 Shaving of epidermal or dermal lesion, single lesion, scalp, neck, hands, feet, genitalia; lesion diameter 0.6 to 1.0 cm

11307 Shaving of epidermal or dermal lesion, single lesion, scalp, neck, hands, feet, genitalia; lesion diameter 1.1 to 2.0 cm

11308 Shaving of epidermal or dermal lesion, single lesion, scalp, neck, hands, feet, genitalia; lesion diameter over 2.0 cm

A raised lesion is removed by shaving from the scalp, neck, hands, feet, or genitalia. The physician applies local anesthesia to the excision site. The scalpel is held parallel to the skin surface and the lesion is removed at its base. Electrocautery or chemical cautery may be used to control bleeding. Code 11305 for a lesion diameter of 0.5 cm or less; 11306 for 0.6 cm to 1.0 cm; 11307 from 1.1 to 2.0 cm; and 11308 for lesions larger than 2.0 cm.

11310-11313

11310 Shaving of epidermal or dermal lesion, single lesion, face, ears, eyelids, nose, lips, mucous membrane; lesion diameter 0.5 cm or less

11311 Shaving of epidermal or dermal lesion, single lesion, face, ears, eyelids, nose, lips, mucous membrane; lesion diameter 0.6 to 1.0 cm

11312 Shaving of epidermal or dermal lesion, single lesion, face, ears, eyelids, nose, lips, mucous membrane; lesion diameter 1.1 to 2.0 cm

11313 Shaving of epidermal or dermal lesion, single lesion, face, ears, eyelids, nose, lips, mucous membrane; lesion diameter over 2.0 cm

A single epidermal or dermal lesion of the face, ears, eyelids, nose, lips, or mucous membrane is removed by shaving. Pedunculated lesions, seborrheic keratoses, fibrous papules or other lesions with a minimal dermal component are commonly removed by shaving. Shaving extends no further than the middle dermis, leaving the subcutaneous layer intact. The area is cleansed and a local anesthetic administered. A blade is used to remove the lesion which is accomplished by transverse incision or by repetitive, horizontal slicing in the same direction. The physician inspects the surrounding tissue to ensure that the entire lesion has been removed. The edges of the wound are then smoothed and bleeding controlled using electrocautery or chemical cautery. The shaved specimen is sent to the laboratory for separately reportable histologic evaluation. Use 11310 for lesion diameter

of 0.5 cm or less, 11311 for lesion diameter of 0.6-1.0 cm, 11312 for lesion diameter of 1.1-2.0 cm, and 11313 for lesion diameter over 2.0 cm.

11400-11406

11400 Excision, benign lesion including margins, except skin tag (unless listed elsewhere), trunk, arms or legs; excised diameter 0.5 cm or less

11401 Excision, benign lesion including margins, except skin tag (unless listed elsewhere), trunk, arms or legs; excised diameter 0.6 to 1.0 cm

11402 Excision, benign lesion including margins, except skin tag (unless listed elsewhere), trunk, arms or legs; excised diameter 1.1 to 2.0 cm

11403 Excision, benign lesion including margins, except skin tag (unless listed elsewhere), trunk, arms or legs; excised diameter 2.1 to 3.0 cm

11404 Excision, benign lesion including margins, except skin tag (unless listed elsewhere), trunk, arms or legs; excised diameter 3.1 to 4.0 cm

11406 Excision, benign lesion including margins, except skin tag (unless listed elsewhere), trunk, arms or legs; excised diameter over 4.0 cm

A benign lesion other than a skin tag of the trunk, arms, or legs is excised along with a margin of normal tissue. Commonly excised benign lesions include: lipomas, dermatofibromas, pyogenic granulomas, epidermoid cysts, and benign nevi. The area is cleansed and a local anesthetic injected. A narrow margin of healthy tissue is identified and a full-thickness incision is made through the dermis. The incision is carried around the lesion and the entire lesion is excised. The lesion is sent to the laboratory for separately reportable histologic evaluation. Bleeding is controlled by electrocautery or chemical cautery. The wound may be closed using simple single layer suture technique. Separately reportable intermediate (layer) closure, complex repair, skin graft, or pedicle flap may also be used to close the surgical wound. Use 11400 for excision diameter 0.5 cm or less, 11401 for excision diameter 0.6-1.0 cm, 11402 for excision diameter of 1.1-2.0 cm, 11403 for excision diameter of 2.1-3.0 cm, 11404 for excision diameter of 3.1-4.0, and 11406 for excision diameter of over 4.0 cm.

11420-11426

11420 Excision, benign lesion including margins, except skin tag (unless listed elsewhere), scalp, neck, hands, feet, genitalia; excised diameter 0.5 cm or less

11421 Excision, benign lesion including margins, except skin tag (unless listed elsewhere), scalp, neck, hands, feet, genitalia; excised diameter 0.6 to 1.0 cm

11422 Excision, benign lesion including margins, except skin tag (unless listed elsewhere), scalp, neck, hands, feet, genitalia; excised diameter 1.1 to 2.0 cm

11423 Excision, benign lesion including margins, except skin tag (unless listed elsewhere), scalp, neck, hands, feet, genitalia; excised diameter 2.1 to 3.0 cm

11424 Excision, benign lesion including margins, except skin tag (unless listed elsewhere), scalp, neck, hands, feet, genitalia; excised diameter 3.1 to 4.0 cm

11426 Excision, benign lesion including margins, except skin tag (unless listed elsewhere), scalp, neck, hands, feet, genitalia; excised diameter over 4.0 cm

A benign lesion other than a skin tag of the scalp, neck, hands, feet, or genitalia is excised along with a margin of normal tissue. Commonly excised benign lesions include: lipomas, dermatofibromas, pyogenic granulomas, epidermoid cysts, and benign nevi. The area is cleansed and a local anesthetic injected. A narrow margin of healthy tissue is identified and a full-thickness incision is made through the dermis. The incision is carried around the lesion and the entire lesion is excised. The lesion is sent to the laboratory for separately reportable histologic evaluation. Bleeding is controlled by electrocautery or chemical cautery. The wound may be closed using simple single layer suture technique. Separately reportable intermediate (layer) closure, complex repair, skin graft, or pedicle flap may also be used to close the surgical wound. Use 11420 for excision diameter 0.5 cm or less, 11421 for excision diameter 0.6-1.0 cm, 11422 for excision diameter of 1.1-2.0 cm, 11423 for excision diameter of 2.1-3.0 cm, 11424 for excision diameter of 3.1-4.0, and 11426 for excision diameter of over 4.0 cm.

● New Code   ▲ Revised Code

11440-11446

11440 Excision, other benign lesion including margins, except skin tag (unless listed elsewhere), face, ears, eyelids, nose, lips, mucous membrane; excised diameter 0.5 cm or less

11441 Excision, other benign lesion including margins, except skin tag (unless listed elsewhere), face, ears, eyelids, nose, lips, mucous membrane; excised diameter 0.6 to 1.0 cm

11442 Excision, other benign lesion including margins, except skin tag (unless listed elsewhere), face, ears, eyelids, nose, lips, mucous membrane; excised diameter 1.1 to 2.0 cm

11443 Excision, other benign lesion including margins, except skin tag (unless listed elsewhere), face, ears, eyelids, nose, lips, mucous membrane; excised diameter 2.1 to 3.0 cm

11444 Excision, other benign lesion including margins, except skin tag (unless listed elsewhere), face, ears, eyelids, nose, lips, mucous membrane; excised diameter 3.1 to 4.0 cm

11446 Excision, other benign lesion including margins, except skin tag (unless listed elsewhere), face, ears, eyelids, nose, lips, mucous membrane; excised diameter over 4.0 cm

A benign lesion other than a skin tag of the face, ears, eyelids, nose, lips, or mucous membrane is excised along with a margin of normal tissue. Commonly excised benign lesions include: lipomas, dermatofibromas, pyogenic granulomas, epidermoid cysts, and benign nevi. The area is cleansed and a local anesthetic injected. A narrow margin of healthy tissue is identified and a full-thickness incision is made through the dermis. The incision is carried around the lesion and the entire lesion is excised. The lesion is sent to the laboratory for separately reportable histologic evaluation. Bleeding is controlled by electrocautery or chemical cautery. The wound may be closed using simple single layer suture technique. Separately reportable intermediate (layer) closure, complex repair, skin graft, or pedicle flap may also be used to close the surgical wound. Use 11440 for excision diameter 0.5 cm or less, 11441 for excision diameter 0.6-1.0 cm, 11442 for excision diameter of 1.1-2.0 cm, 11443 for excision diameter of 2.1-3.0 cm, 11444 for excision diameter of 3.1-4.0, and 11446 for excision diameter of over 4.0 cm.

11450-11451

11450 Excision of skin and subcutaneous tissue for hidradenitis, axillary; with simple or intermediate repair

11451 Excision of skin and subcutaneous tissue for hidradenitis, axillary; with complex repair

Skin and subcutaneous tissue in the axillary region (armpit) is excised to treat hidradenitis. Hidradenitis is a chronic condition characterized by swollen, painful, inflamed lesions of the cutaneous apocrine (sweat) glands. The condition can also affect surrounding subcutaneous tissue and fascia. When suppurative hidradenitis occurs, draining sinus tracts (fistulas) are present in the axilla. Surgical treatment is typically limited to suppurative hidradenitis. The skin and subcutaneous tissue overlying the apocrine glands is excised and any fistulous tracts exposed and removed. Severe suppurative hidradenitis requires extensive removal of all involved skin and subcutaneous tissue. In 11450, the wound is closed with simple single layer repair or intermediate repair involving one or more deeper layers of subcutaneous tissue and superficial fascia. In 11451, a complex repair requiring more than layered closure is required to close the surgical wound. Complex repair includes repair requiring extensive undermining, stents, or retention sutures. Separately reportable skin graft or flap may also be required to close the wound.

11462-11463

11462 Excision of skin and subcutaneous tissue for hidradenitis, inguinal; with simple or intermediate repair

11463 Excision of skin and subcutaneous tissue for hidradenitis, inguinal; with complex repair

Skin and subcutaneous tissue in the inguinal region (groin) is excised to treat hidradenitis. Hidradenitis is a chronic condition characterized by swollen, painful, inflamed lesions of the cutaneous apocrine (sweat) glands. The condition can also affect surrounding subcutaneous tissue and fascia. When suppurative hidradenitis occurs, draining sinus tracts (fistulas) are present in the inguinal region. Surgical treatment is typically limited to suppurative hidradenitis. The skin and subcutaneous tissue overlying the apocrine glands is excised and any fistulous tracts exposed and removed. Severe suppurative hidradenitis requires extensive removal of all involved skin and subcutaneous tissue. In 11462, the wound is closed with simple single layer repair or intermediate repair involving one or more deeper layers of subcutaneous tissue and superficial fascia. In 11463, a complex repair requiring more than layered closure is required. Complex repair includes repair requiring extensive undermining, stents, or retention sutures. Separately reportable skin graft or flap may also be required to close the surgical wound.

11470-11471

11470 Excision of skin and subcutaneous tissue for hidradenitis, perianal, perineal, or umbilical; with simple or intermediate repair

11471 Excision of skin and subcutaneous tissue for hidradenitis, perianal, perineal, or umbilical; with complex repair

Skin and subcutaneous tissue in the perianal, perineal, or umbilical region is excised to treat hidradenitis. Hidradenitis is a chronic condition characterized by swollen, painful, inflamed lesions of the cutaneous apocrine (sweat) glands. The condition can also affect surrounding subcutaneous tissue and fascia. When suppurative hidradenitis occurs, draining sinus tracts (fistulas) are present in the perianal, perineal, or umbilical region. Surgical treatment is typically limited to suppurative hidradenitis. The skin and subcutaneous tissue overlying the apocrine glands is excised and any fistulous tracts exposed and removed. Severe suppurative hidradenitis requires extensive removal of all involved skin and subcutaneous tissue. In 11471, the wound is closed with simple single layer repair or intermediate repair involving one or more deeper layers of subcutaneous tissue and superficial fascia. In 11471, a complex repair requiring more than layered closure is required. Complex repair includes repair requiring extensive undermining, stents, or retention sutures. Separately reportable skin graft or flap may also be required to close the surgical wound.

11600-11606

11600 Excision, malignant lesion including margins, trunk, arms, or legs; excised diameter 0.5 cm or less

11601 Excision, malignant lesion including margins, trunk, arms, or legs; excised diameter 0.6 to 1.0 cm

11602 Excision, malignant lesion including margins, trunk, arms, or legs; excised diameter 1.1 to 2.0 cm

11603 Excision, malignant lesion including margins, trunk, arms, or legs; excised diameter 2.1 to 3.0 cm

11604 Excision, malignant lesion including margins, trunk, arms, or legs; excised diameter 3.1 to 4.0 cm

11606 Excision, malignant lesion including margins, trunk, arms, or legs; excised diameter over 4.0 cm

A malignant lesion of the trunk, arms, or legs is excised along with a margin of normal tissue. Commonly excised malignant lesions include: basal cell carcinoma, squamous cell carcinoma, verrucous carcinoma, and melanoma. The area is cleansed and a local anesthetic injected. A margin of healthy tissue is identified and a full-thickness incision is made through the dermis. The incision is carried around the lesion and the entire lesion is excised. Separately reportable frozen section may be performed at the time of the excision to ensure that an adequate margin has been excised. If malignant tissue is identified at the margin, additional tissue is excised until all margins are clean. The lesion is sent to the laboratory for separately reportable histologic evaluation. Bleeding is controlled by electrocautery or chemical cautery. The wound may be closed using simple single layer suture technique. Separately reportable intermediate (layer) closure, complex repair, skin graft, or pedicle flap may also be used to close the surgical wound. Use 11600 for excision diameter 0.5 cm or less, 11601 for excision diameter 0.6-1.0 cm, 11602 for excision diameter of 1.1-2.0 cm, 11603 for excision diameter of 2.1-3.0 cm, 11604 for excision diameter of 3.1-4.0, and 11606 for excision diameter of over 4.0 cm.

11620-11626

11620 Excision, malignant lesion including margins, scalp, neck, hands, feet, genitalia; excised diameter 0.5 cm or less

11621 Excision, malignant lesion including margins, scalp, neck, hands, feet, genitalia; excised diameter 0.6 to 1.0 cm

11622 Excision, malignant lesion including margins, scalp, neck, hands, feet, genitalia; excised diameter 1.1 to 2.0 cm

11623 Excision, malignant lesion including margins, scalp, neck, hands, feet, genitalia; excised diameter 2.1 to 3.0 cm

11624 Excision, malignant lesion including margins, scalp, neck, hands, feet, genitalia; excised diameter 3.1 to 4.0 cm

11626 Excision, malignant lesion including margins, scalp, neck, hands, feet, genitalia; excised diameter over 4.0 cm

A malignant lesion of the scalp, neck, hands, feet, or genitalia is excised along with a margin of normal tissue. Commonly excised malignant lesions include: basal cell carcinoma, squamous cell carcinoma, verrucous carcinoma, and melanoma. The area is cleansed and a local anesthetic injected. A margin of healthy tissue is identified and a full-thickness incision is made through the dermis. The incision is carried around the lesion and the entire lesion is excised. Separately reportable frozen section may be performed at the time of the excision to ensure that an adequate margin has been excised. If malignant tissue is identified at the margin, additional tissue is excised until all margins are clean. The lesion is sent to the laboratory for separately reportable histologic evaluation. Bleeding is controlled by electrocautery or chemical cautery. The wound may be closed using simple single layer suture technique. Separately reportable intermediate (layer) closure, complex repair, skin graft, or pedicle flap may also be used to close the surgical wound. Use 11620

Integumentary/Skin

for excision diameter 0.5 cm or less, 11621 for excision diameter 0.6-1.0 cm, 11622 for excision diameter of 1.1-2.0 cm, 11623 for excision diameter of 2.1-3.0 cm, 11624 for excision diameter of 3.1-4.0, and 11626 for excision diameter of over 4.0 cm.

11640-11646

11640 **Excision, malignant lesion including margins, face, ears, eyelids, nose, lips; excised diameter 0.5 cm or less**

11641 **Excision, malignant lesion including margins, face, ears, eyelids, nose, lips; excised diameter 0.6 to 1.0 cm**

11642 **Excision, malignant lesion including margins, face, ears, eyelids, nose, lips; excised diameter 1.1 to 2.0 cm**

11643 **Excision, malignant lesion including margins, face, ears, eyelids, nose, lips; excised diameter 2.1 to 3.0 cm**

11644 **Excision, malignant lesion including margins, face, ears, eyelids, nose, lips; excised diameter 3.1 to 4.0 cm**

11646 **Excision, malignant lesion including margins, face, ears, eyelids, nose, lips; excised diameter over 4.0 cm**

A malignant lesion of the face, ears, eyelids, nose, lips, or mucous membrane is excised along with a margin of normal tissue. Commonly excised malignant lesions include: basal cell carcinoma, squamous cell carcinoma, verrucous carcinoma, and melanoma. The area is cleansed and a local anesthetic injected. A margin of healthy tissue is identified and a full-thickness incision is made through the dermis. The incision is carried around the lesion and the entire lesion is excised. Separately reportable frozen section may be performed at the time of the excision to ensure that an adequate margin has been excised. If malignant tissue is identified at the margin, additional tissue is excised until all margins are clean. The lesion is sent to the laboratory for separately reportable histologic evaluation. Bleeding is controlled by electrocautery or chemical cautery. The wound may be closed using simple single layer suture technique. Separately reportable intermediate (layer) closure, complex repair, skin graft, or pedicle flap may also be used to close the surgical wound. Use 11640 for excision diameter 0.5 cm or less, 11641 for excision diameter 0.6-1.0 cm, 11642 for excision diameter of 1.1-2.0 cm, 11643 for excision diameter of 2.1-3.0 cm, 11644 for excision diameter of 3.1-4.0, and 11646 for excision diameter of over 4.0 cm.

Excision, malignant lesion

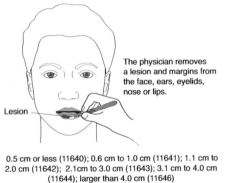

The physician removes a lesion and margins from the face, ears, eyelids, nose or lips.

Lesion

0.5 cm or less (11640); 0.6 cm to 1.0 cm (11641); 1.1 cm to 2.0 cm (11642); 2.1cm to 3.0 cm (11643); 3.1 cm to 4.0 cm (11644); larger than 4.0 cm (11646)

11719

11719 **Trimming of nondystrophic nails, any number**

Healthy, nondystrophic fingernails and/or toenails are trimmed by a physician or other health care professional such as a podiatrist. Patients with diabetes mellitus, chronic thrombophlebitis, or peripheral neuropathies associated with other conditions such as malnutrition, malabsorption, vitamin B12 deficiency, alcoholism, malignant neoplasm, or multiple sclerosis may require the services of a physician or podiatrist for trimming of nails. The nails and skin around the nails are inspected for signs of inflammation, nonhealing wounds, or other disease. One or more nondystrophic nails are then carefully trimmed and shaped using nail cutters or scissors.

11720-11721

11720 **Debridement of nail(s) by any method(s); 1 to 5**

11721 **Debridement of nail(s) by any method(s); 6 or more**

Fingernails or toenails are debrided using any method. Nail debridement is performed to remove the diseased nail bed or plate usually due to a mycotic (fungal) infection of the nail. The nail is trimmed at its tip and then aggressively debrided using a scalpel, file, or electric drill or nail grinder. The nail is thinned as much as possible and then smoothed with the file or abrasive pads. A topical antifungal medication may be painted on the remaining nail. Use 11720 for one to five nails or 11721 for six or more nails.

11730-11732

11730 **Avulsion of nail plate, partial or complete, simple; single**

11732 **Avulsion of nail plate, partial or complete, simple; each additional nail plate (List separately in addition to code for primary procedure)**

A simple avulsion of nail plate, partial or complete, is performed. A freer elevator is inserted under the edge of the nail plate and the nail lifted until a plane of cleavage forms between the nail bed and plate. The cleavage is extended proximally to the matrix. The elevator is then moved in a side-to-side motion to free the lateral margins of the nail. When the lateral margins have been freed, the freer elevator is inserted under the cuticle and again moved from side-to-side. The nail is then grasped with a hemostat and avulsed using a rolling-twisting motion. Use 11730 for a single nail plate avulsion and 11732 for each additional nail plate.

11740

11740 **Evacuation of subungual hematoma**

The physician removes a collection of blood from under the fingernail or toenail. This is often the result of blunt trauma to the nail. An electrocautery unit is used to pierce the nail plate and allow the hematoma to drain. The wound is wrapped so it can continue to drain.

11755

11755 **Biopsy of nail unit (eg, plate, bed, matrix, hyponychium, proximal and lateral nail folds) (separate procedure)**

The nail unit consists of the plate; bed, matrix; proximal, lateral and distal grooves; proximal and lateral folds; and epithelium of the nail bed (hyponychium). The exact technique depends on the portion of the nail unit requiring biopsy. A common technique is a double punch biopsy. A 4-6 mm punch tool is used to remove a circular section of the nail plate. A second smaller punch is then used to obtain a tissue sample. Alternatively, an excisional biopsy may be performed. The area to be biopsied is identified. An incision is made with the preferred site being the lateral margin of the nail. The incision is extended to the underlying bony phalanx. A tissue sample is obtained. The biopsy site may be left open to heal or undermined and closed with sutures.

11760-11762

11760 **Repair of nail bed**

11762 **Reconstruction of nail bed with graft**

The nail is repaired (11760) or reconstructed with a graft (11762) to prevent deformity of the nail bed following laceration. The distal nail plate is avulsed to allow inspection of the nail matrix while leaving as much of the proximal nail plate in place. Alternatively, complex lacerations may require complete nail avulsion prior to repair. The injured nail tissue is irrigated and debrided. In 11760, the nail bed and matrix are carefully reapposed and repaired with absorbable sutures. The avulsed nail is debrided, trimmed and reattached to the nail bed. In 11762, a nail bed avulsion is repaired using a split thickness nail matrix graft from the same nail or from the great toe. Alternatively, split or full thickness nail bed graft, a split thickness skin graft, or a reverse dermal graft may be used. The graft is harvested and configured to the appropriate size and shape. It is then carefully positioned over the injured nail bed and the nail bed reconstructed. The injury is dressed with a nonadherent dressing.

11765

11765 **Wedge excision of skin of nail fold (eg, for ingrown toenail)**

A wedge excision of skin of nail fold is performed to treat an ingrown toenail. Wedge excision is typically performed for chronic infection resulting in diseased tissue along the nail fold. An incision is made at the nail fold and a wedge-shaped excision of the diseased tissue performed. The wound is left open to heal by secondary intention. Antibiotic ointment and a dressing are applied.

11770-11772

11770 **Excision of pilonidal cyst or sinus; simple**

11771 **Excision of pilonidal cyst or sinus; extensive**

11772 **Excision of pilonidal cyst or sinus; complicated**

A pilonidal cyst is located just above the cleft of buttocks and typically contains hair and skin debris. If the cyst becomes infected, draining sinuses may form. For chronic infection of a pilonidal cyst with sinus formation, a number of surgical options are available. In 11770, a simple excision is performed. The extent of the pilonidal cavity is determined by probing or injection of methylene blue dye into the sinus. The sinuses are individually excised and the surgical wounds closed. A lateral incision is then made and the pilonidal cavity curetted. Following curettage, the incision is left open and packed with gauze. In 11771, an extensive excision is performed. The entire anterior aspect of the cyst is excised, the base of the cyst curetted, and the wound packed open. In 11772, a complicated excision is performed. The entire cyst is excised down to the sacral fascia and then packed open. Alternatively, the anterior cyst may be excised and the edges of the cyst exteriorized by suturing the cut edges of the remaining cyst wall to the edges of the skin. This is also referred to as marsupialization. The wound is packed open.

11900-11901

11900   Injection, intralesional; up to and including 7 lesions
11901   Injection, intralesional; more than 7 lesions

Intralesional injection is performed. Corticosteroids are the most commonly used drugs and are used to treat acute or chronic inflammatory processes, hyperplastic and hypertrophic skin disorders, and other conditions. A needle with a syringe attached is filled with the pharmacologic agent. The needle is inserted under the skin at the site of the lesion and the pharmacologic agent is injected. The pharmacologic agent slowly disperses through the dermis over a period of time providing prolonged localized therapy. Use 11900 for up to and including seven lesions or 11901 for more than seven lesions.

11920-11922

11920   Tattooing, intradermal introduction of insoluble opaque pigments to correct color defects of skin, including micropigmentation; 6.0 sq cm or less
11921   Tattooing, intradermal introduction of insoluble opaque pigments to correct color defects of skin, including micropigmentation; 6.1 to 20.0 sq cm
11922   Tattooing, intradermal introduction of insoluble opaque pigments to correct color defects of skin, including micropigmentation; each additional 20.0 sq cm, or part thereof (List separately in addition to code for primary procedure)

The physician outlines the tattoo site with a pen. The area is then injected with colored dye using a tattoo instrument, specifically designed to create artificial pigmentation in an area that has abnormal pigmentation. Use code 11920 for tattooing 6.0 sq cm or less; 11921 for 6.1-20.0 sq cm; and add-on code 11922 for each additional 20.0 sq cm or any number of additional square centimeters within that amount.

11950-11954

11950   Subcutaneous injection of filling material (eg, collagen); 1 cc or less
11951   Subcutaneous injection of filling material (eg, collagen); 1.1 to 5.0 cc
11952   Subcutaneous injection of filling material (eg, collagen); 5.1 to 10.0 cc
11954   Subcutaneous injection of filling material (eg, collagen); over 10.0 cc

The physician injects filling material subcutaneously. This material is often collagen and is used to treat acne scars and facial wrinkles, among other dermatological defects. Code 11950 for injection of 1 cc or less; 11951 for injection of 1.1 to 5.0 cc; 11952 for injection of 5.1 to 10.0 cc; 11954 for injection of over 10.0 cc.

11960

11960   Insertion of tissue expander(s) for other than breast, including subsequent expansion

A tissue expander is utilized for the stretching of skin prior to reconstruction. The tissue expander is similar to a balloon, and the physician fills the expander with saline solution over time to prepare the site for reconstruction. An incision is created at the site and the subcutaneous tissue is separated from the muscle. The expanders are inserted into the prepared space and the site is closed. During subsequent visits, the tissue expander is gradually inflated with saline solution. The expander is left in place until the time of the final reconstruction.

11970

11970   Replacement of tissue expander with permanent prosthesis

The physician removes a previously inserted tissue expander and replaces it with a permanent prosthesis or graft. The expander is deflated. An incision is made at the site and the tissue expander is removed. A permanent prosthesis or graft is inserted and may be stabilized with sutures, screws, or wires. The incision is closed with sutures.

11971

11971   Removal of tissue expander(s) without insertion of prosthesis

The expander is deflated. The physician creates an incision at the site and removes the expander. A prothesis or another expander is not re-introduced. A drain may be placed in the surgical site. The site is closed with sutures.

11976

11976   Removal, implantable contraceptive capsules

The physician removes implantable contraceptive capsules. The physician palpates the implantation site and locates all the capsules. If they cannot be located by palpation, a separately reportable radiograph may be obtained to identify the capsules. A local anesthetic is injected. A small incision is made over the capsules. The capsules are dissected from surrounding tissue and removed. The incision is closed.

11980

11980   Subcutaneous hormone pellet implantation (implantation of estradiol and/or testosterone pellets beneath the skin)

Hormone pellets provide a slow continuous release of hormones into the bloodstream and are usually used for hormone replacement therapy. The pellets are usually comprised of estradiol or testosterone and are used in conjunction with progesterone therapy. Under local anesthesia, hormone pellets are surgically implanted under the skin through a small incision. Pressure is applied to the site until bleeding stops. Steri-strips are used to close the wound. New pellets are added every six months.

11981-11983

11981   Insertion, non-biodegradable drug delivery implant
11982   Removal, non-biodegradable drug delivery implant
11983   Removal with reinsertion, non-biodegradable drug delivery implant

A non-biodegradable drug delivery implant is inserted (11981), removed (11982), or removed and new implant inserted (11983). This type of insert is usually cylindrical and is inserted using an insertion device provided by the drug manufacturer. In 11981, the insertion site, which is usually the inner aspect of the upper arm, is identified and cleansed. A local anesthetic is administered along the tract of the planned insertion site. A small incision is made at the planned insertion site. The tip of the insertion tool which has been previously loaded with the drug cylinder is then inserted into the incision and advanced subcutaneously. Once the drug delivery implant is properly placed, it is released from the insertion tool and insertion device is withdrawn. The physician then palpates the skin over the implant to ensure that it is properly positioned. The incision is closed. In 11982, an incision is made over the proximal tip of the drug delivery implant. If the tissue pseudocapsule overlying the proximal tip is not visible, the distal end of the implant is palpated and the implant is then massaged forward toward the incision line. The tissue pseudocapsule is then nicked, a mosquito clamp inserted and the opening in the pseudocapsule expanded. The tip of the implant is identified, grasped, and removed. In 11983, the existing implant is removed as described in 11982 and then a new implant inserted as described in 11981.

12001-12007

12001   Simple repair of superficial wounds of scalp, neck, axillae, external genitalia, trunk and/or extremities (including hands and feet); 2.5 cm or less
12002   Simple repair of superficial wounds of scalp, neck, axillae, external genitalia, trunk and/or extremities (including hands and feet); 2.6 cm to 7.5 cm
12004   Simple repair of superficial wounds of scalp, neck, axillae, external genitalia, trunk and/or extremities (including hands and feet); 7.6 cm to 12.5 cm
12005   Simple repair of superficial wounds of scalp, neck, axillae, external genitalia, trunk and/or extremities (including hands and feet); 12.6 cm to 20.0 cm
12006   Simple repair of superficial wounds of scalp, neck, axillae, external genitalia, trunk and/or extremities (including hands and feet); 20.1 cm to 30.0 cm
12007   Simple repair of superficial wounds of scalp, neck, axillae, external genitalia, trunk and/or extremities (including hands and feet); over 30.0 cm

Simple repair of superficial wounds of the scalp, neck, axillae, external genitalia, trunk and/or extremities is performed. The wound is cleansed and a local anesthetic administered. The wound is inspected and determined to be superficial involving only the epidermis, dermis or subcutaneous tissue without involvement of deeper tissues and without heavy contamination. A simple one-layer closure using sutures, staples, or tissue adhesive is performed. Alternatively, chemical cautery or electrocautery may be used to treat the wound without closure. Use 12001 for simple repair of a wound 2.5 cm or less, 12002 for a wound 2.6 to 7.5 cm, 12004 for a wound 7.6 to 12.5 cm, 12005 for a wound 12.6 to 20.0 cm, 12006 for a wound 20.1-30.0 cm, or 12007 for a wound over 30.0 cm.

Integumentary/Skin

12011-12018

12011 Simple repair of superficial wounds of face, ears, eyelids, nose, lips and/or mucous membranes; 2.5 cm or less

12013 Simple repair of superficial wounds of face, ears, eyelids, nose, lips and/or mucous membranes; 2.6 cm to 5.0 cm

12014 Simple repair of superficial wounds of face, ears, eyelids, nose, lips and/or mucous membranes; 5.1 cm to 7.5 cm

12015 Simple repair of superficial wounds of face, ears, eyelids, nose, lips and/or mucous membranes; 7.6 cm to 12.5 cm

12016 Simple repair of superficial wounds of face, ears, eyelids, nose, lips and/or mucous membranes; 12.6 cm to 20.0 cm

12017 Simple repair of superficial wounds of face, ears, eyelids, nose, lips and/or mucous membranes; 20.1 cm to 30.0 cm

12018 Simple repair of superficial wounds of face, ears, eyelids, nose, lips and/or mucous membranes; over 30.0 cm

Simple repair of superficial wounds of the face, ears, eyelids, nose, lips, and/or mucous membranes is performed. The wound is cleansed and a local anesthetic administered. The wound is inspected and determined to be superficial involving only the epidermis, dermis or subcutaneous tissue without involvement of deeper tissues and without heavy contamination. A simple one-layer closure using sutures, staples, or tissue adhesive is performed. Alternatively, chemical cautery or electrocautery may be used to treat the wound without closure. Use 12011 for simple repair of a wound 2.5 cm or less, 12013 for a wound 2.6 to 5.0 cm, 12014 for a wound 5.1 to 7.5 cm, 12015 for a wound 7.6 to 12.5 cm, 12016 for a wound 12.6 to 20.0 cm, 12017 for a wound 20.1-30.0 cm, or 12018 for a wound over 30.0 cm.

12020-12021

12020 Treatment of superficial wound dehiscence; simple closure
12021 Treatment of superficial wound dehiscence; with packing

Wound dehiscence is an opening or splitting of a wound along the suture line. The wound is cleansed. The edges of the wound may be trimmed to initiate bleeding. In 12020, a simple single layer wound closure is performed using sutures, staples, or tissue adhesive. In 12021, the wound is left open and packed with sterile gauze. Packing is typically performed on wounds that are infected. A secondary closure may be performed when the infection has resolved.

12031-12037

12031 Repair, intermediate, wounds of scalp, axillae, trunk and/or extremities (excluding hands and feet); 2.5 cm or less

12032 Repair, intermediate, wounds of scalp, axillae, trunk and/or extremities (excluding hands and feet); 2.6 cm to 7.5 cm

12034 Repair, intermediate, wounds of scalp, axillae, trunk and/or extremities (excluding hands and feet); 7.6 cm to 12.5 cm

12035 Repair, intermediate, wounds of scalp, axillae, trunk and/or extremities (excluding hands and feet); 12.6 cm to 20.0 cm

12036 Repair, intermediate, wounds of scalp, axillae, trunk and/or extremities (excluding hands and feet); 20.1 cm to 30.0 cm

12037 Repair, intermediate, wounds of scalp, axillae, trunk and/or extremities (excluding hands and feet); over 30.0 cm

Intermediate repair of wounds of the scalp, axillae, trunk, and/or extremities is performed. The wound is cleansed and a local anesthetic administered. The wound is inspected and determined to involve deeper layers of the subcutaneous tissue and superficial (non-muscle) fascia or to require extensive cleaning and/or removal of particulate matter in a heavily contaminated superficial wound. A layered closure using sutures, staples, and/or tissue adhesive is performed. Tissues are undermined using a scissors or scalpel to minimize tension on the wound. Bleeding is controlled by chemical or electrocautery. The deepest layers are then closed with absorbable sutures and the knot is buried. Alternatively, permanent sutures may be used. The superficial layer is closed taking care to ensure that the wound edges are aligned and everted to prevent depression of the scar. Use 12031 for intermediate repair of a wound 2.5 cm or less, 12032 for a wound 2.6 to 7.5 cm, 12034 for a wound 7.6 to 12.5 cm, 12035 for a wound 12.6 to 20.0 cm, 12036 for a wound 20.1 to 30.0 cm, 12037 for a wound over 30.0 cm.

12041-12047

12041 Repair, intermediate, wounds of neck, hands, feet and/or external genitalia; 2.5 cm or less

12042 Repair, intermediate, wounds of neck, hands, feet and/or external genitalia; 2.6 cm to 7.5 cm

12044 Repair, intermediate, wounds of neck, hands, feet and/or external genitalia; 7.6 cm to 12.5 cm

12045 Repair, intermediate, wounds of neck, hands, feet and/or external genitalia; 12.6 cm to 20.0 cm

12046 Repair, intermediate, wounds of neck, hands, feet and/or external genitalia; 20.1 cm to 30.0 cm

12047 Repair, intermediate, wounds of neck, hands, feet and/or external genitalia; over 30.0 cm

Intermediate repair of wounds of the neck, hands, feet, or external genitalia is performed. The wound is cleansed and a local anesthetic administered. The wound is inspected and determined to involve deeper layers of the subcutaneous tissue and superficial (non-muscle) fascia or to require extensive cleaning and/or removal of particulate matter in a heavily contaminated superficial wound. A layered closure using sutures, staples, and/or tissue adhesive is performed. Tissues are undermined using a scissors or scalpel to minimize tension on the wound. Bleeding is controlled by chemical or electrocautery. The deepest layers are then closed with absorbable sutures and the knot is buried. Alternatively, permanent sutures may be used. The superficial layer is closed taking care to ensure that the wound edges are aligned and everted to prevent depression of the scar. Use 12041 for intermediate repair of a wound 2.5 cm or less, 12042 for a wound 2.6 to 7.5 cm, 12044 for a wound 7.6 to 12.5 cm, 12045 for a wound 12.6 to 20.0 cm, 12046 for a wound 20.1 to 30.0 cm, 12047 for a wound over 30.0 cm.

12051-12057

12051 Repair, intermediate, wounds of face, ears, eyelids, nose, lips and/or mucous membranes; 2.5 cm or less

12052 Repair, intermediate, wounds of face, ears, eyelids, nose, lips and/or mucous membranes; 2.6 cm to 5.0 cm

12053 Repair, intermediate, wounds of face, ears, eyelids, nose, lips and/or mucous membranes; 5.1 cm to 7.5 cm

12054 Repair, intermediate, wounds of face, ears, eyelids, nose, lips and/or mucous membranes; 7.6 cm to 12.5 cm

12055 Repair, intermediate, wounds of face, ears, eyelids, nose, lips and/or mucous membranes; 12.6 cm to 20.0 cm

12056 Repair, intermediate, wounds of face, ears, eyelids, nose, lips and/or mucous membranes; 20.1 cm to 30.0 cm

12057 Repair, intermediate, wounds of face, ears, eyelids, nose, lips and/or mucous membranes; over 30.0 cm

Intermediate repair of wounds of the face, ears, eyelids, nose, lips, and/or mucous membranes is performed. The wound is cleansed and a local anesthetic administered. The wound is inspected and determined to involve deeper layers of the subcutaneous tissue and superficial (non-muscle) fascia or to require extensive cleaning and/or removal of particulate matter in a heavily contaminated superficial wound. A layered closure using sutures, staples, and/or tissue adhesive is performed. Tissues are undermined using a scissors or scalpel to minimize tension on the wound. Bleeding is controlled by chemical or electrocautery. The deepest layers are then closed with absorbable sutures and the knot is buried. Alternatively, permanent sutures may be used. The superficial layer is closed taking care to ensure that the wound edges are aligned and everted to prevent depression of the scar. Use 12051 for intermediate repair or a wound 2.5 cm or less, 12052 for a wound 2.6 to 5.0 cm, 12053 for a wound 5.1 to 7.5 cm, 12054 for a wound 7.6 to 12.5 cm, 12055 for a wound 12.6 to 20.0 cm, 12056 for a wound 20.1-30.0 cm, or 12057 for a wound over 30.0 cm.

13100-13102

13100 Repair, complex, trunk; 1.1 cm to 2.5 cm
13101 Repair, complex, trunk; 2.6 cm to 7.5 cm
13102 Repair, complex, trunk; each additional 5 cm or less (List separately in addition to code for primary procedure)

A complex repair of a wound of the trunk is performed. The wound is cleansed and a local anesthetic administered. The wound is inspected and determined to require more than layered closure. If the complex repair is for scar revision, the scar is excised. If the repair is for a traumatic laceration or avulsion, the wound is cleansed and particulate matter removed. The wound may be debrided using sharp dissection. Tissues may be extensively undermined using a scissors or scalpel to minimize tension on the wound. Bleeding is controlled by chemical or electrocautery. Closure of the wound depends on the site and nature of the injury. The deepest layers may be closed with absorbable sutures and the knot buried followed by closure of superficial layers with non-absorbable sutures. If retention sutures are used to hold the edges of the wound together without tension, they are placed through the entire thickness of the wound, a short length of plastic or rubber tubing is threaded over each suture and each suture is then tied. Stents may also be used to hold tissue in place or maintain the opening of an orifice. Care is taken to carefully align wound edges to prevent scar depression. Use 13100 for complex repair of a wound of the trunk 1.1 to 2.5 cm in length and 13101 for a wound 2.6 to 7.5 cm in length. Use add-on code 13102 for each additional 5 cm or less for wounds over 7.5 cm in length.

Complex repair

Complex suturing of torn, crushed, or deeply lacerated tissue

13120-13122

13120   **Repair, complex, scalp, arms, and/or legs; 1.1 cm to 2.5 cm**
13121   **Repair, complex, scalp, arms, and/or legs; 2.6 cm to 7.5 cm**
13122   **Repair, complex, scalp, arms, and/or legs; each additional 5 cm or less (List separately in addition to code for primary procedure)**

Complex repair occurs when more than one layered closure is needed, which may include scar revision, debridement, extensive undermining, stents, or retention sutures. Under local anesthesia, the wound site is cleaned and the physician performs a complex repair of the subcutaneous tissue, dermis, and epidermis of the scalp, arms and/or legs. Dissolving sutures are used for the suture layers beneath the skin. In the case of multiple wounds of the same complexity in the same anatomical area, the lengths of all the similar wounds are added in order to find the correct code. Code 13120 for repairs 1.1 cm to 2.5 cm; and 13121 for repairs 2.6 cm to 7.5 cm. Code 13122 in addition to 13121 for each 5 cm or less repaired over 7.5 cm.

13131-13133

13131   **Repair, complex, forehead, cheeks, chin, mouth, neck, axillae, genitalia, hands and/or feet; 1.1 cm to 2.5 cm**
13132   **Repair, complex, forehead, cheeks, chin, mouth, neck, axillae, genitalia, hands and/or feet; 2.6 cm to 7.5 cm**
13133   **Repair, complex, forehead, cheeks, chin, mouth, neck, axillae, genitalia, hands and/or feet; each additional 5 cm or less (List separately in addition to code for primary procedure)**

A complex repair of a wound of the forehead, cheeks, chin, mouth, neck, axillae, genitalia, hands and/or feet is performed. The wound is cleansed and a local anesthetic administered. The wound is inspected and determined to require more than layered closure. If the complex repair is for scar revision, the scar is excised. If the repair is for a traumatic laceration or avulsion, the wound is cleansed and particulate matter removed. The wound may be debrided using sharp dissection. Tissues may be extensively undermined using a scissors or scalpel to minimize tension on the wound. Bleeding is controlled by chemical or electrocautery. Closure of the wound depends on the site and nature of the injury. The deepest layers may be closed with absorbable sutures and the knot buried followed by closure of superficial layers with non-absorbable sutures. If retention sutures are used to hold the edges of the wound together without tension, they are placed through the entire thickness of the wound, a short length of plastic or rubber tubing is threaded over each suture and each suture is then tied. Stents may also be used to hold tissue in place or maintain the opening of an orifice. Care is taken to carefully align wound edges to prevent scar depression. Use 13131 for complex repair of a wound of the forehead, cheeks, chin, mouth, neck, axillae, genitalia, hands and/or feet 1.1 to 2.5 cm in length and 13132 for a wound 2.6 to 7.5 cm in length. Use add-on code 13133 for each additional 5 cm or less for wounds over 7.5 cm in length.

13151-13153

13151   **Repair, complex, eyelids, nose, ears and/or lips; 1.1 cm to 2.5 cm**
13152   **Repair, complex, eyelids, nose, ears and/or lips; 2.6 cm to 7.5 cm**
13153   **Repair, complex, eyelids, nose, ears and/or lips; each additional 5 cm or less (List separately in addition to code for primary procedure)**

A complex repair of a wound of the eyelids, nose, ears and/or lips is performed. The wound is cleansed and a local anesthetic administered. The wound is inspected and determined

to require more than layered closure. If the complex repair is for scar revision, the scar is excised. If the repair is for a traumatic laceration or avulsion, the wound is cleansed and particulate matter removed. The wound may be debrided using sharp dissection. Tissues may be extensively undermined using a scissors or scalpel to minimize tension on the wound. Bleeding is controlled by chemical or electrocautery. Closure of the wound depends on the site and nature of the injury. The deepest layers may be closed with absorbable sutures and the knot buried followed by closure of superficial layers with non-absorbable sutures. If retention sutures are used to hold the edges of the wound together without tension, they are placed through the entire thickness of the wound, a short length of plastic or rubber tubing is threaded over each suture and each suture is then tied. Stents may also be used to hold tissue in place or maintain the opening of an orifice. Care is taken to carefully align wound edges to prevent scar depression. Use 13151 for complex repair of a wound of the eyelids, nose, ears and/or lips 1.1 to 2.5 cm in length, and 13152 for a wound 2.6 to 7.5 cm in length. Use add-on code 13153 for each additional 5 cm or less for wounds over 7.5 cm in length.

13160

13160   **Secondary closure of surgical wound or dehiscence, extensive or complicated**

Secondary closure of an extensive or complicated surgical wound or wound dehiscence is performed. This procedure covers two scenarios, one in which the surgical wound is not closed at the time of the original surgical procedure and another in which a surgically closed wound opens along the previous suture line. Secondary surgical wound closure is performed on a date subsequent to the original surgical procedure during a separate surgical session or encounter. The edges of the open surgical wound are trimmed. The deepest layers may be closed with absorbable sutures and the knot buried followed by closure of superficial layers with non-absorbable sutures. If retention sutures are used to hold the edges of the wound together without tension, they are placed through the entire thickness of the wound, a short length of plastic or rubber tubing is threaded over each suture and each suture is then tied. Stents may also be used to hold tissue in place or maintain the opening of an orifice. Care is taken to carefully align wound edges to prevent scar depression. Secondary closure of a wound dehiscence is performed on a wound that has opened at the site of the earlier repair. The extent of the wound dehiscence is evaluated. The wound is irrigated with sterile saline or an antibiotic solution. The previously placed sutures are removed and the edges of the wound are trimmed. Any necrotic tissue is debrided. The wound is then repaired as described above.

14000-14001

14000   **Adjacent tissue transfer or rearrangement, trunk; defect 10 sq cm or less**
14001   **Adjacent tissue transfer or rearrangement, trunk; defect 10.1 sq cm to 30.0 sq cm**

An adjacent tissue transfer or rearrangement is performed to treat a defect of the trunk. The primary defect may be due to a traumatic wound or laceration or a surgically created defect resulting from excision of a lesion or scar. If a lesion or scar is present, it is excised. The primary defect is evaluated to determine the most appropriate type of transfer or rearrangement which may be a Z-plasty, W-plasty, V-Y-plasty, rotation flap, advancement flap or double pedicle flap. Adjacent skin and subcutaneous tissue are incised and elevated leaving one or more of the tissue borders attached. This creates a secondary defect. Surrounding tissue is undermined to allow adequate mobilization of the skin flaps. The tissue is then transferred or rearranged to cover the primary defect. The transfer or rearrangement may be configured to cover the secondary defect as well or the secondary defect may be closed with a separately reportable skin graft. The primary and secondary defects are measured to determine size of the defect. Use 14000 for a defect of 10 sq cm or less and 14001 if the defect measures 10.1 square cm to 30 square cm.

14020-14021

14020   **Adjacent tissue transfer or rearrangement, scalp, arms and/or legs; defect 10 sq cm or less**
14021   **Adjacent tissue transfer or rearrangement, scalp, arms and/or legs; defect 10.1 sq cm to 30.0 sq cm**

An adjacent tissue transfer or rearrangement is performed to treat a defect of the scalp, arms, and/or legs. The primary defect may be due to a traumatic wound or laceration or a surgically created defect resulting from excision of a lesion or scar. If a lesion or scar is present, it is excised. The primary defect is evaluated to determine the most appropriate type of transfer or rearrangement which may be a Z-plasty, W-plasty, V-Y-plasty, rotation flap, advancement flap or double pedicle flap. Adjacent skin and subcutaneous tissue are incised and elevated leaving one or more of the tissue borders attached. This creates a secondary defect. Surrounding tissue is undermined to allow adequate mobilization of the skin flaps. The tissue is then transferred or rearranged to cover the primary defect. The transfer or rearrangement may be configured to cover the secondary defect as well or the secondary defect may be closed with a separately reportable skin graft. The primary and secondary defects are measured to determine size of the defect. Use 14020 for a defect of 10 sq cm or less and 14021 if the defect measures 10.1 square cm to 30 square cm.

  ● New Code   ▲ Revised Code   CPT © 2016 American Medical Association. All Rights Reserved.   © 2017 decisionHealth

Integumentary/Skin

14040-14041

14040 Adjacent tissue transfer or rearrangement, forehead, cheeks, chin, mouth, neck, axillae, genitalia, hands and/or feet; defect 10 sq cm or less

14041 Adjacent tissue transfer or rearrangement, forehead, cheeks, chin, mouth, neck, axillae, genitalia, hands and/or feet; defect 10.1 sq cm to 30.0 sq cm

An adjacent tissue transfer or rearrangement is performed to treat a defect of the forehead, cheeks, chin, mouth, neck, axillae, genitalia, hands, and/or feet. The primary defect may be due to a traumatic wound or laceration or a surgically created defect resulting from excision of a lesion or scar. If a lesion or scar is present, it is excised. The primary defect is evaluated to determine the most appropriate type of transfer or rearrangement which may be a Z-plasty, W-plasty, V-Y-plasty, rotation flap, advancement flap or double pedicle flap. Adjacent skin and subcutaneous tissue are incised and elevated leaving one or more of the tissue borders attached. This creates a secondary defect. Surrounding tissue is undermined to allow adequate mobilization of the skin flaps. The tissue is then transferred or rearranged to cover the primary defect. The transfer or rearrangement may be configured to cover the secondary defect as well as the secondary defect may be closed with a separately reportable skin graft. The primary and secondary defects are measured to determine size of the defect. Use 14040 for a defect of 10 sq cm or less and 14041 if the defect measures 10.1 square cm to 30 square cm.

14060-14061

14060 Adjacent tissue transfer or rearrangement, eyelids, nose, ears and/or lips; defect 10 sq cm or less

14061 Adjacent tissue transfer or rearrangement, eyelids, nose, ears and/or lips; defect 10.1 sq cm to 30.0 sq cm

An adjacent tissue transfer or rearrangement is performed to treat a defect of the eyelids, nose, ears, and/or lips. The primary defect may be due to a traumatic wound or laceration or a surgically created defect resulting from excision of a lesion or scar. If a lesion or scar is present, it is excised. The primary defect is evaluated to determine the most appropriate type of transfer or rearrangement which may be a Z-plasty, W-plasty, V-Y-plasty, rotation flap, advancement flap or double pedicle flap. Adjacent skin and subcutaneous tissue are incised and elevated leaving one or more of the tissue borders attached. This creates a secondary defect. Surrounding tissue is undermined to allow adequate mobilization of the skin flaps. The tissue is then transferred or rearranged to cover the primary defect. The transfer or rearrangement may be configured to cover the secondary defect as well or the secondary defect may be closed with a separately reportable skin graft. The primary and secondary defects are measured to determine size of the defect. Use 14060 for a defect of 10 sq cm or less and 14061 if the defect measures 10.1 square cm to 30 square cm.

14301-14302

14301 Adjacent tissue transfer or rearrangement, any area; defect 30.1 sq cm to 60.0 sq cm

14302 Adjacent tissue transfer or rearrangement, any area; each additional 30.0 sq cm, or part thereof (List separately in addition to code for primary procedure)

The primary defect may be due to a traumatic wound or laceration or a surgically created defect resulting from excision of a lesion or scar. If a lesion or scar is present, it is excised. The primary defect is evaluated to determine the most appropriate type of transfer or rearrangement which may be a Z-plasty, W-plasty, V-Y-plasty, rotation flap, advancement flap or double pedicle flap. Adjacent skin and subcutaneous tissue are incised and elevated leaving one or more of the tissue borders attached. This creates a secondary defect. Surrounding tissue is undermined to allow adequate mobilization of the skin flaps. The tissue is then transferred or rearranged to cover the primary defect. The transfer or rearrangement may be configured to cover the secondary defect as well or the secondary defect may be closed with a separately reportable skin graft. The primary and secondary defects are measured to determine size of the defect. Use 14301 for a defect 30.1-60.0 sq cm and 14302 for each additional 30 sq cm or part thereof.

14350

14350 Filleted finger or toe flap, including preparation of recipient site

A large wound on the hand or foot requires a flap for closure. The physician creates an incision down the middle of the finger or toe and dissects the tissue from the bone. Vascular integrity is retained. The physician prepares the recipient site, rotates the flap to the appropriate position, and closes the wound in sutured layers.

15002-15003

15002 Surgical preparation or creation of recipient site by excision of open wounds, burn eschar, or scar (including subcutaneous tissues), or incisional release of scar contracture, trunk, arms, legs; first 100 sq cm or 1% of body area of infants and children

15003 Surgical preparation or creation of recipient site by excision of open wounds, burn eschar, or scar (including subcutaneous tissues), or incisional release of scar contracture, trunk, arms, legs; each additional 100 sq cm, or part thereof, or each additional 1% of body area of infants and children (List separately in addition to code for primary procedure)

The physician excises an open wound or burn eschar, removes an existing scar, or makes an incision to release the skin contracture caused by the scar. Simple debridement or granulation tissue removal may also be done to create a recipient site for skin grafting to repair the defect. After a healthy bed of vascular tissue is prepared, a separately reportable skin graft can be placed on the site of the trunk, arms, or legs. Code 15002 reports surgical preparation of the first 100 sq cm or 1% of body area of infants or children. Report code 15003 together with code 15002 for each additional 100 sq cm or each additional 1% of body area of infants or children, or any number of additional square centimeters or percentage of child's body area within those measured amounts.

15004-15005

15004 Surgical preparation or creation of recipient site by excision of open wounds, burn eschar, or scar (including subcutaneous tissues), or incisional release of scar contracture, face, scalp, eyelids, mouth, neck, ears, orbits, genitalia, hands, feet and/or multiple digits; first 100 sq cm or 1% of body area of infants and children

15005 Surgical preparation or creation of recipient site by excision of open wounds, burn eschar, or scar (including subcutaneous tissues), or incisional release of scar contracture, face, scalp, eyelids, mouth, neck, ears, orbits, genitalia, hands, feet and/or multiple digits; each additional 100 sq cm, or part thereof, or each additional 1% of body area of infants and children (List separately in addition to code for primary procedure)

The physician excises an open wound or burn eschar, removes an existing scar, or makes an incision to release the skin contracture caused by the scar. Simple debridement or granulation tissue removal may also be done to create a recipient site for skin grafting to repair the defect. After a healthy bed of vascular tissue is prepared, a separately reportable skin graft can be placed on the site of the face, scalp, eyelids, mouth, neck, ears, orbits, genitalia, hands, feet, or multiple digits. Code 15004 reports surgical preparation of the first 100 sq cm or 1% of body area of infants or children. Report code 15005 together with code 15004 for each additional 100 sq cm or each additional 1% of body area of infants or children, or any number of additional square centimeters or percentage of child's body area within those measured amounts.

15040

15040 Harvest of skin for tissue cultured skin autograft, 100 sq cm or less

Skin from the patient is harvested for tissue culture for a skin autograft. This procedure is typically performed on burn patients with burns covering 30% or more of total body surface area (TBSA). The subcutaneous tissue is infiltrated with a solution containing epinephrine to control bleeding. A dermatome is used to harvest a small piece, 100 sq cm or less, of the patient's skin. The harvested skin is then sent to a specialized laboratory where the epithelial cells are separated from dermal cells and placed in an incubator where they are provided with nutrients so that the cells will grow into sheets of skin that can be used as grafts over the burned regions. The dermal cells may also be cultured and the layers of cells combined prior to grafting.

15050

15050 Pinch graft, single or multiple, to cover small ulcer, tip of digit, or other minimal open area (except on face), up to defect size 2 cm diameter

Single or multiple pinch grafts are harvested to cover a small ulcer, the tip of a finger or toe, or other small open area other than one on the face. This code is reported when pinch grafting is used to cover a defect up to 2 cm in size. Pinch grafts are small pieces of skin that are used to cover a wound. The center of the pinch graft contains both dermis and epidermis (full-thickness) while the edges contain only epidermis (split-thickness). A small area of skin similar in texture to the defect area is selected. The donor site is cleansed and a local anesthetic is injected. A needle is then inserted under the skin and used to raise the skin at the donor site. The pinch graft is then excised and transferred to the defect area. This is repeated until the physician has harvested enough tissue to fill the defect.

15100-15101

15100 Split-thickness autograft, trunk, arms, legs; first 100 sq cm or less, or 1% of body area of infants and children (except 15050)

15101 Split-thickness autograft, trunk, arms, legs; each additional 100 sq cm, or each additional 1% of body area of infants and children, or part thereof (List separately in addition to code for primary procedure)

A split-thickness autograft is harvested and used to cover a defect on the trunk, arms, or legs. Split-thickness skin grafts (STSG) consist of the entire epidermis and a partial thickness of the dermis. Common harvest sites include the thigh, buttocks, abdominal wall, or scalp. There are a number of techniques used to harvest the STSG, but the most common involves the use of a dermatome. The donor site is injected with a local anesthetic and epinephrine to control bleeding. The oscillating blade of the dermatome is adjusted to the proper depth. The dermatome is advanced over the skin surface at the donor site in a continuous motion using downward pressure and the graft is harvested. The graft is prepared for transfer to the recipient site which may include use of a meshing device to expand the surface area of the graft. The graft is placed over the prepared wound bed of the recipient site. It is secured with sutures, usually four corner sutures with running suture around the periphery. Alternatively, staples or a fibrin sealant may be used. Use 15100 for the first 100 sq cm or less in adults or 1% of total body surface area (TBSA) in infants and children and 15101 for each additional 100 sq cm (adults) or 1% of TBSA (infants/children) or part thereof.

15110-15111

15110 Epidermal autograft, trunk, arms, legs; first 100 sq cm or less, or 1% of body area of infants and children

15111 Epidermal autograft, trunk, arms, legs; each additional 100 sq cm, or each additional 1% of body area of infants and children, or part thereof (List separately in addition to code for primary procedure)

An epidermal autograft is harvested and used to cover a defect on the trunk, arms, or legs. Epidermal autografts consist only of epidermis. Common harvest sites include the thigh, buttocks, abdominal wall, or scalp. The subcutaneous tissue at the donor site is injected with a local anesthetic and epinephrine to control bleeding. The oscillating blade of the dermatome is adjusted to the proper depth to ensure that only epidermis with little or no dermis is harvested. The dermatome is advanced over the skin surface at the donor site in a continuous motion using downward pressure, and the graft is harvested. The graft is prepared for transfer to the recipient site which may include use of a meshing device to expand the surface area of the graft. The graft is placed over the prepared wound bed of the recipient site. It is secured with sutures, usually four corner sutures with running suture around the periphery. Alternatively staples or fibrin sealant may be used. Use 15110 for the first 100 sq cm or less in adults or 1% of total body surface area (TBSA) in infants and children and 15111 for each additional 100 sq cm (adults) or 1% of TBSA (infants/children) or part thereof.

15115-15116

15115 Epidermal autograft, face, scalp, eyelids, mouth, neck, ears, orbits, genitalia, hands, feet, and/or multiple digits; first 100 sq cm or less, or 1% of body area of infants and children

15116 Epidermal autograft, face, scalp, eyelids, mouth, neck, ears, orbits, genitalia, hands, feet, and/or multiple digits; each additional 100 sq cm, or each additional 1% of body area of infants and children, or part thereof (List separately in addition to code for primary procedure)

Epidermal autografts consist only of epidermis. Common harvest sites include the thigh, buttocks, abdominal wall, or scalp. The subcutaneous tissue at the donor site is injected with a local anesthetic and epinephrine to control bleeding. The oscillating blade of the dermatome is adjusted to the proper depth to ensure that only epidermis with little or no dermis is harvested. The dermatome is advanced over the skin surface at the donor site in a continuous motion using downward pressure, and the graft is harvested. The graft is prepared for transfer to the recipient site which may include use of a meshing device to expand the surface area of the graft. The graft is placed over the prepared wound bed of the recipient site. It is secured with sutures, usually four corner sutures with running suture around the periphery. Alternatively staples or fibrin sealant may be used. Use 15115 for the first 100 sq cm or less in adults or 1% of total body surface area (TBSA) in infants and children and 15116 for each additional 100 sq cm (adults) or 1% of TBSA (infants/children) or part thereof.

15120-15121

15120 Split-thickness autograft, face, scalp, eyelids, mouth, neck, ears, orbits, genitalia, hands, feet, and/or multiple digits; first 100 sq cm or less, or 1% of body area of infants and children (except 15050)

15121 Split-thickness autograft, face, scalp, eyelids, mouth, neck, ears, orbits, genitalia, hands, feet, and/or multiple digits; each additional 100 sq cm, or each additional 1% of body area of infants and children, or part thereof (List separately in addition to code for primary procedure)

Split-thickness skin grafts (STSG) consist of the entire epidermis and a partial thickness of the dermis. Common harvest sites include the thigh, buttocks, abdominal wall, or scalp. There are a number of techniques used to harvest the STSG, but the most common involves the use of a dermatome. The donor site is injected with a local anesthetic and epinephrine to control bleeding. The oscillating blade of the dermatome is adjusted to the proper depth. The dermatome is advanced over the skin surface at the donor site in a continuous motion using downward pressure and the graft is harvested. The graft is prepared for transfer to the recipient site, which may include use of a meshing device to expand the surface area of the graft. The graft is then placed over the prepared wound bed of the recipient site. It is secured with sutures, usually four corner sutures with running suture around the periphery. Use 15120 for the first 100 sq cm or less in adults or 1% of total body surface area (TBSA) in infants and children and 15121 for each additional 100 sq cm (adults) or 1% of TBSA (infants/children) or part thereof.

15130-15131

15130 Dermal autograft, trunk, arms, legs; first 100 sq cm or less, or 1% of body area of infants and children

15131 Dermal autograft, trunk, arms, legs; each additional 100 sq cm, or each additional 1% of body area of infants and children, or part thereof (List separately in addition to code for primary procedure)

Dermal autografts consist only of dermis. Common harvest sites include the thigh, buttocks, abdominal wall, or scalp. The subcutaneous tissue at the donor site is injected with a local anesthetic and epinephrine to control bleeding. The oscillating blade of the dermatome is adjusted to the proper depth and a split thickness skin graft raised but not harvested from the dermal bed. The blade depth is readjusted and a second pass of the dermatome is made over the same site to obtain a dermal graft. The dermal graft is prepared for transfer to the recipient site. The dermal graft is placed over the prepared wound bed of the recipient site. It is secured with sutures, usually four corner sutures with running suture around the periphery. Alternatively staples or fibrin sealant may be used. The split-thickness graft that was raised but not harvested is placed over the donor site and secured with sutures, staples or fibrin glue. Use 15130 for the first 100 sq cm or less in adults or 1% of total body surface area (TBSA) in infants and children and 15131 for each additional 100 sq cm (adults) or 1% of TBSA (infants/children) or part thereof.

15135-15136

15135 Dermal autograft, face, scalp, eyelids, mouth, neck, ears, orbits, genitalia, hands, feet, and/or multiple digits; first 100 sq cm or less, or 1% of body area of infants and children

15136 Dermal autograft, face, scalp, eyelids, mouth, neck, ears, orbits, genitalia, hands, feet, and/or multiple digits; each additional 100 sq cm, or each additional 1% of body area of infants and children, or part thereof (List separately in addition to code for primary procedure)

Dermal autografts consist only of dermis. Common harvest sites include the thigh, buttocks, abdominal wall, or scalp. The subcutaneous tissue at the donor site is injected with a local anesthetic and epinephrine to control bleeding. The oscillating blade of the dermatome is adjusted to the proper depth and a split thickness skin graft raised but not harvested from the dermal bed. The blade depth is readjusted and a second pass of the dermatome is made over the same site to obtain a dermal graft. The dermal graft is prepared for transfer to the recipient site. The dermal graft is placed over the prepared wound bed of the recipient site. It is secured with sutures, usually four corner sutures with running suture around the periphery. Alternatively staples or fibrin sealant may be used. The split-thickness graft that was raised but not harvested is placed over the donor site and secured with sutures, staples or fibrin glue. Use 15135 for the first 100 sq cm or less in adults or 1% of total body surface area (TBSA) in infants and children and 15136 for each additional 100 sq cm (adults) or 1% of TBSA (infants/children) or part thereof.

15150-15152

15150 Tissue cultured skin autograft, trunk, arms, legs; first 25 sq cm or less

15151 Tissue cultured skin autograft, trunk, arms, legs; additional 1 sq cm to 75 sq cm (List separately in addition to code for primary procedure)

15152 Tissue cultured skin autograft, trunk, arms, legs; each additional 100 sq cm, or each additional 1% of body area of infants and children, or part thereof (List separately in addition to code for primary procedure)

A tissue cultured skin autograft is used to cover a defect on the trunk, arms, or legs. Epidermal tissue is harvested from the patient in a separately reportable procedure and then sent to a specialized lab where it is separated from dermal cells and cultured in an incubator. The epidermal cells, also called keratinocytes, are provided with nutrients so that the cells will grow into sheets of skin that can be used as grafts. The tissue cultured graft is placed in transport medium and returned to the facility for the grafting procedure. The physician removes the graft from the transport medium and places it over the prepared wound bed of the recipient site. It is secured with interrupted sutures around the periphery. Alternatively, staples or fibrin sealant may be used. Use 15150 for 25 sq cm or less, 15151 for an additional 1 sq cm to 75 sq cm, and 15152 for each additional 100 sq cm (adults) or 1% of TBSA (infants/children) or part thereof.

15155-15157

15155 Tissue cultured skin autograft, face, scalp, eyelids, mouth, neck, ears, orbits, genitalia, hands, feet, and/or multiple digits; first 25 sq cm or less

15156 Tissue cultured skin autograft, face, scalp, eyelids, mouth, neck, ears, orbits, genitalia, hands, feet, and/or multiple digits; additional 1 sq cm to 75 sq cm (List separately in addition to code for primary procedure)

15157 Tissue cultured skin autograft, face, scalp, eyelids, mouth, neck, ears, orbits, genitalia, hands, feet, and/or multiple digits; each additional 100 sq cm, or each additional 1% of body area of infants and children, or part thereof (List separately in addition to code for primary procedure)

A tissue cultured skin autograft is used to cover a defect on the face, scalp, eyelids, mouth, neck, ears, orbits, genitalia, hands, feet, and/or multiple digits. Epidermal tissue is harvested from the patient in a separately reportable procedure and then sent to a specialized lab where it is separated from dermal cells and cultured in an incubator. The epidermal cells, also called keratinocytes, are provided with nutrients so that the cells will grow into sheets of skin that can be used as grafts. The tissue cultured graft is placed in transport medium and returned to the facility for the grafting procedure. The physician removes the graft from the transport medium and places it over the prepared wound bed of the recipient site. It is secured with interrupted sutures around the periphery. Alternatively, staples or fibrin sealant may be used. Use 15155 for 25 sq cm or less; 15156 for an additional 1 sq cm to 75 sq cm; and 15157 for each additional 100 sq cm (adults) or 1% of TBSA (infants/children) or part thereof.

15200-15201

15200 Full thickness graft, free, including direct closure of donor site, trunk; 20 sq cm or less

15201 Full thickness graft, free, including direct closure of donor site, trunk; each additional 20 sq cm, or part thereof (List separately in addition to code for primary procedure)

A full-thickness free skin graft is harvested from the patient and used to close a wound or other skin defect on the trunk. Full-thickness grafts contain all the skin layers, including blood vessels. The donor site is selected taking into account the characteristics of the recipient site and attempting to match thickness, texture, pigmentation, and the presence or absence of hair. The configuration of the wound is outlined over the donor region enlarging it slightly to allow for contracture. A local anesthetic is injected along with epinephrine to control bleeding. The full-thickness graft is harvested using a scalpel by first incising the skin along the marked edges and then elevating it with a skin hook. As the skin is elevated, the subcutaneous fat is separated from the graft. Once the skin graft has been separated from underlying tissue the donor site is closed with sutures. Any remaining subcutaneous fat is removed and the skin graft is positioned on the defect. The skin graft is secured with sutures and a layered dressing applied including a nonadherent layer, a bulky layer of gauze, a compression layer, and an anti-shear layer. Code 15200 reports a graft to repair a defect on the trunk not exceeding 20.0 sq cm. Use code 15201 together with code 15200 to report each additional 20.0 sq cm or portion thereof.

15220-15221

15220 Full thickness graft, free, including direct closure of donor site, scalp, arms, and/or legs; 20 sq cm or less

15221 Full thickness graft, free, including direct closure of donor site, scalp, arms, and/or legs; each additional 20 sq cm, or part thereof (List separately in addition to code for primary procedure)

The physician harvests a full-thickness graft from a donor site. The graft contains all the skin layers, including blood vessels. The donor site is closed. The subcutaneous fat is removed and the skin graft is positioned on the defect. The defect area and full-thickness graft are closed with sutures. Code 15220 reports a graft to repair a defect on the scalp, arms, and/or legs, not exceeding 20.0 sq cm. Use code 15221 together with code 15220 to report each additional 20.0 sq cm covered on the scalp, arms, or legs or any additional square centimeters within that amount.

15240-15241

15240 Full thickness graft, free, including direct closure of donor site, forehead, cheeks, chin, mouth, neck, axillae, genitalia, hands, and/or feet; 20 sq cm or less

15241 Full thickness graft, free, including direct closure of donor site, forehead, cheeks, chin, mouth, neck, axillae, genitalia, hands, and/or feet; each additional 20 sq cm, or part thereof (List separately in addition to code for primary procedure)

The physician harvests a full-thickness graft from a donor site. The graft contains all the skin layers, including blood vessels. The donor site is closed. The subcutaneous fat is removed and the skin graft is positioned on the defect. The defect area and full-thickness graft are closed with sutures. Code 15240 reports a graft to repair a defect on the forehead, cheeks, chin, mouth, neck, axillae, genitalia, hands, and/or feet, not exceeding 20.0 sq cm. Use code 15241 together with 15240 to report each additional 20.0 sq cm covered or any additional square centimeters within that amount.

15260-15261

15260 Full thickness graft, free, including direct closure of donor site, nose, ears, eyelids, and/or lips; 20 sq cm or less

15261 Full thickness graft, free, including direct closure of donor site, nose, ears, eyelids, and/or lips; each additional 20 sq cm, or part thereof (List separately in addition to code for primary procedure)

The physician harvests a full-thickness graft from a donor site. The graft contains all the skin layers, including blood vessels. The donor site is closed. The subcutaneous fat is removed and the skin graft is positioned on the defect. The defect area and full-thickness graft are closed with sutures. Code 15260 reports a graft to repair a defect on the nose, ears, eyelids, and/or lips, not exceeding 20.0 sq cm. Use code 15261 together with 15260 to report each additional 20.0 sq cm covered or any additional square centimeters within that amount.

15271-15272

15271 Application of skin substitute graft to trunk, arms, legs, total wound surface area up to 100 sq cm; first 25 sq cm or less wound surface area

15272 Application of skin substitute graft to trunk, arms, legs, total wound surface area up to 100 sq cm; each additional 25 sq cm wound surface area, or part thereof (List separately in addition to code for primary procedure)

A skin substitute composed of acellular bioengineered constructs and/or allogeneic cells is used to treat an open wound. Skin substitutes may be used to promote healing of burns, skin donor sites, diabetic or venous ulcers, or other hard-to-heal, chronic, open wounds of the skin and underlying soft tissues. Examples of skin substitutes include acellular dermal allograft, tissue cultured allogeneic skin substitutes, tissue cultured allogenic dermal substitute, and acellular xenograft. An acellular dermal allograft is a chemically treated skin graft from a cadaver donor that has had the antigenic epidermal cellular components removed. Tissue cultured allogeneic skin substitutes consist of two layers. The upper layer is cultured from human keratinocytes that multiply to form the epidermal layer. The lower, dermal layer is composed of human fibroblasts from the same donor cultured on a matrix of collagen from an animal source. Tissue cultured allogeneic dermal substitutes are composed of human fibroblast cells, such as that found in newborn foreskin tissue. The fibroblasts are seeded onto a bioabsorbable mesh scaffold. The dermal substitute is created as the fibroblasts multiply to fill the spaces in the mesh scaffold. As the fibroblasts multiply, they secrete human dermal collagen, matrix proteins, growth factors, and cytokines which are hormone-like proteins that regulate immune response. The resulting dermal substitute contains metabolically active, living cells. A skin xenograft, also referred to as a heterograft, refers to skin or other tissue obtained from another species, usually a pig (porcine) or cow (bovine). An acellular xenograft is one in which the cells, cell debris, DNA, and RNA have been removed. The xenograft is composed of acellular animal collagen along with elastin fibers that have been treated using cross-linking so that the collagen will not be broken down and reabsorbed. The exact procedure depends on the type of skin substitute used. If an acellular dermal allograft is used, the dermal allograft sheets are removed from the packet, rehydrated in an isotonic sodium chloride solution, and trimmed to the appropriate dimensions. The sheets are applied over the prepared wound bed in a single or multiple layers and secured using absorbable sutures. Any excess at the periphery of the wound is trimmed. Tissue cultured allogeneic skin substitute is fenestrated which involves making a series of holes or openings in the skin substitute. The fenestrated skin substitute is then applied to the prepared wound bed and secured with sutures. Tissue cultured allogeneic dermal substitute is applied to the prepared wound bed and secured with sutures or staples. For an acelluar xenograft, the implant sheet is cut to the size and shape of the wound, applied to the prepared wound bed, and secured with sutures. Following application of the skin substitute, a layered dressing is then applied including a nonadherent layer, a bulky layer of gauze, a compression layer, and an anti-shear layer. These codes report treatment of a total wound surface area up to 100 sq cm on the trunk, arms, or legs. Use 15271 for the first 25 sq cm or less and 15272 for each additional 25 sq cm of wound surface area, or part thereof.

Integumentary/Skin

15273-15274

15273 Application of skin substitute graft to trunk, arms, legs, total wound surface area greater than or equal to 100 sq cm; first 100 sq cm wound surface area, or 1% of body area of infants and children

15274 Application of skin substitute graft to trunk, arms, legs, total wound surface area greater than or equal to 100 sq cm; each additional 100 sq cm wound surface area, or part thereof, or each additional 1% of body area of infants and children, or part thereof (List separately in addition to code for primary procedure)

A skin substitute composed of acellular bioengineered constructs and/or allogeneic cells is used to treat an open wound. Skin substitutes may be used to promote healing of burns, skin donor sites, diabetic or venous ulcers, or other hard-to-heal, chronic, open wounds of the skin and underlying soft tissues. Examples of skin substitutes include acellular dermal allograft, tissue cultured allogeneic skin substitutes, tissue cultured allogenic dermal substitute, and acellular xenograft. Acellular dermal allograft is a chemically treated skin graft from a cadaver donor that has had the antigenic epidermal cellular components removed. Tissue cultured allogeneic skin substitutes consist of two layers. The upper layer is cultured from human keratinocytes that multiply to form the epidermal layer. The lower, dermal layer is composed of human fibroblasts from the same donor cultured on a matrix of collagen from an animal source. Tissue cultured allogeneic dermal substitutes are composed of human fibroblast cells, such as that found in newborn foreskin tissue. The fibroblasts are seeded onto a bioabsorbable mesh scaffold. The dermal substitute is created as the fibroblasts multiply to fill the spaces in the mesh scaffold. As the fibroblasts multiply, they secrete human dermal collagen, matrix proteins, growth factors, and cytokines which are hormone-like proteins that regulate immune response. The resulting dermal substitute contains metabolically active, living cells. A skin xenograft, also referred to as a heterograft, refers to skin or other tissue obtained from another species, usually a pig (porcine) or cow (bovine). An acellular xenograft is one in which the cells, cell debris, DNA, and RNA have been removed. The xenograft is composed of acellular animal collagen along with elastin fibers that have been treated using cross-linking so that the collagen will not be broken down and reabsorbed. The exact procedure depends on the type of skin substitute used. If an acellular dermal allograft is used, the dermal allograft sheets are removed from the packet, rehydrated in an isotonic sodium chloride solution, and trimmed to the appropriate dimensions. The sheets are applied over the prepared wound bed in a single or multiple layers and secured using absorbable sutures. Any excess at the periphery of the wound is trimmed. Tissue cultured allogeneic skin substitute is fenestrated which involves making a series of holes or openings in the skin substitute. The fenestrated skin substitute is then applied to the prepared wound bed and secured with sutures. Tissue cultured allogeneic dermal substitute is applied to the prepared wound bed and secured with sutures or staples. For an acelluar xenograft, the implant sheet is cut to the size and shape of the wound, applied to the prepared wound bed, and secured with sutures. Following application of the skin substitute, a layered dressing is then applied including a nonadherent layer, a bulky layer of gauze, a compression layer, and an anti-shear layer. These codes report treatment of a total wound surface area greater than or equal to 100 sq cm of the trunk, arms, or legs. Use 15273 for the first 100 sq cm in adults or 1% of TBSA of infants and children. Use 15274 for each additional 100 sq cm of wound surface area in adults or part thereof, or 1% of TBSA of infants and children, or part thereof.

15275-15276

15275 Application of skin substitute graft to face, scalp, eyelids, mouth, neck, ears, orbits, genitalia, hands, feet, and/or multiple digits, total wound surface area up to 100 sq cm; first 25 sq cm or less wound surface area

15276 Application of skin substitute graft to face, scalp, eyelids, mouth, neck, ears, orbits, genitalia, hands, feet, and/or multiple digits, total wound surface area up to 100 sq cm; each additional 25 sq cm wound surface area, or part thereof (List separately in addition to code for primary procedure)

A skin substitute composed of acellular bioengineered constructs and/or allogeneic cells is used to treat an open wound. Skin substitutes may be used to promote healing of burns, skin donor sites, diabetic or venous ulcers, or other hard-to-heal, chronic, open wounds of the skin and underlying soft tissues. Examples of skin substitutes include acellular dermal allograft, tissue cultured allogeneic skin substitutes, tissue cultured allogenic dermal substitute, and acellular xenograft. Acellular dermal allograft is a chemically treated skin graft from a cadaver donor that has had the antigenic epidermal cellular components removed. Tissue cultured allogeneic skin substitutes consist of two layers. The upper layer is cultured from human keratinocytes that multiply to form the epidermal layer. The lower, dermal layer is composed of human fibroblasts from the same donor cultured on a matrix of collagen from an animal source. Tissue cultured allogeneic dermal substitutes are composed of human fibroblast cells, such as that found in newborn foreskin tissue. The fibroblasts are seeded onto a bioabsorbable mesh scaffold. The dermal substitute is created as the fibroblasts multiply to fill the spaces in the mesh scaffold. As the fibroblasts multiply, they secrete human dermal collagen, matrix proteins, growth factors, and cytokines which are hormone-like proteins that regulate immune response. The resulting dermal substitute contains metabolically active, living cells. A skin xenograft, also referred to as a heterograft, refers to skin or other tissue obtained from another species, usually a pig (porcine) or cow (bovine). An acellular xenograft is one in which the cells, cell debris, DNA, and RNA have been removed. The xenograft is composed of acellular animal collagen along with elastin fibers that have been treated using cross-linking so that the collagen will not be broken down and reabsorbed. The exact procedure depends on the type of skin substitute used. If an acellular dermal allograft is used, the dermal allograft sheets are removed from the packet, rehydrated in an isotonic sodium chloride solution, and trimmed to the appropriate dimensions. The sheets are applied over the prepared wound bed in a single or multiple layers and secured using absorbable sutures. Any excess at the periphery of the wound is trimmed. Tissue cultured allogeneic skin substitute is fenestrated which involves making a series of holes or openings in the skin substitute. The fenestrated skin substitute is then applied to the prepared wound bed and secured with sutures. Tissue cultured allogeneic dermal substitute is applied to the prepared wound bed and secured with sutures or staples. For an acelluar xenograft, the implant sheet is cut to the size and shape of the wound, applied to the prepared wound bed, and secured with sutures. Following application of the skin substitute, a layered dressing is then applied including a nonadherent layer, a bulky layer of gauze, a compression layer, and an anti-shear layer. These codes report treatment of a total wound surface area up to 100 sq cm of the face, scalp, eyelids, mouth, neck, ears, orbits, genitalia, hands, feet, and/or multiple digits. Use 15275 for the first 25 sq cm or less and 15276 for each additional 25 sq cm of the wound surface area, or part thereof.

15277-15278

15277 Application of skin substitute graft to face, scalp, eyelids, mouth, neck, ears, orbits, genitalia, hands, feet, and/or multiple digits, total wound surface area greater than or equal to 100 sq cm; first 100 sq cm wound surface area, or 1% of body area of infants and children

15278 Application of skin substitute graft to face, scalp, eyelids, mouth, neck, ears, orbits, genitalia, hands, feet, and/or multiple digits, total wound surface area greater than or equal to 100 sq cm; each additional 100 sq cm wound surface area, or part thereof, or each additional 1% of body area of infants and children, or part thereof (List separately in addition to code for primary procedure)

A skin substitute composed of acellular bioengineered constructs and/or allogeneic cells is used to treat an open wound. Skin substitutes may be used to promote healing of burns, skin donor sites, diabetic or venous ulcers, or other hard-to-heal, chronic, open wounds of the skin and underlying soft tissues. Examples of skin substitutes include acellular dermal allograft, tissue cultured allogeneic skin substitutes, tissue cultured allogenic dermal substitute, and acellular xenograft. Acellular dermal allograft is a chemically treated skin graft from a cadaver donor that has had the antigenic epidermal cellular components removed. Tissue cultured allogeneic skin substitutes consist of two layers. The upper layer is cultured from human keratinocytes that multiply to form the epidermal layer. The lower, dermal layer is composed of human fibroblasts from the same donor cultured on a matrix of collagen from an animal source. Tissue cultured allogeneic dermal substitutes are composed of human fibroblast cells, such as that found in newborn foreskin tissue. The fibroblasts are seeded onto a bioabsorbable mesh scaffold. The dermal substitute is created as the fibroblasts multiply to fill the spaces in the mesh scaffold. As the fibroblasts multiply, they secrete human dermal collagen, matrix proteins, growth factors, and cytokines which are hormone-like proteins that regulate immune response. The resulting dermal substitute contains metabolically active, living cells. A skin xenograft, also referred to as a heterograft, refers to skin or other tissue obtained from another species, usually a pig (porcine) or cow (bovine). An acellular xenograft is one in which the cells, cell debris, DNA, and RNA have been removed. The xenograft is composed of acellular animal collagen along with elastin fibers that have been treated using cross-linking so that the collagen will not be broken down and reabsorbed. The exact procedure depends on the type of skin substitute used. If an acellular dermal allograft is used, the dermal allograft sheets are removed from the packet, rehydrated in an isotonic sodium chloride solution, and trimmed to the appropriate dimensions. The sheets are applied over the prepared wound bed in a single or multiple layers and secured using absorbable sutures. Any excess at the periphery of the wound is trimmed. Tissue cultured allogeneic skin substitute is fenestrated which involves making a series of holes or openings in the skin substitute. The fenestrated skin substitute is then applied to the prepared wound bed and secured with sutures. Tissue cultured allogeneic dermal substitute is applied to the prepared wound bed and secured with sutures or staples. For an acelluar xenograft, the implant sheet is cut to the size and shape of the wound, applied to the prepared wound bed, and secured with sutures. Following application of the skin substitute, a layered dressing is then applied including a nonadherent layer, a bulky layer of gauze, a compression layer, and an anti-shear layer. These codes report treatment of a total wound surface area greater than or equal to 100 sq cm of the face, scalp, eyelids, mouth, neck, ears, orbits, genitalia, hands, feet, and/or multiple digits. Use 15277 for the first 100 sq cm in adults or 1% of TBSA of infants and children. Use 15278 for each additional 100 sq cm of wound surface area in adults, or part thereof, or 1% of TBSA of infants and children, or part thereof.

15570-15576

15570   Formation of direct or tubed pedicle, with or without transfer; trunk

15572   Formation of direct or tubed pedicle, with or without transfer; scalp, arms, or legs

15574   Formation of direct or tubed pedicle, with or without transfer; forehead, cheeks, chin, mouth, neck, axillae, genitalia, hands or feet

15576   Formation of direct or tubed pedicle, with or without transfer; eyelids, nose, ears, lips, or intraoral

Creation of a direct or tubed pedicle flap is the first stage of a multiple stage procedure. Direct and tubed pedicle flaps are full thickness flaps that are used to cover non-adjacent defects. Pedicle flaps remain attached to their blood supply at the donor site. A direct pedicle flap is developed and transferred to the recipient site at the same surgical session with the donor site approximated to the recipient site. A tubed pedicle flap is developed and transferred to the recipient site with the lateral flap edges sewn together to create a tube. The size and configuration of the flap is determined, the donor site is incised, and a full-thickness flap raised. The flap is sutured to the recipient site in multiple layers. The donor site is closed with sutures. Alternatively, a separately reportable skin graft or local flap may be required to close the donor site. Use 15570 for transfer of a flap to the trunk or when a tubed flap is formed on the trunk for later transfer to another site. Use 15572 for transfer of a flap to the scalp, arms, or legs or when a tubed flap is formed at one of these sites for later transfer to another site. Use 15574 for transfer of a flap to the forehead, cheeks, chin, mouth, neck, axillae, genitalia, hands or feet or when a tubed flap is formed at one of these sites for later transfer to another site. Use 15576 for transfer of a flap to the eyelids, nose, ears, lips, or intraoral repairs or when a tubed flap is formed at one of these sites for later transfer to another site.

15600-15630

15600   Delay of flap or sectioning of flap (division and inset); at trunk

15610   Delay of flap or sectioning of flap (division and inset); at scalp, arms, or legs

15620   Delay of flap or sectioning of flap (division and inset); at forehead, cheeks, chin, neck, axillae, genitalia, hands, or feet

15630   Delay of flap or sectioning of flap (division and inset); at eyelids, nose, ears, or lips

Delay of flap refers to a staged division of the flap to enhance vascular supply. Sectioning of flap refers to division of the flap and inset at the recipient site. If a delay of flap, also referred to as a delay maneuver, is performed, the pedicle is partially divided to encourage more efficient circulation at the recipient site. If a sectioning of flap is performed, the flap is transected and the physician completes inset and closure of defect at the recipient site. Any unused portion of the flap is then returned to the donor site. If the donor site has been closed with a skin graft, the skin graft is removed and replaced with the remainder of the flap. If additional coverage is required at the donor site, a separately reportable skin graft or local flap may be applied. Use 15600 for delay or sectioning of a flap to the trunk. Use 15610 for delay or sectioning of flap to the scalp, arms, or legs. Use 15620 for delay or sectioning of flap to the forehead, cheeks, chin, mouth, neck, axillae, genitalia, hands or feet. Use 15630 for delay or sectioning of flap to the eyelids, nose, ears, or lips.

15650

15650   Transfer, intermediate, of any pedicle flap (eg, abdomen to wrist, Walking tube), any location

The physician moves a previously placed pedicle graft into an intermediate position before the final placement. The procedure is performed after the recipient site is vascularized and viable. The procedure may occur at any location on the body, and may occur more than once before the final placement. This procedure is also known as walking the flap.

15731

15731   Forehead flap with preservation of vascular pedicle (eg, axial pattern flap, paramedian forehead flap)

A forehead flap with preservation of vascular pedicle is done. The paramedian forehead flap, in particular, is used as an excellent, reliable way of repairing severe nasal defects and is the type of forehead flap described here. The cutaneous branch of the supratrochlear artery is first located a couple of centimeters above the orbital rim. This anatomical marker is found by pencil doppler and used to form the forehead skin flap. The base is kept narrow enough that the length of the flap is not limited and it won't strangulate when twisted down to the recipient site and cut off the vascular supply. The shape of the flap is planned using a template and marked. The distance to the defect is measured to ensure that the flap will reach the recipient site. The flap is then elevated in a subgaleal plane above the periosteum inferiorly to preserve the vascular pedicle. The flap is then twisted into position in the defect. The donor site can usually be closed primarily.

15732-15738

15732   Muscle, myocutaneous, or fasciocutaneous flap; head and neck (eg, temporalis, masseter muscle, sternocleidomastoid, levator scapulae)

15734   Muscle, myocutaneous, or fasciocutaneous flap; trunk

15736   Muscle, myocutaneous, or fasciocutaneous flap; upper extremity

15738   Muscle, myocutaneous, or fasciocutaneous flap; lower extremity

The physician utilizes a graft of muscle, muscle and skin, or muscle fascia and a skin flap to repair a defect. The flap is prepared from the donor site and then rotated to cover the defect. The flap is sutured into place and the donor site is closed with sutures or a skin graft. If a skin graft is needed to close the donor site, report this procedure separately. Code 15732 for donor sites on the head and/or neck; 15734 for donor sites on the trunk; 15736 for donor sites on the upper extremities; and 15738 for donor sites on the lower extremities.

15740-15750

15740   Flap; island pedicle requiring identification and dissection of an anatomically named axial vessel

15750   Flap; neurovascular pedicle

A flap is created by incising skin and underlying tissues as needed, leaving the blood supply intact. The tissue is then transferred from the original (donor) site to the recipient site to cover a tissue defect. In 15740, an island pedicle flap is created. The skin and underlying subcutaneous tissues are incised usually in a V or Y configuration. The axial vessel in the subcutaneous or muscle tissue that will supply the flap is identified and protected. Dissection continues to mobilize the tissue flap and axial vessel. The island pedicle flap is then advanced over the defect. This may involve rotating the flap or tunneling the flap underneath adjacent tissue to reach the site of the defect. The flap is then secured with sutures over the primary tissue defect and the secondary defect created by the flap is also repaired. In 15750, a neurovascular pedicle flap is created in the same manner. An incision is made over the neurovascular bundle. The nerve that innervates the tissue, the artery that will supply the flap, as well as the vein that will drain the flap are identified. The skin and subcutaneous tissue are incised to create the flap. The tissue flap and neurovascular structures are mobilized. The neurovascular pedicle flap is then advanced to the recipient site which may involve rotating or tunneling the flap. The flap is secured with sutures over the primary tissue defect and the secondary defect created by the flap is also repaired.

15756

15756   Free muscle or myocutaneous flap with microvascular anastomosis

Under general anesthesia, the physician implants a free muscle or myocutaneous flap into a defect area. The physician also performs microvascular anastomosis to connect the blood vessels to the defect area. To begin the procedure, the physician prepares the donor area and removes the muscle section or myocutaneous flap. The donated muscle or myocutaneous flap is sutured into the appropriate position using half-mattress sutures. Microscopy is used to connect the appropriate vessels from the donor tissue to the recipient bed. The physician may inject fluorescent dye into the vessels to check for accurate joining of the vessels. Adjustments are then made if needed. The wound is sutured closed, and a dressing is applied. Splinting may be necessary to reduce shrinkage of the flap. The donor site is also closed and dressed.

15757

15757   Free skin flap with microvascular anastomosis

Under general anesthesia, the physician implants a free skin flap into a defect area. The physician also performs microvascular anastomosis to connect the blood vessels and nerves to the defect area. To begin the procedure, the physician prepares the donor area and removes the skin flap. The donated skin flap is sutured into the appropriate position using half-mattress sutures. Microscopy is used to connect the appropriate vessels and nerves from the donor tissue to the recipient bed. The physician may inject fluorescent dye into the vessels to check for accurate joining of the vessels. Adjustments are then made if needed. The wound is sutured closed and a dressing is applied. Splinting may be necessary to reduce shrinkage of the skin flap. The donor site is also closed and dressed.

15758

15758   Free fascial flap with microvascular anastomosis

Under general anesthesia, the physician implants a free fascial flap into a defect area. The physician also performs microvascular anastomosis to connect the blood vessels and nerves to the defect area. To begin the procedure, the physician prepares the donor area and removes the fascial flap. The donated fascial flap is sutured into the appropriate position . Microscopy is used to connect the appropriate vessels and nerves from the donor tissue to the recipient bed. The physician may inject fluorescent dye into the vessels to check for accurate joining of the vessels. Adjustments are then made if needed. The wound is sutured closed and a dressing is applied. Splinting may be necessary to reduce shrinkage of the skin flap. The donor site is also closed and dressed.

Integumentary/Skin

15760-15770

15760   **Graft; composite (eg, full thickness of external ear or nasal ala), including primary closure, donor area**
15770   **Graft; derma-fat-fascia**

Composite full-thickness grafts from the ear consist of epidermis, dermis and fat with cartilage sandwiched in between these layers. Derma-fat-fascia grafts consist of fat covered by derma on the surface and fascia at the base of the graft. In 15760, the size and configuration of the graft is determined and traced onto the donor site. Mattress sutures may be placed through the graft prior to excision to hold the tissue layers in place. The graft is then excised and prepared for transfer to the recipient site. Primary suture closure of the donor site is performed. In 15770, the defect is measured and the donor site marked to the size and configuration of the required graft. The graft is harvested and used to fill a soft tissue defect.

15775-15776

15775   **Punch graft for hair transplant; 1 to 15 punch grafts**
15776   **Punch graft for hair transplant; more than 15 punch grafts**

The physician removes small full thickness grafts from the scalp with a circular punch tool. These grafts are then transplanted to another region. This procedure is most commonly used for hair transplantation in balding men or women. Code 15775 for transplantation of 1 to 15 punch grafts, and code 15776 for transplantation of more than 15 punch grafts.

15777

15777   **Implantation of biologic implant (eg, acellular dermal matrix) for soft tissue reinforcement (ie, breast, trunk) (List separately in addition to code for primary procedure)**

A biologic implant such as acellular dermal matrix is implanted for soft tissue reinforcement at the time of a separately reportable repair or reconstruction procedure. Acellular dermal matrix may be derived from human tissue (AlloDerm¬Æ, DermaMatrix¬Æ, Turbplast ¬Æ) or porcine dermis (Strattice ¬Æ). Acellular dermal matrix derived from human tissue is a chemically treated skin graft from a cadaver donor that has had the antigenic epidermal cellular components removed. Removing the epidermis and cells responsible for immune reactions reduces the chance for rejection of the graft. This type of allograft was initially used to treat burn patients, but it is now also used for reconstructive procedures, dental and oral procedures, and plastic and cosmetic procedures as well. Acellular dermal matrix derived from porcine dermis is also treated with a process that removes cells, cell debris, DNA, and RNA to reduce the incidence of rejection. For human acelluar dermal matrix, the implant sheets are removed from the packet, rehydrated in an isotonic sodium chloride solution, and trimmed to the appropriate dimensions. The sheets are applied over the prepared wound bed in multiple layers and secured using absorbable sutures. Any excess at the periphery of the wound is trimmed. For acellular xenograft implants, the implant is removed from the packaging. The implant sheet is then cut to the size and shape of the wound, applied to the prepared wound bed, and secured with sutures. Once the acellular dermal matrix is in place the separately reportable repair or reconstruction procedure is completed.

15780-15783

15780   **Dermabrasion; total face (eg, for acne scarring, fine wrinkling, rhytids, general keratosis)**
15781   **Dermabrasion; segmental, face**
15782   **Dermabrasion; regional, other than face**
15783   **Dermabrasion; superficial, any site (eg, tattoo removal)**

Dermabrasion is the controlled abrasion of the upper layers of skin in order to create smoother skin, remove wrinkles, small scars or foreign bodies (tattoos). Code 15780 for dermabrasion of the total face; 15781 for dermabrasion of a segment of the face; 15782 for regional dermabrasion on areas other than the face; and 15783 for superficial dermabrasion, such as tattoo removal, on any site.

15786-15787

15786   **Abrasion; single lesion (eg, keratosis, scar)**
15787   **Abrasion; each additional 4 lesions or less (List separately in addition to code for primary procedure)**

The physician smooths down, or improves the appearance of a lesion, such as thickening of the skin or a scar. This is achieved via various abrasion techniques. Code 15786 for abrasion of a single lesion and code 15787 for each additional four lesions or less.

15788-15793

15788   **Chemical peel, facial; epidermal**
15789   **Chemical peel, facial; dermal**
15792   **Chemical peel, nonfacial; epidermal**
15793   **Chemical peel, nonfacial; dermal**

The physician applies a chemical agent (e.g., phenol or glycolic acid) to remove the epidermis and/or dermis. This procedure, known as a chemical peel, or chemexfoliation, is used to remove fine lines and wrinkles of the epidermis or dermis. Code 15788 to report a chemical peel of the facial epidermis; 15789 of the facial dermis; 15792 of the non-facial epidermis; and 15793 of the non-facial dermis.

15819

15819   **Cervicoplasty**

Under general anesthesia, the physician removes extraneous skin around the neck . The excess skin is excised and the remaining skin is sutured together in layers.

15820-15821

15820   **Blepharoplasty, lower eyelid**
15821   **Blepharoplasty, lower eyelid; with extensive herniated fat pad**

In 15820, loose or redundant skin of the lower eyelid just below the lashes is grasped, pulled taught, and trimmed away. If the musculature needs support, a stitch may be placed through the tendon at the lateral aspect of the eyelid and secured to the periosteum of the orbital rim. A running suture is placed to close the skin and repair the eyelid. In 15821, an incision is made in the conjunctiva of the lower lid and the underlying fat pad is exposed. The tendon on the lateral aspect of the eyelid is exposed and severed as needed to allow better exposure of the underlying fat pad. The herniated fat pad is dissected free of surrounding tissue. The fat may be removed, or more commonly, a subperiosteal tunnel is created at the medial aspect of the lower lid conjunctiva. The fat is transposed and positioned in the tear trough over the cheekbone. Loose sutures are placed through the skin to secure the fat pad in its new location. The lateral aspect of the eyelid is then incised and a wedge of eyelid is excised to allow tightening of the lower lid. A new tendon is fashioned and attached to the periosteum of the orbital rim using a single suture. Loose or redundant skin just below the lashes is grasped, pulled taught, and trimmed away. A running suture is placed to close the skin.

15822-15823

15822   **Blepharoplasty, upper eyelid**
15823   **Blepharoplasty, upper eyelid; with excessive skin weighting down lid**

The physician creates an incision in the crease of the upper eyelid. Excess/redundant skin is pulled taught and trimmed away. If the musculature needs support, a stitch may be added (15822). For removal of fatty tissue deposits in addition to removal of excess/redundant skin, report 15823. The wound is closed in sutured layers.

15824

15824   **Rhytidectomy; forehead**

The physician performs a rhytidectomy of the forehead by excising excess skin. The physician creates an incision, usually by the hairline of the forehead and dissects the tissue subcutaneously down to the eyebrows. The skin is pulled taught and the excess skin is trimmed. The wound is sutured in multiple layers.

15825

15825   **Rhytidectomy; neck with platysmal tightening (platysmal flap, P-flap)**

The physician performs a rhytidectomy of the neck by excising excess skin. The physician creates an incision, usually in front of the ears. The superficial musculoaponeurotic system (SMAS) is dissected and tightened with sutures in front of the ears. Another incision is created under the chin, through the platysma muscle, creating a flap (P-flap). This flap is pulled up and back and secured with multilayered sutures. The wounds are closed in multiple layers.

15826

15826   **Rhytidectomy; glabellar frown lines**

The physician performs a rhytidectomy of the glabellar frown lines (wrinkles between the eyebrows) by excising excess skin. The physician creates an incision, usually by the hairline of the forehead and dissects the tissue subcutaneously down to the eyebrows. The skin is pulled taught and the excess skin is trimmed. The wound is sutured in multiple layers.

15828

15828   **Rhytidectomy; cheek, chin, and neck**

The physician creates an incision in a naturally occurring wrinkle of the cheek, chin or neck. Excess skin is trimmed. The wound is closed in multiple layers.

   ● New Code   ▲ Revised Code

15829

15829   Rhytidectomy; superficial musculoaponeurotic system (SMAS) flap

The physician makes an incision in front of the ears. The superficial musculoaponeurotic system (SMAS) is dissected and tightened with sutures in front of the ears. The wound is closed in multiple layers.

15830-15839

15830   Excision, excessive skin and subcutaneous tissue (includes lipectomy); abdomen, infraumbilical panniculectomy

15832   Excision, excessive skin and subcutaneous tissue (includes lipectomy); thigh

15833   Excision, excessive skin and subcutaneous tissue (includes lipectomy); leg

15834   Excision, excessive skin and subcutaneous tissue (includes lipectomy); hip

15835   Excision, excessive skin and subcutaneous tissue (includes lipectomy); buttock

15836   Excision, excessive skin and subcutaneous tissue (includes lipectomy); arm

15837   Excision, excessive skin and subcutaneous tissue (includes lipectomy); forearm or hand

15838   Excision, excessive skin and subcutaneous tissue (includes lipectomy); submental fat pad

15839   Excision, excessive skin and subcutaneous tissue (includes lipectomy); other area

Excessive skin and subcutaneous tissue is removed from the abdomen in an infraumbilical panniculectomy, including lipectomy. A panniculectomy removes overhanging fat and skin, such as occurs in cases of extreme weight loss, that can cause a host of skin problems or interfere with movement. An incision is made from below the sternum to the pubic bone. Another incision is made across the pubic area where the excess fat and skin is carefully removed. Fat on the underside of skin may need to be dislodged and removed by scraping it with a cannula, a long hollow needle, inserted under the skin and then suctioned out. The remaining skin is brought back together and closed. A drain is usually inserted and left for a period of healing. Report similar procedures to remove excessive skin and subcutaneous tissue, including fat, from other body areas besides the abdomen by using 15832 for the thigh; 15833 for the leg; 15834 for the hip; 15835 for the buttock; 15836 for the arm; 15837 for the forearm or hand; 15838 for the submental fat pad; and 15839 for another area.

15840-15845

15840   Graft for facial nerve paralysis; free fascia graft (including obtaining fascia)

15841   Graft for facial nerve paralysis; free muscle graft (including obtaining graft)

15842   Graft for facial nerve paralysis; free muscle flap by microsurgical technique

15845   Graft for facial nerve paralysis; regional muscle transfer

The physician obtains a graft used to correct facial paralysis. The fascia is harvested from the donor site, usually the fascia lata in the leg. The graft is transplanted to the face and sutured beneath the skin to partially reanimate the face in areas which were previously paralyzed (15840). Code 15841 if a free muscle graft is utilized; 15842 if a free muscle flap with microsurgical technique is utilized; and 15845 if the physician performs a regional muscle transfer.

15847

15847   Excision, excessive skin and subcutaneous tissue (includes lipectomy), abdomen (eg, abdominoplasty) (includes umbilical transposition and fascial plication) (List separately in addition to code for primary procedure)

Excessive skin and subcutaneous tissue is removed from the abdomen in an abdominoplasty that includes umbilical transposition and fascial placation. This procedure is commonly known as a tummy tuck. A long incision is made above the pubic area from hip to hip. Another incision is made to free the navel from its surrounding tissues. The skin is dissected from the abdominal wall up to the ribs and the large skin flap is retracted to expose the abdominal muscles. These vertical muscles are tightened by being pulled closer together and stitched into position. This slims down the waistline and makes the abdominal wall firmer. Excess fat may need to be scraped loose and removed. The skin flap is then laid down and the extra skin is removed. An opening must be cut for the new positioning of the navel, which is then stitched into place. The incisions are closed and a drain is usually placed for draining fluid from the surgical site.

15850-15851

15850   Removal of sutures under anesthesia (other than local), same surgeon

15851   Removal of sutures under anesthesia (other than local), other surgeon

Sutures that were placed during a previous surgical or traumatic wound closure are removed under regional or general anesthesia. Regional or general anesthesia is not typically required for suture removal unless the patient is a young child or unable to understand and cooperate with the physician during suture removal. A regional or general anesthetic is administered by an anesthesiologist. The surgeon then removes the sutures.

Use 15850 for removal by the surgeon that the performed the original procedure or 15851 if a different surgeon removes the sutures.

15852

15852   Dressing change (for other than burns) under anesthesia (other than local)

A dressing change is performed under regional or general anesthesia for a condition other than a burn. Regional or general anesthesia is not typically required for dressing change unless the patient is a young child or unable to understand and cooperate with the physician during the dressing change. A regional or general anesthetic is administered by an anesthesiologist. The physician then removes the dressing, inspects the wound, and redresses the wound as needed.

15860

15860   Intravenous injection of agent (eg, fluorescein) to test vascular flow in flap or graft

The physician injects a dye agent intravenously, such as fluorescein or methylene blue to test vascular flow in a flap or graft area.

15876-15879

15876   Suction assisted lipectomy; head and neck

15877   Suction assisted lipectomy; trunk

15878   Suction assisted lipectomy; upper extremity

15879   Suction assisted lipectomy; lower extremity

This procedure is most commonly referred to as liposuction. The physician creates incisions into the skin over areas of excessive fat deposits. The physician then inserts a suction curettage cannula through the incision and moves the cannula in rows through the area, evacuating excess fat cells. The incisions are closed with simple closure. Code 15876 for liposuction of the head and neck; 15877 for liposuction of the trunk; 15878 for liposuction of the upper extremity; and 15879 for liposuction of the lower extremity.

15920-15922

15920   Excision, coccygeal pressure ulcer, with coccygectomy; with primary suture

15922   Excision, coccygeal pressure ulcer, with coccygectomy; with flap closure

A coccygeal pressure ulcer may also be referred to as a pressure sore, bedsore, or decubitus ulcer. The coccyx is the triangular bone at the base of the spine formed by fusion of the four coccygeal vertebrae. The patient lies face down and the physician creates an elliptical incision around the coccygeal pressure ulcer. The pressure ulcer is excised. The coccyx is then exposed. A finger is used to elevate the tip of the coccyx and the coccyx is dissected free of underlying tissue up to the level of the sacrum. The coccyx is then severed at the sacrococcygeal joint and removed. Any rough bony surfaces are smoothed with a file. In 15920, the wound is closed in layers using primary suture repair. In 15922, a local skin flap is used to close the wound. Skin adjacent to the wound is incised down to the level of subcutaneous fat and the skin is mobilized. The skin flap is then rotated or advanced and sutured over the wound. The donor site is also repaired with sutures.

15931-15933

15931   Excision, sacral pressure ulcer, with primary suture

15933   Excision, sacral pressure ulcer, with primary suture; with ostectomy

The physician excises a pressure ulcer, commonly known as a bedsore, of the sacral region. The sacrum is the triangular-shaped bone, which lies between the 5th lumbar vertebra and the coccyx. The patient lies face down and the physician creates an elliptical incision over the sacrum. The physician removes the affected skin surrounding the pressure ulcer and irrigates the wound. The sacrum is separated from the surrounding tissue. The site is then sutured closed with primary sutures. Code 15933 if the bone beneath the ulcer is removed prior to closure of the site.

15934-15935

15934   Excision, sacral pressure ulcer, with skin flap closure

15935   Excision, sacral pressure ulcer, with skin flap closure; with ostectomy

A sacral pressure ulcer may also be referred to as a pressure sore, bedsore, or decubitus ulcer. The sacrum is the triangular bone between the 5th lumbar vertebra and the coccyx. The patient lies face down and the physician creates an elliptical incision around the sacral pressure ulcer. The pressure ulcer is excised. In 15934, a local skin flap is used to close the wound. Skin adjacent to the wound is incised down to the level of subcutaneous fat and the skin is mobilized. The skin flap is then rotated or advanced and sutured over the wound. The donor site is also repaired with sutures. In 15935, the sacrum is exposed and sacral bone underlying the pressure ulcer is inspected. Any involved bone or bony protuberances are excised taking care to protect surrounding nerves and blood vessels. Remaining rough bony surfaces are smoothed with a file. The wound is then closed with a local skin flap as described above.

Integumentary/Skin

15936-15937

15936 Excision, sacral pressure ulcer, in preparation for muscle or myocutaneous flap or skin graft closure

15937 Excision, sacral pressure ulcer, in preparation for muscle or myocutaneous flap or skin graft closure; with ostectomy

A sacral pressure ulcer, also referred to as a pressure sore, bedsore, or decubitus ulcer, is excised with or without excision of bone in preparation for closure using a separately reportable muscle or myocutaneous flap or skin graft. The sacrum is the triangular bone between the 5th lumbar vertebra and the coccyx. The patient lies face down and the physician creates an incision around the sacral pressure ulcer and all necrotic tissue is excised, including skin, subcutaneous tissue and muscle. The bursa and any involved bone or bony protuberances are also excised taking care to protect surrounding nerves and blood vessels. Remaining rough bony surfaces are smoothed with a file. The edges of the wound are trimmed and the wound bed prepared for the muscle or myocutaneous flap or skin graft. Common types of flaps used include superior gluteal myocutaneous flap, superior portion of the gluteus maximus muscle, and bilateral V-Y myocutaneous advancement flaps. The muscle or myocutaneous flap or skin graft is developed and prepared for placement in the sacral wound in a separately reportable procedure. Use 15936 if the procedure is performed without removal of bone (ostectomy) and 15937 if ostectomy is performed.

15940-15941

15940 Excision, ischial pressure ulcer, with primary suture

15941 Excision, ischial pressure ulcer, with primary suture; with ostectomy (ischiectomy)

The physician excises a pressure ulcer, commonly known as a bedsore, of the ischial region. The ischium is the ventral and posterior sides of the three principle bones composing either half of the pelvis. The patient lies face down and the physician creates an elliptical incision over the ischial tuberosity to remove the infected tissues. The physician removes the affected skin surrounding the pressure ulcer and irrigates the wound. The wound is irrigated and closed with primary sutures. Code 15941 if any of the bone below the ulcer is removed before closure.

15944-15945

15944 Excision, ischial pressure ulcer, with skin flap closure

15945 Excision, ischial pressure ulcer, with skin flap closure; with ostectomy

An ischial pressure ulcer may also be referred to as a pressure sore, bedsore, or decubitus ulcer. The ischium is located in the lower posterior portion of the bony pelvis. The patient lies face down and the physician creates an elliptical incision around the ischial pressure ulcer. The pressure ulcer is excised and the wound is irrigated. In 15944, a local skin flap is used to close the wound. Skin adjacent to the wound is incised down to the level of subcutaneous fat and the skin is mobilized. The skin flap is then rotated or advanced and sutured over the wound. The donor site is also repaired with sutures. In 15945, the ischium is exposed and bone underlying the pressure ulcer is inspected. Any involved bone or bony protuberances are excised taking care to protect surrounding nerves and blood vessels. Remaining rough bony surfaces are smoothed with a file. The wound is then closed with a local skin flap as described above.

15946

15946 Excision, ischial pressure ulcer, with ostectomy, in preparation for muscle or myocutaneous flap or skin graft closure

A ischial pressure ulcer, also referred to as a pressure sore, bedsore, or decubitus ulcer, is excised with or without excision of bone (ostectomy) in preparation for closure using a separately reportable muscle or myocutaneous flap or skin graft. The ischium is located in the lower posterior portion of the bony pelvis. The patient lies face down and the physician creates an incision around the ischial pressure ulcer and all necrotic tissue is excised, including skin, subcutaneous tissue and muscle. Involved bone or bony protuberances are also excised. Remaining rough bony surfaces are smoothed with a file. The edges of the wound are trimmed and the wound bed prepared for the muscle or myocutaneous flap or skin graft. Common types of flaps used include a gluteal thigh rotation flap, a gluteus maximus muscle flap, or an inferior gluteus maximus myocutaneous flap. The muscle or myocutaneous flap or skin graft is then developed and prepared for placement in the sacral wound in a separately reportable procedure.

15950-15953

15950 Excision, trochanteric pressure ulcer, with primary suture

15951 Excision, trochanteric pressure ulcer, with primary suture; with ostectomy

15952 Excision, trochanteric pressure ulcer, with skin flap closure

15953 Excision, trochanteric pressure ulcer, with skin flap closure; with ostectomy

A trochanteric pressure ulcer may also be referred to as a pressure sore, bedsore, or decubitus ulcer. The trochanters are projections at the proximal end of the femur that serve as attachment points for muscles of the thigh and buttock. The greater trochanter is located on the outer aspect of the femur and the lesser trochanter is on the inner aspect.

Trochanteric pressure ulcers occur over the greater trochanter. The physician creates an elliptical incision around the trochanteric pressure ulcer and all necrotic tissue is excised, including skin, subcutaneous tissue and muscle. In 15950, the wound is closed in layers using primary suture repair. In 15951, the trochanter is exposed and the trochanteric bursa and bone are inspected. The bursa is resected and involved bone or bony protuberances are excised taking care to protect surrounding nerves and blood vessels. Remaining rough bony surfaces are smoothed with a file. The wound is then closed in layers using primary suture repair. In 15952, a local skin flap is used to close the wound. Skin adjacent to the wound is incised down to the level of subcutaneous fat and the skin is mobilized. The skin flap is then rotated or advanced and sutured over the wound. The donor site is also repaired with sutures. In 15953, the trochanter is exposed and the trochanteric bursa and bone are inspected. The bursa is resected and involved bone or bony protuberances are excised taking care to protect surrounding nerves and blood vessels. Remaining rough bony surfaces are smoothed with a file. The wound is then closed with a local skin flap as described above.

15956-15958

15956 Excision, trochanteric pressure ulcer, in preparation for muscle or myocutaneous flap or skin graft closure

15958 Excision, trochanteric pressure ulcer, in preparation for muscle or myocutaneous flap or skin graft closure; with ostectomy

A trochanteric pressure ulcer, also referred to as a pressure sore, bedsore, or decubitus ulcer, is excised with or without excision of bone in preparation for closure using a separately reportable muscle or myocutaneous flap or skin graft. The trochanters are projections at the proximal end of the femur that serve as attachment points for muscles of the thigh and buttock. The greater trochanter is located on the outer aspect of the femur and the lesser trochanter is on the inner aspect. Trochanteric pressure ulcers occur over the greater trochanter. The physician creates an incision around the trochanteric pressure ulcer and all necrotic tissue is excised, including skin, subcutaneous tissue and muscle. The bursa and any involved bone or bony protuberances are excised as needed taking care to protect surrounding nerves and blood vessels. Remaining rough bony surfaces are smoothed with a file. The edges of the wound are trimmed and the wound bed prepared for the muscle or myocutaneous flap or skin graft. Common types of flaps include tensor fascia lata flap, vastus lateralis myocutaneous flap, gluteal thigh flap and anterior thigh flap. The muscle or myocutaneous flap or skin graft is developed and prepared for placement in the sacral wound in a separately reportable procedure. Use 15956 if the procedure is performed without removal of bone (ostectomy) and 15958 if ostectomy is performed.

16000

16000 Initial treatment, first degree burn, when no more than local treatment is required

The physician provides initial local treatment of a first degree burn. Burns are classified by degree. A first degree burn is the least serious type causing injury only to the epidermis, the top layer of skin. The burn area is examined and washed with an antiseptic cleanser. A soothing cream and a sterile dressing is applied as needed. The patient is instructed on the use of pain relievers such as acetaminophen, ibuprofen, or aspirin.

16020-16030

16020 Dressings and/or debridement of partial-thickness burns, initial or subsequent; small (less than 5% total body surface area)

16025 Dressings and/or debridement of partial-thickness burns, initial or subsequent; medium (eg, whole face or whole extremity, or 5% to 10% total body surface area)

16030 Dressings and/or debridement of partial-thickness burns, initial or subsequent; large (eg, more than 1 extremity, or greater than 10% total body surface area)

The physician provides initial or subsequent treatment of a partial thickness burn including debridement of tissue and/or the application of dressings. Burns are classified by the extent of total body surface area (TBSA) involved and by the depth or the degree of the burn. A partial thickness burn is one that injures the epidermis or top layers of skin as well as the dermis or deeper layers of skin. The burn area is examined and the patient queried as to the cause of the burn. The area is washed with an antiseptic cleanser as needed and any foreign material removed. Dead or damaged tissue is also removed as needed. A soothing cream may be applied. The burn may be covered with a sterile dressing. Use code 16020 for a small burn comprising less than five percent of TBSA. Use code 16025 for a medium burn such as a burn of the entire face or the entire surface of one extremity or a burn comprising five to ten percent of TBSA. Use code 16030 for a large burn such as more than one extremity or comprising more than ten percent of TBSA.

Integumentary/Skin

16035-16036

16035 Escharotomy; initial incision
16036 Escharotomy; each additional incision (List separately in addition to code for primary procedure)

The physician performs an escharotomy. Escharotomy is used to treat a third degree burn where the damaged skin or eschar has lost elasticity becoming rigid and hard. A tight eschar of an extremity can interfere with circulation and if left untreated can cause loss of the limb. A tight eschar of the chest can interfere with respiration causing atelectasis or pneumonia. One or more incisions are made in the damaged skin to allow the underlying tissue to expand. The incision is made along the entire length of the eschar and carried down to viable subcutaneous tissue. The incision causes the tissue to gape open. Bleeding is controlled, the escharotomy packed with Slivazine cream and dressings applied as needed. If a limb is involved it is elevated to help limit edema at the burn site. Use code 16035 for the initial escharotomy incision and 16036 for each additional incision.

17000-17004

17000 Destruction (eg, laser surgery, electrosurgery, cryosurgery, chemosurgery, surgical curettement), premalignant lesions (eg, actinic keratoses); first lesion
17003 Destruction (eg, laser surgery, electrosurgery, cryosurgery, chemosurgery, surgical curettement), premalignant lesions (eg, actinic keratoses); second through 14 lesions, each (List separately in addition to code for first lesion)
17004 Destruction (eg, laser surgery, electrosurgery, cryosurgery, chemosurgery, surgical curettement), premalignant lesions (eg, actinic keratoses), 15 or more lesions

A commonly treated type of premalignant lesion is an actinic keratosis (AK), also referred to as solar keratosis. These types of lesions are confined to the epidermis and typically appear as rough, scaly patches on sun exposed skin. The lesion is examined and the most appropriate form of destruction determined. Local anesthesia is administered as needed. Cryosurgery using liquid nitrogen to freeze the lesion is the most common technique. Surgical curettage followed by electrosurgery is another common method of destruction. Multiple lesions are more often treated with a chemical or pharmacologic agents or laser resurfacing with a carbon dioxide laser. Use 17000 for the first lesion and 17003 for each lesion from the second through fourteenth. Use 17004 for 15 or more lesions.

Destruction, premalignant lesions (eg, actinic keratoses); first lesion

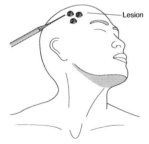
Lesion

The physician destroys a premalignant lesion. Destruction of benign, cutaneous vascular proliferative lesions, or removal of skin tags are not included in this procedure. Local anesthesia is included. Code 17000 for the first lesion; 17003 for each additional lesion destroyed up to 14 lesions; 17004 if 15 or more lesions are destroyed.

17106-17108

17106 Destruction of cutaneous vascular proliferative lesions (eg, laser technique); less than 10 sq cm
17107 Destruction of cutaneous vascular proliferative lesions (eg, laser technique); 10.0 to 50.0 sq cm
17108 Destruction of cutaneous vascular proliferative lesions (eg, laser technique); over 50.0 sq cm

Cutaneous vascular proliferative lesions include conditions such as port wine stain, hemangioma, and telangiectasia. Cutaneous vascular lesions require selective photothermolysis of oxyhemoglobin, which is accomplished with a yellow light laser such as a flash lamp pumped pulsed-dye laser, argon-pumped tunable dye laser, or copper vapor, copper bromide, or krypton laser. The laser is programmed to the appropriate wavelength, pulse duration, and pulse energy for the target lesion. The laser is then activated and the lesion treated. The patient may require multiple laser treatment sessions to achieve the desired results. Use 17106 for lesions less than 10.0 sq cm in size, 17107 for lesions 10.0-50.0 sq cm, and 17108 for lesions over 50.0 sq cm.

17110-17111

17110 Destruction (eg, laser surgery, electrosurgery, cryosurgery, chemosurgery, surgical curettement), of benign lesions other than skin tags or cutaneous vascular proliferative lesions; up to 14 lesions
17111 Destruction (eg, laser surgery, electrosurgery, cryosurgery, chemosurgery, surgical curettement), of benign lesions other than skin tags or cutaneous vascular proliferative lesions; 15 or more lesions

Benign lesions other than skin tags or cutaneous vascular proliferative lesions are destroyed by laser surgery, electrosurgery, cryosurgery, chemosurgery, or surgical curettement. A local anesthetic may be administered. The type of destruction depends on the lesion type and location and may include use of a laser, heat or thermal energy (electrosurgery), cold or freezing (cryosurgery), chemical destruction, or scraping (surgical curettement). Use 17110 to report destruction of up to 14 lesions and 17111 for destruction of 15 or more lesions.

17250

17250 Chemical cauterization of granulation tissue (proud flesh, sinus or fistula)

The physician uses chemical cauterization to destroy granulation tissue such as excess scar tissue, also referred to as proud flesh, or a sinus or fistula. Liquid silver nitrate applied with a Q-tip or a silver nitrate stick is dabbed onto the granulation tissue. This is done during the last stages of healing of an open wound.

17260-17266

17260 Destruction, malignant lesion (eg, laser surgery, electrosurgery, cryosurgery, chemosurgery, surgical curettement), trunk, arms or legs; lesion diameter 0.5 cm or less
17261 Destruction, malignant lesion (eg, laser surgery, electrosurgery, cryosurgery, chemosurgery, surgical curettement), trunk, arms or legs; lesion diameter 0.6 to 1.0 cm
17262 Destruction, malignant lesion (eg, laser surgery, electrosurgery, cryosurgery, chemosurgery, surgical curettement), trunk, arms or legs; lesion diameter 1.1 to 2.0 cm
17263 Destruction, malignant lesion (eg, laser surgery, electrosurgery, cryosurgery, chemosurgery, surgical curettement), trunk, arms or legs; lesion diameter 2.1 to 3.0 cm
17264 Destruction, malignant lesion (eg, laser surgery, electrosurgery, cryosurgery, chemosurgery, surgical curettement), trunk, arms or legs; lesion diameter 3.1 to 4.0 cm
17266 Destruction, malignant lesion (eg, laser surgery, electrosurgery, cryosurgery, chemosurgery, surgical curettement), trunk, arms or legs; lesion diameter over 4.0 cm

Most types of malignant lesions are treated by excision; however, squamous cell carcinoma, verrucous carcinoma, and lesions that have not penetrated deeper layers of the dermis may be treated using destruction. The lesion is examined and the most appropriate form of destruction determined. Local anesthesia is administered as needed. Cryosurgery using liquid nitrogen to freeze the lesion is one destruction technique. Surgical curettage followed by electrosurgery is another common method of destruction. Other techniques include chemosurgery with a chemical or pharmacologic agent or laser destruction with a carbon dioxide laser. Us 17260 for a trunk, arm or leg lesion with a diameter of 0.5 cm or less, 17261 for lesion diameter of 0.6 to 1.0 cm, 17262 for lesion diameter 1.1 to 2.0, 17263 for lesion diameter 2.1 to 3.0, 17264 for lesion diameter 3.1 to 4.0, or 17266 for lesion diameter over 4.0 cm.

17270-17276

17270 Destruction, malignant lesion (eg, laser surgery, electrosurgery, cryosurgery, chemosurgery, surgical curettement), scalp, neck, hands, feet, genitalia; lesion diameter 0.5 cm or less
17271 Destruction, malignant lesion (eg, laser surgery, electrosurgery, cryosurgery, chemosurgery, surgical curettement), scalp, neck, hands, feet, genitalia; lesion diameter 0.6 to 1.0 cm
17272 Destruction, malignant lesion (eg, laser surgery, electrosurgery, cryosurgery, chemosurgery, surgical curettement), scalp, neck, hands, feet, genitalia; lesion diameter 1.1 to 2.0 cm
17273 Destruction, malignant lesion (eg, laser surgery, electrosurgery, cryosurgery, chemosurgery, surgical curettement), scalp, neck, hands, feet, genitalia; lesion diameter 2.1 to 3.0 cm
17274 Destruction, malignant lesion (eg, laser surgery, electrosurgery, cryosurgery, chemosurgery, surgical curettement), scalp, neck, hands, feet, genitalia; lesion diameter 3.1 to 4.0 cm
17276 Destruction, malignant lesion (eg, laser surgery, electrosurgery, cryosurgery, chemosurgery, surgical curettement), scalp, neck, hands, feet, genitalia; lesion diameter over 4.0 cm

Malignant lesions of the skin include basal cell carcinoma, squamous cell carcinoma, and malignant melanoma. The lesion is examined and the most appropriate form of destruction

Integumentary/Skin

determined. A local anesthetic as administered as needed. Cryosurgery is performed with liquid nitrogen to freeze the lesion using a series of freeze thaw cycles. Surgical curettage followed by electrosurgery is another method of destruction. Multiple lesions are more often treated using chemical or pharmacologic agent or laser resurfacing with a carbon dioxide laser. The physician destroys the lesion as well as a surrounding border of normal tissue. Use 17270 for a lesion with diameter of less than 0.5 cm, use 17271 for lesion diameter 0.6-1.0, use 17272 for lesion diameter 1.1-2.0, use 17273 for lesion diameter 2.1-3.0, use 17274 for lesion 3.1-4.0, use 17276 for lesion diameter over 4.0.

17280-17286

17280 **Destruction, malignant lesion (eg, laser surgery, electrosurgery, cryosurgery, chemosurgery, surgical curettement), face, ears, eyelids, nose, lips, mucous membrane; lesion diameter 0.5 cm or less**

17281 **Destruction, malignant lesion (eg, laser surgery, electrosurgery, cryosurgery, chemosurgery, surgical curettement), face, ears, eyelids, nose, lips, mucous membrane; lesion diameter 0.6 to 1.0 cm**

17282 **Destruction, malignant lesion (eg, laser surgery, electrosurgery, cryosurgery, chemosurgery, surgical curettement), face, ears, eyelids, nose, lips, mucous membrane; lesion diameter 1.1 to 2.0 cm**

17283 **Destruction, malignant lesion (eg, laser surgery, electrosurgery, cryosurgery, chemosurgery, surgical curettement), face, ears, eyelids, nose, lips, mucous membrane; lesion diameter 2.1 to 3.0 cm**

17284 **Destruction, malignant lesion (eg, laser surgery, electrosurgery, cryosurgery, chemosurgery, surgical curettement), face, ears, eyelids, nose, lips, mucous membrane; lesion diameter 3.1 to 4.0 cm**

17286 **Destruction, malignant lesion (eg, laser surgery, electrosurgery, cryosurgery, chemosurgery, surgical curettement), face, ears, eyelids, nose, lips, mucous membrane; lesion diameter over 4.0 cm**

The physician destroys a malignant lesion of the using methods such as laser surgery, electrosurgery, cryosurgery, chemosurgery, or surgical curettement. Most types of malignant lesions are treated by excision; however, squamous cell carcinoma, verrucous carcinoma, and lesions that have not penetrated deeper layers of the dermis may be treated using destruction. The lesion is examined and the most appropriate form of destruction determined. Local anesthesia is administered as needed. Cryosurgery using liquid nitrogen to freeze the lesion is one destruction technique. Surgical curettage followed by electrosurgery is another common method of destruction. Other techniques include chemosurgery with a chemical or pharmacologic agent or laser destruction with a carbon dioxide laser. Use 17280 for a face, ear, eyelid, nose, lip or mucous membrane lesion with a diameter of 0.5 cm or less, 17281 for lesion diameter of 0.6 to 1.0 cm, 17282 for lesion diameter 1.1 to 2.0, 17283 for lesion diameter 2.1 to 3.0, 17284 for lesion diameter 3.1 to 4.0, or 17286 for lesion diameter over 4.0 cm.

17311-17312

17311 **Mohs micrographic technique, including removal of all gross tumor, surgical excision of tissue specimens, mapping, color coding of specimens, microscopic examination of specimens by the surgeon, and histopathologic preparation including routine stain(s) (eg, hematoxylin and eosin, toluidine blue), head, neck, hands, feet, genitalia, or any location with surgery directly involving muscle, cartilage, bone, tendon, major nerves, or vessels; first stage, up to 5 tissue blocks**

17312 **Mohs micrographic technique, including removal of all gross tumor, surgical excision of tissue specimens, mapping, color coding of specimens, microscopic examination of specimens by the surgeon, and histopathologic preparation including routine stain(s) (eg, hematoxylin and eosin, toluidine blue), head, neck, hands, feet, genitalia, or any location with surgery directly involving muscle, cartilage, bone, tendon, major nerves, or vessels; each additional stage after the first stage, up to 5 tissue blocks (List separately in addition to code for primary procedure)**

Mohs micrographic surgery technique, is a method of removing complex or ill-defined cancer of the skin in which the physician acts as both the surgeon and the pathologist during the procedure. This technique is an exact and very precise method of tumor removal and has the highest recovery rate. Mohs technique is used to treat two of the most common skin cancers: basal cell carcinoma and squamous cell carcinoma. The surgeon removes the tumor in thin layers of tissue. The excised specimens are stained, or color-coded, and examined immediately under a microscope to track the tumor's removal down to the roots, leaving healthy tissue unharmed. The color coding of the removed specimens allows the surgeon to accurately map out and identify the location of remaining cancer cells in each specimen. Code 17311 for Mohs micrographic removal of tumors of the head, neck, hands, feet, genitalia, or any location with surgery directly involving muscle, cartilage, bone, tendon, major nerves, or vessels; first stage, up to 5 tissue blocks and code 17312 for each additional stage after the first stage, up to 5 tissue blocks.

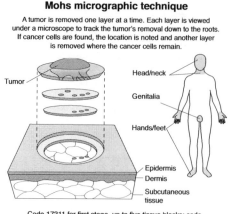

Mohs micrographic technique

A tumor is removed one layer at a time. Each layer is viewed under a microscope to track the tumor's removal down to the roots. If cancer cells are found, the location is noted and another layer is removed where the cancer cells remain.

Tumor

Head/neck
Genitalia
Hands/feet

Epidermis
Dermis
Subcutaneous tissue

Code 17311 for first stage, up to five tissue blocks; code 17312 for each additional stage, up to five tissue blocks

17313-17315

17313 **Mohs micrographic technique, including removal of all gross tumor, surgical excision of tissue specimens, mapping, color coding of specimens, microscopic examination of specimens by the surgeon, and histopathologic preparation including routine stain(s) (eg, hematoxylin and eosin, toluidine blue), of the trunk, arms, or legs; first stage, up to 5 tissue blocks**

17314 **Mohs micrographic technique, including removal of all gross tumor, surgical excision of tissue specimens, mapping, color coding of specimens, microscopic examination of specimens by the surgeon, and histopathologic preparation including routine stain(s) (eg, hematoxylin and eosin, toluidine blue), of the trunk, arms, or legs; each additional stage after the first stage, up to 5 tissue blocks (List separately in addition to code for primary procedure)**

17315 **Mohs micrographic technique, including removal of all gross tumor, surgical excision of tissue specimens, mapping, color coding of specimens, microscopic examination of specimens by the surgeon, and histopathologic preparation including routine stain(s) (eg, hematoxylin and eosin, toluidine blue), each additional block after the first 5 tissue blocks, any stage (List separately in addition to code for primary procedure)**

Mohs micrographic surgery technique is a method of removing complex or ill-defined cancer of the skin, in which the physician acts as both the surgeon and the pathologist during the procedure. This technique is an exact and precise method of tumor removal and has the highest recovery rate. Mohs technique is used to treat two of the most common skin cancers: basal cell carcinoma and squamous cell carcinoma. The surgeon removes the tumor in thin layers of tissue. The excised specimens are stained, or color-coded, and examined immediately under a microscope to track the tumor's removal down to the roots, leaving healthy tissue unharmed. The color coding of the removed specimens allows the surgeon to accurately map out and identify the location of remaining cancer cells in each specimen. Code 17313 for Mohs micrographic removal of tumors of the the of the trunk, arms, or legs; first stage, up to 5 tissue blocks; code 17314 for each additional stage after the first stage, up to 5 tissue blocks; and report 17315 for each additional block after the first 5 tissue blocks of any stage.

17340-17360

17340 **Cryotherapy (CO2 slush, liquid N2) for acne**
17360 **Chemical exfoliation for acne (eg, acne paste, acid)**

Acne is treated using cryotherapy, also referred to as CO_2 slush or liquid N2, or chemical exfoliation, such as acne paste or acid is performed. In 17340, cryotherapy is used. The surface skin lesions are frozen using cryospray, cryoprobe, or a cotton-tipped applicator. Each site is treated for a few seconds. If a double freeze-thaw cycle is required the lesion is treated a second time. Alternatively, the entire surface of the involved area of skin may be exfoliated using a cotton-tipped applicator. In 17360, chemical exfoliation is used. Chemical exfoliation refers to a controlled removal of one or more layers of epidermis and superficial dermis using a wounding agent in patients with active acne. Typically, the physician uses alpha hydroxy acids (AHA) at a concentration of 50%-70% applied over involved areas to exfoliate the surface layers of the skin.

17380

17380 **Electrolysis epilation, each 30 minutes**

The physician inserts an electroneedle into a hair follicle and activates an electric current, which kills the hair follicle. This procedure is repeated throughout a localized area and is useful for permanent hair removal. Code 17380 reports 30 minutes of electrolysis epilation.

● New Code   ▲ Revised Code   CPT © 2016 American Medical Association. All Rights Reserved.   © 2017 DecisionHealth

Breast

19000-19001

19000	Puncture aspiration of cyst of breast
19001	Puncture aspiration of cyst of breast; each additional cyst (List separately in addition to code for primary procedure)

The cyst is palpated. The skin over the cyst is cleansed and a local anesthetic administered as needed. A needle connected to a syringe is inserted into the cyst and the fluid aspirated to collapse the cyst. Pressure is applied to control bleeding. Steristrips and antibiotic ointment are applied to the puncture site as needed. Use 19000 for a single cyst and 19001 for each additional cyst treated.

19020

19020	Mastotomy with exploration or drainage of abscess, deep

The physician performs a mastotomy with deep exploration or drainage of abscess. A radial incision is made in the skin extending outward over the abscess site or site to be explored. The incision is deepened and the area of concern is evaluated. If an abscess is present, the abscess cavity is entered, loculations are broken up by finger dissection, and the abscess is drained. Cultures are taken and sent for separately reportable laboratory analysis. The abscess site is irrigated with saline solution, packed with gauze, and left open to drain.

19030

19030	Injection procedure only for mammary ductogram or galactogram

The physician performs the injection procedure only for a mammary ductogram or galactogram. The physician places a needle or cannula into the duct of the breast and injects contrast media. A dissecting microscope may be necessary for accurate placement. This procedure is used for radiographic study of the area. The needle or cannula is removed.

19081-19082

19081	Biopsy, breast, with placement of breast localization device(s) (eg, clip, metallic pellet), when performed, and imaging of the biopsy specimen, when performed, percutaneous; first lesion, including stereotactic guidance
19082	Biopsy, breast, with placement of breast localization device(s) (eg, clip, metallic pellet), when performed, and imaging of the biopsy specimen, when performed, percutaneous; each additional lesion, including stereotactic guidance (List separately in addition to code for primary procedure)

A percutaneous biopsy of the breast is performed using stereotactic guidance to identify the lesion. The skin is cleansed and a local anesthetic is injected. Stereotactic technique uses a fixed coordinate system to identify the lesion's unique location within the breast by defining it in terms of specific x, y, and z coordinates relative to an original reference point. The breast is positioned between a compression plate and a support in back to keep the lesion in a fixed position. Breast thickness under compression determines the depth dimension. An initial image is obtained perpendicular to the compression plate at 0 degrees angulation and this initial image is used to center the lesion in the biopsy window of the compression plate. Other images are obtained at specified angles to and from the relative 0 position by rotation around the known center. Geometric calculations are used to determine the lesion location in three dimensions. If a needle biopsy is performed, the needle is inserted into the lesion and a tissue sample is obtained. In order to obtain an adequate tissue sample, 3-6 separate core needle insertions are typically required. When an adequate tissue sample has been obtained, it is sent to the laboratory for pathology exam. If an automated vacuum assisted or rotating biopsy device is used, the skin is nicked and a breast probe is placed in the area of the lesion. A vacuum line then draws breast tissue into the sampling chamber of the device. Alternatively, a rotating cutting device is advanced and the tissue sample is carried through the probe and captured by a tissue cassette. The probe is then rotated to a new position and the next tissue sample is obtained until 8-10 samples are taken at rotations of approximately 30 degrees. When the sampling process is complete, the probe is removed and pressure is applied to the biopsy site. Placement of a metallic localization clip or pellet is performed when a more extensive procedure, such as a lumpectomy, is anticipated so that the physician can identify the exact site where tissue has been removed. Following the biopsy procedure, the needle is left in place. A plastic stylette with a metal clip or pellet at the end is inserted through the biopsy needle and advanced to the biopsy site using imaging guidance. The metal clip or pellet is released and the stylette and needle are removed. Additional images of the biopsy specimen may be obtained prior to separately reportable pathology examination of the tissue. Use code 19081 for biopsy of the first lesion and 19082 for biopsy of each additional lesion.

19083-19084

19083	Biopsy, breast, with placement of breast localization device(s) (eg, clip, metallic pellet), when performed, and imaging of the biopsy specimen, when performed, percutaneous; first lesion, including ultrasound guidance
19084	Biopsy, breast, with placement of breast localization device(s) (eg, clip, metallic pellet), when performed, and imaging of the biopsy specimen, when performed, percutaneous; each additional lesion, including ultrasound guidance (List separately in addition to code for primary procedure)

A percutaneous biopsy of the breast is performed using ultrasound guidance. The skin is cleansed and a local anesthetic is injected. A transducer is used to locate the lesion in the breast. The radiologist constantly monitors placement of the biopsy needle, vacuum, or rotating device using the ultrasound probe. If a needle biopsy is performed, the needle is inserted into the lesion and a tissue sample is obtained. In order to obtain an adequate tissue sample, 3-6 separate core needle insertions are typically required. If an automated vacuum assisted or rotating biopsy device is used, the skin is nicked and a breast probe is placed in the area of the lesion. A vacuum line then draws breast tissue into the sampling chamber of the device. Alternatively, a rotating cutting device is advanced and the tissue sample is carried through the probe and captured by a tissue cassette. The probe is then rotated to a new position and the next tissue sample is obtained until 8-10 samples are taken at rotations of approximately 30 degrees. When the sampling process is complete, the probe is removed and pressure is applied to the biopsy site. Placement of a metallic localization clip or pellet is performed when a more extensive procedure, such as a lumpectomy, is anticipated so that the physician can identify the exact site where tissue has been removed. Following the biopsy procedure, the needle is left in place. A plastic stylette with a metal clip or pellet at the end is inserted through the biopsy needle and advanced to the biopsy site using ultrasound guidance. The metal clip or pellet is released and the stylette and needle are removed. Additional images of the biopsy specimen may be obtained prior to separately reportable pathology exam of the tissue. Use code 19083 for biopsy of the first lesion and 19084 for biopsy of each additional lesion.

19085-19086

19085	Biopsy, breast, with placement of breast localization device(s) (eg, clip, metallic pellet), when performed, and imaging of the biopsy specimen, when performed, percutaneous; first lesion, including magnetic resonance guidance
19086	Biopsy, breast, with placement of breast localization device(s) (eg, clip, metallic pellet), when performed, and imaging of the biopsy specimen, when performed, percutaneous; each additional lesion, including magnetic resonance guidance (List separately in addition to code for primary procedure)

A percutaneous biopsy of the breast is performed using magnetic resonance guidance. Magnetic resonance is a noninvasive, non-radiating imaging technique that uses the magnetic properties of hydrogen atoms in the body. The nuclei of hydrogen atoms emit radiofrequency signals when the body is exposed to radiowaves transmitted within a strong magnetic field. The computer processes the signals and converts the data into tomographic, 3D images with very high resolution. The needle being used with MRI guidance may have special metallic ringlets around it; be coated with contrast material; or have a signal receiving coil in its tip. The skin is cleansed. The target area is localized using magnetic resonance and then anesthetized. The biopsy needle, vacuum, or rotating device is inserted under MRI guidance. If a needle biopsy is performed, the needle is inserted into the lesion and a tissue sample is obtained. In order to obtain an adequate tissue sample, 3-6 separate core needle insertions are typically required. If an automated vacuum assisted or rotating biopsy device is used, the skin is nicked and a breast probe is placed in the area of the lesion. A vacuum line then draws breast tissue into the sampling chamber of the device. Alternatively, a rotating cutting device is advanced and the tissue sample is carried through the probe and captured by a tissue cassette. The probe is then rotated to a new position and the next tissue sample is obtained until 8-10 samples are taken at rotations of approximately 30 degrees. When the sampling process is complete, the probe is removed and pressure is applied to the biopsy site. Placement of a metallic localization clip or pellet is performed when a more extensive procedure is anticipated, such as a lumpectomy, so that the physician can identify the exact site where tissue has been removed. Following the biopsy procedure, the needle is left in place. A plastic stylette with a metal clip or pellet at the end is inserted through the biopsy needle and advanced to the biopsy site using imaging guidance. The metal clip or pellet is released and the stylette and needle are removed. Additional images of the biopsy specimen may be obtained prior to separately reportable pathology exam of the tissue. Use code 19085 for biopsy of the first lesion and 19086 for biopsy of each additional lesion.

Breast

19100

19100   Biopsy of breast; percutaneous, needle core, not using imaging guidance (separate procedure)

A percutaneous needle core biopsy of the breast is performed without imaging guidance in a separate procedure. The skin is cleansed and a local anesthetic is injected. The location of the lump is palpated. The physician fixes the lesion with one hand while the needle is inserted into the lesion with the other. In order to obtain an adequate tissue sample, 3-6 separate core needle insertions are typically required. When an adequate tissue sample has been obtained, it is sent to the laboratory for pathology exam.

19101

19101   Biopsy of breast; open, incisional

The physician creates an incision above a suspicious tissue mass in the breast. A sample of tissue from the suspicious mass is removed and reviewed. If the mass is benign, the incision is closed with layered sutures. If malignant, the wound may be closed until more extensive surgery can be completed.

19105

19105   Ablation, cryosurgical, of fibroadenoma, including ultrasound guidance, each fibroadenoma

Cryosurgical ablation is performed on a fibroadenoma of the breast, a benign tumor that may be a palpable mass or seen as a mammographic abnormality. Using ultrasound guidance, the fibroadenoma is located and a probe is inserted into the tumor mass. Through the probe, which usually contains liquid nitrogen, the tissue is cooled down to a temperature below -20 degrees Celsius. The extreme cold temperature is maintained to produce well-demarcated borders of cell destruction and the tumor is ablated in situ.

19110-19112

19110   Nipple exploration, with or without excision of a solitary lactiferous duct or a papilloma lactiferous duct
19112   Excision of lactiferous duct fistula

Nipple exploration is performed to diagnose the cause of bloody discharge from the nipple. The most common cause is a nonpalpable, benign lesion or papilloma. In 19110, following cleansing of the nipple, the breast is massaged from the periphery to the center to locate the affected duct. Expression of bloody fluid indicates that the affected duct has been located. The physician then cannulates and dilates the duct. Once the duct is adequately dilated the duct and its branches are explored using a ductoscope. If a lesion is found, the duct and the lesion are excised. In 19112, a lactiferous duct fistula is excised. A lactiferous duct fistula may occur due to obstruction of the duct with infection and abscess formation, following incision and drainage of a breast abscess, or following excision of a breast lesion. The physician makes an incision over the fistulous tract and excises the fistulous tract along with the entire obstructed duct. Surrounding inflamed tissue including a portion of the skin of the areola and nipple may also be excised.

19120

19120   Excision of cyst, fibroadenoma, or other benign or malignant tumor, aberrant breast tissue, duct lesion, nipple or areolar lesion (except 19300), open, male or female, 1 or more lesions

The physician performs an open excision of one or more masses or lesions of the male or female breast. Types of lesions excised include: cyst, fibroadenoma, or other benign or malignant tumor, aberrant breast tissue, duct lesion, or nipple or areolar lesion. The skin over the planned incision site is cleansed and a local anesthetic injected. The skin is incised and the lesion, mass, or aberrant tissue identified. The lesion, mass or region of aberrant breast tissue is dissected free of surrounding breast tissue and removed in its entirety. Separately reportable frozen sections may be reviewed by a pathologist and additional tissue removed as needed. The lesion, mass, or breast tissue is sent to the laboratory for separately reportable pathological examination. Drains are placed as needed and the wound closed in layers. The procedure may be repeated at additional sites if multiple masses or lesions are present.

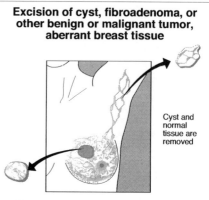

Excision of cyst, fibroadenoma, or other benign or malignant tumor, aberrant breast tissue

Cyst and normal tissue are removed

The physician excises one or more tumors, cysts, lesions, or fibroadenomas from the tissue of the breast.

19125-19126

19125   Excision of breast lesion identified by preoperative placement of radiological marker, open; single lesion
19126   Excision of breast lesion identified by preoperative placement of radiological marker, open; each additional lesion separately identified by a preoperative radiological marker (List separately in addition to code for primary procedure)

Placement of a radiological marker is used for nonpalpable lesions that have been identified on a mammogram or ultrasound of the breast. The physician incises the breast using the radiological marker as guide. The physician then excises the area of concern along with a margin of normal breast tissue. Bleeding is controlled with electrocautery or ligation. A drain may be inserted. The surgical wound is then closed using layered sutures. Use 19125 for excision of the first lesion and 19126 for each additional lesion separately identified by a radiological marker.

19260-19272

19260   Excision of chest wall tumor including ribs
19271   Excision of chest wall tumor involving ribs, with plastic reconstruction; without mediastinal lymphadenectomy
19272   Excision of chest wall tumor involving ribs, with plastic reconstruction; with mediastinal lymphadenectomy

The chest wall refers to the bone and muscle that surrounds the chest cavity and protects the lungs, heart, great vessels and other vital organs. Tumors of the chest wall may be benign or malignant, primary or secondary (metastatic). Benign tumors generally do not invade other tissues or spread to other organs, but due to the size or location may need to be removed. Malignant tumors can spread to adjacent or remote tissue or organs and do require treatment. Primary tumors originate in the chest wall structures while secondary tumors originate elsewhere and spread (metastasize) to the chest wall. In 19260, the chest wall tumor and involved ribs are excised. The skin over the tumor is incised and the chest is opened. The full thickness of the chest wall including the adjacent pleura is resected along with a 4-5 cm margin of healthy tissue. The involved rib and at least one rib above and below the level of the tumor is resected. The chest wall is not reconstructed. In 19271, the chest wall tumor is excised as described above and a chest wall reconstruction is performed. The exact nature of the reconstruction depends on the site and extent of the chest wall defect. Alloplastic material such as stainless steel, titanium, Lucite and fiberglass may be used to repair skeletal defects. Another option for repairing skeletal defect is the use of ribs or bone grafts. Ribs may be harvested whole or split longitudinally and a partial rib graft harvested. Marlex mesh combined with methylmethacrylate provides semirigid support and is another material used in reconstruction. Soft tissue defects may be repaired with latissimus dorsi, pectoralis major, or abdominus rectus muscle flaps, omentum, fasciocutaneous or osteocutaneous flaps. In 19272, the chest wall tumor is excised along with mediastinal lymph nodes and then the chest wall is reconstructed. Following excision of the chest wall tumor, mediastinal lymph nodes are dissected from surrounding tissue and removed. The chest wall is then reconstructed using techniques described above.

19281-19282

19281 Placement of breast localization device(s) (eg, clip, metallic pellet, wire/needle, radioactive seeds), percutaneous; first lesion, including mammographic guidance

19282 Placement of breast localization device(s) (eg, clip, metallic pellet, wire/needle, radioactive seeds), percutaneous; each additional lesion, including mammographic guidance (List separately in addition to code for primary procedure)

Placement of a breast localization device(s), such as a clip, metallic pellet, wire/needle, or radioactive seed, is performed so that the physician can identify the exact site of the lesion prior to a breast biopsy or lumpectomy. The area of concern is marked on the skin and mammogram images of the breast are obtained. Using these images, the needle is advanced into the lesion and additional mammogram images are taken to confirm placement of the needle within the mass. For wire localization, a hooked wire is inserted into the lesion at a perpendicular angle using a needle. The wire remains anchored within the mass when the needle is withdrawn, and a short length of wire extends out through the skin. Alternatively, a plastic stylette with a localization device such as a clip, metallic pellet, or radioactive seed at the end is inserted through the biopsy needle and advanced to the site of the lesion using mammographic guidance. The localization device is released and the stylette and needle are removed. Use 19281 for placement of the localization device in the first lesion and 19282 for each additional lesion.

19283-19284

19283 Placement of breast localization device(s) (eg, clip, metallic pellet, wire/needle, radioactive seeds), percutaneous; first lesion, including stereotactic guidance

19284 Placement of breast localization device(s) (eg, clip, metallic pellet, wire/needle, radioactive seeds), percutaneous; each additional lesion, including stereotactic guidance (List separately in addition to code for primary procedure)

Placement of a breast localization device(s), such as a clip, metallic pellet, wire/needle, or radioactive seed, is performed so that the physician can identify the exact site of the lesion prior to a breast biopsy or lumpectomy. The area of concern is marked on the skin and stereotactic guidance is used to locate the lesion in the breast. Stereotactic technique uses a fixed coordinate system to identify the lesion's unique location within the breast by defining it in terms of specific x, y, and z coordinates relative to an original reference point. The breast is positioned between a compression plate and a support in back to keep the lesion in a fixed position. Breast thickness under compression determines the depth dimension. An initial image is obtained perpendicular to the compression plate at 0 degrees angulation and this initial image is used to center the lesion in the biopsy window of the compression plate. Other images are obtained at specified angles to and from the relative 0 position by rotation around the known center. Geometric calculations are used to determine the lesion location in three dimensions. Using these calculations, the needle is advanced into the lesion and images are taken to confirm placement of the needle within the mass. For wire localization, a hooked wire is inserted into the lesion at a perpendicular angle using a needle. The wire remains anchored within the mass when the needle is withdrawn, and a short length of wire extends out through the skin. Alternatively, a plastic stylette with a localization device such as a clip, metallic pellet, or radioactive seed at the end is inserted through the biopsy needle and advanced to the site of the lesion using stereotactic guidance. The localization device is released and the stylette and needle are removed. Use 19283 for placement of the localization device in the first lesion and 19284 for each additional lesion.

19285-19286

19285 Placement of breast localization device(s) (eg, clip, metallic pellet, wire/needle, radioactive seeds), percutaneous; first lesion, including ultrasound guidance

19286 Placement of breast localization device(s) (eg, clip, metallic pellet, wire/needle, radioactive seeds), percutaneous; each additional lesion, including ultrasound guidance (List separately in addition to code for primary procedure)

Placement of a breast localization device(s), such as a clip, metallic pellet, wire/needle, or radioactive seed, is performed so that the physician can identify the exact site of the lesion prior to a breast biopsy or lumpectomy. The area of concern is marked on the skin and ultrasound images of the breast are obtained. A transducer is used to locate the lesion in the breast. Using these images, the needle is advanced into the lesion and the radiologist constantly monitors and confirms placement of the needle within the mass. For wire localization, a hooked wire is inserted into the lesion at a perpendicular angle using a needle. The wire remains anchored within the mass when the needle is withdrawn, and a short length of wire extends out through the skin. Alternatively, a plastic stylette with a localization device such as a clip, metallic pellet, or radioactive seed at the end is inserted through the biopsy needle and advanced to the site of the lesion using ultrasonic guidance. The localization device is released and the stylette and needle are removed. Use 19285

for placement of the localization device in the first lesion and 19286 for each additional lesion.

19287-19288

19287 Placement of breast localization device(s) (eg clip, metallic pellet, wire/needle, radioactive seeds), percutaneous; first lesion, including magnetic resonance guidance

19288 Placement of breast localization device(s) (eg, clip, metallic pellet, wire/needle, radioactive seeds), percutaneous; each additional lesion, including magnetic resonance guidance (List separately in addition to code for primary procedure)

Placement of a breast localization device(s), such as a clip, metallic pellet, wire/needle, or radioactive seed, is performed so that the physician can identify the exact site of the lesion prior to a breast biopsy or lumpectomy. The area of concern is marked on the skin and magnetic resonance imaging is used to locate the lesion in the breast. Magnetic resonance is a noninvasive, non-radiating imaging technique that uses the magnetic properties of hydrogen atoms in the body. The nuclei of hydrogen atoms emit radiofrequency signals when the body is exposed to radiowaves transmitted within a strong magnetic field. The computer processes the signals and converts the data into tomographic, 3D images with very high resolution. The needle being used with MRI guidance may have special metallic ringlets around it; be coated with contrast material; or have a signal receiving coil in its tip. Using magnetic resonance guidance, the needle is advanced into the lesion and additional images are taken to confirm placement of the needle within the mass. For wire localization, a hooked wire is inserted into the lesion at a perpendicular angle using a needle. The wire remains anchored within the mass when the needle is withdrawn, and a short length of wire extends out through the skin. Alternatively, a plastic stylette with a localization device such as a clip, metallic pellet, or radioactive seed at the end is inserted through the biopsy needle and advanced to the site of the lesion using magnetic resonance guidance. The localization device is released and the stylette and needle are removed. Use 19287 for placement of the localization device in the first lesion and 19288 for each additional lesion.

19296-19297

19296 Placement of radiotherapy afterloading expandable catheter (single or multichannel) into the breast for interstitial radioelement application following partial mastectomy, includes imaging guidance; on date separate from partial mastectomy

19297 Placement of radiotherapy afterloading expandable catheter (single or multichannel) into the breast for interstitial radioelement application following partial mastectomy, includes imaging guidance; concurrent with partial mastectomy (List separately in addition to code for primary procedure)

An expandable radioelement application catheter, either single or multichannel, is placed into a breast cavity for interstitial radiotherapy following tissue-sparing partial mastectomy, lumpectomy, or excisional biopsy. This kind of therapy delivers radiation into the surgical cavity plus a small margin beyond instead of irradiating the entire breast. Treatment is completed in a matter of days instead of weeks. A single incision is made. A trocar is placed into the surgical cavity using ultrasound guidance to create a pathway for the expandable catheter. The trocar is removed and the applicator is inserted through the pathway into the surgical cavity in closed position. The expansion tool is rotated to deploy the catheter, usually consisting of multiple lumens surrounding one central lumen, which expand and conform to fit the size of the cavity. The catheter(s) are then connected to an afterloading device for delivering the radiation source. Multiple catheters that expand individually provide the flexibility to contour and control the dosage through a single access site, combining the benefits of tissue-sparing interstitial brachytherapy with the ease of intracavitary balloon brachytherapy. This therapy may be done on a date that follows the lumpectomy or partial mastectomy (19296) or it may be done on the same day as the surgery (19297).

19298

▲ **19298** Placement of radiotherapy after loading brachytherapy catheters (multiple tube and button type) into the breast for interstitial radioelement application following (at the time of or subsequent to) partial mastectomy, includes imaging guidance

Radiotherapy after loading brachytherapy catheters, multiple tube and button type, are placed into the breast for interstitial radioelement application following partial mastectomy. Placement of the catheters may be performed at the time of or subsequent to the mastectomy procedure. The distribution of the catheters is determined in a separately reportable procedure. Implant needles are then placed into the breast tissue using the previously determined distribution pattern under direct vision or using imaging guidance. Once all needles are placed, the distribution is checked to ensure coverage of the entire area to be treated with brachytherapy. The needles are then replaced with the after loading brachytherapy tube catheters by threading the leader end of the brachytherapy tube catheters through the implant needles. The needles are removed. The catheter has

● New Code ▲ Revised Code

a button-shaped end piece to keep the catheter in place as the needles are removed. A second fixing button is then threaded over the end of the catheter that is protruding from the skin to fix both ends of the catheter in the breast tissue. Any excess catheter protruding from the skin is trimmed. Stiffening devices within the catheters are removed. Each catheter is checked to ensure patency by passing a non-radioactive dummy cable through the catheter. The catheter ends are prepared to accept the radiotherapy after loader connection tubing. Special padding and a dressing is then applied over the breast to prevent kinking of the catheters. The catheters will be loaded and the brachytherapy procedure performed in a separately reportable procedure.

19300

19300   Mastectomy for gynecomastia

A mastectomy is performed for gynecomastia which is an abnormal enlargement of one or both breasts in men. Excisional removal of breast tissue is performed primarily in patients with excess glandular tissue. An incision is made at the base of the areola, or if large amounts of tissue are present, the incision is made in the inframammary fold. Excess tissue around and below the areola and at the sides of the breast is dissected off the pectoral muscle and excised. Excess skin is also removed. The incision is closed. A drain may be inserted through a separate incision to prevent accumulation of fluid. The chest is wrapped to provide compression to the surgical site.

19301-19302

19301   Mastectomy, partial (eg, lumpectomy, tylectomy, quadrantectomy, segmentectomy)

19302   Mastectomy, partial (eg, lumpectomy, tylectomy, quadrantectomy, segmentectomy); with axillary lymphadenectomy

Partial mastectomy is performed to remove a cancerous (malignant) lesion or one that is suspected of being cancerous. An incision is made over the lump or mass which is visually inspected. The lump or mass is removed along with a margin of healthy tissue and sent to the laboratory for histological analysis. The surgical site and surrounding breast tissue are inspected for any additional lesions. If axillary lymphadectomy is also performed, an incision is made in the lowest area of the axilla. The borders of the pectoralis major and latissimus dorsi muscles are identified. The axillary vein is identified and dissected from surrounding tissue. The axillary neural structures are identified and protected. Axillary lymph nodes are excised. Usually 15-25 axillary nodes are removed from under the axillary vein and along the nerves and muscles of the axilla. Once all cancerous or suspicious tissue has been excised, a drain is placed and the surgical wound is closed. Use 19301 when partial mastectomy is performed without axillary lymphadenectomy and 19302 when the procedure is performed with axillary lymphadenectomy.

19303

19303   Mastectomy, simple, complete

A simple, complete mastectomy is done to remove the breast tissue with skin, without lymph nodes or muscle. A curved incision is made under the breast, which includes the breast tissue up into the axillary region, called the tail of Spence. Skin is separated from the breast tissue, which in dissected from the underlying muscle fascia and sternum. All the breast tissue, along with the corresponding skin, including the nipple, is removed. A drain tube may be placed and the skin edges are reapproximated and closed.

19304

19304   Mastectomy, subcutaneous

A subcutaneous mastectomy is performed by making an incision along the inframammary crease and dissecting the breast tissue from the underlying muscle fascia and the skin. The breast tissue is removed and the muscle remains. The skin may be examined first for any pathology that would necessitate removal, and the nipple and areola are sutured back into position. A suction catheter or drainage tube is inserted and a prosthesis may also be placed under the skin before closure.

19305-19306

19305   Mastectomy, radical, including pectoral muscles, axillary lymph nodes
19306   Mastectomy, radical, including pectoral muscles, axillary and internal mammary lymph nodes (Urban type operation)

Radical mastectomy includes removal of the entire breast, nipple, and areola with excision of pectoralis major and minor muscles and axillary lymph nodes. Sometimes a more extensive procedure, referred to as an Urban-type radical mastectomy is performed which in addition to the procedures listed above includes excision of internal mammary lymph nodes. An elliptical incision is made to include the breast and the tissue that extends into the axilla referred to as the tail of Spence. The breast tissue, skin, areola, and nipple are removed en bloc along with the underlying pectoral muscles of the chest. Axillary lymph nodes are dissected from the underlying axillary vein along the neighboring nerves and muscles and removed. If an Urban-type procedure is performed, the internal mammary nodes are dissected free of surrounding tissue and removed as is tissue connected to the sternum, portions of the rectus fascia, latissimus dorsi muscle, and clavicle. The skin is

closed or a separately reportable myocutaneous graft placed for closure when there is not have enough remaining skin to close the surgical site. Alternatively, a separately reportable breast reconstruction procedure or prosthesis placement may be performed prior to closure. Surgical wounds are closed around a suction catheter or drainage tube. Use 19305 for radical mastectomy with excision of pectoral muscles and axillary lymph nodes or 19306 for a more extensive Urban-type procedure that also includes removal of internal mammary lymph nodes and surrounding tissue.

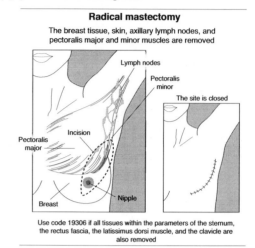

Radical mastectomy

The breast tissue, skin, axillary lymph nodes, and pectoralis major and minor muscles are removed

Use code 19306 if all tissues within the parameters of the sternum, the rectus fascia, the latissimus dorsi muscle, and the clavicle are also removed

19307

19307   Mastectomy, modified radical, including axillary lymph nodes, with or without pectoralis minor muscle, but excluding pectoralis major muscle

A modified radical mastectomy, including axillary lymph nodes, with or without pectoralis minor muscle, but excluding pectoralis major muscle is done. This is a more common type of radical mastectomy procedure. An elliptical incision is made around the breast, including the tissue that extends into the axilla, the tail of Spence. The breast tissue, skin, areola, and nipple are removed enbloc along with the axillary lymph nodes, which are dissected from under the axillary vein and along the neighboring nerves and muscles and removed, as are the intramammary lymph nodes. The pectoralis minor muscle may or may not be removed but the major pectoral muscle of the chest under the breast is left in place. A skin or myocutaneous graft may be necessary for closure in patients who do not have enough remaining skin to close the surgical site. A suction catheter or drainage tube is inserted and a prosthesis may also be placed under the skin before closure.

19316

19316   Mastopexy

The physician performs a mastopexy, commonly known as a breast lift. Depending on the amount of skin laxity, incisions may be made around the areola, around the areola and vertically down to the breast crease, or around the areola, vertically down to the crease and horizontally along the crease. The underlying breast tissue is lifted and reconfigured to improve the contour and firmness of the breast. The nipple and areola are moved to a higher position on the breast. If the areola is enlarged, it is reduced by removing skin along the perimeter. Excess skin is excised. The incisions are then closed in layers beginning deep within the breast tissue to maintain the new breast contour. Subcutaneous tissue and skin are closed with sutures, skin adhesive and tape.

19318

19318   Reduction mammaplasty

The physician performs breast reduction surgery, also known as reduction mammaplasty. The physician creates an incision that circles the areola, extends downward, and follows the natural curve of the crease beneath the breast (anchor shaped incision). The surgeon removes excess glandular tissue, fat, and skin, and moves the nipple and areola into their new position. The physician then brings the skin from both sides of the breast down and around the areola, shaping the new contour of the breast. Liposuction may be used to remove excess fat from the axillary area area. In most cases, the nipple remains attached to its blood vessels and nerves. However, if the breast is very large or pendulous, the nipple and areola may have to be completely removed and grafted into a higher position. Bleeding is controlled via electrocautery and the incision is closed with sutures.

19324-19325

19324   Mammaplasty, augmentation; without prosthetic implant
19325   Mammaplasty, augmentation; with prosthetic implant

Augmentation mammaplasty is performed to enhance the size and/or shape of the breast. In 19324, the procedure is performed without prosthetic implant. An incision is made around the areola and on the underside of the breast. The physician rearranges the existing breast tissue and may use other body tissue to enhance the size or shape of the breast. Any redundant skin is excised. The nipple and areola are sutured in their new position and the site is closed by layered suturing. In 19325, a prosthestic implant is used to enhance the size or shape of the breast. An incision is made either in the crease where the breast meets the chest, around the areola, or in the armpit. The incision is placed so resulting scars will be as inconspicuous as possible. Working through the incision, the surgeon lifts the breast and skin to create a pocket either directly behind the breast tissue or underneath the chest wall (pectoral) muscle. The implant is then centered beneath the nipple. Drainage tubes may be used for several days following surgery. The incisions are closed with sutures and tape may be used to reinforce the sutures. A gauze bandage is placed over the breasts to help with healing.

19328-19330

19328   Removal of intact mammary implant
19330   Removal of mammary implant material

Intact breast implants may be removed when there is a problem with the implant such as a change in size or shape of the implant, shifting or asymmetry of the implant. Intact implants may also be removed due to an adverse reaction to the implant material with symptoms such as bleeding, infection, capsular contraction, necrosis or calcium deposits, or a diagnosis of breast cancer. Implant material is removed when the implant ruptures or leaks. An incision is made under the breast in the inframammary crease, around the areola, or over the scar from the implant procedure. In 19328, an intact implant is removed. If the implant is filled with saline, the saline may be removed. Breast tissue, fat and muscle are dissected away from the implant and the implant is removed. Alternatively, the physician may remove both the implant and the scar tissue capsule that has formed around the implant which is referred to as en bloc removal. The implant cavity is inspected for any remnants of the implant, irrigated with saline, and the incision closed with sutures. In 19330, implant material is removed. Ruptured or leaking implants are removed en bloc with the scar tissue capsule. The implant cavity is inspected for any remnants of the implant and if any implant material such as silicone gel that has migrated beyond the scar tissue capsule it is removed. When all of the implant material has been removed, the implant cavity is flushed with saline, a drain placed if needed, and the incision closed.

19340

19340   Immediate insertion of breast prosthesis following mastopexy, mastectomy or in reconstruction

The physician inserts the breast prosthesis (implant) during the same surgical session as a mastopexy, mastectomy, or other reconstructive breast surgery. Working through the existing incisions, a pocket is created behind remaining muscle, breast tissue, fat, and skin. The implant is placed in the pocket and centered behind the nipple. Overlying tissues are shaped and contoured over the implant and then closed in layers. Drainage tubes are placed if needed. A compression type dressing is applied.

19342

19342   Delayed insertion of breast prosthesis following mastopexy, mastectomy or in reconstruction

The physician inserts a breast prosthesis (implant) after a previous mastopexy, mastectomy or breast reconstruction. The physician creates an incision either in the crease where the breast meets the chest, around the areola, or in the axillary area, usually over the site of the previous incisions. Working through the incision, the surgeon lifts the breast tissue and skin to create a pocket, either directly behind the breast tissue or underneath the chest wall muscle (the pectoral muscle). The implant is then centered beneath the nipple. Drainage tubes may be used for several days following the surgery. Sutures are used to close the incisions, which may also be taped for greater support. A gauze bandage may be applied over the breast to help with healing.

19350

19350   Nipple/areola reconstruction

The physician performs nipple or areola reconstructive surgery. A skin graft is harvested, often from the inner thigh, ear, or vulva. The donor site is closed with sutures. The physician excises tissue from the existing nipple, or obtains another graft from the thigh, ear, or vulva. The donor site is closed with sutures. A circular incision is made over the site of the areola and a thin layer of skin is excised. The skin graft for the areola is positioned in place and sutured closed. A small circular incision is created in the center of the areola for the nipple. The second graft is placed there and the nipple is secured with sutures.

19355

19355   Correction of inverted nipples

The physician corrects inverted nipples by creating radial incisions around the areola and forming the nipples to the normal everted position. Transection of fibrous bands and ducts may be necessary to perform this procedure. Extraneous tissue may be removed. The nipple is secured via sutures, and the incision sites are also closed with sutures.

19357

19357   Breast reconstruction, immediate or delayed, with tissue expander, including subsequent expansion

The physician performs breast reconstruction with a tissue expander. Subsequent expansion is also included. The physician creates an incision at the site of a previous mastectomy and forms a pocket under remaining chest wall tissue. A tissue expander is placed into that pocket, for later expansion. The point of inflation can remain inside the body, or be brought outside the body. Saline is injected into the expander, which is inflated to a size larger than the current breast. The expander is gradually expanded further over time, until the desired size is reached. The expander may be left in place, or removed via a separate procedure.

19361

19361   Breast reconstruction with latissimus dorsi flap, without prosthetic implant

The physician reconstructs a breast using the latissimus dorsi muscle, without a prosthetic implant. Skin and muscle from the back of the patient are transferred to the chest area, after a mastectomy. The physician creates an incision in the back and dissects a portion of the latissimus dorsi, which is transferred to the defect area remaining from the mastectomy. The muscle flap remains connected to a main artery and is rotated under the arm and into place. The donor incision is closed with layered sutures. A thin layer of skin is removed from the breast, and positioned as a graft for the areola. The areola graft is sutured in place. A nipple is created via tissue rearrangement in the center of the areola.

19364

19364   Breast reconstruction with free flap

A free flap of skin, fat, and muscle are harvested from a donor location on the patient's body (often the buttocks or thigh) and transferred to the defect remaining from a mastectomy. The artery and vein are preserved and reattached in the breast region. The donor site is closed with layered sutures. The graft is positioned in the most aesthetically pleasing position, and secured to the chest wall. The site is closed with sutures. A breast implant may be added, if the muscle does not have enough mass to match the existing breast.

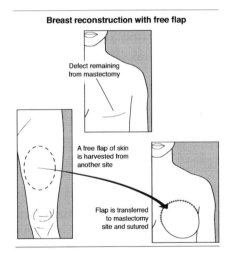

Breast reconstruction with free flap

Defect remaining from mastectomy

A free flap of skin is harvested from another site

Flap is transferred to mastectomy site and sutured

19366

19366   Breast reconstruction with other technique

The physician reconstructs the breast with a technique not covered in another code. This includes the harvesting of muscle from a donor location and the transfer to the defect location. A breast implant may be necessary. The site is closed.

19367-19369

19367   Breast reconstruction with transverse rectus abdominis myocutaneous flap (TRAM), single pedicle, including closure of donor site
19368   Breast reconstruction with transverse rectus abdominis myocutaneous flap (TRAM), single pedicle, including closure of donor site; with microvascular anastomosis (supercharging)
19369   Breast reconstruction with transverse rectus abdominis myocutaneous flap (TRAM), double pedicle, including closure of donor site

The physician performs a TRAM flap procedure to reconstruct the breast after a mastectomy. A TRAM flap stands for transverse rectus abdominis myocutaneous flap. Utilizing microsurgery, the physician repositions a portion of the transverse rectus abdominis muscle (ab muscle) into the defect site, via a subcutaneous tunnel. The arteries and veins remain intact. The TRAM graft is positioned in the form of a breast and sutured in place. All incisions are closed via sutures. Code 19368 if the blood vessels are reconnected using microvascular anastomosis. Code 19369 if the TRAM graft has two pedicles, or if both sides of the rectus abdominis are used.

19370-19371

19370   Open periprosthetic capsulotomy, breast
19371   Periprosthetic capsulectomy, breast

The fibrous capsule that forms around a prosthetic breast implant is incised or excised to release adhesions or remove excessive scar tissue. An incision is usually made over the existing scar, which may be below the areola, under the breast, or in the axilla. The physician cuts through fibrous scar tissue surrounding the previously placed implant. This scarring is known as capsular contraction. In 19370, the physician then creates a larger pocket. In 19371, the physician excises the scar tissue around the implant. The incision is then closed with layered sutures.

19380

19380   Revision of reconstructed breast

A revision of a reconstructed breast is performed. Because the goal of breast reconstruction is to provide an aesthetically reconstructed breast, revision surgery may be required to provide the desired results. Revision is performed to achieve the desired size and shape of the breast, remove excess tissue or revise scars from previous surgeries. Incisions are made over existing scars. Breast tissue is reshaped and contoured. If an implant has been used as part of the previous reconstruction, it may be repositioned or replaced. Excess breast tissue is excised. Redundant skin is removed and scars revised. Drains are placed as needed and the skin is closed in layers.

Revision of reconstructed breast

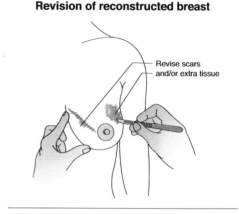

Revise scars and/or extra tissue

19396

19396   Preparation of moulage for custom breast implant

A custom breast implant model is created for the patient. This model will closely resemble the breast which has not been removed via mastectomy. A custom breast implant is created from this model.

Musculoskeletal System

20005

20005 Incision and drainage of soft tissue abscess, subfascial (ie, involves the soft tissue below the deep fascia)

An incision is made over the abscessed area and carried down to the subfascial tissue. Forceps or a closed blunt hemostat is used to open the incision and allow drainage of purulent material. Specimens are obtained for separately reportable culture and sensitivity. A finger is then inserted through the incision to break up and evacuate any pockets of pus. The abscessed cavity is copiously irrigated with sterile saline. A drain is placed or the cavity is packed with gauze.

20100-20103

20100 Exploration of penetrating wound (separate procedure); neck
20101 Exploration of penetrating wound (separate procedure); chest
20102 Exploration of penetrating wound (separate procedure); abdomen/flank/back
20103 Exploration of penetrating wound (separate procedure); extremity

A penetrating traumatic wound, such as that due to gunshot or a stab injury, is explored in a separate procedure. A scalpel is used to extend the wound margins so that underlying tissue can be visualized. The underlying subcutaneous tissue, fascia and muscle is examined and the depth of penetration determined. The wound is irrigated with normal saline to improve visualization and remove debris. The wound is debrided using sharp and blunt dissection and any foreign bodies removed. Bleeding from minor blood vessels in the subcutaneous tissue, muscle fascia, or muscle is controlled by ligation or coagulation. Once it has been determined that the penetrating injury does not involve deeper tissues, that major blood vessels and nerves are intact, and in the case of chest or abdominal wounds that the injury does not extent into the thoracic or abdominal cavity, the wound may be packed open or closed in layers. Use 20100 if exploration is for penetrating wounds of the neck, 20101 for the chest, 20102 for the abdomen, and 20103 for an extremity.

20150

20150 Excision of epiphyseal bar, with or without autogenous soft tissue graft obtained through same fascial incision

The physician excises the epiphyseal bar to correct a partial epiphyseal arrest, where the patient has significant growth remaining in a long bone (e.g., femur, tibia). Under general anesthesia, the patient is placed in the supine position. The physician excises part of the injured epiphyseal plate, to encourage bone growth. This is a major surgery and often requires weeks in the hospital for recovery. An autogenous soft tissue graft may be used to fill in the void after excision. Care is taken to preserve muscle and nerve health during the procedure. The site is closed with sutures and dressed with compressive bandages, to reduce the formation of hematomas. The affected limb is immobilized.

20200-20205

20200 Biopsy, muscle; superficial
20205 Biopsy, muscle; deep

An incisional biopsy is performed on superficial (20200) or deep (20205) muscle tissue. This procedure is typically done to diagnose diseases involving muscle tissue, such as muscular dystrophy, myasthenia gravis, polymyositis, dermatomyositis, amyotrophic lateral sclerosis (ALS), Friedreich's ataxia, and trichinosis or toxoplasmosis parasitic infections of the muscles. The planned biopsy site is cleansed. An incision is then made in the muscle and a tissue sample obtained. The tissue sample is then sent for separately reportable pathology examination. Use 20200 for muscle biopsy involving a superficial incision or 20205 if a deeper incision with tissue dissection must be made to access the site.

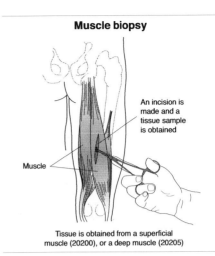

Muscle biopsy

An incision is made and a tissue sample is obtained

Muscle

Tissue is obtained from a superficial muscle (20200), or a deep muscle (20205)

20206

20206 Biopsy, muscle, percutaneous needle

A percutaneous needle muscle biopsy is performed. This procedure is typically done to diagnose diseases involving muscle tissue, such as muscular dystrophy, myasthenia gravis, polymyositis, dermatomyositis, amyotrophic lateral sclerosis (ALS), Friedreich's ataxia, and parasitic infections of the muscles. Common biopsy sites include the bicep, deltoid, or quadriceps muscles. The planned biopsy site is cleansed. A biopsy needle is then inserted into the muscle and a small tissue sample obtained. This may be repeated multiple times at various sites along the muscle to obtain an adequate sample. The tissue sample is then sent for separately reportable pathology examination.

20220-20225

20220 Biopsy, bone, trocar, or needle; superficial (eg, ilium, sternum, spinous process, ribs)
20225 Biopsy, bone, trocar, or needle; deep (eg, vertebral body, femur)

Under local anesthesia (occasionally, general anesthesia) the physician obtains a biopsy of a bone. A large needle is placed into the spinous process or superficial bone and the tissue is removed. If a biopsy of a deep bone is performed (20225), an exploration needle is positioned, and then a smaller one is inserted through the exploration one to obtain a sample. Different approaches are used for vertebral biopsy. No closure is usually necessary.

20240-20245

▲ **20240** Biopsy, bone, open; superficial (eg, sternum, spinous process, rib, patella, olecranon process, calcaneus, tarsal, metatarsal, carpal, metacarpal, phalanx)
▲ **20245** Biopsy, bone, open; deep (eg, humeral shaft, ischium, femoral shaft)

An open bone biopsy removes a small sample of bone for pathological analysis with the patient under regional block or general anesthesia. Bone biopsy may be used to evaluate bone pain or tenderness, confirm a diagnosis found by another test, investigate abnormalities found on radiologic scans, determine between benign bone masses and bone cancer, and/or diagnose bone disease or infection, including osteoporosis, osteomalacia, and osteomyelitis. A skin incision is made over the targeted biopsy site and carried down through subcutaneous tissue and muscle to the bone. A small segment of bone is removed and sent to the laboratory for analysis. Blood vessels are tied off or cauterized to control bleeding. The site is cleansed and the wound is sutured closed and bandaged. Code 20240 reports open biopsy of superficial bone including sternum, spinous process, rib, patella, olecranon process, calcaneus, tarsal, metatarsal, carpal, metacarpal and phalanx. Code 20245 reports open biopsy of deep bone including humeral shaft, ischium and femoral shaft.

20250-20251

20250 Biopsy, vertebral body, open; thoracic
20251 Biopsy, vertebral body, open; lumbar or cervical

Under general anesthesia, the patient is placed in a prone position. An incision is created above the vertebra to be biopsied. The muscles surrounding the vertebra are dissected tested for testing and diagnosis. Tissue is excised and the muscles are repositioned. The

Musculoskeletal System

incision is closed in layers. Code 20250 for a thoracic vertebral biopsy and 20251 for a lumbar or cervical vertebral biopsy.

20500-20501

20500   Injection of sinus tract; therapeutic (separate procedure)
20501   Injection of sinus tract; diagnostic (sinogram)

Sinus tracts in the musculoskeletal system are typically the result of a puncture wound that becomes infected or osteomyelitis following an injury such as an open fracture or following a surgical procedure. In a therapeutic procedure (20500), a sterile catheter is inserted into the sinus tract and advanced until resistance is encountered. Sterile saline may be injected to flush out the fluid and debris. An antibiotic or other therapeutic substance is injected to treat the infection. In a diagnostic procedure (20501), also referred to as a sinogram, a sterile catheter is inserted into the sinus tract under separately reportable radiographic supervision. Contrast is then injected and observed radiographically to determine the size and location of the sinus tract.

20520-20525

20520   Removal of foreign body in muscle or tendon sheath; simple
20525   Removal of foreign body in muscle or tendon sheath; deep or complicated

The physician removes a foreign body from a muscle or tendon sheath. If radiologic imaging is needed to locate the foreign body, report this separately. An incision is made above the affected area. Cutaneous tissue is dissected until the foreign body can be removed. The site is closed if no infection is present. If infection is present, the sight may be packed open with gauze. Code 20520 if the removal is simple and 20525 if the removal is deep or complicated.

20526

20526   Injection, therapeutic (eg, local anesthetic, corticosteroid), carpal tunnel

A therapeutic injection using a local anesthetic or corticosteroid is performed to treat symptoms of carpal tunnel syndrome. This procedure is referred to as a carpal tunnel or median nerve injection. The flexor carpi radialis (FCR) and palmaris longus (PL) tendons are located. The skin over the planned needle insertion site is cleansed. The needle is inserted just proximal to the most proximal wrist crease and medial to the PL tendon. The needle is directed toward the ring finger and advanced until the PL tendon is encountered. The syringe is retrated to ensure that the needle is clear of all blood vessels. The local anesthetic or steroid solution is injected. The needle is removed and the local anesthetic or steroid is allowed to disperse distally using gravity and finger motion.

20527

20527   Injection, enzyme (eg, collagenase), palmar fascial cord (ie, Dupuytren's contracture)

Dupuytren's contracture is caused by thickening and tightening of palmar fibrous tissue due to excessive collagen deposition beneath the skin of the hand and fingers. While painless, the thickening causes a flexion contracture making it difficult or impossible to fully extend one or more fingers. Using separately reportable ultrasound as needed, the soft tissues of the hand are visualized and the flexor tendon is identified. The depth of the skin to the surface of the flexor tendon is measured to insure that the tendon is not accidently injected as only the fibrous tissue (cords) should be injected. A needle with a syringe containing an enzyme such as collagenase is advanced into the fibrous tissue and injected. The enzyme weakens the cords of fibrous tissue. The patient returns the next day for separately reportable manipulation of the hand and fingers and mechanical breakage of the cord which straightens the fingers.

20550-20551

20550   Injection(s); single tendon sheath, or ligament, aponeurosis (eg, plantar "fascia")
20551   Injection(s); single tendon origin/insertion

The physician injects a single tendon sheath, ligament, or aponeurosis (20550) or a single tendon origin or insertion (20551). In 20550, the site of maximum tenderness is identified by palpation. The needle is advanced into the tendon sheath, ligament, or aponeurosis and an anesthetic, steroid, or other therapeutic substance is injected. More than one injection to the same tendon sheath or ligament may be administered. In 20551, the tendon origin or insertion is located. A needle is advanced into the origin or insertion and an anesthetic, steroid, or other therapeutic substance is injected.

20552-20553

20552   Injection(s); single or multiple trigger point(s), 1 or 2 muscle(s)
20553   Injection(s); single or multiple trigger point(s), 3 or more muscle(s)

The physician injects a single or multiple trigger points in one or two muscles (20552) or three or more muscles (20553). Trigger points are tiny contraction knots that develop in a muscle when it is injured or overworked. The physician identifies the trigger points by palpating the muscle. The needle is advanced into the muscle and an anesthetic, steroid, or other therapeutic substance is injected. This is repeated until all trigger points on all involved muscles have been treated.

20555

20555   Placement of needles or catheters into muscle and/or soft tissue for subsequent interstitial radioelement application (at the time of or subsequent to the procedure)

Needles or catheters are placed in the muscle and/or soft tissue for subsequent interstitial radioelement application. This may be performed at the time of or following another separately reportable procedure such as removal of a mass or tumor. This code reports the placement of the needles or catheters only. The interstitial radioelement application (brachytherapy) is reported separately. Tumor margins in the muscle and/or soft tissue are marked. The needle or catheter implant sites are determined and entrance and exit sites are marked on the skin surface. The first needle or catheter is introduced through the previously marked entrance site. Typically, a needle is first introduced and then a catheter is introduced through the needle. The catheter is positioned and secured and the needle is removed through a separate predetermined exit site. This is repeated until all catheters are in place. Drains with multiple drainage holes are then placed perpendicular to the catheters and each catheter is threaded through a drain hole. The stiff leader portion of the catheter is removed and a dressing is applied.

20600-20604

20600   Arthrocentesis, aspiration and/or injection, small joint or bursa (eg, fingers, toes); without ultrasound guidance
20604   Arthrocentesis, aspiration and/or injection, small joint or bursa (eg, fingers, toes); with ultrasound guidance, with permanent recording and reporting

Arthrocentesis and/or aspiration is performed to remove fluid from a joint or bursa in order to diagnose the cause of joint effusion and/or to reduce pain caused by the excess fluid. Injection of a joint or bursa may be performed in conjunction with the arthrocentesis procedure and is typically performed using an anti-inflammatory medication such as a steroid to reduce inflammation of the joint or bursa. The skin over the joint is cleansed. A local anesthetic is injected as needed. A needle with a syringe attached is inserted into the affected joint or bursa. Fluid is removed and sent for separately reportable laboratory analysis. This may be followed by a separate injection of medication into the joint or bursa. Use 20600 for arthrocentesis, aspiration and/or injection of a small joint or bursa, such as in the fingers or toes when no ultrasound guidance is used for needle placement. Report 20604 when ultrasonic guidance is used and a permanent recording is made with a report of the procedure.

20605-20606

20605   Arthrocentesis, aspiration and/or injection, intermediate joint or bursa (eg, temporomandibular, acromioclavicular, wrist, elbow or ankle, olecranon bursa); without ultrasound guidance
20606   Arthrocentesis, aspiration and/or injection, intermediate joint or bursa (eg, temporomandibular, acromioclavicular, wrist, elbow or ankle, olecranon bursa); with ultrasound guidance, with permanent recording and reporting

Arthrocentesis, or aspiration is performed to remove fluid from a joint or bursa in order to diagnose the cause of joint effusion and/or to reduce pain caused by the excess fluid. Injection of a joint or bursa may be performed in conjunction with the arthrocentesis procedure and is typically performed using an anti-inflammatory medication such as a steroid to reduce inflammation of the joint or bursa. The skin over the joint is cleansed. A local anesthetic is injected as needed. A needle with a syringe attached is inserted into the affected joint or bursa. Fluid is removed and sent for separately reportable laboratory analysis. This may be followed by a separate injection of medication into the joint or bursa. Use 20605 for an intermediate joint or bursa, such as the temporomandibular joint, acromioclavicular joint, wrist, elbow, or ankle joint, or the olecranon bursa when no ultrasound guidance is used for needle placement. Report 20606 when ultrasonic guidance is used and a permanent recording is made with a report of the procedure.

20610-20611

20610   Arthrocentesis, aspiration and/or injection, major joint or bursa (eg, shoulder, hip, knee, subacromial bursa); without ultrasound guidance
20611   Arthrocentesis, aspiration and/or injection, major joint or bursa (eg, shoulder, hip, knee, subacromial bursa); with ultrasound guidance, with permanent recording and reporting

Arthrocentesis, aspiration, and/or injection of a joint or bursa is performed. Arthrocentesis and aspiration is performed to remove fluid from a joint or bursa in order to diagnose the cause of joint effusion and/or to reduce pain caused by the excess fluid. Injection of a joint or bursa may be performed in conjunction with the arthrocentesis procedure and is typically performed using an anti-inflammatory medication such as a steroid to reduce inflammation of the joint or bursa. The skin over the joint is cleansed. A local anesthetic is injected as needed. A needle with a syringe attached is inserted into the affected joint or bursa. Fluid is removed and sent for separately reportable laboratory analysis. This may

Musculoskeletal System

be followed by a separate injection of medication into the joint or bursa. Use 20610 for a major joint or bursa, such as the shoulder, knee, or hip joint, or the subacromial bursa when no ultrasound guidance is used for needle placement. Report 20611 when ultrasonic guidance is used and a permanent recording is made with a report of the procedure.

Arthrocentesis

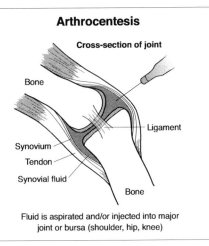

Fluid is aspirated and/or injected into major joint or bursa (shoulder, hip, knee)

20612

20612   Aspiration and/or injection of ganglion cyst(s) any location

The physician administers local anesthesia and inserts a needle into one or more ganglion cysts at any location. Fluid is aspirated and/or injected. A ganglion cyst is a small, benign cystic tumor, composed of ganglion cells, containing viscous fluid and connected either with a joint membrane or a tendon sheath.

20615

20615   Aspiration and injection for treatment of bone cyst

The physician administers local anesthesia and inserts a needle into a bone cyst. Fluid is aspirated and medication is injected. A bone cyst is a one-chambered cyst containing serous fluid and lined with a thin layer of connective tissue. Bone cysts usually occur in the shaft of a long bone in a child.

20650

20650   Insertion of wire or pin with application of skeletal traction, including removal (separate procedure)

The physician inserts a Steinmann pin through a bone so that it is protruding from either side of the bone. A weighted device use for skeletal traction is attached to the Steinmann pin to stabilize the fracture until a more permanent solution can be provided. Removal of the Steinmann pin and skeletal traction device are also included in this code.

20660

20660   Application of cranial tongs, caliper, or stereotactic frame, including removal (separate procedure)

The physician applies cranial tongs, a caliper, or a stereotactic frame for stabilization of the cervical spine. Local anesthesia is applied, after the pin placement locations have been shaved and Betadine has been applied. The pins from the device are simultaneously advanced into the cranial skin. The skull is not pierced. Lock nuts are tightened to maintain the appropriate depth and stability of the device. These nuts are checked every few hours for appropriate stability. The removal of this device is also included in this code.

20661

20661   Application of halo, including removal; cranial

A cranial halo device is applied to stabilize the cervical spine. The four pin insertion sites are shaved and cleansed with an anti-infective agent. Local anesthesia is injected. The halo device is positioned over the skull. The anterior pins are placed first. They are inserted through the skin and advanced until the bone is engaged in the area referred to as the safe zone. This is the region just below the greatest skull circumference. The anterior pins are placed above the supraorbital ridge to prevent penetration into the orbit and lateral to the middle portion of the supraorbital rim to avoid the supratrochlear and supraorbital nerves and the frontal sinus. The posterior pins are then placed. The diagonally opposed pins are tightened simultaneously until the desired penetration of bone has been reached. Lock nuts are tightened to maintain the appropriate depth and stability of the device. Rods are then attached to the halo and to a vest, cast, or traction setup. Removal of the halo is included.

20662-20663

20662   Application of halo, including removal; pelvic
20663   Application of halo, including removal; femoral

A halo device is used to stabilize the bones of the pelvis or femur. In 20662, a pelvic hoop is positioned around the pelvis. The pin insertion sites are cleansed with an anti-infective agent. Local anesthesia is injected. Two straight pins are then advanced through the skin over the anterior superior aspect of the iliac spines. The pins are passed through the bone and exit at the posterior superior aspect of the iliac spines. The pins are connected to the pelvic hoop. The hoop is then connected to four vertical bars that may be connected to a cast or traction setup. In 20663, a femoral hoop is positioned. The pin insertion sites are cleansed with an anti-infective agent and anesthesia is administered. Pins are then advanced through the skin and into the femur. The pins are attached to the femoral hoop. Rods are then attached to a cast or traction setup.

20664

20664   Application of halo, including removal, cranial, 6 or more pins placed, for thin skull osteology (eg, pediatric patients, hydrocephalus, osteogenesis imperfecta)

A cranial halo device with 6 or more pins is applied to stabilize the cervical spine in a patient with thin skull osteology. Pediatric patients as well as individuals with hydrocephalus or bone disorders such as osteogenesis imperfecta commonly require 6 or more pins. The pin insertion sites are shaved and cleansed with an anti-infective agent. A general anesthetic is administered. The halo device is positioned over the skull. The anterior pins are placed first. They are inserted through the skin and advanced until the bone is engaged in the area referred to as the safe zone. This is the region just below the greatest skull circumference. The anterior pins are placed above the supraorbital ridge to prevent penetration into the orbit and lateral to the middle portion of the supraorbital rim to avoid the supratrochlear and supraorbital nerves and the frontal sinus. Lateral pins are placed anterior to the temporalis muscle and fossa to prevent painful mastication and penetration of the thinner bone at the fossa. The posterior pins are then placed. The diagonally opposed pins are tightened simultaneously until the desired penetration of the bone has been reached. Lock nuts are tightened to maintain the appropriate depth and stability of the device. Rods are then attached to the halo and to a vest, cast, or traction setup. Removal of the halo is included.

20665

20665   Removal of tongs or halo applied by another individual

Tongs or a halo previously placed by another individual are removed. While maintaining cervical alignment, the halo or tongs pins are unscrewed. The pin sites are cleansed and may be filled with bone wax to encourage healing of the skull. The pin sites may be closed with sutures. A dressing is applied as needed.

20670-20680

20670   Removal of implant; superficial (eg, buried wire, pin or rod) (separate procedure)
20680   Removal of implant; deep (eg, buried wire, pin, screw, metal band, nail, rod or plate)

An internal fixation device or implant is removed. Internal fixation devices or implants are used to fix and support bones that have been fractured or weakened by a disease process. Some implants are removed while others are left in the bone. The skin is incised at the site of the implant and the implant is exposed. The bone and implant are inspected and the implant is carefully removed. Use 20670 when a superficial implant, such as a buried wire, pin, or rod is removed. Use 20680 when a deep implant, such as a buried wire, pin, screw, metal band, nail, rod, or plate is removed.

20690-20692

20690   Application of a uniplane (pins or wires in 1 plane), unilateral, external fixation system
20692   Application of a multiplane (pins or wires in more than 1 plane), unilateral, external fixation system (eg, Ilizarov, Monticelli type)

The physician applies an external fixation device encourage healing in a fracture or joint injury. Under general anesthesia, a drill is used to creates small holes through the affected bones. Wires or pins are placed through the skin and bone holes and attached to the external fixation device. This device creates stability a the point of injury. Code 20690 for a uniplane, unilateral, external fixation system, and code 20692 for a multiplane, unilateral, external fixation system.

20693

20693   Adjustment or revision of external fixation system requiring anesthesia (eg, new pin[s] or wire[s] and/or new ring[s] or bar[s])

The physician adjusts or revises an external fixation device, which encourages healing in a fracture or joint injury. Under general anesthesia, wires or pins are placed through the skin

CPT © 2016 American Medical Association. All Rights Reserved.

● New Code   ▲ Revised Code

Musculoskeletal System

and bone holes and attached to the external fixation device. Previously inserted pin, wires, plates, etc., may be rearranged or replaced during this procedure.

20694

20694   Removal, under anesthesia, of external fixation system

The physician removes an external fixation device. Under general anesthesia, wires or pins, which have been placed through the skin and bone holes and attached to the external fixation device, are removed. Any incisions are closed with sutures or Steri-strips.

20696-20697

20696   Application of multiplane (pins or wires in more than 1 plane), unilateral, external fixation with stereotactic computer-assisted adjustment (eg, spatial frame), including imaging; initial and subsequent alignment(s), assessment(s), and computation(s) of adjustment schedule(s)

20697   Application of multiplane (pins or wires in more than 1 plane), unilateral, external fixation with stereotactic computer-assisted adjustment (eg, spatial frame), including imaging; exchange (ie, removal and replacement) of strut, each

A multiplane unilateral external fixation device is placed with stereotactic computer-assisted adjustment, including imaging. Multiplane external fixation is particularly useful in treating complex intra-articular fractures or deformities. Computer-assisted application of multiplane external fixation allows simultaneous correction of multiple axes of a fracture or deformity and creates a dynamic type of fixation, allowing mobility of the involved joint. The exact nature of the procedure is dependent on the site and type of fracture or deformity. The external fixator struts, rings, bolts, cubes and/or springs, also referred to as the spatial frame, are positioned externally around the involved bone. The spatial frame is then secured to the bones using pins or wires placed through the rings and/or struts and into the bone. The components of the spatial frame work in concert to manipulate the deformity and bring the bones into anatomic alignment. The spatial frame is adjusted using computer software that allows the physician to make precise adjustments. The physician fine-tunes the alignment of the bone to achieve optimal correction of the deformity using a patient-specific adjustment schedule. Use code 20696 for initial and subsequent alignments, assessments, and computations of the adjustment schedules. Use code 20697 for exchange of a strut. Exchange includes both the removal and replacement of the strut and is reported for each strut exchanged.

20802

20802   Replantation, arm (includes surgical neck of humerus through elbow joint), complete amputation

The physician performs replantation of an arm, which has been completely amputated. Under general anesthesia, any damaged tissue is carefully removed. Then, the ends of the amputated bones are trimmed before they are rejoined. This step makes putting together the soft tissue on either side of the wound easier. Arteries, veins, nerves, muscles, and tendons are sutured together. Areas without skin are covered with a graft. Uncovered nerves, tendons, and joints may be covered by a free-tissue transfer along with its artery and veins. The amputation site is closed in layers.

20805

20805   Replantation, forearm (includes radius and ulna to radial carpal joint), complete amputation

The physician performs replantation of a forearm, which has been amputated between the wrist and elbow. Under general anesthesia, any damaged tissue is carefully removed. Then, the ends of the amputated bones are trimmed before they are rejoined. This step makes putting together the soft tissue on either side of the wound easier. Arteries, veins, nerves, muscles, and tendons are sutured together. Areas without skin are covered with a graft. Uncovered nerves, tendons, and joints may be covered by a free-tissue transfer along with its artery and veins. The amputation site is closed in layers.

20808

20808   Replantation, hand (includes hand through metacarpophalangeal joints), complete amputation

The physician performs replantation of a hand, which has been amputated between the wrist and fingers. Under general anesthesia, any damaged tissue is carefully removed. Then, the ends of the amputated bones are trimmed before they are rejoined. This step makes putting together the soft tissue on either side of the wound easier. Arteries, veins, nerves, muscles, and tendons are sutured together. Areas without skin are covered with a graft. Uncovered nerves, tendons, and joints may be covered by a free-tissue transfer along with its artery and veins. The amputation site is closed in layers.

20816

20816   Replantation, digit, excluding thumb (includes metacarpophalangeal joint to insertion of flexor sublimis tendon), complete amputation

The physician performs replantation of a digit, excluding the thumb, which has been amputated from the hand at its meta carpal joint. Under general anesthesia, any damaged tissue is carefully removed. Then, the ends of the amputated bones are trimmed before they are rejoined. This step makes putting together the soft tissue on either side of the wound easier. Arteries, veins, nerves, muscles, and tendons are sutured together. Areas without skin are covered with a graft. Uncovered nerves, tendons, and joints may be covered by a free-tissue transfer along with its artery and veins. The amputation site is closed in layers.

20822

20822   Replantation, digit, excluding thumb (includes distal tip to sublimis tendon insertion), complete amputation

The physician performs replantation of a digit, excluding the thumb, which has been amputated from the hand between the finger tip and the attachment of the finger to the palm. Under general anesthesia, any damaged tissue is carefully removed. Then, the ends of the amputated bones are trimmed before they are rejoined. This step makes putting together the soft tissue on either side of the wound easier. Arteries, veins, nerves, muscles, and tendons are sutured together. Areas without skin are covered with a graft. Uncovered nerves, tendons, and joints may be covered by a free-tissue transfer along with its artery and veins. The amputation site is closed in layers.

20824

20824   Replantation, thumb (includes carpometacarpal joint to MP joint), complete amputation

The physician performs replantation of a thumb, which has been amputated at the joint of the thumb to the palm. Under general anesthesia, any damaged tissue is carefully removed. Then, the ends of the amputated bones are trimmed before they are rejoined. This step makes putting together the soft tissue on either side of the wound easier. Arteries, veins, nerves, muscles, and tendons are sutured together. Areas without skin are covered with a graft. Uncovered nerves, tendons, and joints may be covered by a free-tissue transfer along with its artery and veins. The amputation site is closed in layers.

20827

20827   Replantation, thumb (includes distal tip to MP joint), complete amputation

The physician performs replantation of a thumb, which has been amputated between the tip of the thumb and the joint of the thumb and palm. Under general anesthesia, any damaged tissue is carefully removed. Then, the ends of the amputated bones are trimmed before they are rejoined. This step makes putting together the soft tissue on either side of the wound easier. Arteries, veins, nerves, muscles, and tendons are sutured together. Areas without skin are covered with a graft. Uncovered nerves, tendons, and joints may be covered by a free-tissue transfer along with its artery and veins. The amputation site is closed in layers.

20838

20838   Replantation, foot, complete amputation

The physician performs replantation of a foot which has been amputated at or near the ankle. Under general anesthesia, any damaged tissue is carefully removed. Then, the ends of the amputated bones are trimmed before they are rejoined. This step makes putting together the soft tissue on either side of the wound easier. Arteries, veins, nerves, muscles, and tendons are sutured together. Areas without skin are covered with a graft. Uncovered nerves, tendons, and joints may be covered by a free-tissue transfer along with its artery and veins. The amputation site is closed in layers.

20900-20902

20900   Bone graft, any donor area; minor or small (eg, dowel or button)
20902   Bone graft, any donor area; major or large

The physician transplants bone from one site to another, usually to promote osteogenesis or provide structural stability. Bone grafts may be used to fill bone defects, promote bone union or provide material for arthrodesis. In an autograft, the transplanted bone is derived from the same person or animal; an allograft (homograft) is derived from another person, and a xenograft (heterograft) is derived from a donor of a different species. The bones used most frequently as donor sites for grafts are the iliac crest, tibia, fibula, greater trochanter, distal end of the radius and posterior portions of the spine. The physician creates an incision over the donor bone and resects the muscles before harvesting a bone graft. Code 20900 for a minor or small graft (e.g., smaller than a dowel or button). Code 20902 for a large or major graft.

Musculoskeletal System

20910-20912

20910   Cartilage graft; costochondral
20912   Cartilage graft; nasal septum

The physician transplants cartilage from one site to another, often for reconstruction of the face to correct TMJ pain. In an autograft, the transplanted cartilage is derived from the same person or animal; an allograft (homograft) is derived from another person; and a xenograft (heterograft) is derived from a donor of a different species. The physician creates an incision over the donor cartilage and resects the muscles before harvesting the cartilage graft. Code 20910 for a costochondral cartilage graft. Code 20912 for a nasal septum cartilage graft.

20920-20922

20920   Fascia lata graft; by stripper
20922   Fascia lata graft; by incision and area exposure, complex or sheet

The physician harvests a fascia lata graft, which is the strong deep fascia of the thigh, for use in a separately reportable reconstruction procedure. In 20920, a stripper device is used to separate the fascia from the muscle. A horizontal incision is made usually above the knee over the ileotibial tract and carried down to the fascial layer. A small incision is made in the fascia and a silk suture placed at the proximal edge to facilitate threading the fascia strip through the stripper. The stripper is engaged and pushed along the fascia in a superior direction while tension is placed on the silk suture. The fascia is pulled through the stripper. When a strip of the desired length is obtained, the stripper is triggered and the strip is cut proximally. Multiple strips may be harvested. In 20922, the fascia lata graft is obtained by incision and surgical exposure of the fascia to obtain a sheet of fascia or for a complex fascia lata harvest. A longitudinal incision up to 10 cm in length is made in the upper or lower thigh. Fat is dissected off the area where the fascia lata will be harvested. The plane of tissue between the fat and fascia lata is undermined and the fascia lata exposed. The graft is cut to the desired size and shape and removed. Following the stripping or excision procedure, the incision is closed, a drain placed, and a pressure dressing applied.

20924

20924   Tendon graft, from a distance (eg, palmaris, toe extensor, plantaris)

The physician obtains a tendon graft from a donor site. The donor site is chosen and an incision is made through the skin and muscle, down to the length of the tendon. A portion of the tendon is excised and held in extended position with a hemostat. The wound is sutured closed and a pressure dressing is applied.

20926

20926   Tissue grafts, other (eg, paratenon, fat, dermis)

The physician harvests a tissue graft, not covered in any other code, such as a paratenon, fat or dermis graft. The paratenon is the fatty or synovial tissue between a tendon and its sheath. The physician creates an incision at the donor site and harvests the tissue. The donor site is closed with layered sutures. Transplantation of this graft is reported separately.

20930-20931

20930   Allograft, morselized, or placement of osteopromotive material, for spine surgery only (List separately in addition to code for primary procedure)
20931   Allograft, structural, for spine surgery only (List separately in addition to code for primary procedure)

A bone allograft or osteopromotive material is placed during a separately reportable surgical procedure on the spine. Bone allograft uses donor bone usually obtained from a cadaver. Bone allograft does not contain any osteoblasts (bone-growing cells) or bone morphogenic proteins (bone growing-proteins), so the graft provides only a calcium scaffolding for new bone to grow on (bone conduction). Osteopromotive materials induce bone growth and may be referred to as osteoinductive materials. These materials contain osteogenic proteins which are natural growth factors that induce bone formation. One type called bone morphogenic proteins (BMP) causes mesenchymal cells to differentiate into chondroblasts and osteoblasts. BMP is combined with an absorbable collagen sponge and implanted into the bone defect to induce new bone growth. Other types include autogenous growth factor concentrate, bovine-derived osteoconductive protein, and recombinant human MP52. Use 20930 to report placement of a morselized bone allograft consisting of donor bone that has been broken into small pieces (crushed), or the placement of osteopromotive material in the bone defect. Use 20931 to report the placement of a structural bone allograft, which is an intact piece of donor bone that has been configured or sculpted to fit into the bone defect.

20936-20938

20936   Autograft for spine surgery only (includes harvesting the graft); local (eg, ribs, spinous process, or laminar fragments) obtained from same incision (List separately in addition to code for primary procedure)
20937   Autograft for spine surgery only (includes harvesting the graft); morselized (through separate skin or fascial incision) (List separately in addition to code for primary procedure)
20938   Autograft for spine surgery only (includes harvesting the graft); structural, bicortical or tricortical (through separate skin or fascial incision) (List separately in addition to code for primary procedure)

A bone autograft is placed during a separately reportable surgical procedure on the spine. An autologous bone graft is taken from the patient's own bone and can be harvested locally from the ribs, spinous process, or lamina through the same incision made for the spinal surgery (20936), or it can be harvested from a remote site, such as the iliac crest, through a separate incision. Autologous bone contains osteoblasts (bone-growing cells) and bone morphogenic proteins (bone-growing proteins) for new bone growth in addition to providing calcium scaffolding for new bone to grow on. In 20937, a moselized bone graft obtained is through a separate incision, such as the iliac crest. An incision is made in the skin over the iliac crest and muscle is stripped to reveal the bone surface. The top portion of the iliac crest is excised and soft cancellous spongy bone is scooped out. The bone is crushed, or morcelized, and then packed into the bone defect in the spine, and compressed to facilitate bone healing. Use 20938 for structural, bicortical, or tricortical bone graft obtained through a separate incision. Both cortical and cancellous bone is harvested, such as from the iliac crest, the bone is configured to fit into the bone defect, and then seated in the prepared space. The structural, bicortical, or tricortical bone graft may be secured using a screw or wire.

20950

20950   Monitoring of interstitial fluid pressure (includes insertion of device, eg, wick catheter technique, needle manometer technique) in detection of muscle compartment syndrome

The physician inserts an interstitial fluid pressure monitoring device into a muscle compartment. This is achieved via wick catheter, needle manometer, or other various techniques. Escalating pressure indicates developing compartment syndrome.

20955-20962

20955   Bone graft with microvascular anastomosis; fibula
20956   Bone graft with microvascular anastomosis; iliac crest
20957   Bone graft with microvascular anastomosis; metatarsal
20962   Bone graft with microvascular anastomosis; other than fibula, iliac crest, or metatarsal

The physician harvests a bone graft from a donor site for the purpose of reconstruction in a future procedure. The donor bone is isolated and dissected with the blood vessels still attached. The donor site is closed in layers. The graft is then used to fill a defect at another site. The blood vessels are attached to the defect area's vessels. The defect area is then closed with layered sutures. Code 20955 for a donor graft from the fibula; code 20956 for a donor graft from the iliac crest; code 20957 for a donor graft from a metatarsal; and code 20962 for a donor graft from a site other than the fibula, iliac crest, or metatarsal.

20969-20973

20969   Free osteocutaneous flap with microvascular anastomosis; other than iliac crest, metatarsal, or great toe
20970   Free osteocutaneous flap with microvascular anastomosis; iliac crest
20972   Free osteocutaneous flap with microvascular anastomosis; metatarsal
20973   Free osteocutaneous flap with microvascular anastomosis; great toe with web space

A free osteocutaneous flap is used to repair a complex soft tissue and bony defect. The exact procedure performed depends on the harvest site and the site of the defect. The defect to be repaired is measured and the dimensions of the cutaneous portion of the flap are determined. The incision lines are drawn onto the skin at the donor site. The skin at the donor site is incised along these lines and dissected from the underlying tissue, taking care to preserve a vascular pedicle. The underlying musculature is exposed and the blood vessels and nerves are preserved. The bone to be harvested is exposed and the amount of bone required to fill the bony defect is harvested, taking care to preserve bony vasculature. The osteocutaneous flap with intact vascular structures is then severed from the donor site and transferred to the prepared recipient bed. The bone is inset into the bony defect and secured. Vascular structures in the flap are anastomosed to blood vessels at the recipient site using microvascular technique. The skin portion of the flap is then positioned in the defect and secured with sutures. The donor site may be closed with sutures or a separately reportable skin graft may be used to repair the donor site. Use 20969 for osteocutaneous flap from a donor site other than the iliac crest, metatarsal, or great toe. For osteocutaneous flap from the iliac crest, use 20970; from the metatarsal, use 20972; from the great toe with web space, use 20973.

Musculoskeletal System

● New Code   ▲ Revised Code

20974-20975

20974 Electrical stimulation to aid bone healing; noninvasive (nonoperative)
20975 Electrical stimulation to aid bone healing; invasive (operative)

Bone typically heals well without the use of bone healing interventions, such as electrical stimulation. However, under some circumstances, normal bone healing may be compromised such as when circulation to the bone fragments is poor or when scar tissue develops at the site of the fracture. Electrical stimulation is a method used for bone healing in such circumstances. In 20974, a noninvasive technique such as pulsed electromagnetic field (PEMF) is used. The PEMF coil is placed on the skin or incorporated into the cast over the fracture site. A separate treatment unit is programmed and attached to the coil. The treatment unit transmits an electrical current along the coil creating an electromagnetic field around the fracture site. Another noninvasive technique uses a capacitive coupling device. Two electrodes are placed on the skin over the fracture site. The electrodes are attached to a battery operated stimulation unit. A low voltage alternating current is used to stimulate bone healing. In 20975, an invasive technique such as direct coupling is used to stimulate bone healing. Cathodes are placed directly into the bone at the fracture site, usually at the time of a separately reported operative procedure to treat the fracture. The cathodes are attached to a small generator that is also implanted. The generator produces a low voltage alternating current which stimulates bone healing.

20979

20979 Low intensity ultrasound stimulation to aid bone healing, noninvasive (nonoperative)

Ultrasound stimulation is applied using a non-invasive device that emits low intensity, pulsed ultrasound through the skin over the site of a fracture to aid in bone healing. The ultrasound stimulator is composed of a battery operated system with an attached transducer. The operating device is programmed. The patient is instructed on at-home use of the device. Coupling gel is applied to the skin at the site of the fracture and the transducer is placed on the skin where the coupling gel has been applied. If the patient has a cast, a small window is created in the cast over the site of the fracture. The transducer is left in place for approximately 20 minutes each day. Many devices have the ability to monitor use. The transducer is used each day for the prescribed amount of time until the fracture has healed.

20982

20982 Ablation therapy for reduction or eradication of 1 or more bone tumors (eg, metastasis) including adjacent soft tissue when involved by tumor extension, percutaneous, including imaging guidance when performed; radiofrequency

Percutaneous radiofrequency ablation (RFA) of a bone tumor uses an interventional radiology technique to destroy tumor cells. Using CT guidance, the bone tumor is identified and an RFA probe is advanced through the skin and into the tumor. The RFA device is activated and a rapidly alternating, heat-generating current is transmitted through the probe. Tumor destruction is monitored, including adjacent soft tissue affected by the tumor, and the probe is repositioned as needed until the entire bone mass has been reduced or destroyed.

20983

20983 Ablation therapy for reduction or eradication of 1 or more bone tumors (eg, metastasis) including adjacent soft tissue when involved by tumor extension, percutaneous, including imaging guidance when performed; cryoablation

Percutaneous cryotherapy ablation technique of a bone tumor(s) uses extreme cold to freeze and destroy tumor cells. The tumor is identified using ultrasound, CT, or MRI guidance. The tumor may require placement of multiple probes to ensure reduction or complete eradication and allow sufficient margins. The entry sites for cryotherapy probe placement are determined and small incisions are made to facilitate placement. The probes are inserted into the center of the lesion using imaging guidance, taking care to avoid major blood vessels. The location of the probe tip is confirmed, the cryoablation unit is activated, and the first freeze-thaw cycle is initiated. The probes are filled with argon gas, resulting in rapid freezing at temperatures as low as -100 degrees centigrade. The ice ball created during the freeze cycle is monitored using imaging guidance to ensure adequate extension of the ice ball beyond the margins of the lesion to include any involved adjacent soft tissue. This is followed by a thawing cycle that is initiated by replacing the argon with helium. Imaging guidance is used to monitor the creation of the cryoablation sphere (ice ball) and assess tumor destruction. Complete eradication typically requires more than one freeze/thaw cycle.

20985

20985 Computer-assisted surgical navigational procedure for musculoskeletal procedures, image-less (List separately in addition to code for primary procedure)

An image-less computer-assisted surgical navigational procedure is performed prior to or during a complex musculoskeletal surgery. Computer-assisted surgical navigational procedures allow surgeons to perform complex procedures through small incisions, such as fixation of a femoral or pelvic fracture. Use of navigational systems provide greater surgical accuracy, reduce surgery time and blood loss, and shorten the postoperative rehabilitation period. The computer-assisted surgical navigation procedure is a three step process involving data acquisition, registration, and tracking. Data acquisition by image-less navigation uses information related to the centers of joint rotation and visual information, such as anatomical landmarks. Registration techniques are then used to relate the image-less anatomic data to the bony anatomy in the surgical field. A computer generated model is prepared from the image-less anatomic information and matched to the surface data points collected during surgery. Tracking is then performed using sensors and measurement devices that provide feedback during surgery regarding correct placement of surgical tools relative to the bony anatomy.

21010

21010 Arthrotomy, temporomandibular joint

A skin incision is made in front of the ear and extended through the subcutaneous tissue to the superficial layer of the deep temporal fascia. The temporal branch of the facial nerve is identified and protected. The temporomandibular joint space is exposed and inspected. Any abnormalities are noted. Tissue samples may be obtained or other minor procedures performed. The incision is closed in layers.

21011-21014

21011 Excision, tumor, soft tissue of face or scalp, subcutaneous; less than 2 cm
21012 Excision, tumor, soft tissue of face or scalp, subcutaneous; 2 cm or greater
21013 Excision, tumor, soft tissue of face and scalp, subfascial (eg, subgaleal, intramuscular); less than 2 cm
21014 Excision, tumor, soft tissue of face and scalp, subfascial (eg, subgaleal, intramuscular); 2 cm or greater

Soft tissues include subcutaneous fat and connective tissue, fascia, muscles, tendons, blood vessels, lymph vessels, nerves, and tissues surrounding the joints. Soft tissue tumors may be benign or malignant. Benign tumors are typically treated by excision, although small malignant or indeterminate tumors, may be excised if the margins are well defined. Depending on the location of the tumor in the soft tissue of the face or scalp, the skin over the tumor may be incised, a skin flap created and elevated, or a series of incisions made along skin creases to allow exposure of the tumor. Overlying tissue is dissected and the soft tissue mass exposed. The tumor is then excised along with a margin of healthy tissue. Separately reportable frozen section may be performed to ensure that all margins are free of tumor cells. Drains are placed as needed and the surgical wound is closed in layers. For tumors in the subcutaneous fat or connective tissue, use 21011 for a mass less than 2 cm and 21012 for a mass 2 cm or greater. For tumors that lie below the fascia, use 21013 for a mass less than 2 cm and 21014 for a mass 2 cm or greater. Subfascial soft tissue tumors include those within muscle tissue and those found in the galea aponeurotica, more commonly referred to as the epicranial aponeurosis. The epicranial aponeurosis is a fibrous sheet of tissue that serves as the attachment for the occipitofrontalis and temporoparietalis muscle fibers.

21015-21016

21015 Radical resection of tumor (eg, sarcoma), soft tissue of face or scalp; less than 2 cm
21016 Radical resection of tumor (eg, sarcoma), soft tissue of face or scalp; 2 cm or greater

Radical resection is typically performed for a malignant neoplasm, such as a sarcoma, although benign tumors and tumors of indeterminate nature may also require radical resection. Depending on the location of the tumor in the face or neck, the skin over the tumor may be incised, a skin flap created and elevated, or a series of incisions made along skin creases to allow exposure of the tumor. Soft tissue surrounding the tumor is dissected and the tumor is exposed. Radical resection involves removal of all involved soft tissue which may include muscles, nerves, and blood vessels. The tumor is resected along with a wide margin of surrounding healthy tissue. Separately reportable frozen section examination is performed to ensure that the margins are free of tumor cells. If margins show evidence of malignancy, additional tissue is removed until all margins are free of tumor cells. The physician then repairs muscle and soft tissues. A separately reportable reconstructive procedure may be performed using muscle, myocutaneous, fascial, or other grafts or flaps at the same or a subsequent surgical session. Drains are placed as needed and the overlying skin closed in layers. Use 21015 for radical resection of a tumor less than 2 cm. Use 21016 for a tumor 2 cm or greater.

● New Code   ▲ Revised Code

21025-21026

21025 Excision of bone (eg, for osteomyelitis or bone abscess); mandible
21026 Excision of bone (eg, for osteomyelitis or bone abscess); facial bone(s)

The physician excises dead or infected bone from the mandible (21025) or facial bones (21026). Drills, osteotomes, and saws are used to excise the dead or infected bone (e.g., for osteomyelitis or bone abscess). Antibiotic beads may be implanted to help stop the spread of infection at the surgical site. Report any bone harvesting or graft separately. The incisions are closed.

21029

21029 Removal by contouring of benign tumor of facial bone (eg, fibrous dysplasia)

The physician removes a benign facial tumor by contouring the defective bone. This procedure is often used for patients diagnosed with fibrous dysplasia. The physician creates an incision and over the tumor and uses files, osteotomes, and other bone shaping tools to create the correct shape for the bone. The incision is closed.

21030

21030 Excision of benign tumor or cyst of maxilla or zygoma by enucleation and curettage

The physician removes a benign tumor or cyst from the maxilla or zygoma bones via enucleation and/or curettage. If the procedure is performed with an external approach, the physician creates an incision on the exterior of the face and dissects the tissue until the tumor can be removed. During an internal approach, the physician makes an incision through the oral cavity to the tumor. In either approach, the tumor is removed intact after being scraped from the bone. Any incision is then sutured closed.

21031-21032

21031 Excision of torus mandibularis
21032 Excision of maxillary torus palatinus

Torus mandibularis and maxillary torus pallatinus are slow-growing, tumor-like bony growths that are considered developmental anomalies even though they do not present until adulthood. Torus mandibularis develops only on the lingual surface of the mandible near the bicuspids and is usually bilateral. Maxillary torus pallatinus develops only in the midline of the hard palate. The bony growths can vary considerably in size and shape. They can be composed of a single nodule or multiple nodules that fuse together. The condition requires surgical treatment only when it interferes with denture placement or when the growths become so large that they are easily injured or ulcerate. An incision is made in the mucosa overlying the bony growth and the bony growth is exposed. The lesion is then chiseled off the bone cortex or removed using a bone bur. Use 21031 for excision of a torus mandibularis. Use 21032 for excision of a maxillary torus pallatinus.

21034

21034 Excision of malignant tumor of maxilla or zygoma

The physician removes a malignant tumor of the maxilla or zygoma. The physician may take several different approaches to dissect the tissue to the level of the tumor. The tumor is excised, including the margins, until the surrounding tissue is free from disease. The physician uses saws, osteotomes, files, and drills to remove the malignant mass. Teeth may or may not be removed. Soft tissue reconstruction may require myocutaneous flaps depending on the approach method and mass of the tumor. All incisions are closed with sutures.

21040

21040 Excision of benign tumor or cyst of mandible, by enucleation and/or curettage

The physician removes a benign tumor or cyst from the mandible via enucleation and/or curettage. If the procedure is performed with an external approach, the physician creates an incision on the exterior of the face and dissects the tissue until the tumor can be removed. During an internal approach, the physician makes an incision through the oral cavity to the tumor. In either approach, the tumor is removed intact after being scraped from the bone. Any incision is then sutured closed.

21044

21044 Excision of malignant tumor of mandible

The physician removes a malignant tumor of the mandible. The physician may take several different approaches to dissect the tissue to the level of the tumor. The tumor is excised, including the margins, until the surrounding tissue is free from disease. The physician uses saws, osteotomes, files, and drills to remove the malignant mass. Teeth may or may not be removed. Soft tissue reconstruction may require myocutaneous flaps depending on the approach method and mass of the tumor. If bone harvesting is required, it should be reported separately. All incisions are closed with sutures.

21045

21045 Excision of malignant tumor of mandible; radical resection

The physician removes a malignant tumor of the mandible through radical resection. The physician uses an intraoral approach to access the tumor. The tumor is excised, including the margins, until the surrounding tissue is free from disease. All or part of the mandible is removed. Teeth may or may not be removed. Reconstruction may require myocutaneous flaps, bone grafts, prostheses, and tissue rearrangement. All incisions are closed with layered sutures.

21046-21047

21046 Excision of benign tumor or cyst of mandible; requiring intra-oral osteotomy (eg, locally aggressive or destructive lesion[s])
21047 Excision of benign tumor or cyst of mandible; requiring extra-oral osteotomy and partial mandibulectomy (eg, locally aggressive or destructive lesion[s])

The physician excises a benign tumor or cyst of the mandible. If the physician uses an intraoral approach, a flap of muscle from within the mouth is incised and reflected. Once the tumor is located it is removed, along with the overlying bone (21046). If an extraoral approach is used, the physician creates an incision outside the mouth and continues incising and reflecting tissue until the tumor can be identified and removed. Additionally part of the mandible is also removed (21047). The area may be packed and closed, or a bone graft may be necessary. Any incisions are then sutured in layers.

21048-21049

21048 Excision of benign tumor or cyst of maxilla; requiring intra-oral osteotomy (eg, locally aggressive or destructive lesion[s])
21049 Excision of benign tumor or cyst of maxilla; requiring extra-oral osteotomy and partial maxillectomy (eg, locally aggressive or destructive lesion[s])

The physician excises a benign tumor or cyst of the maxilla. If the physician uses an intraoral approach, a flap of muscle from within the mouth is incised and reflected. Once the tumor is located it is removed, along with the overlying bone (21048). If an extraoral approach is used, the physician creates an incision outside the mouth and continues incising and reflecting tissue until the tumor can be identified and removed. Additionally part of the maxilla is also removed (21049). The area may be packed and closed, or a bone graft may be necessary. Any incisions are then sutured in layers.

21050

21050 Condylectomy, temporomandibular joint (separate procedure)

The physician excises the condyle of the mandible at the temporomandibular joint. A condyle is a rounded articular surface at the extremity of a bone. Often, the physician creates an incision near the ear and removes all or part of mandibular condyle. Reconstruction of the area is possible, or a prosthetic condyle can be inserted. The incision is closed with layered sutures.

21060

21060 Meniscectomy, partial or complete, temporomandibular joint (separate procedure)

The physician creates an incision near the ear until the meniscus of the joint is exposed. A clamp is placed on the meniscus. All or part of the meniscus is excised. The remaining space may be filled with adjoining tissue or a prosthetic disc. The incision is closed with layered sutures.

21070

21070 Coronoidectomy (separate procedure)

The physician removes the coronoid process of the mandible. The physician creates an intraoral incision. Tissue is reflected from the mandible until the coronoid process can be clamped and excised. The physician utilizes drills, saws, files, and/or osteotomes in the excision process. The incision is closed primarily.

21073

21073 Manipulation of temporomandibular joint(s) (TMJ), therapeutic, requiring an anesthesia service (ie, general or monitored anesthesia care)

A therapeutic temporomandibular joint (TMJ) manipulation is performed under general or monitored anesthesia care. TMJ manipulation is performed to treat TMJ disorders including clicking and popping, pain, and restricted movement. General or monitored anesthesia care is provided and a local anesthetic is also given to the temporomandibular joint, injecting the masseter, temporalis, medial pterygoid, and lateral pterygoid muscles as needed. Once adequate local anesthesia is achieved, manual manipulation of the jaw is performed. The mandible is first manipulated backward (posteriorly) and maintained in this position. The jaw is then gradually manipulated downward (inferiorly) followed by side-to-side motion. This manipulation of the mandible opens the joint space allowing more

Musculoskeletal System

complete range of motion. Range of motion is evaluated and manipulation is repeated until maximum range of motion has been achieved and joint clicking is no longer present.

21076

21076   Impression and custom preparation; surgical obturator prosthesis

A surgical obturator prosthesis is used to close a defect in the hard palate and maxilla due to a congenital or acquired defect, such as cleft palate or a defect caused by resection of a tumor of the hard palate and/or maxilla. This type of prosthesis is prepared prior to surgery and placed at the time of surgery. It is a temporary prosthesis designed to restore continuity of the hard palate during the period immediately following surgery. The obturator is designed to separate the oral and nasal cavities, enable the patient to chew and swallow, provide occlusion with the mandible, support the mandible, reestablish speech, and provide a cosmetically acceptable appearance. Prior to the surgical procedure the prosthetist obtains an impression of the defect and other structures of the mouth. Radiological studies, such as a CT scan may also be obtained to help evaluate the anatomy. A mold is prepared and the custom prosthesis is constructed. The obturator is then placed at the time of the surgical procedure.

21077

21077   Impression and custom preparation; orbital prosthesis

An orbital prosthesis is a removable prosthetic that replaces the eye, eyelids, and surrounding bone and skin. While the orbital prosthesis does not allow movement of the eyelids or eye, it does protect the eye socket and underlying tissues from debris and bacteria and does allow for a more cosmetically acceptable appearance. An impression is made of the orbital defect. A mold is then created from the impression. The orbital prosthesis is created using medical silicone that is color matched to the patient. The eye component is fabricated separately of acrylic and is also color matched to the patient. The eye and orbit components are then connected to create the orbital prosthesis. The orbital prosthesis is attached using adhesives. Alternatively, if a retained orbital prosthesis has been constructed it is placed during a separately reportable surgical procedure.

21079-21080

21079   Impression and custom preparation; interim obturator prosthesis
21080   Impression and custom preparation; definitive obturator prosthesis

An interim obturator prosthesis (21079) is one that is made following surgical resection of a portion or all of one or both maxilla and may include replacement of teeth in the defect area. It replaces the surgical obturator that is used during the immediate postoperative period. The interim obturator may be worn for several months while wound healing continues. A definitive obturator prosthesis (21080) is a permanent prosthesis that is fabricated once the traumatic or surgical defect has completely healed. The obturator is designed to separate the oral and nasal cavities, enable the patient to chew and swallow, provide occlusion with the mandible, support the mandible, r-establish speech, and provide a cosmetically acceptable appearance. In 21079, the prosthetist obtains an impression of the defect and other structures of the mouth after the immediate postoperative period when some healing has occurred. Radiological studies, such as a CT scan, may also be obtained to help evaluate the anatomy. A mold is prepared and the custom prosthesis is constructed. In 21080, the prosthetist obtains an impression of the defect and other structures of the mouth after the surgery wound has completely healed and creates the prosthesis as described above.

21081

21081   Impression and custom preparation; mandibular resection prosthesis

A mandibular resection prosthesis is fabricated to improve occlusal contact of the remaining mandibular dentition with the maxillary dentition following resection of the mandible. Impressions are taken of the mandible and maxilla. A mold is created and the mandibular resection prosthesis fabricated. This type of prosthesis may require use of a flange, guide, or occlusal platform that is incorporated in the prosthesis and that then guides the remaining mandibular segment into optimal occlusal contact with the maxilla.

21082

21082   Impression and custom preparation; palatal augmentation prosthesis

A palatal augmentation prosthesis is used to reshape the hard palate to improve tongue-palate contact during speech and swallowing in patients with impaired tongue mobility due to surgery, trauma, or neurological motor deficits. An impression of the palate, maxillary bone and teeth is obtained. A mold is created and a custom palatal augmentation prosthesis fabricated.

21083

21083   Impression and custom preparation; palatal lift prosthesis

A palatal lift prosthesis is a prosthesis for the soft palate. The soft palate, also referred to as the velum or muscular palate, is located in the back and roof of the mouth and is composed of soft tissue. The soft palate closes off the nasal passages during swallowing and also aids in closing off the trachea. A palatal lift prosthesis is a removable prosthesis

designed to improve function of an incompetent soft palate by elevating the soft tissue and improving velopharyngeal closure. An impression of the upper aspect of the mouth is obtained. A mold is created and a custom palatal lift prosthesis fabricated.

21084

21084   Impression and custom preparation; speech aid prosthesis

A speech aid prosthesis is a removable maxillary prosthesis used in patients with acquired or congenital defects of the soft palate with dysfunction of the palatopharyngeal sphincter. This type of prosthesis is used to improve both speech and swallowing function. The prosthesis covers the soft palate and extends into the pharynx to separate the oropharynx and nasopharynx during speech and swallowing. An impression is taken of the soft palate and a mold created. A custom speech aid prosthesis is fabricated.

21085

21085   Impression and custom preparation; oral surgical splint

The physician creates an oral surgical splint. The physician creates molds of the affected area and creates the splint from these molds. An intra-oral splint (e.g., orthotic) is a plastic prosthetic which is usually made to cover the lower teeth for patients with a temporomandibular disorder. The purpose of the oral splint is to act as a diagnostic aid to help the physician determine the correct position of the jaw and temporomandibular joint.

21086

21086   Impression and custom preparation; auricular prosthesis

An auricular prosthesis replaces all or a portion of the outer ear. An impression of the contralateral outer ear is obtained. Alternatively, an impression of the ear of a morphologically similar individual may be used. A mold is created. A custom prosthetic outer ear is fabricated using medical silicone that is color-matched to the patient. The prosthetic outer ear is attached to the patient using adhesive or an osseointegrated craniofacial implant.

21087

21087   Impression and custom preparation; nasal prosthesis

The physician creates a nasal prosthesis for the patient. Molds are formed of the patient's nose and face. These molds are used in making a latex nasal prosthesis, which is attached to the face via adhesive or magnets. Photographs of the patient help the physician to create a nasal prosthesis which reflects the face of the patient prior to surgery.

21088

21088   Impression and custom preparation; facial prosthesis

The physician creates a facial prosthesis for the patient. Molds are formed of the patient's face. These molds are used in making a latex facial prosthesis, which is attached to the face via adhesive or magnets. Photographs of the patient help the physician to create a nasal prosthesis which reflects the face of the patient prior to surgery.

21100

21100   Application of halo type appliance for maxillofacial fixation, includes removal (separate procedure)

A halo-type fixation device is applied to the head of the patient. Screws are used to secure the device to the skull and maxilla. The device is also attached at the teeth of the patient. If the patient has no teeth, dentures may be fitted. Removal of this device is also included in this code.

21110

21110   Application of interdental fixation device for conditions other than fracture or dislocation, includes removal

Interdental fixation is applied by the physician to wire the jaws together. This procedure is specifically for conditions other than fracture or dislocation. Ivy loops or arch bars may be used for fixation purposes. For patients without teeth, dentures may be wired first, and then wired together. Other orthodontic appliances may be used in conjunction with the devices listed in this description.

21116

21116   Injection procedure for temporomandibular joint arthrography

An injection procedure for temporomandibular joint arthrography is performed. The skin over the injection site is cleansed and a local anesthetic is injected. A needle may be inserted into the joint and fluid aspirated with a syringe. The radiopaque substance is then injected into the temporomandibular joint, which is exercised to help distribute the radiopaque substance. Once the contrast has been distributed throughout the joint, separately reportable radiographic images are obtained.

21120

21120   Genioplasty; augmentation (autograft, allograft, prosthetic material)

Augmentation genioplasty is peformed to correct of the bony contour of the chin. This can be accomplished using prosthetic material such as an alloplastic implant made of medical silicone or other materials, autogenous cartilage or bone grafts, or cadaveric allografts of cartilage or bone. Using a submental or intraoral approach, dissection is carried down to the periosteum of the chin. The midline is marked with a suture and the periosteum is incised taking care to protect the mental nerves on each side of the mandible. If an alloplastic implant is used, it is placed beneath the periosteum taking care to line up the midline of the implant with the midline of the chin. The overlying soft tissues are closed in layers. If cartilage or bone autograft is used, it is harvested through a separate incision. The autograft is then configured to the desired size and shape and implanted as described above. If an allograft is used it is obtained from the tissue bank, configured to the desired size and shape, and implanted as described above.

21121-21123

21121   Genioplasty; sliding osteotomy, single piece
21122   Genioplasty; sliding osteotomies, 2 or more osteotomies (eg, wedge excision or bone wedge reversal for asymmetrical chin)
21123   Genioplasty; sliding, augmentation with interpositional bone grafts (includes obtaining autografts)

Genioplasty is peformed by sliding osteotomy to correct of the bony contour of the chin. An incision is made in the gingivolabial sulcus and the periosteum is exposed. Subperiosteal dissection is performed laterally from the midline until the mental nerves have been identified. Placement of the bone cuts is determined and the mandible is then cut on each side using a sagittal saw. The chin is advanced or retruded depending on whether the patient has a receding or protruding chin. The bone is secured in the desired position using wires or a plate and screw device. The overlying soft tissues are closed in layers. Use 21121 for a single piece sliding osteotomy which involves a single bone cut on each side of the mandible. Use 21122 when two or more bone cuts are required on each side of the face, such as a wedge excision or bone wedge reversal. Multiple bone cuts are typically required for reshaping of an assymetrical chin. Use 21123 for a sliding ostetomy with augmentation using interpositional bone grafts. Osteotomies are performed as described above. The bone autograft is harvested through a separate incision. The autograft is then configured to the desired size and shape and packed in the surgical defect created by the osteotomy. The bone is then secured in the desired position with wires or a plate and screw device.

21125-21127

21125   Augmentation, mandibular body or angle; prosthetic material
21127   Augmentation, mandibular body or angle; with bone graft, onlay or interpositional (includes obtaining autograft)

The physician augments the mandibular body or angle through introduction of prosthetic material (21125) or via a bone graft (21127). In code 21125, the physician creates an incision extraorally or at the angle of the mandible. A synthetic prosthesis is inserted onto the mandible and secured with wire or screws. The prosthesis augments the mandible's contour. In code 21127, the physician harvests bone from the patient's own body, often from the hip or rib. Using both intraoral and skin incisions, the physician reflects surrounding tissue and inserts the bone graft into the desired location. The graft is secured with wires or screws. All incisions are closed.

21137-21139

21137   Reduction forehead; contouring only
21138   Reduction forehead; contouring and application of prosthetic material or bone graft (includes obtaining autograft)
21139   Reduction forehead; contouring and setback of anterior frontal sinus wall

Forehead reduction surgery is performed to reduce and reshape a prominent or asymmetrical frontal bone in the forehead. An incision is made at the junction of the forehead and the hairline. The skin and soft tissues of the forehead are undermined to the level of the brows and the frontal bone is exposed. In 21137, the forehead is reduced by contouring only. The bony prominences are reduced and the frontal bone sculpted using a bur. In 21138, both contouring and prosthetic material or bone grafts are used to reduce bony prominences and improve symmetry of the frontal bone. Countouring is performed as described above on bony prominences. The asymmetry is then addressed. Depressions in the frontal bone are built up using bone cement or bone grafts. If bone cement is used it is placed in the depressed region and carefully sculpted to build up the bone. If a bone allograft is used it is harvested usually from the iliac crest. A skin incision is made over the iliac crest and the muscle is stripped to reveal the bone surface. Cortical and/or cancellous bone is harvested. The bone is configured to the desired size and shape and/or cancellous bone is morcelized and placed into the depressed region of the frontal bone and carefully sculpted to restore symmetry to the frontal bone. In 21139, forehead reduction with contouring and setback of the anterior frontal sinus wall is performed. This procedure is performed for large brow bones caused by overgrowth of the underlying frontal sinus. Contouring is performed as described above. The frontal table of the frontal sinus is

then removed and reshaped. Once the desired shape has been attained, the frontal table of the frontal sinus is setback in the forehead in a flatter, more recessed position and secured using internal fixation. The skin and soft tissues are then replaced over the frontal bone, any excess skin is excised, and the incision is closed in layers.

21141-21143

21141   Reconstruction midface, LeFort I; single piece, segment movement in any direction (eg, for Long Face Syndrome), without bone graft
21142   Reconstruction midface, LeFort I; 2 pieces, segment movement in any direction, without bone graft
21143   Reconstruction midface, LeFort I; 3 or more pieces, segment movement in any direction, without bone graft

The physician reconstructs the midface without the use of bone grafts in a patient with a congenital facial bone deformity or for cosmetic purposes. A Lefort I osteotomy involves the lower maxillary region, which is defined as being below the infraorbital nerve and medial to the zygomatic-maxillary suture. The premolars and last molars are extracted as needed. The palatal mucosa is tunneled to prevent tearing of palatal tissues during the maxillary osteotomy. An incision is made in the buccal sulcus from the 1st molar on one side to the 1st molar on the opposite side. The lateral aspect of the nasal cavity is exposed and the nasal mucosa elevated. Using measurements obtained prior to surgery, the physician marks the planned bone cuts in the maxilla. The lateral wall one side of the maxilla is cut using a bur. A thin osteotome is placed in the cut and gentle pressure applied to fracture the medial and posterior wall of the maxilla. The pterygoid plate is separated from the maxilla using a pterygoid osteotome. The pterygoid hamulus is located and carefully separated from the pterygoid plate. The procedure is repeated on the opposite side of the maxilla. The nasal septum cartilage and vomer are separated from the maxilla using a septal gouge or osteotome. After the anterior nasal spine has been fractured, the gouge or osteotome is angled towards the floor of the nose. The maxilla is downfractured using thumb pressure and then mobilized using the pterygoid osteotome. Once the maxilla is completely detached and mobile, anterior osteotomy is performed at the premolar region bilaterally. The nasal septal cartilage, posterior wall and palatal bone are trimmed. The maxilla is repositioned and stabilized with wires. Measurements are checked to ensure that the desired repositioning of the maxilla has been achieved. Lip position and occlusion are also checked. An intermaxillary fixation device is applied. The buccal incision is closed. Use 21141 if a single bone segment is moved in any direction. Use 21142 if two bone segments are moved in any direction. Use 21143 if three or more bone segments are moved in any direction.

21145-21147

21145   Reconstruction midface, LeFort I; single piece, segment movement in any direction, requiring bone grafts (includes obtaining autografts)
21146   Reconstruction midface, LeFort I; 2 pieces, segment movement in any direction, requiring bone grafts (includes obtaining autografts) (eg, ungrafted unilateral alveolar cleft)
21147   Reconstruction midface, LeFort I; 3 or more pieces, segment movement in any direction, requiring bone grafts (includes obtaining autografts) (eg, ungrafted bilateral alveolar cleft or multiple osteotomies)

The physician reconstructs the midface with the use of bone grafts in a patient with a facial bone deformity or for cosmetic purposes. A Lefort I osteotomy involves the lower maxillary region, which is defined as being below the infraorbital nerve and medial to the zygomatic-maxillary suture. The premolars and last molars are extracted as needed. The palatal mucosa is tunneled to prevent tearing of palatal tissues during the maxillary osteotomy. An incision is made in the buccal sulcus from the 1st molar on one side to the 1st molar on the opposite side. The lateral aspect of the nasal cavity is exposed and the nasal mucosa elevated. Using measurements obtained prior to surgery, the physician marks the planned bone cuts in the maxilla. The lateral wall on one side of the maxilla is cut using a bur. A thin osteotome is placed in the cut and gentle pressure applied to fracture the medial and posterior wall of the maxilla. The pterygoid plate is separated from the maxilla using a pterygoid osteotome. The pterygoid hamulus is located and carefully separated from the pterygoid plate. The procedure is repeated on the opposite side of the maxilla. The nasal septum cartilage and vomer are separated from the maxilla using a septal gouge or osteotome. After the anterior nasal spine has been fractured, the gouge or osteotome is angled towards the floor of the nose. The maxilla is downfractured using thumb pressure and then mobilized using the pterygoid osteotome. Once the maxilla is completely detached and mobile, anterior osteotomy is performed at the premolar region bilaterally. The nasal septal cartilage, posterior wall and palatal bone are trimmed. The maxilla is repositioned and stabilized with wires. Measurements are checked to ensure that the desired repositioning of the maxilla has been achieved. Lip position and occlusion are also checked. Bone grafts are harvested from the iliac crest or other site. If bone is harvested from the iliac crest, a skin incision is made over the iliac crest and the muscle is stripped to reveal the bone surface. Cortical and/or cancellous bone is harvested. The bone is configured to the desired size and shape and/or cancellous bone is morcelized and placed in the defect. An intermaxillary fixation device is applied. The buccal incision is closed. Use 21145 if a single bone segment is moved in any direction. Use 21146 if two

● New Code   ▲ Revised Code

Musculoskeletal System

bone segments are moved in any direction. Use 21147 if three or more bone segments are moved in any direction.

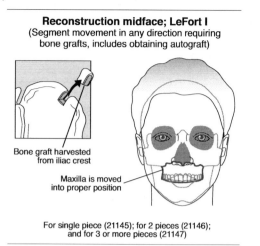

Reconstruction midface; LeFort I
(Segment movement in any direction requiring bone grafts, includes obtaining autograft)

Bone graft harvested from iliac crest

Maxilla is moved into proper position

For single piece (21145); for 2 pieces (21146); and for 3 or more pieces (21147)

21150-21151

21150 Reconstruction midface, LeFort II; anterior intrusion (eg, Treacher-Collins Syndrome)

21151 Reconstruction midface, LeFort II; any direction, requiring bone grafts (includes obtaining autografts)

The physician reconstructs the midface in a patient with a facial bone deformity. A Lefort II osteotomy involves the pyramidal nasoorbitomaxillary region, which in addition to the lower maxillary region includes the following structures: the frontal process of the maxilla to the maxillary-frontal suture, the nasal bone to the nasofrontal suture, total nasal cartilaginous complex, and the infraorbital rim medial to the infraorbital nerve. This procedure requires both intraoral and cutaneous incisions to access the bones of the face. The premolars and last molars are extracted as needed. The palatal mucosa is tunneled to prevent tearing of palatal tissues during the maxillary osteotomy. An incision is made in the buccal sulcus from the 1st molar on one side to the 1st molar on the opposite side. The lateral aspect of the nasal cavity is exposed and the nasal mucosa elevated. Exposure extends from the piriform aperture anteriorly to the pterygomaxillary-palatine fissure posteriorly to the infraorbital osseous rim superiorly to the nasolacrimal duct medially to the lateral orbital rim laterally. Using measurements obtained prior to surgery, the physician marks the planned bone cuts. The periorbita is detached from the anterior orbital rim. Medial and lateral orbital osteotomies are performed on one side of the face. The lateral vertical osteotomy extends through the maxillary buttress and then a horizontal cut is made to the pterygomaxillary-palatine fissure. The anterior orbital floor osteotomy is completed to the infraorbital nerve using from the previously created medial and lateral orbital rim cuts. The procedure is then repeated on the opposite side of the face. The bones are downfractured taking care to ensure all bones are completely mobilized. The bones are then repositioned as needed to correct the facial bone deformity. Measurements are checked to ensure that the desired repositioning of the bones has been achieved. Lip position and occlusion are also checked. If bone allograft is used it is harvested from the iliac crest. A skin incision is made over the iliac crest and the muscle is stripped to reveal the bone surface. Cortical and/or cancellous bone is harvested. The bone is configured to the desired size and shape and/or cancellous bone is morcelized and placed in the defect. Wires, miniplates or screw fixation is used to secure the bones and any bone grafts in the desired position. An intermaxillary fixation device is applied. The buccal incision is closed. Use 21150 if the procedure is performed without bone grafts. Use 21151 if bone grafts are used.

21154-21155

21154 Reconstruction midface, LeFort III (extracranial), any type, requiring bone grafts (includes obtaining autografts); without LeFort I

21155 Reconstruction midface, LeFort III (extracranial), any type, requiring bone grafts (includes obtaining autografts); with LeFort I

Lefort III osteotomy involves the high maxillary region, which in addition to the pyramidal nasoorbitomaxillary region includes the following structures: the zygoma, the lateral orbital rim inferiorly to the frontozygomatic suture, and the zygomatic arch laterally to the zygomatiic process of the temporal bone. Bone cuts are made in a configuration that allows the facial bones to be moved anteriorly and/or superiorly. In 21154, an extracranial approach is used. An incision is made from one ear, carried up along the hairline, across the forehead at the hairline and then down to the opposite ear. Soft tissues are dissected and a coronal flap created. The supraorbital region, nasal bones, and malar complex are exposed. A supplemental orbital floor approach may be used to provide greater exposure. Using measurements obtained prior to surgery, the physician marks the planned bone cuts. Bone cuts are made on one side of the face and repeated on the opposite side.

The bones are completely separated from the cranial base and repositioned as needed to correct the facial bone deformity. Measurements are checked to ensure that the desired repositioning of the bones has been achieved. Bone is harvested from the iliac crest. A skin incision is made over the iliac crest and the muscle is stripped to reveal the bone surface. Cortical and/or cancellous bone is harvested. The bone is configured to the desired size and shape and/or cancellous bone is morcelized and placed. Wires, miniplates or screw fixation is used to secure the bones and bone grafts in the desired position. The incisions are closed. In 21155, there is also a deformity of the lower maxillary region and a Lefort I procedure is performed in conjunction with the Lefort III procedure. An incision is made in the buccal sulcus from the 1st molar on one side to the 1st molar on the opposite side. The lateral aspect of the nasal cavity is exposed and the nasal mucosa elevated. Using measurements obtained prior to surgery, the physician marks the bone and then cuts the lateral wall on one side of the maxilla using a bur. A thin osteotome is placed in the cut and gentle pressure applied to fracture the medial and posterior wall of the maxilla. The pterygoid plate is separated from the maxilla using an osteotome. The pterygoid hamulus is located and carefully separated from the pterygoid plate. The procedure is repeated on the opposite side of the maxilla. The nasal septal cartilage and vomer are separated from the maxilla using a gouge. After the anterior nasal spine has been fractured, the gouge is angled towards the floor of the nose. The maxilla is downfractured using thumb pressure and then mobilized using the pterygoid osteotome. Once the maxilla is completely detached and mobile, anterior osteotomy is performed at the premolar region bilaterally. The nasal septal cartilage, posterior wall and palatal bone are trimmed and the maxilla is repositioned and stabilized with wires. Measurements are checked to ensure that the desired repositioning of the maxilla has been achieved. Lip position and occlusion are also checked. Wires, miniplates, and screws are used to secure the bones and any bone grafts. Incisions are closed.

21159

21159 Reconstruction midface, LeFort III (extra and intracranial) with forehead advancement (eg, mono bloc), requiring bone grafts (includes obtaining autografts); without LeFort I

The physician reconstructs the midface with a LeFort III osteotomy, without a LeFort I procedure. Under general anesthesia, the physician creates various incisions, including transoral, lower eyelid, scalp, etc. The midfacial bones are manipulated and completely disconnected from the cranial base. The midface is moved into the proper position and the bone grafts are inserted into the appropriate sites. Osteotomes, saws and burs are used to correct misshapen areas of bone. Plates, screws, and wires are also used for fixation. An antibiotic solution is used and then the incisions are closed. Intermaxillary fixation may be necessary.

21160

21160 Reconstruction midface, LeFort III (extra and intracranial) with forehead advancement (eg, mono bloc), requiring bone grafts (includes obtaining autografts); with LeFort I

The physician reconstructs the midface with a LeFort III (extra and intracranial) osteotomy, with forehead advancement (e.g., mono bloc), requiring bone grafts, including a LeFort I procedure. Under general anesthesia, the physician harvests bone grafts from the hip, rib, or skull of the patient. The physician then creates various incisions (e.g., transoral, lower eyelid, scalp, etc.) into the face. The midfacial and frontal bones are manipulated, along with the maxilla, and completely disconnected from the cranial base. The midface, attached to the frontal bone, and the maxilla are moved into the proper positions and the bone grafts are inserted into the appropriate sites. Osteotomes, saws and burs are used to correct misshapen areas of bone. Plates, screws, and wires are also used for fixation. An antibiotic solution is used and then the incisions are closed. Intermaxillary fixation may be necessary.

21172

21172 Reconstruction superior-lateral orbital rim and lower forehead, advancement or alteration, with or without grafts (includes obtaining autografts)

The physician reconstructs the superior-lateral orbital rim and lower forehead for correction of skeletal deformities. Bone grafts may or may not be used. If used, they are usually harvested from the hip, rib, or skull of the patient. Under general anesthesia, the physician creates various incisions (e.g., eyelid, scalp, etc.) to gain access to the surgical site. The bones are reshaped and repositioned in the proper position. If bone grafts are necessary, they are inserted in the desired position to augment the forehead or orbital rim. Fixation devices, wires, plates and screws may be used to maintain the proper shape of the facial bones. The incisions are closed.

21175

21175 Reconstruction, bifrontal, superior-lateral orbital rims and lower forehead, advancement or alteration (eg, plagiocephaly, trigonocephaly, brachycephaly), with or without grafts (includes obtaining autografts)

The physician reconstructs both superior-lateral orbital rims and the lower forehead, for correction of skeletal deformities. Bone grafts may or may not be used. If used, they are usually harvested from the hip, rib, or skull of the patient. Under general anesthesia, the physician creates various incisions (e.g., eyelid, scalp, etc.) to gain access to the surgical site. The bones are reshaped and repositioned in the proper position. If bone grafts are necessary, they are inserted in the desired position to augment the forehead or orbital rim. Fixation devices, wires, plates and screws may be used to maintain the proper shape of the facial bones. The incisions are closed.

21179-21180

21179 Reconstruction, entire or majority of forehead and/or supraorbital rims; with grafts (allograft or prosthetic material)

21180 Reconstruction, entire or majority of forehead and/or supraorbital rims; with autograft (includes obtaining grafts)

The physician reconstructs the entire or majority of the forehead and/or the supraorbital rims, for correction of skeletal deformities, with the assistance of bone grafts. Under general anesthesia, the physician creates various incisions (e.g., eyelid, scalp, etc.) to gain access to the surgical site. The bones are reshaped and repositioned in the proper position. The bone grafts are inserted in the desired position to augment the forehead or supraorbital rims. If an allograft or prosthetic is utilized for the graft, Code 21179. If an autograft is utilized, Code 21180. Fixation devices, wires, plates and screws may be used to maintain the proper shape of the facial bones. The incisions are closed.

21181

21181 Reconstruction by contouring of benign tumor of cranial bones (eg, fibrous dysplasia), extracranial

The physician reconstructs the cranial bones, because of a benign tumor (e.g., fibrous dysplasia). This reconstruction is achieved via contouring of the affected area. The physician creates various incisions to access the site of the tumor. Burs, osteotomes, files, and saws are used to contour the cranial bone to the desired shape. The incisions are closed in layers.

21182-21184

21182 Reconstruction of orbital walls, rims, forehead, nasoethmoid complex following intra- and extracranial excision of benign tumor of cranial bone (eg, fibrous dysplasia), with multiple autografts (includes obtaining grafts); total area of bone grafting less than 40 sq cm

21183 Reconstruction of orbital walls, rims, forehead, nasoethmoid complex following intra- and extracranial excision of benign tumor of cranial bone (eg, fibrous dysplasia), with multiple autografts (includes obtaining grafts); total area of bone grafting greater than 40 sq cm but less than 80 sq cm

21184 Reconstruction of orbital walls, rims, forehead, nasoethmoid complex following intra- and extracranial excision of benign tumor of cranial bone (eg, fibrous dysplasia), with multiple autografts (includes obtaining grafts); total area of bone grafting greater than 80 sq cm

The physician reconstructs the orbital walls, rims, forehead, and nasoethmoid complex, after excision of benign tumor(s) of the cranial bone. Multiple autografts are used. Under general anesthesia, the physician creates various incisions (e.g., eyelid, scalp, etc.) to gain access to the surgical site. The tumor(s) are excised via intra and extracranial approaches. The bones are precisely fractured and then repositioned in the proper placement. Bone grafts are harvested from the hip, rib, or skull of the patient, and are then inserted in the desired position to augment and stabilize the sites where tumors have been removed. Fixation devices, wires, plates and screws are used to maintain the proper shape of the facial bones. The incisions are closed in layers. Code 21182 if the total area of bone grafting is less than 40 sq. cm; code 21183 if the total area of bone grafting is greater than 40 sq. cm, but less than 80 sq. cm; and code 21184 if the total area of bone grafting is greater than 80 sq. cm.

21188

21188 Reconstruction midface, osteotomies (other than LeFort type) and bone grafts (includes obtaining autografts)

The physician reconstructs the midface through non-LeFort-style osteotomy. Under general anesthesia, the physician creates various incisions, including transoral, lower eyelid, scalp, etc. The midfacial bones are manipulated and completely disconnected from the cranial base. The midface is moved into the proper position and the bone grafts are inserted into the appropriate sites. Osteotomes, saws and burs are used to correct misshapen areas of bone. Plates, screws, and wires are also used for fixation. The physician harvests bone grafts from the hip, rib, or skull of the patient and places them at appropriate sites in the surgical area. An antibiotic solution is used, and then the incisions are closed. Intermaxillary fixation may be necessary.

21193-21194

21193 Reconstruction of mandibular rami, horizontal, vertical, C, or L osteotomy; without bone graft

21194 Reconstruction of mandibular rami, horizontal, vertical, C, or L osteotomy; with bone graft (includes obtaining graft)

The physician reconstructs the mandibular rami through horizontal, vertical, C, or L osteotomies, for correction of mandibular deformities. Under general anesthesia, the physician creates various incisions into the mandible, including a possible intraoral approach. The mandibular rami are exposed. Osteotomes, saws, and burs are used to create various cuts into the bone. The mandible is separated into parts and manipulated into a new formation. Plates, screws, and wires are also used for fixation. If a bone graft is necessary, the physician harvests bone grafts from the hip, rib, or skull of the patient and places them at appropriate sites in the surgical area. An antibiotic solution is used, and then the incisions are closed. Intermaxillary fixation may be necessary. Code 21193 if no bone graft is necessary and code 21194 if bone grafts are necessary.

21195-21196

21195 Reconstruction of mandibular rami and/or body, sagittal split; without internal rigid fixation

21196 Reconstruction of mandibular rami and/or body, sagittal split; with internal rigid fixation

The physician reconstructs the mandibular rami and/or body using a sagittal split. The physician creates an incision over the mandibular ramus and saws, drills, and osteotomes are used to separate the mandible. When separated, the jaw is moved forward into the desired position. Code 21195 if the mandible is held in place with wires. Code 21196 if the mandible is held in place with an internal rigid fixation device. The incisions are closed.

21198-21199

21198 Osteotomy, mandible, segmental

21199 Osteotomy, mandible, segmental; with genioglossus advancement

The physician corrects a localized deformity of the mandible by performing a segmental osteotomy. The physician creates an incision over the area of the deformity and reflects tissue until the bone segment is isolated. Saws, drills and osteotomes are used to remove the segment of deformed bone. The mandible is held in place with wires, screws, metal plates, or an acrylic splint (21198). Code 21199 if the genioglossus muscle of the tongue is advanced. All incisions are closed.

21206

21206 Osteotomy, maxilla, segmental (eg, Wassmund or Schuchard)

The physician corrects a localized deformity of the maxilla by performing a segmental osteotomy (e.g., Wassmund or Schuchard). The physician creates an incision over the area of the deformity and reflects tissue until the bone segment is isolated. Saws, drills, and osteotomes are used to remove the segment of deformed bone. The maxilla is held in place with wires, screws, metal plates, or an acrylic splint. Internal fixation may or may not be used. All incisions are closed.

21208

21208 Osteoplasty, facial bones; augmentation (autograft, allograft, or prosthetic implant)

The physician augments the facial bones via osteoplasty. The physician harvests bones grafts from the patient's hip, skull, or rib, or uses an allograft or prosthetic to enhance the contour of the face. The physician creates an incision over the bone and inserts the grafts or prosthesis. All incisions are closed.

21209

21209 Osteoplasty, facial bones; reduction

The physician reduces the facial bones via osteoplasty. The physician creates an incision over the bone and uses saws or drills to remove portions of excess or deformed bone. All incisions are closed.

21210

21210 Graft, bone; nasal, maxillary or malar areas (includes obtaining graft)

The physician utilizes a bone graft to augment or aid in the healing of the nasal, maxillary, or malar regions. Under general anesthesia, the physician obtains bone grafts from the patient's rib, skull or hip. An incision is made over the defective area, and the physician plants the graft into the appropriate region. Wires, plates, or screws may be used to hold the graft to the recipient site. All incisions are closed.

Musculoskeletal System

21215

21215   Graft, bone; mandible (includes obtaining graft)

The physician utilizes a bone grafts to augment or aid in the healing of the mandible. Under general anesthesia, the physician obtains bone grafts from the patient's rib, skull or hip. An incision is made over the defective area of the mandible and the physician plants the graft. Wires, plates, or screws may be used to hold the graft to the recipient site. All incisions are closed.

21230-21235

21230   Graft; rib cartilage, autogenous, to face, chin, nose or ear (includes obtaining graft)
21235   Graft; ear cartilage, autogenous, to nose or ear (includes obtaining graft)

A cartilage graft is harvested from the patient for use in a reconstructive procedure. In 21230, a rib (costal) cartilage graft is harvested for use in a reconstructive procedure on the face, chin, nose or ear. Rib cartilage is typically harvested from the eighth or ninth ribs. If more cartilage is required, the tenth rib may also be used. An incision is made over the eighth rib and dissection carried down to the rib perichondrium. Careful dissection is required because the pleura is often adherent to the perichondrium. The rib cartilage is separated from surrounding soft tissue and the cartilage graft excised. Depending on the amount of rib cartilage required, additional cartilage may be obtained from the ninth and tenth ribs. Following the rib cartilage harvest, saline is instilled into the surgical wound, which is inspected for evidence of air bubbles indicating a pleural leak. If the pleura have been torn, it is repaired with sutures. Overlying soft tissues are then closed in layers. The cartilage graft is then configured to the required size and shape and used to reconstruct the deformity of the face, chin, nose or ear. In 21235, ear (auricular or conchal) cartilage is harvested from the patient for use in reconstruction of the nose or ear. An incision is made either behind (postauricular incision) the ear or on the anterior aspect of the ear. The perichondrium is incised and a cartilage graft harvested. The graft is then shaped with a scalpel, placed in the defect in the ear or nose, and secured with sutures.

21240-21242

21240   Arthroplasty, temporomandibular joint, with or without autograft (includes obtaining graft)
21242   Arthroplasty, temporomandibular joint, with allograft

A skin incision is made in front of the ear and extended through the subcutaneous tissue to the superficial layer of the deep temporal fascia. The temporal branch of the facial nerve is identified and protected. The temporomandibular joint space is exposed and inspected. Inflamed or damaged tissue is excised. Osteophytes are excised and articular cartilage is smoothed. The meniscus may be resected or repositioned. If the meniscus is resected or extensive excision of bone or fibrous tissue is required due to ankylosis of the temporomandibular joint, a temporal muscle and fascia flap is developed to reconstruct the joint or replace the meniscus. Alternatively an auricular cartilage graft or an allograft may be used. Once the reconstruction procedure is complete, the joint capsule is repaired and overlying soft tissues are closed in layers. Use 21240 when the procedure is performed with or without an autograft. Use 21242, when an allograft is used.

21243

21243   Arthroplasty, temporomandibular joint, with prosthetic joint replacement

The physician creates an incision by or in the ear to reach the temporomandibular joint and may also create an incision below the jaw. The fossa above the condyle may be replaced with a prosthetic, as well as the condyle itself. The prosthetic is secured with screws to the remaining condylar neck. All incisions are closed.

21244

21244   Reconstruction of mandible, extraoral, with transosteal bone plate (eg, mandibular staple bone plate)

The physician reconstructs the mandible with a transosteal bone plate. This procedure is primarily performed to prepare the jaw for dentures. An extraoral approach is used to dissect the tissue away from the mandible. Holes are drilled through the bone and into the oral cavity. Posts connected to the bone plate are inserted into the drilled holes. The plate is secured with an external fixation device. All incisions are closed.

21245-21246

21245   Reconstruction of mandible or maxilla, subperiosteal implant; partial
21246   Reconstruction of mandible or maxilla, subperiosteal implant; complete

The physician creates an incision over the area of the jaw without teeth. The bone is exposes as much as possible and a custom made implant is inserted. This procedure may span two surgical sessions if the physician creates the implant from molds formed during a prior encounter. Another technique utilizes CT scans of the jaw to form custom implants, and this method only requires one surgical session. The implant is metal and has posts used for dental fixation. The dissected tissue is arranged and sutured around the posts. The metal plate is positioned by the bone. The implant is fixated by the healing and scarring

process. All incisions are closed. Code 21245 for a partial reconstruction and code 21246 for a complete reconstruction.

21247

21247   Reconstruction of mandibular condyle with bone and cartilage autografts (includes obtaining grafts) (eg, for hemifacial microsomia)

The physician uses bone and cartilage grafts to reconstruct the mandibular condyle. The physician obtains bone and cartilage, usually from the ribs, for use in the reconstruction. An incision is made near or in the ear to reach the temporomandibular joint. The joint is isolated and exposed. The bone and cartilage graft is inserted into the recipient bed, with the cartilaginous end replacing the condyle. The graft is fixated with screws, wires, and metal plates. All incisions are closed.

21248-21249

21248   Reconstruction of mandible or maxilla, endosteal implant (eg, blade, cylinder); partial
21249   Reconstruction of mandible or maxilla, endosteal implant (eg, blade, cylinder); complete

The physician reconstructs the mandible or maxilla with an endosteal implant (e.g., blade or cylinder). Code 21248 for a partial reconstruction and 21249 for a complete reconstruction. The physician creates an incision over the area of the jaw without teeth. The bone is exposed as much as possible and an implant is inserted into pre-drilled precision holes. The tissue is arranged and sutured around the post with a blade style implant. With cylindrical implants, the tissue is sutured closed on top of the posts. A later surgery is necessary to attach the dental prosthesis. All incisions are closed.

21255

21255   Reconstruction of zygomatic arch and glenoid fossa with bone and cartilage (includes obtaining autografts)

The physician obtains a bone and cartilage graft from the patient's hip, rib, or skull (usually from the rib). An incision is created near the ear and the zygomatic arch and glenoid fossa are exposed through tissue resection. The graft is inserted into the recipient bed and wires, plates, and/or screws are used to hold the graft in place. All incisions are closed.

21256

21256   Reconstruction of orbit with osteotomies (extracranial) and with bone grafts (includes obtaining autografts) (eg, micro-ophthalmia)

Grafts are taken from the hip, rib, or skull of the patient. The physician can access the orbits through several different incision points, such as through the lower eyelid, eyebrow, or maxillary vestibule, etc. Once the orbit has been accessed, the physician uses drills and saws to create incisions into the orbital rims. The bone is repositioned and secured with wires, screws, and plates. The grafts are placed into the recipient beds. All incisions are closed.

21260

21260   Periorbital osteotomies for orbital hypertelorism, with bone grafts; extracranial approach

Grafts are taken from the hip, rib, or skull of the patient. The physician can access the orbits and nasoorbital region through several different incision points, such as through the lower eyelid, eyebrow, or maxillary vestibule, etc. Once the orbit has been accessed, the physician uses drills and saws to create incisions into the orbital rims. Portions of the nasal and ethmoidal bones are removed. The orbits are repositioned and secured with wires, screws, and plates. The grafts are placed into the recipient beds to fill the defects caused by the orbital repositioning. All incisions are closed.

21261

21261   Periorbital osteotomies for orbital hypertelorism, with bone grafts; combined intra- and extracranial approach

A portion of the frontal bone is temporarily removed, so that intracranial cuts may be made. The brain is retracted during this portion of the procedure. Grafts are taken from the hip, rib, or skull of the patient. The physician can access the orbits and nasoorbital region through several different incision points, such as through the lower eyelid, eyebrow, or maxillary vestibule, etc. Once the orbits have been accessed, the physician uses drills and saws to create incisions into the orbital rims. Portions of the nasal and ethmoidal bones are removed. The orbits are repositioned and secured with wires, screws, and plates. The grafts are placed into the recipient beds to fill the defects caused by the orbital repositioning. The frontal bone is reattached with plates or screws, and the brain returns to its previous position. All incisions are closed.

● New Code   ▲ Revised Code

21263

21263   **Periorbital osteotomies for orbital hypertelorism, with bone grafts; with forehead advancement**

The physician repositions the orbits closer together and moves the forehead forward to improve the contours of the face. A portion of the frontal bone is temporarily removed, so that intracranial cuts may be made. The brain is retracted during this portion of the procedure. Grafts are taken from the hip, rib, or skull of the patient. The physician can access the orbits and nasoorbital region through several different incision points, such as through the lower eyelid, eyebrow, or maxillary vestibule, etc. Once the orbits have been accessed, the physician uses drills and saws to create incisions into the orbital rims. Portions of the nasal and ethmoidal bones are removed. The orbits are repositioned and secured with wires, screws, and plates. The grafts are placed into the recipient beds to fill the defects caused by the orbital repositioning. The frontal bone is reattached in a more forward position, and held in place with plates or screws. The brain returns to its previous position. All incisions are closed.

21267

21267   **Orbital repositioning, periorbital osteotomies, unilateral, with bone grafts; extracranial approach**

The physician repositions one orbit via periorbital osteotomies and bone grafts through an extracranial approach. Grafts are taken from the hip, rib, or skull of the patient. The physician can access the orbit through several different incision points, such as through the lower eyelid, eyebrow, or maxillary vestibule, etc. Once the orbit has been accessed, the physician uses drills and saws to create incisions into the orbital rim. The orbit is repositioned and secured with wires, screws, and plates. Grafts are placed into recipient beds to fill the defects caused by the orbital repositioning. All incisions are closed.

21268

21268   **Orbital repositioning, periorbital osteotomies, unilateral, with bone grafts; combined intra- and extracranial approach**

The physician repositions one orbit via periorbital osteotomies and bone grafts through a combined intra- and extracranial approach. A portion of the frontal bone is temporarily removed, so that intracranial cuts may be made. The brain is retracted during this portion of the procedure. Grafts are taken from the hip, rib, or skull of the patient. The physician can access the orbit through several different incision points, such as through the lower eyelid, eyebrow, or maxillary vestibule, etc. Once the orbit has been accessed, the physician uses drills and saws to create incisions into the orbital rim. The orbit is repositioned and secured with wires, screws, and plates. Grafts are placed into the recipient beds to fill the defects caused by the orbital repositioning. The frontal bone is reattached with plates or screws, and the brain returns to its previous position. All incisions are closed.

21270

21270   **Malar augmentation, prosthetic material**

The physician augments the cheek (malar region) with prosthetic material. The physician creates incisions though the lower eyelids and maxillary buccal vestibule. The malar defect is identified and the prosthetic is implanted to improve the contours of the cheek. It is held in place with wires, plates, or screws. All incisions are closed.

21275

21275   **Secondary revision of orbitocraniofacial reconstruction**

The physician performs a second, follow-up, surgery for the reconstruction of the orbits and face. The physician gains access to affected bones via any type of incision, such as through the lower eyelid, eyebrow, or maxillary vestibule, etc. Grafts may be taken from the hip, rib, or skull of the patient. The physician uses drills and saws to create incisions into the orbitocraniofacial bones. The bones are again positioned in the desired location and secured with wires, plates, and/or screws. If grafts are required, they are placed into the recipient beds to fill the defects caused by the repositioning. All incisions are closed.

21280

21280   **Medial canthopexy (separate procedure)**

The physician reattaches the medial canthal tendon to the corresponding nasal bone. The canthal tendon is isolated via an incision. A steel suture is secured through the tendon and a hole is created in the opposite nasal bone. The suture is passed through the hole and attached to the bone. All incisions are closed.

21282

21282   **Lateral canthopexy**

The physician reattaches the lateral canthal tendon to the zygoma (cheek) bone. The canthal tendon is isolated via an incision. A steel suture is secured through the tendon, and a hole is created in the cheek bone. The suture is passed through the hole and attached to the bone. All incisions are closed.

21295-21296

21295   **Reduction of masseter muscle and bone (eg, for treatment of benign masseteric hypertrophy); extraoral approach**

21296   **Reduction of masseter muscle and bone (eg, for treatment of benign masseteric hypertrophy); intraoral approach**

Benign hypertrophy of the masseter muscle and underlying bone is a rare disorder of unknown cause characterized by bulging of the muscle at the mandibular angle. In 21295, an extraoral preauricular approach is used. In 21296, an intraoral incision is made along the anterior edge of the mandibular ramus. Subperiosteal dissection is performed followed by detachment of the masseter muscle at the inferior posterior border of the mandible. A bur is used to reduce the bony prominence at the mandibular angle. Alternatively a saw may be used to reduce the posterior border of the mandible and create a more obtuse angle. Additional bone contouring is performed as needed using a bur, chisel or osteotome. Once the desired bone contour has been achieved, the masseter muscle is then resected and reduced in size. The muscle is reattached to the mandible and incisions are closed.

21310-21320

21310   **Closed treatment of nasal bone fracture without manipulation**

21315   **Closed treatment of nasal bone fracture; without stabilization**

21320   **Closed treatment of nasal bone fracture; with stabilization**

The two nasal bones project from the frontal processes of the maxilla and the nasal process of the frontal bone and join at the midline. Separately reportable radiographs of the nasal bones are obtained to determine the severity of the injury. In 21310, the nasal fracture is determined to be nondisplaced and no manipulation of the fracture fragments is required. Any nasal bleeding is controlled with internal packing. In 21315, a minimally displaced nasal fracture is reduced. Depressed fragments are reduced using an elevator inserted into the nose. Outward pressure is applied with the elevator while using the thumb to apply counterpressure on the exterior of the nose. Alternatively, forceps may be used to grasp the displaced bone and move it into correct anatomical alignment. Following reduction of the nasal bones, the septum is evaluated to ensure that it is in alignment. Separately reportable radiographs are obtained to confirm anatomic reduction. Internal packing is applied to control bleeding. In 21320, the nasal fracture is reduced as described in 21315 and then stabilized using internal packing and an external splint.

21325

21325   **Open treatment of nasal fracture; uncomplicated**

The physician creates an incision along the nasal septum, in order to visualize the fractured bone(s). Forceps and nasal elevators are used to reposition the bones. Portions of bone may be excised to aid in repositioning. All incisions are closed. Splints are used to stabilize the area.

21330

21330   **Open treatment of nasal fracture; complicated, with internal and/or external skeletal fixation**

The physician treats a nasal fracture in an open environment. The physician creates an incision along the nasal septum, in order to visualize the fractured bone(s). Additional incisions may also be necessary. Forceps and nasal elevators are used to reposition the bones. Portions of bone may be excised to aid in repositioning. The physician utilizes screws, plates, and wires to internally stabilize the fracture. All incisions are closed. Splints may also be used for further fixation.

21335

21335   **Open treatment of nasal fracture; with concomitant open treatment of fractured septum**

The physician treats concomitant nasal and septal fractures in an open environment. The physician creates an incision along the nasal septum, in order to visualize the fractured bones and cartilage. Additional incisions may also be necessary. Forceps and nasal elevators are used to reposition the bones. Portions of bone and cartilage may be excised to aid in repositioning. The physician utilizes transseptal sutures, screws, plates, and wires to internally stabilize the fracture. All incisions are closed. External splints may be necessary to further stabilize the fracture.

21336

21336   **Open treatment of nasal septal fracture, with or without stabilization**

The physician treats a septal fracture in an open environment. The physician creates an incision along the nasal septum, in order to visualize the fractured bone(s). Forceps and nasal elevators are used to reposition the bones. Portions of bone and cartilage may be excised to aid in repositioning. Splints may be used to stabilize the area. All incisions are closed.

Musculoskeletal System

21337

21337   Closed treatment of nasal septal fracture, with or without stabilization

The physician treats a septal fracture in a closed environment. The physician uses forceps or nasal elevators to realign the septal fracture. Septal sutures are used to reduce hematoma formation and splints may also be necessary.

21338-21339

21338   Open treatment of nasoethmoid fracture; without external fixation
21339   Open treatment of nasoethmoid fracture; with external fixation

The physician may use various incisions in order to visualize the fractured bones. The physician uses rigid reduction to stabilize the bones in the correct position. Wires, plates, or screws may be used to accomplish stabilization. Portions of bone may be excised to aid in repositioning. If the medial canthal ligaments are detached, they are reattached in a separately reportable service. All incisions are closed. Code 21338 if no external fixation is necessary. Code 21339 if external fixation is used.

21340

21340   Percutaneous treatment of nasoethmoid complex fracture, with splint, wire or headcap fixation, including repair of canthal ligaments and/or the nasolacrimal apparatus

The physician repairs a nasoethmoid fracture via a percutaneous approach. The physician uses percutaneous pins or screws attached to stable bone and external fixation devices to create stabilized fracture reduction. If the medial canthal ligaments are detached, they are reattached. The nasolacrimal apparatus is repaired using sutures and tubing. All incisions are closed.

21343

21343   Open treatment of depressed frontal sinus fracture

The physician gains access to the fracture through either a bicoronal incision, or incisions directly over the fracture. The physician may remove sinus mucosa and then stabilize the fracture with wires, plates, or screws. All incisions are closed.

21344

21344   Open treatment of complicated (eg, comminuted or involving posterior wall) frontal sinus fracture, via coronal or multiple approaches

The physician repairs a complicated (e.g., comminuted or involving the posterior wall) frontal sinus fracture in an open environment. Any approach method may be used to gain access to the fracture site. The physician removes the sinus mucosa and usually ablates the sinus in order to prevent postoperative infection. If the fracture extends to the posterior wall, the bony wall may be removed, and the nasofrontal duct plugged. Stabilization of the fracture is achieved via screws, plates, and wires. All incisions are closed.

21345

21345   Closed treatment of nasomaxillary complex fracture (LeFort II type), with interdental wire fixation or fixation of denture or splint

The physician repairs a nasomaxillary complex fracture (LeFort II) in a closed environment. This type of fracture is commonly referred to as a pyramidal fracture. Interdental fixation, such as wires, dentures, or splints, is utilized in stabilization of the fracture.

21346

21346   Open treatment of nasomaxillary complex fracture (LeFort II type); with wiring and/or local fixation

The physician repairs a nasomaxillary complex fracture (LeFort II) in an open environment. This type of fracture is commonly referred to as a pyramidal fracture. The physician accesses the fracture via an incision through the cheek. The fractured area is realigned via manipulation. The physician utilizes screws, wires, and/or plates to stabilize the fracture site. All incisions are closed. Intermaxillary fixation may be necessary.

21347

21347   Open treatment of nasomaxillary complex fracture (LeFort II type); requiring multiple open approaches

The physician repairs a nasomaxillary complex fracture (LeFort II) in an open environment. This type of fracture is commonly referred to as a pyramidal fracture. The physician accesses the fracture via multiple incisions. The fractured area is realigned via manipulation. The physician utilizes screws, wires, and/or plates to stabilize the fracture site. All incisions are closed. Intermaxillary fixation may be necessary.

21348

21348   Open treatment of nasomaxillary complex fracture (LeFort II type); with bone grafting (includes obtaining graft)

The physician repairs a nasomaxillary complex fracture (LeFort II) in an open environment. This type of fracture is commonly referred to as a pyramidal fracture. The physician

accesses the fracture via multiple incisions. The physician obtains a bone graft from the patient's hip, rib, or skull. The fractured area is realigned via manipulation, and bone grafts are placed in the defect areas. The physician utilizes screws, wires, and/or plates to stabilize the fracture site. All incisions are closed. Intermaxillary fixation may be necessary.

21355

21355   Percutaneous treatment of fracture of malar area, including zygomatic arch and malar tripod, with manipulation

The physician repairs a fracture of the malar area, including the zygomatic arch and malar tripod, with percutaneous manipulation. The physician makes a stab wound into the cheek and uses a rod or bone hook to move the fractured bone back into place. The instrument is retracted and the incision is closed.

21356

21356   Open treatment of depressed zygomatic arch fracture (eg, Gillies approach)

The physician treats a depressed fracture of the zygomatic arch in an open environment. The Gilles (also Gillies) approach is the most common method, and is a technique for reducing fractures of the zygoma and the zygomatic arch through an incision in the temporal region above the hairline. Regardless of the approach, an instrument is inserted under the muscle fascia and manipulates the fracture into the proper anatomical position. The instrument is removed and all incisions are closed.

21360

21360   Open treatment of depressed malar fracture, including zygomatic arch and malar tripod

The physician treats a depressed malar fracture, including the zygomatic arch and malar tripod, in an open environment. No internal fixation is utilized during this procedure. The physician creates incisions around the face at various locations, including an intraoral incision through the maxillary buccal vestibule. The fracture is reduced to its correct anatomical placement via the use of Carroll-Girard screw or other instrument which lifts the fractured bones into position. Manual reduction is used on the malar complex. All incisions are closed.

21365

21365   Open treatment of complicated (eg, comminuted or involving cranial nerve foramina) fracture(s) of malar area, including zygomatic arch and malar tripod; with internal fixation and multiple surgical approaches

The physician repairs a complicated fracture of the malar area in an open environment. Multiple surgical approaches are used to gain access to the fracture site(s). The fracture is reduced to its correct anatomical placement via the use of Carroll-Girard screw or other instrument which lifts the fractured bones into position. The fracture is stabilized with internal fixation, including screws, wires, and/or plates. Manual reduction is used on the malar complex. All incisions are closed.

21366

21366   Open treatment of complicated (eg, comminuted or involving cranial nerve foramina) fracture(s) of malar area, including zygomatic arch and malar tripod; with bone grafting (includes obtaining graft)

The physician repairs a complicated fracture of the malar area in an open environment. Multiple surgical approaches are used to gain access to the fracture site(s), including a transoral incision through the maxillary buccal vestibule. The fracture is reduced to its correct anatomical placement via the use of Carroll-Girard screw or other instrument which lifts the fractured bones into position. Through another incision, the physician obtains a bone graft from the patient's hip, rib, or skull. Bone grafts are placed in the defect areas. The physician utilizes screws, wires, and/or plates to stabilize the fracture site. All incisions are closed.

21385

21385   Open treatment of orbital floor blowout fracture; transantral approach (Caldwell-Luc type operation)

Open repair of an orbital floor blowout fracture using a transantral approach (Caldwell-Luc procedure) is performed to restore anatomic and functional defects of the globe. Orbital fractures are a common injury sustained with mid-facial trauma and may include extraocular muscle entrapment with impairment of eye movement in addition to aesthetic facial deformity. The upper lip is retracted to expose the gingivobuccal sulcus and a horizontal incision is made superior to the sulcus creating a wide mucosal band. Using a periosteal elevator, the periosteum and overlying soft tissue are elevated from the underlying maxillary bone to the infraorbital foramen. The maxillary sinus is entered via an antral window (Caldwell-Luc antrostomy) and the bone fragment is preserved. The maxillary sinus is visualized and the herniated orbital contents are removed or repositioned back into the orbit. The fracture is reduced and an implant may be inserted if a bony deficit is present. The sinus cavity is checked for hemostasis, the antral wall bone fragment is replaced, and the incision is closed with sutures.

21386

21386   Open treatment of orbital floor blowout fracture; periorbital approach

Open repair of an orbital floor blowout fracture using a periorbital approach is performed to restore anatomic and functional defects of the globe. Orbital fractures are a common injury sustained with mid-facial trauma and may include extraocular muscle entrapment with impairment of eye movement in addition to aesthetic facial deformity. The conjunctiva is incised across the length of the lower eyelid just below the base of the tarsus. Traction sutures are placed and the conjunctiva is pulled superiorly to cover the cornea. The plane between the orbital septum and orbicularis muscle is bluntly dissected to the orbital rim. The periosteum is opened and elevated off the orbital floor. The herniated orbital tissue is removed or repositioned back into the orbit and the fracture is reduced. The surgical area is checked for hemostasis, the traction sutures are cut, the conjunctiva is repositioned, and the incision is closed with sutures.

21387

21387   Open treatment of orbital floor blowout fracture; combined approach

Open repair of an orbital floor blowout fracture using a combined (transconjunctival with lateral canthotomy) approach is performed to restore anatomic and functional defects of the globe. Orbital fractures are a common injury sustained with mid-facial trauma and may include extraocular muscle entrapment with impairment of eye movement in addition to aesthetic facial deformity. Traction sutures are placed in the lower eyelid. A pointed scissor inserted horizontally at the outer lid angle is used to make an incision along the palpebral fissure through the skin, orbicularis oculi muscle, and conjuctiva. The lateral canthal tendon fibers that fan superficially are then transected and the lower lid is everted using the previously placed traction sutures. The lateral canthal tendon is transected using scissors to entirely free the lower eyelid. The conjunctiva is then incised across the length of the lower eyelid just below the base of the tarsus. Traction sutures are placed, and the conjunctiva is pulled superiorly to cover the cornea. The plane between the orbital septum and orbicularis muscle is bluntly dissected to the orbital rim. The periosteum is opened and elevated off the orbital floor. The herniated orbital tissue is removed or repositioned back into the orbit and the fracture is reduced. The surgical area is checked for hemostasis. Sutures are placed into the transected edges of the inferior and superior lateral canthal tendon and provisionally tightened. The traction sutures positioning the conjunctiva superiorly are cut and the conjunctiva is repositioned. The ends of lateral canthal tendon sutures are brought out of the conjunctival incision and that incision is then closed with sutures. The canthal suture is tightened bringing the lower eyelid back to its original position. The lateral canthotomy subcutaneous tissue is closed with sutures followed by closure of the skin incision.

21390

21390   Open treatment of orbital floor blowout fracture; periorbital approach, with alloplastic or other implant

Open repair of an orbital floor blowout fracture using a periorbital approach and alloplastic or other implant is performed to restore anatomic and functional defects of the globe. Orbital fractures are a common injury sustained with mid-facial trauma and may include extraocular muscle entrapment with impairment of eye movement in addition to aesthetic facial deformity. The conjunctiva is incised across the length of the lower eyelid just below the base of the tarsus. Traction sutures are placed and the conjunctiva is pulled superiorly to cover the cornea. The plane between the orbital septum and orbicularis muscle is bluntly dissected to the orbital rim. The periosteum is opened and elevated off the orbital floor. The herniated orbital tissue is removed or repositioned back into the orbit. The fracture is reduced and an orbital implant comprised of porous polyethylene, silicone, Teflon, Supramid, titanium mesh, bioresorbable copolymer plates, or vicryl mesh is inserted to fill the bony deficit. The surgical area is checked for hemostasis, the traction sutures are cut, the conjunctiva is repositioned, and the incision is closed with sutures.

21395

21395   Open treatment of orbital floor blowout fracture; periorbital approach with bone graft (includes obtaining graft)

Open repair of an orbital floor blowout fracture using a periorbital approach with a bone graft is performed to restore anatomic and functional defects of the globe. Orbital fractures are a common injury sustained with mid-facial trauma and may include extraocular muscle entrapment with impairment of eye movement in addition to aesthetic facial deformity. The conjunctiva is incised across the length of the lower eyelid just below the base of the tarsus. Traction sutures are placed and the conjunctiva is pulled superiorly to cover the cornea. The plane between the orbital septum and orbicularis muscle is bluntly dissected to the orbital rim. The periosteum is opened and elevated off the orbital floor. The herniated orbital tissue is removed or repositioned back into the orbit. The fracture is reduced and an autogenous bone graft harvested from the maxillary wall, calvaria, iliac crest, rib, or fibula and shaped to match the contour of the bony deficit is inserted into the orbital space. The surgical area is checked for hemostasis, the traction sutures are cut, the conjunctiva is repositioned, and the incision is closed with sutures.

21400-21401

21400   Closed treatment of fracture of orbit, except blowout; without manipulation
21401   Closed treatment of fracture of orbit, except blowout; with manipulation

Closed treatment of a fracture of the orbit other than an orbital floor (blowout) fracture is performed Separately reportable radiographs are obtained to confirm the fracture. In 21400, a nondisplaced fracture of the orbit is evaluated. A neurovascular exam is performed to ensure that nerves and blood vessels at the site of injury are intact. No manipulation of fracture fragments is required. In 21401, a minimally displaced fracture of the orbit is evaluated. The displaced fracture fragments are manually reduced (manipulated) or a hook/screw is used to manipulate the fragments back to correct anatomic alignment. Separately reportable radiographs are obtained to confirm anatomic reduction.

21406

21406   Open treatment of fracture of orbit, except blowout; without implant

Open repair of a non-blowout orbital fracture, without implant is performed to restore the orbit to its natural shape. The natural skin creases are evaluated and incision lines are marked. A temporary tarsorrhaphy may be performed to protect the cornea by placing a mattress suture through the edges of the upper and lower eyelids to close the lids over the eye. The ends of the suture are grasped with a clamp and traction is applied upwards. The skin is incised along the marked lines to visualize the underlying orbicular muscle. The incision is extended subcutaneously over the pretarsal portion of the orbicularis oculi muscle to create a skin flap the full length of the incision. A dissection plane between the orbicularis oculi muscle and the septum orbitale is then created and suborbicular undermining of the muscle is performed using a slit-like lateral incision over the bony orbital rim. The suborbicular dissection plane is opened, leaving the orbital septum intact. The suborbicular pocket is extended downward over the whole lower palpebral region and the upper portion of the pocket below the tarsus is then opened. The remaining layer of the orbicularis oculi muscle is separated just below the lower border of the tarsus to create a skin muscle flap congruent with the lower eyelid. The eyelid and flap is retracted inferiorly over the anterior edge of the infraorbital rim and a periosteal elevator is employed to strip the periosteum from the bone. The intraorbital nerve is identified and preserved before continuing dissection along the upper facial surface of the anterior maxilla. The borders of the fracture are identified and orbital soft tissue that has herniated through any bony deficit is reduced. The fracture may be repaired with hardware, if indicated. The periosteum is then redraped over the bony surface and secured.

21407

21407   Open treatment of fracture of orbit, except blowout; with implant

Open repair of a non-blowout orbital fracture, with implant is performed to restore the orbit to its natural shape. The natural skin creases are evaluated and incision lines are marked. A temporary tarsorrhaphy may be performed to protect the cornea by placing a mattress suture through the edges of the upper and lower eyelids to close the lids over the eye. The ends of the suture are grasped with a clamp and traction is applied upwards. The skin is incised along the marked lines to visualize the underlying orbicular muscle. The incision is extended subcutaneously over the pretarsal portion of the orbicularis oculi muscle to create a skin flap the full length of the incision. A dissection plane between the orbicularis oculi muscle and the septum orbitale is then created and suborbicular undermining of the muscle is performed using a slit-like lateral incision over the bony orbital rim. The suborbicular dissection plane is opened, leaving the orbital septum intact. The suborbicular pocket is extended downward over the whole lower palpebral region and the upper portion of the pocket below the tarsus is then opened. The remaining layer of the orbicularis oculi muscle is separated just below the lower border of the tarsus to create a skin muscle flap congruent with the lower eyelid. The eyelid and flap is retracted inferiorly over the anterior edge of the infraorbital rim and a periosteal elevator is employed to strip the periosteum from the bone. The intraorbital nerve is identified and preserved before continuing dissection along the upper facial surface of the anterior maxilla. The borders of the fracture are identified and orbital soft tissue that has herniated through any bony deficit is reduced. The fracture is reduced and an orbital implant (porous polyethylene, silicone, Teflon, Supramid, titanium mesh, bioresorbable copolymer plates) is inserted into the remaining bony deficit to prevent orbital soft tissue from prolapsing and restore the natural contour and volume of the orbit. The periosteum is then redraped over the implant and bony surface and secured with sutures.

21408

21408   Open treatment of fracture of orbit, except blowout; with bone grafting (includes obtaining graft)

Open repair of a non-blowout orbital fracture, with bone grafting is performed to restore the orbit to its natural shape. The natural skin creases are evaluated and incision lines are marked. A temporary tarsorrhaphy may be performed to protect the cornea by placing a mattress suture through the edges of the upper and lower eyelids to close the lids over the eye. The ends of the suture are grasped with a clamp and traction is applied upwards. The skin is incised along the marked lines to visualize the underlying orbicular muscle.

Musculoskeletal System

The incision is extended subcutaneously over the pretarsal portion of the orbicularis oculi muscle to create a skin flap the full length of the incision. A dissection plane between the orbicularis oculi muscle and the septum orbitale is then created and suborbicular undermining of the muscle is performed using a slit-like lateral incision over the bony orbital rim. The suborbicular dissection plane is opened, leaving the orbital septum intact. The suborbicular pocket is extended downward over the whole lower palpebral region and the upper portion of the pocket below the tarsus is then opened. The remaining layer of the orbicularis oculi muscle is separated just below the lower border of the tarsus to create a skin muscle flap congruent with the lower eyelid. The eyelid and flap is retracted inferiorly over the anterior edge of the infraorbital rim and a periosteal elevator is employed to strip the periosteum from the bone. The intraorbital nerve is identified and preserved before continuing dissection along the upper facial surface of the anterior maxilla. The borders of the fracture are identified and orbital soft tissue that has herniated through any bony deficit is reduced. The fracture is reduced and an autogenous bone graft harvested from the maxillary wall, calvaria, iliac crest, rib, or fibula and shaped to match the contour of the bony deficit is then inserted to prevent orbital soft tissue from prolapsing and restore the natural contour and volume of the orbit. The periosteum is then redraped over the grafted bony surface and secured with sutures.

21421

21421   Closed treatment of palatal or maxillary fracture (LeFort I type), with interdental wire fixation or fixation of denture or splint

The physician does not create any incisions for this procedure, instead, arches are secured in the patient's mouth with interdental wire. Alternately, dentures or splints may be used to stabilize the maxillary fracture.

21422

21422   Open treatment of palatal or maxillary fracture (LeFort I type)

The physician creates incisions in the maxillary buccal vestibule from within the oral cavity. The maxillary fracture is exposed and the physician repositions the bone segments and stabilizes the area with screws, plates, or pins. The incisions are closed. Intermaxillary or interdental fixation may be used to further stabilize the fracture.

21423

21423   Open treatment of palatal or maxillary fracture (LeFort I type); complicated (comminuted or involving cranial nerve foramina), multiple approaches

This fracture is comminuted or involve the cranial nerve foramina. The physician utilizes both intraoral and lower eyelid approaches in order to visualize the fracture. The maxilla is repositioned and stabilized with screws, plates, or wires. Repositioning of the infraorbital nerve may be performed, which may necessitate bone grafting for support of the nerve. All incisions are closed. The physician may use a customized palatal splint or intermaxillary device for stabilization.

21431-21432

21431   Closed treatment of craniofacial separation (LeFort III type) using interdental wire fixation of denture or splint
21432   Open treatment of craniofacial separation (LeFort III type); with wiring and/or internal fixation

A Le Fort III fracture, also called a craniofacial separation or dysjunction, is a transverse fracture of the midface that starts at the nasofrontal and frontomaxillary sutures and extends posteriorly along the medial wall of the orbit through the nasolacrimal groove and ethmoid bones. The fracture continues along the floor of the orbit at the inferior orbital fissure and then through the lateral orbital wall, zygomaticofrontal junction and zygomatic arch. A branch of the fracture also extends through the base of the perpendicular plate of the ethmoid and vomer and the interface of the pterygoid plates to the base of the sphenoid. In 21431, a closed reduction is performed. Disimpaction of the maxillary bone is accomplished using disimpaction forceps or other intruments inserted intranasally or intraorally. Anatomic reduction is verified radiographically and the fracture is then stabilized using arch bars placed on the upper and lower molars and interdental wire fixation. In 21432, an open reduction with wiring and/or internal fixation is performed. An incision is made intraorally in the buccal sulcus. Alternatively subciliary or transconjunctival incisions may be used. The fracture is reduced and anatomic reduction verified radiographically. The fracture is stabilized using miniplates and monocortical self-tapping screws. For a simple Lefort III fracture bilateral zygomaticofrontal fixation is usually sufficient.

21433-21436

21433   Open treatment of craniofacial separation (LeFort III type); complicated (eg, comminuted or involving cranial nerve foramina), multiple surgical approaches
21435   Open treatment of craniofacial separation (LeFort III type); complicated, utilizing internal and/or external fixation techniques (eg, head cap, halo device, and/or intermaxillary fixation)
21436   Open treatment of craniofacial separation (LeFort III type); complicated, multiple surgical approaches, internal fixation, with bone grafting (includes obtaining graft)

A Le Fort III fracture, also called a craniofacial separation or dysjunction, is a transverse fracture of the midface that starts at the nasofrontal and frontomaxillary sutures and extends posteriorly along the medial wall of the orbit through the nasolacrimal groove and ethmoid bones. The fracture continues along the floor of the orbit at the inferior orbital fissure and then through the lateral orbital wall, zygomaticofrontal junction and zygomatic arch. A branch of the fracture also extends through the base of the perpendicular plate of the ethmoid and vomer and the interface of the pterygoid plates to the base of the sphenoid. In 21433, open reduction of a complicated Lefort III fracture requiring multiple surgical approaches is performed. Complicated fractures are defined as those that are comminuted or involve the cranial nerve foramina. Exposure may be by sublabial incision to expose the maxilla, subciliary or transconjunctival incisions to expose the orbital rim, or by columellar-septal transfixion incisions to expose the piriform aperture and frontmaxillary region. If more exposure is required incisions may be made in the lateral brow glabellar fold or a bicoronal scalp flap may be used to expose the fracture. The fracture is reduced and anatomic reduction verified radiographically. The fracture is stabilized using interdental fixation. In 21435, a complicated fracture is disimpacted and reduced via multiple approaches. Miniplates and screws and/or interosseous wiring are used to stabilize the fracture fragments. External fixation may be used instead of or in addition to internal fixation when there are extensive panfacial fractures. Common types of external fixation include head cap, halo, and intermaxillary fixation. In 21436, a complicated fracture is treated as described in 21435 but bone grafts are also used to stabilize the bone fragments. A bone autograft is harvested, usually from the iliac crest. A skin incision is made over the iliac crest and the muscle is stripped to reveal the bone surface. Cortical and/or cancellous bone is harvested. The bone is configured to the desired size and shape and/or cancellous bone is morcelized and packed into the fracture. Internal fixation is used to stabilize the fracture fragments and bone grafts.

21440

21440   Closed treatment of mandibular or maxillary alveolar ridge fracture (separate procedure)

The physician uses manipulation to reduce the fracture and stabilizes the area using arch bars and dental wire. Alternate stabilization methods include dental bonding, intermaxillary fixation, and creating a custom acrylic splint.

21445

21445   Open treatment of mandibular or maxillary alveolar ridge fracture (separate procedure)

The physician creates incisions in the maxillary buccal vestibule from within the oral cavity. The physician uses manipulation to reduce the fracture and stabilizes the area using plates, screws, and wires. The use of arch bars and dental wire may also be necessary. Alternate stabilization methods include intermaxillary fixation and creating a custom acrylic splint. All incisions are closed.

21450-21451

21450   Closed treatment of mandibular fracture; without manipulation
21451   Closed treatment of mandibular fracture; with manipulation

Separately reportable radiographs are obtained to confirm the fracture of the mandible. In 21450, a nondisplaced mandible fracture is evaluated. No manipulation of fracture fragments is required. No fixation of the fragments is required. In 21451, a minimally displaced fracture is treated. Local anesthesia is administered as needed. The fracture fragments are manually reduced. No fixation of the fragments is required.

21452

21452   Percutaneous treatment of mandibular fracture, with external fixation

Separately reportable radiographs are obtained to confirm the fracture of the mandible. The displaced fracture fragments are manipulated into alignment through a small incision using Kirschner wires placed in the mandible under fluoroscopic visualization. The Kirschner wires are used as "joysticks" to manipulate the bone segments. Once the bone segments are aligned, external fixation is used to stabilize the mandible.

21453

21453   Closed treatment of mandibular fracture with interdental fixation

The physician treats a mandibular fracture with interdental fixation, which does not require any incisions. The physician uses wire and arch bars to stabilize the jaw. For patients who do not have teeth, the physician may create dentures or acrylic splints and attach them to the jaw first, before inserting the arch bars and wires.

21454

21454   Open treatment of mandibular fracture with external fixation

The physician creates an incision either in the oral cavity, or in the skin directly above the fracture. The fracture is isolated, visualized, and manipulated into the correct position. After the mandibular fracture is reduced, the physician drills holes into the mandible through incisions. Rods or pins are placed into the holes. They protrude through the skin and are stabilized by a traction bar. The main incision is closed.

21461-21462

21461   Open treatment of mandibular fracture; without interdental fixation
21462   Open treatment of mandibular fracture; with interdental fixation

The physician creates an incision either directly above the fracture point or intraorally through the mucosa. The fracture is isolated, visualized, and reduced. Plates, wires, and/or screws are used to hold the mandible in the correct position. Code 21461 if intermaxillary fixation is not used. Code 21462 if intermaxillary fixation is necessary, resulting in the jaws being wired together.

21465

21465   Open treatment of mandibular condylar fracture

The physician creates an incision near or through the ear to access the fracture. Occasionally an incision will be made intraorally to access the site. The soft tissue is dissected and the temporomandibular joint and its fractured condyle are exposed. The physician then reduces the fracture and returns the condyle to its appropriate position, securing it with screws, wires, and/or plates. It may also be stable enough not to need internal fixation. All incisions are closed. The physician may choose to use intermaxillary fixation if necessary.

21470

21470   Open treatment of complicated mandibular fracture by multiple surgical approaches including internal fixation, interdental fixation, and/or wiring of dentures or splints

The physician accesses the fracture of the mandible through various incisions in the skin and/or mucosa. The physician reduces the fracture and secures the bones with screws, wires, and/or plates. Interdental fixation is used to immobilize the area during healing. All incisions are closed. The physician may use wire and arch bars to stabilize the jaw. For patients who do not have teeth, the physician may create dentures or acrylic splints and attach them to the jaw first, before inserting the arch bars and wires.

21480-21485

21480   Closed treatment of temporomandibular dislocation; initial or subsequent
21485   Closed treatment of temporomandibular dislocation; complicated (eg, recurrent requiring intermaxillary fixation or splinting), initial or subsequent

The temporomandibular joints (TMJ), located on both sides of the jaw (mandible), are gliding joints formed by the condyles of the mandible and articular eminences of the temporal bone. The articular surfaces of the mandible and temporal bones are separated by an articular disc called the meniscus. Dislocation occurs when the condyle moves too far and gets stuck in front of the articular eminence of the temporal bone. If the surrounding muscles spasm the jaw may remain in a dislocated position with the jaw locked open. Local anesthetics and/or an intravenous muscle relaxant are administered as needed. In 21480, the dentist or physician then pulls the mandible down and tips the chin up to free the condyle. The mandible is then guided back into normal position. In 21485, the dentist or physician manipulates the mandible back into position as described above and then immobilizes the jaw using interdental wire fixation or a splint. Immobilization causes the ligaments to tighten and will help limit movement of the jaw when the immobilization device is removed. Wiring or splinting the jaw is usually reserved for recurrent dislocations. Use codes 21480 and 21485 for initial or subsequent closed treatment of TMJ dislocation.

21490

21490   Open treatment of temporomandibular dislocation

The physician creates an incision near or in the ear and exposes the joint. The condyle and joint are rearticulated using medical instruments. Any ligament damage is repaired and the incision is closed.

21497

21497   Interdental wiring, for condition other than fracture

The physician uses wire and arch bars to stabilize the jaw. For patients who do not have teeth, the physician may create dentures or acrylic splints and attach them to the jaw first, before inserting the arch bars and wires.

21501-21502

21501   Incision and drainage, deep abscess or hematoma, soft tissues of neck or thorax
21502   Incision and drainage, deep abscess or hematoma, soft tissues of neck or thorax; with partial rib ostectomy

The physician drains a deep abscess or hematoma of the soft tissues of the neck or thorax. In 21501, an incision is made in the skin of the neck or thorax over the abscess or hematoma site. The incision is carried down through the soft tissue and the abscess or hematoma is opened. If drainage is performed for an abscess, any loculations are broken up using blunt finger dissection. If drainage is for a hematoma, blood clots are removed by suction. The abscess or hematoma cavity is flushed with saline or antibiotic solution. Drains are placed as needed. The incision may be closed in layers or packed with gauze and left open. In 21502, a partial rib ostectomy is also performed when there is an abscess with involvement of the bone. The rib may also be excised even if there does not appear to be bony involvement when there is a fistulous tract over the rib or when the abscess is near the bone. The abscess is drained as described above. The rib is inspected for evidence of destruction or periosteal granulation tissue. Involved areas of the rib or are resected.

21510

21510   Incision, deep, with opening of bone cortex (eg, for osteomyelitis or bone abscess), thorax

The physician creates an incision into the bone cortex of a bone found in the thorax. This is commonly done to treat osteomyelitis or a bone abscess. The skin above the bone is dissected and the bone is exposed. Any external abscess is removed and holes are drilled into the bone. The area is drained and irrigated thoroughly with an antibiotic solution. Any damaged tissue is removed. The area is either closed with sutures, or packed and left open to continue draining. If left open, the gauze is changed daily and a second surgery closes the site.

21550

21550   Biopsy, soft tissue of neck or thorax

Soft tissue biopsy of the neck or thorax is performed. Soft tissues include muscles, tendons, fat, blood vessels, lymph vessels, nerves, and tissues surrounding the joints. Local, regional, or general anesthesia or conscious sedation is administered depending on the site and depth of the planned biopsy. The area over the planned biopsy site is cleansed. An incision is made and tissue dissected down to the mass or lesion taking care to protect blood vessels and nerves. A tissue sample is obtained and sent to the laboratory for separately reportable histological evaluation. The incision is closed with sutures.

21552-21556

21552   Excision, tumor, soft tissue of neck or anterior thorax, subcutaneous; 3 cm or greater
21554   Excision, tumor, soft tissue of neck or anterior thorax, subfascial (eg, intramuscular); 5 cm or greater
21555   Excision, tumor, soft tissue of neck or anterior thorax, subcutaneous; less than 3 cm
21556   Excision, tumor, soft tissue of neck or anterior thorax, subfascial (eg, intramuscular); less than 5 cm

Soft tissues include subcutaneous fat and connective tissue, fascia, muscles, tendons, blood vessels, lymph vessels, nerves, and tissues surrounding the joints. Soft tissue tumors may be benign or malignant. Benign tumors are typically treated by excision, although small malignant or indeterminate tumors, may be excised if the margins are well defined. Depending on the location of the tumor in the soft tissue of the neck or anterior thorax, the skin over the tumor may be incised, a skin flap created and elevated, or a series of incisions made along skin creases to allow exposure of the tumor. Overlying tissue is dissected and the soft tissue mass exposed. The tumor is then excised along with a margin of healthy tissue. Separately reportable frozen section may be performed to ensure that all margins are free of tumor cells. Drains are placed as needed and the surgical wound is closed in layers. For tumors in the subcutaneous fat or connective tissue, use 21555 for a mass less than 3 cm and 21552 for a mass 3 cm or greater. For tumors that lie below the fascia, use 21556 for a mass less than 5 cm and 21554 for a mass 5 cm or greater. Subfascial soft tissue tumors include those within muscle tissue.

Musculoskeletal System

21557-21558

21557 Radical resection of tumor (eg, sarcoma), soft tissue of neck or anterior thorax; less than 5 cm

21558 Radical resection of tumor (eg, sarcoma), soft tissue of neck or anterior thorax; 5 cm or greater

Radical resection is typically performed for a malignant neoplasm, such as a sarcoma, although benign tumors and tumors of indeterminate nature may also require radical resection. Depending on the location of the tumor in the neck or anterior thorax, the skin over the tumor may be incised, a skin flap created and elevated, or a series of incisions made along skin creases to allow exposure of the tumor. Soft tissue surrounding the tumor is dissected and the tumor is exposed. Radical resection involves removal of all involved soft tissue which may include muscles, nerves, and blood vessels. The tumor is resected along with a wide margin of surrounding healthy tissue. Separately reportable frozen section examination is performed to ensure that the margins are free of tumor cells. If margins show evidence of malignancy, additional tissue is removed until all margins are free of tumor cells. The physician then repairs muscle and soft tissues. A separately reportable reconstructive procedure may be performed using muscle, myocutaneous, fascial, or other grafts or flaps at the same or a subsequent surgical session. Drains are placed as needed and the overlying skin closed in layers. Use 21557 for radical resection of a tumor less than 5 cm; use 21558 for a tumor 5 cm or greater.

21600

21600 Excision of rib, partial

Under general anesthesia, the physician creates an incision down to the rib which is to be removed. The rib is isolated and a saw is used to remove a portion of the rib. The area is irrigated and closed with sutures.

21610

21610 Costotransversectomy (separate procedure)

The physician creates an incision above the costovertebral joint and resects tissue until the joint can be visualized. The transverse process is removed from the vertebral body along with a portion of the adjacent rib. All incisions are closed.

21615-21616

21615 Excision first and/or cervical rib

21616 Excision first and/or cervical rib; with sympathectomy

Under general anesthesia, the physician creates an incision over the clavicle and isolates the rib. Saws and other instruments are used to remove the rib from its articulation. The surgical site is irrigated and all incisions are closed (21615). Code 21616 if in addition to the rib removal, the sympathetic nerve pathway is severed (sympathectomy).

21620

21620 Ostectomy of sternum, partial

The physician removes a portion of the sternum. The physician creates an incision into the chest above the sternum. The sternum is identified and isolated. Surrounding tissue is dissected, and saws and other medical instruments are used to remove a portion of the sternum. The remained bone is made smooth. The site is irrigated, and all incisions are closed.

21627

21627 Sternal debridement

Under general anesthesia, the physician creates an incision in the chest above the sternum. The incision is carried down until the sternum can be visualized. Medical instruments are used to debride the sternum. The area is irrigated. All incisions are closed.

21630-21632

21630 Radical resection of sternum

21632 Radical resection of sternum; with mediastinal lymphadenectomy

Under general anesthesia, the physician creates an incision over the sternum and upper chest. Soft tissue is dissected and the sternum is identified and isolated. Saws and other implements are used to remove the sternum completely. Ribs are detached from the sternum and debrided as necessary. Separately reportable internal fixation devices may be necessary. All incisions are closed (21630). Code 21632 if the physician also performs a mediastinal lymphadenectomy.

21685

21685 Hyoid myotomy and suspension

The physician performs a hyoid myotomy and suspension which is used to treat obstructive sleep apnea syndrome by enlarging the airway behind the tongue (retrolingual) and in the lower pharynx (hypopharyngeal). An incision is made just above the hyoid bone and skin flaps developed to expose the subplatysmal fat and muscles. The subplatysmal fat is partially resected. The fascia between the sternohyoid muscles is incised and the thyroid

cartilage exposed. Lateral exposure is achieved by retracting the muscles on each side of the thyroid cartilage. A needle is used to pierce the lateral aspect of the cartilage on one side. A wire is attached to the end of the needle and the needle and wire are passed through the cartilage on the opposite side. The hyoid bone is exposed and the wire placed around the anterior aspect of the hyoid bone. The wire is then tightened by twisting the two ends together which advances the hyoid bone and opens the airway. The ends of the wire are pinched off and bent into the subplastysmal fat. A drain is placed and the plastysma, subcutaneous fat, and skin closed with sutures.

21700-21705

21700 Division of scalenus anticus; without resection of cervical rib

21705 Division of scalenus anticus; with resection of cervical rib

The physician divides the scalenus anticus muscle with or without resection of cervical rib to treat thoracic outlet syndrome or cervical rib syndrome. These two syndromes are characterized by compression of the brachial plexus by the scalenus anticus muscle alone or by a supernumerary cervical rib arising from the C7 vertebra. The subclavian artery and vein may also be compressed. An incision is made above the clavicle. The sternocleidomastoid is exposed and incised to allow exposure of the scalenus anticus muscle. The scalenus anticus muscle is divided and any fibrous bands that are noted to be compressing the brachial plexus are divided and excised. If there is a supernumerary cervical rib, dissection continues down to the cervical rib. If the rib is exacerbating the brachial plexus compression, it is resected. Use 21700 for division of scalenus anticus muscle alone and 21705 when the scalenus anticus muscle is divided and the cervical rib resected.

21720-21725

21720 Division of sternocleidomastoid for torticollis, open operation; without cast application

21725 Division of sternocleidomastoid for torticollis, open operation; with cast application

Open division of the sternocleidomastoid is typically performed to treat congenital muscular torticollis but may also be performed for acquired torticollis. Depending on the severity of the torticollis a unipolar or bipolar release may be performed. An incision is made above the medial aspect of the clavicle and the sternocleidomastoid tendons of the sternum and clavicle exposed. The tendon sheaths are incised longitudinally and the inferior ends of the tendons are partially resected. The patient's head is then turned to the affected side and the chin depressed. The platysma muscle and adjacent fascia are divided and the surgical wound is explored for any remaining bands of contracted sternocleidomastoid muscle or fascia and these bands are divided. For severe torticollis a bipolar release is performed. The physician first releases the sternocleidomastoid just distal to the tip of the mastoid process through a small incision behind the ear and then releases the muscle at the sternum and clavicle as described above. The patient may be placed in a cervical collar or a cast may be applied to maintain proper alignment of the head and neck. The cast consists of an upper body cast with metal rods on either side of the neck that are attached to the cast and a head immobilizer that goes around the forehead and upper aspect of the skull. Use 21720 when the procedure is performed without cast application and 21725 when a cast is applied.

21740

21740 Reconstructive repair of pectus excavatum or carinatum; open

Under general anesthesia, the physician creates an incision over the sternum and deepens it until the sternum is visible. The physician then views the ribs and removes or repairs any deformed bony or cartilaginous structures. The sternum and ribs are positioned in the anatomically correct positions, and internal fixation is employed to stabilize the area. All incisions are closed.

21742-21743

21742 Reconstructive repair of pectus excavatum or carinatum; minimally invasive approach (Nuss procedure), without thoracoscopy

21743 Reconstructive repair of pectus excavatum or carinatum; minimally invasive approach (Nuss procedure), with thoracoscopy

Under general anesthesia, two lateral incisions are made on either side of the chest. A curved steel bar is inserted under the sternum. In code 21743, a separate incision is made for a thoracoscope for direct visualization as the bar is passed under the sternum. The bar is individually curved for each patient and is used to pop out the depression. It is then fixed to the ribs on either side and the incisions are closed and dressed. A small steel, grooved plate may be used at the end of the bar to help stabilize and fix the bar to the rib. All incisions are closed.

Musculoskeletal System

21750

21750   **Closure of median sternotomy separation with or without debridement (separate procedure)**

Under general anesthesia, the physician creates an incision over the previously separated sternum until the sternum can be visualized. The physician may debride the bone or soft tissue. Internal fixation is used to hold any bone fragments in place and to hold the sternum in the correct position. The incision is closed.

21811-21813

21811   **Open treatment of rib fracture(s) with internal fixation, includes thoracoscopic visualization when performed, unilateral; 1-3 ribs**
21812   **Open treatment of rib fracture(s) with internal fixation, includes thoracoscopic visualization when performed, unilateral; 4-6 ribs**
21813   **Open treatment of rib fracture(s) with internal fixation, includes thoracoscopic visualization when performed, unilateral; 7 or more ribs**

Unilateral rib fracture(s) are repaired using open reduction, internal fixation (ORIF) and may include thoracoscopic visualization of the pleural cavity to assess for bleeding and/or visceral damage. A standard thoracotomy incision is made in the skin over the area of rib injury and carried down through the subcutaneous tissue and fascia. The muscles overlying the ribs are retracted and the intercostal muscles are incised at the superior rib boarders to expose the fracture(s). The fracture sites are cleaned and nonunion fibrous tissue is removed. Care is taken not to disrupt the intercostal neurovascular bundles at the inferior aspect of the ribs. The fractured ends of the rib(s) are mobilized, reduced, and fixed in place with appropriate hardware such as metal plates, intramedullary fixation devices, Judet Struts, absorbable plates, or U-Plates. Thoracoscopic visualization may take place at any point during this procedure. The muscles are reapproximated with a running stitch. The fascia and subcutaneous tissue are closed with interrupted stitches. The skin is closed with staples. Code 21811 is used when the procedure is limited to repair of 1-3 rib fractures; code 21812 is used for 4-6 fractures; and code 21813 is used for 7 or more rib fractures.

21820

21820   **Closed treatment of sternum fracture**

The fracture is determined to be stable and non-displaced via separately reportable x-rays. No braces or splints are used. The patient is placed on reduced activity.

21825

21825   **Open treatment of sternum fracture with or without skeletal fixation**

The physician creates an incision over the sternum and accesses the fractured sternum. The fracture is reduced, and the physician may use internal fixation to maintain stability and reduction. All incisions are closed.

21920-21925

21920   **Biopsy, soft tissue of back or flank; superficial**
21925   **Biopsy, soft tissue of back or flank; deep**

Soft tissue biopsy of the back or flank is performed. Soft tissues include muscles, tendons, fat, blood vessels, lymph vessels, nerves, and tissues surrounding the joints. Local, regional, or general anesthesia or conscious sedation is administered depending on the site and depth of the planned biopsy. The area over the planned biopsy site is cleansed. An incision is made and tissue dissected down to the mass or lesion taking care to protect blood vessels and nerves. A tissue sample is obtained and sent to the laboratory for separately reportable histological evaluation. The incision is closed with sutures. Use 21920 for a superficial biopsy or 21925 for biopsy of deeper tissues requiring more extensive dissection of overlying tissues.

21930-21933

21930   **Excision, tumor, soft tissue of back or flank, subcutaneous; less than 3 cm**
21931   **Excision, tumor, soft tissue of back or flank, subcutaneous; 3 cm or greater**
21932   **Excision, tumor, soft tissue of back or flank, subfascial (eg, intramuscular); less than 5 cm**
21933   **Excision, tumor, soft tissue of back or flank, subfascial (eg, intramuscular); 5 cm or greater**

Soft tissues include subcutaneous fat and connective tissue, fascia, muscles, tendons, blood vessels, lymph vessels, nerves, and tissues surrounding the joints. Soft tissue tumors may be benign or malignant. Benign tumors are typically treated by excision, although small malignant or indeterminate tumors, may be excised if the margins are well defined. A skin incision is made over the tumor in the back or flank or a skin flap created and elevated. Overlying tissue is dissected and the soft tissue mass exposed. The tumor is then excised along with a margin of healthy tissue. Separately reportable frozen section may be performed to ensure that all margins are free of tumor cells. Drains are placed as needed and the surgical wound is closed in layers. For tumors in the subcutaneous fat or connective tissue, use 21930 for a mass less than 2 cm and 21931 for a mass 2 cm or

greater. For tumors below the fascia, use 21932 for a mass less than 5 cm and 21933 for a mass 5.0 cm or greater. Subfascial soft tissue tumors include those within muscle tissue.

21935-21936

21935   **Radical resection of tumor (eg, sarcoma), soft tissue of back or flank; less than 5 cm**
21936   **Radical resection of tumor (eg, sarcoma), soft tissue of back or flank; 5 cm or greater**

Soft tissues include muscles, tendons, fat, blood vessels, lymph vessels, nerves, and tissues surrounding the joints. Soft tissue tumors may be benign or malignant. Radical resection is typically performed for a malignant neoplasm, such as a sarcoma, although benign tumors and tumors of indeterminate nature may also require radical resection. A skin incision is made over the tumor in the back or flank or a skin flap created and elevated. Overlying subcutaneous and soft tissues are dissected and the soft tissue tumor mass exposed. The tumor is removed en bloc along with a wide margin of surrounding tissue. Radical resection involves excision of all involved soft tissue which may include muscles, nerves, and blood vessels. Separately reportable frozen section is performed to ensure that all margins are free of tumor cells. If margins show evidence of malignancy, additional tissue is removed until all margins are free of tumor cells. Drains are placed as needed. The surgical wound may be closed in layers, or separately reportable reconstructive procedures performed. Use 21935 for radical resection of a tumor less than 5 cm; use 21936 for a tumor 5 cm or greater.

22010-22015

22010   **Incision and drainage, open, of deep abscess (subfascial), posterior spine; cervical, thoracic, or cervicothoracic**
22015   **Incision and drainage, open, of deep abscess (subfascial), posterior spine; lumbar, sacral, or lumbosacral**

An incision is made in the skin of the back over the abscess site. The incision is carried down through the soft tissue, the fascia is incised, and the abscess pocket opened. Any loculations are broken up using blunt finger dissection. The abscess cavity is flushed with saline or antibiotic solution. Drains are placed as needed. The incision may be closed in layers or packed with gauze and left open. Use 22010 for incision and drainage of a deep, subfascial abscess in the cervical, thoracic or cervicothoracic spine and 22015 for one located in the lumbar, sacral, or lumbosacral spine.

22100-22103

22100   **Partial excision of posterior vertebral component (eg, spinous process, lamina or facet) for intrinsic bony lesion, single vertebral segment; cervical**
22101   **Partial excision of posterior vertebral component (eg, spinous process, lamina or facet) for intrinsic bony lesion, single vertebral segment; thoracic**
22102   **Partial excision of posterior vertebral component (eg, spinous process, lamina or facet) for intrinsic bony lesion, single vertebral segment; lumbar**
22103   **Partial excision of posterior vertebral component (eg, spinous process, lamina or facet) for intrinsic bony lesion, single vertebral segment; each additional segment (List separately in addition to code for primary procedure)**

The physician partially excises a bony lesion from a vertebral component (e.g., spinous process, lamina, or facet). The physician creates an incision over the vertebral segment containing the bony lesion (e.g., bone spur) and carries the incision through the paravertebral muscles and to the lesion. The physician excises the affected portion of the vertebral segment. The incision is closed. Code 22100 for the cervical segment; 22101 for the thoracic segment; 22102 for the lumbar segment; and 22103 for each additional segment after the first excision.

22110-22116

22110   **Partial excision of vertebral body, for intrinsic bony lesion, without decompression of spinal cord or nerve root(s), single vertebral segment; cervical**
22112   **Partial excision of vertebral body, for intrinsic bony lesion, without decompression of spinal cord or nerve root(s), single vertebral segment; thoracic**
22114   **Partial excision of vertebral body, for intrinsic bony lesion, without decompression of spinal cord or nerve root(s), single vertebral segment; lumbar**
22116   **Partial excision of vertebral body, for intrinsic bony lesion, without decompression of spinal cord or nerve root(s), single vertebral segment; each additional vertebral segment (List separately in addition to code for primary procedure)**

An incision is made over the affected vertebral segment or just lateral to the affected vertebra. The paravertebral muscles are exposed and incised or retracted. The vertebral body is exposed and the lesion located. The extent of the lesion is evaluated visually and radiographically as needed. The amount of bone to be removed from the vertebral body is mapped out. Removal of the bone lesion is accomplished using a high speed bur and/

Musculoskeletal System

CPT © 2016 American Medical Association. All Rights Reserved.   ● New Code   ▲ Revised Code or curette while taking care to protect nerve roots and other vital structures. Following complete removal of the bone lesion, the incision closed in layers. Use 22110 for excision of a bone lesion of one cervical vertebral body; 22112 for a lesion of one thoracic vertebral body; 22214 for a lesion of one lumbar vertebral body; and 22116 for excision of a lesion from each additional vertebral body after the first.

22206-22208

22206 Osteotomy of spine, posterior or posterolateral approach, 3 columns, 1 vertebral segment (eg, pedicle/vertebral body subtraction); thoracic

22207 Osteotomy of spine, posterior or posterolateral approach, 3 columns, 1 vertebral segment (eg, pedicle/vertebral body subtraction); lumbar

22208 Osteotomy of spine, posterior or posterolateral approach, 3 columns, 1 vertebral segment (eg, pedicle/vertebral body subtraction); each additional vertebral segment (List separately in addition to code for primary procedure)

A three column osteotomy of the spine, also referred to as a pedicle subtraction osteotomy, is performed on a single thoracic segment using a posterior or posterolateral approach in 22206. The spine has three columns: anterior, middle, and posterior. The anterior column is composed of the vertebral body, the middle column is composed of two thick pedicles surrounding the vertebral foramen through which the spinal cord passes, and the posterior column is composed of the lamina, two transverse processes, and the spinous process. Thoracic and lumbar procedures for complex spinal deformities typically require osteotomy of all three columns. An incision is made in the skin of the back directly over the deformed vertebral segment or to the side of the vertebral segment requiring reconstruction. The fascia is incised. Subperiosteal dissection is performed along the spinal process, lamina, both transverse processes, and rib head of the vertebral segment. The posterior segment is resected taking care to preserve the pedicles. This includes excision of the lamina (laminectomy), excision of the facets bilaterally (facetectomy), and resection of the ribs bilaterally. A cavity is created under the pedicles, which are resected. A wedge resection of the vertebral body is performed. A curette is used to thin the posterior vertebral wall until it is paper thin. The lateral portions of the vertebra are resected. A reverse angled curette is used to greenstick the posterior cortex of the vertebral body. The lateral vertebral body wall is resected at the level of the pedicles. The osteotomy is closed so that all columns are situated bone-on-bone. Correction of the deformity is evaluated by intraoperative imaging. Use 22207 for a three column osteotomy of a lumbar segment and 22208 for three column osteotomy of each additional vertebral segment.

22210-22216

22210 Osteotomy of spine, posterior or posterolateral approach, 1 vertebral segment; cervical

22212 Osteotomy of spine, posterior or posterolateral approach, 1 vertebral segment; thoracic

22214 Osteotomy of spine, posterior or posterolateral approach, 1 vertebral segment; lumbar

22216 Osteotomy of spine, posterior or posterolateral approach, 1 vertebral segment; each additional vertebral segment (List separately in addition to primary procedure)

A spinal osteotomy involves removing part of the vertebra to correct a deformity, such as a flexion deformity. Excising a portion of the vertebra allows the vertebral segment to be realigned to improve function and stability of the spine and relieve pain. Using a posterior or posterolateral approach, an incision is made directly over the affected vertebral segment(s) or just lateral to the vertebra. The fascia is incised. Subperiosteal dissection is performed along the spinal process, lamina, both transverse processes, and rib head of the vertebral segment as needed. A wedge of bone is resected which may include portions of the supraspinatus and infraspinatus ligaments and spinous processes. The patient is carefully repositioned as manual pressure is applied at the osteotomy site until the opposing ligaments tear. This is accomplished while keeping nerve roots and other vital structures under direct visualization to ensure that no impingement of these structures occurs as the vertebra is manipulated and the bony gap closed. Once the bony gap created by the wedge resection has been closed, separately reportable bone grafts and/or spinal instrumentation may be utilized to stabilize the spine. A body cast or jacket is applied as needed to immobilize the spine. Use 22210 for osteotomy of one cervical vertebral segment, 22212 for one thoracic segment, 22214 for one lumbar segment, and 22216 for each additional vertebral segment after the first.

22220-22226

22220 Osteotomy of spine, including discectomy, anterior approach, single vertebral segment; cervical

22222 Osteotomy of spine, including discectomy, anterior approach, single vertebral segment; thoracic

22224 Osteotomy of spine, including discectomy, anterior approach, single vertebral segment; lumbar

22226 Osteotomy of spine, including discectomy, anterior approach, single vertebral segment; each additional vertebral segment (List separately in addition to code for primary procedure)

A spinal osteotomy involves removing part of the vertebra to correct a deformity, such as a flexion deformity. Excising a portion of the vertebra allows the vertebral segment to be realigned to improve function and stability of the spine and relieve pain. Depending on the level and extent of the deformity, an anterior neck, thoracic, thoracoabdominal, abdominal, retropleural, or retroperitoneal incision is made. Soft tissues are dissected and the vertebrae are exposed. Subperiosteal dissection is performed along the vertebral segment as needed. Depending on the approach, a portion of the lamina may be removed to access the intervertebral disc. A curette is used to remove the intervertebral disc or disc fragments. A wedge of bone from the vertebral body is resected which may include portions of the surrounding ligaments and spinous processes. The patient is carefully repositioned as manual pressure is applied at the osteotomy site until the opposing ligaments tear. This is accomplished while keeping nerve roots and other vital structures under direct visualization to ensure that no impingement of these structures occurs as the vertebra is manipulated and the bony gap closed. Once the bony gap created by the wedge resection has been closed, separately reportable bone grafts and/or spinal instrumentation may be utilized to stabilize the spine. A body cast or jacket is applied as needed to immobilize the spine. Use 22220 for osteotomy of one cervical vertebral segment, 22222 for one thoracic segment, 22224 for one lumbar segment, and 22226 for each additional vertebral segment after the first.

22310-22315

22310 Closed treatment of vertebral body fracture(s), without manipulation, requiring and including casting or bracing

22315 Closed treatment of vertebral fracture(s) and/or dislocation(s) requiring casting or bracing, with and including casting and/or bracing by manipulation or traction

Closed treatment of one or more vertebral body fractures is performed with casting or bracing. The vertebral body is the thick, disc-shaped anterior portion of the vertebra that is the weight-bearing part. Types of fractures typically treated with closed techniques include simple compression fractures and burst fractures. The superior and inferior surfaces attach to the intervertebral discs. A neurovascular exam is performed to ensure that nerves and blood vessels at the site of injury are intact. In 22310, no manipulation of fracture fragments is required. The patient is treated with pain medication and the spine is immobilized with a cervical collar, halo device, thoracic or lumbar corset, or a body cast or brace. In 22315, closed treatment of minimally displaced vertebral fractures and/or dislocations with no neurological deficit is performed using manipulation or traction and casting and/or bracing. The minimally displaced fracture and/or dislocated vertebrae are manually reduced (manipulated) into anatomic alignment. Alternatively, traction may be used to realign the spine. A longitudinal force is applied along the axis of the spine to decompress the fracture. Following reduction, separately reportable radiographs are again obtained to ensure anatomic alignment. The spine is then immobilized and hyperextended using a brace or cast.

22318-22319

22318 Open treatment and/or reduction of odontoid fracture(s) and or dislocation(s) (including os odontoideum), anterior approach, including placement of internal fixation; without grafting

22319 Open treatment and/or reduction of odontoid fracture(s) and or dislocation(s) (including os odontoideum), anterior approach, including placement of internal fixation; with grafting

The os odontoideum, or odontoid process, is the strong toothlike process on the which projects upward from the surface of the axis. The patient is placed in a supine position and the physician creates an incision through the muscle, carefully avoiding the carotid artery, trachea, and esophagus. The surrounding soft tissue is retracted and area vessels may be ligated. Guide wires are used to stabilize the fracture or dislocation. Code 22318 if no bone grafting is necessary. Code 22319 if bone grafting is necessary. A drain may be inserted, and all incisions are closed.

Musculoskeletal System

22325-22328

22325   **Open treatment and/or reduction of vertebral fracture(s) and/or dislocation(s), posterior approach, 1 fractured vertebra or dislocated segment; lumbar**

22326   **Open treatment and/or reduction of vertebral fracture(s) and/or dislocation(s), posterior approach, 1 fractured vertebra or dislocated segment; cervical**

22327   **Open treatment and/or reduction of vertebral fracture(s) and/or dislocation(s), posterior approach, 1 fractured vertebra or dislocated segment; thoracic**

22328   **Open treatment and/or reduction of vertebral fracture(s) and/or dislocation(s), posterior approach, 1 fractured vertebra or dislocated segment; each additional fractured vertebra or dislocated segment (List separately in addition to code for primary procedure)**

The patient is placed in a prone position and the physician creates an incision over the fractured or dislocated vertebra or dislocated segment. The physician uses a rod to stabilize the area. Fusion may be necessary, and is achieved via grafting (separately reportable) or internal fixation. The incision is closed. Code 22325 for a lumbar procedure; 22326 for cervical; 22327 for a thoracic site; and 22328 for each additional fractured or dislocated vertebra or segment in addition to the primary procedure.

22505

22505   **Manipulation of spine requiring anesthesia, any region**

Manipulation under anesthesia (MUA) is the use of manual manipulation of the spine combined with the use of some form of anesthesia (usually general or conscious sedation). MUA allows the physician to manipulate patients, who otherwise cannot tolerate manual techniques because of pain response, spasm, muscle contractures, and guarding. MUA uses a combination of specific short-level arm manipulations, passive stretches, and specific articular and postural kinesthetic integrations to obtain a desired outcome. Daily rehabilitation usually follows an MUA procedure.

22510-22512

22510   **Percutaneous vertebroplasty (bone biopsy included when performed), 1 vertebral body, unilateral or bilateral injection, inclusive of all imaging guidance; cervicothoracic**

22511   **Percutaneous vertebroplasty (bone biopsy included when performed), 1 vertebral body, unilateral or bilateral injection, inclusive of all imaging guidance; lumbosacral**

22512   **Percutaneous vertebroplasty (bone biopsy included when performed), 1 vertebral body, unilateral or bilateral injection, inclusive of all imaging guidance; each additional cervicothoracic or lumbosacral vertebral body (List separately in addition to code for primary procedure)**

Percutaneous vertebroplasty is performed to stabilize a compression fracture caused by osteoporosis of the spine. It may also be used to treat aggressive hemangiomas of the vertebral body and for palliative treatment of pathological fractures caused by benign or malignant neoplasms of the spine. The patient is placed in a prone position. Using fluoroscopic or CT guidance, the vertebral level requiring vertebroplasty is identified. Local anesthesia is administered. A spinal needle is advanced into one side of the vertebral body and deep local and subperiosteal anesthesia is administered. If a biopsy is needed, a small incision is made in the skin. A bone biopsy needle is advanced into the vertebral body, and a bone sample is obtained. The bone sample is sent for separately reportable pathological examination. The percutaneous vertebroplasty is then performed. A spinal needle is advanced into one side the vertebral body in a unilateral procedure using a transpedicular or parapedicular approach. A mixture of polymethylmethacrylate (PMMA) bone cement and contrast medium, such as sterile barium or tungsten powder, is injected into the vertebral body. The bone cement is observed with the aid of the contrast medium as it diffuses throughout the intertrabecular bone marrow space and reinforces the structure of the fractured vertebral body. The needle is withdrawn. A second injection is performed on the opposite side of the vertebral body for bilateral repair procedures. For percutaneous vertebroplasty of a single cervicothoracic vertebral body, use 22510; for a single lumbosacral vertebral body, use 22511; and for each additional cervicothoracic or lumbosacral vertebral body, use 22512.

22513-22515

22513   **Percutaneous vertebral augmentation, including cavity creation (fracture reduction and bone biopsy included when performed) using mechanical device (eg, kyphoplasty), 1 vertebral body, unilateral or bilateral cannulation, inclusive of all imaging guidance; thoracic**

22514   **Percutaneous vertebral augmentation, including cavity creation (fracture reduction and bone biopsy included when performed) using mechanical device (eg, kyphoplasty), 1 vertebral body, unilateral or bilateral cannulation, inclusive of all imaging guidance; lumbar**

22515   **Percutaneous vertebral augmentation, including cavity creation (fracture reduction and bone biopsy included when performed) using mechanical device (eg, kyphoplasty), 1 vertebral body, unilateral or bilateral cannulation, inclusive of all imaging guidance; each additional thoracic or lumbar vertebral body (List separately in addition to code for primary procedure)**

Percutaneous augmentation of the vertebra is performed to treat a compression fracture caused by osteoporosis, multiple myeloma, primary or metastatic malignant lesions, benign lesions, or traumatic injury of the spine. The patient is placed in a prone position. Using image guidance, a small skin incision is made over the affected vertebra. A working channel is created on one side of the vertebra by advancing a needle to the desired location in the vertebra. Needle biopsies are obtained as needed. A guidewire is then advanced through the needle. The needle is withdrawn and a cannula is advanced over the guidewire and the guidewire is removed. This is repeated on the opposite side for bilateral augmentation procedures. A mechanical device, such as a miniature expandable jack or expandable balloon tamp, is then placed through the cannula and expanded to create a cavity as contrast medium is simultaneously instilled. The fracture may also be reduced using the mechanical device. Once the cavity has been created, the mechanical device is removed. The cavity is then filled with morcellized bone graft material, polymethylmethacrylate (PMMA) bone cement, or other bone graft substitute using a bone biopsy needle. The bone graft or cement is mixed with contrast medium so that the physician can observe filling of the cavity. Once the cavity is filled, the needle is withdrawn. A second injection may be performed on the opposite side of the vertebral body. For percutaneous augmentation of a single thoracic vertebral body, use 22513; for a single lumbar vertebral body, use 22514; and for each additional thoracic or lumbar vertebral body, use 22515.

22526-22527

22526   **Percutaneous intradiscal electrothermal annuloplasty, unilateral or bilateral including fluoroscopic guidance; single level**

22527   **Percutaneous intradiscal electrothermal annuloplasty, unilateral or bilateral including fluoroscopic guidance; 1 or more additional levels (List separately in addition to code for primary procedure)**

Percutaneous intradiscal electrothermal annuloplasty is a minimally invasive, catheter-based technique used to treat patients with chronic low back pain from disc pathology. The target disc is first identified with discography. A special spinal catheter with an embedded thermal resistive coil is placed posterolaterally into the disc annulus, or nucleus. The catheter is passed through the disc and back out posteriorly in a circuit-like manner. Electrothermal heat is then generated through the coil and the disc material is heated for about 20 minutes at 90 degrees centigrade. The heat does not destroy, burn, or ablate the tissue. The heat is thought to provide pain relief by shrinking the collagen fibers and thermocoagulating the adjacent nerve tissue or pain receptors. Report 22526 for a single level, either unilateral or bilateral. Code 22527 for one or more levels, either unilateral or bilateral, in addition to the initial, primary level. Fluoroscopic guidance is included.

22532-22534

22532   **Arthrodesis, lateral extracavitary technique, including minimal discectomy to prepare interspace (other than for decompression); thoracic**

22533   **Arthrodesis, lateral extracavitary technique, including minimal discectomy to prepare interspace (other than for decompression); lumbar**

22534   **Arthrodesis, lateral extracavitary technique, including minimal discectomy to prepare interspace (other than for decompression); thoracic or lumbar, each additional vertebral segment (List separately in addition to code for primary procedure)**

Arthrodesis by lateral extracavitary technique including minimal discectomy to prepare the interspace (other than for decompression) is performed. Lateral extracavity approach requires resection of the ribs, and exposure of the pleura, and/or peritoneum. A midline incision is made and extended laterally to expose the paraspinous muscle bundle over the thoracic or lumbar vertebral segment to be fused. The paraspinous muscles are elevated off the spinous processes and laminae. The paraspinous muscle bundle is then divided and elevated off the ribs. The rib is dissected from the intercostal muscles and pleura. The rib is resected and the intercostal nerve identified and protected. A high speed drill is used to remove the associated transverse process and the lateral portion of the facet and pedicle. The dural sac and vertebral body are exposed. If the procedure involves the lumbar spine, the peritoneum is exposed and retracted. The nerve root is retracted to allow better visualization of the vertebral body. Degenerated disc material is removed to prepare the interspace for arthrodesis. Cartilage is removed from vertebral endplates and bone is decorticated. Separately reportable bone allograft or autograft is then placed between the vertebral endplates to facilitate the interbody arthrodesis. Drains are placed as needed and the incisions closed. Use code 22532 to report thoracic arthrodesis by lateral extracavitary technique, code 22533 for lumbar arthrodesis, and code 22534 for arthrodesis of each additional thoracic or lumbar vertebral segment.

22548

22548   Arthrodesis, anterior transoral or extraoral technique, clivus-C1-C2 (atlas-axis), with or without excision of odontoid process

The clivus is the sloping surface at the posterior aspect of the skull that is composed of the body of the sphenoid and the basal part of the occipital bone. The clivus extends from the dorsum sellae to the foramen magnum. In this procedure the clivus is fused to the C1 and C2 vertebrae to stabilize the head. The C1 and C2 vertebrae are also referred to as the atlas and axis respectively. In a transoral approach, the clivus-C1-C2 interspaces are accessed through an incision in the soft palate. The soft palate is split and retracted laterally using suture anchors. Alternatively the clivus-C1-C2 interspaces may be approached via an extraoral, retropharyngeal, or anterolateral approach. The prevertebral fascia is incised and the anterior arch of the atlas, the odontoid process, and the vertebral body of the axis are exposed. The procedure may be performed with or without excision of the odontoid process, also called the dens, which is a peg-like process that projects up from the axis and through the ring of the atlas. To excise the odontoid process, the anterior arch of the atlas is resected first under fluoroscopic guidance and the odontoid exposed. The full length of the odontoid is then excised from its apex to base. Soft tissues, such as the tectorial membrane, that are impinging on the spinal cord are also excised as needed. Fusion of the clivus-C1-C2 is accomplished using separately reportable bone grafts. Structural corticocancellous bone grafts are strategically placed between the clivus-C1-C2 interspaces. Bur holes are created in the inion and foramen magnum on each side of the midline and wire fixation applied to immobilize the clivus-C1-C2. Additional internal fixation devices may also be applied in a separately reportable procedure.

22551-22552

22551   Arthrodesis, anterior interbody, including disc space preparation, discectomy, osteophytectomy and decompression of spinal cord and/or nerve roots; cervical below C2

22552   Arthrodesis, anterior interbody, including disc space preparation, discectomy, osteophytectomy and decompression of spinal cord and/or nerve roots; cervical below C2, each additional interspace (List separately in addition to code for separate procedure)

The damaged cervical vertebra below C2 is approached from the front (ventral) side of the body. The soft tissues and muscles overlying the cervical spine are dissected. The trachea and esophagus are retracted away from the surgical site. The affected portion of the cervical spine is exposed. A groove or channel is created in the vertebral body to expose the intervertebral disc and nerve roots. The intervertebral disc is exposed and carefully removed with the aid of the surgical microscope. Bone spurs and any bone impinging on the nerve roots is also removed along with the ligament that covers the spinal cord. Cartilage is removed from the vertebral endplates above and below the disc space and the bone is decorticated. Separately reportable bone allograft or autograft is then placed between the vertebral endplates to facilitate the interbody arthrodesis. Separately reportable internal fixation may also be used to stabilize the spine. Upon completion of the procedure, bleeding is controlled, drains are placed as needed, and soft tissues and skin are closed in layers. Use 22551 for a single cervical interspace and 22552 for each additional interspace.

22554

22554   Arthrodesis, anterior interbody technique, including minimal discectomy to prepare interspace (other than for decompression); cervical below C2

Spinal surgical immobilization of a joint so the bones grow solidly together is performed for herniated disks, lesions, and stabilization of fractures and dislocations of the spine. Traction is applied to the head. The damaged vertebrae is approached from the front (ventral) side of the body. A cut is made through the neck, avoiding the esophagus, trachea, and thyroid. An instrument is used to hold the intervertebral muscles apart. A drill is inserted in the afflicted vertebrae and the positioning of the drill is confirmed via x-ray. The drill or saw is then used to cut a groove or channel in the front of the vertebrae. The area between the two adjacent vertebrae are cleaned out with spring loaded forceps that are equipped with a sharp blade. The cartilage containing plates above and below the vertebrae to be fused are removed. The physician takes bone procured from a donor or the hip area of the individual undergoing the procedure. The bone graft is packed into the spaces cleaned out and trimmed to fit. The traction to the head is slowly lessened so the bone graft stays in place. The fibrous membranes covering the deep vertebral area are sutured, a drain is placed, and the incision is sutured.

22556

22556   Arthrodesis, anterior interbody technique, including minimal discectomy to prepare interspace (other than for decompression); thoracic

Spinal surgical immobilization of a joint so the bones grow solidly together is performed for herniated disks, lesions, and stabilization of fractures and dislocations of the spine. Traction is applied to the head. The damaged vertebrae is approached from the neck (thoracic). A cut is made through the neck, avoiding the esophagus, trachea, and thyroid. An instrument is used to hold the intervertebral muscles apart. A drill is inserted in the afflicted vertebrae and the positioning of the drill is confirmed via x-ray. The drill or saw is then used to cut a groove or channel in the front of the vertebrae. The area between the two adjacent vertebrae is cleaned out with spring loaded forceps that are equipped with a sharp blade. The cartilage containing plates above and below the vertebrae to be fused are removed. The physician takes bone procured from a donor or the hip area of the individual undergoing the procedure. The bone graft is packed into the spaces cleaned out and trimmed to fit. The traction to the head is slowly lessened so the bone graft stays in place. The fibrous membranes covering the deep vertebral area are sutured, a drain is placed, and the incision is sutured.

22558

22558   Arthrodesis, anterior interbody technique, including minimal discectomy to prepare interspace (other than for decompression); lumbar

Spinal surgical immobilization of a joint so the bones grow solidly together is performed for herniated disks, lesions, and stabilization of fractures and dislocations of the spine. Traction is applied to the head. The damaged vertebrae is approached from the part of the lower back between the thorax and the pelvis (lumbar). A cut is made through the back. An instrument is used to hold the intervertebral muscles apart. A drill is inserted in the afflicted vertebrae and the positioning of the drill is confirmed via x-ray. The drill or saw is then used to cut a groove or channel in the front of the vertebrae. The area between the two adjacent vertebrae is cleaned out with spring loaded forceps that are equipped with a sharp blade. The cartilage containing plates above and below the vertebrae to be fused are removed. The physician takes bone procured from a donor or the hip area of the individual undergoing the procedure. The bone graft is packed into the spaces cleaned out and trimmed to fit. The traction to the head is slowly lessened so the bone graft stays in place. The fibrous membranes covering the deep vertebral area are sutured, a drain is placed, and the incision is sutured.

22585

22585   Arthrodesis, anterior interbody technique, including minimal discectomy to prepare interspace (other than for decompression); each additional interspace (List separately in addition to code for primary procedure)

Spinal surgical immobilization of a joint so the bones grow solidly together is performed for herniated disks, lesions, and stabilization of fractures and dislocations of the spine. Traction is applied to the head. The damaged vertebrae is approached from the front (ventral) side of the body. A cut is made through the neck, avoiding the esophagus, trachea, and thyroid. An instrument is used to hold the intervertebral muscles apart. A drill is inserted in the afflicted vertebrae and the positioning of the drill is confirmed via x-ray. The drill or saw is then used to cut a groove or channel in the front of the vertebrae. The area between the two adjacent vertebrae is cleaned out with spring loaded forceps that are equipped with a sharp blade. The cartilage containing plates above and below the vertebrae to be fused are removed. The physician takes bone procured from a donor or the hip area of the individual undergoing the procedure. The bone graft is packed into the spaces cleaned out and trimmed to fit. The traction to the head is slowly lessened so the bone graft stays in place. The fibrous membranes covering the deep vertebral area are sutured, a drain is placed, and the incision is sutured. This code is for each additional interspace. This code can be added to codes 22554, 22556, or 22558.

22586

22586   Arthrodesis, pre-sacral interbody technique, including disc space preparation, discectomy, with posterior instrumentation, with image guidance, includes bone graft when performed, L5-S1 interspace

Lumbar arthrodesis is performed on the L5-S1 interspace using a pre-sacral interbody technique including discectomy to prepare the interspace, placement of posterior instrumentation, placement of bone grafts as needed, and imaging guidance. The pre-sacral interbody technique, also referred to as transsacral or paracoccygeal, uses a minimally invasive percutaneous approach to the anterior portion of the disc space. The patient is placed in a prone position and a small incision is made at the level of the coccyx slightly lateral to the midline. A trocar is advanced anterior to the sacrum under fluoroscopic guidance. A small presacral channel is created in the L5-S1 disc space. The two adjacent vertebral bodies are distracted, and the disc interspace is prepared by removing the intervertebral disc material and the cartilage from the end plates of the adjacent vertebrae. Separately reportable bone allografts from a donor or autografts are obtained. Spinal fusion (arthrodesis) is accomplished by packing the bone graft material into the disc

Musculoskeletal System

space. The body of the superior vertebra is drilled, and a posterior fixation rod or screw is implanted.

22590

22590 Arthrodesis, posterior technique, craniocervical (occiput-C2)

The patient is immobilized using a halo vest orthosis and a Stryker frame to facilitate the positioning of the patient. The physician makes an incision from the back part of the skull to the C3 vertebra. The fascia is opened, and the paravertebral muscles are retracted. Using a drill, the physician drills through the back part of the skull in a horizontal fashion. The drill is then used to make a hole in the base of the C2 vertebra. Wires are placed through the holes with a third wire placed around C1. Bone grafts from a donor of the hip area of the patient are tied into place using the wires. The fascia is closed, sutured, a drain is placed, and the incision is closed.

22595

22595 Arthrodesis, posterior technique, atlas-axis (C1-C2)

The C1-C2 articulation, also referred to as the atlas-axis, is composed of three joints which include a central atlantoaxial joint and two lateral atlantoaxial joints. These joints allow rotation of the head from side to side. Posterior arthrodesis, also referred to as posterior fusion, of C1-C2 reduces neck rotation and prevents both forward and backward motion of the head. Fusion may be used alone or in conjunction with other procedures to treat fractures or instability of C1-C2. The head is immobilized. An incision is made in the back of the neck over the C1-C2 joint. Soft tissues are dissected and the vertebrae are exposed. Separately reportable fracture treatment or decompression is performed as needed. A separately reportable bone graft is obtained from the iliac crest or other site and prepared. The bone graft is placed. Drill holes are created in the C1-C2 vertebrae and wires are threaded through the vertebrae to immobilize the joint. Alternatively, other reportable internal fixation devices may be placed. A drain may be placed and the surgical wound is then closed in layers.

22600-22614

22600 Arthrodesis, posterior or posterolateral technique, single level; cervical below C2 segment

22610 Arthrodesis, posterior or posterolateral technique, single level; thoracic (with lateral transverse technique, when performed)

22612 Arthrodesis, posterior or posterolateral technique, single level; lumbar (with lateral transverse technique, when performed)

22614 Arthrodesis, posterior or posterolateral technique, single level; each additional vertebral segment (List separately in addition to code for primary procedure)

Posterior or posterolateral arthrodesis, also referred to as fusion, of one or more intervertebral joints is performed to treat a fracture or other instability. Fusion may be used alone or in conjunction with other procedures. If a posterior or posterolateral approach is used, an incision is made in the back of the neck or in the back over the affected vertebral joints. Soft tissues are dissected and the vertebrae are exposed. Separately reportable fracture treatment or decompression is performed as needed. The transverse processes, facet joints, and/or lamina are prepared for bone grafting. A separately reportable bone graft is obtained from the iliac crest or other site and prepared. Allograft bone obtained from a bone bank may also be used. The bone graft is placed. Drill holes are created in the facets or spinous processes of each vertebra and wires are threaded through the vertebrae to immobilize the joint. Alternatively, other reportable internal fixation devices may be placed through the pedicles or facets. A drain may be placed and the surgical wound is then closed in layers. Use 22600 for fusion of a single level of the cervical spine below the C2 segment; use 22610 for fusion of a single level of the thoracic spine; use 22612 for fusion of a single level of the lumbar spine. Use 22614 for fusion of each additional vertebral segment.

22630-22632

22630 Arthrodesis, posterior interbody technique, including laminectomy and/or discectomy to prepare interspace (other than for decompression), single interspace; lumbar

22632 Arthrodesis, posterior interbody technique, including laminectomy and/or discectomy to prepare interspace (other than for decompression), single interspace; each additional interspace (List separately in addition to code for primary procedure)

Posterior interbody arthrodesis, also referred to as interbody fusion, of one or more intervertebral joints is performed to treat a vertebral fracture or instability. Fusion may be used alone or in conjunction with other procedures. An incision is made in the back over the affected lumbar vertebral joints. Soft tissues are dissected and the vertebrae are exposed. Muscle is retracted off the lamina. A bone drill is used to remove part of the lamina. The intervertebral disc is removed and the joint space is prepared for arthrodesis. Separately reportable fracture treatment or decompression may be performed as needed. A separately reportable bone graft is obtained from the iliac crest or other site and prepared. Allograft bone obtained from a bone bank may also be used. The bone graft is placed in the

intervertebral joint space. Drill holes are created in the facets or spinous processes of each vertebra and wires are threaded through the vertebrae to immobilize the joint. Alternatively, other reportable internal fixation devices may be placed through the pedicles or facets. A drain may be placed and the surgical wound is then closed in layers. Use 22630 for fusion of a single lumbar intervertebral joint space. Use 22632 for fusion of each additional intervertebral space.

22633-22634

22633 Arthrodesis, combined posterior or posterolateral technique with posterior interbody technique including laminectomy and/or discectomy sufficient to prepare interspace (other than for decompression), single interspace and segment; lumbar

22634 Arthrodesis, combined posterior or posterolateral technique with posterior interbody technique including laminectomy and/or discectomy sufficient to prepare interspace (other than for decompression), single interspace and segment; each additional interspace and segment (List separately in addition to code for primary procedure)

Fusion of one or more of the lumbar vertebral joints is performed to treat a fracture or other instability using a combined posterior or posterolateral technique with posterior interbody technique. Fusion may be used alone or in conjunction with other procedures. Using a posterior or posterolateral approach, an incision is made in the lower back over the affected lumbar vertebral joint(s). Soft tissues are dissected and the vertebrae are exposed. A bone drill is used to remove part of the lamina. The intervertebral disc is removed and the joint space is prepared for arthrodesis. Separately reportable fracture treatment or decompression may be performed as needed. The transverse processes, facet joints, and/or lamina are prepared for bone grafting. A separately reportable bone graft is obtained from the iliac crest or other site and prepared. Allograft bone obtained from a bone bank may also be used. The bone graft is placed in the intervertebral joint space to facilitate fusion of the vertebral bodies. Additional bone graft material is used as needed to fuse other sites in the vertebral joint such as the transverse processes, facet joints, or lamina. Drill holes are created in the facets or spinous processes of each vertebra and wires are threaded through the vertebrae to immobilize the joint. Alternatively, other separately reportable internal fixation devices may be placed through the pedicles or facets. A drain may be placed and the surgical wound is then closed in layers. Use 22633 for fusion of a single interspace and vertebral segment of the lumbar spine. Use 22634 for fusion of each additional interspace and vertebral segment.

22800-22804

22800 Arthrodesis, posterior, for spinal deformity, with or without cast; up to 6 vertebral segments

22802 Arthrodesis, posterior, for spinal deformity, with or without cast; 7 to 12 vertebral segments

22804 Arthrodesis, posterior, for spinal deformity, with or without cast; 13 or more vertebral segments

Posterior arthrodesis, also referred to as spinal fusion, of two or more vertebral segments is performed to treat spinal deformity such as scoliosis or kyphosis. Fusion may be used alone or in conjunction with other procedures. An incision is made in the back of the neck or in the back over the affected area of the spine. Soft tissues are dissected and the vertebrae are exposed. The facet joints are removed. The vertebral segments are roughened in preparation for bone grafting. A separately reportable autogenous bone graft is obtained from the ribs, iliac crest, or other site and the bone graft is prepared. Allograft bone obtained from a bone bank may also be used. The bone graft is placed along the prepared vertebrae. Separately reportable internal fixation devices are placed through the pedicles or facets. A drain may be placed and the surgical wound is then closed in layers. A body cast is applied is needed. Use 22800 for fusion of up to 6 vertebral segments; use 22802 for fusion of 7-12 vertebral segments; use 22804 for fusion of 13 or more vertebral segments.

22808-22812

22808 Arthrodesis, anterior, for spinal deformity, with or without cast; 2 to 3 vertebral segments

22810 Arthrodesis, anterior, for spinal deformity, with or without cast; 4 to 7 vertebral segments

22812 Arthrodesis, anterior, for spinal deformity, with or without cast; 8 or more vertebral segments

Anterior arthrodesis, also referred to as spinal fusion, of two or more vertebral segments is performed to treat spinal deformity such as kyphosis or scoliosis. Fusion may be used alone or in conjunction with other procedures. Depending on the level and extent of the deformity, an anterior neck, thoracic, thoracoabdominal, abdominal, retropleural, or retroperitoneal incision is made. Soft tissues are dissected and the vertebrae are exposed. The vertebral segments are roughened in preparation for bone grafting. A separately reportable autogentous bone graft is obtained from the ribs, iliac crest, or other site and the bone graft is prepared. Allograft bone obtained from a bone bank may also be used. The bone graft is placed along the prepared vertebrae. Separately reportable internal

Musculoskeletal System

fixation devices are placed through the pedicles or facets. A drain may be placed and the surgical wound is then closed in layers. A body cast is applied is needed. Use 22808 for anterior approach fusion of 2-3 vertebral segments; use 22810 for fusion of 4-7 vertebral segments; use 22812 for fusion of 8 or more vertebral segments.

22818-22819

22818 **Kyphectomy, circumferential exposure of spine and resection of vertebral segment(s) (including body and posterior elements); single or 2 segments**

22819 **Kyphectomy, circumferential exposure of spine and resection of vertebral segment(s) (including body and posterior elements); 3 or more segments**

The physician fixes a condition in which the spine bulges out, causing a hump in the patients' back. Damaged and deformed vertebrae are removed, and the physician uses bone grafts and metal rods and wires to correct the deformity. Code 22818 if one or two vertebrae segments are affected, and 22819 if 3 or more segments are affected.

22830

22830 **Exploration of spinal fusion**

The patient is placed in position (e.g., posterior, posteriolateral, anterior, etc.) , depending on the site of the fusion. The physician examines the joint between two vertebrae that have been fused together for signs of damage or disease. The physician may also examine any instrumentation that had been placed during the fusion. The incision is closed with sutures.

22840

22840 **Posterior non-segmental instrumentation (eg, Harrington rod technique, pedicle fixation across 1 interspace, atlantoaxial transarticular screw fixation, sublaminar wiring at C1, facet screw fixation) (List separately in addition to code for primary procedure)**

Posterior non-segmental spine instrumentation is applied during a separately reportable arthrodesis (fusion) procedure on the spine. Spinal instrumentation is used to treat a deformity or instability of the spine. Posterior non-segmental fixation involves attaching the fixation device to the top and bottom vertebral segments without attaching it to any of the vertebral segments in between. Types of fixation include: Harrington rod technique, pedicle fixation across one interspace, atlantoaxial transarticular screw fixation, sublaminar wiring at C1, and facet screw fixation. Harrington rod technique involves placing a long rod spanning multiple vertebral segments fixed to the spine using hooks at the top and bottom vertebral segments only. Pedicle fixation across a single interspace, also referred to as transpedicular fixation, involves inserting a screw in a posteroanteromedial direction through the pedicle into the vertebral segment above and below one single interspace. The screws are then secured to a plate or other fixator to provide stability. Atlantoaxial transarticular screw fixation involves placing a screw through the C1-2 vertebral bodies. Following preoperative 3D fluoroscopic assessment of anatomy and calculation of correct screw trajectory, a single (unilateral) pedicle screw or two (bilateral) pedicle screws are placed in the atlantoaxial complex-through the pedicle of C2, traversing the C1-2 interspace, and penetrating the lateral mass of C1. C1 sublaminar wiring involves placing a wire through the C1-C2 lamina to provide stability. Facet screw fixation involves placing a short screw horizontally from the inferior articular process of the superior vertebra, traversing the interspace, and penetrating the articular process of the inferior vertebra. Alternatively, the facet screw can be angled and placed in the base of the pedicle or a translaminar facet screw can be placed through the spinous process and lamina of the contralateral side and penetrate the base of the pedicle.

22841

22841 **Internal spinal fixation by wiring of spinous processes (List separately in addition to code for primary procedure)**

Internal spinal fixation by wiring of spinous processes is performed during a separately reportable arthrodesis (fusion) procedure on the spine. A hole is drilled in the base of the spinous process of the cephalad (superior) vertebra and the wire is passed through the hole and beneath the caudad (inferior) vertebra and tied with a wire tightener. Alternatively, a hole can also be drilled in the superior and inferior vertebra, the wire passed through both holes in both vertebra, and tied with a wire tightener.

22842-22844

22842 **Posterior segmental instrumentation (eg, pedicle fixation, dual rods with multiple hooks and sublaminar wires); 3 to 6 vertebral segments (List separately in addition to code for primary procedure)**

22843 **Posterior segmental instrumentation (eg, pedicle fixation, dual rods with multiple hooks and sublaminar wires); 7 to 12 vertebral segments (List separately in addition to code for primary procedure)**

22844 **Posterior segmental instrumentation (eg, pedicle fixation, dual rods with multiple hooks and sublaminar wires); 13 or more vertebral segments (List separately in addition to code for primary procedure)**

Posterior segmental spinal instrumentation is applied during a separately reportable arthrodesis (fusion) procedure on the spine. Spinal instrumentation is used to treat a deformity or instability of the spine. Posterior segmental fixation involves attaching the

fixation device to the top and bottom vertebral segments and at least one additional vertebral segment in between. Types of fixation include pedicle fixation across multiple interspaces and dual rods with multiple hooks and sublaminar wires. Pedicle fixation across multiple interspaces, also referred to as transpedicular fixation, involves inserting a screw in a posteroanteromedial direction through the pedicle into the vertebral body. This is performed across two or more interspaces (three or more vertebrae) and the screws are then secured to a plate or other fixator to provide stability. In dual rod fixation with multiple hooks and sublaminar wires, rods are placed on each side of the affected part of the spine and then fixed to each vertebral segment using hooks and/or sublaminar wires. Hooks may be fixed to the pedicle or lamina. If sublaminar wires are used, the wire loops are placed under the lamina of each vertebral segment and then around the rods and tightened. Use 22842 for posterior segmental instrumentation performed on 3 to 6 vertebral segments, 22843 for 7 to 12 vertebral segments, and 22844 for 13 or more vertebral segments.

22845-22847

22845 **Anterior instrumentation; 2 to 3 vertebral segments (List separately in addition to code for primary procedure)**

22846 **Anterior instrumentation; 4 to 7 vertebral segments (List separately in addition to code for primary procedure)**

22847 **Anterior instrumentation; 8 or more vertebral segments (List separately in addition to code for primary procedure)**

Anterior spinal instrumentation is applied during a separately reportable arthrodesis (fusion) procedure on the spine. Spinal instrumentation is used to treat a deformity or instability of the spine. Anterior spinal instrumentation is placed from the front of the body. Depending on the vertebral level, the access incision may be made in the front of the neck, the thorax, or the abdomen. Anterior instrumentation may also be placed from the side using an anterolateral approach. The appropriate approach is selected, overlying muscles are retracted, and blood vessels are retracted or ligated. The vertebrae are accessed, and prepared, with muscles stripped. Separately reportable discectomy may be performed. A single or dual rod is placed and attached to the spine segments using hooks and/or screws and/or separately reportable intervertebral cage devices. Cages, hooks, and screws may be stabilized using separately reportable bone graft(s). Bone graft material is tightly packed and compressed around the cages, hooks, and/or screws. Use 22845 when anterior instrumentation is applied to 2 to 3 vertebral segments, 22846 for 4 to 7 vertebral segments, and 22847 for 8 or more vertebral segments.

22848

22848 **Pelvic fixation (attachment of caudal end of instrumentation to pelvic bony structures) other than sacrum (List separately in addition to code for primary procedure)**

Pelvic fixation is performed by attachment of the caudal end of spinal instrumentation to pelvic bony structures other than the sacrum during a separately reportable spinal arthrodesis (fusion) procedure. Pelvic fixation may be performed to treat pelvic obliquity caused by scoliosis that prevents balanced postures for sitting and/or standing, or to provide additional stability following severe traumatic injury to the spine or radical procedures for treating spinal neoplasms. There are a number of different fixation devices including L-rod, S-rod, transiliac screws, iliosacral fixation, and iliac screws. The approach may be anterior, posterior, or combined anterior-posterior. After the appropriate approach is made, overlying muscles are retracted, and blood vessels are retracted or ligated. The appropriate pelvic fixation device is selected. Intraoperative halo-femoral traction may be applied to reduce pelvic obliquity in scoliosis patients. A halo traction device is applied to the skull and a femoral pin is placed. These traction devices are then weighted to provide distraction forces to straighten the spinal curvature and bring the higher iliac crest into better alignment with the lower iliac crest. The caudal end of the previously placed spinal instrumentation is then attached to rods and/or screws placed in the pelvis, usually the iliac bones. Separately reportable bone grafts may be used to stabilize the fixation device.

22849

22849 **Reinsertion of spinal fixation device**

This procedure is performed to reattach a device to the spine that has become dislodged.

22850

22850 **Removal of posterior nonsegmental instrumentation (eg, Harrington rod)**

The physician removes a metal device which is attached only at the top and bottom of the device from the spinal column.

22852

22852 **Removal of posterior segmental instrumentation**

The physician removes a metal device which is attached at the top, bottom, and various other places along the device from the spinal column.

● New Code   ▲ Revised Code

22853-22859

- 22853   Insertion of interbody biomechanical device(s) (eg, synthetic cage, mesh) with integral anterior instrumentation for device anchoring (eg, screws, flanges), when performed, to intervertebral disc space in conjunction with interbody arthrodesis, each interspace (List separately in addition to code for primary procedure)
- 22854   Insertion of intervertebral biomechanical device(s) (eg, synthetic cage, mesh) with integral anterior instrumentation for device anchoring (eg, screws, flanges), when performed, to vertebral corpectomy(ies) (vertebral body resection, partial or complete) defect, in conjunction with interbody arthrodesis, each contiguous defect (List separately in addition to code for primary procedure)
- 22859   Insertion of intervertebral biomechanical device(s) (eg, synthetic cage, mesh, methylmethacrylate) to intervertebral disc space or vertebral body defect without interbody arthrodesis, each contiguous defect (List separately in addition to code for primary procedure)

A procedure is performed to decompress the spinal cord and nerves and restore intervertebral disc space and anatomic alignment with insertion of an intervertebral biomechanical device. Surgical immobilization of the spine by fusing adjacent vertebrae (arthrodesis) and/or removing all or part of a vertebral body (corpectomy) may be done for degenerative disc disease, spinal stenosis, or bone spurs (osteophytes). The intervertebral biomechanical device is usually a cylindrical or square shaped synthetic cage or that can be packed with autogenous bone material to promote arthrodesis. For cervical placement, a horizontal incision is made in the side of the neck. The platysma muscle is transected, the plane between the sternocleidomastoid muscle and strap muscles is entered, and the space between the trachea/esophagus and the carotid sheath is accessed. The fascia is dissected away from the disc space. For lumbar placement, an incision is made in the left side of the abdomen and the muscles retracted. The peritoneum is kept intact and retracted to the side as are vascular structures such as the aorta and vena cava. For both approaches, all or part of the intervertebral disc may be removed in a separately reported procedure. The biomechanical device is placed into the intervertebral disc space (22853) or vertebral body defect (22854) in conjunction with interbody arthrodesis. Bone graft material may be inserted into the device, with integral anterior fixation of the device, if performed, accomplished using screws/flanges. Report code 22859 when an intervertebral device, such as a synthetic cage, mesh, or methylmethacrylate is inserted into the intervertebral disc space or vertebral body defect to maintain foraminal height or spinal cord/nerve decompression without arthrodesis, or fusing of adjacent vertebrae.

22855

22855   Removal of anterior instrumentation

The physician removes a metal instrument from the front of the spinal column.

22856-22858

22856   Total disc arthroplasty (artificial disc), anterior approach, including discectomy with end plate preparation (includes osteophytectomy for nerve root or spinal cord decompression and microdissection); single interspace, cervical

22858   Total disc arthroplasty (artificial disc), anterior approach, including discectomy with end plate preparation (includes osteophytectomy for nerve root or spinal cord decompression and microdissection); second level, cervical (List separately in addition to code for primary procedure)

A cervical total disc arthroplasty on a single interspace is performed via an anterior approach using an artificial disc with a discectomy with end plate preparation including osteophytectomy for nerve root or spinal cord decompression and microdissection. An artificial cervical disc is a prosthetic device that is inserted between two cervical vertebrae to replace a severely diseased or damaged cervical disc. Total disc arthroplasty using an artificial disc preserves motion at the disc space and is used as an alternative to spinal fusion which eliminates motion at that space. An incision is made in the front of the neck just off the midline of the spine. The esophagus is retracted. Nerves and arteries are identified and protected as the soft tissues of the neck are dissected and the spine is exposed. The intervertebral muscles are retracted and the diseased or damaged disc is identified. The disc is removed and the disc space is prepared for the artificial disc. The end plates above and below the disc space are milled and shaped to accommodate the artificial disc. Tension is applied to the vertebral bodies above and below the disc space to open the space allowing placement of the artificial disc. The disc is then inserted and the two metal plates that surround the polyurethane core and saline cushion are pressed into the prepared bony end plates. Tension is released from the vertebral bodies above and below the artificial disc which compresses the disc and holds it in place. Following placement of the artificial disc, incisions are closed. A temporary drain may be placed. Use code 22858 to report a second cervical level that is treated in addition to the first interspace.

22857

22857   Total disc arthroplasty (artificial disc), anterior approach, including discectomy to prepare interspace (other than for decompression), single interspace, lumbar

Total disc arthroplasty is done for complete, artificial replacement of an extremely damaged or diseased intervertebral disc. This code reports an anterior approach through an abdominal incision to reach a lumbar vertebra. When the spinal column is reached, the intervertebral muscles are retracted and the target disc is identified using x-ray for confirmation. The pathogenic cartilaginous disc matter is cleaned out with a rongeur to prepare the intervertebral disc space for the artificial implant. There are different designs or types of artifical disc implants, but a common one used has two metal endplates with a convex, weight-bearing polyethylene insert. The metal endplates are inserted into the prepared disc space in a collapsed state; seated into the vertebrae above and below; then opened with distraction. The polyethylene, weight bearing disc material insert is then placed in the space and seated into the endplates by a snap-lock mechanism. When the total disc replacement is assembled, the wounds are closed and a drain is left in place. Code this code for a single, lumbar interspace.

22861

22861   Revision including replacement of total disc arthroplasty (artificial disc), anterior approach, single interspace; cervical

The physician revises a cervical total disc arthroplasty which may include replacement of the artificial disc using an anterior approach. Revision may be required due to pain, degenerative changes, or improper alignment of the spine at the treated or adjacent disc spaces. An incision is made in the front of the neck just off the midline of the spine. The esophagus is retracted. Nerves and arteries are identified and protected as the soft tissues of the neck are dissected and the spine exposed. The intervertebral muscles are retracted and the artificial disc exposed. The existing artificial disc is dissected off the end plates and removed. The amount of bone loss and damage to the vertebral bodies is evaluated. If a new disc can be placed, the disc space is prepared for a new artificial disc. The end plates above and below the disc space are milled and shaped to accommodate the new artificial disc. Tension is applied to the vertebral bodies above and below the disc space to open the space allowing placement of the artificial disc. The new artificial disc is inserted and the two metal plates that surround the polyurethane core and saline cushion are pressed into the prepared bony end plates taking care to ensure that a normal cervical lordotic curvature is maintained. Tension is released from the vertebral bodies above and below the artificial disc which compresses the artificial disc and holds it in place. Following placement of the new artificial disc, incisions are closed. A temporary drain may be placed.

22862

22862   Revision including replacement of total disc arthroplasty (artificial disc), anterior approach, single interspace; lumbar

The physician revises a cervical total disc arthroplasty, which includes replacement of an artificial disc through an incision in the abdomen. Revision may be required due to pain, degenerative changes, or improper alignment of the spine at the treated or adjacent disc spaces. The intervertebral muscles are retracted and the artificial disc exposed. The existing artificial disc is dissected off the end plates and removed. The amount of bone loss and damage to the vertebral bodies is evaluated. If a new disc can be placed, the disc space is prepared for a new artificial disc. The end plates above and below the disc space are milled and shaped to accommodate the new artificial disc. Tension is applied to the vertebral bodies above and below the disc space to open the space allowing placement of the artificial disc. The new artificial disc is inserted and the two metal plates that surround the polyurethane core and saline cushion are pressed into the prepared bony end plates taking care to ensure that normal curvature is present. When replacement is to be done, the failed implant or component is removed and the interspace is explored and prepared for insertion of another prosthesis or component, which is seated into position. The fascia and muscle tissue are repaired and the wound is closed with a drain left in place.

22864

22864   Removal of total disc arthroplasty (artificial disc), anterior approach, single interspace; cervical

The physician removes a cervical artificial disc at a single interspace using an anterior approach. An incision is made in the front of the neck just off the midline of the spine. The esophagus is retracted. Nerves and arteries are identified and protected as the soft tissues of the neck are dissected and the spine exposed. The intervertebral muscles are retracted and the artificial disc exposed. The existing artificial disc is dissected off the end plates and removed. The amount of bone loss and damage to the vertebral bodies is evaluated. Following removal of the artificial disc, additional separately reportable procedures are performed as needed to stabilize the cervical spine. A temporary drain may be placed.

Musculoskeletal System

22865

22865 Removal of total disc arthroplasty (artificial disc), anterior approach, single interspace; lumbar

A previously placed, artificial total disc arthroplasty is removed from a single, lumbar interspace by anterior approach. An incision is made in the abdomen and muscle and tissue are retracted to reach the spinal column. The artificial disc implant is located. Adhesions and fibrous tissue are freed and distraction is applied to open the intervertebral space. The implant is unseated from its position between the vertebrae above and below and removed. The space is explored and debrided. Muscle and tissue is closed in position for wound repair.

22867-22868

● **22867** Insertion of interlaminar/interspinous process stabilization/distraction device, without fusion, including image guidance when performed, with open decompression, lumbar; single level

● **22868** Insertion of interlaminar/interspinous process stabilization/distraction device, without fusion, including image guidance when performed, with open decompression, lumbar; second level (List separately in addition to code for primary procedure)

A procedure is performed to insert one or more interlaminar/interspinous process implant(s) or spacer(s) to stabilize and/or open the neural foramen of the lumbar spine and decompress the spinal nerves. Interlaminar devices are implanted adjacent to the lamina and have 2 sets of wings that are placed around the inferior and superior spinous processes to restrict movement. Interspinous spacers are small devices implanted between the vertebral spinous processes and then expanded to relieve pressure on a nerve(s). These devices may be used in adults with spinal stenosis who have pain and/or neurogenic claudication. A small incision is made over the targeted lumbar disc(s) and carried down through the subcutaneous tissue. Dissection continues through the dorsolumbar fascia lateral to the midline and the multifidus is detached. The supraspinous ligaments attached to the fascia are preserved and the ligamentum flavum is elevated and resected. The superior and inferior laminae are partially resected. The exiting and transversing nerve roots are decompressed using a microscope if necessary. Partial facetectomies and foraminal decompression may be performed using a rongeur and/or drill. Incrementally sized dilators are inserted across the intraspinous space close to the posterior border of the facet joint. A sizing instrument is inserted and the appropriate device is inserted between the spinous processes as anterior to the intralaminar space as possible. The device is secured with screws. Drains may be placed before closure. Code 22867 reports the insertion of interlaminar/interspinous process stabilization/distraction device at a single level of the lumbar spine, with open decompression but without fusion, including image guidance when performed. Code 22868 reports additional device insertion at a second level of the lumbar spine.

22869-22870

● **22869** Insertion of interlaminar/interspinous process stabilization/distraction device, without open decompression or fusion, including image guidance when performed, lumbar; single level

● **22870** Insertion of interlaminar/interspinous process stabilization/distraction device, without open decompression or fusion, including image guidance when performed, lumbar; second level (List separately in addition to code for primary procedure)

A procedure is performed to insert one or more interlaminar/interspinous implant(s) or spacer(s) to stabilize and/or distract (open) the neural foramen of the lumbar spine. Interlaminar devices are implanted adjacent to the lamina and have 2 sets of wings that are placed around the inferior and superior spinous processes to restrict movement. Interspinous spacers are small devices implanted between the vertebral spinous processes and then expanded to relieve pressure on a nerve(s). These devices may be used in adults with spinal stenosis who have pain and/or neurogenic claudication. A small incision is made over the targeted lumbar disc(s) and carried down through the subcutaneous tissue. Dissection continues through the dorsolumbar fascia lateral to the midline and the multifidus is detached. The supraspinous ligaments attached to the fascia are preserved and the ligamentum flavum is elevated and resected. The superior and inferior laminae are partially resected. Incrementally sized dilators are inserted across the intraspinous space close to the posterior border of the facet joint. A sizing instrument is inserted and the appropriate device is inserted between the spinous processes as anterior to the intralaminar space as possible. The device is secured with screws. Drains may be placed before closure. Code 22869 reports the insertion of interlaminar/interspinous process stabilization/distraction device at a single level of the lumbar spine, without open decompression or fusion, including image guidance when performed. Code 22870 reports additional device insertion at a second level of the lumbar spine.

22900-22903

22900 Excision, tumor, soft tissue of abdominal wall, subfascial (eg, intramuscular); less than 5 cm

22901 Excision, tumor, soft tissue of abdominal wall, subfascial (eg, intramuscular); 5 cm or greater

22902 Excision, tumor, soft tissue of abdominal wall, subcutaneous; less than 3 cm

22903 Excision, tumor, soft tissue of abdominal wall, subcutaneous; 3 cm or greater

Soft tissues include subcutaneous fat and connective tissue, fascia, muscles, tendons, blood vessels, lymph vessels, nerves, and tissues surrounding the joints. Soft tissue tumors may be benign or malignant. Benign tumors are typically treated by excision, although small malignant or indeterminate tumors, may be excised if the margins are well defined. Depending on the location of the tumor in the soft tissue of the abdominal wall, the skin over the tumor may be incised or a skin flap created and elevated to allow exposure of the tumor. Overlying tissue is dissected and the soft tissue mass exposed. The tumor is then excised along with a margin of healthy tissue. Separately reportable frozen section may be performed to ensure that all margins are free of tumor cells. Drains are placed as needed and the surgical wound is closed in layers. For tumors in the subcutaneous fat or connective tissue, use 22902 for a mass less than 3 cm and 22903 for a mass 3 cm or greater. For tumors that lie below the fascia, use 22900 for a mass less than 5 cm and 22901 for a mass 5 cm or greater. Subfascial soft tissue tumors include those within muscle tissue.

22904-22905

22904 Radical resection of tumor (eg, sarcoma), soft tissue of abdominal wall; less than 5 cm

22905 Radical resection of tumor (eg, sarcoma), soft tissue of abdominal wall; 5 cm or greater

Soft tissues include muscles, tendons, fat, blood vessels, lymph vessels, nerves, and tissues surrounding the joints. Soft tissue tumors may be benign or malignant. Radical resection is typically performed for a malignant neoplasm, such as a sarcoma, although benign tumors and tumors of indeterminate nature may also require radical resection. A skin incision is made over the tumor in the abdominal wall or a skin flap created and elevated. Overlying subcutaneous and soft tissues are dissected and the soft tissue tumor exposed. The tumor is removed en bloc along with a wide margin of surrounding tissue. Radical resection involves excision of all involved soft tissue which may include muscles, nerves, and blood vessels. Separately reportable frozen section is performed to ensure that all margins are free of tumor cells. If margins show evidence of malignancy, additional tissue is removed until all margins are free of tumor cells. Drains are placed as needed. The surgical wound may be closed in layers, or separately reportable reconstructive procedures performed. Use 22904 for radical resection of a tumor less than 5 cm, and 22905 for a tumor 5 cm or greater.

23000

23000 Removal of subdeltoid calcareous deposits, open

Open removal of one or more subdeltoid calcareous deposits is performed. The skin over the shoulder is incised and the subdeltoid region is exposed through a deltoid incision. A synovectomy of the bursal floor is performed. The calcium deposits typically found in the supraspinatous tendon are located. The tendon is incised and the calcium deposits are removed. Soft, paste-like deposits are removed by milking the calcium deposit from the tendon with the help of a curette. Hard deposits are scraped from the tendon using a curette. The procedure continues until all calcium deposits have been found and removed.

23020

23020 Capsular contracture release (eg, Sever type procedure)

A capsular contracture release, such as a Sever type procedure, is performed on the shoulder. An incision is made in the deltopectoral interval. The clavipectoral fascia is exposed and divided vertically just lateral to the conjoined tendon. Dissection is extended up to the coracoacromial ligament. The subscapularis tendon and lesser tuberosity of the humerus are exposed. The fascia is then divided in a proximal direction just lateral to the coracoids. The incision is extended distally to the level of the anterior circumflex artery. The musculocutaneous and axillary nerves are identified and protected. The deltoid muscle and coracobrachialis are retracted. Scar tissue is divided in the anterior capsule just below the supraspinatus tendon of the biceps with dissection carried down to the superior border of the subscapularis tendon. With the arm in adduction, external rotation is tested and then tested again with the arm in abduction. The glenoid capsule is divided as needed. The shoulder is manipulated to increase range of motion. Internal rotation is tested and if range of motion is inadequate, a posterior capsular release is performed. Gentle manipulation may also be used to increase range of motion. Once optimal range of motion has been achieved, the surgical site is irrigated and incisions are closed.

23030-23031

23030 Incision and drainage, shoulder area; deep abscess or hematoma
23031 Incision and drainage, shoulder area; infected bursa

An incision and drainage of a deep abscess or hematoma in the shoulder area is performed. The soft tissues of the shoulder area are those overlying the clavicle, scapula, humeral head and neck. The approach is dictated by the location of the abscess or hematoma. The soft tissues are dissected and the pocket of pus or blood located. The wall of the abscess or hematoma is incised and the pus or blood drained. A large abscess may require probing of the pus pocket to break down loculations and ensure that all infection has been drained. The abscess or hematoma site is then flushed with antibiotic and/or normal saline solution. The pocket may be left open to drain, packed with gauze, or closed. In 23031, an incision and drainage of an infected bursa is performed. The infected bursa is incised and the fluid drained. The bursal sac may be flushed with antibiotic and/or normal saline solution prior to closure.

Incision and drainage, shoulder area

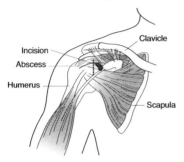

Deep abscess or hematoma (23030), infected bursa (23031)

23035

23035 Incision, bone cortex (eg, osteomyelitis or bone abscess), shoulder area

An incision of the bone cortex of the shoulder is performed for osteomyelitis or a bone abscess. Bones of the shoulder area include the clavicle, scapula, humeral head and neck. An incision is made in the skin and carried down through the soft tissue overlying the site of the osteomyelitis or bone abscess. The periosteum over the lesion is elevated, a button of cortical bone is removed, and the bone marrow is exposed. If frank pus is encountered, the button hole may be enlarged and extended using a chisel or gouge along the bone for one to two inches. If the epiphysis is involved, a section of the epiphyseal cortex may be removed. The bone abscess is drained.

23040-23044

23040 Arthrotomy, glenohumeral joint, including exploration, drainage, or removal of foreign body
23044 Arthrotomy, acromioclavicular, sternoclavicular joint, including exploration, drainage, or removal of foreign body

There are three joints in the shoulders. The glenohumeral joint is a shallow ball and socket type joint formed by the glenoid fossa of the scapula and the head of the humerus. The sternoclavicular joint is the medial articulation between the sternum and clavicle. The acromioclavicular joint is the lateral articulation between the acromion in the scapula and clavicle. In 23040, an open exploration of the glenohumeral joint is performed. Using an anterior approach, a skin incision is made over the deltoid and pectoral muscles. The muscles are divided and the the scapularis tendon is split to expose the glenohumeral joint capsule. The joint capsule is incised and the glenohumeral joint is explored. If infection is present, fluid, blood and purulent material is drained. Any loculations are broken up using blunt dissection. The joint is flushed with sterile saline or antibiotic solution using pulsed lavage to clear debris. If a foreign body is contained within the joint it is located and removed. Drains are placed and the incision closed around the drains. In 23044, an open exploration of the sternoclavicular or acromioclavicular joint is performed. The approach depends on which joint is being explored. Once the joint capsule has been exposed, it is incised and the joint explored. If an infection is present, fluid, blood and purulent material is drained. Any loculations are broken up using blunt dissection. The joint is flushed with sterile saline or antibiotic solution using pulsed lavage to clear debris. If a foreign body is contained within the joint it is located and removed. Drains are placed and the incision closed around the drains.

23065-23066

23065 Biopsy, soft tissue of shoulder area; superficial
23066 Biopsy, soft tissue of shoulder area; deep

Soft tissue biopsy of the shoulder area is performed. Soft tissues include muscles, tendons, fat, blood vessels, lymph vessels, nerves, and tissues surrounding the joints. Local, regional, or general anesthesia or conscious sedation is administered depending on the site and depth of the planned biopsy. The area over the planned biopsy site is cleansed. An incision is made and tissue dissected down to the mass or lesion taking care to protect blood vessels and nerves. A tissue sample is obtained and sent to the laboratory for separately reportable histological evaluation. The incision is closed with sutures. Use 23065 for a superficial biopsy or 23066 for biopsy of deeper tissues requiring more extensive dissection of overlying tissues.

23071-23076

23071 Excision, tumor, soft tissue of shoulder area, subcutaneous; 3 cm or greater
23073 Excision, tumor, soft tissue of shoulder area, subfascial (eg, intramuscular); 5 cm or greater
23075 Excision, tumor, soft tissue of shoulder area, subcutaneous; less than 3 cm
23076 Excision, tumor, soft tissue of shoulder area, subfascial (eg, intramuscular); less than 5 cm

Soft tissues include subcutaneous fat and connective tissue, fascia, muscles, tendons, blood vessels, lymph vessels, nerves, and tissues surrounding the joints. Soft tissue tumors may be benign or malignant. Benign tumors are typically treated by excision, although small malignant or indeterminate tumors may be excised if the margins are well defined. Depending on the location of the tumor in the soft tissue of the shoulder area, the skin over the tumor may be incised or a skin flap created and elevated. Overlying tissue is dissected and the soft tissue mass exposed. The tumor is then excised along with a margin of healthy tissue. Separately reportable frozen section may be performed to ensure that all margins are free of tumor cells. Drains are placed as needed and the surgical wound is closed in layers. For tumors in the subcutaneous fat or connective tissue, use 23075 for a mass less than 3 cm and 23071 for a mass 3 cm or greater. For tumors that lie below the fascia, use 23076 for a mass less than 5 cm and 23073 for a mass 5 cm or greater. Subfascial soft tissue tumors include those within muscle tissue.

23077-23078

23077 Radical resection of tumor (eg, sarcoma), soft tissue of shoulder area; less than 5 cm
23078 Radical resection of tumor (eg, sarcoma), soft tissue of shoulder area; 5 cm or greater

Soft tissues include muscles, tendons, fat, blood vessels, lymph vessels, nerves, and tissues surrounding the joints. Soft tissue tumors may be benign or malignant. Radical resection is typically performed for a malignant neoplasm, such as a sarcoma, although benign tumors and tumors of indeterminate nature may also require radical resection. A skin incision is made over the tumor in the shoulder area or a skin flap created and elevated. Overlying tissue is dissected and the tumor exposed. The tumor is removed en bloc along with a wide margin of surrounding tissue. Radical resection involves excision of all involved soft tissue which may include muscles, nerves, and blood vessels. Separately reportable frozen section is performed to ensure that all margins are free of tumor cells. If margins show evidence of malignancy, additional tissue is removed until all margins are free of tumor cells. Drains are placed as needed. The surgical wound may be closed in layers, or separately reportable reconstructive procedures performed. Use 23077 for radical resection of a tumor less than 5 cm; use 23078 for a tumor 5 cm or greater.

23100-23101

23100 Arthrotomy, glenohumeral joint, including biopsy
23101 Arthrotomy, acromioclavicular joint or sternoclavicular joint, including biopsy and/or excision of torn cartilage

There are three joints in the shoulders. The glenohumeral joint is a shallow ball and socket type joint formed by the glenoid fossa of the scapula and the head of the humerus. The sternoclavicular joint is the medial articulation between the sternum and clavicle. The acromioclavicular joint is the lateral articulation between the acromion in the scapula and clavicle. In 23100, an open biopsy of the glenohumeral joint is performed. Using an anterior approach, a skin incision is made over the deltoid and pectoral muscles. The muscles are divided and the scapularis tendon is split to expose the glenohumeral joint capsule. The joint capsule is incised and the glenohumeral joint is explored for evidence of disease, injury, or other abnormalities. Tissue samples are obtained from the joint cavity and sent for separately reportable laboratory analysis. Following completion of the procedure, the incisions are closed, and a dressing is applied. In 23101, an open exploration of the sternoclavicular or acromioclavicular joint is performed. The approach depends on which joint is being explored. Once the joint capsule has been exposed, it is incised and the joint explored for disease, injuries, or other abnormalities. Tissue samples are obtained from the joint cavity and sent for separately reportable laboratory analysis.

Musculoskeletal System

● New Code   ▲ Revised Code

Torn cartilage is excised as needed. Following completion of the procedure, the incisions are closed, and a dressing is applied.

23105-23106

23105   **Arthrotomy; glenohumeral joint, with synovectomy, with or without biopsy**
23106   **Arthrotomy; sternoclavicular joint, with synovectomy, with or without biopsy**

Synovial tissue lines the glenohumeral and sternoclavicular joints and produces synovial fluid. When synovial tissue becomes inflamed due to rheumatoid arthritis, synovial proliferative disorder, or other condition, the synovium produces excess synovial fluid resulting in joint effusion. In 23105, an open synovectomy of the glenohumeral joint is performed with or without biopsy. The glenohumeral joint is a shallow ball and socket type joint formed by the glenoid fossa of the scapula and the head of the humerus. Using an anterior approach, a skin incision is made over the deltoid and pectoral muscles. The muscles are divided and the scapularis tendon is split to expose the glenohumeral joint capsule. The joint capsule is incised and the glenohumeral joint is explored. Synovial tissue samples are obtained from the joint cavity as needed and sent for separately reportable laboratory analysis. A motorized shaver is then used to remove the synovium. Care is taken to resect all inflamed synovial tissue without damaging underlying vascular or nervous tissue. The joint is flushed with saline to remove any debris. Following completion of the procedure, the incisions are closed, and a dressing is applied. In 23106, an open synovectomy of the sternoclavicular joint is performed. The sternoclavicular joint is the medial articulation between the sternum and clavicle. An incision is made over the sternoclavicular joint. Soft tissues are dissected and the joint capsule is exposed and incised. The joint explored for damage, disease or other abnormalities. Synovial issue samples are obtained as needed and sent for separately reportable laboratory analysis. Synovial tissue is then resected as described above. Following completion of the procedure, the incisions are closed, and a dressing is applied.

23107

23107   **Arthrotomy, glenohumeral joint, with joint exploration, with or without removal of loose or foreign body**

An open exploration of the glenohumeral joint is performed for the presence of disease, injury, or other conditions including loose or foreign bodies. The glenohumeral joint is a shallow ball and socket type joint formed by the glenoid fossa of the scapula and the head of the humerus. Using an anterior approach, a skin incision is made over the deltoid and pectoral muscles. The muscles are divided and the scapularis tendon is split to expose the glenohumeral joint capsule. The joint capsule is incised and the joint is explored. The joint is flushed with normal saline to remove any debris. The humeral head and glenoid fossa are examined for osteochondral defects. Any fraying or instability of the anterior and posterior labrum is evaluated. The anterior joint capsule and subscapularis and glenohumeral ligaments are examined for tears, adhesions, or fraying. The biceps tendon is examined for tears, inflammation, or degenerative disease. Any tearing of the rotator cuff is evaluated. The supraspinatus and infraspinatus tendons are examined as is the subacromial space. The posterior aspect of the glenohumeral joint is then examined including the axillary pouch and posterior recess. Any loose or foreign bodies within the glenohumeral joint are located and removed. The joint is again flushed with normal saline. Following completion of the procedure, the incisions are closed, and a dressing is applied.

23120-23125

23120   **Claviculectomy; partial**
23125   **Claviculectomy; total**

An open partial or total excision of the clavicle is performed. In 23120, a partial claviculectomy is performed. Partial excision may be used to treat a number of conditions including tumor, infection, or vascular compromise. Partial distal claviculectomy, also referred to as a Mumford procedure, is performed to treat pain and loss of motion caused by arthritis or impingement at the acromioclavicular joint. A skin incision is made over the portion f the clavicle to be excised. Soft tissues are dissected and the clavicle exposed and the portion to be excised identified. A burr is used to divide the clavicle and the diseased portion is removed. If a Mumford procedure is performed, the anterior aspect of the acromion is resected using a stone-cutting burr to remove the articular surface. The underside of the acromion is smoothed with an end-cutting shaver. Next, the distal end of the clavicle is exposed and resected using a cutting burr. Approximately one to two cm at the distal end of the clavicle is excised to prevent contact between the articular surfaces of the acromion and the clavicle. In 23125, a total claviculectomy is performed for treatment of tumor, infection, nonunion, or vascular compromise. The entire clavicle is exposed and dissected free of all connective tissue including attachments at the acromioclavicular and sternoclavicular joints. The clavicle is removed in its entirety. Soft tissues are repaired. Drains are placed as needed and the incision closed in layers around the drains.

23130

23130   **Acromioplasty or acromionectomy, partial, with or without coracoacromial ligament release**

The physician performs a partial acromioplasty or acromionectomy with or without release of the coracoacromial ligament. An incision is made in the Langer's lines from the anterior edge of the acromion extending just lateral to the coracoid process of the scapula. The deltoid muscle is split beginning approximately 5 cm distal to the acromioclavicular joint in the direction of its fibers. The undersurface of the anterior aspect of the acromion is shaved. The deltoid is dissected off the anterior aspect of the acromion and the acromioclavicular joint capsule taking care to preserve the stump of the deltoid's tendinous origin. A wedge-shaped piece of bone is then resected from the underside of the acromion. The coracoacromial ligament is released as needed from its attachment on the acromion. The deltoid muscle is then repaired by reattaching it to the acromioclavicular joint capsule, the trapezius, and its tendon of origin.

23140-23146

23140   **Excision or curettage of bone cyst or benign tumor of clavicle or scapula**
23145   **Excision or curettage of bone cyst or benign tumor of clavicle or scapula; with autograft (includes obtaining graft)**
23146   **Excision or curettage of bone cyst or benign tumor of clavicle or scapula; with allograft**

A bone cyst is a fluid filled space within the bone. One common type is a unicameral or simple bone cyst, which is a benign lesion. A less common type is an aneurysmal bone cyst which consists of vascular tissue surrounding a blood filled cystic lesion. There are a number of different types of benign bone tumors including giant cell tumors, chondromixoid fibromas, and enchondromas. In 23140, an incision is made in the skin over the site of lesion in the clavicle or scapula. Soft tissues are dissected and the lesion is exposed. If a cystic lesion is present, the bone is incised and a bone window created to open the cyst. Fluid is aspirated and sent to the laboratory for separately reportable analysis. A curette is inserted through the bone window and the lining of the cystic cavity is completely removed by curettage. Alternatively, some cystic lesions and most benign tumors are treated by excision. The lesion is exposed as described above. The physician then excises the benign lesion along with a margin of surrounding healthy bone. In 23145, the lesion is curetted or excised as described above. The physician then obtains healthy bone locally or from a separate site, such as the iliac crest. The bone autograft is packed into the defect in the proximal humerus. In 23146, the lesion is curetted or excised as described above. The defect is then packed with donor bone (allograft).

23150-23156

23150   **Excision or curettage of bone cyst or benign tumor of proximal humerus**
23155   **Excision or curettage of bone cyst or benign tumor of proximal humerus; with autograft (includes obtaining graft)**
23156   **Excision or curettage of bone cyst or benign tumor of proximal humerus; with allograft**

A bone cyst is a fluid filled space within the bone. One common type is a unicameral or simple bone cyst, which is a benign lesion. A less common type is an aneurysmal bone cyst which consists of vascular tissue surrounding a blood filled cystic lesion. There are a number of different types of benign bone tumors including giant cell tumors, chondromixoid fibromas, and enchondromas. In 23150, an incision is made in the skin over the site of lesion in the proximal humerus. Soft tissues are dissected and the lesion is exposed. If a cystic lesion is present, the bone is incised and a bone window created to open the cyst. Fluid is aspirated and sent to the laboratory for separately reportable analysis. A curette is inserted through the bone window and the lining of the cystic cavity is completely removed by curettage. Alternatively, some cystic lesions and most benign tumors are treated by excision. The lesion is exposed as described above. The physician then excises the benign lesion along with a margin of surrounding healthy bone. In 23155, the lesion is curetted or excised as described above. The physician then obtains healthy bone locally or from a separate site, such as the iliac crest. The bone autograft is packed into the defect in the proximal humerus. In 23156, the lesion is curetted or excised as described above. The defect is then packed with donor bone (allograft).

23170-23174

23170   **Sequestrectomy (eg, for osteomyelitis or bone abscess), clavicle**
23172   **Sequestrectomy (eg, for osteomyelitis or bone abscess), scapula**
23174   **Sequestrectomy (eg, for osteomyelitis or bone abscess), humeral head to surgical neck**

A sequestrectomy is performed for osteomyelitis or bone abscess of the clavicle (23170), scapula (23172), or humeral head to neck (23174). A sequestrum is a piece of necrotic bone that has become separated from healthy surrounding bone. An incision is made in the skin and carried down through the soft tissue overlying the site of the osteomyelitis or bone abscess. If the periosteum is soft and viable, it is elevated off the necrotic sequestrum. The necrotic bone is excised and the ribbon of periosteum that was elevated off the necrotic bone is then approximated over the cortical bone defect. If the periosteum is not viable

● New Code   ▲ Revised Code   CPT © 2016 American Medical Association. All Rights Reserved.   © 2017 DecisionHealth

and new bone, also referred to as involucrum, has formed around the sequestrum, the necrotic bone is removed leaving the involucrum which will form new bone in the cortical bone defect. The incisions in the soft tissue and skin are closed and a dressing applied.

23180-23184

23180 **Partial excision (craterization, saucerization, or diaphysectomy) bone (eg, osteomyelitis), clavicle**

23182 **Partial excision (craterization, saucerization, or diaphysectomy) bone (eg, osteomyelitis), scapula**

23184 **Partial excision (craterization, saucerization, or diaphysectomy) bone (eg, osteomyelitis), proximal humerus**

The physician performs a partial excision of bone, also referred to as craterization, saucerization, or diaphysectomy to treat osteomyelitis of the clavicle (23180), scapula (23182), or proximal humerus (23184). Craterization and saucerization of bone involves removing infected and necrotic bone to form a shallow depression in the bone surface that will allow drainage from the infected area. Diaphysectomy involves removal of the infected portion of the shaft of a long bone. An incision is made in the skin and carried down through the soft tissue overlying the site of the osteomyelitis. Any soft tissue sinus tracts and devitalized soft tissue are resected. The area of necrotic and infected bone is exposed. A series of drill holes are made in the necrotic and infected bone and the bone between the drill holes is excavated to create an oval window using an osteotome. The amount of bone removed is dependent on the extent of the infection. A curette may be used to remove devitalized tissue from the medullary canal. Debridement continues until punctate bleeding is identified in the exposed bony surface. When all devitalized and infected tissue has been removed, the wound is copiously irrigated with sterile saline or antibiotic solution. The surgical wound is loosely closed and a drain placed.

23190

23190 **Ostectomy of scapula, partial (eg, superior medial angle)**

Partial ostectomy of the scapula is performed to treat pain, deformity, lesion, or other disease of the bone. One common site of resection is the superior medial angle. A skin incision is made in the upper aspect of the back over the affected scapula. Soft tissues are dissected and the site of deformity or lesion in the scapula is exposed. Diseased bone or bony overgrowth is then excised and sent for separately reportable pathology exam. The remaining bone is smoothed and overlying soft tissues and skin are closed in layers.

23195

23195 **Resection, humeral head**

A skin incision is made over the shoulder joint to resect bone of the humeral head. Dissection is carried down through soft tissues and the joint capsule is exposed and opened. The humeral head is dislocated from the shoulder joint and inspected. The humeral head is then removed. The remaining bone edges are smoothed. The bone is then positioned in the shoulder socket and soft tissue structures are secured to the bone to maintain the humerus in the joint socket. The joint capsule is closed and overlying soft tissue and skin are closed in layers.

23200

23200 **Radical resection of tumor; clavicle**

Radical resection is typically performed for a malignant neoplasm although benign tumors and tumors of indeterminate nature may also require radical resection. A skin incision is made over the tumor in the clavicle or a skin flap created and elevated. Overlying tissue is dissected and the tumor exposed. All bone and cartilage in the clavicle with tumor involvement is resected. The tumor is removed en bloc along with a wide margin of surrounding tissue. Radical resection of bone includes excision of all involved soft tissue which may include muscles, tendons, fat, blood vessels, lymph vessels, nerves, and tissues surrounding the joints. Separately reportable frozen section is performed to ensure that all margins are free of tumor cells. If margins show evidence of malignancy, additional tissue is removed until all margins are free of tumor cells. Drains are placed as needed. The surgical wound may be closed in layers or separately reportable reconstructive procedures performed.

23210

23210 **Radical resection of tumor; scapula**

Radical resection is typically performed for a malignant neoplasm although benign tumors and tumors of indeterminate nature may also require radical resection. A skin incision is made over the tumor in the scapula or a skin flap created and elevated. Overlying tissue is dissected and the tumor exposed. All bone and cartilage in the scapula with tumor involvement is resected. The tumor is removed en bloc along with a wide margin of surrounding tissue. Radical resection of bone includes excision of all involved soft tissue which may include muscles, tendons, fat, blood vessels, lymph vessels, nerves, and tissues surrounding the joints. Separately reportable frozen section is performed to ensure that all margins are free of tumor cells. If margins show evidence of malignancy, additional tissue is removed until all margins are free of tumor cells. Drains are placed as needed. The

surgical wound may be closed in layers, or separately reportable reconstructive procedures performed.

23220

23220 **Radical resection of tumor, proximal humerus**

Radical resection is typically performed for a malignant neoplasm although benign tumors and tumors of indeterminate nature may also require radical resection. A skin incision is made over the tumor in the proximal humerus or a skin flap created and elevated. Overlying tissue is dissected and the tumor exposed. All bone and cartilage in the proximal humerus with tumor involvement is resected. The tumor is removed en bloc along with a wide margin of surrounding tissue. Radical resection of bone includes excision of all involved soft tissue which may include muscles, tendons, fat, blood vessels, lymph vessels, nerves, and tissues surrounding the joints. Separately reportable frozen section is performed to ensure that all margins are free of tumor cells. If margins show evidence of malignancy, additional tissue is removed until all margins are free of tumor cells. Drains are placed as needed. The surgical wound may be closed in layers, or separately reportable reconstructive procedures performed.

23330

23330 **Removal of foreign body, shoulder; subcutaneous**

A subcutaneous foreign body in the shoulder area is removed. Subcutaneous tissue refers to the fat and connective tissue that lies between the overlying dermis and underlying muscle fascia. The foreign body is located by palpation or separately reportable radiographs. A straight or elliptical incision is made in the skin. The subcutaneous tissue is dissected and the foreign body identified. A hemostat or grasping forceps is then used to remove the foreign body. Alternatively, the physician may need to dissect tissue around the foreign body to remove it. The wound is then flushed with normal saline or antiobiotic solution and the incision is closed with sutures.

23333

23333 **Removal of foreign body, shoulder; deep (subfascial or intramuscular)**

Deep tissue refers to the tissue below the muscle fascia (subfascial) or within the muscle itself (intramuscular). The foreign body is located by palpation or separately reportable radiographs. A straight or elliptical incision is made in the skin over the site of the foreign body. Dissection is carried down through soft tissues and into the deeper subfascial or intramuscular tissue and the foreign body is located. A hemostat or grasping forceps is then used to remove the foreign body. Alternatively, the physician may need to dissect tissues around the foreign body in order to remove it. The wound is then flushed with normal saline or antibiotic solution and the operative wound is closed in layers.

23334-23335

23334 **Removal of prosthesis, includes debridement and synovectomy when performed; humeral or glenoid component**

23335 **Removal of prosthesis, includes debridement and synovectomy when performed; humeral and glenoid components (eg, total shoulder)**

A skin incision is made over the shoulder joint to remove components of a previously placed shoulder prosthesis. Dissection is carried down through soft tissues and the joint capsule is exposed and opened. The humeral head or prosthesis is dislocated and the shoulder joint structures are inspected. In 23334, a hemiprosthesis (partial joint replacement) is removed by carefully freeing the component from the humerus or the glenoid cavity. Bone cement used to secure the prosthesis is also removed. Bony surfaces are smoothed. A new prosthesis may be placed in a separately reportable procedure or in the case of an infection, a drain may be placed and soft tissues closed around the drain. In 23335, a total shoulder prosthesis is removed. This is performed in the same manner described above except that both components (glenoid and humeral) are removed.

23350

23350 **Injection procedure for shoulder arthrography or enhanced CT/MRI shoulder arthrography**

An injection procedure for shoulder arthrography is performed. The skin over the injection site is cleansed and a local anesthetic is injected. A needle may be inserted into the joint and fluid aspirated with a syringe. The radiopaque substance is then injected into the shoulder joint, usually under fluoroscopic guidance and the joint is exercised to help distribute the radiopaque substance. Once the contrast has been distributed throughout the joint, separately reportable radiographic images are obtained, or computed tomography or magnetic resonance imaging techniques may be used.

23395-23397

23395 **Muscle transfer, any type, shoulder or upper arm; single**

23397 **Muscle transfer, any type, shoulder or upper arm; multiple**

Muscle transfer is typically performed to stabilize the shoulder and/or restore function. There are a number of techniques available, including local transfer of one of the existing shoulder muscles to a new site, or free transfer of an expendable muscle, such as the

Musculoskeletal System

gracilis muscle in the thigh. A skin incision is made over the shoulder and the injured or atrophied shoulder muscle is identified. The muscle is excised. If a local muscle is transferred, existing bony attachments are severed and the muscle is reattached at the new site. If a free transfer is performed, a separate incision is made over the muscle to be harvested. The muscle is excised along with its nerve and blood supply in a separately reportable procedure. The muscle is then trimmed as needed and sutured to bones of the shoulder, or in some cases, to the ribs in a manner that stabilizes the joint and/or allows re-innervation of the muscle and restoration of motion. In 23395, a single muscle transfer is performed on the shoulder or upper arm. In 23397, multiple muscle transfers are performed.

23400

23400   Scapulopexy (eg, Sprengels deformity or for paralysis)

The scapula is fixed to the underlying ribs using internal fixation in cases of paralysis or deformity. An incision is made along the medial aspect of the scapula through skin and subcutaneous tissue. The trapezius muscle is exposed. The supraspinatus and infraspinatus muscles are elevated off the scapula and the body of the scapula is exposed. The lateral trapezius muscle is incised as needed to expose the supraspinatus fossa. The scapula is elevated and tension is placed on the rhomboid insertions at the medial border of the scapula. The rhomboids are then detached from the scapula and the subscapularis is separated from the ventral aspect of the scapula and the subscapularis bursa is exposed. The serratus posterior is elevated and the third, fourth, fifth, and sixth ribs are exposed. Subperiosteal dissection is performed to separate the inferior border of the ribs from neurovascular bundles and from the parietal pleura. A small amount of cortical bone is removed from the dorsal aspect of the ribs and the ventral aspect of the scapula. Wires are then passed under each exposed rib. A reconstruction plate is placed at the infraspinatus fossa along the medial aspect of the scapula. Drill holes are then made in the body of the scapula and the previously placed wires are pulled through the holes to secure the scapula to the ribs. Overlying muscle is repaired followed by layered closure of subcutaneous tissue and skin.

23405-23406

23405   Tenotomy, shoulder area; single tendon
23406   Tenotomy, shoulder area; multiple tendons through same incision

A tendon problem in the shoulder such as an injury, tendinitis, or a superior labrum tear, also referred to as a SLAP (superior labrum anterior to posterior) tear, is treated using tenotomy. An incision is made in the skin of the shoulder overlying the tendon or tendons that are to be incised and severed or released. Soft tissues are dissected and the tendon is exposed. The tendon is then incised and severed or released close to the bony attachment site. Bleeding is controlled with electrocautery. This may be repeated on additional tendons of the shoulder. Following completion of the procedure, the operative wound is closed in layers. Use 23405 for tenotomy of a single tendon. Use 23406 if multiple tendons are released through the same incision.

23410-23412

23410   Repair of ruptured musculotendinous cuff (eg, rotator cuff) open; acute
23412   Repair of ruptured musculotendinous cuff (eg, rotator cuff) open; chronic

The physician performs an open repair of a ruptured musculotendinous cuff, also referred to as the rotator cuff, of the shoulder. The rotator cuff is a group of muscles and tendons in the shoulder that control shoulder joint motion. This group of muscles and tendons includes the supraspinatus, infraspinatus, subscapularis, and teres minor. The tendons of these muscles fuse together to form the rotator cuff and attach on the humeral head. An incision is made over the shoulder joint and the rotator cuff is exposed. The underside of the acromion is inspected, smoothed, and flattened as needed using a motorized burr and shaver. The rotator cuff is visualized and the size and pattern of the tear evaluated. Thin or fragmented portions of the rotator cuff are removed. If the defect is repaired by direct tendon to tendon repair, the proximal and distal portions of the ruptured tendon are sutured together. Large defects may require tendon mobilization or advancement of tendon flaps. If a tendon to bone repair is required, the site where the rotator cuff will be reattached to bone is debrided. Side-to-side stitches may be used to initiate closure of a large rotator cuff defect. Next, sutures are passed through the tendon ends and secured. Metallic anchors with sutures are then placed in the humerus at the site where the tendon will be reattached. The anchors are recessed below the bone surface with only the sutures exposed. The sutures are passed through the tendon and tied pulling the tendon down to the prepared bone surface. When the procedure is complete, the incision is closed and a dressing is applied. Use code 23410 for repair of an acute rupture of the rotator cuff and code 23412 for repair of a chronic rotator cuff injury.

23415

23415   Coracoacromial ligament release, with or without acromioplasty

The coracoacromial ligament attaches to the corocoid process on the anterior aspect of the scapula and acromion process on the posterior scapula and helps to stabilize the shoulder joint. A skin incision is made in the superior aspect of the shoulder joint over

the coracoacromial ligament. Soft tissues are dissected and the ligament is exposed. The shoulder joint is explored and impingement of the rotator cuff against the edge of the acromion at the attachment of the coracoacromial ligament is confirmed. The ligament is released by detaching it from the undersurface of the acromion. The ligament is debrided with a shaver. The undersurface of the acromion is inspected to determine whether an acromioplasty is required. If needed, acromioplasty is accomplished by smoothing the undersurface of the acromion with an end-cutting motorized shaver. A burr is then used to remove any remaining ligament fibers and define the anterolateral acromial surface. The surgical site is flushed with sterile saline and incisions are closed in layers.

23420

23420   Reconstruction of complete shoulder (rotator) cuff avulsion, chronic (includes acromioplasty)

The rotator cuff is a group of muscles and tendons in the shoulder that control shoulder joint motion. This group of muscles and tendons includes the supraspinatus, infraspinatus, subscapularis, and teres minor. The tendons of these muscles fuse to form the rotator cuff and attach on the humeral head. An incision is made over the shoulder joint. Soft tissue is dissected and the joint capsule is exposed and incised. Joint structures are inspected. An acromioplasty is performed first by flattening and smoothing the underside using a motorized burr and shaver. The rotator cuff is inspected and the size and pattern of the tear is evaluated. Thin or fragmented portions of the rotator cuff are removed. The defect is reconstructed using direct tendon to tendon repair which involves suturing the proximal and distal portions of the ruptured tendon together. Large defects may require tendon mobilization or advancement of tendon flaps. If a tendon to bone repair is required, the site where the rotator cuff will be reattached to bone is debrided. Side-to-side stitches may be used to initiate closure of a large rotator cuff defect. Sutures are then passed through the ends of the tendons. Metallic anchors with sutures are then placed in the humerus at the site where the tendon will be reattached. The anchors are recessed below the bone surface with only the sutures exposed. The sutures are passed through the tendon and tied pulling the tendon down to the prepared bone surface. The joint is flushed with sterile saline, incisions are closed, and a dressing is applied.

23430

23430   Tenodesis of long tendon of biceps

Biceps tenodesis is performed to treat a tear of the long head of the biceps or to relieve tendonitis. The biceps brachii muscle, more commonly referred to simply as the biceps, has two attachments, also referred to as origins, at the shoulder. The long head of the biceps attaches at the supraglenoid tubercle of the scapula. The short head attaches at the coracoid process of the scapula. To perform tenodesis of the long head, the tendon is detached from the scapula and then transferred and secured to the humerus. An incision is made over the shoulder joint. Soft tissue is dissected and the joint capsule is exposed and incised. Joint structures are inspected. The long head of the biceps is identified and detached from the scapula. Damaged tissue is debrided. The bicipital groove in the humerus is evaluated and if it is flattened, it is deepened using a burr. Two bone anchors are placed in the bicipital groove. Sutures are placed through the long head of the biceps and affixed to the bone anchors in the bicipital groove. Alternatively, a bone tunnel may be created through the humerus and the biceps tendon pulled through the tunnel and affixed using a screw. The joint is flushed with sterile saline, incisions are closed, and a dressing is applied.

23440

23440   Resection or transplantation of long tendon of biceps

Resection or transplantation of the long head of the biceps is performed to treat a tear or to relieve tendonitis. The biceps brachii muscle, more commonly referred to simply as the biceps, has two attachments, also referred to as origins, at the shoulder. The long head of the biceps attaches at the supraglenoid tubercle of the scapula. The short head attaches at the coracoid process of the scapula. An incision is made over the anterior aspect of the shoulder joint. Soft tissue is dissected and the extra-articular aspect of the long head of the biceps is identified and detached from the scapula. If the long head of the biceps is severely damaged, it may be detached from the scapula and completely excised, leaving the biceps attached at the shoulder by the short head only. Alternatively, the long head may be transplanted to another site in the shoulder. The damaged tissue may be debrided or a portion of the long head excised. The joint capsule is exposed and incised as needed. Joint structures are inspected. The transplant site in the shoulder is identified and the bone is prepared. The tendon is then attached using bone anchors and sutures, a bone tunnel with screw fixation, or an alternative technique. The joint is flushed with sterile saline, incisions are closed, and a dressing is applied.

23450

23450   Capsulorrhaphy, anterior; Putti-Platt procedure or Magnuson type operation

An anterior repair of the shoulder capsule is performed to treat instability of the glenohumeral joint and recurrent anterior dislocation of the shoulder. In the Putti-Platt procedure, the subscapularis tendon is shortened to bring the head of the humerus closer to the shoulder blade. The subscapularis muscle has its origin on the subscapular fossa of the scapula and inserts on the anterior aspect of the humerus at the lesser tubercle. The subscapularis tendon fuses with other tendons to form the shoulder joint capsule. An incision is made over the anterior aspect of the shoulder joint. Soft tissue is dissected; the joint capsule is opened; and the insertion of the subscapularis tendon on the lesser tubercle is exposed. The subscapularis tendon is detached from the humerus and divided longitudinally in the midportion. The lateral free end is attached to the anterior rim of the glenoid and the medial free end is sutured over the lateral end. The effect is to shorten and tighten the subscapularis tendon. The Magnuson procedure is performed in a similar fashion except that the subscapularis is detached from the lesser tuberosity and reattached just lateral to the bicipital groove. This produces a tendon sling that helps to hold the humeral head in the glenohumeral joint.

23455

23455   Capsulorrhaphy, anterior; with labral repair (eg, Bankart procedure)

An anterior repair of the shoulder capsule is performed to treat instability of the glenohumeral joint and recurrent anterior dislocation of the shoulder. In the Bankart procedure, a detachment of the anterior joint capsule from the fibro-cartilaginous glenoid ligament, also called a Bankart lesion, is repaired. An incision is made over the anterior aspect of the shoulder joint. The deltopectoral groove is dissected and the cephalic vein is exposed and protected. The coracoid process is excised with an osteotome allowing the attached coracobrachialis and short head of the biceps to retract inferiorly. The subscapularis is exposed and separated from the joint capsule. A vertical incision is made in the suscapularis lateral to the glenoid rim and lateral and medial flaps are created. The humeral head is retracted. The labrum is trimmed and repaired as needed. The rim of the glenoid and anterior neck of the scapula are smoothed using an osteotome. Three holes are drilled in the anterior glenoid rim. A suture is passed through each hole and then through the lateral capsular flap. The sutures are tied, securing the lateral flap to the anterior glenoid rim. The same sutures are then used to tie down the medial capsular flap over the lateral flap. The subscapularis is then reattached to the lesser tuberosity. The coracoid is anchored using sutures at its base. Overlying tissues are closed in layers and a dressing is applied.

23460-23462

23460   Capsulorrhaphy, anterior, any type; with bone block
23462   Capsulorrhaphy, anterior, any type; with coracoid process transfer

An anterior repair of the shoulder capsule is performed to treat instability of the glenohumeral joint and recurrent anterior dislocation of the shoulder. The technique used to repair the glenohumeral joint structures depends on the nature of the injury. Repair of the anterior capsule can be divided into anatomic and nonanatomic repairs. In anatomic repairs, the shoulder structure that has been damaged or disrupted is repaired. In nonanatomic repairs, shoulder structures are shortened and/or tightened to stabilize the joint and prevent dislocation. In 23460, any type of repair is performed using a bone block, also referred to as a bone graft. An incision is made over the anterior aspect of the shoulder joint. Soft tissues are dissected and the joint capsule is exposed and opened. The injury is repaired by shortening and/or tightening the subscapularis or by repairing the joint structures. The area of bone requiring the bone graft is prepared. An autograft is harvested or an allograft is obtained from the bone bank. The bone is then configured and placed into the defect. Soft structures are closed over the joint and the skin is closed in layers. In 23462, any type of repair is performed with coracoid process transfer. The procedure is performed as described above except that at the beginning of the procedure, the coracoid process is excised with an osteotome. After the joint structures are repaired, the coracoid process, along with the attached coracobrachialis and short head of the biceps, is transferred to another site to provide more stability to the shoulder joint. The coracoid is anchored using sutures at its base. Overlying tissues are closed in layers and a dressing is applied.

23465

23465   Capsulorrhaphy, glenohumeral joint, posterior, with or without bone block

A posterior repair of the glenohumeral joint capsule is performed to treat posterior instability and recurrent posterior dislocation of the shoulder joint. Posterior dislocation occurs less frequently than anterior dislocation and typically involves subacromial dislocation of the humeral head, but may also involve subglenoid or subspinous dislocation. A number of surgical techniques are used, depending on whether the condition being treated is a simple posterior dislocation, chronic locked dislocation, or chronic posterior instability. Using a reverse Bankart technique, a skin incision is made posteriorly beginning at the posterolateral border of the acromion and extending to the axilla. Blunt dissection is carried down through the deltoid and then through the infraspinatus and teres minor interval. The joint capsule is opened and the joint structures are exposed. The humeral head is retracted and the posterior rim of the glenoid is exposed. A bone block harvested from the acromion or iliac crest may be used to reshape the glenoid. An osteotomy is performed from the supraglenoid tubercle to the origin of the long triceps tendon. The bone block (graft) is then wedged into the osteotomy site. Suture anchors are placed in the glenoid rim and sutures are used to repair the capsule. Overlying tendons

and muscles are closed in layers, followed by layered closure of subcutaneous tissue and skin. The Neer technique uses the same approach, followed by division of the infraspinatus in an oblique fashion. The joint capsule is incised lateral to the greater tuberosity in a T-shaped configuration, and superior and inferior flaps are created. The humeral neck is prepared with a curette or burr and the superior flap is pulled down and reattached on the humeral neck. The inferior flap is pulled backward and upward over the superior flap and secured. The capsular flaps are reinforced using the superficial infraspinatus tendon which is sutured to the scapula. The deeper aspect of the infraspinatus tendon is sutured over the superficial aspect to preserve external rotation of the shoulder. The Rockwood technique uses the same approach with a vertical incision through the infraspinatus tendon. The joint capsule is incised vertically between the humerus and glenoid, and medial and lateral flaps are created. The medial flap is advanced superiorly and laterally and secured. The lateral flap is placed over the medial repair.

23466

23466   Capsulorrhaphy, glenohumeral joint, any type multi-directional instability

The physician sutures a wound to the rear of the shoulder joint to repair any type of instability in the shoulder joint.

23470-23472

23470   Arthroplasty, glenohumeral joint; hemiarthroplasty
23472   Arthroplasty, glenohumeral joint; total shoulder (glenoid and proximal humeral replacement (eg, total shoulder))

A hemiarthroplasty of the glenohumeral joint involves placement of a prosthetic humeral head, while a total shoulder arthroplasty involves prosthetic replacement of both the glenoid and the humeral head. A deltopectoral approach is used to expose the shoulder joint. The deltopectoral interval and cephalic vein are identified. The conjoint tendon is retracted medially. The subscapularis tendon is incised and the joint capsule is opened. In 23470, the humeral head is exposed and subscapularis attachments on the proximal humeral head are released. The humeral head is dislocated. The arm is externally rotated. The humeral head is cut and removed using an oscillating saw. Any osteophytes on the remaining humeral head are excised. A template is used to size the excised portion of the humeral head. A pilot hole is created in the humeral shaft followed by reaming to the desired width and depth. A trial prosthetic stem and head are then inserted and the joint is reduced. Range of motion is evaluated. The joint is dislocated and the trial implant is removed. The anterior humeral neck is drilled and sutures are placed. The permanent implant is inserted and secured with sutures and bone cement as needed. The subscapularis tendon is secured to the humeral neck. The rotator interval is closed. A suction drain is placed and the deltopectoral interval is closed around the drain. In 23472, the shoulder joint is exposed and the humeral head is removed as described above. The glenoid surface is also prepared by shaving. The prosthetic components are then sized. The humeral head is replaced as described above. The glenoid surface is replaced with a plastic socket which is cemented into the scapula. Closure of the surgical wound is performed as described above.

23473-23474

23473   Revision of total shoulder arthroplasty, including allograft when performed; humeral or glenoid component
23474   Revision of total shoulder arthroplasty, including allograft when performed; humeral and glenoid component

Revision of a total shoulder arthroplasty may be required when there is loosening of the humeral and/or glenoid components. The glenoid component may also require revision if there is severe rotator cuff insufficiency or glenoid bone deficiency. Infection and periprosthetic fracture of the humerus are also indications for revision. A deltopectoral approach is used to expose the shoulder joint. The deltopectoral interval and cephalic vein are identified. The conjoint tendon is retracted medially. Scar tissue is released from surrounding structures; the subscapularis tendon is incised; and the joint capsule is opened. In some patients, the subscapularis may be lengthened using a Z-shaped incision. If the humeral component requires revision, the prosthetic humeral head is exposed and removed as needed. A new humeral head is then placed, or the existing humeral head is repositioned and secured using a press-fit technique or cement, depending on the type of component used. If the glenoid component requires revision, it is removed or repositioned and secured with cement. A bone allograft may also be prepared and placed to repair any bone defects and ensure a secure fit of the glenoid and/or humeral components. The subscapularis tendon is secured to the humeral neck. The rotator interval is closed. A suction drain is placed and the deltopectoral interval is closed around the drain. Use code 23473 when revision arthroplasty is performed on only one component, glenoid or humeral. Use 23474 when revision arthroplasty is performed on both the glenoid and humeral components.

Musculoskeletal System

23480-23485

23480 Osteotomy, clavicle, with or without internal fixation

23485 Osteotomy, clavicle, with or without internal fixation; with bone graft for nonunion or malunion (includes obtaining graft and/or necessary fixation)

An osteotomy of the clavicle is performed to treat a number of conditions including chronic dislocation of the sternoclavicular joint and malunion or nonunion of the clavicle. The location of the osteotomy depends on the condition being treated. In 23480, the procedure is performed without bone grafting. A skin incision is made over the planned osteotomy site on the clavicle. The clavicle is exposed and drill holes are created at the lateral and medial aspects of the planned osteotomy site. A horizontal bone cut is made between the two drill holes. A vertical cut is made at the inferomedial and superolateral aspects of the horizontal cut to form a Z-osteotomy. The clavicle is then lengthened by sliding the cut edges apart. Holes are drilled on each site of the lateral cuts and sutures are threaded through the holes to secure the bones. Alternatively, the cut edges may be secured using screws, a plate and screw device, or another internal fixation device. In 23485, an osteotomy is performed as described above with bone grafting for malunion or nonunion. Bone is harvested locally or from a separate site such as the iliac crest. The clavicle is prepared for grafting. The bone graft is configured and placed at the site of the malunion or nonunion. The surgical wound is closed in layers and a dressing is applied.

23490-23491

23490 Prophylactic treatment (nailing, pinning, plating or wiring) with or without methylmethacrylate; clavicle

23491 Prophylactic treatment (nailing, pinning, plating or wiring) with or without methylmethacrylate; proximal humerus

Prophylactic treatment of the clavicle or proximal humerus is performed to provide additional strength and support to the bone in cases of osteoporosis or osteolytic disease such as that caused by bone metastases. The bone may be reinforced by a variety of techniques. Placement of pins or screws can be performed using a percutaneous technique. A small skin incision is made over the planned screw insertion site. Using radiographic guidance, one or more pins or screws are placed through the clavicle or proximal humerus. A hollow cannulated screw may be placed that allows injection of bone cement (methylmethacrylate) through the screw into the clavicle or proximal humerus. Alternatively, the bone may be drilled and bone cement injected directly into the bone. If plate and screw or wire cerclage is used, an incision is made over the clavicle or proximal humerus. The bone is exposed. Internal fixation devices are then placed to provide support for the damaged bone. Layered closure of the operative wound is then performed. Use 23490 for prophylactic pinning, wiring, plating, or nailing of the clavicle and 23491 for the proximal humerus including injection of methylmethacrylate, when used.

23500-23505

23500 Closed treatment of clavicular fracture; without manipulation

23505 Closed treatment of clavicular fracture; with manipulation

Closed treatment of a fracture of the clavicle is performed. Separately reportable radiographs are obtained to confirm the fracture. In 23500, a nondisplaced fracture of the clavicle is evaluated. A neurovascular exam is performed to ensure that the nerves and blood vessels at the site of the injury are intact. No manipulation of the fracture fragments is required. A figure-of-eight splint may be applied to immobilize the fracture site. In 23505, a minimally displaced fracture of the clavicle is evaluated. The displaced fracture fragments are manually reduced (manipulated) back to proper anatomic alignment. Separately reportable radiographs are obtained to confirm anatomic reduction. The fracture is immobilized using a figure-of-eight splint or other immobilization device.

23515

23515 Open treatment of clavicular fracture, includes internal fixation, when performed

An open reduction of a clavicular fracture is performed including any necessary internal fixation. An incision is made over the fracture site and the fracture ends are debrided and placed in anatomical alignment. If internal fixation is required, a guide pin is passed medially into the clavicle using fluoroscopic guidance and overdrilled to fit the appropriate length screw. The guide pin is removed from the medial clavicle, passed into the lateral clavicle, and overdrilled in the same fashion to fit the appropriate screw length. The guide pin is directed out the back of the clavicle, the drill is attached, and the pin is redirected through the full length of the clavicle. A cannulated screw and washer are placed from the back of the clavicle down the center for internal fixation. Alternatively, a reconstruction locking plate, clavicle hook, or multiple screws may be placed to maintain alignment of the fracture ends.

23520-23525

23520 Closed treatment of sternoclavicular dislocation; without manipulation

23525 Closed treatment of sternoclavicular dislocation; with manipulation

The physician treats a dislocation of the joint between the clavicle and the sternum. In 23520, the shoulder is placed in a sling for stabilization. In 23525, the bone is

manipulated back into position manually or with traction. This procedure can be used to treat a one time dislocation or recurrent dislocation of the joint.

23520-23525

23520 Closed treatment of sternoclavicular dislocation; without manipulation

23525 Closed treatment of sternoclavicular dislocation; with manipulation

The physician treats a dislocation of the joint between the clavicle and the sternum. In 23520, the shoulder is placed in a sling for stabilization. In 23525, the bone is manipulated back into position manually or with traction. This procedure can be used to treat a one time dislocation or recurrent dislocation of the joint.

23530-23532

23530 Open treatment of sternoclavicular dislocation, acute or chronic

23532 Open treatment of sternoclavicular dislocation, acute or chronic; with fascial graft (includes obtaining graft)

The sternoclavicular joint (SCJ) is a saddle-type joint that allows the clavicle to move in nearly all planes, most importantly providing the ability to thrust the arm and shoulder forward. About half of the medial clavicle articulates with the manubrium, which is the upper portion of the sternum. The strength and stability of the SCJ is dependent on the integrity of the joint capsule and supporting ligaments. There are several open reduction techniques for dislocation. A skin incision is made over the SCJ and overlying soft tissue structures are dissected. The joint capsule is exposed. In 23530, the dislocation is reduced and stabilized as needed using sutures. The joint capsule is incised. Two holes are drilled in the medial aspect of the clavicle and another two holes are drilled in the lateral aspect of the manubrium. Sutures are then passed through the clavicle and the manubrium and secured. Alternatively, the clavicle may be secured to the first rib by wrapping the two structures with suture material. In 23532, a fascial graft is used to stabilize the SCJ. The SCJ is exposed as described above and the clavicle and manubrium are drilled in the same manner. A section of the fascia lata is harvested from the thigh and fashioned into a graft. The fascial graft is then passed through the drill holes and secured with sutures or it is wrapped around the clavicle and first rib and secured. Range of motion is tested. Surgical wounds are closed in layers.

23540-23545

23540 Closed treatment of acromioclavicular dislocation; without manipulation

23545 Closed treatment of acromioclavicular dislocation; with manipulation

Closed treatment of an acromioclavicular (AC) dislocation, also referred to as an AC separation or separated shoulder, is performed. The AC joint is a cartilaginous joint with a fibrocartilaginous meniscal disc between the hyaline cartilage of the articular surfaces of the acromial process and clavicle. The joint is stabilized by muscles and ligaments. AC joint dislocations typically occur due to a traumatic event such as a direct blow to the shoulder or a fall on an outstretched hand that disrupts the muscles and ligaments. Separately reportable radiographs are obtained to confirm dislocation. In 23540, the AC dislocation is treated without manipulation using pain medication, anti-inflammatory drugs, and activity modification. Range of motion may be limited using a sling. In 23545, a minimally displaced AC dislocation is manually reduced (manipulated) into anatomic alignment. A second set of radiographs may be obtained to confirm anatomic alignment. A sling is applied and the patient is instructed as to any limitations on activity. Pain medication and anti-inflammatory drugs are prescribed as needed.

23550-23552

23550 Open treatment of acromioclavicular dislocation, acute or chronic

23552 Open treatment of acromioclavicular dislocation, acute or chronic; with fascial graft (includes obtaining graft)

Open treatment of an acute or chronic acromioclavicular (AC) dislocation, also referred to as an AC separation or shoulder separation, is performed. The AC joint is a cartilaginous joint with a fibrocartilaginous meniscal disc between the hyaline cartilage of the articular surfaces of the acromial process and clavicle. The joint is stabilized by muscles and ligaments. AC joint dislocations typically occur due to traumatic event such as a direct blow to the shoulder or a fall on an outstretched hand that disrupts the muscles and ligaments. Separately reportable radiographs are obtained to confirm dislocation. In 23550, an incision is made over the AC joint. The AC articulation is debrided. The torn deltotrapezial fascia is repaired. A bioabsorbable or nonbioabsorbable device may be used to stabilize the joint such as a screw placed through the clavicle and into the coracoid base or a pin placed through the acromion across the AC joint and down the clavicle. Alternatively the coracoacromial ligament may be repositioned over the AC joint to stabilize it. In 23552, a fascial graft is used to stabilize the joint. A strip of fascia is harvested and configured as needed to stabilize the joint. The arm is placed in a sling and the patient is instructed as to any limitations on activity.

23570-23575

23570   Closed treatment of scapular fracture; without manipulation
23575   Closed treatment of scapular fracture; with manipulation, with or without skeletal traction (with or without shoulder joint involvement)

Closed treatment of a fracture of the scapula is performed. Separately reportable radiographs are obtained to confirm the fracture. In 23570, a nondisplaced fracture of the scapula is evaluated. A neurovascular exam is performed to ensure that the nerves and blood vessels at the site of the injury are intact. No manipulation of the fracture fragments is required. The arm may be placed in a sling to immobilize the shoulder until the fracture heals. In 23575, a minimally displaced fracture of the scapula with or without involvement of the shoulder joint is treated with manipulation with or without skeletal traction. The displaced fracture fragments are manually reduced (manipulated) back to proper anatomic alignment. Separately reportable radiographs are obtained to confirm anatomic reduction. The fracture site is immobilized by placing the arm in a sling. For severely comminuted fractures overhead skeletal traction may be used to immobilize the fracture. This is accomplished using a pin inserted into the proximal ulna at the olecranon and applying weighted skeletal traction.

23585

23585   Open treatment of scapular fracture (body, glenoid or acromion) includes internal fixation, when performed

Open treatment of a fracture of the body, glenoid, or acromion of the scapula is performed with or without internal fixation. Separately reportable radiographs are obtained to confirm the fracture. The approach depends on the site and type of scapular fracture: anterior rim fractures are approached anteriorly with the patient in beach chair position; posterior fractures are approached posteriorly or with a combined posterosuperior approach. The most common approach is posterior with an incision extending over the lateral third of the scapular spine to the lateral tip of the acromion and then distally in a midlateral line. The deltoid muscle is dissected off the scapular spine and the acromion and then split. The infraspinatus and teres minor musculotendinous units are exposed and the deltoid is retracted to the level of the inferior margin of the teres minor. The infraspinatus tendon is incised and dissected off the posterior glenohumeral capsule. The glenohumeral joint capsule is opened and the humeral head is retracted to expose the glenoid cavity. The fracture fragments are reduced. If internal fixation is required, temporary K-wire or screw fixation is applied and anatomic alignment of the fracture fragments is confirmed radiographically. Permanent internal fixation such as an interfragmentary compression screw or contoured reconstruction plate is then applied as needed. The shoulder is immobilized by placing the arm in a sling.

23600-23605

23600   Closed treatment of proximal humeral (surgical or anatomical neck) fracture; without manipulation
23605   Closed treatment of proximal humeral (surgical or anatomical neck) fracture; with manipulation, with or without skeletal traction

Closed treatment of a fracture of the surgical or anatomical neck of the proximal humerus is performed. Separately reportable radiographs are obtained to confirm the fracture. In 23600, a nondisplaced proximal humerus fracture is evaluated. No manipulation of the fracture fragments is required. A splint or cast may be applied to immobilize the fracture site. In 23605, a minimally displaced fracture of the proximal humerus is evaluated. The displaced fracture fragments are manually reduced (manipulated) back to proper anatomic alignment. Separately reportable radiographs are obtained to confirm anatomic reduction. The fracture may be immobilized using a splint or cast.

23615

23615   Open treatment of proximal humeral (surgical or anatomical neck) fracture, includes internal fixation, when performed, includes repair of tuberosity(s), when performed

An open reduction of a proximal fracture of the humeral neck, either surgical or anatomical, is performed with repair of tuberosity(s), if needed, and any necessary internal fixation. Accessing the fracture may require detaching the deltoid muscle from the clavicle by creating an osteoperiosteal flap lateral to the acromion. The fracture ends and bone fragments are debrided and placed in anatomical alignment. If internal fixation is required, pins, screws, wires, and/or a plate may be used to maintain alignment of the bone fragments. The technique and fixation devices vary depending on the configuration of the fracture. Screw tension band technique may be used to repair proximal humeral fractures involving the lesser and greater tuberosity. A cancellous lag screw is inserted from the shaft up into the head of the humerus and positioned just below the subchondral bone. Figure of eight tension band wiring is then passed around the rotator cuff origin on the greater tuberosity to a drill hole in the humeral shaft. A second wire is then passed through both the lesser and greater tuberosities. Another technique involves insertion of a T or L dynamic compression (DC) plate. The plate is placed on the anterolateral surface of the humerus, just anterior to the deltoid insertion. Cancellous screws are placed in the proximal fragment and cortical screws in the shaft. Lag screws are then inserted from the proximal

fragment to the distal shaft. Any tuberosity fragments are incorporated into the fixation device or fixed with tension band wiring.

23616

23616   Open treatment of proximal humeral (surgical or anatomical neck) fracture, includes internal fixation, when performed, includes repair of tuberosity(s), when performed; with proximal humeral prosthetic replacement

An open reduction of a proximal fracture of the humeral neck, either surgical or anatomical, is performed with proximal humeral prosthetic replacement, including repair of tuberosity(s) as needed and any necessary internal fixation. An incision is made over the fracture site and the long head of the biceps is identified and tagged, and a tenotomy is performed. The fracture line is exposed and four mattress sutures are placed around the greater tuberosity at the bone-tendon junction of the infraspinatus and teres minor tendons. Stay sutures are placed around the lesser tuberosity at the subscapularis bone-tendon junction. The tuberosities are retracted and the greater tuberosity is measured. The origin of the long head of the biceps is excised and the humeral head bone fragment is removed. The humeral head is measured and a properly sized prosthesis is selected. A bone graft is procured from the bone fragments and the medullary canal of the humeral shaft is prepared for the prosthesis by reaming. A properly sized prosthesis is then selected and placed into the medullary canal to test the fit. Care is taken to ensure that the normal humeral height is recreated. Drill holes are placed in the proximal humeral shaft and sutures are placed in the drill holes in preparation for tuberosity fixation. The stem of the humeral prosthesis is then cemented into place. The lesser and greater tuberosities are reconstructed and fixed to the shaft, to the prosthesis, and to each other. A bone graft is placed in the window of the fracture prosthesis under the greater tuberosity and under the medial edge of the prosthetic head. Two of the previously placed mattress sutures are passed around the prosthetic neck and tied down. The other two previously placed mattress sutures are passed around the humeral neck, through the subscapularis tendon, and tied down. Tension band sutures are placed through the humeral shaft to create vertical tension on the osteosynthesis complex. The rotator cuff is repaired and the biceps tendon is reattached.

23620-23625

23620   Closed treatment of greater humeral tuberosity fracture; without manipulation
23625   Closed treatment of greater humeral tuberosity fracture; with manipulation

Closed treatment of a fracture of a greater humeral tuberosity is performed. Separately reportable radiographs are obtained to confirm the fracture. In 23620, a nondisplaced greater humeral tuberosity fracture is evaluated. No manipulation of the fracture fragments is required. A splint or cast may be applied to immobilize the fracture site. In 23625, a minimally displaced fracture of the greater humeral tuberosity is evaluated. The displaced fracture fragments are manually reduced (manipulated) back to proper anatomic alignment. Separately reportable radiographs are obtained to confirm anatomic reduction. The fracture may be immobilized using a splint or cast.

23630

23630   Open treatment of greater humeral tuberosity fracture, includes internal fixation, when performed

An open reduction of an isolated fracture of the greater tuberosity of the humerus is performed including any necessary internal fixation. Isolated, displaced fractures of the greater humeral tuberosity are rare and are usually accompanied by rotator cuff tears between the supraspinatus and subscapularis tendons. The approach is dictated by the nature of the injury. Small fractures resulting from avulsion of the supraspinatus tendon are usually repaired by an anterosuperior approach. Alternatively, an incision is made over the anterior or anteroinferior shoulder. The deltoid muscle is split by peeling it off the posterior acromion. The greater tuberosity is exposed and the fracture site is identified. The fracture site is debrided and the fragment is positioned in anatomical alignment. The greater tuberosity fragment may be secured using heavy nonabsorbable sutures. If internal fixation is required, wire or cancellous lag screws with washers may be applied. Exposure by a deltopectoral approach may be required for larger fractures to allow for placement of drill holes and suture, wire, or screw fixation. Following repair of the fracture, any injury to the rotator cuff is repaired.

23650-23655

23650   Closed treatment of shoulder dislocation, with manipulation; without anesthesia
23655   Closed treatment of shoulder dislocation, with manipulation; requiring anesthesia

The physician performs closed reduction of a shoulder dislocation with manipulation. Shoulder dislocations are classified as anterior, posterior, or inferior depending on the direction of the dislocation. The exact manipulation technique used depends on the direction of the dislocation and physician preference. A combination of traction and/or coutertraction and internal and/or external rotation is employed to return the humeral head to normal anatomic position in the glenohumeral joint. Following reduction of the

Musculoskeletal System

shoulder dislocation, a neurovascular examination is performed and the shoulder is immobilized in a sling, swathe, or shoulder immobilizer. Use code 23650 when closed reduction of the shoulder dislocation is performed without anesthesia and code 23655 when anesthesia is required.

23660

23660   Open treatment of acute shoulder dislocation

The physician performs open reduction of an acute shoulder dislocation. Open reduction is typically performed when the shoulder dislocation is complicated by blood vessel and/or nerve injury or when multiple attempts at closed reduction fail. An incision is made over the shoulder joint. For open reduction of an anterior shoulder dislocation, the subscapularis and anterior joint capsule are incised near the insertion to the lesser tuberosity of the humerus. Lateral traction is applied and the humerus is then externally rotated to return the humeral head to normal anatomic alignment in the glenohumeral joint. Lateral traction is maintained and the humerus is internally rotated to verify that the humerus has passed by the anterior glenoid lip and into the glenoid fossa. For open reduction of a posterior shoulder dislocation, a deltopectoral approach, posterior approach, or a deltoid splitting approach may be used. The joint capsule is incised at the rotator interval and the humeral head is returned to normal anatomic position under direct vision. The stability of the reduction is evaluated by internal rotation of the shoulder. Incisions are closed and the shoulder is immobilized in a sling, swathe, or immobilizer.

23665

23665   Closed treatment of shoulder dislocation, with fracture of greater humeral tuberosity, with manipulation

Closed reduction of a shoulder dislocation with concomitant fracture of the greater humeral tuberosity is performed with manipulation. In this type of fracture-dislocation injury, the greater humeral tuberosity is fractured and displaced with retraction of the attached rotator cuff musculature, and the humeral head and lesser tuberosity are dislocated. The exact manipulation technique used depends on the direction of the dislocation and physician preference. A combination of traction and/or countertraction and internal and/or external rotation is employed to return the humeral head to normal anatomic alignment in the glenohumeral joint. Following reduction of the shoulder dislocation, radiographs are obtained and anatomic reduction of the dislocation is checked along with the position of fracture fragments of the greater humeral tuberosity. Additional manipulation of fracture fragments is performed as needed. Once anatomic alignment has been achieved, the shoulder is immobilized in a cast.

23670

23670   Open treatment of shoulder dislocation, with fracture of greater humeral tuberosity, includes internal fixation, when performed

An open reduction of a shoulder dislocation with a fracture of the greater tuberosity of the humerus is performed, including any necessary internal fixation. Fracture-dislocation of the greater humeral tuberosity involves displacement of the greater tuberosity with retraction of the attached rotator cuff musculature. The humeral head and lesser tuberosity are dislocated. Exposure by a deltopectoral approach is used. The clavipectoral fascia is divided. The subacromial, subdeltoid, and subcoracoid spaces are developed and the conjoint tendon is retracted. The axillary nerve is located and protected. The long head of the biceps tendon is located distally and followed to the rotator interval, which is opened. The displaced bone fragment containing the greater tuberosity is identified and sutures are placed at the bone-tendon junction. Drill holes may be placed in the humeral shaft with sutures passed through the drill holes to allow for additional figure-of-eight fixation. The humeral head and the attached lesser tuberosity are reduced and fixed with sutures or staples, or internal fixation, such as wire, plates, or screws. The greater tuberosity fracture is then reduced and fixed with sutures supplemented by the previously placed figure-of-eight sutures attached to the humeral shaft. Additional fixation with cancellous screws may be applied. Following repair of the fracture, any injury to the rotator cuff is repaired.

23675

23675   Closed treatment of shoulder dislocation, with surgical or anatomical neck fracture, with manipulation

Closed reduction of a shoulder dislocation with concomitant fracture of the surgical or anatomical neck of the humerus is performed. In this type of fracture-dislocation injury, the greater and lesser tuberosities remain attached to the humeral head which is dislocated, and the surgical or anatomical neck of the humerus is fractured. The exact manipulation technique used depends on the direction of the dislocation and physician preference. A combination of traction and/or countertraction and internal and/or external rotation is employed to return the humeral head to normal anatomic alignment in the glenohumeral joint. Following reduction of the shoulder dislocation, radiographs are obtained and anatomic reduction of the dislocation is checked along with the position of fracture fragments of the surgical or anatomical humeral neck. Additional manipulation of fracture fragments is performed as needed. Once anatomic alignment has been achieved, the shoulder is immobilized in a cast.

23680

23680   Open treatment of shoulder dislocation, with surgical or anatomical neck fracture, includes internal fixation, when performed

Open reduction of a shoulder dislocation with fracture of the surgical or anatomical neck of the humerus is done, including any necessary internal fixation. In surgical neck fracture-dislocations, the greater and lesser tuberosities remain attached to the humeral head. Exposure is by anterior superior or deltopectoral approach. The fracture-dislocation is reduced. A variety of fixation techniques may be used depending on the exact nature of the injury. Unstable oblique or spiral fractures may be fixed using a plate. Other techniques include the use of drill holes in the shaft below the fracture and placement of figure-of-eight sutures. Enders nails with tension suture or wire may also be used.

23700

23700   Manipulation under anesthesia, shoulder joint, including application of fixation apparatus (dislocation excluded)

The physician performs a manipulation of the shoulder joint under anesthesia including application of a fixation apparatus. This procedure is used primarily to treat frozen shoulder which is a condition characterized by thickening and contracture of the joint capsule. Following the administration of anesthesia, the shoulder is moved through a gentle range of motion to separate adhesions. When all adhesions have been separated and the shoulder can be moved through a complete range of motion, the shoulder may be injected with an anti-inflammatory and a local anesthetic. A sling or strapping may be applied. The patient is instructed on range of motion exercises as well as the need to resume physical therapy to maintain range of motion and prevent adhesions from recurring.

23800-23802

23800   Arthrodesis, glenohumeral joint
23802   Arthrodesis, glenohumeral joint; with autogenous graft (includes obtaining graft)

Arthrodesis of the shoulder involves fusion of the glenohumeral joint. A deltopectoral approach is used to expose the shoulder joint. The deltopectoral interval and cephalic vein are identified. The conjoint tendon is retracted medially. The subscapularis tendon is incised and the joint capsule is opened. The shoulder is dislocated. Cortical bone is removed from the joint surfaces of the acromion, glenoid fossa, and humeral head. If a bone autograft is used for the joint fusion, it is harvested locally or from a remote site such as the iliac crest. The bone graft is prepared and placed into the joint space. The humerus is returned to the joint socket. Because of the limited bony surface of the glenoid fossa, the humeral head is subluxated upward to bring it in contact with the acromion. The humerus is abducted; the arm is flexed; and the positioning is assessed before application of fixation devices. A plate is contoured to fit the patient and placed along the spine of the scapula over the acromion extending down on to the humeral shaft. The plate is secured with compression screws placed through the humeral head and into the glenoid fossa. Additional screws are placed as needed to secure the plate. The shoulder is immobilized using a shoulder spica cast. Use 23800 when the procedure is performed without autogenous bone graft. Use 23802 when an autogenous bone graft is used.

23900

23900   Interthoracoscapular amputation (forequarter)

The physician makes removes the shoulder blade, collar bone, and the arm, along with other soft tissue of the shoulder because of disease or injury.

23920-23921

23920   Disarticulation of shoulder
23921   Disarticulation of shoulder; secondary closure or scar revision

Disarticulation (amputation) of the arm at the shoulder is a rarely performed procedure typically limited to conditions such as extensive malignant neoplasms or severe trauma. In 23920, a subclavicular incision along the lateral third of the clavicle is made. The pectoralis major is dissected and a window is created between the pectoralis minor and subclavian muscles. The subclavian vein is exposed, suture ligated, and divided below the entry point of the cephalic vein. The subclavian artery is exposed, suture ligated, and divided at the exit point of the thoracoacromial artery. Alternatively, arteries and veins may be divided more distally at the time through the same incision used in the disarticulation procedure. A skin incision is made at the lateral edge of the pectoralis major and extended over the distal aspect of the deltoid muscle. A second axillary incision is then carried from anterior to posterior. Skin flaps are created. The deltoid, supraspinatus, and infraspinatus muscles are detached from the humerus. The long head of the biceps, long head of the triceps, and teres minor are severed. The pectoralis major is also detached from the humerus. The conjoint tendon and subscapularis are severed and the neurovascular bundle is exposed. The axillary nerve is identified and transected. Posterior structures are then severed, including the long head of the triceps, latissimus dorsi, and teres major muscles. Once the soft tissues and shoulder capsule are completely divided, the arm is removed. The remaining musculature is closed and the deltoid muscle is sutured over underlying musculature. Drains are placed as needed and skin flaps are sutured in place.

Musculoskeletal System

● New Code   ▲ Revised Code

In 23921, secondary closure or scar revision is performed at the site of a previous shoulder disarticulation procedure. Any necrotic or infected tissue is removed. If scar revision is required, scar tissue is excised. The amputation is then closed using grafts or flaps.

23930-23931

23930	**Incision and drainage, upper arm or elbow area; deep abscess or hematoma**
23931	**Incision and drainage, upper arm or elbow area; bursa**

An incision and drainage of a deep abscess or hematoma or an infected bursa is performed. In 23930, the soft tissues of the upper arm or elbow are incised and drained. The soft tissues in this area are those overlying the humeral shaft, distal humerus, and elbow joint. The approach is dictated by the location of the abscess or hematoma. The soft tissues are dissected and the pocket of pus or blood located. The wall of the abscess or hematoma is incised and the pus or blood drained. A large abscess may require probing of the pus pocket to break down loculations and ensure that all infection has been drained. The abscess or hematoma site is then flushed with antibiotic and/or normal saline solution. The pocket may be left open to drain, packed with gauze, or closed. In 23931, an incision and drainage of an infected bursa is performed. Bursa are sacs lined with synovial membrane that contain synovial fluid and are found in areas subject to friction such as prominent body parts, joints or areas where tendons pass over bone. The infected bursa is incised and the fluid drained. The bursal sac may be flushed with antibiotic and/or normal saline solution prior to closure.

23935

23935	**Incision, deep, with opening of bone cortex (eg, for osteomyelitis or bone abscess), humerus or elbow**

The bone cortex of the humeral shaft, distal humerus, radial head or neck or the olecranon process is opened to treat a condition such as osteomyelitis or bone abscess. An incision is made in the skin and carried down through the soft tissue overlying the site of the infected bone. The periosteum over the infected region of the bone is elevated, a button of cortical bone removed, and the bone marrow exposed. Opening the bone cortex relieves pressure caused by inflammation of the bone marrow and prevents restriction of blood flow to the infected bone. If frank pus is encountered, the button hole may be enlarged and extended using a chisel or gouge along the bone for one to two inches. If the epiphysis is involved, a section of the epiphyseal cortex may be removed. The bone abscess is drained.

24000

24000	**Arthrotomy, elbow, including exploration, drainage, or removal of foreign body**

An open exploration of the elbow joint is performed. The joint capsule is opened using a posterior, posterolateral, medial, or anterolateral approach and joint structures are examined. If joint effusion is present, the fluid is drained. If an infection is present, fluid, blood and purulent material is drained. Any loculations are broken up using blunt dissection. The joint is flushed with sterile saline or antibiotic solution using pulsed lavage to clear debris. If a foreign body is contained within the joint, it is located and removed. Drains are placed and the incision is closed around the drains.

24006

24006	**Arthrotomy of the elbow, with capsular excision for capsular release (separate procedure)**

Arthrotomy with excision of the joint capsule is performed to treat capsular contracture of the elbow joint. The joint capsule is exposed using a posterior, posterolateral, medial, or anterolateral approach, depending on the site and type of the contracture. For excision via a posterolateral approach, a proximal incision is made from the lateral supracondylar ridge to the lateral epicondyle and extended distally in a curvilinear fashion to the posterior border of the ulna. The anterior musculature is stripped and the anterior capsule is exposed. The extensor carpi radialis longus (ECRL) is retracted and elevated off the lateral epicondyle. The ECRL, brachioradialis, and brachialis are elevated off the joint capsule. The lateral collateral ligament (LCL) and ulnar nerve are identified and protected. The common extensor tendon is dissected off the LCL and joint capsule. The joint capsule is incised, elevated, and the contracted portion is excised. Range of motion is evaluated by flexing and extending the joint and turning the palm up and down. Additional dissection is performed as needed to free any adhesions that are compromising mobility. Following release of the capsular contracture, the surgical wound is repaired in a layers and dressings are applied.

24065-24066

24065	**Biopsy, soft tissue of upper arm or elbow area; superficial**
24066	**Biopsy, soft tissue of upper arm or elbow area; deep (subfascial or intramuscular)**

Soft tissue biopsy of the upper arm or elbow area is performed. Soft tissues include muscles, tendons, fat, blood vessels, lymph vessels, nerves, and tissues surrounding the joints. Local, regional, or general anesthesia or conscious sedation is administered depending on the site and depth of the planned biopsy. The skin over the biopsy site is cleansed. An incision is made and tissue dissected down to the mass or lesion taking care to protect blood vessels and nerves. A tissue sample is obtained and sent to the laboratory for separately reportable histological evaluation. The incision is closed with sutures. Use 24065 for a superficial biopsy or 24066 for biopsy of deeper tissues requiring more extensive dissection of overlying tissues.

24071-24076

24071	**Excision, tumor, soft tissue of upper arm or elbow area, subcutaneous; 3 cm or greater**
24073	**Excision, tumor, soft tissue of upper arm or elbow area, subfascial (eg, intramuscular); 5 cm or greater**
24075	**Excision, tumor, soft tissue of upper arm or elbow area, subcutaneous; less than 3 cm**
24076	**Excision, tumor, soft tissue of upper arm or elbow area, subfascial (eg, intramuscular); less than 5 cm**

Soft tissues include subcutaneous fat and connective tissue, fascia, muscles, tendons, blood vessels, lymph vessels, nerves, and tissues surrounding the joints. Soft tissue tumors may be benign or malignant. Benign tumors are typically treated by excision, although small malignant or indeterminate tumors may be excised if the margins are well defined. Depending on the location of the tumor in the soft tissue of the upper arm or elbow area, the skin over the tumor may be incised or a skin flap created and elevated. Overlying tissue is dissected and the soft tissue mass exposed. The tumor is then excised along with a margin of healthy tissue. Separately reportable frozen section may be performed to ensure that all margins are free of tumor cells. Drains are placed as needed and the surgical wound is closed in layers. For tumors in the subcutaneous fat or connective tissue, use 24075 for excision of less than 3 cm and 24071 for excision of 3 cm or greater. For tumors that lie below the fascia, use 24076 for excision of less than 5 cm and 24073 for excision of 5 cm or greater. Subfascial soft tissue tumors include those within muscle tissue.

24077-24079

24077	**Radical resection of tumor (eg, sarcoma), soft tissue of upper arm or elbow area; less than 5 cm**
24079	**Radical resection of tumor (eg, sarcoma), soft tissue of upper arm or elbow area; 5 cm or greater**

Soft tissues include muscles, tendons, fat, blood vessels, lymph vessels, nerves, and tissues surrounding the joints. Soft tissue tumors may be benign or malignant. Radical resection is typically performed for a malignant neoplasm, such as a sarcoma, although benign tumors and tumors of indeterminate nature may also require radical resection. A skin incision is made over the tumor in the upper arm or elbow area or a skin flap is created and elevated. Overlying tissue is dissected and the tumor exposed. The tumor is removed en bloc along with a wide margin of surrounding tissue. Radical resection involves excision of all involved soft tissue which may include muscles, nerves, and blood vessels. Separately reportable frozen section is performed to ensure that all margins are free of tumor cells. If margins show evidence of malignancy, additional tissue is removed until all margins are free of tumor cells. Drains are placed as needed. The surgical wound may be closed in layers, or separately reportable reconstructive procedures performed. Use 24077 for radical resection of soft tissue of less than 5 cm; use 24079 for 5 cm or greater.

24100-24102

24100	**Arthrotomy, elbow; with synovial biopsy only**
24101	**Arthrotomy, elbow; with joint exploration, with or without biopsy, with or without removal of loose or foreign body**
24102	**Arthrotomy, elbow; with synovectomy**

The physician performs an arthrotomy of the elbow with synovial biopsy only (24100), with joint exploration including biopsy or removal of loose or foreign body (24101), or with synovectomy (24102). The elbow joint capsule is opened using a posterior, medial, or anterolateral approach. In 24100, synovial fluid is aspirated and synovial tissue samples are obtained and sent for separately reportable laboratory analysis. In 24101, the elbow joint is explored. Biopsies are obtained as needed and sent for separately reportable laboratory analysis. The ulnar nerve is identified and decompressed as needed. Osteophytes (bone spurs) are removed with an osteotome. Loose or foreign bodies are also located and removed. In 24102, the inflamed synovial tissue is removed. If synovectomy is required in the posterior compartment, the synovium around the olecranon fossa is removed using a shaver. The medial gutter is addressed next. Rongeurs are used to clear the gutter. The synovium is then grasped and carefully removed with a shaver while taking care to protect the ulnar nerve. Upon completion of the procedure, the posterior compartment is irrigated with saline solution. Next, the anterior compartment is explored and synovectomy is performed. The shaver is used to remove the synovium at the humerus. Working proximal to distal and medial to lateral, the synovium is removed from the anterior compartment. Once the synovectomy is complete, the compartment is flushed with saline solution and incisions are closed.

Musculoskeletal System

24105

24105   Excision, olecranon bursa

Excision of the olecranon bursa, also referred to as olecranon bursectomy, is performed to treat severe chronic bursitis that has not responded to other less invasive treatments. The olecranon bursa is a fluid filled sac that overlies the olecranon process of the proximal ulna. A midlateral incision is made at the elbow and the triceps tendon is split longitudinally. If the bursa is greatly distended, it is windowed and fluid is released before excision is done. The olecranon bursa is then dissected from surrounding soft tissue and removed. The surgical wound is closed in layers.

24110-24116

24110   Excision or curettage of bone cyst or benign tumor, humerus
24115   Excision or curettage of bone cyst or benign tumor, humerus; with autograft (includes obtaining graft)
24116   Excision or curettage of bone cyst or benign tumor, humerus; with allograft

A bone cyst is a fluid filled space within the bone. One common type is a unicameral or simple bone cyst, which is a benign lesion. A less common type is an aneurysmal bone cyst which consists of vascular tissue surrounding a blood filled cystic lesion. There are a number of different types of benign bone tumors including giant cell tumors, chondromixoid fibromas, and enchondromas. In 24110, an incision is made in the skin over the site of lesion in the humeral shaft or distal humerus. Soft tissues are dissected and the lesion is exposed. If a cystic lesion is present, the bone is incised and a bone window created to open the cyst. Fluid is aspirated and sent to the laboratory for separately reportable analysis. A curette is inserted through the bone window and the lining of the cystic cavity is completely removed by curettage. Alternatively, some cystic lesions and most benign tumors are treated by excision. The lesion is exposed as described above. The physician then excises the benign lesion along with a margin of surrounding healthy bone. In 24115, the lesion is curetted or excised as described above. The physician then obtains healthy bone locally or from a separate site, such as the iliac crest. The bone autograft is packed into the defect in the humeral shaft or distal humerus. In 24116, the lesion is curetted or excised as described above. The defect is then packed with donor bone (allograft).

24120-24126

24120   Excision or curettage of bone cyst or benign tumor of head or neck of radius or olecranon process
24125   Excision or curettage of bone cyst or benign tumor of head or neck of radius or olecranon process; with autograft (includes obtaining graft)
24126   Excision or curettage of bone cyst or benign tumor of head or neck of radius or olecranon process; with allograft

A bone cyst is a fluid filled space within the bone. One common type is a unicameral or simple bone cyst, which is a benign lesion. A less common type is an aneurysmal bone cyst which consists of vascular tissue surrounding a blood filled cystic lesion. There are a number of different types of benign bone tumors including giant cell tumors, chondromixoid fibromas, and enchondromas. In 24120, an incision is made in the skin over the site of lesion in the head or neck of the radius or the olecranon process. Soft tissues are dissected and the lesion is exposed. If a cystic lesion is present, the bone is incised and a bone window created to open the cyst. Fluid is aspirated and sent to the laboratory for separately reportable analysis. A curette is inserted through the bone window and the lining of the cystic cavity is completely removed by curettage. Alternatively, some cystic lesions and most benign tumors are treated by excision. The lesion is exposed as described above. The physician then excises the benign lesion along with a margin of surrounding healthy bone. In 24125, the lesion is curetted or excised as described above. The physician then obtains healthy bone locally or from a separate site, such as the iliac crest. The bone autograft is packed into the defect in the head or neck of the radius or the olecranon process. In 24126, the lesion is curetted or excised as described above. The defect is then packed with donor bone (allograft).

24130

24130   Excision, radial head

Excision of the radial head without a concurrent fracture is typically performed to treat old trauma to the radial head causing pain, instability, or other disability of the elbow joint. A posterolateral skin incision is made over the radial head. Soft tissue structures are dissected taking care to protect the posterior interosseous nerve. The lateral collateral ligament is carefully dissected from the radial head leaving the distal fibers attached to the radius below the radial head. A bone saw is then used to excise the radial head. Bone edges are smoothed and overlying soft tissue and skin are closed in layers.

24134-24138

24134   Sequestrectomy (eg, for osteomyelitis or bone abscess), shaft or distal humerus
24136   Sequestrectomy (eg, for osteomyelitis or bone abscess), radial head or neck
24138   Sequestrectomy (eg, for osteomyelitis or bone abscess), olecranon process

A sequestrectomy is performed for osteomyelitis or bone abscess of the humeral shaft or distal humerus (24134), radial head or neck (24136), or olecranon process (24138). A sequestrum is a piece of necrotic bone that has become separated from healthy surrounding bone. An incision is made in the skin and carried down through the soft tissue overlying the site of the osteomyelitis or bone abscess. If the periosteum is soft and viable, it is elevated off the necrotic sequestrum. The necrotic bone is excised and the ribbon of periosteum that was elevated off the necrotic bone is then approximated over the cortical bone defect. If the periosteum is not viable and an involucrum has formed around the sequestrum, the necrotic bone is removed leaving the involucrum which will form new bone in the cortical bone defect. The incisions in the soft tissue and skin are closed and a dressing applied.

24140-24147

24140   Partial excision (craterization, saucerization, or diaphysectomy) bone (eg, osteomyelitis), humerus
24145   Partial excision (craterization, saucerization, or diaphysectomy) bone (eg, osteomyelitis), radial head or neck
24147   Partial excision (craterization, saucerization, or diaphysectomy) bone (eg, osteomyelitis), olecranon process

The physician performs a partial excision of bone, also referred to as craterization, saucerization, or diaphysectomy to treat osteomyelitis of the humerus (24140), radial head or neck (24145), or olecranon process (24147). Craterization and saucerization of bone involves removing infected and necrotic bone to form a shallow depression in the bone surface that will allow drainage from the infected area. Diaphysectomy involves removal of the infected portion of the shaft of a long bone. An incision is made in the skin and carried down through the soft tissue overlying the site of the osteomyelitis. Any soft tissue sinus tracts and devitalized soft tissue are resected. The area of necrotic and infected bone is exposed. A series of drill holes are made in the necrotic and infected bone and the bone between the drill holes is excavated to create an oval window using an osteotome. The amount of bone removed is dependent on the extent of the infection. A curette may be used to remove devitalized tissue from the medullary canal. Debridement continues until punctate bleeding is identified in the exposed bony surface. When all devitalized and infected tissue has been removed, the wound is copiously irrigated with sterile saline or antibiotic solution. The surgical wound is loosely closed and a drain placed.

24149

24149   Radical resection of capsule, soft tissue, and heterotopic bone, elbow, with contracture release (separate procedure)

A radical resection of the elbow joint capsule is performed to treat an elbow contracture, also referred to as a stiff elbow. Radical resection includes the excision of the contracted capsule, soft tissue, and heterotopic bone. Heterotopic bone is calcified bone that forms within the soft tissue as a result of trauma, head injury, burn, Paget's disease, or other conditions. The joint capsule is exposed using a posterior, posterolateral, medial, or anterolateral approach, depending on the site and type of contracture. To perform excision via a posterolateral approach, a proximal incision is made from the lateral supracondylar ridge to the lateral epicondyle and extended distally in a curvilinear fashion to the posterior border of the ulna. The anterior musculature is stripped and the anterior capsule is exposed. The extensor carpi radialis longus (ECRL) is retracted and elevated off the lateral epicondyle. The ECRL, brachioradialis, and brachialis are elevated off the joint capsule. The lateral collateral ligament (LCL) and ulnar nerve are identified and protected. The common extensor tendon is dissected off the LCL and joint capsule. The joint capsule is incised, elevated, and the contracted portion is excised along with contracted soft tissue and heterotopic bone. Range of motion is evaluated by flexing and extending the joint and turning the palm up and down. Additional dissection and excision is performed as needed until optimal mobility is achieved. The surgical wound is repaired in layers and dressings are applied.

24150

24150   Radical resection of tumor, shaft or distal humerus

Radical resection is typically performed for a malignant neoplasm although benign tumors and tumors of indeterminate nature may also require radical resection. A skin incision is made over the tumor in the shaft or distal humerus, or a skin flap is created and elevated. Overlying tissue is dissected and the tumor exposed. All bone and cartilage in the shaft or distal humerus with tumor involvement is resected. The tumor is removed en bloc along with a wide margin of surrounding tissue. Radical resection of bone includes excision of all involved soft tissue which may include muscles, tendons, fat, blood vessels, lymph vessels, nerves, and tissues surrounding the joints. Separately reportable frozen section is performed to ensure that all margins are free of tumor cells. If margins show evidence of

● New Code   ▲ Revised Code

malignancy, additional tissue is removed until all margins are free of tumor cells. Drains are placed as needed. The surgical wound may be closed in layers, or separately reportable reconstructive procedures performed.

24152

24152   Radical resection of tumor, radial head or neck

Radical resection is typically performed for a malignant neoplasm although benign tumors and tumors of indeterminate nature may also require radical resection. A skin incision is made over the tumor in the radial head or neck, or a skin flap is created and elevated. Overlying tissue is dissected and the tumor exposed. All bone and cartilage in the radial head or neck with tumor involvement is resected. The tumor is removed en bloc along with a wide margin of surrounding tissue. Radical resection of bone includes excision of all involved soft tissue which may include muscles, tendons, fat, blood vessels, lymph vessels, nerves, and tissues surrounding the joints. Separately reportable frozen section is performed to ensure that all margins are free of tumor cells. If margins show evidence of malignancy, additional tissue is removed until all margins are free of tumor cells. Drains are placed as needed. The surgical wound may be closed in layers, or separately reportable reconstructive procedures performed.

24155

24155   Resection of elbow joint (arthrectomy)

Elbow resection, also referred to as elbow arthrectomy or resection arthroplasty, is performed to treat joint immobility due to trauma, infection, or other disease process, or failure of total elbow replacement. The extent of the resection is dependent on the severity of the joint damage and includes partial or complete resection. The joint is exposed using a posterior, posterolateral, medial, or anterolateral approach, depending on the site and type of joint damage. To perform resection via a posterolateral approach, a proximal incision is made from the lateral supracondylar ridge to the lateral epicondyle and extended distally in a curvilinear fashion to the posterior border of the ulna. The anterior musculature is stripped and the anterior capsule is exposed. The extensor carpi radialis longus (ECRL) is retracted and elevated off the lateral epicondyle. The ECRL, brachioradialis, and brachialis are elevated off the joint capsule. The lateral collateral ligament (LCL) and ulnar nerve are identified and protected. The common extensor tendon is dissected off the LCL and joint capsule. The joint capsule is incised and joint structures are examined. An oscillating saw is used to excise the olecranon process which also exposes the articular surface of the posterior humerus. The deteriorated joint surfaces are excised from the humerus and radius as needed. All bone edges are smoothed. Muscles and tendons are reattached to the remaining bony surfaces. A drain may be placed. The joint capsule is closed. The surgical wound is repaired in layers and dressings are applied.

24160-24164

24160   Removal of prosthesis, includes debridement and synovectomy when performed; humeral and ulnar components

24164   Removal of prosthesis, includes debridement and synovectomy when performed; radial head

A skin incision is made over the elbow joint medial or lateral to the olecranon process to remove an implant. In 24160, the humeral and ulnar components of a previously placed joint implant are removed. Soft tissues are dissected and the ulnar nerve is identified and protected. The humeral implant component is exposed. The interval between the anconeus and flexor carpi ulnaris is incised and the triceps is mobilized. The anconeus is elevated off the lateral aspect of the ulnar component. The radial aspect of the elbow joint is exposed next. The implant is removed by carefully freeing each component from the humeral and ulnar bones. Bone cement is also removed. Bony surfaces are smoothed. A new prosthesis may be placed in a separately reportable procedure, or in the case of an infection, a drain may be placed and the surgical wound closed around the drain. In 24164, a lateral or posterolateral approach may be used to remove a previously placed radial head implant. If a lateral approach is used, an incision is made between the carpi radialis brevis and the extensor digitorum muscles. The annular ligament is exposed and freed from surrounding structures. Neurovascular structures are identified and protected. Dissection continues until the radial head implant is exposed. The implant is carefully freed and removed. Bone cement is also removed. A new prosthesis may be placed in a separately reportable procedure, or in the case of an infection, a drain may be placed and the surgical wound closed around the drain.

24200-24201

24200   Removal of foreign body, upper arm or elbow area; subcutaneous

24201   Removal of foreign body, upper arm or elbow area; deep (subfascial or intramuscular)

A subcutaneous (24200) or deep (24201) foreign body in the upper arm or elbow area is removed. Subcutaneous tissue refers to the fat and connective tissue that lies between the overlying dermis and underlying muscle fascia. Deep tissue refers to the tissue below the muscle fascia (subfascial) or within the muscle itself (intramuscular). The foreign body is located by palpation or separately reportable radiographs. A straight or elliptical incision

is made in the skin. In 24200, the subcutaneous tissue is dissected and the foreign body identified. A hemostat or grasping forceps is then used to remove the foreign body. Alternatively, the physician may need to dissect tissues around the foreign body to remove it. The wound is then flushed with normal saline or antibiotic solution and the incision is closed. In 24201, dissection is carried into the deeper subfascial or intramuscular tissue and the foreign body identified and removed.

24220

24220   Injection procedure for elbow arthrography

An injection procedure for elbow arthrography is performed. The skin over the injection site is cleansed and a local anesthetic is injected. A needle may be inserted into the joint and fluid aspirated with a syringe. The radiopaque substance is then injected into the elbow joint, which is exercised to help distribute the radiopaque substance. Once the contrast has been distributed throughout the joint, separately reportable radiographic images are obtained.

24300

24300   Manipulation, elbow, under anesthesia

Manipulation under anesthesia (MUA) of the elbow is performed. This procedure is performed to improve range of motion by rupturing fibrous adhesions (arthrofibrosis) that develop following surgery or fracture of the elbow. An anesthetic is administered. The physician then takes the elbow through a complete range of motion including flexion, extension, supination and pronation. The physician must use sufficient force to rupture the adhesions while taking care not to apply too much force which could injure the joint structures or bones.

24301

24301   Muscle or tendon transfer, any type, upper arm or elbow, single (excluding 24320-24331)

Muscle or tendon transfer is typically performed to stabilize the elbow and/or restore function. There are a number of techniques including local transfer of one of the existing elbow or upper arm muscles to a new site, or free transfer of an expendable muscle, such as the gracilis muscle in the thigh. A skin incision is made over the elbow or upper arm and the injured or atrophied muscle is identified. If a local muscle or tendon is transferred, existing bony attachments are severed and the muscle or tendon is reattached at a new site. If a free transfer is performed, a separate incision is made over the muscle to be harvested. The muscle is excised along with its nerve and blood supply in a separately reportable procedure. The muscle is then trimmed as needed and sutured to bones of the elbow in a manner that stabilizes the joint and/or allows reinnervation of the muscle and restoration of motion. This code reports a single muscle or tendon transfer.

24305

24305   Tendon lengthening, upper arm or elbow, each tendon

Tendon lengthening is performed to treat flexion or extension contractures in the upper arm or elbow. A skin incision is made over the elbow or upper arm and the tendon of the affected muscle is identified. Typically, a Z-plasty incision is used to lengthen the tendon. The tendon is incised and range of motion is checked. Overlying soft tissues and skin are closed in layers. A cast or splint is applied to maintain the tendon length. This code is reported separately for each tendon that is incised and lengthened.

24310

24310   Tenotomy, open, elbow to shoulder, each tendon

Tenotomy, also referred to as tendon release, is performed to treat inflammation or other disorders, such as golfer's elbow or tennis elbow. A skin incision is made over the elbow or upper arm and the affected tendon is identified. The tendon is inspected and the extent of damage is evaluated. The tendon is incised horizontally near its attachment to the bone. The tendon is then split longitudinally and scar tissue is removed. The loose end of the tendon may be sutured to nearby fascial tissue. Overlying soft tissues and skin are closed in layers. A splint is applied to maintain the arm in the proper position. This code is reported separately for each tendon that is treated with tenotomy.

24320

24320   Tenoplasty, with muscle transfer, with or without free graft, elbow to shoulder, single (Seddon-Brookes type procedure)

Muscle transfer combined with tendon repair (tenoplasty) is performed to stabilize the elbow and upper arm and/or restore function. There are a number of techniques including local transfer of one of the existing elbow or upper arm muscles to a new site or free transfer of an expendable muscle, such as the gracilis muscle in the thigh. A skin incision is made over the elbow or upper arm and the injured or atrophied tendon is identified. Neurovascular structures are dissected and protected. The injured tendon is detached and debrided as needed. The tendon may be sliced open and scar tissue removed. The planned attachment site on the shoulder, upper arm, or elbow is drilled. The repaired tendon is attached to the new site by a fixing wire pulled through the drill hole. Alternatively, screw fixation may be used to fix a bone fragment connected to the tendon. If a local muscle is transferred, existing bony attachments are severed and the muscle is reattached at a new site. If a free transfer is performed, a separate incision is made over the muscle to be harvested. The muscle is excised along with its nerve and blood supply in a separately reportable procedure. The muscle is then trimmed as needed and sutured to bones of the shoulder, upper arm, or elbow in a manner that stabilizes the joint and/or allows reinnervation of the muscle and restoration of motion. This code reports a single muscle or tendon transfer.

24330-24331

24330   Flexor-plasty, elbow (eg, Steindler type advancement)
24331   Flexor-plasty, elbow (eg, Steindler type advancement); with extensor advancement

Flexor-plasty of the elbow is performed to repair complete or partial detachment of the flexor-pronator complex at the elbow or to improve flexion. An incision is made over the elbow joint. In 24330, the ulnar nerve is dissected and protected. If the flexor-pronator complex is intact, it is surgically detached along with a portion of the medial epicondyle with a chisel. The flexor group is dissected. The planned attachment site on the humerus is drilled. The freed flexor group is transferred proximally 2-6 cm and attached to the medial or mediovolar surface of the humerus. A fixing wire is pulled through the drill hole and the flexor group is secured. Screw fixation may also be used to fix the epicondyle fragment. In 24331, the flexor-plasty is performed as described above and then the lateral extensor group is also released, transposed proximally 3-7 cm, and fixed to the humerus in the same manner.

24332

24332   Tenolysis, triceps

Tenolysis of the triceps is performed to restore elbow motion by releasing scar tissue resulting from trauma or other injury to the triceps tendon at the elbow. An incision is made over the distal aspect of the triceps. Soft tissues are dissected and the ulnar nerve is identified and protected. The interval between the lateral triceps and the humerus is dissected and the radial nerve is exposed and protected. Adhesions between the triceps tendon and humerus are lysed. Dissection continues distally into the posterior aspect of the elbow joint and adhesions in the area of the elbow joint are also lysed. Range of motion is evaluated. The surgical wound is closed in layers and a dressing is applied.

24340

24340   Tenodesis of biceps tendon at elbow (separate procedure)

Biceps tenodesis at the elbow is performed to treat a tear in the biceps tendon or to relieve tendinitis. The distal aspect of the biceps brachii muscle, more commonly referred to simply as the biceps, inserts on the radial tuberosity at the elbow. An incision is made either medial or lateral to the biceps, carried down over the antecubital fossa, and extended distally over the brachioradialis muscle in the forearm. Neurovascular structures are identified and protected. The tendon is located, inspected, and detached from the radial tuberosity as needed. To treat tendonitis, the tendon is debrided and damaged tendon tissue is excised. Any tears are repaired. The tendon is then reattached to the radial tuberosity with bone anchors. The joint is flushed with sterile saline, incisions are closed, and a dressing is applied.

24341

24341   Repair, tendon or muscle, upper arm or elbow, each tendon or muscle, primary or secondary (excludes rotator cuff)

Muscle or tendon repair is performed to stabilize the elbow and upper arm and/or restore function. A skin incision is made over the elbow or upper arm and the injured or atrophied muscle or tendon is identified. Neurovascular structures are dissected and protected. If a muscle is repaired, the site of the injury is located and inspected. Damaged muscle is excised. The muscle is then suture repaired. If a tendon is repaired, the injured tendon is detached from the bone and debrided as needed. The planned attachment site on the upper arm or elbow is drilled. A fixing wire is pulled through the drill hole and the tendon is secured. Alternatively, screw fixation may be used to fix a bone fragment connected to the tendon. This code reports a single muscle or tendon repair performed at the time of the acute injury as a primary repair or performed after the acute injury as a secondary repair.

24342

24342   Reinsertion of ruptured biceps or triceps tendon, distal, with or without tendon graft

The distal aspect of biceps brachii muscle, more commonly referred to simply as the biceps, inserts on the radial tuberosity at the elbow. The distal aspect of the triceps brachii, more commonly referred to as the triceps, inserts on the olecranon of the ulna. Reinsertion of a distally ruptured biceps tendon at the elbow is performed using a one- or two-incision technique. Using one incision, the cut is made either medial or lateral to the biceps, carried down over the antecubital fossa, and extended distally over the bracioradialis muscle in the forearm. Neurovascular structures are identified and protected. The end of the tendon

is located, retrieved, and debrided. The tendon is then reattached to the radial tuberosity with bone anchors. Using the two-incision technique, a proximal incision is made over the distal biceps tendon sheath. The tendon sheath is opened and the end of the ruptured tendon is located and retracted into the surgical wound. Sutures are placed through the end of the tendon. A second incision is made over the forearm and the radial tuberosity is exposed. Drill holes are placed in the radial tuberosity. The biceps is then retrieved through the distal incision and the previously placed sutures are passed through the drill holes in the radial tuberosity and secured. To reinsert a ruptured distal triceps tendon, an incision is made over the distal aspect of the triceps. Soft tissues are dissected and the ulnar nerve is identified and protected. The end of the tendon is located, retrieved, and debrided. Dissection continues distally into the posterior aspect of the elbow joint and the olecranon is exposed. Suture anchors are placed or holes are drilled in the olecranon. The triceps tendon is secured to the olecranon process. The wound is flushed with sterile saline, closed in layers, and a dressing is applied.

24343-24344

24343   Repair lateral collateral ligament, elbow, with local tissue
24344   Reconstruction lateral collateral ligament, elbow, with tendon graft (includes harvesting of graft)

The elbow joint is covered by a thin, broad fibrous capsule that is reinforced by the collateral ligaments. The lateral collateral ligament (LCL), also referred to as the radial collateral ligament, attaches superiorly to the lateral epicondyle of the humerus and inferiorly by the annular ligament of the radius, in turn attached to the trochlear notch of the ulna and encircling the head of the radius, keeping the head in contact with its notch in the ulna. Injury to the LCL may accompany acute trauma, but is more commonly associated with chronic stress and is often associated with tennis elbow. In 24343, the proximal LCL is repaired. An incision is made over the lateral humeral epicondyle and extended distally across the elbow joint to the proximal ulna. The fascia overlying the anconeus and extensor carpi ulnaris is incised. Tissue is dissected and the joint capsule is exposed. Overlying tendons and muscles are elevated off the joint capsule while taking care to protect neurovascular structures. The LCL is exposed and the joint capsule is incised. The radial head is exposed. The LCL is released from the lateral epicondyle. The LCL is debrided and damaged tissue is excised. Drill holes are placed in the lateral epicondyle and the LCL is reattached with sutures. Local tissue, usually a split anconeus fascia transfer, is used to reinforce the LCL as needed. If a distal repair is required, the LCL is released from the radial head and repaired in the same fashion. In 24344, the LCL is reconstructed using a tendon graft. A tendon graft is harvested, usually from the palmaris longus, but the plantaris, Achilles or hamstring tendons may also be used. The graft tendon is trimmed to the appropriate size and shape and attached to the lateral epicondyle on the humerus and the radial head with a fixation device such as a screw or button.

24345-24346

24345   Repair medial collateral ligament, elbow, with local tissue
24346   Reconstruction medial collateral ligament, elbow, with tendon graft (includes harvesting of graft)

The elbow joint is covered by a thin, broad fibrous capsule that is reinforced by the collateral ligaments. The medial collateral ligament (MCL), also referred to as the ulnar collateral ligament, is composed of three interconnected bands of tissue. The anterior band covers the area between the anterior medial epicondyle of the humerus and the coronoid process of the ulna. The posterior band attaches to the posterior aspect of the medial humeral epicondyle and the medial edge of the ulnar olecranon process. An intermediate band contains a ray of fibers that merges with the anterior and posterior bands. Injury to the MCL may be due to acute trauma or chronic stress to the elbow joint. In 24345, the MCL is repaired. An incision is made over the medial aspect of the elbow joint. Tissue is dissected and the joint capsule is exposed. Overlying tendons and muscles are elevated off the joint capsule while taking care to protect neurovascular structures. The MCL is exposed and the joint capsule is incised. The MCL is released from bony attachments at the site of the injury. The MCL is debrided and damaged tissue is excised. Local tissue is used to reinforce the repair as needed. One or more drill holes are placed at the bony attachment site and the MCL is reattached with sutures. Alternatively, screws or suture anchors may be used. In 24346, the MCL is reconstructed using a free tendon graft. A tendon graft is harvested, usually from the palmaris longus, but the plantaris, Achilles or hamstring tendons may also be used. The tendon is trimmed to the appropriate size and shape and attached to the bone using screws or suture anchors. Alternatively, a docking technique may be used which involves drilling a single hole into the bone, threading the graft through the tunnel and securing the graft with sutures.

24357

24357   Tenotomy, elbow, lateral or medial (eg, epicondylitis, tennis elbow, golfer's elbow); percutaneous

Lateral epicondylitis, also referred to as tennis elbow, is characterized by pain on the outside of the elbow, caused by injury to the wrist extensors, the muscles that pull the hand up. Medial epicondylitis, also referred to as golfer's elbow, is characterized by pain on the inner side of the elbow, caused by injury to the wrist flexors, the muscles that pull the hand down. An incision is made over the lateral or medial epicondyle. In a lateral tenotomy, the extensor carpi radialis brevis tendon that attaches the wrist extensors to the lateral epicondyle is incised. In a medial tenotomy, the common flexor tendon that attaches the wrist flexors to the medial epicondyle is incised. Use 24358 when tenotomy is performed with open debridement of soft tissue and/or bone. The tendon fascia of the affected site is incised. Any degenerated tissue is excised. Soft tissue is removed from the tendon insertion site in the lateral or medial epicondyle. Any bone spurs are removed. Multiple drill holes may be made in the affected epicondyle. Use 24359 when tenotomy is performed with open debridement of soft tissue and/or bone, and an open tendon repair or reattachment is also performed. Bone anchors are placed in the affected epicondyle. The suture material of the bone anchors is passed through the remaining portion of the affected tendon and the tendon is reattached to the epicondyle.

24358-24359

24358 Tenotomy, elbow, lateral or medial (eg, epicondylitis, tennis elbow, golfer's elbow); debridement, soft tissue and/or bone, open

24359 Tenotomy, elbow, lateral or medial (eg, epicondylitis, tennis elbow, golfer's elbow); debridement, soft tissue and/or bone, open with tendon repair or reattachment

Lateral epicondylitis, also referred to as tennis elbow, is characterized by pain on the outside of the elbow, caused by injury to the wrist extensors, the muscles that pull the hand up. Medial epicondylitis, also referred to as golfer's elbow, is characterized by pain on the inner side of the elbow, caused by injury to the wrist flexors, the muscles that pull the hand down. An incision is made over the lateral or medial epicondyle. In a lateral tenotomy, the extensor carpi radialis brevis tendon that attaches the wrist extensors to the lateral epicondyle is incised. In a medial tenotomy, the common flexor tendon that attaches the wrist flexors to the medial epicondyle is incised. Use 24358 when tenotomy is performed with open debridement of soft tissue and/or bone. The tendon fascia of the affected site is incised. Any degenerated tissue is excised. Soft tissue is removed from the tendon insertion site in the lateral or medial epicondyle. Any bone spurs are removed. Multiple drill holes may be made in the affected epicondyle. Use 24359 when tenotomy is performed with open debridement of soft tissue and/or bone, together with an open tendon repair or reattachment. Bone anchors are placed in the affected epicondyle. The suture material of the bone anchors is passed through the remaining portion of the affected tendon and the tendon is reattached to the epicondyle.

24360

24360 Arthroplasty, elbow; with membrane (eg, fascial)

A skin incision is made over the elbow joint medial or lateral to the olecranon process to repair damaged or deteriorated articular cartilage and joint surfaces in an arthroplasty procedure using a fascial membrane. Soft tissues are dissected and the ulnar nerve is identified and protected. The lateral epicondyle of the humerus is exposed. The interval between the anconeus and flexor carpi ulnaris is incised and the triceps is mobilized. The anconeus is elevated off the lateral aspect of the proximal ulna. The radial aspect of the elbow joint is addressed next and tissue is dissected off the lateral epicondyle. The elbow is externally rotated and flexed. The posterior joint capsule is opened. The roof of the olecranon is exposed. The medial collateral ligament is released from the epicondyle. Tissue is dissected off the humerus. All joint surfaces are exposed and deteriorated articular cartilage and bone are removed. A fascial graft is harvested. The joint surfaces are then covered with fascia. Ligaments and tendons, such as the triceps are reattached. A subcutaneous pocket may be created for the ulnar nerve between subcutaneous fat and fascia near the medial epicondyle. Fascia and skin are closed in layers. The arm is fully extended and placed in a splint.

24361-24362

24361 Arthroplasty, elbow; with distal humeral prosthetic replacement

24362 Arthroplasty, elbow; with implant and fascia lata ligament reconstruction

A skin incision is made over the elbow joint medial or lateral to the olecranon process to perform arthroplasty using a distal humeral prosthesis. Soft tissues are dissected and the ulnar nerve is identified and protected. The lateral epicondyle of the humerus is exposed. The interval between the anconeus and flexor carpi ulnaris is incised and the triceps mobilized. The anconeus is elevated off the lateral aspect of the proximal ulna. The radial aspect of the elbow joint is addressed next and tissue is dissected off the lateral epicondyle. The elbow is externally rotated and flexed. The posterior joint capsule is removed. The roof of the olecranon is exposed. The medial collateral ligament is released from the epicondyle. Tissue is dissected off the humerus and the roof of the olecranon fossa is removed down to the level of cancellous bone. The humeral canal is reamed. A cutting guide is placed and the distal aspect of the humerus is removed along the plane of the medial and lateral supracondylar columns. A trial implant is placed to check width and alignment. The articular surfaces of the ulna and radius are smoothed. The permanent humeral implant is placed and bone cement is injected in a retrograde fashion to secure it. Ligaments and tendons are reattached. A fascia lata graft may be harvested and elbow ligament reconstruction also performed before reattachment. The triceps is medialized. A subcutaneous pocket is created for the ulnar nerve and the nerve is placed

between subcutaneous fat and fascia near the medial epicondyle. Fascia and skin are closed in layers. The arm is fully extended and placed in a splint. Use 24361 for humeral prosthetic replacement without fascia lata graft. Use 24362 when fascia lata graft ligament reconstruction is also performed.

24363

24363 Arthroplasty, elbow; with distal humerus and proximal ulnar prosthetic replacement (eg, total elbow)

A skin incision is made over the elbow joint medial or lateral to the olecranon process to perform a total elbow arthroplasty. Soft tissues are dissected and the ulnar nerve is identified and protected. The lateral epicondyle of the humerus is exposed. The interval between the anconeus and flexor carpi ulnaris is incised and the triceps is mobilized. The anconeus is elevated off the lateral aspect of the proximal ulna. The radial aspect of the elbow joint is addressed next and tissue is dissected off the lateral epicondyle. The elbow is externally rotated and flexed. The posterior joint capsule is removed. The roof of the olecranon is exposed. The medial collateral ligament is released from the epicondyle. The tip of the olecranon is removed with a rongeur or oscillating saw. Tissue is dissected off the humerus and the roof of the olecranon fossa is removed down to the level of cancellous bone. The humeral canal is reamed. A cutting guide is placed and the distal aspect of the humerus is removed along the plane of the medial and lateral supracondylar columns. A distal humeral trial implant is placed to check width and alignment. The ulnar canal is established next using a high speed bur followed by a reamer. A proximal ulnar trial implant is placed and tested. The trial implants are removed. The radial head is debrided or resected. The permanent implants are placed and bone cement is injected in a retrograde fashion to secure them. The implants are locked together with a pin which is used to create a hinged prosthetic joint. Ligament and tendons are reattached. The triceps is medialized. A subcutaneous pocket is created for the ulnar nerve and the nerve is placed between subcutaneous fat and fascia near the medial epicondyle. Fascia and skin are closed in layers. The arm is fully extended and placed in a splint.

24365-24366

24365 Arthroplasty, radial head

24366 Arthroplasty, radial head; with implant

Arthroplastic repair of the radial head may be done using a lateral or posterolateral approach. If a lateral approach is used, an incision is made between the carpi radialis brevis and the extensor digitorum muscles. The annular ligament is exposed and freed from surrounding structures. Neurovascular structures are identified and protected. Dissection continues until the radial head and neck are completely exposed. In 24365, the deteriorated joint surface on the radial head is removed. A number of different techniques are available to restore the integrity and function of the joint. The radial head may be covered with fascia to replace the deteriorated cartilage and bone. Alternatively, an interposition arthroplasty may be performed using fascia, cartilage, metal, or plastic to maintain the joint space. A gap arthroplasty may be performed which involves the use of a decompression device placed to maintain the space between the remaining bony surfaces. In 24366, the radial head is replaced with a prosthetic implant. An oscillating saw is used to divide the radial neck at the level of the tuberosity. The bone edges of the remaining radial surface are trimmed and leveled as needed. The radius is reamed in preparation for placement of the radial prosthesis stem. A trial component is placed and fitted, and range of motion is checked. The stem component of the permanent prosthesis is then placed and the distal aspect of the stem is packed with bone chips as needed. Bone cement is injected under pressure and the stem is impacted in the shaft until the rim is properly seated on the resected surface of the radius. The cup component is attached to the stem component. Range of motion and joint stability is checked. The annular ligament is repaired. Muscles and tendons are reapproximated. Subcutaneous tissue and skin is closed in layers.

24370-24371

24370 Revision of total elbow arthroplasty, including allograft when performed; humeral or ulnar component

24371 Revision of total elbow arthroplasty, including allograft when performed; humeral and ulnar component

Revision of total elbow arthroplasty is typically performed for component loosening, joint instability, infection, or periprosthetic fracture. The old incision over the elbow joint is incised. Soft tissues are dissected and the ulnar nerve is identified and protected. The ulnar component is exposed. The subperiosteum is exposed along the ulna to a point just past the tip of the implant. The loose bone cement is removed. The radial nerve is identified and protected and the humeral component is exposed. Loose cement is removed. The ulnar and humeral components are then evaluated and removed as needed. If infection or necrotic bone is present, bone and other tissues are debrided as needed. The components may be exchanged for new components or the existing components may be repositioned. The humeral and ulnar components are then tamped into place and tested. The components are secured using allograft bone, cerclage wires and/or bone cement. The humeral and ulnar components are locked together with a pin to create a hinged prosthetic joint. Ligaments and tendons are reattached. The triceps is medialized. A subcutaneous pocket

Musculoskeletal System

is created for the ulnar nerve and the nerve is placed between subcutaneous fat and fascia near the medial epicondyle. Fascia and skin are closed in layers. The arm is fully extended and placed in a splint. Report 24370 when either the humeral component or the ulnar component is in need of revision, and 24371 when both components are revised.

24400-24410

24400   Osteotomy, humerus, with or without internal fixation

24410   Multiple osteotomies with realignment on intramedullary rod, humeral shaft (Sofield type procedure)

An osteotomy of the humeral shaft or distal humerus is performed to treat a condition such as a rotational deformity caused by malunion or osteogenesis imperfecta. The location of the osteotomy and the type performed is dependent on the site and type of the deformity. Some commonly used osteotomies include transverse, wedge, sliding, right or left angle, V-osteotomy, and Z-osteotomy. An incision is made in the upper arm over the site of the deformity. Soft tissues are dissected and the humerus is exposed. The periosteum is elevated. Using a drill, saw, and/or osteotome, the bone is cut in the previously determined configuration. Pins, screws, a plate and screw device, or other type of internal fixation is applied as needed to secure the cut edges in anatomical alignment. Alternatively, a separately reportable external fixation device may be applied. In 24400, a single osteotomy is performed with or without internal fixation. In 24410, multiple osteotomies of the humeral shaft are performed with insertion and realignment using an intramedullary rod. The osteotomies are performed as described above. The humerus is sized and an appropriately sized intramedullary rod is selected. A drill hole is created in the distal or proximal aspect of the humerus. The intramedullary canal is drilled or reamed through the drill hole. If a cannulated rod is used, a guidewire is placed into the intramedullary canal. The rod is then advanced over the guidewire until it is properly positioned within the canal. The bone is anatomically positioned at each osteotomy site and the rod is secured using screws or pins or other devices.

24420

24420   Osteoplasty, humerus (eg, shortening or lengthening) (excluding 64876)

A plastic procedure is performed on the humerus to lengthen or shorten the bone. The humerus is exposed. If the humerus is to be shortened, the sites of the bone cuts are identified. The bone is cut and a segment of the humerus is excised. The remaining distal and proximal portions of the humerus are then brought into contact with each other and internal fixation is applied to stabilize the reconfigured bone. If the humerus is to be lengthened, cuts are made in the bone and a distraction device is applied. The distraction device is used to very slowly pull the bone apart. As the bone is pulled apart, new bone is deposited at the site of the osteotomy. Once the bone has reached the desired length, distraction is discontinued and the bone is allowed to consolidate and heal.

24430-24435

24430   Repair of nonunion or malunion, humerus; without graft (eg, compression technique)

24435   Repair of nonunion or malunion, humerus; with iliac or other autograft (includes obtaining graft)

Humeral fractures typically heal in about 10 weeks. However, if union of the fracture fragments has not occurred in 8-10 months, the patient is considered to have a nonunion of the fracture. Malunion caused by malalignment of the fracture fragments can cause osseous abnormalities, incongruity of articular surfaces, soft tissue contracture, nerve impingement, and other complications. The original fracture site of the humerus is exposed. The nonunion or malunion is evaluated to determine what type of repair is required. In 24430, the nonunion or malunion of the humerus is treated without a graft using internal fixation such as a compression plate. For a nonunion, a compression plate is placed over the fracture site and secured with lag screws. For a malunion, the humerus may be refractured, realigned, and internal fixation placed to maintain the fracture in anatomical alignment. Following placement of the fixation device, stability of the fracture is checked and alignment is verified radiographically. In 24435, a bone graft is used to fill the bone defect and encourage healing of the nonunion or malunion. The site of the nonunion or malunion is prepared which may include refracture of the bone. A bone autograft is harvested, usually from the iliac crest. A skin incision is made over the iliac crest and the muscle is stripped to reveal the bone surface. Cortical and/or cancellous bone is harvested. The bone is configured to the size and shape of the defect or cancellous bone is morcelized and packed into the defect. Internal fixation, such as a pin or wire is used as needed to secure the bone graft. A compression plate and screws or other internal fixation is used to stabilize the fracture.

24470

24470   Hemiepiphyseal arrest (eg, cubitus varus or valgus, distal humerus)

Hemiepiphyseal arrest is performed to treat an angulation deformity at the elbow such as cubitus varus or valgus. Cubitus varus causes the forearm to deviate toward the midline. Cubitus valgus causes the forearm to deviate away from the midline. This procedure is performed only on children and adolescents who have not attained full bone growth. The

deviation at the joint is treated by hemiepiphyseal arrest which disrupts bone growth at the distal humerus. The epiphysis is also referred to as the growth plate. An incision is made over the distal aspect of the humerus and extended down over the elbow joint. Soft tissues are dissected, taking care to protect blood vessels and nerves. The distal humerus is exposed. Blount staples, transphyseal screws, or a plate and screw device are strategically placed in the epiphysis of the distal humerus to temporarily arrest growth in that region of the bone. The other portion of the epiphysis is not treated and growth continues thereby diminishing or correcting the angulation deformity.

24495

24495   Decompression fasciotomy, forearm, with brachial artery exploration

Decompression fasciotomy is performed to treat compartment syndrome, a condition in which swelling of tissue in the muscle compartment causes compression of the blood vessels and nerves. Muscle compartments are surrounded by fascia that separates groups of muscles from each other. Fascia is a thick layer of connective tissue that does not expand. Swelling of tissue within the compartment can restrict blood supply and cause permanent muscle and nerve damage. In the forearm, damage to the brachial artery may also occur. There are two compartments in the forearm, referred to as the flexor (volar) and extensor (dorsal) compartments. One or both compartments may require decompression. Decompression of the flexor compartment is typically performed first. A curvilinear skin incision is made beginning proximal to the antecubital fossa at the elbow crease and carried down to the middle of the palm. Alternatively, a lazy S type incision may be used that extends from the elbow crease on the ulnar side curving to the radial side at the midforearm and returning to the ulnar side at the wrist. The incision is then extended into the midpalm. Incisions are carried down through the fascia following the same line as the skin incision. Compartment pressure is checked to ensure that the deep flexor muscles have been adequately decompressed. The brachial artery is exposed within the antecubital fossa and followed distally to the point where it divides into the radial and ulnar arteries. The brachial artery may also be explored proximally. If the brachial artery has been damaged, a separately reportable bypass graft procedure may be performed. If the extensor compartment also requires decompression, a dorsal incision is made over the extensor muscles and carried down between the extensor wad and the extensor digitorum communis muscles. The fascia over each of the two dorsal compartments is opened, taking care to incise fascia over each of the superficial and deep muscle bellies. Pressures are checked to ensure extensor muscles have been adequately decompressed. Muscle tissue and nerves are inspected and any nonviable tissue is debrided using sharp excision. The skin and fascial incisions are left open and covered with a dressing. The patient is returned to the operating room for wound closure once the swelling subsides, usually within 24-72 hours.

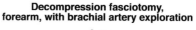

Decompression fasciotomy, forearm, with brachial artery exploration

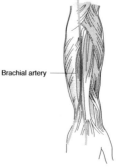

Brachial artery

A portion of the membrane covering the forearm muscle is incised to relieve built-up pressure. The brachial artery is examined for disease/injury after being constricted.

24498

24498   Prophylactic treatment (nailing, pinning, plating or wiring), with or without methylmethacrylate, humeral shaft

Prophylactic treatment is performed to prevent fracture of a humeral shaft that is already weakened as a result of a disease process or neoplasm. Common methods used to maintain bone integrity include nailing, pinning, plating, or wiring with or without the use of methylmethacrylate. The weakened bone is evaluated radiographically and the best form of prophylaxis is determined. An intramedullary implant may be placed using either an antegrade or retrograde approach. In an antegrade approach, an incision is made over the proximal humerus through the rotator cuff or just lateral to the articular surface of the humerus and a hole is drilled in the bone to allow placement of the intramedullary device. In a retrograde approach, the distal triceps is split and a hole is drilled in the olecranon process. A nail or rod is then inserted into the intramedullary space. The nail is secured with locking screws placed distally and proximally. If pins are used, they may be placed transcutaneously through the weakened region of the bone. Plating requires open exposure

Musculoskeletal System

of the bone and placement of a plate that is secured with screws. Wiring involves wrapping a wire cerclage around the bone. When methylmethacrylate is used, it is injected into bony defects.

24500-24505

24500 Closed treatment of humeral shaft fracture; without manipulation
24505 Closed treatment of humeral shaft fracture; with manipulation, with or without skeletal traction

Closed treatment of a fracture of the humeral shaft is performed. Separately reportable radiographs are obtained to confirm the fracture. In 24500, a nondisplaced fracture of the humeral shaft is evaluated. A neurovascular exam is performed to ensure that the nerves and blood vessels at the site of the injury are intact. No manipulation of the fracture fragments is required. The entire arm is immobilized using one of several techniques, including a long arm splint, coaptation splint, hanging arm cast, humeral/shoulder spica cast, Velpeau dressing, sling and swath, or functional brace. In 24505, a minimally displaced fracture of the humerus is treated with manipulation with or without skeletal traction. The displaced fracture fragments are manually reduced (manipulated) back to proper anatomic alignment. Separately reportable radiographs are obtained to confirm anatomic reduction. The fracture site is immobilized by placing the arm in one of the immobilization devices described above. For severely comminuted fractures overhead skeletal traction may be used to immobilize the fracture. This is accomplished using a pin inserted into the proximal ulna at the olecranon and weighted skeletal traction.

24515

24515 Open treatment of humeral shaft fracture with plate/screws, with or without cerclage

Open treatment of a humeral shaft fracture is performed with surgical fixation using plates and screws with or without cerclage. Depending on the site of the fracture, a posterior or anterolateral approach is used. In a posterior approach, an incision is made in the skin over the interval between the lateral and long heads of the triceps. The medial head of the triceps is incised and the posterior aspect of the humeral shaft is exposed. If more exposure is required, the distal aspects of the brachial cutaneous and radial nerves are identified and retracted medially. The medial and lateral heads of the triceps are then elevated off the lateral intermuscular septum and bone to expose the humeral shaft proximally to the axillary nerve. In an anterolateral approach, the incisional plane is developed proximally between the deltoid and pectoralis major muscles and distally between the musculocutaneous and radial nerves. Once the fracture site is exposed, a compression plate is applied and secured with lag screws. Fracture stability is checked and wire cerclage is used, if needed, to further stabilize the fracture. Adequate reduction of fracture fragments may be verified radiographically.

24516

24516 Treatment of humeral shaft fracture, with insertion of intramedullary implant, with or without cerclage and/or locking screws

Open treatment of a humeral shaft fracture is performed with surgical fixation using an intramedullary implant with or without cerclage and/or locking screws. Intramedullary nailing is performed without direct fracture exposure, using either an antegrade or retrograde approach. In an antegrade approach, an incision is made over the proximal humerus either through the rotator cuff or just lateral to the articular surface of the humerus. An intramedullary nail is then inserted into the intramedullary space. The nail is typically secured with locking screws placed both proximally and distally. In a retrograde approach, the distal triceps is split and a hole is drilled in the olecranon process. The nail is inserted and a locking screw is placed at the proximal end of the nail. Fracture stability is checked and wire cerclage is used, if needed, to further stabilize the fracture. Adequate reduction of fracture fragments may be verified radiographically.

24530-24535

24530 Closed treatment of supracondylar or transcondylar humeral fracture, with or without intercondylar extension; without manipulation
24535 Closed treatment of supracondylar or transcondylar humeral fracture, with or without intercondylar extension; with manipulation, with or without skin or skeletal traction

Closed treatment of a supracondylar or transcondylar humeral fracture with or without intercondylar extension is performed. The distal humerus has two projections, the lateral and medial epicondyles. A supracondylar fracture is located immediately above the epicondyles and a transcondylar fracture is one that extends through them. These types of fractures may also extend into the intercondylar region and involve the trachlea and/or olecranon fossa. Separately reportable radiographs are obtained to confirm the fracture. In 24530, a nondisplaced supracondylar or transcondylar fracture of the humerus with or without intercondylar extension is evaluated. A neurovascular exam is performed to ensure that the nerves and blood vessels at the site of the injury are intact. No manipulation of the fracture fragments is required. The arm is initially immobilized using a long arm splint that may be replaced with a cast once any swelling has subsided. In 24535, a minimally displaced supracondylar or transdylar fracture of the humerus with or without intercondylar

extension is treated with manipulation with or without skin or skeletal traction. The displaced fracture fragments are manually reduced (manipulated) back to proper anatomic alignment. Separately reportable radiographs are obtained to confirm anatomic reduction. The fracture site is initially immobilized by placing the arm in long arm splint followed by casting when any swelling has subsided. Alternatively the fracture may be treated with skin or skeletal traction. If skin traction is used, the arm is splinted and the weighted traction device attached to the arm using wraps, tape or straps. A special type of skin traction called Dunlop's traction may be used to maintain a flexed position. If skeletal traction is used, a pin is inserted in the proximal ulna at the olecranon and overhead or side arm weighted traction applied.

24538

24538 Percutaneous skeletal fixation of supracondylar or transcondylar humeral fracture, with or without intercondylar extension

Percutaneous skeletal fixation of a supracondylar or transcondylar humeral fracture with or without intercondylar extension is performed. The distal humerus has two projections, the lateral and medial epicondyles. A supracondylar fracture is located immediately above the epicondyles and a transcondylar fracture is one that extends through them. These types of fractures may also extend into the intercondylar region and involve the trochlea and/or olecranon fossa. Separately reportable radiographs are obtained to confirm the fracture. The fracture fragments are manually reduced (manipulated) back into proper anatomic alignment. Separately reportable radiographs are obtained to confirm anatomic reduction. The ulnar nerve is located and protected. This may require a small incision over the ulnar groove to hold the ulnar nerve out of the way. Next, percutaneous pins or K-wires are inserted to stabilize the fracture fragments. The pin or K-wire is positioned on the drill and inserted. A small incision may be made in the skin to facilitate placement of the pin or K-wire. Two pins are typically used, one inserted laterally and a second one inserted medially. Pins are positioned so that they cross each other proximal to the fracture site at an angle of about 30 degrees. Correct positioning of the pins and anatomic reduction is confirmed radiographically. The pins are trimmed but left protruding from the skin. A long arm cast is applied.

24545-24546

24545 Open treatment of humeral supracondylar or transcondylar fracture, includes internal fixation, when performed; without intercondylar extension
24546 Open treatment of humeral supracondylar or transcondylar fracture, includes internal fixation, when performed; with intercondylar extension

An open reduction of a fracture of the distal humerus, supracondylar or transcondylar, is performed, including any necessary internal fixation. The distal humerus has two projections, the lateral epicondyle and the medial epicondyle. Fractures immediately above the epicondyles are referred to as supracondylar fractures. Fractures through the epicondyles are referred to as transcondylar. These types of fractures may extend into the intercondylar region of the bone and involve the trochlea and/or olecranon fossa. The trochlea is the pulley-like process that receives the ulna and the olecranon fossa is the posterior depression in the distal humerus that articulates with the olecranon in the ulna. Open repair of these types of fractures is usually performed by olecranon osteotomy. An incision is made in the skin over the elbow. The ulnar nerve is released from the cubital tunnel and exposed, retracted, and protected. The olecranon is isolated and a small incision is made into the capsule. A probe is passed into the trochlea and the coronoid process is identified. The osteotomy cut is then made just proximal to the coronoid process. The olecranon with the intact triceps insertion is reflected posteriorly. The entire supracondylar and transcondylar joint surfaces are now easily accessed. Supracondylar and transcondylar fractures are repaired by reconstructing the articular surface and securing the fracture fragments to the humeral shaft. Small fragments may be secured with sutures. Internal fixation, such as pins and/or screws may be used to secure larger fragments. One technique temporarily places pins that are replaced with screws once satisfactory reduction is achieved. Following satisfactory reduction and fixation of the fracture, the olecranon osteotomy is closed. Use 24545 when the fracture does not extend into the intercondylar region (trochlea, olecranon process) and 24546 when fractures in the intercondylar region (trochlea and olecranon fossa) are also repaired.

24560-24565

24560 Closed treatment of humeral epicondylar fracture, medial or lateral; without manipulation
24565 Closed treatment of humeral epicondylar fracture, medial or lateral; with manipulation

Closed treatment of a medial or lateral epicondylar fracture of the humerus is performed. The medial and lateral epicondyles are boney projections at the distal humerus. Epicondylar fractures are extra-articular fractures involving the medial or lateral columns. Separately reportable radiographs are obtained to confirm the fracture. A neurovascular exam is performed to ensure that the nerves and blood vessels at the site of the injury are intact. In 24560, a nondisplaced medial or lateral epicondylar fracture of the humerus is evaluated. No manipulation of the fracture fragments is required. The arm is immobilized using a long arm posterior splint, sugar tong splint, or long arm cast. In 24565, a minimally displaced medial or lateral epicondylar fracture of the humerus is treated. The displaced fracture fragments are manually reduced (manipulated) back to proper anatomic alignment. Separately reportable radiographs are obtained to confirm anatomic reduction. The arm is immobilized as described above.

24566

24566   Percutaneous skeletal fixation of humeral epicondylar fracture, medial or lateral, with manipulation

Percutaneous skeletal fixation of a medial or lateral epicondylar fracture of the humerus is performed. The medial and lateral epicondyles are bony projections at the distal humerus. Epicondylar fractures are extra-articular fractures involving the medial or lateral columns. Separately reportable radiographs are obtained to confirm the fracture. A neurovascular exam is performed to ensure that the nerves and blood vessels at the injury site are intact. The fracture fragments are manually reduced (manipulated) back into proper anatomic alignment. Separately reportable radiographs are obtained to confirm anatomic reduction. The ulnar nerve is located and protected. This may require a small incision over the ulnar groove to hold the ulnar nerve out of the way. Next, percutaneous pins or K-wires are inserted to stabilize the fracture fragments. The pin or K-wire is positioned on the drill and inserted. A small incision may be made in the skin to facilitate placement of the pin or K-wire. Two pins are used, one inserted laterally and one inserted medially, although for some fractures, other pin configurations are used. Correct positioning of the pins and anatomic reduction is confirmed radiographically. The pins are trimmed but left protruding from the skin. A long arm cast is applied.

24575

24575   Open treatment of humeral epicondylar fracture, medial or lateral, includes internal fixation, when performed

An open reduction of a fracture of the medial or lateral epicondyle of the distal humerus is performed including any necessary internal fixation. The distal humerus has two projections, the lateral epicondyle and the medial epicondyle. Epicondylar fractures are extra-articular fractures that involve the medial or lateral columns. This procedure is performed when an isolated displaced fracture of either the medial or lateral epicondyle (not both) is present. The fracture site is exposed, the ulnar nerve is identified and protected, and debris is cleared from the site before the fracture is reduced. Small fragments may be secured with sutures. Internal fixation, such as K-wire, pins, nails, and/or screws may be used to secure larger fragments. The wound is closed and a splint applied.

24576-24577

24576   Closed treatment of humeral condylar fracture, medial or lateral; without manipulation

24577   Closed treatment of humeral condylar fracture, medial or lateral; with manipulation

Closed treatment of a fracture of the medial or lateral condyle of the distal humerus is performed. The distal humerus has two projections, the lateral epicondyle and medial epicondyle. Condylar fractures extend through and separate the medial metaphysis and epicondyle from the rest of the humerus. Condylar fractures also extend in the trochlea and involve the articular surface. This procedure is performed when a fracture of either the medial or lateral condyle (not both) is present. Separately reportable radiographs are obtained to confirm the fracture. A neurovascular exam is performed to ensure that the nerves and blood vessels at the site of the injury are intact. In 24576, a nondisplaced medial or lateral condylar fracture of the humerus is evaluated. No manipulation of the fracture fragments is required. The arm is immobilized using a long arm cast. In 24577, a minimally displaced medial or lateral epicondylar fracture of the humerus is treated. The displaced fracture fragments are manually reduced (manipulated) back to proper anatomic alignment. Separately reportable radiographs are obtained to confirm anatomic reduction. The arm is immobilized as described above.

24579

24579   Open treatment of humeral condylar fracture, medial or lateral, includes internal fixation, when performed

An open reduction of a fracture of the medial or lateral condyle of the distal humerus is performed including any necessary internal fixation. The distal humerus has two projections, the lateral and medial epicondyle. Condylar fractures extend through and separate the medial metaphysis and epicondyle from the rest of the humerus. Condylar fractures also extend into the trochlea and involve the articular surface. This procedure is performed when a fracture of either the medial or lateral condyle (not both) is present. An incision is made in the skin over the elbow. If the medial condyle is fractured, branches of the medial antebrachial cutaneous nerve are identified and protected as is the ulnar nerve. If ulnar nerve transposition is required, the ulnar nerve is released from the cubital tunnel and exposed, then retracted and protected. The isolated fracture in the medial or lateral condyle is identified. Fracture surfaces are cleared of debris and the joint space is irrigated. The medial or lateral condylar fragment is reduced and secured at a minimum of two sites to prevent rotation. Small fragments may be secured with sutures. Internal fixation, such

as K-wires, pins, nails, screws, or plate and screw fixation may be used to secure larger fragments. The wound is closed and a splint is applied.

24582

24582   Percutaneous skeletal fixation of humeral condylar fracture, medial or lateral, with manipulation

Percutaneous skeletal fixation of a medial or lateral condylar fracture of the humerus is performed. The distal humerus has two projections, the lateral and medial epicondyle. Condylar fractures extend through and separate the medial metaphysis and epicondyle from the rest of the humerus. Condylar fractures also extend in the trochlea and involve the articular surface. This procedure is performed when a fracture of either the medial or lateral condyle (not both) is present. Separately reportable radiographs are obtained to confirm the fracture. A neurovascular exam is performed to ensure that the nerves and blood vessels at the injury site are intact. The fracture fragments are manually reduced (manipulated) back to proper anatomic alignment. Separately reportable radiographs are obtained to confirm anatomic reduction. The ulnar nerve is located and protected. This may require a small incision over the ulnar groove to hold the ulnar nerve out of the way. Next, percutaneous pins or K-wires are inserted to stabilize the fracture fragments. The pin or K-wire is positioned on the drill and inserted. A small incision may be made in the skin to facilitate placement of the pin or K-wire. Two pins are typically used, one inserted laterally and one inserted medially, although for some fractures, other pin configurations are used. Correct positioning of the pins and anatomic reduction is confirmed radiographically. The pins are trimmed but left protruding from the skin. A long arm cast is applied.

24586-24587

24586   Open treatment of periarticular fracture and/or dislocation of the elbow (fracture distal humerus and proximal ulna and/or proximal radius)

24587   Open treatment of periarticular fracture and/or dislocation of the elbow (fracture distal humerus and proximal ulna and/or proximal radius); with implant arthroplasty

A displaced periarticular fracture and/or dislocation of the elbow is treated by open reduction (24586) or a prosthetic elbow implant (24587). An incision is made over the posterior aspect of the elbow. The ulnar nerve is exposed and dissected free of surrounding structures from the medial intermuscular septum proximally to the flexor carpi ulnaris distally and protected. The triceps tendon is split in the midline from the distal aspect of humerus to the olecranon process. The radial nerve is exposed and protected. Fracture fragments and debris are cleared from the fracture site. In 24586, fractures of the distal humerus, proximal ulna, and/or proximal radius are reduced. Internal fixation is used to maintain fracture fragments in anatomical alignment or separately reportable external fixation may be applied. Alignment is verified radiographically and the operative wound is closed in layers. In 24587, elbow joint structures are replaced with a prosthetic implant. The lateral epicondyle of the humerus is exposed. The interval between the anconeus and flexor carpi ulnaris is incised and the triceps mobilized. The anconeus is elevated off the lateral aspect of the proximal ulna. The radial aspect of the elbow joint is addressed next and tissue dissected off the lateral epicondyle. The elbow is externally rotated and flexed. The posterior joint capsule is removed. The roof of the olecranon is exposed. The medial collateral ligament is released from the epicondyle. The tip of the olecranon is removed with a rongeur or oscillating saw. Tissue is dissected off the humerus and the roof of the olecranon fossa is removed down to the level of cancellous bone. The humeral canal is reamed. A cutting guide is placed and the distal aspect of the humerus is removed along the plane of the medial and lateral supracondylar columns. A trial implant is placed to check width and alignment. The ulnar canal is established using a high speed bur followed by a reamer. A trial implant is placed and tested. The trial implants are removed. The radial head is debrided or resected. The permanent implants are placed and bone cement injected in a retrograde fashion to secure them. The implants are locked together with a pin which is used to create a hinged prosthetic joint. Ligament and tendons are reattached. The triceps is medialized. A subcutaneous pocket is created for the ulnar nerve and the nerve is placed between subcutaneous fat and fascia near the medial epicondyle. Fascia and skin are closed in layers. The arm is fully extended and placed in a splint.

24600-24605

24600   Treatment of closed elbow dislocation; without anesthesia

24605   Treatment of closed elbow dislocation; requiring anesthesia

The physician treats a closed dislocation of the elbow. For a posterior elbow dislocation the patient is placed in a prone position. With the humerus supported by the examination table, the dislocated elbow is flexed to 90 degrees with the forearm hanging off the table and the fingers pointing to the ground. Manual downward traction is applied to the forearm with one hand while the humerus is grasped with the other hand and downward pressure is applied to the olecranon. Alternatively, the patient may be placed in a supine position with the affected arm extended to the side and the elbow slightly flexed. The humerus is held in position by an assistant while the physician applies in-line traction to the forearm keeping the elbow slightly flexed and supinated. For an anterior elbow dislocation, an assistant applies countertraction to the humerus by grasping it with two hands while the physician applies in-line traction to the forearm. Range of motion is then tested and neurovascular structures reassessed to ensure that there is no entrapment of nerves or blood vessels. A splint is applied as needed. Use code 24600 to report treatment without anesthesia and 24605 if anesthesia is required.

24615

24615   Open treatment of acute or chronic elbow dislocation

Open treatment of acute elbow dislocation is most often performed when there is neurovascular compromise of joint structures or when attempted closed reduction of the elbow fails. Chronic elbow dislocation requires open treatment due to soft tissue contractures or other degeneration of joint structures due to the chronic injury. An incision is made over the elbow. The site of the incision may vary based on the type of dislocation (anterior, posterior, or divergent). The ulnar and radial nerves are identified and protected. Blood vessels are also identified and protected. In chronic dislocation any adhesions are lysed. Soft tissues are debrided as needed. The elbow joint is reduced and range of motion and stability of the joint is evaluated. The operative wound is closed in layers and the elbow is immobilized as needed.

24620

24620   Closed treatment of Monteggia type of fracture dislocation at elbow (fracture proximal end of ulna with dislocation of radial head), with manipulation

Closed treatment of a Monteggia type fracture dislocation at the elbow is performed with manipulation. Monteggia type fracture dislocation is characterized by a fracture of the proximal end of the ulna with dislocation of the radial head. Separately reportable radiographs are obtained to confirm the fracture. A neurovascular exam is performed to ensure that the nerves and blood vessels at the injury site are intact. The dislocated radial head is manually reduced (manipulated) back into proper anatomic alignment. If the ulnar fracture is displaced, it is manipulated back into anatomic alignment. Separately reportable radiographs are obtained to confirm that reduction of the fracture dislocation is in good alignment. The arm is immobilized in a long arm cast.

24635

24635   Open treatment of Monteggia type of fracture dislocation at elbow (fracture proximal end of ulna with dislocation of radial head), includes internal fixation, when performed

An open reduction of a Monteggia type fracture dislocation at the elbow is performed including any necessary internal fixation. This type of injury is characterized by fracture of the proximal end of the ulna with dislocation of the radial head. An incision is made to expose the fracture in the proximal ulna. The ulnar fracture is reduced first. The fracture ends are exposed and cleaned. Fracture fragments are reduced and internal fixation is applied as needed. Internal fixation devices used are typically either dynamic compression plate or limited contact-dynamic compression plate fixed with screws just proximal and distal to the fracture. Once satisfactory reduction of the ulnar fracture has been achieved, the radial head dislocation will usually reduce indirectly. If the radial head does not reduce indirectly, an incision is made over the joint and an open reduction is performed. This may require repair of the annular ligament. When satisfactory reduction has been achieved of both the ulnar fracture and radial head, the wounds are closed and a splint is applied.

24640

24640   Closed treatment of radial head subluxation in child, nursemaid elbow, with manipulation

Closed treatment of a radial head subluxation in a child, also referred to as nursemaid elbow, is performed with manipulation. Nursemaid elbow occurs when the head of the radius slips under the annular ligament, usually resulting from the wrist or hand being pulled, such as when an adult has a hold of the hand or wrist and the child lurches in the opposite direction. Separately reportable radiographs may be obtained to rule-out a fracture. To treat nursemaid elbow, the elbow is first immobilized and the region of the radial head is palpated with one hand. Using the other hand, the radial head is manipulated back into its normal position. This can be accomplished using several different techniques including axial compression applied at the wrist with supination of the forearm and flexion of the elbow. Alternatively, pronation or extension of the forearm may be used to manipulate the radial head back into normal position. As the radial head returns to its normal position, a click or snap is felt at the radial head. Once the radial head subluxation has been reduced, the child is observed until normal arm movement is verified. If the child does not demonstrate normal arm movement within 15 to 30 minutes, separately reportable radiographs may be obtained to verify successful reduction.

24650-24655

24650   Closed treatment of radial head or neck fracture; without manipulation
24655   Closed treatment of radial head or neck fracture; with manipulation

Closed treatment of a radial head or neck fracture is performed. Separately reportable radiographs are obtained to confirm the fracture. A neurovascular exam is performed to ensure that the nerves and blood vessels at the site of the injury are intact. In 24650,

a nondisplaced fracture of the radial head or neck is evaluated. No manipulation of the fracture fragments is required. The arm is immobilized using a long arm splint or cast. In 24655, a minimally displaced fracture of the radial head or neck is treated. The displaced fracture fragments are manually reduced (manipulated) back to proper anatomic alignment. Separately reportable radiographs are obtained to confirm anatomic reduction. A long arm splint or cast is applied to immobilize the arm.

24665-24666

24665   Open treatment of radial head or neck fracture, includes internal fixation or radial head excision, when performed
24666   Open treatment of radial head or neck fracture, includes internal fixation or radial head excision, when performed; with radial head prosthetic replacement

An open reduction of a radial head or neck fracture is performed including any necessary internal fixation or radial head excision. Using a posterior approach, the fracture site in the radial head or neck is exposed. The site is cleared of debris, reduced, and intra-articular fragments are secured to the radial shaft. It is sometimes necessary to remove the radial head and fix the fragments on the back table, although it is preferable to fix the fracture in place so as to preserve soft tissue attachments. Internal fixation is applied as needed, including screws alone or minifragment plates and screws. Internal fixation is typically performed on each individual fragment. If the radial head cannot be repaired, the radial head fragments or the entire radial head may be excised. Use 24666 when radial head prosthetic replacement is performed. The radial neck is divided with an oscillating saw, and then trimmed and leveled using an end-cutting mill. The implant bed is prepared using reamers of increasing diameter. A trial component is placed in the surgically created canal to check the fit and range of motion, and any necessary adjustments are made to the canal, which is then packed with bone chips. Bone cement is inserted and the implant stem is seated in the canal with the implant collar flush with the resected surface of the radius. The cup component is snapped into the joint. Range of motion and the stability of the cup under the condyle are checked and the annular ligament is repaired.

24670-24675

24670   Closed treatment of ulnar fracture, proximal end (eg, olecranon or coronoid process[es]); without manipulation
24675   Closed treatment of ulnar fracture, proximal end (eg, olecranon or coronoid process[es]); with manipulation

Closed treatment of a fracture of the proximal end of the ulna is performed without manipulation in 24670. This procedure includes treatment of fractures of the olecranon or coronoid process. The ulna is the medial bone of the forearm. The proximal end contains the olecranon, the bony prominence at the posterior elbow and the coronoid process, the anterior projection. The olecranon and coronoid processes receive the trochlea of the humerus, forming the articulate elbow joint. A nondisplaced fracture of the proximal end of the ulna is evaluated. Separately reportable x-rays are reviewed. The fracture may be immobilized using a sling or splint. Use 24675 when closed treatment of an ulnar fracture is performed with manipulation. A minimally displaced fracture of the proximal end of the ulna is evaluated and separately reportable x-rays are obtained. The displaced fragments are manually reduced (manipulated) back to proper anatomic alignment, verified by separately reportable x-rays. The fracture may be immobilized using a sling or splint.

24685

24685   Open treatment of ulnar fracture, proximal end (eg, olecranon or coronoid process[es]), includes internal fixation, when performed

Open reduction of a fracture of the proximal end of the ulna is performed including any necessary internal fixation. This procedure includes treatment of fractures of the olecranon or coronoid process. The ulna is the medial bone of the forearm. The proximal end of the ulna contains the olecranon, the bony prominence at the posterior elbow and the coronoid process, the anterior projection. The olecranon and coronoid process receive the trochlea of the humerus forming the elbow joint. An incision is made over the elbow and the fracture site is cleared of debris. The fracture is reduced into proper position and the fragments are fixed using sutures and/or internal fixation, such as a combination of wires, pins and/or screws, or a plate placed under the ulna and around the tip of the elbow fixed with screws. The fracture is immobilized using a sling or splint.

24800-24802

24800   Arthrodesis, elbow joint; local
24802   Arthrodesis, elbow joint; with autogenous graft (includes obtaining graft)

Arthrodesis, also referred to as fusion, is performed primarily to treat severe elbow pain caused by arthritis that is not responding to nonsurgical interventions or for severe trauma to the elbow. A skin incision is made over the posterior aspect of the elbow. Tendons and ligaments are retracted and the joint surface exposed. A bur is used to remove the articular cartilage from the radial head, olecranon process of the ulna and the distal articular surface of the humerus. The elbow is positioned in 90 degrees of flexion and the radius, ulna, and humerus carefully aligned. Bone grafts may be obtained through the same incision (local) or harvested through a separate incision. The bone graft is configured

CPT © 2016 American Medical Association. All Rights Reserved.

● New Code   ▲ Revised Code

Musculoskeletal System

and packed into the joint space. The bones may be immobilized using plate and screw fixation or a separately reportable external fixation device. The incisions are closed. If plate and screw fixation has been used, the arm is placed in a cast or splint. Use 24800 for arthrodesis with a local bone graft. Use 24802, when the bone graft is obtained through a separate incision.

24900-24920

24900   Amputation, arm through humerus; with primary closure
24920   Amputation, arm through humerus; open, circular (guillotine)

An above-elbow amputation may be high (at the proximal metaphysis above the deltoid tuberosity), middle (any site along the diaphysis), or low (supracondylar). The patient is positioned with the shoulder slightly elevated on the operative side. In 24900, skin and muscle flap incision lines are marked on the skin. Typically, an anterior/posterior fishmouth flap is used. The skin and superficial fascia are incised perpendicular to the skin surface. Underlying soft tissue is dissected and blood vessels and nerves exposed. Large blood vessels are mobilized, suture ligated and divided. Nerves are mobilized from the muscular bed, doubly ligated and divided and allowed to retract into the muscle tissue. Muscles are transected along the previously marked flap lines. The humerus is exposed and periosteal flaps are created. The bone is transected at the level of the periosteal flaps. The flaps are sutured over the remaining bone. Antagonistic muscle groups are sutured to each other and anchored to the periosteum in such a way that the remaining portion of the humerus is completely enveloped in muscle. Muscle sutures may be reinforced using synthetic tape that is placed through drill holes in the humerus to prevent movement of the muscle tissue. Drains are placed and subcutaneous fascia and skin closed around the drains. A rigid dressing is applied to reduce pain and prevent edema. In 24920, a circular amputation, also called a guillotine or linear amputation, is performed. Skin incisions are made in a circular (linear) fashion at the predetermined site in the upper arm. Soft tissue is dissected and blood vessels and nerves located, ligated, and transected as described above. The underlying muscle tissue is then transected at a point proximal to the skin incision. Periosteal flaps are created and the humerus is then transected slightly higher than the muscle. The periosteal flaps, muscle and skin are then closed over the bone as described above and a rigid dressing applied.

24925

24925   Amputation, arm through humerus; secondary closure or scar revision

Secondary closure or scar revision of previous above-elbow amputation through the humerus is performed to obtain a pain-free stump covered with normal skin that functions well with a prosthesis. For secondary closure, the raw surface of the stump is debrided and all devitalized tissue is excised. Skin and subcutaneous tissue are fashioned into flaps and used to cover the stump taking care to ensure that there is no undue tension along the suture line. For scar revision, the scar tissue is excised. Skin flaps are fashioned and the edges are undermined to ensure smooth, tension-free approximation along the suture line.

24930

24930   Amputation, arm through humerus; re-amputation

Re-amputation of the arm through the humerus is done at a higher level to remove diseased, infected, or nonviable tissue posing a risk to the patient and/or form a healthy stump for use with a prosthesis. The incision lines for the re-amputation are marked on the skin. The skin and underlying soft tissue are incised. The muscles are exposed, isolated by muscle group, and divided. Nerves and blood vessels are identified and isolated, taking care to ensure that nerves are separated from arteries to prevent pulsatile irritation of the nerves. Nerves are transected and allowed to retract into soft tissue. Blood vessels are suture ligated and transected. The humerus is exposed and periosteal flaps are created. The humerus is transected at the level of the periosteal flaps. The flaps are sutured over the remaining bone. Antagonistic muscle groups are sutured to each other and anchored to the periosteum in such a way that the remaining portion of the humerus is completely enveloped in muscle. Skin flaps are fashioned and sutured over the muscle.

24931

24931   Amputation, arm through humerus; with implant

An above-elbow amputation may be high (at the proximal metaphysis above the deltoid tuberosity), middle (any site along the diaphysis), or low (supracondylar). One of the more common implants is a T-prosthesis which is configured with artificial humeral condyles. The patient is positioned with the shoulder slightly elevated on the operative side. Skin and muscle flap incision lines are marked on the skin taking care that the flap is long enough to cover the prosthetic implant. The skin and superficial fascia are incised perpendicular to the skin surface. Underlying soft tissue is dissected and blood vessels and nerves exposed. Large blood vessels are mobilized, suture ligated and divided. Nerves are mobilized from the muscular bed, doubly ligated and divided and allowed to retract into the muscle tissue. Muscles are transected along the previously marked flap lines. The humerus is exposed and transected. The humerus stump is prepared and sized, and an appropriate prosthetic implant selected. The prosthetic implant is secured to the stump. The flaps are sutured over the remaining bone and implant. Antagonistic muscle groups are sutured to each other and

anchored in such a way that the remaining portion of the humerus and the implant are completely enveloped in muscle. Muscle sutures may be reinforced using synthetic tape that is placed through drill holes in the humerus to prevent movement of the muscle tissue. Drains are placed and subcutaneous fascia and skin closed around the drains. A rigid dressing is applied to reduce pain and prevent edema.

24935

24935   Stump elongation, upper extremity

Stump elongation is typically performed to improve the fit of a prosthesis and to provide greater mobility of the remaining portion of the limb and the prosthesis. The incision lines are marked on the skin. The skin and underlying soft tissue are incised. The muscles are exposed and dissected taking care to protect nerves and blood vessels. The humerus is exposed and the periosteum incised. The bone is then elongated using either vascularized bone flaps or a bone stretching device. If vascularized bone flaps are used, they are harvested and configured to the appropriate size and shape in a separately reportable procedure. The bone is then transected and the vascularized bone flaps are placed between the two bone segments and secured with internal fixation devices. The flaps are sutured over the remaining bone. Antagonistic muscle groups are sutured to each other and anchored to the periosteum in such a way that the remaining portion of the humerus is completely enveloped in muscle. Skin flaps are fashioned and sutured over the muscle. Alternatively, the bone may be transected and a separately reportable bone-lengthening external fixation device applied. As the transected bone segments begin to heal, the external fixation frame is adjusted several times a day moving the bones apart a millimeter at a time to allow new bone to be deposited between the two segments. Once the desired bone length has been achieved, the external fixation device is removed.

24940

24940   Cineplasty, upper extremity, complete procedure

Cineplasty of the upper extremity involves surgically isolating a muscle or muscle group in the chest or arm, applying skin grafts, and then attaching the muscle to a prosthetic limb or device that can be operated by contraction of the muscle. Cineplasty is not commonly performed today; however with new advances in biomechanics and prosthetic technology new techniques for cineplasty are being developed. The exact procedure depends on the level of the amputation and the muscle group to be isolated. The skin is incised and the pectoral, biceps, triceps or forearm muscle(s) is exposed. A loop of muscle is developed in the case of an upper arm (humeral) amputation or a muscle tunnel created in the lower arm. The physician may perform a myoplasty which involves isolating agonist and antagonist residual muscle pairs and tying them off so that they can work together to control the prosthesis. Myodesis which involves attaching the muscle to bone may be performed instead of or in addition to myoplasty. Full thickness skin grafts are harvested usually form the abdomen or upper thigh and prepared for grafting. The skin grafts are configured to the necessary dimensions and sutured over the exposed muscle loop or tunnel. The muscle is then attached to the prosthesis in such a way that the muscle can be used to operate the prosthesis.

25000-25001

25000   Incision, extensor tendon sheath, wrist (eg, deQuervains disease)
25001   Incision, flexor tendon sheath, wrist (eg, flexor carpi radialis)

Tendonitis or tenosynovitis causing pain at the wrist and/or in the hand is treated by incision of the tendon sheath. The skin over the affected tendon(s) in the wrist is incised and the tendon(s) exposed. The tendon sheath of the involved tendon or tendons is inspected and incised longitudinally. The skin is closed with sutures. Use 25000 for incision of the extensor tendon sheath to treat a condition such as DeQuervain's disease. DeQuervain's disease, also referred to as DeQuervain's tenosynovitis or tendonitis, is a painful inflammation of the extensor tendons at the wrist on the thumb side of the arm. Use 25001 for incision of the flexor carpi radialis tendon sheath or other flexor tendons at the wrist.

25020-25023

25020   Decompression fasciotomy, forearm and/or wrist, flexor OR extensor compartment; without debridement of nonviable muscle and/or nerve
25023   Decompression fasciotomy, forearm and/or wrist, flexor OR extensor compartment; with debridement of nonviable muscle and/or nerve

Decompression fasciotomy is performed to treat compartment syndrome, a condition in which swelling of tissue in the muscle compartment causes compression of the blood vessels and nerves. Muscle compartments are surrounded by fascia that separates groups of muscles from each other. Fascia is a thick layer of connective tissue that does not expand. Swelling of tissue within the compartment can restrict blood supply and cause permanent muscle and nerve damage. There are two compartments in the forearm, referred to as the flexor (volar) and extensor (dorsal) compartments. In this procedure, only one compartment of the forearm and/or wrist, either the flexor or extensor, requires decompression. To decompress the flexor compartment, a curvilinear skin incision is made beginning proximal to the antecubital fossa at the elbow crease and carried down to the middle of the palm. Alternatively, a lazy S type incision may be used that extends from the elbow crease on the ulnar side curving to the radial side at the midforearm and returning to the ulnar side at the wrist. The incision is then extended into the midpalm. Incisions are carried down through the fascia following the same line as the skin incision. Compartment pressure is checked to ensure that the deep flexor muscles have been adequately decompressed. If the extensor compartment requires decompression, a dorsal incision is made over the extensor muscles and carried down between the extensor wad and the extensor digitorum communis muscles. The fascia over each of the two dorsal compartments is opened, taking care to incise fascia over each of the superficial and deep muscle bellies. Pressures are checked to ensure extensor muscles have been adequately decompressed. In 25023, muscle tissue and nerves are inspected and any nonviable tissue is also debrided using sharp excision. Use 25020 when decompression of the flexor or extensor compartment is done without debridement. The skin and fascial incisions are left open and covered with a dressing. The patient is returned to the operating room for wound closure once the swelling subsides, usually within 24-72 hours.

25024-25025

25024 Decompression fasciotomy, forearm and/or wrist, flexor AND extensor compartment; without debridement of nonviable muscle and/or nerve

25025 Decompression fasciotomy, forearm and/or wrist, flexor AND extensor compartment; with debridement of nonviable muscle and/or nerve

Decompression fasciotomy is performed to treat compartment syndrome, a condition in which swelling of tissue in the muscle compartment causes compression of the blood vessels and nerves. Muscle compartments are surrounded by fascia that separates groups of muscles from each other. Fascia is a thick layer of connective tissue that does not expand. Swelling of tissue within the compartment can restrict blood supply and cause permanent muscle and nerve damage. There are two compartments in the forearm, referred to as the flexor (volar) and extensor (dorsal) compartments. In this procedure, both the flexor and extensor compartments require decompression. Decompression of the flexor compartment is performed first. A curvilinear skin incision is made beginning proximal to the antecubital fossa at the elbow crease and carried down to the middle of the palm. Alternatively, a lazy S type incision may be used that extends from the elbow crease on the ulnar side curving to the radial side at the midforearm and returning to the ulnar side at the wrist. The incision is then extended into the midpalm. Incisions are carried down through the fascia following the same line as the skin incision. Compartment pressure is checked to ensure that the deep flexor muscles have been adequately decompressed. The extensor compartment is then decompressed using a dorsal incision over the extensor muscles carried down between the extensor wad and the extensor digitorum communis muscles. The fascia over each of the two dorsal compartments is opened, taking care to incise fascia over each of the superficial and deep muscle bellies. Pressures are checked to ensure extensor muscles have been adequately decompressed. In 25025, muscle tissue and nerves are inspected and any nonviable tissue is debrided using sharp excision. Use 25024 for decompression of both the flexor and extensor compartments without debridement. The skin and fascial incisions are left open and covered with a dressing. The patient is returned to the operating room for wound closure once the swelling subsides, usually within 24-72 hours.

25028-25031

25028 Incision and drainage, forearm and/or wrist; deep abscess or hematoma

25031 Incision and drainage, forearm and/or wrist; bursa

An incision and drainage of a deep abscess or hematoma or an infected bursa is performed. In 25028, the soft tissues of the forearm and/or wrist are incised and drained. The soft tissues in this area are those overlying the radius, ulna, and/or carpal bones in the wrist joint. The approach is dictated by the location of the abscess or hematoma. The soft tissues are dissected and the pocket of pus or blood located. The wall of the abscess or hematoma is incised and the pus or blood drained. A large abscess may require probing of the pus pocket to break down loculations and ensure that all infection has been drained. The abscess or hematoma site is then flushed with antibiotic and/or normal saline solution. The pocket may be left open to drain, packed with gauze, or closed. In 25031, an incision and drainage of an infected bursa is performed. Bursa are sacs lined with synovial membrane that contain synovial fluid and are found in areas subject to friction such as prominent body parts, joints or areas where tendons pass over bone. The infected bursa is incised and the fluid drained. The bursal sac may be flushed with antibiotic and/or normal saline solution prior to closure.

25035

25035 Incision, deep, bone cortex, forearm and/or wrist (eg, osteomyelitis or bone abscess)

The bone cortex of the radius, ulna or one of the carpal bones is opened to treat a condition such as osteomyelitis or bone abscess. An incision is made in the skin and carried down through the soft tissue overlying the site of the infected bone. The periosteum over the infected region of the bone is elevated, a button of cortical bone removed, and the bone marrow exposed. Opening the bone cortex relieves pressure caused by inflammation of the bone marrow and prevents restriction of blood flow to the infected bone. If frank

pus is encountered, the buttonhole may be enlarged and extended using a chisel or gouge along the bone for one to two inches. If the epiphysis is involved, a section of the epiphyseal cortex may be removed. The bone abscess is drained.

25040

25040 Arthrotomy, radiocarpal or midcarpal joint, with exploration, drainage, or removal of foreign body

The radiocarpal joint is the region between the radius, the triangular fibrocartilage and the proximal row of carpal bones. The midcarpal joint is the region between the two rows of carpal bones in the wrist. An incision is made over the dorsal or ventral aspect of the wrist depending on whether the condition being explored can be more readily visualized by exposing the dorsal or ventral aspect of the joint. Soft tissues are dissected taking care to protect nerves and blood vessels. Tendons are retracted as needed and the joint capsule is incised. The joint is visually inspected and any abnormalities noted. If an infection is present, any pockets of pus are opened and drained. The joint space is irrigated with sterile saline or antibiotic solution as needed. A temporary drain may be positioned in the joint space. If a foreign body is present, it is located, grasped with forceps and removed. Following completion of the procedure, the joint capsule is closed, and overlying soft tissue and skin are closed in layers.

25065-25066

25065 Biopsy, soft tissue of forearm and/or wrist; superficial

25066 Biopsy, soft tissue of forearm and/or wrist; deep (subfascial or intramuscular)

Soft tissue biopsy of the forearm and/or wrist area is performed. Soft tissues include muscles, tendons, fat, blood vessels, lymph vessels, nerves, and tissues surrounding the joints. Local, regional, or general anesthesia or conscious sedation is administered depending on the site and depth of the planned biopsy. The skin over the biopsy site is cleansed. An incision is made and tissue dissected down to the mass or lesion taking care to protect blood vessels and nerves. A tissue sample is obtained and sent to the laboratory for separately reportable histological evaluation. The incision is closed with sutures. Use 25065 for a superficial biopsy of a mass or lesion in the subcutaneous tissue. Use 25066 for biopsy of deeper tissues requiring more extensive dissection of overlying tissues, such as a biopsy below the muscle fascia (subfascial) or within the muscle itself (intramuscular).

25071-25076

25071 Excision, tumor, soft tissue of forearm and/or wrist area, subcutaneous; 3 cm or greater

25073 Excision, tumor, soft tissue of forearm and/or wrist area, subfascial (eg, intramuscular); 3 cm or greater

25075 Excision, tumor, soft tissue of forearm and/or wrist area, subcutaneous; less than 3 cm

25076 Excision, tumor, soft tissue of forearm and/or wrist area, subfascial (eg, intramuscular); less than 3 cm

Soft tissues include subcutaneous fat and connective tissue, fascia, muscles, tendons, blood vessels, lymph vessels, nerves, and tissues surrounding the joints. Soft tissue tumors may be benign or malignant. Benign tumors are typically treated by excision, although small malignant or indeterminate tumors may be excised if the margins are well defined. Depending on the location of the tumor in the soft tissue of the forearm and/or wrist area, the skin over the tumor may be incised or a skin flap created and elevated. Overlying tissue is dissected and the soft tissue mass exposed. The tumor is then excised along with a margin of healthy tissue. Separately reportable frozen section may be performed to ensure that all margins are free of tumor cells. Drains are placed as needed and the surgical wound is closed in layers. For tumors in the subcutaneous fat or connective tissue, use 25075 for excision of less than 3 cm and 25071 for excision of 3 cm or greater. For tumors that lie below the fascia, use 25076 for excision of less than 3 cm and 25073 for excision of 3 cm or greater. Subfascial soft tissue tumors include those within muscle tissue.

25077-25078

25077 Radical resection of tumor (eg, sarcoma), soft tissue of forearm and/or wrist area; less than 3 cm

25078 Radical resection of tumor (eg, sarcoma), soft tissue of forearm and/or wrist area; 3 cm or greater

Soft tissues include muscles, tendons, fat, blood vessels, lymph vessels, nerves, and tissues surrounding the joints. Soft tissue tumors may be benign or malignant. Radical resection is typically performed for a malignant neoplasm, such as a sarcoma, although benign tumors and tumors of indeterminate nature may also require radical resection. A skin incision is made over the tumor in the forearm and/or wrist area, or a skin flap is created and elevated. Overlying tissue is dissected and the tumor exposed. The tumor is removed en bloc along with a wide margin of surrounding tissue. Radical resection involves excision of all involved soft tissue which may include muscles, nerves, and blood vessels. Separately reportable frozen section is performed to ensure that all margins are free of tumor cells. If margins show evidence of malignancy, additional tissue is removed until all margins are free of tumor cells. Drains are placed as needed. The surgical wound may be closed in layers, or separately reportable reconstructive procedures performed. Use 25077 for radical resection of soft tissue tumor of forearm and wrist less than 3 cm, and 25078 for 3 cm or greater.

25085

25085   Capsulotomy, wrist (eg, contracture)

A longitudinal midline incision or horizontal incision in Langer's lines is made over the dorsal aspect of the wrist depending on the site of the pathology. Full thickness skin flaps are developed down to the extensor retinaculum taking care to protect the superficial radial nerve, the dorsal sensory branch of the ulnar nerve and blood vessels. The retinaculum is incised longitudinally over the third dorsal compartment. If exposure of the ulnar aspect of the wrist is required, the extensor policis longus is retracted radially and the fourth extensor compartment elevated subperiosteally or the septum divided between the third and fourth compartments to create a flap over the ulna. If exposure of the radial aspect of the wrist is required the extensor retinaculum is elevated off Lister's tubercle and the second dorsal compartment released. For ulnar capsulotomy, the dorsal radioulnar ligament is incised longitudinally. For radial capsulotomy, the dorsal radiocarpal and intercarpal ligaments are incised in line with their fibers. The wrist capsule is then incised. Any adhesions are released. The surgical wound is then closed in layers.

25100-25101

25100   Arthrotomy, wrist joint; with biopsy
25101   Arthrotomy, wrist joint; with joint exploration, with or without biopsy, with or without removal of loose or foreign body

A longitudinal midline incision or horizontal incision in Langer's lines is made over the dorsal aspect of the wrist depending on the site of the pathology. Full thickness skin flaps are developed down to the extensor retinaculum taking care to protect the superficial radial nerve, the dorsal sensory branch of the ulnar nerve and blood vessels. The retinaculum is incised longitudinally over the third dorsal compartment. If exposure of the ulnar aspect of the wrist is required, the extensor policis longus is retracted radially and the fourth extensor compartment elevated subperiosteally or the septum divided between the third and fourth compartments to create a flap over the ulna. If exposure of the radial aspect of the wrist is required the extensor retinaculum is elevated off Lister's tubercle and the second dorsal compartment released. For ulnar capsulotomy, the dorsal radioulnar ligament is incised longitudinally. For radial capsulotomy, the dorsal radiocarpal and intercarpal ligaments are incised in line with their fibers. The wrist capsule is then incised and the wrist joint exposed. In 25100, biopsy forceps are used to obtain a tissue sample. In 25101, the joint is explored and any abnormalities noted. Tissue samples are obtained as needed. Any loose or foreign bodies are located and removed. Upon completion of the procedure, the joint is flushed with sterile saline and the surgical wound is then closed in layers.

25105

25105   Arthrotomy, wrist joint; with synovectomy

Synovectomy is performed to treat inflammation of the synovial tissue caused by conditions such as rheumatoid arthritis. The patient is placed in supine position with the shoulder abducted. A pneumatic tourniquet is applied to the upper arm. A longitudinal midline incision or horizontal incision in Langer's lines is made over the dorsal aspect of the wrist depending on the site of the pathology. Full thickness skin flaps are developed down to the extensor retinaculum taking care to protect the superficial radial nerve, the dorsal sensory branch of the ulnar nerve and blood vessels. The retinaculum is incised longitudinally over the third dorsal compartment. If exposure of the ulnar aspect of the wrist is required, the extensor policis longus is retracted radially and the fourth extensor compartment elevated subperiosteally or the septum divided between the third and fourth compartments to create a flap over the ulna. If exposure of the radial aspect of the wrist is required the extensor retinaculum is elevated off Lister's tubercle and the second dorsal compartment released. The wrist capsule is then incised. The wrist is examined and all inflamed synovial tissue is excised. Upon completion of the procedure, the joint is flushed with normal saline and the surgical wound is closed in layers.

25107

25107   Arthrotomy, distal radioulnar joint including repair of triangular cartilage, complex

The triangular fibrocartilage complex (TFCC) is a cushioning structure in the wrist that can be injured by falling on an outstretched hand. The patient is placed in supine position with the shoulder abducted. A pneumatic tourniquet is applied to the upper arm. Full thickness skin flaps are developed down to the extensor retinaculum taking care to protect the superficial radial nerve, the dorsal sensory branch of the ulnar nerve and blood vessels. The retinaculum is incised longitudinally over the third dorsal compartment. The extensor policis longus is retracted radially and the septum divided between the third and fourth compartments to create a flap over the ulna. Dissection continues down to the dorsal radioulnar ligament (DRUL). The DRUL and the periosteum over the lunate fossa are reflected. Drill holes are created in the dorsoulnar aspect of the distal radius. Horizontal

mattress sutures are placed in the triangular fibrocartilage complex and then through the previously created drill holes in the radius. Upon completion of the procedure, the joint is flushed with normal saline incisions are closed in layers.

25109

25109   Excision of tendon, forearm and/or wrist, flexor or extensor, each

A flexor or extensor tendon in the wrist or forearm is excised. Flexor tendons act to bend the wrist or decrease the angle between parts of the limb and extensor tendons straighten the wrist or increase the angle between parts of the limb, bringing them back into alignment. The physician incises the skin over the target tendon, retracting overlying tissue to reach the tendon, which is then dissected free from its attachments. The tendon is freed and both ends are severed. The tendon is removed and The incision is closed with sutures.

25110

25110   Excision, lesion of tendon sheath, forearm and/or wrist

The physician incises the skin over the target flexor or extensor tendon of the forearm or wrist. Overlying tissue is retracted and the tendon is exposed. The tendon sheath lesion is located, carefully dissected free of surrounding healthy tissue, and excised in its entirety. The abnormal tissue is sent for separately reportable pathology evaluation. The surgical wound is closed in layers.

25111-25112

25111   Excision of ganglion, wrist (dorsal or volar); primary
25112   Excision of ganglion, wrist (dorsal or volar); recurrent

A ganglion cyst is a small, benign cystic tumor, composed of ganglion cells, containing viscous fluid and connected either with a joint membrane or a tendon sheath. The physician makes an incision through the skin, subcutaneous and soft tissues. The ganglion cyst is exposed, dissected free of surrounding tissue, and excised from the joint membrane or a tendon on the top or the bottom of the wrist. Use 25111 for the initial excision of a primary ganglion cyst. Code 25112 if a recurrent cyst needs to be re-excised.

25115-25116

25115   Radical excision of bursa, synovia of wrist, or forearm tendon sheaths (eg, tenosynovitis, fungus, Tbc, or other granulomas, rheumatoid arthritis); flexors
25116   Radical excision of bursa, synovia of wrist, or forearm tendon sheaths (eg, tenosynovitis, fungus, Tbc, or other granulomas, rheumatoid arthritis); extensors, with or without transposition of dorsal retinaculum

The physician incises the skin and subcutaneous tissue over the affected bursa, wrist synovia, and/or flexor or extensor tendon of the forearm. In 25115, the volar aspect of the wrist joint and flexor tendons are exposed. Affected bursa, wrist synovia and flexor tendons are examined. If the bursa is greatly distended, it is windowed and fluid is released before excision is done. The fluid is sent for separately reportable laboratory evaluation. Any inflamed synovial tissue is also excised. If the flexor tendon sheath is inflamed it is incised longitudinally and all inflamed or abnormal tissue excised. In 25116, the dorsal aspect of the wrist joint and extensor tendon sheaths are exposed. Full thickness skin flaps are developed down to the extensor retinaculum taking care to protect the superficial radial nerve, the dorsal sensory branch of the ulnar nerve and blood vessels. The retinaculum is incised longitudinally over the third dorsal compartment. If exposure of the ulnar aspect of the wrist is required, the extensor policis longus is retracted radially and the fourth extensor compartment elevated subperiosteally or the septum divided between the third and fourth compartments to create a flap over the ulna. If exposure of the radial aspect of the wrist is required the extensor retinaculum is elevated off Lister's tubercle and the second dorsal compartment released. Affected bursa, wrist synovia and extensor tendons are examined. All inflamed tissue is excised as described above. To maintain stability of the wrist, the dorsal retinaculum may be rearranged or transposed. The surgical wound is then closed in layers. The abnormal tissue is sent for separately reportable pathology evaluation. The surgical wound is closed in layers.

25118-25119

25118   Synovectomy, extensor tendon sheath, wrist, single compartment
25119   Synovectomy, extensor tendon sheath, wrist, single compartment; with resection of distal ulna

This procedure is performed to treat inflammation of the synovial tissue caused by conditions such as rheumatoid arthritis. An incision is made over the posterior aspect of the wrist. The dorsal retinaculum is exposed and transverse incisions made at the proximal and distal borders. A longitudinal incision is made through the sixth compartment over the extensor carpi ulnaris tendon. The retinaculum is elevated and displaced radially to allow exposure the affected extensor tendon compartment. The affected compartment is explored and all inflamed synovial tissue is removed using a motorized suction shaving device. Use code 25118 for synovectomy performed on a single compartment. Use 25119 for a synovectomy performed on a single compartment with resection of the distal ulna. The synovectomy is performed as described above. The distal ulna is exposed taking care to protect the ulnar artery and nerve. The distal 1-2 cm of the ulna is then excised using an osteotome or bone saw. The ulnar styloid process and ulnar collateral ligament are preserved if possible. The remaining bone is smoothed and contoured. The remnants of the wrist capsule are anchored to the distal ulna and the wrist incision is closed in layers.

25120-25126

25120 **Excision or curettage of bone cyst or benign tumor of radius or ulna (excluding head or neck of radius and olecranon process)**

25125 **Excision or curettage of bone cyst or benign tumor of radius or ulna (excluding head or neck of radius and olecranon process); with autograft (includes obtaining graft)**

25126 **Excision or curettage of bone cyst or benign tumor of radius or ulna (excluding head or neck of radius and olecranon process); with allograft**

A bone cyst is a fluid filled space within the bone. One common type is a unicameral or simple bone cyst, which is a benign lesion. A less common type is an aneurysmal bone cyst which consists of vascular tissue surrounding a blood filled cystic lesion. There are a number of different types of benign bone tumors including giant cell tumors, chondromixoid fibromas, and enchondromas. In 25120, an incision is made in the skin over the site of the lesion in the radial or ulnar shaft or distal radius or ulna. Soft tissues are dissected and the lesion is exposed. If a cystic lesion is present, the bone is incised and a bone window created to open the cyst. Fluid is aspirated and sent to the laboratory for separately reportable analysis. A curette is inserted through the bone window and the lining of the cystic cavity is completely removed by curettage. Alternatively, some cystic lesions and most benign tumors are treated by excision. The lesion is exposed as described above. The physician then excises the benign lesion along with a margin of surrounding healthy bone. In 25125, the lesion is curetted or excised as described above. The physician then obtains healthy bone locally or from a separate site, such as the iliac crest. The bone autograft is packed into the defect in the radius or ulna. In 25126, the lesion is curetted or excised as described above. The defect is then packed with donor bone (allograft).

25130-25136

25130 **Excision or curettage of bone cyst or benign tumor of carpal bones**

25135 **Excision or curettage of bone cyst or benign tumor of carpal bones; with autograft (includes obtaining graft)**

25136 **Excision or curettage of bone cyst or benign tumor of carpal bones; with allograft**

The physician removes or scrapes away a cyst or non-cancerous tumor from one of the eight small bones that make up the wrist joint. A bone cyst is a fluid filled space within the bone. One common type is a unicameral or simple bone cyst, which is a benign lesion. A less common type is an aneurysmal bone cyst which consists of vascular tissue surrounding a blood filled cystic lesion. There are a number of different types of benign bone tumors including giant cell tumors, chondromixoid fibromas, and enchondromas. In 25130, an incision is made in the skin over the site of the lesion in carpal bone. Soft tissues are dissected and the lesion is exposed. If a cystic lesion is present, the bone is incised and a bone window created to open the cyst. Fluid is aspirated and sent to the laboratory for separately reportable analysis. A curette is inserted through the bone window and the lining of the cystic cavity is completely removed by curettage. Alternatively, some cystic lesions and most benign tumors are treated by excision. The lesion is exposed as described above. The physician then excises the benign lesion along with a margin of surrounding healthy bone. In 25135, the lesion is curetted or excised as described above. The physician then obtains healthy bone locally or from a separate site, such as the iliac crest. The bone autograft is packed into the defect in the carpal bone. In 25136, the lesion is curetted or excised as described above. The defect is then packed with donor bone (allograft).

25145

25145 **Sequestrectomy (eg, for osteomyelitis or bone abscess), forearm and/or wrist**

A sequestrectomy is performed for osteomyelitis or bone abscess of the forearm and/or wrist. A sequestrum is a piece of necrotic bone that has become separated from healthy surrounding bone. An incision is made in the skin and carried down through the soft tissue overlying the site of the osteomyelitis or bone abscess. If the periosteum is soft and viable, it is elevated off the necrotic sequestrum. The necrotic bone is excised and the ribbon of periosteum that was elevated off the necrotic bone is then approximated over the cortical bone defect. If the periosteum is not viable and an involucrum has formed around the sequestrum, the necrotic bone is removed, leaving the involucrum which will form new bone within the cortical bone defect. The incisions in the soft tissue and skin are closed and a dressing is applied.

25150-25151

25150 **Partial excision (craterization, saucerization, or diaphysectomy) of bone (eg, for osteomyelitis); ulna**

25151 **Partial excision (craterization, saucerization, or diaphysectomy) of bone (eg, for osteomyelitis); radius**

The physician performs a partial excision of bone, also referred to as craterization, saucerization, or diaphysectomy to treat osteomyelitis of the ulna (25150) or ulna (25151). Craterization and saucerization of bone involves removing infected and necrotic bone to form a shallow depression in the bone surface that will allow drainage from the infected area. Diaphysectomy involves removal of the infected portion of the shaft of a long bone. An incision is made in the skin and carried down through the soft tissue overlying the site of the osteomyelitis. Any soft tissue sinus tracts and devitalized soft tissue are resected. The area of necrotic and infected bone is exposed. A series of drill holes are made in the necrotic and infected bone and the bone between the drill holes is excavated to create an oval window using an osteotome. The amount of bone removed is dependent on the extent of the infection. A curette may be used to remove devitalized tissue from the medullary canal. Debridement continues until punctate bleeding is identified in the exposed bony surface. When all devitalized and infected tissue has been removed, the wound is copiously irrigated with sterile saline or antibiotic solution. The surgical wound is loosely closed and a drain placed.

25170

25170 **Radical resection of tumor, radius or ulna**

Radical resection is typically performed for a malignant neoplasm although benign tumors and tumors of indeterminate nature may also require radical resection. A skin incision is made over the tumor in the radius or ulna, or a skin flap is created and elevated. Overlying tissue is dissected and the tumor exposed. All bone and cartilage in the radius or ulna with tumor involvement is resected. The tumor is removed en bloc along with a wide margin of surrounding tissue. Radical resection of bone includes excision of all involved soft tissue which may include muscles, tendons, fat, blood vessels, lymph vessels, nerves, and tissues surrounding the joints. Separately reportable frozen section is performed to ensure that all margins are free of tumor cells. If margins show evidence of malignancy, additional tissue is removed until all margins are free of tumor cells. Drains are placed as needed. The surgical wound may be closed in layers, or separately reportable reconstructive procedures performed.

25210-25215

25210 **Carpectomy; 1 bone**

25215 **Carpectomy; all bones of proximal row**

The carpus or wrist joint consists of eight small bones in two rows with four bones in each row. The proximal row includes the pisiform, triquetrum, lunate, and scaphoid (navicular) bones. The distal row includes the hamate, capitate, trapezoid and trapezium bones. In 25210, a single carpal bone is excised. A longitudinal incision is made in the dorsal aspect of the wrist over the carpal bone that is to be excised. Traction is applied to the fingers. The carpal bone is exposed taking care to preserve the ligament. A rongeur is used to excise the middle portion of the bone causing it to collapse inward. The remaining proximal and distal aspects of the bone are carefully excised. The incision is closed in layers and the wrist immobilized in a cast. In 25215, all four carpal bones in the proximal row are excised. Removal of all four bones is typically performed to treat scapholunate advanced collapse (SLAC). SLAC results from chronic or untreated scapholunate dissociation or chronic scaphoid nonunion causing osteoarthritis and subluxation of the wrist joint. Other indications include dorsiflexion instability, nonunion of scaphoid with carpal instability, failed prosthetic replacement of lunate, and Keinbock's disease. A longitudinal incision is made over the dorsal aspect of the wrist. Traction is applied to the fingers. The proximal carpal bones are exposed taking care to preserve the radioscaphocapitate ligament. A rongeur is used to excise the middle portion of each bone which causes the bones to collapse inward. The remaining proximal and distal aspects of each bone are carefully excised. The incision is closed in layers and the wrist immobilized in a cast.

25230

25230 **Radial styloidectomy (separate procedure)**

Radial styloidectomy is performed to treat pain caused by impingement between the scaphoid bone and the radial styloid process. An incision is made over the radial aspect of the wrist between the first and second extensor tendon compartments taking care to identify and protect sensory branches of the radial nerve and radial artery. Subperiosteal dissection is performed down to bone for 1.5 to 2 cm. The periosteum is elevated off the bone along with the retinaculum. The radioscaphoid joint is exposed and the joint capsule incised. An intra-articular elevator is used to elevate the scaphoid off the radial styloid. An osteotome or bone saw is used to excise the radial styloid. When enough bone has been removed to relieve the impingement, the periosteum is reapproximated, the retinaculum repaired, and overlying soft tissues are closed in layers.

Musculoskeletal System

Musculoskeletal System

25240

25240   Excision distal ulna partial or complete (eg, Darrach type or matched resection)

An incision is made over the posterior aspect of the wrist. The dorsal retinaculum is exposed and transverse incisions made at the proximal and distal borders. A longitudinal incision is made through the sixth compartment over the extensor carpi ulnaris tendon. The retinaculum is elevated and displaced radially. The distal ulna is exposed taking care to protect the ulnar artery and nerve. The distal 1-2 cm of the ulna is then excised using an osteotome or bone saw. The ulnar styloid process and ulnar collateral ligament are preserved if possible. The remaining bone is smoothed and contoured. The remnants of the wrist capsule are anchored to the distal ulna and the wrist incision is closed in layers.

25246

25246   Injection procedure for wrist arthrography

An injection procedure for wrist arthrography is performed. The skin over the injection site is cleansed and a local anesthetic is injected. A needle may be inserted into the joint and fluid aspirated with a syringe. The radiopaque substance is then injected into the wrist joint, which is exercised to help distribute the radiopaque substance. Once the contrast has been distributed throughout the joint, separately reportable radiograph images are obtained.

25248

25248   Exploration with removal of deep foreign body, forearm or wrist

Deep tissue refers to the tissue below the muscle fascia (subfascial) or within the muscle itself (intramuscular). The foreign body in the wrist or forearm is located by palpation or separately reportable radiographs. A straight or elliptical incision is made in the skin and subcutaneous tissue. The muscle fascia is exposed and incised. Dissection continues as needed into the muscle tissue until the foreign body is located. The physician may need to dissect tissues around the foreign body to remove it or a hemostat or grasping forceps may be used to remove the foreign body. The wound is then flushed with normal saline or antibiotic solution and the incision is closed in layers.

25250-25251

25250   Removal of wrist prosthesis; (separate procedure)
25251   Removal of wrist prosthesis; complicated, including total wrist

The physician makes an incision in the area of the wrist and dissects down to the bone. A prosthetic device is removed that had been previously placed. Code 25251 if the procedure is complicated and the prosthetic device that is removed involves the entire wrist.

25259

25259   Manipulation, wrist, under anesthesia

Manipulation under anesthesia (MUA) of the wrist is performed. This procedure is performed to improve range of motion by rupturing fibrous adhesions (arthrofibrosis) that develop following surgery or fracture of the wrist. An anesthetic is administered. The physician then takes the wrist through a complete range of motion including flexion, hyperextension, radial deviation, and ulnar deviation. The physician must use sufficient force to rupture the adhesions while taking care not to apply too much force which could injure the joint structures or bones.

25260-25265

25260   Repair, tendon or muscle, flexor, forearm and/or wrist; primary, single, each tendon or muscle
25263   Repair, tendon or muscle, flexor, forearm and/or wrist; secondary, single, each tendon or muscle
25265   Repair, tendon or muscle, flexor, forearm and/or wrist; secondary, with free graft (includes obtaining graft), each tendon or muscle

The flexor tendons and muscles are located on the palmar aspect of the forearm and wrist and originate from the medial epicondyle of the humerus and the proximal radius and ulna. The flexor tendons and muscles originating from these sites include the flexor carpi radialis, palmaris longus, flexor carpi ulnaris, flexor digitorum superficialis, flexor digitorum profundus, and flexor pollicis longus. These muscles and tendons allow flexion of the wrist, hand, and fingers. The flexor tendons and muscles are common sites of both open and closed injuries. Lacerations and puncture wounds can cause partial or complete transection of one or more flexor tendons. Closed injuries such as avulsion are another type of injury that can occur. An incision is made over the site of the flexor tendon or muscle injury. If the tendon has been completely transected, the severed end of the flexor tendon is located, grasped and pulled distally or proximally. The tendon is then suture repaired. If the tendon has only been partially transected, the transected fibers are repaired. If the muscle itself has been lacerated or torn, the muscle tissue is repaired in layers. Use 25260 to report primary suture repair of a single flexor tendon or muscle. If a functional result is not achieved from the primary repair, secondary repair may be required. Use 25263 to report secondary suture repair of a single flexor tendon or muscle. Use 25265 for a secondary

repair requiring placement of a free graft. A local tendon graft is harvested and attached to the remnants of the severed tendon in the forearm or wrist and then attached at the distal insertion site of the tendon. Range of motion is tested and tension adjusted as needed to allow good range of motion in the wrist, hand, and fingers. The surgical wound is closed in layers. The wrist and hand are immobilized using a splint or cast.

25270-25274

25270   Repair, tendon or muscle, extensor, forearm and/or wrist; primary, single, each tendon or muscle
25272   Repair, tendon or muscle, extensor, forearm and/or wrist; secondary, single, each tendon or muscle
25274   Repair, tendon or muscle, extensor, forearm and/or wrist; secondary, with free graft (includes obtaining graft), each tendon or muscle

The extensor tendons and muscles are located on the dorsal aspect of the forearm and wrist and originate from the lateral epicondyle and lateral supracondylar ridge of the humerus and the proximal dorsal surface of the ulna. The extensor tendons and muscles originating from these sites include the extensor carpi radialis longus, extensor carpi ulnaris, extensor digitorum, and extensor indicis. These muscles and tendons allow extension of the wrist, hand, and fingers. Both open injuries such as laceration or puncture and closed injuries such as rupture or avulsion may require repair. An incision is made over the site of the affected extensor tendon or muscle. If the tendon has been completely transected, the severed end of the extensor tendon is located, grasped and pulled distally or proximally. The tendon is then suture repaired. If the tendon has only been partially transected, the transected fibers are repaired. If the muscle itself has been lacerated or torn, the muscle tissue is repaired in layers. Use 25270 to report primary suture repair of a single extensor tendon or muscle. If a functional result is not achieved from the primary repair, secondary repair may be required. Use 25272 to report secondary suture repair of a single extensor tendon or muscle. Use 25274 for a secondary repair requiring placement of a free graft. A local tendon graft is harvested and attached to the remnants of the severed tendon in the forearm or wrist and then attached at the distal insertion site of the tendon. Range of motion is tested and tension adjusted as needed to allow good range of motion in the wrist, hand and fingers. The surgical wound is closed in layers. The wrist and hand are immobilized using a splint or cast.

25275

25275   Repair, tendon sheath, extensor, forearm and/or wrist, with free graft (includes obtaining graft) (eg, for extensor carpi ulnaris subluxation)

A tear or laceration of an extensor tendon sheath in the forearm or wrist without injury to the extensor tendon itself is repaired. One common site of tendon sheath injury occurs in the extensor carpi ulnaris (ECU) at the wrist due to a partial dislocation of the wrist, also referred to as subluxation, caused by forced supination, palmar flexion, or ulnar deviation. The ECU tendon is located in the sixth dorsal compartment of the wrist. To repair the ECU tendon sheath, an incision is made over the dorsal aspect of the wrist and the distal ulna. Soft tissues are dissected taking care to protect the dorsal branch of the ulnar nerve. The retinaculum of the sixth dorsal compartment is exposed and inspected. The retinaculum is incised and the tendon sheath is exposed. The tear or laceration is located. The tendon sheath is incised and the tendon is examined and determined to be intact. The damaged retinaculum and tendon sheath are debrided. A graft is then harvested from the dorsal retinaculum of the wrist. The retinacular graft is then used to repair the tendon sheath and the retinaculum of the sixth dorsal compartment.

25280

25280   Lengthening or shortening of flexor or extensor tendon, forearm and/or wrist, single, each tendon

A flexion or extension deformity in the wrist is corrected by lengthening or shortening one of the flexor or extensor tendons in the forearm or wrist. Flexion and extension deformities may be due to late effects of injuries or due to disease processes such as severe rheumatoid arthritis or osteoarthritis. To lengthen a flexor or extensor tendon, a skin incision is made over the tendon to be lengthened, soft tissues are dissected, and the tendon is exposed. A Z-shaped incision is made in the tendon which lengthens it by allowing the tendon fibers to slide apart as the wrist is flexed or extended. Tendon sutures are placed to maintain the tendon in the lengthened position. The wrist is immobilized in a splint or cast so that the wrist can be maintained the desired position until the tendon heals. To shorten a tendon, the tendon is divided. The divided ends of the tendon are then overlapped and sutured together. The wrist is immobilized in a splint. This code reports lengthening or shortening of a single tendon. If more than one tendon in the wrist requires shortening or lengthening to achieve the desired result, code 25280 should be reported for each tendon that is lengthened or shortened.

25290

25290   Tenotomy, open, flexor or extensor tendon, forearm and/or wrist, single, each tendon

An incision is made in the skin of the forearm or wrist overlying the flexor or extensor tendon that is to be incised. Soft tissues are dissected and the tendon is exposed. The

● New Code   ▲ Revised Code   CPT © 2016 American Medical Association. All Rights Reserved.   © 2017 DecisionHealth

tendon is then incised and severed or released. Bleeding is controlled with electrocautery. Following completion of the procedure, the operative wound is closed in layers. Report 25290 for each separate tendon on which a tenotomy is performed.

25295

25295   Tenolysis, flexor or extensor tendon, forearm and/or wrist, single, each tendon

Tenolysis of a single flexor or extensor tendon is performed at the level of the forearm or wrist to restore wrist, hand, and finger motion by releasing scar tissue resulting from trauma or a disease process. An incision is made over the affected flexor or extensor tendon. Soft tissues are dissected. For flexor tendon tenolysis, the affected tendon is identified and adhesions are severed. For extensor tendon tenolysis at the wrist, the dorsal retinaculum over the affected compartment is opened. Adhesions are lysed. Range of motion is evaluated. The surgical wound is closed in layers and a dressing is applied. Report 25295 for each flexor or extensor tendon that is released from scar tissue.

25300-25301

25300   Tenodesis at wrist; flexors of fingers
25301   Tenodesis at wrist; extensors of fingers

Tenodesis of finger flexors or extensors is performed to treat a tear or rupture of the tendon. The tendon is located, inspected, and detached from the insertion site as needed. The tendon is debrided and damaged tendon tissue is excised. Any tears along the length of the tendon are repaired. The tendon is then attached to the appropriate bone at the wrist with sutures or bone anchors. The joint is flushed with sterile saline, incisions are closed, and a dressing is applied. Use 25300 for tenodesis of the flexors of the fingers. Use 25301 for tenodesis of the extensors of the fingers.

25310-25312

25310   Tendon transplantation or transfer, flexor or extensor, forearm and/or wrist, single; each tendon
25312   Tendon transplantation or transfer, flexor or extensor, forearm and/or wrist, single; with tendon graft(s) (includes obtaining graft), each tendon

Tendon transplantation or transfer of a single flexor or extensor tendon at the forearm or wrist is performed to restore function usually resulting from a traumatic injury to the nerve, tendon or muscle. Less commonly the loss of function may be due to rheumatoid or gouty arthritis. The procedure varies depending on the function that the surgeon is trying to restore. For example compromised finger flexion may be treated by transfer of the flexor carpi ulnaris tendon and/or flexor carpi radialis tendon. Extension of the fingers may be treated by transfer of the extensor carpi radialis tendon. To accomplish a tendon transplant or transfer, a longitudinal incision is made over the donor tendon and the tendon exposed. The donor tendon is freed from attachments in a manner that will allow it to be secured to the recipient site. This may include harvesting the tendon with a strip of periosteum. The muscle is also freed from fascial attachments to allow maximum mobility and length for the tendon transfer. A second incision is made over the recipient site which is where the tendon will be attached. The donor tendon is then routed to the recipient site and secured with temporary sutures. A neuromuscular stimulator is used to test the donor tendon function. The tension of the donor tendon is adjusted as needed to ensure maximum function and then permanently secured at the recipient site. Following closure of the surgical wounds, the wrist and/or hand is immobilized as needed. Use 25310 for each tendon that is transplanted or transferred without the use of a tendon graft. Use 25312 for each tendon requiring a tendon graft to achieve the desired length. If a tendon graft is needed, the tendon to be used for grafting is exposed and harvested. The tendon graft is anastomosed to the donor tendon and this is then attached to the recipient site.

25315-25316

25315   Flexor origin slide (eg, for cerebral palsy, Volkmann contracture), forearm and/or wrist
25316   Flexor origin slide (eg, for cerebral palsy, Volkmann contracture), forearm and/or wrist; with tendon(s) transfer

This procedure is performed to release flexion contracture of the wrist, hand, and fingers caused by cerebral palsy or ischemic injury to the nerves and soft tissues also referred to as a Volkmann's contracture. In 25315, an incision is made along the ulnar border of the forearm from the wrist to the just above the elbow. The ulnar and median nerves and the brachial artery are identified and protected. The ulnar nerve is decompressed at the point where it enters the cubital tunnel and descends beneath the flexor carpi ulnaris muscle. The flexor carpi ulnaris and flexor carpi radialis muscles are released at their attachments to the ulna and radius. The ulnar nerve is transposed anteriorly. The flexor carpi ulnaris and flexor carpi radialis are then detached from the superficial origin on the medial epicondyle of the humerus. This allows the muscles to displace or slide distally along the forearm. The flexor pollicis longus and flexor digitorum superficialis are also detached from the origins on the radius to allow them to slide distally as well. The distal displacement of these muscles releases the flexion contractures in the wrist and hand. Following closure of the surgical wound, the wrist and hand are immobilized in extension. In 25316, the flexor origin slide is performed as described above along with one or more tendon transfers. To

accomplish a tendon transfer, a longitudinal incision is made over the donor tendon and the tendon exposed. The donor tendon is freed from attachments in a manner that will allow it to be secured to the recipient site. This may include harvesting the tendon with a strip of periosteum. The muscle is also freed from fascial attachments to allow maximum mobility and length for the tendon transfer. A second incision is made over the recipient site which is where the tendon will be attached. The donor tendon is then routed to the recipient site and secured with temporary sutures. A neuromuscular stimulator is used to test the donor tendon function. The tension of the donor tendon is adjusted as needed to ensure maximum function and then permanently secured at the recipient site. Following closure of the surgical wounds, the wrist and/or hand is immobilized in extension.

25320

25320   Capsulorrhaphy or reconstruction, wrist, open (eg, capsulodesis, ligament repair, tendon transfer or graft) (includes synovectomy, capsulotomy and open reduction) for carpal instability

The physician makes an incision over the wrist and dissects soft tissue. Reconstruct ion of ligaments, tendons, or a graft is used to repair wrist instability. The incision is then closed.

25332

25332   Arthroplasty, wrist, with or without interposition, with or without external or internal fixation

The physician makes an incision over the wrist and repairs the interface between the small bones of the wrist joint and the bones of the forearm. Diseased or damaged bone may be removed, remobilize bones that have become locked in place may be performed, or other measures to restore prior function to the joint is completed. The wrist may be immobilized, either inside the skin with pins, or outside the body with a cast or sling.

25335

25335   Centralization of wrist on ulna (eg, radial club hand)

A deformity of the forearm and wrist such as radial club hand is treated by removing the carpal bones and then positioning the hand over the ulna. Radial club hand is a congenital deformity with varying degrees of severity ranging from complete absence of the radius to cases where the radius is just slightly shorter and smaller than normal. There may also be absence of the thumb and deformities of the fingers, elbow joint and soft tissue of the forearm. The severity is also affected by the presence or absence of a bar of fibrous tissue at the distal end of the radius called an anlage that connects the shortened radius to the carpal bones. The fibrous tissue of the anlage has only a limited ability to grow. If an anlage is present, as the ulna of the fetus grows in utero the hand becomes bent or clubbed toward the radial side of the arm and the ulna may also be bowed. A dorsal longitudinal incision is made over the radial aspect of the wrist and forearm. The carpal bones and ulna are exposed. Bone is excised from the distal ulna and the distal ulna squared off. One or more carpal bones are removed as needed to allow the hand to sit over the ulna. A rectangular notch is created in one of the remaining carpal bones and the squared off ulna is inserted into the notch. Internal fixation is applied as needed to secure the ulna to the carpal bone. The surgical wound is closed in layers and the wrist is immobilized in a cast.

25337

25337   Reconstruction for stabilization of unstable distal ulna or distal radioulnar joint, secondary by soft tissue stabilization (eg, tendon transfer, tendon graft or weave, or tenodesis) with or without open reduction of distal radioulnar joint

Reconstruction of the wrist is performed due to continued instability of the wrist at the distal ulna or radioulnar joint after previous surgical attempts to repair a traumatic injury to the wrist or to surgically treat a disease process such as rheumatoid, gouty or osteoarthritis. This procedure uses soft tissue reconstruction techniques which may include tendon transfer, tendon graft or weave, and/or tenodesis and the exact procedure can vary significantly. One procedure used to treat instability is flexor carpi ulnaris tenodesis. An incision is made over the palmar aspect of the distal ulna. The flexor carpi ulnaris is dissected from the pisiform bone and freed from soft tissue connections up to the musculotendinous junction. The tendon is split in half longitudinally and then one half of the tendon is severed at the musculotendinous junction. A window is created deep to the ulnar artery and nerve and the harvested tendon strip is passed through the window. The ulnar head is excised. An oblique drill hole is created on the dorsal aspect of the ulnar neck exiting in the open medullary canal. The tendon strip is passed through the open end of the medullary canal and out the drill hole. A distal incision is made in the interosseous membrane and the tendon strip is passed through the incision in a palmar direction. Traction is applied to the tendon strip as the forearm is supinated and the tendon strip is then sutured to the interosseous membrane. The tendon is then looped around the extensor carpi ulnaris tendon and sutured to itself to keep the extensor carpi ulnaris from subluxing over the resected ulna. Alternatively tendons at the wrist may be released from their insertion sites and transferred to the ulnar or radioulnar joint in a configuration that will increase stability, a tendon may be harvested from another site and used as a graft or interwoven in another tendon, or another type of tenodesis may be used to achieve greater

Musculoskeletal System

stability of these joints. If the radioulnar joint is malpositioned, the physician may also perform a procedure to return the radioulnar joint to its normal anatomic position.

25350-25355

25350   Osteotomy, radius; distal third
25355   Osteotomy, radius; middle or proximal third

An osteotomy of the radius is performed to correct a deformity or realign the bone. The location of the osteotomy and the type performed is dependent on the site and type of the deformity. Some commonly used osteotomies include transverse, wedge, sliding, right or left angle, V-osteotomy, and Z-osteotomy. Using separately reportable radiographic studies, the physician determines where the bone cut will be made to achieve the desired result prior to the start of the surgical procedure. An incision is made over the radius. Soft tissues are dissected and the radius is exposed. The periosteum is elevated. Using a drill, saw, and/or osteotome, the bone is cut in the previously determined configuration. Bone grafts are interposed between the cut bone segments as needed. Pins, screws, a plate and screw device, or other type of internal fixation is applied as needed to secure the cut edges in anatomical alignment. Alternatively, a separately reportable external fixation device may be applied. Use 25350 for osteotomy of the distal radius. Use 25355 for an osteotomy of the middle or proximal radius.

25360-25365

25360   Osteotomy; ulna
25365   Osteotomy; radius AND ulna

An osteotomy of the ulna alone or the radius and the ulna is performed to correct a deformity or realign the bone. The location of the osteotomy and the type performed is dependent on the site and type of the deformity. Some commonly used osteotomies include transverse, wedge, sliding, right or left angle, V-osteotomy, and Z-osteotomy. Using separately reportable radiographic studies, the physician determines where the bone cuts will be made to achieve the desired result prior to the start of the surgical procedure. An incision is made in the forearm over the site of the deformity. In 25360, soft tissues are dissected and the ulna is exposed. The periosteum is elevated. Using a drill, saw, and/or osteotome, the bone is cut in the previously determined configuration. Bone grafts are interposed between the cut bone segments as needed. Pins, screws, a plate and screw device, or other type of internal fixation is applied as needed to secure the cut edges in anatomical alignment. Alternatively, a separately reportable external fixation device may be applied. In 25365, osteotomies are performed as described above on both the radius and ulna.

25370-25375

25370   Multiple osteotomies, with realignment on intramedullary rod (Sofield type procedure); radius OR ulna
25375   Multiple osteotomies, with realignment on intramedullary rod (Sofield type procedure); radius AND ulna

Multiple osteotomies of the radius and/or ulna are performed to correct a deformity or realign the bones. The location of the osteotomies and the type performed is dependent on the site and type of the deformity. Some commonly used osteotomies include transverse, wedge, sliding, right or left angle, V-osteotomy, and Z-osteotomy. Using separately reportable radiographic studies, the physician determines where the bone cuts will be made to achieve the desired result prior to the start of the surgical procedure. A longitudinal incision is made over the forearm. Soft tissues are dissected and the radius is exposed. The periosteum is elevated. Using a drill, saw, and/or osteotome, the bone is cut in the previously determined configuration. The radius and/or ulna is sized and an appropriately sized intramedullary rod is selected. A drill hole is created in the distal or proximal aspect of the radius and/or ulna. The intramedullary canal is drilled or reamed through the drill hole. If a cannulated rod is used, a guidewire is placed into the intramedullary canal. The rod is then advanced over the guidewire until it is properly positioned within the canal. The bone is anatomically positioned at each osteotomy site and the rod is secured using screws, pins or other devices. Use 25370 for multiple osteotomies of the radius alone or the ulna alone. Use 25375 for multiple osteotomies of both the radius and ulna.

25390-25391

25390   Osteoplasty, radius OR ulna; shortening
25391   Osteoplasty, radius OR ulna; lengthening with autograft

A plastic procedure is performed on the radius or ulna to lengthen or shorten the bone. Using separately reportable radiographic studies, the physician determines where the bone cuts will be made to achieve the desired result prior to the start of the surgical procedure. The radius or ulna is exposed. In 25390, the radius or ulna is shortened. The sites of the bone cuts are identified. The bone is cut and a segment of the bone is excised. The remaining distal and proximal portions of the bone are then brought into contact with each other and internal fixation is applied to stabilize the reconfigured bone. Alternatively, a separately reportable external fixation device may be applied. In 25391, the radius or ulna is lengthened. Cuts are made in the bone and the bone is distracted. A bone

autograft is harvested, usually from the iliac crest. A skin incision is made over the iliac crest and the muscle is stripped to reveal the bone surface. Cortical and/or cancellous bone is harvested. The bone is configured to the desired size and shape and/or cancellous bone is morcelized and packed into the defect. Pins, screws, a plate and screw device, or other type of internal fixation is applied as needed to secure the cut edges in anatomical alignment. Alternatively, a separately reportable external fixation device may be applied.

25392-25393

25392   Osteoplasty, radius AND ulna; shortening (excluding 64876)
25393   Osteoplasty, radius AND ulna; lengthening with autograft

A plastic procedure is performed on the radius and ulna to lengthen or shorten the bones. Using separately reportable radiographic studies, the physician determines where the bone cuts will be made to achieve the desired result prior to the start of the surgical procedure. The radius and ulna are exposed. In 25392, the radius and ulna are shortened. The sites of the bone cuts are identified. Each bone is cut and a segment of the bone is excised. The remaining distal and proximal portions of the two bones are then brought into contact with each other and internal fixation is applied to stabilize the reconfigured bones. Alternatively, a separately reportable external fixation device may be applied. In 25393, the radius and ulna are lengthened. Cuts are made in both bones and the bones are distracted. A bone autograft is harvested, usually from the iliac crest. A skin incision is made over the iliac crest and the muscle is stripped to reveal the bone surface. Cortical and/or cancellous bone is harvested. The bone is configured to the desired size and shape and/or cancellous bone is morcelized and packed into the defects. Pins, screws, a plate and screw device, or other type of internal fixation is applied as needed to secure the cut edges of both bones in anatomical alignment. Alternatively, a separately reportable external fixation device may be applied.

25394

25394   Osteoplasty, carpal bone, shortening

One of the carpal bones is shortened to correct a malformation or malalignment in the wrist joint. Using separately reportable radiographic studies, the physician determines where the bone cuts will be made to achieve the desired result prior to the start of the surgical procedure. A dorsal incision is made over the carpal bone to be shortened. The retinaculum is incised and tendons are retracted. The wrist capsule is opened and the affected carpal bone exposed. Kirschner wires may be placed through the carpal bone at the level of the osteotomy and fluoroscopic images obtained to ensure that the wires are in the desired position. A drill, saw, or osteotome is then used to cut the carpal bone and a portion of the carpal bone is excised. The remaining distal and proximal segments are reapproximated and secured using wires, staples or another type of internal fixation device. The joint capsule and overlying soft tissues are closed in layers.

25400-25420

25400   Repair of nonunion or malunion, radius OR ulna; without graft (eg, compression technique)
25405   Repair of nonunion or malunion, radius OR ulna; with autograft (includes obtaining graft)
25415   Repair of nonunion or malunion, radius AND ulna; without graft (eg, compression technique)
25420   Repair of nonunion or malunion, radius AND ulna; with autograft (includes obtaining graft)

When union of the fracture fragments does not occur after sufficient healing time has elapsed, the patient is considered to have a nonunion of the fracture. Malunion with malalignment of the fracture fragments can cause osseous abnormalities, incongruity of articular surfaces, soft tissue contracture, nerve impingement, and other complications. The original fracture sites of the radius and/or ulna are exposed. The nonunion or malunion is evaluated to determine what type of repair is required which may include internal fixation without or with a bone graft. If it is treated without a graft using internal fixation, a compression plate may be used. For a nonunion, a compression plate is placed over the fracture site and secured with lag screws. For a malunion, the radius and ulna may be refractured, realigned, and internal fixation placed to maintain the fracture in anatomical alignment. Following placement of the fixation device, stability of the fracture is checked and alignment is verified radiographically. If a bone graft is used to fill the bone defect and encourage healing, the site of the nonunion or malunion is prepared which may include refracture of the bone. A bone autograft is harvested, usually from the iliac crest. A skin incision is made over the iliac crest and the muscle is stripped to reveal the bone surface. Cortical and/or cancellous bone is harvested. The bone is configured to the size and shape of the defect or cancellous bone is morcelized and packed into the defect. Internal fixation, such as a pin or wire is used as needed to secure the bone graft. A compression plate and screws or other internal fixation is used to stabilize the fracture. Use 25400 for repair of a nonunion or malunion of the radius or ulna without a bone graft or 25405 when a bone graft is required. Use 25415 for repair of a nonunion or malunion of both the radius and ulna without a bone graft or 25420 when a bone graft is also required.

● New Code   ▲ Revised Code

25425-25426

25425 Repair of defect with autograft; radius OR ulna
25426 Repair of defect with autograft; radius AND ulna

A bone defect not due to a nonunion or malunion of a fracture is repaired using an autograft. The site of the defect is prepared. A bone autograft is harvested, usually from the iliac crest. A skin incision is made over the iliac crest and the muscle is stripped to reveal the bone surface. Cortical and/or cancellous bone is harvested. The bone is configured to the size and shape of the defect or cancellous bone is morcelized and packed into the defect. Internal fixation, such as a pin or wire is used as needed to secure the bone graft. A compression plate and screws or other internal fixation is used to stabilize the bone. Use 25425 for repair of a bone defect in the radius or ulna. Use 25426 for repair of a bone defect in both the radius and ulna.

25430

25430 Insertion of vascular pedicle into carpal bone (eg, Hori procedure)

A vascular pedicle is used to restore blood supply to one of the carpal bones. For unknown reasons, the carpal bones, particularly the lunate, sometimes experience a loss of blood supply. If the blood supply is not restored osteonecrosis occurs. An incision is made over the posterior aspect of the wrist over the affected carpal bone. Tendons are retracted. The terminal branches of the interosseous artery and vein are isolated, ligated, and transected distal to the carpal bone. The proximal aspect of the interosseous artery and vein are mobilized. The carpal bone is exposed and a drill hole created extending into the middle of the bone. The interosseous artery and vein are placed in the carpal bone and secured with sutures to the overlying periosteum. The joint capsule is repaired and soft tissues and skin closed in layers.

25431

25431 Repair of nonunion of carpal bone (excluding carpal scaphoid (navicular)) (includes obtaining graft and necessary fixation), each bone

When union of the fracture fragments does not occur after sufficient healing time has elapsed, the patient is considered to have a nonunion of the fracture. An incision is made over the posterior aspect of the wrist. The extensor tendons are retracted and the wrist capsule incised over the affected carpal bone excluding the scaphoid (navicular). The original fracture site is exposed. The nonunion is evaluated to determine what type of repair is required. The fracture site is cleared of scar tissue and the carpal bone debrided until healthy cancellous bone has been exposed. A local bone graft is harvested, usually from the radius. A skin incision is made over the radius. The periosteum is elevated and a cortical window created. Cancellous bone is harvested. The periosteum over the radius is repaired. The bone graft is configured to the size and shape of the defect or morcelized and packed into the defect. Internal fixation, such as a pin or wire is used as needed to secure the bone graft and the carpal bone fragments. Use 25431 for each carpal bone repaired excluding the scaphoid (navicular).

25440

25440 Repair of nonunion, scaphoid carpal (navicular) bone, with or without radial styloidectomy (includes obtaining graft and necessary fixation)

When union of the fracture fragments does not occur after sufficient healing time has elapsed, the patient is considered to have a nonunion of the fracture. Scaphoid nonunion can cause mechanical pain from radial styloid impingement which may be treated by a radial styloidectomy. An incision is made over the posterior aspect of the wrist. The extensor tendons are retracted and the wrist capsule incised over the scaphoid (navicular) bone. The original fracture site is exposed. The nonunion is evaluated to determine what type of repair is required. The fracture site is cleared of scar tissue and the scaphoid bone debrided until healthy cancellous bone has been exposed. A local bone graft is harvested, usually from the radius. A skin incision is made over the radius. The periosteum is elevated and a cortical window created. Cancellous bone is harvested. If the radial styloid is impinging on the scaphoid bone, a bone saw is used to excise enough of the styloid to relieve the impingement. The periosteum over the radius is repaired. The bone graft is configured to the size and shape of the defect or morcelized and packed into the defect. Internal fixation, such as a pin or wire is used as needed to secure the bone graft and the carpal bone fragments.

25441-25442

25441 Arthroplasty with prosthetic replacement; distal radius
25442 Arthroplasty with prosthetic replacement; distal ulna

An incision is made in the midline over the posterior aspect of the wrist from the distal aspect of the forearm to the proximal aspect of the metacarpal . The radiocarpal joint and distal radioulnar joint (DRUJ) are exposed. The retinaculum is released beginning along the ulnar border and the release is extended all the way to the radial border. The radial and ulnar nerves are protected with vessel loops. The tendons are retracted. The dorsal aspect of the joint capsule is elevated as a single layer. In 25441, a prosthetic replacement of the radius is performed. A guide is placed over the distal radius to help identify the amount of bone to be excised. The distal radius is excised using a bone saw or osteotome. The

remaining portion of the distal radius is sized and a trial radial component placed. The trial prosthesis is evaluated and adjustments made as needed. The final prosthetic component is tamped into place. Sutures placed through the triangular fibrocartilage are used to stabilize the prosthesis. The dorsal aspect of the joint capsule is returned to its normal position over the wrist joint and repaired with sutures. The retinaculum is repaired and overlying soft tissues and skin are repaired in layers. In 25442, a prosthetic replacement of the distal ulna is performed. The distal ulna is excised. An appropriately sized prosthesis is selected and tested. Adjustments are made as needed and the final ulnar prosthesis is secured. The joint capsule, retinaculum, soft tissues and skin are closed as described above.

25443-25445

25443 Arthroplasty with prosthetic replacement; scaphoid carpal (navicular)
25444 Arthroplasty with prosthetic replacement; lunate
25445 Arthroplasty with prosthetic replacement; trapezium

Prosthetic replacement of the scaphoid, lunate, or trapezium bone is performed. An incision is made in the midline over the posterior aspect of the wrist from the distal aspect of the forearm to the proximal aspect of the metacarpal . The radiocarpal joint is exposed. The retinaculum is released beginning along the ulnar border and extending all the way to the radial border. The radial and ulnar nerves are protected with vessel loops. The retinaculum is completed released and the tendons are retracted. The dorsal aspect of the joint capsule is elevated as a single layer. The damaged carpal bone is resected using an oscillating saw. A trial carpal component is then secured to the affected carpal bone. The trial prosthesis is evaluated and adjustments made as needed. The final prosthetic components is then tamped into place. Sutures placed through the triangular fibrocartilage are used to stabilize the prosthetic component. The dorsal aspect of the joint capsule is then returned to its normal position over the wrist joint and repaired with sutures. The retinaculum is repaired and overlying soft tissues and skin are repaired in layers. Use code 25443 for prosthetic replacement of the scaphoid (navicular) bone, code 25444 for the lunate, or code 25445 for the trapezium.

25446

25446 Arthroplasty with prosthetic replacement; distal radius and partial or entire carpus (total wrist)

A total wrist replacement is performed. An incision is made in the midline over the posterior aspect of the wrist from the distal aspect of the forearm to the proximal aspect of the metacarpal . The radiocarpal joint and distal radioulnar joint (DRUJ) are exposed. The retinaculum is released beginning along the ulnar border and extended all the way to the radial border. The radial and ulnar nerves are protected with vessel loops. The retinaculum is completely released and the tendons are retracted. The dorsal aspect of the joint capsule is elevated as a single layer. Part or all of the carpal bones are resected using an oscillating saw. A guide is placed over the distal radius to help identify the amount of bone to be removed from the distal radius. The distal radius is excised using a bone saw or osteotome. The remaining portion of the distal radius is then sized and a trial radial component placed. Any remaining carpal bones are stabilized with Kirschner wires. A drill hole is created in one of the remaining carpal bones or if all the carpal bones have been resected a drill hole is created in the third metacarpal bone. The drill holes are used to center the hand over over the radial component of the total wrist prosthesis. A trial carpal component is then secured to the remaining carpal bones or the metacarpals. The trial prosthesis is evaluated and adjustments made as needed. The final prosthetic components are then tamped into place. Sutures placed through the triangular fibrocartilage are used to stabilize the prosthetic components. The dorsal aspect of the joint capsule is returned to its normal position over the wrist joint and repaired with sutures. The retinaculum is repaired and overlying soft tissues and skin are repaired in layers.

25447

25447 Arthroplasty, interposition, intercarpal or carpometacarpal joints

An incision is made over the affected intercarpal or carpometacarpal joint. Soft tissues are dissected. Tendons are retracted. Nerves and blood vessels are protected. The joint capsule is opened. Soft tissue and articular cartilage are debrided. A bur is used to smooth the bone surfaces. A local tendon graft may be harvested for interposition between the bone surfaces. Alternatively an allograft or xenograft may be used. The graft is carefully positioned to span the entire bone surfaces. The graft is anchored with sutures as needed. The joint capsule is closed and overlying soft tissue and skin are closed in layers.

25449

25449 Revision of arthroplasty, including removal of implant, wrist joint

The physician makes an incision over the site of the previous arthroplasty. The damaged or dislocated prothesis is readjusted or removed. A new prothesis may be inserted, if necessary. The incision is then closed.

Musculoskeletal System

● New Code   ▲ Revised Code

25450-25455

25450 Epiphyseal arrest by epiphysiodesis or stapling; distal radius OR ulna
25455 Epiphyseal arrest by epiphysiodesis or stapling; distal radius AND ulna

Epiphyseal arrest is performed to treat an angulation deformity at the wrist or a bone length discrepancy between the radius and ulna. The epiphysis is also referred to as the growth plate. An incision is made over the distal aspect of the radius and/or ulna and extended down over the wrist joint. Soft tissues are dissected, taking care to protect blood vessels and nerves. The distal radius and/or ulna are exposed. Blount staples, transphyseal screws, or a plate and screw device are strategically placed in the epiphysis of the distal radius or ulna to temporarily arrest bone growth. If the procedure is performed to treat an angulation deformity only a portion of the epiphysis is arrested. The other portion of the epiphysis is not treated and growth continues thereby diminishing or correcting the angulation deformity. If the procedure is performed to treat a bone length discrepancy, the entire epiphysis is arrested. Use 25450 for epiphyseal arrest of the radius or ulna. Use 25455 if the procedure is performed on both the radius and ulna.

25490-25492

25490 Prophylactic treatment (nailing, pinning, plating or wiring) with or without methylmethacrylate; radius
25491 Prophylactic treatment (nailing, pinning, plating or wiring) with or without methylmethacrylate; ulna
25492 Prophylactic treatment (nailing, pinning, plating or wiring) with or without methylmethacrylate; radius AND ulna

Prophylactic treatment is performed to prevent fracture of the radius and/or ulna when the bone is weakened as a result of a disease process or neoplasm. Common methods used to maintain bone integrity include nailing, pinning, plating, or wiring with or without the use of methylmethacrylate. The weakened bone is evaluated radiographically and the best form of prophylaxis is determined. An intramedullary nail or rod may be placed using either an antegrade or retrograde approach. An incision is made over the proximal or distal radius or ulna. A nail or rod is then inserted into the intramedullary space. The nail is secured with locking screws placed distally and proximally. If pins are used, they may be placed transcutaneously through the weakened region of the bone. Plating requires open exposure of the bone and placement of a plate that is secured with screws. Wiring involves wrapping a wire cerclage around the bone. When methylmethacrylate is used, it is injected into bony defects. Use 25490 for the radius, 25491 for the ulna, or 25492 when both the radius and ulna are treated.

25500-25505

25500 Closed treatment of radial shaft fracture; without manipulation
25505 Closed treatment of radial shaft fracture; with manipulation

Closed treatment of a radial shaft fracture is performed. Separately reportable radiographs are obtained to confirm the fracture. A neurovascular exam is performed to ensure that the nerves and blood vessels at the site of the injury are intact. In 25500, a nondisplaced fracture of the radial shaft is evaluated. No manipulation of the fracture fragments is required. The arm is immobilized using a long arm splint or cast. In 25505, a minimally displaced fracture of the radial shaft is treated. The displaced fracture fragments are manually reduced (manipulated) back to proper anatomic alignment. Separately reportable radiographs are obtained to confirm anatomic reduction. A long arm splint or cast is applied to immobilize the arm.

25515

25515 Open treatment of radial shaft fracture, includes internal fixation, when performed

Open reduction of a radial shaft fracture is performed, including any necessary internal fixation. The radius is the lateral bone of the forearm and the shaft is the center portion. An isolated radial shaft fracture, without fracture of the ulna or any accompanying joint dislocation, is unusual; however, it typically requires open reduction. An incision is made over the fracture site in the radial shaft and the site is cleared of debris. The fracture is reduced into proper alignment and the fragments are typically fixed using internal fixation, most commonly a plate and screw device. When anatomical alignment has been secured, the wound is closed. An immobilization device may be applied such as a sling, splint, or cast.

25520

25520 Closed treatment of radial shaft fracture and closed treatment of dislocation of distal radioulnar joint (Galeazzi fracture/dislocation)

Closed treatment of a radial shaft fracture with closed treatment of a dislocation of the distal radioulnar joint is performed. This injury is also referred to as a Galeazzi fracture-dislocation. Separately reportable radiographs are obtained to confirm the fracture-dislocation. A neurovascular exam is performed to ensure that the nerves and blood vessels at the injury sites are intact. The fracture of the radial shaft is treated first using longitudinal traction to correct the radial angulation. After the radial shaft fracture has been reduced, the distal radioulnar joint is evaluated radiographically to determine if the dislocation reduced itself spontaneously as the radial shaft fracture was manipulated back into anatomic alignment. If the distal radioulnar joint is still dislocated, it is also manipulated back into alignment. Separately reportable radiographs are obtained to confirm correct reduction of both the radial shaft fracture and the radioulnar joint dislocation. A long arm splint or cast is applied to immobilize the arm.

25525-25526

25525 Open treatment of radial shaft fracture, includes internal fixation, when performed, and closed treatment of distal radioulnar joint dislocation (Galeazzi fracture/ dislocation), includes percutaneous skeletal fixation, when performed
25526 Open treatment of radial shaft fracture, includes internal fixation, when performed, and open treatment of distal radioulnar joint dislocation (Galeazzi fracture/ dislocation), includes internal fixation, when performed, includes repair of triangular fibrocartilage complex

Open reduction of a radial shaft Galeazzi fracture with closed reduction of the distal radioulnar joint (DRUJ) dislocation is performed in 25525, including any necessary internal fixation of the radial shaft and any percutaneous fixation of the DRUJ dislocation. A Galeazzi fracture/dislocation is a solitary fracture of the radial shaft at the junction of the middle and distal thirds with an accompanying subluxation or dislocation of the DRUJ. An incision is made over the fracture site in the radial shaft and the pieces are reduced using fracture reduction forceps and manual traction. Anatomic alignment of the radial shaft is then verified using x-ray. Internal fixation of the radial shaft fracture is typically required, using a compression plate and screws. The DRUJ dislocation is assessed for reduction and stability. If it has not spontaneously reduced following reduction of the radial shaft fracture, a closed reduction is performed. If the reduction is unstable, percutaneous skeletal fixation with K-wires is performed placing the K wires from the ulna into the radius just proximal to the articular surface. The wound is closed and a long arm splint is applied. Use 25526 when the DRUJ dislocation cannot be reduced using closed reduction and open reduction must be performed. Following reduction of the radial shaft fracture, open reduction of the DRUJ is performed through a dorsal incision. Soft tissue of the triangular fibrocartilage complex is debrided and repaired. Stabilization may be required, using internal fixation devices, such as screws or pins. Surgical wounds are closed and a long arm splint is applied.

25530-25535

25530 Closed treatment of ulnar shaft fracture; without manipulation
25535 Closed treatment of ulnar shaft fracture; with manipulation

Closed treatment of an ulnar shaft fracture is performed. Separately reportable radiographs are obtained to confirm the fracture. A neurovascular exam is performed to ensure that the nerves and blood vessels at the site of the injury are intact. In 25530, a nondisplaced fracture of the ulnar shaft is evaluated. No manipulation of the fracture fragments is required. The arm is immobilized using a long arm splint or cast. In 25535, a minimally displaced fracture of the ulnar shaft is treated. The displaced fracture fragments are manually reduced (manipulated) back to proper anatomic alignment. Separately reportable radiographs are obtained to confirm anatomic reduction. A long arm splint or cast is applied to immobilize the arm.

25545

25545 Open treatment of ulnar shaft fracture, includes internal fixation, when performed

Open reduction of a fracture of the ulnar shaft is performed including any necessary internal fixation. The ulna is the lateral bone of the forearm and the shaft is the middle portion. An ulnar shaft fracture is also referred to as a nightstick fracture because it is typically the result of a direct blow to the ulnar border as happens when protecting oneself from a blow. An incision is made over the fracture site and the fascia is dissected. An incision is made through the fascia between the extensor carpi ulnaris and the flexor carpi ulnaris. The fracture site is exposed by incising and elevating the periosteum. The site is cleared of debris and reduced into proper alignment. Internal fixation is applied as needed, most commonly a plate and screw device.

25560-25565

25560 Closed treatment of radial and ulnar shaft fractures; without manipulation
25565 Closed treatment of radial and ulnar shaft fractures; with manipulation

Closed treatment of combined radial and ulnar shaft fractures is performed. Separately reportable radiographs are obtained to confirm the fracture. A neurovascular exam is performed to ensure that the nerves and blood vessels at the site of the injury are intact. In 25560, nondisplaced fractures of the radial and ulnar shafts are evaluated. No manipulation of the fracture fragments is required. The arm is immobilized using a long arm splint or cast. In 25565, minimally displaced fractures of the radial and ulnar shafts are treated. The displaced fracture fragments are manually reduced (manipulated) back to proper anatomic alignment. Separately reportable radiographs are obtained to confirm anatomic reduction. A long arm splint or cast is applied to immobilize the arm.

● New Code   ▲ Revised Code

Musculoskeletal System

25574-25575

25574 Open treatment of radial AND ulnar shaft fractures, with internal fixation, when performed; of radius OR ulna

25575 Open treatment of radial AND ulnar shaft fractures, with internal fixation, when performed; of radius AND ulna

Open treatment of a fracture of both bones in the forearm (radius and ulna) is performed. An incision is made in the skin over the fracture. Overlying fascia is incised and muscle is divided. When the radius is being reduced, the arm is first supinated and the attachment to the supinator is released. The arm is then pronated, the pronator teres identified, and the insertion of the pronator is released. The radial fracture is exposed and cleared of debris, and then reduced into proper alignment. Internal fixation may be applied, usually a plate and screw device. The supinator and pronator teres are reattached. The ulnar fracture is then reduced in a similar manner. Internal fixation may be applied, usually a plate and screw device. Overlying fascia is repaired and the wound is closed. If internal fixation is required, use 25574 when it is applied to either the radial or the ulnar shaft fracture, but not both. Use 25575 if any necessary internal fixation is applied to both the radial and the ulnar fracture after open treatment.

25600-25605

25600 Closed treatment of distal radial fracture (eg, Colles or Smith type) or epiphyseal separation, includes closed treatment of fracture of ulnar styloid, when performed; without manipulation

25605 Closed treatment of distal radial fracture (eg, Colles or Smith type) or epiphyseal separation, includes closed treatment of fracture of ulnar styloid, when performed; with manipulation

Closed treatment of distal radial fracture or epiphyseal separation is performed. This procedure includes closed treatment of a fracture of the ulnar styloid if present . There are three main types of distal forearm fractures or epiphyseal injuries. These include an extension or Colles' fracture, a flexion or Smith's fracture, a push-off or Barton's or Hutchinson's fracture. Epiphyseal separation occurs in children when the cartilaginous epiphysis or growth plate separates or fractures off the bone. Separately reportable radiographs are obtained to confirm the fracture or epiphyseal separation. A neurovascular exam is performed to ensure that the nerves and blood vessels at the site of the injury are intact. In 25600, a nondisplaced fracture of the distal radius with or without a fracture of the ulnar styloid is evaluated. No manipulation of the fracture fragments is required. The arm is immobilized using a splint or cast. In 25605, a minimally displaced fracture of the distal radius with or without a fracture of the ulnar styloid is treated. The displaced fracture fragments are manually reduced back to proper anatomic alignment using traction and manipulation. Separately reportable radiographs are obtained to confirm anatomic reduction. A splint or cast is applied to immobilize the arm.

25606

25606 Percutaneous skeletal fixation of distal radial fracture or epiphyseal separation

Percutaneous skeletal fixation is performed for a fracture of the distal radius, the lower part of the outer bone of the forearm (near the wrist), or an epiphyseal separation. The epiphysis is the growth plate portion at the end of a long bone which continues ossifying from cartilage while the bone is growing. The fracture or separation must first be reduced back into proper alignment. Traction and manipulation may be applied to reduce the fracture. The physician then places a couple of Kirschner wires, called K wires or pins, into the bone to hold the fractured pieces together. K wires are thin, rigid, sharp, stainless steel pins, which are driven into the bone through the skin using a drill for percutaneous skeletal fixation. The K wires are placed through the radius across the fracture into the opposite bone. The K wires are then cut just below the skin and the arm is immobilized. The pins may be removed after a few weeks or are sometimes used for definitive fixation on small fracture fragments.

25607-25609

25607 Open treatment of distal radial extra-articular fracture or epiphyseal separation, with internal fixation

25608 Open treatment of distal radial intra-articular fracture or epiphyseal separation; with internal fixation of 2 fragments

25609 Open treatment of distal radial intra-articular fracture or epiphyseal separation; with internal fixation of 3 or more fragments

Open treatment of a distal radial extra-articular fracture or epiphyseal separation is performed with internal fixation. The distal radius is the lower part of the outer bone of the forearm (near the wrist). An extra-articular fracture line does not extend into the joint or affect how the bone functions with the neighboring structures. The physician makes an incision down the front, lateral side of the distal forearm to expose the wrist fracture. Muscle and tendons are retracted and care is taken to protect the median nerve. The pronator quadratus muscle may be severed from its attachment. The fracture or epiphyseal separation is reduced into proper position and a small metal plate is placed to hold the fractured piece in place and affixed to the bone fragment with screws. Code 25608 when

two fragments are held with internal fixation and 25609 when three or more fragments are affixed using internal fixation devices.

25622-25624

25622 Closed treatment of carpal scaphoid (navicular) fracture; without manipulation

25624 Closed treatment of carpal scaphoid (navicular) fracture; with manipulation

Closed treatment of a carpal scaphoid fracture, also referred to as a navicular fracture, is performed. The scaphoid bone, also called the navicular bone, is one of eight carpal bones that make up the wrist joint. It is located at the base of the thumb and is the most frequently injured bone in the wrist. Separately reportable radiographs are obtained to confirm the fracture, although carpal scaphoid fractures may not be apparent radiographically until one to two weeks following the injury. A neurovascular exam is performed to ensure that the nerves and blood vessels at the site of the injury are intact. In 25622, a nondisplaced fracture of the carpal scaphoid is evaluated. No manipulation of the fracture fragments is required. The arm is immobilized using a short arm splint or cast. In 25624, a minimally displaced fracture of the carpal scaphoid is treated. The displaced fracture fragments are manually reduced (manipulated) back to proper anatomic alignment. Separately reportable radiographs are obtained to confirm anatomic reduction. A short arm splint or cast is applied to immobilize the arm.

25628

25628 Open treatment of carpal scaphoid (navicular) fracture, includes internal fixation, when performed

Open reduction of a carpal scaphoid fracture, also referred to as a navicular fracture, is performed with any necessary internal fixation. Eight separate small bones, called carpal bones, make up the wrist. The scaphoid bone, also called the navicular, is the carpal bone at the base of the thumb and the most commonly injured bone in the wrist. Fracture of the scaphoid bone usually results from a fall onto an outstretched hand. An incision is made in the palm (volar approach) and the fracture site in the scaphoid is identified, cleared of debris, and reduced back into position. Internal fixation may be applied and typically screw fixation is used. The fracture fragments are secured first with a guidewire and then supplemental stabilization wire is placed adjacent to the guidewire. A screw hole is drilled and a screw is inserted from the scaphotrapezial joint through the distal pole of the scaphoid. Anatomic alignment is confirmed and the wound is closed.

25630-25645

25630 Closed treatment of carpal bone fracture (excluding carpal scaphoid [navicular]); without manipulation, each bone

25635 Closed treatment of carpal bone fracture (excluding carpal scaphoid [navicular]); with manipulation, each bone

25645 Open treatment of carpal bone fracture (other than carpal scaphoid [navicular]), each bone

A fracture of one of the carpal bones excluding the carpal scaphoid (navicular) bone is treated using closed treatment without manipulation, closed treatment with manipulation, or open treatment. There are eight carpal bones arranged in two rows at the carpus or wrist joint. The proximal row contains the scaphoid, lunate, triquetrum, and pisiform. The distal row contains the trapezium, trapezoid, capitate,and hamate. If more than one carpal bone is fractured, treatment of each bone is reported separately. Separately reportable radiographs are obtained to confirm the fracture. A neurovascular exam is performed to ensure that the nerves and blood vessels at the site of the injury are intact. In 25630, a nondisplaced or minimally displaced fracture of one of the carpal bones other than the scaphoid is evaluated. No manipulation of the fracture fragments is required. The wrist is immobilized using a short arm splint or cast. In 25635, a displaced fracture of the one of the carpal bones other than the scaphoid is treated with manipulation. The displaced fracture fragments are manually reduced (manipulated) back to proper anatomic alignment. Separately reportable radiographs are obtained to confirm anatomic reduction. A short arm splint or cast is applied to immobilize the wrist. In 25645, a displaced fracture of one of the carpal bones other than the scaphoid is treated by open reduction. An incision is made through the skin, the fracture site is identified, cleared of debris, and fracture fragments reduced. Internal fixation such as a small fragmentation screw or intraosseous wiring is applied as needed. A short arm cast is applied to immobilize the wrist.

25650-25652

25650 Closed treatment of ulnar styloid fracture

25651 Percutaneous skeletal fixation of ulnar styloid fracture

25652 Open treatment of ulnar styloid fracture

A fracture of the ulnar styloid is treated using closed treatment, percutaneous skeletal fixation, or open treatment. Separately reportable radiographs are obtained to confirm the fracture. A neurovascular exam is performed to ensure that the nerves and blood vessels at the site of the injury are intact. In 25650, a nondisplaced or minimally displaced fracture of the ulnar styloid is evaluated. No manipulation of the fracture fragments is required.

Musculoskeletal System

● New Code   ▲ Revised Code

The arm is immobilized using a splint or cast. In 25651, a displaced fracture of the ulnar styloid is treated using percutaneous skeletal fixation. The displaced fracture fragments are manually reduced (manipulated) back to proper anatomic alignment. Separately reportable radiographs are obtained to confirm anatomic reduction. A Kirschner wire, also referred to as K-wire or pin, is then placed through the skin and driven into the bone at the fracture site using a drill. Anatomic reduction is confirmed radiographically. A splint or cast is applied to immobilize the arm. In 25652 a displaced fracture of the ulnar styloid is treated by open reduction. An incision is made through the skin between the extensor and flexor carpi ulnaris (ECU, FCU) tendons. The fracture site is identified, cleared of debris, and fracture fragments reduced. A small fragmentation screw, intraosseous wiring, or tension banding may be placed to maintain proper anatomic alignment of fracture fragments. A cast is applied to immobilize the arm.

25660-25670

25660   Closed treatment of radiocarpal or intercarpal dislocation, 1 or more bones, with manipulation

25670   Open treatment of radiocarpal or intercarpal dislocation, 1 or more bones

Radiocarpal and intercarpal dislocations are rare and complex injuries caused by high-energy impact. Separately reportable radiographs are obtained. The physician then evaluates the extent of the injury to the bones, ligaments, and soft tissues of the wrist. In 25660, a closed reduction is performed and the affected bones are manually manipulated into correct anatomic position. Following closed reduction, a second set of radiographs may be obtained to verify the reduction of the dislocated carpal bones. A cast is typically applied to prevent reinjury and allow ligaments to heal. In 25670, an open reduction is performed. The surgical approach is dependent on which carpal bones are involved. Ligaments are repaired using suture anchors and the bones may be stabilized with pins or K-wires.

25671-25676

25671   Percutaneous skeletal fixation of distal radioulnar dislocation

25675   Closed treatment of distal radioulnar dislocation with manipulation

25676   Open treatment of distal radioulnar dislocation, acute or chronic

A distal radioulnar joint (DRUJ) dislocation is treated using percutaneous skeletal fixation (25671), closed treatment with manipulation (25675), or open treatment (25676). DRUJ dislocation without concomitant fracture is a rare injury. Dislocation may be dorsal which is caused by hyperpronation or volar which is caused by hypersupination. Seprately reportable radiographs are obtained to determine the extent of injury. In 25675, a DRUJ dislocation is reduced manually. For a dorsal dislocation, the forearm is supinated while direct pressure is applied over the ulna. For a volar dislocation, the ulna is mobilized dorsally while the forearm is pronated. The wrist is immobilized in a cast. In 25671, the DRUJ dislocation is reduced manually as described in 25675 and then stabilized with a pin or K-wire inserted percutaneously. In 25676, open treatment of an acute or chronic DRUJ dislocation is performed. Open treatment is required when attempt at closed reduction fails, for recurrent subluxation and dislocations, and when soft tissue is interposed between the bones. Using a dorsal approach, a longitudinal skin incision is made just radial to the extensor carpi ulnaris tendon. The extensor digiti minimi is released from it sheath and retracted in a radial direction to expose the joint space. Interposed tissue is cleared from joint space and the dislocation is reduced. Damaged tissue is debrided and joint structures are repaired. Pins or K-wires may be used to stabilize the joint. The surgical wound is irrigated and incisions closed. The wrist is immobilized in a cast.

25680-25685

25680   Closed treatment of trans-scaphoperilunar type of fracture dislocation, with manipulation

25685   Open treatment of trans-scaphoperilunar type of fracture dislocation

A trans-scaphoperilunar type fracture dislocation may also be referred to as a Mayfield fracture dislocation. This is a rare type of injury resulting from a high energy impact to the wrist that involves fracture of the scaphoid and dislocation of the lunate. Separately reportable radiographs are obtained to verify the fracture. In 25680, closed treatment is used to manually manipulate (reduce) the scaphoid fracture and lunate dislocation into anatomical alignment. A second set of radiographs is obtained to verify anatomic reduction. The wrist is immobilized in a cast. In 25685, an open reduction is performed. An incision is made in the volar aspect of the wrist. The fracture site is irrigated and cleared of bone fragments and debris. The scaphoid fracture is reduced and stabilized with screw fixation, K-wires and/or anchor sutures. The lunate dislocation is reduced. Anatomic alignment is verified radiographically, incisions are closed, and the wrist is immobilized in cast.

25690-25695

25690   Closed treatment of lunate dislocation, with manipulation

25695   Open treatment of lunate dislocation

Lunate dislocation typically results from a backwards fall onto an outstretched hand. Separately reportable radiographs are obtained to verify the fracture. In 25690, closed treatment is used to manually manipulate (reduce) the fracture fragments into anatomical

---

alignment. A second set of radiographs is obtained to verify anatomic reduction. The wrist is immobilized in a cast. In 25695, an open reduction is performed. An incision is made in the lunate. The dislocation is reduced and stabilized with pins or K-wires. Anatomic alignment is verified radiographically, incisions are closed, and the wrist is immobilized in a cast.

25800

25800   Arthrodesis, wrist; complete, without bone graft (includes radiocarpal and/ or intercarpal and/or carpometacarpal joints)

Arthrodesis, also referred to as joint fusion, is performed to relieve pain and restore joint stability in patients with rheumatoid arthritis, osteoarthritis, post-traumatic arthritis, spastic flexion contracture, degenerative scaphoid nonunion, or failed wrist arthroplasty. An incision is made in the midline over the posterior aspect of the wrist from the distal aspect of the forearm to the proximal aspect of the metacarpal. The radiocarpal joint and distal radioulnar joint (DRUJ) are exposed. The retinaculum is released beginning along the ulnar border and extending all the way to the radial border. The radial and ulnar nerves are protected with vessel loops. The tendons are retracted. Articular cartilage is removed using a rongeur or bur. The radiocarpal, intercarpal, and/or carpometacarpal joints are then immobilized using internal fixation devices such as pins, or a plate and screws. For complete fusion using a plate and screws, a plate that extends from the metacarpal of the long finger to the distal radius is used. The plate is secured with a screw to the metacarpal of the long finger, capitate bone, and then to the radius to fuse the wrist. The surgical wound is closed in layers.

25805

25805   Arthrodesis, wrist; with sliding graft

The physician makes an incision over the area of the wrist and dissects down to the bone. The wrist joint is immobilized by sliding bone from the surrounding area into position to block the joint from moving. The incision is then closed.

25810

25810   Arthrodesis, wrist; with iliac or other autograft (includes obtaining graft)

An incision is made in the midline over the posterior aspect of the wrist from the distal aspect of the forearm to the proximal aspect of the metacarpal. The radiocarpal joint and distal radioulnar joint (DRUJ) are exposed. The superficial branch of the radial nerve is identified and protected. The interval between the first and second dorsal compartments is located and dorsal carpal ligament incised leaving the ligament attached to the volar aspect of the radius. Overlying tendons are retracted. The extensor carpi radialis longus is sectioned proximal to the base of the second metacarpal. The joint capsule is incised and the radiocarpal, intercarpal, and second carpometacarpal joints are exposed. Articular cartilage is removed from the radiocarpal joint using a rongeur or bur. A bone autograft is harvested. A skin incision is made over the iliac crest or other site, and the muscle is stripped to reveal the bone surface. Cortical and cancellous bone is harvested. The bone is configured to the size and shape needed for grafting. A slot is cut in the radius, carpal bones, and first and second metacarpals. The bone graft is placed across the radiocarpal, intercarpal, and metacarpal joints. The graft is secured with a Kirschner wire. The dorsal carpal ligament is sutured over the bone graft. The surgical wound is closed in layers and the wrist is placed in a long arm cast.

Arthrodesis, wrist

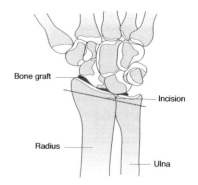

An incison is made into the wrist and the joint is immobilized with an iliac or other autograft to block the wrist from moving

25820-25825

25820   Arthrodesis, wrist; limited, without bone graft (eg, intercarpal or radiocarpal)

25825   Arthrodesis, wrist; with autograft (includes obtaining graft)

Arthrodesis, also referred to as joint fusion, is performed to relieve pain and restore joint stability in patients with rheumatoid arthritis, osteoarthritis, post-traumatic arthritis, spastic flexion contracture, degenerative scaphoid nonunion, or failed wrist arthroplasty. An incision is made in the midline over the posterior aspect of the wrist from the distal aspect of the forearm to the proximal aspect of the metacarpal. The radiocarpal joint and distal radioulnar joint (DRUJ) are exposed. The retinaculum is released beginning along the ulnar border and the release is extended all the way to the radial border. The radial and ulnar nerves are protected with vessel loops. The tendons are retracted. Articular cartilage is removed using a rongeur or bur. In 25820, the radiocarpal or intercarpal joints are immobilized using internal fixation devices such as pins, or a plate and screws. For limited fusion a pin may be placed through the radius and carpal bone or through the affected carpal bones. In 25825, a bone graft is harvested. Usually a local bone graft is used. Cortical bone chips or morcelized cancellous bone is placed in the joint space and secured with pins or wires. The surgical wound is closed in layers and the wrist immobilized in a cast.

25830

25830   Arthrodesis, distal radioulnar joint with segmental resection of ulna, with or without bone graft (eg, Sauve-Kapandji procedure)

An incision is made over the dorsoulnar aspect of the wrist. The distal branch of the ulnar nerve is identified and protected. The extensor retinaculum is divided. Tendons are retracted, the joint capsule divided, and the distal radioulnar joint exposed. A periosteal ulnar flap is created. Articular cartilage at the radioulnar joint is removed with a rongeur or bur. The distal 1 cm of the ulna is excised. A guide pin is placed through the ulna and across the distal radioulnar joint under fluoroscopic guidance. Screws and/or pins are used to secure the radius and ulna to each other. The periosteal flap is repaired and the joint capsule closed. The extensor retinaculum is repaired and overlying soft tissue and skin is closed in layers.

25900-25905

25900   Amputation, forearm, through radius and ulna
25905   Amputation, forearm, through radius and ulna; open, circular (guillotine)

A below-elbow amputation may be high (a few cm below the elbow joint), middle (through the radial and ulnar shafts) or low (a few cm above the wrist). The patient is positioned with the shoulder slightly elevated on the operative side. In 25900, skin and muscle flap incision lines are marked on the skin. Typically, an anterior/posterior fishmouth flap is used. The skin and superficial fascia are incised perpendicular to the skin surface. Underlying soft tissue is dissected and blood vessels and nerves exposed. Large blood vessels are mobilized, suture ligated and divided. Nerves are mobilized from the muscular bed, doubly ligated, divided, and allowed to retract into muscle tissue. The radius and ulna are exposed and periosteal flaps are created. The radius and ulna are transected at the level of the periosteal flaps taking care to ensure that the bones are of equal length. The periosteal flaps are sutured over the remaining bone. Antagonistic muscle groups are sutured to each other and anchored to the periosteum in such a way that the remaining portions of the radius and ulna are completely enveloped in muscle. Muscle sutures may be reinforced using synthetic tape that is placed through drill holes in the radius and ulna to prevent movement of the muscle tissue. Drains are placed and subcutaneous fascia and skin closed around the drains. A rigid dressing is applied to reduce pain and prevent edema. In 25905, a circular amputation, also called a guillotine or linear amputation, is performed. Skin incisions are made in a circular (linear) fashion at the predetermined site in the forearm. Soft tissue is dissected and blood vessels and nerves located, ligated, and transected as described above. The underlying muscle tissue is then transected at a point proximal to the skin incision. Periosteal flaps are created. The radius and ulna are then transected at the level of the periosteal flaps and slightly higher than the remaining muscle tissue. The periosteal flaps, muscle and skin are then closed as described above and a rigid dressing applied.

25907

25907   Amputation, forearm, through radius and ulna; secondary closure or scar revision

Secondary closure or scar revision of a previous below-elbow amputation through the radius and ulna is performed to obtain a pain-free stump covered with normal skin that functions well with a prosthesis. For secondary closure, the raw surface of the stump is debrided and all devitalized tissue is excised. Skin and subcutaneous tissue are fashioned into flaps and used to cover the stump taking care that there is not any undue tension along the suture line. For scar revision, the scar tissue is excised. Skin flaps are fashioned and the edges are undermined to ensure smooth, tension-free approximation along the suture line.

25909

25909   Amputation, forearm, through radius and ulna; re-amputation

Re-amputation of the arm through the radius and ulna is done at a higher level to remove diseased, infected, or nonviable tissue posing a risk to the patient and/or to form a healthy stump for use with a prosthesis. The incision lines for the re-amputation are marked on the skin. The skin and underlying soft tissue are incised. The muscles are exposed, isolated by

muscle group, and divided. Nerves and blood vessels are identified and isolated, taking care to ensure that nerves are separated from arteries to prevent pulsatile irritation of the nerves. Nerves are transected and allowed to retract into soft tissue. Blood vessels are suture ligated and transected. The radius and ulna are exposed and periosteal flaps are created. The bones are transected at the level of the periosteal flaps. The flaps are sutured over the remaining bone segments. Antagonistic muscle groups are sutured to each other and anchored to the periosteum in such a way that the remaining portions of the radius and ulna are completely enveloped in muscle. Skin flaps are fashioned and sutured over the muscle.

25915

25915   Krukenberg procedure

Krukenberg procedure is performed on patients with congenital absence of the hand or a previous traumatic or therapeutic amputation at the wrist. This is a reconstructive procedure that involves separating the radius and ulna, rearranging the muscles, and covering each bone with skin so that the radius and ulna form an innervated, mobile pincer that can be used to manipulate objects. The skin over the anterior aspect of the forearm is incised in the midline and the incision is carried over the stump and the posterior forearm in the midline. Soft tissues are dissected and the overlying muscles divided longitudinally into equal halves. The flexor digitorum sublimis and flexor digitorum profundus are separated using blunt dissection. The interosseous membrane between the radius and ulna is divided taking care to protect the interosseous blood vessels. The lengths of the radius and ulna are evaluated and bone excised as needed. The forearm muscles are rearranged and sutured over the tips of each bone. The radius and ulna are then separately covered with skin from the forearm and skin grafts. Drains are placed as needed in each of the stumps.

25920-25924

25920   Disarticulation through wrist
25922   Disarticulation through wrist; secondary closure or scar revision
25924   Disarticulation through wrist; re-amputation

An amputation through the wrist joint is performed. In 25920, palmar and dorsal flaps are created beginning distal to the radial and ulnar styloid processes. Finger flexor and extensor tendons are divided and allowed to retract. Wrist flexor and extensor tendons are identified and released from the distal insertions and reflected away from the operative site. Median and ulnar nerves are identified and sectioned proximal to the amputation site. Each of the distal branches of the radial nerve is also sectioned in the same manner. The radial and ulnar arteries are ligated at the appropriate level. The hand and wrist are then severed just below the radius and ulna taking care to preserve the triangular fibrocartilage. The radial and ulnar styloids are rounded off as needed. The skin and soft tissue flaps are then configured to cover the distal aspect of the radius and ulna. In 25922, a secondary closure or scar revision of a previous wrist disarticulation is performed to obtain a pain-free stump covered with normal skin that functions well with a prosthesis. For secondary closure, the raw surface of the stump is debrided and all devitalized tissue is excised. Skin and subcutaneous tissue are fashioned into flaps and used to cover the stump. For scar revision, the scar tissue is excised. Skin flaps are fashioned and the edges are undermined to ensure smooth, tension-free approximation along the suture line. In 25924, a re-amputation at the wrist is done to remove diseased, infected, or nonviable tissue posing a risk to the patient and/or to form a healthy stump for use with a prosthesis. The incision lines for the re-amputation are marked on the skin. The skin and underlying soft tissue are incised. The muscles are exposed, isolated by muscle group, and divided. Nerves and blood vessels are identified and isolated, taking care to ensure that nerves are separated from arteries to prevent pulsatile irritation of the nerves. Nerves are transected and allowed to retract into soft tissue. Blood vessels are suture ligated and transected. Bone is removed as needed. Skin flaps are fashioned and sutured over the muscle.

25927-25931

25927   Transmetacarpal amputation
25929   Transmetacarpal amputation; secondary closure or scar revision
25931   Transmetacarpal amputation; re-amputation

The physician amputates the fingers on a hand. The bones that form the fingers are completely removed from the hand. Code 25929 if the physician revisits the site of the procedure to apply a more permanent closure to the resulting wound(s), or removes excess scar tissue. Code 25931 if the site of the procedure is revisited to remove more tissue from the area of the amputation.

26010-26011

26010   Drainage of finger abscess; simple
26011   Drainage of finger abscess; complicated (eg, felon)

The skin is cleansed and local anesthetic injected as needed. A straight or elliptical incision is made over the abscess. Any pockets of pus are opened using blunt dissection. The abscess is drained and then irrigated with sterile solution. Use 26010 for a simple drainage procedure. Use 26011 when the drainage procedure is complicated, such as that

Musculoskeletal System

performed for a felon. A felon is more complicated to drain because it involves the nail fold and undersurface of the nail wall (perionychium).

26020

26020   Drainage of tendon sheath, digit and/or palm, each

Tendons are bundles of fibrous tissue that attach muscles to bone. The tendons in hands and fingers are covered by sheaths lined with synovial tissue that secretes synovial fluid to lubricate the tendons and facilitate movement of the hands and fingers. When a tendon or other structures in the hand or fingers become inflamed or infected, it is sometimes necessary to incise the tendon sheath in order to drain fluid or purulent material trapped beneath the tendon sheath. The skin over the affected tendon is incised. Soft tissues are dissected and the tendon sheath is exposed. The sheath is incised longitudinally and fluid and purulent material drained. Drains are placed as needed and the tendon sheath, soft tissues, and skin closed around the drains.

26025-26030

26025   Drainage of palmar bursa; single, bursa
26030   Drainage of palmar bursa; multiple bursa

Bursa are sacs lined with synovial membrane that contain synovial fluid and are found in areas subject to friction such as prominent body parts, joints or areas where tendons pass over bone. The approach is dictated by the location palmar bursa to be incised. The inflamed or infected bursa is incised and the fluid drained. The bursal sac may be flushed with antibiotic and/or normal saline solution prior to closure. Use 26025 for incision and drainage of the single palmar bursa; use 26030 when multiple palmar bursa are incised and drained.

26034

26034   Incision, bone cortex, hand or finger (eg, osteomyelitis or bone abscess)

The bone cortex of the one of the bones in the hand or fingers is opened to treat a condition such as osteomyelitis or bone abscess. Bones include the metacarpals the hand and the proximal, middle, and distal phalanges in the fingers. An incision is made in the skin and carried down through the soft tissue overlying the site of the infected bone. The periosteum over the infected region of the bone is elevated, a button of cortical bone removed, and the bone marrow exposed. Opening the bone cortex relieves pressure caused by inflammation of the bone marrow and prevents restriction of blood flow to the infected bone. If frank pus is encountered, the button hole may be enlarged and extended using a chisel or gouge along the bone for one to two inches. If the epiphysis is involved, a section of the epiphyseal cortex may be removed. The bone abscess is drained.

26035

26035   Decompression fingers and/or hand, injection injury (eg, grease gun)

The fingers and/or hand are decompressed following an injection injury. An injection injury results when the patient unintentionally injects a substance from a grease gun, spray gun, diesel injector, paint gun, concrete gun, plastic injector, or other high-pressure industrial injection device. The most common site of injury is the nondominant index finger, but other common sites include the long finger, thumb, and palm. Decompression involves incising the skin over the injection site and inspecting deeper tissues. The injected material is removed and necrotic tissue debrided. The wound is irrigated with normal saline and packed open.

26037

26037   Decompressive fasciotomy, hand (excludes 26035)

A decompression fasciotomy of the hand is performed to treat compartment syndrome which may be caused by a crushing injury, burn, or even by accidental infiltration of intravenous medications into the tissues of the hand. There are ten separate osteofascial compartments in the hand and depending on the site of the compartment syndrome release may be accomplished using dorsal incisions of the hand or by carpal tunnel release. For release using dorsal incisions, the hand is incised over the second and fourth metacarpals. Extensor tendons are retracted to allow access to both the dorsal and volar interosseous compartments. Each compartment is opened using a longitudinal incision. The wounds are covered with a sterile dressing until tissue swelling subsides at which time the wounds may be closed with sutures or separately reportable skin grafting procedures performed.

26040-26045

26040   Fasciotomy, palmar (eg, Dupuytren's contracture); percutaneous
26045   Fasciotomy, palmar (eg, Dupuytren's contracture); open, partial

Dupuytren's contracture is caused by thickening and tightening of the fibrous tissue beneath the skin of the hand and fingers. While painless, the thickening causes a flexion contracture making it difficult or impossible to fully extend one or more fingers. In 26040, a percutaneous fasciotomy is performed. A small stab incision is created in the palm over the region of thickening and the fibrous tissue is incised. In 26045, an incision is made in

the palm of the hand. The thickened fibrous tissue is then incised. The wound is closed in layers.

26055

26055   Tendon sheath incision (eg, for trigger finger)

The flexor tendons of the hand extend from the muscles above the wrist to the ends of the fingers. Each tendon passes through a tendon sheath in the finger which is a tunnel that keeps the tendon close to the bone. If the tendon becomes irritated and inflamed or develops nodules it may be difficult for the tendon to slide through the tendon sheath. If nodules are present the nodules may catch temporarily at the mouth of the tendon sheath, and then as the tendon finally passes through the tight area the finger will suddenly pop straight out. This condition is known as trigger finger. A small incision is made in the palm of the hand over the affected finger. The tendon sheath is cut.

26060

26060   Tenotomy, percutaneous, single, each digit

The skin over the affected tendon is cleansed and the anatomical landmarks and percutaneous puncture sites marked. An 18 gauge needle is inserted through the skin and advanced to the selected site under the tendon. The needle is placed with the cutting edge against the tendon and withdrawn to cut the tendon longitudinally. Report 26060 for each digit on which a percutaneous tenotomy is performed.

26070-26080

26070   Arthrotomy, with exploration, drainage, or removal of loose or foreign body; carpometacarpal joint
26075   Arthrotomy, with exploration, drainage, or removal of loose or foreign body; metacarpophalangeal joint, each
26080   Arthrotomy, with exploration, drainage, or removal of loose or foreign body; interphalangeal joint, each

There are five carpometacarpal (CMC) joints in each hand. These five joints are articulations between the distal row of carpal bones at the wrist and the proximal aspect of the metacarpal bones that make up the palm of the hand. In 26070, an incision is made in the skin over the affected carpometacarpal joint. Soft tissues are dissected taking care to protect surrounding nerves and blood vessels. The joint capsule is exposed and incised. The joint capsule is visually inspected. If an infection is present, fluid, blood and purulent material is drained. Any loculations are broken up using blunt dissection. The joint is flushed with sterile saline or antibiotic solution using pulsed lavage to clear debris. If a foreign body is contained within the joint it is located and removed. Drains are placed and the incision closed around the drains. Use 26075 if the procedure is performed on the metacarpophalangeal (MCP) joint. There are five MCP joints which are articulations between the bones of the palm of the hand and the first bone in each finger. Use 26080 if the procedure is performed on the interphalangeal (IP) joint. There are nine IP joints in each hand, one in the thumb and two in each finger. The IP joints are articulations between the phalanges which are the bones in the fingers. These procedures are reported for each separate joint treated.

26100-26110

26100   Arthrotomy with biopsy; carpometacarpal joint, each
26105   Arthrotomy with biopsy; metacarpophalangeal joint, each
26110   Arthrotomy with biopsy; interphalangeal joint, each

There are five carpometacarpal (CMC) joints in each hand. These five joints are articulations between the distal row of carpal bones at the wrist and the proximal aspect of the metacarpal bones that make up the palm of the hand. In 26100, an incision is made in the skin over the affected carpometacarpal joint. Soft tissues are dissected taking care to protect surrounding nerves and blood vessels. The joint capsule is exposed and incised. The joint capsule is visually inspected. Tissue samples are obtained from the joint capsule and/or synovial membrane and sent for separately reportable laboratory evaluation. Use 26105 if the procedure is performed on the metacarpophalangeal (MCP) joint. There are five MCP joints which are articulations between the bones of the palm of the hand and the first bone in each finger. Use 26110 if the procedure is performed on the interphalangeal (IP) joint. There are nine IP joints in each hand, one in the thumb and two in each finger. The IP joints are articulations between the phalanges which are the bones in the fingers. These procedures are reported for each separate joint treated.

● New Code   ▲ Revised Code

26111-26116

26111   Excision, tumor or vascular malformation, soft tissue of hand or finger; subcutaneous; 1.5 cm or greater

26113   Excision, tumor, soft tissue, or vascular malformation, of hand or finger, subfascial (eg, intramuscular); 1.5 cm or greater

26115   Excision, tumor or vascular malformation, soft tissue of hand or finger, subcutaneous; less than 1.5 cm

26116   Excision, tumor, soft tissue, or vascular malformation, of hand or finger, subfascial (eg, intramuscular); less than 1.5 cm

Soft tissues include subcutaneous fat and connective tissue, fascia, muscles, tendons, blood vessels, lymph vessels, nerves, and tissues surrounding the joints. Soft tissue tumors may be benign or malignant. Benign tumors are typically treated by excision, although small malignant or indeterminate tumors may be excised if the margins are well defined. Depending on the location of the tumor or vascular malformation in the soft tissue of the hand or finger, the skin over the tumor may be incised or a skin flap created and elevated. Overlying tissue is dissected and the soft tissue mass exposed. The tumor or vascular malformation is then excised along with a margin of healthy tissue. Separately reportable frozen section may be performed to ensure that all margins are free of tumor cells. Drains are placed as needed and the surgical wound is closed in layers. For tumors or vascular malformations in the subcutaneous fat or connective tissue, use 26115 for excision of less than 1.5 cm and 26111 for excision of 1.5 cm or greater. For tumors or vascular malformations that lie below the fascia, use 26116 for excision of less than 1.5 cm and 26113 for excision of 1.5 cm or greater. Subfascial soft tissue tumors include those within muscle tissue.

26117-26118

26117   Radical resection of tumor (eg, sarcoma), soft tissue of hand or finger; less than 3 cm

26118   Radical resection of tumor (eg, sarcoma), soft tissue of hand or finger; 3 cm or greater

Soft tissues include muscles, tendons, fat, blood vessels, lymph vessels, nerves, and tissues surrounding the joints. Soft tissue tumors may be benign or malignant. Radical resection is typically performed for a malignant neoplasm, such as a sarcoma, although benign tumors and tumors of indeterminate nature may also require radical resection. A skin incision is made over the tumor in the hand or finger, or a skin flap is created and elevated. Overlying tissue is dissected and the tumor exposed. The tumor is removed en bloc along with a wide margin of surrounding tissue. Radical resection involves excision of all involved soft tissue which may include muscles, nerves, and blood vessels. Separately reportable frozen section is performed to ensure that all margins are free of tumor cells. If margins show evidence of malignancy, additional tissue is removed until all margins are free of tumor cells. Drains are placed as needed. The surgical wound may be closed in layers, or separately reportable reconstructive procedures performed. Use 26117 for radical resection of soft tissue tumor of hand or finger less than 3 cm; use 26118 for 3 cm or greater.

26121-26125

26121   Fasciectomy, palm only, with or without Z-plasty, other local tissue rearrangement, or skin grafting (includes obtaining graft)

26123   Fasciectomy, partial palmar with release of single digit including proximal interphalangeal joint, with or without Z-plasty, other local tissue rearrangement, or skin grafting (includes obtaining graft)

26125   Fasciectomy, partial palmar with release of single digit including proximal interphalangeal joint, with or without Z-plasty, other local tissue rearrangement, or skin grafting (includes obtaining graft); each additional digit (List separately in addition to code for primary procedure)

Thickened fascia in the palm only or palm and fingers is excised. Typically, a zigzag incision is made over the palm and affected fingers as needed. In 26121, the skin and subcutaneous tissue is elevated off the palmar fascia and pretendinous fascial cord. At the metacarpal head the soft tissue is carefully dissected and the digital nerves and arteries on either side of the tendon cords identified and protected. The thickened fascia over the affected tendon is then progressively elevated from the proximal aspect of the palm to the head of the metacarpal. Once the fascial cord has been completely freed from digital nerves and vessels, the thickened fascia is excised which frees the underlying tendon and relieves the flexion contracture of the affected finger. Soft tissues in the palm of the hand are rearranged as needed to cover and protect underlying structures. The zigzag incision is closed or a skin graft is harvested and used to close the surgical wound. Use 26123 if the zigzag incision is extended over the proximal interphalangeal joint and the fascial cord in a single finger is removed along with the fascial cord in the palm. Use 26125 for each additional finger from which the fascial cord is excised.

26130-26140

26130   Synovectomy, carpometacarpal joint

26135   Synovectomy, metacarpophalangeal joint including intrinsic release and extensor hood reconstruction, each digit

26140   Synovectomy, proximal interphalangeal joint, including extensor reconstruction, each interphalangeal joint

There are five carpometacarpal (CMC) joints in each hand. These five joints are articulations between the distal row of carpal bones at the wrist and the proximal aspect of the metacarpal bones that make up the palm of the hand. In 26130, an incision is made in the skin over the affected carpometacarpal joint. Soft tissues are dissected taking care to protect surrounding nerves and blood vessels. The joint capsule is exposed and incised. The joint capsule is visually inspected. The inflamed synovial tissue is excised. In 26135, a synovectomy is performed on the metacarpophalangeal (MCP) joint along with release and reconstruction of the extensor hood. There are five MCP joints which are articulations between the bones of the palm of the hand and the first bone in each finger. The extensor tendons that begin in the distal forearm and cross over the wrist become the extensor hood as they travel into the fingers. The extensor hood flattens out and covers the top of the finger and then sends out branches on each side that connect to the middle and distal phalanges. Small ligaments connect the extensor hood to other tendons which work together to provide smooth, balanced motion in the fingers. The synovectomy is performed as described above. The extensor hood is then carefully dissected from surrounding tissue and reconstructed so that interconnected tendons and ligaments can move freely. In 26140, a synovectomy is performed on the proximal interphalangeal (IP) joint along with extensor reconstruction. There are nine IP joints in each hand, one in the thumb and two (proximal and distal) in each finger. The IP joints are articulations between the phalanges which are the bones in the fingers. The synovectomy is performed as described above. The extensor tendon is carefully dissected from surrounding tissue and reconstructed as described above.

26145

26145   Synovectomy, tendon sheath, radical (tenosynovectomy), flexor tendon, palm and/or finger, each tendon

This procedure is performed to treat inflammation of the synovial tissue in the tendon sheath caused by conditions such as rheumatoid arthritis. A skin incision is made over the affected tendon in the palm or finger. Overlying tissues are dissected and the tendon sheath exposed. The tendon sheath is incised and inspected. All inflamed synovial tissue is removed using a motorized suction shaving device. Report 26145 for each separate tendon sheath treated on which a radical tenosynovectomy is performed.

26160

26160   Excision of lesion of tendon sheath or joint capsule (eg, cyst, mucous cyst, or ganglion), hand or finger

The physician incises the skin over the target flexor or extensor tendon or joint capsule of the hand or finger. Overlying tissue is dissected and the tendon or joint is exposed. The tendon sheath or joint capsule lesion is located, carefully dissected free of surrounding healthy tissue, and excised in its entirety. The abnormal tissue is sent for separately reportable pathology evaluation. The surgical wound is closed in layers.

26170-26180

26170   Excision of tendon, palm, flexor or extensor, single, each tendon

26180   Excision of tendon, finger, flexor or extensor, each tendon

A tendon of the palm or hand may need to be removed following traumatic injury or an open wound that is complicated by infection. The affected flexor or extensor tendon in the palm or finger is exposed. The tendon is dissected free of surrounding tissue and released from attachments to bone, ligaments, and other tendons. The tendon is then removed. Report 26170 for each flexor or extensor tendon in the palm that is excised. Report 26180 for each flexor or extensor tendon in the finger that is excised.

26185

26185   Sesamoidectomy, thumb or finger (separate procedure)

Sesamoid bones are small bones embedded in a tendon. The primary functions of sesamoid bones are to modify pressure, diminish friction, and alter the direction of muscle pull. The sesamoid bones in the fingers are not found in all individuals and not all individuals have sesamoid bones in the same locations. However, most people have 5 sesamoid bones in each hand with two located in the metacarpophalangeal (MCP) joint of the thumb, one located in the interphalangeal (IP) joint of the thumb, one at the MCP joint of the index finger and one at the MCP joint of the little finger. Other less common sites include the MCP joints of the middle and ring fingers, and the distal IP joint of the index finger. The surgical approach depends on which sesamoid bone is being excised. An incision is made over the affected joint. Overlying tissue is dissected taking care to identify and protect digital nerves. Surrounding joint structures are visually inspected for injury or disease. The sesamoid bone is located within the tendon by palpation. The tendon is

Musculoskeletal System

incised longitudinally and the sesamoid bone is sharply excised taking care to protect the integrity of the tendon. Incisions are closed and a bulky dressing and splint applied.

26200-26205

26200	**Excision or curettage of bone cyst or benign tumor of metacarpal**
26205	**Excision or curettage of bone cyst or benign tumor of metacarpal; with autograft (includes obtaining graft)**

A bone cyst is a fluid filled space within the bone. One common type is a unicameral or simple bone cyst, which is a benign lesion. A less common type is an aneurysmal bone cyst which consists of vascular tissue surrounding a blood filled cystic lesion. There are a number of different types of benign bone tumors including giant cell tumors, chondromixoid fibromas, and enchondromas. In 26200, an incision is made in the skin over the site of lesion in one of the metacarpal bones. Soft tissues are dissected and the lesion is exposed. If a cystic lesion is present, the bone is incised and a bone window created to open the cyst. Fluid is aspirated and sent to the laboratory for separately reportable analysis. A curette is inserted through the bone window and the lining of the cystic cavity is completely removed by curettage. Alternatively, some cystic lesions and most benign tumors are treated by excision. The lesion is exposed as described above. The physician then excises the benign lesion along with a margin of surrounding healthy bone. In 26205, the lesion is curetted or excised as described above. The physician then obtains healthy bone locally or from a separate site, such as the iliac crest. The bone autograft is packed into the defect in the metacarpal bone.

26210-26215

26210	**Excision or curettage of bone cyst or benign tumor of proximal, middle, or distal phalanx of finger**
26215	**Excision or curettage of bone cyst or benign tumor of proximal, middle, or distal phalanx of finger; with autograft (includes obtaining graft)**

A bone cyst is a fluid filled space within the bone. One common type is a unicameral or simple bone cyst, which is a benign lesion. A less common type is an aneurysmal bone cyst which consists of vascular tissue surrounding a blood filled cystic lesion. There are a number of different types of benign bone tumors including giant cell tumors, chondromixoid fibromas, and enchondromas. In 26210, an incision is made in the skin over the site of lesion in proximal, middle or distal phalanx of one of the fingers. Soft tissues are dissected and the lesion is exposed. If a cystic lesion is present, the bone is incised and a bone window created to open the cyst. Fluid is aspirated and sent to the laboratory for separately reportable analysis. A curette is inserted through the bone window and the lining of the cystic cavity is completely removed by curettage. Alternatively, some cystic lesions and most benign tumors are treated by excision. The lesion is exposed as described above. The physician then excises the benign lesion along with a margin of surrounding healthy bone. In 26215, the lesion is curetted or excised as described above. The physician then obtains healthy bone locally or from a separate site, such as the iliac crest. The bone autograft is packed into the defect in the proximal, middle or distal phalanx.

26230-26236

26230	**Partial excision (craterization, saucerization, or diaphysectomy) bone (eg, osteomyelitis); metacarpal**
26235	**Partial excision (craterization, saucerization, or diaphysectomy) bone (eg, osteomyelitis); proximal or middle phalanx of finger**
26236	**Partial excision (craterization, saucerization, or diaphysectomy) bone (eg, osteomyelitis); distal phalanx of finger**

The physician performs a partial excision of bone, also referred to as craterization, saucerization, or diaphysectomy to treat osteomyelitis of the metacarpal (26230), proximal or middle phalanx of the finger (26235), or distal phalanx of the finger (26236). Craterization and saucerization of bone involves removing infected and necrotic bone to form a shallow depression in the bone surface that will allow drainage from the infected area. Diaphysectomy involves removal of the infected portion of the shaft of a long bone. An incision is made in the skin and carried down through the soft tissue overlying the site of the osteomyelitis. Any soft tissue sinus tracts and devitalized soft tissue are resected. The area of necrotic and infected bone is exposed. A series of drill holes are made in the necrotic and infected bone and the bone between the drill holes is excavated to create an oval window using an osteotome. The amount of bone removed is dependent on the extent of the infection. A curette may be used to remove devitalized tissue from the medullary canal. Debridement continues until punctate bleeding is identified in the exposed bony surface. When all devitalized and infected tissue has been removed, the wound is copiously irrigated with sterile saline or antibiotic solution. The surgical wound is loosely closed and a drain placed.

26250

26250	**Radical resection of tumor, metacarpal**

Radical resection is typically performed for a malignant neoplasm although benign tumors and tumors of indeterminate nature may also require radical resection. A skin incision is made over the tumor in the metacarpal bone, or a skin flap is created and elevated. Overlying tissue is dissected and the tumor exposed. All bone and cartilage in

the metacarpal bone with tumor involvement is resected. The tumor is removed en bloc along with a wide margin of surrounding tissue. Radical resection of bone includes excision of all involved soft tissue which may include muscles, tendons, fat, blood vessels, lymph vessels, nerves, and tissues surrounding the joints. Separately reportable frozen section is performed to ensure that all margins are free of tumor cells. If margins show evidence of malignancy, additional tissue is removed until all margins are free of tumor cells. Drains are placed as needed. The surgical wound may be closed in layers, or separately reportable reconstructive procedures performed.

26260-26262

26260	**Radical resection of tumor, proximal or middle phalanx of finger**
26262	**Radical resection of tumor, distal phalanx of finger**

Radical resection is typically performed for a malignant neoplasm although benign tumors and tumors of indeterminate nature may also require radical resection. A skin incision is made in the finger over the bone tumor in the proximal, middle, or distal phalanx or a skin flap is created and elevated. Overlying tissue is dissected and the tumor exposed. All bone and cartilage with tumor involvement is resected. The bone tumor is removed en bloc along with a wide margin of surrounding tissue. Radical resection of bone includes excision of all involved soft tissue which may include muscles, tendons, fat, blood vessels, lymph vessels, nerves, and tissues surrounding the joints. Separately reportable frozen section is performed to ensure that all margins are free of tumor cells. If margins show evidence of malignancy, additional tissue is removed until all margins are free of tumor cells. Drains are placed as needed. The surgical wound may be closed in layers, or separately reportable reconstructive procedures performed. Use 26260 for radical resection of a tumor in the proximal or middle phalanx and 26262 for a tumor in the distal phalanx.

26320

26320	**Removal of implant from finger or hand**

The most common sites of hand or finger implants are the metacarpophalangeal (MCP) joints and the proximal interphalangeal (PIP) joints. These implants are used to treat arthritic finger joints when more conservative therapy has failed to relieve pain and restore function. These implants sometimes require removal due to infection or mechanical malfunction of the implant. An incision is made in the skin over the region of the hand or finger containing the implant. Soft tissues are dissected and the implant exposed. The implant is then removed. A separately reportable joint reconstruction or fusion procedure may be performed. The soft tissues and skin are closed in layers.

26340

26340	**Manipulation, finger joint, under anesthesia, each joint**

Manipulation under anesthesia (MUA) of a finger joint is performed. This procedure is performed to improve range of motion by rupturing fibrous adhesions (arthrofibrosis) that develop following surgery or traumatic injury to the finger. An anesthetic is administered. The physician then takes a single finger joint through a complete range of motion. The physician must use sufficient force to rupture the adhesions while taking care not to apply too much force which could injure the joint structures or bones. Report 26340 for each finger joint treated.

26341

26341	**Manipulation, palmar fascial cord (ie, Dupuytren's cord), post enzyme injection (eg, collagenase), single cord**

Dupuytren's contracture is caused by thickening and tightening of palmar fibrous tissue due to excessive collagen deposition beneath the skin of the hand and fingers. While painless, the thickening causes a flexion contracture making it difficult or impossible to fully extend one or more fingers. Following a separately reportable enzyme injection into the fibrous tissue to weaken the cord (20527), manipulation of the palmar fascial cord, also called Dupuytren's cord, is performed. The patient returns the day after the injection procedure. The hand and fingers are then manipulated and the flexed finger is extended. This causes mechanical breakage of the weakened cord allowing better range of motion of the affected finger(s). Use 26341 for reporting the manipulation of a single palmar fascial cord.

26350-26352

26350	**Repair or advancement, flexor tendon, not in zone 2 digital flexor tendon sheath (eg, no man's land); primary or secondary without free graft, each tendon**
26352	**Repair or advancement, flexor tendon, not in zone 2 digital flexor tendon sheath (eg, no man's land); secondary with free graft (includes obtaining graft), each tendon**

Injuries of the flexor tendons include partial or complete laceration, tear, or rupture. Flexor tendons in the hand are defined by zone. Repair or advancement procedures performed in zones 1 and 3 are reported with these codes. Zone 1 involves any tendon injury that is distal to the flexor digitorum superficialis (FDS) insertion which would include only injuries to the profundus tendon. Zone 3 is essentially any injury in the palm from the edge distal carpal ligament to the distal palmar crease. Primary repair is typically performed

● New Code	▲ Revised Code

within 24 hours of injury; however if there is gross contamination of the wound primary repair may be delayed for up to 2 weeks. Secondary repair is typically defined as that performed more than two weeks after the initial injury. The tendon is exposed through a volar zigzag or lateral incision. Soft tissues are dissected taking care to protect the neurovascular structures. The distal and proximal ends of the severed tendon are located which may require a separate incision if the proximal end has retracted and cannot be located through the first incision. In 26350, the distal and proximal ends of the tendon are approximated and sutured together. This may be performed as a primary or secondary repair and is reported for each flexor tendon repaired. In 26352, a secondary repair using a free graft is performed. The site of the original tendon injury is exposed. A tendon graft is harvested usually the palmaris longus from the distal forearm. The graft is then attached to the affected flexor muscle usually at the wrist and tunneled to the point where it will be attached. The graft is secured at the attachment site with sutures.

26356-26358

26356   Repair or advancement, flexor tendon, in zone 2 digital flexor tendon sheath (eg, no man's land); primary, without free graft, each tendon

26357   Repair or advancement, flexor tendon, in zone 2 digital flexor tendon sheath (eg, no man's land); secondary, without free graft, each tendon

26358   Repair or advancement, flexor tendon, in zone 2 digital flexor tendon sheath (eg, no man's land); secondary, with free graft (includes obtaining graft), each tendon

Injuries of the flexor tendons include partial or complete laceration, tear, or rupture. Flexor tendons in the hand are defined by zone. Repair or advancement procedures performed in zone 2 are reported with these codes. Zone 2, also referred to as Bunnel's or no man's land, is defined as the area between the insertion of flexor digitorum superficialis tendon to the proximal A1 pulley which is essentially the region from the proximal end of the proximal phalanx to the distal end of the middle phalanx. Primary repair is typically performed within 24 hours of injury; however if there is gross contamination of the wound primary repair may be delayed for up to 2 weeks. Secondary repair is typically defined as that performed more than two weeks after the initial injury. The tendon is exposed through a volar zigzag or lateral incision. Soft tissues are dissected taking care to protect the neurovascular structures. The distal and proximal ends of the severed tendon are located which may require a separate incision if the proximal end has retracted and cannot be located through the first incision. In 26356, a primary suture repair is performed. The distal and proximal ends of the tendon are approximated and sutured together. In 26357, a secondary suture repair is performed in the same manner. In 26358, a secondary repair using a free graft is performed. The site of the original tendon injury is exposed. A tendon graft is harvested usually the palmaris longus from the distal forearm. The graft is then attached to the affected flexor muscle usually at the wrist and tunneled to the point where it will be attached. The graft is secured at the attachment site with sutures.

26370-26373

26370   Repair or advancement of profundus tendon, with intact superficialis tendon; primary, each tendon

26372   Repair or advancement of profundus tendon, with intact superficialis tendon; secondary with free graft (includes obtaining graft), each tendon

26373   Repair or advancement of profundus tendon, with intact superficialis tendon; secondary without free graft, each tendon

The flexor digitorum profundus (FDP) extends from the upper anterior and medial aspects of the ulna to the wrist and then divides at the wrist into four tendons that insert at the palmar base of the distal phalanx of each finger after passing through the flexor digitorum superficialis (FDS) tendon. In 26370, a primary repair or advancement is performed on the FDP when the FDS is still intact. The distal and proximal ends of the FDP are located. Primary repair is typically performed within 24 hours of injury; however if there is gross contamination of the wound primary repair may be delayed for up to 2 weeks. Secondary repair is typically defined as that performed more than two weeks after the initial injury. The tendon is exposed through a volar zigzag or lateral incision. Soft tissues are dissected taking care to protect neurovascular structures. The distal and proximal ends of the severed tendon are located which may require a separate incision if the proximal end has retracted and cannot be located through the first incision. The proximal end is advanced distally and sutured to the distal end. Alternatively, if less than a 1 cm distal stump remains the tendon is advanced and sutured to base of the distal phalanx. In 26372, a secondary repair or advancement of the FDP with an intact FDS is performed using a free graft. The site of the original tendon injury is exposed. A tendon graft is harvested usually the palmaris longus from the distal forearm. The graft is then attached to the affected portion of the FDP muscle and tunneled to the base of the distal phalanx where it is anchored to the phalangeal base. In 26373, a secondary suture repair or advancement is performed without a free graft using the same technique described in 26370.

26390-26392

26390   Excision flexor tendon, with implantation of synthetic rod for delayed tendon graft, hand or finger, each rod

26392   Removal of synthetic rod and insertion of flexor tendon graft, hand or finger (includes obtaining graft), each rod

When a flexor tendon repair fails or is not performed in a timely manner, delayed flexor tendon grafting must be performed using a two stage procedure. In 26390, the first stage of the procedure is performed. This involves excision of the injured tendon and insertion of a synthetic rod. A zigzag incision is made over the affected tendon. Soft tissues are dissected taking care to protect neurovascular structures. The tendon sheath is incised. The injured tendon is dissected free of surrounding tissue. The tendon is excised. A synthetic rod is inserted along the entire length of the tendon sheath. Overlying soft tissues and skin are closed in layers. The synthetic rod remains in place for approximately 10 weeks while the tendon sheath heals around the rod. In 26392, the second stage is performed. A tendon graft is harvested from the forearm or leg. The distal and proximal ends of the old incision are opened. The tendon graft is attached to the synthetic rod at the proximal end. The rod is then removed through the distal end of the old incision and as it is removed the tendon graft is pulled into the newly formed tendon sheath. The tendon graft is sutured to the proximal end of the native tendon. Tension of the tendon graft is adjusted until the desired range of motion is attained. The distal end of the tendon graft is trimmed and anchored to the bone.

26410-26412

26410   Repair, extensor tendon, hand, primary or secondary; without free graft, each tendon

26412   Repair, extensor tendon, hand, primary or secondary; with free graft (includes obtaining graft), each tendon

Injuries of the extensor tendons of the hand include partial or complete laceration, tear, or rupture. Primary repair is typically performed within 24 hours of injury; however if there is gross contamination of the wound primary repair may be delayed for up to 2 weeks. Secondary repair is typically defined as that performed more than two weeks after the initial injury. The tendon is exposed through a dorsal incision. Soft tissues are dissected taking care to protect the neurovascular structures. The distal and proximal ends of the severed tendon are located which may require a separate incision if the proximal end has retracted and cannot be located through the first incision. In 26410, the distal and proximal ends of the tendon are approximated and sutured together. This may be performed as a primary or secondary repair and is reported for each flexor tendon repaired. In 26412, a primary or secondary repair using a free graft is performed. The site of the original tendon injury is exposed. A tendon graft is harvested from the forearm or leg. The graft is then attached to the affected extensor muscle and tunneled to the site where it will be attached. The graft is secured at the attachment site with sutures.

26415-26416

26415   Excision of extensor tendon, with implantation of synthetic rod for delayed tendon graft, hand or finger, each rod

26416   Removal of synthetic rod and insertion of extensor tendon graft (includes obtaining graft), hand or finger, each rod

When an extensor tendon repair fails or is not performed in a timely manner, delayed extensor tendon grafting must be performed using a two stage procedure. In 26415, the first stage of the procedure is performed. This involves excision of the injured tendon and insertion of a synthetic rod. A zigzag incision is made over the affected tendon. Soft tissues are dissected taking care to protect neurovascular structures. The tendon sheath is incised. The injured tendon is dissected free of surrounding tissue. The tendon is excised. A synthetic rod is inserted along the entire length of the tendon sheath. Overlying soft tissues and skin are closed in layers. The synthetic rod remains in place for approximately 10 weeks while the tendon sheath heals around the rod. In 26416, the second stage is performed. A tendon graft is harvested from the forearm or leg. The distal and proximal ends of the old incision are opened. The tendon graft is attached to the synthetic rod at the proximal end. The rod is then removed through the distal end of the old incision and as it is removed the tendon graft is pulled into the newly formed tendon sheath. The tendon graft is sutured to the proximal end of the native tendon. Tension of the tendon graft is adjusted until the desired range of motion is attained. The distal end of the tendon graft is trimmed and anchored to the bone.

26418-26420

26418   Repair, extensor tendon, finger, primary or secondary; without free graft, each tendon

26420   Repair, extensor tendon, finger, primary or secondary; with free graft (includes obtaining graft) each tendon

Injuries of the extensor tendons of the fingers include partial or complete laceration, tear, or rupture. Primary repair is typically performed within 24 hours of injury; however if there is gross contamination of the wound primary repair may be delayed for up to 2 weeks. Secondary repair is typically defined as that performed more than two weeks

Musculoskeletal System

after the initial injury. The tendon is exposed through a dorsal incision. Soft tissues are dissected taking care to protect the neurovascular structures. The distal and proximal ends of the severed tendon are located which may require a separate incision if the proximal end has retracted and cannot be located through the first incision. In 26418, the distal and proximal ends of the tendon are approximated and sutured together. This may be performed as a primary or secondary repair and is reported for each flexor tendon repaired. In 26420, a primary or secondary repair using a free graft is performed. The site of the original tendon injury is exposed. A tendon graft is harvested from the forearm or leg. The graft is then attached to the affected extensor muscle and tunneled to the site where it will be attached. The graft is secured at the attachment site with sutures.

26426-26428

26426   **Repair of extensor tendon, central slip, secondary (eg, boutonniere deformity); using local tissue(s), including lateral band(s), each finger**
26428   **Repair of extensor tendon, central slip, secondary (eg, boutonniere deformity); with free graft (includes obtaining graft), each finger**

The extensor tendons in the fingers are composed of tendons that run along the sides of the finger and another that runs along the top. The tendon that runs over the top attaches to the middle phalanx at a site called the central slip. When the central slip is injured the finger cannot be completely straightened at the proximal interphalangeal joint. This type of injury called a boutonniere deformity is usually caused by a forceful blow to the bent finger or a laceration on the top of the finger that severs the central slip from its attachment to the bone. It can also be caused by rheumatoid arthritis. Repairs of the central slip that require rearrangement of local tissues or free graft are secondary repairs that are performed following a failed primary repair or several weeks after the injury occurred. An incision is made over the top of the finger and the extensor tendon and central slip exposed. There are a number of repair techniques and the one used depends on the exact nature of the injury. In 26426, the tendon and central slip are repaired using local tissue rearrangement. The lateral bands may be repositioned dorsally or the lateral band on one side may be used to reconstruct the central slip and the lateral band on the opposite side elongated to stabilize the joint. The extrinsic and interosseous tendons may be separated from the lumbrical and oblique retinacular ligaments and the lateral band may be centralized. A Kirshner wire is then inserted through the distal phalanx and into the middle phalanx to hold the proximal interphalangeal joint in extension. In 26428, the site of the original tendon injury is exposed. A tendon graft is harvested from the forearm or leg. The graft is then used to repair the extensor tendon and central slip.

26432

26432   **Closed treatment of distal extensor tendon insertion, with or without percutaneous pinning (eg, mallet finger)**

An injury to the distal extensor tendon insertion can cause mallet finger which is a flexion deformity of the distal interphalangeal joint. The affected finger cannot be straightened. This type of injury is usually caused by a blunt force to the end of the finger that causes the tendon to tear or rupture. In some cases a piece of bone may pull away along with the tendon. Closed treatment may involve splinting the finger to keep it fully extended while the damaged distal extensor tendon heals. Alternatively, a Kirschner wire may be placed through the distal phalanx across the distal interphalangeal joint and into the middle phalanx to keep the finger in extension.

26433-26434

26433   **Repair of extensor tendon, distal insertion, primary or secondary; without graft (eg, mallet finger)**
26434   **Repair of extensor tendon, distal insertion, primary or secondary; with free graft (includes obtaining graft)**

An injury to the distal extensor tendon insertion can cause mallet finger which is a flexion deformity of the distal interphalangeal joint. The affected finger cannot be straightened. This type of injury is usually caused by a blunt force to the end of the finger that causes the tendon to tear or rupture. In some cases a piece of bone may pull away along with the tendon. Primary repair is typically performed within 24 hours of injury; however if there is gross contamination of an open wound primary repair may be delayed for up to 2 weeks. Secondary repair is typically defined as that performed more than two weeks after the initial injury. The tendon is exposed through a dorsal incision. Soft tissues are dissected taking care to protect the neurovascular structures. The distal and proximal ends of the ruptured tendon are located which may require a separate incision. In 26433, the distal and proximal ends of the tendon are approximated and sutured together. This may be performed as a primary or secondary repair and is reported for each flexor tendon repaired. If a piece of bone has pulled away, it may be secured to the distal phalanx with a pin or screw. In 26434, a primary or secondary repair using a free graft is performed. The site of the original tendon injury is exposed. A tendon graft is harvested from the forearm or leg. The graft is then sutured to the proximal end of the ruptured tendon and secured to the distal end of the tendon or to the distal phalanx with a pin or screw.

26437

26437   **Realignment of extensor tendon, hand, each tendon**

The extensor tendons that straighten the fingers normally lie over metacarpals and extend over the top of the metacarpophalangeal joint and into the fingers. Ligaments called sagittal bands and intercommunications between the tendons stabilize the extensor tendons and hold them in place. If the stabilizing structures are damaged the extensor tendons can slip to the side of the metacarpophalangeal joint making it difficult to straighten the fingers. Eventually the hand may become permanently flexed or bent at the metacarpophalangeal joint. A dorsal incision is made over the affected extensor tendon. The tendon is returned to normal position and the stabilizing structures repaired with sutures. A drain may be placed. The surgical wound is repaired in layers and a bulky dressing applied. Report 26437 for each extensor tendon that is realigned.

26440-26442

26440   **Tenolysis, flexor tendon; palm OR finger, each tendon**
26442   **Tenolysis, flexor tendon; palm AND finger, each tendon**

Tenolysis of a single flexor tendon in the palm or finger is performed to restore hand and/or finger motion by releasing scar tissue that has resulted from trauma or a disease process. An incision is made over the affected flexor tendon. Soft tissues are dissected. In 26440, the affected flexor tendon is identified and adhesions along the length of the tendon in the palm or finger are severed. Range of motion is evaluated. The surgical wound is closed in layers and a dressing is applied. In 26442, adhesions are severed along the entire length of the tendon in the palm and finger. These codes are reported for each separate tendon treated by tenolysis.

26445-26449

26445   **Tenolysis, extensor tendon, hand OR finger, each tendon**
26449   **Tenolysis, complex, extensor tendon, finger, including forearm, each tendon**

Tenolysis is performed to release the tendon from scar tissue resulting from trauma or a disease process and to restore hand or finger motion. In 26445, tenolysis is performed on a of a single extensor tendon in the hand or finger. An incision is made over the affected extensor tendon. Soft tissues are dissected and the tendon exposed in the hand or finger. Adhesions are lysed. Range of motion is evaluated. The surgical wound is closed in layers and a dressing is applied. Report 26445 for each extensor tendon in the hand or finger that is released from scar tissue. In 26449, a more complex tenolysis is performed on an extensor tendon in the finger. The extensor tendons for the fingers actually begin in the forearm and in this procedure the proximal aspect of the tendon in the forearm is also freed from scar tissue. An incision is made over the dorsal aspect of the affected finger. Soft tissues are dissected and the tendon exposed. Scar tissue is lysed. Range of motion is evaluated and it is determined that additional tenolysis is required on the proximal tendon segment in the forearm. An incision is made in the forearm. The tendon is exposed and adhesions in the forearm lysed. Range of motion is again evaluated. The surgical wounds in the finger and forearm are closed in layers. Report 26449 for each finger tendon treated by complex tenolysis.

26450-26455

26450   **Tenotomy, flexor, palm, open, each tendon**
26455   **Tenotomy, flexor, finger, open, each tendon**

An incision is made in the skin of the palm or finger overlying the flexor tendon. Soft tissues are dissected and the tendon is exposed. The tendon is then incised and severed or released. Bleeding is controlled with electrocautery. Following completion of the procedure, the operative wound is closed in layers. Report 26450 for each separate palmar flexor tendon on which a tenotomy is performed. Report 26455 for each separate finger flexor tendon on which a tenotomy is performed.

26460

26460   **Tenotomy, extensor, hand or finger, open, each tendon**

A dorsal incision is made in the skin of the hand or finger overlying the extensor tendon. Soft tissues are dissected and the tendon is exposed. The tendon is then incised and severed or released. Bleeding is controlled with electrocautery. Following completion of the procedure, the operative wound is closed in layers. Report 26460 for each separate hand or finger extensor tendon on which a tenotomy is performed.

26471-26474

26471   **Tenodesis; of proximal interphalangeal joint, each joint**
26474   **Tenodesis; of distal joint, each joint**

Tenodesis involves stabilizing a joint by anchoring the tendons that move the joint to surrounding structures. In 26471, tenodesis of the proximal interphalangeal (PIP) joint is performed to treat hyperextension deformity at the PIP joint. An incision is made over the flexor digitorum superficialis (FDS) tendon. One slip of the FDS tendon separated from the other and then divided 1.5-2.0 cm proximal to the PIP joint. With the finger held in slight flexion, the divided FDS slip is sutured to the flexor tendon sheath. Report 26471 for each joint treated with tenodesis. In 26474, tenodesis is performed on the distal interphalangeal (DIP) joint to treat loss of function of the flexor digitorum profundus (FDP). Loss of FDP function causes hyperextension of the DIP joint. The FDP tendon is divided. Strips of tendon are inserted into the tendon sheath using tendon weaving forceps and then the tendon strips are secured with sutures. The DIP is placed in 25-30 degrees of flexion and a Kirschner wire is passed through the distal phalanx and into the middle phalanx to maintain the appropriate level of flexion while the tenodesis site heals.

26476-26477

26476   Lengthening of tendon, extensor, hand or finger, each tendon
26477   Shortening of tendon, extensor, hand or finger, each tendon

An extension deformity in the hand or finger is corrected by lengthening or shortening one of the extensor tendons. Extension deformities may be due to late effects of injuries or due to disease processes such as severe rheumatoid arthritis or osteoarthritis. In 26476, the extensor tendon is lengthened. A skin incision is made over the tendon to be lengthened, soft tissues are dissected, and the tendon is exposed. A Z-shaped incision is made in the tendon which lengthens it by allowing the tendon fibers to slide apart as the wrist is flexed or extended. Tendon sutures are placed to maintain the tendon in the lengthened position. The hand or finger is immobilized in a splint or cast so that the desired length can be maintained until the tendon heals. In 26477, the extensor tendon is shortened. To shorten a tendon, the tendon is divided. The divided ends of the tendon are then overlapped and sutured together. The hand or finger is immobilized in a splint. These codes should be reported for each tendon that is lengthened or shortened.

26478-26479

26478   Lengthening of tendon, flexor, hand or finger, each tendon
26479   Shortening of tendon, flexor, hand or finger, each tendon

A flexion deformity in the hand or finger is corrected by lengthening or shortening one of the flexor tendons. Flexion deformities may be due to late effects of injuries or due to disease processes such as severe rheumatoid arthritis or osteoarthritis. In 26478, the flexor tendon is lengthened. A skin incision is made over the tendon to be lengthened, soft tissues are dissected, and the tendon is exposed. A Z-shaped incision is made in the tendon which lengthens it by allowing the tendon fibers to slide apart as the wrist is flexed or extended. Tendon sutures are placed to maintain the tendon in the lengthened position. The hand or finger is immobilized in a splint or cast so that the desired length can be maintained until the tendon heals. In 26479, the flexor tendon is shortened. To shorten a tendon, the tendon is divided. The divided ends of the tendon are then overlapped and sutured together. The hand or finger is immobilized in a splint. These codes should be reported for each tendon that is lengthened or shortened.

26480-26483

26480   Transfer or transplant of tendon, carpometacarpal area or dorsum of hand; without free graft, each tendon
26483   Transfer or transplant of tendon, carpometacarpal area or dorsum of hand; with free tendon graft (includes obtaining graft), each tendon

Tendon transplantation or transfer of a single tendon in the carpometacarpal region or dorsum of hand is performed to restore function usually resulting from a traumatic injury to the nerve, tendon or muscle. Less commonly the loss of function may be due to rheumatoid or gouty arthritis. The procedure varies depending on the function that the surgeon is trying to restore. To accomplish a tendon transplant or transfer, a longitudinal incision is made over the donor tendon and the tendon exposed. The donor tendon is freed from attachments in a manner that will allow it to be secured to the recipient site. This may include harvesting the tendon with a strip of periosteum. Muscle may also be freed from fascial attachments to allow maximum mobility and length for the tendon transfer. A second incision is made over the recipient site which is where the tendon will be attached. The donor tendon is then routed to the recipient site and secured with temporary sutures. A neuromuscular stimulator is used to test the donor tendon function. The tension of the donor tendon is adjusted as needed to ensure maximum function and then permanently secured at the recipient site. Following closure of the surgical wounds, the wrist and/ or hand is immobilized as needed. Use 26480 for each tendon that is transplanted or transferred without the use of a tendon graft. Use 26483 for each tendon requiring a tendon graft to achieve the desired length. If a tendon graft is needed, the tendon to be used for grafting is exposed and harvested. The tendon graft is anastomosed to the donor tendon and this is then attached to the recipient site.

26485-26489

26485   Transfer or transplant of tendon, palmar; without free tendon graft, each tendon
26489   Transfer or transplant of tendon, palmar; with free tendon graft (includes obtaining graft), each tendon

Tendon transplantation or transfer of a single tendon in the palm is performed to restore function usually resulting from a traumatic injury to the nerve, tendon or muscle. Less commonly the loss of function may be due to rheumatoid or gouty arthritis. The procedure

varies depending on the function that the surgeon is trying to restore. To accomplish a tendon transplant or transfer, a longitudinal incision is made over the donor tendon and the tendon exposed. The donor tendon is freed from attachments in a manner that will allow it to be secured to the recipient site. This may include harvesting the tendon with a strip of periosteum. Muscle may also be freed from fascial attachments to allow maximum mobility and length for the tendon transfer. A second incision is made over the recipient site which is where the tendon will be attached. The donor tendon is then routed to the recipient site and secured with temporary sutures. A neuromuscular stimulator is used to test the donor tendon function. The tension of the donor tendon is adjusted as needed to ensure maximum function and then permanently secured at the recipient site. Following closure of the surgical wounds, the wrist and/or hand is immobilized as needed. Use 26485 for each tendon that is transplanted or transferred without the use of a tendon graft. Use 26489 for each tendon requiring a tendon graft to achieve the desired length. If a tendon graft is needed, the tendon to be used for grafting is exposed and harvested. The tendon graft is anastomosed to the donor tendon and this is then attached to the recipient site.

26490-26496

26490   Opponensplasty; superficialis tendon transfer type, each tendon
26492   Opponensplasty; tendon transfer with graft (includes obtaining graft), each tendon
26494   Opponensplasty; hypothenar muscle transfer
26496   Opponensplasty; other methods

Opponensplasty is performed to restore thumb abduction in patients with median nerve damage. There are a number of techniques including transfer of the palmaris longus, superficialis, extensor indicis, extensor digiti minimi, flexor pollicis brevis, as well as others. In 26490, opponensplasty is performed by transfer of the superficialis tendon. This requires creation of a pulley using slips from the flexor carpi ulnaris and extensor carpi ulnaris tendons. An incision is made over the ulnar aspect of the wrist. The flexor carpi ulnaris tendon is exposed, dissected and split longitudinally. The medial slip is divided 4 cm proximal to its insertion on the pisiform bone. The insertion of the extensor carpi ulnaris is exposed. The proximal end of the cut slip of the flexor carpi ulnaris is sutured to the insertion of the extensor carpi ulnaris to create a pulley. The tendon of the superficialis is divided and passed under the remaining portion of the flexor carpi ulnaris and through the pulley. A subcutaneous tunnel is created and the two slips of the superficialis are pulled through. One slip of the superficialis is sutured to the distal part of the first metacarpal. The other is sutured to the insertion of the abductor pollicis brevis or the proximal phalanx. In 26492, a tendon graft is harvested from the forearm or leg and transplanted to muscles and tendons of the palm and thumb to restore abduction of the thumb. The flexor carpi ulnaris is then transferred and extended with the tendon graft. In 26494, the hypothenar muscles are transferred to restore thumb abduction. The hypothenar muscles are a group of three muscles in the palm that control motion of the little finger. The three muscles are the abductor digiti minimi, the flexor digiti minimi, and the opponens digiti minimi. These muscles are mobilized and transferred to muscles and tendons of the thumb to restore abduction. In 26496, opponsplasty is performed by a method other than superficialis transfer, tendon graft, or hypothenar muscle transfer, such as a palmaris longus (Camitz) transfer. An incision is made over the carpal tunnel. The distal palmaris longus is exposed and released along with a strip of palmar fascia. The palmar fascia is fashioned into a tube. A subcutaneous tunnel is created from the distal forearm to the radial aspect of the metacarpophalangeal joint of the thumb and the fascial tube passed through the tunnel and secured to the abductor pollicis brevis tendon. The tension of the transferred tendon is adjusted. Incisions are closed in layers and the thumb is immobilized in opposition with a splint.

26497-26499

26497   Transfer of tendon to restore intrinsic function; ring and small finger
26498   Transfer of tendon to restore intrinsic function; all 4 fingers
26499   Correction claw finger, other methods

Loss of intrinsic function in the fingers causes a condition known as claw hand or claw finger which is caused by an imbalance of the intrinsic and extrinsic muscles of the hand. In 26497, intrinsic function ring and little fingers is enhanced by transfer of the FDS tendon of the ring finger which substitutes for functions normally performed by the interosseous and lumbrical muscles of the ring and little fingers. Transfer of the FDS relieves some of the clawing and improves flexion at the metacarpophalangeal (MCP) joint. The FDS is detached from its insertion on the ring finger and split longitudinally. One half of the FDS is passed dorsally through the first interosseous muscle. The other half is passed volarly and tunneled to lumbrical muscle. In 26498, a similar procedure is performed on all four fingers. In 26499, claw finger is corrected by a method other than tendon transfer to lateral bands.

Musculoskeletal System

26500-26502

26500   Reconstruction of tendon pulley, each tendon; with local tissues (separate procedure)

26502   Reconstruction of tendon pulley, each tendon; with tendon or fascial graft (includes obtaining graft) (separate procedure)

The pulley system in the fingers is critical for finger flexion. The retinacular system for each finger contains 5 annular pulleys and 4 cruciate pulleys, while the thumb has 2 annular pulleys and 1 oblique pulley. In the finger, the second annular (A2) and fourth annular (A4) pulleys are the most critical. The oblique pulley is critical for the thumb. When a critical pulley is injured flexion is compromised unless the pulley is reconstructed using local or free tendon or fascial grafts. In 26500, local tissue such as the flexor digitorum superficialis (FDS) is used to reconstruct the pulley. The injured pulley is exposed and damaged tissue excised. A slip from the FDS or other tissue is harvested or rearranged and secured to the pulley remnant, passed through drill holes in the bone, or wrapped around the phalanx to reconstruct the pulley. Range of motion is checked and tension adjusted to ensure that the desired snugness is achieved. In 26502, a tendon or fascial graft is harvested, usually from the forearm or leg. A new pulley is constructed using techniques similar to those described above. The operative wound is closed in layers and the hand is placed in a bulky dressing and splint. These codes are reported once for each tendon requiring reconstruction of one or more pulleys.

26508

26508   Release of thenar muscle(s) (eg, thumb contracture)

The thenar muscles include the abductor pollicis brevis, flexor pollicis brevis, opponens pollicis, and adductor pollicis. These muscles originate from the flexor retinaculum and carpal bones and insert at the proximal phalanx of the thumb. Release of one or more of these muscles is performed to treat thumb contracture. An incision is made over the palm and proximal phalanx of the thumb. The thenar muscles are exposed and evaluated to determine which muscle(s) require release. The muscle(s) responsible for the contracture are then strategically cut to release the contracture. Range of motion is evaluated and additional release is performed as needed. The incision is closed in layers and the hand immobilized in a splint or cast.

26510

26510   Cross intrinsic transfer, each tendon

The muscles of the hand are divided into two groups, extrinsics and intrinsics. Extrinsic muscles are located in the forearm but have long tendons that extend across the wrist and insert into the hand and fingers. Intrinsic muscles are located totally within the hand and are divided into 4 groups, which include thenar, hypothenar, lumbrical, and interossei. The thenar group consists of four muscles that abduct, flex, and adduct the thumb. The hypothenar group consists of four muscles that move the small finger. The lumbrical muscles assist with flexion of the metacarpophalangeal joint and extension of the interphalangeal joints and also form the lateral bands with the interosseous muscles. The interosseous muscles consist of 3 volar and 4 dorsal muscles that originate in the metacarpals and form the lateral bands with the lumbricals. Crossed intrinsic transfer involves the interosseous muscles and is performed to treat ulnar drift caused by severe rheumatoid arthritis. The finger is incised and the interosseous muscle exposed. The interosseous tendon on the ulnar side of the finger is near the middle of the proximal phalanx and freed from the central and lateral slips. The interosseous muscle is then rerouted across the adjacent web space and attached to the radial extensor hood or anchored to the radial collateral ligament of the adjacent finger to provide radial stability. This procedure is typically performed on the second, third and fourth fingers and is reported for each interosseous tendon that is transferred.

26516-26518

26516   Capsulodesis, metacarpophalangeal joint; single digit

26517   Capsulodesis, metacarpophalangeal joint; 2 digits

26518   Capsulodesis, metacarpophalangeal joint; 3 or 4 digits

Capsulodesis is performed to correct a flexion or extension deformity in the metacarpophalangeal (MCP) joint of the finger. An incision is made over the affected MCP joint. The flexor pollicis longus is exposed and a portion of the tendon sheath excised. The tendon is retracted and the volar plate exposed. The volar plate is incised at its proximal and lateral attachments to divide the intrinsic muscles. Only the distal attachment is left intact. The finger is then positioned in a slightly flexed position to maximize function. The volar plate is placed in direct contact with the metacarpal neck. The bone is drilled and a Kirschner wire placed to hold the volar plate against the metacarpal bone and to maintain the finger in the desired position. Use 26516 for capsulodesis of a one finger, 26517 for two fingers, or 26518 for three or four fingers.

26520-26525

26520   Capsulectomy or capsulotomy; metacarpophalangeal joint, each joint

26525   Capsulectomy or capsulotomy; interphalangeal joint, each joint

Capsulectomy or capsulotomy is performed to relieve extension or flexion contracture in the metacarpophalangeal (MCP) or interphalangeal (IP) joint due to disease, burn, or other injury. In 26520 a contracture of the MCP joint is treated. For an extension contracture of the MCP joint, an incision is made over the dorsal aspect of the affected joint. The retinaculum is incised perpendicular to the common extensor in the direction of the fibers at the joint margin. The retinaculum is freed from the underlying collateral ligament and the joint capsule is incised. A portion of the joint capsule may also be excised to help relieve the contracture and to provide better range of motion. The volar recess is re-established. The joint is then positioned in flexion and a pin used to maintain the joint in this position. For a flexion contracture of the MCP joint, an incision is made over the volar aspect of the affected joint. Subcutaneous fibrous tissue and/or fascial bands are excised as needed. Neurovascular bundles are identified and protected. The lower portion of the collateral ligament along with the overlying retinaculum is then excised. The joint capsule is incised and a portion of the joint capsule excised as needed. Report for each MCP joint treated with capsulectomy or capsulotomy. In 26525, a contracture of the IP joint is treated. For a dorsal capsulotomy or capsulectomy, a curvilinear incision is made over the dorsal aspect of the affected IP joint. The ligaments on both sides of the joint are divided. The retinaculum is divided adjacent to the lateral bands. A portion of the collateral ligament is excised. The collateral ligament is freed from the joint margin. The joint capsule is incised and/or a portion excised as needed to improve range of motion. The volar recess is re-established, the retinaculum repaired and the joint pinned in the desired degree of flexion. For a flexion contracture, lateral incisions are made over both sides of the affected IP joint. The volar retinaculum is excised along with the attachment to the flexor sheath. The fibrous portion of the volar plate is incised and the flexor sheath divided. The joint is pinned in full extension. Report for each IP joint treated with capsulotomy or capsulectomy.

26530-26531

26530   Arthroplasty, metacarpophalangeal joint; each joint

26531   Arthroplasty, metacarpophalangeal joint; with prosthetic implant, each joint

An incision is made over the dorsal aspect of the metacarpophalangeal (MCP) joint. Soft tissues are dissected and the extensor tendons exposed taking care to protect superficial veins and nerves. In 26530, arthroplasty is performed without placement of a prosthetic joint implant. The joint capsule is exposed and incised. Diseased joint tissue and bone spurs are excised. The articular cartilage is smoothed. The joint is flushed with sterile saline to remove debris. The joint capsule is closed followed by overlying soft tissue and skin. Use 26530 for each MCP joint treated with arthroplasty alone. In 26531, the joint is replaced with a prosthetic implant. The extensor mechanism is separated from the joint capsule using blunt dissection. The sagittal band is released as needed. Intrinsic tendons are released and ligaments stripped off the proximal phalanx. The metacarpal head is excised. The joint capsule is elevated and stripped off the proximal phalanx. The bone ends are smoothed. The metacarpal and proximal phalanx bones are sized and the center of each bone drilled in preparation for insertion of the implant stems. A temporary replacement joint is placed to ensure that the correct size has been selected. Adjustments are made as needed until a good fit is achieved. The permanent implant is then inserted. The size, fit, and movement of the permanent implant are again checked before the implant is permanently seated in the joint. Overlying soft tissues and skin are closed in layers. Use 26531 for each joint treated with arthroplasty and prosthetic joint implantation.

26535-26536

26535   Arthroplasty, interphalangeal joint; each joint

26536   Arthroplasty, interphalangeal joint; with prosthetic implant, each joint

An incision is made over the dorsal or volar aspect of the interphalangeal (IP) joint. Soft tissues are dissected and tendons exposed taking care to protect blood vessels and nerves. In 26535, arthroplasty is performed without placement of a prosthetic joint implant. The joint capsule is exposed and incised. Diseased joint tissue and bone spurs are excised. The articular cartilage is smoothed. The joint is flushed with sterile saline to remove debris. The joint capsule is closed followed by overlying soft tissue and skin. Use 26535 for each IP joint treated with arthroplasty alone. In 26536, the joint is replaced with a prosthetic implant. Several types of implants are available, including interpositional, surface, and total joint types. The joint is exposed using either a dorsal or volar approach. The joint is debrided and bone spurs excised. Depending on which IP joint is being replaced, the head of either the proximal or middle phalanx is excised. The proximal and middle or middle and distal phalanges are sized and the center of each bone drilled in preparation for insertion of the implant stems. A temporary prosthetic joint is placed to ensure that the correct size has been selected. Adjustments are made as needed until a good fit is achieved. The permanent implant is then inserted. The size, fit, and movement of the permanent implant are again checked before the implant is permanently seated in the joint. Overlying soft tissues and skin are closed in layers. Use 26536 for each IP joint treated with arthroplasty and prosthetic joint implantation.

Musculoskeletal System

26540

26540   Repair of collateral ligament, metacarpophalangeal or interphalangeal joint

Repair of the collateral ligament of the metacarpophalangeal (MCP) or interphalangeal (IP) joint is typically performed to treat a traumatic injury such as a laceration or rupture. If an open wound is present it is explored, devitalized tissue debrided and any foreign material removed. If there is a closed injury an incision is made on the volar aspect of the affected joint. If the injury has occurred at the MCP joint, subcutaneous tissue and fascia is incised. Neurovascular bundles are identified and protected. The injured collateral ligament is exposed. If the ligament has been severed it is repaired with sutures. If the ligament has ruptured at its attachment to bone it is reattached with a pin or bone anchor. The overlying traumatic or surgical wound is then closed in layers. If the injury has occurred at the IP joint, a dorsal incision is made over the affected joint. The collateral ligament is exposed and repaired with sutures or reattached to the bone using a pin or bone anchor.

26541-26542

26541   Reconstruction, collateral ligament, metacarpophalangeal joint, single; with tendon or fascial graft (includes obtaining graft)

26542   Reconstruction, collateral ligament, metacarpophalangeal joint, single; with local tissue (eg, adductor advancement)

Reconstruction of the collateral ligament of the metacarpophalangeal (MCP) joint is typically performed to treat a traumatic injury such as a laceration or rupture. If an open wound is present it is explored, devitalized tissue debrided and any foreign material removed. If there is a closed injury, a volar incision is made over the affected MCP joint. The subcutaneous tissue and fascia is dissected. Neurovascular bundles are identified and protected. The injured collateral ligament is exposed and the extent of injury evaluated. In 26541, the collateral ligament is repaired with a tendon or fascial graft. The palmaris longus is the most commonly used tendon graft, but other tendons such as the extensor pollicis brevis, plantaris, a slip of the abductor pollicis longus or a portion of the flexor carpi radialis may be used instead. An incision is made over the tendon or fascial graft harvest site. The required length of tendon or fascia is excised. The graft is attached to remnants of the ligament or bony structures using sutures or bone anchors. Range of motion is evaluated and tension of the graft adjusted as needed. The wound is closed in layers. In 26542, the collateral ligament is repaired with local tissue using a technique such as adductor advancement. The adductor tendon is exposed and detached from the bone at the insertion site. The adductor tendon is then relocated distally to increase stability of the MCP joint.

26545

26545   Reconstruction, collateral ligament, interphalangeal joint, single, including graft, each joint

Reconstruction of the collateral ligament of the interphalangeal (IP) joint is typically performed to treat a traumatic injury such as a laceration or rupture. If an open wound is present it is explored, devitalized tissue debrided and any foreign material removed. If there is a closed injury, a dorsal incision is made over the affected IP joint. The injured collateral ligament is exposed and the extent injury evaluated. An incision is made over the tendon or fascial graft harvest site. The required length of tendon or fascia is excised. The graft is attached to remnants of the ligament or bony structures using sutures or bone anchors. Range of motion is evaluated and tension of the graft adjusted as needed. The wound is closed in layers.

26546

26546   Repair non-union, metacarpal or phalanx (includes obtaining bone graft with or without external or internal fixation)

When union of the fracture fragments does not occur after sufficient healing time has elapsed, the patient is considered to have a nonunion of the fracture. The original fracture site in the metacarpal or phalanx is exposed. The nonunion is evaluated to determine what type of repair is required which may include internal and/or external fixation without or with a bone graft. If a bone graft is used to fill the bone defect and encourage healing, the site of the nonunion is prepared for bone grafting. A bone autograft is harvested. A skin incision is made over the iliac crest or other site, and the muscle is stripped to reveal the bone surface. Cortical and/or cancellous bone is harvested. The bone is configured to the size and shape of the defect or cancellous bone is morcelized and packed into the defect. Internal fixation, such as a pin or wire is used as needed to secure the bone graft. Additional internal fixation devices may be used to stabilize the fracture or an external fixation device may be applied.

26548

26548   Repair and reconstruction, finger, volar plate, interphalangeal joint

Volar plate injury typically occurs due to combined hyperextension and longitudinal compression forces that cause avulsion of the volar plate. Lateral incisions are made over both sides of the affected IP joint. A portion of the collateral ligaments are excised. The joint capsule is incised. The finger is hyperextended to allow access to the articular surfaces of the IP joint. The volar recess is re-established by creating a groove in the volar rim. The volar plate is advanced to the surgically created groove. Drill holes are created in the phalanx and the volar plate is secured with sutures. The joint is placed in 20-30 degrees of flexion and Kirschner wires used to immobilize the joint.

26550

26550   Pollicization of a digit

Pollicization involves transfer of one of the fingers, usually the index finger, to the position of the thumb in a patient with traumatic amputation, congenital absence or hypoplasia of the thumb. An incision is made over the metacarpal bone of the metacarpal bone. Soft tissues are dissected taking care to preserve neurovascular structures. The midportion and base of the index finger metacarpal bone is excised while preserving the metacarpal head. The metacarpophalangeal joint of the index finger will function as the carpometacarpal joint of the new thumb and the metacarpal head will function as the trapezium bone. The index finger is then rotated into the thumb position. The lateral slips of the dorsal aponeurosis are mobilized. The two interossei muscles of the index finger are detached and fixed in a shortened position to the lateral slips on both sides of the new thumb. Rearrangement of the index finger interossei muscles improves function allowing full or nearly full opposition and abduction of the new thumb and creates the thenar eminence to give the new thumb a more cosmetically acceptable appearance. A dorsoradial skin flap is created and rotated to cover the gap between the newly created thumb and the middle finger.

26551

26551   Transfer, toe-to-hand with microvascular anastomosis; great toe wrap-around with bone graft

A great toe wrap around procedure involves a partial toe-to-hand transfer using only the nail and pulp of the great toe with or without a portion of the distal phalanx in the transfer. The bony structure of the great toe is left intact on the foot and covered with skin grafts. This procedure may be used for either traumatic or congenital absence of a digit, usually the thumb. The hand is prepared to receive the toe transfer. The recipient site is incised and any scar tissue excised. The bone stump is prepared. The tissues of the hand are dissected and extensor and flexor tendons and nerve ends are identified and isolated. Blood vessels are also located, isolated and prepared for anastomosis. Incision lines are outlined on the skin around the great toe. A dermal flap is elevated taking care to isolate and preserve the dorsalis pedis artery and a large subcutaneous dorsal vein in the foot for the microvascular anastomosis. Dissection of soft tissue around the toe continues until the nail and pulp are completely excised. A portion of the distal phalanx in the toe may also be included in the flap. The toe flap is transferred to the hand and blood vessels in the toe flap anastomosed to blood vessels in the hand. Nerves in the toe are also anastomosed to nerves in the hand. A bone autograft is harvested, usually from the iliac crest. A skin incision is made over the iliac crest and the muscle is stripped to reveal the bone surface. Bone is harvested and configured to the size and shape needed to reconstruct the bony portion of the finger. The bone graft is then attached to the bone stump in the hand and the soft tissue toe flap wrapped around the bone to construct a new thumb. Kirschner wires are used to hold the bone graft in place until osteosynthesis occurs. Full thickness skin grafts or flaps are used as needed to cover the great toe donor site.

26553-26554

26553   Transfer, toe-to-hand with microvascular anastomosis; other than great toe, single

26554   Transfer, toe-to-hand with microvascular anastomosis; other than great toe, double

A single or double toe-to-hand transfer using a toe other than the great toe is performed. The hand is prepared to receive the toe transfer. The recipient site is incised and any scar tissue excised. The bone stump is prepared. The tissues of the hand are dissected and extensor and flexor tendons and nerve ends are identified and isolated. Blood vessels are also located, isolated and prepared for anastomosis. Incision lines are outlined on the skin around the toe that will be transferred. A dermal flap is elevated taking care to isolate and preserve the dorsalis pedis artery and a large subcutaneous dorsal vein in the foot for the microvascular anastomosis. Dissection of soft tissue around the toe continues until bony structures are reached. The toe is then excised taking care to preserve the joint capsule and ligaments at the metarsophalangeal joint. The toe is transferred to the hand and blood vessels in the toe flap anastomosed to blood vessels in the hand. Nerves in the toe are also anastomosed to nerves in the hand. Ligaments and tendons are anastomosed and Kirschner wires are used to hold the bony structures in place until osteosynthesis occurs. Full thickness skin grafts or flaps are used as needed to cover the toe donor site. Use 26553 for a single toe-to-hand transfer. Use 26554 for a double toe-to-hand transfer.

26555

26555   Transfer, finger to another position without microvascular anastomosis

The physician moves a finger from one place to another on the hand without surgically connecting nerves, blood vessels, or other structures.

Musculoskeletal System

26556

26556   Transfer, free toe joint, with microvascular anastomosis

A free toe joint transfer is performed to reconstruct an injured finger joint. There are a number of techniques and the exact procedure depends on whether the joint transfer is performed on the metacarpophalangeal or proximal interphalangeal joint. The finger joint to be replaced is prepared by removing the joint structures while taking care to isolate and preserve blood vessels that supply the joint. A dorsal pedicle flap is developed at the toe joint to be transferred taking care to preserve the blood vessels. Joint structures are harvested keeping blood supply to the dorsal flap intact. The toe joint is transferred to the finger and blood vessels anastomosed. Overlying soft tissues are closed in layers. The transfered joint in the finger is immobilized with a Kirschner wire. The surgical wound in the toe is repaired and Kirschner wires used to stabilize the toe until osteosynthesis occurs.

26560-26562

26560   Repair of syndactyly (web finger) each web space; with skin flaps
26561   Repair of syndactyly (web finger) each web space; with skin flaps and grafts
26562   Repair of syndactyly (web finger) each web space; complex (eg, involving bone, nails)

Syndactaly is a condition in which two or more fingers in the hand are joined. Simple syndactyly involves only the soft tissues of the hand while complex syndactyly involves soft tissue and bone or cartilaginous tissue and/or the nail. In 26560, simple syndactyly is treated by division of the soft tissues and skin flap closure. Zigzag incisions are made over the dorsal and volar aspects of the conjoined fingers. Soft tissues are dissected and the interdigital connective tissue layer identified. Beginning distally the soft tissue is carefully separated taking care to preserve blood supply to both digits. Once the digits are completely separated, the skin flaps are defatted and used to close the zigzag incisions on both fingers. In 26561, simple syndactyly is treated with division of soft tissues and skin flap and graft closure. The procedure is performed as described above except that full thickness skin grafts are used in conjunction with skin flaps to allow complete closure of the zigzag incision. Full thickness skin grafts are harvested usually from the plantar instep and prepared for grafting. The skin grafts are configured to the necessary dimensions and used to help close the zigzag incisions. In 26562, complex syndactyly is treated. Zigzag incisions are made over the volar and dorsal aspects of the conjoined fingers. Soft tissues are dissected as described above. If the nails are joined they are split. The conjoined bony or cartilaginous tissue is carefully dissected taking care to preserve ligaments and tendons. Once the fingers are completely separated, lateral nail folds are created using two horizontal nail flaps or palmar pulp is defatted and advanced dorsally to create the lateral nail folds. The zigzag incisions are then closed using skin flaps and/or grafts.

26565-26567

26565   Osteotomy; metacarpal, each
26567   Osteotomy; phalanx of finger, each

An osteotomy of one of the metacarpal bones or phalanges is performed to correct a deformity or realign the bone. The location of the osteotomy and the type performed is dependent on the site and type of the deformity. Some commonly used osteotomies include transverse, wedge, sliding, right or left angle, V-osteotomy, and Z-osteotomy. Using separately reportable radiographic studies, the physician determines where the bone cut will be made to achieve the desired result prior to the start of the surgical procedure. An incision is made over the metacarpal or phalanx. Soft tissues are dissected and the bone is exposed. The periosteum is elevated. Using a drill, saw, and/or osteotome, the bone is cut in the previously determined configuration. Bone grafts are interposed between the cut bone segments as needed. Pins, screws, a plate and screw device, or other type of internal fixation is applied as needed to secure the cut edges in anatomical alignment. Alternatively, a separately reportable external fixation device may be applied. Use 26565 for osteotomy of a metacarpal bone. Report for each metacarpal bone treated with osteotomy. Use 26567 for an osteotomy of the phalanx. Report for each phalanx treated with osteotomy.

26568

26568   Osteoplasty, lengthening, metacarpal or phalanx

A plastic procedure is performed on the metacarpal or phalanx to lengthen the bone. Using separately reportable radiographic studies, the physician determines where the bone cuts will be made to achieve the desired result prior to the start of the surgical procedure. The metacarpal or phalanx is exposed. Cuts are made in the bone and the bone is distracted. A bone autograft is harvested, usually from the iliac crest. A skin incision is made over the iliac crest and the muscle is stripped to reveal the bone surface. Cortical and/or cancellous bone is harvested. The bone is configured to the desired size and shape and/or cancellous bone is morcelized and packed into the defect. Pins, screws, a plate and screw device, or other type of internal fixation is applied as needed to secure the cut edges in anatomical alignment. Alternatively, a separately reportable external fixation device may be applied.

26580

26580   Repair cleft hand

Cleft hand is a congenital anomaly in which the hand is missing part or all of one or more fingers in the center of the hand. This results in a central V-shaped gap or cleft in the hand. The extent of the anomaly varies. Cleft hand is treated surgically when function of the hand is significantly impaired. The surgical procedure performed depends on the exact nature of the anomaly. Cleft hand repair involves rearrangement of the skin and soft tissue to close the gap at the cleft site. Bones are stabilized or transferred and any deformities of the fingers or thumb are also corrected. One common technique is Snow procedure, which involves deepening the space between the thumb and index finger. Skin from the cleft site is transposed with its blood supply and used to cover the space between the thumb and index finger. The cleft is then closed in layers.

26587

26587   Reconstruction of polydactylous digit, soft tissue and bone

Polydactyly of the hand is a condition in which there are one or more extra digits. Polydactyly is classified as Type I if only soft tissue is involved, Type II if the digit includes bone and/or cartilage, or Type III if the complete digit and metacarpal are duplicated. Polydactyly is also classified as radial or pre-axial when there is an extra thumb, ulnar or postaxial when there is an extra small finger, and central when there is an extra digit in the central part of the hand. This procedure involves reconstruction of the duplicated digit. In pre-axial or post-axial, the duplicated or split thumb or small finger must be reconstructed to create a single digit. This involves excision of bone or cartilage with rearrangement of skin, soft tissue, tendons, joints and ligaments to reconstruct a single digit. Central polydactyly typically requires a more complex reconstruction of both the hand and the fingers.

26590

26590   Repair macrodactylia, each digit

Macrodactyly of the fingers is an overgrowth of bone and soft tissue including nerves, fat, and skin that causes abnormally large digit or digits. Surgery is performed to reduce the size of the enlarged digit which involves debulking the soft tissue and shortening the finger usually by excision of one of the phalanges or the metacarpal bone. The procedure may be performed in a staged fashion. To debulk the soft tissue, the thickened layers of skin are excised. Skin grafts are harvested from healthy tissue in the more proximal aspect of the digit or hand or from the plantar instep. The skin graft is then configured to cover the surgically created defect and secured with sutures. To shorten the finger, the affected digit is incised over the bone that is to be excised. Soft tissues are dissected and the bone exposed. The bone is detached from surrounding structures and excised. Soft tissues are excised and/or rearranged as needed to produce a cosmetically acceptable result.

26591-26593

26591   Repair, intrinsic muscles of hand, each muscle
26593   Release, intrinsic muscles of hand, each muscle

The muscles of the hand are divided into two groups, extrinsics and intrinsics. Extrinsic muscles are located forearm but have long tendons that extend across the wrist and insert into the hand and fingers. Intrinsic muscles are located totally within the hand and are divided into 4 groups, which include thenar, hypothenar, lumbrical, and interossei. The thenar group consists of four muscles that abduct, flex, and adduct the thumb. The hyopthenar group consists of four muscles that move the small finger. The lumbrical muscles assist with flexion of the metacarpophalangeal joint and extension the interphalangeal joints and also form the lateral bands with the interosseous muscles. The interosseous muscles consist of 3 volar and 4 dorsal muscles that originate in the metacarpals and form the lateral bands with the lumbricals. In 26591, the intrinsic muscles of the hand are repaired usually following a traumatic injury such as a laceration. If an open wound is present it is explored, devitalized tissue debrided and any foreign material removed. The intrinsic muscle is then repaired with sutures. Overlying soft tissues and skin are closed in layers. Report for each intrinsic muscle requiring repair. In 26593, intrinsic muscles of the hand are released. Release is performed to treat muscle imbalances, contractures caused by adhesions or scar tissue or other deformities in the hand. An incision is made over the muscle to be released. Soft tissues are dissected and the affected muscle is exposed. Any adhesions or scar tissue are excised. The muscle may be detached from bony attachments to treat an imbalance or contracture. Range of motion is checked to ensure that the abnormality is corrected. Once the desired result has been achieved overlying soft tissues are closed in layers. Report for each intrinsic muscle that is released.

26596

26596   Excision of constricting ring of finger, with multiple Z-plasties

Constriction ring syndrome is a congenital disorder caused by fibrous bands from the amniotic sac wrapping around the developing fetus. The fibrous bands can wrap around any part of the fetus but the fingers are one of the more common sites. These fibrous bands can cause swelling, cut off lymphatic or venous flow, and interfere with development of the

Musculoskeletal System

digit. A zigzag incision is made in the skin over the constricting ring. The constricting fibrous tissue is excised. The skin is rearranged to allow closure of the surgical defect.

26600-26607

26600   **Closed treatment of metacarpal fracture, single; without manipulation, each bone**

26605   **Closed treatment of metacarpal fracture, single; with manipulation, each bone**

26607   **Closed treatment of metacarpal fracture, with manipulation, with external fixation, each bone**

Closed treatment of a single metacarpal fracture is performed. If more than one metacarpal fracture is treated, treatment of each bone is reported separately. Separately reportable radiographs are obtained to confirm the fracture. A neurovascular exam is performed to ensure that the nerves and blood vessels at the site of the injury are intact. In 26600, a nondisplaced or minimally displaced fracture of a single metacarpal bone is evaluated. No manipulation of the fracture fragments is required. The hand is immobilized using a splint or cast. In 26605, a displaced fracture of a single metacarpal bone is treated with manipulation. The displaced fracture fragments are manually reduced (manipulated) back to proper anatomic alignment. Separately reportable radiographs are obtained to confirm anatomic reduction. A splint or cast is applied to immobilize the hand. In 26607, a displaced fracture of a single metacarpal bone is provisionally reduced as described in 26605. A small skin incision is then made on either side of the fracture site. Pin hole tracks are pre-drilled and two pins inserted, one proximal and one distal to the fracture site. The pins are provisionally connected to an external fixation bar. Traction is applied to the pins and the fracture fragments are further manipulated until adequate anatomic reduction is achieved. The pins are then fixed to the connecting bar. The hand is immobilized using a splint or cast.

26608

26608   **Percutaneous skeletal fixation of metacarpal fracture, each bone**

A small skin incision is made proximal to the fracture site in the metacarpal bone. A small drill is used to create a corticotomy proximal to the fracture site. The fracture is reduced and one or more pre-bent Kirschner wires are advanced by hand across the fracture site through the medullary canal. Anatomical reduction is verified radiographically.

26615

26615   **Open treatment of metacarpal fracture, single, includes internal fixation, when performed, each bone**

A dorsal (back of the hand) incision is made over the fractured metacarpal bone. The fracture site is exposed and cleared of any debris. The fracture is reduced and secured with internal fixation as needed. The type of internal fixation varies depending on the nature and site of the fracture. K wires, pins, mini-fragment screws, or a plate and screw device may be used. Anatomic alignment may be verified by fluoroscopy or x-ray. If open treatment of more than one metacarpal fracture is required, report 26615 for each bone treated.

26641

26641   **Closed treatment of carpometacarpal dislocation, thumb, with manipulation**

Closed treatment of a carpometacarpal (CMC) dislocation of the thumb is performed with manipulation. CMC dislocation of the thumb without concomitant fracture is rare due to the strength of the volar ligament. Separately reportable radiographs are obtained to evaluate the injury. The dislocation is manually reduced by combining thumb traction with metacarpal extension, pronation, and abduction. A second set of radiographs may be obtained to confirm anatomic alignment.

26645

26645   **Closed treatment of carpometacarpal fracture dislocation, thumb (Bennett fracture), with manipulation**

Closed treatment of a carpometacarpal fracture dislocation of the thumb, also called a Bennett fracture, is performed with manipulation. A Bennett fracture occurs at the base of the thumb with involvement of the articular surface of the metacarpal bone. Separately reportable radiographs are obtained to evaluate the injury. The fracture dislocation is manually reduced by combining thumb traction with metacarpal extension, pronation, and abduction. A second set of radiographs is obtained to confirm anatomic alignment. The thumb is immobilized in a thumb spica cast.

26650

26650   **Percutaneous skeletal fixation of carpometacarpal fracture dislocation, thumb (Bennett fracture), with manipulation**

A carpometacarpal fracture dislocation of the thumb is fixed by manipulation and percutaneous skeletal fixation. This is also called a Bennett fracture and occurs at the base of the thumb, characterized by involvement of the articular surface of the metacarpal bone often with significant displacement of fracture fragments. The fracture dislocation at the base of the thumb is reduced by combining thumb traction with metacarpal extension,

pronation, and abduction. Two K wires are then placed by drilling through the dorsal radial (thumb) metacarpal base into the reduced volar ulnar fragment, or for a very small fragment, a K wire may be placed from the thumb metacarpal into the trapezium or index metacarpal.

26665

26665   **Open treatment of carpometacarpal fracture dislocation, thumb (Bennett fracture), includes internal fixation, when performed**

A carpometacarpal fracture dislocation of the thumb, also called a Bennett fracture, is treated with open reduction. A Bennett fracture occurs at the base of the thumb and is characterized by involvement of the articular surface of the metacarpal bone, often with significant displacement of fracture fragments. An L-shaped incision is made over the skin and subcutaneous tissue of the thumb metacarpal and carried down to the thenar musculature, which is reflected off the subperiosteal tissue to allow direct visualization of the joint. The fracture site is cleared of debris. Towel-clip forceps are used to reduce the fracture and temporarily maintain alignment of the fragments. Alternatively, temporary wire fixation may be used to secure the fracture fragments prior to internal fixation, which is usually required. Either K wires or mini-fragment screws may be used.

26670-26675

26670   **Closed treatment of carpometacarpal dislocation, other than thumb, with manipulation, each joint; without anesthesia**

26675   **Closed treatment of carpometacarpal dislocation, other than thumb, with manipulation, each joint; requiring anesthesia**

Closed treatment of a carpometacarpal (CMC) dislocation other than the thumb is performed with manipulation. Separately reportable radiographs are obtained to evaluate the injury. The dislocation is manually reduced by using longitudinal traction with manual pressure on the base of the metacarpal. The finger may be immobilized with a splint. If more than one CMC dislocation requires closed treatment, each is reported separately. Use 26670 when the procedure is performed without anesthesia and 26675 when anesthesia is required.

26676

26676   **Percutaneous skeletal fixation of carpometacarpal dislocation, other than thumb, with manipulation, each joint**

A small skin incision is made over the metacarpal bone and a small drill is used to create a corticotomy. The dislocated carpometacarpal bones are reduced and returned to anatomical alignment. One or more pre-bent Kirschner wires are advanced by hand into the metacarpal medullary canal, across the carpometacarpal joint, and into the carpal bone. Anatomical reduction of the dislocation is verified radiographically. Report 26676 for each carpometacarpal joint dislocation treated by percutaneous fixation.

26685-26686

26685   **Open treatment of carpometacarpal dislocation, other than thumb; includes internal fixation, when performed, each joint**

26686   **Open treatment of carpometacarpal dislocation, other than thumb; complex, multiple, or delayed reduction**

A single carpometacarpal (CMC) dislocation other than the thumb is treated with open reduction. In 26685, a dorsal (back of the hand) incision is made over the dislocated carpometacarpal joint and the joint surface is exposed. Extensor tendons are retracted for better exposure. The joint capsule is opened and the dislocation is reduced. Internal fixation is applied as needed and typically wire fixation is used. The joint capsule is repaired and the wound is closed. If open treatment is done on more than one carpometacarpal joint, report 26685 for each joint treated. In 26686, a complex carpopmetacaral dislocation other than the thumb is treated by open reduction in the same manner as described above. Complex carpometacarpal dislocation includes those that have been dislocated multiple times and those with delayed treatment.

26700-26705

26700   **Closed treatment of metacarpophalangeal dislocation, single, with manipulation; without anesthesia**

26705   **Closed treatment of metacarpophalangeal dislocation, single, with manipulation; requiring anesthesia**

Metacarpophalangeal (MCP) dislocation results from hyperextension of the finger. Separately reportable radiographs are obtained to verify the injury. The dislocation is manually reduced by hyperextending the joint to 90 degrees and then pushing the base of the proximal phalanx into flexion. A second set of radiographs may be obtained to confirm reduction. The finger is then buddy-taped to an adjacent finger. If more than one MCP dislocation requires closed treatment, each is reported separately. Use 26700 when the procedure is performed without anesthesia and 26705 when anesthesia is required.

Musculoskeletal System

26706

26706 **Percutaneous skeletal fixation of metacarpophalangeal dislocation, single, with manipulation**

A small skin incision is made over the proximal phalanx and a small drill is used to create a corticotomy. The dislocated metacarpophalangeal bones are reduced and returned to anatomical alignment. One or more pre-bent Kirschner wires are advanced by hand into the phalangeal medullary canal, across the metacarpophalangeal joint, and into the metacarpal bone. Anatomical reduction of the dislocation is verified radiographically. Report 26706 for each metacarpophalangeal joint dislocation treated by percutaneous fixation.

26715

26715 **Open treatment of metacarpophalangeal dislocation, single, includes internal fixation, when performed**

A single metacarpophalangeal (MCP) dislocation is treated openly, including any necessary internal fixation. A dorsal (back of the hand) or volar (palm) incision is made over the dislocated metacarpophalangeal joint. If a volar incision is used, care is taken to avoid digital neurovascular bundles. Tendons and muscles are retracted, the volar plate is teased out of the joint, and the dislocation is reduced. Internal fixation is applied as needed and typically wire fixation is used. The wound is closed. If open treatment of more than one joint is required, report 26715 for each joint treated.

26720-26725

26720 **Closed treatment of phalangeal shaft fracture, proximal or middle phalanx, finger or thumb; without manipulation, each**
26725 **Closed treatment of phalangeal shaft fracture, proximal or middle phalanx, finger or thumb; with manipulation, with or without skin or skeletal traction, each**

Closed treatment of a single phalangeal shaft fracture of the proximal or middle phalanx of the finger or thumb is performed. If more than one fracture is treated, treatment of each bone is reported separately. Separately reportable radiographs are obtained to confirm the fracture. A neurovascular exam is performed to ensure that the nerves and blood vessels at the site of the injury are intact. In 26720, a nondisplaced single proximal or middle phalangeal shaft fracture is evaluated. No manipulation of the fracture fragments is required. The finger is immobilized using a splint. In 26725, a displaced single proximal or middle phalangeal shaft fracture is treated with manipulation with or without skin or skeletal traction. The displaced fracture fragments are manually reduced (manipulated) back to proper anatomic alignment. Separately reportable radiographs are obtained to confirm anatomic reduction. The finger is immobilized using a finger splint, skin traction splint or skeletal traction splint. Skin traction is applied if needed using a malleable plastic or metal splint and taping the finger to the splint to provide skin traction and maintain reduction of the fracture. Skeletal traction is applied if needed by placing a wire through the bone and attaching a rubber band to one end of the transosseous wire. The rubber band is then passed over a hoop and attached to the other end of the wire providing the skeletal traction required to maintain reduction of the fracture.

26727

26727 **Percutaneous skeletal fixation of unstable phalangeal shaft fracture, proximal or middle phalanx, finger or thumb, with manipulation, each**

A small skin incision is made proximal to the fracture site in the phalangeal shaft. A small drill is used to create a corticotomy proximal to the fracture site. The fracture is reduced and one or more pre-bent Kirschner wires are advanced by hand across the fracture site through the medullary canal. Anatomical reduction is verified radiographically. Report 26727 for each phalangeal shaft fracture treated by percutaneous fixation.

26735

26735 **Open treatment of phalangeal shaft fracture, proximal or middle phalanx, finger or thumb, includes internal fixation, when performed, each**

An incision is made over the fractured phalanx and overlying tissue is retracted. The periosteum is elevated and the fracture is identified. The fracture site is cleared of debris and then the fracture is reduced. Internal fixation is applied as needed. Pins, small screws, or a plate and screw device may be used to maintain alignment of the fracture fragments. If open treatment of more than one proximal or middle phalanx shaft fracture is required, report 26735 for each bone treated.

26740-26742

26740 **Closed treatment of articular fracture, involving metacarpophalangeal or interphalangeal joint; without manipulation, each**
26742 **Closed treatment of articular fracture, involving metacarpophalangeal or interphalangeal joint; with manipulation, each**

Closed treatment of an articular fracture involving the metacarpophalanageal or interphalangeal joint is performed. If more than one fracture is treated, treatment of each bone and/or each fracture site is reported separately. Separately reportable radiographs

are obtained to confirm the fracture. A neurovascular exam is performed to ensure that the nerves and blood vessels at the site of the injury are intact. In 26740, a nondisplaced metacarpophalangeal or interphalangeal joint fracture is evaluated. No manipulation of the fracture fragments is required. The finger is immobilized using a splint or buddy taping. In 26745, a displaced metacarpophalangeal or interphalangeal joint fracture is treated with manipulation. The displaced fracture fragments are manually reduced (manipulated) back to proper anatomic alignment. Separately reportable radiographs are obtained to confirm anatomic reduction. The finger is immobilized using a finger splint or buddy taping.

26746

26746 **Open treatment of articular fracture, involving metacarpophalangeal or interphalangeal joint, includes internal fixation, when performed, each**

Separately reportable radiographs are obtained to confirm the fracture. A neurovascular exam is performed to ensure that the nerves and blood vessels at the injury site are intact. An incision is made over the fracture site and overlying tissue is retracted. The joint capsule is incised; the fracture is exposed; and the fragments are reduced. Internal fixation such as a K-wire or pin is placed into the bone as needed to maintain the fragments in position. Separately reportable radiographs are obtained to confirm correct reduction and pin placement. The finger is immobilized using a finger splint. If more than one fracture is treated, each bone or fracture site is reported separately.

26750-26755

26750 **Closed treatment of distal phalangeal fracture, finger or thumb; without manipulation, each**
26755 **Closed treatment of distal phalangeal fracture, finger or thumb; with manipulation, each**

Closed treatment of a single distal phalangeal fracture of the finger or thumb is performed. If more than one fracture is treated, treatment of each bone is reported separately. Separately reportable radiographs are obtained to confirm the fracture. A neurovascular exam is performed to ensure that the nerves and blood vessels at the site of the injury are intact. In 26750, a nondisplaced distal phalangeal fracture is evaluated. No manipulation of the fracture fragments is required. The finger is immobilized using a splint. In 26755, a displaced single distal phalangeal fracture is treated with manipulation. The displaced fracture fragments are manually reduced (manipulated) back to proper anatomic alignment. Separately reportable radiographs are obtained to confirm anatomic reduction. The finger is immobilized using a finger splint.

26756

26756 **Percutaneous skeletal fixation of distal phalangeal fracture, finger or thumb, each**

Separately reportable radiographs are obtained to confirm the fracture. A neurovascular exam is performed to ensure that the nerves and blood vessels at the injury site are intact. The fracture is reduced and a wire or pin is placed through the skin to maintain the fracture fragments in anatomic alignment. Separately reportable radiographs are obtained to confirm proper reduction and pin placement. The finger is immobilized using a finger splint. If more than one fracture is treated, each one is reported separately.

26765

26765 **Open treatment of distal phalangeal fracture, finger or thumb, includes internal fixation, when performed, each**

An incision is made over the fractured phalanx and overlying tissue is retracted. The periosteum is elevated and the fracture is identified. The fracture site is cleared of debris and the fracture is reduced. Internal fixation is applied as needed. Pins, small screws, or a plate and screw device may be used to maintain alignment of the fracture fragments. If open treatment of more than one distal phalanx fracture is required, report 26765 for each bone treated.

26770-26775

26770 **Closed treatment of interphalangeal joint dislocation, single, with manipulation; without anesthesia**
26775 **Closed treatment of interphalangeal joint dislocation, single, with manipulation; requiring anesthesia**

Interphalangeal (IP) joint dislocation results from hyperextension or hyperflexion of the finger. Separately reportable radiographs are obtained to evaluate the injury. With the hand securely braced, the dislocation is manually reduced by grasping the dislocated phalanx and hyperextending the joint slightly for a dorsal dislocation or hyperflexing slightly for a volar dislocation. The dislocated phalanx is then gently pushed into normal anatomical position. Following reduction flexor-extensor function and range of motion are checked. The finger is immobilized in a splint. If more than one IP joint dislocation requires closed treatment, each is reported separately. Use 26770 when the procedure is performed without anesthesia and 26775 when anesthesia is required.

● New Code   ▲ Revised Code

26776

26776   **Percutaneous skeletal fixation of interphalangeal joint dislocation, single, with manipulation**

A small skin incision is made over the more distal phalanx and a small drill is used to create a corticotomy. The dislocated phalangeal bones are reduced and returned to anatomical alignment. One or more pre-bent Kirschner wires are advanced by hand into the phalangeal medullary canal, across the interphalangeal joint, and into the more proximal phalanx. Anatomical reduction of the dislocation is verified radiographically. Report 26776 for each interphalangeal joint dislocation treated by percutaneous fixation.

26785

26785   **Open treatment of interphalangeal joint dislocation, includes internal fixation, when performed, single**

A dislocated interphalangeal joint is reduced openly, with any necessary internal fixation. A curvilinear, dorsal (back of hand) incision is made over the interphalangeal joint and tissue is dissected down to the extensor mechanism. An incision is made between the lateral bands and the central slip. The lateral bands are retracted and the joint is reduced. The central slip is repaired. Internal fixation is applied as needed. A K wire is typically used for stabilization. The extensor mechanism is repaired and the skin is closed. If open treatment of more than one interphalangeal joint is required, report 26785 for each joint treated.

26820

26820   **Fusion in opposition, thumb, with autogenous graft (includes obtaining graft)**

Fusion of the thumb in opposition at the carpometacarpal joint is typically performed to treat arthritis or instability of the joint. Opposition moves the thumb into the palm toward the small finger. An incision is made on the lateral aspect of the thumb over the CMC joint. The joint capsule is incised and the joint surfaces inspected. The articular cartilage is excised from joint surfaces of the metacarpal base and trapezium. The trapezium is rounded and reshaped using a bur so that it will fit into the base of the metacarpal bone. A bone autograft is harvested, usually from the iliac crest. A skin incision is made over the iliac crest and the muscle is stripped to reveal the bone surface. Cortical and/or cancellous bone is harvested. The bone is configured to the size and shape of the defect or cancellous bone is morcelized and packed into the defect. Internal fixation, such as a pin or wire is used as needed to secure the bone graft and maintain the thumb in opposition until the joint has fused. Soft tissues are repaired in layers and a short arm cast is applied.

26841-26842

26841   **Arthrodesis, carpometacarpal joint, thumb, with or without internal fixation**
26842   **Arthrodesis, carpometacarpal joint, thumb, with or without internal fixation; with autograft (includes obtaining graft)**

Arthrodesis of the carpometacarpal joint of the thumb is typically performed to treat arthritis or instability of the joint. An incision is made on the lateral aspect of the thumb over the CMC joint. The joint capsule is incised and the joint surfaces inspected. The articular cartilage is excised from joint surfaces of the metacarpal base and trapezium. The trapezium is smoothed and reshaped using a bur so that it will fit into the base of the metacarpal bone. In 26841, internal fixation, such as a pin or wire is used as needed to maintain the thumb in the desired position until the joint has fused. Soft tissues are repaired in layers and a short arm cast is applied. In 26842, the joint is prepared as described above. A bone autograft is harvested, usually from the iliac crest. A skin incision is made over the iliac crest and the muscle is stripped to reveal the bone surface. Cortical and/or cancellous bone is harvested. The bone is configured to the size and shape of the defect or cancellous bone is morcelized and packed into the defect. Internal fixation, such as a pin or wire is used as needed to secure the bone graft and maintain the thumb in the desired position until the joint has fused. Soft tissues are repaired in layers and a short arm cast is applied.

26843-26844

26843   **Arthrodesis, carpometacarpal joint, digit, other than thumb, each**
26844   **Arthrodesis, carpometacarpal joint, digit, other than thumb, each; with autograft (includes obtaining graft)**

Arthrodesis of a carpometacarpal (CMC) joint other than the thumb is typically performed to treat arthritis or instability of the joint. An incision is made over the CMC joint. The joint capsule is incised and the joint surfaces inspected. The articular cartilage is excised from joint surfaces of the metacarpal base and carpal bone. The carpal is smoothed and reshaped using a bur so that it will fit into the base of the metacarpal bone. In 26843, internal fixation, such as a pin or wire is used as needed to maintain the CMC joint in the desired position until the joint has fused. Soft tissues are repaired in layers and a short arm cast is applied. In 26844, the joint is prepared as described above. A bone autograft is harvested, usually from the iliac crest. A skin incision is made over the iliac crest and the muscle is stripped to reveal the bone surface. Cortical and/or cancellous bone is harvested. The bone is configured to the size and shape of the defect or cancellous bone is morcelized and packed into the defect. Internal fixation, such as a pin or wire is used as

needed to secure the bone graft and maintain the CMC joint in the desired position until the joint has fused. Soft tissues are repaired in layers and a short arm cast is applied.

26850-26852

26850   **Arthrodesis, metacarpophalangeal joint, with or without internal fixation**
26852   **Arthrodesis, metacarpophalangeal joint, with or without internal fixation; with autograft (includes obtaining graft)**

Arthrodesis of a metacarpophalangeal (MCP) joint is typically performed to treat arthritis or instability of the joint. An incision is made over the MCP joint. The joint capsule is incised and the joint surfaces inspected. The articular cartilage is excised from joint surfaces of the metacarpal head and phalanx. The metacarpal is smoothed and reshaped using a bur so that it will fit into the base of the phalanx bone. In 26850, internal fixation, such as a pin or wire is used as needed to maintain the MCP joint in the desired position until the joint has fused. Soft tissues are repaired in layers and a short arm cast is applied. In 26852, the joint is prepared as described above. A bone autograft is harvested, usually from the iliac crest. A skin incision is made over the iliac crest and the muscle is stripped to reveal the bone surface. Cortical and/or cancellous bone is harvested. The bone is configured to the size and shape of the defect or cancellous bone is morcelized and packed into the defect. Internal fixation, such as a pin or wire is used as needed to secure the bone graft and maintain the MCP joint in the desired position until the joint has fused. Soft tissues are repaired in layers and a short arm cast is applied.

26860-26863

26860   **Arthrodesis, interphalangeal joint, with or without internal fixation**
26861   **Arthrodesis, interphalangeal joint, with or without internal fixation; each additional interphalangeal joint (List separately in addition to code for primary procedure)**
26862   **Arthrodesis, interphalangeal joint, with or without internal fixation; with autograft (includes obtaining graft)**
26863   **Arthrodesis, interphalangeal joint, with or without internal fixation; with autograft (includes obtaining graft), each additional joint (List separately in addition to code for primary procedure)**

Arthrodesis of an interphalangeal (IP) joint is typically performed to treat arthritis or instability of the joint. An incision is made over the IP joint. In 26860 and 26861, the joint capsule is incised and the joint surfaces inspected. The articular cartilage is excised from joint surfaces of the phalangeal bones. The articular surfaces of the bones are smoothed and reshaped using a bur so that they can be maintained in the desired position. Internal fixation, such as a pin or wire is used as needed to maintain the IP joint in the desired position until the joint has fused. Soft tissues are repaired in layers and a cast or splint is applied. Use 26860 for a fusion of the single IP joint. Use 26861 for fusion of each additional IP joint. In 26862 and 26863, arthrodesis of the IP joint is performed as described above, but a bone graft taken from the patient is also used to fuse the joint. A bone autograft is harvested, usually from the iliac crest. A skin incision is made over the iliac crest and the muscle is stripped to reveal the bone surface. Cortical and/or cancellous bone is harvested. The bone is configured to the size and shape of the defect or cancellous bone is morcelized and packed into the defect. Internal fixation, such as a pin or wire is used as needed to secure the bone graft and maintain the IP joint in the desired position until the joint has fused. Use 26862 for a fusion of the single IP joint with a bone autograft. Use 26863 for fusion of each additional IP joint with an autograft.

26910

26910   **Amputation, metacarpal, with finger or thumb (ray amputation), single, with or without interosseous transfer**

Occasionally an entire finger or the thumb must be amputated due to severe trauma, infection, or malignant tumor. This is also called a ray amputation and ray amputations generally involve excision of a portion of the metacarpal bone. A V-incision is made over the CMC joint and carried down over the distal aspect metacarpal bone of the injured finger or thumb. Soft tissues are dissected and the distal metacarpal bone exposed. Tendons are detached or divided and reattached as needed to the remaining metacarpal bone. Digital nerves are divided and the nerve end transferred to the interosseous space as needed to prevent neuroma formation. Blood vessels are suture ligated and divided. A small bone saw is used to cut the metacarpal bone at the desired level. Soft tissues are rearranged to cover the metacarpal bone and overlying soft tissues are closed in layers.

26951-26952

26951   **Amputation, finger or thumb, primary or secondary, any joint or phalanx, single, including neurectomies; with direct closure**
26952   **Amputation, finger or thumb, primary or secondary, any joint or phalanx, single, including neurectomies; with local advancement flaps (V-Y, hood)**

An amputation of all or part of the finger or thumb is performed due to severe trauma, infection, or malignant tumor. This procedure may be performed at the level of one of the interphalangeal or the metacarpophalangeal joint or it may be performed through one of the phalanges. A skin incision is made at the level where the amputation will be performed. Soft tissues are dissected and the IP or CMC joint or the phalanx exposed. Tendons are detached or divided and reattached as needed to the remaining bone. Digital nerves are longitudinally distracted distally and transected. This technique is referred to as a traction neurectomy. It allows the nerve end to retract proximally so that it is 1-1.5 cm from the end of the stump which minimizes the risk of neuroma formation. Blood vessels are suture ligated and divided or cauterized. If the amputation is performed at the joint, joint structures are dissected and finger is completed severed. Articular cartilage is not removed from the remaining bone as it provides a cushion for the underlying bone. If the amputation is performed through one of the phalanges, a small bone saw is used to cut the bone at the desired level. The bone end is smoothed using a rongeur or file. In 26951, the overlying soft tissues are closed in layers. In 26952, a local advancement flap is developed and used to cover the stump. Types of flaps used include fillet flap, volar V-Y flap, bilateral V-Y flap, homodigital island flaps.

26990-26991

26990   Incision and drainage, pelvis or hip joint area; deep abscess or hematoma
26991   Incision and drainage, pelvis or hip joint area; infected bursa

In 26990, an incision is made in the skin over the abscess or hematoma site. The incision is carried down through the soft tissue and the abscess or hematoma is opened. If drainage is performed for an abscess, any loculations are broken up using blunt finger dissection. If drainage is for a hematoma, blood clots are removed by suction. The abscess or hematoma cavity is flushed with saline or antibiotic solution. In 26991, an incision is made in the skin over the infected bursa. The infected bursa is opened with a scalpel and drained. The site is flushed with saline or antibiotic solution. Drains are placed as needed. The incision may be closed in layers or packed with gauze and left open.

26992

26992   Incision, bone cortex, pelvis and/or hip joint (eg, osteomyelitis or bone abscess)

The bone cortex of the one of the bones in the pelvis or hip joint, which includes the head or neck of the femur, is opened to treat a condition such as osteomyelitis or bone abscess. An incision is made in the skin and carried down through the soft tissue overlying the site of the infected bone. The periosteum over the infected region of the bone is elevated, a button of cortical bone removed, and the bone marrow exposed. Opening the bone cortex relieves pressure caused by inflammation of the bone marrow and prevents restriction of blood flow to the infected bone. If frank pus is encountered, the button hole may be enlarged and extended using a chisel or gouge along the bone for one to two inches. If the epiphysis is involved, a section of the epiphyseal cortex may be removed. The bone abscess is drained.

27000-27003

27000   Tenotomy, adductor of hip, percutaneous (separate procedure)
27001   Tenotomy, adductor of hip, open
27003   Tenotomy, adductor, subcutaneous, open, with obturator neurectomy

The hip adductor is located on the medial (inner) aspect of the hip joint. Adductor tenotomy may be performed for congenital hip dislocation or adduction contracture with subluxation of hip caused by spastic type cerebral palsy. In 27000, a percutaneous tenotomy is performed. Contrast material is injected into the hip joint and the position of the femoral head is evaluated. The adductor tendon is located and a stab incision is made over the tendon. The adductor tendon is incised. In 27001, an open adductor tenotomy is performed. A small skin incision is made in the medial aspect of the groin. The adductor tendon is exposed and incised. The femoral head is then positioned within the acetabulum. The patient is placed in a hip spica cast. In 27003, an open subcutaneous adductor tenotomy is performed with obturator neurectomy. The skin is incised and subcutaneous tissues are dissected. The adductor tendon is exposed and incised. The anterior branch of the obturator nerve is exposed and a portion of the nerve is excised. The femoral head is then positioned within the acetabulum and a hip spica cast is applied.

27005

27005   Tenotomy, hip flexor(s), open (separate procedure)

Tenotomy of hip flexors is performed to treat severe flexion deformities typically resulting from spastic paraplegia or spastic cerebral palsy. The flexion deformity is evaluated. Contracture of the iliopsoas muscle is often the cause of the flexion deformities. The skin over the iliopsoas tendon is incised and the iliopsoas muscle is exposed. A complete tenotomy is then performed at the lesser trochanter. The hamstring tendons may also be released for knee flexion deformity. This may include incision of the biceps femoris, semitendinosus, and/or semimembranosus tendons at the hip. The operative incisions are closed in layers. Casts or braces are applied as needed.

27006

27006   Tenotomy, abductors and/or extensor(s) of hip, open (separate procedure)

Tenotomy of hip extensors and/or abductors is performed to treat extension and/or abduction contracture in patients with spastic paraplegia or cerebral palsy. The extension and/or abduction deformity is evaluated. For an extension deformity, the skin over the

quadriceps muscle is incised at the hip. The rectus femoris, vastus lateralis, vastus medialis, and vastus intermedius tendons are exposed and tenotomies are performed as needed. For abduction contractures, the insertion sites of the gluteal muscles are exposed and tendons are released at the hip as needed to relieve the contracture. The operative incisions are closed in layers. Casts or braces are applied as needed.

27025

27025   Fasciotomy, hip or thigh, any type

Fascia is a layer of fibrous tissue that lies beneath the skin and envelopes underlying tissue. Fascia also surrounds muscles and separates groups of muscles from each other. Fasciotomy is performed to relieve tightness in the fascia that is causing pain or restricting motion in the hip or thigh. A skin incision is made over the planned fasciotomy site in the hip or thigh. The fascia is exposed and a series of incisions are made to relax the fascia. One common fasciotomy site is the fascia lata. The fascia lata is exposed from the region of the iliac spine to the greater trochanter. The fascia lata is then incised along its entire length as well as between the muscles.

27027

27027   Decompression fasciotomy(ies), pelvic (buttock) compartment(s) (eg, gluteus medius-minimus, gluteus maximus, iliopsoas, and/or tensor fascia lata muscle), unilateral

The physician performs a unilateral decompression fasciotomy in one or more of the four pelvic (buttock) muscle compartments, which include the gluteus medius-minimus, the gluteus maximus, the iliopsoas, and the tensor fascia lata muscle. Compartment syndrome of the pelvic compartments, while rare, does sometimes occur as a complication of trauma or injury to the pelvic ring. There are a number of approach options. A curved incision may be made parallel to the iliac crest, or a posterior incision may be employed from the iliac spine to the greater trochanter. A third option is a double curved incision from the iliac spine, over the greater trochanter and extended down to the gluteal fold. The incision is then carried medially beneath the buttocks and down to the mid-posterior thigh. The tensor fascia lata is exposed and incised. The muscle sheaths of the gluteal muscles and/or iliopsoas are then incised and decompressed as needed. Multiple incisions of the gluteal muscle sheaths may be required. The sciatic nerve may also be exposed and inspected to determine if there is any direct injury.

27030

27030   Arthrotomy, hip, with drainage (eg, infection)

A skin incision is made over the lateral aspect of the hip joint. Soft tissues are dissected and the joint capsule is opened. Fluid is drained from the joint and sent for separately reportable laboratory evaluation. The hip joint is examined for evidence of infection, inflammation, injury, or disease. A cannula is inserted and the joint is flushed with saline solution to remove purulent material or debris. Antibiotic or other solutions may also be instilled. The solutions are then drained from the joint. Upon completion of the arthrotomy, one or more drains may be placed in the hip joint and the incision is closed around the drains.

27033

27033   Arthrotomy, hip, including exploration or removal of loose or foreign body

Loose bodies within the hip joint result from trauma to the joint, which causes pieces of cartilage to become detached. These loose pieces of cartilage then float within the joint space and can become caught during hip movement, causing pain and reduced mobility. To remove the loose bodies, a skin incision is made over the lateral aspect of the hip joint. Soft tissues are dissected and the joint capsule is opened. The hip joint is examined for evidence of injury or disease. Loose or foreign bodies are located and removed. Upon completion of the procedure, the joint is flushed with sterile saline and the incision is closed.

27035

27035   Denervation, hip joint, intrapelvic or extrapelvic intra-articular branches of sciatic, femoral, or obturator nerves

The sciatic nerve arises from the sacral plexus in the pelvis, exits the pelvis at the greater sciatic foramen, and then extends through the thigh along the posterior compartment. The femoral and obturator nerves arise from the lumbar plexus. The femoral nerve traverses the pelvis and enters the thigh through the retroinguinal space beneath the inguinal ligament. The obturator nerve traverses the brim of the pelvis, enters the obturator canal, and extends into the thigh. These nerves can become trapped between the fascia, causing pain and limiting range of motion. An intrapelvic denervation is performed using an extraperitoneal approach. A skin incision is made in the right or left lower quadrant of the abdomen depending on which hip is affected. The external oblique muscle is divided above the inguinal ligament. The internal oblique and transverse abdominis muscles are split. The peritoneum and urinary bladder are retracted to permit exposure of the intrapelvic course of the sciatic, femoral, and/or obturator nerves. The affected nerve is then followed into the intra-articular region of the hip joint and divided, or a portion is destroyed. For an extrapelvic intra-articular denervation, the skin is incised over the lateral aspect of the hip and subcutaneous tissues are dissected. Dissection is carried into the articular region of the hip and the affected nerve is exposed. The nerve is then divided or a portion is destroyed.

27036

27036   Capsulectomy or capsulotomy, hip, with or without excision of heterotopic bone, with release of hip flexor muscles (ie, gluteus medius, gluteus minimus, tensor fascia latae, rectus femoris, sartorius, iliopsoas)

A skin incision is made over the lateral aspect of the hip from the proximal aspect of the greater trochanter to approximately 1 cm distal to the lesser trochanter. The fascia lata is incised longitudinally and the vastus lateralis is divided or retracted laterally. Capsular attachments at the tronchanteric ridge and/or vastus tubercle are exposed. Hip flexor muscles are incised and released as needed, which may include the gluteus minimus, gluteus medius, tensor fascia latae, rectus femoris, sartorius, and/or iliopsoas muscles. A capsulotomy or capsulectomy is then performed. To perform a capsulotomy, the hip joint capsule is incised in line with the neck of the femur to open the proximal aspect and then the incision is carried distally, beginning at the intertrochanteric ridge and creating a T-shaped incision into the joint capsule. To perform a capsulectomy, the joint capsule is opened in the same fashion and a portion of the joint capsule is then excised. If heterotopic ossification has occurred, any heterotopic bone that is impairing mobility or joint function is excised. Heterotopic ossification, also referred to as ectopic bone, refers to formation of new bone within or around a joint or at another site where bone would not normally form. Heterotopic bone formation in the hip joint can compromise range of motion and if severe enough, can affect the ability of the patient to walk or even sit. Heterotopic ossification may result from fracture or other trauma to the pelvis, hip joint, or femur; cerebral palsy or brain injury with significant spasticity; or brain injury with coma lasting longer than 2 weeks.

27040-27041

27040   Biopsy, soft tissue of pelvis and hip area; superficial
27041   Biopsy, soft tissue of pelvis and hip area; deep, subfascial or intramuscular

Soft tissues include muscles, tendons, fat, blood vessels, lymph vessels, nerves, and tissues surrounding the joints. Local, regional, or general anesthesia or conscious sedation is administered depending on the site and depth of the planned biopsy. The area over the planned biopsy site is cleansed. An incision is made and tissue dissected down to the mass or lesion taking care to protect blood vessels and nerves. A tissue sample is obtained and sent to the laboratory for separately reportable histological evaluation. The incision is closed with sutures. Use 27040 for a superficial biopsy or 27041 for biopsy of deeper tissues requiring more extensive dissection of overlying tissues, such as a biopsy below the muscle fascia (subfascial) or within the muscle itself (intramuscular).

27043-27048

27043   Excision, tumor, soft tissue of pelvis and hip area, subcutaneous; 3 cm or greater
27045   Excision, tumor, soft tissue of pelvis and hip area, subfascial (eg, intramuscular); 5 cm or greater
27047   Excision, tumor, soft tissue of pelvis and hip area, subcutaneous; less than 3 cm
27048   Excision, tumor, soft tissue of pelvis and hip area, subfascial (eg, intramuscular); less than 5 cm

Soft tissues include subcutaneous fat and connective tissue, fascia, muscles, tendons, blood vessels, lymph vessels, nerves, and tissues surrounding the joints. Soft tissue tumors may be benign or malignant. Benign tumors are typically treated by excision, although small malignant or indeterminate tumors may be excised if the margins are well defined. Depending on the location of the tumor in the soft tissue of the pelvis and hip area, the skin over the tumor may be incised or a skin flap created and elevated. Overlying tissue is dissected and the soft tissue mass exposed. The tumor is then excised along with a margin of healthy tissue. Separately reportable frozen section may be performed to ensure that all margins are free of tumor cells. Drains are placed as needed and the surgical wound is closed in layers. For tumors in the subcutaneous fat or connective tissue, use 27047 for excision of less than 3 cm and 27043 for excision of 3 cm or greater. For tumors that lie below the fascia, use 27048 for excision of less than 5 cm and 27045 for excision of 5 cm or greater. Subfascial soft tissue tumors include those within muscle tissue.

27049

27049   Radical resection of tumor (eg, sarcoma), soft tissue of pelvis and hip area; less than 5 cm

Soft tissues include muscles, tendons, fat, blood vessels, lymph vessels, nerves, and tissues surrounding the joints. Soft tissue tumors may be benign or malignant. Radical resection is typically performed for a malignant neoplasm, such as a sarcoma, although benign tumors and tumors of indeterminate nature may also require radical resection. A skin incision is made over the tumor in the pelvis and hip area, or a skin flap is created and elevated. Overlying tissue is dissected and the tumor exposed. The tumor is removed en bloc along

with a wide margin of surrounding tissue. Radical resection involves excision of all involved soft tissue which may include muscles, nerves, and blood vessels. Separately reportable frozen section is performed to ensure that all margins are free of tumor cells. If margins show evidence of malignancy, additional tissue is removed until all margins are free of tumor cells. Drains are placed as needed. The surgical wound may be closed in layers, or separately reportable reconstructive procedures performed. Use 27049 for radical resection of soft tissue tumor less than 5 cm in the pelvis and hip.

27050-27052

27050   Arthrotomy, with biopsy; sacroiliac joint
27052   Arthrotomy, with biopsy; hip joint

Tissue samples are obtained to evaluate conditions such as pain, inflammatory disease, infection, lesions, or tumors. In 27050, the sacroiliac joint (SIJ) is approached via a skin incision in the lower back over the right or left SIJ. Soft tissues are divided and the joint is exposed. In 27052, a skin incision is made over the lateral aspect of the hip joint; soft tissues are divided; and the joint capsule is opened. The bone and joint surfaces of the SI or hip joint are examined and any abnormalities are noted. Biopsies are then obtained as needed of lesions, synovial tissue, cartilage, and/or bone. The tissue samples are sent for separately reportable laboratory analysis. Upon completion of the biopsy, the SI or hip joint is flushed with saline solution and the operative wound is closed in layers.

27054

27054   Arthrotomy with synovectomy, hip joint

Synovectomy is performed to remove inflamed synovial tissue. A skin incision is made over the lateral aspect of the hip joint; soft tissues are dissected; and the joint capsule is opened. The hip joint is examined for evidence of injury or disease. The inflamed synovial tissue is removed using a synovial resector. Upon completion of the procedure, the joint is flushed with sterile saline and the incisions are closed.

27057

27057   Decompression fasciotomy(ies), pelvic (buttock) compartment(s) (eg, gluteus medius-minimus, gluteus maximus, iliopsoas, and/or tensor fascia lata muscle) with debridement of nonviable muscle, unilateral

The physician performs a unilateral decompression fasciotomy in one or more of the four pelvic (buttock) compartments with debridement of nonviable muscle. These compartments include the gluteus medius-minimus, the gluteus maximus, the iliopsoas, and the tensor fascia lata muscle. Compartment syndrome of the pelvic compartments, while rare, does sometimes occur as a complication of trauma or injury to the pelvic ring. There are a number of approach options. A curved incision may be made parallel to the iliac crest, or a posterior incision may be employed from the iliac spine to the greater trochanter. A third option is a double curved incision from the iliac spine, over the greater trochanter and extended down to the gluteal fold. The incision is then carried medially beneath the buttocks and down to the mid-posterior thigh. The tensor fascia lata is exposed and incised. The muscle sheaths of the gluteal muscles and/or iliopsoas are then incised and decompressed as needed. Multiple incisions of the gluteal muscle sheaths may be required. The exposed muscle tissue is evaluated and nonviable tissue is excised. Care is taken to preserve as much viable tissue as possible, excising muscle only until capillary bleeding is noted. The sciatic nerve may also be exposed and inspected to determine if there is any direct injury to it.

27059

27059   Radical resection of tumor (eg, sarcoma), soft tissue of pelvis and hip area; 5 cm or greater

Soft tissues include muscles, tendons, fat, blood vessels, lymph vessels, nerves, and tissues surrounding the joints. Soft tissue tumors may be benign or malignant. Radical resection is typically performed for a malignant neoplasm, such as a sarcoma, although benign tumors and tumors of indeterminate nature may also require radical resection. A skin incision is made over the tumor in the pelvis and hip area, or a skin flap is created and elevated. Overlying tissue is dissected and the tumor exposed. The tumor is removed en bloc along with a wide margin of surrounding tissue. Radical resection involves excision of all involved soft tissue which may include muscles, nerves, and blood vessels. Separately reportable frozen section is performed to ensure that all margins are free of tumor cells. If margins show evidence of malignancy, additional tissue is removed until all margins are free of tumor cells. Drains are placed as needed. The surgical wound may be closed in layers, or separately reportable reconstructive procedures performed. Use 27059 for radical resection of soft tissue tumor 5 cm or greater in the pelvis and hip.

27060-27062

27060   Excision; ischial bursa
27062   Excision; trochanteric bursa or calcification

Bursae are fluid filled sacs that protect bony prominences and joints. In 27060, the ischial bursa, a fluid filled sac over the ischial tuberosity, is excised. Injury to the bursa typically results from a blow to the ischial tuberosity. This can result in inflammation, scarring, and

CPT © 2016 American Medical Association. All Rights Reserved.

Musculoskeletal System

bone spur formation. The skin over the ischial bursa is incised and the bursa is exposed. The bursa is dissected from surrounding tissue and excised. The ischial tuberosity is inspected and bone spurs are removed as needed. In 27062, the trochanteric bursa, located over the greater trochanter, is excised. Trochanteric bursitis may result from muscle imbalances, leg length discrepancies, overtraining, or hyperpronation of the foot. The skin over the greater trochanter is incised and the bursa is exposed. The bursa is dissected from surrounding tissue and excised. Bone spurs are removed as needed.

27065-27067

27065 Excision of bone cyst or benign tumor, wing of ilium, symphysis pubis, or greater trochanter of femur; superficial, includes autograft, when performed

27066 Excision of bone cyst or benign tumor, wing of ilium, symphysis pubis, or greater trochanter of femur; deep (subfascial), includes autograft, when performed

27067 Excision of bone cyst or benign tumor, wing of ilium, symphysis pubis, or greater trochanter of femur; with autograft requiring separate incision

A bone cyst is a fluid-filled space within bone. One common type of bone cyst is a unicameral or simple bone cyst, which is a benign lesion. A less common type is an aneurysmal bone cyst which consists of vascular tissue surrounding a blood filled cystic lesion. There are a number of different types of benign bone tumors including giant cell tumors, chondromixoid fibromas, and enchondromas. In 27065, a superficial bone cyst or benign tumor is excised from the pelvis or proximal femur. Superficial lesions are those in the wing of the ilium, symphysis pubis, or greater tronchanter of the femur. An incision is made in the skin over the site of the lesion. Soft tissues are dissected and the lesion is exposed. If a cystic lesion is present, the bone is incised and a bone window is created to open the cyst. Fluid is aspirated and sent to the laboratory for separately reportable analysis. A curette is inserted through the bone window and the lining of the cystic cavity is completely removed by curettage. Alternatively, some cystic lesions and most benign tumors are treated by excision. The lesion is exposed as described above. The physician then excises the benign lesion along with a margin of surrounding healthy bone. The resulting bony defect may be left open or the physician may pack the defect with a bone autograft. If a bone autograft is used, local healthy bone is excised through the same incision and packed into the defect. In 27066, a deep bone cyst or benign tumor of the pelvis or proximal femur is treated as described above. Deeper bony structures require additional soft tissue dissection to expose and remove the lesion. The resulting bony defect may be left open or the physician may pack the defect with a bone autograft obtained through the same incision. In 27067, a deep bone cyst or benign tumor is excised as described above and the defect is packed with a bone autograft obtained from a separate site requiring a separate incision.

27070-27071

27070 Partial excision, wing of ilium, symphysis pubis, or greater trochanter of femur, (craterization, saucerization) (eg, osteomyelitis or bone abscess); superficial

27071 Partial excision, wing of ilium, symphysis pubis, or greater trochanter of femur, (craterization, saucerization) (eg, osteomyelitis or bone abscess); deep (subfascial or intramuscular)

The physician performs a partial excision of bone, also referred to as craterization or saucerization, to treat osteomyelitis or bone abscess of the pelvis and hip joint. Craterization or saucerization of bone involves removing infected and necrotic bone to form a shallow depression in the bone surface that will allow drainage from the infected area. An incision is made in the skin and carried down through the soft tissue overlying the site of the osteomyelitis or bone abscess. Any soft tissue sinus tracts and devitalized soft tissue are resected. The area of necrotic and infected bone is exposed. A series of drill holes are made in the necrotic and infected bone and the bone between the drill holes is excavated to create an oval window using an osteotome. The amount of bone removed is dependent on the extent of the infection. A curette may be used to remove devitalized tissue from the medullary canal. Debridement continues until punctate bleeding is identified in the exposed bony surface. When all devitalized and infected tissue has been removed, the wound is copiously irrigated with sterile saline or antibiotic solution. The surgical wound is loosely closed and a drain placed. Use code 27070 for partial excision of superficial osteomyelitis or bone abscess such as that located in the wing of the ilium, symphysis pubis, or greater trochanter and code 27071 for deep subfascial or submuscular bone of the pelvis and hip joint.

27075

27075 Radical resection of tumor; wing of ilium, 1 pubic or ischial ramus or symphysis pubis

Radical resection is typically performed for a malignant neoplasm although benign tumors and tumors of indeterminate nature may also require radical resection. A skin incision is made over the site of the bone tumor, or a skin flap is created and elevated. Overlying tissue is dissected and the tumor exposed. All bone and cartilage with tumor involvement in the wing of the ilium, a single pubic or ischial ramus, or the symphysis pubis is resected.

The tumor is removed en bloc along with a wide margin of surrounding tissue. Radical resection of bone includes excision of all involved soft tissue which may include muscles, tendons, fat, blood vessels, lymph vessels, nerves, and tissues surrounding the joints. Separately reportable frozen section is performed to ensure that all margins are free of tumor cells. If margins show evidence of malignancy, additional tissue is removed until all margins are free of tumor cells. Drains are placed as needed. The surgical wound may be closed in layers, or separately reportable reconstructive procedures performed.

27076

27076 Radical resection of tumor; ilium, including acetabulum, both pubic rami, or ischium and acetabulum

Radical resection is typically performed for a malignant neoplasm although benign tumors and tumors of indeterminate nature may also require radical resection. A skin incision is made over the site of the bone tumor, or a skin flap is created and elevated. Overlying tissue is dissected and the tumor exposed. All bone and cartilage with tumor involvement in the ilium, both pubic rami, or the ischium and acetabulum is resected. The tumor is removed en bloc along with a wide margin of surrounding tissue. Radical resection of bone includes excision of all involved soft tissue which may include muscles, tendons, fat, blood vessels, lymph vessels, nerves, and tissues surrounding the joints. Separately reportable frozen section is performed to ensure that all margins are free of tumor cells. If margins show evidence of malignancy, additional tissue is removed until all margins are free of tumor cells. Drains are placed as needed. The surgical wound may be closed in layers, or separately reportable reconstructive procedures performed.

27077

27077 Radical resection of tumor; innominate bone, total

Radical resection is typically performed for a malignant neoplasm although benign tumors and tumors of indeterminate nature may also require radical resection. A skin incision is made over the site of the bone tumor, or a skin flap is created and elevated. Overlying tissue is dissected and the tumor exposed. The total innominate bone is resected. The tumor is removed en bloc along with a wide margin of surrounding tissue. Radical resection of bone includes excision of all involved soft tissue which may include muscles, tendons, fat, blood vessels, lymph vessels, nerves, and tissues surrounding the joints. Separately reportable frozen section is performed to ensure that all margins are free of tumor cells. If margins show evidence of malignancy, additional tissue is removed until all margins are free of tumor cells. Drains are placed as needed. The surgical wound may be closed in layers, or separately reportable reconstructive procedures performed.

27078

27078 Radical resection of tumor; ischial tuberosity and greater trochanter of femur

Radical resection is typically performed for a malignant neoplasm although benign tumors and tumors of indeterminate nature may also require radical resection. A skin incision is made over the site of the bone tumor, or a skin flap is created and elevated. Overlying tissue is dissected and the tumor exposed. All bone and cartilage with tumor involvement in the ischial tuberosity or greater trochanter of the femur is resected. The tumor is removed en bloc along with a wide margin of surrounding tissue. Radical resection of bone includes excision of all involved soft tissue which may include muscles, tendons, fat, blood vessels, lymph vessels, nerves, and tissues surrounding the joints. Separately reportable frozen section is performed to ensure that all margins are free of tumor cells. If margins show evidence of malignancy, additional tissue is removed until all margins are free of tumor cells. Drains are placed as needed. The surgical wound may be closed in layers, or separately reportable reconstructive procedures performed.

27080

27080 Coccygectomy, primary

Coccygectomy is performed to treat chronic pain and instability usually resulting from old trauma to the coccyx. The patient is placed in the jack-knife position. A skin incision is made medially beginning just proximal to the sacrococcygeal joint and is carried down over the coccyx to the crease in the buttocks. Soft tissues are dissected and the coccyx is exposed. The distal tip of the coccyx is then elevated and dissected free of tissues around the anus. Blunt dissection is used to separate underlying tissues from the distal tip of the coccyx to the sacrococcygeal joint. The coccyx is then excised. Rough edges at the tip of the sacrum are smoothed using a file. Overlying tissue is then closed in layers.

27086-27087

27086 Removal of foreign body, pelvis or hip; subcutaneous tissue
27087 Removal of foreign body, pelvis or hip; deep (subfascial or intramuscular)

Subcutaneous tissue refers to the fat and connective tissue that lies between the overlying dermis and underlying muscle fascia. Deep tissue refers to the tissue below the muscle fascia (subfascial) or within the muscle itself (intramuscular). The foreign body is located by palpation or separately reportable radiographs. A straight or elliptical incision is made in the skin. In 27086, the subcutaneous tissue is dissected and the foreign body identified.

Musculoskeletal System

A hemostat or grasping forceps is then used to remove the foreign body. Alternatively, the physician may need to dissect tissues around the foreign body to remove it. The wound is then flushed with normal saline or antiobiotic solution and the incision is closed. In 27087 dissection is carried into the deeper subfascial or intramuscular tissue and the foreign body identified and removed.

27090-27091

27090   Removal of hip prosthesis; (separate procedure)
27091   Removal of hip prosthesis; complicated, including total hip prosthesis, methylmethacrylate with or without insertion of spacer

The skin is incised over the old incision line along the lateral aspect of the hip and soft tissue is dissected to reach a previously implanted hip prosthesis. Extensive soft tissue release resulting from scar tissue formation may be required, including partial release of the psoas tendon, partial release of the gluteus maximus insertion, or release of the head of the rectus femoris. The hip is dislocated and the femoral head or femoral head prosthesis is exposed. To remove the acetabular component, the entire pseudocapsule is excised and the acetabular cup is removed. To remove the femoral component, any trochanteric overhang is removed using a high speed burr. Alternatively, a trochanteric osteotomy may be performed. The proximal aspect of the femoral stem is cleared of any visible bone cement or bony overgrowth. Depending on the type of prosthesis, the femoral component may be removed easily using traction or removal may require severing of fibrous or bony ingrowth into the prosthesis using flexible osteotomies or a small burr. Once the femoral component has been sufficiently loosened, it is extracted. The surgical sites are flushed with saline and/or antibiotic solution. Use 27090 for an uncomplicated removal of a hip prosthesis. Use 27091 for a complicated removal, which includes removal of both components of a total hip prosthesis, removal of bone cement (methylmethacrylate), and placement of a spacer when needed. A spacer is typically used when the hip joint has become infected, preventing immediate replacement of the total hip prosthesis.

27093-27095

27093   Injection procedure for hip arthrography; without anesthesia
27095   Injection procedure for hip arthrography; with anesthesia

The skin over the injection site is cleansed and a local anesthetic injected. A needle may be inserted into the joint and fluid aspirated with a syringe. The radiopaque substance is then injected into the hip joint. The joint is exercised to help distribute the radiopaque substance. Once the radiopaque substance has been distributed throughout the joint, separately reportable radiographs are obtained. Use code 27093 if the procedure is performed without anesthesia; use 27095 if anesthesia is used.

27096

27096   Injection procedure for sacroiliac joint, anesthetic/steroid, with image guidance (fluoroscopy or CT) including arthrography when performed

Injection of an anesthetic or steroid into the sacroiliac joint is performed with the use of fluoroscopic or CT guidance and joint arthrography as needed. The skin over the injection site is cleansed and a local anesthetic is injected. Using continuous fluoroscopic or CT guidance, a needle is inserted into the joint and fluid is aspirated as needed. If arthrography is performed, a radiopaque substance is injected into the sacroiliac joint. Once the radiopaque substance has been distributed throughout the joint, separately reportable radiographic images are obtained. An anesthetic or steroid injection is then administered.

27097

27097   Release or recession, hamstring, proximal

Proximal release or recession of the hamstring is performed to treat flexion deformity of the knee in patients with conditions such as cerebral palsy. An incision is made in the gluteal crease over the ischial tuberosity. The gluteus maximus muscle is identified and retracted. The hamstring origins are exposed. The sciatic nerve is identified and protected. The hamstring origins are released from the ischial tuberosity and allowed to slide distally. Bleeding is controlled and the incision is closed in layers. A long leg cast is applied to maintain extension of the knee.

27098

27098   Transfer, adductor to ischium

The adductor longus and brevis are located on the medial (inner) aspect of the hip joint. Transfer of the hip adductors to the ischium may be performed to treat adduction contracture with subluxation of hip caused by spastic type cerebral palsy. A skin incision is made in the medial aspect of the groin. The adductor longus tendon is exposed, divided, and transferred posteriorly to the ischial tuberosity. The adductor brevis may also be divided and/or transferred using the same technique.

27100

27100   Transfer external oblique muscle to greater trochanter including fascial or tendon extension (graft)

Transfer of the external oblique muscle to the greater trochanter is performed to improve abduction of the hip in patients with abductor paralysis. A long oblique skin incision is made from the pubic spine over the iliac crest and up to the costal margin in the posterior axillary line. The aponeurosis of the external oblique muscle is incised parallel to Poupart's ligament and the incision is carried down to the pubis. A second incision is made approximately 2 cm from and parallel to the first incision. These incisions are joined at the pubis. Another incision is carried superiorly along the medial border of the belly of the external oblique muscle to free the muscle fibers from the aponeurosis. The inferior incision is extended laterally to the anterior superior spine of the ilium. The external oblique muscle is then divided at its insertion on the iliac crest. The muscle belly is freed from underlying structures using blunt dissection. The cut edge of the external oblique muscle is folded under and sutured to itself. The gap in the aponeurosis is closed with sutures from the pubis as far laterally as possible. A lateral incision is then made over the greater tronchanter. The fascia and periosteum are incised in two places and two drill holes are made in the greater trochanter. A subcutaneous tunnel is created from the greater trochanter to the lower abdomen. The fascial tendon which has been configured using the aponeurosis of the external oblique muscle is passed through the tunnel to the greater trochanter. The hip is placed in wide abduction and the fascial tendon is passed through the drill holes and secured with sutures. The incisions are closed in layers and a spica cast is applied to maintain the hip in wide abduction.

27105

27105   Transfer paraspinal muscle to hip (includes fascial or tendon extension graft)

The paraspinal muscles are deep muscles along the spine that include the longissimus, iliocostalis, and spinalis. The origin of the paraspinal muscles is from the spinous processes and the iliac crest. The insertion is at the posteromedial aspect of the ribs. To transfer a paraspinal muscle to the hip, the thoracolumbar fascia is incised medially and the serratus posterior inferior muscles are elevated. The paraspinal muscle to be transferred is released from its origin and freed from surrounding tissue. The hip is exposed and the paraspinal muscle is transferred to the hip. A fascial or tendon extension graft may be created to provide the necessary length for attachment to the hip. Incisions are closed in layers.

27110-27111

27110   Transfer iliopsoas; to greater trochanter of femur
27111   Transfer iliopsoas; to femoral neck

Transfer of the iliopsoas muscle to the greater trochanter or femoral neck is performed to treat congenital hip dislocation or paralysis of the hip adductor muscles. The iliopsoas is approached using an anterolateral incision over the insertion site on the lesser trochanter. The ilopsoas is divided at its insertion. A notch is created in the wing of the ilium between the anterior superior and anterior inferior spines. The gluteus medius and minimus muscles are split. The iliopsoas muscle is passed through the notch in the wing of the ilium and then through the split in the gluteus medius and minimus muscles. The iliopsoas is then secured to the greater trochanter or femoral neck. Use 27110 when the iliopsoas is transferred to the greater trochanter. Use 27111 when it is transferred to the femoral neck.

27120

27120   Acetabuloplasty; (eg, Whitman, Colonna, Haygroves, or cup type)

The acetabulum, which is a cup-shaped depression on the external surface of the pelvis, is reshaped to improve function of the hip joint. There are a number of surgical techniques used to reshape the acetabulum and the technique used depends on the nature of the deformity. An incision is made over the lateral aspect of the hip. Soft tissue is dissected and released to allow exposure of the hip joint and dislocation of the femoral head from the acetabulum. The cartilage and bone is removed from the surface of the acetabulum using an osteotome. A prosthetic cup is secured to the acetabulum. The femoral head is relocated within the prosthetic cup that forms the new hip socket. Incisions are closed in layers. Alternatively, for congenital hip deformity, the femoral head is placed deep in the acetabular socket. The rim of the acetabulum is prepared with the osteotome and bone grafting is performed to fill in the gap created by the acetabular osteotomy. The hip is placed in abduction and a hip spica cast is applied. As the acetabulum heals, the femoral head serves as a mold for the socket. As bone callus forms, it conforms to the shape of the femoral head to form a hemispherically shaped socket.

27122

27122   Acetabuloplasty; resection, femoral head (eg, Girdlestone procedure)

An acetabuloplasty with resection of the femoral head, also referred to as a Girdlestone procedure, involves removing cartilage and bone in the acetabulum and resecting the femoral head so that the acetabulum and femur will fuse together. This procedure may be performed for patients with painful, failed total hip procedures, or patients with primary septic arthritis or secondary infection of the hip following hip replacement surgery. An

● New Code   ▲ Revised Code

Musculoskeletal System

Musculoskeletal System

incision is made over the lateral aspect of the hip. Soft tissue is dissected and released to allow exposure of the hip joint and dislocation of the femoral head from the acetabulum. The joint is flushed with sterile saline. The cartilage and bone is removed from the surface of the acetabulum using an osteotome. Part or all of the femoral head and/or neck is also excised. The remaining portion of the femur is then positioned in the acetabulum. A hip spica cast is applied to prevent movement of the hip.

27125

27125   Hemiarthroplasty, hip, partial (eg, femoral stem prosthesis, bipolar arthroplasty)

The physician performs a hemiarthroplasty of the hip, also referred to as a partial hip replacement, femoral stem prosthesis, unipolar arthroplasty, or bipolar arthroplasty. Hemiarthroplasty involves removal of the femoral head and replacement with a unipolar femoral head and stem prosthetic implant. Alternatively, a bipolar hemiprosthesis may be used which includes a femoral head and stem with an acetabular cup component. The acetabular cup component is not fixed in the acetabulum, which allows the bipolar hemiprosthesis to move on two poles. The acetabular cup component rotates in the acetabulum and the smaller ball component that fits in the cup rotates within the cup. An incision is made laterally over the hip joint. The hip capsule is incised to expose the diseased femoral head, which is removed. The acetabulum is inspected and any diseased cartilage is removed. An appropriately sized femoral head prosthesis or bipolar hemiprosthesis is selected. The femoral shaft is reamed to the exact size and shape of the prosthetic stem. The stem is then inserted into the prepared femoral canal. Bone cement may be used to secure the stem. The metal ball that replaces the femoral head is attached to the stem. The prosthetic femoral head or bipolar hemiprosthesis is then manipulated into place in the hip joint and range of motion is evaluated. Once it has been determined that the prosthetic implant is functioning properly, the joint capsule is closed and the skin is reapproximated.

27130

27130   Arthroplasty, acetabular and proximal femoral prosthetic replacement (total hip arthroplasty), with or without autograft or allograft

A total hip replacement involves removal of diseased cartilage and bone from the acetabulum and femur with replacement using a prosthetic ball and socket. An incision is made over the lateral aspect of the hip. Soft tissue is dissected and released to allow exposure of the hip joint and dislocation of the femoral head from the acetabulum. The cartilage and bone is removed from the surface of the acetabulum using an osteotome. A prosthetic cup is secured to the acetabulum. The femoral head is excised and the femoral shaft is reamed to allow insertion of the stem of the ball and stem component of the prosthesis. The stem is inserted into the prepared femoral shaft and secured using bone cement or a press- fit technique. If the ball is not attached to the stem it is attached and the ball component is placed into cup component. The prosthetic hip joint is taken through a full range of motion to ensure adequate stability and motion of hip. A drain is placed and incisions are closed in layers around the drain.

27132

27132   Conversion of previous hip surgery to total hip arthroplasty, with or without autograft or allograft

A hip that has been previously operated upon is converted to a total hip arthroplasty. Conversion involves removal of existing hardware such as pins or screws, correction of any bony abnormalities, implantation of total hip components, and bone grafting. The skin is incised over the old incision line along the lateral aspect of the hip. Soft tissue is dissected. Extensive soft tissue release resulting from scar tissue formation may be required, including partial release of the psoas tendon, partial release of the gluteus maximus insertion, and release of the head of the rectus femoris. The hip is dislocated and the femoral head is exposed. Any existing hardware, such as pins or screws, is removed. The cartilage and bone is removed from the surface of the acetabulum using an osteotome. The acetabulum is evaluated for bone loss and bone allografts and/or autografts are used to reconstitute the hip socket as needed. A prosthetic cup is secured to the acetabulum. The femoral head is excised and the femoral shaft is reamed to allow insertion of the stem of the ball and stem component of the prosthesis. The femoral shaft is evaluated for bone loss and bone allografts and/or autografts are again used to reconstitute the femur as needed. The stem is inserted into the prepared femoral shaft and secured using bone cement or a press- fit technique. If the ball is not already attached to the stem, it is attached next and the ball component is placed into the cup component. The prosthetic hip joint is taken through a full range of motion to ensure adequate stability and mobility of the hip. A drain is placed and incisions are closed in layers around the drain.

27134-27138

27134   Revision of total hip arthroplasty; both components, with or without autograft or allograft

27137   Revision of total hip arthroplasty; acetabular component only, with or without autograft or allograft

27138   Revision of total hip arthroplasty; femoral component only, with or without allograft

A failed total hip arthroplasty is revised. Revision involves removal of existing implants, correction of any bony abnormalities, implantation of new or revised total hip components, and bone grafting. The skin is incised over the old incision line along the lateral aspect of the hip. Soft tissue is dissected. Extensive soft tissue release resulting from scar tissue formation may be required, including partial release of the psoas tendon, partial release of the gluteus maximus insertion, and release of the head of the rectus femoris. The hip is dislocated and the femoral head prosthesis is exposed. To remove the acetabular component, the entire pseudocapsule is excised and the acetabular cup is removed. To remove the femoral component, any trochanteric overhang is removed using a high speed burr. Alternatively, a trochanteric osteotomy may be performed. The proximal aspect of the femoral stem is cleared of any visible bone cement or bony overgrowth. Depending on the type of prosthesis, the femoral component may be removed easily using traction or removal may require severing of fibrous or bony ingrowth into the prosthesis using flexible osteotomies or a small burr. Once the femoral component has been sufficiently loosened, it is extracted. If bone cement has been used to secure the total hip components, it is removed from both the acetabulum and the femoral canal. The surgical sites are flushed with saline and/or antibiotic solution. The acetabulum and femoral shaft are evaluated for bone loss and bone allografts and/or autografts are used to reconstitute the bones as needed. The physician then makes the necessary revisions to the total hip components. The revised components are then implanted. Use 27134 for revision of both the acetabular and femoral components. Use 27137 for revision of the acetabular component of the total hip prosthesis only. Use 27138 for revision of the femoral component only.

27140

27140   Osteotomy and transfer of greater trochanter of femur (separate procedure)

Osteotomy and transfer of the greater trochanter may be performed to improve abductor function and to allow for proper soft tissue tension in patients who have had a previous injury or procedures on the hip joint. A skin incision is made over the lateral aspect of the hip joint. Soft tissues are dissected and the greater trochanter is exposed. The planned osteotomy site is marked and a series of cuts are made in the femur around the greater trochanter until the greater trochanter is completely severed from the femur. The greater trochanter is then repositioned on the femur and secured with wires, cables, and/or a plate and screw fixation device. Hip range of motion is checked and incisions are closed in layers.

27146-27147

27146   Osteotomy, iliac, acetabular or innominate bone
27147   Osteotomy, iliac, acetabular or innominate bone; with open reduction of hip

An osteotomy of the iliac, acetabular, or innominate bone is typically performed to treat a congenital malformation of these bones that results in subluxation or dislocation of the hip. Following careful evaluation of the exact nature of the malformation, the bone requiring reshaping by osteotomy is exposed. The planned osteotomy site is marked and cuts are made in the bone to allow the shape of the bone to be reconfigured. If the femoral head is malpositioned, it may be reduced and the osteotomy performed around the reduced femoral head. This allows the reshaped bones to conform to the size and shape of the femoral head. Wedges created from the cut bone are strategically placed at the osteotomy sites to maintain the proper angles in the cut bone. Internal fixation including pins, screws, wires, or other devices used as needed to maintain the position of the bone. Use 27146 for osteotomy only. Use 27147 when open reduction of the hip is also performed.

27151-27156

27151   Osteotomy, iliac, acetabular or innominate bone; with femoral osteotomy
27156   Osteotomy, iliac, acetabular or innominate bone; with femoral osteotomy and with open reduction of hip

An osteotomy of the iliac, acetabular, or innominate bone with femoral osteotomy is typically performed to treat a congenital malformation of these bones that results in a leg length discrepancy as well as subluxation or dislocation of the hip. Following careful evaluation of the exact nature of the malformation, the affected bones in the pelvis (iliac, acetabular, or innominate) and the femur are exposed. The planned osteotomy sites in the affected pelvic bone are marked and cuts are made in the bone to allow the shape of the bone to be reconfigured. The leg length discrepancy or malformation of the femur is evaluated and cuts are also made in the femur to allow shortening, lengthening and/or reshaping. If the femoral head is malpositioned, it may be reduced and the pelvic osteotomy performed around the reduced femoral head. This allows the reshaped pelvic bones to conform to the size and shape of the femoral head. Wedges created from the cut bone are strategically placed at the osteotomy sites to maintain the proper angles in the cut bone. Internal fixation including pins, screws, wires, or other devices are used as needed to maintain the shape and position of the bones. Use 27151 for pelvic and femoral osteotomy only. Use 27156 when open reduction of the hip is also performed.

27158

27158   Osteotomy, pelvis, bilateral (eg, congenital malformation)

Bilateral osteotomies of the pelvis are typically performed to treat a congenital malformation of pelvis that results in bilateral subluxation or dislocation of the hips. Following careful evaluation of the exact nature of the malformation, the bones requiring reshaping by osteotomy are exposed. The planned osteotomy sites are marked and cuts are made in the bones to allow the shape of the pelvis to be reconfigured. Wedges created from the cut bone are strategically placed at the osteotomy sites to maintain the proper angles in the cut bones. Internal fixation including pins, screws, wires, or other devices are used as needed to maintain the position of the bones.

27161

27161   Osteotomy, femoral neck (separate procedure)

Osteotomy of the femoral neck is performed to treat a short, long, or malformed femoral neck. A skin incision is made over the lateral aspect of the hip joint. Soft tissues are dissected and the femur is exposed. The femoral head is dislocated from the acetabulum. The planned osteotomy sites are marked and a series of cuts are made in the femoral neck to allow shortening, lengthening, or reconfiguring of the bone. Wedges created from the cut bone are strategically placed at the osteotomy sites to maintain the proper angles in the cut bone. Internal fixation including pins, screws, wires, or other devices are used as needed to maintain the shape and position of the bone. The femoral head is replaced in the acetabulum. Hip range of motion is checked and incisions are closed in layers.

27165

27165   Osteotomy, intertrochanteric or subtrochanteric including internal or external fixation and/or cast

Osteotomy of the proximal femur is performed to treat congenital or acquired deformities of the intertrochanteric or subtrochanteric region of the hip. A skin incision is made over the lateral aspect of the hip joint. Soft tissues are dissected and the proximal femur is exposed. The femoral head is dislocated from the acetabulum. The planned osteotomy sites are marked and a series of cuts is made in the trochanteric and/or subtrochanteriic regions. Wedges created from the cut bone are strategically placed at the osteotomy sites to maintain the proper angles in the cut bone. Internal fixation including pins, screws, wires, or other devices are used as needed to maintain the shape and position of the bone. The femoral head is replaced in the acetabulum. Incisions are closed in layers. An external fixation system may be applied instead of or in addition to internal fixation. A hip spica cast is applied as needed.

27170

27170   Bone graft, femoral head, neck, intertrochanteric or subtrochanteric area (includes obtaining bone graft)

A bone graft is placed in the head, neck, intertrochanteric, or subtrochanteric region of the femur. Bone grafts are used to fill bone defects, to promote osteogenesis and union of the bone, to provide structural stability, or for arthrodesis. A lateral skin incision is made over the hip joint. The proximal femur is exposed. The femoral head is dislocated from the acetabulum as needed. The bone defect is inspected and the size and type of bone graft required to repair the defect is determined. The bone harvest site is exposed by dividing and stripping away overlying muscle tissue. Common harvest sites include the iliac crest, tibia, fibula, and greater trochanter of the femur. Cortical and/or cancellous bone may be harvested. If cancellous bone is required, the overlying cortical bone is excised and the soft spongy cancellous bone is scooped out. The bone autograft is then prepared for placement into the bone defect. This may require crushing of cancellous bone or reconfiguration of cortical bone to the appropriate size and shape. The bone graft is then placed in the defect. Incisions at the harvest site and over the femur are closed in layers.

27175-27176

27175   Treatment of slipped femoral epiphysis; by traction, without reduction

27176   Treatment of slipped femoral epiphysis; by single or multiple pinning, in situ

A slipped capital femoral epiphysis (SCFE) is a disorder affecting the adolescent hip in which the growth plate just below the femoral head slips off the femur in a backward direction. This can be a gradual process or it can occur due to trauma. In 27175, the SCFE is treated using traction to gradually return the slipped epiphysis to proper position. A traction pin is placed through the tibial tubercle. The leg is then suspended and weighted longitudinal traction is applied. Traction is maintained until the slipped epiphysis is returned to anatomical alignment. In 27176, the SCFE is treated by in situ placement of one or more pins. Intraoperative radiographs are obtained to identify the center of the SCFE. These radiographs are used to identify pin insertion site(s) and angle(s) of insertion which are marked on the skin. A small incision is made at the first pin entry point. A

guidewire is placed through the skin incision and advanced into the bone by gentle tapping or by drilling. Correct position of the guidewire is confirmed radiographically. The guidewire is removed and a pin or screw is placed into the tract created by the guidewire. Correct position of the pin or screw is again confirmed radiographically. Additional pins or screws are placed as needed using the same technique. Entry incisions are closed with sutures.

27177-27178

27177   Open treatment of slipped femoral epiphysis; single or multiple pinning or bone graft (includes obtaining graft)

27178   Open treatment of slipped femoral epiphysis; closed manipulation with single or multiple pinning

A slipped capital femoral epiphysis (SCFE) is a disorder affecting the adolescent hip in which the growth plate just below the femoral head slips off the femur in a backward direction. This can be a gradual process or it can occur due to trauma. In 27177, the SCFE is treated by open technique with placement of one or more pins or with bone graft. A lateral skin incision is made over the hip joint. Soft tissues are dissected and the femur is exposed. The degree of slippage is evaluated and the appropriate repair technique is determined. If pinning is used, the pin site(s) and angle(s) are determined. A guidewire is placed into the bone at the first insertion site and advanced by gentle tapping or by drilling. Correct position of the guidewire is confirmed radiographically. The guidewire is removed and a pin or screw is placed into the tract created by the guidewire. Correct position of the pin or screw is again confirmed radiographically. Additional pins or screws are placed as needed using the same technique. If bone graft is required, the bone harvest site is exposed by dividing and stripping away overlying muscle tissue. Common harvest sites include the iliac crest, tibia, fibula, and greater trochanter of the femur. Cortical and/or cancellous bone may be harvested. If cancellous bone is required, the overlying cortical bone is excised and the soft spongy cancellous bone is scooped out. The bone autograft is then prepared for placement into the defect in the capital femoral epiphysis. This may require crushing of cancellous bone or reconfiguration of cortical bone to the appropriate size and shape. The bone graft is placed in the defect. Incisions at the harvest site and over the femur are closed in layers. Entry incisions are closed with sutures. In 27178, the SCFE is reduced using a closed technique. Radiographs are obtained to determine the extent of slippage. The femoral head and neck are manually manipulated into anatomical alignment. Alignment is maintained using placement of pins which is performed using an open technique as described above.

27179-27181

27179   Open treatment of slipped femoral epiphysis; osteoplasty of femoral neck (Heyman type procedure)

27181   Open treatment of slipped femoral epiphysis; osteotomy and internal fixation

A slipped capital femoral epiphysis (SCFE) is a disorder affecting the adolescent hip in which the growth plate just below the femoral head slips off the femur in a backward direction. This can be a gradual process or it can occur due to trauma. A lateral skin incision is made over the hip joint. Soft tissues are dissected and the hip joint is exposed. The joint capsule is incised. The degree of slippage is evaluated and the appropriate repair technique is determined. In 27179, the SCFE is treated with femoral neck osteoplasty, also referred to as a Heyman procedure. The hip is moved through a range of motions to determine where the bone prominence resulting from the slippage impinges against the rim of the acetabulum. The periosteum of the femoral neck at the site of the prominence is incised and elevated. The prominence is removed by carefully smoothing and remodeling the bone. Once the prominence has been removed, the periosteum is repaired. The joint capsule is closed, followed by layered closure of soft tissues and skin. In 27181, the SCFE is treated using an osteotomy and internal fixation. To compensate for backward slippage of the femoral capital epiphysis, a wedge of bone is excised from the distal aspect of the femoral neck or proximally at the lower aspect of the head and upper aspect of the neck. This allows realignment of the femoral head, neck, and shaft of the femur. The femoral head, neck, and shaft are repositioned and then secured using internal fixation devices such as pins or screws.

27185

27185   Epiphyseal arrest by epiphysiodesis or stapling, greater trochanter of femur

Epiphyseal arrest of the greater trochanter of the femur is performed to treat or prevent overgrowth of the greater trochanter, which can affect hip movement and alter gait. An incision is made over the lateral aspect of the hip. Soft tissues are dissected and the greater trochanter is exposed. Epiphyseal arrest is accomplished by epiphysiodesis which involves drilling across the greater trochanter physis followed by placement of screws in the drill holes or by stapling around the epiphyseal plate. The incision is closed in layers.

27187

27187   Prophylactic treatment (nailing, pinning, plating or wiring) with or without methylmethacrylate, femoral neck and proximal femur

Prophylactic treatment of the femoral neck or proximal femur is performed to provide additional strength and support to the bone in cases of osteoporosis or osteolytic

Musculoskeletal System

disease such as that caused by bone metastases. The bone may be reinforced by a variety of techniques. Placement of pins or screws can be performed using a percutaneous technique. A small skin incision is made over the planned screw insertion site. Using radiographic guidance, one or more pins or screws are placed through the femoral neck and proximal femur. A hollow cannulated screw may be placed that allows injection of bone cement (methylmethacrylate) through the screw into the femoral neck. Alternatively, the bone may be drilled and bone cement injected directly into the bone. If plate and screw or wire cerclage is used, an incision is made over the lateral aspect of the hip. The proximal femur is exposed. Internal fixation devices are then placed to provide support for the damaged bone. Layered closure of the operative wound is then performed.

27197-27198

- ● **27197** **Closed treatment of posterior pelvic ring fracture(s), dislocation(s), diastasis or subluxation of the ilium, sacroiliac joint, and/or sacrum, with or without anterior pelvic ring fracture(s) and/or dislocation(s) of the pubic symphysis and/or superior/inferior rami, unilateral or bilateral; without manipulation**

- ● **27198** **Closed treatment of posterior pelvic ring fracture(s), dislocation(s), diastasis or subluxation of the ilium, sacroiliac joint, and/or sacrum, with or without anterior pelvic ring fracture(s) and/or dislocation(s) of the pubic symphysis and/or superior/inferior rami, unilateral or bilateral; with manipulation, requiring more than local anesthesia (ie, general anesthesia, moderate sedation, spinal/epidural)**

Closed treatment following posterior pelvic ring injury is performed to align and stabilize the bony structure. A posterior pelvic ring (ilium, sacroiliac joint, and/or sacrum) injury is often unstable and frequently involves injury to the anterior pelvis as well (pubic symphysis and/or superior/inferior pubic rami). An injury may include fracture, dislocation, diastasis, and/or subluxation and usually results from a traumatic, high energy event such as head on or side impact motor vehicle accident or fall from a height. Because of the proximity of pelvic organs, blood vessels, and nerves, an injury to the pelvic ring can cause intra-peritoneal and retro-peritoneal visceral and/or vascular injury. The goal of closed treatment is to minimize injury to soft tissue and internal organs, reduce pain by relieving pressure on nerves, and maintain blood flow circulation. Closed reduction with or without manipulation may be accomplished using a pelvic circumferential compression device (PCCD, binder) or folded sheet centered over the greater trochanters and wrapped securely around the pelvis. To correct lower extremity external rotation, the knees and/or ankles and feet can be taped together. Closed reduction may also be facilitated with the use of a C-clamp applied to the trochanteric region to direct compressive force posteriorly across the sacroiliac joints. Code 27197 reports closed treatment of posterior pelvic ring injury, with or without anterior pelvic ring injury, unilateral or bilateral; without manipulation and code 27198 reports with manipulation, requiring moderate sedation, general anesthesia, or regional anesthesia (spinal, epidural).

27200-27202

27200 **Closed treatment of coccygeal fracture**
27202 **Open treatment of coccygeal fracture**

The coccygeal fracture is evaluated. A rectal exam may be performed. The physician inserts a gloved finger into the rectum to feel for abnormalities including abnormal movement of the coccyx. Separately reportable radiographic studies may be performed. The patient is instructed to rest and pain medication may be prescribed. Pain and tenderness may persist for weeks or months. If severe pain persists after sufficient healing time has elapsed, a separately reportable steroid injection may be administered. Use 27202 for open treatment of coccygeal fracture. An incision is made over the coccyx. The fracture site is cleansed of debris. The displaced fracture fragments are reduced. Alternatively, the coccyx may be excised. The wound is irrigated and closed.

27215

27215 **Open treatment of iliac spine(s), tuberosity avulsion, or iliac wing fracture(s), unilateral, for pelvic bone fracture patterns that do not disrupt the pelvic ring, includes internal fixation, when performed**

The ilium is one of three paired bones that make up the pelvic girdle, or ring. The iliac bones are located in the upper anterior aspect of the pelvic girdle and are divided into four anatomic regions – the anterior iliac spine, the posterior iliac spine, the iliac tuberosity (tubercle), and the iliac wing. In this procedure, a fracture of one of the iliac bones (right or left) that has not disrupted the pelvic ring is treated by open reduction. A separately reportable radiographic study of the pelvis is performed to assess the degree of displacement of the fracture fragments. An incision is made over the fracture site, which is exposed and cleared of debris, and then reduced into proper anatomic alignment. Internal fixation is applied as needed, most often by screw fixation or a plate and screw device. The wound is irrigated and the incision is closed with sutures.

27216

27216 **Percutaneous skeletal fixation of posterior pelvic bone fracture and/or dislocation, for fracture patterns that disrupt the pelvic ring, unilateral (includes ipsilateral ilium, sacroiliac joint and/or sacrum)**

Posterior pelvic ring fractures involve the ilium and/or sacrum. Dislocation or fracture dislocation injuries in the posterior pelvic ring involve the sacroiliac joints. A separately reportable radiographic study of the pelvis is performed to assess the posterior pelvic ring fracture or fracture dislocation. The fracture/dislocation is reduced by applying traction along the femoral axis on the side of the fracture while restraining the contralateral leg and trunk at the same time to prevent movement. When anatomical alignment has been achieved, a threaded guiding pin is inserted under radiographic guidance to help identify the correct placement for screw(s). A bone drill is used to prepare the bone for screw placement. Cannulated screws are then placed percutaneously through the fracture site in the ilium or sacrum. If a fracture dislocation of the sacroiliac joint is present, the screws are placed from the ilium, through the sacroiliac joint, and into the sacrum.

27217

27217 **Open treatment of anterior pelvic bone fracture and/or dislocation for fracture patterns that disrupt the pelvic ring, unilateral, includes internal fixation, when performed (includes pubic symphysis and/or ipsilateral superior/inferior rami)**

Anterior pelvic ring injuries involve fracture of the pubic rami and/or dislocation (diastasis) of the pubic symphysis. A separately reportable radiographic study of the pelvis is performed to assess the anterior pelvic ring fracture and/or dislocation. An incision is made over the fracture/dislocation site. The anterior rectus muscle is identified and any avulsion injury is evaluated. If the anterior rectus is intact, it is incised. Dissection continues, taking care to identify and protect neurovascular structures as well as the spermatic cord and bladder in males. The fracture/dislocation site is exposed and cleared of debris, then reduced by applying pressure over both iliac crests. If pressure alone does not provide adequate reduction of the fracture fragments, pelvic reduction clamps or forceps may be used. When anatomical reduction has been achieved, the bone is prepared for plate and screw fixation. A plate is fixed to the superior surface of the symphysis pubis with cancellous screws inserted through the anterior superior aspect of the pubis on either side of the symphysis. The screws are positioned in a posterior inferior direction penetrating the full depth of the pubis on each side. Anatomic reduction is verified radiographically. The wound is irrigated and closed.

27218

27218 **Open treatment of posterior pelvic bone fracture and/or dislocation, for fracture patterns that disrupt the pelvic ring, unilateral, includes internal fixation, when performed (includes ipsilateral ilium, sacroiliac joint and/or sacrum)**

Posterior pelvic ring fractures involve the ilium and/or sacrum. Dislocation or fracture dislocation injuries in the posterior pelvic ring involve the sacroiliac joints. A separately reportable radiographic study of the pelvis is performed to assess the posterior pelvic ring injury. An incision is made to expose the fracture/dislocation site, which is cleared of debris and then reduced. When anatomical reduction has been achieved, the bone is prepared for an internal fixation device, which may include screws alone, transiliac sacral bar (Harrington rod) fixation, or a plate and screw fixation device. If screws are applied, a temporary pin fixation device is placed and alignment of the fracture fragments is verified radiographically. The bone is prepared using a drill and the screw(s) are placed. If Harrington rods are used, they are positioned and then fixed with threaded nuts. If a plate and screw fixation device is used, the plate is fixed to the dorsum of the sacrum and the posterior iliac spines bilaterally. Anatomic reduction is verified by separately reportable radiographs. The wound is irrigated and closed.

27220-27222

27220 **Closed treatment of acetabulum (hip socket) fracture(s); without manipulation**
27222 **Closed treatment of acetabulum (hip socket) fracture(s); with manipulation, with or without skeletal traction**

The physician treats a fracture of the acetabulum (hip socket). Separately reportable radiographs and/or a CT scan are obtained to evaluate the injury to the hip region. The anterior and posterior pelvic bones and the greater trochanter are palpated. Range of motion of the hip and lumbosacral spine is checked. A neurovascular examination is performed to ensure that there is no nerve impingement. In 27220, the fracture is determined to be nondisplaced or only minimally displaced. The patient is treated may be treated with bed rest. Crutches or a walker may be prescribed so that the patient can ambulate without bearing weight on the side of the fracture. In 27222, the fracture fragments are reduced using manual force. The patient may be placed in skeletal traction to maintain fracture reduction. Skeletal traction is accomplished by inserting a pin at the proximal aspect of the tibia. The traction device is then attached to the pin and weights are used to maintain the fracture reduction.

27226

27226   Open treatment of posterior or anterior acetabular wall fracture, with internal fixation

The acetabulum is composed of an anterior (iliopubic) column, posterior (ilioischial) column, anterior wall, posterior wall, quadrilateral plate (medial wall), and dome. The anterior and posterior walls form the articular surface of the hip and help stabilize the hip joint. An incision is made over the hip joint and the posterior or anterior wall fracture is exposed. The hip joint is debrided, irrigated, and all loose fragments are removed. The fracture is reduced and the fragments are secured with temporary pin or wire fixation. Anatomic reduction is verified radiographically. Permanent fixation devices are then applied. Internal fixation may include lag screw fixation or a plate and screw device. If lag screws are used, the outer cortex of the bone is over-drilled with the drill bit placed perpendicular to the fracture site. Lag screws are inserted into the bone. If plate and screw fixation is used, a buttress plate is placed along the posterior or anterior rim of the acetabulum at the fracture site and secured with lag screws. Separately reportable bone grafts may also be used to secure the fracture fragments.

27227

27227   Open treatment of acetabular fracture(s) involving anterior or posterior (one) column, or a fracture running transversely across the acetabulum, with internal fixation

The acetabulum is composed of an anterior (iliopubic) column, posterior (ilioischial) column, anterior wall, posterior wall, quadrilateral plate (medial wall), and dome. An anterior column fracture extends through the anterior wall and into the ischiopubic segment of the pelvis A posterior column fracture extends through the posterior wall and interrupts the ilioischial line. A transverse acetabular fracture extends through both columns but does not completely disrupt the dome of the acetabulum leaving a portion of the dome attached to the iliac wing. An incision is made over the hip joint to expose the anterior or posterior column fracture or transverse fracture of the acetabulum. The hip joint is debrided, irrigated, and all loose fragments are removed. The fracture is reduced and anatomic reduction is verified radiographically. Permanent fixation devices are then applied. Internal fixation may include a combination of lag screw fixation and plate and screw devices. If lag screws are used, the outer cortex of the bone is over-drilled with the drill bit placed perpendicular to the fracture site. Lag screws are inserted into the bone. If plate and screw fixation is used, a reconstruction plate is placed along the acetabular surface at the fracture site and secured with lag screws. A second plate may be placed from the isichial tuberosity to the lateral ilium in posterior column fractures. Separately reportable bone grafts may also be used to secure the fracture fragments.

27228

27228   Open treatment of acetabular fracture(s) involving anterior and posterior (two) columns, includes T-fracture and both column fracture with complete articular detachment, or single column or transverse fracture with associated acetabular wall fracture, with internal fixation

The acetabulum is composed of an anterior (iliopubic) column, posterior (ilioischial) column, anterior wall, posterior wall, quadrilateral plate (medial wall), and dome. This code reports complex fractures of the acetabulum that involve more than one fracture line. Two column fractures have fracture lines that extend into the ilioischial line posteriorly and iliopubic segment anteriorly resulting in separation of the entire acetabulum from the iliac wing. A two column fracture may be referred to as a floating acetabular fracture. T-fractures are transverse fractures with an additional fracture line that disrupts the quadrilateral surface resulting in separation of the anterior and posterior columns. A single column fracture or transverse fracture that has a second fracture line disrupting the articular surface of the acetabulum is also considered a complex fracture. An incision is made over the hip joint and the fracture sites in the acetabulum are exposed. The hip joint is debrided, irrigated, and all loose fragments are removed. The fracture is reduced and anatomic reduction is verified radiographically. Permanent fixation devices are then applied. Internal fixation may include a combination of lag screw fixation and plate and screw devices. If lag screws are used, the outer cortex of the bone is over-drilled with the drill bit placed perpendicular to the fracture line. Lag screws are inserted into the bone. If plate and screw fixation is used, a reconstruction plate is placed along the acetabular surface at the fracture site and secured with lag screws. A second plate may be placed from the isichial tuberosity to the lateral ilium to secure the posterior column fracture. Separately reportable bone grafts may also be used to secure the fracture fragments.

27230-27232

27230   Closed treatment of femoral fracture, proximal end, neck; without manipulation

27232   Closed treatment of femoral fracture, proximal end, neck; with manipulation, with or without skeletal traction

Closed treatment of a proximal end, neck fracture of the femur is performed. Separately reportable radiographs are obtained to confirm the fracture. A neurovascular exam is performed to ensure that the nerves and blood vessels at the site of the injury are intact.

In 27230, a nondisplaced fracture of the neck of the femur is evaluated. No manipulation of the fracture fragments is required. The patient is instructed on the need to keep weight off the injury and provided with crutches or other walking aid. In 27232, a minimally displaced fracture of the neck of the femur is treated. The displaced fracture fragments are manually reduced (manipulated) back to proper anatomic alignment. Separately reportable radiographs are obtained to confirm anatomic reduction. Following reduction of the fracture fragments, skeletal traction is applied if needed by placing a pin through the distal femur or proximal tibia and applying weighted traction.

27235

27235   Percutaneous skeletal fixation of femoral fracture, proximal end, neck

Separately reportable radiographs are obtained to confirm the fracture. A neurovascular exam is performed to ensure that the nerves and blood vessels at the site of the injury are intact. The fracture fragments are manually reduced (manipulated) back to proper anatomic alignment. Separately reportable radiographs are obtained to confirm proper reduction of the fracture fragments, after which one or more pins or screws are inserted through the skin to stabilize the fracture. Typically three pins or screws are used in an inverted triangle configuration. Using a lateral approach, guide pins are drilled into place traversing the fracture in the neck of the femur. Cannulated pins or screws are then inserted over the guide pins, across the fracture, and into the head of the femur. The guide pins are removed once the fixation screws or pins have traversed the fracture. The fixation pins or screws are tightened to apply compression across the fracture site.

27236

27236   Open treatment of femoral fracture, proximal end, neck, internal fixation or prosthetic replacement

An incision is made laterally over the hip joint. The hip capsule is incised and the fracture site in the femoral neck is exposed and cleared of debris. If internal fixation is to be used, the fracture is first reduced. Guide wires are then inserted to temporarily hold the reduced fracture in place. Typically three guide wires are inserted parallel to each other in an inverted triangle configuration. Appropriately sized screws are selected, the outer cortex of the proximal femur is reamed, and cannulated screws are placed. Optimal screw placement and anatomic reduction of the fracture is confirmed radiographically. If the femoral neck fracture is treated by prosthetic replacement, a hip hemiarthroplasty is typically performed which involves removal of the femoral head and replacement with a prosthetic implant. An appropriate size femoral head prosthesis is selected. The femoral shaft is reamed to the exact size and shape of the prosthetic stem, which is then inserted into the prepared femoral canal. Bone cement may be used to secure the stem. The metal ball that will replace the femoral head is attached to the stem. The prosthetic femoral head is then manipulated into place in the hip joint. Hip range of motion is evaluated. Once it has been determined that the prosthetic implant is functioning properly, the joint capsule is closed and the skin is reapproximated.

27238-27240

27238   Closed treatment of intertrochanteric, peritrochanteric, or subtrochanteric femoral fracture; without manipulation

27240   Closed treatment of intertrochanteric, peritrochanteric, or subtrochanteric femoral fracture; with manipulation, with or without skin or skeletal traction

Intertrochanteric fractures are extracapsular fractures that occur between the greater and lesser trochanters. Peritrochanteric fractures occur around or encircle the greater or lesser trochanter. Subtrochanteric fractures occur just below the greater and lesser trochanters. Separately reportable radiographs are obtained to confirm the fracture. A neurovascular exam is performed to ensure that the nerves and blood vessels at the site of the injury are intact. In 27238, a nondisplaced intertrochanteric, peritrochanteric, or subtrochanteric fracture of the femur is evaluated. No manipulation of the fracture fragments is required. The patient is instructed on the need to keep weight off the injury and provided with crutches or other walking aid. In 27240, a minimally displaced intertrochanteric, peritrochanteric, or subtrochanteric fracture of the femur is treated. The displaced fracture fragments are manually reduced (manipulated) back to proper anatomic alignment. Separately reportable radiographs are obtained to confirm anatomic reduction. Following reduction of the fracture fragments, skin or skeletal traction is applied if needed. If skin traction is used, the leg is splinted and the weighted traction device attached to the leg using wraps, tape or straps. If skeletal traction is used, a pin is inserted through the distal femur or proximal tibia and weighted traction applied.

27244-27245

27244   Treatment of intertrochanteric, peritrochanteric, or subtrochanteric femoral fracture; with plate/screw type implant, with or without cerclage

27245   Treatment of intertrochanteric, peritrochanteric, or subtrochanteric femoral fracture; with intramedullary implant, with or without interlocking screws and/or cerclage

Treatment of an intertrochanteric, peritrochanteric, or subtrochanteric fracture of the femur is performed using a plate and screw type implant with or without cerclage.

CPT © 2016 American Medical Association. All Rights Reserved.

● New Code   ▲ Revised Code

Musculoskeletal System

Intertrochanteric fractures are extracapsular fractures that occur between the greater and lesser trochanters. Peritrochanteric fractures occur around or encircle the greater or lesser trochanter. Subtrochanteric fractures occur just below the greater and lesser trochanters. Separately reportable radiographs are obtained to confirm the fracture. A neurovascular exam is performed to ensure that the nerves and blood vessels at the site of the injury are intact. Closed reduction is performed using longitudinal traction and verified radiographically. If closed reduction is not successful, open reduction is performed. An incision is made from the tip of the greater trochanter and extended proximally to allow exposure of the gluteus maximus muscle which is dissected along its fibers. If greater exposure is required, the incision is extended distally and the iliotibial band incised. A metal plate is placed along the lateral aspect of the femur and secured to the femoral shaft with screws. A large screw is then inserted through the bone, across the fracture site, into the femoral head, and secured to the metal plate. A wire cerclage may also be wrapped around the fracture fragments to provide additional stability. In 27245, the fracture is treated using an intramedullary implant, also referred to as in intramedullary nail or rod, with or without interlocking screws and/or cerclage. Intramedullary implants are inserted down the center of the femoral shaft. The fracture is exposed as described above. A guide wire is inserted into the greater trochanter and advanced into the intramedullary canal of femoral shaft. The femoral shaft is reamed. An appropriately sized implant is selected and mounted on the insertion device. The intramedullary implant is then positioned in the femoral shaft. If interlocking screws are required, they are placed through the intramedullary implant at points proximal and distal to the fracture site. Typically one or more screws are placed at the femoral neck and additional screws are placed in the mid-shaft of the femur. A wire cerclage may also be wrapped around the fracture fragments to provide additional stability.

27246

27246   Closed treatment of greater trochanteric fracture, without manipulation

The greater trochanter is the larger of the two projections just below the neck of the femur. Separately reportable radiographs are obtained to confirm the fracture. A neurovascular exam is performed to ensure that the nerves and blood vessels at the site of the injury are intact. No manipulation of the fracture fragments is required. The patient is given instructions on weight bearing limits and is provided with crutches or other walking aid, if needed.

27248

27248   Open treatment of greater trochanteric fracture, includes internal fixation, when performed

A greater trochanteric fracture is reduced openly, with any necessary internal fixation. The greater trochanter is the larger of the two bony projections just below the neck of the femur that serves as a point of attachment or insertion site for muscles of the thigh and buttocks, including the gluteus medius, gluteus minimus, piriformis, obturator internus, and gemelli muscles. A large fracture fragment that is completely displaced and mechanically significant is typically treated by open reduction. A lateral incision is made over the greater trochanter and dissection is carried down to the fascia lata, which is split longitudinally. The fracture site is exposed and cleared of debris, then reduced. Internal fixation is applied as needed. A tension band technique is commonly applied using wires or cables to secure the fracture fragments. Alternatively, in situ screw fixation may be used.

27250-27252

27250   Closed treatment of hip dislocation, traumatic; without anesthesia
27252   Closed treatment of hip dislocation, traumatic; requiring anesthesia

Traumatic hip dislocation is usually the result of high-energy blunt force trauma such as a motor vehicle accident. While anterior or posterior dislocation can occur, posterior dislocation is the most common. Neurovascular status of the involved leg is first evaluated. Closed treatment involves manual reduction of the dislocated hip using a combination of traction and mechanical forces to return the femoral head to its correct location in the acetabulum. Following closed reduction of the dislocated hip, neurovascular status is again evaluated. Successful reduction is confirmed with separately reportable radiographs. Use 27250 when the procedure is performed without anesthesia. Use 27252 when anesthesia is required.

27253-27254

27253   Open treatment of hip dislocation, traumatic, without internal fixation
27254   Open treatment of hip dislocation, traumatic, with acetabular wall and femoral head fracture, with or without internal or external fixation

Traumatic hip dislocation is usually the result of high-energy blunt force trauma such as a motor vehicle accident. While anterior or posterior dislocation can occur, posterior dislocation is the most common. In 27253, treatment involves open reduction of the dislocated hip without internal fixation. The hip is usually approached through a posterior incision. Soft tissues are divided and the proximal femur and acetabulum are exposed. The joint is irrigated to remove any bone fragments or soft tissue that might impair movement. The femoral head is then reduced using a combination of traction and mechanical forces.

Once the femoral head is properly positioned in the acetabulum, the incision is closed in layers. In 27254, an acetabular wall and/or femoral head fracture is treated in conjunction with open reduction of the dislocated hip. The anterior and posterior acetabular walls form the articular surface of the hip and help stabilize the hip joint. If the acetabulum is fractured, an incision is made over the hip joint and the posterior or anterior wall fracture is exposed. The hip joint is debrided, irrigated, and all loose fragments are removed. The fracture is reduced and the fragments are secured with temporary pin or wire fixation. Anatomic reduction is verified radiographically. Permanent fixation devices are then applied as needed. Internal fixation may include lag screw fixation or a plate and screw device. If lag screws are used, the outer cortex of the bone is over-drilled with the drill bit placed perpendicular to the fracture site. Lag screws are inserted into the bone. If plate and screw fixation is used, a buttress plate is placed along the posterior or anterior rim of the acetabulum at the fracture site and secured with lag screws. If the femoral head is fractured, the fracture is debrided and reduced into normal anatomic position. If internal fixation is required, screws, pins, or other internal fixation are placed below the articular surface of the femoral head. The dislocated hip is then reduced. Alternatively, the fracture-dislocation may be reduced and an external fixation device applied instead of or in addition to the internal fixation.

27256-27257

27256   Treatment of spontaneous hip dislocation (developmental, including congenital or pathological), by abduction, splint or traction; without anesthesia, without manipulation
27257   Treatment of spontaneous hip dislocation (developmental, including congenital or pathological), by abduction, splint or traction; with manipulation, requiring anesthesia

Developmental dysplasia of the hip (DDH) may occur due to congenital malformation or it may occur during development and affect osseous structures, the joint capsule, and/or soft tissue. Closed treatment of spontaneous dislocation caused by DDH may first require manual reduction of the dislocated hip using a combination of traction and mechanical forces to return the femoral head to its correct location in the acetabulum. Depending on the severity and nature of the hip dysplasia, reduction may be maintained using abduction, splint, or traction. Abduction is accomplished by means of a Pavlik harness. The harness has shoulder straps that pass through a chest strap, over the shoulder, and then attach to the leg splint on the opposite leg. This type of splint holds both legs in abduction. Skin traction is used when the harness or splinting is not successful. Traction is applied using a boot or an adhesive strap applied to the medial and lateral aspect of the lower leg. If adhesive strapping is used, a spreader is placed a few inches from the foot. Ace wraps are used to hold the boot or strapping in place. Ropes with weights and counterweights are then used to suspend the leg and apply traction to reduce the dislocated hip. Use 27256 when the procedure is performed without anesthesia and without manipulation. Use 27257 when anesthesia is required and the hip is reduced using manipulation.

27258-27259

27258   Open treatment of spontaneous hip dislocation (developmental, including congenital or pathological), replacement of femoral head in acetabulum (including tenotomy, etc)
27259   Open treatment of spontaneous hip dislocation (developmental, including congenital or pathological), replacement of femoral head in acetabulum (including tenotomy, etc); with femoral shaft shortening

Developmental dysplasia of the hip (DDH) may occur due to congenital malformation of the joint or it may occur during development and affect osseous structures, the joint capsule, and/or soft tissue. Open treatment of spontaneous dislocation caused by DDH includes adductor tenotomy and/or release of other tissues as needed to allow reduction of the dislocation. In 27258, a skin incision is made in the medial aspect of the groin. The adductor tendon is exposed and incised. Other soft tissue structures are released as needed. The femoral head is then repositioned within the acetabulum to reduce the dislocation. Incisions are closed and a splint or hip spica cast is applied to maintain the hip in abduction. In 27259, the physician performs an osteotomy to shorten the femoral shaft in addition to tenotomy and reduction of the spontaneous dislocation as described above. Prior to reduction of the dislocated femoral head, the planned osteotomy sites are marked and a series of cuts are made in the proximal femoral shaft. Bone is excised. Wedges created from the cut bone are strategically placed at the osteotomy sites to maintain the proper angles in the cut bone. Some of the excised bone may also be morsellized and used for bone grafting. Internal fixation including pins, screws, wires, or other devices is used as needed to maintain the shape and position of the bone. The femoral head is replaced in the acetabulum. Incisions are closed in layers. A hip spica cast is applied as needed.

27265-27266

27265 Closed treatment of post hip arthroplasty dislocation; without anesthesia
27266 Closed treatment of post hip arthroplasty dislocation; requiring regional or general anesthesia

Dislocation of the hip following total hip arthroplasty is a fairly common complication. Before attempting reduction, neurovascular status is evaluated. Closed reduction is then performed using a combination of traction and mechanical forces to return the prosthetic femoral head to its correct location in the prosthetic acetabular cup. Following reduction of the dislocated hip, neurovascular status is again evaluated. Successful reduction is confirmed with separately reportable radiographs. Use 27265 when the procedure is performed without anesthesia. Use 27266 when regional or general anesthesia is required.

27267-27268

27267 Closed treatment of femoral fracture, proximal end, head; without manipulation
27268 Closed treatment of femoral fracture, proximal end, head; with manipulation

Closed treatment of a proximal end femoral head fracture is performed without manipulation in 27267. Proximal end femoral head fractures occur most often in younger patients due to trauma. Following separately reportable radiographic studies, a nondisplaced or minimally displaced proximal end hip fracture is evaluated for stability. If the femoral head at the site of the fracture is determined to be in normal anatomic position, range of motion is checked. When evaluating range of motion, any abnormal noise or vibration (crepitation) at the site of the fracture is noted. The patient is instructed on the need to keep weight off the injured leg and provided with crutches or other walking aid. Use 27268 when closed treatment of a proximal end femoral head fracture with manipulation is performed. Following separately reportable radiographic evaluation, a closed reduction of a displaced fracture is performed. The fracture is manually manipulated to reposition the displaced bone fragment back into position for healing.

27269

27269 Open treatment of femoral fracture, proximal end, head, includes internal fixation, when performed

Open treatment of a proximal end femoral head fracture is performed. Proximal end femoral head fractures occur most often in younger patients due to trauma. An incision is made over the anterolateral aspect of the hip joint. Dissection is carried down to the joint capsule, which is incised and the hip is dislocated anteriorly. The fracture is identified and debrided, then reduced into normal anatomic position, verified visually and radiographically. If internal fixation is required, screws, pins, or other internal fixation devices are placed below the articular cartilaginous surface of the femoral head. The fracture is compressed by the fixation device and optimal reduction to normal anatomic position is again confirmed visually and radiographically.

27275

27275 Manipulation, hip joint, requiring general anesthesia

Manipulation of the hip under anesthesia is used to break up fibrous adhesions and scar tissue around the joint. Anesthesia is required when the patient is unable to tolerate manipulation of the joint due to pain, spasm, muscle contractures, or guarding. Following administration of anesthesia, the hip joint is taken through a series of stretches and articular maneuvers to disrupt any adhesions or scar tissue and restore some joint mobility and increase range of motion.

27279

27279 Arthrodesis, sacroiliac joint, percutaneous or minimally invasive (indirect visualization), with image guidance, includes obtaining bone graft when performed, and placement of transfixing device

Sacroiliac (SI) joint arthrodesis is a procedure used to artificially induce ossification between the spine (sacrum) and the pelvis (ilium) in patients with intractable joint pain often caused by fracture or arthritis. Fusion is accomplished by using a bone graft, synthetic bone substitute, or metal implant inserted across the SI joint. The percutaneous or minimally invasive technique uses fluoroscopic guidance to landmark the area and place the graft(s). If an autograft is used, the bone is first harvested from the iliac crest or rib of the patient. Allograft bone is obtained from a bone bank. A small incision is made in the skin and carried down to the fascia of the gluteal muscle. The muscle is penetrated and a Steinmann pin is inserted through the ilium, across the SI joint, and into the lateral sacrum. The uppermost implant is placed first followed by additional implants below. Holes for the implants are made first with a hollow pin. The bone grafting material is then inserted through the pin and the pin is removed. To avoid damage to nerves, additional implants are placed between the foramen openings at S1 and S2. The bone grafting material is packed into place to fuse the SI joint, and the fascia and skin are closed.

27280

27280 Arthrodesis, open, sacroiliac joint, including obtaining bone graft, including instrumentation, when performed

Fusion of the sacroiliac (SI) joint is performed for pain, instability, and/or degenerative disease. Open arthrodesis may be performed by anterior or posterior approach. Using an open anterior approach, an incision is made over the iliac crest to the anterior superior iliac spine. The iliacus muscle is stripped off the iliac wing and the SI joint is exposed. Using a posterior open approach, an incision is made over the posterior iliac crest and carried down to the posterior inferior spine. The gluteus maximus is stripped off the ilium to expose the SI joint. The joint surface is debrided and cancellous bone is exposed. Bone grafts are harvested from the iliac crest or other site. The bone graft is prepared and inserted into the joint space. The physician then applies internal fixation such as pins, screws, or a plate and screw device to stabilize the bone graft and maintain fusion of the joint. Muscles are reattached and incisions are closed in layers.

27282

27282 Arthrodesis, symphysis pubis (including obtaining graft)

Fusion of the symphysis pubis is performed to treat pain, instability, and/or inflammation (osteitis pubis) of the joint. The skin is incised over the lower abdomen and pubis. The incision is carried down through Scarpa's and Camper's fasciae to expose the abdominal fascia. An incision is made along the linea alba. The bladder is protected and the rectus abdominis insertion is lifted off the bone to expose the symphysis pubis. The fibrocartilaginous disc and hyaline cartilage is debrided using a curette or drill until bleeding is encountered in the cancellous bone. The iliac crest is exposed and the cortical bone is incised. A cancellous bone graft is harvested and packed into the symphysis pubis. A plate and screw device is then used to stabilize the joint. A drain may be placed in the retropubic region and incisions are closed in layers.

27284-27286

27284 Arthrodesis, hip joint (including obtaining graft)
27286 Arthrodesis, hip joint (including obtaining graft); with subtrochanteric osteotomy

Although hip fusion is seldom performed today due to the success of hip replacement, it is sometimes performed in young patients who are heavy laborers and patients following failed hip replacement. A lateral incision is made over the hip joint. The femoral head is dislocated from the acetabulum. The articular surfaces of the femoral head and acetabulum are debrided down to bleeding cancellous bone. An incision is made over the iliac crest; the overlying bone is incised; and cancellous bone is harvested. The cancellous bone is prepared and packed into the joint space. The femoral head is returned to the hip socket and a plate and screw device is placed along the femur and pelvis to hold the hip joint stationary. As the bones heal together, they completely obliterate the joint and fuse the femoral head and acetabulum. Use 27284 for hip joint arthrodesis performed without subtrochanteric osteotomy. Use 27286 when subtrochnateric osteotomy is also performed. The hip is fused as described above followed by subtrochanteric osteotomy. The planned osteotomy sites are marked and a series of cuts are made in the subtrochanteric region on the femur. Bone is excised. Wedges created from the cut bone are strategically placed at the osteotomy sites to maintain the proper angles in the cut bone. Some of the excised cancellous bone may also be morsellized and used for bone grafting. Internal fixation including pins, screws, wires, or other devices is used as needed to maintain the shape and position of the bone.

27290

27290 Interpelviabdominal amputation (hindquarter amputation)

An interpelviabdominal amputation, also referred to as a hindquarter amputation, hemipelvectomy, or transpelvic amputation, involves amputation of half the pelvis and the leg on the same side. The procedure is rarely performed, only used in cases of severe trauma, infections such as gas gangrene, or malignant neoplasms such as Ewing's sarcoma, osteosarcoma, and chondrosarcoma that involve the lower extremity and pelvic girdle. The incision lines are marked on the skin over the pelvis, hip, and thigh. The skin and underlying soft tissue is incised. A myocutaneous flap is created from the overlying tissue if possible. Muscles of the abdomen, back, and hip are detached from bone and the bony pelvis and hip are exposed. The extent of the trauma, infection, or malignant neoplasm is assessed and the extent of the pelvectomy is determined. Blood vessels are suture ligated and transected. Bones of the pelvis are cut along the planned amputation site using a bone saw. The pelvis and lower extremity are completely severed and sent for pathological examination. Drains are placed in the pelvis. The previously created myocutaneous flap is used to cover the surgical wound.

27295

27295 Disarticulation of hip

Hip disarticulation is a rarely performed procedure that involves amputation of the leg at the hip joint. The procedure is performed for severe trauma such as crush injuries, infections such as gas gangrene, failed vascular procedures on the lower extremity, or

Musculoskeletal System

● New Code   ▲ Revised Code

for malignant neoplasms such as Ewing's sarcoma, osteosarcoma, and chondrosarcoma involving the proximal femur. The incision lines are marked on the skin over the hip and thigh. The skin and underlying soft tissue are incised beginning at the anteromedial aspect of the hip joint. The incision is carried laterally over the greater trochanter and then over the posterior aspect of the hip joint. A myocutaneous flap is created from the overlying tissue if possible. Femoral vessels are exposed, suture ligated, and transected. The anterior musculature is transected at the level of the greater trochanter. The adductor attachments are transected at their origins on the ischium and pubic rami. The posterior musculature is then transected at the ischium. The sciatic nerve is transected. Gluteal vessels are ligated and transected. The femoral head is then disarticulated and the entire leg is amputated at the hip. Drains are placed in the hip region. The previously created myocutaneous flap is used to cover the surgical wound.

27301

27301   Incision and drainage, deep abscess, bursa, or hematoma, thigh or knee region

To treat an abscess or hematoma in the thigh or knee area, an incision is made in the skin over the abscess or hematoma site and carried down through the soft tissue. The abscess or hematoma is opened. If drainage is performed for an abscess, any loculations are broken up using blunt finger dissection. If drainage is for a hematoma, blood clots are removed by suction. The abscess or hematoma cavity is flushed with saline or antibiotic solution. To treat an infected bursa, an incision is made in the skin over the bursa. The bursa is opened with a scalpel and drained. The site is flushed with saline or antibiotic solution. Drains are placed as needed. The incision may be closed in layers or packed with gauze and left open.

27303

27303   Incision, deep, with opening of bone cortex, femur or knee (eg, osteomyelitis or bone abscess)

The bone cortex of the femoral shaft, distal femur or tibial plateau is opened to treat a condition such as osteomyelitis or bone abscess. An incision is made in the skin and carried down through the soft tissue overlying the site of the infected bone. The periosteum over the infected region of the bone is elevated, a button of cortical bone removed, and the bone marrow exposed. Opening the bone cortex relieves pressure caused by inflammation of the bone marrow and prevents restriction of blood flow to the infected bone. If frank pus is encountered, the button hole may be enlarged and extended using a chisel or gouge along the bone for one to two inches. If the epiphysis is involved, a section of the epiphyseal cortex may be removed. The bone abscess is drained.

27305

27305   Fasciotomy, iliotibial (tenotomy), open

The iliotibial tendon, also referred to as the iliotibial band, is a long tendon that extends from the upper thigh to the lateral aspect of the leg and inserts at the tibia, attaching the tensor fasciae latae muscle at the knee. If the iliotibial tendon becomes contracted, it can cause pain and instability of the knee. An incision is made over the lateral aspect of the knee joint and the iliotibial tendon is exposed. The posterior aspect of the iliotibial band is then incised to relieve excessive tightness affecting knee joint stability. Range of motion is tested to ensure that an adequate release has been achieved. Incisions are closed in layers.

27306-27307

27306   Tenotomy, percutaneous, adductor or hamstring; single tendon (separate procedure)
27307   Tenotomy, percutaneous, adductor or hamstring; multiple tendons

Hamstring tenotomy is used to treat flexion deformities of the knee and adductor tenotomy along with hamstring tenotomy is used to improve gait in patients with cerebral palsy. The hamstring consists of three muscles, the biceps femoris, semitendinosus, and semimembranosus. These muscles extend the knee and flex the thigh. The gracilis muscle flexes and adducts the thigh. In 27306, a percutaneous tenotomy on the gracilis tendon or a single hamstring tendon is performed. A stab incision is made in the popliteal crease over the tendon insertion site in the tibia. Without enlarging the puncture site, the gracilis or hamstring tendon is divided. A long leg or cylinder cast is applied with the knee extended. Use 27307 to report division of multiple tendons in one leg.

27310

27310   Arthrotomy, knee, with exploration, drainage, or removal of foreign body (eg, infection)

A skin incision is made over of the knee joint. Tissues are dissected and the joint capsule is exposed. The joint capsule is opened and the knee joint explored. If an infection is present, fluid including blood and purulent matter is drained from the knee. Cultures are obtained and sent separately reportable laboratory analysis. The knee is flushed with saline solution to remove any debris. Any foreign bodies are located and removed. The knee is again

flushed with saline solution. Drains are placed as needed. The incision closed in layers around the drain. A dressing is applied.

27323-27324

27323   Biopsy, soft tissue of thigh or knee area; superficial
27324   Biopsy, soft tissue of thigh or knee area; deep (subfascial or intramuscular)

Soft tissues include muscles, tendons, fat, blood vessels, lymph vessels, nerves, and tissues surrounding the joints. Local, regional, or general anesthesia or conscious sedation is administered depending on the site and depth of the planned biopsy. The skin over the biopsy site is cleansed. An incision is made and tissue dissected down to the mass or lesion taking care to protect blood vessels and nerves. A tissue sample is obtained and sent to the laboratory for separately reportable histological evaluation. The incision is closed with sutures. Use 27323 for a superficial biopsy or 27324 for biopsy of deeper tissues requiring more extensive dissection of overlying tissues, such as a biopsy below the muscle fascia (subfascial) or within the muscle itself (intramuscular).

27325-27326

27325   Neurectomy, hamstring muscle
27326   Neurectomy, popliteal (gastrocnemius)

The physician excises a segment of nerve innervating the hamstring muscle. This procedure may be done to alleviate cases of clonus or successive spasms of the muscle. An incision is made transversely across the hamstring muscle and the fascia is divided to reach the innervating nerves. The correct nerve is identified by applying electrical current or gentle pressure to produce the muscle spasm. The nerve is then divided to sever the connection of electrical impulses to the muscle and is removed. The wound is then closed. Code 27326 for a similar neurectomy procedure performed on the popliteal or gastrocnemius muscle behind the knee.

27327-27328

27327   Excision, tumor, soft tissue of thigh or knee area, subcutaneous; less than 3 cm
27328   Excision, tumor, soft tissue of thigh or knee area, subfascial (eg, intramuscular); less than 5 cm

Soft tissues include subcutaneous fat and connective tissue, fascia, muscles, tendons, blood vessels, lymph vessels, nerves, and tissues surrounding the joints. Soft tissue tumors may be benign or malignant. Benign tumors are typically treated by excision, although small malignant or indeterminate tumors may be excised if the margins are well defined. Depending on the location of the tumor in the soft tissue of the thigh or knee area, the skin over the tumor may be incised or a skin flap created and elevated. Overlying tissue is dissected and the soft tissue mass exposed. The tumor is then excised along with a margin of healthy tissue. Separately reportable frozen section may be performed to ensure that all margins are free of tumor cells. Drains are placed as needed and the surgical wound is closed in layers. For tumors in the subcutaneous fat or connective tissue, use 27327 for excision of less than 3 cm. For tumors that lie below the fascia, use 27328 for excision of less than 5 cm. Subfascial soft tissue tumors include those within muscle tissue.

27329

27329   Radical resection of tumor (eg, sarcoma), soft tissue of thigh or knee area; less than 5 cm

Soft tissues include muscles, tendons, fat, blood vessels, lymph vessels, nerves, and tissues surrounding the joints. Soft tissue tumors may be benign or malignant. Radical resection is typically performed for a malignant neoplasm, such as a sarcoma, although benign tumors and tumors of indeterminate nature may also require radical resection. A skin incision is made over the tumor in the thigh or knee area, or a skin flap is created and elevated. Overlying tissue is dissected and the tumor exposed. The tumor is removed en bloc along with a wide margin of surrounding tissue. Radical resection involves excision of all involved soft tissue which may include muscles, nerves, and blood vessels. Separately reportable frozen section is performed to ensure that all margins are free of tumor cells. If margins show evidence of malignancy, additional tissue is removed until all margins are free of tumor cells. Drains are placed as needed. The surgical wound may be closed in layers, or separately reportable reconstructive procedures performed. Use 27329 for radical resection of soft tissue tumor in the thigh or knee of less than 5 cm.

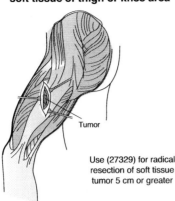

Radical resection of tumor soft tissue of thigh or knee area

Tumor

Use (27329) for radical resection of soft tissue tumor 5 cm or greater

27330-27331

27330   Arthrotomy, knee; with synovial biopsy only
27331   Arthrotomy, knee; including joint exploration, biopsy, or removal of loose or foreign bodies

A skin incision is made over the knee joint. Tissues are dissected and the joint capsule is exposed. The joint capsule is opened. The knee is flushed with saline solution to remove any debris. The knee joint is examined for evidence of injury or disease. In 27330, a synovial biopsy is performed. Synovial tissue lines the knee joint and produces synovial fluid. It can become inflamed due to rheumatoid arthritis, synovial proliferative disorder, or other condition. Synovial tissue samples are taken and sent for separately reportable laboratory analysis. In 27331, the joint is explored. Any loose or foreign bodies are identified and removed. Tissue samples are obtained as needed and sent for separately reportable laboratory analysis. The knee is again flushed with saline solution and the incision closed in layers.

27332-27333

27332   Arthrotomy, with excision of semilunar cartilage (meniscectomy) knee; medial OR lateral
27333   Arthrotomy, with excision of semilunar cartilage (meniscectomy) knee; medial AND lateral

Excision or resection of the meniscus is performed on a torn meniscus that cannot be repaired. Typically resection is performed on tears that extend into the non-vascular region where they are unlikely to heal even if repaired. A skin incision is made over of the knee joint. Tissues are dissected and the joint capsule is exposed. The joint capsule is opened. The knee is flushed with saline solution to remove any debris. The knee joint is examined and the tear is located and probed with a small hook to determine the extent of the tear. The torn fragment is then resected and removed using forceps, motorized shaver, scissors, or knives. Only the damaged portion of the meniscus is removed. The edge of the remaining meniscus is smoothed with a motorized shaver. The knee is flushed with saline solution to remove debris and reinspected. If there are meniscal tears in both the medial and lateral compartments, the tear in the second compartment is addressed next and the meniscus removed in the same manner. Upon completion of the procedure the joint capsule is closed followed by soft tissue and skin which are closed in layers. A compressive dressing is then applied. Use 27332 when only one meniscus, medial or lateral, is resected. Use 27333 when both the medial and lateral menisci are partially or totally resected.

27334-27335

27334   Arthrotomy, with synovectomy, knee; anterior OR posterior
27335   Arthrotomy, with synovectomy, knee; anterior AND posterior including popliteal area

Synovial tissue lines the knee joint and produces synovial fluid. When it becomes inflamed due to rheumatoid arthritis, synovial proliferative disorder, or other condition, the synovium produces excess synovial fluid resulting in joint effusion. A skin incision is made over of the knee joint. Tissues are dissected and the joint capsule is exposed. The joint capsule is opened. The knee is flushed with saline solution to remove any debris. The knee joint is examined for evidence of disease, injury or infection. A motorized shaver is then used to remove the synovium. Care is taken to resect all inflamed synovial tissue without damaging underlying vascular or nervous tissue. Upon completion of the procedure, bleeding is controlled by electrocautery, the joint capsule is closed followed by soft tissue and skin which are closed in layers. A compressive dressing is applied. Use 27334 for a synovectomy of the anterior or posterior compartment. Use 27334 for a synovectomy of the anterior and posterior compartments including the popliteal area.

27337-27339

27337   Excision, tumor, soft tissue of thigh or knee area, subcutaneous; 3 cm or greater
27339   Excision, tumor, soft tissue of thigh or knee area, subfascial (eg, intramuscular); 5 cm or greater

Soft tissues include subcutaneous fat and connective tissue, fascia, muscles, tendons, blood vessels, lymph vessels, nerves, and tissues surrounding the joints. Soft tissue tumors may be benign or malignant. Benign tumors are typically treated by excision, although small malignant or indeterminate tumors may be excised if the margins are well defined. Depending on the location of the tumor in the soft tissue of the thigh or knee area, the skin over the tumor may be incised or a skin flap created and elevated. Overlying tissue is dissected and the soft tissue mass exposed. The tumor is then excised along with a margin of healthy tissue. Separately reportable frozen section may be performed to ensure that all margins are free of tumor cells. Drains are placed as needed and the surgical wound is closed in layers. For tumors in the subcutaneous fat or connective tissue, use 27337 for soft tissue excision of 3 cm or greater. For tumors that lie below the fascia, use 27339 for excision of soft tissue 5 cm or greater. Subfascial soft tissue tumors include those within muscle tissue.

27340

27340   Excision, prepatellar bursa

The prepatellar bursa is a fluid-filled sac located in front of the patella (knee-cap) directly beneath the skin of the knee. The prepatellar bursa allows the patella to slide freely beneath the skin as the knee is bent and straightened. An incision is made in the skin over the top of the knee and the prepatellar bursa is removed (excised). The skin is repaired with sutures.

27345

27345   Excision of synovial cyst of popliteal space (eg, Baker's cyst)

A synovial cyst in the popliteal space, also referred to as a popliteal or Baker's cyst, is excised. A synovial cyst in the popliteal space is characterized by swelling and tightness behind the knee that may be accompanied by pain. An incision is made in the skin at the back of the knee over the popliteal cyst and carried down to the popliteal fossa. The cyst is visualized and is usually found between the medial head of the gastrocnemius and semimembranosus tendons. Blunt and sharp dissection are used to free the cyst down to its communication with the joint capsule. The base of the cyst is excised. The joint capsule where the cyst originated is visualized and any defect in the joint capsule is identified and repaired. The defect may be reinforced using a synthetic patch placed over the joint capsule.

27347

27347   Excision of lesion of meniscus or capsule (eg, cyst, ganglion), knee

A cyst is a cavity or sac that is lined with epithelium and contains liquid or semisolid material. A ganglion is a cyst contained in fibrous tissue, muscle, bone, or cartilage. An incision is made in the skin over the site of the lesion in the meniscus or joint capsule of the knee. The lesion is exposed, dissected free of surrounding tissue, and removed. The incision is closed with sutures.

27350

27350   Patellectomy or hemipatellectomy

A complete or partial removal of the patella, also referred to as the kneecap, is typically performed to treat a non-healing injury, repeated dislocation, or severe arthritis of the patella causing significant pain. A vertical skin incision is made over the patella, soft tissues are dissected, and the patella is exposed and examined. Muscle and tendon attachments to the patella are severed. The physician then removes all or part of the patella. If part of the patella is removed, the remaining portion is smoothed using a motorized shaver. The quadriceps tendon and patellar tendon are then reattached to the remaining portion of the patella. If the patella has been completely removed, the quadriceps tendon and patellar tendon are sutured together to preserve the ability to extend the knee. Overlying soft tissue and skin are closed in layers.

27355-27358

27355   Excision or curettage of bone cyst or benign tumor of femur
27356   Excision or curettage of bone cyst or benign tumor of femur; with allograft
27357   Excision or curettage of bone cyst or benign tumor of femur; with autograft (includes obtaining graft)
27358   Excision or curettage of bone cyst or benign tumor of femur; with internal fixation (List in addition to code for primary procedure)

A bone cyst is a fluid filled space within the bone. Once common type is a unicameral or simple bone cyst, which is a benign lesion. A less common type is an aneurysmal bone cyst which consists of vascular tissue surrounding a blood filled cystic lesion. There are a number of different types of benign bone tumors including giant cell tumors,

Musculoskeletal System

chondromixoid fibromas, and enchondromas. In 27355, an incision is made in the skin over the site of lesion in the femoral shaft or distal femur. Soft tissues are dissected and the femur is exposed. If a cystic lesion is present, the bone is incised and a window created to open the cyst. Fluid is aspirated and sent to the laboratory for separately reportable analysis. A curette is inserted through the bone window and the lining of the cystic cavity is completely removed by curettage. Alternatively, some cystic lesions and most benign tumors are treated by excision. The lesion is exposed as described above. The physician then excises the benign lesion along with a margin of surrounding healthy bone. In 27356, the lesion is curetted or excised as described above. The defect is then packed with donor bone tissue (allograft). In 27357, the lesion is curetted or excised as described above. The physician then obtains healthy bone locally or from a separate site, such as the iliac crest. The bone autograft is packed into the defect in the femur. In 27358, following curettage or excision of the bone cyst or benign tumor performs, the physician then performs separately reportable internal fixation of the femur. Internal fixation may be required due to the size or the location of surgically created bony defect. Plates, screws, or other fixation devices are strategically placed to prevent fracture of the femur and/or secure the bone graft.

27360

27360   Partial excision (craterization, saucerization, or diaphysectomy) bone, femur, proximal tibia and/or fibula (eg, osteomyelitis or bone abscess)

The physician performs a partial excision of bone, also referred to as craterization, saucerization, or diaphysectomy to treat osteomyelitis or bone abscess of the femur, proximal tibia, or proximal fibula. Craterization and saucerization of bone involves removing infected and necrotic bone to form a shallow depression in the bone surface that will allow drainage from the infected area. Diaphysectomy involves removal of the infected portion of the shaft of a long bone. An incision is made in the skin and carried down through the soft tissue overlying the site of the osteomyelitis. Any soft tissue sinus tracts and devitalized soft tissue are resected. The area of nectrotic and infected bone is exposed. A series of drill holes are made in the necrotic and infected bone and the bone between the drill holes is excavated to create an oval window using an osteotome. The amount of bone removed is dependent on the extent of the infection. A curette may be used to remove devitalized tissue from the medullary canal. Debridement continues until punctate bleeding is identified in the exposed bony surface. When all devitalized and infected tissue has been removed, the wound is copiously irrigated with sterile saline or antibiotic solution. The surgical wound is loosely closed and a drain placed.

27364

27364   Radical resection of tumor (eg, sarcoma), soft tissue of thigh or knee area; 5 cm or greater

Soft tissues include muscles, tendons, fat, blood vessels, lymph vessels, nerves, and tissues surrounding the joints. Soft tissue tumors may be benign or malignant. Radical resection is typically performed for a malignant neoplasm, such as a sarcoma, although benign tumors and tumors of indeterminate nature may also require radical resection. A skin incision is made over the tumor in the thigh or knee area, or a skin flap is created and elevated. Overlying tissue is dissected and the tumor exposed. The tumor is removed en bloc along with a wide margin of surrounding tissue. Radical resection involves excision of all involved soft tissue which may include muscles, nerves, and blood vessels. Separately reportable frozen section is performed to ensure that all margins are free of tumor cells. If margins show evidence of malignancy, additional tissue is removed until all margins are free of tumor cells. Drains are placed as needed. The surgical wound may be closed in layers, or separately reportable reconstructive procedures performed. Use 27364 for radical resection of a soft tissue tumor 5 cm or greater in the thigh or knee.

27365

27365   Radical resection of tumor, femur or knee

Radical resection is typically performed for a malignant neoplasm although benign tumors and tumors of indeterminate nature may also require radical resection. A skin incision is made over the site of the bone tumor, or a skin flap is created and elevated. Overlying tissue is dissected and the tumor exposed. All bone and cartilage with tumor involvement in the femur or knee is resected. The tumor is removed en bloc along with a wide margin of surrounding tissue. Radical resection of bone includes excision of all involved soft tissue which may include muscles, tendons, fat, blood vessels, lymph vessels, nerves, and tissues surrounding the joints. Separately reportable frozen section is performed to ensure that all margins are free of tumor cells. If margins show evidence of malignancy, additional tissue is removed until all margins are free of tumor cells. Drains are placed as needed. The surgical wound may be closed in layers, or separately reportable reconstructive procedures performed.

27370

27370   Injection of contrast for knee arthrography

Contrast is injected prior to knee arthrography. The skin over the injection site is cleansed and a local anesthetic is injected. A needle may be inserted into the joint and fluid aspirated with a syringe. The radiopaque substance is then injected into the knee joint,

which is exercised to help distribute the radiopaque substance. Once the contrast has been distributed throughout the joint, separately reportable radiographic images are obtained.

27372

27372   Removal of foreign body, deep, thigh region or knee area

Separately reportable radiographs may be obtained to localize the foreign body. The skin is cleansed and an incision is made over the site. Muscle, tendon, and/or ligaments overlying the foreign object are divided and tissue is dissected until the foreign body can be removed or excised along with any granulomatous tissue encapsulating it.

27380-27381

27380   Suture of infrapatellar tendon; primary
27381   Suture of infrapatellar tendon; secondary reconstruction, including fascial or tendon graft

The infrapatellar tendon is actually a ligament that connects the tibia and patella. The infrapatellar tendon is sometimes referred to as the patellar tendon. A midline incision is made extending from the top of the patella to the medial aspect of the tibial tubercle. Medial and lateral flaps are created to facilitate exploration of the medial and lateral retinacula. The torn infrapatellar tendon is identified and mobilized. The infrapatellar tendon is debrided. Depending on the site of the tear, the tibial tubercle and/or inferior pole of the patella is also debrided. Sutures are placed in the torn tendon. The bony surface of the tibial tubercle and/or inferior pole of the patella are prepared by drilling tunnels or placing suture anchors. The tendon sutures are then passed through the tunnels or suture anchors and the infrapatellar tendon is secured to the bone. A second drill hole may be created in the tibial tubercle and a suture passed from the tibial tubercle through the quadriceps tendon at the upper pole of the patella. Patellar height is evaluated. Once correct patellar height is attained, the infrapatellar tendon sutures are tied. The wound is irrigated and the incision closed. Use 27381 for secondary suture repair of the infrapatellar tendon including any required fascial or tendon grafts. An incision is made over the site of the old infrapatellar tendon defect. Scar tissue is dissected and the injured infrapatellar tendon identified. A fascial or tendon autograft or allograft is fashioned and first secured to the remaining infrapatellar tendon remnant and then to the previously prepared bone tunnels in the tibial tubercle and/or inferior pole of the patella.

27385-27386

27385   Suture of quadriceps or hamstring muscle rupture; primary
27386   Suture of quadriceps or hamstring muscle rupture; secondary reconstruction, including fascial or tendon graft

Tears and ruptures of the quadriceps muscle usually affect the indirect (distal) head of the rectus femoris. Complete rupture of the hamstring muscle requiring surgery is a rare injury that typically occurs proximally near the ischium. In 27385, a ruptured quadriceps or hamstring muscle is repaired. For quadriceps muscle/tendon rupture, an anterior longitudinal incision is made in the midline over the quadriceps muscle and extended over the patella. The patella is exposed and the ruptured ends of the quadriceps muscle are located. Drill holes are created in the patella. Sutures are placed in the torn quadriceps muscle/tendon. The muscle/tendon sutures are then passed through the drill holes and tied over the distal pole of the patella. Range of motion is evaluated. The wound is irrigated and the incision closed. For hamstring rupture, a longitudinal incision is made over the site of the defect. Soft tissues are dissected taking care to protect the sciatic nerve. The ruptured ends of the hamstring muscle/tendon are located and tagged. Sutures are passed through the remaining proximal end of the ruptured tendon or through the ischium and then passed through the proximal aspect of the distal tendon remnant. Use 27386 for secondary suture repair of the quadriceps or hamstring muscle/tendon including any required fascial or tendon grafts. An incision is made over the site of the old muscle/tendon defect. Scar tissue is dissected and the injured muscle/tendon identified. A fascial or tendon autograft or allograft is fashioned and first secured to the remaining quadriceps or hamstring muscle/tendon remnant and then to the passed through the previously prepared bone tunnels the patella and secured.

27390-27392

27390   Tenotomy, open, hamstring, knee to hip; single tendon
27391   Tenotomy, open, hamstring, knee to hip; multiple tendons, 1 leg
27392   Tenotomy, open, hamstring, knee to hip; multiple tendons, bilateral

Hamstring tenotomy is used to treat flexion deformities of the knee. The hamstring consists of three muscles, the biceps femoris, semitendinosus, and semimembranosus. These muscles extend the knee and flex the thigh. In 27390, an open tenotomy on a single hamstring tendon is performed. An incision is made in the popliteal crease over the tendon insertion site in the tibia. Soft tissues are dissected and the tendon to be divided is exposed. The tendon is incised and divided. A long leg or cylinder cast is applied with the knee extended. Use 27392 to report division of multiple hamstring tendons in one leg and 27392 to report division of multiple tendons in both legs.

27393-27395

27393	Lengthening of hamstring tendon; single tendon
27394	Lengthening of hamstring tendon; multiple tendons, 1 leg
27395	Lengthening of hamstring tendon; multiple tendons, bilateral

The physician lengthens the hamstring tendons. Hamstring lenthening is performed to treat spastic cerebral palsy, meningomyelocele, or other neurological disorders that create a muscle imbalance resulting in flexed-knee gait. The hamstring consists of three muscles: the biceps femoris, semitendinosus, and semimembranosus. These muscles extend the knee and flex the thigh. In 27393, a single hamstring tendon is lengthened. An incision is made in the popliteal crease over the tendon insertion site in the tibia. The tendon to be lengthened is exposed. A Z-shaped incision is made in the tendon which lengthens it by allowing the tendon fibers to slide apart as the knee is extended. Tendon sutures are placed to maintain the tendon in the lengthened position. A long leg or cylinder cast is applied with the knee extended. Use 27394 to report lengthening of multiple hamstring tendons in one leg and 27395 to report lengthening of multiple tendons in both legs.

27396-27397

27396	Transplant or transfer (with muscle redirection or rerouting), thigh (eg, extensor to flexor); single tendon
27397	Transplant or transfer (with muscle redirection or rerouting), thigh (eg, extensor to flexor); multiple tendons

Any muscle within the thigh is transplanted or transferred, redirecting or rerouting muscle action to any part of the thigh, including transplant or transfer of any tendon, whether extensor or flexor. Muscular imbalance in the thigh causes knee problems and difficulty walking. Different tendon transfer procedures in the thigh may be done to minimize the dysfunction by redirecting the forces in the muscles. Muscle transfer may also be used to reduce spasticity in certain cases. In 27396, a single tendon/muscle transplant is done. For example, the rectus femoris is one of the four quadriceps muscles attached to the patella as a knee extensor at one end and above the hip on the pelvis at the other end. The muscle acts on behalf of both the knee and hip. If knee function is stifled, the physician may transfer the rectus femoris off the pelvis onto the femur, recessing the muscle and sacrificing one of its actions, so that hip motion is no longer felt or reacted to, and the muscle supplies motion and sensory information only for the knee. In another kind of transfer, the muscle may be given an entirely new function, such as when the physician detaches the distal end of the rectus femoris near the knee and reattaches it behind the knee, to act as a knee flexor. With the muscle reattached to the backside of the knee, the tugs and pulls from the hip movement at the top of the muscle will now cause reactions that flex the knee, rather than extend it. In 27397, multiple tendons/muscles may be transferred or rerouted, such as when the rectus femoris is transferred off the pelvis onto the femur and a hamstring is also transplanted to provide a rotator for the thigh.

27400

27400	Transfer, tendon or muscle, hamstrings to femur (eg, Egger's type procedure)

Tendon or muscle transfer of hamstrings to the distal femur is performed using an Egger's type procedure. This is performed to treat spastic cerebral palsy, meningomyelocele, or other neurological disorders that create a muscle imbalance resulting in flexed-knee gait. The hamstring consists of three muscles: the biceps femoris, semitendinosus, and semimembranosus. These muscles extend the knee and flex the thigh. The insertion of the hamstring tendons on the proximal tibia are first exposed using a horizontal incision at the popliteal crease. The hamstring tendons are then divided and transferred to the proximal aspect of the femoral condyles and anchored into position.

27403

27403	Arthrotomy with meniscus repair, knee

A torn meniscus is repaired when the tear occurs in the outer vascular region of the meniscus where it has the necessary blood supply to heal. A skin incision is made over the involved knee compartment. The joint capsule is incised and the knee inspected to identify evidence of disease, injury, or infection. The tear is located and probed to determine the extent of the tear. The edges of the meniscus tear are prepared using a small rasp or motorized shaver. Blood supply is evaluated. To enhance healing when blood supply is questionable, a blood clot may be placed between opposing edges, small vascular access channels may be created around the periphery of the tear, or the joint lining may be abraded to encourage bleeding. The meniscus is then repaired with sutures, absorbable tacks, or other internal fixation devices. The knee is flushed with saline solution to remove debris. The joint capsule is closed followed by layered closure of overlying soft tissue. A compressive dressing is applied.

27405-27409

27405	Repair, primary, torn ligament and/or capsule, knee; collateral
27407	Repair, primary, torn ligament and/or capsule, knee; cruciate
27409	Repair, primary, torn ligament and/or capsule, knee; collateral and cruciate ligaments

There are four major ligaments that stabilize the knee. The anterior cruciate ligament (ACL) is located in the center of the knee joint connecting the femur to the tibia. The posterior cruciate ligament (PCL) is located in the center of the knee behind the ACL and also connects the femur to the tibia. Both cruciate ligaments provide rotational stability in the knee. Injury to either ligament can cause the knee to buckle. The medial collateral ligament (MCL) is located on the inner aspect of the knee and the lateral collateral ligament (LCL) on the outer aspect. The MCL and LCL are less frequently injured and rarely require surgical repair. Ligament injuries involve tears in the ligament with or without injury to the joint capsule. A skin incision is made over the involved region of the knee. Soft tissues are dissected. If an isolated MCL or LCL tear being repaired, the involved ligament is exposed and inspected. The tear is repaired with sutures. Suture anchors may be used to supplement the repair. If the ACL or PCL is injured, the joint capsule is incised and the knee is inspected. The affected ligament is then repaired with sutures. Any capsular tears are also repaired. Use 27405 for repair of a torn MCL or LCL and/or capsule. Use 27407 for repair of a torn ACL or PCL and/or capsule. Use 27409 for repair multi-ligament injuries involving the collateral and cruciate ligaments. These codes are used only for the primary repair of the ligaments and/or joint capsules.

27412

27412	Autologous chondrocyte implantation, knee

The most common sites in the knee treated using chondrocyte implantation include the distal femoral condyles or trochlea, and the patellofemoral joint. Several weeks or months prior to the implantation procedure, chondrocytes are harvested from the patient in a separately reportable procedure by taking biopsies of the synovial tissue of the knee. The synovial biopsies are then prepared for implantation in the laboratory using cellular expansion technique. Once sufficient chondrocyte expansion has occurred, the patient returns for the implantation procedure. An skin incision is made over the knee and soft tissue dissected. The joint capsule is incised and the defect in the knee exposed. The diseased articular cartilage is excised and a bed created for placement of the prepared chondrocytes. A periosteal patch is harvested and contoured to completely cover the defect. The patch is sutured into place leaving an opening to allow implantation of the chondrocytes. The choncrocytes are implanted under the patch and the unclosed edge of the patch sealed using sutures and glue. The joint capsule is closed with sutures followed by layered closure of the soft tissue and skin.

27415

27415	Osteochondral allograft, knee, open

This procedure uses small, cylindrical osteochondral grafts to smooth and resurface the articular cartilage. A skin incision is made over the involved knee compartment. The joint capsule is incised and the knee is inspected to identify the area of cartilage damage. The damaged area is measured and the number of grafts required to repair the cartilage determined. The damaged cartilage is debrided, drilled, and prepared for implantation of donor osteochondral grafts (allografts) obtained from a bone bank. One or more allografts are prepared to fit the articular surface defect, placed into the defect and stabilized. Range of motion is checked to ensure that the allografts are stable. Upon completion of the procedure, the arthroscope and surgical tools are removed, and portal incisions are closed.

27416

27416	Osteochondral autograft(s), knee, open (eg, mosaicplasty) (includes harvesting of autograft[s])

Osteochondral autografts are harvested from the patient's healthy knee tissue and applied to the damaged articular surface of the knee using an open mosaicplasty technique that involves harvesting a number of small cylindrical osteochondral plugs from non-weight bearing regions of the knee and transplanting them into the site of the osteochondral defect. A skin incision is made over the involved knee compartment. The joint capsule is incised (arthrotomy) and the damaged tissue is debrided and prepared for transplant. The donor site is selected and the harvest device is directed in an exact perpendicular line to the articular surface to harvest osteochondral tissue. The recipient site is prepared by using an appropriate sized drill and matching the size and shape of the drilled tunnel to the harvested tissue. The osteochondral autograft is then inserted into the prepared recipient site. This process is repeated until the defect is filled or there is no more healthy tissue available at the donor site.

27418

27418	Anterior tibial tubercleplasty (eg, Maquet type procedure)

The physician performs an anterior tibial tubercleplasty to treat patellar instability. This procedure may also be referred to as a Maquet or Fulkerson osteotomy. An incision is made lateral to the patella across the tibial tuberosity and carried distally along the anterior ridge of the tibia. Muscles overlying the anterior compartment are elevated. The medial and lateral borders of the patellar tendon and tibial tuberosity are exposed. An incision is made through the periosteum distal to the tuberosity. K-wires are inserted from the anteromedial tibial surface to the posterolateral surface. A medial osteotomy cut is made that follows the plane of the K-wires followed by a lateral osteotomy cut directed anteriorly. The tibial tuberosity is then repositioned and the patella is aligned within the intercondylar groove. Patellar tracking is assessed for any under or over correction. Once proper alignment is achieved, one or more screws are placed to secure the tibial tuberosity.

27420

27420   Reconstruction of dislocating patella; (eg, Hauser type procedure)

The physician performs a reconstruction for a dislocating patella. In 27420, a distal transfer of the tibial tuberosity, also referred to as a Hauser procedure, is performed. An incision is made lateral to the patella across the tibial tuberosity and carried distally along the anterior ridge of the tibia. Muscles overlying the anterior compartment are elevated. The medial and lateral borders of the patellar tendon and tibial tuberosity are exposed. An incision is made through the periosteum distal to the tuberosity. Osteotomy is then performed to free the tibial tuberosity distally, medially, and laterally. A portion of the tuberosity is removed at the distal end and the remainder of the tuberosity is temporarily secured to the underlying bony bed. The patella is aligned within the intercondylar groove. Patellar tracking is assessed for any under or over correction. Once proper alignment is achieved, one or more screws are placed to secure the tibial tuberosity.

27422

27422   Reconstruction of dislocating patella; with extensor realignment and/or muscle advancement or release (eg, Campbell, Goldwaite type procedure)

Reconstruction of a dislocating patella is performed by extensor realignment and/or muscle advancement or release. This procedure may also be referred to as a Campbell or Goldwaite procedure. If extensor realignment is needed, the patellar tendon is split vertically. The lateral half is detached from the tibial tuberosity, pulled under the medial half, and then reattached to the tuberosity. This positions the patella medially and helps prevent lateral shift of the patella. If muscle advancement is required, the quadriceps (vastus medialis) is dissected off the patella and the quadriceps tendon is split. The quadriceps muscle is then advanced onto the patella, and when appropriate tension is achieved, the muscle is secured with suture anchors or periosteal stitches. Osteotomy is then performed and the tibial tubercle is repositioned to allow proper tracking of the patella. Patellar tracking is evaluated, and when optimal alignment is achieved, the tibial tubercle is secured with screws.

27424

27424   Reconstruction of dislocating patella; with patellectomy

Reconstruction of a dislocating patella is performed with patellectomy. A longitudinal, tendon-splitting incision is made over the patella. The quadriceps tendon and patellar ligament are carefully dissected off the patella. The patella is then excised. The patellectomy defect is then closed longitudinally. The quadriceps muscle may be advanced laterally and distally over the defect and plicated to increase the angle of insertion at the sagittal plane which may help to preserve quadriceps strength and function following removal of the patella.

27425

27425   Lateral retinacular release, open

An open lateral retinacular release is performed to treat misalignment of the patella. A longitudinal incision is made just lateral to the patella, extending from the superior pole of the patella to Gerdy's tubercle. The incision is extended down to the lateral retinaculum and a subcutaneous flap is created. The lateral retinaculum is incised longitudinally from the vastus medialis to a point just distal to Gerdy's tubercle. Patellar mobility is evaluated. If further dissection is required, the lateral retinacular flap is dissected off the deep fibers and the deep retinacular tissue is incised parallel to the superficial retinaculum. Patellar mobility is again evaluated. When adequate mobility is achieved, the medial layer of the deep retinaculum is sutured to the lateral edge of the superficial retinaculum.

27427-27429

27427   Ligamentous reconstruction (augmentation), knee; extra-articular
27428   Ligamentous reconstruction (augmentation), knee; intra-articular (open)
27429   Ligamentous reconstruction (augmentation), knee; intra-articular (open) and extra-articular

There are four major ligaments that stabilize the knee. The anterior cruciate ligament (ACL) is located in the center of the knee joint connecting the femur to the tibia. The posterior cruciate ligament (PCL) is located in the center of the knee behind the ACL and also connects the femur to the tibia. The medial collateral ligament (MCL) is located on the inner aspect of the knee and the lateral collateral ligament (LCL) on the outer aspect. The MCL and LCL are less frequently injured and rarely require surgical reconstruction or augmentation. There are two types of reconstruction, extra-articular and intra-articular.

Extra-articular reconstruction uses structures outside the joint to reinforce the ACL and PCL and stabilize the knee. One technique is to tighten the iliotibial tract to prevent lateral movement of the knee. Extra-articular procedures are not commonly performed. To perform intra-articular reconstruction of a damaged ACL, the joint capsule is incised and the ACL inspected. A shaver is introduced and the ACL is removed. The notch where the ACL was located is inspected and widened using a burr. If the patellar tendon is being used to reconstruct the ACL, the central third of the patellar tendon is harvested with a bone block at each end. Sutures are placed through the bone blocks. A drill guide is positioned on the tibia. The guide wire is then drilled into place exiting within the knee joint at the attachment site of the original ACL. The drill hole in the tibia is then made. A femoral drill guide is then passed through the tibial drill hole. The drill guide is positioned on the posterior aspect of the femur. The femoral guide wire is placed and the femoral drill hole made. The patellar tendon or other graft material is placed through the drill holes and secured with screws. An intra-articular reconstruction of a torn PCL is performed in the same manner except that the damaged PCL is removed and the reconstruction may be performed using a tibial tunnel or tibial inlay technique. In addition, a portion of the Achilles tendon may be harvested and used in PCL reconstruction. Use 27427 for extra-articular ligamentous reconstruction or augmentation of the knee, use 27428 for an intra-articular procedure, or use 27429 for a combined intra-articular and extra-articular procedure.

27430

27430   Quadricepsplasty (eg, Bennett or Thompson type)

The quadriceps is a composite muscle that includes the rectus femoris, vastus lateralis, vastus medialis, and vastus intermedius. All four components have insertion sites at the upper border and sides of the patella and the tibial tuberosity through the patellar ligament and serve to extend the knee. The rectus femoris also flexes the thigh. Quadricepsplasty is typically performed on patients with a previous injury to the thigh muscle or bone resulting in severe quadriceps scarring with loss of knee mobility. In a Thompson type quadricepsplasty, an incision is made in the anterior thigh extending from the upper third of the thigh to the lower border of the patella. The fascia is divided on either side of the rectus femoris, which is retracted to expose the vastus lateralis, vastus medialis, and vastus intermedius. The vastus medialis and vastus lateralis are freed and allowed to fall to the medial and lateral sides. The knee joint capsule is divided over the medial and lateral aspects of the patella. The incisions over the joint capsule are extended until the contracture of the capsule is released. The vastus intermedius is exposed. The scar tissue which may involve the entire vastus intermedius is excised leaving only fibrous and periosteal tissue over the anterior femur. The knee is then manipulated to sever any remaining intra-articular adhesions. If the vastus medialis and/or vastus lateralis are normal (free of scar tissue), they are then sutured to the rectus femoris. If the vastus medialis and/or vastus lateralis are badly scarred, they are not attached. Instead, subcutaneous tissue and fat are brought down and sutured to the rectus femoris to create a new intermuscular septum and eliminate all scar tissue from the remaining quadriceps. The skin is then closed. A Bennett type quadricepsplasty differs in that the rectus femoris is not isolated from other components of the quadriceps, and the scarred portions of the quadriceps are lengthened rather than excised.

27435

27435   Capsulotomy, posterior capsular release, knee

A capsulotomy with posterior capsular release is performed on the knee to treat flexion contracture. An incision is made over the posteromedial aspect of the knee. The joint capsule is exposed and incised. Scar tissue is excised and the posterior capsule is detached from the femur. Range of motion is checked and incisions are closed in layers. A cast is applied as needed to maintain the knee in extension.

27437-27438

27437   Arthroplasty, patella; without prosthesis
27438   Arthroplasty, patella; with prosthesis

Arthroplasty of the patella or prosthetic resurfacing of the patella is performed to treat degenerative disease of the patellofemoral joint. An incision is made over the anteromedial aspect of the knee. The joint capsule is exposed and incised. The patellofemoral joint is inspected and any osteophytes along the borders of the intercondylar notch are excised. Patellar tracking is evaluated. In 27437, the patellar cartilage is inspected and any overgrowth is excised. The articular surface of the patella is smoothed. Patellar tracking is again checked. Incisions are closed in layers. In 27438, the patella is exposed as described above. Range of motion is evaluated and the geometric center of the patella is identified. Using an inset technique, cartilage and bone on the articular surface of the patella are resected. An appropriately sized patellar component is selected and affixed to the resurfaced patella. Using an inset technique, a channel is reamed through the full thickness of the patella. The patellar implant is then inset into the channel. Range of motion is again checked to ensure proper tracking of the patella. The surgical wound is closed in layers.

Musculoskeletal System

27440-27441

27440 Arthroplasty, knee, tibial plateau
27441 Arthroplasty, knee, tibial plateau; with debridement and partial synovectomy

Arthroplasty of the medial or lateral tibial plateau is performed to treat degenerative joint disease. The articular surface of proximal tibia is composed of the medial and lateral plateaus and the intercondylar eminence. The medial and lateral plateaus articulate with the medial and lateral femoral condyles respectively. In 27440, an incision is made over the anteromedial or anterolateral aspect of the knee depending on which plateau is affected. The joint capsule is incised and the medial and/or lateral compartment inspected. The proximal tibial surface is then prepared using intramedullary or extramedullary alignment rods to ensure proper alignment of the joint and bone angles. If degenerative joint disease has caused knee ligaments to become contracted, they are released. A trial component is placed and range of motion evaluated. The tibial component which consists of a metal tray and spacer is then placed on the tibia. The metal tray is secured to the bone with bone cement or screws. The spacer is then attached to the metal tray. Range of motion is checked. Overlying soft tissues and skin are repaired in layers. In 27441, debridement and partial synovectomy is performed in conjunction with the prosthetic replacement of one of the tibial plateaus. After the joint capsule has been incised and inspected, all damaged tissue including bone spurs and inflamed synovium is excised. The arthroplasty of the tibial plateau is then performed as described above.

27442-27443

27442 Arthroplasty, femoral condyles or tibial plateau(s), knee
27443 Arthroplasty, femoral condyles or tibial plateau(s), knee; with debridement and partial synovectomy

Arthroplasty of the femoral condyles or tibial plateaus is performed to treat degenerative joint disease. The articular surface of proximal tibia is composed of the medial and lateral plateaus and the intercondylar eminence. The medial and lateral plateaus articulate with the medial and lateral femoral condyles respectively. In 27442, an anterior incision is made over the knee joint. The joint capsule is incised and the knee joint inspected. If arthroplasty is performed on the femoral condyles, the distal femur is exposed and a cutting guide placed on the end of the femur to ensure that the bone cut is made in such a way that proper alignment of the joint and leg angles is maintained. Bone is then cut from the distal end of the femur. The prosthetic femoral component is then placed on the femur. If an uncemented prosthesis is used, it is pushed onto the carefully prepared femur and held in place by friction. If a cemented prosthesis is used, bone cement is used to secure the prosthesis to the bone. If arthroplasty is performed on the tibial plateaus, the proximal tibial surface is then prepared using intramedullary or extramedullary alignment rods to ensure proper alignment of the joint and bone angles. If degenerative joint disease has caused knee ligaments to become contracted, they are released. A trial component is placed and range of motion evaluated. The tibial component which consists of a metal tray and spacer is then placed on the tibia. The metal tray is secured to the bone with bone cement or screws. The spacer is then attached to the metal tray. Range of motion is checked. Overlying soft tissues and skin are repaired in layers. In 27443, debridement and partial synovectomy is performed in conjunction with the prosthetic replacement of the femoral condyles or tibial plateaus. After the joint capsule has been incised and inspected, all damaged tissue including bone spurs and inflamed synovium is excised. The arthroplasty of the femoal condyles or tibial plateaus is then performed as described above.

27445

27445 Arthroplasty, knee, hinge prosthesis (eg, Walldius type)

There are two basic types of knee prostheses, hinged and unlinked. This code reports knee arthroplasty using a hinged prosthesis. The Waldius hinged prosthesis is a first generation prosthesis and has largely been replaced with newer types such as the third generation S-ROM rotating hinged total knee prosthesis. Other hinged prostheses currently in use include the MOST, the Kotz, and the LINK. Hinged prostheses are generally used when there is degenerative joint disease or bone tumor with significant bone loss or when there is failure or other complication such as infection following placement of an unlinked type of prosthesis. An anterior incision is made over the knee joint. The joint capsule is incised and the knee joint inspected. Bone spurs and intra-articular soft tissues are excised. The distal femur is exposed and an intramedullary alignment system placed on the end of the femur to ensure that the bone cut is made in such a way that proper alignment of the joint and leg angles is maintained. Bone is cut from the distal end of the femur. The proximal tibial surface is prepared using intramedullary or extramedullary alignment rods in the same manner. If degenerative joint disease has caused knee ligaments to become contracted, they are released. The femur and tibia are sized and reamed. Trial components are placed and patellofemoral tracking evaluated if the patella has not been previously removed. Lateral release or medial reefing is performed as needed to ensure proper patellofemoral tracking. If there is significant patellofemoral degenerative joint disease, the patella is resurfaced with a polyethylene button. Depending on the type of femoral component being used, the stem is inserted into the femur and is either secured using a

press-fit technique or with bone cement. The tibial stem is secured to the proximal tibia in the same manner. Range of motion is evaluated. Soft tissues and skin are closed in layers.

27446

27446 Arthroplasty, knee, condyle and plateau; medial OR lateral compartment

A partial knee replacement, also called a unicompartmental knee replacement, is performed. An incision is made over the medial or lateral aspect of the knee depending on which compartment is being replaced with prosthetic joint components. Alternatively, an incision may be made over the anterior aspect of the knee so that the whole knee joint can be explored. The joint capsule is incised and the medial and/or lateral compartment inspected. The distal femur is exposed and a cutting guide placed on the end of the lateral or medial aspect of the femur to ensure that the bone cut is made in such a way that proper alignment of the joint and leg angles is maintained. Bone is cut from the distal end of the femur. The lateral or medial tibial surface is prepared using a cutting guide in the same manner. The medial or lateral prosthetic femoral component is placed on the femur. If an uncemented prosthesis is used, it is pushed onto the carefully prepared femur and held in place by friction. If a cemented prosthesis is used, bone cement is used to secure the prosthesis to the bone. The tibial component which consists of a metal tray and spacer is placed on the tibia. The metal tray is secured to the bone with bone cement or screws. The spacer is attached to the metal tray. Range of motion is checked. Overlying soft tissues and skin are repaired in layers.

27447

27447 Arthroplasty, knee, condyle and plateau; medial AND lateral compartments with or without patella resurfacing (total knee arthroplasty)

A total knee replacement is performed. An incision is made over the anterior aspect of the knee. The joint capsule is incised and the knee joint inspected. Bone spurs and intra-articular soft tissues are excised. The distal femur is exposed and an intramedullary alignment system or other cutting guide placed on the end of the femur to ensure that the bone cut is made in such a way that proper alignment of the joint and leg angles is maintained. Bone is cut from the distal end of the femur. The proximal tibial surface is prepared using intramedullary or extramedullary alignment rods in the same manner. If degenerative joint disease has caused knee ligaments to become contracted, they are released. Trial components are placed and patellofemoral tracking evaluated. Lateral release or medial reefing is performed as needed to ensure proper patellofemoral tracking. If there is significant patellofemoral degenerative joint disease, the patella is resurfaced with a polyethylene button. Depending on the type of femoral component being used, it is either secured using a press-fit technique or with bone cement. The tibial component consisting of a metal tray and plastic spacing device is secured to the proximal tibia. The metal tray is secured with screws or bone cement and the spacing device is attached to the metal tray. Range of motion is evaluated. Soft tissues and skin are closed in layers.

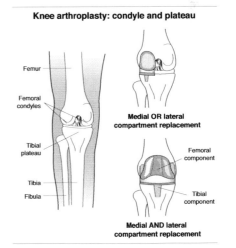

Knee arthroplasty: condyle and plateau

Femur

Femoral condyles

Tibial plateau

Tibia

Fibula

Medial OR lateral compartment replacement

Femoral component

Tibial component

Medial AND lateral compartment replacement

27448-27450

27448 Osteotomy, femur, shaft or supracondylar; without fixation
27450 Osteotomy, femur, shaft or supracondylar; with fixation

An osteotomy of the femoral shaft or supracondylar region is performed to correct a deformity or realign the bone. The location of the osteotomy and the type performed is dependent on the site and type of the deformity. Some commonly used osteotomies include transverse, wedge, sliding, right or left angle, V-osteotomy, and Z-osteotomy. Using separately reportable radiographic studies, the physician determines where the bone cut will be made to achieve the desired result prior to the start of the surgical procedure. An incision is made over the femoral shaft or supracondylar region. Soft tissues are dissected and the femur is exposed. The periosteum is elevated. Using a drill, saw, and/or osteotome, the bone is cut in the previously determined configuration. Bone grafts are interposed between the cut bone segments as needed. Pins, screws, a plate and screw device, or other type of internal fixation is applied as needed to secure the cut edges in anatomical alignment. Alternatively, a separately reportable external fixation device may be applied. Use 27448 when the procedure is performed without internal or external fixation. Use 27450 when a fixation device is used.

27454

27454   Osteotomy, multiple, with realignment on intramedullary rod, femoral shaft (eg, Sofield type procedure)

Multiple osteotomies of the femoral shaft are performed to correct a deformity or realign the bones. The location of the osteotomies and the type performed is dependent on the site and type of the deformity. Some commonly used osteotomies include transverse, wedge, sliding, right or left angle, V-osteotomy, and Z-osteotomy. Using separately reportable radiographic studies, the physician determines where the bone cuts will be made to achieve the desired result prior to the start of the surgical procedure. A longitudinal incision is made over the femoral shaft. Soft tissues are dissected and the femur is exposed. The periosteum is elevated. Using a drill, saw, and/or osteotome, the bone is cut in the previously determined configuration. The femur is sized and an appropriately sized intramedullary rod is selected. A drill hole is created in the distal or proximal aspect of the femur. The intramedullary canal is drilled or reamed through the drill hole. If a cannulated rod is used, a guidewire is placed into the intramedullary canal. The rod is then advanced over the guidewire until it is properly positioned within the canal. The bone is anatomically positioned at each osteotomy site and the rod is secured using screws or pins or other devices.

27455-27457

27455   Osteotomy, proximal tibia, including fibular excision or osteotomy (includes correction of genu varus [bowleg] or genu valgus [knock-knee]); before epiphyseal closure

27457   Osteotomy, proximal tibia, including fibular excision or osteotomy (includes correction of genu varus [bowleg] or genu valgus [knock-knee]); after epiphyseal closure

An osteotomy of the proximal tibia with excision of a portion of the fibula or fibular osteotomy is performed to correct a deformity or realign the bone. This procedure may be performed to correct genu varus, also referred to as bowleg, or genu valgus also referred to as knock-knee. The location of the osteotomy and the type performed is dependent on the site and type of the deformity. Some commonly used osteotomies include transverse, wedge, sliding, right or left angle, V-osteotomy, and Z-osteotomy. Using separately reportable radiographic studies, the physician determines where the bone cut will be made to achieve the desired result prior to the start of the surgical procedure. An incision is made over the lower leg. Soft tissues are dissected and the tibia and fibula are exposed. The tibial periosteum is elevated. Using a drill, saw, and/or osteotome, the bone is cut in the previously determined configuration. A portion of the fibula is excised or a fibular osteotomy is performed in the same manner. Bone grafts are interposed between the cut bone segments as needed. Pins, screws, a plate and screw device, or other type of internal fixation is applied as needed to secure the cut edges in anatomical alignment. Alternatively, a separately reportable external fixation device may be applied. Use 27455 when the procedure is performed on a child or adolescent before epiphyseal closure when the bone is still growing. Use 27457 when the procedure is performed after epiphyseal closure when full bone growth has been attained.

27465-27468

27465   Osteoplasty, femur; shortening (excluding 64876)
27466   Osteoplasty, femur; lengthening
27468   Osteoplasty, femur; combined, lengthening and shortening with femoral segment transfer

A plastic procedure is performed on the femur to lengthen or shorten the bone. Using separately reportable radiographic studies, the physician determines where the bone cuts will be made to achieve the desired result prior to the start of the surgical procedure. The femur is exposed. In 27465, the femur is shortened. The sites of the bone cuts are identified. The bone is cut and a segment of the bone is excised. The remaining distal and proximal portions of the bone are then brought into contact with each other and internal fixation is applied to stabilize the reconfigured bone. Alternatively, a separately reportable external fixation device may be applied. In 27466, the femur is lengthened. Cuts are made in the bone and the bone is distracted. A bone autograft is harvested, usually from the iliac crest. A skin incision is made over the iliac crest and the muscle is stripped to reveal the bone surface. Cortical and/or cancellous bone is harvested. The bone is configured to the desired size and shape and/or cancellous bone is morcelized and packed into the defect. Pins, screws, a plate and screw device, or other type of internal fixation is applied as needed to secure the cut edges in anatomical alignment. Alternatively, a separately reportable external fixation device may be applied. In 27468, a combined lengthening and shortening procedure is performed using the techniques described above. The femoral segment that has been excised during the shortening procedure is then transferred to the

site where the lengthening is being performed and is used to lengthen this portion of the bone.

27470-27472

27470   Repair, nonunion or malunion, femur, distal to head and neck; without graft (eg, compression technique)

27472   Repair, nonunion or malunion, femur, distal to head and neck; with iliac or other autogenous bone graft (includes obtaining graft)

When union of the fracture fragments does not occur after sufficient healing time has elapsed, the patient is considered to have a nonunion of the fracture. Malunion caused by malalignment of the fracture fragments can cause osseous abnormalities, incongruity of articular surfaces, soft tissue contracture, nerve impingement, and other complications. The original fracture site in the femur is exposed. The nonunion or malunion is evaluated to determine what type of repair is required. In 27470, the nonunion or malunion of the femur is treated without a graft using internal fixation, such as a compression plate. For a nonunion, a compression plate is placed over the fracture site and secured with lag screws. For a malunion, the femur may be refractured, realigned, and internal fixation placed to maintain the fracture in anatomical alignment. Following placement of the fixation device, stability of the fracture is checked and alignment is verified radiographically. In 27472, a bone graft is used to fill the bone defect and encourage healing. The site of the nonunion or malunion is prepared which may include refracture of the bone. A bone autograft is harvested, usually from the iliac crest. A skin incision is made over the iliac crest and the muscle is stripped to reveal the bone surface. Cortical and/or cancellous bone is harvested. The bone is configured to the size and shape of the defect or cancellous bone is morcelized and packed into the defect. Internal fixation, such as a pin or wire is used as needed to secure the bone graft. A compression plate and screws or other internal fixation is used to stabilize the fracture.

27475-27479

27475   Arrest, epiphyseal, any method (eg, epiphysiodesis); distal femur
27477   Arrest, epiphyseal, any method (eg, epiphysiodesis); tibia and fibula, proximal
27479   Arrest, epiphyseal, any method (eg, epiphysiodesis); combined distal femur, proximal tibia and fibula

Epiphyseal arrest is performed to treat a bone length discrepancy between the femurs or between the tibia and fibula. The epiphysis is also referred to as the growth plate. An incision is made over the distal aspect of the femur and/or the proximal aspect of the tibia and/or fibula. Soft tissues are dissected, taking care to protect blood vessels and nerves. The distal femur and/or proximal tibia and/or fibula are exposed. Blount staples, transphyseal screws, or a plate and screw device are strategically placed in the epiphysis of the distal femur and/or proximal tibia and/or fibula to temporarily arrest bone growth. Use 27475 for epiphyseal arrest of the distal femur. Use 27477 if the procedure is performed on the proximal tibia and fibula. Use 27479 if epiphyseal arrest is performed on the distal femur and proximal tibia and fibula.

27485

27485   Arrest, hemiepiphyseal, distal femur or proximal tibia or fibula (eg, genu varus or valgus)

Hemiepiphyseal arrest is performed to treat an angulation deformity of the leg such as genu varus (bowleg) or genu valgum (knock-knee). The epiphysis is also referred to as the growth plate. An incision is made over the distal aspect femur or the proximal aspect of the tibia or fibula. Soft tissues are dissected, taking care to protect blood vessels and nerves. The distal femur or proximal tibia or fibula is exposed. Blount staples, transphyseal screws, or a plate and screw device are strategically placed in the epiphysis of the distal femur or proximal tibia or fibula to temporarily arrest bone growth. When an angulation deformity is treated, only a portion of the epiphysis is arrested. The other portion of the epiphysis is not treated and growth continues thereby diminishing or correcting the angulation deformity.

27486-27487

27486   Revision of total knee arthroplasty, with or without allograft; 1 component
27487   Revision of total knee arthroplasty, with or without allograft; femoral and entire tibial component

Revision of a total knee arthroplasty may be performed for mechanical complications or failure of the implant or for other complications such as infection. Revision may involve only the femoral or tibial component or both components may be revised. A long incision is made beginning over the femur, carried down over the knee and extended over the tibia. Soft tissues are dissected taking care to protect nerves and blood vessels. The femoral and/or tibial components are removed. The amount of bone loss is evaluated. If a bone allograft is required, it is obtained from the bone bank. The bone is configured to the size and shape of the defect or cancellous bone is morcelized and packed into the defect. Internal devices such as a metallic cage, plate, and screws may also be used to help restore bone length. Once bone reconstruction has been completed, a new prosthesis is implanted. If knee ligaments are contracted, they are released. Trial components are then placed and patellofemoral tracking evaluated. Lateral release or medial reefing

Musculoskeletal System

is performed as needed to ensure proper patellofemoral tracking. If there is significant patellofemoral degenerative joint disease, the patella is resurfaced with a polyethylene button. If an unlinked type of prosthesis is used, the femoral component is either secured using a press-fit technique or with bone cement. The tibial component consisting of a metal tray and plastic spacing device is then secured to the proximal tibia. The metal tray is secured with screws or bone cement and the spacing device is then attached to the metal tray. If a hinged prosthesis is used, the stem is inserted into the femur and is either secured using a press-fit technique or with bone cement. The tibial stem is then secured to the proximal tibia in the same manner. Range of motion is evaluated. Soft tissues and skin are closed in layers. Use 27486 if only the femoral or tibial component is revised. Use 27487 if both components are revised.

27488

27488 Removal of prosthesis, including total knee prosthesis, methylmethacrylate with or without insertion of spacer, knee

A partial or total knee prosthesis is removed without replacement. Removal without replacement may be performed due to infection or other complication related to the prosthesis. A long incision is made beginning over femur, carried down over the knee and extended over the tibia. Soft tissues are dissected taking care to protect nerves and blood vessels. The femoral and/or tibial components are removed and all infected bone and soft tissue is excised. A spacer may then be placed in the joint space to keep the muscles and other tissues around the knee joint from contracting. The spacer is composed of one or two pieces of bone cement often imbibed with antibiotics. A drain is placed as needed and overlying soft tissues are closed in layers.

27495

27495 Prophylactic treatment (nailing, pinning, plating, or wiring) with or without methylmethacrylate, femur

Prophylactic treatment is performed to prevent fracture of the femur when the bone is weakened as a result of a disease process or neoplasm. Common methods used to maintain bone integrity include nailing, pinning, plating, or wiring with or without the use of methylmethacrylate. The weakened bone is evaluated radiographically and the best form of prophylaxis is determined. An intramedullary nail or rod may be placed using either an antegrade or retrograde approach. A small incision is made over the proximal or distal femur. A nail or rod is then inserted into the intramedullary space. The nail is secured with locking screws placed distally and proximally. If pins are used, they may be placed transcutaneously through the weakened region of the bone. Plating requires open exposure of the bone and placement of a plate that is secured with screws. Wiring involves wrapping a wire cerclage around the bone. When methylmethacrylate is used, it is injected into bony defects.

27496-27497

27496 Decompression fasciotomy, thigh and/or knee, 1 compartment (flexor or extensor or adductor)

27497 Decompression fasciotomy, thigh and/or knee, 1 compartment (flexor or extensor or adductor); with debridement of nonviable muscle and/or nerve

Decompression fasciotomy is performed to treat compartment syndrome, a condition in which swelling of tissue in the muscle compartment causes compression of the blood vessels and nerves. Muscle compartments are surrounded by fascia that separates groups of muscles from each other. Fascia is a thick layer of connective tissue that does not expand. Swelling of tissue within the compartment can restrict blood supply and cause permanent muscle and nerve damage. There are three compartments in the upper leg (thigh) and knee region, referred to as the flexor, extensor, and adductor compartments. In 27496 and 27497, only a single compartment requires decompression. A skin incision is made over the lateral aspect of the thigh beginning just distal to the intertrochanteric line and extending to the lateral epicondyle. Subcutaneous tissue is dissected and the iliotibial band is exposed. The iliotibial band is incised in the direction of its fibers. The vastus lateralis is reflected off the lateral intermuscular septum and the septum is opened proximally and distally along the entire length of the skin incision. Pressures within the anterior or posterior compartment are checked first. If elevated, the anterior or posterior compartment is incised. If the adductor compartment is affected, a medial incision is made to decompress the adductor compartment. Pressure in the affected anterior, posterior, or adductor compartment is again checked to ensure that the muscles have been adequately decompressed. Bleeding is controlled by electrocautery. 27497, muscle tissue and nerves are inspected and any nonviable tissue is also debrided using sharp excision. The skin and fascial incisions are left open and covered with a dressing. The patient is returned to the operating room for wound closure once the swelling subsides, usually within 24-72 hours. Use 27496 for decompression of a single compartment without debridement.

27498-27499

27498 Decompression fasciotomy, thigh and/or knee, multiple compartments

27499 Decompression fasciotomy, thigh and/or knee, multiple compartments; with debridement of nonviable muscle and/or nerve

Decompression fasciotomy is performed to treat compartment syndrome, a condition in which swelling of tissue in the muscle compartment causes compression of the blood vessels and nerves. Muscle compartments are surrounded by fascia that separates groups of muscles from each other. Fascia is a thick layer of connective tissue that does not expand. Swelling of tissue within the compartment can restrict blood supply and cause permanent muscle and nerve damage. There are three compartments in the upper leg (thigh) and knee region, referred to as the flexor, extensor, and adductor (medial) compartments. In 27498 and 27499, multiple compartments require decompression. A skin incision is made over the lateral aspect of the thigh beginning just distal to the intertrochanteric line and extending to the lateral epicondyle. Subcutaneous tissue is dissected and the iliotibial band is exposed. The iliotibial band is incised in the direction of its fibers. The vastus lateralis is reflected off the lateral intermuscular septum and the septum is opened proximally and distally along the entire length of the skin incision. Pressures within the anterior and posterior compartments are checked first. The anterior and/or posterior compartments are incised as needed. Compartment pressures are again checked to ensure that the muscles have been adequately decompressed. Medial compartment pressures are checked and if elevated, a medial incision is made to decompress the adductor compartment. Bleeding is controlled by electrocautery. In 27499, muscle tissue and nerves are inspected and any nonviable tissue is debrided using sharp excision. The skin and fascial incisions are left open and covered with a dressing. The patient is returned to the operating room for wound closure once the swelling subsides, usually within 24-72 hours. Use 27498 for decompression of multiple compartments without debridement.

27500

27500 Closed treatment of femoral shaft fracture, without manipulation

A femoral shaft fracture is treated without manipulation. Separately reportable radiographs are obtained to confirm the fracture. A neurovascular exam is performed to ensure that the nerves and blood vessels at the site of the injury are intact. No manipulation of the fracture fragments is required. A hip spica cast is applied to immobilize the fracture.

27501

27501 Closed treatment of supracondylar or transcondylar femoral fracture with or without intercondylar extension, without manipulation

The distal femur has two projections, the lateral and medial epicondyles. Fractures immediately above the epicondyles are referred to as supracondylar fractures and fractures through the epicondyles are referred to as transcondylar. These types of fractures may extend through the region between the epicondyles and into the intercondylar fossa. Separately reportable radiographs are obtained to confirm the fracture. A neurovascular exam is performed to ensure that the nerves and blood vessels at the site of the injury are intact. No manipulation of the fracture fragments is required. A leg brace is applied to stabilize the fracture.

27502

27502 Closed treatment of femoral shaft fracture, with manipulation, with or without skin or skeletal traction

A femoral shaft fracture is treated with manipulation, with or without skin or skeletal traction. Separately reportable radiographs are obtained to confirm the fracture. A neurovascular exam is performed to ensure that the nerves and blood vessels at the site of the injury are intact. The fracture fragments are manually reduced (manipulated) back to proper anatomic alignment. Separately reportable radiographs are obtained to confirm anatomic reduction. Following reduction of the fracture fragments, skin or skeletal traction is applied, if needed. If skin traction is used, the leg is splinted and the weighted traction device is attached to the leg using wraps, tape, or straps. If skeletal traction is used, a pin is inserted through the distal femur or proximal tibia and weighted traction is applied.

27503

27503 Closed treatment of supracondylar or transcondylar femoral fracture with or without intercondylar extension, with manipulation, with or without skin or skeletal traction

The distal femur has two projections, the lateral and medial epicondyles. Fractures immediately above the epicondyles are referred to as supracondylar and fractures through the epicondyles are referred to as transcondylar. These types of fractures may extend through the region between the epicondyles and into the intercondylar fossa. Separately reportable radiographs are obtained to confirm the fracture. A neurovascular exam is performed to ensure that the nerves and blood vessels at the site of the injury are intact. The fracture fragments are manually reduced (manipulated) back to proper anatomic alignment. Separately reportable radiographs are obtained to confirm anatomic reduction. Following reduction of the fracture fragments, skin or skeletal traction is applied, if needed.

Musculoskeletal System

If skin traction is used, the leg is splinted and the weighted traction device is attached to the leg using wraps, tape, or straps. If skeletal traction is used, a pin is inserted through the proximal tibia and weighted traction is applied.

27506-27507

27506 **Open treatment of femoral shaft fracture, with or without external fixation, with insertion of intramedullary implant, with or without cerclage and/or locking screws**

27507 **Open treatment of femoral shaft fracture with plate/screws, with or without cerclage**

Open treatment of a femoral shaft fracture is performed. In 27506, the fracture is treated with insertion of an intramedullary implant, with or without cerclage and/or locking screws, with or without external fixation. The nail may be placed using an antegrade or retrograde approach, with antegrade approach being the most common. Using an antegrade approach the greater trochanter of the femur is identified and an incision made above the posterior tip of the trochanter. The tensor fascia is incised and the gluteus maximus split. The gluteus medius tendon may be split or the nail may be inserted behind it. An awl is used to create an opening in the femur. A guide pin is inserted through the cannulated awl and advanced into the medullary canal. A properly sized intramedullary implant is selected based on measurements obtained using the guide wire. The intramedullary implant (nail, rod) is driven into the intramedullary canal and secured with interlocking screws distally and proximally. The fracture may also be stabilized using wire cerclage wrapped around the bone at the site of the fracture. If the fracture requires additional stabilization, an external fixation device may be applied in conjunction with the intramedullary implant. External fixator pins are placed through the skin and into the femur at various angles. An external fixator frame is then applied and clamps used to secure the frame to the pins. Alignment of the fracture is checked radiographically and changes made to pin orientation by manipulating the frame. Once the fracture fragments are in anatomical alignment, the clamps are locked in place. In 27507, open treatment of a femoral shaft fracture is performed using plate and screws with or without cerclage. An incision is made over the femoral shaft at the site of the fracture. The fracture site is cleared of debris. Traction or a femoral distraction device is used to reduce the fracture. An appropriorately sized and configured plate is selected based on the exact nature of the fracture. The plate is placed across the fracture site and anchored with screws. A wire cerclage may be wrapped around the bone at the fracture site to provide additional stabilization.

27508

27508 **Closed treatment of femoral fracture, distal end, medial or lateral condyle, without manipulation**

The medial and lateral condyles are two expanded areas of bone lying just below the medial and lateral epicondyles that articulate with the tibia. Separately reportable radiographs are obtained to confirm the fracture. A neurovascular exam is performed to ensure that the nerves and blood vessels at the site of the injury are intact. No manipulation of the fracture fragments is required. A leg brace is applied to stabilize the fracture.

27509

27509 **Percutaneous skeletal fixation of femoral fracture, distal end, medial or lateral condyle, or supracondylar or transcondylar, with or without intercondylar extension, or distal femoral epiphyseal separation**

The distal femur has two projections, the lateral and medial epicondyles. Fractures immediately above the epicondyles are referred to as supracondylar and fractures through the epicondyles are referred to as transcondylar. These types of fractures may extend through the region between the epicondyles and into the intercondylar fossa or they may result in separation of the epiphyseal plate. Separately reportable radiographs are obtained to confirm the fracture. A neurovascular exam is performed to ensure that the nerves and blood vessels at the site of the injury are intact. A small skin incision is made over the distal femur. Using radiographic guidance, a drill is used to create one or more corticotomies at the sites where pins will be placed. The fracture fragments are manually reduced (manipulated) back to proper anatomic alignment and one or more pins are advanced across the fracture site to help maintain the fracture fragments in anatomical alignment. Anatomical reduction is verified radiographically.

27510

27510 **Closed treatment of femoral fracture, distal end, medial or lateral condyle, with manipulation**

The medial and lateral condyles are two expanded areas of bone lying just below the medial and lateral epicondyles that articulate with the tibia. Separately reportable radiographs are obtained to confirm the fracture. A neurovascular exam is performed to ensure that the nerves and blood vessels at the site of the injury are intact. The fracture fragments are manually reduced (manipulated) back to proper anatomic alignment. Separately reportable radiographs are obtained to confirm anatomic reduction and a leg brace is applied to stabilize the fracture.

27511-27513

27511 **Open treatment of femoral supracondylar or transcondylar fracture without intercondylar extension, includes internal fixation, when performed**

27513 **Open treatment of femoral supracondylar or transcondylar fracture with intercondylar extension, includes internal fixation, when performed**

The distal femur has two projections, the lateral epicondyle and the medial epicondyle. Fractures immediately above these epicondyles are referred to as supracondylar. Fractures through the epicondyles are referred to as transcondylar. These types of fractures may extend into the intercondylar region of the bone with fracture of the intercondylar fossa. An incision is made over the lateral aspect of the distal femur extending over the articular surface of the knee. Tissue is dissected down to the fascia lata and it is split. The distal segment of the femur is approached by carefully dissecting the vastus lateralis along its posterior aspect. Arterial bleeding is controlled by electrocautery and ligation of vessels. The fracture site is exposed and cleared of debris. The fracture in the supracondylar or transcondylar region is reduced indirectly by application of longitudinal traction and/or use of a femoral distraction device. Internal fixation is selected based on the exact nature of the fracture. Fixator devices are carefully selected and customized to avoid intersection of fracture lines with the blade, screw, or intramedullary device. Types of internal fixation used for supracondylar or transcondylar fractures include: low-contact dynamic compression (LC-DC) plates, dynamic condylar screws (DCS), condylar blade plates, condylar buttress plates, locking plates, T-buttress plates, intramedullary devices (nails or rods), or cannulated lag screws. After the fracture is reduced and all fragments are secured using one or more fixation devices, x-rays are obtained to verify anatomic reduction. Use 27511 when the fracture does not extend into the intercondylar region (intercondylar fossa). Use 27513 when a fracture of the intercondylar region is also treated and an arthrotomy is done to gain access to the intercondylar fossa. The procedure is performed as described above with additional reconstruction of the intercondylar fracture.

27514

27514 **Open treatment of femoral fracture, distal end, medial or lateral condyle, includes internal fixation, when performed**

The condyles are two expanded areas of the bone that articulate with the tibia and lie just below the medial and lateral epicondyles. For large fragments, a midline incision is made over the knee with parapatellar release and patellar dislocation to allow direct access to the fracture site. For smaller fragments, a medial or lateral incision may be made over the affected condyle. The incision is extended into the joint capsule, the fracture is exposed, cleared of debris and the fragments are reduced. Internal fixation is applied as needed. Temporary fixation is achieved by placement of wires and anatomic alignment is verified by x-ray. Permanent screw or plate and screw fixation is then applied and the wires are removed. Depending on the exact nature of the fracture and the size and number of fracture fragments, one or more fixation devices may be required. Anatomic alignment is again verified by x-ray. Soft tissue is reapproximated and the wound is closed.

27516-27517

27516 **Closed treatment of distal femoral epiphyseal separation; without manipulation**

27517 **Closed treatment of distal femoral epiphyseal separation; with manipulation, with or without skin or skeletal traction**

The epiphysis, also referred to as the epiphyseal or growth plate, is the area where bone growth occurs. Separation of the growth plate occurs due to trauma and must be treated or bone growth will stop. In the femur, this would result in leg length discrepancy. Separately reportable radiographs are obtained to evaluate the epiphyseal injury in the distal femur. In 27516, a nondisplaced distal epiphyseal separation is treated. No manipulation is required. The leg is immobilized in a long leg or hip spica cast. In 27517, a minimally displaced distal epiphyseal separation is treated by closed reduction. Manual force is applied to reduce the fracture fragments so they are situated in normal anatomic alignment. Reduction is checked radiographically to ensure anatomic alignment. Skin or skeletal traction may be used to maintain the bone fragments in anatomic alignment and to preserve leg length. If skin traction is used, a traction strap that extends beyond the foot is secured to the lower leg using a wrap bandage. A sling may be placed under the knee. Weights are attached to a pulley and the traction strap in a manner that allows a longitudinal force to be applied. If skeletal traction is used, a wire, pin, screw, or clamp is placed through the skin and secured to the proximal tibia. The ends of the skeletal traction hardware extend beyond the skin and are attached to a pulley system and weights to provide a longitudinal or distracting force to the leg. If traction is not used, the leg is immobilized in a long leg or hip spica cast.

27519

27519 **Open treatment of distal femoral epiphyseal separation, includes internal fixation, when performed**

This type of injury may also be referred to as a Salter-Harris fracture. The epiphysis, also referred to as the epiphyseal plate or growth plate, is the area where bone growth occurs. The femur continues to lengthen until early adulthood. Epiphyseal separation is an injury to the growth plate that occurs due to trauma and must be treated or growth in the affected leg will stop, causing leg length discrepancies. An incision is made over the lateral aspect of the knee. Dissection is carried down to the fascia lata, which is split. The vastus lateralis is elevated. Careful dissection around the growth plate is then performed and the fracture fragments are exposed. Anatomic alignment is restored by direct visualization and careful manipulation of the fracture fragments so as not to cause additional injury to the growth plate. When anatomic reduction has been achieved, fracture fragments may be secured with internal fixation. Wire fixation is temporarily placed and alignment of fracture fragments is checked radiographically. Permanent fixation is then applied, such as screws and/or pins. Anatomic reduction is again verified radiographically, soft tissue is reapproximated, and the wound is closed.

27520

27520   Closed treatment of patellar fracture, without manipulation

Separately reportable radiographs are obtained to confirm the fracture. A neurovascular exam is performed to ensure that the nerves and blood vessels at the site of the injury are intact. No manipulation of the fracture fragments is required. The knee is immobilized using a knee brace. The patient is given instructions on weight bearing limits and is provided with crutches or other walking aid, if needed.

27524

27524   Open treatment of patellar fracture, with internal fixation and/or partial or complete patellectomy and soft tissue repair

Separately reportable radiographs are obtained to confirm a patellar fracture. A neurovascular exam is performed to ensure that the nerves and blood vessels at the site of the injury are intact. Open reduction of an acute patellar fracture is performed via an anterior approach. The patella is exposed and inspected along with surrounding structures. If there are any loose bodies preventing reduction, they are removed. The patella is then manipulated back into position. Following the reduction, a second set of radiographs may be obtained. Internal fixation devices such as pins, screws, or a plate and screw device may be placed. Alternatively, part or all of the patella may be excised. The muscles and tendons attached to the patella are divided taking care to preserve the quadriceps tendon above the patella and the patellar tendon below. The patella is removed. The quadriceps and patellar tendon are sutured together. Soft tissues and skin are closed in layers. The knee may be protected and immobilized using a compression wrap, or a splint or cast may be applied.

27530-27532

27530   Closed treatment of tibial fracture, proximal (plateau); without manipulation

27532   Closed treatment of tibial fracture, proximal (plateau); with or without manipulation, with skeletal traction

Closed treatment of a proximal tibial fracture, also referred to as a tibial plateau fracture, is performed. Separately reportable radiographs are obtained to confirm the fracture. A neurovascular exam is performed to ensure that the nerves and blood vessels at the site of the injury are intact. In 27530, a nondisplaced or minimally displaced fracture is treated. No manipulation of the fracture fragments is required. The patient is placed in a hinged cast-brace to allow protected mobilization of the knee joint. The patient is given instructions on non-weight bearing requirements and is provided with crutches or other walking aid. In 27532, a nondisplaced or minimally displaced fracture is treated with or without manipulation, with skeletal traction. The displaced fracture fragments are manually reduced (manipulated) back to proper anatomic alignment as needed. Separately reportable radiographs are obtained to confirm anatomic reduction. Following reduction of the fracture fragments, skeletal traction is applied. A pin is inserted through the proximal tibia and weighted traction applied.

27535-27536

27535   Open treatment of tibial fracture, proximal (plateau); unicondylar, includes internal fixation, when performed

27536   Open treatment of tibial fracture, proximal (plateau); bicondylar, with or without internal fixation

The proximal end of the tibia has two condyles, medial and lateral. Tibial plateau fractures occur at the proximal end of the tibia and extend into the articular cartilage of the knee joint. The fracture may involve one or both condyles. Use 27535 for a unicondylar (medial or lateral) tibial plateau fracture. For repair of a medial tibial plateau fracture, an incision is made over the medial femoral condyle and extended anteriorly and distally across the joint line to the medial edge of the patellar tendon, then continued in a posterior distal direction. The tibial flare is exposed, the fracture site is identified and cleared of debris, and the fracture is reduced. Internal fixation is applied as needed. Placement of a plate and screw device in the medial plateau may require division of the pes anserinus-the common tendinous insertion of the sartorius, gracilius, and semitendinosus along the medial aspect of the tibia, to allow adequate exposure of the medial plateau. An arthrotomy may also be performed to examine the articular surface. For repair of a lateral tibial plateau fracture, a limited hockey stick approach may be used, typically when the

fracture fragments can be secured using screws alone: an incision is made over the fibular head and extended to Gerdy's tubercle, then either anteriorly or posteriorly to expose the fracture. Dissection is carried down to the iliotibial (IT) band and the band is split in the direction of its fibers. The joint capsule is visualized and a horizontal inframeniscal incision is made to fully expose the fracture site. The fracture is reduced and the fragments are secured using screw fixation. Alternatively, a longitudinal approach may be used when the fracture fragments are secured with a plate and screw device. Anatomic alignment of fracture fragments is verified radiographically. Use 27536 for open treatment of a bicondylar (both medial and lateral) tibial plateau fracture. An anterior incision is made over the knee joint. The medial plateau fragments are reduced. Temporary fixation of the medial plateau may be performed using a medial buttress plate. Once anatomic alignment has been achieved, fracture fragments in the lateral plateau are reduced. A lateral locking plate is applied with posterior locking screws. The medial buttress plate is removed and the medial plateau fragments are secured with a washer and screw device.

27538

27538   Closed treatment of intercondylar spine(s) and/or tuberosity fracture(s) of knee, with or without manipulation

The intercondylar spines, also referred to as the intercondylar eminences or tibial spines, are two upward projections in the center of the proximal tibial surface between the lateral and medial condyles. The tibial tuberosity is a projection on the anterior proximal tibia and the point of attachment for the patellar ligament. Separately reportable radiographs are obtained to confirm the fracture. A neurovascular exam is performed to ensure that the nerves and blood vessels at the site of the injury are intact. The fracture fragments are manually reduced (manipulated) back to proper anatomic alignment as needed. Separately reportable radiographs are obtained to confirm anatomic reduction. The knee is immobilized using a cast or brace.

27540

27540   Open treatment of intercondylar spine(s) and/or tuberosity fracture(s) of the knee, includes internal fixation, when performed

The intercondylar spine, also referred to as the intercondylar eminence or tibial spine, consists of two upward projections in the center of the proximal tibial surface that lies between the lateral and medial condyles. The tibial tuberosity is a projection on the anterior proximal tibia and the point of attachment for the patellar ligament. For an intercondylar tibial spine fracture, an incision is made over the anterior medial aspect of the knee. The medial joint capsule is incised and the hematoma is evacuated. The fracture is exposed and cleared of debris, then reduced. The fragments may be secured using sutures or internal fixation, including wires, screws, and/or pins. Anatomical alignment is verified radiographically. For a tibial tuberosity fracture, an incision is made over the anterior medial knee just over the proximal tibia. The fracture site is exposed and cleared of debris, then reduced. Fractures that do not involve the articular surface are fixed using one or two screws through the tibial tubercle into the proximal tibia. Fractures involving the articular surface require anterior medial arthrotomy. The fracture is reduced and temporary wire fixation is applied. Alignment is verified radiographically before permanent screw fixation is applied.

27550-27552

27550   Closed treatment of knee dislocation; without anesthesia

27552   Closed treatment of knee dislocation; requiring anesthesia

Knee dislocation is a relatively rare injury that can cause vascular impairment if not recognized and treated without delay. The peripheral pulses are checked to ensure that no vascular impairment is present. If vascular impairment is present, reduction is typically performed without obtaining pre-reduction radiographs. If peripheral pulses are present, separately reportable radiographs may be obtained. The physician uses longitudinal traction to reduce the dislocation. Following the reduction, a second set of radiographs may be obtained. The leg is splinted and the patient is instructed to ice and elevate the knee. Use 27550 when the dislocation is treated without anesthesia and 27552 when anesthesia is required.

27556

27556   Open treatment of knee dislocation, includes internal fixation, when performed; without primary ligamentous repair or augmentation/reconstruction

There are five types of knee dislocation: anterior, posterior, lateral, medial, and rotary. Treatment of a knee dislocation depends on which ligaments are injured and the severity of the injury. An incision is made over the knee and the joint capsule is incised. The injury site is exposed and cleared of debris, such as loose osteochondral fragments. The knee dislocation is reduced and checked radiographically. Then, the stability of the knee is checked. Internal fixation is applied if needed to maintain alignment and stability. The wound is irrigated and The incision is closed with sutures.

Musculoskeletal System

Musculoskeletal System

27557-27558

27557 **Open treatment of knee dislocation, includes internal fixation, when performed; with primary ligamentous repair**

27558 **Open treatment of knee dislocation, includes internal fixation, when performed; with primary ligamentous repair, with augmentation/ reconstruction**

There are five types of knee dislocation: anterior, posterior, lateral, medial, and rotary. Treatment of a knee dislocation depends on which ligaments are injured and the severity of the injury. There are four ligaments in the knee. The medial collateral ligament is on the medial (inner) aspect of the knee and connects the femur and tibia. The lateral collateral ligament is on the lateral (outer) aspect of the knee and connects the femur and fibula. Both collateral ligaments lie outside the joint capsule. The anterior cruciate ligament (ACL) connects the front of the tibia to the back of the lateral femoral condyle. The posterior cruciate ligament (PCL) connects the back of the tibia to the front of the medial femoral condyle. Both cruciate ligaments lie within the joint capsule. An incision is made over the knee and the joint capsule is incised. The injury site is exposed and cleared of debris, such as loose osteochondral fragments. The knee dislocation is reduced and checked radiographically. Torn ligaments are repaired with sutures or staples. Avulsed ligament(s) with large bone fragments may be secured with internal fixation, such as screws and the stability of the knee is checked. Use 27558 when ligament repair requires augmentation and/or reconstruction. If augmentation is performed, the tendon is first repaired with sutures or staples and then augmented with a tendon graft. For instance, to augment the ACL, a tunnel is drilled through the tibia into the knee joint. Then, a second tunnel is drilled from the inside of the knee joint up through the femur. A separate incision is made and a tendon graft harvested and surgically prepared. The end of the graft is placed in the previously drilled tibial and femoral tunnels. Screw fixation is used to secure the graft in both tunnels. The graft runs along the repaired ACL providing additional reinforcement. PCL augmentation is performed in the same manner except that the graft is positioned to run along the length of the repaired PCL tendon to provide additional reinforcement. Reconstruction of the ACL or PCL is performed when the ligament is so severely damaged that it must be excised and a new ACL or PCL reconstructed using a tendon autograft or allograft. Tunnels are prepared as they are for the augmentation procedure. The tissue graft is then positioned and secured in the tunnels. The augmentation/reconstruction is checked radiographically and ligament stability is checked with gentle range of motion.

27560-27562

27560 **Closed treatment of patellar dislocation; without anesthesia**

27562 **Closed treatment of patellar dislocation; requiring anesthesia**

Patellar dislocation may be the result of trauma or due to a biomechanical imbalance of the knee joint, such as a high riding patella (patella alta). Separately reportable radiographs may be obtained. For an acute patellar dislocation that does not reduce spontaneously, the physician manually manipulates the patella into correct anatomical position. Following the reduction, a second set of radiographs may be obtained. The knee may be protected and immobilized using a compression wrap or a splint or cast may be applied. The patient is instructed to ice and elevate the knee. Use 27560 when the dislocation is treated without anesthesia and 27562 when anesthesia is required.

27566

27566 **Open treatment of patellar dislocation, with or without partial or total patellectomy**

Patellar dislocation may be the result of trauma or a biomechanical imbalance of the knee joint, such as a high riding patella (patella alta). Separately reportable radiographs may be obtained. Open reduction of an acute patellar dislocation is performed via an anterior approach. The patella is exposed and inspected along with surrounding structures. If there are any loose bodies preventing reduction, they are removed. The patella is then manipulated back into position. Following the reduction, a second set of radiographs may be obtained. Alternatively, part or all of the patella may be excised. The muscles and tendons attached to the patella are divided taking care to preserve the quadriceps tendon above the patella and the patellar tendon below. The patella is removed. The quadriceps and patellar tendon are sutured together. Soft tissues and skin are closed in layers. The knee may be protected and immobilized using a compression wrap, or a splint or cast may be applied.

27570

27570 **Manipulation of knee joint under general anesthesia (includes application of traction or other fixation devices)**

Manipulation of the knee under anesthesia is performed to break up fibrous adhesions and scar tissue around the joint. Anesthesia is required when the patient is unable to tolerate manipulation of the joint due to pain, spasm, muscle contractures, or guarding. Following administration of anesthesia, the knee joint is taken through a series of stretches and articular maneuvers to disrupt any adhesions or scar tissue and restore some joint mobility and range of motion.

27580

27580 **Arthrodesis, knee, any technique**

Arthrodesis of the knee, also referred to as knee fusion, is performed primarily for failed total knee replacement. There are a number of techniques used including internal fixation, external fixation, and/or bone grafting. If the fusion is performed for failed total knee replacement, the total knee prosthesis is first removed in a separately reportable procedure. Vascular bone is exposed on the femur and tibia. The tibial bone is cut first taking care to place the cuts with proper slope in the coronal and sagittal planes. The joint is aligned in 0-5 degrees of valgus and in 10-15 degrees of flexion. The femur is then cut in a line parallel to the tibial surface. The amount of shortening resulting from preparation of the joint is evaluated. Bone grafts may be used to provide a minimal amount of additional length. An internal or external compression fixator device is then placed. Alternatively, intramedullary nail fixation may be used. Bone grafts are placed around the periphery of the knee joint to improve fusion. If a compression fixator device is used, the device is then tightened. The incision is closed in layers.

27590-27591

27590 **Amputation, thigh, through femur, any level**

27591 **Amputation, thigh, through femur, any level; immediate fitting technique including first cast**

Incision lines are marked on the skin for amputation of the leg through the femur at the appropriate level. The skin and underlying soft tissue are incised. The muscles are exposed, isolated by muscle group, and divided. Nerves and blood vessels are identified and isolated, taking care to ensure that nerves are separated from the arteries to prevent pulsatile irritation of the nerves. Nerves are transected and allowed to retract into soft tissue. Blood vessels are sutured ligated and transected. The femur is exposed and periosteal flaps are created. The femur is transected at the level of the periosteal flaps. The flaps are sutured over the remaining femur. Antagonistic muscle groups are sutured to each other and anchored to the periosteum in such a way that the remaining portion of the femur is completely enveloped in muscle. Skin flaps are fashioned and sutured over muscle. Use 27590 when the extremity is wrapped in an elastic bandage or placed in a plaster splint. Following wound healing, the patient is fitted for a prosthesis. Use 27591 when a cast of the stump is obtained and the patient is immediately fitted for a prosthesis.

27592

27592 **Amputation, thigh, through femur, any level; open, circular (guillotine)**

Guillotine amputation through the femur is performed primarily following trauma with heavily contaminated wounds or on a severely infected leg. The level of amputation is determined based on the extent of injury or infection. The skin is marked to allow skin flaps to be developed as far distally as possible. The skin is incised down to the deep fascia and allowed to retract. Muscle is incised in a circular fashion around the femur and allowed to retract. Nerves are transected as they are encountered. Blood vessels are suture ligated and transected. The femur is transected in line with the retracted muscle. The stump is left open and dressings are applied. When the risk of infection has passed, separately reportable secondary closure or re-amputation at a higher level is performed.

27594

27594 **Amputation, thigh, through femur, any level; secondary closure or scar revision**

Secondary closure or scar revision of previous leg amputation through the femur is performed to obtain a pain-free stump covered with normal skin that functions well with a prosthesis. For secondary closure, the raw surface of the stump is debrided and all devitalized tissue is excised. Skin and subcutaneous tissue are fashioned into flaps and used to cover the stump taking care that there is not any undue tension along the suture line. For scar revision, the scar tissue is excised. Skin flaps are fashioned and the edges are undermined to ensure smooth, tension-free approximation along the suture line.

27596

27596 **Amputation, thigh, through femur, any level; re-amputation**

Re-amputation of the leg through the femur is done at a higher level to remove diseased, infected, or nonviable tissue posing a risk to the patient and/or form a healthy stump for use with a prosthesis. The incision lines for the re-amputation are marked on the skin. The skin and underlying soft tissue are incised. The muscles are exposed, isolated by muscle group, and divided. Nerves and blood vessels are identified and isolated, taking care to ensure that nerves are separated from arteries to prevent pulsatile irritation of the nerves. Nerves are transected and allowed to retract into soft tissue. Blood vessels are suture ligated and transected. The femur is exposed and periosteal flaps are created. The femur is transected at the level of the periosteal flaps. The flaps are sutured over the remaining femur. Antagonistic muscle groups are sutured to each other and anchored to the periosteum in such a way that the remaining portion of the femur is completely enveloped in muscle. Skin flaps are fashioned and sutured over the muscle.

27598

27598   Disarticulation at knee

To remove the leg at the knee joint, a fish-mouth incision line is marked on the skin with an anterior flap extending approximately 4 inches distal to the knee joint and a posterior flap extending approximately 1.5 inches distal to the joint. The skin is incised down to deep fascia which is dissected off the joint capsule. The flaps are reflected upward above the level of the femoral condyle. The patellar tendon is divided. The knee is flexed and the joint capsule and surrounding ligaments are severed. The popliteal vessels are suture ligated and divided. The popliteal nerve is divided. The hamstrings are detached and the patella is dissected from the patellar tendon and removed. Once all connective tissue has been divided, the lower leg is removed. The medial and lateral femoral condyles are partially removed and the corners are smoothed using a rasp. Any protrusions on the posterior surface of the femur are smoothed using an osteotome. The hamstrings and patellar tendon are sutured together over the intercondylar notch. Drains are placed. The flaps are aligned and the deep fascia and skin are closed in layers around the drains. A compression dressing is applied.

27600-27602

27600   Decompression fasciotomy, leg; anterior and/or lateral compartments only

27601   Decompression fasciotomy, leg; posterior compartment(s) only

27602   Decompression fasciotomy, leg; anterior and/or lateral, and posterior compartment(s)

A decompression fasciotomy of the lower leg is performed to treat compartment syndrome. The muscles of the lower leg are divided into anterior, lateral, and posterior muscle compartments. Each compartment contains muscle, blood vessels, and nerves surrounded by a fascial sheath. Long bone fractures, crush injuries and other trauma can cause swelling within the muscle compartment. However, the surrounding fascia does not have the ability to expand. This causes an increase in interstitial pressures that can lead to tissue necrosis with permanent functional impairment of the limb. Treatment consists of decompression fasciotomy of the affected compartments. In 27600, decompression fasciotomy of anterior and/or lateral compartments is performed. A longitudinal incision is made over the intermuscular septum between the anterior and lateral compartments. For decompression of the anterior compartment, a nick is made in the fascia midway between the septum and tibial crest. The fascia is opened proximally and distally with scissors. For decompression of the lateral compartment, the fascia is incised parallel to the fibular shaft taking care to identify and protect the peroneal nerve. In 27601, decompression fasciotomy of the posterior compartment(s) is performed. There are two posterior compartments (deep and superficial) that can be approached via a single posterior longitudinal incision. The deep posterior compartment is approached by undermining tissues anterior to the posterior tibial margin taking care to protect the saphenous vein and nerve. The fascia of the deep posterior compartment is incised longitudinally under the belly of the soleus muscle. The superficial compartment may also be opened by incising the fascia posterior and parallel to the incision in the deep compartment. In 27602, decompression fasciotomy is performed on the posterior compartment(s) and anterior and/or lateral compartments as described above.

27603-27604

27603   Incision and drainage, leg or ankle; deep abscess or hematoma

27604   Incision and drainage, leg or ankle; infected bursa

In 27603, an incision is made in the skin over the abscess or hematoma site. The incision is carried down through the soft tissue and the abscess or hematoma is opened. If drainage is performed for an abscess, any loculations are broken up using blunt finger dissection. If drainage is for a hematoma, blood clots are removed by suction. The abscess or hematoma cavity is flushed with saline or antibiotic solution. In 27604, an incision is made in the skin over the infected bursa. The infected bursa is opened with a scalpel and drained. The site is flushed with saline or antibiotic solution. Drains are placed as needed. The incision may be closed in layers or packed with gauze and left open.

27605-27606

27605   Tenotomy, percutaneous, Achilles tendon (separate procedure); local anesthesia

27606   Tenotomy, percutaneous, Achilles tendon (separate procedure); general anesthesia

A percutaneous tenotomy of the Achilles tendon is performed to treat shortening or contracture of the tendon. Achilles tenotomy is commonly performed to treat clubfoot deformity. A small stab incision is made over the Achilles tendon at the planned tenotomy site. The tendon is then incised. Typically, a Z-plasty incision is used to lengthen the tendon. The small stab incision is closed with sutures or steri-strips. The foot is then placed in a cast to stretch and preserve the length in the tendon. Use 27605 when the procedure is performed under local anesthesia. Use 27606 when general anesthesia is required.

27607

27607   Incision (eg, osteomyelitis or bone abscess), leg or ankle

The bone cortex of the tibia, fibula, talus or calcaneus is opened to treat a condition such as osteomyelitis or bone abscess. An incision is made in the skin and carried down through the soft tissue overlying the site of the infected bone. The periosteum over the infected region of the bone is elevated, a button of cortical bone removed, and the bone marrow exposed. Opening the bone cortex relieves pressure caused by inflammation of the bone marrow and prevents restriction of blood flow to the infected bone. If frank pus is encountered, the button hole may be enlarged and extended using a chisel or gouge along the bone for one to two inches. If the epiphysis is involved, a section of the epiphyseal cortex may be removed. The bone abscess is drained.

27610

27610   Arthrotomy, ankle, including exploration, drainage, or removal of foreign body

The approach to the ankle joint is dependent on the site of the fluid collection, foreign body or other condition requiring exploration of the joint. Tissues are dissected and the joint capsule is exposed. The joint capsule is opened and the ankle joint explored. If an infection is present, fluid including blood and purulent matter is drained from the ankle. Cultures are obtained and sent separately reportable laboratory analysis. The ankle is flushed with saline solution to remove any debris. Any foreign bodies are located and removed. The ankle is again flushed with saline solution. Drains are placed as needed. The incision is closed in layers around the drain. A dressing is applied.

27612

27612   Arthrotomy, posterior capsular release, ankle, with or without Achilles tendon lengthening

In the ankle, the ligaments that surround and stabilize the joint also form part of the joint capsule. When the ligaments and tendons are too tight or when there is a congenital malformation of the foot or ankle such as clubfoot, the joint capsule must be incised and the ligaments released to correct the tightness or malformation. Using a posterior approach to the ankle joint, tissues are dissected and the joint capsule is exposed. The posterior ligaments and joint capsule are incised to increase range of motion and correct any malformation. The Achilles tendon may also be incised using either a Z-plasty configuration or a series of longitudinal incisions. The foot is then placed in a cast to maintain the foot in a more anatomically correct position or to stretch and preserve length in the ligaments and Achilles tendon.

27613-27614

27613   Biopsy, soft tissue of leg or ankle area; superficial

27614   Biopsy, soft tissue of leg or ankle area; deep (subfascial or intramuscular)

Soft tissues include muscles, tendons, fat, blood vessels, lymph vessels, nerves, and tissues surrounding the joints. Local, regional, or general anesthesia or conscious sedation is administered depending on the site and depth of the planned biopsy. The area over the planned biopsy site is cleansed. An incision is made and tissue dissected down to the mass or lesion taking care to protect blood vessels and nerves. A tissue sample is obtained and sent to the laboratory for separately reportable histological evaluation. The incision is closed with sutures. Use 27613 for a superficial biopsy or 27614 for biopsy of deeper tissues requiring more extensive dissection of overlying tissues, such as a biopsy below the muscle fascia (subfascial) or within the muscle itself (intramuscular).

27615-27616

27615   Radical resection of tumor (eg, sarcoma), soft tissue of leg or ankle area; less than 5 cm

27616   Radical resection of tumor (eg, sarcoma), soft tissue of leg or ankle area; 5 cm or greater

Soft tissues include muscles, tendons, fat, blood vessels, lymph vessels, nerves, and tissues surrounding the joints. Soft tissue tumors may be benign or malignant. Radical resection is typically performed for a malignant neoplasm, such as a sarcoma, although benign tumors and tumors of indeterminate nature may also require radical resection. A skin incision is made over the tumor in the lower leg or ankle area, or a skin flap is created and elevated. Overlying tissue is dissected and the tumor exposed. The tumor is removed en bloc along with a wide margin of surrounding tissue. Radical resection involves excision of all involved soft tissue which may include muscles, nerves, and blood vessels. Separately reportable frozen section is performed to ensure that all margins are free of tumor cells. If margins show evidence of malignancy, additional tissue is removed until all margins are free of tumor cells. Drains are placed as needed. The surgical wound may be closed in layers, or separately reportable reconstructive procedures performed. Use 27615 for radical resection of a soft tissue tumor of less than 5 cm in the leg or ankle, and 27616 for a tumor 5 cm or greater.

Musculoskeletal System

27618-27619

27618 Excision, tumor, soft tissue of leg or ankle area, subcutaneous; less than 3 cm

27619 Excision, tumor, soft tissue of leg or ankle area, subfascial (eg, intramuscular); less than 5 cm

Soft tissues include subcutaneous fat and connective tissue, fascia, muscles, tendons, blood vessels, lymph vessels, nerves, and tissues surrounding the joints. Soft tissue tumors may be benign or malignant. Benign tumors are typically treated by excision, although small malignant or indeterminate tumors may be excised if the margins are well defined. Depending on the location of the tumor in the soft tissue of the lower leg or ankle area, the skin over the tumor may be incised or a skin flap created and elevated. Overlying tissue is dissected and the soft tissue mass exposed. The tumor is then excised along with a margin of healthy tissue. Separately reportable frozen section may be performed to ensure that all margins are free of tumor cells. Drains are placed as needed and the surgical wound is closed in layers. For tumors in the subcutaneous fat or connective tissue, use 27618 for excision of less than 3 cm. For tumors that lie below the fascia, use 27619 for excision of less than 5 cm. Subfascial soft tissue tumors include those within muscle tissue.

27620

27620 Arthrotomy, ankle, with joint exploration, with or without biopsy, with or without removal of loose or foreign body

The approach to the ankle joint is dependent on the suspected condition that is being evaluated. An incision is made in the skin and carried down through soft tissues taking care to protect nerves and vascular structures. The ankle joint capsule is incised and the joint inspected for evidence of injury, disease, or infection. Tissue samples are taken as needed and sent for separately reportable laboratory analysis. If a loose or foreign body is located, it is removed. The joint is then flushed with saline to remove any debris. The joint capsule closed followed by layered closure of overlying soft tissue and skin.

27625-27626

27625 Arthrotomy, with synovectomy, ankle

27626 Arthrotomy, with synovectomy, ankle; including tenosynovectomy

Synovial tissue lines the ankle joint and produces synovial fluid. When it becomes inflamed due to rheumatoid arthritis, synovial proliferative disorder, or other condition, the synovium produces excess synovial fluid resulting in joint effusion. The approach to the ankle joint is dependent on the suspected location of the diseased synovial tissue. An incision is made in the skin and carried down through soft tissues taking care to protect nerves and vascular structures. The ankle joint capsule is incised and the joint inspected for evidence of injury, disease, or infection. In 27625, a motorized shaver is then used to remove the synovium. Care is taken to resect all inflamed synovial tissue without damaging underlying vascular or nervous tissue. The joint is flushed with saline to remove any debris. The joint capsule closed followed by layered closure of overlying soft tissue and skin. In 27626, severe tenosynovitis is treated with synovectomy as described above and excision of damaged or diseased extensor tendons, which may also include excision of the tibialis anterior tendon and the tibial and fibular retromalleolar tendons.

27630

27630 Excision of lesion of tendon sheath or capsule (eg, cyst or ganglion), leg and/or ankle

Common types of tendon sheath or joint capsule lesions include cysts or ganglia. Ganglia are multiloculated fluid-filled cysts that arise from fibrous tissue. These types of benign lesions are typically only removed if they are causing significant discomfort while standing or walking. The approach is dependent on the location of the lesion. An incision is made in the skin and carried down through soft tissues taking care to protect nerves and vascular structures. The tendon sheath or joint capsule is exposed and the cyst identified. The cyst is carefully dissected free of tendon sheath or capsule and removed. The incision is closed in a layered fashion.

27632-27634

27632 Excision, tumor, soft tissue of leg or ankle area, subcutaneous; 3 cm or greater

27634 Excision, tumor, soft tissue of leg or ankle area, subfascial (eg, intramuscular); 5 cm or greater

Soft tissues include subcutaneous fat and connective tissue, fascia, muscles, tendons, blood vessels, lymph vessels, nerves, and tissues surrounding the joints. Soft tissue tumors may be benign or malignant. Benign tumors are typically treated by excision, although small malignant or indeterminate tumors may be excised if the margins are well defined. Depending on the location of the tumor in the soft tissue of the lower leg or ankle area, the skin over the tumor may be incised or a skin flap created and elevated. Overlying tissue is dissected and the soft tissue mass exposed. The tumor is then excised along with a margin of healthy tissue. Separately reportable frozen section may be performed to ensure that all margins are free of tumor cells. Drains are placed as needed and the surgical wound is closed in layers. For tumors in the subcutaneous fat or connective tissue, use 27632 for

soft tissue excision of 3 cm or greater. For tumors that lie below the fascia, use 27634 for excision of soft tissue 5 cm or greater. Subfascial soft tissue tumors include those within muscle tissue.

27635-27638

27635 Excision or curettage of bone cyst or benign tumor, tibia or fibula

27637 Excision or curettage of bone cyst or benign tumor, tibia or fibula; with autograft (includes obtaining graft)

27638 Excision or curettage of bone cyst or benign tumor, tibia or fibula; with allograft

A bone cyst is a fluid filled space within the bone. One common type is a unicameral or simple bone cyst, which is a benign lesion. A less common type is an aneurysmal bone cyst, which consists of vascular tissue surrounding a blood filled cystic lesion. There are a number of different types of benign bone tumors including giant cell tumors, chondromixoid fibromas, and enchondromas. In 27635, an incision is made in the skin over the site of lesion in the tibia or fibula. Soft tissues are dissected and the lesion is exposed. If a cystic lesion is present, the bone is incised and a window created to open the cyst. Fluid is aspirated and sent to the laboratory for separately reportable analysis. A curette is inserted through the bone window and the lining of the cystic cavity is completely removed by curettage. Alternatively, some cystic lesions and most benign tumors are treated by excision. The lesion is exposed as described above. The physician then excises the benign lesion along with a margin of surrounding healthy bone. In 27637, the lesion is curetted or excised as described above. The physician then obtains healthy bone locally or from a separate site, such as the iliac crest. The bone autograft is packed into the defect in the tibia or fibula. In 27638, the lesion is curetted or excised as described above. The defect is then packed with donor bone (allograft).

27640-27641

27640 Partial excision (craterization, saucerization, or diaphysectomy), bone (eg, osteomyelitis); tibia

27641 Partial excision (craterization, saucerization, or diaphysectomy), bone (eg, osteomyelitis); fibula

Craterization and saucerization of bone involves removing infected and necrotic bone to form a shallow depression in the bone surface that will allow drainage from the infected area. Diaphysectomy involves removal of the infected portion of the shaft of a long bone. An incision is made in the skin and carried down through the soft tissue overlying the site of the osteomyelitis. Soft tissue sinus tracts and devitalized soft tissue are resected. The area of necrotic and infected bone is exposed. A series of drill holes are made in the necrotic and infected bone and the bone between the drill holes is excavated to create an oval window using an osteotome. The amount of bone removed is dependent on the extent of the infection. A curette may be used to remove devitalized tissue from the medullary canal. Debridement continues until punctate bleeding is identified in the exposed bony surface. When all devitalized and infected tissue has been removed, the wound is copiously irrigated with sterile saline or antibiotic solution. The surgical wound is loosely closed and a drain placed. Use 27640 for partial excision of bone of the tibia, and 27641 for partial excision of bone the fibula.

27645-27647

27645 Radical resection of tumor; tibia

27646 Radical resection of tumor; fibula

27647 Radical resection of tumor; talus or calcaneus

Radical resection is typically performed for a malignant neoplasm although benign tumors and tumors of indeterminate nature may also require radical resection. A skin incision is made over the site of the bone tumor, or a skin flap is created and elevated. Overlying tissue is dissected and the tumor exposed. All bone and cartilage with tumor involvement is resected. The tumor is removed en bloc along with a wide margin of surrounding tissue. Radical resection of bone includes excision of all involved soft tissue which may include muscles, tendons, fat, blood vessels, lymph vessels, nerves, and tissues surrounding the joints. Separately reportable frozen section is performed to ensure that all margins are free of tumor cells. If margins show evidence of malignancy, additional tissue is removed until all margins are free of tumor cells. Drains are placed as needed. The surgical wound may be closed in layers, or separately reportable reconstructive procedures performed. For radical resection of a bone tumor of the tibia, use 27645; fibula, use 27646; talus or calcaneus, use 27647.

27648

27648 Injection procedure for ankle arthrography

The skin over the injection site is cleansed and a local anesthetic is injected. A needle may be inserted into the joint and fluid aspirated with a syringe. The radiopaque substance is then injected into the ankle joint, which is exercised to help distribute the radiopaque substance. Once the contrast has been distributed throughout the joint, separately reportable radiographic images are obtained.

● New Code   ▲ Revised Code

Musculoskeletal System

27650-27654

27650   Repair, primary, open or percutaneous, ruptured Achilles tendon
27652   Repair, primary, open or percutaneous, ruptured Achilles tendon; with graft (includes obtaining graft)
27654   Repair, secondary, Achilles tendon, with or without graft

The Achilles tendon is the largest tendon in the body. It connects the gastrocnemius and soleus muscles in the calf to the calcaneus and is vital for walking, running, and jumping. The Achilles tendon can become weak and thin with age or lack of use which leaves it prone to injury. The most common type of injury is a complete tear or rupture of the Achilles tendon. In 27650, the Achilles tendon is suture repaired. If an open approach is used, a posteromedial longitudinal skin incision is made of over the lower leg and ankle region. Subcutaneous tissue is dissected and the paratenon exposed. The paratenon is divided longitudinally and the ruptured ends of the Achilles tendon exposed. The ruptured ends are debrided and then approximated and repaired with heavy nonabsorbable sutures. If a percutaneous approach is used, the foot is positioned in maximal equinus. Multiple stab wounds are made over the posterior aspect of the ankle and sutures are passed through the distal and proximal ends of the Achilles tendon. The sutures are then cut, tied off, and pushed into the subcutaneous tissue. Overlying soft tissues and skin are repaired. A short leg non-weight bearing cast is applied. In 27652, a graft is used to repair the tendon. This can be accomplished using fascial augmentation with the gastrocnemius aponeurosis or with the plantaris tendon. If the gastrocnemius aponeurosis is used, a rectangular flap 1-2 cm wide and 7-8 cm long is created and raised to within 3 cm of the rupture site. The proximal edge of the flap is flipped distally across the rupture and sutured to the distal aspect of the rupture site. If the plantaris tendon is used it is either woven across the rupture site or fanned out and sutured to the rupture site. Both 27650 and 27652 are used for primary repair of the Achilles tendon. In 27654, a secondary repair of the Achilles tendon is performed when the primary repair has failed, the tendon ruptures again, or when the tendon is surgically repaired several weeks after the original injury occurred. The tendon may be repaired with sutures or with a graft using the same techniques described above.

27656

27656   Repair, fascial defect of leg

Muscle fascia is a sheet of fibrous tissue that covers muscles and muscle groups and separates the lower leg into muscle compartments. A defect in the muscle fascia is a disruption of the fibrous sheet through which muscle tissue can protrude or herniate. The fascial defect is exposed. The defect is repaired with sutures.

27658-27659

27658   Repair, flexor tendon, leg; primary, without graft, each tendon
27659   Repair, flexor tendon, leg; secondary, with or without graft, each tendon

The flexor muscles and tendons of the lower leg include the peroneus longus, peroneus brevis, plantaris, popliteus, flexor digitorum longus, flexor hallucis longus, and tibialis posterior. Lacerations and puncture wounds can cause partial or complete transection of one or more flexor tendons. Closed injuries such as avulsion can also occur. An incision is made over the site of the flexor tendon or muscle injury. If the tendon has been completely transected, the severed end of the flexor tendon is located, grasped and pulled distally or proximally. The tendon is then suture repaired. If the tendon has only been partially transected, the transected fibers are repaired. If the muscle itself has been lacerated or torn, the muscle tissue is repaired in layers. Use 27658 to report primary suture repair of a single flexor tendon or muscle. If a functional result is not achieved from the primary repair, secondary repair may be required. Use 27659 to report secondary suture repair of a single flexor tendon or muscle. Secondary repair may be performed as described above or a graft may be used. A tendon graft is harvested and attached to the remnants of the severed tendon in the lower leg and then attached at the distal insertion site of the tendon. Range of motion is tested and tension adjusted as needed to allow good range of motion in the ankle and toes. The surgical wound is closed in layers. The leg and ankle are immobilized using a splint or cast.

27664-27665

27664   Repair, extensor tendon, leg; primary, without graft, each tendon
27665   Repair, extensor tendon, leg; secondary, with or without graft, each tendon

27664-27665The extensor muscles and tendons of the lower leg include the tibialis anterior, extensor digitorum, peroneus tertius, extensor hallucis longus. Lacerations and puncture wounds can cause partial or complete transection of one or more extensor tendons. Closed injuries such as avulsion are another type of injury that can occur. An incision is made over the site of the extensor tendon or muscle injury. If the tendon has been completely transected, the severed end of the extensor tendon is located, grasped and pulled distally or proximally. The tendon is then suture repaired. If the tendon has only been partially transected, the transected fibers are repaired. If the muscle itself has been lacerated or torn, the muscle tissue is repaired in layers. Use 27664 to report primary suture repair of a single extensor tendon or muscle. If a functional result is not achieved from the primary repair, secondary repair may be required. Use 27665 to report secondary suture repair of a single extensor tendon or muscle. Secondary repair may be performed as

described above or a graft may be used. A tendon graft is harvested and attached to the remnants of the severed tendon in the lower leg and then attached at the distal insertion site of the tendon. Range of motion is tested and tension adjusted as needed to allow good range of motion in the ankle and toes. The surgical wound is closed in layers. The leg and ankle are immobilized using a splint or cast.

27675-27676

27675   Repair, dislocating peroneal tendons; without fibular osteotomy
27676   Repair, dislocating peroneal tendons; with fibular osteotomy

The peroneus longus and peroneus brevis muscles are located in the lateral compartment of the lower leg. The tendons of these two muscles begin prior to crossing the ankle joint. They remain in a common tendon sheath bordered anteriorly by the fibular sulcus, medially by the calcaneofibular and posterior tibiofibular ligaments, and posterolaterally by the superior retinaculum. As these tendons pass distal to the fibula, they are separated by the peroneal tubercle and each enters a separate tendon sheath. The peroneus brevis inserts at the fifth metatarsal base while the peroneus longus passes through the plantar region of the foot and inserts on the first metatarsal. There is also a peroneal groove in the posterior surface of the lateral malleolus that is covered by fibrocartilage and helps to keep the peroneal tendons in the correct location. Dislocation is usually a result of injury to the superior retinaculum. In 27675, the dislocation is treated without fibular osteotomy. An incision is made over the lateral aspect of the ankle. The retinaculum is inspected to determine whether there is sufficient retinaculum to cover the tendons. The tendons are replaced in the peroneal groove and the retinaculum is sutured over the tendons. In some cases the peroneal groove will be deepened first to help prevent dislocation. Other types of repairs involve reinforcement of the retinaculum using the Achilles tendon, rerouting the tendons using the calcaneofibular ligament or repair using part of the external lateral ligament. In 27676, a bone block procedure such as a sliding distal fibular osteotomy is performed. Bone cuts are made in the distal fibula to allow rotation of the bone fragment which serves as a mechanical block to prevent anterior displacement of the tendons. The bone fragment is secured with screws.

27680-27681

27680   Tenolysis, flexor or extensor tendon, leg and/or ankle; single, each tendon
27681   Tenolysis, flexor or extensor tendon, leg and/or ankle; multiple tendons (through separate incision[s])

Tenolysis involves freeing a tendon from surrounding tissue. In 27680, tenolysis of a single flexor or extensor tendon is performed at the level of the lower leg or ankle to restore ankle, foot, and/or toe motion by releasing scar tissue resulting from trauma or a disease process. An incision is made over the affected flexor or extensor tendon. Soft tissues are dissected. The affected tendon is identified and adhesions are severed. Range of motion is evaluated. The surgical wound is closed in layers and a dressing is applied. In 27681, tenolysis of multiple tendons is performed in the same manner, usually through separate incisions.

27685-27686

27685   Lengthening or shortening of tendon, leg or ankle; single tendon (separate procedure)
27686   Lengthening or shortening of tendon, leg or ankle; multiple tendons (through same incision), each

A flexion or extension deformity in the ankle is corrected by lengthening or shortening one of the flexor or extensor tendons in the lower leg or ankle. Flexion and extension deformities may be due to late effects of injuries or due to disease processes such as severe rheumatoid arthritis or osteoarthritis. To lengthen a flexor or extensor tendon, a skin incision is made over the tendon to be lengthened, soft tissues are dissected, and the tendon is exposed. A Z-shaped incision is made in the tendon which lengthens it by allowing the tendon fibers to slide apart as the ankle is flexed or extended. Tendon sutures are placed to maintain the tendon in the lengthened position. The ankle is immobilized in a splint or cast so that the ankle can be maintained in the desired position until the tendon heals. To shorten a tendon, the tendon is divided. The divided ends of the tendon are then overlapped and sutured together. The ankle is immobilized in a splint. Use 27685 for lengthening or shortening of a single tendon in the leg or ankle. Use 27686 for lengthening or shortening of multiple tendons through the same incision.

27687

27687   Gastrocnemius recession (eg, Strayer procedure)

Gastrocnemius recession is performed to treat tightness in the gastrocnemius muscle causing equinus contracture as well as ankle and foot pain. Equinus contracture is characterized by the inability to move the ankle past neutral which is defined as a 90 degree angle between the leg and foot. Equinus contracture is compensated for by greater movement in the transverse tarsal joint of the midfoot which is what causes pain and may also cause plantar fasciitis, acquired flatfoot deformity, and metatarsalgia. A longitudinal posteromedial incision is made over the mid-calf region. Soft tissues are dissected and the gastrocnemius muscle is exposed. A Z-shaped incision is made in the Achilles tendon which

Musculoskeletal System

lengthens it by allowing the tendon fibers to slide apart as the ankle is flexed. The Achilles tendon may be left to heal in the lengthened position or it may be sutured to underlying tissues in the lengthened position. The ankle is immobilized in a cast, splint, or CAM-type walking boot so that the ankle can be maintained in the desired position until the tendon heals.

27690-27692

27690 Transfer or transplant of single tendon (with muscle redirection or rerouting); superficial (eg, anterior tibial extensors into midfoot)

27691 Transfer or transplant of single tendon (with muscle redirection or rerouting); deep (eg, anterior tibial or posterior tibial through interosseous space, flexor digitorum longus, flexor hallucis longus, or peroneal tendon to midfoot or hindfoot)

27692 Transfer or transplant of single tendon (with muscle redirection or rerouting); each additional tendon (List separately in addition to code for primary procedure)

Tendon transplantation or transfer of a single tendon of the lower leg is performed to restore function usually resulting from a traumatic injury to the nerve, tendon or muscle. Less commonly the loss of function may be due to rheumatoid or gouty arthritis. The procedure varies depending on the function that the surgeon is trying to restore. In 27690, superficial transfer or transplant of a single tendon is performed. The most common procedure is transplant of the anterior tibial extensors into the midfoot. To accomplish a tendon transplant or transfer, a longitudinal incision is made over the donor tendon and the tendon exposed. The donor tendon is freed from attachments in a manner that will allow it to be secured to the recipient site. This may include harvesting the tendon with a strip of periosteum. The muscle is also freed from fascial attachments to allow maximum mobility and length for the tendon transfer. A second incision is made over the recipient site which is where the tendon will be attached. The donor tendon is then routed to the recipient site and secured with temporary sutures. A neuromuscular stimulator is used to test the donor tendon function. The tension of the donor tendon is adjusted as needed to ensure maximum function and then permanently secured at the recipient site. Following closure of the surgical wounds, the ankle and foot are immobilized as needed. In 27691, a single deep tendon transfer or transplant is performed. This may involve transfer of the anterior tibial or posterior tibial tendon through the interosseous space or transfer of the flexor digitorum longus, flexor hallucis longus, or peroneal tendon to the midfoot or hindfoot. The procedure is performed as described above except that deeper tissues must be dissected to allow rerouting of the tendon to the recipient site. If more than one tendon is transferred or transplanted during the same surgical session, use 27692 for each additional superficial or deep tendon transfer or transplant after the first.

27695-27696

27695 Repair, primary, disrupted ligament, ankle; collateral
27696 Repair, primary, disrupted ligament, ankle; both collateral ligaments

Ligaments in the ankle joint are divided into three groups including the deltoid or medial collateral ligament which stabilizes the ankle medially, three lateral collateral ligaments (anterior talofibular, posterior talofibular, and calcaneofibular ligament) that stabilize the joint laterally and the syndesmotic ligaments that maintain anterior and posterior alignment. Disruption of any of these ligaments causes instability of the ankle joint. In 27695, only one of the collateral groups of ligaments is disrupted. An incision is made over the lateral or medial aspect of the ankle. The injured ligament is exposed and damaged tissue debrided. The ligament is then repaired with sutures. Alternatively if the ligament has detached from the bone, it is reattached with a bone screw. In 27696, both collateral groups of ligaments are disrupted and each is repaired as described above. Use 27695 or 27696 only for primary repair of the ligament(s).

27698

27698 Repair, secondary, disrupted ligament, ankle, collateral (eg, Watson-Jones procedure)

Ligaments in the ankle joint are divided into three groups including the deltoid or medial collateral ligament which stabilizes the ankle medially, three lateral collateral ligaments (anterior talofibular, posterior talofibular, and calcaneofibular ligament) that stabilize the joint laterally and the syndesmotic ligaments that maintain anterior and posterior alignment. Disruption of any of these ligaments causes instability of the ankle joint. When repair of the collateral ankle ligaments is performed several weeks after the original injury due to failed primary repair or failure of more conservative treatment or for a reinjury following a primary repair, the repair is a secondary repair. There are a number of different techniques, but most involve the use of grafts. One of the more common techniques is the Watson-Jones procedure for secondary repair of the lateral collateral ligaments. An incision is made over the lateral aspect of the ankle joint. Soft tissues are dissected and the joint capsule exposed and incised. The anterior talofibular ligament and calcaneofibular ligament are exposed. A tendon graft is harvested to reconstruct the ligament. Common donor tendons include the peroneus brevis, peroneus longus, Achilles and plantaris. If the peroneus brevis tendon is used, a drill hole is created through the fibula approximately 2 cm from the tip of the lateral malleolus and a second vertical drill hole is made in the

talus. The tendon is passed through the drill hole in the talus from dorsal to plantar and then through the drill hole in the fibula from anterior to posterior and secured with sutures or bone screw to the posterior aspect of the fibula. Ankle stability is evaluated and the tension on the tendon graft adjusted as needed. The tendon is secured with sutures or a bone scre to the posterior aspect of the fibula. Overlying soft tissues are closed in layers. A boot, splint or cast is applied to immobilize the ankle.

27700-27702

27700 Arthroplasty, ankle
27702 Arthroplasty, ankle; with implant (total ankle)

Arthroplasty of the ankle is performed to treat degenerative changes in the ankle including rheumatoid arthritis, osteoarthritis, and traumatic arthropathy. An incision is made over the anterior aspect of the ankle joint. Soft tissues are dissected and the joint capsule exposed and incised. Joint structures are inspected. Loose bodies, bone spurs, and inflamed tissue are excised. In 27700, ankle arthroplasty is performed without use of an implant. One type of procedure is a distraction ankle arthroplasty. Following removal of loose bodies, bone spurs, and damaged tissue, the ankle is distracted using an external distraction device. This type of device is similar to an external fixation device. The device pulls the ankle joint structures apart a minimal amount, usually about 5 mm which is less the α inch. This allows cartilage to rest, heal and regenerate. When ankle joint cartilage has healed, the external distraction device is removed. In 27702, ankle arthroplasty with an implant is performed. Depending on the type of implant used, the distal aspects of the tibia and fibula and the proximal aspect of the talus may be replaced or only the distal fibula and proximal talus may be replaced. A cutting guide is placed over the tibia and the distal aspect of the tibia is excised. A portion of the fibula may also be excised. A cutting guide is then placed over the talus and a portion of the talus is excised. Once the bone has been resected, the joint is debrided which includes a total capsulectomy, excision of osteophytes and release of lateral and medial talomalleolar joint spaces. Drilling guides are placed on the resected bones and fixation holes drilled. Trial implant components are placed and the implant fit evaluated and adjusted as needed. The permanent implant components are then placed and secured with bone screws and bone cement as needed. The tibiofibular joint may be fused to improve ankle stability. The incision is closed over a suction drain.

27703

27703 Arthroplasty, ankle; revision, total ankle

A revision of a total ankle is performed for mechanical complications or failure of the implant or for other complications such as infection. Revision may involve only one component or all components may be revised. A long incision is made over the ankle. Soft tissues are dissected taking care to protect nerves and blood vessels. The implant components are removed. The amount of bone loss is evaluated. If a bone allograft is required, it is obtained from the bone bank. The bone is configured to the size and shape of the defect or cancellous bone is morcelized and packed into the defect. The tibiofibular joint is evaluated and bone graft and fusion performed as needed. Once bone reconstruction has been completed, a new prosthesis is implanted. If ankle ligaments are contracted, they are released. Trial components are then placed and range of motion evaluated. The implant components are either secured using a press-fit technique, with bone screws or with bone cement. Soft tissues and skin are closed in layers over a suction drain.

27704

27704 Removal of ankle implant

Removal of a total ankle implant is performed for pain, mechanical complications or failure of the implant, or for other complications such as infection. A long incision is made over the ankle. Soft tissues are dissected taking care to protect nerves and blood vessels. The implant components are removed. Damaged and infected tissue is debrided. If the procedure is performed for infection, an antibiotic infiltrated spacer may be placed. Alternatively, a separately reportable ankle arthrodesis may be performed. The surgical wound is closed in layers over a suction drain.

27705-27709

27705 Osteotomy; tibia
27707 Osteotomy; fibula
27709 Osteotomy; tibia and fibula

An osteotomy of the tibial and/or fibular shafts and/or distal tibia and/or fibula is performed to correct a deformity or realign the bone. The location of the osteotomy and the type performed is dependent on the site and type of the deformity. Some commonly used osteotomies include transverse, wedge, sliding, right or left angle, V-osteotomy, and Z-osteotomy. Using separately reportable radiographic studies, the physician determines where the bone cuts will be made to achieve the desired result prior to the start of the surgical procedure. An incision is made over the lower leg. Soft tissues are dissected and the tibia and fibula are exposed. The periosteum of the tibia and/or fibula is elevated. Using a drill, saw, and/or osteotome, the bone is cut in the previously determined configuration. Bone grafts are interposed between the cut bone segments as needed. Pins, screws, a plate and screw device, or other type of internal fixation is applied as needed to secure the cut edges in anatomical alignment. Alternatively, a separately reportable external fixation device may be applied. Use 27705 for osteotomy on the tibia alone. Use 27707 for osteotomy on the fibula alone. Use 27709 for osteotomy on both the tibia and fibula.

27712

27712   Osteotomy; multiple, with realignment on intramedullary rod (eg, Sofield type procedure)

Multiple osteotomies of the tibia and/or fibula are performed to correct a deformity or realign the bones. The location of the osteotomies and the type performed is dependent on the site and type of the deformity. Some commonly used osteotomies include transverse, wedge, sliding, right or left angle, V-osteotomy, and Z-osteotomy. Using separately reportable radiographic studies, the physician determines where the bone cuts will be made to achieve the desired result prior to the start of the surgical procedure. A longitudinal incision is made over the lower leg. Soft tissues are dissected and the bone is exposed. The periosteum is elevated. Using a drill, saw, and/or osteotome, the bone is cut in the previously determined configuration. The tibia and/or fibula is sized and an appropriately sized intramedullary rod is selected. A drill hole is created in the distal or proximal aspect of the tibia and/or fibula. The intramedullary canal is drilled or reamed through the drill hole. If a cannulated rod is used, a guidewire is placed into the intramedullary canal. The rod is then advanced over the guidewire until it is properly positioned within the canal. The bone is anatomically positioned at each osteotomy site and the rod is secured using screws, pins or other devices.

27715

27715   Osteoplasty, tibia and fibula, lengthening or shortening

A plastic procedure is performed on the tibia and fibula to lengthen or shorten the bone. Using separately reportable radiographic studies, the physician determines where the bone cuts will be made to achieve the desired result prior to the start of the surgical procedure. The tibia and fibula are exposed. For a shortening procedure, the sites of the bone cuts are identified. The tibia and fibula are cut and segments of the bone are excised. The remaining distal and proximal portions of the bone are then brought into contact with each other and internal fixation is applied to stabilize the reconfigured bones. Alternatively, a separately reportable external fixation device may be applied. For a lengthening procedure, cuts are made in the tibia and fibula, and the bones are distracted. A separately reportable bone autograft is harvested, usually from the iliac crest. A skin incision is made over the iliac crest and the muscle is stripped to reveal the bone surface. Cortical and/or cancellous bone is harvested. The bone is configured to the desired size and shape and/or cancellous bone is morcelized and packed into the defects. Pins, screws, a plate and screw device, or other type of internal fixation is applied as needed to secure the cut edges in anatomical alignment. Alternatively, a separately reportable external fixation device may be applied.

27720-27725

27720   Repair of nonunion or malunion, tibia; without graft, (eg, compression technique)
27722   Repair of nonunion or malunion, tibia; with sliding graft
27724   Repair of nonunion or malunion, tibia; with iliac or other autograft (includes obtaining graft)
27725   Repair of nonunion or malunion, tibia; by synostosis, with fibula, any method

When union of the fracture fragments does not occur after sufficient healing time has elapsed, the patient is considered to have a nonunion of the fracture. Malunion caused by malalignment of the fracture fragments can cause osseous abnormalities, incongruity of articular surfaces, soft tissue contracture, nerve impingement, and other complications. The original fracture site in the tibia is exposed. The nonunion or malunion is evaluated to determine what type of repair is required. In 27720, the nonunion or malunion of the tibia is treated without a graft using internal fixation, such as a compression plate. For a nonunion, a compression plate is placed over the fracture site and secured with lag screws. For a malunion, the tibia may be refractured, realigned, and internal fixation placed to maintain the fracture in anatomical alignment. Following placement of the fixation device, stability of the fracture is checked and alignment is verified radiographically. In 27722, a sliding bone graft is used, usually to treat a malunion. Using a drill, saw, and/or osteotome, the tibia is cut in such a way that the bone segments can be rotated or moved into anatomical alignment. Pins, screws, a plate and screw device, or other type of internal fixation is applied as needed to secure the cut edges in anatomical alignment. The In 27724, a bone graft is used to fill the bone defect and encourage healing. The site of the nonunion or malunion is prepared which may include refracture of the bone. A bone autograft is harvested, usually from the iliac crest. A skin incision is made over the iliac crest and the muscle is stripped to reveal the bone surface. Cortical and/or cancellous bone is harvested. The bone is configured to the size and shape of the defect or cancellous bone is morcelized and packed into the defect. Internal fixation, such as a pin or wire is used as needed to secure the bone graft. A compression plate and screws or other internal fixation is used to stabilize the fracture. In 27725, an osseous union is created between

the tibia and fibula to treat nonunion of the tibia. The tibia and fibula are exposed at the tibial fracture site. A bone graft is harvested as described above. The bone graft is placed between the tibia and fibula and secured with screws to allow the two bones to fuse together at the tibial fracture site.

27726

27726   Repair of fibula nonunion and/or malunion with internal fixation

Fibular fractures that do not fuse (nonunion) or do not heal properly resulting in deformity (malunion) can cause pain and instability as well as fibular shortening with malrotation and derangement of the ankle joint. A lateral incision is made over the site of the old fracture. Dissection is carried down to the site of the nonunion or malunion. An oscillating saw or osteotome is used to cut the bone (osteotomy). Using preoperative measurements, the osteotomy is carried out so that proper length, rotation, and alignment of the bone are restored. Preliminary internal fixation is applied to maintain the bone in proper alignment, which is then verified visually and radiographically. Additional screws, plates, and other internal fixation devices are applied as needed using fluoroscopic guidance as required.

27727

27727   Repair of congenital pseudarthrosis, tibia

Congenital pseudoarthrosis of the tibia is a rare condition characterized by a bony defect that may be cystic, sclerotic, or dysplastic in nature and abnormal movement at the site of the defect. Pseudoarthrosis is a term that means false joint and in the case of congenital tibial pseudoarthrosis there is anterolateral movement or bowing of the tibia. A skin incision is made over the defect in the tibia. Soft tissues are dissected and the bone defect exposed. The bone lesion is excised. There are a number of repair techniques including placement of a compression device, placement of a vascularized free fibular graft, autogenous bone grafting, intermedullary rodding, or other technique and the exact procedure depends on the repair technique performed. Following repair of the tibia, incisions are closed in layers. A cast or splint is applied as needed to immobilize the leg.

27730-27734

27730   Arrest, epiphyseal (epiphysiodesis), open; distal tibia
27732   Arrest, epiphyseal (epiphysiodesis), open; distal fibula
27734   Arrest, epiphyseal (epiphysiodesis), open; distal tibia and fibula

Epiphyseal arrest is performed to treat a bone length discrepancy between the lower legs or between the tibia and fibula. The epiphysis is also referred to as the growth plate. An incision is made over the distal aspect tibia and/or fibula. Soft tissues are dissected, taking care to protect blood vessels and nerves. The distal tibia and/or fibula are exposed. Blount staples, transphyseal screws, or a plate and screw device are strategically placed in the epiphysis of the distal tibia and/or fibula to temporarily arrest bone growth. Use 27730 for epiphyseal arrest of the distal tibia. Use 27732 if the procedure is performed on the distal fibula. Use 27734 if epiphyseal arrest is performed on the distal tibia and fibula.

27740-27742

27740   Arrest, epiphyseal (epiphysiodesis), any method, combined, proximal and distal tibia and fibula
27742   Arrest, epiphyseal (epiphysiodesis), any method, combined, proximal and distal tibia and fibula; and distal femur

Epiphyseal arrest is performed to treat a bone length discrepancy between the lower legs or between the tibia and fibula. The epiphysis is also referred to as the growth plate. In 27740, epiphyseal arrest is performed on both the proximal and distal aspects of the tibia and fibula. Incisions are made over the proximal and distal tibia and fibula. Soft tissues are dissected, taking care to protect blood vessels and nerves. The proximal and distal tibia and fibula are exposed. Blount staples, transphyseal screws, or a plate and screw device are strategically placed in the epiphyses of the proximal and distal tibia and fibula to temporarily arrest bone growth. Use 27742 when epiphyseal arrest is performed on the distal femur in addition to epiphyseal arrest on the proximal and distal tibia and fibula.

27745

27745   Prophylactic treatment (nailing, pinning, plating or wiring) with or without methylmethacrylate, tibia

Prophylactic treatment is performed to prevent fracture of the tibia when the bone is weakened as a result of a disease process or neoplasm. Common methods used to maintain bone integrity include nailing, pinning, plating, or wiring with or without the use of methylmethacrylate. The weakened bone is evaluated radiographically and the best form of prophylaxis is determined. An intramedullary nail or rod may be placed using either an antegrade or retrograde approach. A small incision is made over the proximal or distal tibia. A nail or rod is then inserted into the intramedullary space. The nail is secured with locking screws placed distally and proximally. If pins are used, they may be placed transcutaneously through the weakened region of the bone. Plating requires open exposure of the bone and placement of a plate that is secured with screws. Wiring involves wrapping a wire cerclage around the bone. When methylmethacrylate is used, it is injected into bony defects.

Musculoskeletal System

27750-27752

27750 Closed treatment of tibial shaft fracture (with or without fibular fracture); without manipulation

27752 Closed treatment of tibial shaft fracture (with or without fibular fracture); with manipulation, with or without skeletal traction

Closed treatment of a tibial shaft fracture with or without fibular fracture is performed. Separately reportable radiographs are obtained to confirm the fracture. A neurovascular exam is performed to ensure that the nerves and blood vessels at the site of the injury are intact. In 27750, a nondisplaced or minimally displaced fracture is treated. No manipulation of the fracture fragments is required. A cast is applied to immobilize the fracture. In 27752, a displaced fracture is treated with manipulation, with or without skeletal traction. The displaced fracture fragments are manually reduced (manipulated) back to proper anatomic alignment. Separately reportable radiographs are obtained to confirm anatomic reduction. A cast is applied to immobilize the fracture. Following reduction of the fracture fragments and casting, skeletal traction is applied as needed. A pin is inserted through the calcaneus and weighted traction applied.

27756-27759

27756 Percutaneous skeletal fixation of tibial shaft fracture (with or without fibular fracture) (eg, pins or screws)

27758 Open treatment of tibial shaft fracture (with or without fibular fracture), with plate/screws, with or without cerclage

27759 Treatment of tibial shaft fracture (with or without fibular fracture) by intramedullary implant, with or without interlocking screws and/or cerclage

The tibial shaft fracture which may also include a fracture of the fibula is verified using separately reportable radiological studies. In 27756, percutaneous skeletal fixation is performed. If the fracture fragments are displaced they are manually manipulated into anatomical alignment and additional radiological studies are performed to verify that the fracture fragments have been successfully reduced. Small incisions are made in the skin and pins or screws placed across the fracture site to maintain the alignment of the fracture fragments. A cast or splint is applied as needed. In 27758, open treatment with plate and screw fixation is performed. An incision is made over the fracture site. Following reduction of the fracture, temporary wire fixation is applied and anatomic alignment verified radiographically. A plate is then placed across the tibial shaft fracture and secured with screws and the temporary wire fixation removed. A wire cerclage may also be used which involves wrapping a wire around the bone. In 27759, an intramedullary implant is used to treat the tibial shaft fracture. A small incision is made in the skin proximal or distal to the fracture site. A bone drill is used to gain access to the medullary canal. A nail or rod is inserted into the intramedullary space. The nail may be secured with locking screws placed distal and proximal to the fracture site. A wire cerclage may also be used which involves wrapping a wire around the bone.

27760-27762

27760 Closed treatment of medial malleolus fracture; without manipulation

27762 Closed treatment of medial malleolus fracture; with manipulation, with or without skin or skeletal traction

Closed treatment of a medial malleolus fracture is performed. The medial malleolus is located at the distal end of the tibia forming the bony prominence at the inner aspect of the ankle. The medial malleolus forms part of the ankle joint, articulating with the talus. Separately reportable radiographs are obtained to confirm the fracture. A neurovascular exam is performed to ensure that the nerves and blood vessels at the site of the injury are intact. In 27760, a nondisplaced or minimally displaced fracture is treated. No manipulation of the fracture fragments is required. A cast is applied to immobilize the fracture. In 27762, a displaced fracture is treated with manipulation, with or without skin or skeletal traction. The displaced fracture fragments are manually reduced (manipulated) back to proper anatomic alignment. Separately reportable radiographs are obtained to confirm anatomic reduction. A cast is applied to immobilize the fracture. Following reduction of the fracture fragments and casting, skeletal traction may also be used. A pin is inserted through the calcaneus and weighted traction applied. Alternatively, skin traction may be applied by splinting and taping the foot and applying a weighted traction device.

27766

27766 Open treatment of medial malleolus fracture, includes internal fixation, when performed

The medial malleolus is located at the distal end of the tibia forming the bony prominence at the inner aspect of the ankle. The medial malleolus forms part of the ankle joint, articulating with the talus. An incision is made over the fracture site to expose it and clear the site of debris. The fracture is manipulated back into proper position and internal fixation, such as screws or a plate and screw device, is applied, if needed. The wound is irrigated and incisions closed.

27767-27769

27767 Closed treatment of posterior malleolus fracture; without manipulation

27768 Closed treatment of posterior malleolus fracture; with manipulation

27769 Open treatment of posterior malleolus fracture, includes internal fixation, when performed

Following separately reportable radiographic studies, the physician evaluates a fracture of the posterior malleolus for stability, size, location, and number of bone fragments. In 27767, closed treatment of a posterior malleolus fracture is performed without manipulation on a fracture that is in anatomic alignment. A cast is applied to maintain alignment of the fracture. Use 27768 when closed treatment of a posterior malleolus fracture with manipulation is performed. Following separately reportable radiographic evaluation, a closed reduction of a displaced fracture is performed. The fracture is manually manipulated to reposition the displaced bone fragment(s) in a more optimal position for healing of the fracture. Reduction may be accomplished by dorsiflexion of the foot. Correct anatomical alignment is confirmed radiographically. A cast is applied to maintain alignment of the fracture. Use 27769 when open treatment of a posterior malleolus fracture is performed. A posterolateral incision is made over posterior malleolus taking care to protect the sural nerve. The peroneal and Achilles tendons are retracted and the fracture site located. The fracture is reduced. If internal fixation is required, screws, pins, or other internal fixation devices are placed. Typically one or two cancellous screws are placed in the posterior malleolus from posterior to anterior. Alternatively cancellous screws may be placed anterior to posterior or lag or cortical screws may be placed through a separate anterior incision. Optimal reduction to normal anatomic position is confirmed visually and radiographically.

27780-27781

27780 Closed treatment of proximal fibula or shaft fracture; without manipulation

27781 Closed treatment of proximal fibula or shaft fracture; with manipulation

Closed treatment of a proximal fibula or fibular shaft fracture is performed. Separately reportable radiographs are obtained to confirm the fracture. A neurovascular exam is performed to ensure that the nerves and blood vessels at the site of the injury are intact. In 27780, a nondisplaced or minimally displaced fracture is treated. No manipulation of the fracture fragments is required. A cast or brace is applied to immobilize the fracture. In 27781, a displaced fracture is treated. The displaced fracture fragments are manually reduced (manipulated) back to proper anatomic alignment. Separately reportable radiographs are obtained to confirm anatomic reduction. A cast or brace is applied to immobilize the fracture.

27784

27784 Open treatment of proximal fibula or shaft fracture, includes internal fixation, when performed

The fibula is the smaller bone of the lateral, or outer, aspect of the lower leg. The proximal (upper) fibula articulates with the tibia. The shaft is the middle portion. An incision is made longitudinally over the fracture site in the proximal tibia or the tibial shaft. Dissection is carried down through soft tissue taking care to isolate and protect the peroneal nerve. The fracture site is exposed and cleared of debris, then reduced. Internal fixation, such as a plate and screw device, is applied if needed. The wound is irrigated and the incision closed.

27786-27788

27786 Closed treatment of distal fibular fracture (lateral malleolus); without manipulation

27788 Closed treatment of distal fibular fracture (lateral malleolus); with manipulation

Closed treatment of a distal fibular (lateral malleolus) fracture is performed. The lateral malleolus is a bony projection at the distal fibula that forms the outer prominence at the ankle. Separately reportable radiographs are obtained to confirm the fracture. A neurovascular exam is performed to ensure that the nerves and blood vessels at the site of the injury are intact. In 27786, a nondisplaced or minimally displaced fracture is treated. No manipulation of the fracture fragments is required. A cast or brace is applied to immobilize the fracture. In 27788, a displaced fracture is treated. The displaced fracture fragments are manually reduced (manipulated) back to proper anatomic alignment. Separately reportable radiographs are obtained to confirm anatomic reduction. A cast or brace is applied to immobilize the fracture.

27792

27792 Open treatment of distal fibular fracture (lateral malleolus), includes internal fixation, when performed

The distal fibula's bony projection, the lateral malleolus, forms the outer prominence of the ankle. The distal fibula articulates with the tibia at the fibular notch. Fracture of the distal fibula can cause instability of the ankle syndesmosis comprised of the anterior tibiofibular ligament, interosseous ligament, and posterior-fibular ligament. A lateral incision is made over the fracture site and care is taken to isolate and protect branches of the superficial peroneal and sural nerves. The fracture site is exposed and cleared of debris, then reduced.

Internal fixation, such as a plate and screw device, is applied if needed. Ankle syndesmosis stability is verified. The wound is irrigated and incisions closed.

27808-27810

27808 **Closed treatment of bimalleolar ankle fracture (eg, lateral and medial malleoli, or lateral and posterior malleoli or medial and posterior malleoli); without manipulation**

27810 **Closed treatment of bimalleolar ankle fracture (eg, lateral and medial malleoli, or lateral and posterior malleoli or medial and posterior malleoli); with manipulation**

A nondisplaced bimalleolar ankle fracture involving the lateral and medial malleoli, the lateral and posterior malleoli, or the medial and posterior malleoli is treated. The distal fibula has a bony projection, called the lateral malleolus, that forms the outer prominence of the ankle. The medial malleolus at the distal end of the tibia forms the bony prominence at the inner aspect of the ankle. The posterior malleolus, also referred to as the posterior lip, is the bony process on the back of the tibia. A nondisplaced bimalleolar fracture of the ankle is evaluated. Separately reportable x-rays are reviewed. The fracture may be immobilized using a splint or cast. Use 27810 when closed treatment of the bimalleolar ankle fracture requires manipulation. The displaced fragments are manipulated back into anatomic alignment, which is verified by separately reportable x-rays. The fracture may be immobilized using a splint or cast.

27814

27814 **Open treatment of bimalleolar ankle fracture (eg, lateral and medial malleoli, or lateral and posterior malleoli, or medial and posterior malleoli), includes internal fixation, when performed**

A bimalleolar ankle fracture involving the lateral and medial malleoli, the lateral and posterior malleoli, or the medial and posterior malleoli is treated openly, using any necessary internal fixation. The distal fibula has a bony projection, called the lateral malleolus, that forms the outer prominence of the ankle. The medial malleolus at the distal end of the tibia forms the bony prominence at the inner aspect of the ankle. The posterior malleolus, also referred to as the posterior lip, is the bony process on the back of the tibia. For open treatment of fractures of the lateral and medial malleoli, a lateral incision is made over the fracture site in the distal fibula. Care is taken to isolate and protect branches of the superficial peroneal and sural nerves. Dissection continues until the periosteum is elevated to expose the fracture site, which is cleared of debris. The fracture is reduced and maintained with a bone clamp. Reduction is checked radiographically. If internal fixation is required, a guidewire is inserted through the fracture and internal fixation, such as a plate and screw device, is then applied. A second incision is then made over the fracture site in the medial malleolus, which is exposed and cleared of debris, then reduced. Internal fixation is next applied if needed. If the fracture involves the lateral or medial malleolus with the posterior malleolus, the posterior malleolus may reduce spontaneously once the lateral or medial malleolus fracture is reduced. If it does not, the incision may be extended posteriorly until the posterior malleolus can be actively reduced, and plate and screw fixation applied as needed. Ankle syndesmosis stability is verified following the bimalleolar fracture repair.

27816-27818

27816 **Closed treatment of trimalleolar ankle fracture; without manipulation**
27818 **Closed treatment of trimalleolar ankle fracture; with manipulation**

Closed treatment of a trimalleolar (lateral, medial, and posterior malleoli) ankle fracture is performed. The malleoli are bony projections at the ankle, the lateral malleolus on the fibula forms the outer prominence of the ankle, the medial malleolus on the fibula forms the inner prominence of the ankle, and the posterior malleolus is the bony process on the back of the tibia. Separately reportable radiographs are obtained to confirm the fracture. A neurovascular exam is performed to ensure that the nerves and blood vessels at the site of the injury are intact. In 27816, a nondisplaced or minimally displaced fracture is treated. No manipulation of the fracture fragments is required. A cast or brace is applied to immobilize the fracture. In 27818, a displaced fracture is treated. The displaced fracture fragments are manually reduced (manipulated) back to proper anatomic alignment. Separately reportable radiographs are obtained to confirm anatomic reduction. A cast or brace is applied to immobilize the fracture.

27822-27823

27822 **Open treatment of trimalleolar ankle fracture, includes internal fixation, when performed, medial and/or lateral malleolus; without fixation of posterior lip**

27823 **Open treatment of trimalleolar ankle fracture, includes internal fixation, when performed, medial and/or lateral malleolus; with fixation of posterior lip**

A trimalleolar ankle fracture involving all three malleoli (lateral, medial, and posterior) is repaired, including any necessary internal fixation. The distal fibula has a bony projection, called the lateral malleolus, that forms the outer prominence of the ankle. The medial malleolus at the distal end of the tibia forms the bony prominence at the inner aspect of

the ankle. The posterior malleolus, also referred to as the posterior lip, is the bony process on the back of the tibia. A lateral incision is made over the fracture site in the lateral malleolus. Care is taken to isolate and protect branches of the superficial peroneal and sural nerves. Dissection continues until the periosteum is elevated to expose the fracture site, which is cleared of debris. The fracture is reduced and maintained with a bone clamp. Reduction is checked radiographically. If internal fixation is required, a guidewire is inserted through the fracture and internal fixation, such as a plate and screw device, is then applied. A second incision is then made over the fracture site in the medial malleolus, which is exposed and cleared of debris, then reduced. Internal fixation is next applied if needed. Sometimes open reduction of the lateral or medial malleolus causes spontaneous reduction of the other malleolus and open reduction is not required on both the lateral and medial malleoli. Open reduction of the lateral or medial malleolus may also spontaneously reduce the posterior malleolus. Use 27822 when the posterior lip does not require open reduction and fixation. Use 27823 when the posterior lip must be reduced and fracture fragments fixed separately. The incision over the lateral malleolus is extended posteriorly, soft tissue attachments of the distal fibula are released, and the posterior ankle joint is exposed. The posterior lip is reduced, a temporary guide is placed, and anatomic reduction is confirmed radiographically. Internal fixation, such as a compression screws or a plate and screw device, is applied as needed.

27824-27825

27824 **Closed treatment of fracture of weight bearing articular portion of distal tibia (eg, pilon or tibial plafond), with or without anesthesia; without manipulation**

27825 **Closed treatment of fracture of weight bearing articular portion of distal tibia (eg, pilon or tibial plafond), with or without anesthesia; with skeletal traction and/or requiring manipulation**

Closed treatment of a fracture of the weight bearing articular portion of the distal tibia, also referred to as a tibial pilon or tibial plafond fracture, is performed with or without anesthesia. Separately reportable radiographs are obtained to confirm the fracture. A neurovascular exam is performed to ensure that the nerves and blood vessels at the site of the injury are intact. In 27824, a nondisplaced or minimally displaced fracture is treated. No manipulation of the fracture fragments is required. A cast is applied to immobilize the fracture. In 27825, a displaced fracture is treated with manipulation and/or skeletal traction. The displaced fracture fragments are manually reduced (manipulated) back to proper anatomic alignment. Separately reportable radiographs are obtained to confirm anatomic reduction. A cast is applied to immobilize the fracture. Skeletal traction may also be used in addition to or instead of manual reduction. Skeletal traction is accomplished by inserting a pin through the calcaneus and applying weighted traction.

27826-27828

27826 **Open treatment of fracture of weight bearing articular surface/portion of distal tibia (eg, pilon or tibial plafond), with internal fixation, when performed; of fibula only**

27827 **Open treatment of fracture of weight bearing articular surface/portion of distal tibia (eg, pilon or tibial plafond), with internal fixation, when performed; of tibia only**

27828 **Open treatment of fracture of weight bearing articular surface/portion of distal tibia (eg, pilon or tibial plafond), with internal fixation, when performed; of both tibia and fibula**

A fracture of the weight bearing articular surface of the distal tibia, also referred to as tibial plafond or tibial pilon fracture, is repaired openly, using any necessary internal fixation. Tibial pilon fractures are high energy, compression type injuries frequently associated with severe articular cartilage and soft tissue injury at the ankle joint. At the time of injury, the distal tibia absorbs the impact, shattering when the axial force exceeds the yield point of the bone. Depending on the position of the foot and the degree of force, the fibula may also shatter. The energy is then absorbed by the soft tissues of the ankle causing injury to subcutaneous tissue and skin. Open treatment may include reduction and internal fixation of the fibula only (27826), the tibia only (27827), or both the tibia and fibula (27828). If the fibula is to be treated with open reduction and internal fixation, it is repaired first. An incision is made over the lateral aspect of the ankle. The superficial peroneal and sural nerves are isolated and protected. The fibula fracture is exposed and cleared of debris, the joint is inspected, and stability of the joint surface is assessed. The fracture is reduced and proper length restored. Internal fixation is applied as needed, usually a plate and screw fixation device with additional interfragmentary screws, as needed. If the tibia is treated with open reduction and internal fixation, an anterior or anteromedial incision is made over the ankle joint. Neurovascular structures are isolated and protected. The tibia fracture is exposed and cleared of debris. A femoral distraction device may be used to help reduce the fracture and restore proper length. The articular surface is restored with as little soft tissue dissection as possible. Internal fixation is applied as needed, usually a buttress plate and screws with additional interfragmentary screws applied as needed. Separately reportable bone grafts may be used to restore the metaphysis. Joint stability is checked. The wound is irrigated and the incision closed.

Musculoskeletal System

27829

27829 **Open treatment of distal tibiofibular joint (syndesmosis) disruption, includes internal fixation, when performed**

A distal tibiofibular joint (syndesmosis) disruption is repaired openly using any necessary internal fixation. The distal tibiofibular joint, called a syndesmosis, is a fibrous connection of ligaments made up of an interosseous membrane and three ligaments: the anterior, interosseous, and tibiofibular. An anterior incision is made over the tibiofibular syndesmosis to expose the injury. The disruption of the joint is reduced. If internal fixation is applied, the tibia and fibula are held tightly together and holes are drilled through the fibula across the joint and into the tibia in a posterolateral to anteromedial direction for screw placement. The screws are placed and checked radiographically. Alternatively, wire fixation or a plate and screw device may be applied. The wound is irrigated and the incision closed.

27830-27831

27830 **Closed treatment of proximal tibiofibular joint dislocation; without anesthesia**

27831 **Closed treatment of proximal tibiofibular joint dislocation; requiring anesthesia**

The proximal tibiofibular joint is a synovial joint situated at the posterolateral aspect of the knee between the lateral condyle of the tibia and the head of the fibula. Synovial joints are covered with hyaline cartilage or fibrocartilage, and have a joint cavity lined with synovial membrane that is filled with synovial fluid. Synovial joints are stabilized by a joint capsule and ligaments. Using manual pressure, the tibiofibular joint is returned to anatomic alignment. Successful reduction is verified using separately reportable radiographs. A splint or cast is applied as needed. Use 27830 if the procedure is performed without general anesthesia. Use 27831 if the general anesthesia is required.

27832

27832 **Open treatment of proximal tibiofibular joint dislocation, includes internal fixation, when performed, or with excision of proximal fibula**

The proximal tibiofibular joint is a synovial joint situated at the posterolateral aspect of the knee between the lateral condyle of the tibia and the head of the fibula. Synovial joints are covered with hyaline cartilage or fibrocartilage, have a joint cavity lined with synovial membrane and filled with synovial fluid. Synovial joints are stabilized by a joint capsule and ligaments. An incision is made laterally over the proximal tibiofibular joint. Overlying ligaments and tendons are identified and dissected. The peroneal nerve is identified and protected and dissection is continued down to the joint capsule. The proximal tibiofibular joint is exposed. The dislocation is reduced using bone reduction clamps. Temporary wire fixation is employed and reduction is checked radiographically, then internal fixation is applied as needed. Wires or screws are placed through the fibular head into the proximal tibial metaphysis. Injured ligaments are repaired or stabilized as needed. Alternatively, the proximal fibula may be resected. Following resection of the fibular head, the lateral collateral ligament and biceps femoris tendon are secured to the tibia. The wounds are irrigated and incisions closed.

27840-27842

27840 **Closed treatment of ankle dislocation; without anesthesia**

27842 **Closed treatment of ankle dislocation; requiring anesthesia, with or without percutaneous skeletal fixation**

Closed treatment of an ankle dislocation is performed. Ankle dislocation without concomitant fracture is a relatively rare injury that can cause neurovascular impairment if not recognized and treated without delay. Neurovascular status is the foot is evaluated. If neurovascular compromise as evidenced by cold, discoloration, or lack of a pulse or sensation, reduction is typically performed without obtaining pre-reduction radiographs. If neurovascular status of the foot is good, separately reportable radiographs may be obtained prior to treatment. Posterior dislocation of the talus is the most common type of dislocation injury. Reduction is accomplished by holding the foot in plantar flexion. An assistant then applies axial traction to the ankle by grasping the distal foot and applying a constant force on the foot. The tibia is grasped proximal to the dislocation and posterior traction applied with one hand while the other hand is placed on the heel of the foot and anterior pressure is applied. Reduction typically occurs in a few moments. Anterior dislocations are treated with anterior traction applied with one hand and axial traction combined with a posterior force applied with the other hand. Lateral dislocations are treated with lateral traction applied with one hand and medial pressure with the other. Medial dislocations are treated with medial traction applied with one hand and lateral pressure with the other. Following reduction the neurovascular status is evaluated and a long leg sugar tong posterior splint applied to immobilize the joint and maintain the ankle in 90 degree flexion. A second set of radiographs may be obtained to confirm anatomic alignment of the ankle structures. Use 27840 for closed treatment without anesthesia. Use 27842 when anesthesia is used and treatment is performed with or without percutaneous fixation. Using separately reportable radiologic guidance, pins are placed through the skin and across the ankle joint to stabilize the joint while soft tissue structures heal.

27846-27848

27846 **Open treatment of ankle dislocation, with or without percutaneous skeletal fixation; without repair or internal fixation**

27848 **Open treatment of ankle dislocation, with or without percutaneous skeletal fixation; with repair or internal or external fixation**

Ankle dislocation without concomitant fracture is a relatively rare injury that can cause neurovascular impairment if not recognized and treated without delay. In 27846, the ankle dislocation is treated by open reduction and may include percutaneous skeletal fixation. A skin incision is made over the ankle joint. Soft tissues are dissected and joint structures are exposed taking care to isolate and protect neurovascular structures. The joint capsule and ligaments are inspected and determined to be intact. Using separately reportable radiologic guidance, the dislocation is reduced. Pins are placed as needed through the skin and across the ankle joint to stabilize the joint while soft tissue structures heal. In 27848, following exposure and inspection of joint structures, the dislocation is reduced and injuries to the joint capsule and/or ligaments are repaired or internal or external fixation is applied. Damaged tissues are debrided. The joint capsule and/or ligaments are then repaired with sutures. Alternatively if a ligament has detached from the bone, it is reattached with a bone screw. Internal or external fixation devices may also be used to maintain an unstable ankle dislocation. Internal fixation may involve the use of pins, screws, or a plate and screw fixation device. External fixation involves placement of pins or screws through the skin and ankle bones. The pins or screws are attached to an external frame to immobilize the joint while the soft tissue injuries heal.

27860

27860 **Manipulation of ankle under general anesthesia (includes application of traction or other fixation apparatus)**

Manipulation of the ankle under anesthesia is performed to break up fibrous adhesions and scar tissue around the joint. Anesthesia is required when the patient is unable to tolerate manipulation of the joint due to pain, spasm, muscle contractures, or guarding. Following administration of anesthesia, the ankle joint is taken through a series of stretches and articular maneuvers to disrupt any adhesions or scar tissue and restore joint mobility and range of motion.

27870

27870 **Arthrodesis, ankle, open**

Ankle arthrodesis is performed to treat ankle pain, deformity, and instability caused by arthritis or deformity of the ankle joint. A long skin incision is made over the ankle. Soft tissues are dissected taking care to protect neurovascular structures. The joint capsule is exposed and incised. The articular cartilage on the talar dome, distal tibial plafond, and distal fibula is excised along with any diseased bone. Depending on the amount of bone loss, bone grafts may be required. If a bone allograft is used it is obtained from the bone bank. If a bone autograft is used, it is harvested, usually from the iliac crest. A skin incision is made over the iliac crest and the muscle is stripped to reveal the bone surface. Cortical and/or cancellous bone is harvested. The bone is configured to the desired size and shape and/or cancellous bone is morcelized and packed into the defect. Pins, screws, a plate and screw device, or other type of internal fixation is used to compress the talus, tibia and fibula together so that the bones will fuse together. Alternatively, an external fixation device may be applied. Overlying soft tissues and skin are closed in layers and the ankle is immobilized in a cast or splint.

27871

27871 **Arthrodesis, tibiofibular joint, proximal or distal**

There are two tibiofibular joints. The proximal tibiofibular joint is a synovial joint situated at the posterolateral aspect of the knee between the lateral condyle of the tibia and the head of the fibula. Synovial joints are covered with hyaline cartilage or fibrocartilage, and have a joint cavity lined with synovial membrane that is filled with synovial fluid. Synovial joints are stabilized by a joint capsule and ligaments. The distal tibiofibular joint is a syndesmosis consisting of a fibrous connection of ligaments made up of an interosseous membrane and three ligaments (anterior, interosseous, and tibiofibular). Fusion of the proximal tibiofibular joint involves an incision just below the knee. Fusion of the distal tibiofibular joint involves an incision at the ankle. Soft tissues are dissected and the proximal or distal tibiofibular joint exposed. Articular cartilage is excised from both bones and internal fixation applied to hold the bones together so that they will fuse. Overlying soft tissues and skin are closed in layers and the leg is immobilized in a cast or splint.

27880-27881

27880 **Amputation, leg, through tibia and fibula**

27881 **Amputation, leg, through tibia and fibula; with immediate fitting technique including application of first cast**

Amputation through the tibia and fibula, also referred to as a below knee (BK) amputation is the most frequently performed major limb amputation procedure. Incision lines are marked on the skin for amputation of the leg through the tibia and fibula. The skin and underlying soft tissues are incised. Dissection is carried down to the muscle. Muscle compartments are identified, isolated, and divided. Neurovascular structures are identified including the tibial nerve, artery, and vein; superficial and deep peroneal nerves and the peroneal artery and vein; the sural nerve; and the saphenous nerve and vein. Nerves and blood vessels are isolated taking care to ensure that nerves are separated from the arteries to prevent pulsatile irritation of the nerves. Nerves are transected as high as possible and allowed to retract into soft tissues. The periosteum of the tibia and fibula is incised and lateral and medial osteoperiosteal flaps elevated. The bone is then resected. The medial tibial flap is sutured to the lateral fibular flap and the lateral tibial flap to the medial fibular flap creating a bridge that covers the end of the bones. The mobilized muscles are configured into flaps and brought over the ends of the tibia and fibula and opposing muscles are sutured together. Skin flaps are fashioned and sutured over muscle. Use 27880 when the extremity is wrapped in an elastic bandage or placed in a plaster splint. Following wound healing, the patient is fitted for a prosthesis. Use 27881 when a cast of the stump is obtained and the patient is immediately fitted for a prosthesis.

27882

27882   Amputation, leg, through tibia and fibula; open, circular (guillotine)

Guillotine amputation through the tibia and fibula is typically performed following trauma with heavily contaminated wounds or on a severely infected leg. The level of amputation is determined based on the extent of injury or infection. The skin is marked to allow skin flaps to be developed as far distally as possible. The skin is incised down to the deep fascia and allowed to retract. Muscle is incised in a circular fashion around the tibia and fibula and allowed to retract. Nerves are transected as they are encountered. Blood vessels are suture ligated and transected. The tibia and fibula are transected in line with the retracted muscle. The stump is left open and dressings are applied. When the risk of infection has passed, separately reportable secondary closure or re-amputation at a higher level is performed.

27884

27884   Amputation, leg, through tibia and fibula; secondary closure or scar revision

Secondary closure or scar revision of previous leg amputation through the tibia and fibula is performed to obtain a pain-free stump covered with normal skin that functions well with a prosthesis. For secondary closure, the raw surface of the stump is debrided and all devitalized tissue is excised. Skin and subcutaneous tissue are fashioned into flaps and used to cover the stump taking care that there is not any undue tension along the suture line. For scar revision, the scar tissue is excised. Skin flaps are fashioned and the edges are undermined to ensure smooth, tension-free approximation along the suture line.

27886

27886   Amputation, leg, through tibia and fibula; re-amputation

Re-amputation of the leg through the tibia and fibula is done at a higher level to remove diseased, infected, or nonviable tissue posing a risk to the patient and/or form a healthy stump for use with a prosthesis. The incision lines for the re-amputation are marked on the skin. The skin and underlying soft tissue are incised. The muscles are exposed, isolated by muscle group, and divided. Nerves and blood vessels are identified and isolated, taking care to ensure that nerves are separated from arteries to prevent pulsatile irritation of the nerves. Nerves are transected and allowed to retract into soft tissue. Blood vessels are suture ligated and transected. The tibia and fibula are exposed and periosteal flaps are created. The tibia and fibula are transected at the level of the periosteal flaps. The flaps are sutured over the remaining tibia and fibula. Antagonistic muscle groups are sutured to each other and anchored to the periosteum in such a way that the remaining portion of the tibia and fibula are completely enveloped in muscle. Skin flaps are fashioned and sutured over the muscle.

27888

27888   Amputation, ankle, through malleoli of tibia and fibula (eg, Syme, Pirogoff type procedures), with plastic closure and resection of nerves

Amputation through the malleoli of the tibia and fibula, such as Syme or Pirogoff type procedures, is performed for injury, vascular insufficiency, or infection of the forefoot. Incision lines are marked on the skin. The skin and underlying soft tissues are incised. Dissection is carried down to the muscle. Muscle compartments are identified, isolated, and divided. Neurovascular structures are identified. Nerves and blood vessels are isolated taking care to ensure that nerves are separated from the arteries to prevent pulsatile irritation of the nerves. The forefoot, midfoot, talus, and calcaneus are excised taking care to preserve the heel pad. The periosteum of the tibia and fibula is incised just below the malleoli. Lateral and medial osteoperiosteal flaps elevated. The bone is then resected. The periosteal flaps are sutured over the remaining tibia and fibula. The plantar fat and skin pad is rotated and sutured over the end of the tibia and fibula providing a sensate weight-bearing surface.

27889

27889   Ankle disarticulation

Incision lines are marked on the skin for disarticulation at the ankle. The skin and underlying soft tissues are incised. Dissection is carried down to the muscle. Muscle compartments are identified, isolated, and the muscles divided. Neurovascular structures are identified. Nerves and blood vessels are isolated taking care to ensure that nerves are separated from the arteries to prevent pulsatile irritation of the nerves. Nerves are transected and allowed to retract into soft tissues. Blood vessels are ligated and divided. The forefoot, midfoot, talus, and calcaneus are removed. The articular cartilage of the tibia is excised. Tendon and muscles are reattached to the bone. The heel pad is rotated and sutured over the end of the tibia.

27892-27894

27892   Decompression fasciotomy, leg; anterior and/or lateral compartments only, with debridement of nonviable muscle and/or nerve

27893   Decompression fasciotomy, leg; posterior compartment(s) only, with debridement of nonviable muscle and/or nerve

27894   Decompression fasciotomy, leg; anterior and/or lateral, and posterior compartment(s), with debridement of nonviable muscle and/or nerve

Decompression fasciotomy is performed to treat compartment syndrome, a condition in which swelling of tissue in the muscle compartment causes compression of the blood vessels and nerves. Muscle compartments are surrounded by fascia that separates groups of muscles from each other. Fascia is a thick layer of connective tissue that does not expand. Swelling of tissue within the compartment can restrict blood supply and cause permanent muscle and nerve damage. There are four compartments in the lower leg which include the anterior, lateral, deep posterior, and superficial posterior compartments. In 27892, the anterior and/or lateral compartments are decompressed. A skin incision is made in the lower leg between the lateral and anterior compartments. The peroneal nerve is identified and protected. Incisions are carried down through the fascia of the anterior and/or lateral compartments. Compartment pressure is checked to ensure that the muscles have been adequately decompressed. In 27893, the superficial and deep posterior compartments are decompressed. A skin incision is made in the posteromedial aspect of the lower leg approximately 2 cm from the tibia. The fascia is exposed and the incision is carried down to the tibia, taking care to protect the saphenous vein and nerve. The deep posterior compartment is exposed and opened under the belly of the soleus muscle. The superficial posterior compartment is also opened as needed. Pressures are checked to ensure muscles have been adequately decompressed. In 27894, the anterior and/or lateral, and posterior compartments are decompressed using two incisions and the techniques described above. Muscle tissue and nerves are inspected and nonviable tissue is also debrided using sharp excision. The skin and fascial incisions are left open and covered with a dressing. The patient is returned to the operating room for wound closure once the swelling subsides, usually within 24-72 hours.

28001

28001   Incision and drainage, bursa, foot

An incision and drainage is performed on a bursa of the foot to treat excessive fluid buildup in the bursal sac (bursitis) that is causing pain. Foot bursae are located in areas of high friction including over the heel and metatarsal bones and act as shock absorbers. An incision is made in the tissue overlying the inflamed bursa. The bursal sac is incised and fluid drained. Incisions are closed in layers.

28002-28003

28002   Incision and drainage below fascia, with or without tendon sheath involvement, foot; single bursal space

28003   Incision and drainage below fascia, with or without tendon sheath involvement, foot; multiple areas

An incision is made in the skin over the infected bursa. Soft tissues are dissected and the fascia exposed and incised. The tendon sheath is exposed and inspected. The infected bursal space is opened with a scalpel and drained. The site is flushed with saline or antibiotic solution. Drains are placed as needed. The incision may be closed in layers or packed with gauze and left open. Use 28002 for a single bursal space. Use 28003 for incision and drainage of multiple areas in the foot.

28005

28005   Incision, bone cortex (eg, osteomyelitis or bone abscess), foot

The bone cortex of one of the bones of the foot is opened to treat a condition such as osteomyelitis or bone abscess. Bones of the foot include the tarsals, metatarsals and proximal, middle and distal phalanges. An incision is made in the skin and carried down through the soft tissue overlying the site of the infected bone. The periosteum over the infected region of the bone is elevated, a button of cortical bone removed, and the bone marrow exposed. Opening the bone cortex relieves pressure caused by inflammation of the bone marrow and prevents restriction of blood flow to the infected bone. If frank pus is encountered, the button hole may be enlarged and extended using a chisel or gouge along

● New Code   ▲ Revised Code

Musculoskeletal System

the bone for one to two inches. If the epiphysis is involved, a section of the epiphyseal cortex may be removed. The bone abscess is drained.

28008

28008   Fasciotomy, foot and/or toe

An incision is made over the plantar aspect of the foot and/or toe taking care to avoid the weight-bearing area of the bottom of the foot. Dissection is carried down to the fascia. The fascia is exposed and tight bands are transected. Overlying soft tissues and skin are closed in layers.

28010-28011

28010   Tenotomy, percutaneous, toe; single tendon
28011   Tenotomy, percutaneous, toe; multiple tendons

A small stab incision is made in the toe over the flexor or extensor tendon that is to be incised. The tendon is then incised and severed or released. Range of motion is evaluated. The small stab incision is closed with sutures or steristrips. Use 28010 for tenotomy of a single tendon. Use 28011 for tenotomy of multiple tendons.

28020-28024

28020   Arthrotomy, including exploration, drainage, or removal of loose or foreign body; intertarsal or tarsometatarsal joint
28022   Arthrotomy, including exploration, drainage, or removal of loose or foreign body; metatarsophalangeal joint
28024   Arthrotomy, including exploration, drainage, or removal of loose or foreign body; interphalangeal joint

There are seven tarsal bones which include the talus, calcaneus, cuboid, navicular, and three cuneiform bones that form multiple articulations and make up the intertarsal joints. The cuboid and the three cuneiforms articulate with the metatarsal bones and form the tarsometatarsal joints. The metatarsal bones articulate with the proximal phalanges forming the metatarsophalangeal joints. The proximal phalanges articulate with the middle phalanges and the middle phalanges articulate with the distal phalanges forming the proximal and distal interphalangeal joints respectively. The approach is dependent on the site of the fluid collection, foreign body or other condition requiring exploration of the joint. Tissues are dissected and the joint capsule is exposed. The joint capsule is opened and the joint explored. If an infection is present, fluid including blood and purulent matter is drained. Cultures are obtained and sent for separately reportable laboratory analysis. The joint is flushed with saline solution to remove any debris. Any foreign bodies are located and removed. The joint is again flushed with saline solution. Drains are placed as needed. The incision is closed in layers around the drain. A dressing is applied. Use 28020 when the procedure is performed on an intertarsal or tarsometatarsal joint. Use 28022 for a tarsometatarsal joint. Use 28024 for one of the proximal or distal interphalangeal joints.

28035

28035   Release, tarsal tunnel (posterior tibial nerve decompression)

The fibro-osseous tunnel created by the flexor retinaculum and the tibia anteriorly, talus posteriorly, and calcaneous laterally is called the tarsal tunnel and houses the posterior tibialis, flexor digitorum, and flexor hallucis longus tendons, the posterior artery and vein, and the posterior tibial nerve. A condition called tarsal tunnel syndrome can occur when the posterior tibial nerve becomes entrapped and compressed. An incision is made over the posteromedial aspect of the ankle. The flexor retinaculum is exposed and released from the lateral malleolus to the sustenaculum tali. The tarsal tunnel is followed distally and the fascial arcade around the medial and lateral plantar nerve branches are released to the level of the abductor hallucis. Once the posterior tibial nerve has been completely freed from adhesions and scar tissue the overlying soft tissue is closed in layers.

28039-28045

28039   Excision, tumor, soft tissue of foot or toe, subcutaneous; 1.5 cm or greater
28041   Excision, tumor, soft tissue of foot or toe, subfascial (eg, intramuscular); 1.5 cm or greater
28043   Excision, tumor, soft tissue of foot or toe, subcutaneous; less than 1.5 cm
28045   Excision, tumor, soft tissue of foot or toe, subfascial (eg, intramuscular); less than 1.5 cm

Soft tissues include subcutaneous fat and connective tissue, fascia, muscles, tendons, blood vessels, lymph vessels, nerves, and tissues surrounding the joints. Soft tissue tumors may be benign or malignant. Benign tumors are typically treated by excision, although small malignant or indeterminate tumors may be excised if the margins are well defined. Depending on the location of the tumor in the soft tissue of the foot or toe, the skin over the tumor may be incised or a skin flap created and elevated. Overlying tissue is dissected and the soft tissue mass exposed. The tumor is then excised along with a margin of healthy tissue. Separately reportable frozen section may be performed to ensure that all margins are free of tumor cells. Drains are placed as needed and the surgical wound is closed in layers. For tumors in the subcutaneous fat or connective tissue, use 28043 for excision of less than 1.5 cm and 28039 for excision of 1.5 cm or greater. For tumors that lie below

the fascia, use 28045 for excision of less than 1.5 cm and 28041 for excision of 1.5 cm or greater. Subfascial soft tissue tumors include those within muscle tissue.

28046-28047

28046   Radical resection of tumor (eg, sarcoma), soft tissue of foot or toe; less than 3 cm
28047   Radical resection of tumor (eg, sarcoma), soft tissue of foot or toe; 3 cm or greater

Soft tissues include muscles, tendons, fat, blood vessels, lymph vessels, nerves, and tissues surrounding the joints. Soft tissue tumors may be benign or malignant. Radical resection is typically performed for a malignant neoplasm, such as a sarcoma, although benign tumors and tumors of indeterminate nature may also require radical resection. A skin incision is made over the tumor in the foot or toe, or a skin flap is created and elevated. Overlying tissue is dissected and the tumor exposed. The tumor is removed en bloc along with a wide margin of surrounding tissue. Radical resection involves excision of all involved soft tissue which may include muscles, nerves, and blood vessels. Separately reportable frozen section is performed to ensure that all margins are free of tumor cells. If margins show evidence of malignancy, additional tissue is removed until all margins are free of tumor cells. Drains are placed as needed. The surgical wound may be closed in layers, or separately reportable reconstructive procedures performed. Use 28046 for radical resection of soft tissue tumor less than 3 cm in the foot or toe, and use 28047 for 3 cm or greater.

28050-28054

28050   Arthrotomy with biopsy; intertarsal or tarsometatarsal joint
28052   Arthrotomy with biopsy; metatarsophalangeal joint
28054   Arthrotomy with biopsy; interphalangeal joint

There are seven tarsal bones which include the talus, calcaneus, cuboid, navicular, and three cuneiform bones that form multiple articulations and make up the intertarsal joints. The cuboid and the three cuneiforms articulate with the metatarsal bones and form the tarsometatarsal joints. The metatarsal bones articulate with the proximal phalanges forming the metatarsophalangeal joints. The proximal phalanges articulate with the middle phalanges and the middle phalanges articulate with the distal phalanges forming the proximal and distal interphalangeal joints respectively. The approach is dependent on the joint to be biopsied. Tissues are dissected and the joint capsule is exposed. The joint capsule is opened. Tissue samples are obtained and sent for separately reportable laboratory analysis. The incision is closed in layers. A dressing is applied. Use 28050 when the procedure is performed on an intertarsal or tarsometatarsal joint. Use 28052 for a tarsometatarsal joint. Use 28054 for one of the proximal or distal interphalangeal joints.

28055

28055   Neurectomy, intrinsic musculature of foot

The physician performs a neurectomy on the intrinsic musculature of the foot. Under magnification, a straight midline incision is made on the back of the foot in the affected web space between the metatarsals, starting near the metatarsal heads down to the edge of skin. The underlying tissue is dissected to the fascia and the transverse metatarsal ligament is identified and divided. The metatarsal heads are spread apart and the nerve is located and dissected to its bifurcation. Inflamed bursa may be removed. The nerve is then carefully and cleanly divided to sever its connection of electrical impulses to the muscle tissue and is removed. The wound is cleaned and repaired.

28060-28062

28060   Fasciectomy, plantar fascia; partial (separate procedure)
28062   Fasciectomy, plantar fascia; radical (separate procedure)

A partial plantar fasciectomy is performed. An incision is made over the plantar fascia taking care to avoid the weight-bearing area of the bottom of the foot. The incision is carried down through subcutaneous fatty tissue and the plantar fascia is exposed. The fascia is separated from plantar fat and muscle tissue. A section of fascia is released taking care to protect neuromuscular structures. The fascia is removed with a knife or scissors. Remaining vertical and sagittal bands of fascia are inspected and transected if found to be tight. The skin is then closed. In 28062 a radical plantar fasciectomy is performed. The entire plantar fascia is exposed by a Z-shaped or S-shaped incision. Taking care not to disrupt tissue deep to the fascial band and to protect neuromuscular structures, the plantar fascia is separated from the plantar fat and muscle tissue and excised.

28070-28072

28070   Synovectomy; intertarsal or tarsometatarsal joint, each
28072   Synovectomy; metatarsophalangeal joint, each

This procedure is performed to treat inflammation of the synovial tissue caused by conditions such as rheumatoid arthritis. An incision is made over the affected intertarsal, tarsometatarsal, or metatarsophalangeal joint. Soft tissues are dissected and the joint capsule is incised. All inflamed synovial tissue is removed using a motorized suction shaving device. Use 28070 for each intertarsal or tarsometatarsal joint. Use 28072 for each metatarsophalangeal joint.

● New Code   ▲ Revised Code

28080

28080   Excision, interdigital (Morton) neuroma, single, each

An interdigital neuroma of the foot, also referred to as a Morton's neuroma, is excised. A neuroma is a mass or lesion composed of nerve tissue. A Morton's neuroma typically occurs between the third and fourth toes in the third interspace. The neuroma may be approached via a dorsal or plantar incision. The neuroma is exposed by carefully dissecting overlying tissue. The deep metatarsal ligament may be cut to relieve pressure on the underlying nerve. The neuroma is excised. Incisions are closed in layers. Report 28080 for each neuroma excised.

28086-28088

28086   Synovectomy, tendon sheath, foot; flexor
28088   Synovectomy, tendon sheath, foot; extensor

This procedure is performed to treat inflammation of the synovial tissue caused by conditions such as rheumatoid arthritis. An incision is made over the affected flexor or extensor tendon sheath. Soft tissues are dissected and the tendon sheath is incised. All inflamed synovial tissue is removed using a motorized suction shaving device. Use 28086 for synovectomy of a flexor tendon sheath. Use 28088 for synovectomy of an extensor tendon sheath.

28090-28092

28090   Excision of lesion, tendon, tendon sheath, or capsule (including synovectomy) (eg, cyst or ganglion); foot
28092   Excision of lesion, tendon, tendon sheath, or capsule (including synovectomy) (eg, cyst or ganglion); toe(s), each

A lesion such as a cyst or ganglion in a tendon, tendon sheath, or joint capsule in the foot or toe is excised. An incision is made in the skin over the affected tendon, tendon sheath or joint capsule. Soft tissues are dissected and lesion is exposed, carefully dissected free of surrounding healthy tissue, and excised in its entirety. The abnormal tissue is sent for separately reportable pathology evaluation. Inflamed synovial tissue may also be removed using a motorized suction shaving device. Use 28090 if the procedure is performed on a tendon, tendon sheath, or joint in the foot. Use 28092 if the procedure is performed on one of the toes.

28100-28103

28100   Excision or curettage of bone cyst or benign tumor, talus or calcaneus
28102   Excision or curettage of bone cyst or benign tumor, talus or calcaneus; with iliac or other autograft (includes obtaining graft)
28103   Excision or curettage of bone cyst or benign tumor, talus or calcaneus; with allograft

A bone cyst is a fluid filled space within the bone. One common type is a unicameral or simple bone cyst, which is a benign lesion. A less common type is an aneurysmal bone cyst which consists of vascular tissue surrounding a blood filled cystic lesion. There are a number of different types of benign bone tumors including giant cell tumors, chondromixoid fibromas, and enchondromas. In 28100, an incision is made in the skin over the site of lesion in the talus or calcaneus. Soft tissues are dissected and the lesion is exposed. If a cystic lesion is present, the bone is incised and a window created to open the cyst. Fluid is aspirated and sent to the laboratory for separately reportable analysis. A curette is inserted through the bone window and the lining of the cystic cavity is completely removed by curettage. Alternatively, some cystic lesions and most benign tumors are treated by excision. The lesion is exposed as described above. The physician then excises the benign lesion along with a margin of surrounding healthy bone. In 28102, the lesion is curetted or excised as described above. The physician then obtains healthy bone from a separate site, such as the iliac crest. The bone autograft is packed into the defect in the talus or calcaneus. In 28103, the lesion is curetted or excised as described above. The defect is then packed with donor bone (allograft).

28104-28107

28104   Excision or curettage of bone cyst or benign tumor, tarsal or metatarsal, except talus or calcaneus
28106   Excision or curettage of bone cyst or benign tumor, tarsal or metatarsal, except talus or calcaneus; with iliac or other autograft (includes obtaining graft)
28107   Excision or curettage of bone cyst or benign tumor, tarsal or metatarsal, except talus or calcaneus; with allograft

A bone cyst is a fluid filled space within the bone. One common type is a unicameral or simple bone cyst, which is a benign lesion. A less common type is an aneurysmal bone cyst which consists of vascular tissue surrounding a blood filled cystic lesion. There are a number of different types of benign bone tumors including giant cell tumors, chondromixoid fibromas, and enchondromas. In 28104, an incision is made in the skin over the site of lesion in a tarsal bone (other than the talus or calcaneus), or one of the metatarsal bones. Soft tissues are dissected and the lesion is exposed. If a cystic lesion is present, the bone is incised and a window created to open the cyst. Fluid is aspirated

and sent to the laboratory for separately reportable analysis. A curette is inserted through the bone window and the lining of the cystic cavity is completely removed by curettage. Alternatively, some cystic lesions and most benign tumors are treated by excision. The lesion is exposed as described above. The physician then excises the benign lesion along with a margin of surrounding healthy bone. In 28106, the lesion is curetted or excised as described above. The physician then obtains healthy bone from a separate site, such as the iliac crest. The bone autograft is packed into the defect in the tarsal or metatarsal bone. In 28107, the lesion is curetted or excised as described above. The defect is then packed with donor bone (allograft).

28108

28108   Excision or curettage of bone cyst or benign tumor, phalanges of foot

A bone cyst is a fluid filled space within the bone. One common type is a unicameral or simple bone cyst, which is a benign lesion. A less common type is an aneurysmal bone cyst, which consists of vascular tissue surrounding a blood filled cystic lesion. There are a number of different types of benign bone tumors including giant cell tumors, chondromixoid fibromas, and enchondromas. An incision is made in the skin over the site of lesion in the proximal, middle, or distal phalanx of one of the toes. Soft tissues are dissected and the lesion is exposed. If a cystic lesion is present, the bone is incised and a window created to open the cyst. Fluid is aspirated and sent to the laboratory for separately reportable analysis. A curette is inserted through the bone window and the lining of the cystic cavity is completely removed by curettage. Alternatively, some cystic lesions and most benign tumors are treated by excision. The lesion is exposed as described above. The physician then excises the benign lesion along with a margin of surrounding healthy bone.

28110

28110   Ostectomy, partial excision, fifth metatarsal head (bunionette) (separate procedure)

A bony protuberance on the fifth metatarsal head, also called a bunionette or tailor's bunion is excised. A longitudinal incision is made over the lateral aspect of the fifth metatarsal head. The joint capsule is incised and a capsular flap created. The metatarsal head is exposed and the lateral condyle is excised. Any redundancy in the joint capsule is excised or the joint capsule is plicated. Overlying soft tissues are closed in layers.

28111-28113

28111   Ostectomy, complete excision; first metatarsal head
28112   Ostectomy, complete excision; other metatarsal head (second, third or fourth)
28113   Ostectomy, complete excision; fifth metatarsal head

Bony overgrowth of the metatarsal head is treated by complete excision of the metatarsal head. A longitudinal or lazy-S incision is made over the dorsal aspect of the affected metatarsal head. Soft tissues are dissected taking care to protect superficial blood vessels. The long extensor tendons are identified and detached and transferred as needed. The joint capsule is incised and a capsular flap created. The metatarsal head is exposed and completely excised. The phalangeal base is preserved. A Kirschner wire is advanced through the proximal phalanx and into the metatarsal medullary canal to stabilize the joint. Any redundancy in the joint capsule is excised or the joint capsule is plicated. Overlying soft tissues are closed in layers. Use 28111 for complete excision of the first metatarsal head. Use 28112 for complete excision of the second, third, or fourth metatarsal heads. Use 28113 for complete excision of the fifth metatarsal head.

28114

28114   Ostectomy, complete excision; all metatarsal heads, with partial proximal phalangectomy, excluding first metatarsal (eg, Clayton type procedure)

Bony overgrowth of the second, third, fourth and fifth metatarsal heads is treated by complete excision of all metatarsal heads. Longitudinal or lazy-S incisions are made over the dorsal aspects of the metatarsal heads. Soft tissues are dissected taking care to protect superficial blood vessels. The long extensor tendons are identified and tenectomies performed as needed. The joint capsules are incised and capsular flaps created. The metatarsal heads are exposed and completely excised. The phalangeal bases are excised. Kirschner wires are advanced through the proximal phalanges and into the metatarsal medullary canal to stabilize the joints. Any redundancy in the joint capsules is excised or the joint capsules are plicated. Overlying soft tissues are closed in layers.

28116

28116   Ostectomy, excision of tarsal coalition

A tarsal coalition is an abnormal connection or fusion between two or more of the tarsal bones that limits motion of the foot. The bones may be joined by bone, cartilage or fibrous tissue. Tarsal coalition is most often a congenital condition, but may also be an acquired condition caused by infection, arthritis, or injury. Symptoms include pain when walking or standing, tired legs, muscle spasms in the leg, flatfoot, walking with a limp, and stiffness of the foot and ankle. The approach depends on which tarsal bones are connected. The bone, cartilage, and fibrous connections are excised. Surrounding fat and/or muscle tissue

Musculoskeletal System

is interposed between the bones. Overlying soft tissues are closed in layers. The foot is immobilized in a cast.

28118-28119

28118   Ostectomy, calcaneus
28119   Ostectomy, calcaneus; for spur, with or without plantar fascial release

Excision of bone from the calcaneus may be performed to treat pain due to retrocalcaneal bursitis or to remove a bone spur. In 28118, bone is excised from the calcaneus usually to treat retrocalcaneal bursitis. An incision is made over the posterior aspect of the heel. Soft tissues are dissected and the calcaneus is exposed. The periosteum over the posterior aspect of the calcaneus is incised and a periosteal flap is elevated. The calcaneus is then resected. The periosteal flap is sutured over the remaining calcaneus. Overlying soft tissue and skin is closed in layers. In 28119, a bone spur is removed usually from the plantar aspect of the calcaneus. Because bone spurs are often accompanied by plantar fasciitis, release of the plantar fascia may also be performed. An incision is made over the plantar aspect of the foot taking care to avoid the weight-bearing area of the bottom of the foot. Dissection is carried down to the fascia. The fascia is exposed, inspected, and any tight bands are transected. The calcaneus is exposed and the bone spur is excised.

28120-28124

28120   Partial excision (craterization, saucerization, sequestrectomy, or diaphysectomy) bone (eg, osteomyelitis or bossing); talus or calcaneus
28122   Partial excision (craterization, saucerization, sequestrectomy, or diaphysectomy) bone (eg, osteomyelitis or bossing); tarsal or metatarsal bone, except talus or calcaneus
28124   Partial excision (craterization, saucerization, sequestrectomy, or diaphysectomy) bone (eg, osteomyelitis or bossing); phalanx of toe

The physician performs a partial excision of bone, also referred to as craterization, saucerization, sequestrectomy, or diaphysectomy for osteomyelitis or bossing of the talus or calcaneus (28120) other tarsal bone (28122), or phalanx of the toe (28124). Osteomyelitis is a pyogenic or pus producing infection of the bone. A boss or bossing is a boney protruberance. Craterization and saucerization of bone involves removing infected and necrotic bone to form a shallow depression in the bone surface that will allow drainage from the infected area. Sequestrectomy is the excision of a piece of necrotic bone that has become separated from healthy surrounding bone. Diaphysectomy involves removal of the infected portion of the shaft of a long bone. If the procedure is performed for osteomyelitis, an incision is made in the skin and carried down through the soft tissue overlying the site of the osteomyelitis. Any soft tissue sinus tracts and devitalized soft tissue are resected. The area of necrotic and infected bone is exposed. A series of drill holes are made in the necrotic and infected bone and the bone between the drill holes is excavated to create an oval window using an osteotome. Any sequestra are excised. The amount of bone removed is dependent on the location of sequestra and the extent of the infection. A curette may be used to remove devitalized tissue from the medullary canal. Debridement continues until punctate bleeding is identified in the exposed bony surface. When all devitalized and infected tissue has been removed, the wound is copiously irrigated with sterile saline or antibiotic solution. The surgical wound is loosely closed and a drain placed. If a boss is removed, the boney protruberance is exposed and excised using an osteotome to chip away the boney overgrowth.

28126

28126   Resection, partial or complete, phalangeal base, each toe

A partial or complete resection is performed on the phalangeal base of the toe. An incision is made over the affected toe joint extending from the midshaft of the proximal phalanx to the midshaft of the metatarsal. The joint capsule is incised. The base of the affected proximal phalanx is underscored and partially or completely resected using an oscillating saw. The resected base is then grasped and peeled out of the joint capsule. Report 28126 for each toe.

28130

28130   Talectomy (astragalectomy)

A talectomy, also referred to as an astragalectomy, is performed. The talus is one of seven tarsal bones that form the ankle. It is the uppermost tarsal bone and the only tarsal bone that articulates with the tibia and fibula. The talus is exposed using an anterolateral approach over the lateral, intermediate, and medial malleoli. The extensor tendons and surrounding blood vessels are mobilized. All ligamentous and capsular attachments of the talus are released. The talus is removed and the calcaneus is displaced posteriorly. The surgical site is carefully inspected to assure that no talar remnants remain. The calcaneus is aligned with the distal tibia and the foot is placed in balanced plantigrade position. Alignment is maintained by placement of a pin across the calcaneus and into the tibia. A cast is applied to immobilize the foot and ankle.

28140

28140   Metatarsectomy

The entire metatarsal bone is excised. A dorsal incision is made in the skin over the affected metatarsal and extended over the metatarsophalangeal joint. Soft tissues are dissected taking care to protect the digital neurovascular bundle. The metatarsal bone is severed from all attachments and excised. If the procedure is performed for an injury or infection, all damaged or septic tissue is debrided. Soft tissues and skin are closed in layers over a drain and a dressing applied.

28150

28150   Phalangectomy, toe, each toe

This procedure is typically performed to correct severe malalignment of the metatarsophalangeal joint causing underlapping, overlapping, or cock-up of the toe. To correct underlapping of the toe, a dorsal Z-type incision is made. To correct overlapping or cockup toe, a volar elliptical incision is made. Typically the proximal phalanx is excised. This is not an amputation. The bone of the phalanx is removed, not the soft tissue. The metatarsophalangeal and proximal interphalangeal joint capsules are incised. The phalanx is removed. Flexor and extensor tendons are released as needed. An intramedullary K-wire may be inserted into the remaining middle and distal phalanges and into the metatarsal bone to maintain proper alignment of these bones. Report 28150 for each toe.

28153

28153   Resection, condyle(s), distal end of phalanx, each toe

A longitudinal incision is made over the affected phalanx. The joint capsule is incised and a capsular flap created. The distal aspect of the phalanx is exposed and the medial and/or lateral condyle is excised. Any redundancy in the joint capsule is excised or the joint capsule is plicated. Overlying soft tissues are closed in layers. Report code 28153 for each toe on which resection of the condyles is performed.

28160

28160   Hemiphalangectomy or interphalangeal joint excision, toe, proximal end of phalanx, each

A partial excision of the proximal aspect of the phalanx of the toe or an interphalangeal joint excision is performed. An incision is made over the affected phalanx and interphalangeal joint. If the proximal end of the phalanx is excised, the joint capsule is incised. The affected phalanx is underscored at the site where the bone will be transected and the proximal end of the phalanx excised using an oscillating saw. The resected portion of the phalanx is then grasped and peeled out of the joint capsule. If the entire joint is excised, flexor and extensor tendons are released as needed. The ligaments connecting the phalangeal bones at the joint are severed and the joint capsule is completely excised along with all articular cartilage. An intramedullary K-wire may be inserted through the phalanges and into the metatarsal bone to maintain proper alignment of these bones. Report 28160 for each toe on which the procedure is performed.

28171-28175

28171   Radical resection of tumor; tarsal (except talus or calcaneus)
28173   Radical resection of tumor; metatarsal
28175   Radical resection of tumor; phalanx of toe

Radical resection is typically performed for a malignant neoplasm although benign tumors and tumors of indeterminate nature may also require radical resection. A skin incision is made over the site of the bone tumor, or a skin flap is created and elevated. Overlying tissue is dissected and the tumor exposed. All bone and cartilage with tumor involvement is resected. The tumor is removed en bloc along with a wide margin of surrounding tissue. Radical resection of bone includes excision of all involved soft tissue which may include muscles, tendons, fat, blood vessels, lymph vessels, nerves, and tissues surrounding the joints. Separately reportable frozen section is performed to ensure that all margins are free of tumor cells. If margins show evidence of malignancy, additional tissue is removed until all margins are free of tumor cells. Drains are placed as needed. The surgical wound may be closed in layers, or separately reportable reconstructive procedures performed. For radical resection of a bone tumor of one of the tarsal bones excluding the talus or calcaneus, use 28171; metatarsal, use 28173; phalanx of toe, use 28175.

28190-28193

28190   Removal of foreign body, foot; subcutaneous
28192   Removal of foreign body, foot; deep
28193   Removal of foreign body, foot; complicated

Treatment depends on the type of foreign body and depth of penetration. The physician inspects the foot for evidence of a puncture site. If no puncture site is present, the foreign body may be located by palpation or separately reportable radiographs. In 28190, a subcutaneous foreign body is removed. Subcutaneous tissue refers to the fat and connective tissue that lies between the overlying dermis and underlying muscle fascia. The skin is incised and the foreign body located. A hemostat or grasping forceps is used

Musculoskeletal System

to remove it. Alternatively, the physician may need to dissect tissues around the foreign body to remove it. The wound is then flushed with normal saline or antibiotic solution and the incision is closed or left open to heal by secondary intention. In 28192, dissection is carried down to deep tissue which includes tissue below the muscle fascia (subfascial) or within the muscle itself (intramuscular). The foreign body is located and removed. In 28193, a complicated foreign body removal is performed. Complicated foreign bodies are those that are in deeper tissues requiring extensive dissection, those that have been retained causing infection, and/or those that are in regions that are difficult to access. The foot is incised and tissue dissected taking care to protect vital structures, such as ligaments, tendons, nerves and blood vessels. The foreign body is located and removed. The wound is debrided as needed and copiously flushed with normal saline to remove debris. Depending on the exact nature of the injury, the wound may be closed or packed open to drain.

Removal of foreign body, foot

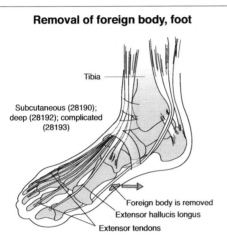

Tibia

Subcutaneous (28190); deep (28192); complicated (28193)

Foreign body is removed
Extensor hallucis longus
Extensor tendons

28200-28202

28200   Repair, tendon, flexor, foot; primary or secondary, without free graft, each tendon

28202   Repair, tendon, flexor, foot; secondary with free graft, each tendon (includes obtaining graft)

The flexor muscles and tendons of the foot include the peroneus longus, peroneus brevis, plantaris, popliteus, flexor digitorum longus, flexor hallucis longus, and tibialis posterior. Lacerations and puncture wounds can cause partial or complete transection of one or more flexor tendons. Closed injuries such as avulsion can also occur. An incision is made over the site of the flexor tendon or muscle injury. If the tendon has been completely transected, the severed end of the flexor tendon is located, grasped and pulled distally or proximally. The tendon is then suture repaired. If the tendon has only been partially transected, the transected fibers are repaired. If the muscle itself has been lacerated or torn, the muscle tissue is repaired in layers. Use 28200 to report primary or secondary suture repair of a single flexor tendon or muscle. Use 28202 to report secondary graft repair of a single flexor tendon or muscle. A tendon graft is harvested and attached to the remnants of the severed tendon. The tendon graft is then attached at the distal insertion site of the tendon. Range of motion is tested and tension adjusted as needed to allow good range of motion in the foot and toes. The surgical wound is closed in layers. The lower leg, ankle and foot are immobilized using a splint or cast.

28208-28210

28208   Repair, tendon, extensor, foot; primary or secondary, each tendon

28210   Repair, tendon, extensor, foot; secondary with free graft, each tendon (includes obtaining graft)

The extensor muscles and tendons of the foot include the tibialis anterior, extensor digitorum, peroneus tertius, and extensor hallucis longus. Lacerations and puncture wounds can cause partial or complete transection of one or more extensor tendons. Closed injuries such as avulsion can also occur. An incision is made over the site of the extensor tendon or muscle injury. If the tendon has been completely transected, the severed end of the extensor tendon is located, grasped and pulled distally or proximally. The tendon is then suture repaired. If the tendon has only been partially transected, the transected fibers are repaired. If the muscle itself has been lacerated or torn, the muscle tissue is repaired in layers. Use 28208 to report primary or secondary suture repair of a single extensor tendon or muscle. Use 28210 to report secondary graft repair of a single extensor tendon or muscle. A tendon graft is harvested and attached to the remnants of the severed tendon in the lower leg. The tendon graft is then attached at the distal insertion site of the tendon. Range of motion is tested and tension adjusted as needed to allow good range of motion in the foot and toes. The surgical wound is closed in layers. The lower leg, ankle, and foot are immobilized using a splint or cast.

28220-28222

28220   Tenolysis, flexor, foot; single tendon

28222   Tenolysis, flexor, foot; multiple tendons

Tenolysis involves freeing a tendon from surrounding tissue. In 28220, tenolysis of a single flexor tendon is performed at the level of the foot to restore foot and/or toe motion by releasing scar tissue resulting from trauma or a disease process. An incision is made over the affected flexor tendon. Soft tissues are dissected. The affected tendon is identified and adhesions are severed. Range of motion is evaluated. The surgical wound is closed in layers and a dressing is applied. In 28222, tenolysis of multiple flexor tendons is performed in the same manner, usually through separate incisions.

28225-28226

28225   Tenolysis, extensor, foot; single tendon

28226   Tenolysis, extensor, foot; multiple tendons

Tenolysis involves freeing a tendon from surrounding tissue. In 28225, tenolysis of a single extensor tendon is performed at the level of the foot to restore foot and/or toe motion by releasing scar tissue resulting from trauma or a disease process. An incision is made over the affected extensor tendon. Soft tissues are dissected. The affected tendon is identified and adhesions are severed. Range of motion is evaluated. The surgical wound is closed in layers and a dressing is applied. In 28226, tenolysis of multiple extensor tendons is performed in the same manner, usually through separate incisions.

28230-28232

28230   Tenotomy, open, tendon flexor; foot, single or multiple tendon(s) (separate procedure)

28232   Tenotomy, open, tendon flexor; toe, single tendon (separate procedure)

An incision is made in the skin of the foot or toe overlying the flexor tendon that is to be incised. Soft tissues are dissected and the tendon is exposed. The tendon is then incised and severed or released. Bleeding is controlled with electrocautery. Following completion of the procedure, the operative wound is closed in layers. Use 28230 for an open tenotomy of one or more flexor tendons of the foot. Use 28232 for an open tenotomy of a single toe tendon.

28234

28234   Tenotomy, open, extensor, foot or toe, each tendon

An incision is made in the skin of the foot or toe overlying the extensor tendon that is to be incised. Soft tissues are dissected and the tendon is exposed. The tendon is then incised and severed or released. Bleeding is controlled with electrocautery. Following completion of the procedure, the operative wound is closed in layers. Report 28234 for tenotomy of each extensor tendon in the foot or toe.

28238

28238   Reconstruction (advancement), posterior tibial tendon with excision of accessory tarsal navicular bone (eg, Kidner type procedure)

Some individuals have an accessory navicular bone, which is an extra tarsal bone on the medial side of the foot and proximal to the navicular bone. The tibialis posterior tendon may insert on the accessory navicular bone. This can result in displacement of the tendon causing the foot to deviate into a valgus position. This accessory navicular bone may also become enlarged or be injured causing pain when walking. A painful accessory navicular bone is treated surgically. A skin incision is made over the medial side of the foot dorsal to the navicular prominence. The incision is extended from the first cuneiform to the sustenaculum tali. The tibialis posterior tendon is exposed and stripped away from the accessory navicular bone leaving a small piece of bone attached to the tendon. The entire accessory navicular bone is excised. The prominent portion of the navicular bone is excised. The tibialis posterior tendon is attached to the plantar surface of the navicular bone by suturing the small piece of bone attached to the tendon to the navicular bone. The incision is closed in layers.

28240

28240   Tenotomy, lengthening, or release, abductor hallucis muscle

Abductor hallucis release or lengthening is performed to treat clubfoot deformity. An incision is made medially from the midportion of the first metatarsal bone to the interphalangeal joint. Soft tissues are dissected and the abductor hallucis tendon is exposed. If release is performed, the abductor hallucis is detached from its insertion site on the proximal phalanx of the great toe. If lengthening procedure is performed, a Z-shaped incision is made in the tendon which lengthens it by allowing the tendon fibers to slide apart as the foot is abducted. Tendon sutures are placed to maintain the tendon in the lengthened position.

28250

28250   Division of plantar fascia and muscle (eg, Steindler stripping) (separate procedure)

This procedure may be referred to as a Steindler stripping and may be performed using either a lateral or medial approach. If a lateral approach is used, a skin incision is developed from the calcaneal tuberosity to the base of the fifth metatarsal. The plantar fascia and muscle adjacent to the calcaneal tuberosity are exposed. The plantar fascia is then divided in a lateral to medial direction just distal to the calcaneal attachment using a blade or scissors. If a medial approach is used, an anterior incision is made curving over the medial side of the foot to the base of the first metatarsal taking care to avoid the weight-bearing area of the foot. The abductor pollicis is released off the calcaneus. Neuromuscular structures are identified and protected. The plantar fascia is exposed and dissected free of adjacent fat. The plantar fascia and muscles are divided just distal to the calcaneal attachment. Plantar and calcaneonavicular ligaments are released as needed. A cast may be applied to immobilize the foot.

28260-28262

28260   Capsulotomy, midfoot; medial release only (separate procedure)
28261   Capsulotomy, midfoot; with tendon lengthening
28262   Capsulotomy, midfoot; extensive, including posterior talotibial capsulotomy and tendon(s) lengthening (eg, resistant clubfoot deformity)

The physician makes an incision in the inward side of the fibrous covering of the ankle joint. This procedure keeps the foot from twisting inward (clubfoot). Code 28261 is the tendons on the inward side of the ankle are lengthened. Code 28262 if incisions must be made in multiple sides of the ankle joint, and many tendons must be lengthened on multiple sides of the foot.

28270-28272

28270   Capsulotomy; metatarsophalangeal joint, with or without tenorrhaphy, each joint (separate procedure)
28272   Capsulotomy; interphalangeal joint, each joint (separate procedure)

Capsulotomy of the metatarsophalangeal or interphalangeal joint is usually performed to release a joint contracture. An incision is made over the affected metatarsophalangeal or interphalangeal joint. Soft tissues are dissected and the joint capsule exposed. Fibrous tissue is dissected and the contracture released. Use 28270 for capsulotomy of the metatarsophalangeal joint. This procedure may be performed with or without suture repair of one or more tendons. Use 28272 for capsulotomy of the interphalangeal joint.

28280

28280   Syndactylization, toes (eg, webbing or Kelikian type procedure)

A syndactylization procedure, also referred to as a webbing or Kelikian procedure, is performed on the toes. The planned skin incisions are outlined on the toes to ensure they will be mirror images of each other. An island of tissue is then created by carefully dissecting the skin free of subcutaneous tissue. Bleeding is controlled using a needle-tipped electrocautery device. Bone remodeling and tendon balancing is performed as needed. The toes are then sutured together by approximating the skin of one toe to the skin of the adjacent toe. A splint is applied to the toes.

28285

28285   Correction, hammertoe (eg, interphalangeal fusion, partial or total phalangectomy)

A hammertoe deformity is corrected by interphalangeal fusion or partial or total phalangectomy. A hammertoe is a flexion deformity of the proximal interphalangeal (PIP) joint that causes the toe to curl downward. A dorsal incision is made over the affected PIP joint. The extensor tendon is split and retracted and the PIP joint capsule is exposed. Wedge-shaped pieces of bone at the base of the middle phalanx and the head of the proximal phalanx are resected. Alternatively, the entire middle or proximal phalanx may be removed. A K-wire or absorbable wire may be inserted through the middle and proximal phalanges to maintain proper alignment and promote fusion of the joint. The dorsal incisions in the PIP joint capsule and skin are suture repaired.

28286

28286   Correction, cock-up fifth toe, with plastic skin closure (eg, Ruiz-Mora type procedure)

A cock-up fifth toe is corrected with a plastic skin closure. This procedure may also be referred to as a Ruiz-Mora procedure. A dorsal incision is made over the proximal interphalangeal (PIP) joint of the fifth toe and an ellipse of skin is removed below the proximal phalanx slightly medial to the margin of the incision. The flexor tendons are dissected and retracted and the PIP joint is exposed. The joint capsule is incised and the collateral ligaments are released. The head of the proximal phalanx is excised. Alternatively, the entire proximal phalanx may be removed. If all or a large section of the proximal phalanx is excised, the flexor and extensor tendons are joined together with purse-string

sutures. A plastic repair of the skin is then performed so that the toe will be maintained in the correct plantar-medial direction.

28288

28288   Ostectomy, partial, exostectomy or condylectomy, metatarsal head, each metatarsal head

An incision is made over the metatarsophalangeal joint. Soft tissues are dissected and the joint capsule exposed. Tendons and neurovascular structures are retracted and protected. The soft tissue attachments at the metatarsal head are mobilized. The metatarsal head is exposed. Bony exostoses are excised. If a condylectomy is performed, a sagittal saw is used to excise the bony prominences. The bone is then smoothed with a rasp. The incision is closed in layers.

28289-28291

▲ **28289   Hallux rigidus correction with cheilectomy, debridement and capsular release of the first metatarsophalangeal joint; without implant**
▲ **28289   28291 Hallux rigidus correction with cheilectomy, debridement and capsular release of the first metatarsophalangeal joint; with implant**

Hallux rigidus is a condition characterized by pain, swelling, stiffness, and decreased range of motion, especially dorsiflexion in the great toe. Hallux rigidus is caused by degenerative changes and inflammation, arthritis, cartilage erosion, joint space narrowing, and bone spurs around the first metatarsophalangeal (MTP) joint. An incision is made in the dorsal midline over the MTP joint of the great toe. The dorsomedial cutaneous nerve is identified and protected. The soft tissue is dissected longitudinally to expose the joint capsule. Excessive synovial tissue is debrided and the joint capsule is explored for loose bodies and abnormalities. Bone spur(s) are shaved (cheilectomy) using an osteotome until flush with the joint. Range of motion is checked and planter adhesions between the metatarsal head and sesamoid bones are released as necessary. If a large amount of bone and/or tissue is removed, an implant of prosthetic material (ceramic, titanium), biologic material (tendon, capsule tissue) or a combination of both may be inserted into the joint space. The implant helps to restore alignment, maintain range of motion, lengthen and strengthen the digit. The site is checked for bleeding, irrigated, and the Incision closed. Code 28289 reports cheilectomy, debridement, and capsular release of the first metatarsophalangeal joint to correct hallux rigidus without insertion of an implant and code 28291 with implant insertion.

28292

▲ **28292   Correction, hallux valgus (bunionectomy), with sesamoidectomy, when performed; with resection of proximal phalanx base, when performed, any method**

A bunionectomy is performed to correct hallux valgus by removing the medial eminence of the metatarsal bone and resecting the base of the proximal phalanx. An incision is made over the medial aspect of the metatarsophalangeal joint. Soft tissues are dissected and the joint capsule is exposed. The joint capsule is incised and the medial eminence is exposed. The eminence is excised in line with the metatarsal shaft. The base of the proximal phalanx is resected. The two sesamoid bones located on either side of the metatarsal head may also be excised if they are fractured or inflamed. A skin incision is made over the sesamoid bone. Soft tissues are dissected around the sesamoid bone and the bone is excised. Two K-wires are placed through the distal phalanx, proximal phalanx and into the distal aspect of the metatarsal bone to maintain the position of the toe. The redundant joint capsule is plicated and closed. Soft tissue and skin are closed in layers.

28295

● **28295   Correction, hallux valgus (bunionectomy), with sesamoidectomy, when performed; with proximal metatarsal osteotomy, any method**

A first metatarsal osteotomy is performed to correct hallux valgus in a bunionectomy procedure. The osteotomy site is distal in 28296 or proximal in 28295. (Mitchell and Chevron procedures are both distal osteotomies.) A medial incision is made just proximal to the medial eminence and extended over the metatarsophalangeal joint. Soft tissues are dissected and the joint capsule is exposed. The metatarsophalangeal joint capsule is incised and the medial eminence is exposed. The medial eminence is excised in line with the metatarsal shaft. The bone cuts are outlined on the metatarsal bone and the section of bone is excised. The metatarsal head is then shifted in a lateral direction 3-5 mm. This is accomplished using a skin hook or towel clamps on the proximal bone segment and then shifting the capital segment. The osteotomy is stabilized with a single Kirschner wire. The two sesamoid bones located on either side of the metatarsal head may also be excised if they are fractured or inflamed. A skin incision is made over the sesamoid bone. Soft tissues are dissected around the sesamoid bone and the bone is excised. Soft tissue and skin are closed in layers.

28296

28296 **Correction, hallux valgus (bunion), with or without sesamoidectomy; with metatarsal osteotomy (eg, Mitchell, Chevron, or concentric type procedures)**

A first metatarsal osteotomy is performed to correct hallux valgus. The osteotomy site may be distal or proximal. Mitchell and Chevron procedures are both distal osteotomies. A medial incision is made just proximal to the medial eminence and extended over the metatarsophalangeal joint. Soft tissues are dissected and the joint capsule exposed. The metatarsophalangeal joint capsule is incised and the medial eminence is exposed. The medial eminence is excised in line with the metatarsal shaft. The bone cuts are outlined on the metatarsal bone and the section of bone is excised. The metatarsal head is then shifted in a lateral direction 3-5 mm. This is accomplished using a skin hook or towel clamps on the proximal bone segment and then shifting the capital segment. The osteotomy is stabilized with a single Kirschner wire. The two sesamoid bones located on either side of the metatarsal head may also be excised if they are fractured or inflamed. A skin incision is made over the sesamoid bone. Soft tissues are dissected around the sesamoid bone and the bone is excised. Soft tissue and skin is closed in layers.

28297

▲ 28297 **Correction, hallux valgus (bunionectomy), with sesamoidectomy, when performed; with first metatarsal and medial cuneiform joint arthrodesis, any method**

A bunionectomy involving excision of the medial eminence, tenotomy, and joint fusion of the first metatarsal bone to the first cuneiform bone is performed to correct hallux valgus. A dorsal incision is made over the metatarsophalangeal joint. Soft tissues are dissected and the joint capsule is exposed. The metatarsophalangeal joint capsule is incised and the medial eminence is exposed. The medial eminence is excised in line with the metatarsal shaft. The tendon on the lateral aspect of the great toe is divided. The first metatarsocuneiform joint is resected and the metatarsal bone is realigned. Screw or other suitable arthrodesis fixation is placed across the first metatarsocuneiform joint to maintain the joint in the corrected position and to allow the bones to fuse. The joint capsule is plicated and repaired. The two sesamoid bones located on either side of the metatarsal head may also be excised if they are fractured or inflamed. A skin incision is made over the sesamoid bone. Soft tissues are dissected around the sesamoid bone and the bone is excised. Soft tissue and skin are closed in layers.

28298-28299

▲ 28298 **Correction, hallux valgus (bunionectomy), with sesamoidectomy, when performed; with proximal phalanx osteotomy, any method**

▲ 28299 **Correction, hallux valgus (bunionectomy), with sesamoidectomy, when performed; with double osteotomy, any method**

A proximal phalanx osteotomy or double osteotomy is performed to correct hallux valgus in a bunionectomy procedure. In 28298, a proximal phalanx osteotomy, also referred to as an Akin procedure, is performed. A medial incision is made just proximal to the medial eminence and extended just distal to the interphalangeal joint. Soft tissues are dissected and the joint capsule is exposed. The metatarsophalangeal joint capsule is incised and the medial eminence is exposed. The medial eminence is excised in line with the metatarsal shaft. A medial wedge osteotomy of the proximal phalanx is completed just distal to the phalangeal base. The redundant joint capsule is plicated and closed. In 28299, a double osteotomy is performed which involves excision of the medial eminence, osteotomy of the proximal phalanx, and an osteotomy of the first metatarsal in addition. Following repair of the joint capsule, the amount of correction needed for the first metatarsal is determined, and the osteotomy on the first metatarsal is then also performed. The two sesamoid bones located on either side of the metatarsal head may also be excised if they are fractured or inflamed. A skin incision is made over the sesamoid bone. Soft tissues are dissected around the sesamoid bone and the bone is excised. Osteotomies are stabilized with Kirschner wires or sutures placed through the distal phalanx, proximal phalanx, and into the distal aspect of the metatarsal bone to maintain the position of the toe.

28300

28300 **Osteotomy; calcaneus (eg, Dwyer or Chambers type procedure), with or without internal fixation**

An osteotomy of the calcaneus is performed with or without internal fixation. This procedure may also be referred to as a Dwyer or Chambers wedge osteotomy. A lateral skin or medial skin incision is made depending on the nature of the calcaneal deformity. The calcaneus is exposed taking care to protect underlying tendons. To perform a closing wedge osteotomy, a wedge of bone is removed from the calcaneus using a saw or osteotome. The heel is then aligned by closing the wedge. Pins or a screw fixation device are then applied as needed to maintain the heel alignment. If an opening wedge osteotomy is performed, the wedge of bone is removed using a saw or osteotome. A laminar spreader is then placed in the surgically created opening and the heel is aligned. A bone allograft or autograft is placed in the bone defect and pin fixation is applied as needed to maintain heel alignment.

28302

28302 **Osteotomy; talus**

Osteotomy of the talus is performed to treat a congenital or acquired deformity of the foot. A skin incision is made over the lateral or medial aspect of the talus. The talus is exposed taking care to protect underlying nerves, blood vessels, and tendons. To perform a closing wedge osteotomy, a wedge of bone is removed from the talus using a saw or osteotome. The hindfoot is then aligned by closing the wedge. Pin or screw fixation is applied as needed to maintain the hindfoot alignment. If an opening wedge osteotomy is performed, a wedge of bone is removed on one side of the talus. The bone is cut on the opposite side and spread using a laminar spreader. The wedge of bone that was removed from one side is placed in the surgically created opening on the opposite side. Additional bone allograft or autograft may also be placed in the bone defect. Pin or screw fixation is applied to maintain the hindfoot in alignment.

28304-28305

28304 **Osteotomy, tarsal bones, other than calcaneus or talus**

28305 **Osteotomy, tarsal bones, other than calcaneus or talus; with autograft (includes obtaining graft) (eg, Fowler type)**

Osteotomy of the navicular, cuboid, and/or cuneiform bones is performed to treat a congenital or acquired deformity of the foot. A procedure on these bones is sometimes referred to as a midtarsal osteotomy. The exact procedure performed depends on the type of foot deformity. In 28304, an osteotomy that does not require bone autograft is performed. The midtarsal V-osteotomy performed for a pes cavus deformity is an example of this type of procedure. The navicular, cuboid, and cuneiform bones are exposed taking care to protect underlying nerves, blood vessels, and tendons. The apex of the V is oriented at the apex of the pes cavus which usually occurs at the navicular bone. The lateral limb of the bone cut extends through the cuboid and the medial limb through the first cuneiform bone. Once the cuts have been made, the forefoot is shifted in a dorsal direction which elevates the forefoot and corrects the pes cavus deformity. Alignment is verified radiographically and pins are placed to maintain the foot in alignment. In 28305, osteotomy with bone autograft is performed. An opening wedge osteotomy is an example of this type of procedure. The tarsal bone is cut and spread using a laminar spreader. A bone autograft consisting of cortical and/or cancellous bone is harvested. The cortical bone autograft is configured to the desired size and shape and/or cancellous bone is morcelized and packed into the surgically created defect in the tarsal. Alignment of the foot is evaluated radiographically. Once the correct position has been attained, pins or screws are used to maintain the cut edges in anatomical alignment. The incision is closed and a short leg cast is applied.

28306-28309

28306 **Osteotomy, with or without lengthening, shortening or angular correction, metatarsal; first metatarsal**

28307 **Osteotomy, with or without lengthening, shortening or angular correction, metatarsal; first metatarsal with autograft (other than first toe)**

28308 **Osteotomy, with or without lengthening, shortening or angular correction, metatarsal; other than first metatarsal, each**

28309 **Osteotomy, with or without lengthening, shortening or angular correction, metatarsal; multiple (eg, Swanson type cavus foot procedure)**

An osteotomy of the first metatarsal with or without lengthening, shortening or angular correction is performed. Osteotomy of the first metatarsal is performed to treat acquired or congenital angular deformities such as hallux valgus, metatarsus primus varus, hallux varus, or dorsal bunion. The first metatarsal is exposed. Depending on the site of the osteotomy and the specific deformity being corrected, the excision may extend over the proximal phalanx and/or medial cuneiform bones. The metatarsophalangeal (MTP) joint capsule may be incised and tendons divided as needed. If a closing wedge osteotomy is performed, the metatarsal bone is cut and bone is removed from the metatarsal base, neck, and/or head using a saw or osteotome. The wedge is closed by cracking the metatarsal and manipulating the bone into anatomic alignment. Internal fixation such as a screw or K-wire is applied as needed to maintain alignment of the bones. If an opening wedge osteotomy is performed, the bone is cut and a laminar spreader used to open and align the bone. Bone autograft is then placed at the osteotomy site. Use code 28306 if no bone autograft or a bone autograft from the first toe is used. Use code 28307, if an autograft is harvested from a site other than the first toe. Autografts may be placed at the osteotomy site or used for joint fusion, such as fusion of the first metatarsal with the first cuneiform bone. Use code 28308 for osteotomy of each metatarsal other than the first metatarsal and code 28309 for ostetomy of multiple metatarsals, such as a Swanson type procedure for a cavus deformity of the foot.

28310-28312

28310 Osteotomy, shortening, angular or rotational correction; proximal phalanx, first toe (separate procedure)

28312 Osteotomy, shortening, angular or rotational correction; other phalanges, any toe

A shortening osteotomy is performed on one of the toes to correct an angular or rotational deformity. The phalanx that is to be shortened is exposed. The sites of the bone cuts are identified. The bone is cut and a segment of the bone is excised. The remaining distal and proximal portions of the bone are then brought into contact with each other and internal fixation is applied to stabilize the reconfigured bone. Use 28310 for shortening osteotomy on the first toe. Use 28312 for shortening osteotomy on phalanges of the second, third, fourth or fifth toe.

28313

28313 Reconstruction, angular deformity of toe, soft tissue procedures only (eg, overlapping second toe, fifth toe, curly toes)

Reconstruction of an angular deformity of the toe involving only soft tissue is performed when there is no bone component to the deformity. The reconstruction procedure depends on the exact nature of the angular deformity. A skin incision is made over the affected toe. Soft tissues are dissected and the structures causing the deformity identified. The extensor tendon may be incised and lengthened, the joint capsule may be opened, or the flexor tendon may be released. Once the deformity has been corrected the overlying soft tissue and skin are repaired in layers. The toe is then splinted to maintain the toe in the correct position until soft tissue healing has occurred.

28315

28315 Sesamoidectomy, first toe (separate procedure)

There are two sesamoid bones on the plantar aspect of the forefoot near the great toe, one on either side of the first metatarsal head. The sesamoid bones act as pulleys providing a smooth surface over which tendons slide. The sesamoid bones in the forefoot also assist in weightbearing and help elevate the bones of the great toe. If these bones fracture or become inflamed, it is sometimes necessary to remove them. A skin incision is made over the sesamoid bone. Soft tissues are dissected around the sesamoid bone and the bone is excised.

28320-28322

28320 Repair, nonunion or malunion; tarsal bones

28322 Repair, nonunion or malunion; metatarsal, with or without bone graft (includes obtaining graft)

When union of the fracture fragments does not occur after sufficient healing time has elapsed, the patient is considered to have a nonunion of the fracture. Malunion caused by malalignment of the fracture fragments can cause osseous abnormalities, incongruity of articular surfaces, soft tissue contracture, nerve impingement, and other complications. The original fracture sites of the tarsal or metatarsal bone are exposed. The nonunion or malunion is evaluated to determine what type of repair is required which may include internal fixation without or with a bone graft. If it is treated without a graft internal fixation may be used. For a nonunion, pins or screws may be placed through the fracture site. For a malunion, the tarsal or metatarsal bone may be refractured, realigned, and internal fixation placed to maintain the fracture in anatomical alignment. Following placement of the fixation device, stability of the fracture is checked and alignment is verified radiographically. If a bone graft is used to fill the bone defect and encourage healing, the site of the nonunion or malunion is prepared which may include refracture of the bone. Cortical and/or cancellous bone is harvested. The bone is configured to the size and shape of the defect or cancellous bone is morcelized and packed into the defect. Internal fixation, such as a pin or wire is used as needed to secure the bone graft. A compression plate and screws or other internal fixation is used to stabilize the fracture. Use 28320 for repair of a nonunion or malunion of a tarsal bone. Use 28322 for repair of a nonunion or malunion of a metatarsal bone.

28340-28341

28340 Reconstruction, toe, macrodactyly; soft tissue resection

28341 Reconstruction, toe, macrodactyly; requiring bone resection

Macrodactyly of the toe is an overgrowth of bone and soft tissue including nerves, fat, and skin that causes an abnormally large digit or digits. Surgery is performed to reduce the size of the enlarged digit which involves debulking the soft tissue and/or shortening the toe usually by excision of one of the phalanges or the metacarpal bone. The procedure may be performed in a staged fashion. In 28340, soft tissue resection of the toe is performed. To debulk the soft tissue, the thickened layers of skin are excised. Skin grafts are harvested from healthy tissue in the more proximal aspect of the digit or hand or from the plantar instep. The skin graft is then configured to cover the surgically created defect and secured with sutures. In 28341, bone resection is performed. To shorten the toe, the affected digit is incised over the bone that is to be excised. Soft tissues are dissected and the bone exposed. The bone is detached from surrounding structures and part or all of the bone

excised. Soft tissues are excised and/or rearranged as needed to produce a cosmetically acceptable result.

28344

28344 Reconstruction, toe(s); polydactyly

Polydactyly of the foot is a condition in which there are one or more extra toes. Polydactyly is classified as Type I if only soft tissue is involved, Type II if the digit includes bone and/or cartilage, or Type III if the complete digit and metacarpal are duplicated. Polydactyly is also classified as pre-axial when there is an extra great toe, postaxial when there is an extra little toe, and central when there is an extra toe in the central part of the foot. This procedure involves reconstruction of the duplicated digit. In pre-axial or post-axial polydactyly, the duplicated or split great toe or little toe must be reconstructed to create a single digit. This involves excision of bone or cartilage with rearrangement of skin, soft tissue, tendons, joints and ligaments to reconstruct a single digit. Central polydactyly typically requires a more complex reconstruction of both the forefoot and the toes.

28345

28345 Reconstruction, toe(s); syndactyly, with or without skin graft(s), each web

Syndactaly is a condition in which two or more toes in the foot are joined. Simple syndactyly involves only the soft tissues of the foot while complex syndactyly involves soft tissue and bone or cartilaginous tissue and/or the nail. Simple syndactyly is treated by division of the soft tissues and skin flap closure. Zigzag incisions are made over the dorsal and volar aspects of the conjoined toes. Soft tissues are dissected and the interdigital connective tissue layer identified. Beginning distally the soft tissue is carefully separated taking care to preserve blood supply to both toes. Once the toes are completely separated, the skin flaps are defatted and used to close the zigzag incisions on both toes. Alternatively skin flap and graft closure may be required. The procedure is performed as described above except that full thickness skin grafts are used in conjunction with skin flaps to allow complete closure of the zigzag incision. Full thickness skin grafts are harvested usually from the plantar instep and prepared for grafting. The skin grafts are configured to the necessary dimensions and used to help close the zigzag incisions. Complex syndactyly requires separation of the conjoined nails, bone, and/or cartilaginous tissue. If the nails are joined they are split. The conjoined bony or cartilaginous tissue is carefully dissected taking care to preserve ligaments and tendons. Once the toes are completely separated, lateral nail folds are created using two horizontal nail flaps or palmar pulp is defatted and advanced dorsally to create the lateral nail folds. The zigzag incisions are then closed using skin flaps and/or grafts.

28360

28360 Reconstruction, cleft foot

Cleft foot is a congenital anomaly in which the foot is missing part or all of one or more toes in the center of the foot. This results in a central V-shaped gap or cleft in the foot. The extent of the anomaly varies. Cleft foot is treated surgically when function of the foot is significantly impaired. The surgical procedure performed depends on the exact nature of the anomaly. Cleft foot repair involves rearrangement of the skin and soft tissue to close the gap at the cleft site. Bones are stabilized or transferred and any deformities of the toes are also corrected. One common technique involves deepening the space between the toes. Skin from the cleft site is transposed with its blood supply and used to cover the space between the toes. The cleft is then closed in layers.

28400-28405

28400 Closed treatment of calcaneal fracture; without manipulation

28405 Closed treatment of calcaneal fracture; with manipulation

Closed treatment of a calcaneal fracture is performed. The calcaneus is the largest of the tarsal bones and forms the heel. It articulates with the cuboid anteriorly and the talus superiorly. Separately reportable radiographs are obtained to confirm the fracture. A neurovascular exam is performed to ensure that the nerves and blood vessels at the site of the injury are intact. In 28400, a nondisplaced or minimally displaced fracture is treated. No manipulation of the fracture fragments is required. A cast or brace is applied to immobilize the fracture. In 28405, a displaced fracture is treated. The displaced fracture fragments are manually reduced (manipulated) back to proper anatomic alignment. Separately reportable radiographs are obtained to confirm anatomic reduction. A cast or brace is applied to immobilize the fracture.

28406

28406 Percutaneous skeletal fixation of calcaneal fracture, with manipulation

Calcaneal fractures are classified as either extra-articular or intra-articular. Percutaneous fixation of a calcaneal fracture is typically performed for intra-articular fractures when there are contraindications to open reduction such as significant comorbidities, soft-tissue injury, vascular insufficiency, or other conditions that would impair healing. If the fracture fragments are displaced they are manually manipulated into anatomical alignment and additional radiological studies are performed to verify that the fracture(s) have been successfully reduced. A small incision is made in the skin, and a Steinman pin is placed through the posterior superior portion of the calcaneal tuberosity while traction is applied across the pin to maintain the calcaneus in anatomical alignment. A second small incision is made and a threaded Steinman pin is inserted through the posterior inferior corner of the calcaneus and into the talar body to stabilize the reduction. A third incision is made and a Steinman pin is placed through the posterior calcaneus and into the cuboid. A cast or splint is applied as needed.

28415-28420

28415   Open treatment of calcaneal fracture, includes internal fixation, when performed

28420   Open treatment of calcaneal fracture, includes internal fixation, when performed; with primary iliac or other autogenous bone graft (includes obtaining graft)

The calcaneus is the largest of the tarsal bones and forms the heel. It articulates with the cuboid anteriorly and the talus superiorly. Fracture of the calcaneus is usually the result of a high impact force to the heel such as a fall or motor vehicle accident. Calcaneal fractures may also be associated with injuries to the subtalar joint, causing limitation of inward (inversion) and outward (eversion) motion. An L-shaped incision is made over the posterolateral aspect of the foot, behind and below the lateral malleolus. The fracture site is exposed and the subtalar joint is inspected. Bone elevators are used to reduce the fracture. Reduction is maintained by temporary placement of wire fixation and anatomic reduction is checked radiographically. Internal fixation, such as screws or a plate and screw device, is applied as needed. Use 28420 when autogenous bone grafting is also done. An incision is made over the iliac crest or another donor site and a bone graft is excised. The graft material is packed into the fracture prior to placement of a plate and screw device, which is secured over the bone graft at the fracture site. The wound is irrigated and The incision is closed with sutures.

28430-28435

28430   Closed treatment of talus fracture; without manipulation
28435   Closed treatment of talus fracture; with manipulation

Closed treatment of a talus fracture is performed. The talus articulates with the tibia and fibula superiorly at the ankle joint and the calcaneus inferiorly at the subtalar joint. Separately reportable radiographs are obtained to confirm the fracture. A neurovascular exam is performed to ensure that the nerves and blood vessels at the site of the injury are intact. In 28430, a nondisplaced or minimally displaced fracture is treated. No manipulation of the fracture fragments is required. A cast or brace is applied to immobilize the fracture. In 28435, a displaced fracture is treated. The displaced fracture fragments are manually reduced (manipulated) back to proper anatomic alignment. Separately reportable radiographs are obtained to confirm anatomic reduction. A cast or brace is applied to immobilize the fracture.

28436

28436   Percutaneous skeletal fixation of talus fracture, with manipulation

This procedure is performed to treat a fracture of the talus. If the fracture is displaced, the fracture is reduced and successful reduction verified by separately reportable radiographs. One or more small skin incisions are made over the planned pin or Kirschner wire insertion sites. A small drill is used to create a corticotomy into which the percutaneous pin or wire will be placed. One or more pins or wires are advanced across the fracture site. Once all pins or wires have been placed, anatomical reduction is again verified by separately reportable radiographs.

28445

28445   Open treatment of talus fracture, includes internal fixation, when performed

A talus fracture is repaired openly, using any necessary internal fixation. The talus is the bone in the foot that articulates with the tibia and fibula superiorly at the ankle joint and with the calcaneus inferiorly at the subtalar joint. Fractures of the talus are typically high impact injuries caused by a fall or motor vehicle accident. The fracture site is exposed and the ankle and/or subtalar joint are inspected. The fracture is cleared of debris and the talar fragments are reduced. Traction may be applied with a talar pin. Severely comminuted fractures may require a second incision to ensure anatomic alignment of all fracture fragments. Temporary wire fixation is applied and anatomic reduction is confirmed radiographically. Internal fixation, such a pins or screws, is applied as needed. The wound is irrigated and incisions are closed.

28446

28446   Open osteochondral autograft, talus (includes obtaining graft[s])

An osteochrondral autograft is harvested locally or from a separate site in the patient and applied to the talus in an open procedure. The most common indication for osteochondral autografting of the talus is osteochondritis dissecans, characterized by deep aching pain in the ankle joint that worsens with activity. An incision is made over the site of the bone lesion in the ankle and the joint capsule is incised (arthrotomy). An osteotomy of the medial or lateral malleolus may be performed to gain access to the site of the lesion on

the talus. The damaged tissue is debrided and prepared for transplant. The osteochondral autografts are harvested from healthy tissue in the patient's knee or less commonly from healthy tissue in the talar articular facet near the lesion. If the healthy tissue is harvested from the knee, an arthroscopy or arthrotomy of the knee is performed. The harvest device is directed in an exact perpendicular line to the articular surface to retrieve osteochondral tissue. The recipient site is prepared by using an appropriate sized drill and matching the size and shape of the drilled tunnel to the harvested tissue. The osteochondral autograft is then inserted into the prepared recipient site. This process is repeated until the defect is filled or there is no more healthy tissue available at the donor site.

28450-28455

28450   Treatment of tarsal bone fracture (except talus and calcaneus); without manipulation, each

28455   Treatment of tarsal bone fracture (except talus and calcaneus); with manipulation, each

Closed treatment of a tarsal bone fracture other than the talus or calcaneus is performed. The anterior tarsal bones include the cuboid, navicular, and three cuneiform bones. If more than one of these tarsal bones are fractured, each bone treated is reported separately. Separately reportable radiographs are obtained to confirm the fracture. A neurovascular exam is performed to ensure that the nerves and blood vessels at the site of the injury are intact. In 28450, a nondisplaced or minimally displaced fracture of one of anterior tarsal bones is treated. No manipulation of the fracture fragments is required. A cast or brace is applied to immobilize the fracture. In 28455, a displaced fracture of one of the anterior tarsal bones is treated. The displaced fracture fragments are manually reduced (manipulated) back to proper anatomic alignment. Separately reportable radiographs are obtained to confirm anatomic reduction. A cast or brace is applied to immobilize the fracture.

28456

28456   Percutaneous skeletal fixation of tarsal bone fracture (except talus and calcaneus), with manipulation, each

This procedure is performed to treat a fracture of the navicular, cuboid, or one of the three cuneiform bones. If the fracture is displaced, the fracture is reduced and successful reduction verified by separately reportable radiographs. One or more small skin incisions are made over the planned pin or Kirschner wire insertion sites. A small drill is used to create a corticotomy into which the percutaneous pin or wire will be placed. One or more pins or wires are advanced across the fracture site. Once all pins or wires have been placed, anatomical reduction is again verified by separately reportable radiographs.

28465

28465   Open treatment of tarsal bone fracture (except talus and calcaneus), includes internal fixation, when performed, each

There are five anterior tarsal bones, which include the cuboid, navicular, and three cuneiform bones. The approach varies depending on which bone is fractured and the fracture location in the affected bone. The fracture site is exposed and inspected, debris is cleared, and the fracture fragments are reduced. Internal fixation, such as pins or screws, is applied as needed. The wound is irrigated and The incision is closed with sutures.

28470-28475

28470   Closed treatment of metatarsal fracture; without manipulation, each
28475   Closed treatment of metatarsal fracture; with manipulation, each

Closed treatment of a metatarsal fracture is performed. There are five metatarsal bones that articulate proximally with the cuboid and cuneiform bones and distally with the proximal row of phalanges. If more than one of the metatarsal bones are fractured, each bone treated is reported separately. Separately reportable radiographs are obtained to confirm the fracture. A neurovascular exam is performed to ensure that the nerves and blood vessels at the site of the injury are intact. In 28470, a nondisplaced or minimally displaced fracture of one of metatarsal bones is treated. No manipulation of the fracture fragments is required. A cast or boot is applied to immobilize the fracture. In 28475, a displaced fracture of one of the metatarsal bones is treated. The displaced fracture fragments are manually reduced (manipulated) back to proper anatomic alignment. Separately reportable radiographs are obtained to confirm anatomic reduction. A cast or boot is applied to immobilize the fracture.

28476

28476   Percutaneous skeletal fixation of metatarsal fracture, with manipulation, each

A small skin incision is made proximal to the fracture site in the metatarsal bone. A small drill is used to create a corticotomy proximal to the fracture site. The fracture is reduced and one or more pre-bent Kirschner wires are advanced by hand across the fracture site through the medullary canal. Anatomical reduction is verified radiographically.

● New Code   ▲ Revised Code

Musculoskeletal System

Musculoskeletal System

28485

28485   Open treatment of metatarsal fracture, includes internal fixation, when performed, each

A single metatarsal bone fracture is repaired openly, using any necessary internal fixation. There are five metatarsal bones that articulate proximally with the cuboid and cuneiform bones and distally with the proximal row of phalanges. An incision is made over the fracture site in the metatarsal bone. The fracture site is exposed and cleared of debris, then the bone fragments are reduced back into position. Internal fixation, such as pins, screws, or a multifragment plate and screw device, is applied as needed. The wound is irrigated and The incision is closed with sutures. If multiple metatarsal bones are repaired using an open technique, report 28485 for each metatarsal treated.

28490-28495

28490   Closed treatment of fracture great toe, phalanx or phalanges; without manipulation
28495   Closed treatment of fracture great toe, phalanx or phalanges; with manipulation

Separately reportable radiographs are obtained to confirm the fracture. A neurovascular exam is performed to ensure that the nerves and blood vessels at the site of the injury are intact. In 28490, a nondisplaced or minimally displaced fracture of one or both phalanges of the great toe is treated. No manipulation of the fracture fragments is required. A cast or boot is applied as needed to immobilize the fracture. In 28495, a displaced fracture is treated. The displaced fracture fragments are manually reduced (manipulated) back to proper anatomic alignment. Separately reportable radiographs are obtained to confirm anatomic reduction. A cast or boot is applied as needed to immobilize the fracture.

28496

28496   Percutaneous skeletal fixation of fracture great toe, phalanx or phalanges, with manipulation

A small skin incision is made proximal to the fracture site in the phalangeal shaft of the great toe. A small drill is used to create a corticotomy proximal to the fracture site. The fracture is reduced and one or more pre-bent Kirschner wires are advanced by hand across the fracture site through the medullary canal. If both phalanges of the great toe are broken, the wires are advanced through both the proximal and distal phalanges. Anatomical reduction is verified radiographically.

28505

28505   Open treatment of fracture, great toe, phalanx or phalanges, includes internal fixation, when performed

An incision is made over the fracture site in the phalanx/phalanges of the great toe. The fracture site is exposed and cleared of debris, and the fracture is reduced. Internal fixation, such as wires, pins, screws, or a minifragment plate and screw device, is applied as needed. The wound is irrigated and The incision is closed with sutures.

28510-28515

28510   Closed treatment of fracture, phalanx or phalanges, other than great toe; without manipulation, each
28515   Closed treatment of fracture, phalanx or phalanges, other than great toe; with manipulation, each

Closed treatment of a fracture of the phalanx or phalanges of a single toe other than the great toe is performed. Separately reportable radiographs are obtained to confirm the fracture. A neurovascular exam is performed to ensure that the nerves and blood vessels at the site of the injury are intact. In 28510, a nondisplaced or minimally displaced fracture of one of the toes other than the great toe is treated. No manipulation of the fracture fragments is required. The fractured toe is buddy taped to an uninjured adjacent toe and immobilization by a rigid, flat shoe recommended. In 28515, a displaced fracture is treated. The displaced fracture fragments are manually reduced (manipulated) back to proper anatomic alignment. Separately reportable radiographs are obtained to confirm anatomic reduction. The fractured toe is buddy taped to an uninjured adjacent toe and immobilization by a rigid, flat shoe recommended. Less commonly, a cast or boot may be applied to immobilize the fracture. If more than one toe other than the great toe is treated, report 28510 or 28515 for each toe treated.

28525

28525   Open treatment of fracture, phalanx or phalanges, other than great toe, includes internal fixation, when performed, each

An incision is made in the toe to expose the fracture site, which is cleared of debris, and then the fracture fragments are reduced. Internal fixation, such as pins, screws, or a minifragment plate and screw device, is applied as needed. The wound is irrigated and The incision is closed with sutures. If phalangeal fractures in multiple toes are repaired using an open technique, report 28525 for each toe treated.

28530-28531

28530   Closed treatment of sesamoid fracture
28531   Open treatment of sesamoid fracture, with or without internal fixation

A sesamoid fracture of the foot is treated. Sesamoid bones are small bones embedded in a tendon. In the foot, two sesamoid bones are located under the great toe joint in the ball of the foot. Separately reportable radiographs are obtained to confirm the fracture. A neurovascular exam is performed to ensure that the nerves and blood vessels at the site of the injury are intact. In 28530, closed treatment of a nondisplaced or minimally displaced sesamoid fracture is performed. If the fracture is nondisplaced, no manipulation of the fracture fragments is required. If the fracture fragments are displaced, they may be reduced (manipulated) back to proper anatomic alignment. Separately reportable radiographs are obtained to confirm anatomic reduction. Padding, strapping, or taping may be used to relieve pressure and tension on the fracture site. A cast or boot may be applied to immobilize the fracture. In 28531, the sesamoid fracture is treated by open reduction with or without internal fixation. The fractured sesamoid bone is exposed. The fracture fragments are excised. Less commonly, the bone is reduced (manipulated) back to proper anatomic alignment and fracture fragments secured using pins or wires inserted into the bone.

28540-28545

28540   Closed treatment of tarsal bone dislocation, other than talotarsal; without anesthesia
28545   Closed treatment of tarsal bone dislocation, other than talotarsal; requiring anesthesia

There are seven tarsal bones including the talus. The six other bones are the calcaneus, cuboid, navicular, and the three cuneiform bones (medial, intermediate, and lateral). Dislocation of the tarsal bones is a rare injury. The neurovascular status of the foot is evaluated. If no pulse is present, emergent reduction of the affected mid-foot joint without pre-reduction radiographs is performed. If neurovascular status is intact, separately reportable radiographs are obtained. With the knee flexed, longitudinal traction is applied to the foot along with pressure on the involved bones to reduce a dislocation. Following reduction, neurovascular status is again evaluated and a second set of radiographs obtained. The foot is immobilized in a splint and the patient is instructed to ice and elevate the foot. Use 28540 when the dislocation is treated without anesthesia and 28545 when anesthesia is required.

28546

28546   Percutaneous skeletal fixation of tarsal bone dislocation, other than talotarsal, with manipulation

A small skin incision is made over the dislocated tarsal joint other than the talotarsal. The dislocated tarsal bones are reduced and anatomical alignment verified by separately reportable radiographs. One or more small skin incisions are made over the planned pin or Kirschner wire insertion sites. A small drill is used to create a corticotomy into which the percutaneous pin or wire will be placed. One or more pins or wires are advanced through one of the involved tarsal bones across the joint and into the second tarsal bone to stabilize the joint. Once all pins or wires have been placed, anatomical reduction is again verified by separately reportable radiographs.

28555

28555   Open treatment of tarsal bone dislocation, includes internal fixation, when performed

A tarsal bone dislocation is treated openly, using any necessary internal fixation. There are seven tarsal bones, two posterior (talus and calcaneus) and five anterior (navicular, cuboid, and three cuneiform). An incision is made over the dislocated joint and the dislocation is reduced. Internal fixation, such as pins or screws, are applied as needed. The wound is irrigated and The incision is closed with sutures.

28570-28575

28570   Closed treatment of talotarsal joint dislocation; without anesthesia
28575   Closed treatment of talotarsal joint dislocation; requiring anesthesia

The talus is one of seven tarsal bones and it articulates superiorly with the tibia and fibula and inferiorly with the calcaneus and navicular bones. Talotarsal dislocation is a rare injury that involves the talocalcaneal and/or talonavicular joints. The neurovascular status of the foot is evaluated. If no pulse is present, emergent reduction of the affected joint(s) without pre-reduction radiographs is performed. If neurovascular status is intact, separately reportable radiographs are obtained. With the knee flexed, reduction is accomplished by applying longitudinal traction to the foot along with pressure on the talus. Following reduction, neurovascular status is again evaluated and a second set of radiographs obtained. The foot is immobilized in a splint and the patient is instructed to ice and elevate the foot. Use 28570 when the dislocation is treated without anesthesia and 28575 when anesthesia is required.

28576

28576   Percutaneous skeletal fixation of talotarsal joint dislocation, with manipulation

A small skin incision is made over the dislocated talotarsal joint. The dislocated tarsal bones are reduced and anatomical alignment verified by separately reportable radiographs. One or more small skin incisions are made over the planned pin or Kirschner wire insertion sites. A small drill is used to create a corticotomy into which the percutaneous pin or wire will be placed. One or more pins or wires are advanced through the talus across the joint and into the tarsal bone to stabilize the joint. Once all pins or wires have been placed, anatomical reduction is again verified by separately reportable radiographs.

28585

28585   Open treatment of talotarsal joint dislocation, includes internal fixation, when performed

A talotarsal joint dislocation is repaired openly, using any necessary internal fixation. The talus articulates with the navicular tarsal bone anteriorly. An incision is made over the dislocated joint and it is reduced. Internal fixation, such as pins or screws, is applied as needed. The wound is irrigated and The incision is closed with sutures.

28600-28605

28600   Closed treatment of tarsometatarsal joint dislocation; without anesthesia
28605   Closed treatment of tarsometatarsal joint dislocation; requiring anesthesia

Tarsometatarsal joint dislocation may also be referred to as a Lisfranc dislocation. The neurovascular status of the foot is evaluated. If no pulse is present, emergent reduction of the joint without pre-reduction radiographs is performed. If neurovascular status is intact, separately reportable radiographs are obtained. Closed reduction is accomplished by longitudinal traction applied to the foot along with pressure on the involved bones. Following reduction, neurovascular status is again evaluated and a second set of radiographs obtained. The toe is immobilized in a splint and the patient is instructed to ice and elevate the foot. Use 28600 when the dislocation is treated without anesthesia and 28605 when anesthesia is required.

28606

28606   Percutaneous skeletal fixation of tarsometatarsal joint dislocation, with manipulation

A small skin incision is made over the metatarsal bone and a small drill is used to create a corticotomy. The dislocated tarsometatarsal bone is reduced and returned to anatomical alignment. One or more pre-bent Kirschner wires are advanced by hand into the metatarsal medullary canal, across the tarsometatarsal joint, and into the tarsal bone. Anatomical reduction of the dislocation is verified by separately reportable radiographs.

28615

28615   Open treatment of tarsometatarsal joint dislocation, includes internal fixation, when performed

There are seven tarsal bones, two posterior (talus and calcaneus) and five anterior (navicular, cuboid, and three cuneiform). The cuboid and the three cuneiform bones articulate anteriorly with the metatarsal bones. An incision is made over the dislocated joint and it is reduced. Internal fixation, such as pins or screws, is applied as needed. The wound is irrigated and The incision is closed with sutures.

28630-28635

28630   Closed treatment of metatarsophalangeal joint dislocation; without anesthesia
28635   Closed treatment of metatarsophalangeal joint dislocation; requiring anesthesia

The neurovascular status of the foot and toes is evaluated. Separately reportable radiographs are obtained. Closed reduction is accomplished using longitudinal traction applied to the toe along with pressure on the involved metatarsal and phalangeal bones. Following reduction, neurovascular status is again evaluated and a second set of radiographs obtained. The foot is immobilized in a splint and the patient is instructed to ice and elevate the foot. Use 28630 when the dislocation is treated without anesthesia and 28635 when anesthesia is required.

28636

28636   Percutaneous skeletal fixation of metatarsophalangeal joint dislocation, with manipulation

A small skin incision is made over the metatarsal or phalangeal bone and a small drill is used to create a corticotomy. The dislocated bones in the metatarsophalangeal joint are reduced and returned to anatomical alignment. One or more pre-bent Kirschner wires are advanced by hand through the medullary canals of the metatarsal and phalangeal bones to maintain the joint in anatomic alignment. Successful reduction of the dislocation is verified by separately reportable radiographs.

28645

28645   Open treatment of metatarsophalangeal joint dislocation, includes internal fixation, when performed

There are five metatarsal bones in the midfoot that articulate anteriorly with the proximal phalanges in the toes. An incision is made over the dislocated joint and it is reduced. Internal fixation, such as wires or pins, is applied as needed. The wound is irrigated and The incision is closed with sutures.

28660-28665

28660   Closed treatment of interphalangeal joint dislocation; without anesthesia
28665   Closed treatment of interphalangeal joint dislocation; requiring anesthesia

The neurovascular status of the toes is evaluated. Separately reportable radiographs are obtained. Closed reduction of the interphalangeal joint dislocation is accomplished using longitudinal traction applied to the toe along with pressure on the involved phalangeal bones. Following reduction, neurovascular status is again evaluated and a second set of radiographs obtained. The foot is immobilized in a splint and the patient is instructed to ice and elevate the foot. Use 28660 when the dislocation is treated without anesthesia and 28665 when anesthesia is required.

28666

28666   Percutaneous skeletal fixation of interphalangeal joint dislocation, with manipulation

A small skin incision is made over the middle or distal phalanx and a small drill is used to create a corticotomy. The dislocated phalangeal bones are reduced and returned to anatomical alignment. One or more pre-bent Kirschner wires are advanced by hand through the medullary canals of the phalangeal bones to maintain the joint in alignment. Successful reduction of the dislocation is verified by separately reportable radiographs.

28675

28675   Open treatment of interphalangeal joint dislocation, includes internal fixation, when performed

The great toe has two phalangeal bones (proximal and distal) and the other four toes have three phalangeal bones (proximal, middle, and distal). An incision is made over the dislocated joint, which is reduced and held in place with internal fixation, such as wires or pins, if needed. The wound is irrigated and The incision is closed with sutures.

28705-28725

28705   Arthrodesis; pantalar
28715   Arthrodesis; triple
28725   Arthrodesis; subtalar

Arthrodesis of the ankle is performed to treat severe arthritis, avascular necrosis of the bones forming the ankle joint, failed total ankle arthroplasty, deformities due to trauma, congenital anomalies such as severe untreated club foot, or deformities due to neuromuscular disease. In 28705, a pantalar arthrodesis is performed which involves fusion of the talus with all bones that it articulates with which include the distal tibia, calcaneus, tarsonavicular, and cuboid. A long longitudinal incision is made over the lateral aspect of the ankle. Soft tissues are dissected and the superficial peroneal and sural nerves are identified and protected. The distal fibula is excised using an oscillating saw just proximal to the tibiotalar joint. A second incision is made over the anteromedial aspect of the ankle. Soft tissues are dissected and the greater saphenous vein and cuticular nerve identified and protected. The articular cartilage is denuded and subchondral bone removed using a sharp bone chisel. The subtalar and transverse tarsal joints are exposed using a laminar spreader and the articular cartilage denuded from these joints. Bone wedges are excised as needed to allow the foot to be placed in plantigrade position. Using the contralateral extremity as the guide the ankle is carefully aligned to allow optimal function. Autogenous bone grafts from the distal tibia or iliac crest are harvested and packed into the joint spaces. Internal fixation, such as threaded guide wires and cannulated screws are placed to immobilize the joint. In 28715, a triple arthrodesis is performed which involves fusion of the talocalcaneal, talonavicular, and calcaneocuboid joints. These joints allow side-to-side movement of the foot. Lateral and medial longitudinal incisions are made just below the ankle. The articular cartilage is removed and the position of the hindfoot is corrected. The joints are stabilized using screws, wires, or staples. Bone grafts may also be placed in the joint spaces. In 28725, a subtalar arthrodesis is performed which involves fusion of the talus and calcaneus. An incision is made over the talocalaneal joint. The posterior facet is exposed. Articular cartilage is excised and bone excised as needed. The foot is placed in the desired position and the talus and calcaneus stabilized using screw fixation. A bone graft may also be placed in the joint space. Incisions are closed and the foot is placed in the short leg cast or cast boot.

Musculoskeletal System

28730-28735

28730 Arthrodesis, midtarsal or tarsometatarsal, multiple or transverse
28735 Arthrodesis, midtarsal or tarsometatarsal, multiple or transverse; with osteotomy (eg, flatfoot correction)

Fusion of multiple midtarsal or tarsometatarsal joints is performed to treat severe, painful arthritis or congenital or acquired deformity of the midfoot. A longitudinal incision is made over the affected midtarsal and/or tarsometatarsal joints taking care to protect superficial nerves and blood vessels. The joint is exposed and all fibrous tissue and articular cartilage is excised. For severe deformity, resection of bone may also be required. The articular surfaces of the bone are carefully scaled using an osteotome. If a bone graft is required it is harvested locally or from the iliac crest or medial malleolus. Bone grafts are configured to the size and shape needed and placed in the joint space. Internal fixation, such as Steinman pins, interfragmentary screws, or plate and screws are placed to stabilize the joints. Incisions are closed in layers. A bulky dressing and splint are applied. Use 28730 when the procedure is performed without an osteotomy. Use 28735 when an osteotomy is also performed to correct a condition such as flatfoot deformity.

28737

28737 Arthrodesis, with tendon lengthening and advancement, midtarsal, tarsal navicular-cuneiform (eg, Miller type procedure)

Midtarsal, tarsal navicular-cuneiform fusion is performed to treat malalignment or sagging of the navicular-cuneiform joint which is commonly associated with flatfoot deformity or severe pronation. An incision is made over the midfoot. Soft tissues are dissected taking care to protect nerves and blood vessels. The midtarsal, tarsal navicular-cuneiform joints are exposed. Cartilage is excised and bone scaled using an osteotome to expose cancellous bone. In a Miller type procedure, the tibialis anterior tendon is lengthened or advanced. A Z-shaped incision is made in the anterior tibialis tendon which lengthens it by allowing the tendon fibers to slide apart as the foot is extended. To perform tendon advancement, the anterior tibialis tendon is detached from the insertion sites on the first metatarsal base and medial plantar surface of the first cuneiform and advanced distally and secured with sutures. Midtarsal, navicular and cuneiform bones are repositioned anatomically. Autogenous bone grafts are harvested locally. Alternatively an iliac bone graft may be harvested through a separate incision. The joints are stabilized with pins or screws inserted across the joints. Incisions are closed in layers, a bulky dressing is applied, and the foot is immobilized in cast, splint or boot.

28740

28740 Arthrodesis, midtarsal or tarsometatarsal, single joint

Fusion of a single midtarsal or tarsometatarsal joint is performed to treat severe, painful arthritis or congenital or acquired deformity of the midfoot. A longitudinal incision is made over the affected midtarsal or tarsometatarsal joint taking care to protect superficial nerves and blood vessels. The joint is exposed and all fibrous tissue and articular cartilage is excised. The articular surfaces of the bone are carefully scaled using an osteotome. If a bone graft is required it is harvested locally or from the iliac crest or medial malleolus. Bone grafts are configured to the size and shape needed and placed in the joint space. Internal fixation, such as Steinman pins, interfragmentary screws, or plate and screws are placed to stabilize the joint. Incisions are closed in layers. A bulky dressing and splint are applied.

28750-28755

28750 Arthrodesis, great toe; metatarsophalangeal joint
28755 Arthrodesis, great toe; interphalangeal joint

An incision is made over the lateral aspect of the great toe taking care to protect nerves and blood vessels. The joint is exposed and articular cartilage excised. The articular surfaces of the metatarsal head and proximal phalanx or the proximal phalanx and distal phalanx are scaled using an osteotome and cancellous bone is exposed. Internal fixation, such as a pin, screws, staples or a small plate, is placed through the bones and across the joint to stabilize the joint. The incision is closed and a bulky dressing applied. Use 28750 for fusion of the metatarsophalangeal joint of the great toe. Use 28755 for fusion of the interphalangeal joint.

28760

28760 Arthrodesis, with extensor hallucis longus transfer to first metatarsal neck, great toe, interphalangeal joint (eg, Jones type procedure)

An incision is made over the lateral aspect of the interphalangeal joint of the great toe taking care to protect nerves and blood vessels. The joint is exposed and articular cartilage excised. The articular surfaces of the proximal and distal phalanx are scaled using an osteotome and cancellous bone is exposed. The extensor hallucis longus is detached and transferred to the first metatarsal neck. Internal fixation, such as a pin, screws, staples or a small plate, is placed through the bones and across the joint to stabilize the joint. The incision is closed and a bulky dressing applied.

28800-28805

28800 Amputation, foot; midtarsal (eg, Chopart type procedure)
28805 Amputation, foot; transmetatarsal

Partial foot amputations can be performed at the midtarsal level or through the metatarsal bones. Midfoot amputations are typically performed for infection, ischemia, or trauma. In 28800, a midtarsal amputation through the talonavicular and calcaneocuboid joints is performed. This procedure may also be called a midtarsal disarticulation or Chopart procedure. Flap configuration is determined and incision lines drawn. The skin is incised. Deeper tissues are then incised and a multilayer soft tissue flap of plantar skin, subcutaneous tissue, and investing fascia is configured. Dissection continues to the level of the talonavicular and calcaneocuboid joints. Fibrous tissue is dissected and the joint capsule incised. Blood vessels are suture ligated and divided. Nerves are severed and allowed to retract into the soft tissue. The ankle dorsiflexor tendons are divided. The remaining proximal segments of the ankle dorsiflexors are attached to either the anterior tibial tendon with sutures or the talus through a drill hole in the talar head or with sutures or staples. Additional tendon transfers are performed as needed to restore balance of the dorsiflexors and plantar flexors . The flap is closed in layers. A cast is applied with the hindfoot in slight dorsiflexion. Alternatively, a separate external fixation device may be used to maintain the foot in the desired position until the tendons have healed. In 28805, a transmetatarsal amputation is performed. The skin is incised and dorsal and plantar flaps are created. The flexor and extensor muscles are elevated and a musculofascial flap created. Blood vessels are ligated and divided. Digital nerves are ligated at a more proximal level. Osteoperiosteal flaps are elevated and the metatarsals transected. The remaining bone is smoothed with a file to ensure that there are no bony prominences. The osteoperiosteal flaps are sutured over the exposed diaphyses of the metatarsals. The flexor and extensor muscle groups are sutured to each other. The dorsal and plantar soft tissues flaps are closed and a bulky dressing is applied.

28810

28810 Amputation, metatarsal, with toe, single

Amputation of the toe with all or a portion of the metatarsal is also referred to as a ray amputation. This is one of the most common types of amputation performed on diabetic patients with vascular complications including ulceration and infection. An incision is made over the affected metatarsal and toe. Soft tissues are dissected and the bones exposed. If the entire metatarsal is removed, the tarsometatarsal joint capsule is incised and the metatarsal is completely detached. If only a portion of the metatarsal is excised, an osteoperiosteal flap is elevated and the metatarsal transected. The remaining bone is smoothed with a file to ensure that there are no bony prominences. The osteoperiosteal flap is sutured over the exposed diaphysis of the metatarsal. Soft tissues are rearranged as needed to provide coverage to the remaining portion of the metatarsal and closed in layers. The skin incision is closed and a soft bulky dressing applied.

28820-28825

28820 Amputation, toe; metatarsophalangeal joint
28825 Amputation, toe; interphalangeal joint

An amputation of the toe is performed through the metatarsophalangeal joint, also referred to as a toe disarticulation, or through the interphalangeal joint, also known as a partial toe amputation. In 28820, an amputation through the metatarsophageal joint is performed. Flap configuration is determined and incision lines drawn. The skin is incised. Deeper tissues are then incised and a multilayer soft tissue flap configured. Dissection continues to the level of the metatarsophageal joint. Fibrous tissue is dissected and the joint capsule incised. Blood vessels are suture ligated and divided. Nerves are severed proximal to blood vessels and allowed to retract into the soft tissue. The metatarsophalangeal joint capsule is incised and the toe is severed. The metatarsal bone is smoothed and the flap closed in layers over the metatarsal bone. In 28825, an amputation through the proximal or distal interphalangeal joint is performed using the same technique described above.

28890

28890 Extracorporeal shock wave, high energy, performed by a physician or other qualified health care professional, requiring anesthesia other than local, including ultrasound guidance, involving the plantar fascia

High energy extracorporeal shock wave (ESW) therapy requiring regional or general anesthesia is performed on the plantar fascia using ultrasound guidance. The foot is examined and the point of maximal heel tenderness is identified. The planned site of ESW therapy is marked. The heel is prepped and either a heel block (regional anesthesia) or general anesthesia is administered. High energy shock waves are then administered per the ESW manufacturer's instructions to the previously identified area of the heel.

29000

29000 Application of halo type body cast (see 20661-20663 for insertion)

Application of a body cast is typically performed 2-3 days before the cranial halo is placed. A stockinette is applied over the area to the casted followed by padding over the stockinette. A plaster or fiberglass roll is then immersed in water and saturated. Excess water is gently squeezed out of the plaster or fiberglass. The plaster is then wrapped around the torso, smoothed and molded. Anterior and posterior halo brackets are incorporated into the cast structure.

29010-29015

29010   **Application of Risser jacket, localizer, body; only**
29015   **Application of Risser jacket, localizer, body; including head**

A Risser jacket is a body cast that extends from the patient's hip to the neck and sometimes includes a portion of the head. Risser jackets are rarely used today. A stockinette is applied over the torso and neck and extended up over the head as needed. Padding is placed over the stockinette. A plaster or fiberglass roll is then immersed in water and saturated. Excess water is gently squeezed out of the plaster or fiberglass. The plaster or fiberglass is then wrapped around the torso, neck and head. As casting material is wrapped it is simultaneously smoothed and molded. Use 29010 for a Risser jacket of the body only. Use 29015 if the Risser jacket extends up the neck and includes a portion of the head.

29035-29046

29035   **Application of body cast, shoulder to hips**
29040   **Application of body cast, shoulder to hips; including head, Minerva type**
29044   **Application of body cast, shoulder to hips; including 1 thigh**
29046   **Application of body cast, shoulder to hips; including both thighs**

A body cast is applied. Depending on the condition being treated, the cast may extend only from the shoulder to hips, may include the head, or may include one or both thighs. A stockinette is applied over the region to be casted. Padding is placed over the stockinette. A plaster or fiberglass roll is then immersed in water and saturated. Excess water is gently squeezed out of the plaster or fiberglass. The plaster or fiberglass is then wrapped around the torso and extended over the neck and head and/or one or both thighs as needed. As casting material is wrapped it is simultaneously smoothed and molded. Use 29035 for application of a shoulder to hip cast. Use 29040 for a Minerva type cast that includes the torso and head. Use 29044 for a body cast that includes one thigh. Use 29046 for a body cast that includes both thighs.

29049

29049   **Application, cast; figure-of-eight**

The physician applies a cast that wraps around the shoulders in a figure-eight fashion. The cast is wrapped around the shoulder under the axillary area and back around the other axillary area behind the neck.

29055

29055   **Application, cast; shoulder spica**

A shoulder spica cast covers the torso and one shoulder extending down the arm to the mid-forearm. A stockinette is applied over the torso and the injured shoulder and arm. Padding is placed over the stockinette. A plaster or fiberglass roll is then immersed in water and saturated. Excess water is gently squeezed out of the plaster or fiberglass. The plaster or fiberglass is then wrapped around the torso, shoulder and arm. As casting material starts to set it is smoothed and molded.

29058

29058   **Application, cast; plaster Velpeau**

A Velpeau cast is applied to immobilize the shoulder. The injured arm is placed across the chest. The arm is immobilized with a swaddling bandage beginning under the axilla on the uninjured side, wrapped around the back, over the injured shoulder, over the injured arm passing just below the elbow and then back under the uninjured axilla and around the chest. The wrap continues until the arm is secured against the chest. The physician then applies a plaster or fiberglass cast over the bandage to completely immobilize the shoulder.

29065-29085

29065   **Application, cast; shoulder to hand (long arm)**
29075   **Application, cast; elbow to finger (short arm)**
29085   **Application, cast; hand and lower forearm (gauntlet)**

A stockinette is applied over the area to be casted followed by padding over the stockinette. A plaster or fiberglass roll is then immersed in water and saturated. Excess water is gently squeezed out of the plaster or fiberglass. The plaster or fiberglass is wrapped around the arm usually from distal to proximal aspects. The plaster or fiberglass is smoothed and molded to the arm. In 29065, a long arm cast extending from the shoulder or mid-humerus to the hand is applied to immobilize distal humeral fractures, elbow fractures and dislocations, and middle to proximal forearm fractures. In 29075, a short arm cast extending from the elbow to fingers is applied to immobilize distal forearm fractures, wrist sprains, carpal fractures, and some metacarpal fractures. Another type of short arm cast is the thumb spica cast that extends from the elbow and covers the thumb

and is used for scaphoid fractures and some thumb fractures. In 29085, a gauntlet cast extending from lower forearm to hand is applied to immobilize distal forearm fractures and wrist injuries.

29086

29086   **Application, cast; finger (eg, contracture)**

A cast is applied to the finger. The finger may be coated with petroleum jelly to protect the skin. Casting tape is then wrapped around the finger. The cast material is then prepared. Quickcast must be heated before and while applying while plaster and fiberglass must be immersed in water. The casting material is wrapped around and molded to the finger.

29105

29105   **Application of long arm splint (shoulder to hand)**

A long arm splint is applied from the shoulder to the hand. Splints stabilize injuries by decreasing movement and providing support to the posterior aspect of the extremity. A stockinette is applied over the arm from the axilla to the wrist followed by padding over the stockinette. The arm is typically positioned with the elbow flexed from 45 to 90 degrees. Plaster sheets cut to the appropriate length are then immersed in water and saturated. Excess water is gently squeezed out of the plaster. The plaster is applied to the posterior aspect of the arm and smoothed and molded. An elastic bandage is wrapped around the arm to secure the splint. The arm is then placed in a sling.

29125-29126

29125   **Application of short arm splint (forearm to hand); static**
29126   **Application of short arm splint (forearm to hand); dynamic**

A static splint (29125) is applied to stabilize an injury by decreasing movement and providing support to the posterior aspect of the forearm, wrist, and hand. A stockinette is applied over the arm from the elbow to the wrist followed by padding over the stockinette. Plaster sheets cut to the appropriate length are then immersed in water and saturated. Excess water is gently squeezed out of the plaster. The plaster is applied to the posterior aspect of the forearm, wrist, and hand. The plaster is smoothed and molded. An elastic bandage is wrapped around the arm to secure the splint. The forearm may be placed in a sling. In 29126, a dynamic splint is applied. A dynamic splint allows movement of the forearm and wrist by placing a gentle sustained force on the wrist. The patient can tighten tubing on the outside of the splint to stretch the forearm and wrist, which improves flexibility of the joints.

29130-29131

29130   **Application of finger splint; static**
29131   **Application of finger splint; dynamic**

A static splint (29130) is applied to stabilize an injury by decreasing movement and providing support to the posterior aspect of the finger. The finger may be coated with petroleum jelly to protect the skin. Casting tape is then wrapped around the finger. The cast material is then prepared. Plaster sheets cut to the appropriate length are then immersed in water and saturated. Excess water is gently squeezed out of the plaster. The plaster is applied to the posterior aspect of the finger. The plaster is smoothed and molded. An elastic bandage or tape is then wrapped around the finger splint. In 29131, a dynamic splint is applied. A dynamic splint allows movement of the finger by placing a gentle sustained force on it. The type of dynamic splint used will depend on the type of injury or condition being treated.

29200

29200   **Strapping; thorax**

Strapping is applied to the thorax to treat a soft tissue injury or provide support to a vulnerable area of the thorax. The physician or physical therapist evaluates the mechanism of injury and areas of weakness or vulnerability to determine where taping is needed. The thoracic area is then taped in a configuration to provide protection and support to the injured or vulnerable areas.

29240-29280

29240   **Strapping; shoulder (eg, Velpeau)**
29260   **Strapping; elbow or wrist**
29280   **Strapping; hand or finger**

Strapping is applied to the shoulder, elbow or wrist, or hand or finger to treat a soft tissue injury or provide support to an area of weakness or vulnerability. The physician or physical therapist evaluates the mechanism of injury and areas of weakness or vulnerability to determine where taping is needed. In 29240, the shoulder is immobilized with the elbow bent and secured with tape or a wrap to the torso. This may be referred to as Velpeau strapping. In 29260, the elbow or wrist is taped in a configuration to provide protection and support to the injured or vulnerable areas. In 29280, the hand or finger is taped.

Musculoskeletal System

29305-29325

29305   Application of hip spica cast; 1 leg
29325   Application of hip spica cast; 1 and one-half spica or both legs

A hip spica cast is applied to immobilize one or both hips. A stockinette is applied beginning at the ribs and extending over one or both legs. Padding is placed over the stockinette with a thick pad at the top around the ribs and over the sacrum and other pressure points. A plaster or fiberglass roll is then immersed in water and saturated. Excess water is gently squeezed out of the plaster or fiberglass. The plaster or fiberglass is then wrapped around the torso and extended over one or both legs. The cast may extend only to the knee or it may extend all the way to the toes. As the casting material sets it is smoothed and molded. A bar covered with cast material may also be attached between the legs at the thigh level to provide additional support. Use 29305 for a hip spica covering one leg. Use 29325 for a hip spica covering one leg and half of the other or both legs.

29345-29355

29345   Application of long leg cast (thigh to toes)
29355   Application of long leg cast (thigh to toes); walker or ambulatory type

A stockinette is applied over the area to be cast followed by padding over the stockinette. A plaster or fiberglass roll is then immersed in water and saturated. Excess water is gently squeezed out of the plaster or fiberglass. The plaster or fiberglass is wrapped around the leg usually from distal to proximal aspects. The plaster or fiberglass is smoothed and molded to the leg. Use 29345 for a long leg cast that is not a walking or ambulatory type and 29355 for one that is a walking or ambulatory type. Walking casts use a prefabricated heel made of a non-slip material that is attached to the bottom of the cast over the heel. Several strips of plaster are applied to the bottom of the cast. The walker is then carefully positioned on the bottom of the cast and the plaster molded around the walker to attach it to the cast. A second strip of plaster is placed in a groove in middle of the walker and then wrapped around the top of the cast over the foot to secure the walker to the cast.

29358

29358   Application of long leg cast brace

A long leg cast-brace is applied to immobilize a fracture of the middle or distal femur. The cast-brace is comprised of a patellar weight bearing cast on the lower leg with an ischial weight bearing cast on the thigh that are connected to each other by external hinges medial and lateral to the knee. A stockinette is applied over the entire leg from thigh to toes followed by padding over the stockinette. A plaster or fiberglass roll is then immersed in water and saturated. Excess water is gently squeezed out of the plaster or fiberglass. The plaster or fiberglass is wrapped around the leg usually from distal to proximal aspects. Plastic sockets are incorporated into the upper portion of the cast for attachment of the external hinges. The plaster or fiberglass is smoothed and molded to the leg. The center portion of the cast over the knee is then cut out and the hinges attached to allow mobility of both the knee and the hip.

29365

29365   Application of cylinder cast (thigh to ankle)

A cylinder or stovepipe cast extending from the thigh to the ankle is applied. This type of cast is used for fractures of the patella and some fractures of the distal femur. A stockinette is applied over the area to be casted followed by padding over the stockinette. A plaster or fiberglass roll is then immersed in water and saturated. Excess water is gently squeezed out of the plaster or fiberglass. The plaster or fiberglass is wrapped around the leg usually from distal to proximal aspects. The plaster or fiberglass is smoothed and molded to the leg.

29405-29425

29405   Application of short leg cast (below knee to toes)
29425   Application of short leg cast (below knee to toes); walking or ambulatory type

The physician applies a cast to the patient's leg. The cast extends from just below the knee to the toes. Code 29425 if padding or a brace is added to the bottom of the cast to allow the patient to walk.

29440

29440   Adding walker to previously applied cast

A walker is added to a previously applied short or long leg cast to allow the patient to walk on the cast. The walker is a prefabricated heel made of a non-slip material that is attached to the bottom of the cast over the heel. Several strips of plaster are applied to the bottom of the cast. The walker is then carefully positioned on the bottom of the cast and the plaster molded around the walker to attach it to the cast. A second strip of plaster is placed in a groove in middle of the walker and then wrapped around the top of the cast over the foot to secure the walker to the cast.

29445

29445   Application of rigid total contact leg cast

A rigid total contact leg cast extending from below the knee to the toes is applied. This type of cast is used to treat plantar ulcers in patients with peripheral neuropathy. The plantar ulcers are caused by sensory loss in combination with repetitive walking stress. The total contact leg cast relieves the plantar stress which promotes healing of the ulcers. A stockinette is applied to over the area to be casted followed by padding over the stockinette. A single layer of plaster is wrapped around the leg usually from distal to proximal aspects followed a layer of fiberglass tape.

29450

29450   Application of clubfoot cast with molding or manipulation, long or short leg

A long or short leg clubfoot cast is applied with molding or manipulation. This type of cast is used to treat a clubfoot deformity characterized by inward rotation with supination of the foot. A series of corrective casts are applied on an infant or young child to progressively stretch the contracted soft tissues and move the foot into a more normal position. A stockinette is applied to over the area to be casted followed by padding over the stockinette. A plaster or fiberglass roll is then immersed in water and saturated. Excess water is gently squeezed out of the plaster or fiberglass. The plaster or fiberglass is wrapped around the leg usually from distal to proximal aspects. The plaster or fiberglass is smoothed and shaped at the ankle and foot to stretch the soft tissues and hold the foot in a more normal position.

29505-29515

29505   Application of long leg splint (thigh to ankle or toes)
29515   Application of short leg splint (calf to foot)

Splints stabilize injuries by decreasing movement and providing support to the posterior aspect of the extremity. A stockinette is applied over the leg followed by padding over the stockinette. Plaster sheets cut to the appropriate length are then immersed in water and saturated. Excess water is gently squeezed out of the plaster. The plaster is applied to the posterior aspect of the leg and smoothed and molded. An elastic bandage is then wrapped around the leg to secure the splint. Use 29505 for a long leg splint extending from the thigh to the ankle or toes. Use 29515 for a short leg splint extending from the calf to the foot.

29520

29520   Strapping; hip

Strapping is applied to the hip to treat a soft tissue injury or to provide support to an area of weakness or vulnerability. The physician or physical therapist evaluates the mechanism of injury and areas of weakness or vulnerability to determine where taping is needed. The hip is then taped in a configuration to provide protection and support to the injured or vulnerable areas.

29530

29530   Strapping; knee

Strapping is applied to the knee to treat a soft tissue injury or provide support to an area of weakness or vulnerability. The physician or physical therapist evaluates the mechanism of injury and areas of weakness or vulnerability to determine where taping is needed. The knee is taped in a configuration to provide protection and support to the injured or vulnerable areas.

29540-29550

29540   Strapping; ankle and/or foot
29550   Strapping; toes

The physician applies tightly wrapped tape to the ankle or foot to stabilize the muscles in that area. Code 29550 if the tape is applied to the toes.

29580

29580   Strapping; Unna boot

An Unna boot strapping is applied to the lower leg to treat a venous ulcer. An Unna boot consists of a moist, gauze bandage impregnated with zinc oxide, calamine lotion, and glycerine that is wrapped from the toes to a point just below the knee coveriing the ulcer. Following application, the gauze dries and hardens. An elastic bandage is also wrapped snuggly around the Unna boot to promote blood return from the extremity to the heart.

29581-29582

29581   Application of multi-layer compression system; leg (below knee), including ankle and foot
29582   Application of multi-layer compression system; thigh and leg, including ankle and foot, when performed

A multi-layer compression system is used to treat and prevent the recurrence of venous ulcers. It consists of two, three, or four layers. There are a number of manufacturers who

Musculoskeletal System

● New Code   ▲ Revised Code

package complete two, three, or four layer compression systems. The venous ulcer is inspected and the type of compression system is selected based on the severity of the ulcer and the type of venous disease. A wound layer is applied over any existing venous ulcers followed by padding, short-stretch, and long-stretch layers. Use 29581 for a compression system that extends from the foot and ankle to the knee. Use 29582 for one that extends from the foot and ankle, over the lower leg and thigh. The compression system is changed periodically, usually at one-week intervals, so that the venous ulcer can be inspected and the extent of healing determined. Report the appropriate code each time the compression system is applied or changed.

29583-29584

29583 **Application of multi-layer compression system; upper arm and forearm**
29584 **Application of multi-layer compression system; upper arm, forearm, hand, and fingers**

A multi-layer compression system is used to treat and prevent the recurrence of venous ulcers. It consists of two, three, or four layers. There are a number of manufacturers who package complete two, three, or four layer compression systems. The venous ulcer is inspected and the type of compression system is selected based on the severity of the ulcer and the type of venous disease. A wound layer is applied over any existing venous ulcers followed by padding, short-stretch, and long-stretch layers. Use 29583 for a compression system that extends over the forearm and upper arm. Use 29584 for one that extends over the fingers and hand, forearm, and upper arm. The compression system is changed periodically, usually at one-week intervals, so that the venous ulcer can be inspected and the extent of healing determined. Report the appropriate code each time the compression system is applied or changed.

29700-29710

29700 **Removal or bivalving; gauntlet, boot or body cast**
29705 **Removal or bivalving; full arm or full leg cast**
29710 **Removal or bivalving; shoulder or hip spica, Minerva, or Risser jacket, etc.**

Bivalving a cast involves opening the cast on both sides to relieve excessive pressure on the casted body part due to swelling or distension. An oscillating saw is used to cut the cast and padding. The cuts are made in a manner that still allows good support of the injured body part. Elastic wrap is then applied over the cast. The elastic wrap may be tightened as the swelling or distension subsides. Removal of the cast involves using an oscillating cast saw to cut the cast on both sides. Underlying padding and stockinette is then cut with scissors and the cast is removed. The skin is inspected for breakdown. Use 29700 for bivalving or removal of a gauntlet, boot, or body cast; use 29705 for a full arm or leg cast; use 29710 for a shoulder or hip spica, Minerva cast, or Risser jacket.

29720

29720 **Repair of spica, body cast or jacket**

A damaged spica, body cast or jacket is evaluated to determine whether the cast can be repaired. The damaged cast material is trimmed as needed. If new stockinette and padding are needed they are applied. The damaged area is then repaired or reinforced by applying additional plaster or fiberglass.

29730

29730 **Windowing of cast**

Windowing of the cast is performed to allow the physician to examine a pressure point or to expose an open wound. The area of cast to be removed is marked. The plaster is cut and removed. The lining material (stockinette and padding) is then carefully removed. The physician examines the open wound or area of exposed skin. A dressing may be applied over an open wound or the cut out window replaced

29740-29750

29740 **Wedging of cast (except clubfoot casts)**
29750 **Wedging of clubfoot cast**

Wedging of the cast is performed to realign the bones. Wedging may be used to open or close the cast and the type of wedge depends on the nature of the malalignment. The area to be wedged is marked. The physician cuts through whole circumference of the plaster or fiberglass excluding a 2-3 cm portion on the opposite side which will be the hinge on which the wedge is opened or closed. The padding is left in place. The cast is then bent to open or close the cast. The cast is repaired with plaster or fiberglass wrap and separately reportable radiographs are obtained to check alignment of the bones. Use 29740 for wedging of any cast other than a clubfoot cast and 29750 for wedging of a clubfoot cast.

29800-29804

29800 **Arthroscopy, temporomandibular joint, diagnostic, with or without synovial biopsy (separate procedure)**
29804 **Arthroscopy, temporomandibular joint, surgical**

An arthroscopy is performed on the temporomandibular joint (TMJ) to diagnose and/or treat structural disorders. Two entry points are marked using the posterior border of

the tragus of the ear and the lateral canthus of the eye as reference points. The skin is punctured with a needle at the anterior entry point until contact with the zygomatic bone is achieved. The needle is then passed downward into the superior joint space. A trocar contained in a cannula is inserted at the posterior entry point using an inferolateral approach toward the glenoid fossa. The joint capsule is punctured. The trocar is withdrawn and the arthroscope is introduced through the cannula. In 29800, a diagnostic procedure is performed with or without synovial biopsy. The TMJ is examined for evidence of injury or disease including fibrous adhesion, floating debris, or disc displacement. Synovial tissue samples are obtained as needed and sent for laboratory analysis. In 29804, following complete examination of the TMJ, a surgical procedure is also performed. The most common procedure is lysis of fibrous adhesions using a blunt trocar—often successful in treating persistent anterior disc displacement. An additional portal may also be created to allow introduction of surgical instruments such as knives or motorized shavers to release fibrous adhesions and retrieve floating debris. Upon completion, the arthroscope and surgical instruments are removed and the incisions are closed.

29805

29805 **Arthroscopy, shoulder, diagnostic, with or without synovial biopsy (separate procedure)**

A diagnostic arthroscopy of the shoulder is performed with or without synovial biopsy. The patient is placed in lateral decubitus position with the arm suspended or in beach chair position. Skin traction is applied to the arm. Anterior and posterior portal incisions are made over the shoulder joint. Sterile saline solution is pumped into the joint to expand the joint space. Arthroscopic instruments are inserted and a diagnostic exam of the shoulder joint is performed. The humeral head and glenoid fossa are examined for osteochondral defects. The anterior and posterior labrum are examined for fraying and evaluated for instability. The anterior joint capsule along with the subscapularis and glenohumeral ligaments are examined for tears, adhesions, and fraying. The biceps tendon is examined for tears, inflammation, or degenerative disease. The rotator cuff is examined for tears. The supraspinatus and infraspinatus tendons are examined as well as the subacromial space. The posterior aspect of the glenohumeral joint is then examined, including the axillary pouch and posterior recess. Following completion of the procedure, instruments are removed, fluid is drained, incisions are closed, and a dressing is applied.

29806

29806 **Arthroscopy, shoulder, surgical; capsulorrhaphy**

The physician performs a surgical arthroscopic capsulorrhaphy of the shoulder. Capsulorrhaphy procedures are done to treat shoulder instability typically caused by a defective or loose capsule. The exact nature of the capsulorrhaphy procedure depends on the cause and location of the capsule defect. The patient is placed in lateral decubitus position with the arm suspended or in beach chair position. Skin traction is applied to the arm. Anterior and posterior portal incisions are made over the shoulder joint. Sterile saline solution is pumped into the joint to expand the joint space. Arthroscopic instruments are inserted and a diagnostic arthroscopy of the shoulder joint is first done to determine the cause of the shoulder instability. Additional portal incisions may be made for placing surgical instruments. If a Bankart lesion is present, the rim of the glenoid is repaired by using bioabsorbable tacks and suture anchors. If the capsule is loose, the rotator interval is closed in a capsular reefing procedure. The physician may also perform a bone block procedure or capsular tightening using a capsular shift. When the surgical procedure is complete, instruments are removed, fluid is drained, incisions are closed, and a dressing is applied.

29807

29807 **Arthroscopy, shoulder, surgical; repair of SLAP lesion**

A surgical arthroscopy of the shoulder is performed to repair a SLAP lesion, a tear on the superior labrum with involvement of the biceps tendon anchor site on the labrum. The patient is placed in lateral decubitus position with the arm suspended or in beach chair position. Skin traction is applied to the arm. Anterior and posterior portal incisions are made over the shoulder joint. Sterile saline solution is pumped into the shoulder joint to expand the joint space. Arthroscopic instruments are inserted and a diagnostic arthroscopy of the shoulder joint is first done to confirm the presence of a SLAP lesion. Additional portal incisions may be made for placing surgical instruments. A shaver is introduced and the fibrous membrane over the superior glenoid neck is debrided. The torn labral tissue and the biceps tissue are also debrided. Next a burr is used to decorticate the bone beneath the superior labrum and the biceps tendon anchor site. The SLAP lesion may be repaired with direct suture or a drill hole may be created below the normal biceps tendon insertion site and a suture anchor implanted for the SLAP lesion repair. When repair of the labral tear is complete, instruments are removed, fluid is drained, incisions are closed, and a dressing is applied.

29819

29819   Arthroscopy, shoulder, surgical; with removal of loose body or foreign body

A surgical arthroscopy of the shoulder is performed with removal of one or more loose/foreign bodies. The patient is placed in lateral decubitus position with the arm suspended or in beach chair position. Skin traction is applied to the arm. Anterior and posterior portal incisions are made over the shoulder joint. Sterile saline solution is pumped into the joint to expand the joint space. Arthroscopic instruments are inserted and a diagnostic arthroscopy of the shoulder joint is first done to locate the loose or foreign body. Additional portal incisions may be made to access the loose or foreign body. A grasping instrument is introduced and the object is removed. When the surgical procedure is complete, instruments are removed, fluid is drained, incisions are closed, and a dressing is applied.

29820-29821

29820   Arthroscopy, shoulder, surgical; synovectomy, partial
29821   Arthroscopy, shoulder, surgical; synovectomy, complete

A surgical arthroscopy of the shoulder with a partial or complete synovectomy is performed. The patient is placed in lateral decubitus position with the arm suspended or in beach chair position. Skin traction is applied to the arm. Anterior and posterior portal incisions are made over the shoulder joint. Sterile saline solution is pumped into the shoulder joint using an infusion pump to expand the joint space. A diagnostic arthroscopy of the shoulder joint is performed and the synovial disease or defect explored. Additional portal incisions are made as needed to introduce surgical tools and access the surgical site. The synovial membrane is then removed using a resector. Bleeding is controlled by radiofrequency or electrocautery. When all the damaged synovium has been resected, the fluid is drained from the shoulder, the incisions are closed, and a dressing is applied. Use code 29820 when partial synovectomy of the shoulder is performed and code 29821 for complete synovectomy.

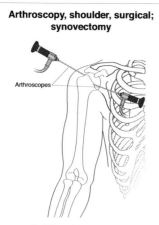

Arthroscopy, shoulder, surgical; synovectomy

Arthroscopes

Partial (29820), complete (29821)

29822-29823

29822   Arthroscopy, shoulder, surgical; debridement, limited
29823   Arthroscopy, shoulder, surgical; debridement, extensive

A surgical arthroscopy of the shoulder with limited or extensive debridement is performed. The patient is placed in lateral decubitus position with the arm suspended or in beach chair position. Skin traction is applied to the arm. Anterior and posterior portal incisions are made over the shoulder joint. Sterile saline solution is pumped into the shoulder joint using an infusion pump to expand the joint space. A diagnostic arthroscopy of the shoulder joint is performed and the articular cartilage defect identified. Additional portal incisions are made as needed to introduce surgical tools and access the surgical site. A shaver is introduced and the articular cartilage is debrided. Use code 29822 when limited debridement of the shoulder is performed and code 29823 for extensive debridement.

29824

29824   Arthroscopy, shoulder, surgical; distal claviculectomy including distal articular surface (Mumford procedure)

This procedure may also be referred to as an arthroscopic Mumford procedure. The patient is placed in lateral decubitus position with the arm suspended or in beach chair position. Skin traction is applied to the arm. Anterior and posterior portal incisions are made over the shoulder joint. Sterile saline solution is pumped into the joint to expand the joint space. Arthroscopic instruments are inserted and a diagnostic exam of the joint is first done to evaluate the glenohumeral joint and subacromial space. Additional portal incisions are made as needed to introduce surgical tools and access the site. The anterior aspect of the acromion is resected using a stone-cutting burr to remove approximately 10 mm or one-half to two-thirds of the anterior acromion. The underside of the acromion is smoothed

with an end-cutting shaver. Next, the distal end of the clavicle is exposed and resected using a stone-cutting burr. Approximately 1-2 cm of the distal end of the clavicle is excised, eliminating contact between the articular surfaces of the acromion and the clavicle. When the procedure is complete, instruments are removed, fluid is drained, incisions are closed, and a dressing is applied.

29825

29825   Arthroscopy, shoulder, surgical; with lysis and resection of adhesions, with or without manipulation

The patient is placed in lateral decubitus position with the arm suspended or in beach chair position. Skin traction is applied to the arm. Anterior and posterior portal incisions are made over the shoulder joint. Sterile saline solution is pumped into the joint to expand the joint space. Arthroscopic instruments are inserted and a diagnostic arthroscopy of the joint is first done to identify adhesions and rule out other pathology. Additional portal incisions are made as needed to introduce surgical tools and access the site. The shoulder is moved through a gentle range of motion to separate adhesions. Adhesions and areas of thickening and contracture that were not relieved by manipulation are cut. The shoulder is again moved through a range of motion. When all adhesions have been severed and the shoulder can be moved through a complete range of motion, the shoulder is injected with an anti-inflammatory and a local anesthetic, instruments are removed, fluid is drained, incisions are closed, and a dressing is applied.

29826

29826   Arthroscopy, shoulder, surgical; decompression of subacromial space with partial acromioplasty, with coracoacromial ligament (ie, arch) release, when performed (List separately in addition to code for primary procedure)

This procedure may also be referred to as an arthroscopic subacromial decompression (ASAD) procedure. The patient is placed in lateral decubitus position with the arm suspended or in beach chair position. Skin traction is applied to the arm. Anterior and posterior portal incisions are made over the shoulder joint. Sterile saline solution is pumped into the joint to expand the joint space. Arthroscopic instruments are inserted and a diagnostic exam of the shoulder is first done to confirm impingement of the rotator cuff against the edge of the acromion at the attachment of the coracoacromial ligament. Additional portal incisions are made as needed to introduce surgical tools and access the site. If a coracoacromial ligament release is required, it is performed first by detaching the ligament from the undersurface of the acromion. The ligament is debrided with a shaver. Subacromial decompression is accomplished by removing the subacromial bursa. The undersurface of the acromion is then cleaned with an end-cutting motorized shaver. A burr is used to remove any remaining ligament fibers and define the anterolateral acromial surface. The acromion is then resected from posterior to anterior. When the procedure is complete, instruments are removed, fluid is drained, incisions are closed, and a dressing is applied.

29827

29827   Arthroscopy, shoulder, surgical; with rotator cuff repair

The rotator cuff is a group of muscles and tendons in the shoulder that control joint motion and includes the supraspinatus, infraspinatus, subscapularis, and teres minor. The tendons of these muscles fuse together to form the rotator cuff with attachment on the humeral head. The patient is placed in lateral decubitus position with the arm suspended or in beach chair position. Skin traction is applied to the arm. Anterior and posterior portal incisions are made over the shoulder joint. Sterile saline solution is pumped into the joint to expand the joint space. Arthroscopic instruments are inserted and a diagnostic arthroscopy of the joint is first done with inspection of the subacromial bursa (bursoscopy). Additional portal incisions are made as needed to introduce surgical tools and access the site. The underside of the acromion is flattened and smoothed using a motorized burr and shaver. The rotator cuff is visualized and the size and pattern of the tear is evaluated. Thin or fragmented portions of the rotator cuff are removed. If the defect is repaired by direct tendon to tendon repair, the proximal and distal portions of the ruptured tendon are sutured together. Large defects may require tendon mobilization or advancement of tendon flaps. If a tendon to bone repair is required, the site where the rotator cuff will be reattached to bone is debrided. Side-to-side stitches may be used to initiate closure of a large rotator cuff defect. Next, a stitch passer and grasper are introduced and the stitches are passed through the tendon ends. The sutures are secured using a knot tying instrument. Metallic anchors with sutures are then placed in the humerus at the site where the tendon will be reattached. The anchors are recessed below the bone surface with only the sutures exposed. The sutures are passed through the tendon and tied, pulling the tendon down to the prepared bone surface. When the procedure is complete, instruments are removed, fluid is drained, incisions are closed, and a dressing is applied.

29828

29828   Arthroscopy, shoulder, surgical; biceps tenodesis

A posterior portal is made for access to the glenohumeral joint. The joint is visualized and the biceps tendon is examined for fraying, inflammation, and tears. The rotator cuff is

Musculoskeletal System

examined for injuries. A probe is placed in a second anterior portal and traction is exerted on the tendon to bring the extra-articular tendon into view before it is debrided. A spinal needle is introduced percutaneously and passed through the biceps tendon and lodged in the bone. Alternatively, the tendon may be captured following insertion of the spinal needle by placing a stitch through the needle and pulling the stitch through the anterior portal. The tendon is then cut and delivered through the anterior portal. The arthroscope is removed and redirected so that the subacromial space can be visualized. The spinal needle is identified. A lateral portal is made to accommodate additional instruments used to divide capsular tissue of the rotator interval and expose the biceps tendon and the bicipital groove. If the bicipital groove is flattened, it is deepened with a round burr. Two anchors are inserted and fixed to the humerus at the bicipital groove. Sutures are then placed through the biceps tendon and affixed to the anchors. Alternatively, a bone tunnel may be created. The end of the biceps tendon is then brought into the subacromial space and placed in the bone tunnel. A screw is used to fix the tendon in the tunnel.

29830

29830   Arthroscopy, elbow, diagnostic, with or without synovial biopsy (separate procedure)

A diagnostic arthroscopy of the elbow with or without synovial biopsy is performed. The patient is placed in lateral decubitus position with the upper arm supported allowing the forearm to swing free. Midlateral and posterior portal incisions are made. The posterior compartment is explored first. Synovial tissue samples are obtained as needed. Next, anterior portal incisions are made. A retractor is placed in the proximal anterolateral portal to allow visualization of the anterior compartment. The scope and surgical instruments are inserted through the anterolateral and proximal anteromedial portals. The anterior compartment is explored and synovial tissue samples are obtained as needed. Upon completion, the elbow joint is flushed with saline solution, the scope and surgical instruments are removed, and the portal incisions are closed.

29834

29834   Arthroscopy, elbow, surgical; with removal of loose body or foreign body

A surgical arthroscopy of the elbow with removal of loose or foreign body is performed. The patient is placed in lateral decubitus position with the upper arm supported allowing the forearm to swing free. Midlateral and posterior portal incisions are made. The posterior compartment is explored first. If a loose or foreign body is in the posterior compartment, an arthroscopic grasper is inserted through one of the portal incisions. The loose or foreign body is rotated so that it can be extracted longitudinally and then removed. Following removal, the compartment is visualized and any additional loose or foreign bodies or fragments are removed in the same manner. Next, anterior portal incisions are made. A retractor is placed in the proximal anterolateral portal to allow visualization of the anterior compartment. The scope and surgical instruments are inserted through the anterolateral and proximal anteromedial portals. The anterior compartment is explored and any loose or foreign bodies are removed as described above. Alternately, it may be possible to push large anterior compartment foreign bodies out with the scope sheath. Once all loose or foreign bodies have been removed, the elbow joint is flushed with saline solution, the scope and surgical instruments are removed, and the portal incisions are closed.

29835-29836

29835   Arthroscopy, elbow, surgical; synovectomy, partial
29836   Arthroscopy, elbow, surgical; synovectomy, complete

A surgical arthroscopy of the elbow with synovectomy is performed. The patient is placed in lateral decubitus position with the upper arm supported allowing the forearm to swing free. Midlateral and posterior portal incisions are made. The posterior compartment is explored first. If synovectomy is required in the posterior compartment, the synovium around the olecranon fossa is removed using an arthroscopic shaver. The medial gutter is addressed next. Small rongeurs are used to clear the gutter. The synovium is then grasped and carefully removed with a shaver while taking care to protect the ulnar nerve. Upon completion of the procedure, the posterior compartment is irrigated with saline solution. Next, anterior portal incisions are made. A retractor is placed in the proximal anterolateral portal to allow visualization of the anterior compartment. The scope and surgical instruments are inserted through the anterolateral and proximal anteromedial portals. The anterior compartment is explored and synovectomy is performed. The shaver is used to remove the synovium at the humerus. Working proximal to distal and medial to lateral, the synovium is removed from the anterior compartment. Once the synovectomy is complete, the compartment is flushed with saline solution, the scope and surgical instruments are removed, and the portal incisions are closed. Use 29835 for a synovectomy of a single compartment (partial synovectomy) and 29836 for a synovectomy of both compartments (complete synovectomy).

29837-29838

29837   Arthroscopy, elbow, surgical; debridement, limited
29838   Arthroscopy, elbow, surgical; debridement, extensive

A surgical arthroscopy of the elbow with debridement is performed. The patient is placed in lateral decubitus position with the upper arm supported allowing the forearm to swing free. Midlateral and posterior portal incisions are made. The posterior compartment is explored first. If debridement is required in the posterior compartment, osteophytes (bone spurs) are removed and the articular cartilage is smoothed using arthroscopic shavers and rongeurs. Upon completion of the procedure, the posterior compartment is irrigated with saline solution. Next, anterior portal incisions are made. A retractor is placed in the proximal anterolateral portal to allow visualization of the anterior compartment. The scope and surgical instruments are inserted through the anterolateral and proximal anteromedial portals. The anterior compartment is explored and debridement is again performed. Once debridement is complete, the anterior compartment is flushed with saline solution, the scope and surgical instruments are removed, and the portal incisions are closed. Use 29837 for debridement of a single compartment (partial debridement) and 29838 for debridement of both compartments (complete debridement).

29840

29840   Arthroscopy, wrist, diagnostic, with or without synovial biopsy (separate procedure)

Diagnostic arthroscopy of the wrist is performed with or without synovial biopsy. A pneumatic tourniquet is applied to the upper arm. The forearm is suspended in a wrist traction device and the second and third fingers are weighted with 7-10 lbs of traction which distracts the wrist joint allowing better visualization of joint structures. A portal incision is made over the posterior aspect of the wrist and the arthroscope is introduced. The arthroscope has a camera that magnifies and projects images onto a video screen. Another portal incision is made and an irrigation cannula is inserted. Fluid is introduced to further expand the joint. Additional small incisions are made as needed to allow visualization of the wrist joint from different angles. The wrist is examined for evidence of injury or disease. Synovial tissue biopsies are taken as needed and sent for laboratory analysis. Following completion of the arthroscopy, the wrist is flushed with saline solution, the instruments are removed, and the portal incisions are closed.

29843

29843   Arthroscopy, wrist, surgical; for infection, lavage and drainage

Surgical arthroscopy of the wrist is performed with lavage and drainage to treat an infection. The patient is placed in supine position with the shoulder abducted. A pneumatic tourniquet is applied to the upper arm. The forearm is suspended in a wrist traction device and the second and third fingers are weighted with 7-10 lbs of traction which distracts the wrist joint allowing better visualization of joint structures. A portal incision is made over the posterior aspect of the wrist and the arthroscope is introduced. Another portal incision is made and a cannula is introduced. Fluid and pus are drained from the wrist joint, which is then flushed with sterile saline or antibiotic solution. Additional portal incisions are made as needed to allow access to the midcarpal joint. Drainage and lavage are performed in the same manner. Upon completion of the procedure, the arthroscope and surgical instruments are removed, and the portal incisions are closed.

29844-29845

29844   Arthroscopy, wrist, surgical; synovectomy, partial
29845   Arthroscopy, wrist, surgical; synovectomy, complete

Surgical arthroscopy of the wrist is performed with synovectomy. This procedure is performed to treat inflammation of the synovial tissue caused by conditions such as rheumatoid arthritis. The patient is placed in supine position with the shoulder abducted. A pneumatic tourniquet is applied to the upper arm. The forearm is suspended in a wrist traction device and the second and third fingers are weighted with 7-10 lbs of traction which distracts the wrist joint allowing better visualization of joint structures. A portal incision is made over the posterior aspect of the wrist and the arthroscope is introduced. Another portal incision is made and a cannula is introduced. The wrist is examined and all inflamed synovial tissue is removed using a motorized suction shaving device. Additional portal incisions are made as needed to allow access to the midcarpal joint and inflamed tissue is removed in the same manner. Upon completion of the procedure, the joint is flushed with normal saline, the arthroscope and surgical instruments are removed, and the portal incisions are closed. Use code 29844 when a partial synovectomy is performed and 29845 for a complete synovectomy.

29846

29846   Arthroscopy, wrist, surgical; excision and/or repair of triangular fibrocartilage and/or joint debridement

Surgical arthroscopy of the wrist is performed with excision and/or repair of the triangular fibrocartilage and/or joint debridement. The triangular fibrocartilage complex (TFCC) is a cushioning structure in the wrist that can be injured by falling on an outstretched hand. The patient is placed in supine position with the shoulder abducted. A pneumatic tourniquet

Musculoskeletal System

                   ● New Code   ▲ Revised Code

is applied to the upper arm. The forearm is suspended in a wrist traction device and the second and third fingers are weighted with 7-10 lbs of traction which distracts the wrist joint allowing better visualization of joint structures. A portal incision is made over the posterior aspect of the wrist and the arthroscope is introduced. Another portal incision is made and a cannula is introduced. Additional portal incisions are made as needed. The wrist is examined and the TFCC is probed to determine the extent of the injury. If peripheral tears are present, they are repaired. Injury to the central disc may be treated with debridement of frayed edges and repair or by excision. Upon completion of the procedure, the joint is flushed with normal saline, the arthroscope and surgical instruments are removed, and the portal incisions are closed.

29847

29847   Arthroscopy, wrist, surgical; internal fixation for fracture or instability

Surgical arthroscopy of the wrist is performed with internal fixation to treat fracture or instability of the wrist. The patient is placed in supine position with the shoulder abducted. A pneumatic tourniquet is applied to the upper arm. The forearm is suspended in a wrist traction device and the second and third fingers are weighted with 7-10 lbs of traction which distracts the wrist joint allowing better visualization of joint structures. A portal incision is made over the posterior aspect of the wrist and the arthroscope is introduced. Another portal incision is made and a cannula is introduced. Additional portal incisions are made as needed. The wrist is examined. If a fracture is present, fracture fragments are removed and the bones at the fracture site are aligned. Pins, wires, or screws are inserted to stabilize the fracture. Upon completion of the procedure, the joint is flushed with normal saline, the arthroscope and surgical instruments are removed, and the portal incisions are closed.

29848

29848   Endoscopy, wrist, surgical, with release of transverse carpal ligament

Surgical endoscopy is performed on the wrist with release of the transverse carpal ligament. This procedure is performed to treat carpal tunnel syndrome (CTS). The carpal tunnel is a space in the wrist that contains the median nerve and nine tendons that pass from the forearm to the hand. When the carpal tunnel swells, the median nerve can become compressed causing numbness, tingling, and pain in the hand and fingers. Two small incisions are made, one over the anterior aspect of the wrist and a second in the palm. An endoscope is introduced and the carpal ligament is visualized. Using direct visualization, a small blade in introduced and the carpal ligament is cut. The endoscope is removed and the incisions are closed.

29850-29851

29850   Arthroscopically aided treatment of intercondylar spine(s) and/or tuberosity fracture(s) of the knee, with or without manipulation; without internal or external fixation (includes arthroscopy)

29851   Arthroscopically aided treatment of intercondylar spine(s) and/or tuberosity fracture(s) of the knee, with or without manipulation; with internal or external fixation (includes arthroscopy)

The physician performs arthroscopically aided treatment of intercondylar spine(s) or tuberosity fractures of the knee with or without manipulation. This type of injury usually occurs primarily in children and may be referred to as a fracture of the tibial eminence. The intercondylar spines are two upward projections in the center of the proximal tibial surface lying between the lateral and medial condyles. The tibial tuberosity is a projection on the anterior proximal tibia and is the point of attachment for the patellar ligament. Portal incisions are made over the anterior knee joint at the medial and lateral aspects. An arthroscope and cannula are introduced and the knee joint is visualized. Any blood or fluid is evacuated. The fracture is identified. To repair an intercondylar spine fracture, a small incision is made just medial to the tibial tubercle. Two guide pins are inserted on either side of the anterior cruciate ligament and passed through the intercondylar fracture fragment. The guide wires are then removed. In 29850, a cannulated suture passer is inserted. Suture material is placed in the mouth of the suture passer and then drawn out of the joint. Tension on the sutures is used to reduce the fracture fragments and the sutures are then tied over the bony bridge to secure the fracture fragments. In 29851, the fracture fragments are secured using internal or external fixation. Internal fixation is accomplished using K-wires or screws placed under arthroscopic guidance to secure the fracture fragments. An external fixation device may be applied instead of or in addition to internal fixation. Tuberosity fractures are repaired in the same manner using suture material (29850) or K-wire or screw fixation with or without external fixation (29851).

29855-29856

29855   Arthroscopically aided treatment of tibial fracture, proximal (plateau); unicondylar, includes internal fixation, when performed (includes arthroscopy)

29856   Arthroscopically aided treatment of tibial fracture, proximal (plateau); bicondylar, includes internal fixation, when performed (includes arthroscopy)

A proximal tibial plateau fracture is treated using an arthroscope and any necessary internal fixation. The proximal end of the tibia has two condyles, medial and lateral. Tibial plateau fractures occur at the proximal end of the tibia and extend into the articular cartilage of the knee joint. The fracture may involve one or both condyles. The exact nature of the arthroscopically aided treatment, also referred to as a limited open technique, varies depending on the configuration of the fracture. Portal incisions are made over the knee joint and instruments are inserted. The joint is visualized arthroscopically and the extent of the tibial plateau injury assessed. If it is determined that the tibial plateau fracture can be reduced arthroscopically, a small incision is made to perform a limited open reduction and internal fixation with the aid of an arthroscope. The fracture site is visualized arthroscopically and cleared of debris. Fracture fragments are reduced using a tenaculum clamp. Alternatively, a femoral distraction device may be used and reduction accomplished by ligamentotaxis. Internal fixation, such as screws or a buttress plate, is applied as needed to stabilize the fracture fragments. The wound is irrigated and incisions are closed. Use 29855 when a unicondylar fracture of the proximal tibia is treated and 29856 when a bicondylar fracture is treated.

29860

29860   Arthroscopy, hip, diagnostic with or without synovial biopsy (separate procedure)

A diagnostic arthroscopy of the hip is performed with or without synovial biopsy. Diagnostic arthroscopy of the hip is performed to evaluate hip pain as well as functional limitations with nonspecific radiological findings. A small portal incision is made on the lateral aspect of the hip joint for introduction of the arthroscope and a second anterolateral portal incision is made for introduction of surgical instruments. Additional portal incisions are made as needed to provide visualization and access. Using fluoroscopic guidance, a catheter is placed into the hip joint through the lateral portal and sterile saline is introduced to distract the joint. The catheter is withdrawn and the arthroscope is introduced. The arthroscope has a camera that projects images onto a video screen. The hip joint is examined for evidence of injury or disease. Synovial tissue samples are taken as needed and sent for laboratory analysis. Following completion of the diagnostic arthroscopy, the hip is flushed with saline solution, the instruments are removed, and the portal incisions are closed.

29861

29861   Arthroscopy, hip, surgical; with removal of loose body or foreign body

A surgical arthroscopy of the hip is performed to remove loose or foreign bodies, resulting from trauma to the hip joint which causes pieces of cartilage to become detached. These then float within the joint space and can become caught during hip movement causing pain and reduced mobility. A small portal incision is made on the lateral aspect of the hip joint for introducing the arthroscope and a second anterolateral portal incision is made for introducing surgical instruments. Additional portal incisions are made as needed to provide visualization and access to hip joint structures. Using fluoroscopic guidance, a catheter is placed into the hip joint through the lateral portal and sterile saline is introduced to distract the joint. The catheter is withdrawn and the arthroscope is introduced. The arthroscope has a camera that projects images onto a video screen. The hip joint is examined for evidence of injury or disease. Loose or foreign bodies are located and retrieved using an arthroscopic grasper. Upon completion of the procedure, the arthroscope and surgical instruments are removed, the joint is flushed with sterile saline, and the portal incisions are closed.

29862

29862   Arthroscopy, hip, surgical; with debridement/shaving of articular cartilage (chondroplasty), abrasion arthroplasty, and/or resection of labrum

A surgical arthroscopy of the hip is performed with debridement and/or shaving of the articular cartilage (chondroplasty), abrasion arthroplasty, or resection of the labrum. This procedure is performed to treat degenerative disease of the articular cartilage, articular cartilage injuries, or labral tears. A small portal incision is made on the lateral aspect of the hip joint for introducing the arthroscope and a second anterolateral portal incision is made for introducing surgical instruments. Additional portal incisions are made as needed to provide visualization and access to hip joint structures. Using fluoroscopic guidance, a catheter is placed into the hip joint through the lateral portal and sterile saline is introduced to distract the joint. The catheter is withdrawn and the arthroscope is introduced. The arthroscope has a camera that projects images onto a video screen. The hip joint is examined for evidence of injury or disease. Chondroplasty is performed using an arthroscopic shaver blade to remove the damaged cartilage and leave a smooth stable surface. Abrasion arthroplasty is performed using a burr to remove tissue from the head and neck of the femur as well as the acetabulum. Tissue is removed to a depth of approximately 1 mm. As the bone heals, it exudes a substance that replaces the lost cartilage. A labral tear is resected using arthroscopic shaver blades or radiofrequency energy. Radiofrequency probes are inserted and used to remove torn tissue and smooth the damaged labrum. Alternatively, the labrum may be repaired. Sutures are passed through the labral tissue and anchored to the bone with bone anchors. Upon completion of the procedure, the arthroscope and surgical instruments are removed, the joint is flushed with sterile saline, and the portal incisions are closed.

29863

29863   Arthroscopy, hip, surgical; with synovectomy

A surgical arthroscopy of the hip is performed with synovectomy. This procedure is performed to remove inflamed synovial tissue. A small portal incision is made on the lateral aspect of the hip joint for introduction of the arthroscope and a second anterolateral portal incision is made for introducing surgical instruments. Additional portal incisions are made as needed to provide visualization and access to hip joint structures. Using fluoroscopic guidance, a catheter is placed into the hip joint through the lateral portal and sterile saline is introduced to distract the joint. The catheter is withdrawn and the arthroscope is inserted. The arthroscope has a camera that projects images onto a video screen. The hip joint is examined for evidence of injury or disease. The inflamed synovial tissue is removed using a synovial resector. Alternatively, radiofrequency probes are inserted and used to remove the inflamed synovial tissue. Upon completion of the procedure, the arthroscope and surgical instruments are removed, the joint is flushed with sterile saline, and the portal incisions are closed.

29866-29867

29866   Arthroscopy, knee, surgical; osteochondral autograft(s) (eg, mosaicplasty) (includes harvesting of the autograft[s])
29867   Arthroscopy, knee, surgical; osteochondral allograft (eg, mosaicplasty)

A surgical arthroscopy of the knee is performed with osteochondral autografts (29866) or allografts (29867), also referred to as mosaicplasty, which is performed to treat chondral and osteochondral defects of the weight bearing articular surfaces of the knee joint. The procedure uses small, cylindrical osteochondral grafts to smooth and resurface the articular cartilage. The knee is first inspected arthroscopically to identify the area of cartilage damage. The damaged area is measured and the number of grafts required to repair the damaged area is determined. In 29866, cylindrical grafts are harvested from a nonweightbearing surface, usually the femoral trochlea or the medial or lateral walls of the intercondylar notch. A tubular chisel is driven into the donor site to obtain carefully sized cylindrical grafts. A tunnel is then drilled at the recipient site and the graft is inserted using a plunger. This process is repeated until the entire damaged area is filled with autogenous grafts. Range of motion is tested to ensure that the graft sites are stable. In 29867, the damaged area is debrided and prepared for implantation of allografts obtained from a bone bank. The allograft is prepared to fit into the articular surface defect. One or more allografts are then placed into the defect and stabilized. Range of motion is checked to ensure that the allografts are stable. Upon completion of the procedure, the arthroscope and surgical tools are removed, and portal incisions are closed.

29868

29868   Arthroscopy, knee, surgical; meniscal transplantation (includes arthrotomy for meniscal insertion), medial or lateral

A surgical arthroscopy of the knee is performed with meniscal transplantation in the medial or lateral compartments. This procedure requires a mini-arthrotomy for insertion of the meniscal graft. The knee is inspected arthroscopically, any meniscal remnant is removed, and the meniscal bed is prepared. If a medial meniscal transplant is performed, two tibial bone tunnels are typically created. If a lateral meniscal transplant is performed, a tibial trough is created. The allograft is then configured to fit into the prepared transplant site. A mini-arthrotomy is performed and the meniscal allograft is introduced and positioned at the transplant site. The arthrotomy is closed and the meniscal transplant is then sutured arthroscopic ally to the meniscocapsular junction. Upon completion of the procedure, the arthroscope and surgical tools are removed and the portal incisions are closed.

29870

29870   Arthroscopy, knee, diagnostic, with or without synovial biopsy (separate procedure)

A diagnostic arthroscopy of the knee is performed with or without synovial biopsy. Two portal incisions are made, one medial and one lateral, at the knee joint. The arthroscope is inserted into the joint cavity through one of these incisions and an irrigation cannula is inserted through the other. The knee is flushed with saline solution to remove any cloudy fluid or debris. The arthroscope has a camera that projects the images onto a video screen. The knee joint is examined for evidence of injury or disease. Synovial tissue samples are taken as needed and sent for laboratory analysis. Following completion of the diagnostic

arthroscopy, the knee is again flushed with saline solution, the instruments are removed, and the portal incisions are closed.

29871

29871   Arthroscopy, knee, surgical; for infection, lavage and drainage

A surgical arthroscopy of the knee is performed with lavage and drainage. This procedure is performed to treat infection, also referred to as septic joint, or severe arthritis. Portal incisions are made medially and laterally over the knee joint. The arthroscope is introduced through one of the portals. A cannula is inserted through a second portal and the joint is flushed with saline solution. The knee is examined for evidence of disease, injury, or infection. Antibiotic or other solutions are instilled as needed to treat infection and remove any debris. The solutions are then drained from the joint. Upon completion of the procedure, the arthroscope, cannula, and other instruments are removed and the portal incisions are closed or a drain may be placed through one or more of the portals.

29873

29873   Arthroscopy, knee, surgical; with lateral release

The physician performs a surgical arthroscopy of the knee with lateral release. Lateral release is performed to treat misalignment of the patella caused by tightness of the lateral retinaculum. Prior to performing the lateral release, a complete arthroscopic examination of the knee is first performed. Portal incisions are made over the anterolateral and anteromedial aspects of the knee. The arthroscope is introduced through the anterolateral portal and the knee is examined. The arthroscope is then switched to the anteromedial portal. Scissors are introduced through the anterolateral portal and a small opening is made in the retinaculum. The tight ligaments on the lateral aspect of the patella are then cut which allows the patella to slide medially toward the center of the femoral groove. Upon completion of the procedure, the arthroscope and surgical tools are removed and the portal incisions are closed.

29874

29874   Arthroscopy, knee, surgical; for removal of loose body or foreign body (eg, osteochondritis dissecans fragmentation, chondral fragmentation)

A surgical arthroscopy of the knee is performed with removal of loose or foreign bodies. Loose bodies include cartilage, meniscal or bone fragments, or hardware that has dislodged and is floating within the knee joint. Foreign bodies include bullets, broken hardware or surgical instruments, or any other body not normally found in the knee. Portal incisions are made medially and laterally over the knee joint. The arthroscope is introduced through one of the portals. A cannula is inserted through a second portal and the joint is flushed with saline solution. The knee is examined for evidence of disease, injury, or infection. The loose or foreign bodies are located and removed with a grasper. Larger loose bodies may be fragmented using an osteotome and suctioned out with a motorized shaver. Upon completion of the procedure, the arthroscope, cannula, and other instruments are removed and portal incisions are closed.

29875-29876

29875   Arthroscopy, knee, surgical; synovectomy, limited (eg, plica or shelf resection) (separate procedure)
29876   Arthroscopy, knee, surgical; synovectomy, major, 2 or more compartments (eg, medial or lateral)

A surgical arthroscopy of the knee is performed with synovectomy. Synovial tissue lines the knee joint and produces synovial fluid. When it becomes inflamed due to rheumatoid arthritis, synovial proliferative disorder, or other condition, the synovium produces excess synovial fluid, resulting in joint effusion. Portal incisions are made medially and laterally over the knee joint. The arthroscope is introduced through one of the portals. A cannula is inserted through a second portal and the joint is flushed with saline solution. The knee is examined for evidence of disease, injury, or infection. A motorized shaver is then used to remove the synovium. Care is taken to resect all inflamed synovial tissue without damaging underlying vascular or nervous tissue. Use 29875 for a partial synovectomy, defined as the removal of synovium from a single compartment, or for removal of the plica or shelf, which is an extension of the synovium in the knee capsule. Use 29876 for a complete synovectomy, which is the removal of synovial tissue from two or more compartments (medial, lateral, patellofemoral). Upon completion of the procedure, bleeding is controlled by electrocautery the arthroscope, cannula, other instruments are removed, and portal incisions are closed. A compressive dressing is then applied.

29877

29877   Arthroscopy, knee, surgical; debridement/shaving of articular cartilage (chondroplasty)

A surgical arthroscopy of the knee is performed with debridement or shaving of the articular cartilage, also referred to as chondroplasty. Chondroplasty is performed to treat early arthritic changes, arthritic condyle, chondral fracture, and chondromalacia. Portal incisions are made medially and laterally over the knee joint. The arthroscope is introduced through one of the portals. A cannula is inserted through a second portal and the joint is flushed with saline solution. The knee is examined for evidence of disease, injury, or infection. A motorized shaver is then used to debride the articular cartilage, removing irregularities and leaving a smooth articular surface. Upon completion of the procedure, the arthroscope, cannula, and other instruments are removed and portal incisions are closed. A compressive dressing is then applied.

29879

29879   Arthroscopy, knee, surgical; abrasion arthroplasty (includes chondroplasty where necessary) or multiple drilling or microfracture

A surgical arthroscopy of the knee is performed with abrasion arthroplasty including chondroplasty. Abrasion arthroplasty is performed to treat severe arthritis or osteochondral fracture. Portal incisions are made medially and laterally over the knee joint. The arthroscope is introduced through one of the portals. A cannula is inserted through a second portal and the joint is flushed with saline solution. The knee is examined for evidence of disease, injury, or infection. Articular cartilage is removed using a motorized shaver. An abrader or burr is then used to remove necrotic (dead) bone. This continues until bleeding is present indicating that all necrotic bone has been removed. Multiple holes may also be drilled into the middle of the bone to induce bleeding and promote scab formation on the bone. As the bone heals it exudes a substance that replaces the lost cartilage. Upon completion of the procedure, the arthroscope, cannula and other instruments are removed and portal incisions are closed. A compressive dressing is then applied.

29880-29881

29880   Arthroscopy, knee, surgical; with meniscectomy (medial AND lateral, including any meniscal shaving) including debridement/shaving of articular cartilage (chondroplasty), same or separate compartment(s), when performed

29881   Arthroscopy, knee, surgical; with meniscectomy (medial OR lateral, including any meniscal shaving) including debridement/shaving of articular cartilage (chondroplasty), same or separate compartment(s), when performed

A surgical arthroscopy of the knee is performed with meniscectomy. A meniscectomy, also referred to as resection, is performed on a torn meniscus that cannot be repaired and typically involves tears that extend into the non-vascular region where they are unlikely to heal even if repaired. Portal incisions are made medially and laterally over the knee joint. The arthroscope is introduced through one of the portals. A cannula is inserted through a second portal and the joint is flushed with saline solution. The knee is examined for evidence of disease, injury, or infection. The tear is located and probed with a small hook to determine the extent of the tear. The torn fragment is then resected and removed using basket forceps, motorized shaver, scissors, or knives. Only the damaged portion of the meniscus is removed. The edge of the remaining meniscus is debrided and smoothed with a motorized shaver. The knee is flushed with saline solution to remove debris and re-inspected. If there are meniscal tears in both the medial and lateral compartments, the tear in the second compartment is addressed next and the meniscus is removed in the same manner. Articular cartilage may also be debrided using a motorized shaver to smooth the joint surfaces in one or both compartments. Upon completion of the procedure, the arthroscope, cannula, and other instruments are removed and portal incisions are closed. A compressive dressing is then applied. Use 29880 when both the medial and lateral menisci are partially or totally resected. Use 29881 when only one meniscus, medial or lateral, is resected.

29882-29883

29882   Arthroscopy, knee, surgical; with meniscus repair (medial OR lateral)
29883   Arthroscopy, knee, surgical; with meniscus repair (medial AND lateral)

A surgical arthroscopy of the knee is performed with meniscus repair. The meniscus is repaired when the tear occurs in the outer vascular region of the meniscus where it has the necessary blood supply to heal. Portal incisions are made medially and laterally over the knee joint. The arthroscope is introduced through one of the portals. A cannula is inserted through a second portal and the joint is flushed with saline solution. The knee is examined for evidence of disease, injury, or infection. The tear is located and probed with a small hook to determine the extent of the tear. The edges of the meniscus tear are prepared using a small rasp or motorized shaver. Blood supply is evaluated. To enhance healing when blood supply is questionable, a blood clot may be placed between opposing edges, small vascular access channels may be created around the periphery of the tear, or the joint lining may be abraded to encourage bleeding. The meniscus is then repaired with sutures, absorbable tacks, or other internal fixation devices. The knee is flushed with saline solution to remove debris and re- inspected. If there are meniscus tears in both the medial and lateral compartments, the tear in the second compartment is addressed next and the meniscus is inspected and repaired in the same manner. Upon completion of the procedure, the arthroscope, cannula and other instruments are removed and the portal incisions are closed. A compressive dressing is then applied. Use 29882 when only one meniscus, medial or lateral, is repaired. Use 29883 when both menisci, medial and lateral, are repaired.

29884

29884   Arthroscopy, knee, surgical; with lysis of adhesions, with or without manipulation (separate procedure)

A surgical arthroscopy of the knee is performed with lysis of adhesions with or without manipulation. Adhesions may be a complication of prior knee surgery such as anterior cruciate ligament repair or total knee arthroplasty, or they may occur following an intra-articular fracture. Portal incisions are made medially and laterally over the knee joint. The arthroscope is introduced through one of the portals. A cannula is inserted through a second portal and the joint is flushed with saline solution. The knee is examined for evidence of disease, injury, or infection. The adhesions are cut and fibrous bands or scar tissue is removed. The knee is flushed with saline solution to remove debris and re-inspected. Upon completion of the procedure, the arthroscope, cannula, and other instruments are removed and the portal incisions are closed. The knee is then manually extended and flexed while the patient is still under anesthesia to promote good range of motion of the knee.

29885-29887

29885   Arthroscopy, knee, surgical; drilling for osteochondritis dissecans with bone grafting, with or without internal fixation (including debridement of base of lesion)

29886   Arthroscopy, knee, surgical; drilling for intact osteochondritis dissecans lesion

29887   Arthroscopy, knee, surgical; drilling for intact osteochondritis dissecans lesion with internal fixation

A surgical arthroscopy of the knee is performed with drilling for osteochondritis dissecans. Osteochondritis dissecans is a condition in which a piece of bone and the overlying joint cartilage separate from the underlying bone of the proximal femur in the knee joint. The cartilage and bone fragment may become completely separated and present as a loose body in the knee joint or the bone may crack without complete separation of the fragment. Epiphyseal aseptic necrosis may also be present. Portal incisions are made medially and laterally over the knee joint. The arthroscope is introduced through one of the portals. A cannula is inserted through a second portal and the joint is flushed with saline solution. The knee is examined for evidence of disease, injury, or infection. The dissecans fragment is located. The base of the lesion is debrided as needed. Multiple small drill holes are then made through the articular cartilage passing through both the diseased or necrotic bone into the normal bone. Drilling creates tunnels that blood vessels can infiltrate allowing dead bone to be replaced with living tissue. When the osteochondritis dissecans lesion is large or when the condition has become chronic, it may be necessary to place bone grafts into the drill holes. The bone graft is usually harvested from the proximal tibia. It is then packed into the drill holes. Internal fixation may also be used alone or in addition to bone grafting to compress and stabilize the dissecans fragment. The knee is then flushed with saline solution to remove debris and is re-inspected. Upon completion of the procedure, the arthroscope, cannula, and other instruments are removed and the portal incisions are closed. Use 29885 when drilling and bone grafts are used with or without internal fixation. Use 29886 when drilling alone is used to treat an intact osteochondritis dissecans lesion. Use 29887 when drilling and internal fixation are required to treat an intact lesion.

29888-29889

29888   Arthroscopically aided anterior cruciate ligament repair/augmentation or reconstruction

29889   Arthroscopically aided posterior cruciate ligament repair/augmentation or reconstruction

The physician performs an arthroscopically aided anterior or posterior cruciate ligament repair, augmentation, or reconstruction. The anterior cruciate ligament (ACL) is located in the center of the knee joint connecting the femur to the tibia. The posterior cruciate ligament (PCL) is located in the center of the knee behind the ACL and also connects the femur to the tibia. Both cruciate ligaments provide rotational stability in the knee. Injury to either ligament can cause the knee to buckle. Three or more portal incisions are made for introduction of the arthroscope and surgical tools. The arthroscope is inserted into the joint cavity through one of these incisions and an irrigation cannula through another. The knee is flushed with saline solution to remove any cloudy fluid or debris. Using a video camera attached to the arthroscope, the physician examines the knee joint. The meniscal cartilage is examined using a probe. If the meniscal tissue is normal, the physician then examines the ACL and PCL. In 29888, a torn ACL is repaired or reconstructed. A shaver is introduced and the damaged ACL is removed. The notch where the ACL is located is inspected and widened as needed using a burr. If the patellar tendon is being used to reconstruct the ACL, two small incisions are made, one over the tibial tubercle and one over the inferior aspect of the patella. The central third of the patellar tendon is harvested with a bone block at each end. The patellar tendon graft is passed beneath the skin and retrieved. Sutures are placed through the bone blocks. Using arthroscopic assistance, a drill guide is positioned on the tibia. The guide wire is then drilled into place exiting within the knee joint at the attachment site of the original ACL. The drill hole in the tibia is then made. A femoral drill guide is then passed through the tibial drill hole using arthroscopic guidance. The drill guide is positioned on the posterior aspect of the femur. The femoral guide wire is then placed and the femoral drill hole made. The drill holes are inspected using the arthroscope. The patellar tendon or other graft material is then placed through the drill holes and secured with screws. The ACL graft is inspected, the arthroscope and surgical instruments are removed, and the incisions are closed. In 29889, a torn PCL is repaired or reconstructed. The procedure is performed in a similar manner to ACL reconstruction except that the damaged PCL is removed and the reconstruction may be performed using a tibial tunnel or tibial inlay technique. In addition, a portion of the Achilles tendon may be harvested and used in PCL reconstruction.

29891

29891   Arthroscopy, ankle, surgical, excision of osteochondral defect of talus and/or tibia, including drilling of the defect

Surgical arthroscopy of the ankle is performed with excision of an osteochondral defect of the talus and/or tibia including drilling of the defect. Osteochondral defects are localized areas of joint damage seen as a section where the cartilage and underlying bone have been disrupted. In the ankle, these occur most frequently on the talus or tibia. The leg is positioned on an L-shaped bar with the thigh supported, the knee bent, and the lower leg allowed to swing freely. The foot is placed in a bracelet and the ankle joint is distracted. A needle is inserted into the joint at the anteromedial aspect and the joint is inflated with saline. The needle is withdrawn and an anteromedial portal is created. A trocar is placed in the anteromedial portal and the arthroscope is inserted through the trocar. The joint is inspected for evidence of injury, disease, or infection. The osteochondral defect in the talus or tibia is located. An anterolateral portal is created. The bone and cartilage fragment is removed. The bony defect is then drilled using fine wires which will allow growth factors to be released and new bone and fibrocartilage to be formed to fill the defect. The joint is then flushed with saline to remove any debris. Upon completion of the procedure, the arthroscope and surgical tools are removed, and the portal incisions are closed.

29892

29892   Arthroscopically aided repair of large osteochondritis dissecans lesion, talar dome fracture, or tibial plafond fracture, with or without internal fixation (includes arthroscopy)

Arthroscopically-aided repair of a large osteochondritis dissecans lesion, talar dome fracture, or tibial plafond fracture is performed with or without internal fixation. Osteochondritis dissecans is a condition in which a piece of bone and the overlying joint cartilage separate from the underlying bone of the proximal tibia in the ankle joint. The cartilage and bone fragment may become completely separated and present as a loose body in the ankle joint or the bone may crack without complete separation of the fragment. The talar dome is the rounded portion on the top of the talus that articulates with the tibia and fibula. The tibial plafond, also referred to as the tibial pilon, is the weight bearing articular surface of the distal tibia. The leg is positioned on an L-shaped bar with the thigh supported, the knee bent, and the lower leg allowed to swing freely. The foot is placed in a bracelet and the ankle joint is distracted. A needle is inserted into the joint at the anteromedial aspect and the joint is inflated with saline. The needle is withdrawn and an anteromedial portal is created. A trocar is placed in the anteromedial portal and the arthroscope is inserted through the trocar. The joint is inspected for evidence of injury, disease, or infection. The dissecans lesion or fracture in the talus or tibia is located. An anterolateral portal is created. Bone fragments are removed and the damaged bone and cartilage are debrided. Subchondral drilling of the tibia or talus may be performed to stimulate blood flow and aid healing of the lesion or fracture site. Depending on the size of the dissecans lesion or the severity of the tibial plafond or talar dome fracture, separately reportable bone grafting may be needed. Internal fixation, such as wires, pins, or screws, may also be required to secure the dissecans lesion or fracture fragments. Bone grafting or internal fixation may necessitate drilling through the medial malleolus for medial dome lesions/fractures, or opening the joint to complete the procedure. The joint is then flushed with saline to remove any debris. Upon completion of the procedure, the arthroscope and surgical tools are removed and the portal and arthrotomy incisions are closed.

29893

29893   Endoscopic plantar fasciotomy

The physician performs endoscopic plantar fasciotomy. This procedure is performed to treat severe strain and inflammation of the plantar fascia which is a band of ligament-like tissue running along the bottom of the foot. A vertical incision is made at the medial aspect of the heel just anterior and inferior to the medial calcaneal tubercle. Blunt dissection is performed to expose the fascia. An obturator/cannula system is introduced and advanced laterally. The endoscope is introduced medially and the medial fascial band is inspected. A knife is used to sever the medial band. The endoscope is then introduced laterally and the probe medially. Any remaining fibers are severed. The medial band is completely released. The lateral fascial band is left intact. The area is then irrigated, the cannula is removed, and the incision is closed.

29894

29894   Arthroscopy, ankle (tibiotalar and fibulotalar joints), surgical; with removal of loose body or foreign body

Surgical arthroscopy of the ankle (tibiotalar and fibulotalar) is performed with removal of loose or foreign bodies. The leg is positioned on an L-shaped bar with the thigh supported, the knee bent, and the lower leg allowed to swing freely. The foot is placed in a bracelet and the ankle joint is distracted. A needle is inserted into the joint at the anteromedial aspect and the joint is inflated with saline. The needle is withdrawn and an anteromedial portal is created. A trocar is placed in the anteromedial portal and the arthroscope is inserted through the trocar. The joint is inspected for evidence of injury, disease, or infection. An anterolateral portal is created. The loose or foreign body is located and removed. The joint is then flushed with saline to remove any debris. Upon completion of the procedure, the arthroscope and surgical tools are removed and the portal incisions are closed.

29895

29895   Arthroscopy, ankle (tibiotalar and fibulotalar joints), surgical; synovectomy, partial

Surgical arthroscopy of the ankle (tibiotalar and fibulotalar) is performed with synovectomy. Synovial tissue lines the ankle joint and produces synovial fluid. When it becomes inflamed due to rheumatoid arthritis, synovial proliferative disorder, or other condition, the synovium produces excess synovial fluid resulting in joint effusion. The leg is positioned on an L-shaped bar with the thigh supported, the knee bent, and the lower leg allowed to swing freely. The foot is placed in a bracelet and the ankle joint is distracted. A needle is inserted into the joint at the anteromedial aspect and the joint is inflated with saline. The needle is withdrawn and an anteromedial portal is created. A trocar is placed in the anteromedial portal and the arthroscope is inserted through the trocar. The joint is inspected for evidence of injury, disease, or infection. An anterolateral portal is created. A motorized shaver is then used to remove the synovium. Care is taken to resect all inflamed synovial tissue without damaging underlying vascular or nervous tissue. The joint is then flushed with saline to remove any debris. Upon completion of the procedure, the arthroscope and surgical tools are removed, and the portal incisions are closed.

29897-29898

29897   Arthroscopy, ankle (tibiotalar and fibulotalar joints), surgical; debridement, limited

29898   Arthroscopy, ankle (tibiotalar and fibulotalar joints), surgical; debridement, extensive

Surgical arthroscopy of the ankle (tibiotalar and fibulotalar) is done with debridement, which is performed primarily to treat arthritis. The leg is positioned on an L-shaped bar with the thigh supported, the knee bent, and the lower leg allowed to swing freely. The foot is placed in a bracelet and the ankle joint is distracted. A needle is inserted into the joint at the anteromedial aspect and the joint is inflated with saline. The needle is withdrawn and an anteromedial portal is created. A trocar is placed in the anteromedial portal and the arthroscope is inserted through the trocar. The joint is inspected for evidence of injury, disease, or infection. An anterolateral portal is created. A motorized shaver is then used to remove redundant cartilage, inflamed tissue, and bone spurs (osteophytes) from the joint surfaces, leaving a smooth surface. Loose fragments are also removed. The joint is then flushed with saline to remove any debris. Upon completion of the procedure, the arthroscope and surgical tools are removed, and the portal incisions are closed. Use 29897 for limited debridement and 29898 for extensive debridement.

29899

29899   Arthroscopy, ankle (tibiotalar and fibulotalar joints), surgical; with ankle arthrodesis

Surgical arthroscopy of the ankle is performed with ankle arthrodesis, also referred to as ankle fusion, performed to treat ankle instability. The leg is positioned on an L-shaped bar with the thigh supported, the knee bent, and the lower leg allowed to swing freely. The foot is placed in a bracelet and the ankle joint is distracted. A needle is inserted into the joint at the anteromedial aspect and the joint is inflated with saline. The needle is withdrawn and an anteromedial portal is created. A trocar is placed in the anteromedial portal and the arthroscope is inserted through the trocar. The joint is inspected for evidence of injury, disease, or infection. An anterolateral portal is created. A motorized shaver is then used to remove redundant cartilage, inflamed tissue, and bone spurs (osteophytes) from the joint surfaces, leaving a smooth surface. Loose fragments are also removed. Two guide wires are placed across the ankle through the medial tibia and talus. Hollow (cannulated) screws are then secured over the guide wires and the guide wires are removed. The joint is then flushed with saline to remove any debris. Upon completion of the procedure, the arthroscope and surgical tools are removed and the portal incisions are closed.

Musculoskeletal System

29900

29900   Arthroscopy, metacarpophalangeal joint, diagnostic, includes synovial biopsy

Diagnostic arthroscopy of the metacarpophalangeal joint is performed, including synovial biopsy. Portal incisions are made overlying the metacarpophalangeal joint in the dorsal-ulnar and dorsal-radial aspects. Blunt dissection is performed to the level of the joint capsule using a small hemostat, which is then used to spread the joint capsule and enter the joint. The arthroscope is introduced through one of the portals and the joint is inspected for evidence of injury, disease, or infection. Synovial tissue samples are taken as needed and sent for laboratory analysis. Upon completion of the procedure, the arthroscope and surgical tools are removed, and the portal incisions are closed.

29901

29901   Arthroscopy, metacarpophalangeal joint, surgical; with debridement

Surgical arthroscopy of the metacarpophalangeal joint is done with debridement, which is performed primarily to treat arthritis. Portal incisions are made overlying the metacarpophalangeal joint in the dorsal-ulnar and dorsal-radial aspects. Blunt dissection is performed to the level of the joint capsule using a small hemostat, which is then used to spread the joint capsule and enter the joint. The arthroscope is introduced through one of the portals and the joint is inspected for evidence of injury, disease, or infection. A motorized shaver is then used to remove redundant cartilage, inflamed tissue, and bone spurs (osteophytes) from the joint surfaces, leaving a smooth surface. Loose fragments are also removed. The joint is then flushed with saline to remove any debris. Upon completion of the procedure, the arthroscope and surgical tools are removed, and the portal incisions are closed.

29902

29902   Arthroscopy, metacarpophalangeal joint, surgical; with reduction of displaced ulnar collateral ligament (eg, Stener lesion)

Surgical arthroscopy of the metacarpophalangeal joint is performed with reduction of a displaced ulnar collateral ligament (UCL), also referred to as a Stener lesion, skier's thumb, or gamekeeper's thumb. The UCL provides stability to the thumb. Injuries to the UCL may present as avulsion fractures or tears within the ligament or at its insertion on the proximal phalanx. A Stener lesion is characterized by interposition of the aponeurosis of the thumb adductor between the distal aspect of the avulsed UCL and its insertion into the base of the proximal phalanx. A finger trap is applied and traction is placed on the thumb. Portal incisions are made overlying the metacarpophalangeal joint in the dorsal-ulnar and dorsal-radial aspects. Blunt dissection is performed to the level of the joint capsule using a small hemostat, which is then used to spread the joint capsule and enter the joint. The arthroscope is introduced through the dorsal-radial portal and the joint is inspected. A motorized shaver is introduced and any hematoma or bone fragments are removed. Synovectomy is then performed so that the UCL injury can be clearly identified. A probe is inserted through the ulnar portal and the UCL is retrieved and reduced. A shaver is introduced and the fracture site is debrided. K-wire is then introduced into the joint just proximal to the bony fragment and attached to the UCL. The K-wire is then placed through the bony fragment and the UCL is secured to the proximal phalanx using a K-wire driver. Proper alignment is verified arthroscopically and radiographically and the wire is cut just below the skin. The joint is then flushed with saline to remove any debris. Upon completion of the procedure, the arthroscope and surgical tools are removed, and the portal incisions are closed.

29904

29904   Arthroscopy, subtalar joint, surgical; with removal of loose body or foreign body

The subtalar joint is the lower ankle joint between the talus and the calcaneus; it is a compound joint divided into two distinct compartments by a space containing the talocalcaneal and cervical ligaments. Prior to insertion of the arthroscope and surgical instruments, the joint is distracted to separate the joint surfaces and allow visualization of the entire joint. Two or three portals are established for access and the entire joint is examined. The loose or foreign body is identified and a grasper is inserted to retrieve the loose or foreign body(s). The joint is irrigated and inspected. A large loose or foreign body that cannot be removed through a portal requires an additional small accessory incision for removal.

29905

29905   Arthroscopy, subtalar joint, surgical; with synovectomy

The subtalar joint is the lower ankle joint between the talus and the calcaneus; it is a compound joint divided into two distinct compartments by a space containing the talocalcaneal and cervical ligaments. Prior to insertion of the arthroscope and surgical instruments, the joint is distracted to separate the joint surfaces and allow visualization of the entire joint. Two or three portals are established for access and the entire joint is examined. The diseased or hypertrophic synovium is identified and a shaver is inserted through one of the portals to excise the abnormal synovium. The joint is irrigated and

debris is removed. The foot is placed in a neutral plantigrade position with the heel in five to ten degrees of valgus to facilitate healing and a brace or splint is applied.

29906

29906   Arthroscopy, subtalar joint, surgical; with debridement

The subtalar joint is the lower ankle joint between the talus and the calcaneus; it is a compound joint divided into two distinct compartments by a space containing the talocalcaneal and cervical ligaments. Prior to insertion of the arthroscope and surgical instruments, the joint is distracted to separate the joint surfaces and allow visualization of the entire joint. Two or three portals are established for access and the entire joint is examined. Abnormal articular cartilage is identified. If abnormalities are not readily apparent, the cartilage is probed to evaluate its texture. Softened cartilage is identified and all abnormal tissue is removed from the talus and calcaneus with a burr. The joint is irrigated to remove debris and the arthroscope is removed. The foot is placed in a neutral plantigrade position with the heel in five to ten degrees of valgus to facilitate healing and a brace or splint is applied.

29907

29907   Arthroscopy, subtalar joint, surgical; with subtalar arthrodesis

The subtalar joint is the lower ankle joint between the talus and the calcaneus; it is a compound joint divided into two distinct compartments by a space containing the talocalcaneal and cervical ligaments. Prior to insertion of the arthroscope and surgical instruments, the joint is distracted to separate the joint surfaces and allow visualization of the entire joint. Two or three portals are established for access and the entire joint is examined. An abrader is inserted and all abnormal cartilage is removed. Following removal of abnormal tissue, all remaining cartilage is removed from adjacent talar and calcaneal surfaces. The bone is shaped so that the surfaces of both bones will be in full contact and fusion can occur. The bones are stabilized using a temporary fixation device. Radiographs are obtained to check alignment of the foot and joint. Permanent internal fixation is applied. Allografting may be required if the bone surfaces are not in full contact. The joint is irrigated to remove debris and the arthroscope is removed. The foot is placed in a neutral plantigrade position with the heel in five to ten degrees of valgus to facilitate healing and a brace or splint is applied.

29914

29914   Arthroscopy, hip, surgical; with femoroplasty (ie, treatment of cam lesion)

A femoroplasty is performed to treat damage to the femoral head caused by abnormal contact and friction between the femoral head and acetabulum. This condition is referred to as femoroacetabular impingement which can cause two types of lesions, one of which is a cam lesion. Cam lesions occur when the relationship between the femoral head and neck is aspherical or not perfectly round. The loss of roundness causes abnormal contact between the femoral head and acetabulum. A small portal incision is made on the lateral aspect of the hip joint for introduction of the arthroscope. A second small incision is made over the anterolateral aspect of the joint for introduction of surgical instruments. Additional incisions are made as needed to provide visualization and access to hip joint structures. Using fluoroscopic guidance, a catheter is placed into the hip through the lateral incision and sterile saline is introduced to distract the joint. The catheter is withdrawn and the arthroscope is introduced. The hip is examined and the extent of the cam lesion is determined. Damaged cartilage at the femoral head is debrided and the articular surface is smoothed and rounded. Microfractures are made in the femoral head to stimulate new cartilage growth. Upon completion of the procedure, the arthroscope is removed, the joint is flushed with sterile saline, and the portal incisions are closed.

29915

29915   Arthroscopy, hip, surgical; with acetabuloplasty (ie, treatment of pincer lesion)

An acetabuloplasty is performed to treat damage to the acetabulum caused by abnormal contact and friction between the femoral head and neck and acetabulum of the hip joint. This condition is referred to as femoroacetabular impingement which can cause two types of lesions, one of which is a pincer lesion within the ball and socket hip joint. Pincer lesions occur when the acetabulum (socket) extends too far over the femoral head (ball) usually at the front top rim of the acetabulum. This over-coverage results in pinching of the labrum between the rim of the acetabulum and the anterior femoral head and neck. The labrum is the cartilage lining the socket that acts as a kind of bumper, providing greater stability and flexible range of motion. A small portal incision is made on the lateral aspect of the hip joint for introduction of the arthroscope. A second small incision is made over the anterolateral aspect of the joint for introduction of surgical instruments. Additional incisions are made as needed to provide visualization and access to hip joint structures. Using fluoroscopic guidance, a catheter is placed into the hip through the lateral incision and sterile saline is introduced to distract the joint. The catheter is withdrawn and the arthroscope is introduced. The hip is examined and the extent of the pincer lesion is determined. Damaged acetabular cartilage is debrided and the articular surface is smoothed and reshaped. Microfractures are made in the acetabulum to stimulate new cartilage growth. Upon completion of the procedure, the arthroscope is removed, the joint is flushed with sterile saline, and the portal incisions are closed.

29916

29916   Arthroscopy, hip, surgical; with labral repair

A labral repair is performed to treat a tear in the cartilage along the acetabular rim. The labrum is a type of cartilage found in ball and socket joints. It covers the rim of the acetabulum in the hip, deepening the socket to provide greater stability of the hip joint while at the same time allowing greater flexibility and increasing range of motion in the joint. Labral tears may occur as a result of an injury or be due to structural abnormalities in the hip joint. A small portal incision is made on the lateral aspect of the hip joint for introduction of the arthroscope. A second small incision is made over the anterolateral aspect of the joint for introduction of surgical instruments. Additional incisions are made as needed to provide visualization and access to hip joint structures. Using fluoroscopic guidance, a catheter is placed into the hip through the lateral incision and sterile saline is introduced to distract the joint. The catheter is withdrawn and the arthroscope is introduced. The hip is examined and the extent of the labral injury is determined. The damaged portion of the labrum is debrided and the articular surface is smoothed using an athroscopic shaver. The tear is then repaired with sutures. Upon completion of the procedure, the arthroscope is removed, the joint is flushed with sterile saline, and the portal incisions are closed.

● New Code   ▲ Revised Code

Respiratory System

30000-30020

30000   Drainage abscess or hematoma, nasal, internal approach
30020   Drainage abscess or hematoma, nasal septum

The abscess or hematoma is approached through an incision inside the nose. The incision is carried down through the soft tissue and the abscess or hematoma is opened. If drainage is performed for an abscess, any loculations are broken up using blunt dissection. If drainage is for a hematoma, blood clots are removed by suction. The abscess or hematoma cavity is flushed with saline or antibiotic solution. Use 30000 if the abscess or hematoma is in the internal nose at a site other than the nasal septum and 30020 if the site is the nasal septum.

30100

30100   Biopsy, intranasal

The physician performs an intranasal biopsy of a lesion or other tissue in the inner lining of the nasal passage. The area to the biopsied is cleansed and a local anesthetic injected. One or more tissue samples are obtained using a scalpel, biopsy forceps, or other technique. The tissue samples are sent to the laboratory for separately reportable histological evaluation. Following the biopsy, the nose may be packed to control bleeding.

30110-30115

30110   Excision, nasal polyp(s), simple
30115   Excision, nasal polyp(s), extensive

Nasal polyps are benign growths on the lining of the nasal passages or sinuses that usually have a teardrop shape. Polyps are removed using a mechanical suction device or microdebrider. Use 30110 for simple polypectomy performed in an office setting using a local anesthetic and 30115 for complicated polypectomy requiring general anesthesia in an outpatient surgical facility.

30117-30118

30117   Excision or destruction (eg, laser), intranasal lesion; internal approach
30118   Excision or destruction (eg, laser), intranasal lesion; external approach (lateral rhinotomy)

An intranasal lesion is excised or destroyed. In 30117, an intranasal approach is used. The area is cleansed and a local anesthetic injected. The lesion is approached through the nostril. If the lesion is excised, a narrow margin of healthy tissue is identified and a full-thickness incision is made through the nasal muscosa. The incision is carried around the lesion and the entire lesion is excised. The lesion is sent to the laboratory for separately reportable histologic evaluation. Bleeding is controlled by electrocautery or chemical cautery. The wound may be left open to heal or closed using simple single layer suture technique. If the lesion is destroyed, the lesion is examined and the most appropriate form of destruction determined. Local anesthesia is administered as needed. Cryosurgery using liquid nitrogen to freeze the lesion is one destruction technique. Surgical curettage followed by electrosurgery is another common method. Other techniques include chemical or laser destruction. In 30118, an external approach via a lateral rhinotomy is used. The incision begins just below the inner aspect of the eyebrow and descends along the lateral wall of the nose to the nasolabial fold where it is carried around the alar margin. Soft tissue is dissected and freed from the ethmoid bone, anteromedial antral wall, and the nasal pyramid. The nasal cavity is then exposed. The lesion is excised or destroyed as described above.

30120

30120   Excision or surgical planing of skin of nose for rhinophyma

The physician excises or planes the skin of the nose to treat rhinophyma, a condition in which there is significant overgrowth (hyperplasia) of the sebaceous glands of the nose. The hyperplastic sebaceous glands are carefully excised or shaved (planed) using a scalpel, dermabrasion, electrocautery, laser, or a combination of these methods. The physician must make sure that an adequate amount of adnexal skin structures remain at the wound base to allow re-epitheliazation of the skin. Upon completion of the excision or planing procedure bleeding is controlled by cautery and an ointment is applied to the wound.

30124-30125

30124   Excision dermoid cyst, nose; simple, skin, subcutaneous
30125   Excision dermoid cyst, nose; complex, under bone or cartilage

A dermoid cyst of the nose is excised. A dermoid cyst is a pocket or cavity under the skin that is composed of epidermis and dermis (skin tissues). In 30124, simple excision is performed on a dermoid cyst located in the skin and subcutaneous tissues. An incision is made in the skin and subcutaneous tissue over cyst and the cyst is exposed. The cyst is then carefully dissected from surrounding soft tissue and excised in its entirety. In 30125, a complex excision is performed on a cyst located under bone or cartilage. An incision is made through the skin and subcutaneous tissue to the overlying bone or cartilage. The overlying bone or cartilage is removed, which may be accomplished by making a small window in the bone or cartilage. The cyst is exposed, carefully dissected from surrounding tissue, and removed in its entirety. The excised bone or cartilage is replaced and secured with sutures. Soft tissue and skin is closed in layers.

30130-30140

30130   Excision inferior turbinate, partial or complete, any method
30140   Submucous resection inferior turbinate, partial or complete, any method

The physician performs a partial or complete excision (30130) or submucous resection (30140) of the inferior turbinate to treat a nasal obstruction caused by enlargement of the soft tissue or bone of the turbinate. There are three sets of turbinates or conchae on each side of the nasal vestibule which are designated by their location as inferior, middle or superior. The turbinates are bony plates or ridges covered by spongy mucosa. The inferior turbinate is located on the lower lateral wall on each side of the nasal cavity. The turbinate is approached through the nostril. In 30130, the physician excises the turbinate mucosa and underlying bone either partially or completely. In 30140, the physician removes the outer aspect of the turbinate mucosa and then removes part or all of the turbinate bone. The inner part of the mucosa is then folded over the surgical wound and any remaining bone and secured with sutures.

30150-30160

30150   Rhinectomy; partial
30160   Rhinectomy; total

A rhinectomy is performed. Partial or total rhinectomy is performed primarily for invasive squamous or basal cell carcinoma or other malignant lesion of the nose. The nasal cavities are examined using a nasal endoscope to locate any visible lesions. The skin and subcutaneous tissue over the area of the nose to be removed is incised and the incision is carried down to cartilage and bone. Random biopsies may be obtained to determine the extent of the malignancy. Involved skin, soft tissue, cartilage, and bone is excised and sent for separately reportable frozen section examination. Following frozen section examination, additional tissue is removed until all margins are free of malignant tissue. A separately reportable reconstructive procedure may be performed subsequent to the rhinectomy or the wound may be dressed with Xeroform gauze and a delayed reconstruction performed at a subsequent surgical session. Use 30150 for a partial rhinectomy and 30160 for a total rhinectomy.

30200

30200   Injection into turbinate(s), therapeutic

A therapeutic injection of one or more nasal turbinate bones is performed. There three turbinate bones, also referred to as the nasal concha, on each side of the nose. These three thin, spongy, bony plates are designated as the inferior, middle, and superior turbinates. The inferior turbinate separates the middle meatus from the inferior meatus. The middle turbinate separates the superior meatus from the middle meatus. The superior nasal turbinate separates the superior meatus from the sphenoethmoid recess. Therapeutic injection of a corticosteroid into the mucosa of the turbinate bone is performed to treat allergic or vasomotor rhinitis. The injection forms a bleb over the turbinate bone that allows for slow release of the medication into the surrounding tissue.

30210

30210   Displacement therapy (Proetz type)

Proetz-type displacement therapy is performed to treat chronic sinus infection. The sinuses communicate with the nasal cavity through small openings called ostia. In healthy individuals the ostia permit free exchange of air and fluids. However, in individuals which chronic sinusitis, the ostia become obstructed. Displacement therapy removes air and mucous from the sinuses and allows the sinuses to fill with saline solution. The patient is placed supine with the head tilted back. Several drops of epinephrine are instilled into each nasal cavity to constrict inflamed nasal tissue. A mixture of epinephrine and saline solution is then instilled into the nasal cavities to displace pus and mucous. Intermittent negative pressure is applied using suction to remove air and fluid from the sinuses. When the negative pressure is released, the sinus cavities fill with the epinephrine and saline solution. This is repeated several times to flush pus and mucous from the sinuses.

30220

30220   Insertion, nasal septal prosthesis (button)

The physician inserts a nasal septal prosthesis, also referred to as a button prosthesis, to close of a nasal septal perforation. The button prosthesis may be used for temporary closure of the nasal septal defect until a definitive procedure can be performed. For patients who are not good surgical risks, it may be used for long-term closure. A topical nasal decongestant is administered and a local anesthetic applied to defect area. If a prefabricated button is used, the perforation is measured. The prefabricated button is trimmed leaving it slightly larger than the defect. A lubricant is applied to the button and it is placed in the defect with the flanges against the upper lateral cartilage and septal junction. If a custom-made button is used, the physician obtains an intranasal cast and then fabricates the button out of silicone. The custom button is then placed in the defect as described above.

30300-30320

30300   Removal foreign body, intranasal; office type procedure
30310   Removal foreign body, intranasal; requiring general anesthesia
30320   Removal foreign body, intranasal; by lateral rhinotomy

Most patients seen for nasal foreign bodies are children between 1 to 8 years of age. Treatment depends on the location of the foreign body in the nose and the object being removed. Removal techniques include gentle suction, long tweezers, or surgical instruments with a loop or hook at the tip. If the object is metallic a magnetized instrument may be used. A soft rubber catheter with an uninflated balloon at the tip may be passed to a site just beyond the foreign body, the balloon inflated, and the catheter removed along with the captured foreign body. Use 30300 when the procedure is performed in the office without anesthesia or 30310 when it is performed in a surgical center under anesthesia. Use 30320 when the foreign body is removed by lateral rhinotomy. An incision is made through the skin on the affected side of the nose. Tissue is dissected to expose the nasal cavity. The foreign body is located and removed. Incisions are closed in a layered fashion.

30400-30420

30400   Rhinoplasty, primary; lateral and alar cartilages and/or elevation of nasal tip
30410   Rhinoplasty, primary; complete, external parts including bony pyramid, lateral and alar cartilages, and/or elevation of nasal tip
30420   Rhinoplasty, primary; including major septal repair

A primary rhinoplasty is performed to reshape the nose. Prior to the surgery, the physician takes photographs and determines the surgical plan. The procedure may be performed entirely through incisions inside the nose (closed technique) or through incisions inside the nose with an additional incision across the columella (open technique). The skin of the nose is marked using the photographs as a guide. The physician then reshapes the nose. In 30400, the lateral and alar cartilages are reshaped and/or the nasal tip is elevated. Cartilage is removed from the sides of the nose if the nose is too wide. The nasal tip is reshaped so that it projects gracefully from the dorsal bridge line. In 30410, a complete rhinoplasty is performed with reshaping of external parts including bony pyramid. The columella and rims of the nose are incised and skin and soft tissue elevated off the lateral cartilages and bony dorsum of the nose. The septum is incised and a mucopericondrial flap opened. Cartilage and bone is removed using shavers and chisels. The bony pyramid may be fractured and reshaped to correct bony deformities. Cartilage grafts obtained during contouring may be used to support and reshape other parts of the nose. In 30420, a rhinoplasty with major septal repair, also referred to as a rhinoseptoplasty, is performed. An incision is made inside the nostril and the mucosa is elevated to expose the underlying bone and cartilage. The nasal septum is then reshaped. Cartilage and bone is removed as needed including any spurs. If a cartilage graft is required, it is usually created using cartilage that has been removed from the septum. If the septum is deviated it is repositioned to the center of the nose. Rhinoplasty is then performed as described above. Upon completion of the procedure, the incision is closed and splints placed inside the nose as needed to maintain the position of the septum. Nasal packing may also be used to control bleeding.

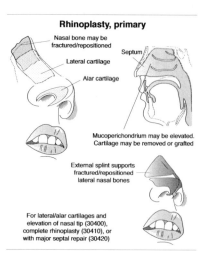

Rhinoplasty, primary

Nasal bone may be fractured/repositioned

Septum

Lateral cartilage

Alar cartilage

Mucoperichondrium may be elevated.
Cartilage may be removed or grafted

External splint supports
fractured/repositioned
lateral nasal bones

For lateral/alar cartilages and
elevation of nasal tip (30400),
complete rhinoplasty (30410), or
with major septal repair (30420)

30430-30450

30430   Rhinoplasty, secondary; minor revision (small amount of nasal tip work)
30435   Rhinoplasty, secondary; intermediate revision (bony work with osteotomies)
30450   Rhinoplasty, secondary; major revision (nasal tip work and osteotomies)

A secondary rhinoplasty, also referred to as a revision rhinoplasty, is performed. Prior to the surgery, the physician evaluates the results of the first rhinoplasty procedure and determines the surgical plan. The procedure may be performed entirely through incisions inside the nose (closed technique) or through incisions inside the nose with an additional incision across the columella (open technique). The skin of the nose is marked using the photographs as a guide. The physician then reshapes the nose. In 30430, a minor revision such as a small amount of nasal tip work is performed. The nasal tip is reshaped so that it projects gracefully from the dorsal bridge line. This may involve removing some cartilage using a shaver or placing a cartilage graft. Secondary procedures often require use of cartilage graft from the ear or rib. In 30435, an intermediate revision is performed which includes bony work with osteotomies. The columella and rims of the nose are incised and skin and soft tissue elevated off the lateral cartilages and bony dorsum of the nose. The septum is incised and a mucopericondrial flap opened. Cartilage and bone is removed using shavers and chisels. The bony pyramid may be fractured and reshaped to correct bony deformities. Cartilage grafts obtained from the ear or rib may be used to support and reshape the nose. In 30450, a major revision is performed which includes nasal tip work and bony work. An incision is made inside the nostril and the mucosa is elevated to expose the underlying bone and cartilage. The lateral cartilage and nasal tip are trimmed and/or augmented by grafting. Nasal bones are refracted using chisels, manually repositioned, and bony dorsum augmented using grafts. Upon completion of the procedure, the incision is closed and splints placed inside the nose as needed. Nasal packing may also be used to control bleeding.

30460-30462

30460   Rhinoplasty for nasal deformity secondary to congenital cleft lip and/or palate, including columellar lengthening; tip only
30462   Rhinoplasty for nasal deformity secondary to congenital cleft lip and/or palate, including columellar lengthening; tip, septum, osteotomies

A rhinoplasty including columellar lengthening is performed for nasal deformity secondary to congenital cleft lip and/or palate. The nasal deformity may involve the tip only or it may involve tip, septum, and bone. Prior to the surgery, the physician takes photographs and determines the surgical plan. The procedure may be performed entirely through incisions inside the nose or through external skin incisions. The skin of the nose is marked using the photographs as a guide. The physician then reshapes the nose. In 30460, the columella is lengthened as needed, asymmetrical nasal alae are reshaped, and the nasal tip is augmented. If an external incision is used, the columella, floor of the nose and upper lip are opened and elevated to expose the nasal tip and columella. The columella is lengthened using an alar flap and/or a cartilage graft from the ear or other site. The nasal tip is augmented so that it projects gracefully from the dorsal bridge line. In 30462, the columella is lengthed, asymmetrical nasal alae are reshaped, the nasal tip is augmented, and a septoplasty and osteotomies performed. The columella and rims of the nose are incised and skin and soft tissue elevated off the lateral cartilages and bony dorsum of the nose. The septum is incised and a mucopericondrial flap opened. Cartilage and bone are removed using shavers and chisels. The bony pyramid may be fractured and reshaped to correct bony deformities. Cartilage grafts obtained during contouring may be used to support and reshape other parts of the nose. The nasal septum is then reshaped. Cartilage and bone is removed as needed. If a cartilage graft is required, cartilage from the septum may be used or a cartilage graft harvested from the ribs or ear. If the septum is deviated it is repositioned to the center of the nose. The columella is lengthened using an alar flap and/or a cartilage graft from the ear or other site. The nasal tip is augmented so that it projects gracefully from the dorsal bridge line. Upon completion of the procedure, the

● New Code   ▲ Revised Code

Respiratory System

incision is closed and splints placed inside the nose as needed to maintain the position of the septum. Nasal packing may also be used to control bleeding.

30465

30465   Repair of nasal vestibular stenosis (eg, spreader grafting, lateral nasal wall reconstruction)

The physician repairs nasal vestibular stenosis that may include spreader grafting, lateral wall reconstruction, and/or elevation of the nasal tip. This procedure is performed to treat nasal obstruction caused by narrowing of the nasal inlets. If cartilage grafts are needed, they are first obtained in a separately reportable procedure. The nasal bone and upper lateral cartilage are exposed. The cartilage and nasal bone are then incised and cartilage spreader grafts are placed bilaterally in the upper lateral wall and nasal bone. Alternatively, the lateral nasal walls may be reconstructed bilaterally by resecting thickened cartilage and reshaping the lateral wall. Flaring sutures may be placed to lift the upper lateral walls and/or the nasal tip may be elevated using nonabsorbable suture material. Any excessive nasal skin is resected.

30520

30520   Septoplasty or submucous resection, with or without cartilage scoring, contouring or replacement with graft

The physician performs a septoplasty or submucous resection with or without cartilage scoring, contouring or replacement with a graft. The nasal septum is the cartilage partition that supports the nose and separates the two nasal passages. Septoplasty is performed to correct a severely deviated or dislocated septum that is obstructing the flow of air through the nose. It is typically performed by submucous resection which involves making an incision inside the nostril and elevating the mucosa to expose the underlying bone and cartilage. The nasal septum is then reshaped. Cartilage and bone is removed as needed including any spurs. If a cartilage graft is required, it is usually created using cartilage that has been removed from the septum. If the septum is deviated it is repositioned to the center of the nose. Upon completion of the procedure, the incision is closed and splints placed inside the nose as needed to maintain the position of the septum. Nasal packing may also be used to control bleeding.

30540-30545

30540   Repair choanal atresia; intranasal
30545   Repair choanal atresia; transpalatine

The physician repairs choanal atresia, a congenital anomaly of the anterior skull base in which one or both posterior nasal passages are closed. In 30540, an intranasal approach is used to repair the atresia. A local anesthetic is injected into the nose. A speculum is inserted into the nose and positioned so that the site of atresia can be visualized. An operating microscope is inserted and the atretic membrane visualized and palpated. A curved incision is made in the mucosa and an anterior mucosal flap created. The mucosal flap is elevated and the bone removed by drilling parallel to the hard palate taking care not to damage surrounding structures. The atretic plate is penetrated to expose the nasopharyngeal mucosa. The opening is enlarged by drilling into the vomer, pterygoid plate and hard palate. Posterior mucosal flaps are created, rotated and laid down adjacent to the previously created anterior flaps and imbricated. Stents are placed and secured to maintain the new choanal opening. In 30545, a transpalatine approach is used to repair a bilateral atresia, a thick bony atresia, or an atresia associated with other anomalies of the anterior nasal cavities or nasopharynx. A curved incision is made in the mucosa of the hard palate. The mucosa is elevated and an anterior flap created. The muscular layer of the soft palate is exposed and incised at its insertion into the posterior edge of the hard palate. The bone along the posterior edge of the hard palate, vomer, and pterygoid region is removed using a drill. Nasal mucosal flaps are created, laid down adjacent to the anterior mucosal flap, and imbricated. Stents are placed in the new choanal openings and the anterior ends secured.

30560

30560   Lysis intranasal synechia

The physician performs a lysis of intranasal synechia. Intranasal synechia refers to the formation of scar tissue or adhesions inside the nasal passage. The scar tissue or adhesions are destroyed using any technique including incision, electrocautery, or laser cautery. A temporary stent may be placed to maintain patency of the nasal opening.

30580

30580   Repair fistula; oromaxillary (combine with 31030 if antrotomy is included)

The physician repairs an oromaxillary fistula, an abnormal passageway between one of the maxillary sinuses located on either side of the nose and the roof of the mouth. A curved incision is made in the mucosa overlying the hard palate or cheek and a mucosal flap is created and then rotated over the abnormal opening to close the fistula. The flap may be reinforced by first applying a piece of medical grade foil over the fistula and then suturing the mucosal flap over the foil.

30600

30600   Repair fistula; oronasal

The physician repairs an oronasal fistula, an abnormal passageway between the mouth and the nose. One technique used involves a three layer repair. First, a septal mucosal flap is created from the nasal floor consisting of septal mucosa from the side opposite the fistula. A slit is made in the remaining layers of nasal septum; the flap is delivered into the defect; and the nasal side of the defect is closed. Bone and cartilage are harvested from the exposed nasal septum. A second flap is developed using the palatal mucosa. The bone and cartilage are placed in the defect; the palatal mucosal flap is positioned over the bone and cartilage; and the oral defect is closed.

30620

30620   Septal or other intranasal dermatoplasty (does not include obtaining graft)

A septal or other intranasal dermatoplasty is performed. This procedure is typically performed to treat severe nose bleeds (epistaxis) such as those occurring due to Rendu-Osler-Weber syndrome also known as hereditary hemorrhagic telangiectasia (HHT). HHT is rare genetic disorder with one symptom being severe recurrent epistaxis caused by telangiectasia of the nasal mucosa. The physician removes the diseased nasal mucosa at the nasal septum or other site in the internal nose using a scalpel taking care to preserve the underlying perichondrium. A separately reportable split-thickness skin graft is then obtained from a separate donor site, usually the thigh. The graft is trimmed, prepared for placement in the nose, and sutured into place over the mucosal defects.

30630

30630   Repair nasal septal perforations

There are a number of techniques available including the use of prosthetic devices, local mucosal flaps with interposition grafts of connective tissue, tunneled sublabial mucosal flap, and free flap repair. If a local flap is used it is taken from adjacent healthy septal tissue or from the inferior turbinate. This may be combined with an interposition graft of mastoid periosteum, cartilage or ethmoid bone. If a sublabial mucosal flap is used, the mucoperichondrium on the side to be repaired is elevated around the perforation and the edges of the perforation debrided until bleeding occurs. The upper lip is exposed and the buccal mucosa on the same side raised and a pedicle flap created just lateral to the frenulum. The flap is then tunneled through a surgically created sublabial-nasal fistula. The flap is placed over the septal perforation and the perforation is closed.

30801-30802

30801   Ablation, soft tissue of inferior turbinates, unilateral or bilateral, any method (eg, electrocautery, radiofrequency ablation, or tissue volume reduction); superficial
30802   Ablation, soft tissue of inferior turbinates, unilateral or bilateral, any method (eg, electrocautery, radiofrequency ablation, or tissue volume reduction); intramural (ie, submucosal)

Ablation may be performed with an electrosurgical probe or a laser. The probe or laser device is inserted into the nostril and advanced to the inferior turbinate. The probe or laser device is then activated and the desired amount of tissue destroyed. The procedure is repeated on the opposite side as needed. In 30801, superficial or surface tissue is destroyed. In 30802, the deeper intramural (submucosal) tissue is destroyed.

30901-30906

30901   Control nasal hemorrhage, anterior, simple (limited cautery and/or packing) any method
30903   Control nasal hemorrhage, anterior, complex (extensive cautery and/or packing) any method
30905   Control nasal hemorrhage, posterior, with posterior nasal packs and/or cautery, any method; initial
30906   Control nasal hemorrhage, posterior, with posterior nasal packs and/or cautery, any method; subsequent

Nasal hemorrhage is also referred to as epistaxis. The most common sites of bleeding are the anterior portion of the nasal septum at the plexus of vessels known as the Kiesselbach's plexus or the ethmoidal vessels also located in the anterior region of the nasal cavity. Less common is bleeding from the sphenopalatine artery located posteriorly. Pledgets soaked in an anesthetic-vasoconstrictor solution are inserted into the nasal cavity for 10-15 minutes to anesthetize and shrink the nasal mucosa. Following removal of the pledgets, the nasal cavity is examined. If the bleeding point can be identified, bleeding is controlled with pressure followed by chemical cautery using a silver nitrate stick applied to the bleeding point. Alternatively, electrocautery may be used. If pressure and electrocautery or chemical cautery fails, Vaseline gauze packing, a nasal tampon or sponge, or an epistaxis balloon may be used. Use 30901 for treatment of a simple anterior nasal hemorrhage by any method and 30902 for a complex anterior nasal hemorrhage. Use 30905 for treatment of a simple posterior nasal hemorrhage and 30906 for a complex posterior nasal hemorrhage.

Respiratory System

● New Code   ▲ Revised Code

30915-30920

30915   Ligation arteries; ethmoidal
30920   Ligation arteries; internal maxillary artery, transantral

The physician ligates the ethmoidal arteries (30915) or internal maxillary artery (30920) usually to treat severe, epistaxis (nose bleed) that cannot be controlled by other methods. In 30915, the ethmoid arteries are approached via an incision between the inner canthus of the eye and midline of the nose. The periosteium is incised and elevated. The suture line between the ethmoid and frontal bones is identified at the superior aspect of the lacrimal bone. The periosteum is elevated off the medial wall of the orbit along the suture line. The anterior and posterior ethmoid arteries are identified and ligated with sutures or vascular clips placed. In 30920, the internal maxillary artery is ligated via a transantral approach. An incision is made through the buccal mucosa. The anterior wall of the maxillary sinus is exposed and removed to provide access to the posterior wall which is also incised and along the lateral aspect and a mucosal flap elevated. A section of the posterior wall is removed and the pterygopalatine fossa exposed. The branches of the maxillary artery are identified and ligated with sutures or vascular clips placed.

30930

30930   Fracture nasal inferior turbinate(s), therapeutic

This procedure is performed to treat nasal obstruction caused by overgrowth (hypertrophy) of the inferior turbinates. An elevator is inserted into the nose to the level of the inferior turbinate. The physician then applies force in a lateral and inferior direction and displaces the inferior turbinate. Alternatively, the elevator may first be placed in the inferior meatus and the turbinate infractured followed by outfracture as described above. The procedure is repeated on the opposite side as needed.

31000-31002

31000   Lavage by cannulation; maxillary sinus (antrum puncture or natural ostium)
31002   Lavage by cannulation; sphenoid sinus

Lavage of the maxillary or sphenoid sinus is performed to treat a sinus infection. The maxillary sinuses are paired sinuses that lie within the maxilla (cheekbone) on each side of the nose. The sphenoid sinuses lie deep within the skull behind the ethmoid sinuses. In 31000, lavage of the maxillary sinus is performed using a cannula inserted through a puncture in the antrum or through the natural ostium. If the cannula is inserted through a puncture in the antrum, a local anesthetic is administered at the inferior meatus. A trocar is placed against the lateral nasal wall just below the inferior turbinate. The antrum is punctured and the cannula is passed into the maxillary sinus. If the cannula is inserted through the natural ostium, the cannula is advanced into the middle meatus, the maxillary ostium identified and a blunt curved catheter advanced through the ostium. The infected maxillary sinus is then flushed with saline solution to remove pus and mucous. In 31002, lavage of the sphenoid sinus is performed using a cannula. The approach varies, but one approach is through the maxillary sinus. From there the nasoantral wall is opened. The cannula is passed through the maxillary sinus and nasoantral wall opening into the middle turbinate and then advanced to the sphenoid ostium. The anterior sphenoid wall is punctured and the cannula inserted into the sphenoid sinus which is flushed with saline solution to remove pus and mucous.

31020

31020   Sinusotomy, maxillary (antrotomy); intranasal

A local anesthetic and vasoconstrictor are injected through the nose along the lateral nasal wall below the inferior turbinate. The maxillary sinus is punctured via the same intranasal route using a trocar. The opening is enlarged with through-cutting forceps. The maxillary sinus is drained and specimens are obtained for culture and sensitivity, then the sinus is irrigated.

31030-31032

31030   Sinusotomy, maxillary (antrotomy); radical (Caldwell-Luc) without removal of antrochoanal polyps
31032   Sinusotomy, maxillary (antrotomy); radical (Caldwell-Luc) with removal of antrochoanal polyps

A radical maxillary sinusotomy(antrostomy), also referred to as a Caldwell-Luc procedure, is performed. An incision is made in the mouth over the canine tooth extending to the first premolar. Electrocautery dissection is carried down through the soft tissue and periosteum to the bone. The periosteum is elevated from the anterior wall of the maxilla taking care to protect the infraorbital nerve. The maxillary sinus is accessed via the canine fossa using a mallet and osteotome. The opening is enlarged using rongeurs. The maxillary sinus is drained and specimens obtained for culture and sensitivity. The maxillary sinus is irrigated. Code 31030 is used when a radical maxillary sinusotomy is performed without removal of antrochoanal polyps. Code 31032 is used when radical maxillary sinusotomy is performed with removal of antrochoanal polyps. Antrochoanal polyps are solitary polyps that originate in the maxillary sinus. As the polyp enlarges, it may prolapse through the natural or accessory ostium into the nasal canal. Further enlargement moves the polyp toward the posterior choana and into the nasopharynx. An antrochoanal polyp can cause

nasal obstruction and serous otitis media if it obstructs the Eustachian tube. The maxillary sinusotomy is performed as described above. The choanal portion of the polyp is removed via a transoral excision. The antral portion of the polyp is removed through the previously created canine fossa opening to the maxillary sinus. The polyp is removed using forceps and surrounding maxillary sinus tissue is debrided and removed as needed.

31040

31040   Pterygomaxillary fossa surgery, any approach

The pterygomaxillary fossa, more commonly referred to as the pterygopalatine fossa, is a small pyramid-shaped space between the pterygoid process, maxilla, and palatine bone that contains the pterygopalatine ganglion and the third part of the maxillary artery. Surgery of the pterygomaxillary fossa is performed for tumors originating in or extending into the fossa. Tumors of this region are rare, however nerve sheath tumors and juvenile angiofibromas do sometimes occur. Other tumors originating in surrounding structures and invading the pterygomaxillary fossa include osteomas, hemangiomas, neurofibromas, adamanitinomas, congenital cysts, and parotid mixed tumors. There are a number of approaches with anterior transmaxillary being one of the more common. Other approaches include lateral, retrosubmandibular, and transnasal endoscopic. Once the fossa has been entered, the tumor is dissected from surrounding vascular structures and nerves. Blood vessels are ligated as needed. The tumor is removed. Any defects in surrounding structures are repaired.

31050-31051

31050   Sinusotomy, sphenoid, with or without biopsy
31051   Sinusotomy, sphenoid, with or without biopsy; with mucosal stripping or removal of polyp(s)

The sphenoid sinus is the most posterior of all the paranasal sinuses, located in the center of the skull base. There are three open approaches that are used for evaluation of lesions or masses in the sphenoid sinus, transpalatal approach, transnasal transseptal approach, external transorbital transethmoidal approach. The transpalatal approach involves incising the palate and elevating a palatal flap off the hard palate. The soft palate musculature is separated from the hard palate and the nasopharynx and floor of the sphenoid sinus exposed. A drill or rongeur is then used to remove portions of the hard palate and vomer and open the sphenoid sinus. The transnasal transseptal approach is through the nostril with exposure augmented when needed with a sublabial incision. Once the superior turbinate is exposed and attachments to the anterior sphenoid wall severed, the sphenoid is entered using fine rongeurs or a sphenoid punch. An external transorbital transethmoidal requires an external incision through the orbit and an ethmoidectomy for access to the sphenoid sinus. In 31050, the sinus may be drained or a biopsy obtained. If a biopsy is needed, biopsy forceps are passed into the sphenoid sinus and a tissue sample obtained. In 31051, mucosal stripping or removal of polyps is performed with or without biopsy. If mucosal stripping is performed, the sinus mucosa is elevated and removed. If a polypectomy is performed, the polyp is grasped with forceps and removed in its entirety.

31070

31070   Sinusotomy frontal; external, simple (trephine operation)

A skin incision is made above the eye on the inner aspect just under the eyebrow. The frontal bone is exposed. A trephine or perforator is used to remove a small disc of bone for access to the frontal sinus. One or more catheters are advanced into the sinus to facilitate drainage. The catheters are left in place and subcutaneous tissue and skin closed around the catheters.

31075

31075   Sinusotomy frontal; transorbital, unilateral (for mucocele or osteoma, Lynch type)

A unilateral frontal sinusotomy is performed by a transorbital approach to remove a mucocele, osteoma, or other mass lesion. This is also referred to as a Lynch-type procedure. An incision is made immediately below the eyebrow on the affected side. The incision is carried down through the subcutaneous tissue to the periosteum. Tissues are then elevated off the underlying frontal bone. An oscillating saw or drill is used to cut through the bone immediately over the frontal sinus. The bone may be left hinged on one side or removed entirely. The mucocele, osteoma, or other mass lesion is located and removed. The bone flap is replaced and secured with plates and screws. Soft tissues and skin are closed in layers.

31080-31085

31080   Sinusotomy frontal; obliterative without osteoplastic flap, brow incision (includes ablation)
31081   Sinusotomy frontal; obliterative, without osteoplastic flap, coronal incision (includes ablation)
31084   Sinusotomy frontal; obliterative, with osteoplastic flap, brow incision
31085   Sinusotomy frontal; obliterative, with osteoplastic flap, coronal incision

Obliterative frontal sinusotomy is less common today, but was performed in the past for intractable frontal sinusitis. It may still be performed for failed endoscopic treatment,

Respiratory System

mucopyocele, late complications of previous open obliteration procedures or failed open obliteration. In 31080, the procedure is performed through a brow incison without an osteoplastic flap. A skin incision just below the eyebrow in the medial aspect is made and carried down through subcutaneous tissue and periosteum. The medial floor of the sinus is opened using a burr and the opening enlarged to allow passage of surgical instruments. The frontal sinus mucosa is elevated and removed in its entirety using a drill and the aid of an endoscope. When the mucosa has been completely ablated, the frontal sinus ostium is plugged with cellulose or other material and the sinus is completely obliterated by filling the cavity with abdominal fat. In 31081, the procedure is performed through a coronal incision without an osteoplastic flap. An incision is made along the hairline and a burr is used to access the medial aspect of the upper wall of the frontal sinus. The sinus is then obliterated as described in 31080. In 31084, the procedure is performed through a brow incision with an osteoplastic flap. An incision is made immediately below the eyebrow, carried across the upper aspect of the nose and extended below the other eyebrow (seagull shaped incision). The incision is carried down through the subcutaneous tissue to the periosteium. Tissues are then elevated off the underlying frontal bone. An oscillating saw or drill is used to cut through the bone immediately over the frontal sinus. The bone may be left hinged on one side or removed entirely. The sinus is then obliterated as described above. The bone flap is replaced and secured with plates and screws. Soft tissues and skin are closed in layers. In 31085, the procedure is performed through a coronal incision beginning at one ear and carried along the hairline to the opposite ear. The incision is carried down through the skin and soft tissues. The superficial layer of the temporalis fascia is elevated along with the fat pad taking care to protect the facial nerve branches. The frontal bone is opened along the superior termporal line and elevated anteriorly along the supraorbital rim and nasofrontal suture and the frontal sinus exposed. The frontal sinus is obliterated as described above. The bone flap is replaced and secured with plates and screws. Soft tissues and skin are closed in layers.

31086-31087

31086   Sinusotomy frontal; nonobliterative, with osteoplastic flap, brow incision
31087   Sinusotomy frontal; nonobliterative, with osteoplastic flap, coronal incision

In 31086, the nonobliterative frontal sinusostomy is performed through a brow incision with an osteoplastic flap. An incision is made immediately below the eyebrow, carried across the upper aspect of the nose and extended below the other eyebrow (seagull shaped incision). The incision is carried down through the subcutaneous tissue to the periosteum. Tissues are then elevated off the underlying frontal bone. An oscillating saw or drill is used to cut through the bone immediately over the frontal sinus. The bone may be left hinged on one side or removed entirely. All purulent material and diseased tissue is removed. The mucosa is completely ablated. The bone flap is replaced and secured with plates and screws. Soft tissues and skin are closed in layers. In 31087, the procedure is performed through a coronal incision beginning at one ear and carried along the hairline to the opposite ear. The incision is carried down through the skin and soft tissues. The superficial layer of the temporalis fascia is elevated along with the fat pad taking care to protect the facial nerve branches. The frontal bone is opened along the superior temporal line and elevated anteriorly along the supraorbital rim and nasofrontal suture and the frontal sinus exposed. Purulent material and diseased tissue is removed. The mucosa is completely ablated. The bone flap is replaced and secured with plates and screws. Soft tissues and skin are closed in layers.

31090

31090   Sinusotomy, unilateral, 3 or more paranasal sinuses (frontal, maxillary, ethmoid, sphenoid)

Unilateral sinusotomies are performed on three or more of the paranasal sinuses which include the frontal, maxillary, ethmoid, and sphenoid. The frontal sinuses are located in the frontal bone (forehead) and there is one on each side. The maxillary sinuses are located in the maxilla (cheek bones) and there is one on each side. The ethmoid sinuses are located in the skull behind the nose and between the eyes and are composed of 6-12 small sinuses or cells on each side. The sphenoid sinus is the most posterior of all the paranasal sinuses, located in the center of the skull base with one sinus on each side. There are a number of approaches that can be used to access each of these sinuses. Unilateral access to the frontal sinuses is typically accomplished by a transorbital approach. The maxillary sinuses may be accessed using an intranasal approach or an intraoral approach through the canine fossa. The ethmoid sinuses may be accessed using an intranasal or extranasal approach. There are three open approaches that are used for access to the sphenoid sinuses, transpalatal approach, transnasal transseptal approach, and external transorbital transethmoidal approach. Three or more of these sinuses on one side (unilateral) are explored and purulent material, diseased tissue, or mucoceles removed.

31200-31201

31200   Ethmoidectomy; intranasal, anterior
31201   Ethmoidectomy; intranasal, total

An intranasal ethmoidectomy is performed. In 31200, diseased tissue is removed in the anterior ethmoid cells. Topical vasoconstrictive agents are appled to the nasal mucosa and a local anesthetic is injected. The sinus ostium (opening) is accessed by moving the middle

turbinate forward. A curette is inserted through the ostium and inflamed and diseased tissue removed. All mucosal tissue in the anterior cells is removed (ablated) down to the bone. In 31201, a total ethmoidectomy is performed which involves removal of diseased tissue from both the anterior and posterior ethmoid cells. The sinus ostium (opening) is accessed by moving the middle turbinate forward. The uncinate process is removed using a curette. The anterior sinuses are cleared of inflamed and diseased tissue. The posterior cells are opened using blunt forceps and inflamed and diseased tissue removed using a curette. All mucosal tissue in the anterior and posterior ethmoid cells is removed (ablated) down to bone.

31205

31205   Ethmoidectomy; extranasal, total

An extranasal total ethmoidectomy is performed. The ethmoid sinus is approached by lateral rhinotomy which involves making an incision along the side of the nose and then drilling through the bone to access the anterior and posterior ethmoid cells. The ethmoid cells are inspected and purulent material and mucoceles evacuated. The mucosa is then removed (ablated) down to the bone. If the ethmoid ostiu is obstructed, an opening is created into the nasal cavity to allow drainage of fluid from the ethmoid cells.

31225-31230

31225   Maxillectomy; without orbital exenteration
31230   Maxillectomy; with orbital exenteration (en bloc)

The physician performs a maxillectomy with or without en bloc orbital exenteration. This type of radical maxillectomy is typically performed for malignant tumors of the maxillary sinus. Orbital structures are removed when the tumor has invaded the periorbital region. In 31225, a maxillectomy is performed with orbital preservation. The maxillary sinus is exposed using a lateral rhinotomy or intraoral approach through the canine fossa depending on the location of the mass. Mucosa and bone of the maxillary sinus are completely resected (removed). The orbital floor is reconstructed. In 31230, the procedure is performed with en bloc orbital exenteration. The maxillectomy is performed as described above. Traction sutures are placed posterior to the margins of the closed lids. An incision is made in the superior aspect through the skin of the eyelid behind the eye lashes. The full-thickness skin incision is carried around the entire circumference of the eye and includes the skin around the outer and inner canthi. The incision is carried through the subcutaneous tissues and into the periosteum around the orbital rim. Periorbital elevators are used to free the periosteum from underlying bone. The eyeball and the entire contents of the orbit are removed en bloc. The skin above and below the eye socket is approximated with sutures.

31231

31231   Nasal endoscopy, diagnostic, unilateral or bilateral (separate procedure)

A topical nasal decongestant and local anesthetic with a vasoconstrictor are applied as needed. A nasal telescope, rigid endoscope, or flexible endoscope is inserted into the nose. The nasal cavity is inspected for disease or abnormalities beginning at the vestibule, proceeding to the floor and inferior meatus, and then to the inferior choana. The sphenoethmoid recess is examined if it is accessible. The frontal recess, middle and superior meatus, middle and superior choana, internal nares, and nasopharynnx may also be examined. The endoscopic exam may be supplemented by a camera with images displayed on a video monitor, recorded on a VCR, or made digitally.

31233

31233   Nasal/sinus endoscopy, diagnostic with maxillary sinusoscopy (via inferior meatus or canine fossa puncture)

The maxillary sinuses are the largest of the paranasal sinuses and are located on either side of the nose in the body of the maxilla. The inferior meatus is one of four passages in the nasal cavity lying just below the inferior concha. The canine fossa is a depression at the front of the maxilla below the infraorbital opening and to the side of the elevation made by the socket of the canine tooth. A topical nasal decongestant and local anesthetic with a vasoconstrictor are applied as needed. The inferior meatus of the nasal cavity is punctured or a trocar is placed through the anterior face of the maxilla at the canine fossa. The endoscope is introduced and the nasal cavity and maxillary sinus are evaluated for disease or abnormalities. The endoscopic exam may be supplemented by a camera with images displayed on a video monitor, recorded on a VCR, or made digitally.

31235

31235   Nasal/sinus endoscopy, diagnostic with sphenoid sinusoscopy (via puncture of sphenoidal face or cannulation of ostium)

A diagnostic nasal endoscopy with sphenoid sinusoscopy via puncture of the sphenoid face or cannulation of the ostium is performed. The sphenoid sinuses are paired sinuses on each side of the head within the sphenoid bone that communicate with the upper posterior nasal cavity or sphenoethmoidal recess. A topical nasal decongestant and local anesthetic with a vasoconstrictor are applied as needed. The endoscope is introduced and the nasal cavity evaluated for disease or abnormalities. The vomer and face of the sphenoid sinus is visualized. The sphenoid sinus may be entered medial to the middle turbinate by enlargement and cannulation of the natural ostium or by puncture of the sphenoidal face (sphenoidotomy). The sphenoidal sinus is evaluated for disease or abnormalities. The endoscopic exam may be supplemented by a camera with images displayed on a video monitor, recorded on a VCR, or made digitally.

31237

31237   Nasal/sinus endoscopy, surgical; with biopsy, polypectomy or debridement (separate procedure)

A topical nasal decongestant and local anesthetic with a vasoconstrictor are applied as needed. An endoscope is introduced through the nose. The nasal cavity and paranasal sinuses are inspected for disease or abnormalities. Tissue samples may be taken and sent to the laboratory. Any polyps are removed using a suction device, grasping forceps, or a microdebrider. Debris and devitalized tissue are removed from the nasal cavity and the maxillary, ethmoid, and sphenoid sinuses. Bleeding is controlled using nasal packing. Plastic splints may be placed in the nose to facilitate healing. The endoscopic exam may be supplemented by a camera with images displayed on a video monitor, recorded on a VCR, or made digitally.

31238

31238   Nasal/sinus endoscopy, surgical; with control of nasal hemorrhage

A topical nasal decongestant and local anesthetic with a vasoconstrictor are applied as needed. An endoscope is introduced through the nose. The nasal cavity is inspected and bleeding sites are identified. Bleeding is controlled using cautery and nasal packing. The endoscopic exam may be supplemented by a camera with images displayed on a video monitor, recorded on a VCR, or made digitally.

31239

31239   Nasal/sinus endoscopy, surgical; with dacryocystorhinostomy

This procedure is done when the nasolacrimal duct is blocked and the flow of tears needs to be restored through the creation of a new tear duct canal. A topical nasal decongestant and local anesthetic with a vasoconstrictor are applied as needed. A fiberoptic light probe is introduced through the upper or lower canaliculus and passed into the lacrimal sac. An endoscope is introduced through the nose and the light probe is located endoscopically on the lateral wall of the nose and its position is noted. A small circle of mucosa is removed at the site of transillumination and the underlying bone is exposed. A portion of the uncinate process may be removed to gain access to the underlying bone, which is removed using a drill or YAG laser. The light probe is removed and replaced with a metal probe. Tenting of the medial wall of the lacrimal sac is observed with the nasal endoscope and the lacrimal sac is opened using cutting forceps. The opening is enlarged to approximately 1 cm. Stents attached to silastic tubing are inserted through the upper and lower canaliculi and the stent is passed into the nose, and removed from the tubing, then the tubing is secured forming a continuous loop around the canaliculi.

31240

31240   Nasal/sinus endoscopy, surgical; with concha bullosa resection

Concha bullosa is a condition where the middle turbinate becomes filled with air (pneumatized), interfering with normal ventilation of the sinus ostia and causing recurrent sinusitis. A topical nasal decongestant and local anesthetic with a vasoconstrictor are applied as needed. An endoscope is introduced through the nose. The nasal cavity and paranasal sinuses are inspected for disease or abnormalities. Microscissors are introduced and a resection of the meatal surface of the middle turbinate is performed. Care is taken to preserve the lateral lamella to provide stability. Resection of the anterior and/or posterior portion of the middle turbinate may also be performed using microscissors.

31254-31255

31254   Nasal/sinus endoscopy, surgical; with ethmoidectomy, partial (anterior)
31255   Nasal/sinus endoscopy, surgical; with ethmoidectomy, total (anterior and posterior)

A surgical nasal/sinus endoscopy is performed with ethmoidectomy. A topical nasal decongestant and local anesthetic with a vasoconstrictor are applied as needed. An endoscope is introduced through the nose. The nasal cavity and paranasal sinuses are inspected for disease or abnormalities. In 31254, an anterior (partial) ethmoidectomy is performed. The anterior ethmoid cells are approached by first removing the uncinate process (uncinectomy). The lower lip of the hiatus semilunaris is then removed and the infundibulum exposed. The anterior wall of the bulla ethmoidalis is then removed to expose the anterior ethmoid cells. The anterior ethmoid cells are removed using through-cutting forceps or a microdebrider. In 31255, an anterior and posterior (complete) ethmoidectomy is performed. The anterior ethmoid cells are removed as described above. The posterior ethmoid cell is then accessed by first perforating the basal lamella in the middle turbinate. The basal lamella is dissected until the posterior ethmoid cell is exposed. Dissection is in an inferior direction taking care not to damage the sphenopalatine area. Superior bony

partitions of the posterior ethmoid cell are removed in a posterior to anterior direction using upbiting through-cutting forceps.

31256-31267

31256   Nasal/sinus endoscopy, surgical, with maxillary antrostomy
31267   Nasal/sinus endoscopy, surgical, with maxillary antrostomy; with removal of tissue from maxillary sinus

A surgical nasal/sinus endoscopy is performed with maxillary antrostomy. A topical nasal decongestant and local anesthetic with a vasoconstrictor are applied as needed. An endoscope is introduced through the nose. The nasal cavity and paranasal sinuses are inspected for disease or abnormalities. In 31256, the maxillary sinus is approached by first removing the uncinate process (uncinectomy). A maxillary ostium seeker is placed behind the uncinate process and the free edge displaced in an anterior direction. Upbiting forceps are used to grasp the uncinate process and the uncinate process is removed. A microdebrider is used to remove any remaining fragments of the uncinate process so that the natural maxillary sinus ostium can be visualized. The ostium seeker is placed through the ostium and the maxillary sinus ostium enlarged. Maxillary antrostomy is completed using through-cutting forceps. In 31267, a maxillary antrostomy is performed as described above followed by removal of tissue from the maxillary sinus. The diseased, moist tissue lining the maxillary sinus is removed using a microdebrider.

31276

31276   Nasal/sinus endoscopy, surgical with frontal sinus exploration, with or without removal of tissue from frontal sinus

A surgical nasal/sinus endoscopy is performed with exploration of the frontal sinus with or without the removal of any frontal sinus tissue. A topical nasal decongestant and local anesthetic with a vasoconstrictor are applied as needed. An endoscope is introduced through the nose. The nasal cavity and paranasal sinuses are inspected for disease or abnormalities. The superior and anterior ethmoid air cells in the frontal recess are opened. The nasofrontal duct or ostium is cleared of any obstruction. When the frontal sinus is reached, curved forceps are employed and the frontal sinus is explored. Diseased or infected tissue is removed as needed.

31287-31288

31287   Nasal/sinus endoscopy, surgical, with sphenoidotomy
31288   Nasal/sinus endoscopy, surgical, with sphenoidotomy; with removal of tissue from the sphenoid sinus

A surgical nasal/sinus endoscopy is performed with sphenoidotomy is performed. A topical nasal decongestant and local anesthetic with a vasoconstrictor are applied as needed. An endoscope is introduced through the nose. The nasal cavity and paranasal sinuses are inspected for disease or abnormalities. In 31287, the sphenoid sinus is approached endoscopically via a medial or lateral approach to the middle turbinate, via middle turbinate removal, or via a transseptal approach. In a medial approach to the middle turbinate, the endoscope is introduced into the middle turbinate and the middle turbinate is pushed laterally to expose the superior turbinate. A probe is then introduced into the superior turbinate and placed at the sphenoid ostium. The lower third of the superior turbinate is removed and the sphenoid sinus opened. The opening is enlarged. The sphenoid sinus is drained and specimens sent for culture and sensitivity. The sphenoid sinus is irrigated. In 31288, a spenoidotomy is performed as described above followed by removal of tissue from the sphenoid sinus. The diseased moist tissue lining the sphenoid sinus is removed using a microdebrider.

31290-31291

31290   Nasal/sinus endoscopy, surgical, with repair of cerebrospinal fluid leak; ethmoid region
31291   Nasal/sinus endoscopy, surgical, with repair of cerebrospinal fluid leak; sphenoid region

A surgical nasal/sinus endoscopy is performed with repair of a cerebrospinal fluid (CSF) leak in the ethmoid or sphenoid sinus. This condition is also referred to as CSF rhinorrhea. A topical nasal decongestant and local anesthetic with a vasoconstrictor are applied as needed. An endoscope is introduced through the nose. The nasal cavity and paranasal sinuses are inspected for disease or abnormalities. The site of the CSF leak is identified. The CSF leak is repaired using fat or muscle tissue to plug the defect. The fat or muscle plug is then covered with fascia. Large CSF leaks may require a cartilage autograft to further strengthen the repair. Code 31290 is used to report repair of a CSF leak in the ethmoid region which includes leaks through the cribiform plate. Code 31291 is used to report repair of a CSF leak in the sphenoid region.

Respiratory System

31292-31293

31292 Nasal/sinus endoscopy, surgical; with medial or inferior orbital wall decompression

31293 Nasal/sinus endoscopy, surgical; with medial orbital wall and inferior orbital wall decompression

A surgical nasal/sinus endoscopy is performed with decompression of the medial and/or inferior orbital wall. A topical nasal decongestant and local anesthetic with a vasoconstrictor are applied as needed. An endoscope is introduced through the nose. The nasal cavity and paranasal sinuses are inspected for disease or abnormalities. The ethmoidal air cells are cleared. The medial orbital wall is exposed and thinned out using a burr. Elevators are then used to open the medial orbital wall and the lamina papyracea is removed. The inferior orbital wall may also be removed. The lamina papyracea is followed to the roof of the maxillary sinus. The floor of the orbit (inferior orbital wall) is then removed in the same manner by first thinning the floor with a burr and then opening the floor using an elevator. Incisions in the orbital periosteum allow orbital fat to prolapse which provides additional decompression of orbital contents. Code 31292 is used when a medial or inferior orbital wall decompression is performed. Code 31293 is used when both the medial and inferior orbital walls are decompressed.

31294

31294 Nasal/sinus endoscopy, surgical; with optic nerve decompression

A surgical nasal/sinus endoscopy is performed with optic nerve decompression. A topical nasal decongestant and local anesthetic with a vasoconstrictor are applied as needed. An endoscope is introduced through the nose. The nasal cavity and paranasal sinuses are inspected for disease or abnormalities. The anterior and posterior ethmoid cells are cleared. The anterior wall of the sphenoid sinus is removed and the bony channel of the optic nerve is exposed. The optic nerve channel and the tip of the orbit are decompressed by using a burr in a posterior to anterior direction. Bony fragments or blood clot impinging on the optic nerve are removed to relieve pressure, thereby decompressing the nerve.

31295-31297

31295 Nasal/sinus endoscopy, surgical; with dilation of maxillary sinus ostium (eg, balloon dilation), transnasal or via canine fossa

31296 Nasal/sinus endoscopy, surgical; with dilation of frontal sinus ostium (eg, balloon dilation)

31297 Nasal/sinus endoscopy, surgical; with dilation of sphenoid sinus ostium (eg, balloon dilation)

Endoscopic dilation of the sinus ostium (opening) is performed to treat chronic sinusitis with obstruction of the sinus ostium. Dilating the ostium opens the sinus by compressing the mucosa and displacing bony structures and restoring normal sinus drainage. A topical nasal decongestant and local anesthetic with a vasoconstrictor are applied as needed. An endoscope is introduced through the nose and advanced to the affected paranasal sinus. Alternatively, for dilation of the maxillary sinus, the canine fossa may be punctured using a trocar. The canine fossa is a depression at the front of the maxilla below the infraorbital opening and to the side of the elevation made by the socket of the canine tooth. A guidewire catheter with a tiny balloon is introduced and advanced into the ostium of the blocked sinus. The balloon is inflated and deflated. The ostium is inspected with the endoscope. Inflation and deflation of the balloon is repeated until the ostium is adequately dilated. The endoscope is removed. Use 31295 for balloon dilation of the maxillary sinus ostium; use 31296 for dilation of the frontal sinus ostium; use 31297 for dilation of the sphenoid sinus ostium.

31300-31320

31300 Laryngotomy (thyrotomy, laryngofissure); with removal of tumor or laryngocele, cordectomy

31320 Laryngotomy (thyrotomy, laryngofissure); diagnostic

A laryngotomy, also referred to as a thyrotomy or laryngofissure, is performed to remove a tumor, a cystic dilation of the laryngeal saccule (laryngocele), or the vocal cord(s) (cordectomy). An incision is made in the skin over the thyroid cartilage. The thyroid cartilage is split in the midline with an oscillating saw. The larynx is exposed. The tumor is identified and excised with a margin of healthy tissue. If the vocal cord is involved, the entire vocal cord is removed along with a margin of healthy tissue. Removal of a laryngocele involves excision of the saccule at its neck. The surgical wound in the larynx is closed by suture. Code 31320 is used when a diagnostic laryngotomy is performed. The larynx is exposed as described above. The larynx is inspected and any disease or abnormalities noted. The surgical wound is closed by suture.

31360-31365

31360 Laryngectomy; total, without radical neck dissection

31365 Laryngectomy; total, with radical neck dissection

The physician removes the entire larynx (voice box). A horizontal incision is made in the skin of the neck at the level of the thyroid cartilage. Subplatysmal flaps are raised and the larynx is exposed and dissected free of surrounding tissue. The delphian node is removed,

the thyroid resected, the hyoid bone removed, and the thyroid cartilage skeletonized. The larynx is then entered with the site of entry dictated by the location and extent of the disease. The larynx is removed in its entirety. The surgical wound is closed. Following the removal of the larynx, a laryngostoma is created. A separate incision is made below the incision for the laryngectomy. The trachea is externalized and sutured to the skin at the sternal notch to create a permanent stoma is in the larynx through which the patient breathes. Code 31360 is used when total laryngectomy is performed without radical neck dissection (RND). Code 31365 is used when RND is also performed. RND is typically performed prior to the total laryngectomy. Lymph node groups levels I-V are dissected free of surrounding tissue and excised. The sternocleidomastoid muscle and the internal jugular vein are removed. The submandibular gland is removed. The anterior belly of the digastric muscle as well as the sternohyoid and sternothyroid muscles may also be removed.

31367-31368

31367 Laryngectomy; subtotal supraglottic, without radical neck dissection

31368 Laryngectomy; subtotal supraglottic, with radical neck dissection

The physician performs a subtotal, supraglottic laryngectomy (SGL). SGL is designed to remove cancer arising from the epiglottis, aryepiglottic folds, and the false vocal cords while preserving primary laryngeal functions, including airway protection, respiration, and phonation. A tracheostomy is performed prior to SGL taking care to keep the tracheostomy incision separate from the SGL incision. A horizontal incision is then made in the skin of the neck at the level of the thyroid cartilage. Subplatysmal flaps are raised. The suprahyoid muscles are released from the hyoid and the infrahyoid muscles divided. The greater conu is skeletonized bilaterally taking care to preserve the hypoglossal nerves. The thyroid is incised such that the true vocal cords are preserved. The pharynx is entered through the vallecula or contralateral pyriform sinus. The mucosa is incised anterior to the arytenoid. An incision is made perpendicularly across the aryepiglottic fold to the level of the ventricle and then turned in a horizontal direction and the larynx opened in a booklike fashion. The portion of the larynx containing the tumor is then removed. The surgical wound is closed by reapproximating the thyroid cartilage to the tongue base. Drains are placed and the skin incisions closed. Code 31367 is used when subtotal, subglottic laryngectomy is performed without radical neck dissection (RND). Code 31368 is used when RND is also performed. RND is typically performed prior to the laryngectomy procedure. Lymph node groups levels I-V are dissected free of surrounding tissue and excised. The sternocleidomastoid muscle and the internal jugular vein are removed. The submandibular gland is removed. The anterior belly of the digastric muscle as well as the sternohyoid and sternothyroid muscles may also be removed.

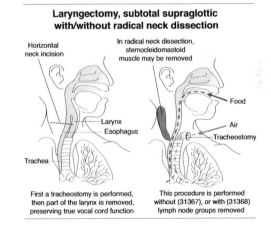

Laryngectomy, subtotal supraglottic with/without radical neck dissection

Horizontal neck incision

In radical neck dissection, sternocleidomastoid muscle may be removed

Food

Larynx
Esophagus

Air
Tracheostomy

Trachea

First a tracheostomy is performed, then part of the larynx is removed, preserving true vocal cord function

This procedure is performed without (31367), or with (31368) lymph node groups removed

31370-31382

31370 Partial laryngectomy (hemilaryngectomy); horizontal

31375 Partial laryngectomy (hemilaryngectomy); laterovertical

31380 Partial laryngectomy (hemilaryngectomy); anterovertical

31382 Partial laryngectomy (hemilaryngectomy); antero-latero-vertical

A partial laryngectomy, also referred to as a hemilaryngectomy is performed. Partial laryngectomy may be performed in a horizontal plane (31370) or vertical plane (31375, 31380, 31382). In the horizontal plane, the procedure is performed for supraglottic cancer involving only one side (unilateral). In the vertical plane, the procedure is performed for cancers of the anterior commissure, vocal processes of the arytenoid cartilage, or glottic cancer. Prior to the procedure, a tracheostomy may be performed for administration of anesthesia. In 31370, a horizontal hemilaryngectomy is performed. A transverse incision is made in the skin of the neck at the level of the thyroid cartilage. Subplatysmal flaps are raised. The suprahyoid muscles are released from the hyoid and the infrahyoid muscles divided. The greater conu is skeletonized bilaterally taking care to preserve the hypoglossal nerves. The thyroid is incised above the true vocal cords. The pharynx is entered through the vallecula or contralateral piriform sinus. The mucosa is incised anterior to the arytenoid. An incision is made perpendicularly across the aryepiglottic fold to the level of the ventricle

Respiratory System

and then turned in a horizontal direction and the larynx opened in a booklike fashion. The involved side of the larynx above the vocal cord is then removed. The surgical wound is closed by reapproximating the thyroid cartilage to the tongue base. Drains are placed and the skin incisions closed. In 31375, a latero-vertical hemilaryngectomy is performed which involves removal of part or all of one vocal cord up to but not including the anterior commissure. The neck is incised as described above with a vertical incision extending inferiorly from the midline of the transverse incision to allow adequate exposure in the vertical plane below the glottis. The larynx is entered below the glottis using a transverse incision through the cricothyroid membrane. The laryngeal incision is extended superiorly up to the thyroid notch. The physician then resects tissue from the midline back to the body of the arytenoid process and from the cricoid process to the vocal cord on the affected side. In 31380, an antero-vertical hemilaryngectomy is performed. The procedure is similar to 31375 except that additional tissue in the anterior aspect of the larynx is excised including the anterior commissure. Part of the contralateral vocal cord may also be excised. In 31382, an antero-latero-vertical hemilaryngectomy is performed. This procedure is the most extensive of the hemilaryngectomy procedures with resection of tissue on one side as described in 31375 along with the anterior commissure, the entire vocal cord on the opposite side, and underlying cartilage.

31390-31395

31390   Pharyngolaryngectomy, with radical neck dissection; without reconstruction
31395   Pharyngolaryngectomy, with radical neck dissection; with reconstruction

The physician performs a pharyngolaryngectomy with radical neck dissection (RND) with or without reconstruction. A pharyngolaryngectomy involves excision of the larynx (voice box) along with a portion of the pharynx. It is typically performed for laryngeal cancers that extend into or have metastasized to the pharynx. Less commonly a severe injury to the throat or neck or disease other than cancer may necessitate removal of the pharynx and larynx. A tracheostomy is performed prior to pharyngolaryngectomy for administration of anesthesia. A horizontal incision is then made in the skin of the neck at the level of the thyroid cartilage. Subplatysmal flaps are raised and the larynx is exposed and dissected free of surrounding tissue. The delphian node is removed, the thyroid resected, the hyoid bone removed, and the thyroid cartilage skeletonized. RND is typically performed prior to the total laryngectomy. Lymph node groups levels I-V are dissected free of surrounding tissue and excised. The sternocleidomastoid muscle and the internal jugular vein are removed. The submandibular gland is removed. The anterior belly of the digastric muscle as well as the sternohyoid and sternothyroid muscles may also be removed. The larynx is then entered with the site of entry dictated by the location and extent of the disease. The larynx is removed. An incision is made in the esophagus. The region of the pharynx to be resected is identified and excised. Following the removal of the pharynx and larynx, a tracheostoma is created. A separate incision is made below the incision for the pharyngolaryngectomy. The trachea is externalized and sutured to the skin at the sternal notch to create a permanent stoma in the larynx through which the patient breathes. In 31390, the pharynx and larynx are not reconstructed. A subsequent (staged) reconstruction procedure may be performed at a later date. In 31395, the pharynx and larynx are reconstructed during the same surgical session. An advancement flap from any remaining pharyngeal tissue and/or myocutaneous flaps are developed from the chest, back or forearm. If an advancement flap is used to close the pharynx, the lateral and posterior walls are mobilized and the edges are approximated and closed with sutures. Commonly used myocutaneous flaps include latissimus dorsi and pectoralis major. If a pectoralis major flap is used, the size of the defect is measured and the skin over the planned flap site marked. Vessels supplying the flap are identified. The skin and muscle are incised and the flap developed. The myocutaneous flap is rotated into the neck with the skin side facing inward. The flap is sutured to any remaining pharyngeal or laryngeal structures to close the defect. Overlying subcutaneous tissue and skin are then closed over the flap.

31400

31400   Arytenoidectomy or arytenoidopexy, external approach

An arytenoidectomy or arytenoidopexy is performed by an external approach. The term arytenoid refers to the cartilage and muscles of the larynx. Arytenoidectomy refers to an excision or laser vaporization of the arytenoid cartilage. Arytenoidopexy refers to fixation or suspension of the arytenoid cartilage. These procedures are performed to open the airway and improve breathing in patients with bilateral vocal cord paralysis. A horizontal skin incision is made over the larynx at the level of the cricothyroid membrane. A subplatysmal apron flap is created to the level of the thyroid notch and elevated. The strap muscles are divided in the midline and retracted laterally and the larynx exposed. The arytenoids and corniculate cartilage are exposed by incising the larynx and dissecting the overlying mucosa. If arytenoidectomy is performed, part or all of the arytenoid cartilage is then removed. If arytenoidopexy is performed, the cartilage is sutured to surrounding laryngeal tissue. The larynx is closed, a drain is placed in the neck, and overlying soft tissue and skin is closed in layers.

31420

31420   Epiglottidectomy

An epiglottidectomy is performed, which involves excision of part or all of the epiglottis. The epiglottis is located at the root of the tongue and covers the larynx when swallowing. It is composed of elastic fibrocartilage covered by mucous membrane. A horizontal skin incision is made in the neck at the level of the hyoid. Dissection is carried down through subcutaneous tissue. The platysma is incised and the hyoid exposed. Hyoid muscles are released. The pharynx is incised just above the hyoid and the vallecular space entered. The epiglottis is exposed and inspected. For removal of a lesion, the mucosa may be removed and the perichondrium stripped from the underlying fibrocartilage of the epiglottis. The pharynx is then closed in layers. Overlying muscle, soft tissue, and skin is then closed and a drain placed in the subplatysmal space.

31500

31500   Intubation, endotracheal, emergency procedure

The mouth is opened and any dentures are removed. A laryngoscope is passed into the hypopharynx and the glottis and vocal cords are visualized. A properly sized endotracheal tube is selected and the balloon is inflated. A stylet is inserted into the endotracheal tube and the tube and stylet are bent into a crescent shape. The endotracheal tube and stylet are inserted alongside the laryngoscope into the trachea and positioned with the balloon lying just beyond the vocal cords. The stylet is removed and the endotracheal tube is connected to the ventilation device and secured with tape. Breath sounds are checked using a stethoscope to ensure that the endotracheal tube is properly positioned.

31502

31502   Tracheotomy tube change prior to establishment of fistula tract

A tracheotomy tube is changed prior to establishment of a fistula tract. An obturator and inner cannula are selected that fit the outer cannula of the existing tracheotomy tube. The obturator is placed in the outer cannula. The cuff of the tube to be removed is deflated, the ties cut, and the tube and inner cannula removed. A new tube is immediately inserted while securely holding the obturator inside the outer cannula. Once the new tube has been inserted, the obturator is removed. The new tube is secured. The inner cannula is inserted and locked into place. The tracheotomy cuff is inflated.

31505-31512

31505   Laryngoscopy, indirect; diagnostic (separate procedure)
31510   Laryngoscopy, indirect; with biopsy
31511   Laryngoscopy, indirect; with removal of foreign body
31512   Laryngoscopy, indirect; with removal of lesion

The physician performs an indirect diagnostic laryngoscopy. The patient sits in a chair and is instructed to stick out his/her tongue. While holding down the tongue, the physician positions a small round mirror at the back of the throat, and shines a light into the mouth. The physician wears a head mirror that reflects light to the back of the throat. Alternatively, indirect laryngoscopy may be performed using a rigid endoscope. The vocal cords, tongue, and top of the throat are examined for signs of disease or injury. The patient may be asked to make a high pitched "eee" sound during the examination for better visualization of the vocal cords. In 31510, an indirect laryngoscopy with biopsy is performed. The vocal cords, tongue, and top of the throat are examined and a tissue sample is obtained. In 31511, an indirect laryngoscopy with removal of foreign body is performed. The foreign body is visualized, grasped with forceps and extracted. In 31512, an indirect laryngoscopy with removal of a lesion is performed. The lesion is identified by indirect laryngoscopy and removed in its entirety.

31513

31513   Laryngoscopy, indirect; with vocal cord injection

Vocal cord injection is performed to provide support to a vocal fold that lacks bulk or mobility caused by atrophy or paralysis. The patient sits in a chair and is instructed to stick out his/her tongue. While holding down the tongue, the physician positions a small round mirror at the back of the throat, and shines a light into the mouth. The physician wears a head mirror that reflects light to the back of the throat. Alternatively, indirect laryngoscopy may be performed using a rigid endoscope. The vocal cords, tongue, and top of the throat are examined for signs of disease or injury. The patient may be asked to make a high pitched sound during the examination for better visualization of the vocal cords. Using a curved needle inserted through the mouth, the vocal fold is then injected with a substance selected to treat the atrophy or paralysis. The vocal cord is visualized through the laryngoscope while being injected. When sufficient rebulking has been attained and/or when the vocal cord has moved medially, coming in contact with the opposite vocal cord for speaking, the needle is removed and the patient is asked to speak so that the effect of the injection procedure can be evaluated. Additional injection is performed as needed until the desired results are attained.

31515

31515   Laryngoscopy direct, with or without tracheoscopy; for aspiration

A direct laryngoscopy with or without tracheoscopy is performed for aspiration. A direct laryngoscope allows the physician to visualize structures directly using fiberoptics. There are two types of direct scopes, a rigid angled scope and a flexible scope. If a flexible scope is used, it is inserted through the nostril. If a rigid scope is used, it is inserted through the mouth. The nasopharynx, oral cavity, oropharynx, hypopharynx, and larynx are examined for evidence of abnormality or injury, such as lacerations, lesions, strictures, or other conditions. The scope may be advanced into the trachea which is also examined. The physician then aspirates fluid from the larynx or trachea which is sent to the laboratory for separately reportable tests.

31520-31526

31520   Laryngoscopy direct, with or without tracheoscopy; diagnostic, newborn
31525   Laryngoscopy direct, with or without tracheoscopy; diagnostic, except newborn
31526   Laryngoscopy direct, with or without tracheoscopy; diagnostic, with operating microscope or telescope

A direct laryngoscope allows the physician to visualize structures directly using fiberoptics. There are two types of direct scopes, a rigid angled scope and a flexible scope. If a flexible scope is used, it is inserted through the nostril. If a rigid scope is used, it is inserted through the mouth. The nasopharynx, oral cavity, oropharynx, hypopharynx, and larynx are examined for evidence of abnormality or injury, such as lacerations, lesions, strictures, or other conditions. The scope may be advanced into the trachea which is also examined. Use 31520 for a diagnostic laryngoscopy on a newborn and 31525 when the procedure is performed on a patient other than a newborn. Use 31526 when an operating microscope or telescope is also used at the time of the diagnostic laryngoscopy to provide better visualization and detailed examination of tissues, lesions, or other abnormalities.

31527

31527   Laryngoscopy direct, with or without tracheoscopy; with insertion of obturator

A direct laryngoscopy with insertion of an obturator with or without tracheoscopy is performed. A direct laryngoscope allows the physician to visualize structures directly using fiberoptics. There are two types of direct scopes, a rigid angled scope and a flexible scope. If a flexible scope is used, it is inserted through the nostril. If a rigid scope is used, it is inserted through the mouth. The nasopharynx, oral cavity, oropharynx, hypopharynx, and larynx are examined for evidence of abnormality or injury, such as lacerations, lesions, strictures, or other conditions. The scope may be advanced into the trachea which is then examined. The physician inserts an obturator to maintain an open airway.

31528-31529

31528   Laryngoscopy direct, with or without tracheoscopy; with dilation, initial
31529   Laryngoscopy direct, with or without tracheoscopy; with dilation, subsequent

A direct laryngoscope allows the physician to visualize structures directly using fiberoptics. There are two types of direct scopes, a rigid angled scope and a flexible scope. If a flexible scope is used, it is inserted through the nostril. If a rigid scope is used, it is inserted through the mouth. The nasopharynx, oral cavity, oropharynx, hypopharynx, and larynx are examined for evidence of abnormality or injury. The scope may be advanced into the trachea, which is examined. The site of the stenosis is identified and the length and width of the stricture is determined. Any areas of malacia or scarring (granulation tissue) are also identified. A dilation laryngoscope or tracheoscope is then advanced to the site of the stenosis and the conical tip is advanced through the stenotic region, left in place for 5 to 10 minutes, and then removed. Use 31528 for the initial dilation procedure and 31529 for subsequent procedures.

31530-31531

31530   Laryngoscopy, direct, operative, with foreign body removal
31531   Laryngoscopy, direct, operative, with foreign body removal; with operating microscope or telescope

A direct laryngoscope allows the physician to visualize structures directly using fiberoptics. There are two types of direct scopes, a rigid angled scope and a flexible scope. An insufflation catheter is placed through the nose and advanced into the hypopharynx to allow administration of anesthesia and oxygen. The oral cavity, oropharynx, hypopharynx, larynx, and trachea are examined with the direct laryngoscope. The foreign body is located and removed with forceps. If a sharp foreign body is embedded in the mucosa, it is grasped with the forceps, disengaged from the mucosa and carefully removed. An operating microscope or telescope may also be used during the procedure to locate the foreign body and to examine the mucosa for evidence of tearing or other injury following removal. Use 31530 when the procedure is performed without the use of an operating microscope or telescope and 31531 when an operating microscope and/or telescope are used.

31535-31536

31535   Laryngoscopy, direct, operative, with biopsy
31536   Laryngoscopy, direct, operative, with biopsy; with operating microscope or telescope

A direct laryngoscope allows the physician to visualize structures directly using fiberoptics. There are two types of direct scopes, a rigid angled scope and a flexible scope. The oral cavity, oropharynx, hypopharynx, larynx, and trachea are examined with the direct laryngoscope. The lesion is located and biopsy forceps used to obtain a tissue sample. An operating microscope and/or telescope may also be used during the procedure to allow better visualization and evaluation of the mucosa and any mucosal lesions. Use 31535 when the procedure is performed without the use of an operating microscope or telescope and 31536 when an operating microscope and/or telescope are used.

31540-31541

31540   Laryngoscopy, direct, operative, with excision of tumor and/or stripping of vocal cords or epiglottis
31541   Laryngoscopy, direct, operative, with excision of tumor and/or stripping of vocal cords or epiglottis; with operating microscope or telescope

A direct laryngoscope allows the physician to visualize structures directly using fiberoptics. There are two types of direct scopes, a rigid angled scope and a flexible scope. The oral cavity, oropharynx, hypopharynx, larynx, and trachea are examined with the direct laryngoscope. The tumor is located and excised along with a margin of healthy tissue. Alternatively, lesions on the vocal cords or epiglottis may be removed by stripping away the superficial tissue. An operating microscope and/or telescope may also be used during the procedure to allow better visualization and evaluation of the tumors or lesions and to allow more meticulous dissection of tissues. Use 31540 when the procedure is performed without the use of an operating microscope or telescope and 31541 when an operating microscope and/or telescope are used.

31545-31546

31545   Laryngoscopy, direct, operative, with operating microscope or telescope, with submucosal removal of non-neoplastic lesion(s) of vocal cord; reconstruction with local tissue flap(s)
31546   Laryngoscopy, direct, operative, with operating microscope or telescope, with submucosal removal of non-neoplastic lesion(s) of vocal cord; reconstruction with graft(s) (includes obtaining autograft)

A direct laryngoscope allows the physician to visualize structures directly using fiberoptics. There are two types of direct scopes, a rigid angled scope and a flexible scope. The oral cavity, oropharynx, hypopharynx, and trachea are examined with the direct laryngoscope. The vocal cords are visualized and the laryngoscope is suspended. An operating microscope and/or telescope are used to examine the lesion and determine its extent. A micro-knife and/or micro-scissors are used to incise the vocal cord tissue. Blunt and sharp dissection is used to separate and remove the lesion from surrounding healthy tissue. In 31545, the surgical defect is closed using a local tissue flap. A tissue flap is developed, trimmed and advanced or rotated over the surgical defect. The flap is secured with sutures. In 31546, the lesion involves deeper tissues and an autograft is used to reconstruct the soft tissue defect resulting from the removal of the lesion. A tissue graft such as fat is harvested from a remote site and prepared for transfer to soft tissue defect. The graft is placed beneath a mucosal flap, which is secured with sutures.

31551-31554

● **31551   Laryngoplasty; for laryngeal stenosis, with graft, without indwelling stent placement, younger than 12 years of age**
● **31552   Laryngoplasty; for laryngeal stenosis, with graft, without indwelling stent placement, age 12 years or older**
● **31553   Laryngoplasty; for laryngeal stenosis, with graft, with indwelling stent placement, younger than 12 years of age**
● **31554   Laryngoplasty; for laryngeal stenosis, with graft, with indwelling stent placement, age 12 years or older**

A procedure is performed to correct laryngeal stenosis, characterized by partial or circumferential airway narrowing of the supraglottis, glottis, or subglottis. Congenital laryngeal stenosis is most commonly found in the subglottic area caused by failure of the laryngeal lumen to recanalize after the epithelial lamina forms. The stenosis may be membranous, circumferential and symmetric, or cartilaginous with deformity of the cricoid cartilage or tracheal ring protruding symmetrically or asymmetrically into the lumen. Congenital laryngeal webs are most often in the glottis. Acquired laryngeal stenosis may be caused by trauma during endotracheal intubation, gastroesophageal reflux, infection, autoimmune disorders, malignancy, amyloidosis, inhalation burns, or radiation. Symptoms include inspiratory or biphasic stridor, apnea, tachypnea, dyspnea, voice hoarseness, aphonia, and dysphagia. Laryngoplasty is done to develop an adequate airway with voice preservation or quality improvement. With an endotracheal tube in place, an incision is made at the level of the larynx to expose the thyroid cartilage. Using a burr, a window is drilled in the cartilage posterior to the midline above the lower edge of the thyroid. The

Respiratory System

perichondrium is undermined posterior and inferior to the window and an endoscope is used to visualize the larynx, including the glottis and cricoarytenoid joints. The area of stenosis is dissected to remove membranous webs or tissue and excess cartilage. A graft is fashioned from autogenous costal cartilage, auricular cartilage, thyroid cartilage or buccal mucosa obtained during a separately reported procedure and sutured in place. A stent made of molded silicone or Teflon may be placed in the airway to secure the graft and expand the reconstructed area and/or an endotracheal tube may be left in place to stent the airway. The endoscope is removed and the incision is closed. Codes 31551 and 31552 report laryngoplasty with graft but without stent placement in a patient younger than 12 years of age (31551) or age 12 years and older (31552). Codes 31553 and 31554 report laryngoplasty with graft and indwelling stent placement in a patient younger than 12 years of age (31553) or age 12 years and older (31554).

31560-31561

31560 Laryngoscopy, direct, operative, with arytenoidectomy
31561 Laryngoscopy, direct, operative, with arytenoidectomy; with operating microscope or telescope

The term arytenoid refers to the cartilage and muscles of the larynx. Arytenoidectomy refers to an excision or laser vaporization of the arytenoid cartilage with laser vaporization being the preferred technique. This procedure is performed to open the airway and improve breathing in patients with bilateral vocal cord paralysis. A direct laryngoscope allows the physician to visualize structures directly using fiberoptics. There are two types of direct scopes, a rigid angled scope and a flexible scope. The oral cavity, oropharynx, hypopharynx, larynx, and trachea are examined with the direct laryngoscope. The larynx is exposed and a suspension device employed to achieve adequate exposure of the glottis. The mucosa overlying the arytenoids and corniculate cartilage is vaporized with a laser to expose the arytenoids. Part of all of the arytenoid cartilage is then vaporized. An operating microscope and/or telescope may also be used during the procedure to allow better visualization and more meticulous vaporization of tissues. Use 31560 when the procedure is performed without the use of an operating microscope or telescope and 31561 when an operating microscope and/or telescope are used.

31570-31571

31570 Laryngoscopy, direct, with injection into vocal cord(s), therapeutic
31571 Laryngoscopy, direct, with injection into vocal cord(s), therapeutic; with operating microscope or telescope

This procedure, also referred to as injection medialization laryngoplasty, is performed to treat vocal cord atrophy or paralysis. A direct laryngoscope allows the physician to visualize structures directly using fiberoptics. There are two types of direct scopes, a rigid angled scope and a flexible scope. The oral cavity, oropharynx, hypopharynx, larynx, and trachea are examined with the direct laryngoscope. The vocal cords are visualized and the laryngoscope is suspended. An operating microscope and/or telescope may be used to examine the vocal cords and perform the injection procedure. The vocal cord is injected lateral to the thyroarytenoid muscle in the paraglottic space with a resorbable material for temporary treatment or an implant material for more permanent treatment. The injection bulks up the vocal cord and moves it to a more normal position. After the injection, the physician evaluates the patient and determines whether the desired result has been achieved or whether additional injections are required. The physician performs additional injections as needed. The procedure may be performed as a unilateral or bilateral procedure. Use 31570 when the procedure is performed without the use of an operating microscope or telescope and 31571 when an operating microscope and/or telescope are used.

31572

● **31572** Laryngoscopy, flexible; with ablation or destruction of lesion(s) with laser, unilateral

A procedure is performed using a flexible laryngoscope and laser to ablate or destroy one or more unilateral lesions including granulomas and polyps in the larynx/vocal cords. A topical anesthetic is instilled into the nasal cavity and onto the palate and posterior pharynx. A laryngoscope is introduced though the nose and topical anesthetic is dripped onto the base of the tongue and the larynx using fiberoptic guidance. The scope is withdrawn. After adequate anesthetic effect has been attained, the flexible laryngoscope with working channel is reinserted through the nose, advanced into the pharynx until the larynx and the lesion(s) are visualized. The laser fiber is advanced though the working channel and ablative energy is delivered to the lesion(s). Once the lesion(s) are adequately destroyed, the laser and scope are removed.

31573-31574

● **31573** Laryngoscopy, flexible; with therapeutic injection(s) (eg, chemodenervation agent or corticosteroid, injected percutaneous, transoral, or via endoscope channel), unilateral
● **31574** Laryngoscopy, flexible; with injection(s) for augmentation (eg, percutaneous, transoral), unilateral

A procedure is performed using a flexible laryngoscope to inject a material into a unilateral vocal fold for therapeutic purposes or augmentation. Therapeutic injection (31573) may be

performed to reduce vocal cord scars, edema, or muscle spasms. Augmentation (31574) may be used to treat unilateral paralysis or vocal cord bowing caused by muscle atrophy, paresis, or presbylaryngis. Materials injected may include steroids, chemodenervation agent (botulinum toxin), gelfoam, collagen, micronized AlloDerm, Teflon and calcium hydroxyapatite. A topical anesthetic is instilled into the nasal cavity and onto the palate and posterior pharynx. A laryngoscope is introduced though the nose and topical anesthetic is dripped onto the base of the tongue and the larynx using fiberoptic guidance. If a percutaneous injection is to be performed, the area of the neck over the thyroid is also injected to anesthetize the skin and deep tissue. The scope is withdrawn. After adequate anesthetic effect, a flexible laryngoscope with working channel is reinserted through the nose and advanced into the pharynx until the larynx and vocal cords are visualized. For a transoral approach, the needle is advanced through the mouth to the larynx/vocal cord and injection of the selected material is administered under endoscopic visualization and the needle is removed. For endoscopic injection, the needle is advanced through a working channel in the endoscope and the vocal cord is injected with the selected material and the needle is removed. For a percutaneous approach, a needle is inserted through the thyroid cartilage and thyrohyoid membrane and angled to reach the vocal cord. The selected material is then injected under endoscopic visualization and the needle is removed. After completion of the procedure, the flexible laryngoscope is removed.

31575-31577

▲ **31575** Laryngoscopy, flexible; diagnostic
▲ **31576** Laryngoscopy, flexible; with biopsy(ies)
▲ **31577** Laryngoscopy, flexible; with removal of foreign body(s)

A diagnostic laryngoscopy is performed using a flexible laryngoscope in 31575. A topical anesthetic is instilled into the nasal cavity and onto the palate and posterior pharynx. A laryngoscope is introduced though the nose and topical anesthetic is dripped onto the base of the tongue and the larynx using fiberoptic guidance. The scope is withdrawn. After adequate anesthetic effect has been attained, the flexible laryngoscope is reinserted through the nose, advanced into the pharynx and the vocal cords, tongue base, and hypopharynx are examined diagnostically for signs of disease or injury. The patient may be asked to sing or speak during the examination for better visualization of the vocal cords. In 31576, biopsy(ies) is performed. A fine biopsy instrument is advanced though the working channel of the scope and one or more tissue samples of suspicious areas are obtained and removed for pathological examination, taking care not to disturb normal tissue. In 31577, removal of foreign body(ies) is performed. The foreign body is visualized, grasped with forceps, and extracted through the scope.

31578

▲ **31578** Laryngoscopy, flexible; with removal of lesion(s), non-laser

A procedure is performed using a flexible laryngoscope to remove one or more unilateral lesions including granulomas and polyps in the larynx/vocal cords with non-laser excision. A topical anesthetic is instilled into the nasal cavity and onto the palate and posterior pharynx. A flexible laryngoscope is introduced though the nose and topical anesthetic is dripped onto the base of the tongue and the larynx using fiberoptic guidance. The scope is withdrawn. After adequate anesthetic effect has been attained, the flexible laryngoscope with working channel is reinserted through the nose, and advanced into the pharynx until the larynx and the lesion(s) are visualized. The micro cutting/extraction device is advanced though the working channel and used to excise and remove the lesion(s).

31579

▲ **31579** Laryngoscopy, flexible or rigid telescopic, with stroboscopy

The physician performs a flexible or rigid telescopic laryngoscopy with stroboscopy. A rigid laryngoscope is passed through the mouth or a flexible laryngoscope may be passed through the nose. The laryngoscope is used in conjunction with a tiny strobe light and video camera to obtain detailed magnified views of the vocal cords. The patient may be asked to sing or speak during the examination for better visualization of the vibrating vocal cords. The tongue and top of the throat are also examined for signs of disease or injury.

31580

▲ **31580** Laryngoplasty; for laryngeal web, with indwelling keel or stent insertion

A laryngeal web is an abnormal sheet of tissue that connects the vocal cords. The condition is usually congenital but may also be acquired following tracheostomy. Small tissue webs may be asymptomatic; however more extensive webs can cause voice changes and respiratory problems. If a previous tracheostomy has not been performed, a separately reportable tracheostomy is performed prior to the laryngoplasty. A horizontal incision is made above the tracheostoma through the plastysma to expose the cervical fascia. A subplastysmal flap is created to the level of the thyroid notch and elevated to allow adequate exposure of the vocal cords. The thyroid and cricoid cartilages and upper trachea are exposed by dividing the strap muscles in the midline and retracting them laterally. A midline laryngofissure incision is made and the vocal cords are exposed. The laryngeal web is divided. A laryngeal keel, which is a type of stent, is placed between the cut edges of the vocal cords to allow epithelialization of the cut edges and prevent reformation of the laryngeal web. The incision is closed in layers. Approximately three weeks later, the incision is reopened and the keel is removed.

31584

▲ **31584   Laryngoplasty; with open reduction and fixation of (eg, plating) of fracture, includes tracheostomy, if performed**

Laryngoplasty with open reduction and fixation of fracture is performed. Fracture of the larynx results from direct trauma to the neck region. A horizontal skin incision is made over the larynx at the level of the cricothyroid membrane. A subplatysmal apron flap is created to the level of the thyroid notch and elevated to allow adequate exposure of the larynx. The strap muscles are divided in the midline and retracted laterally and the larynx is exposed. Depending on the level of the fracture, the thyroid cartilage may need to be opened using an oscillating saw. The larynx is opened and the inside examined to determine the extent of the injury. Any vocal cord or mucosal lacerations are repaired with sutures. Laryngeal cartilage fractures are debrided and returned to normal anatomic position. The fracture site is immobilized with wire sutures, metal alloy miniplates, or absorbable miniplates. The neck incision is closed in layers. Any tracheotomy performed is included.

31587

▲ **31587   Laryngoplasty, cricoid split, without graft placement**

A laryngoplasty is performed using cricoid cartilage split technique without graft placement. The cricoid cartilage is a ring of cartilage that completely surrounds the trachea. This procedure is performed primarily to treat congenital subglottic stenosis due to a small cricoid ring. The patient is typically already intubated due to the stenosis. A horizontal skin incision is made over the larynx at the level of the cricothyroid membrane. A subplatysmal apron flap is created to the level of the thyroid notch and elevated to allow adequate exposure of the cricoid cartilage. The cricoid cartilage and upper trachea are exposed by dividing the strap muscles in the midline and retracting them laterally. A vertical midline incision is made through the inferior two-thirds of the thyroid cartilage, the cricoid, and the first two tracheal rings to relieve the stenosis. Incisions are closed with layers. The patient remains intubated throughout the procedure and for approximately 10 days following the procedure.

31590

31590   Laryngeal reinnervation by neuromuscular pedicle

Laryngeal reinnervation is performed using a neuromuscular pedicle. This procedure is used to treat unilateral vocal cord paralysis. Typical indications for the procedure include involvement of the superior and recurrent laryngeal nerves, a glottis defect less than 3-4 cm, and a bowed vocal cord. A horizontal skin incision is made in the neck at the level of the hyoid. Dissection is carried down through subcutaneous tissue. The platysma is incised and the hyoid exposed. A neuromuscular pedicle is harvested from the omohyoid muscle and consists of a 1 cm block of muscle enervated by the hypoglossal nerve. The thyrocartilage is incised and a window created on the affected side. The neuromuscular pedicle is placed into thyroarytenoid muscle and secured with sutures. The neck incision is closed in layers and drain placed as needed.

31591

● **31591   Laryngoplasty, medialization, unilateral**

Unilateral medialization laryngoplasty restores laryngeal function by moving the paralyzed vocal fold to the midline, allowing the vocal cords to close completely. Normal functioning vocal cords open during breathing and close during speech, coughing, and swallowing. Vocal cord paralysis may result from surgery, malignancy, trauma, neurologic disorders, or idiopathic causes. Symptoms of unilateral vocal cord paralysis include a weak, breathy quality to the voice and impairment of swallowing and cough reflexes that may lead to choking and/or aspiration of food and liquids. With the patient under sedation, the skin overlying the larynx is anesthetized and a small incision is made to expose the thyroid cartilage. Using a burr, a window is drilled in the cartilage posterior to the midline above the lower edge of the thyroid. The perichondrium is undermined posterior and inferior to the window and an endoscope is used to visualize the vocal cords. An implant fashioned from silastic block, Gore-Tex, or other similar material is contoured to fit three dimensionally along the medial-lateral, superior-inferior, and anterior-posterior spaces. The implant is positioned in place and the patient is awakened just enough to vocalize. Once the implant is sized appropriately, the patient is again sedated and the implant sutured in place. The endoscope is removed and the incision is closed.

31592

● **31592   Cricotracheal resection**

Cricotracheal resection is done to remove a narrowed, scarred section of airway just below the larynx with laryngeal reattachment to healthy tracheal tissue. Narrowing or scarring of the trachea may result from injury during intubation or tracheostomy, a tracheal tumor or other abnormal tissue growth, inflammatory disease, or radiation to the chest or neck. An endotracheal tube is inserted to deliver anesthesia and maintain a patent airway. A horizontal incision is made along the base of the neck (standard low collar line) and mucosal flaps are developed in the subplatysmal plane to expose the airway from the

hyoid bone superiorly to the manubrium inferiorly. The strap muscles are retracted and the thyroid isthmus is divided in the midline. The distal end of the stenosis is identified and the trachea is circumferentially mobilized to the inferior border of the cricoid cartilage. Using blunt dissection along the anterior wall of the trachea to the level of the aortic arch/carina allows for further mobilization of the trachea and reduces the tension of the anastomosis. The vascular supply is preserved with minimal lateral dissection. The cricoid muscle is then identified and reflected superiorly. The perichondrium on the upper and lower border of the cricoid cartilage is incised and the anterior segment is excised. Dissection continues along the inner aspect of the cricoid cartilage with careful preservation of the laryngeal nerves. The stenosis is excised from within the cricoid lumen while preserving the outer perichrondrium of the cricoid plate. The cricoid plate is thinned posteriorly. The distal and proximal margins of the stenosis are identified and the tissue is resected en bloc. The transected normal trachea is then telescoped into the posterior cricoid plate and sutured to the mucosal flap and thyroid cartilage. A T-tube may be inserted into the trachea to maintain a patent airway. The incision is closed in layers and chin to chest fixation sutures may be placed to prevent flexion of the neck during the first postoperative week.

31595

31595   Section recurrent laryngeal nerve, therapeutic (separate procedure), unilateral

A therapeutic unilateral section of the recurrent laryngeal nerve is performed in a separate procedure. This procedure is performed to treat spastic dysphonia, a severe vocal disability in which the vocal cords are spaced too closely together. Sectioning of the recurrent laryngeal nerve on one side causes nerve paralysis and retracts the involved vocal cord away from the midline resulting in improved voice quality. The skin of the neck is incised on the right or left side and soft tissues dissected. The right or left lobe of the thyroid is mobilized and the recurrent laryngeal nerve identified in the tracheoesophageal groove. The nerve is divided (sectioned). Overlying soft tissues and skin are then closed in layers.

31600-31610

31600   Tracheostomy, planned (separate procedure)
31601   Tracheostomy, planned (separate procedure); younger than 2 years
31603   Tracheostomy, emergency procedure; transtracheal
31605   Tracheostomy, emergency procedure; cricothyroid membrane
31610   Tracheostomy, fenestration procedure with skin flaps

The physician performs a planned tracheostomy on a patient two years or older (31600) or younger than two years (31601). The patient is positioned with the neck extended. Landmarks are identified and marked. A local anesthetic is injected along the planned incision line. The skin is incised and subcutaneous fat removed. Dissection continues down through the platysma until the midline raphe between the strap muscles is exposed. The strap muscles are separated and retracted to expose the pretracheal fascia and thyroid isthmus. The thyroid isthmus is retracted or divided as needed. Fascia is removed from the anterior face of the trachea. The trachea is incised in a T, H, or U shaped configuration and the trachea reflected. Stay sutures are placed. The tracheostomy tube is then inserted and secured with sutures. A tracheostomy collar is applied. In 31603, an emergency transtracheal tracheostomy is performed as described above. In 31605, an emergency cricothyroid membrane tracheostomy is peformed. The cricoid cartilage is palpated and an incision made horizontally above its superior border. The cricothyroid membrane is exposed and punctured at the midline with the blade directed inferiorly to prevent damage to the true vocal cords. The incision is widened and a cannula inserted for ventilation. In 31610, a tracheostomy is performed using a fenestration procedure with skin flaps. Following creation of the tracheostomy as described in 31600 and 31602, the anterior portion of the tracheal rings are removed to create a more permanent opening in the trachea. Skin flaps are then developed and sutured to the tracheal opening.

31611

31611   Construction of tracheoesophageal fistula and subsequent insertion of an alaryngeal speech prosthesis (eg, voice button, Blom-Singer prosthesis)

The physician constructs a tracheoesophageal (TE) fistula and subsequently inserts an alaryngeal speech prosthesis commonly known as a voice button or Blom-Singer prosthesis. A TE voice prosthesis allows patients who have undergone removal of the larynx (laryngectomy) to produce speech by shunting air from the lungs to the esophagus and vibrating esophageal tissue. A rigid bronchoscope is inserted into the pharynx. Using the bronchoscope for visualization and insertion of surgical tools, the posterior wall of the trachea is punctured along with the anterior wall of the esophagus to create a tract (fistula) between the two structures. The tract is dilated and a 16 French catheter inserted. The fistula is allowed to mature for approximately one week and then a tracheoesophageal prosthesis is inserted through an existing tracheostoma. Alternatively, the procedure can be performed at the time of the laryngectomy under direct visualization.

Respiratory System

31612

31612   Tracheal puncture, percutaneous with transtracheal aspiration and/or injection

A percutaneous tracheal puncture is performed for transtracheal aspiration and/or injection procedure. A small stab incision is made over the trachea at the level of the cricoid. A needle or catheter is then advanced through the thyroid and into the trachea. Fluid is aspirated and/or medication or other pharmacological substance injected. The needle or catheter is then withdrawn and the stab incision closed with sutures or an adhesive patch.

31613-31614

31613   Tracheostoma revision; simple, without flap rotation
31614   Tracheostoma revision; complex, with flap rotation

The physician revises an existing tracheostoma. This procedure is performed to treat stenosis of the stoma. In 31613, a simple revision is performed without flap rotation. The trachea is isolated for a length of 2-3 rings. The tracheostoma scar tissue causing the stenosis is then excised. In 31614, a complex revision is performed with flap rotation. Scar tissue is excised as described above. One or more skin flaps are then developed and inserted into the stoma. The skin and subcutaneous tissues are incised to create the flap. The incision in the trachea may be extended vertically. The skin flap is then sutured to the trachea.

31615

31615   Tracheobronchoscopy through established tracheostomy incision

A tracheobronchoscopy is performed through an established tracheostomy incision. The bronchoscope is inserted through the tracheostoma and into the trachea. The trachea is examined. The bronchoscope is then advanced into the main right and left bronchi which are also examined and any abnormalities are noted. The bronchoscope is withdrawn and the main right and left bronchi, carina, and trachea are again carefully inspected for evidence of disease or injury.

31622-31623

31622   Bronchoscopy, rigid or flexible, including fluoroscopic guidance, when performed; diagnostic, with cell washing, when performed (separate procedure)
31623   Bronchoscopy, rigid or flexible, including fluoroscopic guidance, when performed; with brushing or protected brushings

A bronchoscopy is performed with or without fluoroscopic guidance with or without cell washing (31622) or with brushing or protected brushings (31623). A rigid or flexible bronchoscope is inserted through the nose or mouth and advanced into the oropharynx under fluoroscopic guidance as needed. The oropharynx is examined. The vocal cords are visualized and examined. The bronchoscope is advanced into the trachea which is also examined before the scope is advanced into the right and left mainstem bronchi. Any abnormalities are noted. If a rigid bronchoscope is used, a telescope or flexible bronchoscope may be inserted through the rigid bronchoscope to visualize the distal segment of each mainstem bronchus. In 31622, if cell washing is performed, normal sterile saline solution is injected into the lung and aspirated to obtain cell samples. In 31623, a cytology brush is advanced through the scope and cell brushing is performed to obtain cell samples. Cell samples are sent to the laboratory for separately reportable cytology examination. The bronchoscope is withdrawn.

31624

31624   Bronchoscopy, rigid or flexible, including fluoroscopic guidance, when performed; with bronchial alveolar lavage

A rigid or flexible bronchoscope is inserted through the nose or mouth and advanced into the oropharynx with or without fluoroscopic guidance. The oropharynx is examined. The vocal cords are visualized and examined. The bronchoscope is then advanced into the trachea, which is also examined before the scope is advanced into each mainstem bronchus and any abnormalities are noted. If a rigid bronchoscope is used, a telescope or flexible bronchoscope may be inserted through the rigid bronchoscope to visualize the distal segment of each mainstem bronchus. Broncheoalveolar secretions from the lower respiratory tract are obtained by bronchial alveolar lavage (BAL). The bronchoscope is wedged into the subsegmental bronchus containing the lung lesion. If diffuse lung disease is present, the scope is wedged into the right middle lobe bronchus. Sterile normal saline is instilled through the scope and aspirated back into the specimen trap using suction.

31625

31625   Bronchoscopy, rigid or flexible, including fluoroscopic guidance, when performed; with bronchial or endobronchial biopsy(s), single or multiple sites

A rigid or flexible bronchoscope is inserted through the nose or mouth and advanced into the oropharynx with or without fluoroscopic guidance. The oropharynx is examined. The vocal cords are visualized and examined. The bronchoscope is then advanced into the trachea, which is also examined before the scope is advanced into each mainstem bronchus and any abnormalities are noted. If a rigid bronchoscope is used, a telescope or flexible bronchoscope may be inserted through the rigid bronchoscope to visualize the distal segment of each mainstem bronchus. Biopsy forceps are advanced and one or more bronchial or endobronchial tissue samples are obtained.

31626

31626   Bronchoscopy, rigid or flexible, including fluoroscopic guidance, when performed; with placement of fiducial markers, single or multiple

Fiducial markers are placed using a bronchoscope prior to stereotactic radiosurgical treatment of a thoracic tumor. A rigid or flexible bronchoscope is inserted through the nose or mouth and advanced into the oropharynx. Fluoroscopic guidance is used as needed. The oropharynx is examined. The vocal cords are visualized and examined. The bronchoscope is advanced into the trachea which is also examined before the scope is advanced into the right and left mainstem bronchi. Any abnormalities are noted. If a rigid bronchoscope is used, a telescope or flexible bronchoscope may be inserted through the rigid bronchoscope to visualize the distal segment of each mainstem bronchus. A sterile gold fiducial marker is placed in a specially designed transbronchial needle composed of a needle and sheath. The needle containing the fiducial marker is then retracted into the sheath and the sheath passed through the working chamber of the bronchoscope to the desired location. The needle and fiducial marker are then unsheathed, passed into the tumor, and the fiducial marker is deployed. This is repeated until all fiducial markers have been placed.

31627

31627   Bronchoscopy, rigid or flexible, including fluoroscopic guidance, when performed; with computer-assisted, image-guided navigation (List separately in addition to code for primary procedure[s])

Navigated bronchoscopy uses a computer-assisted, image-guided navigation system to help perform the primary bronchoscopy procedure. In a separately reportable bronchoscopy procedure, a rigid or flexible bronchoscope is inserted through the nose or mouth and advanced into the oropharynx. Fluoroscopic guidance is used as needed. The oropharynx is examined. The vocal cords are visualized and examined. The bronchoscope is advanced into the trachea which is also examined before the scope is advanced into the right and left mainstem bronchi. Any abnormalities are noted. If a rigid bronchoscope is used, a telescope or flexible bronchoscope may be inserted through the rigid bronchoscope to visualize the distal segment of each mainstem bronchus. During the procedure, the navigation system uses computer data and images to track the position and orientation of the bronchoscope and surgical tools in relation to lesions or defects identified during the examination of the airways. The computer system registers data related to anatomic landmarks allowing the physician more precision and accuracy during the performance of the primary bronchoscopy procedure.

31628

31628   Bronchoscopy, rigid or flexible, including fluoroscopic guidance, when performed; with transbronchial lung biopsy(s), single lobe

A rigid or flexible bronchoscope is inserted through the nose or mouth and advanced into the oropharynx with or without fluoroscopic guidance. The oropharynx is examined. The vocal cords are visualized and examined. The bronchoscope is then advanced into the trachea, which is also examined before the scope is advanced into each mainstem bronchus and any abnormalities are noted. If a rigid bronchoscope is used, a telescope or flexible bronchoscope may be inserted through the rigid bronchoscope to visualize the distal segment of each mainstem bronchus. Tiny transbronchial biopsy forceps are passed out of the bronchoscope into the smaller bronchi and tissue samples are obtained from the outer part of the lung. One or more tissue samples may be obtained from a single lobe.

31629

31629   Bronchoscopy, rigid or flexible, including fluoroscopic guidance, when performed; with transbronchial needle aspiration biopsy(s), trachea, main stem and/or lobar bronchus(i)

A rigid or flexible bronchoscope is inserted through the nose or mouth and advanced into the oropharynx with or without fluoroscopic guidance. The oropharynx is examined. The vocal cords are visualized and examined. The bronchoscope is then advanced into the trachea, which is also examined before the scope is advanced into each mainstem bronchus and any abnormalities are noted. If a rigid bronchoscope is used, a telescope or flexible bronchoscope may be inserted through the rigid bronchoscope to visualize the distal segment of each mainstem bronchus. A catheter with a flexible needle tip is introduced to perform transbronchial needle aspiration (TBNA) biopsy of the trachea, main stem bronchus, or lobar bronchus. The TBNA needle is passed through the trachea or bronchus to the biopsy site. Suction is applied while the needle is agitated back and forth across the tissue or lesion to sheer off cells for biopsy(s) and the catheter is withdrawn.

Respiratory System

● New Code   ▲ Revised Code

31630-31631

31630 Bronchoscopy, rigid or flexible, including fluoroscopic guidance, when performed; with tracheal/bronchial dilation or closed reduction of fracture

31631 Bronchoscopy, rigid or flexible, including fluoroscopic guidance, when performed; with placement of tracheal stent(s) (includes tracheal/bronchial dilation as required)

A rigid or flexible bronchoscope is inserted through the nose or mouth and advanced into the oropharynx with or without fluoroscopic guidance. The oropharynx is examined. The vocal cords are visualized and examined. The bronchoscope is advanced into the trachea and it is examined. The site of the tracheal fracture or stenosis is identified. If a rigid bronchoscope is used, the fracture or stenosis can be treated directly with the rigid bronchoscope. The tracheal fracture is reduced (returned to normal position) or the narrowed (stenosed) area is dilated as the rigid bronchoscope is passed through the trachea. If complete reduction or opening of the stenotic site is not achieved by the first pass of the bronchoscope, serially larger rigid bronchoscopes are passed until the cartilage rings in the trachea are in correct anatomical position or the stenotic site is enlarged. If a flexible bronchoscope is used, a balloon catheter is inserted to reduce the fracture or dilate the stenosis. The balloon is serially inflated and deflated until the fracture is reduced or the stenotic site enlarged. Use 31631 if a stent is placed following dilation to maintain an open airway. A stent delivery catheter or other stent delivery device is advanced through the bronchoscope to the site of the obstruction or stenosis. The stent is placed at the site of the tracheal fracture or stenosis to maintain an open airway.

31632

31632 Bronchoscopy, rigid or flexible, including fluoroscopic guidance, when performed; with transbronchial lung biopsy(s), each additional lobe (List separately in addition to code for primary procedure)

A rigid or flexible bronchoscope is inserted through the nose or mouth and advanced into the oropharynx with or without fluoroscopic guidance. The oropharynx is examined. The vocal cords are visualized and examined. The bronchoscope is then advanced into the trachea, which is also examined before the scope is advanced into each mainstem bronchus and any abnormalities are noted. If a rigid bronchoscope is used, a telescope or flexible bronchoscope may be inserted through the rigid bronchoscope to visualize the distal segment of each mainstem bronchus. Tiny transbronchial biopsy forceps are passed out of the bronchoscope into the smaller bronchi and tissue samples are obtained from the outer part of the lung. This procedure reports one or more tissue samples obtained from each additional lobe following the primary tissue sample(s) taken from the first lobe (reported separately).

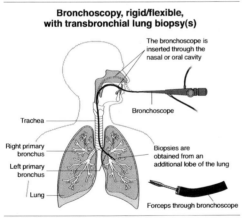

Bronchoscopy, rigid/flexible, with transbronchial lung biopsy(s)

The bronchoscope is inserted through the nasal or oral cavity.

Bronchoscope

Trachea

Right primary bronchus

Left primary bronchus

Lung

Biopsies are obtained from an additional lobe of the lung

Forceps through bronchoscope

31633

31633 Bronchoscopy, rigid or flexible, including fluoroscopic guidance, when performed; with transbronchial needle aspiration biopsy(s), each additional lobe (List separately in addition to code for primary procedure)

A rigid or flexible bronchoscope is inserted through the nose or mouth and advanced into the oropharynx with or without fluoroscopic guidance. The oropharynx is examined. The vocal cords are visualized and examined. The bronchoscope is then advanced into the trachea, which is also examined before the scope is advanced into each mainstem bronchus and any abnormalities are noted. If a rigid bronchoscope is used, a telescope or flexible bronchoscope may be inserted through the rigid bronchoscope to visualize the distal segment of each mainstem bronchus. A catheter with a flexible needle tip is introduced to perform transbronchial needle aspiration (TBNA) biopsy of the trachea, main stem bronchus, or lobar bronchus. The TBNA needle is passed through the trachea or bronchus to the biopsy site. Suction is applied while the needle is agitated back and forth across the tissue or lesion to sheer off cells for biopsy(s) and the catheter is withdrawn.

This procedure reports one or more tissue samples obtained from each additional lobe following the primary tissue sample(s) taken from the first lobe (reported separately).

31634

31634 Bronchoscopy, rigid or flexible, including fluoroscopic guidance, when performed; with balloon occlusion, with assessment of air leak, with administration of occlusive substance (eg, fibrin glue), if performed

A rigid or flexible bronchoscope is inserted through the nose or mouth and advanced into the oropharynx. Fluoroscopic guidance is used as needed. The oropharynx, vocal cords, and trachea are examined as the fluoroscope is advanced. The mainstem bronchus is examined. If a rigid bronchoscope is used, a telescope or flexible bronchoscope may be inserted through the rigid bronchoscope to visualize the distal segment of the mainstem bronchus. The site of the air leak is identified. A balloon catheter is introduced. The balloon is inflated at the site of the air leak. The leak is occluded and then evaluated. Closure of the air leak may be attempted using fibrin sealant or glue, gelfoam, silicone plug, albumin gluteraldehyde tissue adhesive, or other substance. The bronchoscope is withdrawn and a more thorough examination of the bronchus, trachea, vocal cords, and oropharynx is performed as the bronchoscope is withdrawn.

31635

31635 Bronchoscopy, rigid or flexible, including fluoroscopic guidance, when performed; with removal of foreign body

A rigid or flexible bronchoscope is inserted through the nose or mouth and advanced into the oropharynx with or without fluoroscopic guidance and a foreign body is removed. The oropharynx is examined. The vocal cords are visualized and examined. The bronchoscope is then advanced into the trachea, which is also examined before the scope is advanced into each mainstem bronchus and any abnormalities are noted. If a rigid bronchoscope is used, a telescope or flexible bronchoscope may be inserted through the rigid bronchoscope to visualize the distal segment of each mainstem bronchus. Once the foreign body is visualized, extraction forceps are advanced, and the foreign body is grasped and extracted. The bronchus is then re-examined to verify that all foreign body remnants have been removed.

31636-31637

31636 Bronchoscopy, rigid or flexible, including fluoroscopic guidance, when performed; with placement of bronchial stent(s) (includes tracheal/bronchial dilation as required), initial bronchus

31637 Bronchoscopy, rigid or flexible, including fluoroscopic guidance, when performed; each additional major bronchus stented (List separately in addition to code for primary procedure)

A rigid or flexible bronchoscope is inserted through the nose or mouth and advanced into the oropharynx with or without fluoroscopic guidance. The oropharynx is examined. The vocal cords are visualized and examined. The bronchoscope is then advanced into the trachea, which is also examined before the scope is advanced into each mainstem bronchus and any abnormalities are noted. If a rigid bronchoscope is used, a telescope or flexible bronchoscope may be inserted through the rigid bronchoscope to visualize the distal segment of each mainstem bronchus. The site of an obstruction or stenosis is identified and assessed. If dilation is required prior to stent placement, a balloon catheter is advanced to the obstructed or stenosed area and the balloon is inflated one or more times to open the lumen. A stent delivery catheter or other stent delivery device is advanced through the bronchoscope to the target site and a bronchial stent is placed within the obstructed or stenosed lumen to open the airway. Use 31637 for each additional major bronchus stent placement.

31638

31638 Bronchoscopy, rigid or flexible, including fluoroscopic guidance, when performed; with revision of tracheal or bronchial stent inserted at previous session (includes tracheal/bronchial dilation as required)

A rigid or flexible bronchoscope is inserted through the nose or mouth and advanced into the oropharynx with or without fluoroscopic guidance. The oropharynx is examined. The vocal cords are visualized and examined. The bronchoscope is then advanced into the trachea, which is also examined before the scope is advanced into each mainstem bronchus and any abnormalities are noted. If a rigid bronchoscope is used, a telescope or flexible bronchoscope may be inserted through the rigid bronchoscope to visualize the distal segment of each mainstem bronchus. A previously placed stent that was not properly positioned on initial placement or has migrated is located. The stent may be retrieved and a new stent placed or the existing stent may be retrieved and repositioned. If dilation is required prior to stent revision, a balloon catheter is advanced to the obstruction or stenosis and the balloon is inflated one or more times to open the lumen. A stent delivery catheter or other stent delivery device is advanced through the bronchoscope to the target site and the tracheal or bronchial stent is placed within the obstructed or stenosed lumen to open the airway.

31640

31640 **Bronchoscopy, rigid or flexible, including fluoroscopic guidance, when performed; with excision of tumor**

A rigid or flexible bronchoscope is inserted through the nose or mouth and advanced into the oropharynx with or without fluoroscopic guidance and a tumor is excised. The oropharynx is examined. The vocal cords are visualized and examined. The bronchoscope is then advanced into the trachea, which is also examined before the scope is advanced into each mainstem bronchus and any abnormalities are noted. If a rigid bronchoscope is used, a telescope or flexible bronchoscope may be inserted through the rigid bronchoscope to visualize the distal segment of each mainstem bronchus. Once the tumor has been visualized, a suction catheter and surgical instruments are introduced and the tumor is excised.

31641

31641 **Bronchoscopy, rigid or flexible, including fluoroscopic guidance, when performed; with destruction of tumor or relief of stenosis by any method other than excision (eg, laser therapy, cryotherapy)**

A rigid or flexible bronchoscope is inserted through the nose or mouth and advanced into the oropharynx. Fluoroscopic guidance is used as needed. The oropharynx is examined. The vocal cords are visualized and examined. The bronchoscope is advanced into the trachea and it is examined. It is then advanced into each mainstem bronchus and any abnormalities are noted. If a rigid bronchoscope is used, a telescope or flexible bronchoscope may be inserted through the rigid bronchoscope to visualize the distal segment of each mainstem bronchus. Once the tumor has been visualized, a suction catheter and laser fiber, quartz fiber (for photodynamic therapy), cryotherapy, electrocautery, or argon plasma coagulation (APC) device are inserted. Technique differs slightly depending on the type of device used. If a laser device is employed, the laser is fired and the lesion destroyed while continuous suction is applied. If cryotherapy is used, repetitive freeze/thaw cycles are used to destroy the lesion. If endobronchial electrocautery (thermal destruction) is employed, direct contact is made with the lesion and thermal probes or forceps are used to destroy the lesion. APC, another form of thermal destruction) does not require direct contact with the lesion. Argon plasma is used to conduct the electric current. When gas is released an arc is created that generates heat and destroys the lesion. If photodynamic therapy is employed, a photosensitizer is administered intravenously and a light source is delivered via a quartz fiber which is delivered through the bronchoscope.

31643

31643 **Bronchoscopy, rigid or flexible, including fluoroscopic guidance, when performed; with placement of catheter(s) for intracavitary radioelement application**

A rigid or flexible bronchoscope is inserted through the nose or mouth and advanced into the oropharynx. Fluoroscopic guidance is used as needed. The oropharynx is examined. The vocal cords are visualized and examined. The bronchoscope is advanced into the trachea and it is examined. It is then advanced into each mainstem bronchus and any abnormalities are noted. If a rigid bronchoscope is used, a telescope or flexible bronchoscope may be inserted through the rigid bronchoscope to visualize the distal segment of each mainstem bronchus. The afterloading catheter is advanced through the bronchoscope to the tumor area. If additional catheters are required the procedure is repeated. Catheter position is confirmed by fluoroscopy. The patient is moved to a shielded room where the radioactive source is afterloaded using a remote device. The afterloading (intracavitary radioelement application) is performed by a radiation oncologist and reported separately. Intracavitary radioelement application is also referred to as brachytherapy.

31645-31646

31645 **Bronchoscopy, rigid or flexible, including fluoroscopic guidance, when performed; with therapeutic aspiration of tracheobronchial tree, initial (eg, drainage of lung abscess)**

31646 **Bronchoscopy, rigid or flexible, including fluoroscopic guidance, when performed; with therapeutic aspiration of tracheobronchial tree, subsequent**

A rigid or flexible bronchoscope is inserted through the nose or mouth and advanced into the oropharynx with or without fluoroscopic guidance. Fluoroscopic guidance is used as needed. The oropharynx is examined. The vocal cords are visualized and examined. The bronchoscope is advanced into the trachea and it is examined. It is then advanced into each mainstem bronchus and any abnormalities are noted. If a rigid bronchoscope is used, a telescope or flexible bronchoscope may be inserted through the rigid bronchoscope to visualize the distal segment of each mainstem bronchus. The bronchoscope is advanced to the site of the lung abscess for initial drainage (aspiration) of the lung abscess. A suction catheter is advanced to the site of the abscess and the fluid is drained (aspirated). Use 31646 for subsequent procedures to drain the lung abscess.

31647

31647 **Bronchoscopy, rigid or flexible, including fluoroscopic guidance, when performed; with balloon occlusion, when performed, assessment of air leak, airway sizing, and insertion of bronchial valve(s), initial lobe**

Bronchoscopy with balloon occlusion is used to assess airways for size and air leaks and to insert a bronchial valve. A rigid or flexible bronchoscope is inserted through the mouth and advanced into the oropharynx, trachea, and then into the right or left mainstem bronchus using fluoroscopic guidance as needed. The bronchoscope is advanced into the segmental or subsegmental bronchus of the lobe containing the air leak. Structures are visualized and evaluated. Airway sizing is done with a calibrated balloon catheter. Airways leading to the air leakage are identified using intermittent balloon occlusion. The balloon catheter is advanced and inflated while observing the air leak in the water seal chamber. Once reduction or cessation of air leakage is observed, a delivery catheter is advanced through the bronchoscope and a valve is placed. The bronchoscope is again passed into the segmental or subsegmental bronchus which is examined for evidence of injury. The bronchoscope is withdrawn and the bronchi, trachea, and oropharynx are examined. Report code 31647 for valve placement in the initial lobe.

31648-31649

31648 **Bronchoscopy, rigid or flexible, including fluoroscopic guidance, when performed; with removal of bronchial valve(s), initial lobe**

31649 **Bronchoscopy, rigid or flexible, including fluoroscopic guidance, when performed; with removal of bronchial valve(s), each additional lobe (List separately in addition to code for primary procedure)**

A bronchial valve is removed due to complications or lack of patient benefit from the device. A rigid or flexible bronchoscope is inserted through the nose or mouth and advanced into the oropharynx, trachea, and then into the right or left mainstem bronchus using fluoroscopic guidance as needed. The bronchoscope is advanced into the segmental or subsegmental bronchus containing the valve. The valve and surrounding structures are visualized and evaluated. The central rod of the valve is grasped with biopsy forceps, which causes the valve to collapse so that it can be removed. The valve is then removed. The bronchoscope is again passed into the segmental or subsegmental bronchus which is examined for evidence of injury. The bronchoscope is withdrawn and the bronchi, trachea, and oropharynx are examined. Use 31648 for removal of one or more bronchial valves from a single initial lobe. Use 31649 for removal of one or more valves from each additional lobe.

31651

31651 **Bronchoscopy, rigid or flexible, including fluoroscopic guidance, when performed; with balloon occlusion, when performed, assessment of air leak, airway sizing, and insertion of bronchial valve(s), each additional lobe (List separately in addition to code for primary procedure[s])**

Bronchoscopy with balloon occlusion is used to assess airways for size and air leaks and to insert a bronchial valve. A rigid or flexible bronchoscope is inserted through the mouth and advanced into the oropharynx, trachea, and then into the right or left mainstem bronchus using fluoroscopic guidance as needed. The bronchoscope is advanced into the segmental or subsegmental bronchus of the lobe containing the air leak. Structures are visualized and evaluated. Airway sizing is done with a calibrated balloon catheter. Airways leading to the air leakage are identified using intermittent balloon occlusion. The balloon catheter is advanced and inflated while observing the air leak in the water seal chamber. Once reduction or cessation of air leakage is observed, a delivery catheter is advanced through the bronchoscope and a valve is placed. The bronchoscope is again passed into the segmental or subsegmental bronchus which is examined for evidence of injury. The bronchoscope is withdrawn and the bronchi, trachea, and oropharynx are examined. Report code 31651 for each additional lobe treated after treatment of the initial lobe (31647).

31652-31653

31652 **Bronchoscopy, rigid or flexible, including fluoroscopic guidance, when performed; with endobronchial ultrasound (EBUS) guided transtracheal and/or transbronchial sampling (eg, aspiration[s]/biopsy[ies]), one or two mediastinal and/or hilar lymph node stations or structures**

31653 **Bronchoscopy, rigid or flexible, including fluoroscopic guidance, when performed; with endobronchial ultrasound (EBUS) guided transtracheal and/or transbronchial sampling (eg, aspiration[s]/biopsy[ies]), 3 or more mediastinal and/or hilar lymph node stations or structures**

Bronchoscopy is performed with endobronchial ultrasound (EBUS) guidance to obtain transtracheal and/or transbronchial tissue samples of mediastinal and/or hilar lymph node structures, which may aid in diagnosing and staging carcinoma and lymphoma, and other conditions like sarcoidosis, silicosis, histoplasmosis, and tuberculosis. The hila are the lung roots through which the major bronchi pass on each side before branching out into the lungs. Mediastinal nodes are located around the tracheobronchial tree between the sternum and spine. Using a transoral or transnasal approach, a rigid or flexible bronchoscope is inserted and the vocal cords, trachea, and carina are examined. The scope is advanced into the left main bronchus and its branches, followed by the right main

Respiratory System

bronchus, right upper lobe bronchus, and bronchus intermedius between the right middle and lower lobes. EBUS is used to visualize the tracheobronchial wall and the surrounding pulmonary structures, enhancing the quality of samples obtained. A transducer may be incorporated into the tip of a specially designed flexible bronchoscope, or a miniature probe transducer with a balloon tip may be inserted through the working channel of a conventional rigid or flexible bronchoscope. For transtracheal or transbronchial biopsy, the bronchoscope is wedged into the wall segment at the desired location and biopsy forceps are passed through the working channel of the scope. The tissue sample is grasped with the forceps and brought up through the channel. The procedure may be repeated at the same location or other sites until adequate tissue samples have been obtained. For needle aspiration, the needle assembly unit is introduced through the working channel of the bronchoscope and the tracheobronchial wall is penetrated by the needle at the desired location(s) until an adequate amount of tissue has been removed. The entire endobronchial tree is carefully inspected again, and the scope is then removed. Code 31652 is used when tissue samples are obtained from one or two mediastinal and/or hilar lymph node stations or structures and code 31653 is used for 3 or more.

31654

31654   Bronchoscopy, rigid or flexible, including fluoroscopic guidance, when performed; with transendoscopic endobronchial ultrasound (EBUS) during bronchoscopic diagnostic or therapeutic intervention(s) for peripheral lesion(s) (List separately in addition to code for primary procedure[s])

A rigid or flexible bronchoscope is inserted through the nose or mouth and advanced into the oropharynx, trachea, and each mainstem bronchus, with or without fluoroscopic guidance. Any abnormalities are noted. A miniaturized ultrasound probe is inserted through a flexible bronchoscope with a biopsy channel at the time of another primary diagnostic bronchoscopy or therapeutic bronchoscopic intervention for peripheral lesions, reported separately. The probe is used to evaluate the airway walls, the surrounding mediastinum, and the lungs. When the probe has been advanced and is inside the airway, a balloon at the tip of the catheter is inflated until full circular contact with the airway wall is achieved and the structures of the wall and surrounding mediastinum become visible with ultrasonic images. The probe is then moved along the airway to visualize and evaluate the airway and surrounding structures in their entirety.

31660-31661

31660   Bronchoscopy, rigid or flexible, including fluoroscopic guidance, when performed; with bronchial thermoplasty, 1 lobe

31661   Bronchoscopy, rigid or flexible, including fluoroscopic guidance, when performed; with bronchial thermoplasty, 2 or more lobes

Bronchial thermoplasty is performed to treat severe, persistent asthma in patients not well controlled with inhaled corticosteroids and long-acting beta-agonists. A rigid or flexible bronchoscope is introduced through the nose or mouth and advanced into the oropharynx using fluoroscopic guidance as needed. The bronchoscope is advanced into the trachea and then into the right or left mainstem bronchus. Any abnormalities are noted. If a rigid bronchoscope is used, a telescope or flexible bronchoscope may be inserted through the rigid bronchoscope to visualize the distal segment of each mainstem bronchus. A catheter containing the thermoplasty device is then introduced through the bronchoscope and positioned in the airway at the first target treatment site which is usually the most distal airway in the targeted lobe. An electrode array is positioned against the wall of the airway. The device is activated and low-power, temperature controlled radiofrequency (RF) energy is delivered to the airway wall for a maximum of 10 seconds at each location. The RF energy heats the wall of that portion of the airway, destroying excessive smooth muscle tissue and decreasing the ability of the airways to constrict and become narrow. The electrodes are repositioned and activated along all accessible airways distal to the mainstem bronchus in the lobe being treated. Use 31660 for treatment of one lobe in a single session. Use 31661 for treatment of 2 or more lobes in a single session. Typically several bronchial thermoplasty sessions are required because only a portion of the lungs (1-2 lobes) is treated at each session.

31717

31717   Catheterization with bronchial brush biopsy

The physician inserts a catheter into the bronchi and obtains a bronchial brush biopsy. A local anesthetic is sprayed in the back of the throat. Using separately reportable radiological guidance, a catheter is advanced through the nose or mouth, into the throat and then into the trachea and bronchi. The catheter contains a brush that is used to obtain a biopsy. Cell samples are obtained by brushing the lining of the bronchi. The catheter is then withdrawn and the cell samples are sent to the laboratory for separately reportable cytology evaluation.

31720-31725

31720   Catheter aspiration (separate procedure); nasotracheal

31725   Catheter aspiration (separate procedure); tracheobronchial with fiberscope, bedside

In 31720, a suction catheter is inserted through the nose and advanced through the pharynx and into the trachea. Accumulated saliva, pulmonary secretions, blood, vomitus, or other foreign material is then aspirated from the trachea and nasopharyngeal area. In 31725, a tracheobronchial catheter aspiration is performed with a fiberscope at the bedside. Conscious sedation is provided as needed. The catheter is introduced through the mouth or a previously established tracheostomy and advanced through the trachea and into the main bronchus under fiberscopic guidance. The catheter is advanced into the right and/or left bronchi as needed. Pulmonary secretions or foreign material is aspirated from the bronchi and trachea using intermittent suction.

31730

31730   Transtracheal (percutaneous) introduction of needle wire dilator/stent or indwelling tube for oxygen therapy

A needle wire dilator or stent or an indwelling tube for oxygen therapy is placed by transtracheal (percutaneous) technique. Percutaneous placement of an indwelling tube for oxygen therapy is also referred to as transtracheal oxygen therapy (TTOT). TTOT is performed on patients requiring long-term oxygen therapy. Tracheal cartilage landmarks are identified and the skin prepped. A superficial incision is made over the entry site usually below the first and above the third tracheal ring. A guidewire is placed. The opening is dilated and a stent is placed. The stent is left in place for approximately a week while the tract matures. When the tract is mature, the stent is removed and an oxygen delivery catheter is inserted.

31750

31750   Tracheoplasty; cervical

A cervical tracheoplasty is performed to repair a defect in the proximal or middle third of the trachea. The exact procedure performed depends on the site and type of defect. The thyroid isthmus is divided and the innominate vessels retracted to expose the trachea. Once the trachea is exposed the defect is located. If the injury or defect is in the tracheal lumen, the trachea is incised. Tracheal tissue may be excised and the defect closed using a patch or graft. Once the repair is complete, the surgical incisions are closed.

31755

31755   Tracheoplasty; tracheopharyngeal fistulization, each stage

The physician performs a tracheoplasty to construct tracheopharyngeal fistula which is an internal tract (opening) between these two structures and is performed in patients who have undergone laryngectomy. The procedure allows the patient to produce speech. This procedure may be performed alone or during a separately reportable laryngectomy. Tracheopharyngeal fistulization used to require multiple procedures and the use of local or remote muscle flaps and grafts. However, some newer techniques allow the procedure to be performed in a single session. There are multiple techniques for creating the fistula and the exact procedure also depends on whether it is performed at the time of the laryngectomy or at a subsequent procedure. If the procedure is performed in a separate surgical session subsequent to the laryngectomy, the larynx first must be exposed. Following exposure of the larynx, the procedure then proceeds in the same manner as when it is performed at the time of the laryngectomy. An incision is made in the cricopharyngeal muscle and extended vertically into the inferior constrictor muscle. The muscular coat of the pharynx and upper esophagus is stretched by placing stay sutures at the edge of the pharyngeal wall and then inserting a finger into the pharyngoesophageal lumen to stretch the muscular coat. The muscular coat is divided leaving the mucosal layer intact. A hollow metal tube is inserted into the pharyngeal lumen with the bevel turned towards the posterior wall of the trachea. A trocar and cannula is inserted through the upper aspect of the posterior tracheal wall and passed through the metal tube into the pharyngeal lumen. A catheter is inserted through the mouth into the pharynx and through the cannula into the surgical wound. A voice prosthesis may be inserted. Alternatively, a tube may be created using the mucosa of the posterior tracheal wall or a muscle flaps or grafts and the tube is then implanted into the pharynx. If the procedure is performed in stages, report 31755 for each stage of the procedure.

31760

31760   Tracheoplasty; intrathoracic

An intrathoracic tracheoplasty is performed to repair a defect in the distal third of the trachea. The exact procedure depends on the site and type of defect. An anterior or posterior approach may be used to expose the trachea. For an anterior approach, a median sternotomy is used. The anterior pericardium is incised. Blood vessels are retracted to expose the trachea and carina. The superior vena cava is retracted to the right, the aorta to the left, the right main pulmonary artery inferiorly, and the innominate vessels superiorly. For a posterior approach, a right posterolateral thoracotomy is used. The posterior mediastinal pleura is dissected up to the thoracic inlet. The azygous vein is divided. The esophagus is dissected free of surrounding tissue and mobilized to allow access to the

Respiratory System

trachea. The trachea is exposed taking care to protect the vagus and laryngeal nerves. Once the trachea is exposed the defect is located. If the defect is in the tracheal lumen, the trachea is incised. Tracheal tissue may be excised and the defect closed using a patch or graft. A muscle flap or other tissue flap or patch may be used to reinforce the repair. Once the repair is complete, the surgical incisions are closed.

31766

31766   Carinal reconstruction

A carinal reconstruction is performed. The carina is the ridge or projection at the distal-most aspect of the trachea where the right and left main bronchi join with the trachea. Carinal reconstruction may be performed for malignancy or tumor invasion of the carina or an injury or defect of the carina. An anterior or posterior approach may be used to expose the carina. For an anterior approach, a median sternotomy is used. The anterior pericardium is incised. Blood vessels are retracted to expose the trachea and carina. The superior vena cava is retracted to the right, the aorta to the left, the right main pulmonary artery inferiorly, and the innominate vessels superiorly. For a posterior approach, a right posterolateral thoracotomy is used. The posterior mediastinal pleura is dissected up to the thoracic inlet. The azygous vein is divided. The esophagus is dissected free of surrounding tissue and mobilized to allow access to the carina. The carina is exposed taking care to protect the vagus and laryngeal nerves. The main right and left bronchus are separated from the carina. Any diseased or damaged carinal tissue is excised which may include a segment of the trachea above the carina. The carina is then reconstructed by creating anastomosis sites for the main right and left bronchus. The left bronchus is anastomosed in an end-to-end fashion and the right bronchus in an end-to-side fashion. A muscle flap or other tissue flap or patch may be used to reinforce the repair. Once the repair is completed, the surgical incisions are closed.

31770-31775

31770   Bronchoplasty; graft repair
31775   Bronchoplasty; excision stenosis and anastomosis

A bronchoplasty is performed with graft repair (31770) or excision of a stenosis with anastomosis (31775). An anterior intercostal incision is made and carried around the chest to the scapula. A rib spreader is used to expose the lung and bronchus and a rib may be removed for better access to the bronchus. The lung is deflated and the bronchus is exposed. In 31770, the bronchus is repaired with a graft. One method is to use a pericardial patch graft. The phrenic nerve is identified and protected. A section of pericardium is excised, fixed in glutaraldehyde solution, washed with normal saline, and configured to repair the defect in the bronchus. The patch is stretched and sutured to the margins of the bronchial defect. The pericardial defect is sutured closed. In 31775, a stenotic (narrowed) segment is excised and the remaining segments anastomosed. The bronchus is mobilized and clamped above and below the narrowed segment. The bronchus is divided and the narrowed segment removed. Traction sutures are placed at the midlateral position of the proximal and distal segment to approximate the airway and reduce tension as proximal and distal bronchial segments are sutured together (anastomosed). Any difference in the circumference of the two segments is addressed by creating small folds (plicating) the segment with the wider diameter. The anastomosis site is reinforced by wrapping it with pericardial fat or pleura. Following completion of the graft repair or anastomosis, saline solution is instilled in the pleural cavity, the lung re-expanded, and the graft or anastomosis checked for air leaks. Chest tubes are placed as needed and chest incisions are closed in layers.

31780-31781

31780   Excision tracheal stenosis and anastomosis; cervical
31781   Excision tracheal stenosis and anastomosis; cervicothoracic

A stenosis of the trachea is excised and the remaining proximal and distal segments are anastomosed. In 31780, the stenosis is in the proximal or middle third of the trachea and a cervical approach is used. The thyroid isthmus is divided and the innominate vessels retracted to expose the trachea. In 31781, the stenosis extends into the distal third of the trachea and a cervicothoracic approach is used. The proximal and middle thirds of the trachea are exposed as described above. A median sternotomy is used to expose the distal third of the trachea. The anterior pericardium is incised. Blood vessels are retracted to expose the trachea and carina. The superior vena cava is retracted to the right, the aorta to the left, the right main pulmonary artery inferiorly, and the innominate vessels superiorly. Once the trachea is exposed the narrowed segment is dissected free of surrounding tissues. The trachea is divided immediately proximal and distal to the narrowed segment and the narrowed segment removed. The remaining distal and proximal segments are mobilized and sutured together (anastomosed). If a sliding tracheoplasty is performed for stenosis, the trachea is divided at the midpoint of the stenosis. The narrowed segment is then split longitudinally with one incision being on the anterior aspect and the other incision on the posterior aspect. The narrowed segments are slid together and the sides sutured together to create a shorter wider trachea. The surgical incisions are closed.

31785-31786

31785   Excision of tracheal tumor or carcinoma; cervical
31786   Excision of tracheal tumor or carcinoma; thoracic

A tumor or carcinoma of the trachea is excised. In 31785, the lesion is in the proximal or middle third of the trachea and a cervical approach is used. The thyroid isthmus is divided and the innominate vessels retracted to expose the trachea. In 31786, the lesion is in the distal third of the trachea and an anterior or posterior intrathoracic approach is used. For an anterior approach, a median sternotomy is used. The anterior pericardium is incised. Blood vessels are retracted to expose the trachea and carina. The superior vena cava is retracted to the right, the aorta to the left, the right main pulmonary artery inferiorly, and the innominate vessels superiorly. For a posterior approach, a right posterolateral thoracotomy is used. The posterior mediastinal pleura is dissected up to the thoracic inlet. The azygous vein is divided. The esophagus is dissected free of surrounding tissue and mobilized to allow access to the trachea. The trachea is exposed taking care to protect the vagus and laryngeal nerves. Once the trachea is exposed the site of the lesion is located and explored. The lesion is excised along with a margin of healthy tissue. The trachea is repaired with sutures. Once the repair is completed, the surgical incisions are closed.

31800-31805

31800   Suture of tracheal wound or injury; cervical
31805   Suture of tracheal wound or injury; intrathoracic

A tracheal wound or injury is repaired with sutures. The exact procedure performed depends on the site and nature of the wound or injury. In 31800, the wound or injury is in the proximal or middle third of the trachea and a cervical approach is used. The thyroid isthmus is divided and the innominate vessels retracted to expose the trachea. In 31805, the wound or injury is in the distal third of the trachea and an anterior or posterior intrathoracic approach is used. For an anterior approach, a median sternotomy is used. The anterior pericardium is incised. Blood vessels are retracted to expose the trachea and carina. The superior vena cava is retracted to the right, the aorta to the left, the right main pulmonary artery inferiorly, and the innominate vessels superiorly. . For a posterior approach, a right posterolateral thoracotomy is used. The posterior mediastinal pleura is dissected up to the thoracic inlet. The azygous vein is divided. The esophagus is dissected free of surrounding tissue and mobilized to allow access to the trachea. The trachea is exposed taking care to protect the vagus and laryngeal nerves. Once the trachea is exposed the wound or injury is located and explored. Bleeding is controlled. The site is cleared of debris and any foreign bodies are removed. If the injury or defect is in the tracheal lumen, the trachea is incised. The edges of the injury or wound are debrided, approximated and repaired with sutures. Once the repair is completed, the surgical incisions are closed.

31820-31825

31820   Surgical closure tracheostomy or fistula; without plastic repair
31825   Surgical closure tracheostomy or fistula; with plastic repair

A tracheostomy or tracheal fistula is surgically closed. Tracheostomies and tracheal fistulas typically close spontaneously following removal of the tracheostomy tube. However, when the opening does not close on its own, it must be surgically closed. In 31820, direct closure is performed without plastic repair. The epithelialized skin tract is excised. The edges of the wound are sutured together in layers. In 31825, closure is performed using plastic surgery techniques. The trachea is closed with sutures or by interposition of a perichondrial flap. The epithelialized skin tract is excised. The skin around the opening is incised and undermined to release tension. Plastic techniques are then used to minimize scarring and scar depression, such as de-epitheliazation, dermal-fat-fascia grafts, acellular dermal grafts. De-epithelization is performed by trimming skin edges and removing epithelium. The de-epethialized tissue is turned under to fill the depression and the skin that has not been de-epithelialized is sutured together. If a dermal-fat-fascia graft is used it is harvested in a separate procedure or an acellular dermal graft is obtained from the tissue bank. The graft is configured to the required dimensions, placed in the defect, and the edges secured with sutures. Adjacent skin is undermined and secured over the graft. The repair is performed so that the scar is located along an existing skin fold if possible.

31830

31830   Revision of tracheostomy scar

The physician revised a tracheostomy scar. Placement and removal of a tracheostomy leaves a visible depressed scar in the center of the neck. The depression is caused by loss of soft tissue between the skin and the underlying strap muscles and trachea. The skin around the scar is incised to release tension, referred to as tracheal tug, and contracted scar tissue excised. There are several techniques that can be used to treat the scar depression, including scar de-epitheliazation, dermal-fat-fascia grafts, or acellular dermal grafts. Scar de-epithelization is performed for a shallow depression. The skin edges are trimmed and the epithelium removed. The de-epethialized tissue is then turned under to fill the depression and the skin that has not been de-epithelialized is sutured together. Deeper defects require placement of a graft to fill the depression. A dermal-fat-fascia graft is harvested in a separate procedure or an acellular dermal graft is obtained from the tissue bank. The graft is configured to the required dimensions, placed in the defect, and the

● New Code   ▲ Revised Code

Respiratory System

edges secured with sutures. Adjacent skin is undermined and secured over the graft. The repair is performed so that the new scar is located along an existing skin fold if possible.

32035-32036

32035   **Thoracostomy; with rib resection for empyema**
32036   **Thoracostomy; with open flap drainage for empyema**

The physician removes part of a rib and creates a hole in the chest cavity to allow drainage of an abscess in the pleural space in 32035. A small incision is made in the chest wall directly overlying the rib above the abscess in the pleural space, also referred to as an empyema collection. A short segment of rib is excised and the pleural space is entered. The pleural space cavities (loculations) are broken down (dissected) using a fingertip or suction tip. The empyema collection is aspirated and the space is irrigated with antibiotic solution. A large bore chest tube is placed into the pocket through a separate incision site. In 32036, an open, U-shaped skin flap is created over the empyema site in the chest to drain the fluid and keep it open for further drainage. A flap of skin and subcutaneous tissue is created long enough to reach the pleural cavity without tension. A section of rib is removed. The tip of the flap is turned in and sutured to the parietal pleura (the pleura lining the chest wall), allowing open drainage of the empyema collection.

32096-32097

32096   **Thoracotomy, with diagnostic biopsy(ies) of lung infiltrate(s) (eg, wedge, incisional), unilateral**
32097   **Thoracotomy, with diagnostic biopsy(ies) of lung nodule(s) or mass(es) (eg, wedge, incisional), unilateral**

The physician performs a thoracotomy for biopsy of the lung. In 32096, a biopsy for lung infiltrates is performed. A lung or pulmonary infiltrate refers to any substance in the lung that causes opacification of the lungs as seen on a chest xray and may be caused by infection, inflammation, fluid accumulation, hemorrhage, or other conditions. In 32097, a lung nodule, which is a small mass in the lung, is biopsied. A small anterior incision is made between the ribs typically in the second, third, fourth, or fifth interspace depending on the site to be biopsied. Pectoralis and intercostal muscles are divided and the pleura is exposed. The ribs are spread. The pleura is incised, the lung is collapsed as needed, and pleural fluid is aspirated. The exposed area of the lung is examined. The lung is reinflated. Clamps are applied to the area to be biopsied. The lung is incised and one or more tissue samples are obtained from the area containing the infiltrates or nodules. Alternatively, a triangular wedge may be excised from the lung. The biopsy area is closed using mattress sutures. A chest tube or catheter is placed within the pleural space as needed. The lung is fully inflated and the chest incision is closed in layers around the chest tube.

32098

32098   **Thoracotomy, with biopsy(ies) of pleura**

The physician performs a thoracotomy for biopsy of the pleura. A small anterior incision is made between the ribs typically in the second, third, fourth, or fifth interspace depending on the site to be biopsied. Pectoralis and intercostal muscles are divided and the pleura is exposed. The ribs are spread. One or more tissue samples are taken from the pleura. A chest tube or catheter is placed within the pleural space as needed. The chest incision is closed in layers around the chest tube.

32100

32100   **Thoracotomy; with exploration**

A thoracotomy is performed for exploration. A large incision is made in the chest which may include splitting the sternum or removing a portion of one or more ribs. If the sternum is split, a chest spreader is placed and the chest cavity is exposed. If an incision is made in the anterolateral or posterolateral chest wall, pectoralis and intercostal muscles are divided and the pleura is exposed. The ribs are spread or a portion of one or more ribs is excised. The pleura is opened and the heart, lungs, and mediastinal structures are examined. Any abnormalities are noted. Following the exploration, a chest tube or catheter is placed within the pleural space as needed. The spreaders are removed and the chest incision is closed in layers around the chest tube.

32110

32110   **Thoracotomy; with control of traumatic hemorrhage and/or repair of lung tear**

A thoracotomy is performed with control of traumatic hemorrhage and/or repair of lung tear. The injured side of the chest is incised at the fifth intercostal space from the sternum to the axilla. Once the intercostal muscles are exposed, they are incised using blunt and sharp dissection taking care not to cause any additional injury to the lung. A rib spreader is inserted and the chest cavity explored. If further exposure is required, incision of the opposite side of the chest is performed in the same manner and the sternum is divided. The site of the bleeding is identified and initial control established using finger pressure, packing, and/or clamps. Once initial control has been established vascular injuries are treated using a combination of ligation and coagulation. If a lung tear is identified, the

injury is repaired using staples or sutures. When all bleeding sites have been identified and the bleeding has been controlled, chest tubes are placed and the chest is closed.

32120

32120   **Thoracotomy; for postoperative complications**

A thoracotomy is performed for postoperative complications. The previous chest incision is reopened. If additional exposure is required both sides of the chest may be opened. A rib or sternal spreader is inserted and chest cavity is explored. The previous surgical site and surrounding tissue is carefully examined for evidence of bleeding, fluid accumulations, or other complications. Any bleeding is initially controlled using finger pressure, packing, and/or clamps. Once initial control has been established vascular injuries are treated using a combination of ligation and coagulation. Any fluid accumulations are aspirated and specimens sent for separately reportable laboratory analysis. Any other complications are addressed. Chest tubes are then placed and the chest incision closed.

32124

32124   **Thoracotomy; with open intrapleural pneumonolysis**

The physician performs a thoracotomy with an open intrapleural pneumonolysis to surgically create a pneumothorax (collapsed lung). This procedure is also referred to as collapse therapy and is used primarily in the treatment of cavitary tuberculosis. An incision is made in the side of the chest. The pleural space is accessed and adhesions between the visceral (pulmonary) pleura and the parietal pleura are cut causing the lung to collapse.

32140

32140   **Thoracotomy; with cyst(s) removal, includes pleural procedure when performed**

The physician performs a thoracotomy and removes one or more cysts in the thoracic cavity. An incision is made in the chest wall overlying the site of the cyst. Following exposure of the cyst, it may be aspirated and decompressed. Any adhesions to intrathoracic structures are severed. The cyst is then excised. If the physician is unable to remove the cyst in its entirety, any remaining cystic tissue may be cauterized to prevent recurrence. A procedure on the pleura may be performed, if necessary, a chest tube is placed, and the incision site is closed.

32141

32141   **Thoracotomy; with resection-plication of bullae, includes any pleural procedure when performed**

The physician performs a thoracotomy and removes one or more bullae from the lung by excision-plication. This procedure may also be referred to as a bullectomy or staple bullectomy. Bullae are complications of emphysema and chronic obstructive pulmonary disease (COPD) in which air pockets develop that become larger over time and severely compromise lung function. An incision is made in the chest wall on the side of the affected lung. The lung is collapsed and one-lung ventilation is initiated. Any pleural adhesions are cut. The bulla is identified and excised (removed) or stapled (plicated). Large bullae may be punctured and collapsed before being excised or stapled. The pleural cavity is irrigated and the lung is reinflated. One or more chest tubes are placed and the incision site is closed.

32150-32151

32150   **Thoracotomy; with removal of intrapleural foreign body or fibrin deposit**
32151   **Thoracotomy; with removal of intrapulmonary foreign body**

The physician performs a thoracotomy and removes a foreign body or protein (fibrin) deposit from the membrane that surrounds the lungs and lines the chest cavity. An incision is made in the chest wall over the site of the foreign body or fibrin deposit and it is identified and removed. The pleural cavity is irrigated. One or more chest tubes may be placed and the incision site is closed. Use 32151 if the foreign body must be removed from the lung tissue. The lung may first be collapsed and one-lung ventilation initiated before the foreign body is identified and removed. The pleural cavity is irrigated and the lung is reinflated. One or more chest tubes are placed and the incision site is closed.

32160

32160   **Thoracotomy; with cardiac massage**

The physician performs an emergency thoracotomy to expose the heart for direct cardiac massage. An incision is made through the left anterolateral skin and subcutaneous tissues to the intercostal musculature. The chest is entered with a finger through the intercostal muscles. The incision is extended with scissors or blunt dissection. The ribs are spread with rib spreaders. If cardiac massage is performed following traumatic injury to the chest, the right side of the chest may also be opened or the physician may divide the sternum. If the chest is opened for massage due to cardiac arrest without injury to the chest, cardiac massage is performed through the left chest incision. The heart is exposed and directly massaged to facilitate blood flow. The descending aorta may be cross clamped so that blood is distributed to the heart, lungs, and brain. As soon as cardiac function has been restored, the patient is transferred to the operating room for definitive treatment of the underlying condition.

32200

32200   Pneumonostomy, with open drainage of abscess or cyst

The physician drains fluid from a cyst or pus-filled sac (abscess) within the lung tissue. A small skin incision is made over the site of the abscess and carried down through deeper tissues in the chest wall. A pneumonostomy tube is advanced into the cyst or abscess in the lung and fluid and/or pus is drained. The cyst or abscess cavity may be flushed with normal saline or an antibiotic solution. A soft drain is placed in the cyst or abscess cavity and secured with sutures to allow for continuous drainage. The incision is closed around the drain.

32215

32215   Pleural scarification for repeat pneumothorax

The physician treats a condition in which air repeatedly builds up in the space between the lungs and the inside of the chest wall. Scar tissue is created which binds the surface of the lung to the inside of the chest wall, preventing the buildup of air.

32220-32225

32220   Decortication, pulmonary (separate procedure); total
32225   Decortication, pulmonary (separate procedure); partial

The physician removes or strips the thickened fibrin layer, also called the rind or peel, from the outer pleural surface of the entire lung to allow the lung to fully expand. This is also called a total pulmonary decortication. A posterolateral incision is made in the chest at the fifth or sixth intercostal space and the lung is exposed. An incision is made into the thickened fibrin layer and the correct decortication plane is identified. The fibrin layer is then grasped and dissected from the underlying visceral pleura. All portions of the lung encased by the thickened fibrin layer are addressed. One or more chest tubes are placed and the incision site is closed. Use 32225, if the thickened layer of fibrin tissue removed involves only a portion of the lung.

32310-32320

32310   Pleurectomy, parietal (separate procedure)
32320   Decortication and parietal pleurectomy

The physician performs a parietal pleurectomy (32310) or a decortication and parietal pleurectomy (32320). The pleura is the serous membrane that surrounds the lungs and lines of the walls of pulmonary cavity. The parietal pleura is the outer layer that lines chest wall including the ribs, mediastinum, pericardium, and diaphragm. The visceral (pulmonary) pleura is the inner layer that covers the lungs. The visceral pleura can become encased in a thick fibrin layer that constricts the lungs. This thickened layer is stripped or decorticated to allow better lung expansion. A posterolateral incision is made in the chest at the fifth or sixth intercostal space and the lung is exposed. In 32310, the parietal pleura is removed. An incision is made in the parietal pleura, which is then stripped off the chest wall using blunt and sharp dissection. In 32320, the parietal pleura is removed and the physician also strips the thickened fibrin layer covering the visceral pleura to decorticate the lung. An incision is made into the thickened fibrin layer and the correct decortication plane identified. The fibrin layer is grasped and dissected from the underlying visceral pleura. All portions of lung encased by the thickened fibrin layer are addressed. One or more chest tubes are placed and the chest incision is closed.

32400

32400   Biopsy, pleura; percutaneous needle

A needle is inserted into the pleural cavity to obtain a tissue sample from the pleura, the membrane that lines the surface of the lungs and the chest wall cavity. The access site is selected and the skin is cleansed. A local anesthetic is administered from the skin to the pleural level. A small incision is made to accommodate the biopsy needle, which is inserted into the pleural space. The cutting edge of the needle is seated in the pleura and a tissue sample is obtained. More than one pass with the needle may be required to obtain an adequate tissue sample.

32405

32405   Biopsy, lung or mediastinum, percutaneous needle

A local anesthetic is administered. If the lesion cannot be palpated, separately reportable fluoroscopic, ultrasound, CT or MR guidance is used to locate the lesion and place the needle. Tissue samples are obtained from the lung or mediastinum using a needle or core biopsy and sent for pathology examination.

32440-32445

32440   Removal of lung, pneumonectomy
32442   Removal of lung, pneumonectomy; with resection of segment of trachea followed by broncho-tracheal anastomosis (sleeve pneumonectomy)
32445   Removal of lung, pneumonectomy; extrapleural

A posterolateral thoracic incision is made in the intercostal space beginning just below the shoulder blade and extending around to the front of the chest. If better access is required a rib is removed. In 32440, a pneumonectomy is performed. The lung is deflated and major blood vessels are ligated and divided. The main bronchus is clamped and incised. The lung is removed. The remaining segment of bronchus is stapled or sutured closed. A chest tube is placed and the chest incision closed. In 32442, pneumonectomy is performed with resection of a segment of trachea followed by broncho-tracheal anastomosis. This procedure is also referred to as a sleeve pneumonectomy. The lung is deflated and major blood vessels are ligated and divided. The trachea is mobilized and a section of trachea excised along with the main bronchus and the diseased or damaged lung. The main bronchus of the remaining lung is then attached to the remaining trachea. In 32445, an extrapleural pneumonectomy is performed which involves removal of the lung and the parietal pleura, pericardium, and part of the diaphragm. The lung is deflated and major blood vessels are ligated and divided. The main bronchus is clamped and incised. Tissue surrounding the lung is dissected taking care not to enter the pleural cavity. The lung is removed along with the parietal pleura. Any involved portion of the pericardium is excised and replaced with a synthetic patch. A portion of the diaphragm is also removed and replaced with a synthetic patch. The remaining segment of bronchus is stapled or sutured closed.

32480-32482

32480   Removal of lung, other than pneumonectomy; single lobe (lobectomy)
32482   Removal of lung, other than pneumonectomy; 2 lobes (bilobectomy)

An intercostal incision is made in the anterior chest and extended around to the posterior chest at the level of the affected lobe or lobes. If more exposure is needed, a rib is removed. The lung is deflated. The main arteries and veins that supply the lobe or lobes are ligated and divided. The secondary bronchi are clamped and divided. The diseased lobe or lobes are dissected from the remaining lung tissue and removed. The remaining portions of the secondary bronchi are stapled or sutured closed. The remaining portion of the lung will often expand to fill the chest cavity. Chest tubes are inserted into the pleural space and the chest incision is closed. Use 32480 if a single lobe is removed and 32482 if two lobes are removed.

32484

32484   Removal of lung, other than pneumonectomy; single segment (segmentectomy)

A lung segmentectomy involves removal of a small portion of the lung. The procedure is typically performed for early stage lung cancer that involves only a small portion of the lung as opposed to an entire lobe. An incision is made at the level of the affected lung segment in the front of the chest and extended around the back to a point under the shoulder blade. The chest cavity is entered through the exposed ribs and sometimes a rib is removed to provide better access to the lung. The diseased or damaged lung tissue is identified and excised. A temporary drainage tube may be inserted into the pleural space to remove air, fluid, and blood from the surgical site. The chest incision is closed.

32486

32486   Removal of lung, other than pneumonectomy; with circumferential resection of segment of bronchus followed by broncho-bronchial anastomosis (sleeve lobectomy)

Sleeve lobectomy involves removal of one lobe of the lung along with a circumferential segment of the bronchus that feeds the affected lobe. The intermediate bronchus in the remaining lobe(s) of the lung is(are) then reconnected to the remaining main bronchus. An incision is generally made at the level of the affected lung segment in the front of the chest and extended around the back to a point under the shoulder blade. The chest cavity is entered through the exposed ribs and sometimes a rib is removed to provide better access to the lung. The lung is then deflated and major blood vessels are tied off. The main bronchus of the affected lung is clamped and incised and the affected lobe is removed along with the diseased or damaged portion of bronchus. The bronchus that feeds the remaining portion of the lung is reconnected to the main bronchus. Although sleeve lobectomy can be done on any lobe and segmental bronchus, it is most commonly done for centrally located right upper lobe tumors that cannot be removed completely by lobectomy alone. If the right upper lobe is removed, the intermediate bronchus is reimplanted in the proximal main bronchus. If the left upper lobe is removed and the lower lobe salvaged, the intermediate bronchus is reimplanted in the proximal left main bronchus. A temporary drainage tube may be inserted into the pleural space to remove air, fluid, and blood from the surgical site. The chest incision is closed.

● New Code   ▲ Revised Code

32488

32488   Removal of lung, other than pneumonectomy; with all remaining lung following previous removal of a portion of lung (completion pneumonectomy)

Completion pneumonectomy involves removal of the remaining portion the lung in a patient who has had a previous lung surgery in which a portion of the lung was removed. An incision is made at the level of the remaining portion of lung in the front of the chest and possibly extended around the back to a point under the shoulder blade. The chest cavity is entered through the exposed ribs and sometimes a rib is removed to provide better access to the lung. The remaining portion of lung is then deflated and major blood vessels are tied off. The main bronchus is clamped and incised and the remaining portion of lung is removed. The end of the bronchus is stapled or sutured closed. A temporary drainage tube may be inserted into the pleural space to remove air, fluid, and blood from the surgical site. The chest incision is closed.

32491

32491   Removal of lung, other than pneumonectomy; with resection-plication of emphysematous lung(s) (bullous or non-bullous) for lung volume reduction, sternal split or transthoracic approach, includes any pleural procedure, when performed

This procedure is also referred to as lung volume reduction surgery (LVRS). When LVRS is performed on both lungs, an incision is made in the center of the chest and the sternum is split. If surgery is performed on only one lung, a transthoracic incision between the ribs may be used. Damaged areas of lung tissue, bullous or nonbullous, are cut away and the tissue surrounding the excision sites is sutured or stapled together (plicated). Bullae are a complication of emphysema in which large air pockets develop that severely compromise lung function. The physician may remove as much as 30% of emphysematous lung using this technique. LVRS may be performed in conjunction with a pleural procedure, which is included, if performed.

32501

32501   Resection and repair of portion of bronchus (bronchoplasty) when performed at time of lobectomy or segmentectomy (List separately in addition to code for primary procedure)

The diseased or damaged section of bronchus is excised. The bronchus is then repaired using one of several techniques. If only a small section of bronchus is removed, a flap of remaining bronchus may be used to repair the defect. When a larger section of bronchus is removed or if there is a large discrepancy in the lumen size between the main bronchus and the segmental bronchus of the remaining lobe, the larger main bronchus may be plicated (folded) and an end-to-end anastomosis performed.

32503-32504

32503   Resection of apical lung tumor (eg, Pancoast tumor), including chest wall resection, rib(s) resection(s), neurovascular dissection, when performed; without chest wall reconstruction(s)

32504   Resection of apical lung tumor (eg, Pancoast tumor), including chest wall resection, rib(s) resection(s), neurovascular dissection, when performed; with chest wall reconstruction

The physician resects a tumor in the apex (top) of the lung that has invaded the chest wall. Apical tumors, also known as Pancoast or pulmonary sulcus tumors, invade chest wall structures and may also infiltrate lymph vessels, the lower roots of the brachial plexus, intercostal nerves between the top three ribs, the stellate ganglion, the sympathetic nerve chain of the vertebral column, and cervical and thoracic vertebrae. The physician may make a posterolateral thoracotomy incision in the back at a point below the shoulder blade that extends around the side along the curvature of the ribs to the front of the chest. Depending on the extent of vertebral involvement, the incision may be extended to include the neck. The lung apex is exposed. The posterior aspect of the first, second, and sometimes the third ribs are removed. If neurological structures are involved, the nerve roots (usually T1 and C8 levels and sometimes C7 level) and lower trunk of the brachial plexus are dissected and severed. If the tumor extends into the intervertebral foramen, a separately reportable hemilaminectomy or vertebral body resection with instrumentation may be performed. The apical lung mass is then mobilized and resected. Depending on the extent of the tumor, the apical lung segment, upper lobe, or rarely, even the entire lung may be removed, including the affected chest wall. Chest tubes are placed and The incision is closed with sutures. If chest wall reconstruction is performed following the tumor resection, report 32504.

32505-32506

32505   Thoracotomy; with therapeutic wedge resection (eg, mass, nodule), initial

32506   Thoracotomy; with therapeutic wedge resection (eg, mass or nodule), each additional resection, ipsilateral (List separately in addition to code for primary procedure)

A skin incision is made over the front of the chest at the level of a mass or nodule in the lung. The incision is extended around the back to a point under the shoulder blade as needed. Soft tissues are dissected and the ribs are exposed. The chest cavity is entered through the intercostal space and sometimes a rib is removed to provide better access to the lung. The section of lung tissue containing the mass or nodule is identified and excised along with a margin of normal lung tissue. Separately reportable pathology exam is performed to ensure that the margins of the excised wedge are free of abnormal tissue. If abnormal tissue is found at the margins, additional lung tissue is removed until the margins are clean. A temporary drainage tube may be inserted into the pleural space to remove air, fluid, and blood from the surgical site. The chest incision is closed. Use 32505 for the first wedge of lung tissue excised for therapeutic purposes. Use 32506 for each additional therapeutic wedge resection of tissue removed from a different site in the same lung.

32507

32507   Thoracotomy; with diagnostic wedge resection followed by anatomic lung resection (List separately in addition to code for primary procedure)

Diagnostic wedge resection is performed to evaluate diseased or damaged lung tissue and to help determine how much of the lung should be removed in a separately reportable anatomic resection of the lung which will be performed during the same surgical session. A skin incision is made in the front of the chest at the level of the diseased or damaged lung tissue. The incision is extended around the back to a point under the shoulder blade as needed. Soft tissues are dissected and the ribs are exposed. The chest cavity is entered through the intercostal space and sometimes a rib is removed to provide better access to the lung. The section of lung containing the abnormal tissue is identified and a wedge of tissue is excised for diagnostic examination. A separately reportable pathology exam is performed and the results are used to determine what definitive lung procedure should then be performed.

32540

32540   Extrapleural enucleation of empyema (empyemectomy)

The physician performs an extrapleural enucleation of empyema. Empyema is a collection of inflammatory fluid and debris in the pleural space resulting from an untreated pleural space infection. An extrapleural enucleation is performed when the empyema has extended through the visceral and parietal pleura and has adhered to adjacent tissue. The chest is incised over the empyema and the extent of extrapleural tissue involvement evaluated. The empyema sac is then dissected along with involved extrapleural tissue and removed in its entirety without rupturing the empyema sac. Chest tubes are placed as needed and the chest incision is closed.

32550

32550   Insertion of indwelling tunneled pleural catheter with cuff

The physician places an indwelling tunneled pleural catheter with a cuff for intermittent drainage of pleural fluid. The skin is cleansed and a local anesthetic is administered. A small incision is made and the catheter is tunneled through the chest and into the pleural space. The catheter is then attached to a vacuum drainage bottle and fluid is drained at the time of insertion. The catheter is capped but remains in place, possibly for several months, to allow for intermittent drainage of pleural fluid, performed as often as three times a week. The catheter is removed when there is no longer an excessive accumulation of fluid in the pleural space.

32551

32551   Tube thoracostomy, includes connection to drainage system (eg, water seal), when performed, open (separate procedure)

The physician inserts a plastic tube into the pleural space to drain fluid from around the lungs. The skin is cleansed and a local anesthetic is administered. A small incision is made between the ribs on the side or the front of the chest and a trocar is used to puncture into the pleural cavity. A small track is then made through the chest wall and a tube is inserted into the pleural cavity. The tube may be connected to a thoracic drainage and collection system. A water seal system may be used to prevent leakage into the chest cavity. Suction is applied to the collection system to drain air or fluid from the pleural space. The chest tube remains in place until drainage is complete, and the lungs have re-expanded.

32552

32552   Removal of indwelling tunneled pleural catheter with cuff

Removal of an indwelling tunneled pleural catheter with a cuff is performed when pleurodesis has been achieved or when there is a mechanical complication such as migration of the catheter away from the fluid or occlusion of the catheter. The skin around the catheter insertion site is cleansed and a local anesthetic administered. The sutures securing the catheter are removed. The cuff is dissected free of the ingrown tissue surrounding the cuff. The cuff is then inspected to ensure that it is completely free of all tissue within the tunnel. The catheter is grasped and removed using firm, constant pressure. Bleeding is controlled using pressure and a dressing placed over the insertion site.

Respiratory System

32553

32553   Placement of interstitial device(s) for radiation therapy guidance (eg, fiducial markers, dosimeter), percutaneous, intra-thoracic, single or multiple

Fiducial markers are gold seeds that are implanted in or around a soft tissue tumor in the thorax prior to stereotactic radiosurgical treatment of a thoracic tumor. The fiducial marker acts as a landmark and allows the lesion and its borders to be precisely defined. The most common type of intrathoracic lesions treated by stereotactic radiosurgery (CyberKnife) are malignant neoplasms of the lung. Separately reportable imaging is performed to locate the lesion and identify the best location for the approach and puncture site. The skin is cleansed and a local anesthetic administered. Using separately reportable CT guidance, a sterile gold fiducial marker is placed in a specially designed thin-walled biopsy needle. The needle is then passed through the skin and to the desired location in or around the lesion. The fiducial marker is deployed. This is repeated until all fiducial markers have been placed.

32554-32555

32554   Thoracentesis, needle or catheter, aspiration of the pleural space; without imaging guidance
32555   Thoracentesis, needle or catheter, aspiration of the pleural space; with imaging guidance

Thoracentesis is performed to remove excessive amounts of fluid from the pleural space between the parietal and visceral pleura that surround the lungs. With the patient seated and the head and arms resting on a table, the skin around the procedure site is cleansed and the area is draped. The skin is prepped and a local anesthetic is administered. The physician inserts a needle between the ribs into the space between the lining of the lungs and the wall of the chest (pleural cavity) and withdraws fluid. Use code 32554 when the procedure is performed without imaging guidance. Code 32555 is reported when ultrasound, fluoroscopy, or CT guidance is used to facilitate placement of the needle.

32556-32557

32556   Pleural drainage, percutaneous, with insertion of indwelling catheter; without imaging guidance
32557   Pleural drainage, percutaneous, with insertion of indwelling catheter; with imaging guidance

A chest tube is inserted to remove air and/or fluid from the chest cavity. The physician inserts an introducer needle into the pleural cavity. An introducer wire is then inserted through the needle and the needle is removed. A dilator is placed over the wire and advanced into the pleural cavity and the puncture site is dilated. The dilator is removed and a catheter is inserted over the wire. The wire is removed. Alternatively, a small incision may be made at the 4th or 5th intercostal space and carried down to the pleura. A Kelly clamp is inserted through the pleura and opened to create a pneumothorax. The chest tube is then inserted. The catheter or tube is secured with sutures and attached to a suction unit. The suction unit may have a water seal chamber to prevent air from entering the pleural cavity. Use 32556 when the procedure is performed without imaging guidance. If ultrasound, fluoroscopy, or CT guidance is used to facilitate placement of the chest tube, code 32557 is reported.

32560

32560   Instillation, via chest tube/catheter, agent for pleurodesis (eg, talc for recurrent or persistent pneumothorax)

The skin is cleansed and a local anesthetic administered. A small incision is made and a chest tube or catheter is inserted into the pleural space. If fluid is present, it is drained from the pleural space. A sclerosing agent such as talc is instilled through the chest tube or catheter to treat recurrent or persistent pneumothorax. The chest tube is temporarily closed allowing the sclerosing agent to spread through the pleural space. The chemical sclerosing agent causes irritation and inflammation of the pleurae that results in the pleurae adhering to each other. Once the sclerosing agent has spread throughout the pleural space, the chest tube is opened and the sclerosing agent suctioned out of the pleural space. The chest tube may be left in place for several days to allow fluid to drain from the chest.

32561-32562

32561   Instillation(s), via chest tube/catheter, agent for fibrinolysis (eg, fibrinolytic agent for break up of multiloculated effusion); initial day
32562   Instillation(s), via chest tube/catheter, agent for fibrinolysis (eg, fibrinolytic agent for break up of multiloculated effusion); subsequent day

The skin is cleansed and a local anesthetic administered. A small incision is made and a chest tube or catheter is inserted into the pleural space. If fluid is present, it is drained from the pleural space. A fibrinolytic agent, such as streptokinase or urokinase, is instilled through the chest tube or catheter. Fibrinolytic agents help to break up fibrinous bands or loculations and facilitate better drainage of purulent material from the pleural space. The chest tube is temporarily closed allowing the fibrinolytic agent to spread through the pleural space. Once the fibrinolytic agent has spread throughout the pleural space, the

chest tube is opened and the fibrinolytic agent and purulent material suctioned out of the pleural space. The chest tube may be left in place for several days to allow fluid to drain from the chest. Use 32561 for instillation of the fibrinolytic agent on the initial day. Use 32562 for instillation of the fibrinolytic agent on each subsequent day.

32601

32601   Thoracoscopy, diagnostic (separate procedure); lungs, pericardial sac, mediastinal or pleural space, without biopsy

There are several different techniques employed in diagnostic thoracoscopy. One technique for evaluation of the lungs and pleura involves blunt entry by passing a clamp over the rib and through the pleura. The pleural space is digitally inspected at the entry site to ensure adequate space for insertion of the scope, which is then inserted under direct vision into the pleural space. The pleura and lung are inspected and abnormalities are noted. Fluid may be evacuated using suction catheters. Using another technique, a small intercostal incision may be made in the chest and a trocar inserted in the intercostal space (the space between two ribs). Following entry into the pleural space, air is injected and an artificial pneumothorax is induced for better visualization of the lung and pleura. An endoscope is inserted through the trocar and the lung and pleura are inspected. Additional small incisions may be made for introducing other surgical instruments; however, diagnostic procedures on the lungs and pleura are often performed through a single incision. Fluid is drained from the chest and the lungs and pleura are inspected again. Any abnormalities are noted. Lesions may be photographed. To examine the mediastinum or pericardial sac, the thoracoscope is introduced at the right or left midaxillary line and the VI or VII intercostal space. Alternatively, for evaluation of mediastinal disease, the thoracoscope may be introduced through a port placed in the subxiphoid region. Additional small chest incisions may be made for the introduction of surgical instruments. The mediastinum or pericardial sac is visualized and examined. Any abnormalities are noted. If the mediastinal space is being evaluated, the carina and main bronchi are examined along with other mediastinal structures, including lymph nodes. To evaluate the pericardial sac, an incision is made in the pericardium and fluid is aspirated and sent for laboratory analysis. The cardiac chambers, epicardium, and pericardium are inspected for lesions or implants. Photographs may be obtained. Once the examination is complete, the scope is withdrawn, air is evacuated, and a chest tube is placed.

32604

32604   Thoracoscopy, diagnostic (separate procedure); pericardial sac, with biopsy

Diagnostic thoracoscopy is performed to visualize the pericardial sac and obtain tissue samples. The thoracoscope is introduced at the right or left midaxillary line and the VI or VII intercostal space. Additional small chest incisions may be made for the introduction of surgical instruments. The pericardial sac is visualized and examined. Any abnormalities are noted. An incision is made in the pericardial sac and fluid is aspirated and sent for laboratory analysis as needed. The cardiac chambers, epicardium, and pericardium are inspected for lesions or implants and tissue samples are obtained. Tissue samples may also be obtained to identify the cause of pericardial effusion, pericarditis, or pericardial constriction. Photographs are obtained as needed.

32606

32606   Thoracoscopy, diagnostic (separate procedure); mediastinal space, with biopsy

Diagnostic thoracoscopy is performed to visualize the mediastinal space and obtain tissue samples. The patient is placed in lateral decubitus position. Using one lung ventilation, the contralateral lung is collapsed. Two or three small incisions are made in the chest for introduction of the thoracoscope and surgical instruments. The thoracoscope may be placed at the VI or VII intercostal space at the middle axillary line or at the anterior or posterior axillary lines. The thoracic cavity is visualized and examined. The mediastinal pleura is then opened and mediastinal space examined. Fluid may be aspirated. Any abnormalities are noted. Photographs are obtained as needed. Tissue samples are then obtained as needed from any of the mediastinal structures, which may include the thymus, lymph nodes, or any masses or lesions in the mediastinal space.

32607-32608

32607   Thoracoscopy; with diagnostic biopsy(ies) of lung infiltrate(s) (eg, wedge, incisional), unilateral
32608   Thoracoscopy; with diagnostic biopsy(ies) of lung nodule(s) or mass(es) (eg, wedge, incisional), unilateral

There are several different techniques employed in thoracoscopy of the lungs with diagnostic biopsy. One technique involves blunt entry by passing a clamp over the rib and through the pleura. The pleural space is digitally inspected at the entry site to ensure adequate space for insertion of the scope, which is then inserted under direct vision into the pleural space. Fluid may be evacuated using suction catheters. The lung is inspected and the site of the infiltrate or nodule is identified. Clamps are applied to the area to be biopsied. The lung is incised and one or more tissue samples are obtained from the area containing the infiltrates or nodules. Using another technique, a small intercostal incision is made in the chest and a trocar is inserted in the intercostal space. Following

Respiratory System

entry into the pleural space, air is injected and an artificial pneumothorax is induced for better visualization of the lung and pleura. An endoscope is inserted through the trocar and the lung is inspected. Additional small incisions may be made for introducing other surgical instruments; however, diagnostic procedures such as biopsies on the lung are often performed through a single incision. Fluid is drained from the chest and the lungs are inspected again. Any abnormalities are noted. Lesions may be photographed prior to biopsy. The lung is reinflated. Clamps are applied to the area to be biopsied. The lung is incised and one or more tissue samples are obtained from the area containing the infiltrates or nodules. Alternatively, a triangular wedge may be excised from the lung. The biopsy area is closed using mattress sutures. A chest tube or catheter is placed within the pleural space as needed. The lung is fully inflated and the portal incisions are closed. Use 32607 for biopsy of one or more lung infiltrates, which refers to any substance in the lung that causes opacification as seen on a chest x-ray and may be caused by infection, inflammation, fluid accumulation, hemorrhage, or other conditions. Use 32608 for biopsy of one or more lung nodules, which is a small mass in the lung.

Thoracoscopy; with diagnostic biopsy(ies) of lung

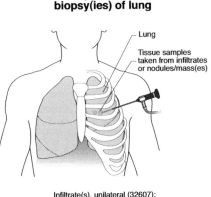

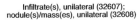

Infiltrate(s), unilateral (32607);
nodule(s)/mass(es), unilateral (32608)

32609

32609   Thoracoscopy; with biopsy(ies) of pleura

There are several different techniques employed in diagnostic thoracoscopy of the pleura with biopsy. One technique for evaluation of the pleura involves blunt entry by passing a clamp over the rib and through the pleura. The pleural space is digitally inspected at the entry site to ensure adequate space for insertion of the scope, which is then inserted under direct vision into the pleural space. The pleura is inspected and abnormalities are noted. Fluid may be evacuated using suction catheters. One or more tissue samples are taken from the pleura. Using another technique, a small intercostal incision may be made in the chest and a trocar inserted in the intercostal space (the space between two ribs). Following entry into the pleural space, air is injected and an artificial pneumothorax is induced for better visualization. An endoscope is inserted through the trocar and the pleura is inspected. Additional small incisions may be made for introducing other surgical instruments; however, diagnostic procedures on the pleura are often performed through a single incision. Fluid is drained from the chest and the pleura is inspected again. Any abnormalities are noted. Lesions may be photographed prior to biopsy. One or more tissue samples are taken from the pleura. A chest tube or catheter is placed within the pleural space as needed. Once the examination is complete, the scope is withdrawn, air is evacuated, portal incisions are closed, a chest tube is placed as needed, and portal incisions are closed.

32650

32650   Thoracoscopy, surgical; with pleurodesis (eg, mechanical or chemical)

Surgical thoracoscopy, also referred to as video assisted thoracoscopic surgery (VATS), is performed for mechanical or chemical pleurodesis. Three small incisions are made, one at the 7th or 8th intercostal space along the mid-axillary line, one in the posterior chest wall under the tip of the scapula, and one in the anterior chest wall at the 5th or 6th intercostal space. A videothoracoscope is inserted through one of the incisions and surgical instruments are inserted through the other incisions. Alternatively, the procedure is sometimes performed through a single incision. When a single incision technique is used, the procedure may be referred to as a pleuroscopy and both the scope and surgical instruments are passed through the single incision. The pleura is inspected, a chest tube is placed, and the pleural space is injected with a chemical sclerosing agent that causes irritation and inflammation of the pleurae, causing them to adhere to each other. The chest tube is temporarily closed, allowing the sclerosing agent to spread through the pleural space. The chest tube is then opened and the sclerosing agent is suctioned out of the chest tube. Alternatively, the pleura can be mechanically abraded, which also causes

inflammation resulting in the pleurae adhering to each other. The chest tube may be left in place for several days to allow fluid to drain from the chest.

32651-32652

32651   Thoracoscopy, surgical; with partial pulmonary decortication
32652   Thoracoscopy, surgical; with total pulmonary decortication, including intrapleural pneumonolysis

Partial pulmonary decortication (32651) or total pulmonary decortication including intrapleural pneumonolysis (32652) is performed by surgical thoracoscopy, also referred to as video assisted thoracoscopic surgery (VATS). A small posterolateral incision is made between the ribs usually at the fifth or sixth intercostal space just below the tip of the scapula. The pleura is identified by digital palpation, a trocar inserted, and the thoracoscope introduced into the pleural space. Fluid is aspirated and the pleural space explored. Two or more additional portal incisions are made for the introduction of surgical instruments. The physician then removes or strips the thickened fibrin layer, also called the rind or peel, from the outer pleural surface of part of the lung in 32651 or the entire lung in 32652. The fibrin layer is incised and the correct decortication plane determined. The fibrin layer is then grasped and dissected from the underlying visceral pleura. All portions of the lung encased by the thickened fibrin layer are addressed. In 32652, adhesions between the lung and the chest wall are also lysed. This is accomplished by the introduction of a cautery device which is used to severe the adhesions. Following completion of the procedure, one or more chest tubes are placed and the incisions are closed.

32653

32653   Thoracoscopy, surgical; with removal of intrapleural foreign body or fibrin deposit

Removal of intrapleural foreign body or fibrin deposit is performed by surgical thoracoscopy, also referred to as video assisted thoracoscopic surgery (VATS). A small posterolateral incision is made between the ribs usually at the fifth or sixth intercostal space just below the tip of the scapula. The pleura is identified by digital palpation; a trocar is inserted; and the thoracoscope is introduced. Fluid is aspirated and the thoracic cavity is explored. The foreign body or fibrin deposit is located. Two or more additional portal incisions are made for the introduction of surgical instruments to grasp and remove the foreign body or fibrin deposit. The pleural space is flushed with saline. A large bore chest tube is introduced as needed for drainage.

32654

32654   Thoracoscopy, surgical; with control of traumatic hemorrhage

Control of traumatic hemorrhage of the thorax is performed by surgical thoracoscopy, also referred to as video assisted thoracoscopic surgery (VATS). A small posterolateral incision is made between the ribs usually at the fifth or sixth intercostal space just below the tip of the scapula. A trocar is inserted and the thoracoscope is introduced. Blood and fluid are aspirated from the thorax and the thoracic cavity is explored to rule out cardiovascular or other injury requiring thoracotomy. The bleeding site is located. In the case of blunt trauma, the bleeding is usually found to be from an injury to intercostal vessels or from a lung laceration. Perforating trauma may result in injury to tissues of the mediastinum or other sites. Two or more additional portal incisions are made for the introduction of surgical instruments. The bleeding is controlled using diathermy, clips, and or staples. Chest tubes are placed as needed and the incisions are closed.

32655-32656

32655   Thoracoscopy, surgical; with resection-plication of bullae, includes any pleural procedure when performed
32656   Thoracoscopy, surgical; with parietal pleurectomy

Surgical thoracoscopy may also be referred to as video assisted thoracoscopic surgery (VATS). A small posterolateral incision is made between the ribs usually at the fifth or sixth intercostal space just below the tip of the scapula. The pleura is identified by digital palpation, a trocar inserted, and the thoracoscope introduced. Two or more additional portal incisions are made for the introduction of surgical instruments. In 32655, one or more bleb(s) or bulla(e) are treated by resection-plication. The pleura is inspected thoracoscopically and any pleural adhesions taken down using diathermy or sharp and blunt dissection. Sterile saline is instilled to identify the leaking bleb or bulla. The bleb or bulla is grasped using an endoscopic grasper or forceps and a linear endoscopic stapler and cutter inserted. Resection-plication of the bleb or bulla is accomplished by placing several lines of staples at the site of the bleb or bulla. Following the resection-plication procedure, the physician may need to perform additional pleural procedures such as a parietal pleurectomy which are included in 32655. In 32656, a parietal pleurectomy is performed alone by surgical thoracoscopy. A forceps is inserted through the anterior incision into the extrapleural plane under video control. The portion of parietal pleura to be removed is identified. The forceps are used to grasp the parietal pleura and strip it off the chest wall. The pleura is then wrapped around the forceps using a twisting motion and gentle traction is employed to remove the sheet of pleura through the portal incision.

Respiratory System

32658

32658   Thoracoscopy, surgical; with removal of clot or foreign body from pericardial sac

The physician removes a clot or foreign body from the pericardial sac using surgical thoracoscopy, also referred to as video assisted thoracoscopic surgery (VATS). The pericardium is the fibrous membrane that covers the heart. A small incision is made between the ribs usually at the sixth or seventh intercostal space along the anterior axillary line and the videothoracoscope is introduced. Two additional portal incisions are made for the introduction of surgical instruments at the posterior axillary line usually at the fifth and eighth intercostal spaces. One lung is collapsed. The inferior pulmonary ligament is divided. The phrenic nerve is identified and protected. In the case of blunt trauma resulting in pericardial blood clot, the pericardium is grasped and retracted away from the heart. Endoscopic scissors are introduced; the pericardium is nicked; and blood and fluid are evacuated. The pericardium is examined and the blood clot is located and removed or a foreign body is identified and removed. Bleeding is controlled, chest tubes are placed as needed, and the incisions are closed.

32659

32659   Thoracoscopy, surgical; with creation of pericardial window or partial resection of pericardial sac for drainage

The physician creates a pericardial window or performs a partial resection of the pericardial sac for drainage using surgical thoracoscopy, also referred to as video assisted thoracoscopic surgery (VATS). The pericardium is the fibrous membrane that covers the heart. A small incision is made between the ribs usually at the sixth or seventh intercostal space along the anterior axillary line and the videothoracoscope is introduced. Two additional portal incisions are made for the introduction of surgical instruments at the posterior axillary line usually at the fifth and eighth intercostal spaces. The inferior pulmonary ligament is divided. The phrenic nerve is identified and protected. The pericardium is grasped and retracted away from the heart. Endoscopic scissors are introduced and the pericardium is nicked and blood and fluid are evacuated. A pericardial window or partial resection of the pericardial sac is then performed. This is accomplished by resecting a 3-4 cm section of the pericardial sac. The pericardium is examined and a sponge is introduced to break up loculations. A second window may be created in the same manner. A chest tube is placed into the pericardial window to drain the pericardial space. A second chest tube is placed in the pleural space.

32661

32661   Thoracoscopy, surgical; with excision of pericardial cyst, tumor, or mass

The physician excises a pericardial cyst, tumor, or mass using surgical thoracoscopy, also referred to as video assisted thoracoscopic surgery (VATS). The pericardium is the fibrous membrane that covers the heart. A small incision is made between the ribs usually at the sixth or seventh intercostal space along the anterior axillary line and the videothoracoscope is introduced. The thoracic cavity is inspected and the cyst, tumor, or mass located. Two additional portal incisions are made for the introduction of surgical instruments at the posterior axillary line usually at the fifth and eighth intercostal spaces. The inferior pulmonary ligament is divided. The phrenic nerve is identified and protected. If the lesion is a cyst, it may be opened and fluid and debris evacuated. The cyst, tumor, or mass is then dissected free of surrounding tissue and removed along with a margin of healthy pericardium. The defect in the pericardium may be covered with a synthetic patch or left open to drain. If it is left open, a chest tube is placed into the defect. A second chest tube is placed in the pleural space.

32662

32662   Thoracoscopy, surgical; with excision of mediastinal cyst, tumor, or mass

An excision of a mediastinal cyst, tumor, or mass is performed by surgical thoracoscopy, also referred to as video assisted thoracoscopic surgery (VATS). The patient is placed in lateral decubitus position and three or more trocars are placed depending on the location of the lesion. A pneumothorax is created to aid in visualization. With the thoracoscope in place, the cyst, tumor, or mass is evaluated as to its site and relationship to adjacent structures. The pleura over the cyst, tumor, or mass is incised and the lesion is dissected off the pleura. If the procedure is performed to excise a cyst, the cystic cavities are opened, aspirated, and decompressed. Complete excision of the cyst wall is then performed using blunt dissection and traction. If it is necessary to leave small remnants of the cyst that are adherent to vital structures, the cyst mucosa is cauterized to help prevent recurrence. If the procedure is for a solid tumor, it is dissected free of surrounding structures; the chest incision is widened, and the mass is placed in an extracting bag to prevent contamination of the chest wall with tumor cells. A chest tube is then placed; trocars are removed; and incisions are closed.

32663

32663   Thoracoscopy, surgical; with lobectomy (single lobe)

Surgical thoracoscopy may also be referred to as video assisted thoracoscopic surgery (VATS). Single lung ventilation is initiated and the thoracoscope is placed at the anterior or posterior axillary line depending on whether the lobe being removed is on the right or left side. Additional trocars are placed for the introduction of surgical instruments. A lung clamp is used to retract the lung and allow visualization of the pulmonary vein and artery. A larger utility incision is made over the superior pulmonary vein for an upper lobe lobectomy or over the third or fourth interspace for a middle or lower lobe lobectomy. The pulmonary vein is dissected free of overlying pleura and divided. The main pulmonary artery is identified and the arterial branch for the lobe being removed is located. Lymph nodes overlying that artery are excised to allow better access and the artery is then clamped and transected using a vascular stapler. The bronchus is exposed and transected. Once all the structures attached to the lobe have been divided, the fissure is exposed and the lung is divided along both minor and major fissures. The excised lobe is placed in a surgical extraction bag, and removed through the utility incision.

32664

32664   Thoracoscopy, surgical; with thoracic sympathectomy

A thoracic sympathectomy is performed by surgical thoracoscopy, also referred to as video assisted thoracoscopic surgery (VATS). The patient is placed in semi-Fowler's position with arms abducted and a roll behind the shoulder to allow access to the upper sympathetic chain. Using one lung ventilation, the contralateral lung is collapsed. Gravity causes the lung to fall downwards and away from the chest wall. One or two small incisions are made in the chest and the thoracoscope is inserted. The sympathetic chain is visualized under the parietal pleura running vertically over the necks of the ribs in the upper vertebral region. The sympathetic chain is divided using hook cautery to cut and coagulate the chain. Alternatively, a segment of chain may be removed. The ganglia is completely obliterated with complete severance of the sympathetic chain. The pleura is divided lateral to the chain and any aberrant nerve bundles are located and severed. The sympathetic nerve bundles are separated and the ends are cauterized to prevent regrowth. The level of the transection is dependent on the condition being treated with division for hyperhidrosis at levels T2-T5, for thoracic outlet syndrome and reflex sympathetic dystrophy at levels T1-T3, and for chronic pancreatic pain at levels T4-T10. When the transection is complete, a chest tube is placed and the subcutaneous tissue is closed. The lungs are expanded, the chest tube is removed, and a subcuticular suture is placed. The procedure is then repeated on the opposite side.

32665

32665   Thoracoscopy, surgical; with esophagomyotomy (Heller type)

Esophagomyotomy is performed by surgical thoracoscopy, also referred to as video assisted thoracoscopic surgery (VATS). A small posterolateral incision is made between the ribs usually at the fourth, fifth or sixth intercostal space at a point near the posterior aspect of the axillary line and the videothoracoscope is introduced. This placement allows the physician to visualize the esophagus from above looking downward. Two additional portal incisions are made for the introduction of surgical instruments, one anterior and one posterior to the line of the esophagus. Additional portal incisions are made and retractors are introduced to retract the lung and diaphragm. The pleural space is entered and air is injected to create an artificial pneumothorax and collapse the lung. The distal esophagus is identified and retracted using a flexible esophagoscope. The muscular layer of the esophagus is incised longitudinally down to the submucosa using endoscopic scissors or hook cautery. The incision is extended approximately 0.5 cm into the stomach. Following completion of the esophagomyotomy, a chest tube is placed through one of the existing portal incisions and the lung is re-expanded. Portal incisions are closed and a nasogastric tube is placed.

32666-32667

32666   Thoracoscopy, surgical; with therapeutic wedge resection (eg, mass, nodule), initial unilateral

32667   Thoracoscopy, surgical; with therapeutic wedge resection (eg, mass or nodule), each additional resection, ipsilateral (List separately in addition to code for primary procedure)

Surgical thoracoscopy may also be referred to as video-assisted thoracoscopic surgery (VATS). Therapeutic wedge resection may be performed through a single portal incision. The incision site and placement of the thoracoscope are dependent on the site of the lesion. Under thoracoscopic control, the lesion is identified and an endograsper is introduced. The lesion is grasped and suspended. An endostapler is then introduced deeply into the lung parenchyma containing the lesion, which is positioned between the jaws of the endostapler using the endograsper. The jaws are then closed around the lung lesion and the endostapler is fired. The jaws are opened and this process is repeated until the entire wedge of parenchyma has been separated from the lung. Endoscissors may also be used to separate the lung tissue. Once the wedge of lung tissue has been resected, an endobag is introduced and the wedge is removed after being placed in the bag. Bleeding is controlled; instruments are removed; and a chest tube is placed through the same portal incision. The physician may perform single or multiple wedge resections on one of the lungs. Use 32666 for the first wedge of lung tissue excised. Use 32667 for each additional wedge of tissue removed from a different site in the same lung.

● New Code   ▲ Revised Code

Respiratory System

32668

32668   Thoracoscopy, surgical; with diagnostic wedge resection followed by anatomic lung resection (List separately in addition to code for primary procedure)

Thoracoscopic diagnostic wedge resection is performed to evaluate diseased or damaged lung tissue and to help determine how much of the lung should be removed in a separately reportable anatomic resection of the lung which will be performed during the same surgical session. The wedge resection may be performed through a single portal incision. The incision site and placement of the thoracoscope are dependent on the site of the lesion. Under thoracoscopic control, the lesion is identified and an endograsper is introduced. The lesion is grasped and suspended. An endostapler is then introduced deeply into the lung parenchyma containing the lesion, which is positioned between the jaws of the endostapler using the endograsper. The jaws are then closed around the lung lesion and the endostapler is fired. The jaws are opened and this process is repeated until the entire wedge of parenchyma has been separated from the lung. Endoscissors may also be used to separate the lung tissue. Once the wedge of lung tissue has been resected, an endobag is introduced and the wedge is removed after being placed in the bag. Bleeding is controlled; instruments are removed; and a chest tube is placed through the same portal incision. Separately reportable pathology exam is performed and the results are used to determine what definitive lung procedure should then be performed.

32669

32669   Thoracoscopy, surgical; with removal of a single lung segment (segmentectomy)

Surgical thoracoscopy may also be referred to as video-assisted thoracoscopic surgery (VATS). A lung segmentectomy involves removal of a small portion of the lung. The procedure is typically performed for early stage lung cancer that involves only a small portion of the lung as opposed to an entire lobe. A 1 cm portal incision is made at the 7th or 8th intercostal space in the posterior axillary line for the camera. A second 4 cm access incision is made at the 5th or 6th intercostal space anteriorly. Following entry into the pleural space, air is injected and an artificial pneumothorax is induced for better visualization. The pleura and lung are explored for evidence of metastatic disease and to determine resectability of the lesion. The pleura is divided at the pleural-parenchymal reflection and hilar structures are explored. The segmental pulmonary vein in the lung segment of interest is identified and staple ligated. Additional pleural dissection is performed as needed. The segmental arteries are identified and divided. The segmental bronchus is encircled, stapled, and divided. The lung may be temporarily reinflated to enhance identification of the segment of lung to be removed. The lung parenchyma is then resected using a stapling device. Once the lung segment has been resected, an endobag is introduced and the segment is removed after being placed in the bag. Bleeding is controlled, instruments are removed, the lung is reinflated, and a chest tube is placed.

32670

32670   Thoracoscopy, surgical; with removal of two lobes (bilobectomy)

Surgical thoracoscopy may also be referred to as video-assisted thoracoscopic surgery (VATS). A bilobectomy involves removal of two lobes of the right lung. Single left lung ventilation is established. A 1 cm portal incision is made at the 7th or 8th intercostal space in the anerior axillary line for the camera. A second portal incision is made at the 7th or 8th intercostal space posteriorly. A 4 cm access incision is made over the 3rd, 4th, or 5th interspace depending on which lobes are being resected. Following entry into the pleural space, air is injected, and an artificial pneumothorax is induced for better visualization. The pleura and lung are explored for evidence of metastatic disease and to determine resectability of the lesion. The pleura are divided at the pleural-parenchymal reflection, hilar structures are explored and the pulmonary veins in the lobes of interest are identified and staple ligated. Additional pleural dissection is performed as needed. The lobar arteries are identified and divided. The lobar bronchi are encircled, stapled, and divided. The lung parenchyma is then resected along the fissure using a stapling device. Once the lobes have been resected, an endopouch is introduced and the lobes are removed after being placed in the pouch. Bleeding is controlled, instruments are removed, the remaining lobe of the right lung is reinflated, and a chest tube is placed.

32671

32671   Thoracoscopy, surgical; with removal of lung (pneumonectomy)

Surgical thoracoscopy may also be referred to as video-assisted thoracoscopic surgery (VATS). The thoracoscope is placed in the 7th or 8th intercostal space over the mid to anterior axillary line on the affected side and thoracic structures are inspected. A working incision is made in the anterolateral chest wall at the 4th intercostal space to provide access to the thoracic cavity. Following entry into the pleural space, air is injected, and an artificial pneumothorax is induced. The pleura and lung are explored for evidence of metastatic disease and to determine resectability of the lung. The pleura is divided at the pleural-parenchymal reflection, hilar structures are explored, and the pulmonary veins are identified and staple ligated. Additional pleural dissection is performed as needed. The pulmonary arteries are identified and divided. The main bronchus is encircled, stapled, and

divided. Dissection continues until the entire lung is mobilized. An endopouch is introduced and the lung is removed through the working incision after being placed in the pouch. Bleeding is controlled, instruments are removed, a chest tube is placed, and incisions are closed.

32672

32672   Thoracoscopy, surgical; with resection-plication for emphysematous lung (bullous or non-bullous) for lung volume reduction (LVRS), unilateral includes any pleural procedure, when performed

Surgical thoracoscopy may also be referred to as video-assisted thoracoscopic surgery (VATS). Resection-plication of emphysematous lung for lung volume reduction surgery (LVRS) is performed on patients with emphysema to improve exercise tolerance and quality of life and is typically performed on the upper lobe. Single lung ventilation is initiated on the non-operative side. A portal incision is made in the 7th intercostal space just anterior to the anterior superior iliac spine (ASIS) on the right or just posterior to the ASIS on the left. A 5 cm access incision is made in the 5th intercostal space just lateral to the left midclavicular line which collapses the lung. A third portal incision may be made in the posterior aspect of the 5th intercostal space. The mediastinal pleura around the hilum is mobilized. The upper lobe is grasped with a ring clamp at its apex and retracted superiorly and laterally. The upper lobe is inspected and the resection lines are identified. An endostapler is introduced and the upper lobe is maneuvered into the jaws of the stapler. Multiple staple firings are used to resect up to 70% of the upper lobe. The resected upper lobe is removed through the access incision. A pleural tent is then created and draped over the staple line to seal any air leaks that may develop. Other pleural procedures are performed as needed. Bleeding is controlled by electrocautery. Chest tubes are placed anteriorly and posteriorly. The lung is inflated while the thoracoscope is still in place and complete expansion of the remaining lung parenchyma is verified. The thoracoscope is removed and portal and access incisions are closed. This code reports a unilateral procedure.

32673

32673   Thoracoscopy, surgical; with resection of thymus, unilateral or bilateral

There are several minimally invasive thoracoscopic approaches for thymectomy which include: transcervical subxiphoid videothoracoscopic thymectomy, subxiphoid video-assisted thoracoscopic extended thymectomy, video-assisted thoracoscopic extended thymectomy, transcervical thoracoscopically assisted thymectomy. Port placement and surgical technique are dependent on the approach used. A left-sided approach uses a camera port placed at the 5th intercostal space and two additional thoracic ports—one through a separate portal incision in the intercostal space and one on the midclavicular line in the 3rd intercostal space. The hemithorax is inflated through the camera port and the left lung is deflated. The mediastinal pleural space is inspected and dissection of fat begins inferiorly at the left pericardiophrenic angle. The thymic gland is dissected from the retrosternal chest wall and the left inferior horn of the thymus is isolated and dissected from the pericardium. The pleura is incised at the superior aspect of the mediastinum, the thymus is mobilized upwards, and thymic tissue is dissected from the plane of the aortopulmonary window. Under thoracoscopic visualization, the thymus is dissected from the right mediastinal pleura and right inferior horn. Cervical fat is dissected from the retrosternal and jugular region and the upper horns of the thymus are exposed. The innominate vein is located on the left and the superior horns of the thymus are dissected. The thymus veins are exposed and doubly clipped and ligated. The thymus gland and fatty tissue of the mediastinum and cervical neck are completely resected, placed in an endobag, and removed through the working port at the 5th intercostal space. Bleeding is controlled. The left lung is inflated, chest tubes are placed as needed, and the portal wounds are closed.

32674

32674   Thoracoscopy, surgical; with mediastinal and regional lymphadenectomy (List separately in addition to code for primary procedure)

Mediastinal lymph nodes are resected during a separately reportable thoracoscopic procedure. Lymph node dissection is typically performed to evaluate metastatic spread to the lymph nodes on patients undergoing lobectomy procedures for malignancies. The exact procedure depends on whether the malignancy is in the right or left lung and what lobes were involved. Following the lobectomy or pneumonectomy, any remaining lobe(s) is(are) retracted away from the mediastinum. A curved ring forceps is placed through the posterior port and used to retract tissue at the medial aspect to expose the mediastinal nodes. The mediastinal pleura overlying this area is incised using electrocautery. The nodal tissue is dissected off surrounding structures and the inferior aspect of the nodal tissue is grasped with ring forceps. Dissection is carried superiorly until all regional nodes or all mediastinal nodes have been completely mobilized. The mobilization is performed while simultaneously using electrocautery and endoclips to control bleeding and lymphatic vessels. The tissue is placed in an endobag and removed through the access port.

Respiratory System

32701

32701   Thoracic target(s) delineation for stereotactic body radiation therapy (SRS/SBRT), (photon or particle beam), entire course of treatment

Stereotactic radiosurgery (SRS) and stereotactic body radiotherapy (SBRT) are image-guided radiation therapies involving focused radiation delivery to destroy tumor cells while sparing the normal tissues. Complex imaging technology is used to map the precise location and size of a tumor. Target delineation, treatment planning, and treatment delivery are the key components of a SRS/SBRT procedure. Code 32701 reports target delineation for radiation therapy of conditions involving the thorax. Pre-treatment target delineation is done to ensure accurate definition of the primary tumor targets. SRS/SBRT is typically delivered in multiple sessions over a course of days (i.e., fractionated), rather than in a single session. Target re-delineation may be required to ensure accurate coverage throughout treatment if significant changes occur in tumor position or size in response to treatment.

32800

32800   Repair lung hernia through chest wall

The physician repairs a lung hernia through the chest wall. Herniation of the lung through the chest wall is a rare condition that may result from thoracic trauma, infection in the thoracic wall, a congenital weakness, or a weakness caused by a prior thoracostomy tube. The majority of lung hernias occur through the intercostal spaces. Congenital hernias can also occur in the cervical region through the thoracic inlet. The least common site is a diaphragmatic lung hernia. To repair an intercostal lung hernia, an incision is made in the skin of the chest over the intercostal space where the lung hernia is located. The incision is carried down through subcutaneous tissue and chest wall musculature. The hernia sac is exposed and dissected free of adjacent tissues. The pleura is freed from the periosteum of the adjacent ribs. The periosteum covering adjacent ribs is then incised and elevated to create periosteal flaps. The periosteal flap of the upper rib is turned downward and that of the lower rib is turned upward. The flaps are then sutured together to obliterate the hernia defect. The periosteal flap repair may be reinforced by wiring the adjacent ribs together. The repair can also be accomplished using muscle or synthetic material instead of or in addition to periosteum. Chest tubes are placed as needed and the chest incision is closed in layered fashion.

32810

32810   Closure of chest wall following open flap drainage for empyema (Clagett type procedure)

The physician closes the chest wall following open flap for drainage of empyema. The empyema cavity is inspected and when it is found to be free of gross infection, the cavity is debrided of any remaining necrotic or inflamed tissue and filled with antibiotic solution. The previously created skin flap is taken down and the physician then determines which of several closure options will be used to cover the chest wall defect. The simplest closure is coverage by a local pleural or intercostal muscle flap. Other muscle flap options include the serratus anterior or latissimus dorsi muscles. Another option is the use of a separately reportable omental flap harvested via an open or laparoscopic approach and passed through the diaphragm and used to fill a part or all of the empyema cavity. The selected flap is then developed, transposed, and secured over the empyema site and chest wall defect is closed.

32815

32815   Open closure of major bronchial fistula

The physician performs an open closure of a major bronchial fistula. The fistula is approached through an anterior incision between one of the ribs. Pectoralis and intercostal muscles are divided and the pleura is exposed. The ribs are spread. Alternatively, if greater exposure is required, the sternum may be split or one or more ribs removed. The fistula is located, debrided of necrotic and inflammatory material, then closed using sutures or staples which may be reinforced with a local flap of pleura, pericardium, or mediastinal fatty tissue. The fistula repair may require development of a vascularized muscle flap that is then transposed to cover the bronchial leak site. Reinforcement may also be accomplished using omentum that is harvested through an abdominal incision and passed through the diaphragm to the fistula site. Chest tubes are placed as needed and chest incisions are closed.

32820

32820   Major reconstruction, chest wall (posttraumatic)

The physician reconstructs the chest wall following a serious, disfiguring injury that has resulted in loss of soft tissue from a portion of the chest. If the physician is repairing an acute injury, devitalized tissue is debrided and any foreign bodies are removed. Depending on the extent of soft tissue damage, surrounding tissues may be mobilized and used to close the wound. Larger acute wounds may require separately reportable rotational or free musculocutaneous flaps or omental flaps. Commonly used muscle flaps include the pectoralis, latissimus dorsi, external oblique, or rectus abdominus. If the chest wall is being

reconstructed after the acute injury has healed, the soft tissue reconstruction may be performed using synthetic materials such as mesh or methylmethacrylate.

32850

32850   Donor pneumonectomy(s) (including cold preservation), from cadaver donor

One or both lungs are removed from a brain-dead patient and perfused with cold preservation solution in preparation for transplant. Typically the lungs are removed en bloc with the heart. A long incision is made in the chest and the thorax is opened. The great vessels and trachea are dissected free of surrounding tissue. Systemic heparin is administered. The pulmonary arteries are cannulated and the pulmonary vasculature is flushed with a cold solution. The heart is stopped along with the respiration. The superior and inferior vena cava, the aorta, and the trachea are divided. The heart and lung block is removed. The heart is separated from the lungs and removed with the attached portions of the superior and inferior vena cava and the aorta. The lungs may also be separated from each other. The harvested lungs are placed in crystalloid solution, packed in ice, and transported to the recipient transplant site.

32851-32852

32851   Lung transplant, single; without cardiopulmonary bypass
32852   Lung transplant, single; with cardiopulmonary bypass

A single lung transplant is performed. The thorax is opened and the lung exposed via a posterolateral incision through the fourth or fifth intercostal space. The fifth rib may be excised to facilitate access to the lung. A second incision may be made in the groin in the event that cardiopulmonary bypass is required and thoracic vessels cannot be cannulated. The lung with the poorest pulmonary function is removed from the transplant recipient. The donor lung is then placed in the thoracic cavity. There are a number of different lung transplant techniques and anastomosis of the bronchus, pulmonary artery, and pulmonary vein may be done in a different order than described here. Bronchial anastomosis is accomplished by telescoping the smaller bronchus into the larger bronchus and suturing the two together. The bronchial anastomosis site is then covered with local peribronchial tissue, thymic tissue pedicle flaps, or pericardial fat. The donor and recipient pulmonary arteries are then carefully approximated to avoid kinking and anastomosed. The left atrium is clamped in preparation for anastomosis of the donor and recipient pulmonary veins. The recipient pulmonary vein is incised, a left atrial cuff created, and the pulmonary vein orifices anastomosed. The lung is reinflated, air evacuated from the pulmonary vasculature at the left atrial suture line, and lung perfusion reestablished. The suture lines are evaluated and reinforced with sutures as needed. Chest tubes are placed as needed and the chest closed. The bronchial anastomosis is inspected by flexible bronchoscopy and the airway is cleared of blood and secretions. If the lung transplant is performed without cardiopulmonary bypass, use code 32851. If cardiopulmonary bypass is required, use code 32852.

32853-32854

32853   Lung transplant, double (bilateral sequential or en bloc); without cardiopulmonary bypass
32854   Lung transplant, double (bilateral sequential or en bloc); with cardiopulmonary bypass

A double lung transplant is performed using either a bilateral sequential or en bloc technique. Bilateral sequential lung transplant is the most commonly used technique. The thorax is opened and the lungs exposed via bilateral anterolateral incision through the fourth or fifth intercostal space. Another incision may be made in the groin in the event that cardiopulmonary bypass is required and thoracic vessels cannot be cannulated. The first lung is removed from the transplant recipient. The donor lung is then placed in the thoracic cavity. There are a number of different lung transplant techniques and anastomosis of the bronchus, pulmonary artery, and pulmonary vein may be done in a different order than described here. Bronchial anastomosis is accomplished by telescoping the smaller bronchus into the larger bronchus and suturing the two together. The bronchial anastomosis site is covered with local peribronchial tissue, mediastinal tissue, thymic tissue pedicle flaps, or pericardial fat. The donor and recipient pulmonary arteries are then carefully approximated to avoid kinking and anastomosed. The left atrium is clamped in preparation for anastomosis of the donor and recipient pulmonary veins. The recipient pulmonary vein is incised, a left atrial cuff created, and the pulmonary vein orifices anastomosed. The lung is reinflated, air evacuated from the pulmonary vasculature at the left atrial suture line, and lung perfusion reestablished. The suture lines are evaluated and reinforced with sutures as needed. Chest tubes are placed as needed and the chest closed. The bronchial anastomosis is inspected by flexible bronchoscopy and the airway is cleared of blood and secretions. This second lung is then removed from the transplant recipient and the second donor lung transplanted using the same technique. If the bilateral lung transplant is performed without cardiopulmonary bypass, use code 32853. To accomplish bilateral lung transplant without cardiopulmonary bypass, the patient is ventilated through the native lung during the first lung transplant and then through the newly transplanted lung while the second lung is transplanted. If cardiopulmonary bypass is required, use code 32854. En bloc transplant is performed through a pleural and pericardial window and requires cardiopulmonary bypass.

Respiratory System

32855-32856

32855   Backbench standard preparation of cadaver donor lung allograft prior to transplantation, including dissection of allograft from surrounding soft tissues to prepare pulmonary venous/atrial cuff, pulmonary artery, and bronchus; unilateral

32856   Backbench standard preparation of cadaver donor lung allograft prior to transplantation, including dissection of allograft from surrounding soft tissues to prepare pulmonary venous/atrial cuff, pulmonary artery, and bronchus; bilateral

A cadaver donor lung is prepared for transplant in a standard backbench (backtable) procedure. The external surface of the lung is examined for tissue damage and abnormalities. The pulmonary veins and left atrial cuff are inspected for length and the presence of any injuries. The pulmonary artery is also checked for length and injuries and is then checked for thrombus. If any thrombus is present it is removed and sent for laboratory examination and culture. The pulmonary artery is then dissected free of surrounding tissue. The bronchial staples are removed and specimens taken of the bronchial secretions which are sent to the lab for cultures. The bronchus is trimmed to the desired length. The bronchial and lobar orifices are suctioned and irrigated with saline as needed. The lung is placed in a sterile basin and packed in ice and/or bathed in cold saline until the recipient transplant team is ready to begin the transplant procedure. In 32855, a standard backbench preparation is performed on a single lung. In 32856, both lungs are prepared for a double lung transplant. In a double lung transplant in addition to the preparation described above, attached pericardium may need to be excised. Next, the posterior wall of the left atrium is divided between the left and right pulmonary veins. Non-vascular staples are placed along the bronchial-carinal junction of the first lung to be transplanted and the main bronchus is divided distal to the staple line. The first lung to be transplanted is prepared as described above and delivered to the transplant recipient team. While the first lung is being transplanted, the second lung is prepared in the same fashion and when preparation is complete, it is also delivered to the transplant recipient team.

32900

32900   Resection of ribs, extrapleural, all stages

The physician performs an extrapleural rib resection to cause collapse of one side of the chest. This procedure is performed to treat pulmonary tuberculosis and chronic empyema. One of several different resection techniques is used. A small section or short portion of rib may be resected or a long posterolateral rib resection is performed. Using a long posterolateral resection technique, the skin is incised over the third rib and the incision is carried down through subcutaneous tissue. The trapezius and rhomboid muscles are incised to expose the rib. A subperiosteal resection is performed without disturbing the pleura and a long section of the third rib is removed. To produce the required collapse of the chest wall and compression of the lung, removal of a smaller portion of the fourth rib and sometimes additional ribs using the same extrapleural subperiosteal technique may be necessary. Because patients undergoing this type of procedure are usually seriously ill, the procedure is often done in stages over several operative sessions. Code 32900 is used to report all stages.

32905-32906

32905   Thoracoplasty, Schede type or extrapleural (all stages)

32906   Thoracoplasty, Schede type or extrapleural (all stages); with closure of bronchopleural fistula

The physician performs a Schede type or extrapleural thoracoplasty. Thoracoplasty is the operative removal of a varying number of ribs to remove the skeletal support from one side of the chest causing the chest wall to collapse. Thoracoplasty may be performed as a single or multiple stage procedure. This procedure is performed to treat chronic thoracic empyema and pulmonary tuberculosis by obliterating the pleural space. There are a number of different approaches but the standard approach is by a parascapular incision. Subperiosteal resection of multiple ribs is then performed. Usually the first through the seventh ribs are resected but as many as eleven may require resection. The intercostal muscles are sectioned. The intercostal nerve is identified and sectioned. An extensive skin and muscle flap is raised and the lung dissected off the entire chest wall. The costotransverse ligament may be divided allowing the scapula and extracostal musculature to drop into the space and help maintain the collapse. Extracostal muscle and skin is then partially closed over gauze packing which causes fresh granulation tissue to form that will eventually obliterate the cavitary or empyema space. In 32905, the thoracoplasty does not require closure of a bronchopleural fistula. In 32906, the thoracoplasty is performed with closure of a bronchopleural fistula. The fistula is debrided of necrotic and inflammatory material. The fistula is then closed using sutures or staples which may be reinforced with a local flap of pleura, pericardium, or mediastinal fatty tissue. The fistula repair may also require development of a vascularized muscle flap or omental flap that is then transposed to cover the bronchial leak site.

32940

32940   Pneumonolysis, extraperiosteal, including filling or packing procedures

The physician performs an extraperiosteal pneumonolysis including filling or packing to cause collapse of one side of the chest. This procedure is performed to treat pulmonary tuberculosis. A long posterolateral skin incision is made over the third rib and the incision is carried down through subcutaneous tissue. The trapezius and rhomboid muscles are incised to expose the rib. A long section of the third rib is removed. A smaller portion of the fourth rib may also be removed. The intercostal muscles are sectioned. The intercostal nerve is identified and sectioned. The adherent, diseased portion of the lung is then dissected free from the chest wall using forceps and scissors, followed by finger dissection. The pneumonolysis typically extends from the third rib down to the sixth rib and from the axillary region to the mediastinum. When sufficient collapse of the lung has been achieved, the collapse is maintained by filling the intrathoracic space with air or packing it with gauze or other packing material.

32960

32960   Pneumothorax, therapeutic, intrapleural injection of air

A therapeutic pneumothorax, also referred to as an artificial pneumothorax, is created by injecting air into the pleural space. This reversible surgical collapse procedure is performed to treat pulmonary tuberculosis. A small intercostal incision is made in the chest. A trocar is inserted into the intercostal space and advanced into the pleural space where air is injected to create an artificial pneumothorax. If the lung does not completely collapse, intrapleural adhesions may be lysed.

32997

32997   Total lung lavage (unilateral)

The physician performs a unilateral total lung lavage, also referred to as a whole lung lavage, which is performed to treat pulmonary alveolar proteinosis, a rare disorder characterized by accumulation of surfactant in the alveoli. Oxygen is administered immediately prior to the procedure to improve oxygen saturation. A general anesthetic is then administered and the patient is intubated with a double lumen endotracheal tube that will allow one-lung ventilation of the untreated lung while whole lung lavage is performed on the other. The baseline compliance of each lung is measured. The lung to be treated is clamped for several minutes to allow oxygen absorption. The lung is then filled with normal saline heated to body temperature. Chest percussion is performed during the saline instillation. The saline is drained from the lung and chest percussion is performed during the recovery cycle. The instillation and recovery cycles are repeated multiple times. Following the final instillation and recovery cycle, a Valsalva maneuver is performed accompanied by aggressive bronchial suctioning. Lung compliance is measured to verify that it has returned to baseline. When end tidal CO2 and pulse oxygen saturation has returned to normal, the patient is extubated.

32998

32998   Ablation therapy for reduction or eradication of 1 or more pulmonary tumor(s) including pleura or chest wall when involved by tumor extension, percutaneous, radiofrequency, unilateral

Percutaneous radiofrequency tumor ablation therapy is done on one lung for reduction or eradication of one or more pulmonary tumor(s), including the pleura or chest wall when involved. Tumor location determines the approach, whether anterior in supine position or posterior in prone position. Steel mesh grounding pads are placed on the patient's lower back and/or gluteal region. CT scanning is used to plan the path of the needle track and the optimal percutaneous placement of the needle. Radiofrequency ablation is carried out with a 17-gauge internally cooled tip electrode needle, selected for tumor size. Twelve minute treatment time ensures complete necrotic coagulation of the tumor volume corresponding to the diameter of the exposed, uninsulated portion of the needle. Using CT guidance, the electrode needle is introduced into the tumor. Electrodes are attached to a generator that produces up to 200 W output. The tip is cooled after applying radiofrequency by infusing cooled saline solution through the cooling lumen of the electrode. Every attempt is made to use only one electrode pass for insertion. Since large tumors require repositioning of the needle for complete ablation, the needle angle is repositioned and reinserted without complete withdrawal using CT guidance. CT scanning is used throughout the procedure in short intervals to detect and manage complications and needle position. When ablation is complete, the needle is withdrawn without cauterizing the probe tract.

Respiratory System

33010-33011

33010   Pericardiocentesis; initial
33011   Pericardiocentesis; subsequent

The physician drains fluid from the pericardium. Under local anesthesia, a long needle is inserted below the sternum into the pericardial space and fluid is aspirated, or withdrawn. The needle or catheter is then removed and a dressing is placed on the wound. Code 33010 for the initial pericardiocentesis. Code 33011 for each subsequent pericardiocentesis.

33015

33015   Tube pericardiostomy

The physician performs a percutaneous tube pericardiostomy under local or general anesthetic. The skin, subxiphoid area, soft tissues of the chest, and the pericardium are infiltrated with local anesthetic. The pericardium is penetrated; fluid is aspirated from the pericardial cavity; and a guidewire is introduced and positioned in the pericardial cavity under fluoroscopic guidance. The skin is then incised and an introducer is placed over the guidewire into the pericardial cavity. Proper location of the introducer is verified fluoroscopically and a chest tube is then threaded into the pericardium. The introducer is removed and the chest tube is secured to the skin with sutures and connected to a chest drainage bag and suction device.

33020

33020   Pericardiotomy for removal of clot or foreign body (primary procedure)

The physician performs a pericardiotomy to remove a blood clot or foreign body from the pericardium via an open approach. The pericardium is the fibrous membrane that covers the heart. The heart is exposed by a subxiphoid approach, median sternotomy, or anterior thoracotomy depending on the planned pericardiotomy site. In the case of blunt trauma resulting in pericardial blood clot, the pericardium is grasped and retracted away from the heart. The pericardium is nicked and blood and fluid are evacuated. The pericardial space is examined, and the blood clot is located and removed. In the case of a foreign body, it is located, grasped with forceps, and removed. A chest tube is placed into the pericardial cavity to drain the pericardial space and additional chest tubes are placed as needed.

33025

33025   Creation of pericardial window or partial resection for drainage

The physician creates a pericardial window or performs a partial resection of the pericardium for drainage using an open approach which includes subxiphoid approach, median sternotomy, or anterior thoracotomy. Using the preferred subxiphoid approach, the linea alba is divided just below the xiphoid process, which is excised if needed. The peritoneum is retracted and the pericardium is exposed and incised. Fluid is aspirated and sent to the laboratory for culture. A pericardial window or partial resection of the pericardial sac is then performed by resecting a 3-4 cm section of the pericardial sac. The pericardium is examined and a sponge is introduced to break up loculations. A second window may be created in the same manner. A chest tube is placed into the pericardial window to drain the pericardial space.

33030-33031

33030   Pericardiectomy, subtotal or complete; without cardiopulmonary bypass
33031   Pericardiectomy, subtotal or complete; with cardiopulmonary bypass

The physician performs a subtotal or complete pericardiectomy via an open approach. Excision of most or all of the pericardium is typically performed to treat constrictive pericarditis, which is a chronic inflammatory process leading to thickening and fibrosis of the pericardium. A median sternotomy or anterolateral thoracotomy is used to expose the heart. The thickened fibrotic pericardium is incised and anterior dissection of the pericardium is initiated taking care to identify and protect the right and left phrenic nerves. Beginning at the ascending aorta the pericardium is excised using blunt and sharp dissection. Dissection continues over the lateral and posterior walls of the left ventricle, the pulmonary veins, and the pulmonary artery. The diaphragmatic surface of the heart is addressed next followed by resection over the free wall of the right ventricle, right atrium and vena cava. Use code 33030 if the procedure is performed without cardiopulmonary bypass. Code 33031 is used when cardiopulmonary bypass is required.

33050

33050   Resection of pericardial cyst or tumor

The physician resects a pericardial cyst or tumor via an open approach. The pericardium is the fibrous membrane that covers the heart. A median sternotomy or anterolateral thoracotomy is used to expose the heart. The thoracic cavity is inspected and the cyst or tumor is located. The right and left phrenic nerves are identified and protected. If the lesion is a cyst, it may be opened with fluid and debris evacuated. The cyst, tumor, or mass is then dissected free of surrounding tissue and removed along with a margin of healthy pericardium. The defect in the pericardium may be covered with a synthetic patch or left open to drain. If it is left open, a chest tube is placed into the defect and an additional chest tube is placed in the pleural space.

33120

33120   Excision of intracardiac tumor, resection with cardiopulmonary bypass

A tumor is removed from the inside of the heart (intracardiac) and any defects caused by the removal are repaired. An incision is made in the skin of the chest and the heart is exposed by median sternotomy. Cardiopulmonary bypass is initiated by cannulating the aorta and the inferior and superior vena cava. Systemic hypothermia is also initiated and the heart is stopped. An incision is made into the involved heart chamber (atriotomy and/or ventriculotomy) and the tumor is exposed and resected. If it is possible to resect the tumor in its entirety and obtain a clear margin of tumor-free heart tissue, then this is done. If this is not possible, as much of the tumor is excised as possible. The heart defect caused by the tumor excision is then repaired. The patient is weaned off cardiopulmonary bypass, chest tubes are placed as needed, and the chest incision is closed.

33130

33130   Resection of external cardiac tumor

An external cardiac tumor is resected. Cardiac neoplasms may be benign or malignant and may involve the endocardium, myocardium, and/or epicardium. External cardiac tumors are those that lie below the parietal pericardium (the fibrous membrane that surrounds the heart) and involve the epicardium or external surface of the heart muscle. An incision is made in the skin of the chest and the heart is exposed by median sternotomy. The thorax is inspected. The pericardium is incised at the site of the external cardiac tumor, which is exposed and resected. If it is possible to resect the tumor in its entirety and to obtain a clear margin of tumor-free heart tissue, this is done. If this is not possible, as much of the tumor is excised as is possible. The heart defect caused by the tumor excision is then repaired. Chest tubes are placed as needed and the chest incision is closed.

33140-33141

33140   Transmyocardial laser revascularization, by thoracotomy; (separate procedure)
33141   Transmyocardial laser revascularization, by thoracotomy; performed at the time of other open cardiac procedure(s) (List separately in addition to code for primary procedure)

Transmyocardial laser revascularization (TMR or TMLR) is performed using an open approach. TMR is performed to improve blood flow in the myocardium (heart muscle). General anesthesia is administered and a double lumen endotracheal tube inserted so that right lung ventilation can be employed allowing better exposure of the heart. The heart is exposed using either a midline sternotomy or anterolateral thoracotomy and the pericardium is incised. The energy level and pulse duration of the laser is set. The laser probe is positioned over the left ventricle in contact with the epicardium. With the aid of a computer the laser beam is directed to the appropriate area of the heart and the laser is fired between heartbeats. The laser creates a one-millimeter channel in the left ventricle that extends from the surface of the heart to internal ventricular chamber. This is repeated 20 to 40 times. The channels on the external surface of the heart typically close quickly. If bleeding from the epicardial surface continues, local pressure or sutures are used to control the bleeding. The channels inside the left ventricle remain open and as the left ventricle pumps oxygen rich blood into the aorta it also sends blood through the laser channels restoring blood flow to the heart muscle. Following completion of TMR, the pericardium is reapproximated and one or more chest tubes placed in the pericardial cavity. Use code 33140 when TMR is performed alone as a separate procedure. Use code 33141 when TMR is performed at the time of another open cardiac procedure.

Cardiovascular System

33202-33203

33202   Insertion of epicardial electrode(s); open incision (eg, thoracotomy, median sternotomy, subxiphoid approach)

33203   Insertion of epicardial electrode(s); endoscopic approach (eg, thoracoscopy, pericardioscopy)

Epicardial electrode(s) or lead(s) are inserted through open chest incision in 33202, such as a thoracotomy, median sternotomy, subxiphoid approach. Epicardial leads are placed on the outer surface of the heart muscle to be stimulated electrically. The chest cavity is opened and the heart is exposed. The electrode(s) are positioned in the appropriate area(s) of heart muscle and affixed there, depending on which device the lead(s) are placed for-whether a single or dual chamber permanent pacemaker or pacing cardioverter defibrillator. Single chamber devices require one electrode inserted into either the atrium or the ventricle. Dual chamber devices require one electrode in the atrium and one in the ventricle. A subcutaneous tunnel is then created from the heart to the pocket under the skin where the device's generator is located, which is usually in the chest under the clavicle or in the upper abdomen under the costal margin. After the lead(s) are placed on the heart muscle, they are tested, guided through the subcutaneous tunnel, connected to the generator, and tested again before incision is closed. These codes report insertion of the epicardial electrode lead(s) only, not the generator. Code 33203 when the lead(s) are placed using an endoscopic approach such as thoracoscopy or pericardioscopy as opposed to an open chest incision.

33206-33208

33206   Insertion of new or replacement of permanent pacemaker with transvenous electrode(s); atrial

33207   Insertion of new or replacement of permanent pacemaker with transvenous electrode(s); ventricular

33208   Insertion of new or replacement of permanent pacemaker with transvenous electrode(s); atrial and ventricular

A permanent cardiac pacemaker system is inserted or replaced, including subcutaneous insertion of the pulse generator and transvenous placement of the endocardial electrodes (leads). Cardiac pacemakers deliver an electronic impulse to the heart at a programmed rate to help the heart maintain a normal heart rhythm. Permanent pacemaker systems may be single chamber (atrial or ventricular) or dual chamber (atrial and ventricular) systems and the leads may be placed either on the surface of the heart (epicardial) or within the heart chamber (endocardial). An incision is made in the skin of the upper chest and the cephalic, subclavian, or jugular vein is exposed. A sheath is inserted into the selected vessel and the pacemaker wire is advanced under radiological guidance into the selected heart chamber. The lead is positioned against the wall of the heart chamber. If a dual chamber device is required, the second wire is threaded to the selected chamber and the lead positioned against the heart wall. The leads are then tested to verify that they are functioning properly. Next, an incision is made in the skin, typically in the left pectoral region, and a subcutaneous pocket is fashioned. The lead(s) is(are) then connected to the pulse generator and the pulse generator is tested. Once it has been determined that the leads and generator are working as desired, the pulse generator is placed into the pocket, sutured to underlying tissue, and the pocket is closed. Code 33206 is used for a single chamber pacemaker with the lead in the right atrium and 33207 for a single chamber pacemaker with the lead in the right ventricle. Code 33208 is used for a dual-chamber pacemaker with leads in both the right atrium and right ventricle.

33210-33211

33210   Insertion or replacement of temporary transvenous single chamber cardiac electrode or pacemaker catheter (separate procedure)

33211   Insertion or replacement of temporary transvenous dual chamber pacing electrodes (separate procedure)

A temporary cardiac pacemaker transvenous electrode or catheter is inserted or replaced. Cardiac pacemakers deliver an electronic impulse to the heart at a programmed rate to help the heart maintain a normal heart rhythm. Temporary pacemakers are used to treat temporary arrhythmias that are expected to resolve or they are used until a permanent pacemaker can be placed. Temporary pacemaker systems may be single chamber (atrial or ventricular) or dual chamber (atrial and ventricular) systems and the leads may be placed either on the surface of the heart (epicardial) or within the heart chamber (endocardial). Transvenous electrode or catheter placement is used when the leads are placed within the heart chamber (endocardial). An incision is made in the skin of the upper chest and the cephalic, subclavian or jugular vein exposed. A sheath is inserted into the selected vessel and the pacemaker wire is advanced under radiological guidance into the selected heart chamber. The lead is positioned against the wall of the heart chamber. If a dual chamber device is required, the second wire is threaded to the selected chamber and the lead positioned against the heart wall. The leads are then tested to verify that they are functioning properly. The lead(s) is(are) then connected to the pulse generator and the pulse generator is tested. Once it has been determined that the leads and generator are working as desired, the temporary pulse generator is taped to the skin or attached to a belt worn by the patient. Code 33210 is used for a single chamber pacemaker with the

lead placed in the right atrium or right ventricle. Code 33211 is used for a dual chamber pacemaker with leads in both the right atrium and right ventricle.

33212-33213

33212   Insertion of pacemaker pulse generator only; with existing single lead

33213   Insertion of pacemaker pulse generator only; with existing dual leads

A permanent cardiac pacemaker pulse generator is inserted and attached to an existing lead(s). Cardiac pacemakers deliver an electronic impulse to the heart at a programmed rate to help the heart maintain a normal rhythm. Permanent pacemaker systems have a single lead, dual leads, or multiple leads. The leads may be placed either on the surface of the heart (epicardial) or within the heart chamber (endocardial). For insertion of the pacemaker generator performed alone or at the time of a separately reportable epicardial lead insertion, an incision is made in the skin, typically in the left pectoral region, and a subcutaneous pocket is fashioned. The lead(s) is(are) then connected to the pulse generator and the pulse generator is tested. Once it has been determined that the leads and generator are working as desired, the pulse generator is placed into the pocket, sutured to underlying tissue, and the pocket is closed. Code 33212 is used for insertion of a pacemaker pulse generator with an existing single lead and 33213 is for insertion of the pulse generator only with existing dual leads.

33214

33214   Upgrade of implanted pacemaker system, conversion of single chamber system to dual chamber system (includes removal of previously placed pulse generator, testing of existing lead, insertion of new lead, insertion of new pulse generator)

The physician upgrades a previously implanted pacemaker system by converting a single chamber system to a dual chamber system. This procedure is typically performed with an existing single chamber ventricular system. Upgrade of the pacemaker system may be performed for a condition referred to as pacemaker syndrome, in which the patient presents with symptoms of heart failure due to retrograde P wave conduction, or for idiopathic hypertrophic subaortic stenosis initially treated with a ventricular pacemaker that needs to be converted to a dual chamber. The pacemaker pocket is opened and the single chamber pulse generator is removed. An incision is made in the skin of the upper chest and the cephalic, subclavian, or jugular vein is exposed. A sheath is inserted into the selected vessel and the pacemaker wire is advanced under radiological guidance into the right atrium. The lead is positioned against the wall of right atrium. The new right atrial lead is tested to verify that it is functioning properly. The existing right ventricular lead is also tested. The leads are then connected to the pulse generator, and the generator is tested. Once it has been determined that the leads and generator are working properly, the pulse generator is placed into the pocket and sutured to underlying tissue, and the pocket is closed.

33215

33215   Repositioning of previously implanted transvenous pacemaker or implantable defibrillator (right atrial or right ventricular) electrode

Using separately reportable fluoroscopic guidance, a previously placed transvenous pacemaker or implantable defibrillator that has become malpositioned is manipulated into correct position against the wall of the right atrium or right ventricle. Once it has been determined that the leads and generator are working as desired, the pulse generator pocket is closed.

33216-33217

33216   Insertion of a single transvenous electrode, permanent pacemaker or implantable defibrillator

33217   Insertion of 2 transvenous electrodes, permanent pacemaker or implantable defibrillator

The existing electrode wire(s) of a permanent pacemaker or implantable defibrillator is(are) first tested and then removed, if defective, and a new wire is inserted and positioned in either the right atrium and/or right ventricle and reattached to the old, existing generator. Code 33216 is for a single chamber permanent pacemaker or implantable defibrillator electrode and code 33217 is for a dual chambered device with two transvenous electrode wires in the right atrium and the right ventricle. An incision is made in the skin of the upper chest to expose the appropriate vein, such as the cephalic, subclavian, or jugular vein. A sheath is inserted into the selected vessel and the pacemaker wire is advanced under radiological guidance into the selected heart chamber. The lead is positioned against the wall of the heart chamber. If a dual chamber device is required, the second wire is threaded to the selected chamber and the lead positioned against the heart wall. The leads are then tested to verify that they are functioning properly. The lead(s) is(are) then connected to the pulse generator and the pulse generator is tested.

● New Code   ▲ Revised Code   CPT © 2016 American Medical Association. All Rights Reserved.   © 2017 DecisionHealth

Cardiovascular System

33218-33220

33218 Repair of single transvenous electrode, permanent pacemaker or implantable defibrillator

33220 Repair of 2 transvenous electrodes for permanent pacemaker or implantable defibrillator

A transvenous electrode for a permanent pacemaker or implantable defibrillator is repaired. The electrode wire is first tested. If it is found to malfunction, then the electrode wire is repaired. Types of problems that can be repaired include an electrode fracture, an insulation defect, or a terminal pin defect. An incision is made in the skin of the upper chest and the malfunctioning electrode wire is located. In the case of an electrode fracture, an in-situ repair is performed by placing a sheath and inserting a guide-wire into the blood vessel containing the electrode wire. The broken section is then bypassed with a new section of wire. In situ repair of insulation defects or terminal pin defect are performed in a similar fashion by passing a guide wire and then bypassing or repairing the defect. The lead is then tested to verify that it is functioning properly. Code 33218 is used for repair of a single electrode. Code 33220 is used for repair of two transvenous electrodes.

33221

33221 Insertion of pacemaker pulse generator only; with existing multiple leads

A permanent cardiac pacemaker pulse generator is inserted and attached to multiple existing leads. Cardiac pacemakers deliver an electronic impulse to the heart at a programmed rate to help the heart maintain a normal rhythm. Permanent pacemaker systems may have a single lead, dual leads, or multiple leads. The leads may be placed either on the surface of the heart (epicardial) or within the heart chamber (endocardial). If this is the initial insertion of the pacemaker generator performed alone or at the time of a separately reportable epicardial lead insertion, an incision is made in the skin, typically in the left pectoral region, and a subcutaneous pocket is fashioned. The multiple leads are then connected to the pulse generator and the pulse generator is tested. Once it has been determined that the leads and generator are working as desired, the pulse generator is placed into the pocket, sutured to underlying tissue, and the pocket is closed.

33222-33223

33222 Relocation of skin pocket for pacemaker
33223 Relocation of skin pocket for implantable defibrillator

The skin pocket for the generator of a cardiac device may need to be relocated due to pain or discomfort at the existing site caused by pressure, necrosis, or erosion of the surrounding tissue, a skin pocket hematoma, or an infection. An incision is made over the pacemaker or implantable defibrillator generator and the skin pocket is opened. The generator is removed and the skin pocket is inspected. If a hematoma is present it is evacuated. If an infection is present, the skin pocket may be flushed with an antibiotic solution. The skin and subcutaneous tissue may be debrided. The old skin pocket is then closed. A new site is selected and a skin pocket is fashioned. The leads are connected to the pulse generator and it is tested. Once it has been determined that the leads and generator are functioning properly, the generator is inserted into the new pocket and sutured to underlying tissue. The new skin pocket is closed over the generator. Use 33222 for relocation of the skin pocket for a pacemaker. Use 33223 for relocation of the skin pocket for an implantable defibrillator.

33224-33226

33224 Insertion of pacing electrode, cardiac venous system, for left ventricular pacing, with attachment to previously placed pacemaker or implantable defibrillator pulse generator (including revision of pocket, removal, insertion, and/or replacement of existing generator)

33225 Insertion of pacing electrode, cardiac venous system, for left ventricular pacing, at time of insertion of implantable defibrillator or pacemaker pulse generator (eg, for upgrade to dual chamber system) (List separately in addition to code for primary procedure)

33226 Repositioning of previously implanted cardiac venous system (left ventricular) electrode (including removal, insertion and/or replacement of existing generator)

The physician inserts a pacing electrode in the cardiac venous system for left ventricular pacing and attaches it to a pacemaker or implantable defibrillator. A pacing electrode is placed in the cardiac venous system to pace the left ventricle to treat patients with advanced heart failure. This type of therapy is sometimes referred to as cardiac resynchronization therapy (CRT) or biventricular pacing. Advanced heart failure with a bundle branch block can cause a delay in contraction of the right and left ventricles as well as asynchronous contraction. CRT improves heart function by causing the walls of the right and left ventricles to contract together in a synchronous fashion. In 33224, a pacing electrode is placed into the coronary sinus vein to pace the left ventricle and attached to a previously placed pacemaker or implantable defibrillator pulse generator. The existing pacemaker or implantable defibrillator generator skin pocket is opened. If the existing generator needs to be replaced, the existing atrial and/or ventricular electrodes are disconnected from the generator, and the existing generator is removed. An incision

is made in the skin of the upper chest and the cephalic, subclavian, or jugular vein is exposed. A sheath is inserted into the selected vessel and the pacemaker wire is advanced under radiological guidance into the coronary sinus vein. The lead is then tested to verify that it is functioning properly. The new coronary sinus vein lead and the existing atrial and/or ventricular leads are connected to the new or existing pulse generator, and the pulse generator is tested. Once it has been determined that the leads and generator are working as desired, the pulse generator is placed into the pocket, sutured to underlying tissue, and the pocket is closed. In 33225, a pacing electrode is placed in the coronary sinus vein and a pacemaker or implantable defibrillator generator is inserted at the same encounter. The pacing electrode may be placed at the same encounter as the initial insertion of the generator or when the pacing system is upgraded. In 33226, a malpositioned pacing electrode in the coronary sinus vein is repositioned using separately reportable fluoroscopic guidance.

33227-33229

33227 Removal of permanent pacemaker pulse generator with replacement of pacemaker pulse generator; single lead system

33228 Removal of permanent pacemaker pulse generator with replacement of pacemaker pulse generator; dual lead system

33229 Removal of permanent pacemaker pulse generator with replacement of pacemaker pulse generator; multiple lead system

A permanent pacemaker pulse generator is removed, usually due to malfunction or because the generator battery is nearing its end of life, and a new pulse generator is inserted. An incision is made in the skin overlying the existing pulse generator, and the skin pocket is opened. The electrodes are disconnected and the pulse generator is dissected free of surrounding tissue and removed. The new pacemaker pulse generator is then attached to the existing lead(s) and tested. Once it has been determined that the leads and new pulse generator are working as desired, the new pulse generator is placed into the pocket, sutured to underlying tissue, and the pocket is closed. Use 33227 for replacement of the pulse generator in a single lead system. Use 33228 for replacement of the pulse generator in a dual lead system. Use 33229 for replacement of a pulse generator in a multiple lead system.

33230-33231

33230 Insertion of implantable defibrillator pulse generator only; with existing dual leads

33231 Insertion of implantable defibrillator pulse generator only; with existing multiple leads

The physician inserts an implantable defibrillator pulse generator, also referred to as an automatic implantable cardioverter-defibrillator (AICD or ICD), in a patient with dual or multiple existing leads. An AICD is used to monitor the heart's electrical activity continuously as well as provide anti-tachycardia pacing to prevent rapid irregular heart rhythm, backup pacing to maintain a healthy heart rhythm, cardioversion using a mild shock to convert an abnormal heart rhythm to a normal rhythm, or defibrillation using a stronger shock to convert a dangerously abnormal rhythm or restore the heart beat when cardiac arrest has occurred. For insertion of the implantable defibrillator pulse generator only, performed alone or at the time of a separately reportable epicardial lead insertion, an incision is made in the skin, typically in the left pectoral region, and a subcutaneous pocket is fashioned. The leads are then connected to the pulse generator and the generator is tested. Once it has been determined that the leads and generator are working, the pulse generator is placed into the pocket and sutured to underlying tissue, and the pocket is closed. Use 33230 for insertion of an AICD pulse generator only with existing dual leads. Use 33231 for insertion of an AICD pulse generator only with existing multiple leads.

33233

33233 Removal of permanent pacemaker pulse generator only

A permanent pacemaker pulse generator is removed without replacement. The pulse generator may be removed due to pressure necrosis, skin pocket hematoma, or infection. An incision is made in the skin overlying the existing pulse generator, and the skin pocket is opened. The electrodes are disconnected and the pulse generator is dissected free of surrounding tissue and removed. If the pulse generator is being removed because of malfunction or because the battery needs to be replaced, a new pulse generator is inserted. If the pulse generator is being removed for another reason, the skin pocket may be debrided, left open to drain, or closed.

Cardiovascular System

Removal of permanent pacemaker pulse generator

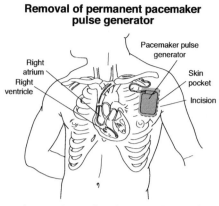

Right atrium
Right ventricle
Pacemaker pulse generator
Skin pocket
Incision

A permanent pacemaker pulse generator is removed, typically when the battery is nearing the end of its life

33234-33235

33234   Removal of transvenous pacemaker electrode(s); single lead system, atrial or ventricular

33235   Removal of transvenous pacemaker electrode(s); dual lead system

One or both transvenous pacemaker electrode wires are removed in an atrial or ventricular single lead system (33234) or a dual lead system (33235). One or both electrode wires may need to be removed because of damage to or malfunction of the lead(s), an infection at the site of the generator or lead(s), or interference of blood flow caused by the lead(s). An incision is made in the chest over the pacemaker generator and the lead is disconnected from the generator. There are several techniques used to remove electrodes and the technique selected depends on the amount of scar tissue present and whether the lead has become embedded in the heart muscle (myocardium). If there is not a great deal of scar tissue, an incision is made in the vein containing the electrode and the electrode is extracted by tugging on the lead. If the lead is embedded in the myocardium, the physician may attach a weight to the end of the lead to provide traction that will free the lead from the myocardium. If a great deal of scar tissue is present, a sheath is inserted into the vein containing the electrode wire. The sheath is then threaded over the existing electrode wire and guided to the tip under separately reportable fluoroscopic control. The lead is extracted. If both leads are removed the extraction procedure is repeated using one of the techniques described above.

33236-33237

33236   Removal of permanent epicardial pacemaker and electrodes by thoracotomy; single lead system, atrial or ventricular

33237   Removal of permanent epicardial pacemaker and electrodes by thoracotomy; dual lead system

The pacemaker pocket is opened and the epicardial electrode (lead, wire) disconnected from the generator. The generator is removed and the pocket closed. The physician then opens the chest using a thoracotomy, median sternotomy, subxiphoid, or subcostal approach. The heart is exposed. The epicardial pacemaker electrode is dissected free of any adherent tissue along its course through the thorax and at its attachment to the pericardium. The electrode is removed. Chest tubes are placed as needed and the chest is closed. Use 33236 when a single lead (atrial or ventricular) system is removed and 33237 when a dual lead system is removed.

33238

33238   Removal of permanent transvenous electrode(s) by thoracotomy

The physician removes one or more permanent transvenous (endocardial) electrodes by thoracotomy. Electrode wires may need to be removed because of damage to or malfunction of the lead(s), an infection at the site of the generator or lead(s), or interference of blood flow caused by the lead(s). Thoracotomy is performed when the electrodes cannot be removed via a transvenous approach due to dense scar tissue and adhesions, or because they are deeply embedded in the heart muscle (myocardium). An incision is made in the chest over the pacemaker generator and the lead is disconnected. The heart is exposed by median sternotomy. If cardiopulmonary bypass is required, the aorta is cannulated followed by the superior and inferior vena cava. To remove an atrial electrode, the right atrium is incised. The electrode is dissected free of adhesive scar tissue and removed. If the electrode is in the right ventricle, it may be approached through the right atrium or through an incision in the right ventricle. If the right atrial approach is used, the right ventricle is inverted and the electrode is dissected free of adhesive scar tissue. Heart wall incisions are closed, chest tubes are placed as needed, and the chest is closed.

33240

33240   Insertion of implantable defibrillator pulse generator only; with existing single lead

The physician inserts an implantable defibrillator pulse generator, also referred to as an automatic implantable cardioverter-defibrillator (AICD or ICD) in a patient with an existing single lead. An AICD is used to monitor the heart's electrical activity continuously as well as provide anti-tachycardia pacing to prevent rapid irregular heart rhythm, backup pacing to maintain a healthy heart rhythm, cardioversion using a mild shock to convert an abnormal heart rhythm to a normal rhythm, or defibrillation using a stronger shock to convert a dangerously abnormal rhythm or restore the heart beat when cardiac arrest has occurred. For insertion of the implantable defibrillator pulse generator only, performed alone or at the time of a separately reportable epicardial lead insertion, an incision is made in the skin, typically in the left pectoral region, and a subcutaneous pocket is fashioned. The existing lead is then connected to the pulse generator and the generator is tested. Once it has been determined that the lead and generator are working, the pulse generator is placed into the pocket and sutured to underlying tissue, and the pocket is closed.

33241

33241   Removal of implantable defibrillator pulse generator only

An implantable defibrillator pulse generator is removed without replacement. The pulse generator may be removed due to pressure necrosis, skin pocket hematoma, or infection. An incision is made in the skin overlying the existing pulse generator, and the skin pocket is opened. The electrodes are disconnected and the generator is dissected free of surrounding tissue and removed. Depending on the reason for the generator removal, the skin pocket may be debrided, left open to drain, or closed.

33243-33244

33243   Removal of single or dual chamber implantable defibrillator electrode(s); by thoracotomy

33244   Removal of single or dual chamber implantable defibrillator electrode(s); by transvenous extraction

The physician removes one or more single or dual chamber implantable defibrillator electrodes by thoracotomy (33243) or by transvenous extraction (33244). Electrode wires may need to be removed because of damage to or malfunction of the lead(s), an infection at the site of the generator or lead(s), or interference of blood flow caused by the lead(s). In 33243, thoracotomy is performed to remove epicardial leads or to remove endocardial leads that cannot be removed via a transvenous approach due to dense scar tissue and adhesions or because they are deeply embedded in the heart muscle (myocardium). An incision is made in the chest over the pacemaker generator and the lead is disconnected from the generator. The heart is exposed by median sternotomy. If cardiopulmonary bypass is required, the aorta is cannulated followed by the superior and inferior vena cava. To remove epicardial leads, the lead is dissected free of the epicardium and removed. To remove an endocardial atrial electrode, the right atrium is incised. The electrode is dissected free of adhesive scar tissue and removed. If the endocardial electrode is in the right ventricle it may be approached through the right atrium or through an incision in the right ventricle. If the right atrial approach is used, the right ventricle is inverted and the electrode is dissected free of adhesive scar tissue. Heart wall incisions are closed, chest tubes are placed as needed, and the chest is closed. In 33244, one or more transvenous (endocardial) electrode wires are removed. An incision is made in the chest over the pacemaker generator and the lead is disconnected from the generator. There are several transvenous techniques used to remove electrodes and the technique selected depends on the amount of scar tissue present and whether the lead has become embedded in the heart muscle (myocardium). If there is not a great deal of scar tissue, an incision is made in the vein containing the electrode and the electrode is extracted by tugging on the lead. If the lead is embedded in the myocardium, the physician may attach a weight to the end of the lead to provide sustained traction that will free the lead from the myocardium. If a great deal of scar tissue is present, a sheath is inserted into the vein containing the electrode wire. The sheath is then threaded over the existing electrode wire and guided to the tip under separately reportable fluoroscopic control. The lead is extracted. If both leads are removed, the extraction procedure is repeated using one of the techniques described above.

33249

33249   Insertion or replacement of permanent implantable defibrillator system, with transvenous lead(s), single or dual chamber

The physician inserts or replaces one or more electrode leads for a single or dual chamber permanent implantable defibrillator with a pulse generator. This device may also be referred to as an automatic implantable cardioverter-defibrillator (AICD or ICD). An AICD is used to monitor the heart's electrical activity continuously as well as provide anti-tachycardia pacing (ATP) to prevent rapid irregular heart rhythm, backup pacing to maintain a healthy heart rhythm, cardioversion using a mild shock to convert an abnormal heart rhythm to a normal rhythm, or defibrillation using a stronger shock to convert a dangerously abnormal rhythm or restore the heart beat when cardiac arrest has occurred.

Cardiovascular System

● New Code   ▲ Revised Code   CPT © 2016 American Medical Association. All Rights Reserved.   © 2017 DecisionHealth

An incision is made in the skin of the upper chest and the cephalic, subclavian, or jugular vein is exposed. A sheath is inserted into the selected vessel and the AICD wire is advanced under radiological guidance into the selected heart chamber. The lead is positioned against the wall of the chamber. If a dual chamber device is required, the second wire is threaded to the selected chamber and the lead is positioned against the heart wall. The leads are then tested to verify that they are functioning properly. Next, an incision is made in the skin, typically in the left pectoral region, and a subcutaneous pocket is fashioned. The leads are then connected to the pulse generator and the generator is tested. Once it has been determined that the leads and generator are working, the pulse generator is placed into the pocket, sutured to underlying tissue, and the pocket is closed.

33250-33251

33250 **Operative ablation of supraventricular arrhythmogenic focus or pathway (eg, Wolff-Parkinson-White, atrioventricular node re-entry), tract(s) and/or focus (foci); without cardiopulmonary bypass**

33251 **Operative ablation of supraventricular arrhythmogenic focus or pathway (eg, Wolff-Parkinson-White, atrioventricular node re-entry), tract(s) and/or focus (foci); with cardiopulmonary bypass**

In Wolff-Parkinson-White syndrome and other similar disorders, there is one or more extra electrical pathways between the atria and ventricles which cause episodes of supraventricular tachycardia. A midline sternotomy is used to access the heart. Epicardial and endocardial electrodes are placed on the beating heart. Separately reportable epicardial and endocardial pacing and mapping is performed to localize the focus, tract, or pathway that is causing of the arrhythmia. If cardiopulmonary bypass is needed, it is established and cardioplegic arrest initiated. The right atrium is incised. The abnormal accessory electrical pathways are destroyed either by surgical incision to interrupt the electrical impulses or by cryoablation or radiofrequency ablation to destroy the pathways. The heart incision is closed. If cardiopulmonary bypass has been used, it is discontinued. Chest tubes are placed as needed and the chest incision is closed. Use 33250 when the ablation procedure is performed on the beating heart without cardiopulmonary bypass and 33251 when the heart is stopped and cardiopulmonary bypass is used.

33254

33254 **Operative tissue ablation and reconstruction of atria, limited (eg, modified maze procedure)**

The surgeon performs a modified maze procedure for limited operative tissue ablation and reconstruction of atria. This is done to correct chronic atrial fibrillation-rapid, uncoordinated muscle contractions of the upper heart chambers causing irregular, rapid heart beat. The maze procedure creates new pathways or circuits for electrical impulses to travel through the heart. A midline sternotomy is made to access the chest. The atrium is incised through the interatrial groove and the atrial appendage is excised. Precise atrial incisions are made and ablation lines are created to interrupt the conduction of abnormal impulses, allowing electrical impulses to travel normally from the sinoatrial node to the atrioventricular node and restore the atria to a more normal size. A maze procedure may need to be done only on the left atrium or on both atria. Incision sites are sutured. A modified maze may include altered atriotomies made to avoid disrupting the sinus node artery; the use of cryo- or radiofrequency ablation to simplify the procedure by creating tissue lesions or ablation lines instead of many incisions which must be sutured; or electrophysiologically excluding the atrial appendage instead of anatomically removing it.

33255-33256

33255 **Operative tissue ablation and reconstruction of atria, extensive (eg, maze procedure); without cardiopulmonary bypass**

33256 **Operative tissue ablation and reconstruction of atria, extensive (eg, maze procedure); with cardiopulmonary bypass**

Extensive operative tissue ablation and reconstruction of atria is done in a maze procedure without cardiopulmonary bypass in 33255 and with bypass in 33256. This is done to correct chronic atrial fibrillation-rapid, uncoordinated muscle contractions of the upper heart chambers causing irregular, rapid heart beat. The maze procedure creates new pathways or circuits for electrical impulses to travel through the heart. A midline sternotomy is made to access the chest and cardiopulmonary bypass is established, if used. Both vena cavae are cannulated for venous return. After cardioplegic arrest, the left atrium is incised through the interatrial groove. A sling is used around the inferior vena cava to lift and turn the heart for better exposure. The atrial appendage is excised and precise atrial incisions are made to interrupt the conduction of abnormal impulses, allowing electrical impulses to travel normally from the sinoatrial node to the atrioventricular node and restore the atria to a more normal size. Incision sites are sutured and a pericardial strip is used for suture line reinforcement. The atrium can hold and pump blood to the ventricle, but the electrical impulses cannot cross the incisions, so the atria no longer fibrillate. A maze procedure may need to be done only on the left atrium or on both atria.

33257

33257 **Operative tissue ablation and reconstruction of atria, performed at the time of other cardiac procedure(s), limited (eg, modified maze procedure) (List separately in addition to code for primary procedure)**

The surgeon performs a modified maze procedure for limited operative tissue ablation and reconstruction of the atria to correct chronic atrial fibrillation-rapid, uncoordinated muscle contractions of the upper heart chambers causing irregular, rapid heart beat. The maze procedure creates new pathways or circuits for electrical impulses to travel through the heart and interrupts irregular pathways. This is done at the time of another separately reportable cardiac procedure. The atrium is incised through the interatrial groove and the atrial appendage is excised. Precise atrial incisions are made and ablation lines are created to interrupt the conduction of abnormal impulses, allowing electrical impulses to travel normally from the sinoatrial node to the atrioventricular node and restore the atria to normal contractions and a more normal size. A maze procedure may need to be done only on the left atrium or on both atria. Incision sites are sutured. A modified maze procedure may include altered atriotomies to avoid disrupting the sinus node artery; the use of cryo- or radiofrequency ablation instead of many incisions which must be sutured, to simplify the procedure by creating tissue lesions or ablation lines; or electrophysiologically excluding the atrial appendage instead of anatomically removing it.

33258-33259

33258 **Operative tissue ablation and reconstruction of atria, performed at the time of other cardiac procedure(s), extensive (eg, maze procedure), without cardiopulmonary bypass (List separately in addition to code for primary procedure)**

33259 **Operative tissue ablation and reconstruction of atria, performed at the time of other cardiac procedure(s), extensive (eg, maze procedure), with cardiopulmonary bypass (List separately in addition to code for primary procedure)**

Extensive operative tissue ablation and reconstruction of atria is done in a maze procedure to correct chronic atrial fibrillation-rapid, uncoordinated muscle contractions of the upper heart chambers causing irregular, rapid heart beat. The maze procedure creates new pathways or circuits for electrical impulses to travel through the heart and interrupts irregular pathways. This is done at the time of another separately reportable cardiac procedure without cardiopulmonary bypass in 33258 and with bypass in 33259. After cardiopulmonary bypass is established, if used, both vena cavae are cannulated for venous return. After cardioplegic arrest, the left atrium is incised through the interatrial groove. A sling is used around the inferior vena cava to lift and turn the heart for better exposure. The atrial appendage is excised and precise atrial incisions are made to interrupt the conduction of abnormal impulses, allowing electrical impulses to travel normally from the sinoatrial node to the atrioventricular node and restore the atria to normal contractions and a more normal size. Incision sites are sutured and a pericardial strip is used for suture line reinforcement. The atrium can hold and pump blood to the ventricle, but the electrical impulses cannot cross the incisions, so the atria no longer fibrillate. A maze procedure may need to be done only on the left atrium or on both atria.

33261

33261 **Operative ablation of ventricular arrhythmogenic focus with cardiopulmonary bypass**

The physician performs an open operative ablation of a ventricular arrhythmogenic focus with cardiopulmonary bypass. Ventricular arrhythmogenic focus is an abnormal or accessory electrical conduction site located below the atria in the ventricles which causes episodes of ventricular tachycardia. A midline sternotomy is used to access the heart. Epicardial and endocardial electrodes are placed on the beating heart. Separately reportable epicardial and endocardial pacing and mapping is performed to localize the focus, tract, or pathway that is causing of the arrhythmia. Cardiopulmonary bypass is established and cardioplegic arrest initiated. The heart is incised over the site of the arrhythmogenic focus. The focus is interrupted by surgical incision or destroyed by cryoablation or radiofrequency ablation. The heart incision is closed. Cardiopulmonary bypass is discontinued. Chest tubes are placed as needed and the chest incision is closed.

33262-33264

33262 **Removal of implantable defibrillator pulse generator with replacement of implantable defibrillator pulse generator; single lead system**

33263 **Removal of implantable defibrillator pulse generator with replacement of implantable defibrillator pulse generator; dual lead system**

33264 **Removal of implantable defibrillator pulse generator with replacement of implantable defibrillator pulse generator; multiple lead system**

The physician removes an existing implantable defibrillator pulse generator, also referred to as an automatic implantable cardioverter-defibrillator (AICD or ICD), and replaces it with a new one usually due to malfunction or because the generator battery is nearing its end of life. An AICD is used to monitor the heart's electrical activity continuously as well as provide anti-tachycardia pacing to prevent rapid irregular heart rhythm, backup pacing to maintain a healthy heart rhythm, cardioversion using a mild shock to convert an abnormal heart

Cardiovascular System

rhythm to a normal rhythm, or defibrillation using a stronger shock to convert a dangerously abnormal rhythm or restore the heart beat when cardiac arrest has occurred. To replace the pulse generator, the skin pocket is opened and the existing generator is removed. The new pulse generator is attached to the existing lead(s) and tested. Once it has been determined that the lead(s) and new pulse generator are working, the new generator is placed into the pocket, sutured to underlying tissue, and the pocket is closed. Use 33262 for a single lead system, 33263 for a dual lead system, or 33264 for a multiple lead system.

33265-33266

33265   Endoscopy, surgical; operative tissue ablation and reconstruction of atria, limited (eg, modified maze procedure), without cardiopulmonary bypass

33266   Endoscopy, surgical; operative tissue ablation and reconstruction of atria, extensive (eg, maze procedure), without cardiopulmonary bypass

Endoscopic operative tissue ablation and reconstruction of atria is performed in a limited fashion with a modified maze procedure (33265) or extensively in a maze procedure (33266), without cardiopulmonary bypass. This is done to correct chronic atrial fibrillation-rapid, uncoordinated muscle contractions of the upper heart chambers causing irregular, rapid heart beat. Patients with lone atrial fibrillation (without other cardiac disease) are candidates for endoscopic, or "keyhole" approach maze procedure, called the beating heart version of surgical atrial fibrillation ablation. This is a robotics applied procedure in which the abnormal atrial pathways of electrical conduction are ablated through small puncture wounds in the chest, including atrial appendage resection, without stopping the heart. The normal conduction pathway is then restored and the atria no longer fibrillate.

33270

33270   Insertion or replacement of permanent subcutaneous implantable defibrillator system, with subcutaneous electrode, including defibrillation threshold evaluation, induction of arrhythmia, evaluation of sensing for arrhythmia termination, and programming or reprogramming of sensing or therapeutic parameters, when performed

A permanent subcutaneous implantable defibrillator system consists of a pulse generator and a lead wire containing sensing electrodes and a defibrillator (shocking) coil. The electrode captures the cardiac rhythm and sends the information to the pulse generator. The pulse generator identifies an arrhythmia such as ventricular tachycardia or fibrillation and deploys an electrical shock along the shocking coil to terminate the arrhythmia. To insert the device, anatomical landmarks are identified and marked on the left chest at the 6th rib between the mid-axillary and anterior axillary lines, along the left sternal border at the 2nd intercostal space for distal lead placement, and at the xiphoid process for proximal lead placement. Small skin incisions are made at the site of the distal and proximal lead wire placements and the lead wire is tunneled from the distal site to the proximal site. The lead wire is suture anchored to the patient's fascia at the distal site. Next, an incision is made in the skin in the previously marked left lateral chest and a subcutaneous pocket large enough to hold the pulse generator is fashioned. The lead wire is then tunneled from the proximal site at the left sternal border to the left lateral pocket and connected to the preprogrammed pulse generator. The unit is tested by inducing an arrhythmia and monitoring termination response. Defibrillation threshold evaluation and reprogramming for sensing or therapeutic levels may also be done. Once the unit is determined to be functioning optimally, the generator is placed within the subcutaneous pocket, secured to the patient's fascia, and the incision is closed.

33271

33271   Insertion of subcutaneous implantable defibrillator electrode

The subcutaneous implantable defibrillator electrode is a multi-lumen polymeric tube lead wire containing sensing electrodes and a defibrillator shocking coil. To insert the electrode, anatomical landmarks are identified and marked on the left chest at the 6th rib between the mid-axillary and anterior axillary lines, along the left sternal border at the 2nd intercostal space for distal lead placement, and at the xiphoid process for proximal lead placement. Small skin incisions are made at the site of the distal and proximal lead wire placements. Using a non-traumatic tool, the lead wire is tunneled from the distal site to the proximal site. Using sutures, the lead wire is anchored to the patient's fascia at the distal site. Next, an incision is made in the skin in the previously marked left lateral chest and the lead wire is tunneled from the proximal site at the left sternal border to the left lateral chest. If the pulse generator has not been inserted, the lead wire is secured to the fascia at the left lateral chest and the incision is closed. If the pulse generator has been inserted, the lead wire is connected to the preprogrammed pulse generator. The unit is tested by inducing an arrhythmia and monitoring the response. Once the unit is determined to be functioning optimally, the lead wire is secured to the patient's fascia and the incision is closed.

33272

33272   Removal of subcutaneous implantable defibrillator electrode

The subcutaneous implantable defibrillator electrode is a multi-lumen polymeric tube lead wire containing sensing electrodes and a defibrillator shocking coil. To remove an electrode, the previous anatomical landmarks are identified on the left chest at the 6th

rib between the mid-axillary and anterior axillary lines, along the left sternal border at the 2nd intercostal space for distal lead placement and at the xiphoid process for proximal lead placement. Skin incisions are made at the distal site, proximal site, and the left lateral chest site, and the electrode is identified. If the pulse generator is in place, the unit is programmed off and the electrode is disconnected. A non-traumatic tunneling tool may be employed to free the electrode from subcutaneous tissue. Once the electrode has been successfully dissected from the tissue, it is disconnected at the proximal site and the securing sutures at the distal and lateral chest sites are cut. The electrode is removed in two sections and the incisions are closed with sutures.

33273

33273   Repositioning of previously implanted subcutaneous implantable defibrillator electrode

Repositioning of a previously implanted subcutaneous implantable defibrillator electrode may be required in the event of electrode movement. Skin incisions are made at the distal and proximal lead insertion site and/or the pulse generator pocket and the electrode is identified. A tunneling tool may be employed to free the electrode from subcutaneous tissue and the electrode may need to be disconnected from the pulse generator to facilitate manipulation and repositioning. Once the electrode has been manipulated back into optimal position and the unit is determined to be functioning, the incisions are closed with sutures.

33282-33284

33282   Implantation of patient-activated cardiac event recorder

33284   Removal of an implantable, patient-activated cardiac event recorder

A patient-activated cardiac event recorder, also referred to as an implantable loop recorder (ILR), is inserted in a subcutaneous pocket in the chest. The patient-activated cardiac event recorder is a device that records heart rhythm for several minutes following activation by the patient at the onset of cardiac symptoms such as heart palpitations, dizziness, or fainting spells. Sensing electrodes are contained within the device. The device continuously monitors and records heart rhythm in a looping memory. The patient uses a hand-held device to activate the device and permanently record events in the device memory. The patient-activated cardiac event recorder can also be programmed to auto-record events. Prior to implanting the cardiac event recorder, the device is tested and programmed. The physician selects the number of patient-activated and auto-activated events to store and sets the electrocardiogram (ECG) storage capacity. Parameters are set for recording of auto-activated events and the optimal sensitivity of the device settings is determined and programmed. An incision is made in the skin, typically in the left pectoral region, and a subcutaneous pocket fashioned. The device is then placed into the pocket and sutured to underlying tissue. The incision is closed over the device. The device is tested to verify that it is working properly. The patient is instructed on the use of the device. In 33284, the physician removes a previously implanted patient-activated event recorder. An incision is made in the skin overlying the device. The device is removed from the subcutaneous pocket. The skin is incision is closed.

33300-33305

33300   Repair of cardiac wound; without bypass

33305   Repair of cardiac wound; with cardiopulmonary bypass

A cardiac wound is repaired. In 33300, the cardiac wound is repaired without cardiopulmonary bypass, also referred to as off-pump cardiac wound repair. The chest is opened to control bleeding and evaluate the site and severity of the cardiac wound. Blood is evacuated from the thorax. The pericardium may be incised to release fluids from the pericardial cavity. An apical traction suture, also referred to as a Beck's suture is placed to allow control of the beating heart. The site of the cardiac wound is located. If the wound is small, bleeding may be controlled using digital pressure and temporary suture. Alternatively, pressure may be applied using a Foley catheter inserted through the cardiac wound with the balloon positioned in the cardiac chamber. The balloon is inflated with normal saline and traction applied to occlude the wound and slow bleeding. A temporary purse-string suture is then placed and the foley catheter removed. The purse-string suture is tied and additional sutures placed as needed. If the wound is large, the inferior and superior vena cava may be clamped to provide a bloodless surgical field. Once bleeding has been controlled, the cardiac wound is further evaluated to determine if there is damage to coronary arteries or other heart structures. If no additional cardiac injuries are identified, permanent closure of the cardiac wound is accomplished using mattress sutures reinforced with pledgets. Care is taken to avoid injury to coronary vessels. The traction suture is removed, chest tubes are placed as needed, and the chest is closed. In 33305, cardiac wound repair is performed with cardiopulmonary bypass using the same surgical techniques described above. Cardiopulmonary bypass, also referred to as on-pump repair, involves cannulating the aorta and superior and inferior vena cava or other vessels and using a machine to circulate the blood. Systemic hypothermia may be initiated prior to stopping the heart (cardioplegia).

33310-33315

33310 Cardiotomy, exploratory (includes removal of foreign body, atrial or ventricular thrombus); without bypass

33315 Cardiotomy, exploratory (includes removal of foreign body, atrial or ventricular thrombus); with cardiopulmonary bypass

An exploratory cardiotomy is performed and any foreign body or atrial or ventricular thrombus is removed. This procedure may also be referred to as an exploratory atriotomy or ventriculotomy. A midline sternotomy is performed to expose the heart. If cardiopulmonary bypass is required, the aorta is cannulated followed by the superior and inferior vena cava. Cardioplegic arrest is then initiated. The heart wall is incised (atriotomy, ventriculotomy) to access the interior aspect of the heart chamber (right atrium, left atrium, right ventricle, left ventricle) that has been injured. The heart chamber is inspected. If a foreign body or thrombus is present it is removed. Heart wall incisions are closed. If cardiopulmonary bypass has been used, it is terminated. Chest tubes are placed as needed, and the chest wall incision is closed. Use code 33310 for exploratory cardiotomy performed without cardiopulmonary bypass. Use code 33315 when cardiopulmonary bypass is used.

33320-33322

33320 Suture repair of aorta or great vessels; without shunt or cardiopulmonary bypass

33321 Suture repair of aorta or great vessels; with shunt bypass

33322 Suture repair of aorta or great vessels; with cardiopulmonary bypass

An injury to the aorta or great vessels is repaired with sutures. Injury to the aorta or great vessels requiring suture repair can occur with either blunt or penetrating trauma which can result in aortic or great vessel transection, rupture, tear, or laceration. Suture repair of the aorta or great vessels can be performed without shunt or cardiopulmonary bypass (33320), also referred to as clamp and sew technique; with shunt bypass (33321) which provides distal aortic perfusion using cannulation of the left ventricular apex, ascending aorta, or left subclavian artery and distal aorta to allow perfusion of distal arteries; or with complete cardiopulmonary bypass (33322). A thoracotomy is performed and the injured blood vessels exposed. To repair an injury to the aorta, the pleura is incised and the left superior pulmonary vein isolated. The phrenic nerves are identified, mobilized, and protected. The anterior surface of the aorta is exposed and the innominate, left common carotid, and left subclavian arteries are identified. The area proximal and distal to the injury is surrounded with umbilical tape to control bleeding in case of hemorrhage. Tissue adherent to the inferior surface of the aorta is divided. The aortic arch is separated from the pulmonary artery, left common carotid, and left subclavian arteries using blunt and sharp dissection. At this point, the aorta may be cross-clamped or shunt bypass or cardiopulmonary bypass initiated. The mediastinal pleura is opened and the aorta fully exposed. The aortic injury is then suture repaired. Injuries to other great vessels are repaired in a similar fashion with dissection of the injured vessel from surrounding tissue and suture repair. Following suture repair, shunt or cardiopulmonary bypass is terminated if used. Chest tubes are placed as needed and the chest incision is closed.

33330-33335

33330 Insertion of graft, aorta or great vessels; without shunt, or cardiopulmonary bypass

33335 Insertion of graft, aorta or great vessels; with cardiopulmonary bypass

An injury to the aorta or great vessels is repaired with synthetic graft insertion. Injury to the aorta or great vessels requiring graft repair can occur with either blunt or penetrating trauma which can result in aortic or great vessel transection, rupture, tear, or laceration. Graft repair of the aorta or great vessels can be performed without shunt or cardiopulmonary bypass (33330), also referred to as clamp and sew technique, or with complete cardiopulmonary bypass (33335). A thoracotomy is performed and the injured blood vessels exposed. To repair an injury to the aorta, the pleura is incised and the left superior pulmonary vein isolated. The phrenic nerves are identified, mobilized, and protected. The anterior surface of the aorta is exposed and the innominate, left common carotid, and left subclavian arteries are identified. The area proximal and distal to the injury is surrounded with umbilical tape to control bleeding in case of hemorrhage. Tissue adherent to the inferior surface of the aorta is divided. The aortic arch is separated from the pulmonary artery, left common carotid, and left subclavian arteries using blunt and sharp dissection. At this point, the aorta may be cross-clamped or cardiopulmonary bypass initiated. The mediastinal pleura is opened and the aorta is fully exposed. The aortic injury is then repaired using a synthetic graft. Proximal anastomosis of the synthetic graft is performed first. A clamp is placed on the graft below the anastomosis site, the proximal clamp released, and the integrity of the proximal anastomosis evaluated. Any leaks are reinforced with additional sutures. Distal anastomosis of the graft is performed in the same fashion. Injuries to other great vessels are repaired in a similar fashion with dissection of the injured vessel from surrounding tissue and graft repair. Following graft repair, cardiopulmonary bypass is terminated if used. Chest tubes are placed as needed and the chest incision is closed.

33340

● **33340** Percutaneous transcatheter closure of the left atrial appendage with endocardial implant, including fluoroscopy, transseptal puncture, catheter placement(s), left atrial angiography, left atrial appendage angiography, when performed, and radiological supervision and interpretation

Percutaneous transcatheter closure of the left atrial appendage (LAA) using an endocardial implant may be performed on a patient with non-valvular atrial fibrillation (NVAF) at high risk for thrombus formation or stroke when oral anticoagulation therapy is contraindicated. The LAA is a highly variable anatomic structure with four morphological groups: LAA with a bend in the proximal end of the dominant lobe (chicken wing); LAA with a long (>4 cm) main lobe as the primary structure (windsock); LAA with limited length (<4 cm) and without forked lobes (cauliflower); and LAA with a dominant central lobe and secondary extension lobes (cactus). The ostium and neck of the LAA also have distinct morphologies with one possibly wider than the other, or both having similar dimensions. The size and configuration of the LAA along with pressure or loading status and presence of sinus rhythm or atrial fibrillation (AF) influence the choice of endocardial implant device. The femoral vein is accessed using a large needle replaced with a vascular sheath. A guidewire is threaded through the sheath and advanced to the right atrium under fluoroscopy. A catheter is inserted over the guidewire and the atrial septum is punctured inferoposteriorly to access the LAA. Heparin bolus is given. A pigtail catheter is advanced into the LAA and angiography is used to assess the LAA anatomy. A J-tipped guidewire is advanced into the left upper pulmonary vein. A sheath containing a delivery cable is advanced into the LAA ostium and navigated over the pigtail catheter until it is aligned in the LAA. Once the position, anchor, size, and seal (PASS) criteria are verified, the selected endocardial implant is released from the delivery cable and pulled back in a tug test to determine filling of the LAA or sealing of the ostium. The delivery cable is removed and angiography of the left atrium and/or LAA is performed. The device is adjusted as necessary. Catheters and guidewires are removed and a purse string suture may be placed in the vessel around the vascular sheath prior to removal to control local bleeding.

33361

33361 Transcatheter aortic valve replacement (TAVR/TAVI) with prosthetic valve; percutaneous femoral artery approach

Aortic valve replacement is a common treatment for symptomatic aortic stenosis. Transcatheter aortic valve replacement/implantation (TAVR/TAVI) is an alternative to open heart aortic valve replacement. Pulmonary and radial artery catheters are inserted as needed for hemodynamic monitoring. Transthoracic echocardiography is performed to confirm aortic valve diameter and is included in the procedure. Alternatively, separately reportable transesophageal echocardiography may be used. Transcatheter aortic valve replacement requires the use of multiple catheters including a reference catheter that is placed first via a separate arterial access site. The reference pigtail catheter is placed percutaneously through the selected artery under fluoroscopic guidance and a root aortogram is performed. A balloon catheter is then advanced from this access site to the aortic valve and inflated to increase the diameter of the stenotic valve so that the prosthetic valve can be placed. The skin over the femoral access artery is prepped. Arterial access is accomplished by needle puncture. A mapping angiogram is performed to ensure that the femoral and iliac arteries are large enough to accommodate the larger caliber catheters. The femoral access artery is sequentially dilated to allow introduction of the large caliber catheter required for placement of the prosthetic aortic valve. A guidewire is inserted and advanced from the access artery through the aorta and positioned at the aortic valve. A catheter containing a compressed aortic valve within a valve cage is advanced over the guidewire to the aortic valve. During prosthesis placement, rapid right ventricular pacing is used to facilitate placement of the valve. The compressed valve is positioned in the native diseased aortic valve and deployed. The valve cage is removed. A balloon tip catheter is positioned in the prosthetic valve and the balloon is inflated to seat the aortic valve. Contrast is injected and a completion angiography is performed to ensure that the valve is functioning properly. All catheters are removed. The vascular access site in the femoral artery is repaired with sutures. Pressure is applied to other vascular access sites and pressure dressings are applied.

33362-33364

33362 Transcatheter aortic valve replacement (TAVR/TAVI) with prosthetic valve; open femoral artery approach

33363 Transcatheter aortic valve replacement (TAVR/TAVI) with prosthetic valve; open axillary artery approach

33364 Transcatheter aortic valve replacement (TAVR/TAVI) with prosthetic valve; open iliac artery approach

Aortic valve replacement is a common treatment for symptomatic aortic stenosis. Transcatheter aortic valve replacement/implantation (TAVR/TAVI) is an alternative to open heart aortic valve replacement and may be performed via an open femoral, axillary, or iliac artery approach. Pulmonary and radial artery catheters are inserted as needed for hemodynamic monitoring. Transthoracic echocardiography is performed to confirm aortic valve diameter and is included in the procedure. Alternatively, separately reportable transesophageal echocardiography may be used. Transcatheter aortic valve replacement

Cardiovascular System

requires the use of multiple catheters including a reference catheter that is placed first via a separate arterial access site. The reference pigtail catheter is placed percutaneously under fluoroscopic guidance and a root aortogram is performed. A balloon catheter is then advanced from this access site to the aortic valve and inflated to increase the diameter of the stenotic valve so that the prosthetic valve can be placed. The skin over the access artery through which the valve will be inserted is prepped. Electrocautery is used to dissect the subcutaneous tissue down to the level of the fascia and sharp dissection is used to expose the femoral, axillary, or iliac artery. With the vessel exposed, an 18 gauge needle is inserted into the artery and the Seldinger technique is used to insert the sheath which is then advanced from the access artery to the aorta. A guidewire is inserted and advanced from the access artery through the aorta and positioned at the aortic valve. A catheter containing a compressed aortic valve within a valve cage is advanced over the guidewire to the aortic valve. During prosthesis placement, rapid right ventricular pacing is used to facilitate placement of the valve. The compressed valve is positioned in the native diseased aortic valve and deployed. The valve cage is removed. A balloon tip catheter is positioned in the prosthetic valve and the balloon is inflated to seat the aortic valve. Contrast is injected and a completion angiography is performed to ensure that the valve is functioning properly. All catheters are removed. The vascular access site in the femoral, axillary, or iliac artery is repaired with sutures. Pressure is applied to other vascular access sites and pressure dressings are applied. Use 33362 for TAVR/TAVI performed via open femoral artery approach, 33363 for open axillary artery approach, and 33364 for open iliac artery approach.

33365

33365   Transcatheter aortic valve replacement (TAVR/TAVI) with prosthetic valve; transaortic approach (eg, median sternotomy, mediastinotomy)

Transcatheter aortic valve implantation (TAVI) is performed to replace a stenotic aortic heart valve with a prosthetic valve using a catheter through transthoracic cardiac exposure. The heart is exposed by sternotomy, thoracotomy, or subxiphoid approach. The pericardium is incised. A small incision is made in the aorta or left ventricle to accommodate the catheter and the collapsed prosthetic aortic valve. The native aortic valve may be dilated using a balloon catheter. The prosthetic aortic valve is then positioned within the native aortic valve and deployed. A balloon catheter is used to seat the valve. Contrast is injected and angiograms are obtained to check position and function of the prosthetic valve. Chest tubes are placed as needed and the chest incision is closed.

33366

33366   Transcatheter aortic valve replacement (TAVR/TAVI) with prosthetic valve; transapical exposure (eg, left thoracotomy)

A stenotic aortic heart valve is replaced with a prosthetic valve using a catheter delivered via a left thoracotomy and transapical stab incision. A limited anterolateral left thoracotomy is performed at the sixth intercostal space to access the apex of the heart. The pericardium is opened. The left ventricle is entered via needle puncture and the opening is serially dilated until the valve delivery catheter can be introduced. The catheter is threaded over a guidewire, through the left ventricle to the native aortic valve. Epicardial pacing wires are placed on the left ventricle as needed to pace the heart during valve delivery. The native aortic valve may be dilated using a balloon catheter prior to placing the prosthetic valve. A catheter containing the compressed aortic valve which is contained within a valve cage is advanced over the guidewire to the native aortic valve. The compressed valve is positioned in the native diseased aortic valve and deployed. The valve cage is removed. A balloon tip catheter is used to seat the aortic valve. The balloon is positioned in the prosthetic valve and inflated. Position and function of the valve is verified. The catheter is removed and the transapical puncture site and chest incisions are closed with sutures.

33367-33369

33367   Transcatheter aortic valve replacement (TAVR/TAVI) with prosthetic valve; cardiopulmonary bypass support with percutaneous peripheral arterial and venous cannulation (eg, femoral vessels) (List separately in addition to code for primary procedure)

33368   Transcatheter aortic valve replacement (TAVR/TAVI) with prosthetic valve; cardiopulmonary bypass support with open peripheral arterial and venous cannulation (eg, femoral, iliac, axillary vessels) (List separately in addition to code for primary procedure)

33369   Transcatheter aortic valve replacement (TAVR/TAVI) with prosthetic valve; cardiopulmonary bypass support with central arterial and venous cannulation (eg, aorta, right atrium, pulmonary artery) (List separately in addition to code for primary procedure)

Transcatheter aortic valve replacement or implantation (TAVR/TAVI) is performed to treat a stenotic aortic heart valve by replacing it with a prosthetic valve. When the procedure is performed with cardiopulmonary bypass (CPB), the CPB is reported additionally. To perform CPB, a venous cannula is inserted into the right atrial appendage and an arterial cannula is placed in the ascending aorta. A cardioplegia cannula is placed in the coronary sinus via a stab incision in the right atrium and a second cannula is placed in the ascending aorta. A left ventricular vent is placed in the right superior pulmonary vein. CPB is established and

cardioplegic arrest is initiated. The TAVR/TAVI is then performed and reported separately. After the TAVR/TAVI procedure is completed, the patient is weaned off bypass. Chest tubes are placed as needed and the chest incision is closed. When cardiopulmonary bypass support is provided during transcatheter aortic valve replacement, cannulation for cardiopulmonary bypass can be complicated by patient's vascular anatomy or body habitus. As a result, different cannulation methods have been developed. Percutaneous peripheral cannulation is the usual route for connecting the pump-oxygenator to the patient's vasculature to establish partial or complete cardiopulmonary bypass but open peripheral cannulation through the femoral, iliac, or axillary vessels, or central cannulation are also used. For percutaneous peripheral arterial and venous cannulation using the femoral vessels, report code 33367. Open peripheral arterial and venous cannulation using the femoral, iliac, and axillary vessels is reported with code 33368, and central arterial and venous cannulation using the aorta, right atrium, and pulmonary artery is reported with code 33369.

33390-33391

● **33390   Valvuloplasty, aortic valve, open, with cardiopulmonary bypass; simple (ie, valvotomy, debridement, debulking, and/or simple commissural resuspension)**

● **33391   Valvuloplasty, aortic valve, open, with cardiopulmonary bypass; complex (eg, leaflet extension, leaflet resection, leaflet reconstruction, or annuloplasty)**

The aortic valve is repaired through an open chest incision with cardiopulmonary bypass. The aortic valve has three cusps or leaflets and is the outlet valve from the left ventricle to the aorta. Infection, age, and congenital defects may cause the valve to become stiff and narrowed or stenotic, limiting blood flow; or the leaflets may be loose and floppy, allowing regurgitation of blood back into the ventricle. The heart is accessed through an anterior midline incision in the chest with the sternum opened, or an intercostal incision on the left side of the chest between two ribs spread open to expose the heart. Cardiopulmonary bypass is initiated with placement of a venous cannula in the right atrium, vena cava or femoral vein, and an atrial cannula in the aorta, femoral or axillary artery, or apex of the heart. The heart is cooled and/or injected with a drug to stop muscle contractions. For simple valvuloplasty (33390), an incision is made in the heart to expose the aortic valve. When stenosis is present, the surgeon may dilate and open the commissures between the leaflets. Calcium deposits and blood clots are identified and removed by debridement or debulking. Simple commissural resuspension to treat valvular regurgitation is accomplished using commissuroplasty. Mattress sutures are placed into the aorta closing the top 1 cm of the commissures and narrowing the diameter of the valve orifice. For complex valvuloplasty (33391), leaflet extension is accomplished by suturing a piece of pericardium to the edge of one or more leaflets. A leaflet hole may be repaired using pericardial tissue or synthetic material sutured in place to form a patch. Leaflet plication or resection is accomplished by tucking and suturing tissue over and onto itself, or removing a wedge of tissue from the center of the leaflet and suturing the gap respectively. Chordae or papillary muscles are inspected and repaired as indicated. Annuloplasty may be performed by suturing a rigid, semi-rigid, or flexible ring to the leaflets forming an annulus of the desired size. Tension from heart muscle contractions and movement of blood through the valve is absorbed by the ring making the valve work more efficiently. Annuloplasty may also be accomplished by tacking one or more valve leaflets to the atrium using sutures or tucks to strengthen and tighten the muscles around the annulus. Muscle contractions are restarted in the heart and the valve is checked for bleeding. The patient is weaned off cardiopulmonary bypass. Drainage tubes are placed before the chest cavity is closed.

33404

33404   Construction of apical-aortic conduit

The physician constructs an apical-aortic conduit to treat aortic stenosis by allowing blood to bypass the stenosed aortic valve. Blood flows from the left ventricle through the conduit to the aorta. A left lateral incision is made through the sixth intercostal space. The inferior pulmonary ligament is divided and the lung is retracted to expose the cardiac apex and aorta. A synthetic tube graft is anastomosed to the aorta in an end-to-side fashion and connected end-to-end to a porcine valve. The pericardium is then incised and the apex of the heart is exposed. A needle is passed through the heart apex into the left ventricle. A guide-wire and dilators are used to create an opening in the ventricle that is temporarily occluded using an occlusion balloon passed over the guidewire. A ventricular coring device is threaded over the catheter and a core of ventricular muscle is removed at the apex. With the occlusion balloon in place, a connector is inserted into the surgically created opening in the ventricle. Sutures are placed through the ventricle muscle, around the opening in the apex, and into the external cuff of the connector. The ventricle connector is then sutured to the valved conduit. Following completion of the procedure, chest tubes are placed as needed and the chest incision is closed.

Cardiovascular System

33405-33410

▲ **33405** Replacement, aortic valve, open, with cardiopulmonary bypass; with prosthetic valve other than a homograft or stentless valve

▲ **33406** Replacement, aortic valve, open, with cardiopulmonary bypass; with allograft valve (freehand)

▲ **33410** Replacement, aortic valve, open, with cardiopulmonary bypass; with stentless tissue valve

An open aortic valve replacement is performed with cardiopulmonary bypass using a prosthetic valve other than a homograft of stentless valve (33405), an allograft valve (33406), or a stentless tissue valve (33410). A mechanical valve is an example of a prosthetic valve other than a homograft or stentless valve. An allograft valve is one obtained from a human cadaver donor. A stentless tissue aortic valve is a normal aortic valve obtained from a pig or cow (porcine valve/xenograft, bovine valve/xenograft). The heart is exposed using a median sternotomy or upper hemisternotomy. A venous cannula is inserted in the right atrial appendage and an arterial cannula in the ascending aorta. One cardioplegia cannula is placed in the coronary sinus via a stab incision in the right atrium and a second in the ascending aorta. A left ventricular vent is placed in the right superior pulmonary vein. Cardiopulmonary bypass is established and cardioplegic arrest is initiated. A transverse incision is made in the aorta and the ascending aorta is transected. The valve annulus is elevated with sutures placed at each commissure and pledgetted sutures placed in the right and non-coronary cusps. The stenosed aortic valve is excised. The aortic annulus and aortic wall are debrided. In 33405, a mechanical or artificial valve is used. The exact surgical technique is dependent on the mechanical or artificial valve selected. In 33406, the aortic allograft (homograft) is attached to the outflow tract after the sinus aorta has been trimmed away. The allograft is positioned in the aortic root and sutured into place. When the allograft is securely attached, the ascending aorta is sutured to the aortic root. In 33410, the stentless tissue valve is aligned and proximal sutures are placed in the subannular position. The commissural posts of the prosthetic stentless valve are each attached with a single suture. A distal row of sutures is placed extending from each cusp outward to the tip of each commissural post taking care to avoid obstruction of the coronary ostia. The aortic wall is then sutured to the prosthetic valve. The incision in the aorta is closed. The aortic cross-clamp is removed and the patient is weaned off cardiopulmonary bypass. Chest tubes are placed as needed and the chest incision is closed.

33411-33412

33411 Replacement, aortic valve; with aortic annulus enlargement, noncoronary sinus

33412 Replacement, aortic valve; with transventricular aortic annulus enlargement (Konno procedure)

Replacement of the aortic valve with aortic annulus enlargement of a noncoronary sinus is performed to treat aortic annular hypoplasia with or without associated aortic valve disease. The heart is exposed using a median sternotomy or upper hemisternotomy. A venous cannula is inserted in the right atrial appendage and an arterial cannula in the ascending aorta. One cardioplegia cannula is placed in the coronary sinus via a stab incision in the right atrium and a second in the ascending aorta. A ventricular vent is placed in the right superior pulmonary vein. Cardiopulmonary bypass is established and cardioplegic arrest is initiated. In 33411, a transverse incision is made in the ascending aorta and extended inferiorly toward the posterior commissure. The aortic annulus is enlarged by separating the adventitia of the aorta from the middle layer using blunt dissection and separating the left atrial wall from the posterior aortic annulus. The posterior commissure is resected. The incised ends of the left coronary and noncoronary annulus are then widely separated. A synthetic patch is used to close the surgically created defect and an aortic valve prosthesis is sutured to the patch. The incision in the aorta is closed. The aortic cross-clamp is removed and the patient is weaned off cardiopulmonary bypass. Chest tubes are placed as needed and the chest incision is closed. In 33412, replacement of the aortic valve is performed with transventricular aortic annulus enlargement to treat severe left ventricular outflow tract obstruction (LVOTO) with aortic annular hypoplasia. The aortic annulus is enlarged as described above. The left ventricular outflow tract is enlarged by incising down the left ventricular septum and placing a synthetic patch graft. The aortic valve is replaced as described above.

33413

33413 Replacement, aortic valve; by translocation of autologous pulmonary valve with allograft replacement of pulmonary valve (Ross procedure)

The aortic valve is replaced by translocation of the patient's pulmonary valve and the pulmonary valve is replaced with a pulmonary valve allograft from a cadaver donor. This procedure may also be referred to as a Ross procedure and is used to treat aortic stenosis. The heart is accessed by opening the sternum. Cardiopulmonary bypass is initiated to maintain heart function. The aorta is incised and the stenotic aortic valve leaflets excised taking care to preserve the coronary arteries. The aortic valve annulus is prepared for the translocation of the pulmonary valve and the annulus (opening) measured. The patient's pulmonary valve is harvested and sutured to the aortic valve annulus. The pulmonary valve annulus is prepared for the cadaver donor allograft pulmonary valve, which is then sutured

into place. Cardiopulmonary bypass is discontinued, chest tubes placed as needed, and the chest is closed.

33414

33414 Repair of left ventricular outflow tract obstruction by patch enlargement of the outflow tract

The physician repairs a left ventricular outflow tract obstruction (LVOTO) by patch enlargement of the outflow tract. This procedure is performed to treat left ventricular outflow tract obstruction involving subvalvular tissue only without involvement of the aortic valve or the left ventricle-aortic junction. The stenosis prevents normal outflow of blood from the left ventricle causing an increased workload on the heart which can result in left ventricular hypertrophy and failure. The heart is accessed by a median sternotomy. Cardiopulmonary bypass is initiated to maintain heart function. The ventricular septum is approached through an incision in the right ventricle. The ventricular septum is then incised. A synthetic patch is used to enlarge the left ventricle. The incision in the right ventricle is closed with a pericardial patch. Cardiopulmonary bypass is discontinued and chest incisions closed.

33415

33415 Resection or incision of subvalvular tissue for discrete subvalvular aortic stenosis

Resection or incision of subvalvular tissue for discrete subvalvular aortic stenosis is performed. This type of aortic stenosis occurs within the left ventricle below the aortic valve. The aortic valve and left ventricular-aortic junction are of normal caliber. The subvalvular stenosis prevents normal outflow of blood from the left ventricle causing an increased workload on the heart which can result in left ventricular hypertrophy and failure. The heart is accessed by a median sternotomy. Cardiopulmonary bypass is initiated to maintain heart function. The ventricular septum may be approached through an incision in the right ventricle with incision of the ventricular septum or through an incision in the aorta. If the obstruction is caused by a ridge or collar of tissue it is incised to widen the outflow tract. Alternatively, the ridge or collar of tissue may be resected. If a right ventricular approach is used, the incision in the septum is closed with sutures and the right ventricle is closed with a pericardial patch. If the approach is through the aorta, the incision in the aorta is closed with sutures. Cardiopulmonary bypass is discontinued and chest incisions closed.

33416

33416 Ventriculomyotomy (-myectomy) for idiopathic hypertrophic subaortic stenosis (eg, asymmetric septal hypertrophy)

Ventriculomyotomy or ventriculomyectomy is performed for idiopathic hypertrophic subaortic stenosis. This condition is more commonly referred to as hypertrophic cardiomyopathy with the most common manifestation being asymmetric enlargement of the left side of heart. This type of aortic stenosis occurs within the left ventricle below the aortic valve. The aortic valve and left ventricular-aortic junction are of normal caliber. The stenosis is due to an overgrowth of muscle tissue most often in the interventricular septum. Treatment involves incising the heart muscle in the left ventricle (ventriculomyotomy) or excising the muscle (ventriculomyectomy). The heart is accessed by a median sternotomy. Cardiopulmonary bypass is initiated to maintain heart function. The left ventricle is approached through an incision in the aorta (aortotomy). One or more deep incisions into the heart muscle are made over the area of hypertrophy. Small amounts of myocardial tissue may be excised to relieve the obstruction. Myocardial tissue is removed until outflow gradients have been reduced to a normal level. The incision in the aorta is closed. Cardiopulmonary bypass is discontinued and chest incision closed.

33417

33417 Aortoplasty (gusset) for supravalvular stenosis

An aortoplasty using a gusset is performed for supravalvular stenosis. Supravalvular stenosis is a type of congenital left ventricular outflow tract obstruction with narrowing of the ascending aorta immediately above the superior margin of the sinuses of Valsalva. The heart is exposed via a median sternotomy. Cardiopulmonary bypass is initiated. An inverted Y-shaped incision is made in the ascending aorta with the two arms of the Y extending across the supravalvular ring. The incision is carried across the area of stenosis into the noncoronary and right sinuses of Valsalva. A synthetic patch (gusset) is placed over the incision in the aorta to increase the diameter of the stenotic region. Once the patch has been sutured to the aorta, cardiopulmonary bypass is discontinued and chest incisions closed.

Cardiovascular System

 ● New Code   ▲ Revised Code

33418-33419

33418 Transcatheter mitral valve repair, percutaneous approach, including transseptal puncture when performed; initial prosthesis

33419 Transcatheter mitral valve repair, percutaneous approach, including transseptal puncture when performed; additional prosthesis(es) during same session (List separately in addition to code for primary procedure)

The transcatheter percutaneous approach to mitral valve repair is used to correct mitral valve regurgitation, which occurs when the anterior and posterior leaflets of the valve fail to close fully during ventricular systole allowing blood to flow back into the left atrium. An edge to edge leaflet repair using a prosthesis such as MitraClip can improve physiologic function of the mitral valve and reduce regurgitation with a minimally invasive technique. Utilizing fluoroscopy and transesophageal echocardiography (TEE), a steerable guide catheter is introduced into the vascular system using standard technique. A dilator is advanced over the guide catheter and across the septum into the left atrium to dilate the vascular pathway and decrease the chance of damage to the walls when the large bore catheter is introduced. The dilator is removed. The prosthesis and delivery catheter are introduced into the left atrium and the prosthesis is positioned above the leak with arms open. When optimal regurgitation reduction is visualized, the prosthesis is advanced into the left ventricle below the valve leaflets. The clip is then attached to each leaflet and the clip arms are closed creating a double orifice opening that allows blood flow on either side. The catheter is removed and the polyester covered metal clip is retained. Code 33418 is used for the initial procedure/prosthesis and code 33419 is added when the surgical procedure requires additional prosthesis(es) to be used.

33420-33422

33420 Valvotomy, mitral valve; closed heart

33422 Valvotomy, mitral valve; open heart, with cardiopulmonary bypass

Mitral valvotomy, also referred to as a commissurotomy, is performed to treat mitral stenosis. The mitral valve is located between the left atrium and left ventricle. Mitral stenosis is a narrowing of the valve orifice that obstructs blood flow from the left atrium into the left ventricle. The most common cause of mitral stenosis is rheumatic heart disease, but other common causes include calcification of the mitral annulus, infective endocarditis, systemic lupus erythematosus, rheumatoid arthritis, and carcinoid heart disease. In 33420, a closed heart mitral valve commissurotomy is performed. A right anterolateral thoracotomy is performed at the fifth intercostal space. The heart is exposed and the pericardium incised anterior to the phrenic nerve between the superior and inferior vena cava. The pericardium is retracted to allow visualization of the right atrium, left atrium, and pulmonary veins. A small incision is made at the interatrial groove at the level of the pulmonary veins. A pursestring suture is placed in the fatty tissue. The interatrial incision is carried into the left atrium and the index finger is inserted. The mitral valve is palpated and the stenosis dilated by passing the index finger into the mitral valve and separating the valve leaflets. The index finger is removed and the pursestring suture tied. In 33422, an open heart mitral valve commissurotomy is performed with cardiopulmonary bypass. The heart is exposed by median sternotomy or right anterolateral thoracotomy. Cardiopulmonary bypass is established and cardioplegia initiated. An incision is made in the left atrium and the mitral valve examined. Localized calcification of the commissures is debrided with a rongeur. The commisures between the leaflets are then incised to release the fusion or scar tissue. The heart is closed and cardiopulmonary bypass discontinued. Chest tubes are placed as needed and the chest is closed.

33425-33427

33425 Valvuloplasty, mitral valve, with cardiopulmonary bypass

33426 Valvuloplasty, mitral valve, with cardiopulmonary bypass; with prosthetic ring

33427 Valvuloplasty, mitral valve, with cardiopulmonary bypass; radical reconstruction, with or without ring

Mitral valvuloplasty is performed to treat mitral valve prolapse and regurgitation. The mitral valve is located between the left atrium and left ventricle. Mitral valve prolapse and regurgitation occur when the valve does not close tightly. When the left ventricle contracts the valve leaflets bulge (prolapse) upward into the left atrium and blood from the left ventricle may leak (regurgitate)back into the left atrium. The heart is exposed by median sternotomy or right anterolateral thoracotomy. Cardiopulmonary bypass is established and cardioplegia initiated. An incision is made in the left atrium and the mitral valve exposed. The type of repair performed depends on the type and extent of damage or malformation of the valve. If the valve annulus is dilated, an annuloplasty may be performed to reduce the size of the orifice. This is accomplished by plicating (folding) the edges of the valve to reduce the diameter of the valve orifice. If a ring annuloplasty device is used the annulus is sized and an appropriately sized ring is placed in the annulus and secured with sutures. The valve leaflets may also be repaired using an autologous pericardial patch. If the chordea have ruptured or elongated, the chordea may be resected, followed by plication to narrow the diameter of the valve and reconstruction of the valve leaflet. If the chordea is broken, they may be replaced with special sutures that replace the chordea. Other techniques to repair chordea include transfer or transposition from one leaflet to another. Upon completion of the repair, the heart incision is closed and the patient is weaned from

cardiopulmonary bypass. Chest tubes are placed as needed and the chest is closed. In 33425, the mitral valve is repaired using a technique such as annuloplasty without the use of a prosthetic ring or a single repair technique. In 33426, the mitral valve is repaired using a ring annuloplasty device. In 33427, radical reconstruction is performed with or without a ring. This involves using multiple repair techniques to reconstruct damaged valve.

33430

33430 Replacement, mitral valve, with cardiopulmonary bypass

The physician performs a mitral valve replacement with cardiopulmonary bypass for mitral stenosis, prolapse, or regurgitation. Replacement is required when the valve is too severely damaged to repair by other techniques. The valve may be replaced with either a non-biological mechanical valve composed of metal and pyrolytic carbon or a biological valve made from animal tissue, such as a porcine valve. The mitral valve is located between the left atrium and left ventricle. Mitral stenosis is a narrowing of the valve orifice that obstructs blood flow from the left atrium into the left ventricle. Mitral valve prolapse and regurgitation occur when the valve does not close tightly. When the left ventricle contracts the valve leaflets bulge (prolapse) upward into the left atrium and blood from the left ventricle may leak (regurgitate) back into the left atrium. The heart is exposed by median sternotomy or right anterolateral thoracotomy. Cardiopulmonary bypass is established and cardioplegia initiated. An incision is made in the left atrium and the mitral valve exposed. The damaged mitral valve is excised. An artificial valve is then sutured into place using non-absorbable sutures or pledgets. The valve is tested to ensure that it is opening and closing properly. The heart is closed and the patient is weaned off of cardiopulmonary bypass. Chest tubes are placed as needed and the chest is closed.

33460

33460 Valvectomy, tricuspid valve, with cardiopulmonary bypass

Valvectomy of the tricuspid valve is performed with cardiopulmonary bypass. The tricuspid valve is located between the right atrium and right ventricle. Excision of the tricuspid valve without replacement is performed when the patient has a severely damaged tricuspid valve due to infective endocarditis. The valve is not replaced when there is a risk of re-infection, which is a particular risk in intravenous drug users. The heart is exposed by median sternotomy. Cardiopulmonary bypass is established and cardioplegia initiated. An incision is made in the right atrium and the tricuspid valve exposed. The entire tricuspid valve is excised including valve leaflets, chordea tendinea, and papillary muscles. The heart incision is closed, and the patient is weaned from cardiopulmonary bypass. Chest tubes are placed as needed and the chest is closed.

33463-33464

33463 Valvuloplasty, tricuspid valve; without ring insertion

33464 Valvuloplasty, tricuspid valve; with ring insertion

The physician performs a valvuloplasty on the tricuspid valve with cardiopulmonary bypass for tricuspid valve regurgitation, insufficiency, or incompetence.. The tricuspid valve is located between the right atrium and right ventricle. Tricuspid valve regurgitation occurs when the valve does not close tightly. When the right ventricle contracts the valve leaflets bulge (prolapse) upward into the right atrium and blood from the right ventricle may leak (regurgitate) back into the right atrium. Tricuspid valve regurgitation occurs due to structural alterations of one or more of the valve components, which include the leaflets, chordea tendinae, annulus, or papillary muscles. The heart is exposed by median sternotomy. Cardiopulmonary bypass is established and cardioplegia initiated. An incision is made in the right atrium and the tricuspid valve exposed. The type of repair performed depends on the type and extent of damage or malformation of the valve. If the valve annulus is dilated, an annuloplasty may be performed to reduce the size of the orifice. This is accomplished by plicating (folding) the edges of the valve to reduce the diameter of the orifice. If a ring annuloplasty device is used the annulus is sized and an appropriately sized ring is placed in the annulus and secured with sutures. If the chordea have ruptured or elongated, the chordea may be resected and then plicated to narrow the diameter of the valve. The valve leaflet may be reconstructed. Broken chordea may be replaced with nonabsorbable synthetic sutures. Other techniques to repair chordea include transfer or transposition from one leaflet to another. Upon completion of the repair, the heart incision is closed, and the patient is weaned from cardiopulmonary bypass. Chest tubes are placed as needed and the chest is closed. Use 33463 when the tricuspid valve is repaired without the use of a prosthetic ring and 33464 when a ring annuloplasty device is used to repair the valve.

33465

33465 Replacement, tricuspid valve, with cardiopulmonary bypass

The physician performs a tricuspid valve replacement with cardiopulmonary bypass for tricuspid valve regurgitation, insufficiency, or incompetence. Replacement is required when the valve is too severely damaged to repair by other techniques. The valve may be replaced with either a non-biological mechanical valve composed of metal and pyrolytic carbon or a biological valve made from animal tissue, such as a porcine valve. The tricuspid valve is located between the right atrium and right ventricle. Tricuspid valve regurgitation occurs

Cardiovascular System

when the valve does not close tightly. When the right ventricle contracts the valve leaflets bulge (prolapse) upward into the right atrium and blood from the right ventricle may leak (regurgitate) back into the left atrium. Tricuspid valve regurgitation occurs due to structural alterations of one or more of the valve components, which include the leaflets, chordea tendinae, annulus, or papillary muscles. The heart is exposed by median sternotomy. Cardiopulmonary bypass is established and cardioplegia initiated. An incision is made in the right atrium and the tricuspid valve exposed. The damaged tricuspid valve is excised. An artificial valve is then sutured into place using non-absorbable sutures or pledgets. The valve is tested to ensure that it is opening and closing properly. The heart is closed and the patient is weaned off cardiopulmonary bypass. Chest tubes are placed as needed and the chest is closed.

33468

33468   Tricuspid valve repositioning and plication for Ebstein anomaly

The physician repositions the tricuspid valve leaflets and plicates the right ventricle to treat Ebstein's anomaly. The tricuspid valve is located between the right atrium and right ventricle and regulates blood flow from the atrium to the ventricle. Ebstein's anomaly is an abnormality of the tricuscpid valve characterized by downward displacement of two of its leaflets. The third leaflet is elongated and may be adherent to the right ventricle. These abnormalities cause blood to leak backward (regurgitate) from the right ventricle into the right atrium, which can result in right atrial enlargement and congestive heart failure in severe cases. The right atrium is opened parallel to the atrioventricular groove. Beginning near the anteroseptal commisure, the anterior leaflet is detached from the tricuspid annulus leaving the anterior attachment of the leaflet intact at the level of the commisure. Detachment of the posterior leaflet continues in one contiguous piece along with the anterior leaflet until the posterior leaflet is completely detached. Fibrous bands between the leaflets and the ventricular wall are then cut and papillary muscle attachments are dissected from the ventricular wall. Longitudinal plication of the atrialized right ventricle is then performed. One line of sutures is placed along a line from the apex of the atrialized portion of the right ventricle to the coronary sinus and includes the septal leaflet attachment, leaving the septal leaflet itself or leaflet remnants untouched. A second line of sutures is placed running in the opposite direction toward the apex of the ventricle. This line of sutures runs along the diaphragmatic endocardial surface of the atrialized chamber and includes the original attachments of the posterior leaflet. The anterior and posterior leaflets are then repositioned on the newly created tricuspid annulus.

33470-33471

33470   Valvotomy, pulmonary valve, closed heart; transventricular
33471   Valvotomy, pulmonary valve, closed heart; via pulmonary artery

Pulmonary valvotomy, also referred to as a commissurotomy, is performed to treat pulmonary atresia or stenosis. The pulmonary valve is located between the right ventricle and pulmonary artery. Pulmonary atresia is a congenital heart defect in which the pulmonary valve has failed to form or the valve leaflets do not open preventing blood from flowing from the right ventricle to the lungs. Pulmonary stenosis is a narrowing of the valve orifice. The heart is approached by median sternotomy. The thymus is partially resected to allow exposure of the heart. In 33471, the main pulmonary artery is incised above the level of the pulmonary valve. The valve is inspected. If the valve annulus is of adequate size, the physician can open the three commissures using sharp dissection. The pulmonary artery incision is then closed. In 33470, the pulmonary valvotomy is performed by a tranventricular approach. A pursestring suture is placed immediately below the pulmonary valve in the right ventricular wall. A small incision is made in the ventricle within the pursestring suture. A mosquito clamp is introduced into the heart and passed through the narrow opening in the valve. The clamp is used to open the valve by causing tearing of the fused the commissures. The clamp is removed and a series of dilators are then passed into the right ventricle and through the pulmonary valve until the pulmonary valve orifice has been dilated to a sufficient diameter. Surgical instruments are removed and the incision closed by tightening the previously placed pursestring suture.

33474

33474   Valvotomy, pulmonary valve, open heart, with cardiopulmonary bypass

Pulmonary valvotomy, also referred to as commissurotomy, is performed to treat pulmonary atresia or stenosis. The pulmonary valve is located between the right ventricle and pulmonary artery. Pulmonary atresia is a congenital heart defect in which the pulmonary valve has failed to form or the valve leaflets do not open, preventing blood from flowing from the right ventricle to the lungs. Pulmonary stenosis is a narrowing of the valve orifice. The heart is approached by median sternotomy. The thymus is partially resected to allow exposure of the heart. The patient is placed on cardiopulmonary bypass. The ascending aorta is cannulated along with the right atrial appendage. The arterial duct is exposed and ligated. Once cardiopulmonary bypass has been initiated, the main pulmonary artery is incised above the level of the pulmonary valve, and the valve is inspected. If the valve annulus is of adequate size, the physician can open the three commissures using sharp dissection. If the annulus is not large enough to allow valvotomy using the main pulmonary artery approach, the incision is extended and the right ventricle is opened to allow repair using a transventricular approach. The commissures are opened using sharp dissection.

Once the valve orifice is opened, incisions in the right ventricle and main pulmonary artery are closed and cardiopulmonary bypass is discontinued. Chest tubes are placed as needed and the chest is closed.

33475

33475   Replacement, pulmonary valve

The physician performs a pulmonary valve replacement. Replacement is required when the valve is too severely damaged to repair by other techniques. The valve may be replaced with either a non-biological mechanical valve composed of plastic, metal and pyrolytic carbon or a biological valve made from animal tissue, such as a porcine valve, or a cadaver donor. The heart is exposed by median sternotomy. Cardiopulmonary bypass is established. The main pulmonary artery is incised above the level of the pulmonary valve. The valve is inspected. If the valve annulus is of adequate size, the replacement may be performed through the pulmonary artery. If the annulus is not large enough to allow replacement using the main pulmonary artery approach, the incision is extended and the right ventricle opened to allow repair using a transventricular approach. The pulmonary valve leaflets are excised. The valve annulus is debrided and measured. An artificial valve is then sutured into place using non-absorbable sutures or pledgets. The valve is tested to ensure that it is opening and closing properly. The heart is closed and the patient is weaned off of cardiopulmonary bypass. Chest tubes are placed as needed and the chest is closed.

33476

33476   Right ventricular resection for infundibular stenosis, with or without commissurotomy

The physician performs a right ventricular resection for infundibular pulmonary stenosis with or without commissurotomy. Infundibular pulmonary stenosis is an obstruction of the outflow of blood in the right ventricle. The obstruction may be due to a fibrous muscle band at the junction of the main cavity of the right ventricle and the infundibulum that divides the right ventricle into two cavities or a hypertrophied infundibulum that narrows the right ventricular outlet. The heart is exposed by median sternotomy. Cardiopulmonary bypass is established. The right ventricle is incised. The obstructive fibrous muscle band is excised to relieve the obstruction. Alternatively, tissue is removed from the thickened muscular infundibulum to enlarge the outflow tract. The pulmonary valve is inspected and if the commissures are fused, the physician opens the three commissures using sharp dissection. The heart is closed and the patient is weaned off of cardiopulmonary bypass. Chest tubes are placed as needed and the chest is closed.

33477

33477   Transcatheter pulmonary valve implantation, percutaneous approach, including pre-stenting of the valve delivery site, when performed

Percutaneous transcatheter pulmonary valve implantation may be used to treat patients with right ventricular outflow tract (RVOT) dysfunction including stenotic or regurgitant right ventricle-to-pulmonary artery conduit, Tetralogy of Fallot without a conduit, and Tetrology of Fallot with failing pulmonic bioprosthetic valves, truncus arteriosus, pulmonary atresia with ventricular septal defects (VSD), or transposition of great arteries with VSD and pulmonic stenosis. The pulmonary valve consists of a delivery sheath with a balloon in balloon catheter that the valve is front-loaded into after crimping and a polytetrafluoroethylene sheath that covers the valve. The access site is selected (femoral vein, subclavian vein, or internal jugular vein) and a large bore needle is inserted through the skin into the vein. A guide wire is introduced through the needle and a catheter sheath is inserted over the wire, which is then threaded to the heart under fluoroscopic guidance. Angiography may be performed to determine the size and anatomy of the RVOT and right ventricular function. If pre-stenting is required to reinforce the conduit, the stent is deployed on a balloon in balloon catheter over the guide wire to the right pulmonary artery and wedged into place. The stent delivery catheter is removed and the valve delivery catheter is then eased over the guide wire to the desired location. The valve is delivered across the pre-stented (or unstented) outflow tract in the pulmonary artery. The placement site and function of the valve are evaluated with angiography and/or intracardiac echocardiography. The catheter, guide wire, and needle are removed and the site is monitored for bleeding. A suture may be required for closure and the area is covered with a dressing.

33478

33478   Outflow tract augmentation (gusset), with or without commissurotomy or infundibular resection

The physician performs a right ventricular outflow tract augmentation using a gusset or patch with or without commissurotomy or infundibular resection. This procedure is performed to treat infundibular pulmonary stenosis, which is an obstruction of the outflow of blood in the right ventricle. The obstruction may be due to a fibrous muscle band at the junction of the main cavity of the right ventricle and the infundibulum that divides the right ventricle into two cavities or a hypertrophied infundibulum that narrows the right ventricular outlet. The heart is exposed by median sternotomy. Cardiopulmonary bypass is established. The pericardium is incised and a patch of pericardium may be harvested to use as a patch graft. The right ventricle is incised along the right ventricular outflow tract.

Cardiovascular System

If there is an obstructive fibrous muscle band it is excised. Alternatively, tissue is removed from the thickened muscular infundibulum to enlarge the outflow tract. The outflow tract is enlarged using an autologous pericardial patch graft or a synthetic patch. The pulmonary valve is inspected and if the commissures are fused, the physician opens the three commissures using sharp dissection. The heart is closed and the patient is weaned off of cardiopulmonary bypass. Chest tubes are placed as needed and the chest is closed.

33496

33496 **Repair of non-structural prosthetic valve dysfunction with cardiopulmonary bypass (separate procedure)**

The physician repairs a non-structural prosthetic valve dysfunction using cardiopulmonary bypass. In non-structural prosthetic valve dysfunction, the dysfunction is due to a condition such as thrombus formation or fibrous tissue ingrowth rather than failure of the prosthetic valve itself. The thrombus or tissue ingrowth causes obstruction of the valve. The heart is exposed by median sternotomy. Cardiopulmonary bypass is established. The heart is incised and the prosthetic valve exposed. If a thrombus is present it is removed. If there is tissue ingrowth, the obstructing tissue is excised. Valve function is tested. The heart is closed and cardiopulmonary bypass discontinued. Chest tubes are placed as needed and the chest is closed.

33500-33501

33500 **Repair of coronary arteriovenous or arteriocardiac chamber fistula; with cardiopulmonary bypass**
33501 **Repair of coronary arteriovenous or arteriocardiac chamber fistula; without cardiopulmonary bypass**

The physician repairs a coronary arteriovenous or arteriocardiac chamber fistula. A coronary arteriovenous fistula is an anomalous communication between a coronary artery and a systemic or pulmonary vein. A coronary arteriocardiac chamber fistula is an anomalous communication between a coronary artery and heart chamber. The heart is exposed by median sternotomy. The feeding coronary artery and the site of fistula insertion in the feeding artery are identified. The course of the fistula and drainage site in the vein or cardiac chamber is also identified. If cardiopulmonary bypass is used it is initiated. If the fistula drains into a vein, the venous end of the fistula is closed with sutures. If the fistula drains into a cardiac chamber, the chamber is opened and the drainage site is closed with sutures or a patch is placed. If the feeding vessel is large, the coronary artery is also incised and the opening to the fistula is closed with sutures. The incision in the coronary artery is then closed. Use 33500, when the procedure is performed with cardiopulmonary bypass and 33501 if the procedure does not require cardiopulmonary bypass.

33502-33504

33502 **Repair of anomalous coronary artery from pulmonary artery origin; by ligation**
33503 **Repair of anomalous coronary artery from pulmonary artery origin; by graft, without cardiopulmonary bypass**
33504 **Repair of anomalous coronary artery from pulmonary artery origin; by graft, with cardiopulmonary bypass**

The coronary arteries normally arise from the ascending aorta just above the aortic valve from the facing sinuses of Valsalva. Coronary arteries do not normally arise from a nonfacing or distant sinus. There are a number of anomalous variants that occur when the coronary artery arises from a pulmonary artery origin and the procedure performed depends on the exact nature of the anomaly. A median sternotomy or posterolateral thoracotomy is used to expose the heart. In 33502, the physician ligates the anomalous coronary artery. The anomalous coronary artery is identified and two ligatures placed immediately above (proximal to) the origin in the pulmonary artery to stop the flow of blood through the anomalous coronary artery. In 33503, the physician repairs the anomalous coronary artery using a bypass graft without cardiopulmonary bypass, also referred to as off-pump coronary artery bypass. An injection is given to slow heart rate. An internal mammary artery or saphenous vein graft is typically used. If a saphenous vein graft is used, an incision is made in the skin of the leg over the section of saphenous vein to be harvested. Soft tissue is dissected off the vein and branches ligated and divided. The section of saphenous vein to be used is then ligated proximally and distally, divided and removed from the leg. The aorta is incised and the bypass graft is anastomosed to the aorta just above the aortic valve. The coronary artery is incised and the graft anastomosed. Once the coronary artery is receiving its blood supply from the aorta instead of the pulmonary artery the anomalous communication between the coronary artery and pulmonary artery is ligated just above the pulmonary artery origin. In 33504, the physician repairs the anomalous coronary artery using cardiopulmonary bypass. Once cardiopulmonary bypass has been initiated, the procedure is performed as described in 33503.

33505

33505 **Repair of anomalous coronary artery from pulmonary artery origin; with construction of intrapulmonary artery tunnel (Takeuchi procedure)**

The physician repairs an anomalous coronary artery with a pulmonary artery origin by construction of an intrapulmonary artery tunnel, also referred to as a Takeuchi procedure.

The heart is accessed by median sternotomy. The procedure may be performed using cardiopulmonary bypass or on the beating heart using off-pump technique. The pericardium is incised and a section of pericardium harvested to use in the tunnel construction. An aortopulmonary window is created in the wall of the aorta and pulmonary artery. A tunnel is fashioned from the section of pericardium and attached to the anomalous coronary artery origin within the pulmonary artery and then passed through the pulmonary artery to the aortopulmonary window and attached to the aorta. If cardiopulmonary bypass has been used, it is discontinued. Chest tubes are placed as needed and the chest is closed.

33506

33506 **Repair of anomalous coronary artery from pulmonary artery origin; by translocation from pulmonary artery to aorta**

The physician repairs an anomalous coronary artery with a pulmonary artery origin by translocation of anomalous coronary artery from the pulmonary artery to the aorta. The heart is accessed by median sternotomy. The procedure may be performed using cardiopulmonary bypass or on the beating heart using off-pump technique. The pericardium is incised and a pericardial patch harvested. The pulmonary artery is incised and the anomalous origin of the coronary artery excised with a button of pulmonary artery tissue. The anomalous coronary artery is mobilized and the aorta incised. The anomalous coronary artery is anastomosed with the pulmonary artery button to the aorta. The defect in the pulmonary artery is repaired using the previously harvested pericardial patch. If cardiopulmonary bypass has been used, it is discontinued. Chest tubes are placed as needed and the chest is closed.

33507

33507 **Repair of anomalous (eg, intramural) aortic origin of coronary artery by unroofing or translocation**

The physician repairs a coronary artery with an anomalous origin in the aorta. The chest is opened using a median sternotomy. Cardiac cannulas are placed and cardiopulmonary bypass initiated. An aortic cross clamp is applied and cardioplegic arrest obtained. The aorta is incised and the ostia (opening) of the anomalous coronary artery identified beside the commissure between the right and left cusps of the aortic valve. The initial portion of the coronary artery is located along an intramural and proximal course between the pulmonary artery and aortic wall. The intramural coronary artery is unroofed which involves transecting (cutting) the anterior wall of the coronary artery horizontally through the uppermost portion of the aortic valve commissure. The commissure is resuspended as needed. The intimal surface of the aorta is attached to the coronary artery with sutures and the coronary artery enlarged as needed. Alternatively, the coronary artery may be translocated (moved) to the correct anatomical position in the aorta. A window is made in the intima of the aorta and the anomalous coronary artery repositioned. The incision in the aorta is closed. Air is removed from the heart and aorta, the cross clamp is removed and the patient is warmed and removed from bypass. Chest tubes are inserted and temporary pacing wires placed. The sternum is closed.

33508

33508 **Endoscopy, surgical, including video-assisted harvest of vein(s) for coronary artery bypass procedure (List separately in addition to code for primary procedure)**

A vein graft is harvested for use in a separately reportable coronary artery bypass procedure using video-assisted endoscopy. A small incision is made over the vein to be harvested, usually the greater saphenous vein. An endoscopic dissection system including a camera and trocar is introduced. If the saphenous vein is being harvested, an incision is made at the knee. The dissection system is first passed along the anterior surface of the vein toward the groin and the vein dissected for several cm. A balloon trocar is inserted, the balloon inflated, and tissues separated by insufflation of air. Dissection continues to the groin. The trocar and camera are removed. The dissection system is then reinserted at the knee and passed along the vein toward the ankle and distal dissection performed in the same manner. The camera and trocar are removed and the trocar tip replaced with bipolar scissors. The camera and bipolar scissors are reinserted and passed first distally and then proximally. The saphenous vein is carefully inspected and side branches ligated. The endoscopic system is removed. Small incisions are made at the groin and ankle and the saphenous vein is ligated and divided proximally and distally. The vein is removed from the leg and prepared for coronary artery bypass.

33510-33516

33510 **Coronary artery bypass, vein only; single coronary venous graft**
33511 **Coronary artery bypass, vein only; 2 coronary venous grafts**
33512 **Coronary artery bypass, vein only; 3 coronary venous grafts**
33513 **Coronary artery bypass, vein only; 4 coronary venous grafts**
33514 **Coronary artery bypass, vein only; 5 coronary venous grafts**
33516 **Coronary artery bypass, vein only; 6 or more coronary venous grafts**

The coronary arteries supply the heart with oxygen and nutrients. Narrowing or blockage of one or more coronary arteries can cause ischemic heart disease and myocardial infarction.

CABG is used to reroute blood around a narrowed or blocked artery. Prior to exposing the heart, one or more veins, usually the greater saphenous veins from the legs, are harvested. If the saphenous veins are used, one or more incisions are made in the thigh or calf of one or both legs. The vein is prepared for grafting. An incision is made in the chest. The sternum is divided and the ribs retracted to expose the heart. The procedure may be performed using off-pump coronary artery bypass (OPCAB) technique or cardiopulmonary bypass may be initiated. If OPCAB technique is used, the surgery is performed on the beating heart after injection of medication to slow the heart rate. If cardiopulmonary bypass is initiated, the patient is connected to the cardiopulmonary bypass pump and cardioplegia initiated. The prepared vein grafts are sewn into place attaching one end of the vein to the ascending aorta and the other end to the diseased coronary artery at a point beyond the blockage. If cardiopulmonary bypass has been used, it is discontinued. When only venous bypass grafts are used, use 33510 to report a single venous graft; 33511 to report two venous grafts; 33512 to report three venous grafts; 33513, to report four venous grafts; 33514 to report five venous grafts, and 33516 to report six or more venous grafts.

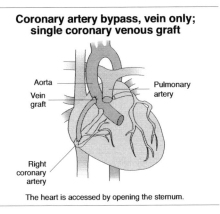

Coronary artery bypass, vein only; single coronary venous graft

Aorta
Vein graft
Pulmonary artery
Right coronary artery

The heart is accessed by opening the sternum.

33517-33523

33517   Coronary artery bypass, using venous graft(s) and arterial graft(s); single vein graft (List separately in addition to code for primary procedure)

33518   Coronary artery bypass, using venous graft(s) and arterial graft(s); 2 venous grafts (List separately in addition to code for primary procedure)

33519   Coronary artery bypass, using venous graft(s) and arterial graft(s); 3 venous grafts (List separately in addition to code for primary procedure)

33521   Coronary artery bypass, using venous graft(s) and arterial graft(s); 4 venous grafts (List separately in addition to code for primary procedure)

33522   Coronary artery bypass, using venous graft(s) and arterial graft(s); 5 venous grafts (List separately in addition to code for primary procedure)

33523   Coronary artery bypass, using venous graft(s) and arterial graft(s); 6 or more venous grafts (List separately in addition to code for primary procedure)

Coronary artery bypass graft (CABG) is performed using a combination of venous and arterial grafts. These codes report the venous grafting only. The coronary arteries supply the heart with oxygen and nutrients. Narrowing or blockage of one of more coronary arteries can cause ischemic heart disease and myocardial infarction. CABG is used to reroute blood around a narrowed or blocked artery. Prior to exposing the heart, one or more veins, usually the greater saphenous veins from the legs, are harvested and prepared for grafting. An incision is made in the chest. The sternum is divided and the ribs are retracted to expose the heart. The procedure may be performed using off-pump coronary artery bypass (OPCAB) technique or cardiopulmonary bypass may be initiated. If OPCAB technique is used, the surgery is performed on the beating heart after injection of medication to slow the heart rate. The prepared vein grafts are sewn into place, attaching one end of the vein to the ascending aorta and the other end to the diseased coronary artery at a point beyond the blockage. When venous grafts are used in conjunction with separately reportable arterial grafts, use 33517 to report a single venous graft; 33518 to report two venous grafts; 33519 to report three venous grafts; 33521, to report four venous grafts; 33522 to report five venous grafts, and 33523 to report six or more venous grafts.

33530

33530   Reoperation, coronary artery bypass procedure or valve procedure, more than 1 month after original operation (List separately in addition to code for primary procedure)

The heart is accessed by reopening the sternum. Special care must be taken because of scar tissues that may have formed from the previous surgery. Cardiopulmonary bypass is initiated to maintain heart function and the reoperation for coronary artery bypass or valve

procedure is completed. Cardiopulmonary bypass is discontinued and the chest is closed. Report when the operation is done more than one month after the original procedure.

33533-33536

33533   Coronary artery bypass, using arterial graft(s); single arterial graft

33534   Coronary artery bypass, using arterial graft(s); 2 coronary arterial grafts

33535   Coronary artery bypass, using arterial graft(s); 3 coronary arterial grafts

33536   Coronary artery bypass, using arterial graft(s); 4 or more coronary arterial grafts

Coronary artery bypass graft (CABG) surgery is performed using arterial bypass grafts. The coronary arteries supply the heart with oxygen and nutrients. Narrowing or blockage of one or more coronary arteries can cause ischemic heart disease and myocardial infarction. CABG is used to reroute blood around a narrowed or blocked artery. Prior to exposing the heart one or more arteries are harvested. Arterial conduits most frequently used include the internal mammary artery (IMA) in the chest, the inferior epigastric artery (IEA) in the abdomen, and the radial artery in the forearm. The gastroepiploic artery, or arterial conduits from other sites may also be used. Arterial conduits may be harvested as pedicle grafts that include satellite veins and surrounding tissues or they may be skeletonized with all surrounding tissue removed leaving the adventitia as the outermost layer of the graft. If the IMA is used, a median sternotomy is employed to access the thoracic cavity. The pleura is displaced laterally to allow access to the IMA. The segment of IMA to be harvested is identified. The IMA segment is typically harvested as a pedicle graft and includes satellite veins and endothoracic fascia. Soft tissue incision sites are marked on each side of the IMA segment. The IMA is separated from the chest wall at the third or fourth intercostal space. Collateral branches in the distal portion of the IMA are divided. The proximal portion of the IMA, including the pericardiacophrenic and thymic arteries, is inspected and collateral branches divided. Following dissection of the IMA graft, placement of the coronary artery bypass graft(s) may be performed using off-pump coronary artery bypass (OPCAB) technique or cardiopulmonary bypass (on pump technique) may be initiated. If OPCAB technique is used, the surgery is performed on the beating heart after injection of medication to slow the heart rate. If cardiopulmonary bypass is initiated, the patient is connected to the cardiopulmonary bypass pump and cardioplegia initiated. The pericardium is incised and the aorta cannulated. The distal end of the IMA is divided and the IMA pedicle rotated. The endothoracic fascia is retracted, incised along the entire length of the graft, and the inferior surface of the IMA exposed. The proximal end of the IMA graft is clamped and the distal end prepared for anastomosis using papaverine solution flush and a papaverine-soaked gauze wrap. If the GEA is used, the abdomen is incised and the omentum exposed. If the IEA is used, the anterior rectus sheath is opened, the rectus muscle retracted medially, and the IEA exposed. The IEA may be harvested as a pedicle graft with satellite veins and surrounding fatty tissues or skeletonized. The IEA segment is clip ligated, collateral branches divided, and the distal and proximal ends of the graft segment divided. If an upper extremity artery is used, such as the radial artery, it is harvested in a separately reportable procedure. The prepared arterial graft(s) are sewn into place attaching one end of the artery to the ascending aorta and the other end to the diseased coronary artery at a point beyond the blockage. When arterial bypass grafts are used, use 33533 to report a single arterial graft; 33534 to report two arterial grafts; 33535 to report three arterial grafts; and 33536 to report four or more arterial grafts. If cardiopulmonary bypass has been used, it is discontinued.

33542-33545

33542   Myocardial resection (eg, ventricular aneurysmectomy)

33545   Repair of postinfarction ventricular septal defect, with or without myocardial resection

The physician performs a myocardial resection. This procedure is typically performed for a ventricular aneurysm resulting from an extensive transmural myocardial infarction and may also be referred to as a ventricular aneurysmectomy. Myocardial resection may also be performed in conjunction with repair of a postinfarction ventricular septal defect (VSD). In 33542, the heart is exposed by median sternotomy. Cardiopulmonary bypass is established followed by cardioplegic arrest. The left ventricle is incised. The non-contractile, scarred area is exposed and assessed. Damaged heart muscle including the area containing the ventricular aneurysm is excised. The heart tissue is reapproximated and closed with sutures. The patient is weaned off cardiopulmonary bypass. Chest tubes are placed as needed and the chest incision is closed. In 33545, the physician repairs a post-infarction VSD with or without myocardial resection. The left ventricle is incised close to the septal margin. A second incision is made in the right ventricle close to the septal margin. The post-infarction VSD is exposed and evaluated. Following the myocardial resection, the VSD is repaired. There are a number of different techniques of VSD repair, including a single or double patch. If a double patch technique is used, two synthetic patches are placed over the defect with the right side of the septum being patched first. The right patch is positioned and held in place with two or three stay sutures. The second patch is then placed over the left side of the septum. Both patches are secured using a running suture placed at the periphery of the patches. Glue may be injected between the patches to reinforce friable septal tissue. If myocardial resection is required it is performed as described above. Strips of felt are placed on the exterior of the heart next to

● New Code   ▲ Revised Code

Cardiovascular System

the ventriculotomies. The ventriculotomies are closed with heavy mattress sutures placed through the felt strips and the ventricle incisions are closed without tension. The patient is weaned off cardiopulmonary bypass. Chest tubes are placed as needed and the chest incision is closed.

33548

33548   Surgical ventricular restoration procedure, includes prosthetic patch, when performed (eg, ventricular remodeling, SVR, SAVER, Dor procedures)

This procedure may also be referred to as ventricular remodeling, surgical anterior ventricular endocardial restoration (SAVER), or a Dor procedure. SVR is performed to treat congestive heart failure due to myocardial infarction which has caused scarring or an aneurysm that has resulted in an enlarged rounded heart and to restore the heart to a more normal size and shape. The remodeling of the heart is performed using a plastic model that has been selected based on the person's body surface area. The heart is exposed by median sternotomy. Cardiopulmonary bypass is established followed by cardioplegic arrest. The left ventricle is incised and retraction sutures placed. The non-contractile, scarred area in the anteroseptal segment is identified and assessed. The sizing device is seated in the apex. The size of the ventricle is assessed. An encircling suture is placed to exclude the non-contractile, scarred tissue. The suture is tightened to form an oval rim with a raised edge and the ventricular reduction is assessed. The opening is measured and an appropriately sized patch selected. The anterior wall is reconstructed by seating the patch in the opening and securing it with sutures. The heart wall is then closed over the patch. The patient is weaned off cardiopulmonary bypass. Chest tubes are placed as needed and the chest incision is closed.

33572

33572   Coronary endarterectomy, open, any method, of left anterior descending, circumflex, or right coronary artery performed in conjunction with coronary artery bypass graft procedure, each vessel (List separately in addition to primary procedure)

An open coronary endarterectomy is performed by any method on the left anterior descending, circumflex, or right coronary artery at the time of a separately reportable coronary artery bypass graft (CABG) procedure. Coronary endarterectomy may be performed in conjunction with CABG when there is diffuse atherosclerotic coronary artery disease. The coronary artery is explored using finger palpation and the extent of disease is estimated. The arterial wall is incised and the atheromatous core is removed. The arteriotomy is extended as needed to inspect major branches of the affected arteries and remove plaque. The atheromatous core may be removed using several different techniques including eversion-type endarterectomy using blind traction or by distal extension of the arteriotomy until normal appearing intima is encountered and removal of the plaque under direct vision. Following removal of plaque, the arteriotomy is closed with sutures or a saphenous vein patch. If more than one of the listed vessels is treated, report coronary endarterectomy once for each vessel treated.

33600-33602

33600   Closure of atrioventricular valve (mitral or tricuspid) by suture or patch
33602   Closure of semilunar valve (aortic or pulmonary) by suture or patch

Valve closure is performed on patients with single ventricle cardiac anomalies. The normal heart has two ventricles, the left pumps blood into the aorta and systemic circulation while the right pumps blood into the pulmonary arteries and lungs. In a single ventricle heart, one ventricle may be absent or poorly developed. This means that only a single ventricle is large enough to pump blood into the aorta and throughout the body. Surgical procedures are performed to maximize the efficiency of the single ventricle in pumping blood into the aorta as well as getting blood to the lungs. Usually multiple procedures are performed in stages. For some single ventricle cardiac anomalies, one part of the surgical process is to close one of the atrioventricular or semilunar valves so that blood is directed into the aorta. The heart is accessed by median sternotomy. If closure is to be accomplished using a pericardial patch, the pericardium is incised and a patch harvested. Cardiopulmonary bypass is initiated. In 33600, either the mitral or tricuspid valve is closed. In 33602 either the aortic or pulmonary valve is closed. The valve to be closed is exposed. If a pericardial patch is used, it is placed over the valve. If the valve is closed with sutures, the valve leaflets are sutured together to completely close the valve.

33606

33606   Anastomosis of pulmonary artery to aorta (Damus-Kaye-Stansel procedure)

The physician performs anastomosis of the pulmonary artery to the aorta, also referred to as Damus-Kaye-Stansel procedure. This procedure is used to treat double inlet left ventricle, tricuspid atresia with transposition of great vessels, and transposition of the great vessels with hypoplastic right ventricle. A median sternotomy is used to access the heart. The procedure varies somewhat depending on the cardiac anomaly being treated. Cardiopulmonary bypass is established and cardioplegia initiated. The aorta is dissected away from the pulmonary artery and completely mobilized. The pulmonary artery is mobilized. A patch graft of pulmonary artery from a cadaver donor is prepared. The right atrium is incised and the atrial septum resected. The underside of the aorta is opened. The

aorta is anastomosed to the proximal pulmonary artery in an end-to-side fashion. If the pulmonary artery is too short for direct anastomosis a cadaver donor pulmonary artery graft is used to achieve the necessary length. The distal end of the divided pulmonary artery is patched using a cadaver donor or synthetic patch. The heart is closed and cardiopulmonary bypass discontinued. Chest tubes are placed and the chest is closed.

33608

33608   Repair of complex cardiac anomaly other than pulmonary atresia with ventricular septal defect by construction or replacement of conduit from right or left ventricle to pulmonary artery

A conduit is a tubular graft that may be made of synthetic material or a cadaver donor aortic or arterial graft. The conduit may be valved or valveless. This procedure is used to treat ventricular outflow tract anomalies or complications from previous surgeries that result in obstruction of the right or left ventricular outflow tract. Median sternotomy is used to access the heart. Cardiopulmonary bypass is established and cardioplegia initiated. The right or left ventricle is incised and the outflow tract examined. A conduit is sutured to the ventricle at the ventriculotomy site. The main pulmonary artery is incised and the conduit is sutured to the pulmonary artery. The heart is closed and cardiopulmonary bypass discontinued. Chest tubes are placed and the chest incision is closed.

33610

33610   Repair of complex cardiac anomalies (eg, single ventricle with subaortic obstruction) by surgical enlargement of ventricular septal defect

A ventricular septal defect (VSD) is an abnormal opening in the interventricular septum that allows oxygenated blood in the left ventricle to mix with unoxygenated blood in the right ventricle. Patients with some complex cardiac anomalies, such as a single functioning ventricle with a smaller under developed ventricle and a small VSD require surgical enlargement the VSD to allow mixing of blood so that enough oxygenated blood reaches the heart and systemic circulation. A median sternotomy is used to access the heart. Cardiopulmonary bypass is initiated. The ventricle is incised. The VSD is enlarged by incising the interventricular septum. The incision in the ventricle is then closed and cardiopulmonary bypass discontinued. Chest tubes are placed and the chest incision is closed.

33611-33612

33611   Repair of double outlet right ventricle with intraventricular tunnel repair
33612   Repair of double outlet right ventricle with intraventricular tunnel repair; with repair of right ventricular outflow tract obstruction

The physician repairs a double outlet right ventricle (DORV) using an intraventricular tunnel, also referred to as a patch or tube graft. DORV is a relatively rare congenital heart defect in which both the aorta and pulmonary artery arise from the right ventricle. A ventricular septal defect (VSD) is also present and provides the only outlet from the left ventricle. Creation of an intraventricular tunnel channels blood from the left ventricle through the VSD to the aorta. Cardiopulmonary bypass is established using bicaval cannulation and cardioplegic arrest is initiated. The right atrium is incised and the heart anatomy inspected. The VSD is visualized through the tricuspid valve and the relationship to the aorta determined. The VSD may be approached through the tricuspid valve or the right ventricle may be incised. If the circumference of the VSD is smaller than the tunnel, the VSD is enlarged by incising the ventricular septum superiorly and anteriorly taking care to avoid the conduction tissue running inferior to the defect. A tunnel matching the circumference of the aorta is created using pericardium, polytetrafluoroethylene (PTFE), or other synthetic material. The tunnel is situated running from the anterior-most portion of the aorta to the VSD. A suture is placed through the base of the tricuspid valve leaflet (anteroseptal commissure) and then through the midportion of the tunnel. Additional sutures are placed on the atrial side of the septal leaflet of the tricuspid valve. Sutures are also placed along the inferior and posterior rim of the VSD and then passed through the tunnel to seat the tunnel down into the defect. The sutures are tied. If the VSD is larger than the tunnel, the remaining VSD opening is closed. The right atrial and right ventricle incisions are closed. In 33612, the physician first performs the above described intraventricular tunnel repair and then corrects right ventricular outflow tract obstruction caused by bulging of the intraventricular tunnel into the outflow tract. This is accomplished by enlarging the right ventricle using an autologous pericardial patch. The right ventriculotomy is closed with the patch.

33615

33615   Repair of complex cardiac anomalies (eg, tricuspid atresia) by closure of atrial septal defect and anastomosis of atria or vena cava to pulmonary artery (simple Fontan procedure)

A complex cardiac anomaly such as tricuspid atresia is treated by closure of the atrial septal defect and simple Fontan procedure which involves anastomosis of the atria or vena cava to the pulmonary artery. Tricuspid atresia is a condition in which the tricuspid valve between the right atrium and right ventricle, is either absent or imperforate. Patients with tricuspid atresia may also have an atrial septal defect (ASD). An ASD is an abnormal opening in the interatrial septum. Blood returning from caval veins to the right

● New Code   ▲ Revised Code   CPT © 2016 American Medical Association. All Rights Reserved.   © 2017 DecisionHealth

Cardiovascular System

atrium crosses the ASD into the left atrium and then enters the left ventricle. The heart is accessed by median sternotomy. The pericardium is incised and a pericardial patch harvested as needed. Cardiopulmonary bypass is initiated. The physician then connects both caval veins to the pulmonary circulation completely bypassing the right ventricle. The superior vena cava is divided at the right atrium and anastomosed to the right pulmonary artery using an end-to-end anastomosis. Two valved synthetic or cadaver donor grafts are then used to reroute blood from the inferior vena cava to the left pulmonary artery. The inferior vena cava is divided at the right atrium and one end of the valved graft anastomosed to the inferior vena cava and the other end is connected to the right atrium. One end of the second valved graft is anastomosed the right atrium. The left pulmonary artery is incised and the other end of the graft is anastomosed to the left pulmonary artery. The ASD is repaired with sutures or the previously harvested pericardial patch. The heart is closed and cardiopulmonary bypass discontinued. Chest tubes are placed and the chest incision closed.

33617

33617   Repair of complex cardiac anomalies (eg, single ventricle) by modified Fontan procedure

In a single ventricle heart, one ventricle may be absent or poorly developed. This means that only a single ventricle is large enough to pump blood into the aorta and throughout the body. Surgical procedures, such as a modified Fontan procedure, are performed to maximize the efficiency of the single ventricle in pumping blood into the aorta as well as getting blood to the lungs. A number of modifications have been made to the original Fontan procedure over the years. The lateral tunnel Fontan procedure is one that is commonly used. The heart is exposed by median sternotomy. Cardiopulmonary bypass is initiated. Two incisions are made in the right atrium one near the atrioventricular groove and a trap-door incision in the roof (superior) aspect. The main pulmonary artery is incised inferiorly and the incision carried out toward the first right hilar branch on one side and the left pulmonary artery on the other. The trap-door incision in the right atrium is sutured to the pulmonary artery incision. A lateral-tunnel is then created in the right atrium using a synthetic tube graft to direct blood flow from the inferior and superior vena cavae into the pulmonary arteries.

33619

33619   Repair of single ventricle with aortic outflow obstruction and aortic arch hypoplasia (hypoplastic left heart syndrome) (eg, Norwood procedure)

The physician performs the Norwood procedure to repair hypoplastic left heart syndrome which is a congenital cardiac anomaly characterized by a single ventricle with aortic outflow obstruction and aortic arch hypoplasia. In this type of cardiac anomaly, the left ventricle and aortic arch fail to develop adequately so the pulmonary artery must supply both the systemic and pulmonary circulations. Surgical intervention is necessary so that there is a balance between blood going to the lungs (pulmonary circulation) as well as to the body (systemic circulation). The heart is exposed by median sternotomy. Cardiopulmonary bypass is established along with hypothermic circulatory arrest. The upper aspect of the heart is incised and the atrial septum completely excised. The ductus arteriosus is ligated, divided and completely excised. The main pulmonary artery is divided proximal to the bifurcation of the pulmonary arteries and the distal pulmonary artery stump closed with a pericardial patch or synthetic or cadaver donor graft. The undersurface of the aortic arch is opened beginning at the ductus arteriosus and continuing distally along the descending aorta to the point where the aorta is of normal diameter and normal in appearance. The aortic incision is also extended proximally along the aortic arch to the level of the main pulmonary artery. A cadaver donor pulmonary graft is prepared for anastomosis. The graft is used to enlarge the hypoplastic aortic arch and connect the proximal aspect of the main pulmonary artery to the aorta. An aortopulmonary shunt or right ventricle to pulmonary artery conduit is then created for lung perfusion. The shunt is created using a synthetic graft placed from either the innominate artery or right ventricle to the central pulmonary artery. The patient is rewarmed and weaned from cardiopulmonary bypass. Chest tubes are placed and the chest incision is closed.

33620

33620   Application of right and left pulmonary artery bands (eg, hybrid approach stage 1)

Application of individual right and left pulmonary artery bands is performed to reduce excessive pulmonary blood flow that can lead to hypertrophy of pulmonary vasculature and irreversible pulmonary hypertension. This procedure is performed as part of a hybrid approach in a staged procedure in patients with certain cardiac anomalies such as hypoplastic left heart syndrome. Banding of the pulmonary arteries is performed as an initial measure to prepare the heart prior to definitive repair of the cardiac anomaly. The heart is exposed through a limited left anterior or lateral thoracotomy or less commonly through a median sternotomy. The pericardium is incised and the thymus is retracted to expose the aorta and pulmonary arteries. An adjustable pulmonary band is prepared by marking the estimated circumference on the band material. The band is placed around the right or left pulmonary artery and then through a snare to secure the ends of the band. The band is adjusted until pulmonary artery pressure distal to the band is within normal levels.

The band is sutured to the arterial adventitia to prevent migration. This is repeated on the contralateral pulmonary artery.

33621

33621   Transthoracic insertion of catheter for stent placement with catheter removal and closure (eg, hybrid approach stage 1)

Transthoracic insertion of a catheter with stent placement in the ductus arteriosus is performed as part of a hybrid approach in a staged procedure in patients with certain cardiac anomalies such as hypoplastic left heart syndrome. It is typically performed in conjunction with separately reportable banding of the right and left pulmonary arteries. The heart is exposed through a limited left anterior or lateral thoracotomy or less commonly through a median sternotomy. The pericardium is incised and the thymus is retracted to expose the aorta and pulmonary arteries. A small incision is made in the main pulmonary artery. A balloon catheter with a stent covered with a sheath is advanced through the main pulmonary artery and into the ductus arteriosus. The stent is carefully positioned; the sheath is removed; and the stent is deployed. The balloon catheter is inflated to ensure full expansion of the stent and secure it in place across the ductus arteriosus. The stent provides a conduit to the aorta until definitive repair of the heart defect can be performed.

33622

33622   Reconstruction of complex cardiac anomaly (eg, single ventricle or hypoplastic left heart) with palliation of single ventricle with aortic outflow obstruction and aortic arch hypoplasia, creation of cavopulmonary anastomosis, and removal of right and left pulmonary bands (eg, hybrid approach stage 2, Norwood, bidirectional Glenn, pulmonary artery debanding)

Reconstruction of a complex cardiac anomaly is performed as stage 2 of a hybrid approach. This type of hybrid approach is used to repair conditions such as hypoplastic left heart syndrome which is a congenital cardiac anomaly characterized by a single ventricle with aortic outflow obstruction and aortic arch hypoplasia. In this type of cardiac anomaly, the left ventricle and aortic arch fail to develop adequately so the pulmonary artery must supply both the systemic and pulmonary circulations. Surgical intervention is necessary so that there is a balance between blood going to the lungs (pulmonary circulation) as well as to the body (systemic circulation). The heart is exposed by median sternotomy. Cardiopulmonary bypass is established along with hypothermic circulatory arrest. The upper aspect of the heart is incised and the atrial septum is completely excised. The previously placed ductus arteriosus stent is removed. The ductus arteriosus is ligated, divided, and completely excised. The main pulmonary artery is divided proximal to the bifurcation of the pulmonary arteries and the distal pulmonary artery stump is closed with a pericardial patch or a synthetic or cadaver donor graft. The undersurface of the aortic arch is opened beginning at the ductus arteriosus and continuing distally along the descending aorta to the point where the aorta is of normal diameter and appearance. The aortic incision is also extended proximally along the aortic arch to the level of the main pulmonary artery. A cadaver donor pulmonary graft is prepared for anastomosis. The graft is used to enlarge the hypoplastic aortic arch and connect the proximal aspect of the main pulmonary artery to the aorta. An aortopulmonary shunt or right ventricle to pulmonary artery conduit is then created for lung perfusion. The shunt is created using a synthetic graft placed from either the innominate artery or right ventricle to the central pulmonary artery. The previously placed pulmonary artery bands are removed. The patient is rewarmed and weaned from cardiopulmonary bypass. Chest tubes are placed and the chest incision is closed.

33641

33641   Repair atrial septal defect, secundum, with cardiopulmonary bypass, with or without patch

The physician repairs an atrial septal secundum defect with or without a patch graft using cardiopulmonary bypass. This type of atrial septal defect (ASD) is also referred to as an ostium sedundum defect and is the most common type of ASD. During fetal development there is a normal opening in the atrial septum called the foramen ovale that allows oxygenated blood from the mother to pass to the left side of the heart. This opening in the atrial septum normally closes after birth but results in ASD when it doesn't close. An ostium secundum type defect is a mid-septal defect that typically extends into the fossa ovalis in the lower portion of the atrial septum. The size and shape varies. The heart is exposed using a median sternotomy or upper hemisternotomy. Venous and arterial cannulas are inserted, cardiopulmonary bypass is established, and cardioplegic arrest is initiated. The right atrium is incised (atriotomy) and the hole in the atrial septum is exposed. If the hole is small, it is repaired with sutures. Larger defects require closure using a pericardial tissue or synthetic patch graft. Following repair of the ASD, the right atrial incision is closed. The patient is then weaned off cardiopulmonary bypass, chest tubes are placed as needed, and the chest incision is closed.

Cardiovascular System

33645

33645   Direct or patch closure, sinus venosus, with or without anomalous pulmonary venous drainage

Direct or patch closure of a sinus venosus type defect is performed with or without repair of anomalous pulmonary venous drainage. There are several types of sinus venosus atrial septal defects (SVASD). The most common type occurs in the upper atrial septum contiguous with the superior vena cava. The defect is almost always associated with anomalous pulmonary venous drainage involving the right upper pulmonary vein draining into the superior vena cava. A less common defect occurs at the junction of the right atrium and inferior vena cava with anomalous venous drainage of the right lower pulmonary vein to the inferior vena cava. The least common defect occurs posterior to the fossa ovalis without involvement of the superior or inferior vena cava and without associated anomalous pulmonary drainage. The heart is exposed using a median sternotomy or upper hemisternotomy. Venous and arterial cannulas are inserted; cardiopulmonary bypass is established; and cardioplegic arrest is initiated. The right atrium is incised (atriotomy) and the sinus venosus defect is exposed. If the defect is small and does not involve the superior or inferior vena cava, it is repaired with sutures. Larger defects with vena cava involvement require closure using a pericardial tissue or synthetic patch graft. The patch is placed over the defect and configured to redirect blood flow from the pulmonary vein into the left atrium. This type of patch closes the septal defect and corrects the anomalous pulmonary venous drainage. The azygous vein may be ligated to prevent it from draining into the left atrium. Following repair of the sinus venosus defect, the right atrial incision is closed. The patient is then weaned off cardiopulmonary bypass; chest tubes are placed as needed; and the chest incision is closed.

33647

33647   Repair of atrial septal defect and ventricular septal defect, with direct or patch closure

An ASD is an abnormal opening in the interatrial septum that allows blood from the right and left atrium (upper chambers of the heart) to mix. A VSD is an abnormal opening in the interventricular septum that allows oxygenated blood in the left ventricle to mix with unoxygenated blood in the right ventricle (lower chambers of the heart). The heart is accessed by opening the sternum. The pericardium is incised and a graft of pericardium harvested as needed. Cardiopulmonary bypass is initiated. The right atrium is opened and the defect in the interatrial septum is closed with sutures or a patch is sutured over the opening. If a patch is used, the physician may use a pericardial patch harvested from the patient or synthetic material. The physician then repairs the VSD through an incision in the right atrium, an incision in the pulmonary artery, or for a supracisternal defect through an incision in the outflow tract (infundibulum) of the right ventricle. The physician sutures the defect or applies a patch as described above. The heart incisions are closed and cardiopulmonary bypass discontinued. Chest tubes are placed and the chest incision is closed.

33660-33670

33660   Repair of incomplete or partial atrioventricular canal (ostium primum atrial septal defect), with or without atrioventricular valve repair

33665   Repair of intermediate or transitional atrioventricular canal, with or without atrioventricular valve repair

33670   Repair of complete atrioventricular canal, with or without prosthetic valve

The physician repairs an atrioventricular septal defect (AVSD) also referred to as an endocardial cushion defect. The endocardial cushions are an embryonic structure that separate the central part of the heart near the tricuspid and atrial valves and also separate the atria from the ventricles. Structures at the central part of the heart that develop from the endocardial cusions include the lower part of the atrial septum and the ventricular septum just below the tricuspid and mitral valves. AVSDs are classified as partial (incomplete), transitional, or complete. A partial or incomplete AVSD , also referred to as an ostium primum atrial septal defect, is one in which part of the ventricular septum is filled in with tissue from the atrioventricular valves or from endocardial cushion tissue and the tricuspid and mitral valves are divided into two distinct valves . A transitional AVSD is one in which the valve leaflets from the common atrioventricular valve are fused to the ventricular septum resulting in closure of most of the septum and division of the common valve into two valves. A complete AVSD has defects in all central heart structures with holes in both the atrial and ventricular septa and an undivided or common atrioventricular valve. The heart is exposed using a median sternotomy. Bicaval and aortic cannulas are inserted, cardiopulmonary bypass is established, and cardioplegic arrest is initiated. The pericardium is incised and a patch harvested for repair of the septal defect. The right atrium is incised (atriotomy) and the AVSD exposed. In 33660, the tricuspid and mitral valves are inspected for size and competence. The cleft in the mitral valve is repaired first through the septal defect. Additional tailoring of the mitral valve is performed as needed to ensure competence of the valve and prevent stenosis. Any defects in the tricuspid valve are also repaired. The atrial septal defect (ASD) is then closed using a patch of pericardium or in the case of a small ASD closed with sutures. In 33665, the small ventricular septal defect (VSD) is closed with sutures, the cleft in the atrioventricular valve is repaired to form two separate valves, and the ASD is closed with a pericardial patch graft. In 33670,

the VSD is repaired using a synthetic patch. The common atrioventricular valve is elevated and valve competence and structure evaluated. If the common valve can be separated, this is done and the valve structures are tailored to ensure competence and prevent stenosis. If two separate valves cannot be constructed, one or both may be replaced with a prosthetic valve. Following repair of the valves, the ASD is closed with a pericardial patch. Following repair of the AVSD, the right atrial incision is closed. The patient is then weaned off cardiopulmonary bypass, chest tubes are placed as needed, and the chest incision is closed.

33675-33677

33675   Closure of multiple ventricular septal defects

33676   Closure of multiple ventricular septal defects; with pulmonary valvotomy or infundibular resection (acyanotic)

33677   Closure of multiple ventricular septal defects; with removal of pulmonary artery band, with or without gusset

A ventricular septal defect (VSD) is a congenital anomaly in which there are one or more abnormal openings in the septum. An incision is made in the chest to access the heart. The pericardium is incised and a patch harvested as needed. Cardiopulmonary bypass is initiated. In 33675, multiple VSDs are repaired through an incision in the right atrium, pulmonary artery, or in the outflow tract (infundibulum) of the right ventricle. The defects are repaired with sutures or a patch. If a patch is used, synthetic material or the previously harvested patch of pericardium is sutured over the defects. The access incision is closed and cardiopulmonary bypass discontinued. Chest tubes are placed and the chest incision is closed. In 33676, multiple VSDs are closed and pulmonary valvotomy or infundibular resection is also performed. This type of repair is performed when the VSD occurs in combination with obstruction of right ventricular outflow tract, such as that occurring with a mild (acyanotic) Tetralogy of Fallot. An incision is made in the right ventricle or pulmonary artery. The obstructive fibrous or muscle band is excised. Alternatively, tissue is removed from the thickened muscular infundibulum to enlarge the outflow tract. The pulmonary valve is inspected and if the commissures are fused, they are opened using sharp dissection. The VSDs are repaired as described above. In 33677, multiple VSDs are closed and a previously placed pulmonary artery band is removed with or without placement of a gusset. Pulmonary artery banding is used as a staged intervention to control pulmonary over circulation and prevent pulmonary artery hypertension and hypertrophy. The pulmonary artery is exposed and a pressure transducer probe used to evaluate the existing pulmonary artery stenosis and pressures. The band is dissected free and removed. The VSDs are repaired as described above. Pulmonary artery pressures are again evaluated and if they are too high, the narrowed area is incised and a patch (gusset) placed to increase the diameter of the pulmonary artery.

33681-33688

33681   Closure of single ventricular septal defect, with or without patch

33684   Closure of single ventricular septal defect, with or without patch; with pulmonary valvotomy or infundibular resection (acyanotic)

33688   Closure of single ventricular septal defect, with or without patch; with removal of pulmonary artery band, with or without gusset

A ventricular septal defect (VSD) is a congenital anomaly in which there are one or more abnormal opening in the septum. An incision is made in the chest to access the heart. The pericardium is incised and a patch harvested as needed. Cardiopulmonary bypass is initiated. In 33681, a single VSD is repaired through an incision in the right atrium, pulmonary artery, or in the outflow tract (infundibulum) of the right ventricle. The defect is repaired with sutures or a patch. If a patch is used, synthetic material or the previously harvested patch of pericardium is sutured over the defect. The access incision is closed and cardiopulmonary bypass discontinued. Chest tubes are placed and the chest incision is closed. In 33684, a single VSD is closed and pulmonary valvotomy or infundibular resection is also performed. This type of repair is performed when the VSD occurs in combination with obstruction of right ventricular outflow, such as that occurring with a mild (acyanotic) Tetralogy of Fallot. An incision is made in the right ventricle or pulmonary artery. The obstructive fibrous or muscle band is excised. Alternatively, tissue is removed from the thickened muscular infundibulum to enlarge the outflow tract. The pulmonary valve is inspected and if the commissures are fused, they are opened using sharp dissection. The VSD is repaired as described above. In 33688, a single VSD is closed and a previously placed pulmonary artery band is removed with or without placement of a gusset. Pulmonary artery banding is used as a staged intervention to control pulmonary over circulation and prevent pulmonary artery hypertension and hypertrophy. The pulmonary artery is exposed and a pressure transducer probe used to evaluate the existing pulmonary artery stenosis and pressures. The band is dissected free and removed. The VSD is repaired as described above. Pulmonary artery pressures are again evaluated and if they are too high, the narrowed area is incised and a patch (gusset) placed to increase the diameter of the pulmonary artery.

33690

33690   Banding of pulmonary artery

Pulmonary artery banding (PAB) is performed is a surgical therapy sometimes used as an initial intervention for congenital cardiac defects with left-to-right shunting and pulmonary overcirculation. PAB reduces excessive pulmonary blood flow and helps prevent hypertrophy of pulmonary vasculature and irreversible pulmonary hypertension. The pulmonary artery is approached through an anterior left thoracotomy in the second or third interspace or a median sternotomy. The pericardium is incised anterior to the left phrenic nerve and the thymus is retracted. The main pulmonary artery and aorta are exposed. The required band circumference is estimated. The band placement site in the mid-portion of the main pulmonary artery is selected and the adventitia between the aorta and main pulmonary artery is dissected at this site. The band is passed through the transverse sinus encircling both the aorta and main pulmonary artery and then is delivered between the two vessels at the dissection site. The band is snared and fixed with hemoclips. A felt or pericardial pledget is placed beneath the snare and the main pulmonary artery. The pledget and band material are then anchored to the main pulmonary artery. The band is tightened. Pulmonary artery pressures, blood pressure, and arterial oxygen saturation are checked to ensure that they are within desired limits. When optimal pressures and oxygen saturation are attained, chest tubes are placed and incisions are closed.

33692-33697

33692   Complete repair tetralogy of Fallot without pulmonary atresia
33694   Complete repair tetralogy of Fallot without pulmonary atresia; with transannular patch
33697   Complete repair tetralogy of Fallot with pulmonary atresia including construction of conduit from right ventricle to pulmonary artery and closure of ventricular septal defect

The physician repairs all heart defects in a neonate with tetralogy of Fallot. Tetralogy of Fallot (TOF) is a congential cardiac anomaly that consists of a combination of four related heart defects which include pulmonary stenosis, right ventricular hypertrophy, ventricular septal defect (VSD), and overriding aorta. Pulmonary stenosis is a narrowing of the pulmonary valve and outflow tract that partially obstructs blood flow from the right ventricle. The pulmonary stenosis causes right ventricular hypertrophy which is a thickening of the muscular walls of the right ventricle resulting from increased pumping pressure required to expel blood from the right ventricle into the pulmonary artery. Ventricular septal defect refers to one or more holes in the ventricular septum. Overriding aorta is a defect in which the aortic valve is enlarged and is shifted slightly to the right lying just above the VSD. In this position, the aorta receives unoxygenated blood from the right ventricle along with oxygenated blood from the left. Some neonates also have pulmonary atresia associated with TOF. Pulmonary atresia is a complete obstruction of blood flow from the right ventricle to the pulmonary artery. The heart is exposed by median sternotomy. Cardiopulmonary bypass is established and cardioplegic arrest initiated. The VSD is repaired with a synthetic patch. Patching the VSD corrects the problem associated with the overriding aorta and prevents mixing of unoxygenated blood in the right ventricle with the oxygenated blood in the left ventricle. The narrowed (stenosed) pulmonary valve is enlarged by resecting obstructive tissue in the right ventricle. In the process of resecting the obstructive tissue a transannular patch may be placed. If a transannular patch is used, a long incision is made traversing the pulmonary artery and valve and a patch is used to enlarge the outflow tract. If pulmonary atresia is present a conduit from the right ventricle to the pulmonary artery is placed. This is accomplished by incising the front surface of the right ventricle taking care to avoid the coronary artery. One end of a synthetic tube is then sutured to the right ventricle. An incision is made at the bifurcation of the pulmonary arteries and the other end of the tube is sutured at the bifurcation to provide a conduit through which blood can flow from the right ventricle to the pulmonary arteries and lungs. Use code 33692 for complete repair of tetralogy of Fallot without pulmonary atresia and without placement of a transannular patch or code 33694 if a transannular patch is required to correct the pulmonary stenosis. Use code 33697 if the neonate has tetraology of Fallot with pulmonary atresia and the repair includes construction of conduit from the right ventricle to the pulmonary artery and closure of the VSD.

33702-33710

33702   Repair sinus of Valsalva fistula, with cardiopulmonary bypass
33710   Repair sinus of Valsalva fistula, with cardiopulmonary bypass; with repair of ventricular septal defect

The physician performs repair of a sinus of Valsalva fistula with cardiopulmonary bypass. The three sinuses of Valsalva are contained in the pericardium and located in the proximal-most portion of the aorta. They correspond to the three cusps of the aortic valve. A sinus of Valsalva fistula is most often due to a congenital anomaly. However, these fistulas may also be a result of penetrating or non-penetrating chest trauma, a complication of a surgical intervention, or a complication of endocarditis. Cardiopulmonary bypass is accomplished using bicaval or other venous and arterial cannulation and cardioplegia initiated. The ascending aorta is clamped, the aorta is opened and the defect in the sinus of Valsalva identified. The aortic valve cusps and coronary ostia are inspected. The sinus of Valsalva

fistula is repaired using sutures or a pericardial or synthetic patch. The ascending aorta is closed. In 33710, a ventricular septal defect (VSD) is also repaired. The VSD may be closed through the aorta or a through a separate incision of the right atrium, right ventricle, or left ventricle. The ventricular defect is repaired by suture closure or with a pericardial or synthetic patch.

33720

33720   Repair sinus of Valsalva aneurysm, with cardiopulmonary bypass

A sinus of Valsalva aneurysm is repaired with cardiopulmonary bypass. The three sinuses of Valsalva, also referred to as the aortic sinuses, are contained in the pericardium in the most proximal portion of the aorta just above the cusps of the aortic valve. An aneurysm of one or more of the sinuses of Valsalva can be either a congenital or acquired defect. Congenital aneurysms usually occur in only a single sinus and are a rare cardiac defect. Acquired defects may occur due to Marfan syndrome, syphilitic aortitis, cystic medial necrosis, atherosclerosis, aging, or chest trauma. The heart is exposed by median sternotomy. Venous and arterial cannulas are inserted and cardiopulmonary bypass is established. The aorta is cross-clamped and cardioplegic arrest is initiated. The aorta is transected and the aneurysm is exposed and explored. Any thrombus contained within the aneurysm is removed. The aneurysm is closed with sutures that may be reinforced with buttresses. Alternatively, a tissue or synthetic patch graft may be used to repair the aneurysmal defect. The aorta is reunited by direct anastomosis or an interposition graft is placed. The patient is then weaned off cardiopulmonary bypass; chest tubes are placed as needed; and the chest incision is closed.

33722

33722   Closure of aortico-left ventricular tunnel

The physician repairs a congenital aortico-left ventricular tunnel (ALVT), a rare cardiac anomaly in which the aortic valve is bypassed by a paravalvular connection (tunnel) between the left ventricle and aorta. The tunnel typically arises from the right aortic sinus but may also arise from the left aortic sinus. The heart is accessed by median sternotomy or thoracotomy. Cardiopulmonary bypass is established. The aorta is cross-clamped and cardioplegic arrest is initiated. A horizontal incision is made in the aorta. The aortic wall is inspected and the exact location of the tunnel is determined. The tunnel orifice (opening) at the aorta is closed with sutures or a patch graft and the tunnel is obliterated. The incision in the aorta is closed; aortic clamps are removed; and the patient is weaned off pulmonary bypass. Chest tubes are placed as needed and the chest incision is closed.

33724

33724   Repair of isolated partial anomalous pulmonary venous return (eg, Scimitar Syndrome)

The surgeon performs repair of isolated partial anomalous pulmonary venous return, a rare congenital heart defect in which some of the pulmonary veins (not all four) return abnormally to the right side of the heart, most commonly right pulmonary veins to the superior vena cava, right atrium, or inferior vena cava, sometimes associated with atrial septal defect. Pulmonary venous blood flow returns to the systemic venous (right) side of the circulatory system before circulating the oxygenated blood through the body. This may not be apparent until middle age. Usually, a midline sternotomy is made to open the chest and access the heart. Cardiopulmonary bypass is initiated and the heart is retracted to the right. The abnormally draining pulmonary veins are visualized and dissected from their anomalous insertion with appropriate repair of the site. The veins are redirected so as to drain into the left atrium and sutured into position. Any atrial septal defect is also closed with a patch sutured over the hole.

33726

33726   Repair of pulmonary venous stenosis

Pulmonary venous stenosis is repaired using living autologous atrial tissue, or the sutureless neoatrium technique described here. Pulmonary venous blood flow is restricted in its return to the heart, which may be initial congenital presentation or following anomalous pulmonary vein connection repair. After initiation of cardiopulmonary bypass and sternotomy to access the heart, the pulmonary veins are visualized by incision through the atrium. For patients who have already undergone repair, access is through the right atrium across the septum to see the extent and location of stenosis, which may be localized to the previous anastomic area. For initial repair, the approach is through the left atrium to the edge of the septum. The common pulmonary vein (confluence) is then incised across its length and the incision is carried into each pulmonary vein by cutting distally into the lung as far as necessary to get beyond the stenotic area. The adventitia is left intact. The divided edge of the left atrial wall is then sutured to the adventitia of the pericardium remote from the divided edge of the pulmonary veins using a running absorbable suture in a circle around the pulmonary veins, staying away from the actual edge of the pulmonary veins. This controls pulmonary venous bleed into the left atrium without any direct suturing of the veins. This may be performed unilaterally for isolated left or right stenosis. After the divided edge of the left atrial wall is sutured to the pericardium

● New Code   ▲ Revised Code

Cardiovascular System

over the incised pulmonary veins, the suture line is routed inward in the direction of the common vein or confluence for hemostasis in the anastomosis.

33730

33730   Complete repair of anomalous pulmonary venous return (supracardiac, intracardiac, or infracardiac types)

The physician performs a complete repair of total anomalous pulmonary venous return (TAPVR), a rare congenital defect in which all four pulmonary veins drain into the right atrium via an abnormal connection instead of into the left atrium as they should do normally. TAPVR is classified based on the location of the abnormal pulmonary vein connection. In supracardiac TAPVR, the pulmonary veins join behind the heart and form an abnormal vertical vein that joins the innominate vein. The innominate vein connects to the superior vena cava and drains into the right atrium. In intracardiac TAPVR, the pulmonary veins join behind the heart and drain directly into the right atrium or through the coronary sinus. The coronary sinus is the vein that returns blood from the heart back to the right atrium. In infracardiac TAPVR, the pulmonary veins join behind the heart and connect with the hepatic veins. The hepatic veins (portal vein system) drain through the vascular liver bed, empty into the inferior vena cava, and then drain into the right atrium. In addition to the anomalous pulmonary venous return, all patients with TAPVR have an atrial septal defect (ASD). The heart is accessed by midline sternotomy or left anterolateral thoracotomy. Cardiopulmonary bypass is established and cardioplegic arrest is initiated. If there is a supracardiac or infracardiac connection and the pulmonary veins are joined in a common confluence, the abnormal connection is severed and the common pulmonary vein confluence is connected to the left atrium. If there is an intracardiac connection to the right atrium or coronary sinus, the atrial septum is partially resected and a new septum is created using a patch graft that directs the flow of blood from the pulmonary veins to the left atrium. Alternatively, if drainage is to a coronary sinus, a tunnel may be created to drain the pulmonary veins to the left atrium. Abnormal vessels that carried pulmonary venous blood to supracardiac, intracardiac, or infracardiac locations are ligated (tied off). The atrial septal defect is then repaired in a separately reportable procedure.

33732

33732   Repair of cor triatriatum or supravalvular mitral ring by resection of left atrial membrane

The physician repairs cor triatriatum or supravalvular mitral ring by resecting the left atrial membrane. Cor triatriatum, also referred to as cor triatriatum sinister, is a congenital heart defect in which the left atrium is divided into an upper and lower chamber by a membrane of tissue, with the pulmonary veins draining into the proximal chamber. Supravalvular mitral ring is a congenital heart defect characterized by an abnormal ridge of tissue on the atrial side of the mitral valve. Both defects restrict the flow of blood from the left atrium to the left ventricle. The heat is accessed by a median sternotomy or thoracotomy. Cardiopulmonary bypass is established and cardioplegic arrest is initiated. An incision is made in the left atrium. In cor triatriatum, the accessory tissue membrane (diaphragm) in the left atrium is excised. In supravalvular mitral ring, the ring is carefully dissected free of any adherent mitral valve leaflets and excised. If repair or replacement of the mitral valve is necessary, this is also performed in a separately reportable procedure. The patient is weaned of cardiopulmonary bypass; chest tubes placed as needed; and the chest incision is closed.

33735-33737

33735   Atrial septectomy or septostomy; closed heart (Blalock-Hanlon type operation)
33736   Atrial septectomy or septostomy; open heart with cardiopulmonary bypass
33737   Atrial septectomy or septostomy; open heart, with inflow occlusion

The physician performs an atrial septectomy or septostomy using a closed heart technique (33735), an open heart technique with cardiopulmonary bypass (33736), or an open heart technique with inflow occlusion (33737). Closed heart atrial septectomy or septostomy may also be referred to as a Blalock-Hanlon atrial septectomy. Atrial septectomy or septostomy is a palliative procedure performed to improve oxygen saturation in patients with complete transposition of the great vessels. The heart is exposed by a right lateral thoracotomy. In 33735, clamps are placed on a small portion of the right and left atria to occlude blood flow. Two parallel incisions, one in the right atrium and one in the left, are made between the clamps close to the septum. The intra-atrial septum is grasped, pulled up and the posterior aspect excised. The clamp is repositioned so that the septum falls back into the atrial cavity. Atrial incisions are closed. In 33736, cardiopulmonary bypass is used. The aorta is cannulated followed by the superior and inferior vena cava and cardiopulmonary bypass established. In 33737, inflow occlusion may be used to temporarily interrupt venous blood flow to the heart. Inflow occlusion involves occluding the superior and inferior vena cava with snares and allowing the heart to empty of blood. Cardiopulmonary bypass or inflow occlusion is typically used in patients with a thick atrial septum. The heart is accessed by median sternotomy. Following initiation of cardiopulmonary bypass or inflow occlusion, the atria are incised and the entire atrial septum within the fossa ovalis is excised taking care to avoid injury to the atrioventricular node. Atrial incisions are closed, chest tubes placed, and the chest incision closed.

33750

33750   Shunt; subclavian to pulmonary artery (Blalock-Taussig type operation)

The physician creates a shunt connecting the subclavian artery to the pulmonary artery, also referred to as a Blalock-Taussig operation. This type of shunt is a closed heart procedure typically performed as a temporary measure to alleviate symptoms of cyanosis associated with cardiac anomalies such as Tetralogy of Fallot. The heart and blood vessels are exposed by a posterolateral incision at the fourth intercostal space. The apex of the lung is retracted. The mediastinal pleura over the subclavian artery is incised. If a direct anastomosis is performed, the subclavian artery is divided and connected to the right or left pulmonary artery in an end-to-side fashion. If a synthetic graft is used, the subclavian artery is mobilized followed by mobilization of the pulmonary artery. The subclavian artery is clamped and a synthetic graft is anastomosed to the subclavian artery just distal to its origin. The pulmonary artery is then clamped and the synthetic graft is anastomosed to the pulmonary artery in an end-to-side fashion just proximal to the lobar branches. The clamps are released and blood flow through the shunt is confirmed.

33755-33762

33755   Shunt; ascending aorta to pulmonary artery (Waterston type operation)
33762   Shunt; descending aorta to pulmonary artery (Potts-Smith type operation)

The physician creates a shunt connecting the ascending aorta to the pulmonary artery (33755), also referred to as a Waterston operation, or the descending aorta to the pulmonary artery (33762), also referred to as a Potts or Potts-Smith operation. These two types of shunts have largely been abandoned due to complications associated with the procedures. They used to be performed as a temporary measure to alleviate symptoms of cyanosis associated with cardiac anomalies such as tetralogy of Fallot. The heart and blood vessels are exposed by median sternotomy or thoracotomy. In 33755, the ascending aorta and right pulmonary artery are incised and connected to each other in a side-to-side fashion. In 33762, the descending aorta and left pulmonary artery are incised and connected to each other in a side-to-side fashion.

33764

33764   Shunt; central, with prosthetic graft

The physician creates a central shunt between the ascending aorta and the main pulmonary artery using a prosthetic graft. This type of shunt is a closed heart procedure typically performed as a temporary measure to alleviate symptoms of cyanosis associated with cardiac anomalies such as tetralogy of Fallot. The heart and blood vessels are exposed by median sternotomy. The thymus is resected. The pericardium is incised vertically and suspended. The ascending aorta and main pulmonary artery are prepared for anastomosis. If cardiopulmonary bypass is required, cannulas are placed and it is initiated. If the procedure is performed without cardiopulmonary bypass, vascular clamps are applied. A short synthetic tube graft with beveled ends is inserted into the ascending aorta and the proximal aspect of the main pulmonary artery and sutured to these vessels. The clamps are released. If cardiopulmonary bypass has been used, the patient is weaned off bypass. The pericardium is reapproximated; chest tubes placed as needed; and the chest incision is closed.

33766-33768

33766   Shunt; superior vena cava to pulmonary artery for flow to 1 lung (classical Glenn procedure)
33767   Shunt; superior vena cava to pulmonary artery for flow to both lungs (bidirectional Glenn procedure)
33768   Anastomosis, cavopulmonary, second superior vena cava (List separately in addition to primary procedure)

The physician creates a superior vena cava to pulmonary artery shunt for flow to one lung (33766), also referred to as classical or unidirectional Glenn procedure, or for flow to both lungs (33767), also referred to as bidirectional Glenn procedure. This type of shunt is a closed heart procedure that is typically performed as a temporary measure to alleviate symptoms of cyanosis associated with cardiac anomalies such as tetralogy of Fallot. The heart and blood vessels are exposed by median sternotomy. Cardiopulmonary bypass is established. In 33766, the right pulmonary artery is transected and connected to the superior vena cava using an end-to-side anastomosis. In 33767, the superior vena cava is connected to the right pulmonary artery which remains connected to the main pulmonary artery allowing blood from the superior vena cava to enter both pulmonary arteries. The azygos and hemiazygos veins are ligated. The superior vena cava is clamped and transected between the clamps. The cardiac end is sutured in two layers. The right pulmonary artery is incised longitudinally and the superior vena cava anastomosed in an end-to-side fashion to the right pulmonary artery. The clamps are released. The patient is weaned off cardiopulmonary bypass, chest tubes are placed as needed, and the chest incision closed. In 33768, a second superior vena cava is anastomosed to the adjacent pulmonary artery at the time of a separately reportable bidirectional Glenn procedure, outflow tract augmentation, or Fontan procedure. This procedure is performed on patients with bilateral superior vena cava. The second vena cava is prepared for insertion of the bypass cannula. The azygous and hemiazygous veins are ligated. The bypass cannula is inserted into the

● New Code   ▲ Revised Code

second superior vena cava which is then clamped and divided between the clamps. The cardiac end is oversewn. An incision is made in the adjacent pulmonary artery. The second superior vena cava is anastomosed to the pulmonary artery in an end-to-side fashion.

33770-33771

33770 Repair of transposition of the great arteries with ventricular septal defect and subpulmonary stenosis; without surgical enlargement of ventricular septal defect

33771 Repair of transposition of the great arteries with ventricular septal defect and subpulmonary stenosis; with surgical enlargement of ventricular septal defect

The physician repairs transposition of the great arteries with ventricular septal defect and subpulmonary stenosis without surgical enlargement of the ventricular septal defect (VSD) in 33770 or with enlargement of the VSD in 33771. Transposition of the great arteries is a congenital anomaly in which the aorta arises from the right ventricle instead of the left as it does in a normal heart and the pulmonary arteries arise from the left instead of the right. This means that the oxygen poor blood returning from the systemic circulation is returned to the body without circulating through the lungs while the oxygen rich blood instead of circulating through the body returns to the lungs. Transposition is often associated with other cardiac anomalies including VSD and subpulmonary stenosis. VSD is an abnormal opening in the ventricular septum that allows oxygen rich and oxygen poor blood to mix. Subpulmonary stenosis is a narrowing in the main pulmonary artery immediately below the pulmonary valve. Transposition of the great arteries complicated by subpulmonary stenosis requires an individualized operative plan and the procedure may vary significantly from one individual to another. The heart is accessed by median sternotomy or thoracotomy. The thymus is resected. The pericardium is incised and a section harvested for later use as a patch graft. The aorta and superior and inferior vena cava are cannulated. Cardiopulmonary bypass is established and the aorta is cross clamped. The right atrium is incised. The VSD is approached through the infundibulum. A baffle is constructed to divert blood flow through the VSD to the aorta using synthetic material, autologous pericardium, an allograft, or a xenograft (bovine pericardium or dura). If the VSD is not large enough to allow construction of the baffle, it is enlarged. The atrial septum is then resected. A patch of synthetic material, autologous pericardium, or a xenograft is used to redirect the systemic venous blood from the superior and inferior vena cava to the orifice of the mitral valve. The pulmonary venous blood is excluded and flows around the baffle to the tricuspid valve. Alternatively, flaps of native atrial septum and atrial wall may be used to construct the intra-atrial baffles. The atrial wall is then patched using the previously harvested section of pericardium. The subpulmonic stenosis may be addressed by removing any obstructive tissue and/or enlarging the main pulmonary artery using a patch graft. Following completion of the repair, the sternum may be closed or left open and closed in a subsequent procedure. Chest tubes are placed as needed.

33774-33777

33774 Repair of transposition of the great arteries, atrial baffle procedure (eg, Mustard or Senning type) with cardiopulmonary bypass

33775 Repair of transposition of the great arteries, atrial baffle procedure (eg, Mustard or Senning type) with cardiopulmonary bypass; with removal of pulmonary band

33776 Repair of transposition of the great arteries, atrial baffle procedure (eg, Mustard or Senning type) with cardiopulmonary bypass; with closure of ventricular septal defect

33777 Repair of transposition of the great arteries, atrial baffle procedure (eg, Mustard or Senning type) with cardiopulmonary bypass; with repair of subpulmonic obstruction

The physician repairs transposition of the great arteries using an atrial baffle technique also referred to as a Mustard or Senning procedure. Transposition of the great arteries is a congenital anomaly in which the aorta arises from the right ventricle instead of the left as it does in a normal heart and the pulmonary arteries arise from the left instead of the right. This means that the oxygen poor blood returning from the systemic circulation is returned to the body without circulating through the lungs while the oxygen rich blood instead of circulating through the body returns to the lungs. Transposition is often associated with other cardiac anomalies including ventricular septal defect (VSD) and subpulmonary stenosis. VSD is an abnormal opening in the ventricular septum that allows oxygen rich and oxygen poor blood to mix. Subpulmonary stenosis is a narrowing of the main pulmonary artery immediately below the pulmonary valve. Transposition of the great arteries complicated by subpulmonary stenosis requires an individualized operative plan and the procedure may vary significantly from one individual to another. The heart is accessed by median sternotomy or thoracotomy. The thymus is resected. The pericardium is incised and a large section harvested for later use as a patch graft. The aorta and superior and inferior vena cava are cannulated. Cardiopulmonary bypass is established and the aorta is cross clamped. The right atrium is incised. The atrial septum is resected. A patch of synthetic material, autologous pericardium, or an allograft is used to redirect the systemic venous blood from the superior and inferior vena cava to the orifice of the mitral valve (Mustard type procedure). The pulmonary venous blood is excluded and flows around the baffle to the tricuspid valve. Alternatively, flaps of native atrial septum and atrial wall may

be used to construct the intra-atrial baffles (Senning type procedure). The atrial wall is then patched using the previously harvested section of pericardium. Use code 33774 when only an atrial baffle procedure is performed. Use code 33775 when atrial baffle procedure is performed with removal of a previously placed pulmonary band. The band is dissected free and removed. Pulmonary artery stenosis is assessed using a transducer and probe. The pulmonary artery is dilated as needed. Use code 33776 when atrial baffle procedure is performed with closure of the VSD. The VSD is approached through the right atrium and an incision made in the infundibulum. The VSD is repaired using a synthetic, pericardial, or xenograft patch. Use code 33777 when the baffle procedure is performed with repair of subpulmonic obstruction. The obstructive tissue below the pulmonary valve is removed. Following completion of the repair, the sternum may be closed or left open and closed in a subsequent procedure. Chest tubes are placed as needed.

33778-33781

33778 Repair of transposition of the great arteries, aortic pulmonary artery reconstruction (eg, Jatene type)

33779 Repair of transposition of the great arteries, aortic pulmonary artery reconstruction (eg, Jatene type); with removal of pulmonary band

33780 Repair of transposition of the great arteries, aortic pulmonary artery reconstruction (eg, Jatene type); with closure of ventricular septal defect

33781 Repair of transposition of the great arteries, aortic pulmonary artery reconstruction (eg, Jatene type); with repair of subpulmonic obstruction

The physician repairs transposition of the great arteries using aortic and pulmonary artery reconstruction, also referred to as a Jatene procedure. Transposition of the great arteries is a congenital anomaly in which the aorta arises from the right ventricle instead of the left as it does in a normal heart and the pulmonary arteries arise from the left instead of the right. This means that the oxygen poor blood returning from the systemic circulation is returned to the body without circulating through the lungs while the oxygen rich blood instead of circulating through the body returns to the lungs. Transposition is often associated with other cardiac anomalies including VSD and subpulmonary stenosis. VSD is an abnormal opening in the ventricular septum that allows oxygen rich and oxygen poor blood to mix. Subpulmonary stenosis is a narrowing of the main pulmonary artery immediately below the pulmonary valve. The heart is accessed by median sternotomy or thoracotomy. The thymus is resected. The pericardium is incised and a section harvested for later use as a patch graft. The ascending aorta and main pulmonary artery and pulmonary branches are dissected free of surrounding tissue. The aorta and superior and inferior vena cava are cannulated. Cardiopulmonary bypass is established and the aorta is cross clamped. The ascending aorta and main pulmonary artery are transected. The ostia (openings) of left and right coronary arteries at the anomalous aortic root in the right ventricle are visualized and excised with the adjacent aortic wall. The coronary artery ostia are transferred as buttons to the anomalous main pulmonary artery root sinuses in the left ventricle. The distal main pulmonary artery and its branches are then brought forward to the right ventricle and the aorta is moved posteriorly to the left ventricle. The distal aorta is anastomosed to the newly created aortic root in the left ventricle. The coronary arteries are also anastomosed to the newly created aortic outflow tract. Use code 33778 when only an aortic and pulmonary artery reconstruction procedure is performed. Use code 33779 when the procedure is performed with removal of a previously placed pulmonary band. The band is dissected free and removed. Pulmonary artery stenosis is assessed using a transducer and probe. The pulmonary artery is dilated as needed. Use code 33780 when the procedure is performed with closure of the VSD. The VSD is approached through the right atrium and an incision made in the infundibulum. The VSD is repaired using a synthetic, pericardial, or xenograft patch. Use code 33781 when the baffle procedure is performed with repair of subpulmonic obstruction. The obstructive tissue below the pulmonary valve is removed. Following completion of the repair, the sternum may be closed or left open and closed in a subsequent procedure. Chest tubes are placed as needed.

33782-33783

33782 Aortic root translocation with ventricular septal defect and pulmonary stenosis repair (ie, Nikaidoh procedure); without coronary ostium reimplantation

33783 Aortic root translocation with ventricular septal defect and pulmonary stenosis repair (ie, Nikaidoh procedure); with reimplantation of 1 or both coronary ostia

The Nikaidoh procedure is performed to treat a complex cardiac anomaly that includes transposition of the great arteries (TGA), ventricular septal defect (VSD), and pulmonary stenosis (PS). A median sternotomy is performed to access the heart and great vessels. A patch graft is harvested from the pericardium. Cardiopulmonary bypass is accomplished using bicaval cannulation. Cardioplegia is initiated. The proximal coronary arteries are mobilized, the right ventricle is incised and the aortic root is separated from the right ventricle. The pulmonary artery is transected and the infundibular septum divided. The posterior aspect of the aortic root is sutured to the pulmonary valve annulus and the anterior aspect is sutured over the VSD. The ascending aorta is transected, a small section removed, and the ascending aorta reconfigured to prevent bowing. A Lecompte maneuver is performed to position the ascending aorta behind the pulmonary artery. The

Cardiovascular System

transected ends of the ascending aorta are then sutured together. The anterior aspect of the hypoplastic main pulmonary artery is incised longitudinally. The posterior aspect of the main pulmonary artery is sutured to the right ventricular outflow tract. A pericardial patch graft is used to reconstruct the right ventricular outflow tract and enlarge the hypoplastic main pulmonary artery. Use 33782 when the procedure is performed without coronary ostium reimplantation. Use 33783 when one or both coronary ostia are individually reimplanted during the translocation. Reimplantation of coronary ostia is performed when the coronary arteries are malpositioned on the aorta compromising blood flow to the heart muscle.

33786

33786   Total repair, truncus arteriosus (Rastelli type operation)

Truncus arteriosus is a congenital cardiac anomaly characterized by a large ventricular septal defect (VSD) with a single heart valve and great vessel (truncus) that override the VSD. This single vessel carries blood to the body (systemic circulation), heart (cardiac circulation), and the lungs (pulmonary circulation). The heart is accessed by median sternotomy or thoracotomy. The thymus is resected. The pericardium is incised and a section is harvested for later use as a patch graft. The single great vessel and its branches are dissected free of surrounding tissue. The aorta and superior and inferior vena cava are cannulated. Cardiopulmonary bypass is established and the aorta is cross-clamped. The right ventricle is incised and the VSD is visualized. Obstructive right ventricular muscle is excised. The orifice of the pulmonary arteries is closed from inside without detachment of the pulmonary artery. An intra-ventricular baffle constructed from the previously harvested pericardium or from synthetic material is sutured into place to close the VSD and redirect blood flow to the aortic valve. Right ventricular to pulmonary artery continuity is achieved using an extra-cardiac, valved homograft conduit or a synthetic, nonvalved tube graft. When using a valved homograft conduit, a tube graft extension may be required to span the distance between the ventriculotomy and the anastomosis site on the main pulmonary artery. The valved conduit and/or tube graft is sutured to the right ventricle to the left of the aorta, taking care to avoid papillary muscles. The valved conduit is then sutured to the main pulmonary artery. The sternum may be closed or left open and closed in a subsequent procedure. Chest tubes are placed as needed.

33788

33788   Reimplantation of an anomalous pulmonary artery

An anomalous pulmonary artery arising from the aorta is reimplanted in the main pulmonary artery. The heart is accessed by median sternotomy or thoracotomy. The thymus is resected and the pericardium is incised. The ascending aorta, anomalous pulmonary artery, and main pulmonary artery are dissected free of surrounding tissue. The anomalous pulmonary artery is ligated and divided. The main pulmonary artery is incised and the anomalous pulmonary artery is anastomosed to the main pulmonary artery. An interposition graft may be placed if the anomalous pulmonary artery cannot be directly anastomosed to the main pulmonary artery. Chest incisions are closed and chest tubes are placed as needed.

33800

33800   Aortic suspension (aortopexy) for tracheal decompression (eg, for tracheomalacia) (separate procedure)

An aortopexy (aortic suspension) is performed for tracheal decompression. This procedure may be performed to treat tracheomalacia, a weakness of the supporting tracheal cartilage with widening of the posterior membranous wall. This can cause tracheal collapse and respiratory difficulties. The aorta is approached via a left anterior thoracotomy. The thymus is resected and the apex of the left upper lobe is retracted inferiorly and posteriorly. The vascular ring is located and the esophagus is examined. Dissection of the aorta from surrounding tissue is avoided. A single row of sutures is placed through the aorta at the aortic arch. The sutures are placed deep enough in the aorta to include the media and adventitia. These sutures are then passed to the undersurface of the sternum and the aorta is anchored to the sternum. Alternatively, the sutures may be passed through the sternum to a subcutaneous pocket and tied. This displaces the arch anteriorly and pulls the anterior wall of the trachea forward preventing collapse.

33802-33803

33802   Division of aberrant vessel (vascular ring)
33803   Division of aberrant vessel (vascular ring); with reanastomosis

The physician repairs a vascular ring by dividing the aberrant vessel. The term vascular ring refers to a collection of vascular compression anomalies characterized by one or more aberrant blood vessels that encircle and compress the trachea and esophagus. The two most common variations are a double aortic arch and a right aortic arch with an anomalous left subclavian artery. The aorta arch normally consists of a single branch that curves to the left after leaving the heart. In a double aortic arch, the arch consists of two branches that surround the esophagus and trachea. These two branches then merge into a single vessel, the descending aorta, to deliver blood to the torso and lower extremies. The right aortic arch configuration causes the left subclavian artery to wrap around the

trachea as it passes from the aorta to the left arm. With a right aortic arch, there may also be a Kommerell's diverticulum which is an aneurysm of the left subclavian artery wall. The ligamentum arteriosum which connects the pulmonary artery to the anomalous left subclavian artery causes constriction of the trachea. To divide a double aortic arch, a left thoracotomy is performed followed by incision of the pleura overlying the vascular ring. Soft tissues are carefully dissected and the vascular structures evaluated. The smaller of the two arches is clamped and blood flow evaluated by checking the right and left radial and carotid pulses. Strong pulses indicate that there is good blood flow through the larger arch. A second vascular clamp is then placed on the smaller arch which is divided between the two clamps. The divided stumps are oversewn with sutures. Adhesive bands surrounding the esophagus are transected. The thoracotomy is closed and air evacuated from the pleural space using a small suction catheter. To treat compression syndrome resulting from a right aortic arch, a left thoracotomy is performed through the fourth intercostal space. Two vascular clamps are placed on the ligamentum arteriosum, which is divided between the descending aorta and pulmonary artery. The stumps are oversewn. Adhesive bands surrounding the esophagus are divided. In 33803, the aberrant vessel is divided and reanastomosed. To treat a right aortic arch, the aorta is clamped and divided as described above. The retroesophageal portion of the aorta is then mobilized. A graft may used to lengthen the aorta, and the ascending and descending portions are then reanastomosed.

33813-33814

33813   Obliteration of aortopulmonary septal defect; without cardiopulmonary bypass
33814   Obliteration of aortopulmonary septal defect; with cardiopulmonary bypass

An aortopulmonary septal defect is a rare congenital cardiac defect in which the septum dividing the aorta and pulmonary artery fails to close as it should during early embryonic development. The heart is accessed by median sternotomy or thoracotomy. The thymus is resected. The pericardium is incised and a section harvested for later use as a patch graft. The aorta and main pulmonary artery are dissected free of surrounding tissue. If cardiopulmonary bypass is used, the aorta and superior and inferior vena cava are cannulated. Cardiopulmonary bypass is then established and the aorta is cross-clamped. The aorta and pulmonary artery are divided and the defect repaired with suture or a pericardial patch graft. Larger defects may require repair with an allograft (homograft), xenograft, or synthetic material. When the repair is complete, chest incisions are closed and chest tubes placed as needed. Use code 33813 if the APSD is repaired without cardiopulmonary bypass and code 33814 if cardiopulmonary bypass is used.

33820-33824

33820   Repair of patent ductus arteriosus; by ligation
33822   Repair of patent ductus arteriosus; by division, younger than 18 years
33824   Repair of patent ductus arteriosus; by division, 18 years and older

The physician repairs patent ductus arteriosus (PDA). Before birth the descending aorta and left pulmonary artery are connected by a blood vessel called the ductus arteriosus. The ductus is essential to fetal circulation. After birth, the ductus normally closes within a few days. In PDA, the duct fails to close after birth which can damage the heart and lungs. The ductus arteriosus is exposed by a posterolateral thoracotomy. In 33820, the ductus is suture ligated (tied) or closed with clips. Alternatively, the ductus may be suture ligated and then divided (cut). If the ductus is divided, use code 33822 for a patient younger than 18 years and 33824 for a patient 18 years or older.

33840-33851

33840   Excision of coarctation of aorta, with or without associated patent ductus arteriosus; with direct anastomosis
33845   Excision of coarctation of aorta, with or without associated patent ductus arteriosus; with graft
33851   Excision of coarctation of aorta, with or without associated patent ductus arteriosus; repair using either left subclavian artery or prosthetic material as gusset for enlargement

Coarctation of the aorta is a narrowing of the aorta between the arterial branches that deliver blood to the upper body and those that deliver blood to the lower body. This defect causes an increased flow of blood to the upper body and reduced flow to the lower body. The narrowed section of the aorta is accessed by posterolateral thoracotomy. The parietal pleura is incised. The transverse aortic arch, left subclavian artery, ligamentum or ductus arteriosus, descending aorta, and intercostal collateral vessels are exposed by careful dissection of surrounding tissue. Proximal and distal control of the aorta is accomplished with vascular clamps. The subclavian artery is also clamped and the intercostal collaterals controlled using vessel loops. If present, the patent ductus arteriosus is controlled with transfixing sutures and a stay suture is placed in the aortic isthmus. The ductus is then ligated. In 33840, the narrowed segment of the aorta is resected (removed) and the proximal and distal aortic segments connected by direct end-to-end anastomosis. In 33845, the aorta is resected and a synthetic tube graft inserted between the upper and lower aortic segments. In 33851, the aorta is resected and either a patch aortoplasty or left subclavian flap aortoplasty (angioplasty) is performed. Patch aortoplasty is accomplished by making a longitudinal incision extending beyond the narrowed section of the aorta. A synthetic patch is trimmed in an elliptical fashion and sutured in place with the widest portion positioned at the coarctation site. The patch typically extends from the subclavian orifice to the intercostal collateral arteries. The parietal pleura is closed over the patch. Left subclavian flap aortoplasty is accomplished by ligating and dividing the distal subclavian artery at the first branch. The flap is created using the proximal subclavian artery. A longitudinal incision is made over the narrowed segment of the aorta and along the proximal subclavian artery to create a flap. The posterior wall of the narrowed segment of the aorta is resected and the subclavian artery flap transposed to cover and enlarge the narrowed segment of the aorta. The parietal pleura is closed, chest incisions are closed, and chest tubes placed as needed.

33852-33853

33852 Repair of hypoplastic or interrupted aortic arch using autogenous or prosthetic material; without cardiopulmonary bypass

33853 Repair of hypoplastic or interrupted aortic arch using autogenous or prosthetic material; with cardiopulmonary bypass

The physician repairs a hypoplastic or interrupted aortic arch using autogenous or prosthetic material. Hypoplastic aortic arch, also referred to as diffuse long-segment coarctation, is a narrowing of the aorta along the entire arch. Interrupted aortic arch is the complete absence of a segment of the aortic arch. Hypoplastic or interrupted aortic arch may occur in conjunction with other cardiac anomalies including ventricular septal defect (VSD), patent ductus arteriosus (PDA), aortopulmonary window, and truncus arteriosus. A posterolateral incision is made to access the aortic arch. The parietal pleura is incised. The ascending aorta, aortic arch and its branches, ductus arteriosus, and descending aorta are mobilized. Care is taken to protect the recurrent laryngeal and phrenic nerves. Lymphatic vessels are controlled with hemoclips. The ductus arteriosus is ligated. If the procedure is performed without cardiopulmonary bypass a partial occluding clamp is applied across the aortic arch. If cardiopulmonary bypass is used, the aorta and superior and inferior vena cava are cannulated, cardiopulmonary bypass is established, and the aorta is cross clamped. The hypoplastic or interrupted arch segment is then repaired using a patch graft or tubular graft. Patch aortoplasty is accomplished by making a longitudinal incision extending beyond the narrowed section of the aorta. A synthetic patch is trimmed in an elliptical fashion and sutured in place with the widest portion positioned at the narrowest segment of the hypoplastic arch. The parietal pleura is closed over the patch. Alternatively, a tube graft may be used to replace a missing segment of the aortic arch. A third technique is placement an autogenous graft, such as left subclavian artery flap graft. Following repair of the arch, the parietal pleura is closed over the graft, the chest incisions are closed, and chest tubes placed as needed.

33860-33863

33860 Ascending aorta graft, with cardiopulmonary bypass, includes valve suspension, when performed

33863 Ascending aorta graft, with cardiopulmonary bypass, with aortic root replacement using valved conduit and coronary reconstruction (eg, Bentall)

A thoracic aortic aneurysm in the ascending aorta is repaired using a graft with cardiopulmonary bypass. A median sternotomy is performed to expose the heart and ascending aorta. Cardiopulmonary bypass is initiated and the ascending aorta is cross-clamped. Following cardioplegic arrest, the ascending aorta is transected above the cross-clamp. In 33860, the ascending aorta graft is sized and modeled to correspond to the right cusp so that the graft will sit upright in the chest. Sub-annular stitches are passed through the graft and tied to secure the graft to the aortic annulus. A Hagar's dilator is used to size the aortic annulus. The aortic valve is evaluated. If valve suspension is needed, the three commissures are suspended. Careful attention to both the height of each suspension and the distance between each suspension is required to avoid distortion of the aortic valve leaflet positioning. The valve is tested to confirm that it is functioning properly. The distal portion of the graft is sewn to the remaining normal ascending aorta. Air is evacuated from the heart; the clamp is removed; and the heart is reperfused. Temporary pacing wires are placed and pacing is begun if needed. Cardiopulmonary bypass is terminated. All cannulas are removed; drains are placed; and the chest is closed. In 33863, the graft repair of the ascending aorta includes replacement of the aortic root using a composite prosthesis as well as coronary artery reconstruction. The aortic root is the portion of the aorta that is connected to the heart. The root contains the aortic annulus, the leaflets of the aortic valve, and the coronary artery ostia (openings). Following transection of the aorta performed as described above, the physician inspects the aortic valve and coronary ostia. Scissor dissection is used to detach the coronary ostia from the aorta along with a rim of aortic tissue. The aortic valve leaflets are excised. The aortic annulus is sized and an appropriately sized composite, valved prosthesis is selected. The proximal (valved) end of the composite prosthesis is inserted into the annulus and secured with sutures. The coronary ostia with the rim of aortic tissue are implanted into the prosthesis. The distal end of the prosthesis is then anastomosed to the distal aorta. The procedure is completed as described above.

33864

33864 Ascending aorta graft, with cardiopulmonary bypass with valve suspension, with coronary reconstruction and valve-sparing aortic root remodeling (eg, David Procedure, Yacoub Procedure)

A thoracic aortic aneurysm in the ascending aorta with involvement of the aortic root is repaired with cardiopulmonary bypass using an ascending aorta graft with aortic valve suspension, coronary artery reconstruction, and valve-sparing aortic annulus remodeling. This is also called a David or Yacoub Procedure. The approach is a standard median sternotomy. Cardiopulmonary bypass is initiated. Following cardioplegic arrest, the ascending aorta is transected above the cross clamp and both the right and left aortic buttons are dissected out. The aortic root and valve are evaluated and the aortic annulus is sized. The right ventricular fibers are separated from the left ventricular outflow track (LVOT) at the level of the right commissure. The aortic valve leaflets are pushed aside and sub-annular stitches are placed with pledgets on the ventricular side, taking care to avoid injury to the conduction system. The stitches exit outside the aorta at the junction of the aorta and LVOT. The ascending aorta graft is then sized and modeled to correspond to the right cusp so that the graft will sit upright in the chest. Sub-annular stitches are passed through the graft and tied to secure the graft to the aortic annulus. A Hagar's dilator is used to size the aortic annulus. The three commissures are resuspended. Careful attention to both the height of each resuspension and the distance between each resuspension is required to avoid distortion of the aortic valve leaflet positioning. The aortic valve is reimplanted and tested to confirm that it is functioning properly. The coronary buttons are reimplanted. The distal portion of the graft is sewn to the remaining normal ascending aorta. Air is evacuated from the heart, the clamp is removed, and the heart is reperfused. Temporary pacing wires are placed and pacing is begun, if needed. Cardiopulmonary bypass is terminated and all cannulas are removed before the chest is closed.

33870

33870 Transverse arch graft, with cardiopulmonary bypass

A transverse arch aortic aneurysm is repaired using a graft with cardiopulmonary bypass. The right subclavian and right femoral artery are cannulated. The heart is accessed by median sternotomy and the brachiocephalic, left common carotid, and left subclavian arteries are exposed. Cardiopulmonary bypass is established and retrograde cold blood cardioplegia is initiated. The femoral cannula is clamped and cerebral perfusion is initiated via the subclavian cannula. Alternatively, cerebral perfusion may be initiated after anastomosis of the left carotid artery. The aortic arch and branches are mobilized and the aorta is transected to replace the diseased section of the aorta using either an en bloc or separated graft technique. Aortic thrombus and plaque are removed. If an en bloc technique is used, a tube graft is placed and the brachiocephalic, left common carotid, and left subclavian arteries are reconstructed and attached to the tube graft. If a separated graft technique is used, a prefabricated four-branched aortic arch prosthesis is used. Three of the four branches correspond to the brachiocephalic, left common carotid, and left subclavian arteries. The fourth branch is used for cerebral perfusion once the distal aortic anastomosis and left common carotid anastomosis have been completed. The branched aortic arch prosthesis is inserted and the distal end is anastomosed to the aorta. The left common carotid artery is sutured to the prosthesis. Cerebral perfusion is then administered through the fourth branch of the prosthesis and the right subclavian artery. The left subclavian and brachiocephalic arteries are sutured to the prosthesis. The proximal end of the prosthesis is then anastomosed to the aorta. Cardiopulmonary bypass is terminated and the fourth branch of the prosthesis is resected. Chest tubes are placed as needed and the chest is closed.

33875-33877

33875 Descending thoracic aorta graft, with or without bypass

33877 Repair of thoracoabdominal aortic aneurysm with graft, with or without cardiopulmonary bypass

Descending thoracic aneurysms originate below the left subclavian artery and extend distally. Thoracoabdominal aneurysms involve the descending thoracic aorta and extend into the abdominal aorta. In 33875, the chest is incised and the descending aorta exposed. If cardiopulmonary bypass is used, cannulas are placed and cardiopulmonary bypass is established. If cardiopulmonary bypass is not used, a partial exclusion clamp is placed across the aorta. The aneurysm sac is opened and aortic thrombus and plaque removed. A synthetic tube graft or conduit is sutured to the healthy aorta distal and proximal to the site of the aneurysm. The aneurysm sac is then closed over the graft, clamps are released, and blood flow re-established. Chest tubes are placed as needed and chest incisions closed. In 33877, a thoracoabdominal approach is used. The duodenum is dissected off the abdominal aorta and the aorta exposed. Proximal control is established below the level of the left subclavian or more distally depending on the extent of involvement of the thoracic aorta. Distal control is established above the iliac arteries. Following diuresis and administration of anti-coagulant, the iliac arteries are clamped. The aorta is also clamped. The aneurysm sac is opened longitudinally and aortic thrombus and plaque removed. The lumbar arteries are oversewn as is the inferior mesenteric artery. A synthetic tube graft or conduit is sutured to healthy aorta proximal to the site of the aneurysm. If the aneurysm extends to the renal arteries, the distal anastomosis may be beveled to incorporate visceral and renal vessels. If the aneurysm extends to the iliac bifurcation, the visceral and renal vessels are reattached to the tube graft or conduit. The distal aorta is then anastomosed to the tube graft or conduit. Following placement of the tube graft or conduit, the aneurysm sac is closed over the graft, clamps are released, and blood flow re-established. The retroperitoneum is repaired and the abdomen closed.

33880-33881

33880 Endovascular repair of descending thoracic aorta (eg, aneurysm, pseudoaneurysm, dissection, penetrating ulcer, intramural hematoma, or traumatic disruption); involving coverage of left subclavian artery origin, initial endoprosthesis plus descending thoracic aortic extension(s), if required, to level of celiac artery origin

33881 Endovascular repair of descending thoracic aorta (eg, aneurysm, pseudoaneurysm, dissection, penetrating ulcer, intramural hematoma, or traumatic disruption); not involving coverage of left subclavian artery origin, initial endoprosthesis plus descending thoracic aortic extension(s), if required, to level of celiac artery origin

The procedure includes placement of the initial endoprosthesis plus descending thoracic aorta extensions to the level of the celiac artery if needed. Endovascular repair of the descending thoracic aorta may be used to treat an aneurysm, pseudoaneurysm, dissection, penetrating ulcer, intramural hematoma or traumatic disruption. An access artery, usually the femoral or iliac, is punctured and a flexible guidewire passed in a retrograde fashion into the ascending aorta using separately reportable fluoroscopic guidance. The contralateral femoral or iliac artery, is punctured, a sheath placed and a second guidewire passed into the ascending aorta. An aortogram is obtained and the aneurysm evaluated. An ultrasound probe is introduced and the aneurysm measured. A properly sized stent-graft (endoprosthesis) is selected. One of the flexible guidewires is removed and exchanged for a stiff guidewire. One of the sheaths is removed and exchanged for an introducer sheath. The stent-graft is loaded and maneuvered into position. Another aortogram is obtained to verify correct positioning of the stent-graft. The stent-graft is deployed. The distal and proximal ends of the stent-graft are ballooned and sealed. Stent-graft extensions to the level of the celiac artery are loaded, positioned and deployed as needed. The overlapping segments of stent-graft extensions are ballooned and sealed. Another aortogram is obtained to verify complete exclusion of the defect in the descending thoracic aorta and to check for leakage at the distal and proximal ends of the graft or stent. In 33880, the aneurysm extends beyond the origin of the subclavian artery and the stent-graft covers and occludes the left subclavian artery. In 33881, the aneurysm does not extend to the level of the subclavian artery and the subclavian artery is not occluded by the stent-graft.

33883-33884

33883 Placement of proximal extension prosthesis for endovascular repair of descending thoracic aorta (eg, aneurysm, pseudoaneurysm, dissection, penetrating ulcer, intramural hematoma, or traumatic disruption); initial extension

33884 Placement of proximal extension prosthesis for endovascular repair of descending thoracic aorta (eg, aneurysm, pseudoaneurysm, dissection, penetrating ulcer, intramural hematoma, or traumatic disruption); each additional proximal extension (List separately in addition to code for primary procedure)

Endovascular repair of the descending thoracic aorta may be used to treat an aneurysm, pseudoaneurysm, dissection, penetrating ulcer, intramural hematoma or traumatic disruption. An access artery, usually the femoral or iliac, is punctured and a flexible guidewire passed in a retrograde fashion into the ascending aorta using separately reportable fluoroscopic guidance. Separately reportable brachial artery access may also be required to assist in placement of the proximal extension components. The contralateral femoral or iliac artery, is punctured, a sheath is placed and a second guidewire passed into the ascending aorta. An aortogram is obtained and the proximal aspect of the aneurysm evaluated. An ultrasound probe is introduced and the proximal extension site measured. A properly sized stent-graft extension prosthesis is selected. One of the flexible guidewires is removed and exchanged for a stiff guidewire. One of the sheaths is removed and exchanged for an introducer sheath. The stent-graft extension prosthesis is loaded and maneuvered into position. Another aortogram is obtained to verify correct positioning of the extension prosthesis which is then deployed. The overlapping segment of the stent-graft and the proximal extension prosthesis are ballooned and sealed. The proximal end of the extension prosthesis is ballooned and sealed to the aorta. Report 33883 for placement of the initial proximal extension prosthesis and 33884 for each additional proximal extension component. When all proximal extensions are in place, another aortogram is obtained to verify complete exclusion of the defect in the thoracic aorta and to check for leakage.

33886

33886 Placement of distal extension prosthesis(s) delayed after endovascular repair of descending thoracic aorta

Delayed placement of a distal prosthesis is performed when there is evidence of an endoleak, when there is migration of the endovascular components with the threat of an endoleak, or when distal aneurysm extension occurs. An access artery, usually the femoral or iliac, is punctured and a flexible guidewire passed in a retrograde fashion into the ascending aorta using separately reportable fluoroscopic guidance. The contralateral femoral or iliac artery, is punctured, a sheath is placed and a second guidewire passed into the ascending aorta. An aortogram is obtained and the aneurysm evaluated. An ultrasound probe is introduced and the distal extension site measured. A properly sized stent-graft extension prosthesis is selected. One of the flexible guidewires is removed and exchanged for a stiff guidewire. One of the sheaths is removed and exchanged for an introducer sheath. The stent-graft extension prosthesis is loaded and maneuvered into position. Another aortogram is obtained to verify correct positioning of the extension prosthesis which is then deployed. The overlapping segment of the original stent-graft and the distal extension prosthesis are ballooned and sealed. The distal end of the extension prosthesis is ballooned and sealed to the aorta. Additional segments are added as needed, ballooned, and sealed. When all distal extensions are in place, another aortogram is obtained to verify complete exclusion of the defect in the descending thoracic aorta and to check for leakage.

33889

33889 Open subclavian to carotid artery transposition performed in conjunction with endovascular repair of descending thoracic aorta, by neck incision, unilateral

The neck is incised and the incision is extended toward the arm along the supraclavicular space. The carotid and subclavian arteries are exposed by soft tissue dissection while mobilizing and protecting surrounding vessels and nerves. The subclavian artery is dissected under the clavicle and exposed as close to the aorta as possible. The arteries are controlled by passing soft rubber loops proximally and distally. An anticoagulant is administered intravenously. Proximal and distal clamps are applied to the subclavian artery, which is divided and the proximal stump is oversewn. The proximal clamp is released and additional sutures are placed as needed to control bleeding. The common carotid artery is then clamped proximally and distally. The subclavian artery is mobilized. The common carotid artery is incised and the subclavian artery is anastomosed to the common carotid in an end-to-side fashion. Vascular clamps are released and additional sutures are placed as needed to control bleeding. Pulses are checked and blood flow is confirmed by Doppler. The neck incision is closed.

33891

33891 Bypass graft, with other than vein, transcervical retropharyngeal carotid-carotid, performed in conjunction with endovascular repair of descending thoracic aorta, by neck incision

The neck is incised bilaterally. The carotid arteries are exposed by soft tissue dissection while mobilizing and protecting surrounding vessels and nerves. The common carotid arteries are controlled by passing soft rubber loops proximally and distally. A tunnel is created behind the pharynx from one side of the neck to the other. A synthetic conduit is then passed through the tunnel. An anticoagulant is administered intravenously. One of the common carotids is clamped proximally and distally. The artery is incised longitudinally and the bypass conduit is anastomosed to the carotid artery. The bypass conduit is then clamped and the common carotid clamps are released. Additional sutures are placed to control bleeding at the first anastomosis site. The second common carotid is then clamped proximally and distally; the artery is incised; and the synthetic conduit is anastomosed. All clamps are removed and any bleeding at the anastomosis site is controlled with additional sutures. Pulses are checked and blood flow is confirmed by Doppler. The neck incisions are closed.

33910-33915

33910 Pulmonary artery embolectomy; with cardiopulmonary bypass
33915 Pulmonary artery embolectomy; without cardiopulmonary bypass

The pulmonary arteries are accessed by median sternotomy or thoracotomy. The main pulmonary artery and pulmonary branches are dissected free of surrounding tissue. If cardiopulmonary bypass is used, the aorta and superior and inferior vena cava are cannulated. Cardiopulmonary bypass is established. The pericardium is incised and the main pulmonary artery is opened. The incision is extended as needed into the right and/or left pulmonary arteries. The embolus is located and removed. Use code 33910 if the procedure is performed with cardiopulmonary bypass and 33915 if cardiopulmonary bypass is not used.

Cardiovascular System

33916

33916   Pulmonary endarterectomy, with or without embolectomy, with cardiopulmonary bypass

Pulmonary endarterectomy is performed to treat chronic thromboembolic pulmonary hypertension. The heart is exposed by median sternotomy or thoracotomy. The pericardium is incised and the proximal main pulmonary artery is exposed. The aorta and superior and inferior vena cava are cannulated. Cardiopulmonary bypass is established and the aorta is cross-clamped. The main pulmonary artery is incised and the incision is extended as needed. If an embolus is present, it is removed. The correct endarterectomy plane is then established. The fibrous obstructive tissue is removed from the main, right, and left pulmonary arteries and lobar, segmental, and subsegmental pulmonary artery branches as needed. The endarterectomy procedure is performed on the pulmonary artery and branches in one lung at a time. When endarterectomy is completed on the first lung, the lung is reperfused. Following reperfusion, a second period of cardiac arrest is established and endarterectomy is performed on the contralateral side. Following completion of the endarterectomy procedure, incisions in the pulmonary arteries are closed; chest tubes are placed as needed; and the chest incision is closed.

33917

33917   Repair of pulmonary artery stenosis by reconstruction with patch or graft

Pulmonary artery stenosis is a narrowing of the artery that may occur in the main pulmonary artery and/or in the right or left pulmonary artery branches. The heart is exposed by median sternotomy. The pericardium is incised and a patch of pericardium is harvested for later use as a patch graft. The main pulmonary artery is dissected free of surrounding tissue, followed by dissection of the right and left pulmonary arteries. The arteries are controlled by the placement of rubber loops which are used to gently occlude the vessels. The narrowed section of pulmonary artery is incised longitudinally. A patch or graft of autologous pericardium, an allograft (homograft), xenograft, or synthetic material is inserted to enlarge the narrowed section of artery. Chest tubes are placed as needed and the chest incision is closed.

33920

33920   Repair of pulmonary atresia with ventricular septal defect, by construction or replacement of conduit from right or left ventricle to pulmonary artery

Pulmonary atresia is a congenital anomaly in which the pulmonary valve fails to develop properly, preventing the leaflets from opening which in turn prevents blood from flowing from the right ventricle to the lungs. In some cases, the patient also has a VSD, which is an opening in the septum between the right and left ventricles. This procedure is performed on patients with both pulmonary atresia and a VSD. Because the anomalous anatomy can vary significantly, the procedure must be individualized for each patient. One technique is described here, but the technique will vary for each patient. The repair is often performed in stages. The heart is exposed by median sternotomy. The pericardium is incised and a patch of pericardium is harvested for later use as a patch graft. Cardiopulmonary bypass is established. The main pulmonary artery and branches as well as the external heart anatomy are evaluated to identify the optimal location for the conduit. The main pulmonary artery is dissected free of surrounding tissue followed by dissection of the right and left pulmonary arteries, which are controlled by the placement of rubber loops used to gently occlude the vessels. The main pulmonary artery is incised longitudinally. A conduit using autologous pericardium, an allograft (homograft), xenograft, or synthetic material is constructed and sutured to the arteriotomy site in the main pulmonary artery. The incision is extended into the right ventricle and the conduit is inserted into the right ventricle and secured with sutures. Depending on the patient's anatomy, the conduit may be attached to the left ventricle instead. If the VSD is repaired during the same surgical session, it is reported separately. The patient is then weaned off cardiopulmonary bypass; chest tubes are placed as needed; and the chest incision is closed.

33922

33922   Transection of pulmonary artery with cardiopulmonary bypass

Transection of the pulmonary artery is performed in newborns with certain cardiac and great vessel anomalies as a palliative procedure until a more extensive repair of the anomaly can be performed. Transection is performed when there is another vascular connection to the lungs that allows the flow of deoxygenated blood into the lungs and the return of oxygenated blood to the heart. An incision is made in the chest to access the heart and pulmonary artery. Cardiopulmonary bypass is initiated. The main pulmonary artery (trunk) is clamped above and below the planned incision site and the artery is transected. The distal and proximal pulmonary artery stumps are repaired with sutures. Chest tubes are placed and the chest incision is closed.

33924

33924   Ligation and takedown of a systemic-to-pulmonary artery shunt, performed in conjunction with a congenital heart procedure (List separately in addition to code for primary procedure)

The heart is exposed by median sternotomy or thoracotomy. The previously created shunt is exposed by careful dissection of surrounding tissue and adhesions. Control of the shunt is accomplished by placing soft rubber tubing proximally and distally. Suture ligatures (ties) are placed at the proximal and distal aspects of the shunt, which is divided and removed.

33925-33926

33925   Repair of pulmonary artery arborization anomalies by unifocalization; without cardiopulmonary bypass

33926   Repair of pulmonary artery arborization anomalies by unifocalization; with cardiopulmonary bypass

Arborization anomalies typically occur in conjunction with pulmonary atresia and a ventricular septal defect (VSD). The arborization anomalies are collateral arteries also referred to as major aorto-pulmonary collateral arteries (MAPCAs) that connect the aorta and pulmonary arteries in the lungs. These collateral arteries must be connected and brought to a more central confluence, a procedure referred to as unifocalization. The multiple cardiac anomalies are typically repaired in a staged fashion with the unifocalization procedure being the first procedure performed. The heart is approached by median sternotomy or thoracotomy. If cardiopulmonary bypass is required, the aorta and superior and inferior vena cava are cannulated. Cardiopulmonary bypass is established and the aorta is cross-clamped. The collaterals (MAPCAs) are dissected free of surrounding tissue and mobilized at their origins in the aorta or brachiocephalic branches. The intraparenchymal or hilar pulmonary artery segment is mobilized. Control of the branch vessels is achieved by placing clamps on the pulmonary artery branches and collaterals. The collateral arteries (MAPCAs) are divided off the aorta. The aortic ends are oversewn. The distal ends of the collaterals are then attached to the pulmonary artery. Clamps are released and additional sutures placed to control bleeding at the anastomosis sites. If cardiopulmonary bypass has been used, the patient is weaned off bypass. Chest tubes are placed and the chest incision is closed. Use code 33925 if the procedure is performed without cardiopulmonary bypass and code 33926 if cardiopulmonary bypass is used.

33930

33930   Donor cardiectomy-pneumonectomy (including cold preservation)

Following confirmation of brain death, the donor is examined by the organ procurement team. A bronchoscopy is performed. The heart and lungs are exposed by median sternotomy and the incision is extended to expose abdominal organs as well. The heart and lungs are inspected. Preliminary dissection of the lungs and heart is performed. The pulmonary artery and aorta are cannulated. The aorta is cross clamped and the body is perfused with cold saline. The heart and both lungs are removed and placed in sterile bags that are then placed in ice. The heart and lungs are then transported to the recipient site.

33933

33933   Backbench standard preparation of cadaver donor heart/lung allograft prior to transplantation, including dissection of allograft from surrounding soft tissues to prepare aorta, superior vena cava, inferior vena cava, and trachea for implantation

The heart with lungs allograft is removed from the sterile container and placed on a sterile table. The heart and lungs are kept on ice and continuously bathed in cold preservation solution. The heart is inspected first. The coronary arteries are inspected and palpated. If any repair is required, this is performed in a separately reportable procedure. The aorta is inspected and the cannulation site is identified and repaired or excised. The superior vena cava is inspected and the azygous vein orifice is excised or oversewn, if present. Any thrombus is removed and sent for culture. The inferior vena cava is inspected and the distance between the division of the vein and the coronary sinus is evaluated. The atrial septum is inspected. If defects are noted, they are repaired in a separately reportable procedure. The aorta is trimmed. The left atrial appendage is inspected and the amputation site is oversewn as needed. The heart is perfused with cardioplegia solution as needed. Attention is then turned to the lungs. The external surface of the lungs is examined and any defects are repaired in separately reportable procedures. Attached pericardium is excised. The tracheal staple line is removed and secretions in the airway are cultured. The trachea is trimmed. The right and left bronchial orifices are suctioned and irrigated with saline as needed. The heart with lungs allograft is wrapped in an iced pad, placed in a basin, and maintained in cold saline until the transplantation procedure begins.

33935

33935   Heart-lung transplant with recipient cardiectomy-pneumonectomy

The heart and lungs are exposed by median sternotomy. Cardiopulmonary bypass is established. The patient's diseased heart and lungs are removed taking care to preserve the phrenic nerves. If an orthotopic heart transplant procedure is performed, the lungs are removed in their entirety and most of the heart is removed leaving the posterior aspect of the recipient's right or both the right and left atria (upper chambers) intact. To perform orthotopic heart transplant, the right atrium of the recipient heart is opened along the atrioventricular groove anteriorly. The incision is extended to the coronary sinus inferiorly and to the right atrial appendage posteriorly. The aorta and main pulmonary artery are divided at the valve commissures. The roof of the left atrium is incised between the aorta and the superior vena cava. The atrial incisions are connected and extended to the left atrial appendage. The heart and lungs are then inserted. The donor and recipient trachea are anastomosed. The donor heart is then anastomosed to the remaining portion of the right or both the left and right atria of the recipient heart. The donor aorta is then connected to the recipient aorta. The patient is weaned off cardiopulmonary bypass, chest tubes are placed, and chest incisions are closed.

33940

33940   Donor cardiectomy (including cold preservation)

Following confirmation of brain death, the donor is examined by the organ procurement team. A bronchoscopy is performed. The heart and lungs are exposed by median sternotomy and the incision is extended to expose abdominal organs as well. The heart is inspected. Preliminary dissection of the lungs and heart is performed. The pulmonary artery and aorta are cannulated. The superior vena cava is divided followed by the left pulmonary vein and inferior vena cava. The aorta is cross clamped and the body is perfused with cold saline. The pulmonary artery and aorta are divided and the heart is removed and placed in a sterile bag that is then placed in ice. The heart is transported to the recipient site.

33944

33944   Backbench standard preparation of cadaver donor heart allograft prior to transplantation, including dissection of allograft from surrounding soft tissues to prepare aorta, superior vena cava, inferior vena cava, pulmonary artery, and left atrium for implantation

The heart allograft is removed from the sterile container and placed on a sterile table. The heart is kept on ice and continuously bathed in cold preservation solution. The external surface of the heart is inspected. The coronary arteries are inspected and palpated. If any repair is required, this is performed in a separately reportable procedure. The aorta is inspected and the cannulation site is identified and repaired or excised. The superior vena cava is inspected and the azygous vein orifice is excised or oversewn, if present. Any thrombus is removed and sent for culture. The inferior vena cava is inspected and the distance between the division of the vein and the coronary sinus is evaluated. The pulmonary artery is separated from the aorta and the pulmonary valve is inspected. The pulmonary vein orifices are joined. The mitral valve and atrial septum are inspected. If defects are noted, they are repaired in a separately reportable procedure. Excess left atrial tissue is excised and a left atrial cuff is created. The aorta is trimmed and the aortic valve is inspected. The left atrial appendage is inspected and the amputation site is oversewn as needed. The heart is perfused with cardioplegia solution as needed. The heart allograft is wrapped in an iced pad, placed in a basin, and maintained in cold saline until the transplantation procedure begins.

33945

33945   Heart transplant, with or without recipient cardiectomy

The heart is exposed by median sternotomy. Cardiopulmonary bypass is established. The patient's diseased heart may be removed (cardiectomy) or more commonly, an orthotopic procedure is performed in which most of the heart is removed leaving the posterior aspect of the right or both the right and left atria (upper chambers) intact. To perform orthotopic transplant, the right atrium of the recipient heart is opened along the atrioventricular groove anteriorly. The incision is extended to the coronary sinus inferiorly and to the right atrial appendage posteriorly. The aorta and main pulmonary artery are divided at the valve commissures. The roof of the left atrium is incised between the aorta and the superior vena cava. The atrial incisions are connected and extended to the left atrial appendage. The donor pulmonary veins are connected to form the left atrial cuff. The donor heart is then anastomosed to the remaining portion of the right or both the left and right atria of the recipient heart. The donor aorta and pulmonary arteries are connected to the recipient aorta and pulmonary arteries. The patient is weaned off cardiopulmonary bypass; chest tubes are placed; and chest incisions are closed.

33946-33947

33946   Extracorporeal membrane oxygenation (ECMO)/extracorporeal life support (ECLS) provided by physician; initiation, veno-venous

33947   Extracorporeal membrane oxygenation (ECMO)/extracorporeal life support (ECLS) provided by physician; initiation, veno-arterial

Extracorporeal membrane oxygenation (ECMO) and extracorporeal life support (ECLS) are interchangeable terms describing long term (usually 3-10 days) heart and lung bypass support that circulates blood outside the body through an artificial lung and returns it back to the bloodstream. In veno-venous (V-V) ECMO/ECLS, venous blood is accessed from a large central vein and returned to the venous system after oxygenation. In veno-arterial (V-A) ECMO/ECLS, venous blood is accessed from a large central vein and returned to a major artery after oxygenation. ECMO/ECLS initiation requires a complex evaluation

of the patient and his or her injury and disease process. This includes laboratory tests, x-rays, cardiograms/echocardiograms, head ultrasound in neonates, and a neurological evaluation. Informed consent must be obtained from the patient and/or family. The equipment is set up including the ECMO pump, ACT machine and tubing, and ECMO bed. Medications are ordered and blood products obtained from the blood bank. Once the ECMO circuit is prepared, the patient and room are ready, and the perfusion team is in position, cannulation of the vessels can then take place and ECMO/ECLS therapy can begin. V-V ECMO/ECLS and V-A ECMO/ECLS may be initiated by a neonatologist, pediatric intensivist, surgeon, or interventional cardiologist, and the patient must be monitored 24/7 by a perfusion specialist. Code 33946 is used to bill for physician services related to V-V ECMO/ECLS initiation. Code 33947 is used to bill for physician services related to V-A ECMO/ECLS initiation.

33948

33948   Extracorporeal membrane oxygenation (ECMO)/extracorporeal life support (ECLS) provided by physician; daily management, each day, veno-venous

Extracorporeal membrane oxygenation (ECMO) and extracorporeal life support (ECLS) are interchangeable terms describing long term (usually 3-10 days) heart and lung bypass support that circulates blood outside the body through an artificial lung and returns it back to the bloodstream. In veno-venous (V-V) ECMO/ECLS, venous blood is accessed from a large central vein and returned to the venous system after oxygenation. V-V ECMO/ECLS is most often used to support a patient who is in respiratory failure with no concurrent major cardiac dysfunction present. This technique increases circulating blood oxygen (O2) levels while decreasing carbon dioxide (CO2) levels. It allows for a lower level of ventilator support, which in turn may lower the incidence of ventilator induced lung injury. Medical oversight of V-V ECMO/ECLS is most often provided by an ICU intensivist and the patient is monitored 24/7 by a team of perfusion specialists.

33949

33949   Extracorporeal membrane oxygenation (ECMO)/extracorporeal life support (ECLS) provided by physician; daily management, each day, veno-arterial

Extracorporeal membrane oxygenation (ECMO) and extracorporeal life support (ECLS) are interchangeable terms describing long term (usually 3-10 days) heart and lung bypass support that circulates blood outside the body through an artificial lung and returns it back to the bloodstream. In veno-arterial (V-A) ECMO/ECLS, venous blood is accessed from a large central vein and returned to a major artery after oxygenation. V-A ECMO/ECLS is most often used to support a patient with severe cardiac failure, usually associated with respiratory failure or following surgical cardiac repair or injury. Medical oversight of V-A ECMO/ECLS is most often provided by an ICU intensivist and the patient is monitored 24/7 by a team of perfusion specialists. Physician services related to V-A ECMO/ECLS daily management can include sedation, anticoagulation, temperature management, hemodynamic stability, electrolyte and blood gas analysis, and respiratory or ventilator support.

33951-33952

33951   Extracorporeal membrane oxygenation (ECMO)/extracorporeal life support (ECLS) provided by physician; insertion of peripheral (arterial and/or venous) cannula(e), percutaneous, birth through 5 years of age (includes fluoroscopic guidance, when performed)

33952   Extracorporeal membrane oxygenation (ECMO)/extracorporeal life support (ECLS) provided by physician; insertion of peripheral (arterial and/or venous) cannula(e), percutaneous, 6 years and older (includes fluoroscopic guidance, when performed)

Extracorporeal membrane oxygenation (ECMO) and extracorporeal life support (ECLS) are interchangeable terms describing long term (usually 3-10 days) heart and lung bypass support that circulates blood outside the body through an artificial lung and returns it back to the bloodstream. In ECMO/ECLS, venous blood is drained from a large central vein and returned either to the venous system or a major artery after oxygenation. ECMO/ECLS in neonates and children is often performed via percutaneous insertion of a dual lumen cannula into the right jugular vein with the drainage holes located between the inferior vena cava (IVC) and the superior vena cava (SVC) and the return holes at the right atrium (RA). ECMO/ECLS can also be accomplished via a two cannulae system with the drainage catheter inserted into the right femoral vein and advanced into the IVC and the return catheter in the right internal jugular vein at the RA/SVC junction. The procedure for cannulation is nearly identical for both techniques. The jugular/femoral vein may be located using ultrasound. The vein is punctured with a hollow needle and a guidewire is introduced into the vessel with placement confirmed using fluoroscopy. The vessel is serially dilated until the cannula/introducer unit can be advanced over the guidewire. Once the correct position is confirmed using fluoroscopy, the guidewire and introducer are removed and the cannula is clamped. The previously primed EMCO/ECLS circuit is then connected and the treatment begins. Code 33951 is used for percutaneous peripheral cannula(e) insertion when the patient is a newborn up to 5 years old, and code 33952 is used for patients age 6 years and older.

● New Code   ▲ Revised Code

33953-33954

33953 Extracorporeal membrane oxygenation (ECMO)/extracorporeal life support (ECLS) provided by physician; insertion of peripheral (arterial and/or venous) cannula(e), open, birth through 5 years of age

33954 Extracorporeal membrane oxygenation (ECMO)/extracorporeal life support (ECLS) provided by physician; insertion of peripheral (arterial and/or venous) cannula(e), open, 6 years and older

Extracorporeal membrane oxygenation (ECMO) and extracorporeal life support (ECLS) are interchangeable terms describing long term (usually 3-10 days) heart and lung bypass support that circulates blood outside the body through an artificial lung and returns it back to the bloodstream. Venous blood is drained from a large central vein and returned either to the venous system a major artery after oxygenation. Peripheral insertion of arterial and/or venous cannula(e) using an open, surgical cut down technique is accomplished by making an incision in the skin over the vessel to be cannulated, such as the femoral or jugular vein, and dissecting the underlying tissue to expose the vessel. A small incision is made in the vessel and a guidewire is introduced and advanced to the correct position with placement confirmed using fluoroscopy. The vessel is then serially dilated until the cannula/introducer unit can be advanced over the guidewire. Once the correct position is confirmed, the guidewire and introducer are removed and the cannula is clamped. The previously primed EMCO/ECLS circuit is then connected to the cannula and treatment begins. The incisions are closed and tubing is secured. Code 33953 is used for open peripheral cannula(s) insertion when the patient is a newborn through 5 years old, and code 33954 is used for patients age 6 years and older.

33955-33956

33955 Extracorporeal membrane oxygenation (ECMO)/extracorporeal life support (ECLS) provided by physician; insertion of central cannula(e) by sternotomy or thoracotomy, birth through 5 years of age

33956 Extracorporeal membrane oxygenation (ECMO)/extracorporeal life support (ECLS) provided by physician; insertion of central cannula(e) by sternotomy or thoracotomy, 6 years and older

Extracorporeal membrane oxygenation (ECMO) and extracorporeal life support (ECLS) are interchangeable terms describing long term (usually 3-10 days) heart and lung bypass support that circulates blood outside the body through an artificial lung and returns it back to the bloodstream. Insertion of a central cannula(e) using a transthoracic approach (sternotomy, thoracotomy) is most often performed during cardiac surgery when the patient fails to wean from cardiopulmonary bypass. The surgeon makes a cut between ribs to open the chest wall, spreads the ribs apart, and enters the chest cavity, or a vertical incision is made along the sternum, and the bone is separated to allow access to the heart. The right atrial appendage and the aortic arch/ascending aorta are cannulated, or in the event of primary left heart failure, the left atrium is cannulated to provide left heart decompression. The tubing is connected to the EMCO/ECLS circuit, the chest is closed and tubing is secured. Code 33955 is used for insertion of a central cannula(e) by sternotomy or thoracotomy when the patient is a newborn through 5 years old, and code 33956 is used for patients age 6 years and older.

33957-33958

33957 Extracorporeal membrane oxygenation (ECMO)/extracorporeal life support (ECLS) provided by physician; reposition peripheral (arterial and/or venous) cannula(e), percutaneous, birth through 5 years of age (includes fluoroscopic guidance, when performed)

33958 Extracorporeal membrane oxygenation (ECMO)/extracorporeal life support (ECLS) provided by physician; reposition peripheral (arterial and/or venous) cannula(e), percutaneous, 6 years and older (includes fluoroscopic guidance, when performed)

Extracorporeal membrane oxygenation (ECMO) and extracorporeal life support (ECLS) are interchangeable terms describing long term heart and lung bypass support that circulates blood outside the body through an artificial lung and returns it back to the bloodstream. The peripheral arterial and/or venous cannula(e) used for ECMO/ECLS is usually placed in the vena cava with desaturated blood flowing out to the ECMO/ECLS circuit from the inferior vena cava (IVC) and oxygenated blood returning to the superior vena cava at the level of the right atrium with flow directed towards the tricuspid valve. Recirculation is a dynamic event and cannula migration can cause suboptimal ECMO/ECLS support. To reposition the cannula(e) percutaneously, the dressing and/or sutures securing the tubing to the skin are removed. Under fluoroscopic guidance, the cannula(e) are pulled back with gentle pressure or grasped with a snare and manipulated until optimal placement is confirmed. The ECMO/ECLS circuit is reconnected and the tubing is then secured to the skin using sutures and/or dressings. Code 33957 is used when the patient is a newborn through 5 years of age, and code 33958 is used for percutaneous peripheral cannula(e) reposition in patients age 6 years and older.

33959-33962

33959 Extracorporeal membrane oxygenation (ECMO)/extracorporeal life support (ECLS) provided by physician; reposition peripheral (arterial and/or venous) cannula(e), open, birth through 5 years of age (includes fluoroscopic guidance, when performed)

33962 Extracorporeal membrane oxygenation (ECMO)/extracorporeal life support (ECLS) provided by physician; reposition peripheral (arterial and/or venous) cannula(e), open, 6 years and older (includes fluoroscopic guidance, when performed)

Extracorporeal membrane oxygenation (ECMO) and extracorporeal life support (ECLS) are interchangeable terms describing long term heart and lung bypass support that circulates blood outside the body through an artificial lung and returns it back to the bloodstream. The peripheral arterial and/or venous cannula(e) used for ECMO/ECLS is usually placed in the vena cava with desaturated blood flowing out to the ECMO/ECLS circuit from the inferior vena cava (IVC) and oxygenated blood returning to the superior vena cava at the level of the right atrium with flow directed towards the tricuspid valve. Recirculation is a dynamic event and cannula migration can cause suboptimal ECMO/ECLS support. To reposition the cannula(e) using an open technique, the dressing and/or sutures securing the tubing to the skin are removed. The vessel is accessed by incising the skin or opening the previous incision if the cannula was inserted using open technique. The sutures securing the cannula to the vessel are cut. Under fluoroscopic guidance, the cannula(e) are pulled back gently or grasped with a snare through the open incision and manipulated until optimal placement is confirmed. The cannula is secured in the vessel using sutures and the incision is closed. The ECMO/ECLS circuit is reconnected and the tubing is then secured to the skin using sutures and/or dressings. Code 33959 is used when the patient is a newborn through 5 years of age, and code 33962 is used for open peripheral cannula(e) reposition in patients age 6 years and older.

33963-33964

33963 Extracorporeal membrane oxygenation (ECMO)/extracorporeal life support (ECLS) provided by physician; reposition of central cannula(e) by sternotomy or thoracotomy, birth through 5 years of age (includes fluoroscopic guidance, when performed)

33964 Extracorporeal membrane oxygenation (ECMO)/extracorporeal life support (ECLS) provided by physician; reposition central cannula(e) by sternotomy or thoracotomy, 6 years and older (includes fluoroscopic guidance, when performed)

Extracorporeal membrane oxygenation (ECMO) and extracorporeal life support (ECLS) are interchangeable terms describing long term heart and lung bypass support that circulates blood outside the body through an artificial lung and returns it back to the bloodstream. Repositioning of a central cannula(e) using a transthoracic approach (sternotomy, thoracotomy) is most often performed when the right atrial appendage and the aortic arch/ascending aorta have been cannulated, or in the event of primary left heart failure, the left atrium has been cannulated to provide left heart decompression. The chest is opened using a standard vertical sternotomy incision through the sternum bone, or thoracotomy approach through the ribs, and the cannula(e) and vessel(s) are identified. Under fluoroscopy guidance, the cannula(e) are repositioned in the vessel(s) by gentle manual pressure or use of a snare until optimal placement is confirmed. The cannula(s) is secured in the vessel using sutures and the incision is closed. The ECMO/ECLS circuit is reconnected and the tubing is then secured to the skin using sutures and/or dressings. Code 33963 is used when the patient is a newborn through 5 years of age, and code 33964 is used for open chest reposition of cannula(e) in patients age 6 years and older.

33965-33966

33965 Extracorporeal membrane oxygenation (ECMO)/extracorporeal life support (ECLS) provided by physician; removal of peripheral (arterial and/or venous) cannula(e), percutaneous, birth through 5 years of age

33966 Extracorporeal membrane oxygenation (ECMO)/extracorporeal life support (ECLS) provided by physician; removal of peripheral (arterial and/or venous) cannula(e), percutaneous, 6 years and older

Extracorporeal membrane oxygenation (ECMO) and extracorporeal life support (ECLS) are interchangeable terms describing long term heart and lung bypass support that circulates blood outside the body through an artificial lung and returns it back to the bloodstream. To remove a peripheral arterial and/or venous cannula(e), the patient is placed in slight trendelenburg or supine position. The ECMO/ECLS circuit tubing is clamped and the dressing and/or sutures securing the cannula(e)/tubing to the skin are removed. The cannula(e) is withdrawn from the vessel using rapid, steady pressure in a parallel line to the skin. To reduce the risk of air embolism, removal should be done during the inspiratory ventilator phase on an intubated patient. If the patient is conscious and able to follow directions, the cannula should be withdrawn during exhalation or Valsalva. Pressure is applied to control bleeding and a sterile dressing is placed over the wound. Code 33965 is used when the patient is a newborn through 5 years of age, and code 33966 is used for patients age 6 years and older.

Cardiovascular System

33967-33968

33967 Insertion of intra-aortic balloon assist device, percutaneous
33968 Removal of intra-aortic balloon assist device, percutaneous

The femoral artery is punctured and a J-shaped guidewire inserted to the level of the aortic arch. Alternatively, the subclavian, axillary, or iliac arteries may be used for percutaneous placement of the IABP. The needle is removed and the arterial puncture site is enlarged using a dilator/sheath combination. The dilator is removed and the balloon is threaded over the guidewire. The balloon is advanced through the descending aorta to just below the left subclavian artery. The sheath is removed from the artery and the leak proof cuff on the balloon hub connected to the balloon pump console. The balloon inflates at the start of diastole to augment coronary perfusion and deflates at systole to assist in the ejection of blood from the left ventricle thereby increasing cardiac output and decreasing left ventricular stroke work and oxygen requirements. In 33968, percutaneous removal of the IAB P is performed. The balloon is deflated and the IABP withdrawn. Pressure is applied to the artery to control bleeding and a sterile pressure dressing applied.

33969

33969 Extracorporeal membrane oxygenation (ECMO)/extracorporeal life support (ECLS) provided by physician; removal of peripheral (arterial and/or venous) cannula(e), open, birth through 5 years of age

Extracorporeal membrane oxygenation (ECMO) and extracorporeal life support (ECLS) are interchangeable terms describing long term heart and lung bypass support that circulates blood outside the body through an artificial lung and returns it back to the bloodstream. To remove peripheral arterial and/or venous cannula(e) using an open technique, the patient is placed in slight trendelenburg or supine position. The ECMO/ECLS circuit tubing is clamped and the dressing and/or sutures securing the cannula(e)/tubing to the skin are removed. The vessel is accessed by incising the skin, or opening the previous incision if the cannula was inserted using open technique. The sutures securing the cannula(e) to the vessel are cut. The cannula(e) is withdrawn from the vessel using rapid, steady pressure in a parallel line to the skin. To reduce the risk of air embolism, removal should be done during the inspiratory ventilator phase on an intubated patient. If the patient is conscious and able to follow directions, the cannula(e) should be withdrawn during exhalation or Valsalva. The opening in the vessel is closed with sutures, followed by closure of the skin using sutures or staples, and a sterile dressing is applied.

33970-33971

33970 Insertion of intra-aortic balloon assist device through the femoral artery, open approach
33971 Removal of intra-aortic balloon assist device including repair of femoral artery, with or without graft

A longitudinal incision is made in the groin over the femoral artery. The femoral artery is exposed and controlled. A vascular graft is sutured to the common femoral artery in an end-to-side fashion. The balloon is introduced into the femoral artery via the graft advanced through the descending aorta to just below the left subclavian artery. The graft is secured to the distal end of the balloon catheter. The IABP catheter is then attached to the balloon pump console. The balloon inflates at the start of diastole to augment coronary perfusion and deflates at systole to assist in the ejection of blood from the left ventricle thereby increasing cardiac output and decreasing left ventricular stroke work and oxygen requirements. In 33971, the IABP is removed and the femoral artery repaired with or without a graft. The femoral artery is opened, the balloon is deflated and the IABP is removed. The femoral artery is then repaired with sutures or a patch or tube graft is placed in the femoral artery.

33973-33974

33973 Insertion of intra-aortic balloon assist device through the ascending aorta
33974 Removal of intra-aortic balloon assist device from the ascending aorta, including repair of the ascending aorta, with or without graft

The aorta is exposed by median sternotomy. A side-biting clamp is placed on the ascending aorta and the aorta is incised. The IAPB is introduced using Seldinger technique, positioned distal to the left subclavian artery, and secured with pursestring sutures. Alternatively, a synthetic graft may be anastomosed to the aorta in an end-to side fashion. The IABP is then introduced through the graft and balloon positioned distal to the left subclavian artery. The IABP catheter is secured to the graft. The catheter is allowed to extend out through the lower edge of the sternal incision. The distal end of the catheter is then attached to the balloon pump console, and the sternal incision is closed around the catheter. The balloon inflates at the start of diastole to augment coronary perfusion and deflates at systole to assist in the ejection of blood from the left ventricle thereby increasing cardiac output and decreasing left ventricular stroke work and oxygen requirements. In 33974, the IABP is removed and the ascending aorta repaired with or without a graft. If the IABP has been placed using Seldinger technique, the chest is reopened and the balloon deflated. The balloon pump is then removed and the previously placed pursestring sutures tied to close the opening in the aorta. Alternatively, the aorta is repaired by placing a patch or tube graft. If the IABP has been placed using a synthetic graft, a small incision is made at the site

where the IABP catheter protrudes from the sternum. The balloon is deflated and the IABP catheter is removed. The previously placed synthetic graft is then sutured closed.

33975-33976

33975 Insertion of ventricular assist device; extracorporeal, single ventricle
33976 Insertion of ventricular assist device; extracorporeal, biventricular

An extracorporeal ventricular assist device (VAD) is inserted in one or both ventricles to assist the heart in pumping blood. The device consists of a mechanical pump, control system, and energy supply. An extracorporeal device uses pumps that are external to the body and connected to the heart by cannulas. VADs are used in patients waiting for a heart transplant or to prolong life in patients with severe heart failure. VADs are also used following heart surgery to allow recovery of one or both ventricles. A median sternotomy is used to expose the heart. Cardiopulmonary bypass is initiated. If a left VAD is being inserted a partial occluding clamp is placed on the aorta. The aorta is incised and an outflow graft sutured to the aorta. The left ventricular apex is elevated and double pursestring sutures reinforced with bovine pericardial pledgets are placed around the planned insertion site in the left ventricle. A cruciate incision is then made at the apex within the surrounding suture line. The inflow cannula is inserted and the pursestring sutures tightened around the cannula. The device is allowed to fill with blood and the inflow cannula and outflow graft are connected to the pump. The pump is connected to the battery pack. The patient is weaned off cardiopulmonary bypass. The VAD flow is checked and adjusted as needed. Hemostasis at the cannula and graft site is checked. Pacing wires are placed. A chest tube is inserted. Chest incisions are closed. If the patient requires a right VAD, the procedure is performed in the same manner except that an inflow graft is placed in the pulmonary artery and an outflow cannula is placed in the right ventricle. Use 33975 for placement of a single ventricle VAD and 33976 when the VAD is placed in both ventricles (biventricular).

33977-33978

33977 Removal of ventricular assist device; extracorporeal, single ventricle
33978 Removal of ventricular assist device; extracorporeal, biventricular

The physician removes an extracorporeal ventricular assist device (VAD). The previous sternal incision is reopened and the chest cavity exposed. The patient is weaned from the VAD to ensure that heart function is adequate. If a left VAD is being removed the aortic outflow graft is divided and the graft site closed with sutures. The inflow cannula is removed from the left ventricle and the cannula site closed with pursestring sutures. If a right VAD is being removed the pulmonary artery inflow graft is divided and the graft site closed. The outflow cannula is removed from the right ventricle and the cannula site closed with pursestring sutures. The suture sites are inspected for hemostasis. Ventricular function is evaluated using transesophageal echocardiography. Pacing wires and chest tubes are placed as needed and the chest is closed. Use 33977 when a single ventricle VAD (right or left) is removed and 33978 when a biventricular device (right and left) is removed.

33979

33979 Insertion of ventricular assist device, implantable intracorporeal, single ventricle

The device consists of a mechanical pump, control system, and energy supply. An implantable intracorporeal device uses a pump that is inside the body. VADs are used in patients waiting for a heart transplant or to prolong life in patients with severe heart failure. VADs are also used following heart surgery to allow recovery of one or both ventricles. A midline chest incision is made and extended to the upper abdomen. A device pocket is created in the upper abdomen. The VAD is placed in the pocket and the driveline tunneled from the abdominal pocket to thoracic cavity. The patient is placed on cardiopulmonary bypass and cardioplegia induced. If a left VAD is placed, the apex of the left ventricle is cored and the inflow cuff attached to the apex using pledgeted mattress sutures. The cuff is then secured to the VAD. The outflow graft length is determined. The aorta is partially clamped and incised and an appropriately sized graft sutured to the aorta. The clamp is released and the VAD filled with blood. The outflow graft is then secured to the VAD. If the patient requires a right VAD, the procedure is performed in the same manner except that an inflow graft is placed in the pulmonary artery and an outflow cuff is placed in the right ventricle. The patient is weaned from cardiopulmonary bypass. Suture sites are checked for hemostasis. Pacing wires are placed on the heart and chest tubes inserted. Drains are placed in the abdominal pocket. The chest and abdominal incisions are closed.

33980

33980 Removal of ventricular assist device, implantable intracorporeal, single ventricle

The previous sternal incision is reopened and the chest cavity exposed. The VAD pocket in the abdomen is also opened. If a left VAD is being removed, the outflow graft and right atrium are cannulated. Cardiopulmonary bypass is initiated and cardioplegia induced. Adhesions around the heart and VAD are carefully dissected. The VAD is detached from the inflow component. The driveline is dissected from surrounding tissue and the VAD removed. The inflow cuff is removed from the left ventricle. The cored hole in the apex of the ventricle is closed with sutures and reinforced with a synthetic patch. The patient is weaned from cardiopulmonary bypass. The cannula is removed from the aortic outflow graft, the graft divided close to the aorta, and the graft stump sutured closed. Suture sites are checked for hemostasis and reinforced as needed. Pacing wires are placed on the heart and chest tubes inserted. A drain is placed in the abdominal pocket. Chest and abdominal incisions are closed. If a right VAD is being removed, the procedure is performed in the same manner except that the VAD is detached from the outflow component in the right ventricle. The pulmonary artery inflow graft is divided and the graft stump closed. The outflow cuff is removed from the right ventricle and the cored hole in the right ventricle is closed with sutures reinforced with a synthetic patch.

33981

33981   **Replacement of extracorporeal ventricular assist device, single or biventricular, pump(s), single or each pump**

An extracorporeal ventricular assist device (VAD) consists of a mechanical pump, control system, and energy supply. An extracorporeal device uses pumps that are external to the body and connected to the heart by an inflow cannula and outflow graft. The pump may need to be replaced due to mechanical failure. The pump is disconnected from the battery pack and from the inflow cannula and outflow graft. A new pump is connected to the inflow cannula and outflow graft and the pump is allowed to fill with blood. The pump is connected to the battery pack and pump function checked.

33982-33983

33982   **Replacement of ventricular assist device pump(s); implantable intracorporeal, single ventricle, without cardiopulmonary bypass**

33983   **Replacement of ventricular assist device pump(s); implantable intracorporeal, single ventricle, with cardiopulmonary bypass**

An implantable intracorporeal single ventricle assist device (VAD) consists of a mechanical pump, control system, and energy supply. An implantable intracorporeal device uses a pump that is inside the body. The pump may need to be replaced due to mechanical failure. A midline chest incision is made and extended to the upper abdomen. The pump pocket in the upper abdomen is opened. If cardiopulmonary bypass is required it is initiated. Following initiation of cardiopulmonary bypass, cardioplegia is initiated as needed. The anterior surface of the heart insertion site of the VAD cannula is inspected. The drive line is located, inspected, and repaired or replaced as needed. The inflow and outflow conduits are dissected and separated from the pump housing. The existing pump is dissected free of surrounding tissue and removed. A new drive line tunnel is created as needed from the thoracic cavity to the abdominal pocket. A new pump is placed in the pocket and connected to the inflow and outflow conduits. The drive line is connected to the pump. If cardiopulmonary bypass has been used, the heart is reperfused and cardioplegia reversed. Air is removed from the VAD and the new pump is started. Pump function is evaluated. Suture sites are checked for hemostasis. Pacing wires are placed on the heart and chest tubes inserted. Drains are placed in the abdominal pocket. The chest and abdominal incisions are closed. Use 33982 when VAD pump replacement is performed without cardiopulmonary bypass. Use 33983 when cardiopulmonary bypass is required.

33984

33984   **Extracorporeal membrane oxygenation (ECMO)/extracorporeal life support (ECLS) provided by physician; removal of peripheral (arterial and/or venous) cannula(e), open, 6 years and older**

Extracorporeal membrane oxygenation (ECMO) and extracorporeal life support (ECLS) are interchangeable terms describing long term heart and lung bypass support that circulates blood outside the body through an artificial lung and returns it back to the bloodstream. To remove peripheral arterial and/or venous cannula(e) using an open technique, the patient is placed in slight trendelenburg or supine position. The ECMO/ECLS circuit tubing is clamped and the dressing and/or sutures securing the cannula(e)/tubing to the skin are removed. The vessel is accessed by incising the skin, or opening the previous incision if the cannula was inserted using open technique. The sutures securing the cannula(e) to the vessel are cut. The cannula(e) is withdrawn from the vessel using rapid, steady pressure in a parallel line to the skin. To reduce the risk of air embolism, removal should be done during the inspiratory ventilator phase on an intubated patient. If the patient is conscious and able to follow directions, the cannula should be withdrawn during exhalation or Valsalva. The opening in the vessel is closed with sutures, followed by closure of the skin using sutures or staples, and a sterile dressing is applied.

33985-33986

33985   **Extracorporeal membrane oxygenation (ECMO)/extracorporeal life support (ECLS) provided by physician; removal of central cannula(e) by sternotomy or thoracotomy, birth through 5 years of age**

33986   **Extracorporeal membrane oxygenation (ECMO)/extracorporeal life support (ECLS) provided by physician; removal of central cannula(e) by sternotomy or thoracotomy, 6 years and older**

Extracorporeal membrane oxygenation (ECMO) and extracorporeal life support (ECLS) are interchangeable terms describing long term heart and lung bypass support that circulates blood outside the body through an artificial lung and returns it back to the bloodstream.

To removal a central cannula(e) using a transthoracic approach (sternotomy, thoracotomy), the patient is placed in slight trendelenburg or supine position. The ECMO/ECLS circuit tubing is clamped and the previous chest incision is opened. The cannula(e) and vessel(s) are identified and the stay sutures are cut. The cannula(e) is then withdrawn from the vessel by using rapid, steady pressure. If the patient is intubated and receiving ventilator support, the cannula(e) should be withdrawn during the inspiratory phase to reduce the risk of air embolism. Once the cannula(e) have been removed, the vessel is closed with vascular suture; the fascia is closed with absorbable suture; and the skin is closed with sutures or staples. A sterile dressing is applied. Code 33985 is used when the patient is a newborn through 5 years of age, and code 33986 is used for patients age 6 years and older.

33987

33987   **Arterial exposure with creation of graft conduit (eg, chimney graft) to facilitate arterial perfusion for ECMO/ECLS (List separately in addition to code for primary procedure)**

A graft conduit such as chimney graft may be used to facilitate arterial perfusion when a patient is receiving ECMO/ECLS support. It is most often employed when the arterial vessel(s) are small and/or when limb ischemia develops with cannulation. Antegrade and retrograde blood flow is facilitated by deployment of a covered stent parallel to the EMCO/ECLS cannula(e) in the femoral or axillary vessel(s). The stent protrudes proximally to preserve blood flow to the side branches of the main vessel. A graft conduit can be performed as a planned operation during initial insertion of the ECMO/ECLS cannula(e) or as a rescue procedure to salvage side branches later in therapy. Insertion of a graft conduit usually requires an open (cut down) technique to access the vessel and placement the graft conduit/stent is confirmed using fluoroscopy and/or transesophageal echocardiography (TEE).

33988-33989

33988   **Insertion of left heart vent by thoracic incision (eg, sternotomy, thoracotomy) for ECMO/ECLS**

33989   **Removal of left heart vent by thoracic incision (eg, sternotomy, thoracotomy) for ECMO/ECLS**

Insertion of a left heart vent during ECMO/ECLS (33988) may be necessary to decompress the left ventricle of the heart. During ECMO/ECLS, the inflow comes from the right heart and left ventricle unloading may be incomplete. An incision is made between the ribs to open the chest wall. The ribs are spread apart, and the chest cavity is entered. Likewise, a vertical incision may be made along the sternum, and the bone separated to allow access to the heart and locate the left ventricle. A cannula is inserted into the apex of the left ventricle and secured. The cannula is then connected via tubing to the venous outflow of the ECMO/ECLS circuit. The incision is closed and a sterile dressing is applied. To remove a left heart vent (33989) that has been inserted via sternotomy or thoracotomy, the tubing connecting the vent to the ECMO/ECLS circuit is clamped and the dressing is removed. The previous skin incision is opened to expose the heart. The cannula is removed from the apex of the left ventricle and the opening in the left ventricle is closed with sutures and checked for bleeding. Once adequate hemostasis has been achieved, the muscle, fascia, and skin are closed and a dressing is applied.

33990-33991

33990   **Insertion of ventricular assist device, percutaneous including radiological supervision and interpretation; arterial access only**

33991   **Insertion of ventricular assist device, percutaneous including radiological supervision and interpretation; both arterial and venous access, with transseptal puncture**

A ventricular assist device (VAD) is a mechanical pump that provides circulatory support for patients with heart failure. A VAD functions as a bridge in patients with reversible cardiac output conditions and patients awaiting heart transplantation. It is used as therapy with end-stage heart disease patients who are not candidates for heart transplantation. VADs are most often used to support the left ventricle. VAD insertion can be performed using either a percutaneous or transthoracic approach and the device can be located within the body (intracorporeal) or outside the body (extracorporeally). In 33990, a VAD is placed percutaneously into the left ventricle using a catheter that is introduced through the femoral artery. Using radiological supervision, a catheter containing a very small pump at the tip is advanced from the femoral artery to the aorta, across the aortic valve, and into the left ventricle. Once the VAD is properly positioned in the left ventricle, the small internal pump assists the heart in forcing blood from the left ventricle into the ascending aorta and the peripheral circulatory system. In 33991, a VAD is placed percutaneously using dual cannulation through the femoral vein and femoral artery. Using fluoroscopic guidance, a cannula is threaded from the femoral vein into the right atrium. A transseptal puncture is made between the right and left atria and the cannula is positioned in the left atrium. A second cannula is placed into the right or left femoral artery and secured with sutures. Both cannulas are attached to an external pump. The pump withdraws oxygenated blood from the left atrium, propels it through an outflow port, and returns it to the femoral artery

Cardiovascular System

via the arterial cannula. This allows oxygenated blood to be pumped from the left atrium into the peripheral arterial system via the femoral artery.

33992

33992   Removal of percutaneous ventricular assist device at separate and distinct session from insertion

Before removing a percutaneous ventricular assist device (VAD), the patient is weaned off the device by reducing the blood pump flow rate in measured increments over several hours. Once the rate has been reduced to the minimum allowed, and the patient is observed to be stable, the pump is turned off and the VAD is removed. The exact procedure performed depends on the type of percutaneous VAD. For a percutaneous VAD placed into the left ventricle via the femoral artery, the insertion site is cleansed and prepped and the sutures are clipped. The catheter is pulled back from the left ventricle into the ascending aorta and then completely withdrawn. The arterial sheath can be removed separately, or the catheter and sheath can be removed simultaneously. Hemostasis is achieved at the arterial access site using either manual or mechanical compression. Alternatively, a cutdown may be performed, and the device is removed as described above. Arterial repair is done along with layered closure of the skin and subcutaneous tissue. The incision is covered with a sterile dressing. For a VAD with an external pump and transseptal and femoral artery cannulas, the cannulas are first clamped. The inflow and outflow lines are disconnected from the external pump. The transseptal line is removed, followed by the arterial cannula. Compression is applied to the venous and arterial puncture sites until hemostasis is attained and dressings are applied.

33993

33993   Repositioning of percutaneous ventricular assist device with imaging guidance at separate and distinct session from insertion

A percutaneous ventricular assist device (VAD) supports the heart using a catheter to intercept the blood flow and pump it through an external device which then pumps the blood back into the patient's vessels. Repositioning of a percutaneous ventricular assist device is performed, for example, if the device advances too far and both the inflow and outflow areas are fully in the left ventricle. In these cases, the physician repositions the device by pulling it back slightly. Repositioning is usually performed under fluoroscopic guidance; however some ventricular assist devices include a repositioning sheath for bedside repositioning of the VAD.

34001-34051

34001   Embolectomy or thrombectomy, with or without catheter; carotid, subclavian or innominate artery, by neck incision

34051   Embolectomy or thrombectomy, with or without catheter; innominate, subclavian artery, by thoracic incision

Embolectomy or thrombectomy is performed through a neck incision on the carotid, subclavian, or innominate artery (34001) or the innominate or subclavian artery through a thoracic incision (34051). The procedure may be performed with or without the use of a catheter. An embolus forms at a site remote to the area of obstruction and travels along the artery until it becomes lodged in a smaller vessel. Most emboli in innominate or subclavian arteries arise from the heart and are often associated with a previous myocardial infarction or rheumatic heart disease. A thrombus forms in a narrowed or stenotic portion of the artery. In 34001, an incision is made in the neck to access the affected artery. Vessel loops are placed proximal and distal to embolus or thrombus to control blood flow. The artery is incised and the clot removed directly using arterial backpressure and/or manual massage. Alternatively, remote removal may be performed using a balloon catheter inserted through an arteriotomy distal to the embolus or thrombus. The uninflated balloon catheter is passed beyond the clot, inflated, and then withdrawn capturing and removing the embolus or thrombus. In 34051, an embolus or thrombus in the proximal aspect of the innominate or subclavian artery is removed using a thoracic approach. The affected artery is exposed by median sternotomy. The embolus or thrombus is removed as described above using either a direct approach or a catheter while taking care not to dislodge the clot into the cerebral circulation. Following removal of the embolus or thrombus, an angiography may be performed to ensure that the entire clot has been removed and that the artery is patent.

34101-34111

34101   Embolectomy or thrombectomy, with or without catheter; axillary, brachial, innominate, subclavian artery, by arm incision

34111   Embolectomy or thrombectomy, with or without catheter; radial or ulnar artery, by arm incision

Embolectomy or thrombectomy is performed through an arm incision on the axillary, brachial, innominate or subclavian artery (34101) or the radial or ulnar artery (34111). The procedure may be performed with or without the use of a catheter. An embolus forms at a site remote to the area of obstruction and travels along the artery until it becomes lodged in a smaller vessel. Most emboli in the axillary, brachial, innominate or subclavian arteries arise from the heart and are often associated with a previous myocardial infarction or rheumatic heart disease. A thrombus forms in a narrowed or stenotic portion of the artery. A thrombus in the axillary and brachial arteries may form due to stenosis

or following puncture of the artery for aortography. An incision is made in the arm to access the affected artery. Vessel loops are placed proximal and distal to embolus or thrombus to control blood flow. The artery is incised and the clot removed directly using arterial backpressure and/or manual massage. Alternatively, remote removal may be performed using a balloon catheter inserted through an arteriotomy distal to the embolus or thrombus. The uninflated balloon catheter is passed beyond the clot, inflated, and then withdrawn capturing and removing the embolus or thrombus. Following removal of the embolus or thrombus, an angiography may be performed to ensure that the entire clot has been removed and that the artery is patent.

34151

34151   Embolectomy or thrombectomy, with or without catheter; renal, celiac, mesentery, aortoiliac artery, by abdominal incision

The procedure may be performed with or without the use of a catheter. An embolus forms at a site remote to the area of obstruction and travels along the artery until it becomes lodged in a smaller vessel. A thrombus forms in a narrowed or stenotic portion of the artery. An incision is made in the abdomen and the affected artery exposed and dissected free of surrounding tissue. Vessel loops are placed proximal and distal to embolus or thrombus to control blood flow. The artery is incised and the clot removed directly using arterial backpressure and/or manual massage. Alternatively, remote removal may be performed using a balloon catheter inserted through an arteriotomy distal to the embolus or thrombus. The uninflated balloon catheter is passed beyond the clot, inflated, and then withdrawn capturing and removing the embolus or thrombus. Following removal of the embolus or thrombus, an angiography may be performed to ensure that the entire clot has been removed and that the artery is patent.

34201-34203

34201   Embolectomy or thrombectomy, with or without catheter; femoropopliteal, aortoiliac artery, by leg incision

34203   Embolectomy or thrombectomy, with or without catheter; popliteal-tibio-peroneal artery, by leg incision

Embolectomy or thrombectomy is performed on the femoropopliteal or aortoiliac artery (34201) or the popliteal-tibio-peroneal artery (34203) through a leg incision. The procedure may be performed with or without the use of a catheter. An embolus forms at a site remote to the area of obstruction and travels along the artery until it becomes lodged in a smaller vessel. A thrombus forms in a narrowed or stenotic portion of the artery. An incision is made in the leg or groin to access the affected artery. Vessel loops are placed proximal and distal to embolus or thrombus to control blood flow. The artery is incised and the clot removed directly using arterial backpressure and/or manual massage. Alternatively, remote removal may be performed using a balloon catheter inserted through an arteriotomy distal to the embolus or thrombus. The uninflated balloon catheter is passed beyond the clot, inflated, and then withdrawn capturing and removing the embolus or thrombus. Following removal of the embolus or thrombus, an angiography may be performed to ensure that the entire clot has been removed and that the artery is patent.

34401-34451

34401   Thrombectomy, direct or with catheter; vena cava, iliac vein, by abdominal incision

34421   Thrombectomy, direct or with catheter; vena cava, iliac, femoropopliteal vein, by leg incision

34451   Thrombectomy, direct or with catheter; vena cava, iliac, femoropopliteal vein, by abdominal and leg incision

Thrombectomy is performed on the vena cava, iliac vein, or femoropopliteal vein using an abdominal and/or leg incision. The procedure may be performed with or without the use of a catheter. A thrombus forms in a narrowed or stenotic portion of the artery. An incision in made in the abdomen and/or leg or groin to expose and access the planned venotomy site. Vessel loops are placed proximal and distal to the thrombus to control blood flow. The vein is incised and thrombus removed by direct exposure. Alternatively, remote removal may be performed using a balloon catheter inserted through a venotomy at a site beyond the thrombus. The uninflated balloon catheter is passed beyond the clot, inflated, and then withdrawn capturing and removing thrombus. Following removal of the thrombus, a venography may be performed to ensure that the entire clot has been removed and that the vein is patent. Use 34401 when a thrombus in the vena cava or iliac vein is removed via an abdominal incision. When the thrombus is in the vena cava, iliac vein, or femoropopliteal vein, use 34421 when a leg incision is used to access the thrombus, and 34451 when both abdominal and leg incisions are used.

34471-34490

34471   Thrombectomy, direct or with catheter; subclavian vein, by neck incision

34490   Thrombectomy, direct or with catheter; axillary and subclavian vein, by arm incision

Thrombectomy is performed on the subclavian or axillary vein using a neck or arm incision. The procedure may be performed with or without the use of a catheter. A thrombus forms in a narrowed or stenotic portion of the artery. An incision in made in the neck or arm

Cardiovascular System

to expose and access the planned venotomy site. Vessel loops are placed proximal and distal to the thrombus to control blood flow. The vein is incised and the thrombus removed by direct exposure. Alternatively, remote removal may be performed using a balloon catheter inserted through a venotomy at a site beyond the thrombus. The uninflated balloon catheter is passed beyond the clot, inflated, and then withdrawn capturing and removing thrombus. Following removal of the thrombus, a venography may be performed to ensure that the entire clot has been removed and that the vein is patent. Use 34471 when a thrombus in the subclavian vein is removed via a neck incision and 34490 when a thrombus in the subclavian or axillary vein is removed by an arm incision.

34501

34501   Valvuloplasty, femoral vein

This procedure is used in patients with valvular incompetence and resulting venous ulceration. The femoral vein is exposed and the adventitia dissected so that the location of valve commissures can be identified. A marking suture is placed in the commissure of the faulty valve. A longitudinal incision is made in the vein from a point distal to the valve and carried through the marking sulture to a point proximal to the valve. The vein is laid open and retention sutures placed in the four corners to provide traction and maintain exposure of the valve. The incompetent valve leaflets are repaired restoring the normal cup-like configuration. The femoral vein is closed and overlying tissues repaired with sutures.

34502

34502   Reconstruction of vena cava, any method

Malignant invasion of the vena cava is the most frequent indication for resection and reconstruction. Other indications include saccular aneurysms, primary malformations, and traumatic injury. The approach depends on whether the superior or inferior vena cava is being reconstructed and on the exact location of the lesion, defect, malformation or injury. Resection and reconstruction may involve direct suture repair for a minimal defect, an interposition graft for a longitudinal resection or a tubular graft if a segment of the vessel is excised. The vena cava is exposed. If the resection is for malignant invasion, the lesion is excised along with a margin of healthy tissue. If there is an aneurysm, malformation, or traumatic injury the involved segment of vena cava is excised. The vena cava is then repaired using running suture or a vascular stapler, or a patch or tubular graft composed of synthetic material, bovine pericardium, or a pericardium from the patient.

34510

34510   Venous valve transposition, any vein donor

Venous valve transposition is performed using any vein donor to treat severe venous insufficiency. An incision is made, usually in the arm, over the healthy vein to obtain a portion containing a normal functioning valve. A segment of vein containing one or two normal functioning valves is dissected free of surrounding tissue. The vein is suture ligated and divided proximal and distal to the healthy vein segment which is removed and prepared for transposition. An incision is made over the affected vein which is usually in the leg. The vein is dissected free of surrounding tissue. Vascular clamps are placed above and below the segment containing the malfunctioning valve and the diseased vein segment is divided and removed. The healthy segment of vein containing the functioning valve is then sutured to the remaining ends of the vein that had the malfunctioning valve. Vascular clamps are released and blood flow evaluated. The skin incision is then repaired in layers.

34520

34520   Cross-over vein graft to venous system

A cross-over vein graft to the venous system is used to shunt blood around obstructed veins in one leg to patent veins in the other. An incision is made below the region of obstruction over the affected vein on the symptomatic side. A second incision is made in the groin on the opposite side and a subcutaneous tunnel is the created across the suprapubic region and extended as needed along the subsartorial region of the symptomatic side. The saphenous vein on the patent side is then dissected free of surrounding tissue and its tributaries ligated. Once a sufficient length of saphenous vein has been freed, the distal aspect is divided. The saphenous vein on the patent side is tunneled to a point below the obstruction on the symptomatic side. The obstructed vein is clamped and incised at a point below the obstruction. An end-to-side anastomosis of the saphenous vein to the obstructed vein is performed.

34530

34530   Saphenopopliteal vein anastomosis

A saphenopopliteal vein anastomosis is performed. An incision is made in the skin over the saphenous vein. The saphenous vein is dissected free of surrounding tissue and its tributies ligated. Once a sufficient length of saphenous vein has been freed, the distal aspect is divided. The saphenous vein is tunneled to the popliteal vein. The obstructed popliteal vein is clamped and incised at a point below the obstruction. An end-to-side anastomosis of the saphenous vein to the obstructed popliteal vein is performed.

34800

34800   Endovascular repair of infrarenal abdominal aortic aneurysm or dissection; using aorto-aortic tube prosthesis

Endovascular repair of an infrarenal abdominal aortic aneurysm or dissection is performed using an aorto-aortic tube prosthesis. This type of prosthesis is comprised of a single component that covers only the aorta. An incision is made in the groin over the femoral artery. A trocar is placed and a guide wire is advanced from the femoral artery through the external and common iliac arteries into the aorta. The guide wire is then advanced through the aneurysm to a point just above the renal arteries. A second guide wire and catheter may be introduced to mark the lower renal artery. An introducer sheath containing the compressed aorto-aortic tube prosthesis is then advanced over the guide wire and positioned in the aorta with the proximal edge below the renal arteries but above the top of the aneurysm defect with the distal edge below the bottom of the defect. If a second catheter has been placed at the lower renal artery, it is withdrawn. The prosthesis is then deployed (expanded) under separately reportable fluoroscopic guidance. Correct placement is verified fluoroscopically. The introducer sheath is removed and a balloon catheter is introduced and expanded to seat (secure) the proximal and distal ends of the prosthesis. The balloon catheter is removed and a pigtail or sidehole catheter is introduced over the guide wire. Angiography is performed to evaluate endograft position, patency of the renal and hypogastric arteries, and to ensure that there are no endoleaks. Patency of lumbar and inferior mesenteric arteries is also checked. Catheters and guide wires are removed and the groin incision is closed.

34802-34803

34802   Endovascular repair of infrarenal abdominal aortic aneurysm or dissection; using modular bifurcated prosthesis (1 docking limb)
34803   Endovascular repair of infrarenal abdominal aortic aneurysm or dissection; using modular bifurcated prosthesis (2 docking limbs)

Endovascular repair of an infrarenal abdominal aortic aneurysm or dissection is performed using a modular bifurcated prosthesis with one (34802) or two (34803) docking limbs. The prosthesis described by 34802 has two separate pieces. The main component covers the aorta and one iliac artery, and a separate component (docking limb) joined to the main component covers the contralateral iliac artery. The prosthesis described by 34803 has three separate pieces: a main component that covers the aorta, and two separate components (docking limbs) joined to the main component and cover the iliac arteries. An incision is made in the groin over the femoral artery. A trocar is placed and a guide wire is advanced from the femoral artery through the external and common iliac arteries into the aorta. The guide wire is then advanced through the aneurysm to a point just above the renal arteries. A second guide wire and catheter may be introduced to mark the lower renal artery. A roadmapping angiogram is obtained prior to introduction of the prosthesis. The contralateral femoral artery is exposed, and a sheath and catheter with a snare system are placed to facilitate placement of the docking limb. An introducer sheath containing the compressed main component of the bifurcated prosthesis is then advanced over the guide wire and positioned in the aorta with the proximal edge below the renal arteries but above the top of the aneurysm defect with the distal edge below the bottom of the defect. If a second catheter has been placed at the lower renal artery, it is withdrawn. The main component is then deployed (expanded) under separately reportable fluoroscopic guidance. Correct placement is verified fluoroscopically. The introducer sheath is removed and a balloon catheter is introduced and expanded to seat (secure) the proximal and distal ends of the prosthesis. The guide wire is left in place within the endograft on the ipsilateral side while the docking limb is placed on the contralateral side. In 34802, a single docking limb is placed on the contralateral side. The guide wire in the contralateral groin is advanced into the docking port. The introducer sheath containing the docking limb is introduced over the contralateral guide wire and firmly seated in the docking port. The distal end of the limb is positioned in the iliac artery just beyond the aneurysm in a segment of normal diameter. Correct position is confirmed fluoroscopically, the sheath is removed, and the limb is deployed. In 34803, a second docking limb is placed on the ipsilateral side using the same technique. The balloon catheter is removed and a pigtail or sidehole catheter is introduced over the guide wire. Angiography is performed to evaluate endograft position, patency of renal and hypogastric arteries, and to ensure that there are no endoleaks. Patency of lumbar and inferior mesenteric arteries is also checked. Catheters and guide wires are removed and the groin incisions are closed.

34804

34804   Endovascular repair of infrarenal abdominal aortic aneurysm or dissection; using unibody bifurcated prosthesis

Endovascular repair of an infrarenal abdominal aortic aneurysm or dissection is performed using a unibody bifurcated prosthesis. An incision is made in the groin over the femoral artery. A trocar is placed and a guide wire is advanced from the femoral artery through the external and common iliac arteries into the aorta. The guide wire is then advanced through the aneurysm to a point just above the renal arteries. A second guide wire and catheter may be introduced to mark the lower renal artery. A roadmapping angiogram is obtained prior to introducing the prosthesis. The contralateral femoral artery is exposed, and a sheath and catheter with a snare system is placed to facilitate capture of the contralateral

Cardiovascular System

iliac limb. An introducer sheath containing the compressed unibody bifurcated prosthesis is then introduced. Introduction of the sheath requires a large incision in the femoral artery due to the size of the unibody sheath, which is advanced over the guide wire and positioned in the aorta with the proximal edge below the renal arteries but above the top of the aneurysm defect. The distal edge should lie below the bottom of the aneurysm defect in the ipsilateral iliac artery. If a second catheter has been placed at the lower renal artery, it is withdrawn. The main component is then deployed (expanded) under separately reportable fluoroscopic guidance. Correct placement is verified fluoroscopically. The introducer sheath is removed and a balloon catheter is introduced and expanded to seat (secure) the proximal and distal ends of the prosthesis. The guide wire in the contralateral groin has already been snared and exits on the ipsilateral side. This wire is retracted and the iliac limb is pulled across the aortic bifurcation into the iliac artery. The distal end of the limb is positioned in the iliac artery just beyond the aneurysm in a segment of normal diameter. Correct position is confirmed fluoroscopically. The contralateral iliac limb is deployed and then seated using a balloon catheter, which is then removed. A pigtail or sidehole catheter is introduced over the guide wire. Angiography is performed to evaluate endograft position, patency of renal and hypogastric arteries, and to ensure that there are no endoleaks. Patency of lumbar and inferior mesenteric arteries is also checked. Catheters and guide wires are removed and the groin incisions are closed.

34805

34805   Endovascular repair of infrarenal abdominal aortic aneurysm or dissection; using aorto-uniiliac or aorto-unifemoral prosthesis

Endovascular repair of an infrarenal abdominal aortic aneurysm or dissection is performed using an aorto-uni-iliac or aorto-unifemoral prosthesis. These types of prostheses are used to treat an aortic aneurysm that extends into a single iliac artery or into both the iliac and femoral arteries on one side. The shapes of these prostheses are similar to an aorto-aortic tube prosthesis except that they are longer and tapered to provide coverage of the defect in the iliac and femoral arteries. An incision is made in the groin over the femoral artery. A trocar is placed and a guide wire is advanced from the femoral artery through the external and common iliac arteries into the aorta. The guide wire is then advanced through the aneurysm to a point just above the renal arteries. A second guide wire and catheter may be introduced to mark the lower renal artery. An introducer sheath containing the compressed aorto-uni-iliac or aorto-unifemoral prosthesis is then advanced over the guide wire and positioned in the aorta with the proximal edge below the renal arteries but above the top of the aneurysm defect. The distal edge should lie below the bottom of the defect in either the iliac or femoral artery. If a second catheter has been placed at the lower renal artery, it is withdrawn. The prosthesis is then deployed (expanded) under separately reportable fluoroscopic guidance. Deployment is performed in sections beginning in the aorta. Once that portion has been deployed and coverage of the aortic aneurysm is verified, the iliac and femoral portions are deployed. Correct placement is verified fluoroscopically. The introducer sheath is removed and a balloon catheter is introduced and expanded to seat (secure) the proximal and distal ends of the prosthesis. The balloon catheter is removed and a pigtail or sidehole catheter is introduced over the guide wire. Angiography is performed to evaluate endograft position, patency of renal and hypogastric arteries, and to ensure that there are no endoleaks. Patency of lumbar and inferior mesenteric arteries is also checked. Catheters and guide wires are removed and the groin incision is closed.

34806

34806   Transcatheter placement of wireless physiologic sensor in aneurysmal sac during endovascular repair, including radiological supervision and interpretation, instrument calibration, and collection of pressure data (List separately in addition to code for primary procedure)

A highly specialized wireless physiologic sensor the size of a grain of rice is placed in the aneurysmal sac during separately reportable transcatheter endovascular repair of an abdominal aortic aneurysm (AAA). This sensor measures pressure inside the aorta following the AAA repair. Even after repair, complications can arise when the aneurysmal sac is not completely isolated. This can cause recurrent pressurization and endoleaks. The sensor measures pressure, flow, and temperature, and allows for direct, noninvasive monitoring for the risk of rupture. The device uses acoustic waves, which transmit effectively through soft tissue, bone, and fluid without being absorbed, and requires very little energy for a high signal-to-noise ratio when accessing deep locations in the body. There is no battery, no antenna, and no connecting leads. The device incorporates a special external unit that powers the implant and receives information directly from the implant. The sensor is placed using an introducer catheter and guidewire. The guidewire is positioned outside the main body of the endograft. The sensor delivery system is advanced over the guidewire and the sensor is carefully positioned in the aneurysmal sac under fluoroscopic guidance. The delivery system is withdrawn. The sensor is maintained in position by a tether and then calibrated. Two measurements are taken. The pre-exclusion measurement is taken prior to placement of the endovascular stent. Following stent placement, the sensor is released from the tether and the post-exclusion measurement is taken. The position of the sensor is again checked to verify that it is still in the correct location at the top of the aneurysmal sac. This code included the necessary radiological supervision and interpretation,

instrument calibration, and collection of pressure data related to placing the physiological sensor.

34808

34808   Endovascular placement of iliac artery occlusion device (List separately in addition to code for primary procedure)

Endovascular placement of an iliac artery occlusion device is performed prior to endovascular repair of an abdominal aortic aneurysm. This procedure is performed when one iliac artery is patent and the other has occlusive disease. The occluded artery is first treated with a separately reportable femoral-femoral prosthetic graft at a previous or the current surgical session. An occlusion device must then be placed to prevent retrograde flow from the diseased bypassed iliac artery into the aneurysm sac. The introducer device with the occluder is advanced under fluoroscopic guidance over a previously placed guide wire into the diseased artery. The occluder device is deployed after the correct position is verified. Hand injection of contrast is performed to verify its correct position as well as complete arterial occlusion. Additional embolization materials are injected as needed until complete occlusion of the artery is accomplished. The introducer is removed and separately reportable endovascular repair of the abdominal aortic aneurysm is then performed.

34812

34812   Open femoral artery exposure for delivery of endovascular prosthesis, by groin incision, unilateral

The femoral artery is exposed to allow delivery of the endovascular device using a unilateral groin incision. The skin over the groin is incised. Subcutaneous tissue is dissected down to the common femoral artery taking care to protect the femoral nerve and vein. The common, superficial, and deep femoral arteries are dissected free of surrounding tissue and captured with vessel loops. The distal external iliac artery may also be dissected which requires retraction and/or division of the inguinal ligament. Small branch arteries are ligated or cauterized. The femoral artery is clamped and incised to allow introduction of guide wires and sheaths. This is a unilateral procedure.

34813

34813   Placement of femoral-femoral prosthetic graft during endovascular aortic aneurysm repair (List separately in addition to code for primary procedure)

A femoral-femoral prosthetic graft is placed at the time of a separately reportable abdominal aortic aneurysm endovascular repair. This procedure is performed when one iliac artery is patent and the other has occlusive disease. A tunneling device is used to create an arched subcutaneous tunnel extending from the patent femoral artery, across the abdomen, to the occluded femoral artery. An appropriate sized conduit is selected and pulled through the tunnel. Following administration of heparin, the femoral arteries are clamped bilaterally. The common femoral artery is incised on one side and the conduit is anastomosed. The common femoral artery is incised on the opposite side and the graft is again anastomosed. Vascular clamps are removed and blood flow through the graft is checked with handheld Doppler.

34820

34820   Open iliac artery exposure for delivery of endovascular prosthesis or iliac occlusion during endovascular therapy, by abdominal or retroperitoneal incision, unilateral

The iliac artery is exposed by abdominal or retroperitoneal incision for separately reportable delivery of endovascular prosthesis or iliac occlusion device during endovascular abdominal aortic aneurysm repair. The skin is incised in the lower abdomen or retroperitoneum and tissue is dissected into the pelvis to expose the iliac artery, taking care to protect veins, nerves, and the ureter. Arterial branches are dissected and bleeding is controlled with ligation or electrocautery. The iliac artery is dissected free of surrounding tissue and secured with vessel loops. The iliac artery is then clamped and incised to allow introduction of guide wires and sheaths. Following completion of the endovascular or iliac occlusion procedure, the artery is repaired and the skin and soft tissue incision is closed in layers. This is a unilateral procedure.

34825-34826

34825   Placement of proximal or distal extension prosthesis for endovascular repair of infrarenal abdominal aortic or iliac aneurysm, false aneurysm, or dissection; initial vessel

34826   Placement of proximal or distal extension prosthesis for endovascular repair of infrarenal abdominal aortic or iliac aneurysm, false aneurysm, or dissection; each additional vessel (List separately in addition to code for primary procedure)

A proximal or distal extension prosthesis is placed in the aorta or iliac artery for endovascular repair of an aortic or iliac aneurysm, false aneurysm, or dissection. An extension prosthesis is used when the main endograft component(s) are found to be too short. This is typically identified as an endoleak during the endograft repair and the extension components are placed during the same surgical session; however, endoleaks

Cardiovascular System

may also be identified postoperatively and the extension prostheses placed during a separate surgical session. The sheath containing the extension prosthesis is advanced over a guide wire and the extension prosthesis is positioned at the site of the endoleak. Correct placement is first confirmed using fluoroscopy and then the extension prosthesis is deployed and seated using a balloon catheter. Contrast is injected to verify that the endoleak is sealed. Use 34825 for placement of an extension prosthesis in the initial vessel and code 34826 for each additional vessel treated.

34830-34832

34830 Open repair of infrarenal aortic aneurysm or dissection, plus repair of associated arterial trauma, following unsuccessful endovascular repair; tube prosthesis

34831 Open repair of infrarenal aortic aneurysm or dissection, plus repair of associated arterial trauma, following unsuccessful endovascular repair; aorto-bi-iliac prosthesis

34832 Open repair of infrarenal aortic aneurysm or dissection, plus repair of associated arterial trauma, following unsuccessful endovascular repair; aorto-bifemoral prosthesis

Open repair of an infrarenal aortic aneurysm or dissection including repair of associated arterial trauma is performed following unsuccessful endovascular repair. Complications related to previous endovascular repair include: endoleaks, dissection, occlusion of major aortic branches or occlusion of aortic or iliac blood flow. An abdominal incision is made and the aorta and iliac/femoral vessels are exposed to points above and below the level of the prosthesis. After administration of intravenous heparin and placement of vascular clamps, the aneurysm is opened and any thrombus is removed. Lodged pieces of the endograft are removed. The prosthesis is then sutured to untraumatized aorta above the aneurysm at the proximal end. Vascular flow is checked and additional sutures are placed as needed. The distal end of the prosthesis in the aorta or iliac/femoral artery(s) is repaired in the same fashion; vascular flow is checked; and additional sutures are placed as needed. Vascular clamps are removed; anticoagulation is reversed; bleeding is controlled; and the surgical wound is closed. Use code 34830 for open repair of a tube prosthesis, 34831 for an aorto-bi-iliac prosthesis, and 34832 for an aorto-bifemoral prosthesis.

34833

34833 Open iliac artery exposure with creation of conduit for delivery of aortic or iliac endovascular prosthesis, by abdominal or retroperitoneal incision, unilateral

The iliac artery is exposed and a conduit is created for delivery of an aortic or iliac endovascular prosthesis by abdominal or retroperitoneal incision. The skin is incised in the lower abdomen or retroperitoneum and tissue is dissected into the pelvis to expose the iliac artery, taking care to protect veins, nerves, and the ureter. Arterial branches are dissected and bleeding is controlled with ligation or electrocautery. The iliac artery is dissected free of surrounding tissue for a length of 5-6 cm and secured with vessel loops. The iliac artery is clamped and incised longitudinally. A conduit is selected and tailored to the appropriate configurations and anastomosed to the iliac artery. The conduit is then clamped; the previously placed clamps are removed from the iliac artery; and any vascular leaks at the anastomosis site are reinforced with sutures. Following completion of the endovascular procedure, the conduit may be left in place and the distal end anastomosed to the iliac artery or the conduit may be removed and the iliac artery repaired. This is a unilateral procedure.

34834

34834 Open brachial artery exposure to assist in the deployment of aortic or iliac endovascular prosthesis by arm incision, unilateral

The brachial artery is exposed by an arm incision to assist in the deployment of an aortic or iliac endovascular prosthesis. The upper arm is incised, taking care to protect and mobilize surrounding nerves and blood vessels. The brachial artery is dissected free of surrounding tissue for a length of 5-6 cm and secured with vessel loops. The brachial artery is incised and guide wires, sheaths, and catheters are placed as needed to assist with deployment of the aortic or iliac endovascular prosthesis. Following completion of the procedure, the brachial artery is repaired and the surgical wound is repaired in layers. This is a unilateral procedure.

34839

34839 Physician planning of a patient-specific fenestrated visceral aortic endograft requiring a minimum of 90 minutes of physician time

Fenestrated visceral aortic endograft placement is a complex procedure used for aortic aneurysm repair. The vascular surgeon, interventional radiologist, general surgeon, or interventional cardiologist must carefully review angiograms and other available diagnostic tests on the patient, select the proper graft for the individual physiology, and plan the procedure accordingly. Endograft repair of an aortic aneurysm is a minimally invasive technique that provides a more stable repair when compared to operating directly on the vessel. The size and location of the aortic disease has to be identified. The size and type of endograft must be carefully selected so that the fenestrations (holes) match up with the natural visceral ostia or openings that branch into other vessels, including the renal arteries, internal iliac arteries, and/or the aortic arch. A minimum of 90 physician minutes is spent in patient-specific planning.

34841-34844

34841 Endovascular repair of visceral aorta (eg, aneurysm, pseudoaneurysm, dissection, penetrating ulcer, intramural hematoma, or traumatic disruption) by deployment of a fenestrated visceral aortic endograft and all associated radiological supervision and interpretation, including target zone angioplasty, when performed; including one visceral artery endoprosthesis (superior mesenteric, celiac or renal artery)

34842 Endovascular repair of visceral aorta (eg, aneurysm, pseudoaneurysm, dissection, penetrating ulcer, intramural hematoma, or traumatic disruption) by deployment of a fenestrated visceral aortic endograft and all associated radiological supervision and interpretation, including target zone angioplasty, when performed; including two visceral artery endoprostheses (superior mesenteric, celiac and/or renal artery[s])

34843 Endovascular repair of visceral aorta (eg, aneurysm, pseudoaneurysm, dissection, penetrating ulcer, intramural hematoma, or traumatic disruption) by deployment of a fenestrated visceral aortic endograft and all associated radiological supervision and interpretation, including target zone angioplasty, when performed; including three visceral artery endoprostheses (superior mesenteric, celiac and/or renal artery[s])

34844 Endovascular repair of visceral aorta (eg, aneurysm, pseudoaneurysm, dissection, penetrating ulcer, intramural hematoma, or traumatic disruption) by deployment of a fenestrated visceral aortic endograft and all associated radiological supervision and interpretation, including target zone angioplasty, when performed; including four or more visceral artery endoprostheses (superior mesenteric, celiac and/or renal artery[s])

Endovascular repair of the visceral abdominal aorta is performed using a fenestrated aortic endograft. These types of prostheses are used to treat an aortic defect that extends into or above the visceral artery branches. Fenestrated endografts have holes at the ostia of the superior mesenteric, celiac and/or renal arteries to allow blood flow into these branches. An incision is made in the groin over the femoral artery. A trocar is placed and a guide wire is advanced from the femoral artery through the external and common iliac arteries into the aorta. The guide wire is then advanced through the defect to a point just above the proximal aspect of the defect. A second guide wire and catheter may be introduced. An introducer sheath containing the compressed aortic endograft is then advanced over the guide wire and positioned in the aorta with the proximal edge above the involved visceral arteries and above the top of the defect. The distal edge of the endograft should lie below the bottom of the defect in the aorta. If a second catheter has been placed, it is withdrawn. The prosthesis is then deployed (expanded) under separately reportable fluoroscopic guidance taking care to ensure that the fenestrations in the endograft lie over the involved visceral vessels. The aortic portion is deployed and coverage of the aortic defect is verified fluoroscopically. The introducer sheath is removed and a balloon catheter is introduced and expanded to seat (secure) the proximal and distal ends of the prosthesis. Stents are then placed through the ostia of the involved visceral arteries and a balloon catheter is used to seat the stents. The balloon catheter is removed and a pigtail or sidehole catheter is introduced over the guide wire. Angiography is performed to evaluate endograft and stent position, patency of superior mesenteric, celiac, and renal arteries, and to ensure that there are no endoleaks. Catheters and guide wires are removed and the groin incision is closed. Use 34841 for placement of an aortic endograft and a single visceral artery endoprosthesis (stent); use 34842 when two visceral arteries are involved with stent placement; use 34843 when three visceral arteries require stent placement; and 34844 for four or more visceral artery endoprostheses.

Cardiovascular System

34845-34848

34845 Endovascular repair of visceral aorta and infrarenal abdominal aorta (eg, aneurysm, pseudoaneurysm, dissection, penetrating ulcer, intramural hematoma, or traumatic disruption) with a fenestrated visceral aortic endograft and concomitant unibody or modular infrarenal aortic endograft and all associated radiological supervision and interpretation, including target zone angioplasty, when performed; including one visceral artery endoprosthesis (superior mesenteric, celiac or renal artery)

34846 Endovascular repair of visceral aorta and infrarenal abdominal aorta (eg, aneurysm, pseudoaneurysm, dissection, penetrating ulcer, intramural hematoma, or traumatic disruption) with a fenestrated visceral aortic endograft and concomitant unibody or modular infrarenal aortic endograft and all associated radiological supervision and interpretation, including target zone angioplasty, when performed; including two visceral artery endoprostheses (superior mesenteric, celiac and/or renal artery[s])

34847 Endovascular repair of visceral aorta and infrarenal abdominal aorta (eg, aneurysm, pseudoaneurysm, dissection, penetrating ulcer, intramural hematoma, or traumatic disruption) with a fenestrated visceral aortic endograft and concomitant unibody or modular infrarenal aortic endograft and all associated radiological supervision and interpretation, including target zone angioplasty, when performed; including three visceral artery endoprostheses (superior mesenteric, celiac and/or renal artery[s])

34848 Endovascular repair of visceral aorta and infrarenal abdominal aorta (eg, aneurysm, pseudoaneurysm, dissection, penetrating ulcer, intramural hematoma, or traumatic disruption) with a fenestrated visceral aortic endograft and concomitant unibody or modular infrarenal aortic endograft and all associated radiological supervision and interpretation, including target zone angioplasty, when performed; including four or more visceral artery endoprostheses (superior mesenteric, celiac and/or renal artery[s])

Endovascular repair of the visceral aorta and infrarenal abdominal aorta is performed using a fenestrated visceral aortic endograft and concomitant unibody or modular infrarenal aortic endograft. Fenestrated endografts have holes at the ostia of the superior mesenteric, celiac, and/or renal arteries to allow blood flow into these branches. An incision is made in the groin over the femoral artery. A trocar is placed and a guide wire is advanced from the femoral artery through the external and common iliac arteries into the aorta. The guide wire is then advanced through the defect to a point just above the proximal aspect of the defect. A second guide wire and catheter may be introduced. An introducer sheath containing the compressed aortic endograft is then advanced over the guide wire and positioned in the aorta with the proximal edge above the involved visceral arteries and above the top of the defect. The distal edge of the endograft should lie below the bottom of the defect in the visceral aorta. Both a visceral aortic endograft and another unibody or modular infrarenal endograft placed in the same manner are used to completely cover the entire defect. If a second catheter has been placed, it is withdrawn. The prosthesis is then deployed (expanded) under separately reportable fluoroscopic guidance taking care to ensure that the fenestrations in the visceral portion of the endograft lie over the involved visceral vessels. Deployment is performed in sections beginning in the visceral aorta. Once that portion has been deployed and coverage of the visceral aortic defect is verified, the infrarenal portion is deployed. Complete coverage of the aortic defect is verified fluoroscopically. The introducer sheath is removed and a balloon catheter is introduced and expanded to seat (secure) the proximal and distal portions of the prostheses. Stents are then placed through the ostia of the involved visceral arteries and a balloon catheter is used to seat the stents. The balloon catheter is removed and a pigtail or sidehole catheter is introduced over the guide wire. Angiography is performed to evaluate endograft and stent position, patency of superior mesenteric, celiac, and renal arteries, and to ensure that there are no endoleaks. Patency of lumbar and inferior mesenteric arteries is also checked. Catheters and guide wires are removed and the groin incision is closed. Use 34845 for placement of a visceral aortic endograft together with an infrarenal abdominal aortic endograft and a single visceral artery endoprosthesis (stent). Use 34846 when two visceral arteries also require stent placement; use 34847 when three visceral arteries are involved; and 34848 for four or more visceral artery endoprostheses.

34900

34900 Endovascular repair of iliac artery (eg, aneurysm, pseudoaneurysm, arteriovenous malformation, trauma) using ilio-iliac tube endoprosthesis

Endovascular graft placement is performed to repair an isolated iliac artery aneurysm, false aneurysm, arteriovenous malformation, or traumatic injury. The ipsilateral (same side) femoral artery is exposed and incised. A guide wire is introduced and advanced to a point just above the proximal aspect of the iliac artery defect. An introducer sheath containing the endovascular graft is advanced over the guide wire and positioned over the iliac artery defect under fluoroscopic guidance. Correct position of the endograft is verified fluoroscopically and the guide wire is removed. The sheath is then removed and the endograft is deployed. A balloon catheter is used as needed to seat the endograft. The balloon catheter is removed and a pigtail or sidehole catheter is introduced over the guide wire. Angiography is performed to evaluate endograft position and to ensure that there are no endoleaks. Catheters and guide wires are removed and the groin incision is closed.

35001-35002

35001 Direct repair of aneurysm, pseudoaneurysm, or excision (partial or total) and graft insertion, with or without patch graft; for aneurysm and associated occlusive disease, carotid, subclavian artery, by neck incision

35002 Direct repair of aneurysm, pseudoaneurysm, or excision (partial or total) and graft insertion, with or without patch graft; for ruptured aneurysm, carotid, subclavian artery, by neck incision

A carotid or subclavian artery aneurysm or pseudoaneurysm including any associated occlusive disease is surgically repaired using direct repair or excision with graft insertion with or without a patch graft via a neck incision. An aneurysm is an abnormal enlargement or dilatation of an artery. Aneurysms may be caused by arteriosclerosis, a mechanical obstruction of the artery such as thoracic outlet syndrome, or malposition of the artery. Other less common causes include syphilis, tuberculosis, and abnormalities of the vessel wall such as fibromuscular dysplasia. A pseudoaneurysm differs from a true aneurysm in that it does not involve all three layers of the artery wall. A pseudoaneurysm is typically the result of blunt or penetrating trauma or a complication of a procedure such as a puncture during a catheterization procedure. The trauma results in formation of a pulsating, encapsulated hematoma in direct communication with the wall of the artery. If a saphenous vein graft is to be used, the lower leg is prepped and the vein graft harvested. An incision is made in the neck. When repairing the subclavian artery, a portion of the clavicle may be excised to allow better access to the artery. Overlying soft tissues (platysma and/or scalene muscles) are divided taking care to protect the phrenic nerve. The underlying common carotid, internal carotid, external carotid, or subclavian artery is exposed. The subclavian, common carotid, and innominate arteries are clamped as needed. The aneurysm sac is opened and thrombus and plaque removed. The artery walls are suture repaired and an autogenous (saphenous vein) or synthetic patch graft applied as needed. Another technique is to excise the aneurysm with direct repair by end-to-end anastomosis of the distal and proximal vessel ends with or without insertion of a patch graft. A third technique is to place an autogenous (saphenous vein) or synthetic tube graft. A longitudinal incision is made in the artery. The tube graft is inserted and sutured to healthy artery distal and proximal to the aneurysm. The aneurysm sac is then closed over the graft. When the repair is completed, the clamps are released and blood flow re-established. In 35001, an aneurysm or pseudoaneurysm is repaired in a nonemergent, elective procedure. In 35002 a ruptured aneurysm is repaired which differs in that an emergency procedure is performed and bleeding from the ruptured aneurysm must be isolated and controlled prior to the aneurysm repair.

35005

35005 Direct repair of aneurysm, pseudoaneurysm, or excision (partial or total) and graft insertion, with or without patch graft; for aneurysm, pseudoaneurysm, and associated occlusive disease, vertebral artery

A vertebral artery aneurysm or pseudoaneurysm, including any associated occlusive disease, is surgically repaired using direct repair or excision with graft insertion with or without a patch graft via an arm incision. An aneurysm is an abnormal enlargement or dilatation of an artery that may be caused by arteriosclerosis, mechanical obstruction, or malposition of the artery. Other less common causes include syphilis, tuberculosis, and abnormalities of the vessel wall such as fibromuscular dysplasia. A pseudoaneurysm differs from a true aneurysm in that it does not involve all three layers of the arterial wall. A pseudoaneurysm is typically the result of blunt or penetrating trauma or a complication of a procedure such as a puncture during catheterization. The trauma results in formation of a pulsating, encapsulated hematoma in direct communication with the wall of the artery. If a saphenous vein graft is to be used, the lower leg is prepped and the vein graft is harvested. Repair of the proximal vertebral artery may be performed through a supraclavicular incision carried down to the sternal notch. The clavicle is divided as needed. The anterior scalene muscle is exposed and divided taking care to protect the phrenic nerve. Vertebral nerve fibers are divided and the vertebral artery is exposed and mobilized. Repair of the distal vertebral artery may be performed through an anterolateral approach in which the sternocleidomastoid is detached from the mastoid process and wide exposure of the vertebral artery is achieved by extension of the incision to the sternal notch. An anterior approach may also be used in which the mandible is retracted. Soft tissues are meticulously dissected to allow preservation of the parotid gland as well as the facial and spinal accessory nerves. The segment of vertebral artery to be repaired is exposed. The vertebral artery and segmental branches are clamped as needed. The aneurysm sac is opened and thrombus and plaque are removed. The artery walls are suture repaired and an autogenous (saphenous vein) or synthetic patch graft is applied as needed. Another technique is to excise the aneurysm with direct repair by end-to-end anastomosis of the distal and proximal vessel ends with or without insertion of a patch graft. A third technique is to place an autogenous or synthetic tube graft. A longitudinal incision is made in the artery. The tube graft is inserted and sutured to healthy artery distal and proximal to the aneurysm. The aneurysm sac is then closed over the graft. When the repair is completed, the clamps are released and blood flow is re-established.

Cardiovascular System

● New Code   ▲ Revised Code

35011-35013

35011 Direct repair of aneurysm, pseudoaneurysm, or excision (partial or total) and graft insertion, with or without patch graft; for aneurysm and associated occlusive disease, axillary-brachial artery, by arm incision

35013 Direct repair of aneurysm, pseudoaneurysm, or excision (partial or total) and graft insertion, with or without patch graft; for ruptured aneurysm, axillary-brachial artery, by arm incision

An axillary-brachial artery aneurysm or pseudoaneurysm including any associated occlusive disease is surgically repaired using direct repair or excision with graft insertion with or without a patch graft via an arm incision. An aneurysm is an abnormal enlargement or dilatation of an artery. Aneurysms may be caused by arteriosclerosis, a mechanical obstruction of the artery such as thoracic outlet syndrome, or malposition of the artery. Other less common causes include syphilis, tuberculosis, and abnormalities of the vessel wall such as fibromuscular dysplasia. A pseudoaneurysm differs from a true aneurysm in that it does not involve all three layers of the artery wall. A pseudoaneurysm is typically the result of blunt or penetrating trauma or a complication of a procedure such as a puncture during a catheterization procedure. The trauma results in formation of a pulsating, encapsulated hematoma in direct communication with the wall of the artery. If a saphenous vein graft is to be used, the lower leg is prepped and the vein graft harvested. An incision is made in the arm over the section of artery to be repaired. Overlying soft tissues are divided. The underlying axillary-brachial artery is exposed. The artery is clamped as needed. The aneurysm sac is opened and thrombus and plaque removed. The artery walls are suture repaired and an autogenous (saphenous vein) or synthetic patch graft applied as needed. Another technique is to excise the aneurysm with direct repair by end-to-end anastomosis of the distal and proximal vessel ends with or without insertion of a patch graft. A third technique is to place an autogenous (saphenous vein) or synthetic tube graft. A longitudinal incision is made in the artery. The tube graft is inserted and sutured to healthy artery distal and proximal to the aneurysm. The aneurysm sac is then closed over the graft. When the repair is completed, the clamps are released and blood flow re-established. In 35011, an aneurysm or pseudoaneurysm is repaired in a nonemergent, elective procedure. In 35013, a ruptured aneurysm is repaired in an emergency procedure. Bleeding from the ruptured aneurysm must be isolated and controlled prior to the aneurysm repair.

35021-35022

35021 Direct repair of aneurysm, pseudoaneurysm, or excision (partial or total) and graft insertion, with or without patch graft; for aneurysm, pseudoaneurysm, and associated occlusive disease, innominate, subclavian artery, by thoracic incision

35022 Direct repair of aneurysm, pseudoaneurysm, or excision (partial or total) and graft insertion, with or without patch graft; for ruptured aneurysm, innominate, subclavian artery, by thoracic incision

An innominate or subclavian artery aneurysm or pseudoaneurysm including any associated occlusive disease is surgically repaired using direct repair or excision with graft insertion with or without a patch graft via a thoracic approach. An aneurysm is an abnormal enlargement or dilatation of an artery. Aneurysms may be caused by arteriosclerosis, a mechanical obstruction of the artery such as thoracic outlet syndrome, or malposition of the artery. Other less common causes include syphilis, tuberculosis, and abnormalities of the vessel wall such as fibromuscular dysplasia. A pseudoaneurysm differs from a true aneurysm in that it does not involve all three layers of the artery wall. A pseudoaneurysm is typically the result of blunt or penetrating trauma or a complication of a procedure such as a puncture during a catheterization procedure. The trauma results in formation of a pulsating, encapsulated hematoma in direct communication with the wall of the artery. If a saphenous vein graft is to be used, the lower leg is also prepped and the vein graft harvested. A median sternotomy is performed and the incision extended as needed into the supraclavicular region or neck. Remnants of the thymus gland are excised as needed. The left brachiocephalic vein is divided or mobilized. The innominate or subclavian artery is exposed and clamped. The aneurysm sac is opened and thrombus and plaque removed. The artery walls are suture repaired and an autogenous (saphenous vein) or synthetic patch graft applied as needed. Another technique is to excise the aneurysm with direct repair by end-to-end anastomosis of the distal and proximal vessel ends with or without insertion of a patch graft. A third technique is to place an autogenous (saphenous vein) or synthetic tube graft. A longitudinal incision is made in the artery. The tube graft is inserted and sutured to healthy artery distal and proximal to the aneurysm. The aneurysm sac is then closed over the graft. When the repair is completed, the clamps are released and blood flow re-established. In 35021, an aneurysm is repaired in a nonemergent, elective procedure. In 35022, a ruptured aneurysm is repaired in an emergency procedure. Bleeding from the ruptured aneurysm must be isolated and controlled prior to the aneurysm repair.

35045

35045 Direct repair of aneurysm, pseudoaneurysm, or excision (partial or total) and graft insertion, with or without patch graft; for aneurysm, pseudoaneurysm, and associated occlusive disease, radial or ulnar artery

A radial or ulnar artery aneurysm or pseudoaneurysm, including any associated occlusive disease, is surgically repaired using direct repair or excision with graft insertion with or without a patch graft via an arm incision. An aneurysm is an abnormal enlargement or dilatation of an artery that may be caused by arteriosclerosis, mechanical obstruction, or malposition of the artery. Other less common causes include syphilis, tuberculosis, and abnormalities of the vessel wall such as fibromuscular dysplasia. A pseudoaneurysm differs from a true aneurysm in that it does not involve all three layers of the arterial wall. A pseudoaneurysm is typically the result of blunt or penetrating trauma or a complication of a procedure such as a puncture during catheterization. The trauma results in formation of a pulsating, encapsulated hematoma in direct communication with the wall of the artery. If a saphenous vein graft is to be used, the lower leg is also prepped, and the vein graft is harvested. An incision is made in the arm over the section of artery to be repaired. Overlying soft tissues are divided. The underlying radial or ulnar artery is exposed and clamped above and below the aneurysm. The aneurysm sac is opened and thrombus and plaque are removed. The artery walls are suture repaired and an autogenous (saphenous vein) or synthetic patch graft is applied as needed. Another technique is to excise the aneurysm with direct repair by end-to-end anastomosis of the distal and proximal vessel ends with or without insertion of a patch graft. A third technique is to place an autogenous or synthetic tube graft. A longitudinal incision is made in the artery. The tube graft is inserted and sutured to healthy artery distal and proximal to the aneurysm. The aneurysm sac is then closed over the graft. When the repair is completed, the clamps are released and blood flow is re-established.

35081-35082

35081 Direct repair of aneurysm, pseudoaneurysm, or excision (partial or total) and graft insertion, with or without patch graft; for aneurysm, pseudoaneurysm, and associated occlusive disease, abdominal aorta

35082 Direct repair of aneurysm, pseudoaneurysm, or excision (partial or total) and graft insertion, with or without patch graft; for ruptured aneurysm, abdominal aorta

An abdominal aortic aneurysm or pseudoaneurysm including any associated occlusive disease is surgically repaired using direct repair or excision with graft insertion with or without a patch graft. An aneurysm is an abnormal enlargement or dilatation of an artery. Aneurysms may be caused by arteriosclerosis, a mechanical obstruction of the artery such as thoracic outlet syndrome, or malposition of the artery. Other less common causes include syphilis, tuberculosis, and abnormalities of the vessel wall such as fibromuscular dysplasia. A pseudoaneurysm differs from a true aneurysm in that it does not involve all three layers of the artery wall. A pseudoaneurysm is typically the result of blunt or penetrating trauma or a complication of a procedure such as a puncture during a catheterization procedure. The trauma results in formation of a pulsating, encapsulated hematoma in direct communication with the wall of the artery. The abdominal aorta is a continuation of the thoracic aorta, lying in the abdominal cavity and eventually dividing into the two iliac arteries that carry blood to the pelvis and legs. A midline abdominal, transverse, or retroperitoneal flank incision is made to access the abdominal aorta. Overlying soft tissues are divided. The duodenum is dissected off the aorta and the aorta exposed. Proximal control is established below the level of the renal arteries and distal control above the iliac arteries. Following diuresis and administration of anti-coagulant, the iliac arteries are clamped. The proximal aorta is also clamped. The aneurysm sac is opened longitudinally and aortic thrombus and plaque removed. The lumbar arteries are oversewn as is the inferior mesenteric artery. A synthetic tube graft or conduit is sutured to healthy aorta distal and proximal to the site of the aneurysm. Following placement of the tube graft or conduit, the aneurysm sac is closed over the graft, clamps are released, and blood flow re-established. The retroperitoneum is repaired and the abdomen closed. In 35081, an aortic aneurysm or pseudoaneurysm is typically repaired in a nonemergent, elective procedure. In 35082, a ruptured aneurysm is repaired in an emergency procedure. Bleeding from the ruptured aneurysm must be isolated and controlled prior to the aneurysm repair.

35091-35092

35091 Direct repair of aneurysm, pseudoaneurysm, or excision (partial or total) and graft insertion, with or without patch graft; for aneurysm, pseudoaneurysm, and associated occlusive disease, abdominal aorta involving visceral vessels (mesenteric, celiac, renal)

35092 Direct repair of aneurysm, pseudoaneurysm, or excision (partial or total) and graft insertion, with or without patch graft; for ruptured aneurysm, abdominal aorta involving visceral vessels (mesenteric, celiac, renal)

An abdominal aortic aneurysm or pseudoaneurysm with visceral vessel involvement (mesenteric, celiac, and/or renal arteries) including any associated occlusive disease is surgically repaired using direct repair or excision with graft insertion with or without a patch graft via. An aneurysm is an abnormal enlargement or dilatation of an artery.

Cardiovascular System

● New Code   ▲ Revised Code

Aneurysms may be caused by arteriosclerosis, a mechanical obstruction of the artery such as thoracic outlet syndrome, or malposition of the artery. Other less common causes include syphilis, tuberculosis, and abnormalities of the vessel wall such as fibromuscular dysplasia. A pseudoaneurysm differs from a true aneurysm in that it does not involve all three layers of the artery wall. A pseudoaneurysm is typically the result of blunt or penetrating trauma or a complication of a procedure such as a puncture during a catheterization procedure. The trauma results in formation of a pulsating, encapsulated hematoma in direct communication with the wall of the artery. The abdominal aorta is a continuation of the thoracic aorta, lying in the abdominal cavity and eventually dividing into the two iliac arteries that carry blood to the pelvis and legs. If a saphenous vein graft is used to repair the visceral vessel, the lower leg is prepped and the vein graft harvested. A midline abdominal, transverse, or retroperitoneal flank incision is made to access the abdominal aorta and visceral vessels. Overlying soft tissues are divided. The duodenum is dissected off the aorta and the aorta exposed. Proximal control is established above the level of the celiac arteries and distal control above the iliac arteries. Supraceliac aortic control is accomplished by dividing ligaments to the left lateral segment of the liver and retracting this portion of the liver. The fibromuscular bands (crura) of the diaphragm are separated and the aorta mobilized. Following diuresis and administration of anti-coagulant, the iliac arteries are clamped. The proximal aorta is also clamped. The aneurysm sac is opened longitudinally and aortic thrombus removed. The lumbar arteries are oversewn as is the inferior mesenteric artery. A synthetic tube graft is sutured to healthy aorta distal and proximal to the site of the aneurysm. The visceral artery is also repaired using an autogenous (saphenvous vein) or synthetic patch or tube graft. Following placement of the tube graft, the aneurysm sac is closed over the graft, clamps are released, and blood flow re-established. The retroperitoneum is repaired and the abdomen closed. In 35091, an aortic aneurysm or pseudoaneurysm with involvement of the visceral vessels (mesenteric, celiac, and/or renal arteries) is repaired in a nonemergent, elective procedure. In 35092, a ruptured aortic aneurysm with involvement of the visceral vessels is repaired in an emergency procedure. Bleeding from the ruptured aneurysm must be isolated and controlled prior to the aneurysm repair.

35102-35103

35102 **Direct repair of aneurysm, pseudoaneurysm, or excision (partial or total) and graft insertion, with or without patch graft; for aneurysm, pseudoaneurysm, and associated occlusive disease, abdominal aorta involving iliac vessels (common, hypogastric, external)**

35103 **Direct repair of aneurysm, pseudoaneurysm, or excision (partial or total) and graft insertion, with or without patch graft; for ruptured aneurysm, abdominal aorta involving iliac vessels (common, hypogastric, external)**

An abdominal aortic aneurysm or pseudoaneurysm with iliac vessel involvement including any associated occlusive disease is surgically repaired using direct repair or excision with graft insertion with or without a patch graft via. An aneurysm is an abnormal enlargement or dilatation of an artery. Aneurysms may be caused by arteriosclerosis, a mechanical obstruction of the artery such as thoracic outlet syndrome, or malposition of the artery. Other less common causes include syphilis, tuberculosis, and abnormalities of the vessel wall such as fibromuscular dysplasia. A pseudoaneurysm differs from a true aneurysm in that it does not involve all three layers of the artery wall. A pseudoaneurysm is typically the result of blunt or penetrating trauma or a complication of a procedure such as a puncture during a catheterization procedure. The trauma results in formation of a pulsating, encapsulated hematoma in direct communication with the wall of the artery. The abdominal aorta is a continuation of the thoracic aorta, lying in the abdominal cavity and eventually dividing into the two iliac arteries that carry blood to the pelvis and legs. A midline abdominal, transverse, or retroperitoneal flank incision is made to access the abdominal aorta. Overlying soft tissues are divided. The duodenum is dissected off the aorta and the aorta exposed. Proximal control is established below the level of the renal arteries and distal control to a level beyond the iliac artery aneurysm. Following diuresis and administration of anti-coagulant, the iliac arteries are clamped below the level of the iliac involvement. The proximal aorta is also clamped. The aneurysm sac is opened longitudinally and aortic thrombus removed. The lumbar arteries are oversewn as is the inferior mesenteric artery. A synthetic iliac bifucation graft is sutured to healthy aorta proximal to the aneurysm and healthy iliac artery distal to the aneurysm. Following placement of the graft, the aneurysm sac is closed over the graft, clamps are released, and blood flow re-established. The retroperitoneum is repaired and the abdomen closed. In 35102, an aortic aneurysm or pseudoaneurysm with involvement of the iliac vessels is repaired in a nonemergent, elective procedure. In 35103, a ruptured aortic aneurysm with involvement of the iliac vessels is repaired in an emergency procedure. Bleeding from the ruptured aneurysm must be isolated and controlled prior to the aneurysm repair.

35111-35112

35111 **Direct repair of aneurysm, pseudoaneurysm, or excision (partial or total) and graft insertion, with or without patch graft; for aneurysm, pseudoaneurysm, and associated occlusive disease, splenic artery**

35112 **Direct repair of aneurysm, pseudoaneurysm, or excision (partial or total) and graft insertion, with or without patch graft; for ruptured aneurysm, splenic artery**

A splenic artery aneurysm or pseudoaneurysm including any associated occlusive disease is surgically repaired using direct repair or excision with graft insertion with or without a patch graft. An aneurysm is an abnormal enlargement or dilatation of an artery. Aneurysms may be caused by arteriosclerosis, a mechanical obstruction of the artery, or malposition of the artery. Other less common causes include syphilis, tuberculosis, and abnormalities of the vessel wall such as fibromuscular dysplasia. A pseudoaneurysm differs from a true aneurysm in that it does not involve all three layers of the artery wall. A pseudoaneurysm is typically the result of blunt or penetrating trauma or a complication of a procedure such as a puncture during a catheterization procedure. The trauma results in formation of a pulsating, encapsulated hematoma in direct communication with the wall of the artery. Pseudoaneurysm of the splenic artery may also be caused by pancreatitis, septic emboli, or arteritis. The splenic artery arises from the celiac trunk which in turn arises from the abdominal aorta just below the diaphragm. If a saphenous vein graft is to be used, the lower leg is prepped and the vein graft harvested. A midline abdominal, transverse, or retroperitoneal flank incision is made to access the splenic artery. Overlying soft tissues are divided. The duodenum is dissected off the aorta and the aorta exposed. Proximal control is established above the level of the celiac arteries and distal control above the iliac arteries. Supraceliac aortic control is accomplished by dividing ligaments to the left lateral segment of the liver and retracting this portion of the liver. The fibromuscular bands (crura) of the diaphragm are separated and the aorta mobilized. Following administration of anti-coagulant, the iliac arteries are clamped. The proximal aorta is also clamped. The aneurysm sac in the splenic artery is opened longitudinally and thrombus removed. The splenic artery is repaired using an autogenous (saphenous vein) or synthetic patch or tube graft. If a tube graft is placed, the aneurysm sac is closed over the graft. Clamps are released and blood flow re-established. The retroperitoneum is repaired and the abdomen closed. In 35111, a splenic aneurysm or pseudoaneurysm is repaired in a nonemergent, elective procedure. In 35112, a ruptured splenic aneurysm is repaired in an emergency procedure. Bleeding from the ruptured aneurysm must be isolated and controlled prior to the aneurysm repair.

35121-35122

35121 **Direct repair of aneurysm, pseudoaneurysm, or excision (partial or total) and graft insertion, with or without patch graft; for aneurysm, pseudoaneurysm, and associated occlusive disease, hepatic, celiac, renal, or mesenteric artery**

35122 **Direct repair of aneurysm, pseudoaneurysm, or excision (partial or total) and graft insertion, with or without patch graft; for ruptured aneurysm, hepatic, celiac, renal, or mesenteric artery**

An aneurysm or pseudoaneurysm including any associated occlusive disease of the celiac, hepatic, renal, or mesenteric artery is surgically repaired using direct repair or excision with graft insertion with or without a patch graft. An aneurysm is an abnormal enlargement or dilatation of an artery. Aneurysms may be caused by arteriosclerosis, a mechanical obstruction of the artery, or malposition of the artery. Other less common causes include syphilis, tuberculosis, and abnormalities of the vessel wall such as fibromuscular dysplasia. A pseudoaneurysm differs from a true aneurysm in that it does not involve all three layers of the artery wall. A pseudoaneurysm is typically the result of blunt or penetrating trauma or a complication of a procedure such as a puncture during a catheterization procedure. The trauma results in formation of a pulsating, encapsulated hematoma in direct communication with the wall of the artery. Pseudoaneurysm of the splenic artery may also be caused by pancreatitis, septic emboli, or arteritis. The celiac artery or trunk arises from the abdominal aorta just below the diaphragm. The hepatic artery arises from the celiac trunk. The paired renal arteries and superior and inferior mesenteric arteries are visceral branches off the aorta. If a saphenous vein graft is to be used, the lower leg is prepped and the vein graft harvested. A midline abdominal, transverse, or retroperitoneal flank incision is made to access the splenic artery. Overlying soft tissues are divided. The duodenum is dissected off the aorta and the aorta exposed. Proximal control is established above the level of the celiac arteries and distal control above the iliac arteries. Supraceliac aortic control is accomplished by dividing ligaments to the left lateral segment of the liver and retracting this portion of the liver. The fibromuscular bands (crura) of the diaphragm are separated and the aorta mobilized. Following administration of anti-coagulant, the vascular clamps are placed to isolate the aneurysm. The aneurysm sac is opened and thrombus and plaque removed. The artery walls are suture repaired and an autogenous (saphenous vein) or synthetic patch graft applied as needed. Another technique is to excise the aneurysm with direct repair by end-to-end anastomosis of the distal and proximal vessel ends with or without insertion of a patch graft. A third technique is to place an autogenous (saphenous vein) or synthetic tube graft. A longitudinal incision is made in the artery. The tube graft is inserted and sutured to healthy artery distal and proximal to the aneurysm. The aneurysm sac is then closed over the graft. Clamps are released and blood flow re-established. The retroperitoneum is repaired and the abdomen closed. In 35121, a celiac, hepatic, renal or mesenteric aneurysm or pseudoaneurysm is repaired in a nonemergent, elective procedure. In 35122, a ruptured aneurysm is repaired in an emergency procedure. Bleeding from the ruptured aneurysm must be isolated and controlled prior to the aneurysm repair.

35131-35132

35131   Direct repair of aneurysm, pseudoaneurysm, or excision (partial or total) and graft insertion, with or without patch graft; for aneurysm, pseudoaneurysm, and associated occlusive disease, iliac artery (common, hypogastric, external)

35132   Direct repair of aneurysm, pseudoaneurysm, or excision (partial or total) and graft insertion, with or without patch graft; for ruptured aneurysm, iliac artery (common, hypogastric, external)

An aneurysm or pseudoaneurysm including any associated occlusive disease of the common iliac artery or the internal (hypogastric) or external iliac branches is surgically repaired using direct repair or excision with graft insertion with or without a patch graft. An aneurysm is an abnormal enlargement or dilatation of an artery. Aneurysms may be caused by arteriosclerosis, a mechanical obstruction of the artery, or malposition of the artery. Other less common causes include syphilis, tuberculosis, and abnormalities of the vessel wall such as fibromuscular dysplasia. A pseudoaneurysm differs from a true aneurysm in that it does not involve all three layers of the artery wall. A pseudoaneurysm is typically the result of blunt or penetrating trauma or a complication of a procedure such as a puncture during a catheterization procedure. The trauma results in formation of a pulsating, encapsulated hematoma in direct communication with the wall of the artery. The paired common iliac arteries form the two terminal branches of the abdominal aorta and then branch into the internal (hypogastric) and external iliac arteries. A lower abdominal and/or leg incision is made to access the affected portion of the iliac artery. Overlying soft tissues are divided and the iliac artery is exposed. Iliac artery control is established above and below the level of the aneurysm. Following administration of anti-coagulant, the iliac artery is clamped above and below the aneurysm. The aneurysm sac is opened and thrombus and plaque removed. The artery walls are suture repaired and an autogenous (saphenous vein) or synthetic patch graft applied as needed. Another technique is to excise the aneurysm with direct repair by end-to-end anastomosis of the distal and proximal vessel ends with or without insertion of a patch graft. A third technique is to place an autogenous (saphenous vein) or synthetic tube graft. A longitudinal incision is made in the artery. The tube graft is inserted and sutured to healthy artery distal and proximal to the aneurysm. The aneurysm sac is then closed over the graft. Clamps are released and blood flow re-established. In 35131, an aneurysm or pseudoaneurysm of the iliac artery is repaired in a nonemergent, elective procedure. In 35132, a ruptured aneurysm is repaired in an emergency procedure. Bleeding from the ruptured aneurysm must be isolated and controlled prior to the aneurysm repair.

35141-35142

35141   Direct repair of aneurysm, pseudoaneurysm, or excision (partial or total) and graft insertion, with or without patch graft; for aneurysm, pseudoaneurysm, and associated occlusive disease, common femoral artery (profunda femoris, superficial femoral)

35142   Direct repair of aneurysm, pseudoaneurysm, or excision (partial or total) and graft insertion, with or without patch graft; for ruptured aneurysm, common femoral artery (profunda femoris, superficial femoral)

An aneurysm or pseudoaneurysm including any associated occlusive disease of the common femoral artery, also referred to as the superficial femoral artery or profunda femoris, is surgically repaired using direct repair or excision with graft insertion with or without a patch graft via. An aneurysm is an abnormal enlargement or dilatation of an artery. Aneurysms may be caused by arteriosclerosis, a mechanical obstruction of the artery, or malposition of the artery. Other less common causes include syphilis, tuberculosis, and abnormalities of the vessel wall such as fibromuscular dysplasia. A pseudoaneurysm differs from a true aneurysm in that it does not involve all three layers of the artery wall. A pseudoaneurysm is typically the result of blunt or penetrating trauma or a complication of a procedure such as a puncture during a catheterization procedure. The trauma results in formation of a pulsating, encapsulated hematoma in direct communication with the wall of the artery. The common femoral arteries are a continuation of the external iliac arteries extending from the inguinal ligament to popliteal artery. A leg incision is made to access the femoral artery. Overlying soft tissues are divided and the femoral artery is exposed. Femoral artery control is established above and below the level of the aneurysm. Following administration of anti-coagulant, the femoral artery is clamped above and below the aneurysm. The aneurysm sac is opened and thrombus and plaque removed. The artery walls are suture repaired and an autogenous (saphenous vein) or synthetic patch graft applied as needed. Another technique is to excise the aneurysm with direct repair by end-to-end anastomosis of the distal and proximal vessel ends with or without insertion of a patch graft. A third technique is to place an autogenous (saphenous vein) or synthetic tube graft. A longitudinal incision is made in the artery. The tube graft is inserted and sutured to healthy artery distal and proximal to the aneurysm. The aneurysm sac is then closed over the graft. Clamps are released and blood flow re-established. In 35141, an aneurysm or

pseudoaneurysm of the femoral artery is repaired in a nonemergent, elective procedure. In 35142, a ruptured aneurysm is repaired in an emergency procedure. Bleeding from the ruptured aneurysm must be isolated and controlled prior to the aneurysm repair.

35151-35152

35151   Direct repair of aneurysm, pseudoaneurysm, or excision (partial or total) and graft insertion, with or without patch graft; for aneurysm, pseudoaneurysm, and associated occlusive disease, popliteal artery

35152   Direct repair of aneurysm, pseudoaneurysm, or excision (partial or total) and graft insertion, with or without patch graft; for ruptured aneurysm, popliteal artery

An aneurysm or pseudoaneurysm including any associated occlusive disease of the popliteal artery is surgically repaired using direct repair or excision with graft insertion with or without a patch graft. An aneurysm is an abnormal enlargement or dilatation of an artery. Aneurysms may be caused by arteriosclerosis, a mechanical obstruction of the artery, or malposition of the artery. Other less common causes include syphilis, tuberculosis, and abnormalities of the vessel wall such as fibromuscular dysplasia. A pseudoaneurysm differs from a true aneurysm in that it does not involve all three layers of the artery wall. A pseudoaneurysm is typically the result of blunt or penetrating trauma or a complication of a procedure such as a puncture during a catheterization procedure. The trauma results in formation of a pulsating, encapsulated hematoma in direct communication with the wall of the artery. The popliteal arteries are a continuation of the common femoral arteries beginning at the popliteal space behind the knee and then bifurcating into the anterior and posterior tibial arteries. A leg incision is made to access the popliteal artery. Overlying soft tissues are divided and the popliteal artery is exposed. Popliteal artery control is established above and below the level of the aneurysm. Following administration of anti-coagulant, the popliteal artery is clamped above and below the aneurysm. The aneurysm sac is opened and thrombus and plaque removed. The artery walls are suture repaired and an autogenous (saphenous vein) or synthetic patch graft applied as needed. Another technique is to excise the aneurysm with direct repair by end-to-end anastomosis of the distal and proximal vessel ends with or without insertion of a patch graft. A third technique is to place an autogenous (saphenous vein) or synthetic tube graft. A longitudinal incision is made in the artery. The tube graft is inserted and sutured to healthy artery distal and proximal to the aneurysm. The aneurysm sac is then closed over the graft. Clamps are released and blood flow re-established. In 35151, an aneurysm or pseudoaneurysm of the popliteal artery is repaired in a nonemergent, elective procedure. In 35152, a ruptured aneurysm is repaired in an emergency procedure. Bleeding from the ruptured aneurysm must be isolated and controlled prior to the aneurysm repair.

35180-35184

35180   Repair, congenital arteriovenous fistula; head and neck
35182   Repair, congenital arteriovenous fistula; thorax and abdomen
35184   Repair, congenital arteriovenous fistula; extremities

A congenital arteriovenous fistula is repaired. A congenital arteriovenous fistula is an abnormal communication between an artery and vein that is present at birth. These types of fistulas can occur anywhere in the vascular system and vary considerably in size and length. The abnormal communication allows blood to flow under high pressure from the artery into the vein. Because venous walls are not strong enough to withstand high pressure arterial blood flow, the venous walls stretch causing enlargement of the venous component. This causes more blood to flow into the venous component and can eventually cause other cardiovascular complications. Most congenital arteriovenous fistulas are difficult to repair because they often extend into adjacent structures. Separately reportable angiography is performed to delineate the course of the arteriovenous fistula. The physician then exposes the fistula and dissects it free of surrounding tissues. Clamps are placed on the artery and vein to isolate the fistula. The fistulous communication is severed and the artery and vein repaired with sutures. Alternatively, a synthetic patch or vein graft may be used to repair the vessels. The clamps are removed and hemostasis of the repair checked. Overlying tissues are closed in layers. Use 35180 for repair of an arteriovenous fistula in the head and neck, 35182 for the thorax and abdomen, and 35184 for the extremities.

35188-35190

35188   Repair, acquired or traumatic arteriovenous fistula; head and neck
35189   Repair, acquired or traumatic arteriovenous fistula; thorax and abdomen
35190   Repair, acquired or traumatic arteriovenous fistula; extremities

An acquired or traumatic arteriovenous fistula is repaired. An acquired arteriovenous fistula is an abnormal communication between an artery and a vein resulting from trauma to blood vessels. It may be evident immediately after the injury or may develop over time. The abnormal communication allows blood to flow under high pressure from the artery into the vein. Because venous walls are not strong enough to withstand high pressure arterial blood flow, the venous walls stretch causing enlargement of the venous component. This causes more blood to flow into the venous component and can eventually cause other cardiovascular complications. Separately reportable angiography is performed to delineate the course of the arteriovenous fistula. The physician then exposes the fistula and dissects it free of surrounding tissues. Clamps are placed on the artery and vein to isolate the

Cardiovascular System

fistula. The fistulous communication is severed and the artery and vein repaired with sutures. Alternatively, a synthetic patch or vein graft may be used to repair the vessels. The clamps are removed and hemostasis of the repair checked. Overlying tissues are closed in layers. Use 35188 for repair of an arteriovenous fistula in the head and neck, 35189 for the thorax and abdomen, and 35190 for the extremities.

35201

35201   Repair blood vessel, direct; neck

The approach depends on which vessel is injured. The injured blood vessel in the neck is exposed and clamped proximal and distal to the injury to control bleeding. Perfusion may be maintained by placement of a temporary shunt. The extent of the injury is evaluated. The edges of the injured blood vessel are debrided and reapproximated in an end-to-end fashion with sutures. The temporary shunt is removed. The clamps are released and hemostasis checked along the suture line. Overlying tissues are suture repaired in layers.

35206-35207

35206   Repair blood vessel, direct; upper extremity
35207   Repair blood vessel, direct; hand, finger

A direct repair of a blood vessel in the upper extremity (35206) or hand or finger (35207) is performed. The approach depends on which vessel is injured. The injured blood vessel is exposed and clamped proximal and distal to the injury to control bleeding. Perfusion may be maintained by placement of a temporary shunt. The extent of the injury is evaluated. The edges of the injured blood vessel are debrided and reapproximated in an end-to-end fashion with sutures. The clamps are released and hemostasis checked along the suture line. Overlying tissues are suture repaired in layers.

35211-35216

35211   Repair blood vessel, direct; intrathoracic, with bypass
35216   Repair blood vessel, direct; intrathoracic, without bypass

A direct repair of an intrathoracic blood vessel is performed. The chest is opened by median sternotomy or other approach. Depending on the nature of the intrathoracic blood vessel injury cardiopulmonary bypass may be initiated. The injured blood vessel is exposed and clamped proximal and distal to the injury to control bleeding. The extent of the injury is evaluated. The edges of the injured blood vessel are debrided and reapproximated in an end-to-end fashion with sutures. The clamps are released and hemostasis checked along the suture line. If cardiopulmonary bypass has been used, the patient is taken off bypass. Overlying tissues are suture repaired in layers. Use 35211 for repair performed with cardiopulmonary bypass and 35216 for repair performed without cardiopulmonary bypass.

35221

35221   Repair blood vessel, direct; intra-abdominal

The approach depends on which vessel is injured. The injured blood vessel is exposed and clamped proximal and distal to the injury to control bleeding. Perfusion may be maintained by placement of a temporary shunt. The extent of the injury is evaluated. The edges of the injured blood vessel are debrided and reapproximated in an end-to-end fashion with sutures. The shunt is removed. The clamps are released and hemostasis checked along the suture line. Overlying tissues are suture repaired in layers.

35226

35226   Repair blood vessel, direct; lower extremity

The approach depends on which vessel is injured. The injured blood vessel is exposed and clamped proximal and distal to the injury to control bleeding. Perfusion may be maintained by placement of a temporary shunt. The extent of the injury is evaluated. The edges of the injured blood vessel are debrided and reapproximated in an end-to-end fashion with sutures. The shunt is removed. The clamps are released and hemostasis checked along the suture line. Overlying tissues are suture repaired in layers.

35231

35231   Repair blood vessel with vein graft; neck

A blood vessel in the neck is repaired with a vein graft. The approach depends on which vessel is injured. The injured blood vessel in the neck is exposed and clamped proximal and distal to the injury to control bleeding. Perfusion may be maintained by placement of a temporary shunt. The extent of the injury is evaluated. A length of vein, usually the saphenous vein in the lower leg, is harvested and prepared for grafting. The edges of the injured blood vessel are debrided and the prepared vein graft sewn to the proximal and distal ends of the injured blood vessel. The temporary shunt is removed. The clamps are released and hemostasis checked along the suture line. Overlying tissues are suture repaired in layers.

35236

35236   Repair blood vessel with vein graft; upper extremity

A blood vessel in the upper extremity is repaired with a vein graft. The approach depends on which vessel is injured. The injured blood vessel in the arm is exposed and clamped proximal and distal to the injury to control bleeding. Perfusion may be maintained by placement of a temporary shunt. The extent of the injury is evaluated. A length of vein, usually the saphenous vein in the lower leg, is harvested and prepared for grafting. The edges of the injured blood vessel are debrided and the prepared vein graft sewn to the proximal and distal ends of the injured blood vessel. The temporary shunt is removed. The clamps are released and hemostasis checked along the suture line. Overlying tissues are suture repaired in layers.

35241-35246

35241   Repair blood vessel with vein graft; intrathoracic, with bypass
35246   Repair blood vessel with vein graft; intrathoracic, without bypass

An intrathoracic blood vessel is repaired with a vein graft. The chest is opened by median sternotomy or other approach. Depending on the nature of the intrathoracic blood vessel injury cardiopulmonary bypass may be initiated. The injured blood vessel is exposed and clamped proximal and distal to the injury to control bleeding. The extent of the injury is evaluated. A length of vein, usually the saphenous vein in the lower leg, is harvested and prepared for grafting. The edges of the injured blood vessel are debrided and the prepared vein graft sewn to the proximal and distal ends of the injured blood vessel. The clamps are released and hemostasis checked along the suture line. If cardiopulmonary bypass has been used, the patient is taken off bypass. Overlying tissues are suture repaired in layers. Use 35241 for repair performed with cardiopulmonary bypass and 35246 for repair performed without cardiopulmonary bypass.

35251

35251   Repair blood vessel with vein graft; intra-abdominal

An intra-abdominal blood vessel is repaired with a vein graft. The approach depends on which vessel is injured. The injured blood vessel is exposed and clamped proximal and distal to the injury to control bleeding. The extent of the injury is evaluated. A length of vein, usually the saphenous vein in the lower leg, is harvested and prepared for grafting. The edges of the injured blood vessel are debrided and the prepared vein graft sewn to the proximal and distal ends of the injured blood vessel. The clamps are released and hemostasis checked along the suture line. Overlying tissues are suture repaired in layers.

35256

35256   Repair blood vessel with vein graft; lower extremity

A blood vessel in the lower extremity is repaired with a vein graft. The approach depends on which vessel is injured. The injured blood vessel in the leg is exposed and clamped proximal and distal to the injury to control bleeding. Perfusion may be maintained by placement of a temporary shunt. The extent of the injury is evaluated. A length of vein, usually the saphenous vein in the lower leg, is harvested and prepared for grafting. The edges of the injured blood vessel are debrided and the prepared vein graft sewn to the proximal and distal ends of the injured blood vessel. The temporary shunt is removed. The clamps are released and hemostasis checked along the suture line. Overlying tissues are suture repaired in layers.

35261

35261   Repair blood vessel with graft other than vein; neck

A blood vessel in the neck is repaired with a graft other than a vein. The approach depends on which vessel is injured. The injured blood vessel in the neck is exposed and clamped proximal and distal to the injury to control bleeding. Perfusion may be maintained by placement of a temporary shunt. The extent of the injury is evaluated. If an arterial graft is used, a length of artery is harvested and prepared for grafting. Alternatively, a synthetic graft may be used. The edges of the injured blood vessel are debrided and the prepared arterial or synthetic graft sewn to the proximal and distal ends of the injured blood vessel. The temporary shunt is removed. The clamps are released and hemostasis checked along the suture line. Overlying tissues are suture repaired in layers.

35266

35266   Repair blood vessel with graft other than vein; upper extremity

A blood vessel in the upper extremity is repaired with a graft other than a vein. The approach depends on which vessel is injured. The injured blood vessel in the arm is exposed and clamped proximal and distal to the injury to control bleeding. Perfusion may be maintained by placement of a temporary shunt. The extent of the injury is evaluated. If an arterial graft is used, a length of artery is harvested and prepared for grafting. Alternatively, a synthetic graft may be used. The edges of the injured blood vessel are debrided and the prepared arterial or synthetic graft sewn to the proximal and distal ends of the injured blood vessel. The temporary shunt is removed. The clamps are released and hemostasis checked along the suture line. Overlying tissues are suture repaired in layers.

Cardiovascular System

● New Code   ▲ Revised Code   © 2017 DecisionHealth

35271-35276

35271 Repair blood vessel with graft other than vein; intrathoracic, with bypass

35276 Repair blood vessel with graft other than vein; intrathoracic, without bypass

An intrathoracic blood vessel is repaired with a graft other than a vein. The chest is opened by median sternotomy or other approach. Depending on the nature of the intrathoracic blood vessel injury cardiopulmonary bypass may be initiated. The injured blood vessel is exposed and clamped proximal and distal to the injury to control bleeding. The extent of the injury is evaluated. If an arterial graft is used, a length of artery is harvested and prepared for grafting. Alternatively, a synthetic graft may be used. The edges of the injured blood vessel are debrided and the prepared arterial or synthetic graft sewn to the proximal and distal ends of the injured blood vessel. If cardiopulmonary bypass has been used, the patient is taken off bypass. Overlying tissues are suture repaired in layers. Use 35271 for repair performed with cardiopulmonary bypass and 35276 for repair performed without cardiopulmonary bypass.

35281

35281 Repair blood vessel with graft other than vein; intra-abdominal

An intra-abdominal blood vessel is repaired with a graft other than a vein. The approach depends on which vessel is injured. The injured blood vessel is exposed and clamped proximal and distal to the injury to control bleeding. The extent of the injury is evaluated. If an arterial graft is used, a length of artery is harvested and prepared for grafting. Alternatively, a synthetic graft may be used. The edges of the injured blood vessel are debrided and the prepared arterial or synthetic graft sewn to the proximal and distal ends of the injured blood vessel. The clamps are released and hemostasis checked along the suture line. Overlying tissues are suture repaired in layers.

35286

35286 Repair blood vessel with graft other than vein; lower extremity

A blood vessel in the lower extremity is repaired with a graft other than a vein. The approach depends on which vessel is injured. The injured blood vessel in the leg is exposed and clamped proximal and distal to the injury to control bleeding. Perfusion may be maintained by placement of a temporary shunt. The extent of the injury is evaluated. If an arterial graft is used, a length of artery is harvested and prepared for grafting. Alternatively, a synthetic graft may be used. The edges of the injured blood vessel are debrided and the prepared arterial or synthetic graft sewn to the proximal and distal ends of the injured blood vessel. The temporary shunt is removed. The clamps are released and hemostasis checked along the suture line. Overlying tissues are suture repaired in layers.

35301

35301 Thromboendarterectomy, including patch graft, if performed; carotid, vertebral, subclavian, by neck incision

Thromboendarterectomy is performed on the carotid, vertebral or subclavian artery via a neck incision. This procedure removes a thrombus, such as a blood clot or atherosclerotic plaque that has adhered to vessels walls, along with the vessel intima from an occluded artery. An access incision is made in the neck over the affected artery. The thrombosed portion of the artery is isolated and dissected away from adjacent structures. Cerebral perfusion may be maintained by placement of a temporary shunt. Clamps are placed proximal and distal to the obstructed portion of the artery. The artery is incised and plaque and blood clot debris are removed. The artery lining (intima) is separated from the arterial walls and removed to increase the diameter of the artery. The edges of the remaining normal intima are sutured to the vessel walls. The artery is repaired primarily with sutures or a venous or synthetic patch graft is applied to enlarge the diameter of the artery. If a shunt has been placed it is removed. The vascular clamps are removed and blood flow through the affected artery reinitiated. The arterial suture line is checked for hemostasis. Overlying tissues are then closed in layers.

35302

35302 Thromboendarterectomy, including patch graft, if performed; superficial femoral artery

Thromboendarterectomy is performed in the superficial femoral artery. This procedure removes a thrombus, such as a blood clot or atherosclerotic plaque adhering to vessel walls, along with the vessel intima, from an occluded artery. The superficial femoral artery is the continuation of the common femoral artery distal to the branching of the deep femoral artery in the upper thigh. An access incision is made in the upper leg. The thrombosed portion of the superficial femoral artery is isolated and dissected away from adjacent structures. Clamps are applied proximally and distally. An incision is made into the blood vessel and plaque and blood clot debris are removed. The vessel lining is separated from the arterial walls and removed, increasing the luminal diameter of the artery. Sutures secure the edges of the normal intima to the vessel walls to prevent separation with resumed blood flow. After the obstruction and vessel intima are removed, a patch graft may be taken from the patient or another donor, or one made of synthetic material may be

sutured to the vessel for repair. After the vessel is closed, the clamps are removed, and the incision is repaired.

35303

35303 Thromboendarterectomy, including patch graft, if performed; popliteal artery

Thromboendarterectomy is performed in the popliteal artery. This procedure removes a thrombus, such as a blood clot or atherosclerotic plaque adhering to vessel walls, along with the vessel intima, from an occluded artery. The popliteal artery is the continuation of the femoral artery down in the knee area. An access incision is made over the knee. The thrombosed portion of the popliteal artery is isolated and dissected away from adjacent structures. Clamps are applied proximally and distally. An incision is made into the blood vessel and plaque and blood clot debris are removed. The vessel lining is separated from the arterial walls and removed, increasing the luminal diameter of the artery. Sutures secure the edges of the normal intima to the vessel walls to prevent separation with resumed blood flow. After the obstruction and vessel intima are removed, a patch graft may be taken from the patient or another donor, or one made of synthetic material may be sutured to the vessel for repair. After the vessel is closed, the clamps are removed, and the incision is repaired.

35304

35304 Thromboendarterectomy, including patch graft, if performed; tibioperoneal trunk artery

This procedure removes a thrombus, such as a blood clot or atherosclerotic plaque adhering to vessel walls, along with the vessel intima, from an occluded artery. The tibioperoneal trunk is the extension of the terminal popliteal artery located in the upper part of the lower leg, from which both the fibular and posterior tibial arteries branch. An access incision is made by extending the standard incision made to expose the popliteal artery below the knee. The medial head of the gastrocnemius muscle and the popliteal vein are retracted. The soleus muscle on the tibia is divided to reach the tibioperoneal trunk. The thrombosed portion is isolated and dissected away from adjacent structures. Clamps are applied proximally and distally. An incision is made into the blood vessel and plaque and blood clot debris are removed. The vessel lining is separated from the arterial walls and removed, increasing the luminal diameter of the artery. Sutures secure the edges of the normal intima to the vessel walls to prevent separation with resumed blood flow. After the obstruction and vessel intima are removed, a patch graft may be taken from the patient or another donor, or one made of synthetic material may be sutured to the vessel for repair. After the vessel is closed, the clamps are removed, and the incision is repaired.

35305-35306

35305 Thromboendarterectomy, including patch graft, if performed; tibial or peroneal artery, initial vessel

35306 Thromboendarterectomy, including patch graft, if performed; each additional tibial or peroneal artery (List separately in addition to code for primary procedure)

This procedure removes a thrombus, such as a blood clot or atherosclerotic plaque adhering to vessel walls, along with the vessel intima, from an occluded artery. The peroneal artery is also known as the fibular artery and branches from the tibioperoneal trunk along with the posterior tibial artery to supply the lower leg. Both the posterior tibial artery and the peroneal artery can be accessed by an incision approximately 2 cm posterior to the tibia. The soleus muscle fibers originating on the tibia are divided to reach the posterior tibial artery, which lies in the deep posterior compartment on the surface of the tibialis posterior muscle. The peroneal artery is exposed by retracted the posterior tibial vessels and continuing laterally to the flexor hallucis longus muscle just medial to the fibula. The thrombosed portion of the target artery is isolated and dissected away from adjacent structures. Clamps are applied proximally and distally. An incision is made into the blood vessel and plaque and blood clot debris are removed. The vessel lining is separated from the arterial walls and removed, increasing the luminal diameter of the artery. Sutures secure the edges of the normal intima to the vessel walls to prevent separation with resumed blood flow. After the obstruction and vessel intima are removed, a patch graft may be taken from the patient or another donor, or one made of synthetic material may be sutured to the vessel for repair. After the vessel is closed, the clamps are removed, and the incision is repaired. Code 35305 for the initial tibial or peroneal artery and 35306 for each additional artery.

35311

35311 Thromboendarterectomy, including patch graft, if performed; subclavian, innominate, by thoracic incision

Thromboendarterectomy is performed on the subclavian or innominate artery via a thoracic approach. This procedure removes a thrombus, such as a blood clot or atherosclerotic plaque that has adhered to vessels walls, along with the vessel intima from an occluded artery. An access incision is made in the chest over the affected artery. The thrombosed portion of the artery is isolated and dissected away from adjacent structures. Perfusion may be maintained by placement of a temporary shunt. Clamps are placed proximal and

Cardiovascular System

distal to the obstructed portion of the artery. The artery is incised and plaque and blood clot debris are removed. The artery lining (intima) is separated from the arterial walls and removed to increase the diameter of the artery. The edges of the remaining normal intima are sutured to the arterial walls. The artery is repaired primarily with sutures or a venous or synthetic patch graft is applied to enlarge the diameter of the artery. If a shunt has been placed it is removed. The vascular clamps are removed and blood flow through the affected artery reinitiated. The arterial suture line is checked for hemostasis. Overlying tissues are then closed in layers.

35321

35321   Thromboendarterectomy, including patch graft, if performed; axillary-brachial

Thromboendarterectomy is performed on the axillary-brachial artery. This procedure removes a thrombus, such as a blood clot or atherosclerotic plaque that has adhered to vessels walls, along with the vessel intima from an occluded artery. An access incision is made in the arm over the affected artery. The thrombosed portion of the artery is isolated and dissected away from adjacent structures. Perfusion may be maintained by placement of a temporary shunt. Clamps are placed proximal and distal to the obstructed portion of the artery. The artery is incised and plaque and blood clot debris are removed. The artery lining (intima) is separated from the arterial walls and removed to increase the diameter of the artery. The edges of the remaining normal intima are sutured to the arterial walls. The artery is repaired primarily with sutures or a venous or synthetic patch graft is applied to enlarge the diameter of the artery. If a shunt has been placed it is removed. The vascular clamps are removed and blood flow through the affected artery reinitiated. The arterial suture line is checked for hemostasis. Overlying tissues are then closed in layers.

35331-35341

35331   Thromboendarterectomy, including patch graft, if performed; abdominal aorta

35341   Thromboendarterectomy, including patch graft, if performed; mesenteric, celiac, or renal

Thromboendarterectomy is performed on the abdominal aorta (35331) or mesenteric, celiac, or renal artery (35341). This procedure removes a thrombus, such as a blood clot or atherosclerotic plaque that has adhered to vessels walls, along with the vessel intima from an occluded artery. An access incision is made in the abdomen and the affected blood vessel exposed. The thrombosed portion of the aorta, mesenteric, celiac, or renal artery is isolated and dissected away from adjacent structures. Perfusion may be maintained by placement of a temporary shunt. Clamps are placed proximal and distal to the obstructed portion of the aorta or other artery. The aorta or other artery is incised and plaque and blood clot debris are removed. The artery lining (intima) is separated from the aorta or other artery walls and removed to increase the diameter of the blood vessel. The edges of the remaining normal intima are sutured to the blood vessel walls. The aorta or other artery is repaired primarily with sutures or a venous or synthetic patch graft is applied to enlarge the diameter. If a shunt has been placed it is removed. The vascular clamps are removed and blood flow through the blood vessel reinitiated. The aortic or other arterial suture line is checked for hemostasis. Overlying tissues are then closed in layers.

35351-35355

35351   Thromboendarterectomy, including patch graft, if performed; iliac
35355   Thromboendarterectomy, including patch graft, if performed; iliofemoral

Thromboendarterectomy is performed on the iliac (35351) or iliofemoral (35355) artery. This procedure removes a thrombus, such as a blood clot or atherosclerotic plaque that has adhered to vessels walls, along with the vessel intima from an occluded artery. An access incision is made in the abdomen for the iliac artery. To expose the iliofemoral artery an abdoiminal and leg incision is used. The thrombosed portion of the artery is isolated and dissected away from adjacent structures. Perfusion may be maintained by placement of a temporary shunt. Clamps are placed proximal and distal to the obstructed portion of the artery. The artery is incised and plaque and blood clot debris are removed. The artery lining (intima) is separated from the artery walls and removed to increase the diameter of the artery. The edges of the remaining normal intima are sutured to the artery walls. The artery is repaired primarily with sutures or a venous or synthetic patch graft is applied to enlarge the diameter. If a shunt has been placed it is removed. The vascular clamps are removed and blood flow through the artery reinitiated. The arterial suture line is checked for hemostasis. Overlying tissues are then closed in layers.

35361-35363

35361   Thromboendarterectomy, including patch graft, if performed; combined aortoiliac
35363   Thromboendarterectomy, including patch graft, if performed; combined aortoiliofemoral

Thromboendarterectomy is performed on the abdominal aorta and iliac artery (35361) or on the abdominal aorta, iliac and femoral artery (35363). This procedure removes a thrombus, such as a blood clot or atherosclerotic plaque that has adhered t o vessels walls, along with the vessel intima from an occluded artery. An access incision is made

in the abdomen and the aorta and iliac artery exposed. If a combined aortoiliofemoral thromboendarterectomy is performed, a leg incision is also made to expose the femoral artery. The thrombosed portions of the affected blood vessels are isolated and dissected away from adjacent structures. Perfusion may be maintained by placement of a temporary shunt. Clamps are placed proximal to the obstructed portion of the aorta and distal to the obstructed portion of the iliac or femoral artery. The affected portions of the blood vessels are incised and plaque and blood clot debris are removed. The artery lining (intima) is separated from the aorta, iliac and femoral artery walls and removed to increase the diameter of the blood vessel. The edges of the remaining normal intima are sutured to the blood vessel walls. The aorta, iliac and femoral arteries are repaired primarily with sutures or a venous or synthetic patch graft is applied to enlarge the diameter of the blood vessels. If a shunt has been placed, it is removed. The vascular clamps are removed and blood flow through the blood vessels reinitiated. The aortic, iliac and femoral artery suture lines are checked for hemostasis. Overlying tissues are then closed in layers.

35371-35372

35371   Thromboendarterectomy, including patch graft, if performed; common femoral
35372   Thromboendarterectomy, including patch graft, if performed; deep (profunda) femoral

Thromboendarterectomy is performed on the common femoral (35371) or deep (profunda) femoral artery (35372). This procedure removes a thrombus, such as a blood clot or atherosclerotic plaque that has adhered t o vessels walls, along with the vessel intima from an occluded artery. An access incision is made in the leg to expose the common or deep femoral artery. The thrombosed portions of the affected blood vessel is isolated and dissected away from adjacent structures. Perfusion may be maintained by placement of a temporary shunt. Clamps are placed proximal to the obstructed portion of the affected artery. The blood vessel is incised and plaque and blood clot debris are removed. The artery lining (intima) is separated from the artery walls and removed to increase the diameter of the blood vessel. The edges of the remaining normal intima are sutured to the artery walls. The affected artery is repaired primarily with sutures or a venous or synthetic patch graft is applied to enlarge the diameter of the blood vessels. If a shunt has been placed, it is removed. The vascular clamps are removed and blood flow through the blood vessels reinitiated. The arterial suture lines are checked for hemostasis. Overlying tissues are then closed in layers.

35390

35390   Reoperation, carotid, thromboendarterectomy, more than 1 month after original operation (List separately in addition to code for primary procedure)

A reoperation is performed on the carotid artery for thromboendarterectomy more than one month following the original operation. This procedure removes a thrombus, such as a blood clot or atherosclerotic plaque that has adhered to vessels walls, along with the vessel intima from an occluded artery. An access incision is made in the neck over the carotid artery. The thrombosed portion of the artery is isolated and dissected away from adjacent structures. Cerebral perfusion may be maintained by placement of a temporary shunt. Clamps are placed proximal and distal to the obstructed portion of the artery. The artery is incised and plaque and blood clot debris are removed. The artery lining (intima) is separated from the arterial walls and removed to increase the diameter of the artery. The edges of the remaining normal intima are sutured to the vessel walls. The artery is repaired primarily with sutures or a venous or synthetic patch graft is applied to enlarge the diameter of the artery. If a shunt has been placed it is removed. The vascular clamps are removed and blood flow through the artery reinitiated. The arterial suture line is checked for hemostasis. Overlying tissues are then closed in layers.

35400

35400   Angioscopy (non-coronary vessels or grafts) during therapeutic intervention (List separately in addition to code for primary procedure)

An angioscopy of non-coronary vessels or grafts is performed during a separately reportable therapeutic intervention. Angioscopy allows visualization of the interior of a blood vessel using a fiberoptic imaging system. The imaging system is composed of illumination fibers, imaging fibers, a video camera and monitor, and a videotape recorder. The skin over the access vessel is cleansed and the vessel punctured. A sheath is placed in the vessel and a guidewire advanced to the non-coronary vessel or graft of interest. The angioscopy catheter is then advanced over the guidewire to a point just proximal to the region to the imaged. An occlusion balloon on the catheter is inflated. The vessel is flushed with lactated Ringers solution. The imaging bundle is then advanced over the guidewire to the region to be examined. Images of the interior of the blood vessel are obtained. The images are displayed on the monitor. The physician reviews and interprets the images and provides a written report.

35500

35500 Harvest of upper extremity vein, 1 segment, for lower extremity or coronary artery bypass procedure (List separately in addition to code for primary procedure)

Upper extremity veins that are commonly used for bypass include the brachial and basilic veins. A deep incision is made in the medial aspect of the upper arm and the brachial or basilic vein exposed. Soft tissue is dissected off the vein and branches ligated and divided. The section of vein to be used is then ligated proximally and distally, divided and removed from the arm. The arm incision is closed and the vein is prepared for bypass grafting.

35501

35501 Bypass graft, with vein; common carotid-ipsilateral internal carotid

A bypass graft is created around a diseased or obstructed portion of the common carotid artery to the internal carotid artery on the same side using a vein harvested from the patient or another donor. Through an incision in the neck, the common carotid is exposed and clamps are applied proximal to the diseased portion. The artery may be tied off above the diseased or obstructed area and then one end of the harvested vein graft is sutured to the common carotid. A vessel clamp is applied to the venous graft while the arterial clamp is released to test for leaks at the anastomosis site. The internal carotid artery on the same side is exposed and then clamped distal to the site. Through an incision, the other end of the venous graft is sutured into place in the internal carotid artery and the grafted site is checked again for leaks and patency before closing the neck wound. This provides a new route for blood to bypass the blocked portion of the common carotid artery.

35506

35506 Bypass graft, with vein; carotid-subclavian or subclavian-carotid

A carotid-subclavian or subclavian-carotid bypass graft using vein is created around a diseased or obstructed portion of the artery. An incision is made above the clavicle (supraclavicular) to expose the subclavian artery. The scalene fat pad is dissected and the anterior scalene muscle divided. An incision is made over the carotid artery and it is exposed. Both arteries are controlled by passing rubber loops proximal and distal to the planned arteriotomy sites. A vein graft is harvested. If a saphenous vein graft is used, an incision is made in the skin of the leg over the section of saphenous vein to be harvested. Soft tissue is dissected off the vein and branches ligated and divided. The section of saphenous vein to be used is then ligated proximally and distally, divided and removed from the leg. The subclavian artery is clamped and incised. The saphenous vein graft is sutured to the subclavian artery. The carotid artery is incised or a window created for placement of the vein graft which is sutured to the artery. The vascular clamps are removed. Blood flow through the graft is checked using Doppler and distal pulses are evaluated to ensure patency of the bypass graft.

35508

35508 Bypass graft, with vein; carotid-vertebral

A carotid-vertebral bypass graft using vein is created around a diseased or obstructed portion of vertebral artery. The vertebral arteries arise from the brachiocephalic artery on the right and the subclavian artery on the left. These arteries enter the C6 transverse process, traveling through the C6-C2 processes exiting at the base of the skull. There is an extracranial segment between C2 and the base of the skull. The intracranial segment begins at the atlanto-occipital membrane and continues until the two vertebral arteries join to form the basilar artery. The vertebrobasilar arteries supply the brainstem, cerebellum, and occipital lobes of the brain. An incision is made over the vertebral artery below the obstructed segment and the vertebral artery is dissected free of surrounding tissue. A vein graft is harvested. If a saphenous vein graft is used, an incision is made in the skin of the leg over the section of saphenous vein to be harvested. Soft tissue is dissected off the vein and branches ligated and divided. The section of saphenous vein to be used is then ligated proximally and distally, divided and removed from the leg. The vertebral artery is clamped and incised. The saphenous vein graft is sutured to the vertebral artery. An incision is made over the common carotid artery and the artery exposed. The carotid artery is incised or a window created for placement of the vein graft which is sutured to the artery. The vascular clamps are removed. Blood flow through the graft is checked using Doppler and distal pulses are evaluated to ensure patency of the bypass graft.

35509

35509 Bypass graft, with vein; carotid-contralateral carotid

A carotid-contralateral carotid bypass graft is created using vein around a diseased or obstructed portion of carotid artery. An incision is made over the common carotid artery on one side of the neck. Soft tissues are carefully dissected and nerves and veins mobilized. The carotid artery is dissected free of surrounding tissue for a length of 5-6 cm. Exposure of the opposite carotid is performed in the same manner. Both carotids are controlled by passing soft rubber loops distal and proximal to the planned arteriotomy sites. A tunnel is created from one side of the neck to the other. A vein graft is harvested. If a saphenous vein graft is used, an incision is made in the skin of the leg over the section of saphenous vein to be harvested. Soft tissue is dissected off the vein and branches ligated and divided. The

section of saphenous vein to be used is then ligated proximally and distally, divided and removed from the leg. The healthy carotid artery is clamped and incised. The saphenous vein graft is sutured to the healthy carotid artery. The diseased contralateral carotid artery is clamped, incised and the vein graft is sutured to the artery. The vascular clamps are removed. Blood flow through the graft is checked using Doppler and distal pulses are evaluated to ensure patency of the bypass graft.

35510

35510 Bypass graft, with vein; carotid-brachial

A carotid-brachial bypass graft is created around a diseased or obstructed portion of artery involving some combination of the distal subclavian, axillary, and brachial arteries. An incision is made in the neck; soft tissue is dissected; and the common carotid artery is exposed. A second incision is made in the arm over the brachial artery, typically just above the elbow. Soft tissue is dissected and the brachial artery is exposed. A tunnel is created beginning at the exposed section of carotid artery, passing through the axillary region and down the arm, and terminating at the exposed section of brachial artery. A vein graft is harvested. If a saphenous vein graft is used, an incision is made in the leg over the section of saphenous vein to be harvested. Soft tissue is dissected off the vein and its branches are ligated and divided. The section of vein to be used is then ligated proximally and distally, divided, and removed from the leg. Vascular clamps are applied to the carotid artery and the artery is incised. The vein graft is sutured to the carotid artery then passed through the previously created tunnel. The brachial artery is clamped and incised and the other end of the vein graft is sutured to the brachial artery. The vascular clamps are removed. Blood flow through the graft is checked using Doppler. Distal pulses are evaluated to ensure patency of the bypass graft.

35511-35512

35511 Bypass graft, with vein; subclavian-subclavian
35512 Bypass graft, with vein; subclavian-brachial

A subclavian-subclavian or subclavian-brachial bypass graft is created around a diseased or obstructed portion of artery. In 35511, the proximal subclavian artery is diseased or obstructed and a subclavian-subclavian bypass graft is performed. This procedure treats disease or obstruction of the contralateral (opposite) subclavian artery. An incision is made at the base of the neck just above the clavicle and the first subclavian artery is exposed. This is repeated on the opposite side and the second subclavian artery is exposed. A tunnel is created across the chest from one subclavian artery to the other. A vein graft is harvested. If a saphenous vein graft is used, an incision is made in the skin of the leg over the section of saphenous vein to be harvested. Soft tissue is dissected off the saphenous vein and saphenous vein branches ligated and divided. The section of saphenous vein to be used is then ligated proximally and distally, divided, and removed from the leg. Vascular clamps are applied to the first subclavian artery and the artery is incised. The vein graft is sutured to the first subclavian artery. The vein graft is then passed through the previously created tunnel. The subclavian artery on the opposite side is clamped and incised. The vein graft is sutured to the opposite subclavian artery. The vascular clamps are removed. Blood flow through the graft is checked using Doppler and distal pulses are evaluated to ensure patency of the bypass graft. In 35512, subclavian-brachial bypass graft is performed to reroute blood around an occlusion in the in the axillary or proximal brachial artery on the ipsilateral side (same side) of the body. Less commonly, subclavian-brachial bypass graft may be performed to treat severe vascular trauma involving the chest wall, shoulder and upper arm. An incision is made at the base of the neck just above the clavicle and the subclavian artery is exposed. A second incision is made in the arm over the brachial artery, typically just above the elbow. Soft tissue is dissected and the brachial artery exposed. A tunnel is created beginning at the exposed section of subclavian artery and passing under the clavicle. The tunnel continues through the axillary region and down the arm, and terminates at the planned anastomosis site in the brachial artery. A saphenous vein graft is harvested as described above. Vascular clamps are applied to the subclavian artery and the artery is incised. The vein graft is sutured to the subclavian artery. The vein graft is then passed through the previously created tunnel. The brachial artery is clamped and incised. The vein graft is sutured to the brachial artery. The vascular clamps are removed. Blood flow through the graft is checked using Doppler and distal pulses are evaluated to ensure patency of the bypass graft.

35515

35515 Bypass graft, with vein; subclavian-vertebral

A subclavian-vertebral bypass graft is created around a diseased or obstructed portion of the vertebral artery. An incision is made at the base of the neck just above the clavicle and the subclavian artery is exposed. Exposure of the proximal vertebral artery may be performed through the same supraclavicular incision carried down to the sternal notch. The clavicle is divided as needed. The anterior scalene muscle is exposed and divided taking care to protect the phrenic nerve. Vertebral nerve fibers are divided and the proximal vertebral artery is exposed. Exposure of the distal vertebral artery may be performed through an anterolateral in which the sternocleidomastoid is detached from the mastoid process and wide exposure of the vertebral artery is achieved by extension of the incision to the sternal notch. A vein graft is harvested. If a saphenous vein graft is used, an incision

● New Code ▲ Revised Code

Cardiovascular System

is made in the leg over the section of saphenous vein to be harvested. Soft tissue is dissected off the vein and its branches are ligated and divided. The section of vein to be used is then ligated proximally and distally, divided, and removed from the leg. Vascular clamps are applied to the subclavian artery and the artery is incised. The vein graft is sutured to the subclavian artery then tunneled through the neck to the vertebral artery, which is clamped and incised. The other end of the vein graft is sutured to the vertebral artery and the vascular clamps are removed. Blood flow through the graft is checked using Doppler.

35516

35516   Bypass graft, with vein; subclavian-axillary

A subclavian-axillary bypass graft is created around a diseased or obstructed portion of the axillary artery on the ipsilateral side (same side) of the body. An incision is made at the base of the neck just above the clavicle and the subclavian artery is exposed. A second incision is made in the chest just below the collar bone over the axillary artery. Soft tissue is dissected and the axillary artery is exposed. A tunnel is created beginning at the exposed section of subclavian artery, passing under the clavicle, and continuing to the exposed portion of axillary artery. A vein graft is harvested. If a saphenous vein graft is used, an incision is made in the leg over the section of saphenous vein to be harvested. Soft tissue is dissected off the vein and its branches are ligated and divided. The section of vein to be used is then ligated proximally and distally, divided, and removed from the leg. Vascular clamps are applied to the subclavian artery and the artery is incised. The vein graft is sutured to the subclavian artery then passed through the previously created tunnel. The axillary artery is clamped and incised and the other end of the vein graft is sutured to the axillary artery. The vascular clamps are removed. Blood flow through the graft is checked using Doppler. Distal pulses are evaluated to ensure patency of the bypass graft.

35518

35518   Bypass graft, with vein; axillary-axillary

An axillary-axillary bypass graft is created around a diseased or obstructed portion of the axillary artery on the contralateral (opposite) side. A skin incision is made in chest just below the clavicle; soft tissue is dissected; and the proximal aspect of the first axillary artery is exposed. This is repeated on the opposite side. A tunnel is created across the chest from one axillary artery to the other. A vein graft is harvested. If a saphenous vein graft is used, an incision is made in the leg over the section of saphenous vein to be harvested. Soft tissue is dissected off the vein and its branches are ligated and divided. The section of vein to be used is then ligated proximally and distally, divided, and removed from the leg. Vascular clamps are applied to the first axillary artery and the artery is incised. The vein graft is sutured to the axillary artery then passed through the previously created tunnel to the second axillary artery, which is clamped and incised. The other end of the vein graft is sutured to the second axillary artery. The vascular clamps are removed. Blood flow through the graft is checked using Doppler. Distal pulses are evaluated to ensure patency of the bypass graft.

35521

35521   Bypass graft, with vein; axillary-femoral

An axillary-femoral bypass graft is created to reroute blood flow around a diseased or obstructed portion of the aorta and/or iliac artery. A skin incision is made in chest just below the clavicle; soft tissue is dissected; and the proximal axillary artery is exposed. A second incision is made in the groin over the common femoral artery, which is also exposed. A tunnel is created beginning at the exposed section of axillary artery, passing down the chest and abdomen, under the inguinal ligament, and terminating at the exposed section of common femoral artery. A vein graft is harvested. If a saphenous vein graft is used, an incision is made in the leg over the section of saphenous vein to be harvested. Soft tissue is dissected off the vein and its branches are ligated and divided. The section of vein to be used is then ligated proximally and distally, divided, and removed from the leg. Vascular clamps are applied to the axillary artery and the artery is incised. The vein graft is sutured to the axillary artery then passed through the previously created tunnel. The common femoral artery is clamped and incised and the other end of the vein graft is sutured to the common femoral artery. The vascular clamps are removed. Blood flow through the graft is checked using Doppler. Distal pulses are evaluated to ensure patency of the bypass graft.

35522

35522   Bypass graft, with vein; axillary-brachial

An axillary-brachial bypass graft is created around a diseased or obstructed portion of the axillary and brachial arteries on the ipsilateral side (same side) of the body. A skin incision is made in chest just below the clavicle; soft tissue is dissected; and the proximal axillary artery is exposed. A second incision is made in the arm over the brachial artery, typically just above the elbow. Soft tissue is dissected and the brachial artery is exposed. A tunnel is created beginning at the exposed section of axillary artery, passing down the arm, and terminating at the exposed section of brachial artery. A vein graft is harvested. If a saphenous vein graft is used, an incision is made in the leg over the section of saphenous

vein to be harvested. Soft tissue is dissected off the vein and its branches are ligated and divided. The section of vein to be used is then ligated proximally and distally, divided, and removed from the leg. Vascular clamps are applied to the axillary artery and the artery is incised. The vein graft is sutured to the axillary artery then passed through the previously created tunnel. The brachial artery is clamped and incised. The other end of the vein graft is sutured to the brachial artery and vascular clamps are removed. Blood flow through the graft is checked using Doppler. Distal pulses are evaluated to ensure patency of the bypass graft.

35523

35523   Bypass graft, with vein; brachial-ulnar or -radial

A stenotic or occluded section of artery in the arm extending from the brachial artery to the ulnar or radial artery is replaced with a venous bypass graft. Brachial-ulnar or brachial-radial bypass procedures are typically performed to treat chronic arterial occlusive disease and ischemia of the upper extremity, often associated with immunosuppression or renal failure. An incision is made in the upper arm over the brachial artery for exposure. Soft tissue is dissected off the artery for several centimeters and rubber loops are placed around the artery to isolate it. Attention is then directed to the lower arm and an incision is made over the ulnar or radial artery, usually at the wrist and the artery is exposed. A section of the ulnar or radial artery is dissected free of soft tissue and isolated with soft rubber loops. A section of saphenous vein is harvested from the leg. Vascular clamps are then applied to the brachial artery, which is incised and the venous graft is sutured to it. The graft is then tunneled through to the ulnar or radial artery. An incision is made in the selected artery and the graft is cut to the correct length and sutured to the selected artery. Vascular clamps are removed, hemostasis is verified, and patency of the graft is checked by Doppler and palpating distal pulses.

35525

35525   Bypass graft, with vein; brachial-brachial

A brachial-brachial bypass graft is created around a diseased or obstructed portion of the brachial artery on the ipsilateral side (same side) of the body. A skin incision is made in the upper arm over the proximal portion of the brachial artery. A second skin incision is made in the arm over the distal brachial artery. A tunnel is created from the proximal to the distal section. A vein graft is harvested. If a saphenous vein graft is used, an incision is made in the leg over the section of saphenous vein to be harvested. Soft tissue is dissected off the vein and its branches are ligated and divided. The section of vein to be used is then ligated proximally and distally, divided, and removed from the leg. Vascular clamps are applied to the proximal brachial artery and the artery is incised. The vein graft is sutured to the proximal brachial artery then passed through the previously created tunnel. The distal brachial artery is clamped and incised and the other end of the vein graft is sutured to the distal brachial artery. The vascular clamps are removed. Blood flow through the graft is checked using Doppler. Distal pulses are evaluated to ensure patency of the bypass graft.

35526

35526   Bypass graft, with vein; aortosubclavian, aortoinnominate, or aortocarotid

An aortosubclavian, aortoinnominate, or aortocarotid bypass graft using a vein is created around a diseased or obstructed portion of the subclavian, innominate, or carotid artery. To perform an aortocarotid artery bypass, an incision is made in the side of the neck over the common carotid artery. Soft tissues are carefully dissected and nerves and veins are mobilized. The carotid artery is dissected free of surrounding tissue. To perform an aortosubclavian or aortoinnominate artery graft, a separate supraclavicular incision may be made, or the affected artery may be exposed along with the aorta by median sternotomy. A tunnel is created from the aorta to the affected artery. A vein graft is harvested. If a saphenous vein graft is used, an incision is made in the skin of the leg over the section of saphenous vein to be harvested. Soft tissue is dissected off the vein and branches are ligated and divided. The section of saphenous vein to be used is then ligated proximally and distally, divided, and removed from the leg. Vascular clamps are placed on the subclavian or carotid artery above and below the planned incision site. The artery is incised and the venous graft is sutured to the artery. A side-biting clamp is placed on the aorta at the planned incision site. The aorta is incised and the venous graft is sutured to the aorta. Vascular clamps are released and suture lines are checked for hemostasis.

35531

35531   Bypass graft, with vein; aortoceliac or aortomesenteric

An aortoceliac or aortomesenteric bypass graft is created using vein around a diseased or obstructed portion of celiac or mesenteric artery. The celiac artery, also referred to as the celiac trunk, arises from the aorta and is the first aortic branch located below the diaphragm. The celiac trunk has three branches, the hepatic artery which supplies the liver, the left gastric artery which supplies the stomach, and the splenic artery which supplies the spleen, pancreas, and stomach. There are two mesenteric arteries. The superior mesenteric artery distributes blood to the small intestines and the upper portion of the large intestine and the inferior mesenteric artery distributes blood to the lower portion of the large intestines and rectum. If the celiac trunk or superior mesenteric artery is obstructed or diseased, the upper abdomen is incised and the lesser omentum opened. The diaphragmatic crura are sharply dissected and the upper abdominal aorta exposed. The celiac artery and its branches or the superior mesenteric artery are exposed and dissected free of surrounding tissues. If the inferior mesenteric artery requires bypass grafting, an incision is made in the lower abdomen and the lower abdominal aorta is exposed. The inferior mesenteric artery is dissected free of surrounding tissues. A vein graft is harvested. If a saphenous vein graft is used, an incision is made in the skin of the leg over the section of saphenous vein to be harvested. Soft tissue is dissected off the vein and branches ligated and divided. The section of saphenous vein to be used is then ligated proximally and distally, divided and removed from the leg. A side-biting clamp is placed on the aorta at the base of the affected artery. The aorta is incised and the venous graft sutured to the aorta. The affected artery is also incised at a point beyond the area of obstruction or disease and the vein graft sutured to the affected artery. The vascular clamp is released and suture lines checked for hemostasis.

35533

35533   **Bypass graft, with vein; axillary-femoral-femoral**

An axillary-femoral-femoral bypass graft is created to reroute blood flow around a diseased or obstructed portion of the aorta and/or iliac arteries. A skin incision is made in the chest just below the clavicle; soft tissue is dissected; and the proximal axillary artery is exposed. Two additional incisions are made in the groin over the common femoral arteries. Soft tissue is dissected and both common femoral arteries are exposed. A tunnel is created beginning at the exposed section of axillary artery, passing down the chest and abdomen, under the inguinal ligament, and terminating at the exposed section of ipsilateral (same side) common femoral artery. A second side tunnel is created from the lower abdomen to the contralateral (opposite side) common femoral artery. A vein graft is harvested. If a saphenous vein graft is used, an incision is made in the leg over the section of saphenous vein to be harvested. Soft tissue is dissected off the vein and its branches are ligated and divided. The section of vein to be used is then ligated proximally and distally, divided, and removed from the leg. Vascular clamps are applied to the axillary artery and the artery is incised. The vein graft is sutured to the axillary artery then passed through the previously created tunnel to the ipsilateral common femoral artery, which is clamped and incised. The vein graft is sutured to the ipsilateral common femoral artery. The contralateral femoral artery is clamped and incised and the graft vein graft is sutured to the contralateral femoral artery. The vascular clamps are removed. Blood flow through the graft is checked using Doppler. Distal pulses are evaluated to ensure patency of the bypass graft.

35535

35535   **Bypass graft, with vein; hepatorenal**

A hepatorenal vein bypass graft is created around a diseased or obstructed portion of the right or left renal artery to restore blood flow to the kidney. The abdomen is incised. The omentum is separated from the transverse colon and the celiac axis is exposed. Celiac axis arteries (hepatic, left gastric, and splenic) are evaluated and the common hepatic artery is isolated. The descending duodenum is mobilized and the inferior vena cava and renal vein are located. The inferior vena cava is mobilized and the renal artery is isolated. A vein graft is harvested. If a saphenous vein graft is used, an incision is made in the skin of the leg over the section of saphenous vein to be harvested. Soft tissue is dissected off the vein and its branches are ligated and divided. The section of saphenous vein to be used is then ligated proximally and distally, divided, and removed from the leg. Vascular clamps are applied to the hepatic artery, which is incised. The vein graft is sutured in an end-to-side configuration to the hepatic artery. The renal artery is then clamped and incised and the vein graft is anastomosed, again in an end-to-side fashion, bypassing the diseased or obstructed portion of the renal artery. The clamps are released and blood flow through the graft is checked using Doppler.

35536

35536   **Bypass graft, with vein; splenorenal**

A splenorenal vein bypass graft is created around a diseased or obstructed portion of the right or left renal artery to restore blood flow to the kidney. The abdomen is incised, the omentum separated from the transverse colon, and the celiac axis exposed. Celiac axis arteries (hepatic, left gastric, and splenic) are evaluated and the splenic artery isolated. The descending duodenum is mobilized and the inferior vena cava and renal vein are located. The inferior vena cava is mobilized and the renal artery isolated. A vein graft is harvested. If a saphenous vein graft is used, an incision is made in the skin of the leg over the section of saphenous vein to be harvested. Soft tissue is dissected off the saphenous vein and saphenous vein branches are ligated and divided. The section of saphenous vein to be used is then ligated proximally and distally, divided and removed from the leg. Vascular clamps are applied to the splenic artery and the artery is incised. The vein graft is sutured in an end-to-side configuration to the splenic artery. The renal artery is clamped and incised and the vein graft is anastomosed end-to-side bypassing the diseased or obstructed portion of the renal artery. The clamps are released and blood flow through the graft checked using Doppler.

35537-35538

35537   **Bypass graft, with vein; aortoiliac**
35538   **Bypass graft, with vein; aortobi-iliac**

A bypass graft is created around a diseased or obstructed portion of the lower aorta to one or both iliac arteries using a vein harvested from the patient or another donor. Through a lower abdominal incision, the aorta is exposed and clamps are applied above the diseased portion. The aorta may be tied off above the diseased or obstructed area and then one end of the harvested vein graft is sutured to the aorta. A vessel clamp is applied to the venous graft while the aortic clamp is released to test for leaks at the anastomosis site. The exposed iliac artery is then clamped distal to the site. Through an incision, the other end of the venous graft is sutured into place in the iliac artery and the grafted site is checked again for leaks and patency before closing the abdominal wound. This provides a new route for blood to bypass the blocked portion of aorta. Code 35537 for a bypass graft from the aorta to one iliac vessel (aortoiliac) and 35538 for bypass grafting from the aorta to both iliac vessels (aortobi-iliac).

35539-35540

35539   **Bypass graft, with vein; aortofemoral**
35540   **Bypass graft, with vein; aortobifemoral**

A bypass graft is created around a diseased or obstructed portion of the lower aorta to one or both femoral arteries using a vein harvested from the patient or another donor. Through a lower abdominal incision, the aorta is exposed and clamps are applied above the diseased portion. The aorta may be tied off above the diseased or obstructed area and then one end of the harvested vein graft is sutured to the aorta. A vessel clamp is applied to the venous graft while the aortic clamp is released to test for leaks at the anastomosis site. The exposed femoral artery is then clamped distal to the site. Through an incision, the other end of the venous graft is sutured into place in the iliac artery and the grafted site is checked again for leaks and patency before closing the abdominal wound. This provides a new route for blood to bypass the blocked portion of aorta. Code 35539 for a bypass graft from the aorta to the femoral artery and 35540 for bypass grafting from the aorta to both femoral vessels.

35556

35556   **Bypass graft, with vein; femoral-popliteal**

A femoral-popliteal vein bypass graft is placed. A groin incision is made on the affected side and the femoral artery exposed. The popliteal artery is also exposed through an incision behind the knee. A tunnel is created from femoral artery to the popliteal artery. A vein graft is harvested. If a saphenous vein graft is used, an incision is made in the skin of the leg over the section of saphenous vein to be harvested. Soft tissue is dissected off the vein and branches ligated and divided. The section of saphenous vein to be used is then ligated proximally and distally, divided and removed from the leg. The vein graft is anastomosed to the femoral artery and then passed through the tunnel to the popliteal artery. The femoral artery is clamped, incised and the proximal end of the graft anastomosed. The popliteal artery is clamped, incised and the distal end of the graft anastomosed. Vascular clamps are released and hemostasis of all anastomosis sites checked. Blood flow through the graft is checked using Doppler and distal pulses are evaluated to ensure patency of the bypass graft.

35558

35558   **Bypass graft, with vein; femoral-femoral**

Incisions are made in the groin bilaterally over the common femoral arteries. Soft tissue is dissected and the common femoral arteries are exposed. An abdominal tunnel is created for placement of a cross-over graft from one femoral artery to the other. A vein graft is harvested. If a saphenous vein graft is used, an incision is made in the skin of the leg over the section of saphenous vein to be harvested. Soft tissue is dissected off the vein and branches ligated and divided. The section of saphenous vein to be used is then ligated proximally and distally, divided and removed from the leg. The common femoral artery on the unobstructed side is clamped, incised and the cross-over graft is sutured to artery. The cross-over graft is passed through the tunnel to the contralateral femoral artery. The contralateral femoral artery is clamped, incised and the graft sutured to the artery. The vascular clamps are removed. Blood flow through the graft is checked using Doppler and distal pulses are evaluated to ensure patency of the bypass graft.

35560

35560   **Bypass graft, with vein; aortorenal**

The upper abdomen is incised and the lesser omentum opened. The diaphragmatic crura are sharply dissected and the upper abdominal aorta exposed. The renal artery is exposed and dissected free of surrounding tissues. A vein graft is harvested. If a saphenous vein graft is used, an incision is made in the skin of the leg over the section of saphenous vein to be harvested. Soft tissue is dissected off the vein and branches ligated and divided. The section of saphenous vein to be used is then ligated proximally and distally, divided and removed from the leg. A side-biting clamp is placed on the aorta at the base of the renal artery. The aorta is incised and the venous graft sutured to the aorta. The renal artery is

Cardiovascular System

● New Code   ▲ Revised Code

incised at a point beyond the area of obstruction or disease and the vein graft sutured to it. The vascular clamp is released and suture lines checked for hemostasis.

35563-35565

35563   Bypass graft, with vein; ilioiliac
35565   Bypass graft, with vein; iliofemoral

An ilioiliac or iliofemoral bypass graft using vein is performed. The abdomen is opened to expose the iliac arteries. In 35563, both iliac arteries are exposed and dissected free of surrounding tissue. An abdominal tunnel is created for placement of a cross-over graft from one iliac artery to the other. A vein graft is harvested. If a saphenous vein graft is used, an incision is made in the skin of the leg over the section of saphenous vein to be harvested. Soft tissue is dissected off the vein and branches ligated and divided. The section of saphenous vein to be used is then ligated proximally and distally, divided and removed from the leg. The iliac artery on the unobstructed side is clamped, incised and the cross-over graft is sutured to artery. The cross-over graft is passed through the tunnel to the contralateral iliac artery. The contralateral iliac artery is clamped, incised and the graft sutured to the artery. Vascular clamps are released and suture lines checked for hemostasis. Blood flow through the graft is checked using Doppler and distal pulses are evaluated to ensure patency of the bypass graft. In 35565, the iliac artery is exposed. An incision is made on the ipsilateral (same) side in the groin over the common femoral artery. Soft tissue is dissected and the common femoral artery is exposed. A tunnel is created from the iliac artery to the femoral artery. The iliac artery is clamped, incised and the proximal end of the vein graft sutured to the iliac artery. The vein graft is passed through the tunnel to the femoral artery. The femoral artery is clamped, incised, and the distal end of the graft sutured to it. Vascular clamps are released and suture lines checked for hemostasis. Blood flow through the graft is checked using Doppler and distal pulses are evaluated to ensure patency of the bypass graft.

35566

35566   Bypass graft, with vein; femoral-anterior tibial, posterior tibial, peroneal artery or other distal vessels

A groin incision is made on the affected side and the femoral artery exposed. The distal anastomosis site on the anterior tibial, posterior tibial, peroneal, or other artery is also exposed. A tunnel is created from femoral artery to the distal anastomosis site. A vein graft is harvested. If a saphenous vein graft is used, an incision is made in the skin of the leg over the section of saphenous vein to be harvested. Soft tissue is dissected off the vein and branches ligated and divided. The section of saphenous vein to be used is then ligated proximally and distally, divided and removed from the leg. The vein graft is anastomosed to the femoral artery and then passed through the tunnel to the distal anastomosis site. The femoral artery is clamped, incised and the proximal end of the graft anastomosed. The distal artery is clamped, incised and the distal end of the graft anastomosed. Vascular clamps are released and hemostasis of all anastomosis sites checked. Blood flow through the graft is checked using Doppler and distal pulses are evaluated to ensure patency of the bypass graft.

35570

35570   Bypass graft, with vein; tibial-tibial, peroneal-tibial, or tibial/peroneal trunk-tibial

A tibial-tibial, peroneal-tibial, tibial/peroneal trunk-tibial vein bypass graft is created around a diseased or obstructed portion of artery to restore blood flow to the lower leg. The leg is incised over the planned proximal anastomosis site in the lower leg. Soft tissue is dissected and muscle fascia is exposed and incised. Muscle bundles are separated and the affected artery (tibial/peroneal trunk, tibial, or peroneal) is exposed. After dissecting soft tissue off the affected artery, control is achieved by passing a rubber loop around the vessel. Adequate blood inflow is verified. Exposure of the planned distal anastomosis site is accomplished in the same manner. A tunnel is then created for placement of the bypass graft. A vein graft is harvested. If a saphenous vein graft is used, an incision is made in the skin of the leg over the section of saphenous vein to be harvested. Soft tissue is dissected off the vein and its branches are ligated and divided. The section of saphenous vein to be used is then ligated proximally and distally, divided, and removed from the leg. Vascular clamps are applied above the diseased or obstructed portion of the artery to be bypassed, and the proximal aspect (inflow) of the artery is incised. The vein graft is then sutured to the artery and passed through the tunnel. The distal anastomosis site in the tibial artery is incised. The vein graft is anastomosed, bypassing the diseased artery segment. The clamps are released. Blood flow through the graft is checked using Doppler, and distal pulses are evaluated to ensure patency of the bypass graft.

35571

35571   Bypass graft, with vein; popliteal-tibial, -peroneal artery or other distal vessels

An incision is made on the affected side behind the knee and the popliteal artery exposed. The distal anastomosis site on the anterior tibial, posterior tibial, peroneal, or other artery is also exposed. A tunnel is created from popliteal artery to the distal anastomosis site.

A vein graft is harvested. If a saphenous vein graft is used, an incision is made in the skin of the leg over the section of saphenous vein to be harvested. Soft tissue is dissected off the vein and branches ligated and divided. The section of saphenous vein to be used is then ligated proximally and distally, divided and removed from the leg. The vein graft is anastomosed to the femoral artery and then passed through the tunnel to the distal anastomosis site. The popliteal artery is clamped, incised and the proximal end of the graft anastomosed. The distal artery is clamped, incised and the distal end of the graft anastomosed. Vascular clamps are released and hemostasis of all anastomosis sites checked. Blood flow through the graft is checked using Doppler and distal pulses are evaluated to ensure patency of the bypass graft.

35572

35572   Harvest of femoropopliteal vein, 1 segment, for vascular reconstruction procedure (eg, aortic, vena caval, coronary, peripheral artery) (List separately in addition to code for primary procedure)

The superficial femoral-popliteal vein (SFPV) is primarily used in reconstruction of aortic grafts due to infection, other infected vascular grafts, limb salvage procedures, and large venous reconstructions. An incision is made along the lateral border of the sartorius muscle. The sartorius muscle is reflected medially and the SFPV exposed and mobilized. The SFPV is ligated and divided at the junction of the deep and common femoral veins. The distal transection site is dependent on the length of vein required for the reconstruction procedure. The SFPV is prepared for use in the reconstruction procedure which includes valvotomy to allow placement of the vein graft in a non-reversed position.

35583-35587

35583   In-situ vein bypass; femoral-popliteal
35585   In-situ vein bypass; femoral-anterior tibial, posterior tibial, or peroneal artery
35587   In-situ vein bypass; popliteal-tibial, peroneal

An in-situ vein bypass is performed using the saphenous vein to bypass occluded lower extremity arteries. An incision is made in the leg and the saphenous vein exposed and evaluated. The proximal and distal aspects are mobilized leaving the rest of the saphenous vein in place. The saphenous vein is ligated, and divided proximally at the saphenofemoral junction with a cuff of femoral vein. The saphenous vein is then anastomosed to the common femoral, proximal superficial femoral or popliteal artery. The venous valves are destroyed using a valvulotome that renders them incompetent so that arterial blood will flow down through the saphenous vein. Saphenous vein tributaries are identified and ligated. The distal aspect of the saphenous vein is ligated and divided and anastomosed to the popliteal, anterior tibial, posterior tibial or peroneal artery. Vascular clamps are released and hemostasis of all anastomosis sites checked. Blood flow through is checked using Doppler and distal pulses are evaluated to ensure patency of the in-situ bypass. Use 35583 for in-situ vein bypass of the femoral-popliteal arteries. Use 35585 if the in-situ vein bypass involves the femoral-anterior tibial, femoral-posterior tibial, or femoral-peroneal arteries. Use 35587 for in-situ vein bypass of the popliteal-tibial or popliteal-peroneal arteries.

35600

35600   Harvest of upper extremity artery, 1 segment, for coronary artery bypass procedure (List separately in addition to code for primary procedure)

One segment of an upper extremity artery, usually the radial artery, is harvested for grafting in a separately reportable coronary artery bypass procedure. An incision is made in the arm over the radial artery beginning just below the antecubital (elbow) crease and extending to the wrist crease. The fascial sheath overlying the superficial muscles of the forearm is divided taking care to protect the lateral cutaneous nerve. The brachioradialis and flexor carpi radialis muscles are retracted to expose the entire length of the radial artery. The radial artery is dissected and side branches clipped or ligated. When the radial artery is completely mobilized, the proximal and distal ends are suture ligated and divided. The radial artery graft is flushed with papaverine and wrapped in papaverine-soaked gauze. Electrocautery is used to control bleeding at the radial artery harvest site. The forearm is closed in layers. The radial artery is prepared for grafting.

35601

35601   Bypass graft, with other than vein; common carotid-ipsilateral internal carotid

A bypass graft is created around a diseased or obstructed portion of the common carotid artery to the internal carotid artery on the same side using a graft other than harvested vein, such as a synthetic graft. Through an incision in the neck, the common carotid is exposed and clamps are applied proximal to the diseased portion. The artery may be tied off above the diseased or obstructed area and then one end of the graft is sutured to the common carotid. A vessel clamp is applied to the graft portion while the arterial clamp is released to test for leaks at the anastomosis site. The internal carotid artery on the same side is exposed and then clamped distal to the site. Through an incision, the other end of the graft is sutured into place in the internal carotid artery and the grafted site is checked

Cardiovascular System

again for leaks and patency before closing the neck wound. This provides a new route for blood to bypass the blocked portion of the common carotid artery.

35606

35606   Bypass graft, with other than vein; carotid-subclavian

A carotid-subclavian bypass graft using other than vein is created around a diseased or obstructed portion of artery. An incision is made above the clavicle (supraclavicular) to expose the subclavian artery. The scalene fat pad is dissected and the anterior scalene muscle divided. An incision is made over the carotid artery and it is exposed. Both arteries are controlled by passing rubber loops proximal and distal to the planned arteriotomy sites. An appropriately sized tubular synthetic graft is selected and prepared. The subclavian artery is clamped and incised. The synthetic graft is sutured to the subclavian artery. The carotid artery is incised or a window created for placement of the graft which is sutured to the artery. The vascular clamps are removed. Blood flow through the graft is checked using Doppler and distal pulses are evaluated to ensure patency of the bypass graft.

35612-35616

35612   Bypass graft, with other than vein; subclavian-subclavian
35616   Bypass graft, with other than vein; subclavian-axillary

A subclavian-subclavian or subclavian-axillary bypass graft is created with other than vein around a diseased or obstructed portion of artery. In 35612, the proximal subclavian artery is diseased or obstructed and a subclavian-subclavian bypass graft is performed. This procedure treats disease or obstruction of the contralateral (opposite) subclavian artery. An incision is made at the base of the neck just above the clavicle and the first subclavian artery is exposed. This is repeated on the opposite side and the second subclavian artery is exposed. A tunnel is created across the chest from one subclavian artery to the other. An appropriately sized tubular synthetic graft is selected and prepared. Vascular clamps are applied to the first subclavian artery and the artery is incised. The synthetic graft is sutured to the first subclavian artery. The graft is then passed through the previously created tunnel. The subclavian artery on the opposite side is clamped and incised. The graft is sutured to the opposite subclavian artery. The vascular clamps are removed. Blood flow through the graft is checked using Doppler and distal pulses are evaluated to ensure patency of the bypass graft. In 35616, subclavian-axillary bypass graft is performed to reroute blood around an occlusion in the axillary artery on the ipsilateral (same) side of the body. An incision is made at the base of the neck just above the clavicle and the subclavian artery exposed. A second incision is made in the arm over the axillary artery. A tunnel is created beginning at the exposed section of subclavian artery and passed under the clavicle. The tunnel continues to the planned anastomosis site in the axillary artery. The synthetic graft is sutured to the axillary artery. The vascular clamps are removed. Blood flow through the graft is checked using Doppler and distal pulses are evaluated to ensure patency of the bypass graft.

35621-35623

35621   Bypass graft, with other than vein; axillary-femoral
35623   Bypass graft, with other than vein; axillary-popliteal or -tibial

An axillary-femoral or axillary-popliteal /-tibial bypass graft with other than vein is created to reroute blood flow around a diseased or obstructed portion of the aorta, iliac, and/or femoral artery. A skin incision is made in the chest just below the clavicle, soft tissue dissected, and the proximal axillary artery is exposed. A second incision is made in the groin over the common femoral artery or in the leg over the popliteal or tibial artery. Soft tissue is dissected and the common femoral, popliteal, or tibial artery exposed. A tunnel is created beginning at the exposed section of axillary artery, passing down the chest and abdomen, passing under the inguinal ligament, and terminating at the exposed section of common femoral artery for an axillary-femoral bypass. If an axillary-popliteal/- tibial bypass is performed the tunnel is extended along the leg to the exposed section of popliteal or tibial artery. An appropriately sized tubular synthetic graft is selected and prepared. Vascular clamps are applied to the axillary artery and the artery is incised. The synthetic graft is sutured to the axillary artery. The graft is then passed through the previously created tunnel. The common femoral, popliteal, or iliac artery is clamped and incised and the graft is sutured to artery. The vascular clamps are removed. Blood flow through the graft is checked using Doppler and distal pulses are evaluated to ensure patency of the bypass graft. Use 35621 for an axillary-femoral bypass graft and 35623 for an axillary-popliteal/-tibial graft.

35626

35626   Bypass graft, with other than vein; aortosubclavian, aortoinnominate, or aortocarotid

An aortosubclavian, aortoinnominate, or aortocarotid bypass graft using material other than a vein is created around a diseased or obstructed portion of the subclavian or carotid artery. To perform an aortocarotid artery bypass, an incision is made in the side of the neck over the common carotid artery. Soft tissues are carefully dissected and nerves and veins are mobilized. The carotid artery is dissected free of surrounding tissue. To perform

an aortosubclavian or aortoinnominate artery graft, a separate supraclavicular incision may be made, or the affected artery may be exposed along with the aorta by median sternotomy. A tunnel is created from the aorta to the affected artery. An appropriately sized tubular synthetic graft is selected and prepared. A side-biting clamp is placed on the aorta at the planned incision site. The aorta is incised and the synthetic graft is sutured to the aorta. Vascular clamps are placed on the subclavian or carotid artery above and below the planned incision site. The artery is incised and the synthetic graft is sutured to the artery. Vascular clamps are released and suture lines are checked for hemostasis. Blood flow through the graft is checked using Doppler and distal pulses are evaluated to ensure patency of the bypass graft.

35631

35631   Bypass graft, with other than vein; aortoceliac, aortomesenteric, aortorenal

An aortoceliac, aortomesenteric, or aortorenal bypass graft is created around a diseased or obstructed portion of the celiac, mesenteric, or renal artery using grafting material from a source other than a vein. The celiac artery, also referred to as the celiac trunk, arises from the aorta and is the first aortic branch located below the diaphragm. The celiac trunk has three branches, the hepatic artery which supplies the liver, the left gastric artery which supplies the stomach, and the splenic artery which supplies the spleen, pancreas, and stomach. There are two mesenteric arteries. The superior mesenteric artery distributes blood to the small intestines and the upper portion of the large intestine and the inferior mesenteric artery distributes blood to the lower portion of the large intestines and rectum. The renal arteries supply blood to the kidneys. If the celiac trunk, superior mesenteric artery, or renal artery is obstructed or diseased, the upper abdomen is incised and the lesser omentum opened. The diaphragmatic crura are sharply dissected and the upper abdominal aorta exposed. The celiac artery and its branches, the superior mesenteric artery, or the renal artery are exposed and dissected free of surrounding tissues. If the inferior mesenteric artery requires bypass grafting, an incision is made in the lower abdomen and the lower abdominal aorta is exposed. The inferior mesenteric artery is dissected free of surrounding tissues. An appropriately sized tubular synthetic graft is selected and prepared. A side-biting clamp is placed on the aorta at the base of the affected artery. The aorta is incised and the synthetic graft sutured to the aorta. The affected artery is also incised at a point beyond the area of obstruction or disease and the synthetic graft sutured to the affected artery. Vascular clamps are released and suture lines checked for hemostasis. Blood flow through the graft is checked using Doppler to ensure patency of the bypass graft.

35632-35634

35632   Bypass graft, with other than vein; ilio-celiac
35633   Bypass graft, with other than vein; ilio-mesenteric
35634   Bypass graft, with other than vein; iliorenal

An ilio-celiac (35632), ilio-mesenteric (35633), or ilio-renal (35634) bypass graft using other than a vein (synthetic conduit) is created around a diseased or obstructed portion of the celiac axis to restore blood flow to the liver, stomach, esophagus, spleen, and pancreas. The common iliac artery on either the right or left side is exposed and isolated. In 35632, the abdomen is incised, the omentum is separated from the transverse colon, and the celiac axis is exposed. Celiac axis arteries (hepatic, left gastric, and splenic) are evaluated. A properly sized synthetic bypass graft is selected. Vascular clamps are applied to the iliac artery and it is incised. The synthetic bypass graft is sutured in an end-to-side configuration to the iliac artery. The celiac artery is clamped and incised and the synthetic bypass graft is anastomosed to it in an end-to-side fashion, bypassing the diseased or obstructed portion of the celiac artery. The clamps are released and blood flow through the graft is checked using Doppler. In 35633, the superior mesenteric artery is exposed and isolated. A properly sized synthetic bypass graft is selected. Vascular clamps are applied to the iliac artery and it is incised. The synthetic bypass graft is sutured in an end-to-side configuration to the iliac artery. The superior mesenteric artery is clamped and incised and the synthetic bypass graft is anastomosed to it in an end-to-side fashion, bypassing the diseased or obstructed portion of the mesenteric artery. The clamps are released and blood flow through the graft is checked using Doppler. In 35634, the descending duodenum is mobilized and the inferior vena cava and renal vein are located. The inferior vena cava is mobilized and the renal artery is isolated. A properly sized synthetic bypass graft is selected. Vascular clamps are applied to the iliac artery and it is incised. The synthetic bypass graft is sutured in an end-to-side configuration to the iliac artery. The renal artery is clamped and incised and the synthetic bypass graft is anastomosed to it in an end-to-side fashion, bypassing the diseased or obstructed portion of the renal artery. The clamps are released and blood flow through the graft is checked using Doppler.

35636

35636   Bypass graft, with other than vein; splenorenal (splenic to renal arterial anastomosis)

A splenorenal bypass graft using other than vein is created around a diseased or obstructed portion of the right or left renal artery to restore blood flow to the kidney. The abdomen is incised, the omentum separated from the transverse colon, and the celiac axis exposed. Celiac axis arteries (hepatic, left gastric, and splenic) are evaluated and the

Cardiovascular System

splenic artery isolated. The descending duodenum is mobilized and the inferior vena cava and renal vein located. The inferior vena cava is mobilized and the renal artery isolated. An appropriately sized tubular synthetic graft is selected and prepared for grafting. Vascular clamps are applied to the splenic artery and the artery is incised. The synthetic graft is sutured in an end-to-side configuration to the splenic artery. The renal artery is clamped and incised and the synthetic graft is anastomosed end-to-side bypassing the diseased or obstructed portion of the renal artery. The clamps are released and blood flow through the graft checked using Doppler.

35637-35638

35637   Bypass graft, with other than vein; aortoiliac
35638   Bypass graft, with other than vein; aortobi-iliac

A bypass graft is created around a diseased or obstructed portion of the lower aorta to one or both iliac arteries using a graft other than harvested vein. The use of artificial grafts made of special synthetic materials is sometimes preferred to natural vein material since the luminal diameter of the synthetic grafts are more accommodating for the larger arteries. Through a lower abdominal incision, the aorta is exposed and clamps are applied above the diseased portion. The aorta may be tied off above the diseased or obstructed area and then one end of the graft is sutured to the aorta. The clamp is released to test for leaks at the anastomosis site. The exposed iliac artery is then clamped distal to the site. Through an incision, the other end of the graft is sutured into place in the iliac artery and the grafted site is checked again for leaks and patency before closing the abdominal wound. This provides a new route for blood to bypass the blocked portion of aorta. Code 35637 for a bypass graft from the aorta to one iliac vessel (aortoiliac) and 35638 for bypass grafting from the aorta to both iliac vessels (aortobi-iliac).

35642-35645

35642   Bypass graft, with other than vein; carotid-vertebral
35645   Bypass graft, with other than vein; subclavian-vertebral

A carotid-vertebral or subclavian-vertebral bypass graft using other than vein is created around a diseased or obstructed portion of vertebral artery. The vertebral arteries arise from the brachiocephalic artery on the right and the subclavian artery on the left. These arteries enter the C6 transverse process, traveling through the C6-C2 processes exiting at the base of the skull. There is an extracranial segment between C2 and the base of the skull. The intracranial segment begins at the atlanto-occipital membrane and continues until the two vertebral arteries join to form the basilar artery. The vertebrobasilar arteries supply the brainstem, cerebellum, and occipital lobes of the brain. An incision is made over the vertebral artery below the obstructed segment and the vertebral artery is dissected free of surrounding tissue. An appropriately sized tubular synthetic graft is selected and prepared. The vertebral artery is clamped and incised. The synthetic graft is sutured to the vertebral artery. In 35642, a carotid-vertebral bypass graft is performed. An incision is made in the neck over the common carotid artery and the artery exposed. The carotid artery is incised or a window created for placement of the synthetic graft which is sutured to the artery. In 35645, a subclavian-vertebral bypass graft is performed. An incision is made below the clavicle and the subclavian artery is exposed, incised, and the synthetic bypass graft sutured to the subclavian artery. The vascular clamps are removed. Blood flow through the graft is checked using Doppler and distal pulses are evaluated to ensure patency of the bypass graft.

35646-35647

35646   Bypass graft, with other than vein; aortobifemoral
35647   Bypass graft, with other than vein; aortofemoral

An aortobifemoral or aortofemoral bypass graft with other than vein is created to bypass a diseased or obstructed portion of the aorta and one or both iliac arteries. In 35646, bypass of both iliac arteries is performed using a synthetic bifurcated graft. The abdomen is opened and small intestine mobilized. The retroperitoneum is opened to expose the aorta. The proximal aorta above the obstructed region is dissected free of surrounding tissue to allow placement of a vascular cross clamp. The iliac arteries are also dissected free of surrounding tissue. The retroperitoneum is elevated and tunnels created to over the iliac arteries for placement of the graft limbs. Incisions are then made over the groin bilaterally to expose the femoral arteries. Tunnels are extended bilaterally to the femoral arteries. The aorta is cross clamped and the aortic portion of the bifurcated graft anastomosed to the aorta. One graft limb is passed through each tunnel to the femoral arteries, the arteries are incised, and the graft limb anastomosed to each femoral artery. Vascular clamps are released and hemostasis of all anastomosis sites checked. Blood flow to the lower extremities is verified. The retroperitoneum is closed as are the abdomen and groin incisions. In 35647, a bypass of the obstructed portion of the aorta and a single iliac artery is performed. The aorta is exposed in the same manner. The obstructed iliac artery is dissected free of surrounding tissue and a tunnel created from the aorta over the iliac artery. A groin incision is made on the affected side and the femoral artery exposed. The tunnel is extended to the femoral artery from the iliac artery. A tubular synthetic graft is anastomosed to the aorta, passed through the tunnel to the femoral artery, and anastomosed to the femoral artery. Clamps are removed, hemostasis of the suture sites verified, and blood flow to the extremity checked. Incisions are closed as described above.

35650

35650   Bypass graft, with other than vein; axillary-axillary

An axillary-axillary bypass graft is created around a diseased or obstructed portion of the axillary artery. This procedure treats disease or obstruction of the contralateral (opposite) axillary artery. A skin incision is made in chest just below the clavicle, soft tissue dissected, and the proximal aspect of the first axillary artery is exposed. This is repeated on the opposite side and the second axillary artery is exposed. A tunnel is created across the chest from one axillary artery to the other. An appropriately sized tubular synthetic graft is selected and prepared for grafting. Vascular clamps are applied to the first axillary artery and the artery is incised. The synthetic graft is sutured to the axillary artery. The graft is then passed through the previously created tunnel. The second axillary artery is clamped and incised. The graft is sutured to the second axillary artery. The vascular clamps are removed. Blood flow through the graft is checked using Doppler and distal pulses are evaluated to ensure patency of the bypass graft.

35654

35654   Bypass graft, with other than vein; axillary-femoral-femoral

A skin incision is made in the chest just below the clavicle, soft tissue dissected, and the proximal axillary artery is exposed. Two additional incisions are made in the groin bilaterally over the common femoral arteries. Soft tissue is dissected and the common femoral arteries are exposed. A tunnel is created beginning at the exposed section of axillary artery, passing down the chest and abdomen, passing under the inguinal ligament, and terminating at the exposed section of common femoral artery on the same side (ipsilateral). An abdominal tunnel is also created for placement of a cross-over graft from the ipsilateral femoral artery to the contralateral femoral artery. An appropriately configured synthetic graft is selected and prepared. Vascular clamps are applied to the axillary artery and the artery is incised. The synthetic graft is sutured to the axillary artery. The graft is then passed through the previously created axillary to groin tunnel. The common femoral artery is clamped and incised and the graft is sutured to artery. The cross-over graft is attached to the synthetic graft in the abdomen and tunneled through the abdomen to the contralateral femoral artery. The contralateral femoral artery is clamped, incised and the graft sutured to the artery. The vascular clamps are removed. Blood flow through the graft is checked using Doppler and distal pulses are evaluated to ensure patency of the bypass graft.

35656

35656   Bypass graft, with other than vein; femoral-popliteal

A groin incision is made on the affected side and the femoral artery exposed. The popliteal artery is also exposed through an incision behind the knee. A tunnel is created from femoral artery to the popliteal artery. An appropriately sized tubular synthetic graft is selected and prepared for grafting. The synthetic graft is passed through the tunnel to the popliteal artery. The femoral artery is clamped, incised and the proximal end of the graft anastomosed. The popliteal artery is clamped, incised and the distal end of the graft anastomosed. Vascular clamps are released and hemostasis of all anastomosis sites checked. Blood flow through the graft is checked using Doppler and distal pulses are evaluated to ensure patency of the bypass graft.

35661

35661   Bypass graft, with other than vein; femoral-femoral

Incisions are made in the groin bilaterally over the common femoral arteries. Soft tissue is dissected and the common femoral arteries are exposed. An abdominal tunnel is created for placement of a cross-over graft from one femoral artery to the other. An appropriately sized tubular synthetic graft is selected and prepared for grafting. The common femoral artery on the unobstructed side is clamped, incised and the cross-over graft is sutured to the artery. The cross-over graft is passed through the tunnel to the contralateral femoral artery. The contralateral femoral artery is clamped, incised and the graft sutured to the artery. The vascular clamps are removed. Blood flow through the graft is checked using Doppler and distal pulses are evaluated to ensure patency of the bypass graft.

35663-35665

35663   Bypass graft, with other than vein; ilioiliac
35665   Bypass graft, with other than vein; iliofemoral

An ilioiliac or iliofemoral bypass graft using other than vein is performed. The abdomen is opened to expose the iliac arteries. In 35663, both iliac arteries are exposed and dissected free of surrounding tissue. An abdominal tunnel is created for placement of a cross-over graft from one iliac artery to the other. An appropriately sized tubular synthetic graft is selected and prepared for grafting. The iliac artery on the unobstructed side is clamped, incised and the cross-over graft is sutured to artery. The cross-over graft is passed through the tunnel to the contralateral iliac artery. The contralateral iliac artery is clamped, incised and the graft sutured to the artery. The vascular clamps are released and suture lines checked for hemostasis. Blood flow through the graft is checked using Doppler and distal pulses are evaluated to ensure patency of the bypass graft. In 35665, the iliac artery is exposed. An incision is made on the ipsilateral (same) side in the groin over the common femoral artery. Soft tissue is dissected and the common femoral artery is exposed. A tunnel is created from the iliac artery to the femoral artery. An appropriately sized tubular synthetic graft is selected and prepared for grafting. The iliac artery is clamped, incised and the proximal end of the synthetic graft sutured to the iliac artery. The synthetic graft is passed through the tunnel to the femoral artery. The femoral artery is clamped, incised, and the distal end of the graft sutured to it. The vascular clamps are released and suture lines checked for hemostasis. Blood flow through the graft is checked using Doppler and distal pulses are evaluated to ensure patency of the bypass graft.

35666-35671

35666   Bypass graft, with other than vein; femoral-anterior tibial, posterior tibial, or peroneal artery

35671   Bypass graft, with other than vein; popliteal-tibial or -peroneal artery

A bypass graft using other than vein is performed on a lower extremity artery. In, 35666, a femoral-anterior tibial, posterior tibial, or peroneal artery bypass graft is performed. A groin incision is made on the affected side and the femoral artery exposed. The distal anastomosis site on the anterior tibial, posterior tibial, or peroneal artery is also exposed. In 35671, a popliteal-tibial or peroneal artery bypass graft is performed. An incision is made on the affected side behind the knee and the popliteal artery exposed. The distal anastomosis site on the anterior tibial, posterior tibial or peroneal artery is also exposed. A tunnel is created from the proximal anastomosis site to the distal anastomosis site. An appropriately sized tubular synthetic graft is selected and prepared for grafting. The synthetic graft is anastomosed to the proximal anastomosis site and then passed through the tunnel to the distal anastomosis site. The proximal artery is clamped, incised and the proximal end of the graft anastomosed. The distal artery is clamped, incised and the distal end of the graft anastomosed. Vascular clamps are released and hemostasis of all anastomosis sites checked. Blood flow through the graft is checked using Doppler and distal pulses are evaluated to ensure patency of the bypass graft.

35681-35683

35681   Bypass graft; composite, prosthetic and vein (List separately in addition to code for primary procedure)

35682   Bypass graft; autogenous composite, 2 segments of veins from 2 locations (List separately in addition to code for primary procedure)

35683   Bypass graft; autogenous composite, 3 or more segments of vein from 2 or more locations (List separately in addition to code for primary procedure)

In 35681, the physician constructs a composite bypass graft using prosthetic material and either a segment of autogenous vein harvested from the patient or less commonly a vein allograft that has been harvested from an organ donor. Composite prosthetic and vein bypass grafts are used when the patient does not have an adequate segment of vein available for the bypass graft procedure. The physician harvests a segment of the ipsilateral greater saphenous vein, contralateral greater saphenous vein, cephalic or basilic arm vein, lesser saphenous vein, or superficial femoral vein. Alternatively, the physician may use a vein allograft. A prosthetic vein segment is also obtained and the vein autograft or allograft is then anastomosed to form a conduit of the required length for the bypass procedure. In 35682 and 35683, the physician constructs an autogenous composite vein bypass graft using two segments (35682) or three or more segments (35683) of vein harvested from two or more locations from a limb other than the one undergoing the bypass procedure. Composite vein bypass grafts are used when the patient does not have an adequate segment of vein available in the limb undergoing the graft procedure to perform the bypass graft procedure. The physician harvests segments of vein from the contralateral greater saphenous vein, lesser saphenous vein or superficial femoral vein or from the cephalic or basilic arm veins. The vein segments are then anastomosed to form a conduit of the required length for the bypass procedure.

35685

35685   Placement of vein patch or cuff at distal anastomosis of bypass graft, synthetic conduit (List separately in addition to code for primary procedure)

The physician places a vein patch or cuff at the distal anastomosis site at the time of a separately reportable arterial bypass procedure and attaches the patch or cuff to a synthetic conduit. Placement of the vein patch or cuff at the distal anastomosis site is performed as an additional service to help improve patency of the synthetic bypass graft. Two techniques are commonly employed, either the Taylor patch technique or the Miller cuff technique. A small piece of autogenous vein is harvested. Using the Taylor patch technique, an incision is made in the artery at the distal anastomosis site. The harvested patch graft is then sutured to the artery. The synthetic graft is sutured to the vein patch. Using the Miller cuff technique, an incision is made in the artery at the distal anastomosis site. The short autogenous vein graft is then sutured to the distal anastomosis site to form a short cuff. The synthetic graft is sutured to the cuff.

35686

35686   Creation of distal arteriovenous fistula during lower extremity bypass surgery (non-hemodialysis) (List separately in addition to code for primary procedure)

Creation of a fistula is performed on bypassed arteries when there is poor outflow from the bypass graft to the remaining portion of native artery. The fistula increases blood flow in the graft by adding a venous outflow tract to the lower extremity artery. The affected artery and a section of adjacent vein are dissected free of surrounding tissue. The vein branches are ligated. The distal end of the vein being used to create the fistula is also ligated. The native vein is incised and a modified venous bypass graft anastomosed to the native artery and the native vein creating a distal arteriovenous fistula.

35691-35693

35691   Transposition and/or reimplantation; vertebral to carotid artery

35693   Transposition and/or reimplantation; vertebral to subclavian artery

The physician performs transposition and/or reimplantation of the vertebral artery to the carotid artery (35691) or to the subclavian artery (35693). An incision is made in the neck and the vertebral artery exposed. A systemic anticoagulant is administered intravenously. The available length of vertebral artery is determined. In 35691, the anastomosis site on the common carotid artery marked. The vertebral artery is clamped just below the longus colli muscle. A ligature is then placed at the origin of the vertebral artery. The vertebral artery is transected above the ligature, pulled through the surrounding loop of the cervical sympathetic ganglia, and brought into proximity of the planned anastomosis site. The vertebral artery is then anastomosed in an end-to-side fashion to the common carotid artery. Prior to complete closure, the vessels are backbled, sutures are tied, and blood flow re-established first to the common carotid artery and then to the vertebral artery. In 35693, a redundant vertebral artery is transposed and reimplanted to the subclavian artery. The anastomosis site on the subclavian artery is marked. The redundant vertebral artery is clamped and divided above the level of the stenosis or occlusion and brought into proximity of the planned anastomosis site. The vertebral artery is anatomosed to the subclavian artery. Prior to complete closure, the vessels are backbled. Sutures are then tied and blood flow re-established.

35694-35695

35694   Transposition and/or reimplantation; subclavian to carotid artery

35695   Transposition and/or reimplantation; carotid to subclavian artery

The physician performs transposition and/or reimplantation of the subclavian artery to the carotid artery (35694) or the carotid artery to the subclavian artery (35695). A supraclavicular incision is made at the base of the neck. The clavicular head is incised and the scalene fat pad mobilized and reflected superiorly. The thoracic duct may be preserved or ligated. The phrenic nerve is identified and protected. The anterior scalene muscle is transected. In 35694, the subclavian artery is exposed and dissected free of surrounding tissue. Subclavian artery branches are divided and ligated. The carotid artery is then exposed through the same incision and dissected free of surrounding tissue. The vagus nerve is identified and protected. A tunnel is created posterior to the jugular vein. A systemic anticoagulant is administered intravenously. The subclavian artery is divided, the proximal stump oversewn, and the artery is then pulled through the previously created tunnel bringing it into proximity with the planned anastomosis site in the carotid artery. The carotid artery is incised. The end of the subclavian artery is then sutured to the side of the carotid artery. In 35695, following exposure of the subclavian and carotid arteries as described above, the proximal common carotid artery is dissected into the mediastinum to obtain an adequate length of carotid artery. A tunnel is created behind the sternocleidomastoid muscle and jugular vein. The carotid artery is clamped distally and proximally and the artery is divided. The proximal stump of the carotid is oversewn. The carotid artery is then pulled through the previously created tunnel bringing it into proximity with the planned anastomosis site in the subclavian artery. The subclavian artery is incised and the end of the carotid artery sutured to the side of the subclavian artery.

35697

35697   Reimplantation, visceral artery to infrarenal aortic prosthesis, each artery (List separately in addition to code for primary procedure)

The physician reimplants a visceral artery to the infrarenal aortic prosthesis. During a separately reportable open procedure on the aorta, the visceral vessel to be reimplanted is dissected free of surrounding soft tissue. A button of aortic tissue is cut from the origin of the visceral vessel to use as a patch. This type of patch technique may be referred to as a Carrel patch. The button is examined to ensure that it is smooth and patent. The planned reimplantation site on the aortic prosthesis is then clamped using a side-biting clamp. A hole is cut in the aortic prosthesis matching the size of the aortic button. The button (Carrel patch) is then sutured to the previously created hole in the aortic prosthesis. Clamps are removed and the anastomosis site is checked for leakage. Additional sutures are applied at the patch site as needed. This procedure is most often performed to re-establish blood supply to the colon by reimplanting the inferior mesenteric artery into the

Cardiovascular System

infrarenal aortic prosthesis but may also be performed on other visceral arteries. Report 35697 for each visceral artery reimplantation performed.

35700

35700   **Reoperation, femoral-popliteal or femoral (popliteal)-anterior tibial, posterior tibial, peroneal artery, or other distal vessels, more than 1 month after original operation (List separately in addition to code for primary procedure)**

After arterial bypass, the graft, inflow artery, or outflow artery may develop a stenosis resulting in re-occlusion and graft failure. The physician incises the leg over the previously placed bypass graft. The graft and inflow and outflow arteries are carefully dissected from surrounding tissues. A new inflow site is identified and mobilized proximal to the original anastomosis site. A new outflow site is identified and mobilized distal to the original anastomosis site. The new bypass graft is placed or in-situ bypass performed in a separately reportable procedure. Re-operation is reported additionally for redo bypass or in-situ grafting of the femoral-popliteal, femoral-anterior tibial, femoral-posterior tibial, femoral-peroneal, femoral-other distal artery, popliteal-anterior tibial, popliteal-posterior tibial, popliteal-peroneal, or popliteal-other distal artery.

35701-35761

35701   **Exploration (not followed by surgical repair), with or without lysis of artery; carotid artery**

35721   **Exploration (not followed by surgical repair), with or without lysis of artery; femoral artery**

35741   **Exploration (not followed by surgical repair), with or without lysis of artery; popliteal artery**

35761   **Exploration (not followed by surgical repair), with or without lysis of artery; other vessels**

An exploration with or without lysis of the artery is performed without surgical repair. An incision is made over the affected artery. Surrounding soft tissue is dissected to allow visualization of the artery. The artery is inspected for evidence of disease or injury. If the artery is constricted due to adhesions, they are lysed. Kinking of the artery may also require lysis of surrounding tissue to allow straightening of the artery and to improve blood flow. After the exploration procedure is completed the incision is closed in layers. Use 35701 for exploration of the carotid artery, 35721 for exploration of the femoral artery, 35741 for exploration of the popliteal artery, and 35761 for exploration of other vessels.

35800-35860

35800   **Exploration for postoperative hemorrhage, thrombosis or infection; neck**
35820   **Exploration for postoperative hemorrhage, thrombosis or infection; chest**
35840   **Exploration for postoperative hemorrhage, thrombosis or infection; abdomen**
35860   **Exploration for postoperative hemorrhage, thrombosis or infection; extremity**

Following a previously performed surgical procedure, the operative wound is re-opened and the surgical site explored for post-operative hemorrhage, thrombosis, or infection. A patient with symptoms indicative of a post-operative hemorrhage, such as low red blood count; thrombosis, such as pain, redness, swelling, shortness of breath; or infection, such as fever, redness, swelling, and/or tenderness over the surgical site is evaluated. If non-surgical measures fail to resolve the symptoms, the patient is returned to the operating room for exploration of the surgical site. The surgical incision is re-opened and thoroughly inspected. Any bleeding is controlled by ligation or cautery. Any blood clots are evacuated. Any evidence of infection is treated by opening abscess pockets and draining pus and fluid. The surgical wound is flushed with normal saline or antibiotic solution. Drains are placed as needed. The surgical wound may be closed or packed with gauze. Use 35800 for post-operative exploration of the neck, 35820 for the chest, 35840 for the abdomen, and 35860 for an extremity.

35870

35870   **Repair of graft-enteric fistula**

Graft-enteric fistulas occur most frequently between an abdominal aortic graft and duodenum but can also occur between other abdominal artery grafts and bowel. The abdomen is opened and explored. The bowel is carefully dissected away from the entire length of the aortic or arterial graft. The fistula is identified. Separately reportable aortic or arterial bypass procedure is typically performed prior to removal of the graft and closure of the fistulous tract. The bowel is separated from the original graft and the graft removed. The bowel is repaired. Omentum may be placed between the repaired bowel and the new graft to prevent a new fistula from forming.

35875-35876

35875   **Thrombectomy of arterial or venous graft (other than hemodialysis graft or fistula)**

35876   **Thrombectomy of arterial or venous graft (other than hemodialysis graft or fistula); with revision of arterial or venous graft**

An open thrombectomy of an arterial or venous graft other than a hemodialysis graft or fistula is performed with or without revision of the graft. Following arterial or venous graft placement, the graft may develop a stenosis with thrombosis formation and re-occlusion which may require open surgical removal of the thrombus with or without revision of the graft. An incision is made in the skin over the arterial or venous graft and the graft. Vessel loops are placed proximal and distal to the thrombus to control blood flow. The graft is opened and the thrombus (clot) removed by direct exposure. The physician may use arterial back pressure or massage to expel the thrombus. Following removal of the thrombus, an angiography may be performed to ensure that the entire clot has been removed and that the arterial or venous graft is patent. Stenosis of the graft may require graft revision. The stenosed area may be enlarged using a patch graft or excised and replaced with a tubular graft segment. Use 35875 when open thrombectomy is performed without revision of the graft and 35876 when open thrombectomy with graft revision is performed.

35879-35881

35879   **Revision, lower extremity arterial bypass, without thrombectomy, open; with vein patch angioplasty**

35881   **Revision, lower extremity arterial bypass, without thrombectomy, open; with segmental vein interposition**

An open revision of a lower extremity arterial bypass is performed without thrombectomy using vein patch angioplasty (35879) or segmental vein interposition (35881). After arterial bypass, the graft, inflow artery, or outflow artery may develop a stenosis. To prevent re-occlusion and graft failure a revision of the bypass graft is performed. In 35879, vein patch angioplasty is performed. An incision is made in skin and soft tissue over the stenosed area of the previously placed lower extremity arterial bypass graft and the graft exposed and dissected free of surrounding tissue. Vessel loops are placed proximal and distal to the stenosed area of the graft to control blood flow. A segment of vein is harvested, usually a segment of saphenous vein, and an elliptical patch tailored to fit over the stenosed segment of the graft. A longitudinal incision is made in the stenosed segment of the graft. The patch graft is inserted within the longitudinal incision and sutured to the previously placed bypass graft. This increases the diameter of the stenosed segment improving blood flow through the graft. Vessel loops are released and a completion angiography performed to ensure that the revised segment of the arterial graft is patent. In 35881, segmental vein interposition is performed. The stenosed segment is exposed and mobilized as described above. Vessel loops are placed proximal and distal to the stenosed area of the graft to control blood flow. A segment of vein is harvested, usually a segment of saphenous vein. The stenosed segment of the previously bypass graft is excised. The tubular segment of new vein graft is trimmed to the proper length and sutured to the remaining proximal and distal segments of the previously placed bypass graft. The vein segment replaces the stenosed segment that has been removed. Vessel loops are released, hemostasis checked, and a completion angiography performed to ensure that the revised segment of the arterial graft is patent.

35883-35884

35883   **Revision, femoral anastomosis of synthetic arterial bypass graft in groin, open; with nonautogenous patch graft (eg, Dacron, ePTFE, bovine pericardium)**

35884   **Revision, femoral anastomosis of synthetic arterial bypass graft in groin, open; with autogenous vein patch graft**

The surgeon openly revises a previous femoral anastomosis of a synthetic arterial bypass graft. An incision is made over the groin area and dissection is carried out down to the previously placed arterial bypass graft anastomosed to the femoral artery. The bypass graft diverts blood flow to or from another artery, such as the aorta, iliac, or popliteal artery, in cases of blocked or diseases vessels. Open revision may be done for stenosis that threatens patency of the graft. The anastomosis site is assessed for leaks, stenosis, or other problems. Clamps are placed and the graft anastomosis site is incised. The stenotic area or problematic portion of the graft is excised and then repaired using another nonautogenous patch graft such as synthetic Dacron, or bovine pericardium in 35883 or a section of harvested vein taken from the patient in 35884. The new patch graft is sutured into place to restore the graft viability and reanastomosed to the femoral artery. Clamps are removed. The patch graft revision and anastomosis are tested before closing the wound.

● New Code   ▲ Revised Code

35901-35907

35901 Excision of infected graft; neck
35903 Excision of infected graft; extremity
35905 Excision of infected graft; thorax
35907 Excision of infected graft; abdomen

An infected vascular graft is excised. A separately reportable re-vascularization procedure with placement of a new graft is typically required prior to removal of the infected graft to ensure that the affected organ or limb is adequately perfused. The infected graft is then exposed and dissected free of surrounding tissues. The inflow and outflow arteries are clamped above and below the graft and the graft is excised. The inflow and outflow arterial walls are debrided at the proximal and distal anastomosis sites until normal non-inflamed artery is encountered. Any inflamed tissue around the graft site is also debrided. The arterial defect is repaired with sutures. Use 35901 for excision of an infected vascular graft in the neck, 35903 for an extremity graft, 35905 for a thoracic graft, and 35907 for an abdominal graft.

36000

36000 Introduction of needle or intracatheter, vein

The physician may place a metal needle, such as a butterfly or scalp needle; a plastic catheter mounted on a metal needle, also referred to as a plastic needle; or an intracatheter, which is a catheter inserted through a needle. The planned puncture site is selected and cleansed. The selected device is then introduced into the vein. A butterfly needle can be introduced into smaller veins in the hand. The butterfly shape stabilizes the hub on the skin surface. If a plastic needle is used, the metal tip is introduced into the vein and then removed. The plastic catheter is advanced into the vein. If an intracatheter is used, the metal needle is used to puncture the vein. The catheter is then introduced through the needle into the vein. The needle or intracatheter is secured to the skin with tape.

36002

36002 Injection procedures (eg, thrombin) for percutaneous treatment of extremity pseudoaneurysm

An injection procedure is performed for percutaneous treatment of an extremity pseudoaneurysm, which is usually complication of arterial puncture following percutaneous diagnostic or therapeutic vascular procedures. The pseudoaneurysm develops when the puncture site fails to seal. Blood then leaks into the surrounding soft tissue and is contained in a cavity that develops adjacent to the puncture site in the artery. Unlike a hematoma, the pseudoaneurysm cavity fills and empties with each heart beat. Using separately reportable imaging guidance, a catheter is introduced into the pseudoaneurysm and a blood clotting agent, such as thrombin solution, is then injected until thrombosis of the pseudoaneurysm occurs. Following the occlusion procedure, the native blood vessels are checked to ensure that they are patent.

36005

36005 Injection procedure for extremity venography (including introduction of needle or intracatheter)

A venogram is performed to diagnose or evaluate a number of conditions including swelling and pain in an extremity, deep vein thrombosis, the source of pulmonary emboli, congenital venous malformation, and other causes of venous obstruction. The procedure may also be used to locate a vein for arterial bypass surgery. The area over the planned puncture site, usually the foot or hand, is cleansed. A needle or intracatheter is placed in the vein. Radiopaque contrast material is injected. A tourniquet may be placed above the ankle or on the lower arm to slow blood flow and allow filling of deep veins. Separately reportable radiographs are obtained at timed intervals during the procedure. Upon completion of the procedure, the intravenous access is flushed with heparin and saline solution. The needle or intracatheter is removed from the vein and pressure applied.

36010

36010 Introduction of catheter, superior or inferior vena cava

Common access veins include the brachial and cephalic veins. A small incision is made over the planned puncture site and an introducer sheath placed in the vein. A guidewire is advanced through the access vein and into the superior or inferior vena cava. The catheter is then advanced over the guidewire into the superior or inferior vena cava. If the puncture site is the brachial or cephalic vein, the inferior vena cava is accessed by advancing the guidewire and catheter into the superior vena cava, through the right atrium and into the inferior vena cava. Injection of medication and/or radiopaque contrast is performed as needed.

36011-36012

36011 Selective catheter placement, venous system; first order branch (eg, renal vein, jugular vein)
36012 Selective catheter placement, venous system; second order, or more selective, branch (eg, left adrenal vein, petrosal sinus)

A selective venous catheterization procedure is performed. Common access veins include the brachial and cephalic veins. A small incision is made over the planned puncture site and an introducer sheath placed in the vein. From the brachial or cephalic vein, a guidewire is advanced through the access vein and into the superior vena cava. From there, the catheter is advanced into a venous branch off the superior vena cava, such as the jugular vein, or the catheter may be advanced through the right atrium and into the inferior vena cava and then into a branch off the inferior vena cava, such as the hepatic or renal vein. The catheter may remain in the first order branch which is any vein that drains directly into the vena cava or the catheter may be advanced into a second order or more selective branch, such as the petrosal sinus or left adrenal vein. Injection of medication and/or radiopaque contrast is performed as needed. Use 36011 for selective catheter placement in a first order vein branch and 36012 for a second order or more selective vein branch.

36013-36015

36013 Introduction of catheter, right heart or main pulmonary artery
36014 Selective catheter placement, left or right pulmonary artery
36015 Selective catheter placement, segmental or subsegmental pulmonary artery

A catheter is introduced into the right heart or main pulmonary artery (36013) or selective catheterization is performed with placement of the catheter in the left or right pulmonary artery (36014) or a segmental or subsegmental pulmonary artery (36015). The catheter is introduced into an extremity vein, with the preferred introduction site being the right femoral vein, although the left femoral vein or an upper extremity vein may also be used. A small skin incision is made over the planned venous insertion site. An introducer sheath is placed in the vein and a guidewire inserted. If the right femoral vein is used, the guidewire is manipulated through the femoral and iliac veins and into the inferior vena cava and advanced to the right atrium. A pigtail catheter with a tip deflecting wire is advanced over the guidewire and into the right atrium. The guidewire is removed. The catheter may remain in the right atrium or a tip deflecting wire may be used to advance the catheter into the right ventricle and main pulmonary artery. In 36014, selective catheterization of the left or right pulmonary artery is performed. The catheter is introduced into the right atrium, advanced into the right ventricle and then into the pulmonary artery as described above. The physician then selectively manipulates the catheter into the left or right pulmonary arteries. In 36015, selective catheterization of a segmental or subsegmental pulmonary artery is performed. The catheter is placed in the left or right pulmonary artery as described above and then manipulated into a segmental or subsegmental pulmonary artery. The segmental and subsegmental arteries are the branches that divide and subdivide within the lungs. Injection of medication and/or radiopaque contrast is performed as needed.

36100

36100 Introduction of needle or intracatheter, carotid or vertebral artery

To place a needle or intracatheter in the carotid artery, the artery is first located by palpation. The carotid artery is stabilized between the index and middle fingers and the needle or intracatheter introduced through the skin, advanced toward the artery until the tip touches the artery wall, and the artery is then punctured. The needle or intracatheter is advanced in a cephalad direction taking care not to injure the carotid artery intima (inner lining). To place a needle or intracatheter in the vertebral artery, the vertebral artery is approached laterally and the needle or intracatheter advanced between one of the cervical interspaces. The skin of the neck is compressed against the cervical spine using the index and middle fingers. The skin is punctured and the needle or intracatheter advanced until it touches the intervertebral foramina at the anterior tubercle of the transverse process. The needle or intracatheter is advanced into the vertebral artery. Blood is aspirated to ensure that the needle or intracatheter is properly placed within the carotid or vertebral artery. Injection of medication and/or radiopaque contrast media is performed as needed.

36120-36140

36120 Introduction of needle or intracatheter; retrograde brachial artery
36140 Introduction of needle or intracatheter; extremity artery

A needle or intracatheter is introduced into the brachial artery in a retrograde fashion or into another extremity artery. In 36120, retrograde introduction of a needle or intracatheter into the brachial artery is performed. To place a needle or intracatheter in the brachial artery, the artery is first located by palpation. The brachial artery is stabilized between the index and middle fingers and the needle or intracatheter introduced through the skin, advanced toward the artery until the tip touches the artery wall, and the artery is then punctured. The needle may be left in the brachial artery or an intracatheter may be advanced in a retrograde fashion through the brachial artery and into the axillary, subclavian or innominate arteries. In 36140, a needle or intracatheter is placed in another extremity artery, such as the radial artery in the arm or the femoral artery in the leg. If

Cardiovascular System

the femoral artery is punctured, the intracatheter may be advanced into the iliac artery. Injection of medication and/or radiopaque contrast is performed as needed.

36160

36160   Introduction of needle or intracatheter, aortic, translumbar

The translumbar approach is rarely used. The patient is placed in a prone position. A long hollow needle contained in a sheath is advanced directly into the aorta using a left flank approach. The needle is then withdrawn leaving the sheath in place. Injection of medication and/or radiopaque contrast media is performed as needed and the sheath is removed. The patient is placed supine with a bed of gauze underneath the left flank to control external bleeding. The patient is carefully monitored for any evidence of internal hemorrhage.

36200

36200   Introduction of catheter, aorta

The catheter is introduced into an extremity artery, with the preferred introduction site being the femoral arteries. A small skin incision is made over the planned insertion site. An introduction sheath is placed in the artery and a guidewire inserted. If one of the femoral arteries is used, the guidewire is manipulated through the femoral and iliac arteries and into the aorta. The catheter is manipulated up and down the aorta as needed and may be moved to the openings of aortic branches but does not enter the branch. Injection of medication and/or radiopaque contrast media is performed as needed.

36215-36218

36215   Selective catheter placement, arterial system; each first order thoracic or brachiocephalic branch, within a vascular family

36216   Selective catheter placement, arterial system; initial second order thoracic or brachiocephalic branch, within a vascular family

36217   Selective catheter placement, arterial system; initial third order or more selective thoracic or brachiocephalic branch, within a vascular family

36218   Selective catheter placement, arterial system; additional second order, third order, and beyond, thoracic or brachiocephalic branch, within a vascular family (List in addition to code for initial second or third order vessel as appropriate)

A selective catheter placement in a thoracic or brachiocephalic branch of a single vascular family of the arterial system is performed. A catheter is introduced into an extremity artery, with the preferred introduction site being a femoral artery, although an upper extremity artery may also be used. A small skin incision is made over the planned insertion site. An introducer sheath is placed in the artery and a guidewire inserted. If the right femoral artery is used, the guidewire is manipulated through the femoral and iliac arteries and into the aorta. A catheter is advanced over the guidewire into the aorta. The guidewire is advanced as needed and the physician then manipulates the catheter over the guidewire into a first order thoracic or brachiocephalic branch off the aorta. The physician continues to selectively advance the guidewire and catheter through higher order branches (second, third, and beyond) until the catheter is situated in the highest order branch requiring evaluation. The guidewire is removed. Injection of medication and/or radiopaque contrast media is performed as needed. Use 36215 if a first order branch is the highest order branch catheterized within the vascular family, 36216 if a second order branch if the highest order branch catheterized, 36217 if a third or higher order branch is the highest order branch catheterized. Use 36218 for catheterization of each additional second, third, or higher order thoracic or brachiocephalic branch within the same vascular family.

36221

36221   Non-selective catheter placement, thoracic aorta, with angiography of the extracranial carotid, vertebral, and/or intracranial vessels, unilateral or bilateral, and all associated radiological supervision and interpretation, includes angiography of the cervicocerebral arch, when performed

Thoracic aorta angiography is a procedure involving nonselective catheter placement into the ascending aorta. In a nonselective access procedure, the catheter is placed in the aorta and is not advanced into higher order branches (second, third, etc.) Vascular access is obtained via a single-wall puncture of either the common femoral artery or the ipsilateral brachial artery. A guidewire is inserted and under fluoroscopic guidance, a catheter is advanced into the thoracic aorta. After confirming the catheter position, radiopaque contrast media is injected into the aorta through the catheter while digital angiographic imaging is performed. The catheter is manipulated up and down the aorta as needed and may be moved to the openings of aortic branches to image the extracranial carotid, vertebral, and/or intracranial vessels. The catheter is not advanced into any of these branches. Upon completion of the procedure, a written interpretation of findings is provided.

36222-36223

36222   Selective catheter placement, common carotid or innominate artery, unilateral, any approach, with angiography of the ipsilateral extracranial carotid circulation and all associated radiological supervision and interpretation, includes angiography of the cervicocerebral arch, when performed

36223   Selective catheter placement, common carotid or innominate artery, unilateral, any approach, with angiography of the ipsilateral intracranial carotid circulation and all associated radiological supervision and interpretation, includes angiography of the extracranial carotid and cervicocerebral arch, when performed

Selective catheter placement in the right or left common carotid or right innominate (brachiocephalic) artery is performed by any approach including percutaneous placement via the femoral, axillary, brachial, or radial artery. A retrograde femoral artery approach is the most common. A small skin incision is made over the planned insertion site. An introducer sheath is placed in the artery and a guidewire is inserted. If the femoral artery is used, the guidewire is manipulated through the femoral and iliac arteries and into the aorta and along the aorta into the aortic arch to a point beyond the left common carotid artery or right innominate artery under continuous fluoroscopic guidance. A catheter is advanced over the guidewire into the aortic arch and positioned at the left common carotid or right innominate artery. The guidewire is retracted and manipulated into the left common carotid or right innominate artery/right common carotid artery. The catheter is again advanced over the guidewire and positioned 2-3 cm below the carotid bifurcation. The guidewire is removed. Radiopaque contrast media is injected. Angiography of the ipsilateral (same side) extracranial carotid circulation, including the cervicocerebral arch is performed (36222). Arterial contrast injections with arterial, capillary, and venous phase imaging are also included when performed. Upon completion of the procedure, the catheter is removed and hemostasis is achieved by applying pressure to the arteriotomy site or using another closure technique. A written interpretation of findings is provided. Use 36223 when angiography of the ipsilateral intracranial carotid circulation, cervicocerebral arch, and the extracranial carotid circulation is performed.

36224

36224   Selective catheter placement, internal carotid artery, unilateral, with angiography of the ipsilateral intracranial carotid circulation and all associated radiological supervision and interpretation, includes angiography of the extracranial carotid and cervicocerebral arch, when performed

Selective catheter placement in the right or left internal carotid artery is performed by percutaneous catheter placement via the femoral, axillary, brachial, or radial artery. A retrograde femoral artery approach is the most common. A small skin incision is made over the planned insertion site. An introducer sheath is placed in the artery and a guidewire is inserted. If the femoral artery is used, the guidewire is manipulated through the femoral and iliac arteries and into the aorta. The guidewire is advanced along the aorta into the aortic arch to a point beyond the left common carotid artery or right innominate artery under continuous fluoroscopic guidance. A catheter is advanced over the guidewire into the aortic arch and positioned at the left common carotid or right innominate artery. The guidewire is retracted and manipulated into the left common carotid or right innominate artery/right common carotid artery. The catheter is again advanced over the guidewire and positioned below the carotid bifurcation. The guidewire is then manipulated into the right or left internal carotid artery, followed by the catheter which is positioned within the internal carotid artery. The guidewire is removed. Radiopaque contrast media is injected. Angiography of the ipsilateral (same side) intracranial carotid circulation including the cervicocerebral arch is performed. Angiography of the external carotid artery may also be performed. Arterial contrast injections with arterial, capillary, and venous phase imaging are also included when performed. Upon completion of the procedure, the catheter is removed and hemostasis is achieved by applying pressure to the arteriotomy site or using another closure technique. A written interpretation of findings is provided.

36225-36226

36225   Selective catheter placement, subclavian or innominate artery, unilateral, with angiography of the ipsilateral vertebral circulation and all associated radiological supervision and interpretation, includes angiography of the cervicocerebral arch, when performed

36226   Selective catheter placement, vertebral artery, unilateral, with angiography of the ipsilateral vertebral circulation and all associated radiological supervision and interpretation, includes angiography of the cervicocerebral arch, when performed

Selective catheter placement in the right innominate (brachiocephalic)/ subclavian artery or left subclavian artery is performed by percutaneous catheter placement via the femoral, axillary, brachial, or radial artery. A retrograde femoral artery approach is the most common. A small skin incision is made over the planned insertion site. An introducer sheath is placed in the artery and a guidewire is inserted. If the femoral artery is used, the guidewire is manipulated through the femoral and iliac arteries into the aorta. The guidewire is advanced along the aorta into the aortic arch to a point beyond the left subclavian artery or right innominate artery under continuous fluoroscopic guidance. A catheter is advanced over the guidewire into the aortic arch and positioned at the left subclavian or right subclavian/innominate artery. The guidewire is retracted and manipulated into the left subclavian or right innominate/right subclavian artery. The catheter is again advanced over the guidewire and positioned below the vertebral artery branch. Use code 36225 when the catheter is not advanced beyond the right innominate/right subclavian artery or left subclavian artery Use 36226 when the catheter is advanced into the vertebral artery. The guidewire is removed. Radiopaque contrast media is injected. Angiography of the ipsilateral (same side) vertebral circulation is performed. Angiography of the cervicocerebral arch may also be performed. Arterial contrast injections with arterial, capillary, and venous phase imaging are also included when performed. Upon completion of the procedure, the catheter is removed and hemostasis is achieved by applying pressure to the arteriotomy site or using another closure technique. A written interpretation of findings is provided.

36227

36227 Selective catheter placement, external carotid artery, unilateral, with angiography of the ipsilateral external carotid circulation and all associated radiological supervision and interpretation (List separately in addition to code for primary procedure)

Selective catheter placement in the right or left external carotid artery is performed by percutaneous catheter placement via the femoral, axillary, brachial, or radial artery. A retrograde femoral artery approach is the most common. A small skin incision is made over the planned insertion site. An introducer sheath is placed in the artery and a guidewire is inserted. If the femoral artery is used, the guidewire is manipulated through the femoral and iliac arteries into the aorta. The guidewire is advanced along the aorta into the aortic arch to a point beyond the left common carotid artery or right innominate artery under continuous fluoroscopic guidance. A catheter is advanced over the guidewire into the aortic arch and positioned at the left common carotid or right innominate artery. The guidewire is retracted and manipulated into the left common carotid or right innominate/common carotid artery. The catheter is again advanced over the guidewire and positioned below the carotid bifurcation. The guidewire is then manipulated into the right or left external carotid artery, followed by the catheter which is positioned within the external carotid artery. The guidewire is removed. Radiopaque contrast media is injected. Angiography of the ipsilateral (same side) external carotid circulation is performed. Arterial contrast injections with arterial, capillary, and venous phase imaging are also included when performed. Upon completion of the procedure, the catheter is removed and hemostasis is achieved by applying pressure to the arteriotomy site or using another closure technique. A written interpretation of findings is provided.

36228

36228 Selective catheter placement, each intracranial branch of the internal carotid or vertebral arteries, unilateral, with angiography of the selected vessel circulation and all associated radiological supervision and interpretation (eg, middle cerebral artery, posterior inferior cerebellar artery) (List separately in addition to code for primary procedure)

Selective catheter placement in intracranial branches beyond the internal carotid arteries or vertebral arteries is performed which may include the middle cerebral artery, posterior inferior cerebellar artery, or other higher level branches. Selective catheter placement to the level of the internal carotid or vertebral arteries is reported separately. If catheterization and angiography for evaluation of circulation of a higher level artery is needed, the guidewire and catheter are advanced into the selected higher level artery or arteries. The guidewire is removed. Radiopaque contrast media is injected. Angiography of the selected higher level vessel circulation is performed. Arterial contrast injections with arterial, capillary, and venous phase imaging are also included when performed. Upon completion of the procedure the catheter is removed and a written report of findings is provided. Report 36228 for each additional higher level artery on which selective catheterization and angiography are performed.

36245-36248

36245 Selective catheter placement, arterial system; each first order abdominal, pelvic, or lower extremity artery branch, within a vascular family

36246 Selective catheter placement, arterial system; initial second order abdominal, pelvic, or lower extremity artery branch, within a vascular family

36247 Selective catheter placement, arterial system; initial third order or more selective abdominal, pelvic, or lower extremity artery branch, within a vascular family

36248 Selective catheter placement, arterial system; additional second order, third order, and beyond, abdominal, pelvic, or lower extremity artery branch, within a vascular family (List in addition to code for initial second or third order vessel as appropriate)

A selective catheter placement in an abdominal, pelvic, or lower extremity branch of a single vascular family of the arterial system is performed. A catheter is introduced into an extremity artery, with the preferred introduction site being a femoral artery, although an

upper extremity artery may also be used. A small skin incision is made over the planned insertion site. An introducer sheath is placed in the artery and a guidewire inserted. If the right femoral artery is used, the guidewire is manipulated through the femoral and iliac arteries and into the aorta. A catheter is advanced over the guidewire into the aorta. The guidewire is advanced as needed and the physician then manipulates the catheter over the guidewire into a first order abdominal, pelvic, or lower extremity branch off the aorta. The physician continues to selectively advance the guidewire and catheter through higher order branches (second, third, and beyond) until the catheter is situated in the highest order branch requiring evaluation. The guidewire is removed. Injection of medication and/or radiopaque contrast media is performed as needed. Use 36245 if a first order branch is the highest order branch catheterized within the vascular family, 36246 if a second order branch if the highest order branch catheterized, 36247 if a third or higher order branch is the highest order branch catheterized. Use 36248 for catheterization of each additional second, third, or higher order abdominal or pelvic, or lower extremity branch within the same vascular family.

36251-36252

36251 Selective catheter placement (first-order), main renal artery and any accessory renal artery(s) for renal angiography, including arterial puncture and catheter placement(s), fluoroscopy, contrast injection(s), image postprocessing, permanent recording of images, and radiological supervision and interpretation, including pressure gradient measurements when performed, and flush aortogram when performed; unilateral

36252 Selective catheter placement (first-order), main renal artery and any accessory renal artery(s) for renal angiography, including arterial puncture and catheter placement(s), fluoroscopy, contrast injection(s), image postprocessing, permanent recording of images, and radiological supervision and interpretation, including pressure gradient measurements when performed, and flush aortogram when performed; bilateral

A selective catheter placement in the main renal artery and any accessory renal arteries is performed for renal angiography. A catheter is introduced into an extremity artery, with the preferred introduction site being a femoral artery in the groin. A small skin incision is made over the planned insertion site. An introducer sheath is placed in the artery and a guidewire is inserted. If the right femoral artery is used, the guidewire is manipulated through the femoral and iliac arteries and into the aorta under fluoroscopic guidance. A catheter is advanced over the guidewire into the aorta. The guidewire is then advanced into the main renal artery and any accessory renal arteries and the physician then manipulates the catheter over the guidewire until the catheter is situated at the desired location. The guidewire is removed. Injection of medication and/or radiopaque contrast media is performed as needed. Pressure gradient measurements may also be obtained to determine if any visualized narrowing in the renal arteries is affecting blood flow to the kidneys. Images are obtained, processed, and permanent recordings are made as needed. The physician reviews the images and recordings and provides a written report of findings. Use 36251 for a selective unilateral renal angiogram. Use 36252 for a selective bilateral study.

36253-36254

36253 Superselective catheter placement (one or more second order or higher renal artery branches) renal artery and any accessory renal artery(s) for renal angiography, including arterial puncture, catheterization, fluoroscopy, contrast injection(s), image postprocessing, permanent recording of images, and radiological supervision and interpretation, including pressure gradient measurements when performed, and flush aortogram when performed; unilateral

36254 Superselective catheter placement (one or more second order or higher renal artery branches) renal artery and any accessory renal artery(s) for renal angiography, including arterial puncture, catheterization, fluoroscopy, contrast injection(s), image postprocessing, permanent recording of images, and radiological supervision and interpretation, including pressure gradient measurements when performed, and flush aortogram when performed; bilateral

A super-selective catheter placement in one or more second order or higher renal branches is performed for renal angiography. A catheter is introduced into an extremity artery, with the preferred introduction site being a femoral artery in the groin. A small skin incision is made over the planned insertion site. An introducer sheath is placed in the artery and a guidewire is inserted. If the right femoral artery is used, the guidewire is manipulated through the femoral and iliac arteries and into the aorta under fluoroscopic guidance. A catheter is advanced over the guidewire into the aorta. The guidewire is then advanced into the main renal artery and the physician manipulates the catheter over the guidewire into the main renal artery. The physician continues to selectively advance the guidewire and catheter through higher order branches (second, third, and beyond) until the catheter is situated in the highest order branch requiring evaluation. The guidewire is removed. Injection of medication and/or radiopaque contrast media is performed as needed. Pressure gradient measurements may also be obtained to determine if any visualized narrowing in the renal arteries is affecting blood flow to the kidneys. Images are obtained, processed, and permanent recordings are made as needed. The physician reviews the

Cardiovascular System

images and recordings and provides a written report of findings. Use 36253 for a super-selective unilateral renal angiogram. Use 36254 for a super-selective bilateral study.

36260-36262

36260 Insertion of implantable intra-arterial infusion pump (eg, for chemotherapy of liver)
36261 Revision of implanted intra-arterial infusion pump
36262 Removal of implanted intra-arterial infusion pump

A subcutaneously placed totally implantable intra-arterial infusion pump is inserted, revised, or removed. Intra-arterial infusion pumps are commonly used to treat metastatic liver cancer. To place the pump (36260) for intra-arterial infusion of chemotherapy into the liver, a right-sided abdominal incision is made in the skin below the ribs. The abdominal wall is opened and the abdomen explored and vascular anatomy evaluated. If hepatic vasculature is normal, the catheter is placed in the gastroduodenal artery (GDA) with the tip positioned at the origin of the (GDA). The proximal GDA is ligated. A separate skin incision is made below the first, and a subcutaneous pocket fashioned between the skin and fascia. The catheter is tunneled to the pump and connected. Pump function is evaluated using fluoroscein dye. The pump may be filled with the chemotherapeutic agent or with heparinized saline to prevent clotting of the catheter. The implantable pump delivers chemotherapy at a slow fixed rate over a two week period at which time the patient returns to the physician's office for refilling of the pump. In 36261, the pump is revised. The subcutaneous pocket is opened and the pump and catheter are evaluated. Any malfunctioning components are replaced or revised. In 36262, the pump is removed. The subcutaneous pocket is opened and the pump disconnected from the catheter and removed. The abdomen is opened and the catheter in the GDA is removed. The subcutaneous pocket is closed as is the abdominal incision.

36400-36406

36400 Venipuncture, younger than age 3 years, necessitating the skill of a physician or other qualified health care professional, not to be used for routine venipuncture; femoral or jugular vein
36405 Venipuncture, younger than age 3 years, necessitating the skill of a physician or other qualified health care professional, not to be used for routine venipuncture; scalp vein
36406 Venipuncture, younger than age 3 years, necessitating the skill of a physician or other qualified health care professional, not to be used for routine venipuncture; other vein

The most common sites for venipuncture in infants and young children include the scalp, external jugular, femoral, saphenous, dorsal veins of the hand, or dorsal arch of the foot. The circumstances necessitating the skill of a physician or other qualified health care professional for the venipuncture procedure are documented and the required consents obtained from the parent or guardian. The most appropriate site for the venipuncture is selected. The site is prepped for sterile entry. The selected vein is punctured and the necessary blood samples obtained for separately reportable laboratory studies. Use 36400 for venipuncture of a jugular or femoral vein, 36405 for a scalp vein, and 36406 for any other vein.

36410

36410 Venipuncture, age 3 years or older, necessitating the skill of a physician or other qualified health care professional (separate procedure), for diagnostic or therapeutic purposes (not to be used for routine venipuncture)

The circumstances necessitating the skill of a physician or other qualified health care professional for the venipuncture procedure are documented and the required consents obtained from the patient, parent or guardian. The most appropriate site for the venipuncture is selected. The site is prepped for sterile entry. The selected vein is punctured and the necessary blood samples obtained or medication administered. Blood specimens are sent to the laboratory for separately reportable laboratory studies.

36415

36415 Collection of venous blood by venipuncture

An appropriate vein is selected, usually one of the larger antecubital veins such as the median cubital, basilic, or cephalic veins. A tourniquet is placed above the planned puncture site. The site is disinfected with an alcohol pad. A needle is attached to a hub and the vein punctured. A vacutainer tube is attached to the hub and the blood specimen collected. The vacutainer tube is removed. Depending on the specific blood tests required, multiple vacutainers may be filled from the same puncture site.

36416

36416 Collection of capillary blood specimen (eg, finger, heel, ear stick)

A blood sample is obtained by capillary puncture usually performed on the finger tip, ear lobe, heel or toe. Heel and toe sites are typically used only on neonates and infants. The planned puncture site is cleaned with an alcohol pad. A lancet is used to puncture the skin.

A drop of blood is allowed to form at the puncture site and is then touched with a capillary tube to collect the specimen.

36420-36425

36420 Venipuncture, cutdown; younger than age 1 year
36425 Venipuncture, cutdown; age 1 or over

Venipuncture is accomplished using a cutdown procedure to access a deep or small vein. The site is prepped for sterile entry. The skin is nicked and the vein carefully exposed. A needle is inserted into the vein and the necessary blood samples obtained or medication administered. Use 36420 for a child younger than age 1. Use 36420 for patients age 1 or over.

36430

36430 Transfusion, blood or blood components

Blood and blood components include whole blood, platelets, packed red blood cells, and plasma products. Transfusions are performed to replace blood that is lost or depleted due to an injury, surgery, sickle cell disease, or treatment for a malignant neoplasm. Red blood cells are given to increase the number of blood cells that transport oxygen and nutrients throughout the body, platelets to control bleeding and improve blood clotting, and plasma to replace total blood volume and provide blood factors that improve blood clotting. The skin is prepped over the planned transfusion site and an intravenous line inserted. Any medication ordered by the physician is administered prior to the transfusion. The blood and/or blood components are administered. The patient is monitored during the transfusion for any signs of adverse reaction.

36440

36440 Push transfusion, blood, 2 years or younger

Transfusions are performed to replace blood that is lost or depleted due to an injury, surgery, sickle cell disease, or treatment for a malignant neoplasm. Push transfusion may be performed through a previously established intravenous line or a new intravenous line may be placed. Any medication ordered by the physician is administered prior to the transfusion. The blood is then administered using a push technique over a relatively short period of time, usually less than 15 minutes. The child is monitored during and after the transfusion for any signs of adverse reaction.

36450-36455

36450 Exchange transfusion, blood; newborn
36455 Exchange transfusion, blood; other than newborn

The exchange equipment is set up. In 36450 the exchange transfusion is performed on a newborn using either a one or two catheter push-pull technique. Using a two catheter technique, the physician selects an appropriate artery and vein. Blood is removed from the selected artery while being infused at the same rate through a vein. A one catheter technique is performed using either an umbilical vein or less frequently an umbilical artery catheter. Placement of the tip of the umbilical catheter is checked by separately reportable radiographs ensure that it is in the inferior vena cava or right atrium. Blood is withdrawn over two minutes and the same volume of donor blood infused at a slightly faster rate. The physician exchanges as much blood as possible. One volume typically exchanges 65% percent of red blood cells, while two volumes exchanges 88%. In 36455, the exchange transfusion is performed on a patient other than a newborn using a two catheter push-pull technique. The physician selects an appropriate artery and vein. Using this technique, blood is removed from the selected artery while being infused at the same rate through a vein.

36456

● **36456** Partial exchange transfusion, blood, plasma or crystalloid necessitating the skill of a physician or other qualified health care professional, newborn

Partial exchange transfusion of blood, plasma, or crystalloid fluid may be performed on a newborn to correct polycythemia or anemia in the absence of hypovolemia and to treat hyperbilirubinemia. Conditions that may increase a newborns risk of polycythemia, anemia, and hyperbilirubinemia include large or small for gestational age, intrauterine growth retardation, Trisomy 21, twin-to-twin transfusion syndrome, Beckwith-Wiedemann syndrome, delayed cord clamping, and maternal diabetes. During a partial exchange transfusion, small amounts of blood are removed through thin catheters placed into blood vessel(s) and replaced with warmed blood, plasma, or crystalloid fluid. Partial exchange transfusion may be accomplished using a push-pull technique through a single catheter placed in either the umbilical artery or umbilical vein or a two catheter method using the umbilical vein and umbilical artery, or one umbilical vessel and a peripheral vein. Following catheter placement, a calculated volume of blood is withdrawn from the umbilical vessel over 2-3 minutes and discarded. The same volume of warmed blood, plasma, or crystalloid fluid is then slowly infused via the same vessel (push-pull) or the second umbilical catheter. The cycle repeats until the desired volume has been exchanged. When using an umbilical vessel and peripheral vein technique, the calculated volume of blood is withdrawn from the umbilical vessel over 2-3 minutes while the same volume of warmed blood, plasma, or crystalloid fluid is infused simultaneously through the peripheral vein.

● New Code   ▲ Revised Code

36460

36460   Transfusion, intrauterine, fetal

There are several indications for fetal transfusion with the most common being when fetal red blood cells of an Rh-positive fetus are destroyed by the Rh-sensitized mother's immune system. Another indication for transfusion is neonatal alloimmune thrombocytopenia (NAIT) caused by maternal antibodies directed against platelet-specific antigens. Prior to the transfusion, an abdominal ultrasound of the pregnant uterus is performed to determine the position of the fetus and locate the placenta and umbilical vein. Amniotic fluid level is also evaluated. Separately reportable ultrasound imaging is then used continuously to monitor proper placement of the needle in the umbilical vein at the placental insertion. Alternatively, transfusion may be performed with the needle inserted into the fetal abdomen. The blood transfusion procedure is performed. The mother and fetus are carefully monitored during and after the transfusion procedure.

36468

36468   Single or multiple injections of sclerosing solutions, spider veins (telangiectasia), limb or trunk

Telangiectasia, also referred to as spider veins, are small branched or clustered red, blue, or purple veins often having the appearance of a spider's web that typically occur on the leg or trunk. The spider veins may be photographed to document the sites and extensiveness of the condition. The skin over the spider veins is cleansed with an antiseptic. The physician then stretches the skin taut using one hand and injects the sclerosing solution with the other. The sclerosing solution causes the spider veins to become inflamed, the vein walls to stick together, and then close. This causes the spider vein to disappear or become less noticeable over time as the body reabsorbs the tissue. Typically the physician will perform anywhere from 5 to 40 injections during a single session.

36470-36471

36470   Injection of sclerosing solution; single vein
36471   Injection of sclerosing solution; multiple veins, same leg

The varicose veins may be photographed to document the sites and extensiveness of the varicosities. The skin over the varicose veins is cleansed with an antiseptic. The physician then stretches the skin taut using one hand and injects the sclerosing solution with the other along the length of the vein. Multiple injections are typically performed for each vein treated. The sclerosing solution causes the varicose veins to become inflamed, the vein walls to stick together and then close permanently. This causes the varicose veins to disappear or become less noticeable over time as the body reabsorbs the tissue. The body reroutes venous blood flow to deeper veins. Use 36470 for sclerotherapy on a single vein and 36471 for multiple veins in the same leg.

36475-36476

36475   Endovenous ablation therapy of incompetent vein, extremity, inclusive of all imaging guidance and monitoring, percutaneous, radiofrequency; first vein treated
36476   Endovenous ablation therapy of incompetent vein, extremity, inclusive of all imaging guidance and monitoring, percutaneous, radiofrequency; second and subsequent veins treated in a single extremity, each through separate access sites (List separately in addition to code for primary procedure)

The physician prepares the site to be treated, sets up the radiofrequency ablation catheter, and tests the equipment. Imaging guidance is used to find the targeted vein and to map and mark the entire length of the vein. Local anesthetic is administered at the vein access site. The skin is incised and a venotomy performed. A guidewire is introduced into the vein and a dilator advanced over the guidewire. The dilator is exchanged for a sheath and the sheath secured with a suture. The guidewire is removed and the radiofrequency probe introduced and advanced along the vein using imaging guidance. An anesthetic is infiltrated into the perivenous space along the entire length of the vein. With the physician continuously monitoring impedance, power, and vein wall temperature, radiofrequency energy is applied as the probe is withdrawn under imaging guidance. Use 36475 for the first vein treated and 36476 for second and subsequent veins in the same extremity accessed through a separate venotomy site.

36478-36479

36478   Endovenous ablation therapy of incompetent vein, extremity, inclusive of all imaging guidance and monitoring, percutaneous, laser; first vein treated
36479   Endovenous ablation therapy of incompetent vein, extremity, inclusive of all imaging guidance and monitoring, percutaneous, laser; second and subsequent veins treated in a single extremity, each through separate access sites (List separately in addition to code for primary procedure)

The physician prepares the site to be treated, sets up the laser ablation catheter, and tests the equipment. Imaging guidance is used to find the targeted vein and to map and mark the entire length of the vein. Local anesthetic is administered at the vein access site. The skin is incised and a venotomy performed. A guidewire is introduced into the vein and a dilator advanced over the guidewire. The dilator is exchanged for a sheath and the sheath secured a suture. The guidewire is removed and the laser fiber introduced and advanced along the vein using imaging guidance. An anesthetic is infiltrated into the perivenous space along the entire length of the vein. With the physician continuously monitoring impedance, power, and vein wall temperature, laser energy is applied as the fiber is withdrawn under imaging guidance. Use 36478 for the first vein treated and 36479 for second and subsequent veins in the same extremity accessed through a separate venotomy site.

36481

36481   Percutaneous portal vein catheterization by any method

Portal vein catheterization is typically performed to place a catheter for separately reportable portography and may include a hemodynamic evaluation. The portal vein delivers deoxygenated blood from the digestive organs to the liver. The portal blood contains nutrients, such as glucose, and other substances that have been absorbed from the digestive tract. The liver monitors the nutrients and other substances contained in the portal blood, stores some of these nutrients, modifies others so that they can be absorbed more easily by the cells, and detoxifies harmful substances. Using separately reportable imaging guidance, a catheter is placed through the skin of the abdomen, guided through the liver, and inserted into the portal vein. Portal blood pressure may be measure, flow gradients evaluated, and separately reportable injection of radiopaque material performed. Following completion of the procedure, a gel-foam sponge may be introduced through the outer sheath of the catheter to plug the transhepatic puncture site and prevent intraperitoneal bleeding.

36500

36500   Venous catheterization for selective organ blood sampling

The vein catheterized depends on the specific organ blood being evaluated. Veins that are most often used for organ blood sampling include the renal veins, hepatic veins, coronary sinus, internal jugular vein, left adrenal vein and deep muscular veins. The selected vein is identified and a catheter placed in the vein using separately reportable imaging guidance. A single blood sample may be obtained or the catheter may be left in place so that multiple blood samples may be obtained.

36510

36510   Catheterization of umbilical vein for diagnosis or therapy, newborn

The umbilical cord stump and surrounding area are cleansed with bactericidal solution. The stump is tied at the base with a pursestring suture or umbilical tape to control bleeding. The cord is cut horizontally and the umbilical vein and two arteries are identified. Thrombi are cleared from the vein and the vein is dilated. An appropriately sized catheter is selected, flushed with heparin solution and closed with a stopcock. The catheter is then inserted through the umbilical vein and advanced until good blood return is obtained. The catheter is secured with the previously placed pursestring suture or umbilical tape. Correct positioning of the catheter is verified with separately reportable radiographs.

36511-36513

36511   Therapeutic apheresis; for white blood cells
36512   Therapeutic apheresis; for red blood cells
36513   Therapeutic apheresis; for platelets

Therapeutic apheresis is performed using a blood processing machine. The machine separates blood into components (white cells, red cells, platelets, plasma) on the basis of weight. Therapeutic apheresis uses the blood processing machine to remove a component of the blood that is contributing to a disease state. The physician evaluates the patient and determines the need for therapeutic apheresis. A previously placed central venous catheter is used or venous catheters are placed and blood tubing connected to the catheters and the apheresis machine. The physician determines the apheresis parameters and programs the machine. Apheresis is initiated. Blood is removed from the body and enters the apheresis machine through one of the venous catheters. The blood is separated into components by the machine, the component causing the disease state is removed, and the remaining blood components returned to the body through a second catheter. The machine may be operated by the physician or the physician may attend the patient while a nurse operates the machine. The physician monitors the patient throughout the procedure which may include cardiac monitoring and pulse oximetry. Upon completion of the procedure, the patient is disconnected from the machine and the patient is re-evaluated. Use 36511 for white cell apheresis, 36512 for red blood cell apheresis, and 36513 for platelet apheresis.

36514-36516

36514   Therapeutic apheresis; for plasma pheresis
36515   Therapeutic apheresis; with extracorporeal immunoadsorption and plasma reinfusion
36516   Therapeutic apheresis; with extracorporeal selective adsorption or selective filtration and plasma reinfusion

Therapeutic apheresis is performed using a blood processing machine to remove plasma or plasma constituents that are contributing to a disease state. The machine separates

Cardiovascular System

blood into components (white cells, red cells, platelets, plasma) on the basis of weight. The physician evaluates the patient and determines the need for plasmapheresis. Plasmapheresis is typically performed using a dual lumen, dialysis-type catheter. The physician determines the plasmapheresis parameters and programs the machine. Plasmapheresis is initiated. Blood is removed from the body and enters the apheresis machine through one lumen of the dialysis-type catheters. The machine may be operated by the physician or the physician may attend the patient while a nurse operates the machine. The physician monitors the patient throughout the procedure which may include cardiac monitoring and pulse oximetry. Upon completion of the procedure, the patient is disconnected from the machine and the patient is re-evaluated. In 36514, the plasma is separated from other blood components and collected in a bag. The cells are returned to the patient with a biologic replacement fluid, such as allogeneic plasma or human serum albumin, through the second lumen of the catheter. In 36515, therapeutic apheresis is performed to remove specific antibodies or proteins from the blood using extracorporeal immunoadsorption and plasma reinfusion. The apheresis machine separates the patient plasma from other blood components. The plasma is adsorbed using an affinity column which removes only the antibody or protein causing the disease state. The rest of the plasma constituents pass through the affinity column and are returned to the body. In 36516, therapeutic apheresis is performed to remove a specific blood constituent, such as lipids, from the blood using extracorporeal selective adsorption or filtration with plasma reinfusion. The specific constituent causing the disease state is separated using an affinity column or filter. The plasma may require treatment post-adsorption or post-filtration before it is reinfused into the patient.

36522

36522   Photopheresis, extracorporeal

Extracorporeal photophoresis (ECP), also referred to as extracorporeal photochemotherapy, is performed. ECP is a form of therapeutic leukapheresis (white blood cell apheresis) that is used to treat cutaneous T-cell lymphoma (CTCL), other types of blood and bone marrow neoplasms and diseases, and patients with chronic graft versus host disease (GVHD). Venous access is established with a peripheral or central venous access line. A specific volume of blood is then passed through three to six cycles of leukapheresis. The volume of blood and the number of cycles is determined by the patient's hematicrit value and size. At the end of each cycle, the red blood cells and plasma are reinfused into the patient. The collected white blood cells are then mixed with heparin, saline and a chemotherapeutic agent. This mixture is exposed to ultraviolet A light (UVA) which causes the mixture to be absorbed into the DNA of the lymphocytes. This causes the treated T-cells to die. The treated white blood cell mixture is then reinfused in the patient. It also appears to that ECP causes additional cell changes that have a further therapeutic effect against circulating abnormal blood cells that have not been treated when the mixture is reinfused.

36555-36556

36555   Insertion of non-tunneled centrally inserted central venous catheter; younger than 5 years of age

36556   Insertion of non-tunneled centrally inserted central venous catheter; age 5 years or older

A non-tunneled centrally inserted central venous catheter (CVC) is placed. A CVC must terminate in the subclavian, brachiocephalic, or iliac veins, the superior or inferior vena cava, or right atrium. A non-tunneled CVC is placed directly into the jugular, subclavian, or femoral vein or the inferior vena cava. Separately reportable imaging guidance may be used to access the venous entry site and/or to manipulate the catheter tip to the final central position. Local anesthesia is administered at the planned puncture site. There are two techniques for insertion. Using a peel-away cannula technique, a cannula with a stylet is inserted into the selected vein. The stylet is removed. The catheter is advanced through the cannula into the vein and advanced into the brachiocephalic vein, subclavian vein, superior vena cava, or right atrium or the iliac vein or inferior vena cava. Using a Seldinger technique, the skin and vein are punctured with a needle. A guidewire is inserted through the needle and advanced several centimeters. An introducer sheath and dilator are advanced over the guidewire and the guidewire and dilator removed. The catheter is then advanced through the introducer sheath and into the brachiocephalic vein, subclavian vein, superior vena cava or right atrium, or iliac vein or inferior vena cava. Placement is checked by separately reportable radiographs. The CVC is secured with sutures and a dressing applied over the insertion site. Use 36555 for non-tunneled CVC placement in a child younger than age 5 and 36556 for a patient age 5 or older.

36557-36558

36557   Insertion of tunneled centrally inserted central venous catheter, without subcutaneous port or pump; younger than 5 years of age

36558   Insertion of tunneled centrally inserted central venous catheter, without subcutaneous port or pump; age 5 years or older

A tunneled centrally inserted central venous catheter (CVC) is placed. A CVC must terminate in the subclavian, brachiocephalic, or iliac veins, the superior or inferior vena cava, or right atrium. A tunneled CVC is placed through a subcutaneous tunnel into the jugular, subclavian, or femoral vein or the inferior vena cava with the most common venous access

site for tunneled devices being the jugular vein. Separately reportable imaging guidance may be used to access the venous entry site and/or to manipulate the catheter tip to the final central position. Local anesthesia is administered at the planned puncture site. Using a Seldinger technique to access the jugular vein, the skin and vein are punctured with a needle. A guidewire is inserted through the needle and advanced several centimeters. An incision is made in the chest wall and a subcutaneous tunnel is created. An introducer sheath and dilator are advanced over the guidewire and the guidewire and dilator removed. The catheter is then advanced through the tunnel to the introducer sheath in the jugular vein and into the brachiocephalic vein, subclavian vein, superior vena cava or right atrium. Placement is checked by separately reportable radiographs. The CVC is secured with sutures, the incision in the chest wall closed with sutures, and a dressing applied over the insertion site. Use 36557 for tunneled CVC placement in a child younger than age 5 and 36558 for a patient age 5 or older.

36560-36561

36560   Insertion of tunneled centrally inserted central venous access device, with subcutaneous port; younger than 5 years of age

36561   Insertion of tunneled centrally inserted central venous access device, with subcutaneous port; age 5 years or older

A tunneled centrally inserted central venous catheter (CVC) with a subcutaneous port is placed. A CVC must terminate in the subclavian, brachiocephalic, or iliac veins, the superior or inferior vena cava, or right atrium. A tunneled CVC is placed through a subcutaneous tunnel into the jugular, subclavian, or femoral vein or the inferior vena cava with the most common venous access site for tunneled devices being the jugular vein. Separately reportable imaging guidance may be used to access the venous entry site and/or to manipulate the catheter tip to the final central position. Local anesthesia is administered at the planned puncture site. Using a Seldinger technique to access the jugular vein, the skin and vein are punctured with a needle. A guidewire is inserted through the needle and advanced several centimeters. A subcutaneous pocket is then created for placement of the port. A subcutaneous tunnel is created from the venous access site to the subcutaneous pocket. An introducer sheath and dilator are advanced over the guidewire and the guidewire and dilator removed. The catheter is then advanced through the tunnel to the introducer sheath in the jugular vein and into the brachiocephalic vein, subclavian vein, superior vena cava or right atrium. Placement is checked by separately reportable radiographs. The catheter and port are connected and the port is placed in the subcutaneous pocket. The incision over the venous access site is closed. The port is sutured into place and the pocket is closed. Use 36560 for tunneled CVC placement with subcutaneous port in a child younger than age 5 and 36561 for a patient age 5 or older.

36563

36563   Insertion of tunneled centrally inserted central venous access device with subcutaneous pump

A central venous catheter (CVC) must terminate in the subclavian, brachiocephalic, or iliac veins, the superior or inferior vena cava, or right atrium. A tunneled CVC is placed through a subcutaneous tunnel into the jugular, subclavian, or femoral vein or the inferior vena cava with the most common venous access site for tunneled devices being the jugular vein. Separately reportable imaging guidance may be used to access the venous entry site and/or to manipulate the catheter tip to the final central position. Local anesthesia is administered at the planned puncture site. Using a Seldinger technique to access the jugular vein, the skin and vein are punctured with a needle. A guidewire is inserted through the needle and advanced several centimeters. A subcutaneous pocket is then created for placement of the pump. A subcutaneous tunnel is created from the venous access site to the subcutaneous pocket. An introducer sheath and dilator are advanced over the guidewire and the guidewire and dilator removed. The catheter is then advanced through the tunnel to the introducer sheath in the jugular vein and into the brachiocephalic vein, subclavian vein, superior vena cava or right atrium. Placement is checked by separately reportable radiographs. The catheter and pump are connected and the pump placed in the subcutaneous pocket. The incision over the venous access site is closed. The pump is sutured into place and the pocket is closed.

36565-36566

36565   Insertion of tunneled centrally inserted central venous access device, requiring 2 catheters via 2 separate venous access sites; without subcutaneous port or pump (eg, Tesio type catheter)

36566   Insertion of tunneled centrally inserted central venous access device, requiring 2 catheters via 2 separate venous access sites; with subcutaneous port(s)

Two tunneled centrally inserted central venous catheters (CVC) are placed via two separate venous access sites. A CVC must terminate in the subclavian, brachiocephalic, or iliac veins, the superior or inferior vena cava, or right atrium. A tunneled CVC is placed through a subcutaneous tunnel into the jugular, subclavian, or femoral vein or the inferior vena cava with the most common venous access site for tunneled devices being the jugular vein. Separately reportable imaging guidance may be used to access the venous entry site and/or to manipulate the catheter tip to the final central position. Local anesthesia is administered at the planned puncture site. In 36565, two tunneled CVCs are placed without connection to a subcutaneous port or pump. Using a Seldinger technique to access the jugular vein, the skin and vein are punctured with a needle. A guidewire is inserted through the needle and advanced several centimeters. An incision is made in the chest wall and a subcutaneous tunnel is created. An introducer sheath and dilator are advanced over the guidewire and the guidewire and dilator removed. The catheter is then advanced through the tunnel to the introducer sheath in the jugular vein and into the brachiocephalic vein, subclavian vein, superior vena cava or right atrium. Placement is checked by separately reportable radiographs. The CVC is secured with sutures, the incision in the chest wall closed with sutures, and a dressing applied over the insertion site. A second tunneled CVC is placed in the same manner via a separately venous access site. In 36566, two tunneled CVCs are placed with connection to a subcutaneous port. Placement of the tunneled catheter is performed as described above. A subcutaneous pocket is then created for placement of the port. A subcutaneous tunnel is created from the venous access site to the subcutaneous pocket. The catheter and port are connected and the port is placed in the subcutaneous pocket. The incision over the venous access site is closed. The port is sutured into place and the pocket is closed. A second catheter and port are placed in the same manner.

36568-36569

36568 **Insertion of peripherally inserted central venous catheter (PICC), without subcutaneous port or pump; younger than 5 years of age**

36569 **Insertion of peripherally inserted central venous catheter (PICC), without subcutaneous port or pump; age 5 years or older**

A peripherally inserted central venous catheter (PICC) is similar to an intravenous line and is used for the delivery of medication or fluids over a prolonged period of time. Ultrasound is used as needed to identify a suitable large vein in the arm. Typically, one of the deeper veins located above the elbow is used, such as the basilic, cephalic, or brachial vein. The planned inserted site is cleansed with bactericidal solution. A tourniquet is placed on the arm and a local anesthetic injected at the planned insertion site. There are two techniques for insertion. Using a peel-away cannula technique, a cannula with a stylet is inserted into the selected vein. The stylet is removed. The PICC line is advanced through the cannula into the vein and advanced into the brachiocephalic vein, subclavian vein, or superior vena cava. Using a Seldinger technique, the skin and vein are punctured with a needle. A guidewire is inserted through the needle and advanced several centimeters. An introducer sheath and dilator are advanced over the guidewire and the guidewire and dilator removed. The PICC line is then advanced through the introducer sheath and into the brachiocephalic vein, subclavian vein, or superior vena cava. Separately reportable radiographs check placement. The PICC is secured with sutures and a dressing applied over the insertion site in the arm. Use 36568 for PICC placement in a child younger than age 5 and 36569 for a patient age 5 or older.

36570-36571

36570 **Insertion of peripherally inserted central venous access device, with subcutaneous port; younger than 5 years of age**

36571 **Insertion of peripherally inserted central venous access device, with subcutaneous port; age 5 years or older**

This type of device includes a port inserted under the skin that is attached to a catheter placed in a peripheral vein and advanced into the superior vena cava. Ultrasound is used as needed to identify a suitable large vein in the arm. Typically, one of the deeper veins located above the elbow is used, such as the basilic, cephalic, or brachial vein. The planned catheter insertion site is incised and the selected vein exposed. Using a Seldinger technique, the vein is punctured with a needle. A guidewire is inserted through the needle and advanced several centimeters. An introducer sheath and dilator are advanced over the guidewire and the guidewire and dilator removed. The catheter is advanced through the introducer sheath and into the brachiocephalic vein, subclavian vein, or superior vena cava. Separately reportable radiographs check placement. The catheter is anchored in the subcutaneous tissue. A subcutaneous pocket is then created for placement of the port. The catheter is tunneled to the port and the catheter and port connected. The incision over the venous access site is closed. The port is sutured into place and the pocket is closed. Use 36570 for peripherally inserted central venous access device (VAD) with port placement in a child younger than age 5 and 36571 for a patient age 5 or older.

36575-36576

36575 **Repair of tunneled or non-tunneled central venous access catheter, without subcutaneous port or pump, central or peripheral insertion site**

36576 **Repair of central venous access device, with subcutaneous port or pump, central or peripheral insertion site**

A previously placed tunneled or non-tunneled central venous access catheter is repaired. This procedure is performed when a portion of the catheter external to the vein is damaged. The repair may be performed on a peripherally or centrally placed catheter. In 36575, the damage to the catheter is evaluated. A non-tunneled catheter that has been cut can be repaired by trimming the remaining catheter and splicing a new catheter hub segment onto the existing catheter. The repair is then checked using an injection of

intravenous fluid. A tunneled catheter may be repaired as described above if the external portion of catheter is damaged. If the catheter contained in the tunnel requires repair, the tunneled portion of the catheter may be exposed by incising the skin and subcutaneous tissue. The necessary catheter repairs are then completed and a new subcutaneous tunnel created as needed. The repaired catheter is secured with sutures. In 36576, a tunneled catheter with a subcutaneous port or pump is repaired. Repair of a catheter leak is one of the more common types of repairs. The port or pump pocket is opened. The catheter is disconnected and the damaged section identified. The damaged section of catheter is removed by trimming the catheter at a point proximal to the damage. The catheter is then reconnected to the port or pump. The repaired catheter is tested to ensure there are no leaks by injecting intravenous fluid. The port or pump is returned to the subcutaneous pocket and secured with sutures. The pocket is closed.

36578

36578 **Replacement, catheter only, of central venous access device, with subcutaneous port or pump, central or peripheral insertion site**

Catheter replacement may be performed on a peripherally or centrally placed catheter. The subcutaneous pocket is opened and the port or pump examined to ensure proper function of that component. Separately reportable radiographs are obtained to verify that the tip of the existing PICC or CVC is correctly positioned. The catheter is then inspected and found to be occluded or damaged. A guidewire is placed through the existing catheter which is withdrawn over the guidewire. A new catheter is then advanced over the guidewire and the tip positioned in the subclavian, brachiocephalic, or iliac vein, the superior or inferior vena cava, or right atrium. The catheter is attached to the port or pump device and the connection checked for leaks using an injection of intravenous fluid. The port or pump is returned to the subcutaneous pocket and secured with sutures. The pocket is closed.

36580-36581

36580 **Replacement, complete, of a non-tunneled centrally inserted central venous catheter, without subcutaneous port or pump, through same venous access**

36581 **Replacement, complete, of a tunneled centrally inserted central venous catheter, without subcutaneous port or pump, through same venous access**

Complete replacement of a centrally inserted central venous catheter (CVC) without a subcutaneous port or pump is performed through the same venous access site. Replacement is performed when a catheter becomes partially or completed obstructed or when another malfunction occurs. Separately reportable radiographs are obtained to verify that the tip of the CVC is correctly positioned. In 36580, a non-tunneled CVC is replaced. A guidewire is placed through the existing catheter which is withdrawn over the guidewire. A new catheter is then advanced over the guidewire and the tip positioned in the subclavian, brachiocephalic, or iliac vein, the superior or inferior vena cava, or right atrium. The new catheter is secured with sutures and flushed with heparin or attached to tubing for administration of intravenous fluids or medication. In 36581, a tunneled CVC is replaced. The indwelling catheter is dissected free of subcutaneous tissue. A guidewire is placed through the existing catheter which is withdrawn over the guidewire. A new catheter is then advanced over the guidewire and the tip positioned in the subclavian, brachiocephalic, or iliac vein, the superior or inferior vena cava, or right atrium. The new catheter is secured within the tunnel with sutures and flushed with heparin or attached to tubing for administration of intravenous fluids or medication.

36582-36583

36582 **Replacement, complete, of a tunneled centrally inserted central venous access device, with subcutaneous port, through same venous access**

36583 **Replacement, complete, of a tunneled centrally inserted central venous access device, with subcutaneous pump, through same venous access**

Complete replacement of a centrally inserted central venous catheter (CVC) with a subcutaneous port or pump is performed through the same venous access site. Replacement is performed when malfunction of the port or pump as well as the CVC occurs. Separately reportable radiographs are obtained to verify that the tip of the CVC is correctly positioned. The subcutaneous pocket is opened and the catheter separated from the port or pump. The port or pump are examined and determined to require replacement. The port or pump is removed. The catheter is also inspected and found to be occluded or damaged. A guidewire is placed through the existing catheter which is withdrawn over the guidewire. A new catheter is then advanced over the guidewire and the tip positioned in the subclavian, brachiocephalic, or iliac vein, the superior or inferior vena cava, or right atrium. A new port or pump is placed in the subcutaneous pocket. The new catheter is attached to the port or pump device and the connection checked for leaks using an injection of intravenous fluid. The pocket is closed. Use 36582 for complete replacement of a CVC and subcutaneous port and 36583 for complete replacement of a CVC and subcutaneous pump.

36584-36585

36584 Replacement, complete, of a peripherally inserted central venous catheter (PICC), without subcutaneous port or pump, through same venous access

36585 Replacement, complete, of a peripherally inserted central venous access device, with subcutaneous port, through same venous access

In 36584, the venous access site is inspected to ensure that it can be used for the replacement PICC line. The site is cleansed with bactericidal solution. A local anesthetic injected at the insertion site. The new catheter is primed with flush solution. The existing catheter is grasped and partially removed leaving several centimeters still within the vein. The existing catheter is trimmed leaving approximately 10 cm outside the vein. The existing catheter is secured with a hemostat to prevent catheter migration. The introducer is advanced into the vein over the trimmed end of the existing catheter. Once the introducer is in place, the existing catheter is completely removed from the vein. The PICC line is inserted through the introducer into the vein and advanced into the brachiocephalic vein, subclavian vein or superior vena cava. Placement is checked by separately reportable radiographs. The PICC is secured with sutures and a dressing applied over the insertion site in the arm. In 36585, the subcutaneous pocket is opened and the port site inspected. The port is separated from the catheter and the port removed from the pocket. The existing catheter is dissected free of the subcutaneous tissue and the existing venous access site exposed. The existing catheter is then partially removed and secured with a hemostat. An introducer sheath is advanced into the vein over the existing catheter and then the existing catheter is removed. The new catheter is advanced through the introducer sheath and into the brachiocephalic vein, subclavian vein, superior vena cava. Placement is checked by separately reportable radiographs. The new catheter is anchored in the subcutaneous tissue. The new port is placed in the subcutaneous pocket. The new catheter is tunneled to the new port and the two components connected. The incision over the venous access site is closed. The port is sutured into place and the pocket is closed.

36589-36590

36589 Removal of tunneled central venous catheter, without subcutaneous port or pump

36590 Removal of tunneled central venous access device, with subcutaneous port or pump, central or peripheral insertion

A tunneled central venous catheter (CVC) is removed. A local anesthetic is injected. In 36589, a tunneled CVC without a subcutaneous port or pump is removed. The skin over the venous access site is incised and sutures removed. The CVC is dissected free of the tunnel and removed. Bleeding is controlled with manual pressure over the venous access site. The incision is closed and a dressing applied. In 36590, a tunneled CVC with a subcutaneous port or pump is removed. The subcutaneous pocket is incised and the port of pump dissected free. The CVC is dissected free of the tunnel and the port or pump and catheter are removed. Bleeding is controlled with manual pressure over the venous access site. The incision is closed and a dressing applied.

36591

36591 Collection of blood specimen from a completely implantable venous access device

The septum of the IVAD is located by palpating the skin over the IVAD. The skin over the IVAD is cleansed and a Huber needle (special side-holed needle) with attached syringe and extension tubing primed with normal saline is inserted into the IVAD at a 90 degree angle. A small amount of blood is aspirated into the syringe and the IVAD is flushed with normal saline. The extension tubing is clamped. The syringe is then disconnected and an intermittent injection cap is attached. A vacutainer is inserted into the injection cap. A discard tube is inserted onto the vacutainer needle. The tubing is unclamped and the discard tube is filled. The extension tubing is clamped and the discard tube is removed and discarded. A blood specimen tube is then inserted onto the vacutainer needle, the extension tubing is again unclamped, and the blood specimen is collected. One or more blood specimen tubes may be filled in this manner, then the vacutainer is removed, and the line is flushed with 20 ml of normal saline. If no other procedures are to be performed, such as infusion of medications, the syringe is disconnected and the extension tubing is flushed with heparin. The Huber needle is then removed.

36592

36592 Collection of blood specimen using established central or peripheral catheter, venous, not otherwise specified

The catheter hub is cleansed and a syringe is attached. The catheter is flushed with normal saline. Blood is then allowed to fill the central line and five ml of blood is aspirated into the syringe and discarded. If a vacutainer system is used, it is attached. Labeled blood tubes are attached to the vacutainer and filled. The vacutainer system is removed and the central line is flushed with normal saline if an infusion procedure is to follow the blood collection. The line is flushed with heparin, otherwise. Alternatively, a syringe without a vacutainer system can also be used to collect a blood specimen.

36593

36593 Declotting by thrombolytic agent of implanted vascular access device or catheter

A thrombolytic agent, such as streptokinase, tissue-type palminogen activator (t-PA), urokinase, or heparin, is instilled into an implanted vascular access device (IVAD) or central venous catheter (CVC) to dissolve a thrombus (blood clot) obstructing the IVAD or catheter. The thrombolytic agent is prepared using the drug manufacturer's protocol. The skin over the IVAD or the catheter hub is cleansed. The thrombolytic agent is instilled into the IVAD or into each lumen of the CVC. The thrombolytic agent is left in the catheter for the required dwell time as indicated by the drug manufacturer. Dwell time may be from 30 to 60 minutes. Patency is checked by attempting to draw blood or infuse fluids. If the IVAD or catheter is still obstructed, a second instillation of the thrombolytic agent may be attempted.

36595

36595 Mechanical removal of pericatheter obstructive material (eg, fibrin sheath) from central venous device via separate venous access

One common complication of a semi-permanent CVC is the formation of a fibrin sheath at the tip of the catheter that causes obstruction or reduced flow through the CVC. A separately reportable venogram is performed and the existence of a fibrin sheath or other pericatheter obstructive material confirmed. A separate venous access site is prepped. The vein is incised and a sheath placed. A guidewire is placed and a snareguiding catheter introduced over the guidewire using separately reportable radiological guidance. The snareguiding catheter is advanced to the site of the pericatheter obstruction at the tip of the existing CVC. The guidewire is removed and a snare advanced to the site of the obstruction. The fibrin sheath or other obstructive material is mechanically removed by stripping it away with the snare. Patency of the CVC is evaluated by injecting intravenous fluid. The snare and snareguiding catheter are removed. The separate venous access site is closed with sutures.

36596

36596 Mechanical removal of intraluminal (intracatheter) obstructive material from central venous device through device lumen

One common complication of a semi-permanent CVC is the accumulation of intraluminal obstructive material that causes complete occlusion or reduced flow through the CVC. A CVC without a subcutaneous port is accessed using a guidewire. A CVC with a port or pump is accessed using a Huber needle. A guidewire is then advanced into the port or pump reservoir. A snareguiding catheter or balloon catheter is advanced over the guidewire through the existing catheter lumen or the port or pump. The guidewire is removed. A snare is then used to strip away the obstructive material or the balloon catheter is inflated to open the obstruction. The snare and snareguiding catheter or the balloon catheter are removed. Patency of the CVC is evaluated by injecting intravenous fluid.

36597

36597 Repositioning of previously placed central venous catheter under fluoroscopic guidance

A separately reportable chest radiograph is obtained and the CVC tip is determined to be improperly positioned. Any sutures anchoring the CVC to the skin are removed. The physician then manipulates the catheter tip into the desired location under separately reportable fluoroscopic guidance. The catheter is secured with sutures and a dressing applied.

36598

36598 Contrast injection(s) for radiologic evaluation of existing central venous access device, including fluoroscopy, image documentation and report

Fluoroscopic evaluation is performed to confirm that the tip is properly positioned and that the catheter has not fractured or kinked. A CVC without a subcutaneous port is accessed by inserting a needle through the catheter hub. A CVC with a port or pump is accessed using a Huber needle. Contrast is injected. Fluoroscopic images are obtained of the catheter tip and along the course of the catheter to evaluate patency of the catheter and determine if there are any leaks. Upon completion of the contrast evaluation, the catheter is flushed with saline followed by an anticoagulant solution.

36600

36600 Arterial puncture, withdrawal of blood for diagnosis

The radial artery is the most common site for arterial puncture with alternative sites being the axillary and femoral arteries. The arterial puncture site is selected. The skin is prepped for sterile entry. The selected artery is punctured and the necessary blood samples obtained for separately reportable laboratory studies. The needle is withdrawn and pressure applied to the puncture site.

● New Code   ▲ Revised Code

36620-36625

36620 Arterial catheterization or cannulation for sampling, monitoring or transfusion (separate procedure); percutaneous

36625 Arterial catheterization or cannulation for sampling, monitoring or transfusion (separate procedure); cutdown

Arterial catheterization or cannulation is performed for sampling, monitoring or transfusion. This procedure may be performed to obtain arterial blood samples for blood gas monitoring, to monitor blood pressure, or for blood transfusion. The radial artery is the most common site for arterial catheterization or cannulation with alternative sites being the axillary and femoral arteries. The insertion site is selected, the skin is prepped for sterile entry, and a local anesthetic injected. Using a Seldinger technique, the skin and artery are punctured with a needle or a cutdown is performed to expose the artery followed by needle puncture. A guidewire is inserted through the needle and advanced several centimeters. An introducer sheath and dilator are advanced over the guidewire and the guidewire and dilator removed. The arterial line is then advanced through the introducer sheath and into the artery. Placement is checked as needed by separately reportable radiographs. The catheter or cannula is secured with tape and a dressing applied over the insertion site. Use 36620 for percutaneous insertion by puncturing the skin and artery. Use 36625 for cutdown, which involves incising the skin over the artery and then dissecting the artery free of surrounding tissue prior to needle puncture.

36640

36640 Arterial catheterization for prolonged infusion therapy (chemotherapy), cutdown

The radial artery is the most common site for arterial catheterization with other common sites being the axillary and femoral arteries. The insertion site is selected, the skin is prepped for sterile entry, and a local anesthetic is injected. The skin over the artery is incised and then the artery is dissected free of surrounding tissue followed by needle puncture of the artery. Using a Seldinger technique a guidewire is inserted through the needle and advanced several centimeters. An introducer sheath and dilator are advanced over the guidewire and the guidewire and dilator removed. The arterial line is advanced through the introducer sheath and into the artery. Placement is checked by separately reportable radiographs. The catheter is secured with tape or sutures and a dressing applied over the insertion site in the arm.

36660

36660 Catheterization, umbilical artery, newborn, for diagnosis or therapy

Umbilical artery catheters (UAC) are used primarily for monitoring blood pressure and obtaining blood gases. The depth of the planned catheter insertion is estimated. The newborn's abdomen and cord are cleansed with alcohol. The area is draped with only the cord exposed and a piece of umbilical tape is tied around the base of the cord to minimize blood loss. Using a surgical blade, the cord is cut 1.0 to 2.0 cm from the skin and stabilized with forceps or hemostat and vessels are identified. One of the two arteries is selected and closed curved iris forceps are inserted into the lumen of the artery up to the bend in the forceps, which are then spread to dilate the artery. The catheter is next inserted into the artery using gentle steady pressure to manipulate it beyond the anterior abdominal wall. After the catheter has been advanced to the desired position in the artery and confirmed by x-ray, a purse string suture is placed around the umbilicus to secure the catheter.

36680

36680 Placement of needle for intraosseous infusion

Intraosseous needle placement is used primarily in infants and young children who have suffered circulatory collapse due to trauma or dehydration. The most common site of needle placement is the proximal tibia, but the distal tibia or distal femur may also be used. To place the needle in the proximal tibia, the physician first palpates the tibial tuberosity and then locates a flat area of bone below the tuberosity taking care to avoid the growth plate. The area is cleansed and a local anesthetic injected. The needle is inserted through the skin and subcutaneous tissue. When bone is reached, constant pressure along with a twisting motion is used to advance the needle through the bone cortex and into the marrow space. The inner trocar is removed from the intraosseous needle and a syringe attached to the needle. Bone marrow is aspirated to confirm proper placement.

36800

36800 Insertion of cannula for hemodialysis, other purpose (separate procedure); vein to vein

Two suitable veins are selected. The blood vessels are exposed and incised. One cannula is inserted into the first vein and another into the second vein. The cannulas are secured with sutures. The distal segments of the selected veins are ligated. The two cannulas are connected with synthetic material which may be partially or completely buried. During dialysis the cannulas are connected to tubing that is directly connected to the dialysis machine.

36810-36815

36810 Insertion of cannula for hemodialysis, other purpose (separate procedure); arteriovenous, external (Scribner type)

36815 Insertion of cannula for hemodialysis, other purpose (separate procedure); arteriovenous, external revision, or closure

An external Scribner-type arteriovenous cannula is inserted for hemodialysis or other purpose. The Scribner-type cannula is a semi-permanent arteriovenous hemodialysis shunt that is rarely used today. A suitable peripheral artery and vein are selected, usually the radial artery and cephalic vein at the wrist or the tibial artery and saphenous vein at the ankle. The blood vessels are exposed and incised. One cannula is inserted into the selected artery and another into the selected vein. The cannulas are secured with sutures. The distal segment of the selected artery and vein are ligated. The two cannulas are externally connected with a rigid piece of Teflon or other synthetic material placed over a stainless steel arm plate when not in use. During dialysis the Teflon segment is removed and the cannulas are connected to tubing that is directly connected to the dialysis machine. Use 36810 for the initial placement of the shunt. Use 36815 for external revision or closure of the shunt. If the shunt is revised, one or both cannulas are removed and new cannulas inserted. To close the shunt, the skin over the cannulas is opened and the cannulas exposed. Securing sutures are cut and the cannulas removed. The vessels sutured closed and the skin over the cannula sites is closed.

36818-36820

36818 Arteriovenous anastomosis, open; by upper arm cephalic vein transposition

36819 Arteriovenous anastomosis, open; by upper arm basilic vein transposition

36820 Arteriovenous anastomosis, open; by forearm vein transposition

An open arteriovenous anastomosis is performed to provide hemodialysis access by upper arm cephalic vein transposition (36818), upper arm basilic vein transposition (36819), or forearm vein transposition (36820). In 36818, an incision is made medially in the upper arm to expose the brachial artery and a second incision is made laterally to expose the cephalic vein. The cephalic vein is assessed to ensure that it is patent and of adequate size. A subcutaneous tunnel is then created between the two incisions. The cephalic vein is mobilized and branches ligated. The mobilized segment of cephalic vein is transected taking care to ensure that it is of adequate length for transposition to a more superficial location and tunneling to the brachial artery. The cephalic vein is pulled through the tunnel. An incision is made in the brachial artery and the segment of cephalic vein sutured (anastomosed) to the brachial artery at the arteriotomy site. In 36819, an incision is made in the medial upper arm and the basilic vein and brachial artery exposed. The basilic vein is assessed and if it is found to be patent and of adequate size, the excision is extended exposing the entire basilic vein up to the point where it joins the axillary vein. The basilic vein is then transected near the elbow, branches are ligated, and the basilic vein is transposed and tunneled subcutaneously to the point where it will be connected to the brachial artery. An incision is made in the brachial artery and the transposed segment of basilic vein is anastomosed to the brachial artery at the arteriotomy site. In 36820, the basilic vein is mobilized from the level of the wrist to the middle of the forearm, transposed and tunneled subcutaneously, and then connected to the radial artery or less commonly to the ulnar artery.

36821

36821 Arteriovenous anastomosis, open; direct, any site (eg, Cimino type) (separate procedure)

A direct arteriovenous anastomosis is performed using an open technique to provide hemodialysis access. This procedure may also be referred to as a Cimino-type arteriovenous anastomosis or Cimino fistula. The most common site for construction of a Cimino fistula is at the wrist, but other sites in the arm may be used. This procedure is typically performed using a local infiltration anesthetic or a brachial plexus nerve block. The arm pulses are palpated and a blood pressure cuff is applied to the upper arm to restrict blood flow. The veins are marked using indelible ink. A longitudinal incision is made in the skin to expose the radial artery. The cephalic vein is dissected free of subcutaneous fat and any tributaries are ligated. The vein is positioned next to the radial artery, which is then mobilized. The artery and vein are then connected (anastomosed) in one of four configurations including side-to-side, arterial end to vein side, vein end to arterial side, or end-to-end. A fistula is created by incising the vein and/or artery depending on the configuration used and suturing the vein and artery together.

36823

36823 Insertion of arterial and venous cannula(s) for isolated extracorporeal circulation including regional chemotherapy perfusion to an extremity, with or without hyperthermia, with removal of cannula(s) and repair of arteriotomy and venotomy sites

A systemic anticoagulant is administered. The major inflow and outflow vessels are identified. The skin over the vessels is incised and the vessels exposed. The vessels are incised and inflow (arterial) and outflow (venous) cannulas inserted. Alternatively, blood vessels may be accessed using percutaneous technique. A tourniquet is applied to

CPT © 2016 American Medical Association. All Rights Reserved.   ● New Code   ▲ Revised Code

Cardiovascular System

temporarily control outflow from collateral vessels. Isolation of the extremity from systemic circulation is confirmed using one of several techniques such injection of contrast material or radiolabeled red blood cells or serum. The chemotherapy agent is then perfused Temperature probes are placed if hyperthermia is to be used and the extremity is heated to the desired temperature. Upon completion of the procedure, the cannulas are removed and the arteriotomy and venotomy sites are repaired.

36825-36830

36825   **Creation of arteriovenous fistula by other than direct arteriovenous anastomosis (separate procedure); autogenous graft**

36830   **Creation of arteriovenous fistula by other than direct arteriovenous anastomosis (separate procedure); nonautogenous graft (eg, biological collagen, thermoplastic graft)**

The physician creates an arteriovenous (AV) fistula using a technique other than direct arteriovenous anastomosis. An AV fistula is an artificial connection between a vein and an artery, which is created to allow repeated long-term access to the vascular system for hemodialysis. An incision is made in the forearm over the planned AV fistula site. An artery and vein are selected, exposed, and dissected free of surrounding tissue. Vessel loops are placed around the vein and artery to control blood flow. If an autogenous graft is used, a vein segment is harvested, usually from the saphenous vein. An incision is made in the skin of the leg over the section of saphenous vein to be harvested. Soft tissue is dissected off the vein and branches ligated and divided. The section of saphenous vein to be used is then ligated proximally and distally, divided and removed from the leg. Alternatively, a non-autogenous graft, such as biological collagen or thermoplastic graft material, may be used. The artery is incised and the graft sutured to the artery. The vein is then incised and the other end of the graft is sutured to the vein. Vessel loops are released and hemostasis checked. Once the artery and vein are joined by the graft, blood flow to the through the vein will increase causing it to become larger and thicker so that it can withstand repeated punctures for vascular access. Use 36825 for AV fistula creation using an autogenous graft and 36830 when a non-autogenous graft is used.

36831

36831   **Thrombectomy, open, arteriovenous fistula without revision, autogenous or nonautogenous dialysis graft (separate procedure)**

Following creation of an AV fistula, a thrombus may form causing occlusion. An incision is made over the AV fistula and the artery and vein. The blood vessels and graft are exposed. Vessel loops are placed proximal and distal to the thrombus to control blood flow. The artery, vein, and/or graft is opened and the thrombus (clot) removed by direct exposure. The physician may use arterial back pressure or massage to expel the thrombus. Following removal of the thrombus, a completion angiography may be performed to ensure that the entire clot has been removed and that the AV fistula is patent.

36832-36833

36832   **Revision, open, arteriovenous fistula; without thrombectomy, autogenous or nonautogenous dialysis graft (separate procedure)**

36833   **Revision, open, arteriovenous fistula; with thrombectomy, autogenous or nonautogenous dialysis graft (separate procedure)**

An open revision of an arteriovenous (AV) fistula is performed with or without thrombectomy. Stenosis, thrombus formation, and occlusion of an AV fistula created using a graft is a complication requiring operative treatment. An incision is made in skin and soft tissue over the area of stenosis. The graft, artery, and vein are exposed. The blood vessels and graft are dissected free of surrounding tissue. Vessel loops are placed proximal and distal to the stenosed area to control blood flow. If a thrombus is present, it is removed by direct exposure. The artery, vein, and/or graft is opened and the thrombus (clot) removed using arterial back pressure or massage to expel the thrombus. The graft is then revised. Revision may involve incision and placement of a vein patch or excision of the stenosed area with placement of a new segment of autogenous vein or non-autogenous graft material. If the AV fistula is revised using a patch graft, a segment of vein, usually the saphenous, is harvested. An elliptical patch is tailored to fit over the stenosed segment of the graft. The patch graft is inserted within the longitudinal incision and sutured into place. This increases the diameter of the stenosed segment improving blood flow through the graft. Alternatively, the stenosed segment of the AV fistula may be excised. A tubular segment of new vein is harvested or a non-autogenous graft is prepared and sutured to the remaining proximal and distal segments of graft or blood vessels. Vessel loops are released, hemostasis checked, and a completion angiography performed to ensure that the revised AV fistula is patent.

36835

36835   **Insertion of Thomas shunt (separate procedure)**

A Thomas shunt is inserted to allow repeated long-term access to the vascular system for hemodialysis. The Thomas shunt is a transcutaneously placed external shunt consisting of two silastic cannulas with a Dacron patch at one end. Separate small incisions are made over the femoral artery and vein and the vessels are exposed. The vessels are incised. The Dacron patch at the end of one silastic cannula is sutured to the femoral artery and the

other silastic cannula is sutured to the femoral vein using the Dacron patch. Suturing the Dacron patches to the vessels prevents the cannula from occluding the vessels. The two cannulas are tunneled subcutaneously to the anterointernal aspect of the thigh, exiting through two skin incisions. The two external cannula tips are joined with a Teflon connector to form a closed loop. The Teflon connector is removed during the dialysis procedure and the cannulas are connected to the hemodialysis tubing. When hemodialysis is not in use, the Teflon connector is replaced on the silastic cannulas.

36838

36838   **Distal revascularization and interval ligation (DRIL), upper extremity hemodialysis access (steal syndrome)**

Steal syndrome is a complication in which the hemodialysis access diverts blood flow from the hand causing ischemia and hand pain. The physician places a bypass graft in the arm with the proximal anastomosis site above the hemodialysis access site and the distal anastomosis below it. The bypass graft will divert blood around the hemodialysis access site allowing better perfusion of the hand. An incision is made in the upper arm over the brachial artery which is exposed and dissected free of surrounding tissue. A second incision is made in the lower arm distal to the hemodialysis access site and the brachial artery exposed. A subcutaneous tunnel is created from the proximal skin incision to the distal skin incision. Vessel loops are placed around the exposed brachial artery. A vein graft is harvested. If a saphenous vein graft is used, an incision is made in the skin of the leg over the section of saphenous vein to be harvested. Soft tissue is dissected off the vein and branches ligated and divided. The section of saphenous vein to be used is then ligated proximally and distally, divided and removed from the leg. Vascular clamps are placed on the brachial artery in the upper arm. The artery is incised and the vein graft anastomosed. The vein graft is tunneled to the lower arm and anastomosed to distal aspect of the brachial artery. A segment of brachial artery is isolated above the distal anastomosis of the just completed bypass graft but below the hemodialysis access. The brachial artery is suture ligated to prevent blood from flowing retrograde into the hemodialysis access. The vascular clamps are removed and hemostasis verified. Blood flow through the graft and hemodialysis access is checked using Doppler and distal pulses are evaluated to ensure patency of the bypass graft.

36860-36861

36860   **External cannula declotting (separate procedure); without balloon catheter**

36861   **External cannula declotting (separate procedure); with balloon catheter**

The physician performs external cannula declotting either without a balloon catheter (36860) or with a balloon catheter (36861). The external cannula is examined and palpated to determine whether the occlusion is due to a thrombus. If the occlusion is due to a small thrombus, the physician first attempts to remove the thrombus by digital manipulation and the injection of a thrombolytic agent (36860). The thrombolytic agent may be administered either in a pulse-spray or a small amount may be injected using a lyse-and-wait technique. In 36861, the physician uses a balloon catheter to declot the cannula. A combination multipurpose catheter and guidewire is passed to the site of the obstruction. The multipurpose catheter is exchanged for a balloon catheter. The balloon catheter is then inflated at the site of the blood clot (thrombus). The balloon catheter is then deflated and blood flow evaluated. The balloon catheter may be inflated-deflated several times and is removed when adequate blood flow is observed.

● New Code   ▲ Revised Code

36901-36903

- ● 36901   Introduction of needle(s) and/or catheter(s), dialysis circuit, with diagnostic angiography of the dialysis circuit, including all direct puncture(s) and catheter placement(s), injection(s) of contrast, all necessary imaging from the arterial anastomosis and adjacent artery through entire venous outflow including the inferior or superior vena cava, fluoroscopic guidance, radiological supervision and interpretation and image documentation and report
- ● 36902   Introduction of needle(s) and/or catheter(s), dialysis circuit, with diagnostic angiography of the dialysis circuit, including all direct puncture(s) and catheter placement(s), injection(s) of contrast, all necessary imaging from the arterial anastomosis and adjacent artery through entire venous outflow including the inferior or superior vena cava, fluoroscopic guidance, radiological supervision and interpretation and image documentation and report; with transluminal balloon angioplasty, peripheral dialysis segment, including all imaging and radiological supervision and interpretation necessary to perform the angioplasty
- ● 36903   Introduction of needle(s) and/or catheter(s), dialysis circuit, with diagnostic angiography of the dialysis circuit, including all direct puncture(s) and catheter placement(s), injection(s) of contrast, all necessary imaging from the arterial anastomosis and adjacent artery through entire venous outflow including the inferior or superior vena cava, fluoroscopic guidance, radiological supervision and interpretation and image documentation and report; with transcatheter placement of intravascular stent(s), peripheral dialysis segment, including all imaging and radiological supervision and interpretation necessary to perform the stenting, and all angioplasty within the peripheral dialysis segment

A procedure is performed using diagnostic angiography to visualize the hemodialysis circuit, including adjacent artery through the entire venous outflow for stenosis or obstruction causing low blood flow, elevated pre-pump arterial pressure, or high venous return pressure. The dialysis circuit may consist of a central venous catheter (CVC), an arteriovenous (AV) fistula, or a synthetic AV graft. For CVC, a double lumen or 2 separate catheters are inserted into a large vein (vena cava, internal jugular, femoral vein). Blood is withdrawn from one lumen for filtration outside the body and returned via a second lumen. An AV fistula is created by anastomosing an artery to a vein and bypassing the capillaries. A synthetic graft also creates an arteriovenous anastomosis using synthetic material when the vessels are not in close proximity. To facilitate dialysis through an AV fistula or graft, a needle placed "upstream" withdraws blood, circulates it through the dialysis machine, and returns the filtered blood through a needle placed "downstream". The AV fistula and graft may become narrowed over time due to intimal hyperplasia and/or thrombosis. For diagnostic angiography of the entire dialysis circuit (36901), an AV fistula or AV graft is accessed with a small needle, a CVC through the port/catheter lumen. A guidewire is threaded through the needle or port/lumen and the needle exchanged for a vascular sheath. A catheter is placed over the guidewire and contrast dye is injected to visualize the vessels through the entire venous outflow using fluoroscopy. If stenosis is present in the peripheral dialysis segment, balloon angioplasty (36902) may be performed. A balloon tipped catheter is inserted over the guidewire through the area of stenosis. The balloon is inflated with dilute radiopaque contrast and visualized with fluoroscopy. At the end of the prescribed time, the balloon is deflated and the catheter is removed. A vascular catheter with a working channel is then threaded over the guidewire and angiography is repeated to evaluate for resistant or residual stenosis. If stenosis remains, a fine mesh/wire stent is delivered to the area of stenosis through the working channel of the vascular catheter (36903). The stent expands, placing pressure on the walls of the blood vessel to keep it open. The catheter is removed and a purse string suture may be placed to control bleeding before the vascular sheath is removed. Stent placement in the peripheral dialysis segment includes the angioplasty.

36904-36906

- ● 36904   Percutaneous transluminal mechanical thrombectomy and/or infusion for thrombolysis, dialysis circuit, any method, including all imaging and radiological supervision and interpretation, diagnostic angiography, fluoroscopic guidance, catheter placement(s), and intraprocedural pharmacological thrombolytic injection(s)
- ● 36905   Percutaneous transluminal mechanical thrombectomy and/or infusion for thrombolysis, dialysis circuit, any method, including all imaging and radiological supervision and interpretation, diagnostic angiography, fluoroscopic guidance, catheter placement(s), and intraprocedural pharmacological thrombolytic injection(s); with transluminal balloon angioplasty, peripheral dialysis segment, including all imaging and radiological supervision and interpretation necessary to perform the angioplasty
- ● 36906   Percutaneous transluminal mechanical thrombectomy and/or infusion for thrombolysis, dialysis circuit, any method, including all imaging and radiological supervision and interpretation, diagnostic angiography, fluoroscopic guidance, catheter placement(s), and intraprocedural pharmacological thrombolytic injection(s); with transcatheter placement of intravascular stent(s), peripheral dialysis segment, including all imaging and radiological supervision and interpretation necessary to perform the stenting, and all angioplasty within the peripheral dialysis circuit

A procedure is performed to dissolve or remove blood clots within the dialysis circuit using percutaneous transluminal mechanical thrombectomy and/or infusion of clot dissolving pharmaceutical agents. The dialysis circuit may consist of a central venous catheter (CVC), an arteriovenous (AV) fistula, or a synthetic AV graft. The incidence of thrombosis is highest with an AV graft and also common with an AV fistula. Symptoms of dialysis circuit thrombosis include absence of thrill or pulse at the fistula/graft site, vessel swelling or distention and/or absence of blood flash with needle insertion. Ultrasound or duplex Doppler study may be used to define the length of the thrombus if the vessel is not well distended. To perform thrombectomy (36904) on an AV fistula, needles are placed at either end of the thrombus and guidewires are inserted in a crossed fashion. Crossing sheaths are then placed over the guidewires and the needles are removed. A thrombolytic pharmaceutical agent (heparin, TPA) is injected into the fistula. After a prescribed period of time, if resistant clot remains, a thrombectomy catheter is inserted over the guidewire and the clot is evacuated mechanically. To perform thrombectomy (36904) on an AV graft, the venous segment is accessed first, then the arterial segment, using a needle in downstream venous direction followed by a guidewire threaded through the clot. The needle is exchanged with a vascular sheath and a thrombolytic pharmaceutical agent is injected through the sheath. After a prescribed period of time, if residual clot remains, an embolectomy catheter is inserted over a guidewire and the clot is evacuated mechanically. This procedure is repeated on the arterial side of the graft with the needle directed upstream. Angiography of the dialysis circuit is then performed to visualize residual blood clot and/or vessel stenosis. If stenosis is present in the peripheral dialysis circuit, balloon angioplasty (36905) may be performed. A balloon tipped catheter is inserted over a guidewire through the stenosed area. The balloon is inflated with dilute radiopaque contrast and visualized with fluoroscopy. The balloon is deflated and the catheter is removed. A vascular catheter with a working channel is then threaded over the guidewire and angiography is repeated to evaluate for resistant or residual stenosis. If stenosis remains, a fine mesh/wire stent is delivered to the area of stenosis through the working channel of the vascular catheter (36906). The stent expands, placing pressure on the walls of the blood vessel to keep it open. The catheter is removed and a purse string suture may be placed to control bleeding before the vascular sheath is removed. Stent placement in the peripheral dialysis segment includes the angioplasty.

36907-36908

- ● 36907   Transluminal balloon angioplasty, central dialysis segment, performed through dialysis circuit, including all imaging and radiological supervision and interpretation required to perform the angioplasty (List separately in addition to code for primary procedure)
- ● 36908   Transcatheter placement of intravascular stent(s), central dialysis segment, performed through dialysis circuit, including all imaging radiological supervision and interpretation required to perform the stenting, and all angioplasty in the central dialysis segment (List separately in addition to code for primary procedure)

A procedure is performed to restore blood flow through a narrowed or obstructed central venous dialysis segment (axillary vein, subclavian vein, innominate vein, vena cava). Symptoms of hemodialysis-related central venous occlusive disease (CVOD) include elevated urea recirculation, elevated venous dialysis pressure, and arm edema. The central venous dialysis segment is accessed via the AV graft/fistula. The AV graft/fistula is punctured with a needle, a guidewire is threaded through the needle, and the needle is exchanged for a vascular sheath. A catheter is placed over the guidewire and angiography is performed to visualize the central venous segments. Transluminal balloon angioplasty (36907) is performed when stenosis of the central vein(s) is identified. A balloon tipped catheter is inserted over the guidewire through the stenosed area. The balloon is inflated with dilute radiopaque contrast and visualized with fluoroscopy. At the end of the prescribed time, the balloon is deflated and the catheter is removed. A vascular catheter with a working channel is then threaded over the guidewire and angiography is repeated to evaluate for resistant or residual stenosis. If stenosis remains, a fine mesh/wire stent is delivered to the area of stenosis in the central venous segment through the working channel of the vascular catheter (36908). The stent expands, placing pressure on the walls of the blood vessel to keep it open. The catheter is removed and a purse string suture may be placed to control bleeding before the vascular sheath is removed. Stent placement in the central dialysis segment includes the angioplasty.

36909

- ● **36909**   **Dialysis circuit permanent vascular embolization or occlusion (including main circuit or any accessory veins), endovascular, including all imaging and radiological supervision and interpretation necessary to complete the intervention (List separately in addition to code for primary procedure)**

Permanent vascular embolization or occlusion of the main dialysis circuit or accessory veins may be used to treat dialysis related steal syndrome, critical hand ischemia, venous aneurysm, central venous occlusion syndrome not amenable to endovascular recanalization, or hyperdynamic heart failure. The dialysis circuit is accessed using a needle and a guidewire is placed through the needle into the vessel. A vascular sheath replaces the needle and a catheter is introduced through the vascular sheath. Contrast dye is injected and the target area of the dialysis circuit/accessory veins is identified using fluoroscopy. An embolization agent (gelfoam, particulate agent, liquid sclerosing agent, liquid glue) or occlusion device (metallic plug/coil) is delivered to the target area through the catheter. Post procedure angiography is obtained to verify that the embolization or occlusion procedure has been successful. The catheter is removed and a purse string suture may be placed to control bleeding before the vascular sheath is removed. Code 36909 includes all imaging and radiological supervision and interpretation necessary to complete the intervention and is reported in addition to the primary procedure.

37140

37140   **Venous anastomosis, open; portocaval**

The physician performs an open portocaval venous anastomosis, also referred to as a portocaval shunt procedure to divert blood from the portal vein into the infrahepatic vena cava. An extended right subcostal incision is made; the hepatoduodenal ligament identified; and the portal vein is exposed from the hilum of the liver to the pancreas. If additional exposure of the portal vein is required, the gastroduodenal and right gastric branches are divided. The peritoneum is then incised just below the hepatic triad and the inferior vena cava is exposed. The portal vein is clamped distal and proximal to the planned anastomosis site and a side biting clamp is placed on the inferior vena cava. For an end-to-side anastomosis, the portal vein is divided and the proximal end is oversewn. The distal end of the portal vein is then anastomosed to the side of the inferior vena cava. For a side-to-side anastomosis, the portal vein is incised and anastomosed to the side of the inferior vena cava.

37145

37145   **Venous anastomosis, open; renoportal**

The physician performs an open renoportal venous anastomosis, also referred to as a renoportal or portorenal shunt procedure. Renoportal shunts are rarely used. An incision is made in the abdomen; the hepatoduodenal ligament is identified; and the portal vein is exposed from the hilum of the liver to the pancreas. If additional exposure of the portal vein is required, the gastroduodenal and right gastric branches are divided. The selected renal vein is then exposed and the portal vein is anastomosed to the renal vein.

37160

37160   **Venous anastomosis, open; caval-mesenteric**

The physician performs an open caval-mesenteric venous anastomosis, also referred to as a mesocaval shunt procedure. A vertical midline incision is made in the abdomen and the colon is retracted toward the head to expose the superior mesenteric vein at the root of the mesentery. A section of the superior mesenteric vein is isolated. The duodenum is mobilized and the inferior vena cava is exposed anteriorly and laterally at the level of the iliac bifurcation. A side-biting clamp is placed on the inferior vena cava and the proximal portion of the superior mesenteric vein is anastomosed to the side of the inferior vena cava. Alternatively, a synthetic graft may be used. The synthetic graft is first anastomosed to the side of the inferior vena cava and then to the side of the superior mesenteric vein.

37180-37181

37180   **Venous anastomosis, open; splenorenal, proximal**
37181   **Venous anastomosis, open; splenorenal, distal (selective decompression of esophagogastric varices, any technique)**

The physician performs an open proximal (37180) or distal (37181) splenorenal venous anastomosis, also referred to as a proximal or distal splenorenal shunt procedure. In 37180, a thoracoabdominal or transabdominal incision is made, the spleen is exposed.

The splenic vein is divided at the splenic porta so that maximum splenic vein length is obtained for anastomosis. The spleen is then removed. The splenic vein is dissected free of the pancreatic bed. Small pancreatic branches draining the splenic vein are isolated and individually ligated. The left renal vein is exposed and isolated. The end of the splenic vein is then anastomosed to the side of the left renal vein. In 37181, an open distal splenorenal venous anastomosis using any technique is performed for selective decompression of esophagogastric varices. A left subcostal approach is used. The coronary vein and right gastroepiploic vein are ligated to reduce blood flow to the esophageal varices. The splenic flexure of the colon is mobilized. The stomach is retracted cephalad and the peritoneum incised over the inferior aspect of the pancreas. The splenic vein is divided and the proximal portion oversewn. The distal portion of the splenic vein is then dissected free of the pancreatic bed. The left renal vein is identified and isolated. The end of the distal splenic vein is then anastomosed to the side of the left renal vein (end-to-side anastomosis) to drain blood from the esophageal varices through the short gastric vessels and into the system circulation.

37182-37183

37182   **Insertion of transvenous intrahepatic portosystemic shunt(s) (TIPS) (includes venous access, hepatic and portal vein catheterization, portography with hemodynamic evaluation, intrahepatic tract formation/dilatation, stent placement and all associated imaging guidance and documentation)**
37183   **Revision of transvenous intrahepatic portosystemic shunt(s) (TIPS) (includes venous access, hepatic and portal vein catheterization, portography with hemodynamic evaluation, intrahepatic tract recanulization/dilatation, stent placement and all associated imaging guidance and documentation)**

The physician inserts one or more transvenous intrahepatic portosystemic shunt(s) (TIPS). Venous access is typically via the right internal jugular vein. The jugular is punctured with a needle and a guidewire is introduced under fluoroscopic guidance. The needle is then exchanged for a vascular introducer and a catheter is advanced over the guidewire and into one of the hepatic veins. Contrast material is injected and portography performed to define and evaluate the portal system for optimal placement of the intrahepatic portosystemic shunt(s). Pressure gradients are obtained. The catheter is advanced into the selected hepatic vein. A needle is then guided through the catheter and advanced into the selected portal vein to create a path for the stent. A guidewire is then passed into the selected portal vein and the needle removed. A balloon tipped catheter is advanced over the guidewire and the tract between the hepatic and portal veins dilated. One or more stents are then placed over the balloon tipped catheter and positioned in the dilated tract. The balloon is inflated to expand the stent(s). Following placement of the stent(s), pressure gradients are again obtained to evaluate the effectiveness of the shunt. A post-procedure venography may also be performed. All guidewires, catheters, and the vascular introducer are removed and direct pressure applied to the puncture site to control bleeding. In 37183, a malfunctioning TIPS is evaluated and revised. Transvenous access to the hepatic and portal veins is accomplished as described in 37182. Contrast material is injected and portography performed to evaluate the stent. Pressure gradients are obtained. The stent is then revised as needed which may include recanalization or dilatation of the tract, revision of the stent by extending the stent or placing additional stents, or removal of the existing stent and replacing it with a new stent. Following the revision procedure, pressure gradients are obtained and venography performed to evaluate results of the revision.

37184-37186

37184   **Primary percutaneous transluminal mechanical thrombectomy, noncoronary, non-intracranial, arterial or arterial bypass graft, including fluoroscopic guidance and intraprocedural pharmacological thrombolytic injection(s); initial vessel**
37185   **Primary percutaneous transluminal mechanical thrombectomy, noncoronary, non-intracranial, arterial or arterial bypass graft, including fluoroscopic guidance and intraprocedural pharmacological thrombolytic injection(s); second and all subsequent vessel(s) within the same vascular family (List separately in addition to code for primary mechanical thrombectomy procedure)**
37186   **Secondary percutaneous transluminal thrombectomy (eg, nonprimary mechanical, snare basket, suction technique), noncoronary, non-intracranial, arterial or arterial bypass graft, including fluoroscopic guidance and intraprocedural pharmacological thrombolytic injections, provided in conjunction with another percutaneous intervention other than primary mechanical thrombectomy (List separately in addition to code for primary procedure)**

The physician performs primary or secondary percutaneous transluminal mechanical thrombectomy in a noncoronary, non-intracranial artery or arterial bypass graft. This procedure is performed using an arterial catheter and a mechanical device that simply breaks ups the blood clot; breaks up the clot in a manner for immediate removal; or snares and retrieves the thrombus. Devices that break up the thrombus include rotating wires or brushes. Devices that break up and remove the thrombus deliver a rapid stream of fluid, using hydrodynamic forces to break up the clot, in conjunction with aspiration to remove it. Retriever devices such as microsnares and snare baskets allow the physician to grasp and remove the thrombus. The technique used varies slightly depending on the type of mechanical device used and the location of the thrombus. The skin over the access artery is prepped, the artery is punctured, and a sheath is placed. A guiding catheter is introduced under fluoroscopic guidance. A microcatheter is then advanced over a microguidewire and passed through the thrombus. The guidewire is then removed and the mechanical thrombectomy device is advanced through the microcatheter to the thrombus. If a rotating wire or brush device is used, it is activated and the thrombus is fragmented. If hydrodynamic forces are used, a stream of fluid is delivered to break up the thrombus which is then aspirated. If a retriever device is used, it is passed beyond the level of the clot, deployed, and the clot is captured by the device and retracted along with the microcatheter. Several passes of the mechanical device may be required to break up and remove the clot. A thrombolytic agent may also be injected during the procedure to help dissolve the clot. Once the procedure is complete, the mechanical device, microcatheter, and guiding catheter are removed. Use code 37184 for primary percutaneous transluminal mechanical thrombectomy in the initial noncoronary, non-intracranial artery or arterial bypass graft, and 37185 for thrombectomy done in a second or all subsequent vessels within the same vascular family. Use code 37186 for a secondary type of percutaneous transluminal thrombectomy for smaller emboli/thrombi provided during other percutaneous interventions (other than a primary mechanical thrombectomy).

37187-37188

37187 **Percutaneous transluminal mechanical thrombectomy, vein(s), including intraprocedural pharmacological thrombolytic injections and fluoroscopic guidance**

37188 **Percutaneous transluminal mechanical thrombectomy, vein(s), including intraprocedural pharmacological thrombolytic injections and fluoroscopic guidance, repeat treatment on subsequent day during course of thrombolytic therapy**

The physician performs percutaneous transluminal mechanical thrombectomy on a vein including fluoroscopic guidance and intraprocedural injection of thrombolytic agent. Percutaneous transluminal mechanical thrombectomy is performed using a catheter and a mechanical device that either breaks ups the thrombus (blood clot), breaks up and removes the thrombus, or snares and retrieves the thrombus. Devices that break up the thrombus include rotating wires or brushes. Devices that break up and retrieve the thrombus include those that deliver a rapid stream of fluid and use hydrodynamic forces to break up the clot in conjunction with aspiration to remove the clot. Retriever type devices such as a microsnare, snare basket, or other retriever device allow the physician to capture or grasp and remove the thrombus. The technique varies slightly depending on the type of mechanical device used and the location of the thrombus. The skin over the blood vessel that will be used to approach the thrombus is prepped, the blood vessel punctured, and a sheath placed. A guiding catheter is introduced under fluoroscopic guidance. A microcatheter is then advanced over a microguidewire and passed through the thrombus. The guidewire is then removed and the mechanical thrombectomy device advanced through the microcatheter to the thrombus. If a rotating wire or brush device is used, it is activated and the thrombus fragmented. If hydrodynamic forces are used, a stream of fluid is delivered to break up the thrombus which is then aspirated. If a retriever device is used, it is passed beyond the level of the clot, deployed, and the clot captured by the device. The retriever device is then retracted along with the microcatheter. Several passes of the mechanical device may be required to break up and remove the clot. A thrombolytic agent may be injected during to the procedure to help dissolve the clot. Once the procedure is complete, the mechanical device, microcatheter, and guiding catheter are removed. Use code 37187 for venous percutaneous transluminal mechanical thrombectomy on the first day and 37188 for repeat treatment on a subsequent day during a multiple day course of thrombolytic therapy.

37191

37191 **Insertion of intravascular vena cava filter, endovascular approach including vascular access, vessel selection, and radiological supervision and interpretation, intraprocedural roadmapping, and imaging guidance (ultrasound and fluoroscopy), when performed**

The physician performs a procedure to filter blood flow in the vena cava (VC) to prevent pulmonary embolism due to migration of deep vein thromboses (blood clots), usually from the pelvis or lower extremity to the lungs. A filter is placed within the lumen of the VC using an endovascular technique. Intravascular filters are umbrella shaped devices that capture blood clots, preventing them from traveling to the lungs. Prior to interruption of the VC, a cavogram is performed so that the vascular anatomy can be evaluated and the presence of a thrombus in the VC ruled out. The femoral or jugular vein is exposed. An introducer sheath is placed in the blood vessel. Under radiological guidance, a guidewire is inserted and advanced through the femoral and iliac veins into the VC. If a jugular vein approach is used, the guidewire is advanced through the jugular and brachiocephalic veins, superior vena cava, right atrium, and into the inferior vena cava as needed. A catheter is advanced over the guidewire and positioned at the site where the filter is to be placed, usually just in the

inferior vena cava below the level of the renal veins. The guidewire is removed. Contrast is injected as needed so that any anatomical variations in the vena cava can be evaluated. A second catheter containing the collapsed IVC filter is then advanced to the target site and deployed when properly positioned. The catheter insertion device is removed, additional cavograms are obtained as needed, and the incision in the neck or groin is closed.

37192

37192 **Repositioning of intravascular vena cava filter, endovascular approach including vascular access, vessel selection, and radiological supervision and interpretation, intraprocedural roadmapping, and imaging guidance (ultrasound and fluoroscopy), when performed**

The physician repositions a vena cava filter that has migrated or one that is being used temporarily to prevent fibrosis and permanent fixation of the filter to the wall of the vena cava. A cavogram is obtained to locate the filter and ensure that there are no clots trapped at the filter site. The femoral or jugular vein is exposed. An introducer sheath is placed in the blood vessel. Under radiological guidance, a guidewire is inserted and advanced through the femoral and iliac veins into the VC. If a jugular vein approach is used, the guidewire is advanced through the jugular and brachiocephalic veins, superior vena cava, right atrium, and into the inferior vena cava as needed. A filter retrieval catheter is advanced over the guidewire to the filter. The guidewire is removed. The hook at the apex of the filter is snared. The outer sheath is advanced over the anchoring hooks of the filter struts until they are disengaged from the wall of the vena cava. The sheath continues to be advanced until the filter is completely collapsed but not completely covered by the sheath. The filter is repositioned and redeployed. The loop snare is disengaged from the hook at the apex of the filter and the retrieval set is removed. Additional cavograms are obtained as needed to evaluate positioning of the filter, and the incision in the neck or groin is closed.

37193

37193 **Retrieval (removal) of intravascular vena cava filter, endovascular approach including vascular access, vessel selection, and radiological supervision and interpretation, intraprocedural roadmapping, and imaging guidance (ultrasound and fluoroscopy), when performed**

The physician removes a vena cava filter. A cavogram is obtained to locate the filter and ensure that there are no clots trapped at the filter site. The femoral or jugular vein is exposed. An introducer sheath is placed in the blood vessel. Under radiological guidance, a guidewire is inserted and advanced through the femoral and iliac veins and into the VC. If a jugular vein approach is used, the guidewire is advanced through the jugular and brachiocephalic veins, superior vena cava, right atrium, and into the inferior vena cava as needed. A filter retrieval catheter is advanced over the guidewire to the filter. The guidewire is removed. The hook at the apex of the filter is snared. The outer sheath is advanced over the anchoring hooks of the filter struts until they are disengaged from the wall of the vena cava. The sheath continues to be advanced until the filter is completely collapsed and enclosed within the sheath. The filter and the retrieval set are removed. Additional cavograms are obtained as needed to evaluate blood flow and ensure that there is no trauma to the vena cava or other structures. The incision in the neck or groin is closed.

37195

37195 **Thrombolysis, cerebral, by intravenous infusion**

The physician performs cerebral thrombolysis by intravenous infusion of a thrombolytic agent. A venous access device, such as a needle or catheter, is placed and a thrombolytic agent is infused with continuous monitoring of the patient's neurologic function. Following infusion of the thrombolytic agent, the physician continues to monitor the patient's neurologic function and additional intravenous medication is administered as needed.

37197

37197 **Transcatheter retrieval, percutaneous, of intravascular foreign body (eg, fractured venous or arterial catheter), includes radiological supervision and interpretation, and imaging guidance (ultrasound or fluoroscopy), when performed**

Transcatheter retrieval of foreign bodies such as fragments of catheters or guidewires from systemic and pulmonary vessels, is performed using snares or retrieval baskets. The physician determines the best vascular access site for the retrieval procedure after identifying the exact location of the intravascular foreign body using angiography. The selected blood vessel is nicked and an introducer sheath is inserted. The retrieval device is selected based on the type of intravascular foreign body and may include a snare, basket, pigtail or recurved catheter, and/or forceps. An introducer catheter of sufficient gauge (8 or 11 French) is inserted and advanced to the site of the foreign body under radiologic guidance (e.g., fluoroscopy, ultrasound). The retrieval device is inserted through the introducer catheter and the foreign body is captured by the device and removed. The introducer catheter is removed and the blood vessel is repaired.

Cardiovascular System

37200

37200   Transcatheter biopsy

The access vessel is selected and exposed. The blood vessel is nicked and an introducer sheath inserted. Using separately reportable radiological supervision and interpretation, a guidewire is advanced to the biopsy site. A biopsy catheter is advanced over the guidewire and the guidewire withdrawn. A tissue sample is obtained from the blood vessel lumen. The biopsy catheter is removed and the tissue sample sent to the laboratory for separately reportable histological analysis. The blood vessel is repaired.

37211-37212

37211   Transcatheter therapy, arterial infusion for thrombolysis other than coronary or intracranial, any method, including radiological supervision and interpretation, initial treatment day

37212   Transcatheter therapy, venous infusion for thrombolysis, any method, including radiological supervision and interpretation, initial treatment day

Transcatheter therapy with infusion of medication for thrombolysis is performed on a vessel other than a coronary or intracranial vessel. To initiate thrombolytic infusion, the skin over the access artery is punctured with a needle. The usual puncture site for arterial infusion thrombolysis (37211) procedures is the common femoral artery. Other puncture sites include the axillary and distal brachial arteries. Venous infusion thrombolysis (37212) is commonly done for deep vein thrombosis, which may use a leg vessel access, and then advance the catheter into the inferior vena cava before infusion. Using radiologic imaging, a guidewire is inserted through the needle into the access vessel and threaded to the site of the obstructing blood clot. An infusion catheter is then advanced over the guidewire to the target site and the guidewire is removed. The catheter is secured across the entire area of thrombosis and the thrombolytic agent is then infused, often over several hours, to break up the clot and relieve the obstruction. Arterial or venous infusion for thrombolysis may be performed over multiple days. Codes 37211 and 37212 report services on the initial day of treatment only and include radiological guidance and supervision with interpretation of images, including venography or arteriography to verify therapy effectiveness, and any catheter repositioning or exchanging.

37213-37214

37213   Transcatheter therapy, arterial or venous infusion for thrombolysis other than coronary, any method, including radiological supervision and interpretation, continued treatment on subsequent day during course of thrombolytic therapy, including follow-up catheter contrast injection, position change, or exchange, when performed

37214   Transcatheter therapy, arterial or venous infusion for thrombolysis other than coronary, any method, including radiological supervision and interpretation, continued treatment on subsequent day during course of thrombolytic therapy, including follow-up catheter contrast injection, position change, or exchange, when performed; cessation of thrombolysis including removal of catheter and vessel closure by any method

After transcatheter arterial or venous infusion for thrombolysis on a vessel other than a coronary vessel is initiated (the initial day of thrombolytic therapy is reported separately), transcatheter therapy is continued for one or more days as needed until the thrombolysis is complete. Using the existing catheter, follow-up diagnostic angiography with contrast is used to evaluate the effects of the thrombolytic infusion. If the position of the catheter must be changed, a guidewire is inserted into the existing catheter and advanced to a more optimal position. The catheter is advanced over the guidewire to the new site. Alternatively, after inserting the guidewire through the existing catheter to the thrombus site, the existing catheter may be removed and a new catheter advanced to the site of the thrombus. Infusion of the thrombolytic agent continues until the desired results are achieved. Treatment is discontinued upon complete lysis with restoration of flow or after lysis of all amenable thrombi and occlusions. The thrombolytic catheter is removed. A closure device may be used to close the vessel, or sheath access may be maintained to allow time for the thrombolytic and adjunctive agents to clear before being removed and manual compression applied for hemostasis. Use 37213 for continued transcatheter thrombolytic therapy on a subsequent day beyond the initial day. Use code 37214 for subsequent day thrombolytic therapy that also includes cessation of thrombolysis, removal of the catheter, and vessel closure.

37215-37216

37215   Transcatheter placement of intravascular stent(s), cervical carotid artery, open or percutaneous, including angioplasty, when performed, and radiological supervision and interpretation; with distal embolic protection

37216   Transcatheter placement of intravascular stent(s), cervical carotid artery, open or percutaneous, including angioplasty, when performed, and radiological supervision and interpretation; without distal embolic protection

Transcatheter placement of intravascular stent(s) in a stenosed cervical carotid artery is performed. For a percutaneous approach, the femoral or other artery is punctured and the introducer sheath is inserted. A guidewire is introduced and advanced into the aortic arch. A carotid configuration catheter is advanced over the guidewire into the aortic arch. Roadmapping angiograms are obtained of the common carotid artery. The guidewire is removed and a hydrophilic wire is introduced. The carotid configuration catheter is inserted over the hydrophilic wire and configured at the aortic arch to conform to the patient's anatomy. The catheter is advanced into the common carotid artery. For the open approach, the introducer sheath is inserted through a surgically exposed common carotid artery via a small skin incision. The open approach is best employed in cases of severe arteriosclerotic disease of the femoral or iliac arteries, or the aorta. Roadmapping angiography is performed on the cervical carotid artery and measurements are made of the artery and area of stenosis. The hydrophilic wire is advanced into the external carotid artery and the carotid catheter is advanced over the wire. The hydrophilic wire is removed and a stiff wire is advanced to the site of the stenosis. A long guiding sheath is advanced over the carotid catheter and stiff wire. The carotid catheter and stiff wire are removed, leaving the long guiding sheath in place. In 37215, a distal embolic protection device is used. The deployment device is advanced across the lesion and positioned in the extracranial aspect of the internal carotid artery. The umbrella filter is opened and the embolic protection deployment device is removed. Angioplasty may then be performed before placing the stent. A balloon catheter is advanced to the site of the lesion and inflated. The area of stenosis is dilated, and the balloon catheter is removed. The stent delivery catheter is then advanced to the site of the lesion and carefully positioned. The stent is deployed and the delivery catheter is removed. A balloon catheter may again be advanced and inflated to seat the stent. All catheters are removed and pressure is applied to the venous access site. Use 37215 when cervical carotid artery stent(s) are placed with a distal embolic protection device and 37216 when the procedure is performed without a distal embolic protection device.

37217

37217   Transcatheter placement of intravascular stent(s), intrathoracic common carotid artery or innominate artery by retrograde treatment, open ipsilateral cervical carotid artery exposure, including angioplasty, when performed, and radiological supervision and interpretation

Transcatheter placement of an intravascular stent(s) in the intrathoracic common carotid artery or the innominate artery is performed. The ipsilateral (same side) cervical carotid artery is exposed with a small skin incision and the introducer sheath is inserted. A guide wire is introduced and advanced retrograde into the intrathoracic common carotid artery or innominate artery. A catheter is advanced over the guide wire. Roadmapping angiography is performed and measurements are made of the artery and area of stenosis. A stiff wire is advanced to the site of the stenosis. A guiding sheath is advanced over the catheter and stiff wire to the stenosed portion of the artery. Angioplasty may then be done before placing the stent. A balloon catheter is advanced to the site of the lesion and inflated, and the stenosed area is dilated. The balloon catheter is removed. The stent delivery catheter is then advanced to the site of the lesion, carefully positioned, and deployed. The stent delivery catheter is removed. A balloon catheter may again be advanced and inflated to seat the stent. Additional angiograms are obtained to evaluate stent placement and patency of the artery. All catheters are removed. The cervical carotid artery is repaired and the operative wound in the neck is closed in layers.

37218

37218   Transcatheter placement of intravascular stent(s), intrathoracic common carotid artery or innominate artery, open or percutaneous antegrade approach, including angioplasty, when performed, and radiological supervision and interpretation

The transcatheter placement of an intravascular stent(s) into the intrathoracic common carotid artery or innominate artery (brachiocehalic trunk) using an open or percutaneous antegrade approach is performed by entering the femoral vein in the area of the groin. If an open technique is employed the skin is incised and fascia separated to expose the femoral vein which is then incised to introduce a catheter sheath. If a percutaneous method is employed, the femoral vein is punctured with a needle and an introducer sheath is inserted. In both techniques, a guide wire is then introduced into the femoral vein and advanced toward the heart where the wire is looped in a clockwise fashion through the left atrium and into the ascending aorta. The left common carotid artery originates along the aortic arch to supply oxygenated blood to the head and neck. The innominate artery (brachiocephalic trunk) also arises from the aortic arch and supplies oxygenated blood to the right arm, head and neck. A catheter is then advanced over the guide wire and roadmapping angiography is performed to identify areas of stenosis in the vessel(s). A stiff wire is advanced to the site of stenosis and a guiding sheath is advanced over the catheter and stiff wire. A balloon catheter is advanced to the site of stenosis and inflated to dilate the narrowing. The balloon catheter is removed and the stent delivery catheter is advanced to the site of the lesion. The stent is carefully positioned and deployed and the stent delivery catheter is removed. If necessary, the balloon catheter may be reintroduced, advanced and inflated to seat the stent. Additional angiography is performed to evaluate the placement of the stent(s) and patency of the artery. The catheters are removed and the femoral site monitored for bleeding. If an open technique was employed the cut down in the femoral vein is closed with vascular suture followed by closure of the skin incision.

● New Code   ▲ Revised Code   © 2017 decisionHealth

37220-37223

37220 Revascularization, endovascular, open or percutaneous, iliac artery, unilateral, initial vessel; with transluminal angioplasty

37221 Revascularization, endovascular, open or percutaneous, iliac artery, unilateral, initial vessel; with transluminal stent placement(s), includes angioplasty within the same vessel, when performed

37222 Revascularization, endovascular, open or percutaneous, iliac artery, each additional ipsilateral iliac vessel; with transluminal angioplasty (List separately in addition to code for primary procedure)

37223 Revascularization, endovascular, open or percutaneous, iliac artery, each additional ipsilateral iliac vessel; with transluminal stent placement(s), includes angioplasty within the same vessel, when performed (List separately in addition to code for primary procedure)

The physician revascularizes an occluded or stenosed iliac artery using angioplasty and/or transluminal stent placement. If an open approach is used, the skin over the access artery is prepped and incised. The artery is exposed and nicked. A sheath is placed. If a percutaneous approach is used, the skin over the access artery, usually one of the femoral arteries, is prepped. The artery is punctured with a needle and a sheath is placed. Using radiological supervision as needed, a guidewire is inserted and advanced from the access artery into the occluded iliac artery. Roadmapping angiograms are obtained. A catheter with a balloon tip is advanced over the guidewire to the site of the occlusion. The balloon is inflated and the plaque is compressed against the wall of the artery. The balloon may be inflated several times to achieve the desired result. The angioplasty catheter is exchanged for a guidewire. An angiography catheter is advanced over the guidewire and the guidewire is withdrawn. Contrast is injected and a completion angiography is performed to ensure that the artery is patent. If an intravascular stent is needed to maintain patency of the artery, the stent delivery catheter is advanced to the site of the lesion. The stent is carefully positioned and deployed. The stent delivery catheter is removed. A balloon catheter may again be advanced and inflated to seat the stent. All catheters are removed. If an open approach has been used, the access artery is repaired and the skin incision is closed. If a percutaneous approach has been used, pressure is applied to the vascular access site and a pressure dressing is applied. Use 37220 for the initial iliac artery treated and 37222 for each additional ipsilateral (same side) iliac artery treated with angioplasty only. Use 37221 for the initial iliac artery treated and 37223 for each additional ipsilateral iliac artery treated with stent placement including angioplasty as needed.

37224-37227

37224 Revascularization, endovascular, open or percutaneous, femoral, popliteal artery(s), unilateral; with transluminal angioplasty

37225 Revascularization, endovascular, open or percutaneous, femoral, popliteal artery(s), unilateral; with atherectomy, includes angioplasty within the same vessel, when performed

37226 Revascularization, endovascular, open or percutaneous, femoral, popliteal artery(s), unilateral; with transluminal stent placement(s), includes angioplasty within the same vessel, when performed

37227 Revascularization, endovascular, open or percutaneous, femoral, popliteal artery(s), unilateral; with transluminal stent placement(s) and atherectomy, includes angioplasty within the same vessel, when performed

The physician revascularizes an occluded or stenosed femoral or popliteal artery using angioplasty, atherectomy, and/or transluminal stent placement. If an open approach is used, the skin over the access artery is prepped and incised. The artery is exposed and nicked. A sheath is placed. If a percutaneous approach is used, the skin over the access artery, usually one of the femoral arteries, is prepped. The artery is punctured with a needle and a sheath is placed. Using radiological supervision, a guidewire is inserted and advanced from the access artery into the occluded femoral or popliteal artery. Roadmapping angiograms are obtained. A catheter with a balloon tip is advanced over the guidewire to the site of the occlusion. The balloon is inflated and the plaque is compressed against the wall of the artery. The balloon may be inflated several times to achieve the desired result. Alternatively, an atherectomy may be performed with or without angioplasty. Atherectomy is performed using a specialized balloon catheter that has a window on one side through which a cutting piston is advanced. The cutting piston shaves plaque from the arterial wall. As the plaque is shaved, it is pushed into the nose of the atherectomy device and removed upon completion of the procedure when the catheter is withdrawn. The physician may make several passes with the atherectomy device to achieve the desired result. The angioplasty or atheretectomy device is exchanged for a guidewire. An angiography catheter is advanced over the guidewire and the guidewire is withdrawn. Contrast is injected and a completion angiography is performed to ensure that the artery is patent. If an intravascular stent is needed to maintain patency of the artery, the stent delivery catheter is advanced to the site of the lesion. The stent is carefully positioned and deployed. The stent delivery catheter is removed. A balloon catheter may again be advanced and inflated to seat the stent. All catheters are removed. If an open approach has been used, the access artery is repaired and the skin incision is closed. If a percutaneous approach has been used, pressure is applied to the vascular access site and a pressure dressing is applied. Use 37224 for the initial femoral or popliteal artery treated

with angioplasty only. Use 37225 for the initial femoral or popliteal artery treated with atherectomy including angioplasty as needed. Use 37226 for the initial femoral or popliteal artery treated with stent placement and angioplasty as needed. Use 37227 for the initial femoral or popliteal artery treated with stent placement and atherectomy, including angioplasty as needed.

37228-37231

37228 Revascularization, endovascular, open or percutaneous, tibial, peroneal artery, unilateral, initial vessel; with transluminal angioplasty

37229 Revascularization, endovascular, open or percutaneous, tibial, peroneal artery, unilateral, initial vessel; with atherectomy, includes angioplasty within the same vessel, when performed

37230 Revascularization, endovascular, open or percutaneous, tibial, peroneal artery, unilateral, initial vessel; with transluminal stent placement(s), includes angioplasty within the same vessel, when performed

37231 Revascularization, endovascular, open or percutaneous, tibial, peroneal artery, unilateral, initial vessel; with transluminal stent placement(s) and atherectomy, includes angioplasty within the same vessel, when performed

The physician revascularizes an occluded or stenosed tibial or peroneal artery using angioplasty, atherectomy, and/or transluminal stent placement. If an open approach is used, the skin over the access artery is prepped and incised. The artery is exposed and nicked. A sheath is placed. If a percutaneous approach is used, the skin over the access artery, usually one of the femoral arteries, is prepped. The artery is punctured with a needle and a sheath is placed. Using radiological supervision, a guidewire is inserted and advanced from the access artery into the occluded tibial or peroneal artery. Roadmapping angiograms are obtained. A catheter with a balloon tip is advanced over the guidewire to the site of the occlusion. The balloon is inflated and the plaque is compressed against the wall of the artery. The balloon may be inflated several times to achieve the desired result. Alternatively, an atherectomy may be performed with or without angioplasty. Atherectomy is performed using a specialized balloon catheter that has a window on one side through which a cutting piston is advanced. The cutting piston shaves plaque from the arterial wall. As the plaque is shaved, it is pushed into the nose of the atherectomy device and removed upon completion of the procedure when the catheter is withdrawn. The physician may make several passes with the atherectomy device to achieve the desired result. The angioplasty or atherectomy device is exchanged for a guidewire. An angiography catheter is advanced over the guidewire and the guidewire is withdrawn. Contrast is injected and a completion angiography is performed to ensure that the artery is patent. If an intravascular stent is needed to maintain patency of the artery, the stent delivery catheter is advanced to the site of the lesion. The stent is carefully positioned and deployed. The stent delivery catheter is removed. A balloon catheter may again be advanced and inflated to seat the stent. All catheters are removed. If an open approach has been used, the access artery is repaired and the skin incision is closed. If a percutaneous approach has been used, pressure is applied to the vascular access site and a pressure dressing is applied. Use 37228 for the initial tibial or peroneal artery treated with angioplasty only. Use 37229 for the initial tibial or peroneal artery treated with atherectomy including angioplasty as needed. Use 37230 for the initial tibial or peroneal artery treated with stent placement and angioplasty as needed. Use 37231 for the initial peroneal or tibial artery treated with stent placement and atherectomy, including angioplasty as needed.

37232-37235

37232 Revascularization, endovascular, open or percutaneous, tibial/peroneal artery, unilateral, each additional vessel; with transluminal angioplasty (List separately in addition to code for primary procedure)

37233 Revascularization, endovascular, open or percutaneous, tibial/peroneal artery, unilateral, each additional vessel; with atherectomy, includes angioplasty within the same vessel, when performed (List separately in addition to code for primary procedure)

37234 Revascularization, endovascular, open or percutaneous, tibial/peroneal artery, unilateral, each additional vessel; with transluminal stent placement(s), includes angioplasty within the same vessel, when performed (List separately in addition to code for primary procedure)

37235 Revascularization, endovascular, open or percutaneous, tibial/peroneal artery, unilateral, each additional vessel; with transluminal stent placement(s) and atherectomy, includes angioplasty within the same vessel, when performed (List separately in addition to code for primary procedure)

The physician revascularizes an additional ipsilateral (same side) occluded or stenosed tibial or peroneal artery using angioplasty, atherectomy, and/or transluminal stent placement. Using the same access artery, the catheter with a balloon tip is advanced over the guidewire to the site of another ipsilateral occluded tibial or peroneal artery. The balloon is inflated and the plaque is compressed against the wall of the artery. The balloon may be inflated several times to achieve the desired result. Alternatively, an atherectomy may be performed with or without angioplasty. Atherectomy is performed using a specialized balloon catheter that has a window on one side through which a cutting piston is advanced. The cutting piston shaves plaque from the arterial wall. As the plaque is shaved, it is pushed into the nose of the atherectomy device and removed upon

Cardiovascular System

completion of the procedure when the catheter is withdrawn. The physician may make several passes with the atherectomy device to achieve the desired result. The angioplasty or atherectomy device is exchanged for a guidewire. An angiography catheter is advanced over the guidewire and the guidewire is withdrawn. Contrast is injected and a completion angiography is performed to ensure that the artery is patent. If an intravascular stent is needed to maintain patency of the artery, the stent delivery catheter is advanced to the site of the lesion. The stent is carefully positioned and deployed. The stent delivery catheter is removed. A balloon catheter may again be advanced and inflated to seat the stent. Use 37232 for each additional tibial or peroneal artery treated with angioplasty only. Use 37233 for each additional tibial or peroneal artery treated with atherectomy including angioplasty as needed. Use 37234 for each additional tibial or peroneal artery treated with stent placement and angioplasty as needed. Use 37235 for each additional peroneal or tibial artery treated with stent placement and atherectomy, including angioplasty as needed.

37236-37237

37236   **Transcatheter placement of an intravascular stent(s) (except lower extremity artery(s) for occlusive disease, cervical carotid, extracranial vertebral or intrathoracic carotid, intracranial, or coronary), open or percutaneous, including radiological supervision and interpretation and including all angioplasty within the same vessel, when performed; initial artery**

37237   **Transcatheter placement of an intravascular stent(s) (except lower extremity artery(s) for occlusive disease, cervical carotid, extracranial vertebral or intrathoracic carotid, intracranial, or coronary), open or percutaneous, including radiological supervision and interpretation and including all angioplasty within the same vessel, when performed; each additional artery (List separately in addition to code for primary procedure)**

Transcatheter placement of an intravascular stent is done in any vessel other than a coronary, cervical carotid, intrathoracic carotid, extracranial vertebral, intracranial, or lower extremity vessel. For percutaneous approach, the femoral or other access artery is punctured and the introducer sheath is inserted. For the open approach, the introducer sheath is inserted through a surgically exposed artery via a small skin incision. The open approach is best employed in cases of severe arteriosclerotic disease affecting the femoral or iliac arteries. A guide wire is introduced and advanced to the site of the stenosis. A catheter is advanced over the guide wire. Roadmapping angiograms are obtained. A stiff wire is advanced to the site of the stenosis. A long guiding sheath is advanced over the catheter and stiff wire. The catheter and stiff wire are removed, leaving the long guiding sheath in place. Angioplasty may then be performed before stent placement. A balloon catheter is advanced to the site of the lesion and inflated to dilate the stenotic area. The balloon catheter is removed. The stent delivery catheter is then advanced to the site of the lesion. The stent is carefully positioned and deployed, and the stent delivery catheter is removed. A balloon catheter may again be advanced and inflated to seat the stent. Additional angiograms are obtained to evaluate stent placement and patency of the artery. All catheters are removed and pressure is applied to the vascular access site. Use 37236 for the initial artery treated and 37237 for each additional artery. These codes also include all radiological supervision and interpretation.

37238-37239

37238   **Transcatheter placement of an intravascular stent(s), open or percutaneous, including radiological supervision and interpretation and including angioplasty within the same vessel, when performed; initial vein**

37239   **Transcatheter placement of an intravascular stent(s), open or percutaneous, including radiological supervision and interpretation and including angioplasty within the same vessel, when performed; each additional vein (List separately in addition to code for primary procedure)**

Percutaneous transcatheter placement of an intravascular stent in a vein is performed. Venous stents may be placed in any vein but are most commonly used in the iliac vein and sometimes extend from the abdominal vena cava through the iliac vein and into the femoral vein. For placement of a stent in the femoral or iliac veins, the femoral vein is punctured and an introducer sheath is inserted. A guide wire is introduced and advanced to the site of the stenosis. A catheter is advanced over the guide wire. Roadmapping venograms are obtained. A balloon catheter is advanced to the site of the lesion and inflated to dilate the lesion. The balloon catheter is removed. The stent delivery catheter is then advanced to the site of the lesion. The stent is carefully positioned and deployed. The stent delivery catheter is removed. A balloon catheter may again be advanced and inflated to seat the stent. Additional venograms are obtained to evaluate stent placement and patency of the vein. All catheters are removed and pressure is applied to the vascular access site. Use 37238 for the initial vein treated and 37239 for each additional vein. These codes also include transcatheter intravascular venous stent placement done using an open approach.

37241-37242

37241   **Vascular embolization or occlusion, inclusive of all radiological supervision and interpretation, intraprocedural roadmapping, and imaging guidance necessary to complete the intervention; venous, other than hemorrhage (eg, congenital or acquired venous malformations, venous and capillary hemangiomas, varices, varicoceles)**

37242   **Vascular embolization or occlusion, inclusive of all radiological supervision and interpretation, intraprocedural roadmapping, and imaging guidance necessary to complete the intervention; arterial, other than hemorrhage or tumor (eg, congenital or acquired arterial malformations, arteriovenous malformations, arteriovenous fistulas, aneurysms, pseudoaneurysms)**

This procedure may be performed to occlude a vascular malformation, arteriovenous fistula, aneurysm, or pseudoaneurysm. The affected blood vessel is identified using angiography. The physician determines the best vascular access site for the occlusion or embolization procedure. The selected blood vessel is nicked and an introducer sheath is inserted. A guide wire is introduced through the sheath and advanced to the planned occlusion or embolization site. A catheter is advanced over the guide wire and the guide wire is withdrawn. Angiography is again performed to delineate the vasculature at the site of the vessel malformation, arteriovenous fistula, aneurysm, or pseudoaneurysm. Occlusive or embolic material is then introduced which might include a viscous collagen agent, polyvinyl alcohol particles, or ethiodized oil. Following the introduction of the occlusive or embolic material, angiograms are obtained to ensure that the treated blood vessel is completely occluded. Upon completion of the procedure, the catheter is removed and pressure is applied to the vascular access site to control bleeding. Use 37241 for venous embolization or occlusion and 37242 for arterial embolization or occlusion.

37243

37243   **Vascular embolization or occlusion, inclusive of all radiological supervision and interpretation, intraprocedural roadmapping, and imaging guidance necessary to complete the intervention; for tumors, organ ischemia, or infarction**

Vascular embolization or occlusion is performed for tumor destruction, organ ischemia, or infarction. Initial angiograms are obtained to identify the feeding blood vessels for the tumor or organ. The physician determines the best vascular access site for the occlusion or embolization procedure. The selected blood vessel is nicked and an introducer sheath is inserted. A guide wire is introduced through the sheath and advanced to the planned occlusion or embolization site. A catheter is advanced over the guide wire and the guide wire is withdrawn. Angiography is again performed to delineate vasculature at the site of the tumor or organ. Occlusive or embolic material is then introduced which might include a viscous collagen agent, polyvinyl alcohol particles, or ethiodized oil. Following the introduction of the occlusive or embolic material, angiograms are obtained to ensure that treated blood vessel is completely occluded. Additional feeding vessels may be catheterized and embolic/occlusive material introduced until all feeding vessels are completely occluded. Upon completion of the procedure, the catheter is removed and pressure is applied to the vascular access site to control bleeding.

37244

37244   **Vascular embolization or occlusion, inclusive of all radiological supervision and interpretation, intraprocedural roadmapping, and imaging guidance necessary to complete the intervention; for arterial or venous hemorrhage or lymphatic extravasation**

This procedure may be performed to control arterial or venous hemorrhaging or lymphatic extravasation. Initial angiograms are obtained to identify the feeding blood vessels for the hemorrhage or lymph vessels for the lymphatic extravasation. The physician determines the best vascular access site for the occlusion or embolization procedure. The selected blood or lymphatic vessel is nicked and an introducer sheath is inserted. A guide wire is introduced through the sheath and advanced to the planned occlusion or embolization site. A catheter is advanced over the guide wire and the guide wire is withdrawn. Angiography is again performed to delineate blood or lymph vessels at the site of the hemorrhage or extravasation. Occlusive or embolic material is then introduced which might include a viscous collagen agent, polyvinyl alcohol particles, or ethiodized oil. Following the introduction of the occlusive or embolic material, angiograms are obtained to ensure that the treated blood or lymph vessel is completely occluded. Additional feeding vessels may be catheterized and embolic/occlusive material introduced until all feeding vessels are completely occluded. Upon completion of the procedure, the catheter is removed and pressure is applied to the vascular access site to control bleeding.

Cardiovascular System

37246-37247

- **37246** Transluminal balloon angioplasty (except lower extremity artery(ies) for occlusive disease, intracranial, coronary, pulmonary, or dialysis circuit), open or percutaneous, including all imaging and radiological supervision and interpretation necessary to perform the angioplasty within the same artery; initial artery
- **37247** Transluminal balloon angioplasty (except lower extremity artery(ies) for occlusive disease, intracranial, coronary, pulmonary, or dialysis circuit), open or percutaneous, including all imaging and radiological supervision and interpretation necessary to perform the angioplasty within the same artery; each additional artery (List separately in addition to code for primary procedure)

Transluminal balloon angioplasty is an endovascular procedure that uses fluoroscopy to visualize one or more arteries and treat narrowing or obstruction with a balloon tipped catheter. To access the artery percutaneously, a needle is placed through the skin into an access vessel in the groin, arm, or neck. A guidewire is threaded through the needle and the needle is replaced with a vascular sheath. For open access, an incision is made in the skin over the vessel. When located, an incision is made into the vessel and a vascular sheath is introduced. For both methods, a vascular catheter is inserted over the guidewire and contrast dye is injected to visualize the artery(ies) and identify areas of stenosis or occlusion. The vascular catheter is replaced with a balloon catheter which is advanced to the narrowed area of the artery(ies). The balloon is inflated with dilute contrast dye to expand the vessel for a prescribed period of time before the balloon is deflated and withdrawn. A vascular catheter is reinserted and angiography is repeated to evaluate for successful opening of the blocked or narrowed artery or any residual stenosis requiring more balloon inflation. Code 37246 reports balloon angioplasty on the initial artery (except those in the brain, coronary, pulmonary, dialysis circuit, or lower extremities for occlusive disease), either open or percutaneous, and includes all imaging and radiological supervision and interpretation necessary to perform the angioplasty within the same artery. Code 37247 reports each additional artery.

37248-37249

- **37248** Transluminal balloon angioplasty (except dialysis circuit), open or percutaneous, including all imaging and radiological supervision and interpretation necessary to perform the angioplasty within the same vein; initial vein
- **37249** Transluminal balloon angioplasty (except dialysis circuit), open or percutaneous, including all imaging and radiological supervision and interpretation necessary to perform the angioplasty within the same vein; each additional vein (List separately in addition to code for primary procedure)

Transluminal balloon angioplasty is an endovascular procedure that uses fluoroscopy to visualize one or more veins and treat narrowing or obstruction with a balloon tipped catheter. To access the vein percutaneously, a needle is placed through the skin into an access vessel in the groin, arm, or neck. A guidewire is threaded through the needle and the needle is replaced with a vascular sheath. For open access, an incision is made in the skin over the vessel. When located, an incision is made into the vessel and a vascular sheath is introduced. For both methods, a vascular catheter is inserted over the guidewire and contrast dye is injected to visualize the vein(s) and identify areas of narrowing or disease. The vascular catheter is replaced with a balloon catheter which is advanced to the narrowed area. The balloon is inflated with dilute contrast dye to expand the vessel for a prescribed period of time before the balloon is deflated and withdrawn. A vascular catheter is reinserted and angiography is repeated to evaluate for successful opening of the blocked or narrowed vein or any residual stenosis requiring more balloon inflation. Code 37248 reports balloon angioplasty on the initial vein (except in the dialysis circuit), either open or percutaneous, and includes all imaging and radiological supervision and interpretation necessary to perform the angioplasty within the same vein. Code 37249 reports each additional vein.

37252-37253

- **37252** Intravascular ultrasound (noncoronary vessel) during diagnostic evaluation and/or therapeutic intervention, including radiological supervision and interpretation; initial noncoronary vessel (List separately in addition to code for primary procedure)
- **37253** Intravascular ultrasound (noncoronary vessel) during diagnostic evaluation and/or therapeutic intervention, including radiological supervision and interpretation; each additional noncoronary vessel (List separately in addition to code for primary procedure)

Intravascular ultrasound (IVUS) is performed on a non-coronary vessel during a separately reportable diagnostic and/or therapeutic vascular procedure. IVUS allows visualization of the blood vessel from the inside with a cross sectional view of the vessel showing the circular layers which include the outer covering (adventitia), the vessel wall (media), the inner endothelial layer (intima), and the open channel through which blood flows (lumen). During the separately reportable intravascular procedure, an IVUS catheter with a miniaturized transducer is advanced over a guidewire to the site requiring ultrasound evaluation. Ultrasound images are then obtained. Radiological supervision for catheter placement, imaging of the appropriate site, review of the ultrasound images, and interpretation with a written report of IVUS findings is included. Use 37252 for the initial vessel evaluated with IVUS and 37253 for each additional vessel.

37500

- **37500** Vascular endoscopy, surgical, with ligation of perforator veins, subfascial (SEPS)

The perforator veins connect the femoral and popliteal veins (deep venous system) of the legs with the superficial saphenous veins. SEPS involves endoscopic ligation of the perforator veins and is performed to treat incompetent perforator veins in patients with severe, chronic venous insufficiency and venous ulcerations by interrupting blood flow between the deep and superficial veins. Ultrasound guidance is used to locate the perforator veins. The leg is exsanguinated. Two small portal incisions are made in the skin of the calf at sites remote from any venous ulceration and carried down to the subfascial space. A space-maker balloon is introduced into the subfascial space and inflated to improve access to the perforator veins. The subfascial space is insufflated with carbon dioxide. The incompetent perforator veins are clipped or divided using endoscopic scissors. Alternatively, a harmonic scalpel may be used coagulate and divide the perforators. Upon completion of the procedure, the surgical instruments are removed, carbon dioxide is released from the subfascial space, and the portal incisions are closed.

37565

- **37565** Ligation, internal jugular vein

The physician ligates the internal jugular vein. The procedure may be performed for a variety of indications including penetrating trauma or injury to the vein, infection, thrombosis, or tinnitus causing hearing loss. A longitudinal incision is made through the skin and platysma to expose the sternocleidomastoid muscle and retracted it to expose the internal jugular vein. The vein is tied off (ligated) using a suture or thin wire.

37600

- **37600** Ligation; external carotid artery

The procedure may be performed for a variety of indications including penetrating trauma and injury to the artery, infection and thrombosis, severe nasal or other hemorrhage, tumor invasion, or vascular malformation. A longitudinal incision is made through the skin and soft tissue. The external carotid artery is exposed. The artery is tied off (ligated) using a suture or thin wire.

37605-37606

- **37605** Ligation; internal or common carotid artery
- **37606** Ligation; internal or common carotid artery, with gradual occlusion, as with Selverstone or Crutchfield clamp

The internal or common carotid artery is ligated. The skin over the carotid artery bifurcation is incised and soft tissues dissected to expose both the common and internal carotid arteries. The internal carotid artery is punctured and a pressure recording device inserted and advanced to the base of the skull for monitoring of internal carotid pressures during the procedure. The common carotid artery is the preferred site of ligation. In 37605, the common carotid artery is clamped and cerebral blood flow evaluated. If cerebral blood flow is adequate, the artery is ligated (tied off) using a suture or thin wire. If cerebral blood is severely compromised, ligation of the internal carotid artery is attempted. The internal carotid artery is clamped and cerebral blood flow evaluated. If cerebral blood flow is adequate, the internal carotid artery is ligated. In 37606, ligation of the internal or common carotid artery is performed using gradual occlusion with a Selverstone or Crutchfield clamp. The clamp is positioned on the internal or common carotid artery and partially closed until blood flow is reduced by approximately 50%. If the patient tolerates the reduced blood flow, the clamp is left in place and controlled occlusion performed over a period days. This is accomplished using a handle attached to the clamp that exits the skin. The clamp can be incrementally tightened at the bedside while monitoring neurovascular status. When the desired amount of occlusion has been accomplished the handle is removed leaving the clamp in place.

37607

- **37607** Ligation or banding of angioaccess arteriovenous fistula

Ligation or banding is performed to treat steal syndrome. Steal syndrome is a complication in which the hemodialysis access diverts blood flow from the hand causing ischemia and hand pain. An incision is made in the lower arm over the AVF and the AVF is exposed. The arterial component of the AVF is dissected free of surrounding tissue and a segment isolated. The AVF is partially ligated or a banded to decrease the amount of blood flowing to through the AVF and increase the amount of blood flowing to the hand. Blood flow through the AVF and hand is checked using Doppler and distal pulses are evaluated to ensure sufficient blood flow to the hand.

Cardiovascular System

37609

37609   Ligation or biopsy, temporal artery

The temporal arteries are located on the temples on each side of the head. Biopsy is performed to diagnose temporal arteritis which is a condition where the temporal arteries and sometimes arteries of the neck and arms become inflamed causing narrowing and reduced blood flow. It is also referred to as giant cell or cranial arteritis. Temporal arteritis can cause sudden permanent bilateral blindness if left untreated. The skin over the temporal artery is disinfected and a small incision made over the artery. The artery is mobilized and suture ligated proximal and distal to the planned biopsy site. A segment of the temporal artery is removed and sent to the laboratory for separately reportable histological studies. Ligation without biopsy is performed in the same manner except that a segment of artery is not removed. Ligation is performed for conditions such as arteriovenous malformation, aneurysm, or hemorrhage.

37615-37618

37615   Ligation, major artery (eg, post-traumatic, rupture); neck
37616   Ligation, major artery (eg, post-traumatic, rupture); chest
37617   Ligation, major artery (eg, post-traumatic, rupture); abdomen
37618   Ligation, major artery (eg, post-traumatic, rupture); extremity

The physician performs a ligation of a major artery to control bleeding following rupture or other traumatic injury to the blood vessel. The site of the injury is opened and explored. Blood is evacuated and the source of the bleeding identified. A vascular clamp is applied to control bleeding and the site thoroughly explored for evidence of other injuries. The artery is dissected free of surrounding tissue to allow placement of a suture ligature or wire band. The artery is tied off with sutures or a thin wire at a point proximal to the rupture. Use 37615, when a major artery in the neck is ligated. Use 37616 when an exploratory thoracotomy is performed and a major artery in the chest is ligated. Use 37617 when an exploratory laparotomy is performed and a major artery in the abdomen is ligated. Use 37618, when a major artery in an extremity (arm or leg) is ligated.

37619

37619   Ligation of inferior vena cava

The physician performs a ligation procedure to interrupt blood flow in the inferior vena cava (IVC) to prevent pulmonary embolism due to migration of deep vein thromboses (blood clots) from the pelvis or lower extremity to the lungs. The procedure is performed using an extravascular ligation technique. Prior to interruption of the IVC, a separately reportable cavogram is performed to evaluate the vascular anatomy and rule out the presence of any thrombus in the IVC. An incision is made in the abdomen. The IVC is exposed and dissected free of surrounding tissue. Blood flow is then partially or completed interrupted. A suture ligature is placed around the IVC. The wall of the vessel may also be plicated which involves making a series of folds around the circumference of the IVC to narrow the lumen. The abdominal wound is then closed in layers.

37650-37660

37650   Ligation of femoral vein
37660   Ligation of common iliac vein

The physician ligates the femoral or common iliac vein. Ligation involves tying off the vein using silk suture or a fine wire to interrupt blood flow. Interruption of blood flow in the femoral or common iliac vein is performed to prevent pulmonary embolism in patients with thromboembolism of the femoral or iliac veins. A separately reportable venography is performed to identify the exact location of the thromboembolism. In 37650, the femoral vein is ligated. A skin incision is made over the superficial or common femoral vein at a point proximal to the thromboembolism and the vein is exposed. The vein is then dissected free of surrounding tissue and ligated. In 37660, the common iliac vein is ligated. A skin incision is made over the common iliac vein at a point proximal to the thromboembolism and the vein is exposed. The vein is then dissected free of surrounding tissue and ligated.

37700

37700   Ligation and division of long saphenous vein at saphenofemoral junction, or distal interruptions

To ligate and divide the long saphenous vein at the saphenofemoral junction, an incision is made in the groin crease and the long saphenous vein and its tributaries exposed. The tributaries are dissected and suture ligated. The saphenofemoral junction is exposed. The long saphenous vein is ligated and divided flush with the femoral vein. To ligate and divide the long saphenous vein at a point distal to the saphenfemoral junction, an incision is made in the thigh over the long saphenous vein at the level where it is to be interrupted. The long saphenous vein is exposed, dissected free of surrounding tissue, ligated, and divided.

37718-37735

37718   Ligation, division, and stripping, short saphenous vein
37722   Ligation, division, and stripping, long (greater) saphenous veins from saphenofemoral junction to knee or below
37735   Ligation and division and complete stripping of long or short saphenous veins with radical excision of ulcer and skin graft and/or interruption of communicating veins of lower leg, with excision of deep fascia

The physician performs ligation, division and stripping of the short or long saphenous vein. In 37718, the short saphenous vein is ligated, divided and stripped. An incision is made over the saphenopopliteal junction and the short saphenous vein exposed. Venous branches along the short saphenous vein are dissected and suture ligated and divided. A second incision is made in the calf over the distal aspect short saphenous vein. The short saphenous vein is clamped proximally and distally. The distal end is ligated and divided below the clamp. The clamp is opened and a stripper inserted into the vein. The stripper is advanced to the saphenopopliteal junction. The proximal aspect of the short saphenous vein is divided below the clamp and suture ligated. The stripper head is tied to the proximal end of the divided short saphenous vein and the vein is pulled out through the calf incision. In 37722, the long saphenous vein is stripped from the saphenofemoral junction to the knee or below. An incision is made in the groin crease and the long saphenous vein and its tributaries exposed. The tributaries are dissected and suture ligated. The saphenofemoral junction is exposed. The long saphenous vein is ligated and divided flush with the femoral vein. A second incision is made at or just below the knee and the long saphenous vein exposed. The vein is stripped using the same technique described above. In 37735, long or short saphenous vein are removed as described above followed by radical excision of an ulcer with skin grafting and/or interruption of communicating veins of the lower leg with excision of deep fascia. If venous ulcers are present they are excised. The physician then harvests skin from a separate donor site. The skin graft is configured to cover the defect and sutured over the defect. The donor site is repaired with sutures. The physician may also dissect and suture ligate communicating veins and remove the deep fascia surrounding the communicating veins.

37760-37761

37760   Ligation of perforator veins, subfascial, radical (Linton type), including skin graft, when performed, open,1 leg
37761   Ligation of perforator vein(s), subfascial, open, including ultrasound guidance, when performed, 1 leg

The perforator veins connect the femoral and popliteal veins (deep venous system) of the legs with the superficial saphenous veins. Ligation is performed to treat incompetent perforator veins in patients with severe, chronic venous insufficiency and venous ulcerations. In 37760, the physician performs an open radical Linton-type procedure to ligate subfascial perforator veins. A long hockey stick incision is made along the medial calf extending posteriorly to the medial malleolus. Subfascial posterior and anterior skin flaps are developed. All posterior medial and paramedial perforators are exposed and clipped or divided to interrupt blood flow between the deep and superficial veins. Upon completion of the ligation procedure, tissues are closed with layered sutures or a skin graft is applied. If a skin graft is needed, the physician harvests skin from a separate donor site. The skin graft is configured to cover the defect and sutured over the defect. The donor site is repaired with sutures. In 37761, perforator veins are ligated using an open subfascial technique. The procedure is performed as described above except that the procedure is performed through a smaller incision and ultrasound guidance may be used to help locate and ligate perforator veins. Upon completion of the procedure, the incision is closed with layered sutures.

37765-37766

37765   Stab phlebectomy of varicose veins, 1 extremity; 10-20 stab incisions
37766   Stab phlebectomy of varicose veins, 1 extremity; more than 20 incisions

Stab phlebectomy is performed on one extremity. This procedure is performed to remove incompetent veins below the saphenofemoral and saphenopopliteal junction not including the proximal great and short saphenous veins. The physician makes multiple small skin incisions or needle punctures along the length of the varicose vein. The varicose vein is undermined and dissected along it course using the stem of a phlebotomy hook. The freed vein is then grasped using the hook and removed with mosquito forceps. The vein is progressively extracted from one incision to the next. Local compression over the venous network is used to control bleeding. Use 37765 for stab phlebectomy performed through 10 to 20 stab incisions and 37766 when more than 20 stab incisions are required.

37780

37780   Ligation and division of short saphenous vein at saphenopopliteal junction (separate procedure)

An incision is made over the saphenopopliteal junction and the short saphenous vein exposed. Venous branches along the short saphenous vein are dissected and suture ligated and divided. The short saphenous vein is clamped at the saphenopopliteal junction, divided

● New Code   ▲ Revised Code

below the clamp and suture ligated. Incisions over the short saphenous vein are closed in a layered fashion.

37785

37785   Ligation, division, and/or excision of varicose vein cluster(s), 1 leg

Varicose vein clusters are small groups of enlarged veins that make a winding pattern or form a knot that is visible through the skin. These varicose vein clusters may be tender to the touch or cause heaviness, aching, pain, skin rashes or sores in the legs. An incision is made over the varicose vein cluster and the cluster exposed. Venous branches at the cluster are dissected and suture ligated and divided. The vein is suture ligated above and below the cluster. The vein may be divided above and below the cluster or it may be dissected free of surrounding and tissue and removed. Incisions over vein cluster are closed in a layered fashion. This procedure is repeated until all symptomatic varicose vein clusters in the leg are treated.

37788

37788   Penile revascularization, artery, with or without vein graft

Penile revascularization is performed with or without vein graft to increase the cavernosal arterial blood supply to the penis. This procedure is performed on patients with penile arterial insufficiency and resulting erectile dysfunction. Penile arterial insufficiency may be caused by arteriosclerotic disease, trauma to the pelvis or perineum, or other organic disease processes. A number of surgical techniques are used to perform revascularization which may include direct anastomosis of the inferior epigastric artery to the corpus cavernosum or placement of a saphenous or basilic vein graft between the inferior epigastric or femoral artery and the corpus cavernosum. To perform direct anastomosis of the inferior epigastric artery to the corpus cavernosum, the artery is exposed, dissected free of surrounding tissue up to the level of the umbilicus, and transected. It is then passed through a subcutaneous tunnel to the base of the penis. The tunica albuginea is then exposed and a plug excised. Using microsurgical technique, the artery is anastomosed to the endothelium of the corpus cavernosum. Following anastomosis, the penis is observed for evidence of erection. Surgical incisions are then closed in a layered fashion. If a vein graft is used, the selected vein is harvested. If a saphenous vein graft is used, an incision is made in the skin of the leg over the section of saphenous vein to be harvested. Soft tissue is dissected off the vein and branches ligated and divided. The section of saphenous vein to be used is then ligated proximally and distally, divided and removed from the leg. The vein graft is then anastomosed in an end-to-side fashion to the inferior epigastric or femoral vein and tunneled to the base of the penis where it is anastomosed to the corpus cavernosum using the same technique described above.

37790

37790   Penile venous occlusive procedure

A penile venous occlusive procedure is performed on a patient with penile venous leakage, penile veno-occlusive insufficiency or venous occlusive dysfunction. Veno-occlusive dysfunction is a cause of erectile dysfunction that results from a greater outflow of venous blood than inflow. Storage of a sufficient amount of blood in the corpora cavernosa is necessary for penile rigidity and leakage causes insufficient storage of blood resulting in erectile dysfunction. Veno-occlusive dysfunction may be a result of trauma or due to a congenital disorder. Penile venous ligation is performed on the cavernosal and crural veins. Using microsurgical technique, the penile veins exhibiting leakage are exposed and carefully dissected free of surrounding tissue. The dorsal arteries and nerves are identified and protected. The penile veins exhibiting leakage are individually suture ligated. Following completion of the ligation procedure the penis is observed for evidence of erection. Surgical wound are closed in a layered fashion.

Cardiovascular System

38100-38102

38100 Splenectomy; total (separate procedure)
38101 Splenectomy; partial (separate procedure)
38102 Splenectomy; total, en bloc for extensive disease, in conjunction with other procedure (List in addition to code for primary procedure)

A total splenectomy (38100) is performed. An incision is made in the abdomen and the spleen exposed. The spleen is mobilized and displaced medially to expose the splenorenal, splenocolic, and gastrosplenic ligaments. If the spleen is significantly enlarged or if it has ruptured, the splenic artery is located first and ligated to reduce the size the spleen or prevent further hemorrhage. Otherwise, the splenorenal, splenocolic, and gastrosplenic ligaments are ligated and divided prior to tying off the splenic artery. The splenic artery and vein are then visualized, ligated and divided. The spleen is removed and the surgery site inspected for bleeding with particular attention being paid to the splenic pedicle and retroperitoneal space. Any bleeding is controlled by electrocautery or by suture ligation of blood vessels. The wound is irrigated and the abdomen closed. In 38101, a partial splenectomy is performed. The diseased or damaged portion of the spleen is visualized. Following mobilization of the spleen, the spleen is incised and the diseased or damaged portion excised. The remaining spleen segment is repaired by sutures or staples. The splenic artery may be ligated if bleeding is not controlled by sutures and staples alone. The remaining spleen segment may be wrapped in omentum or synthetic mesh. A drain may be inserted. The abdomen is then closed around the drain. In 38102, an en bloc total splenectomy is performed for extensive disease in conjunction with another procedure. The en bloc total splenectomy is performed as described above.

38115

38115 Repair of ruptured spleen (splenorrhaphy) with or without partial splenectomy

A ruptured spleen is repaired (splenorrhaphy) with or without partial splenectomy. An incision is made in the abdomen and the spleen is exposed, mobilized, and displaced medially. Actively bleeding vessels are ligated. Damaged or devitalized splenic tissue is first debrided. The rupture is then repaired with sutures or staples. If damage is extensive, a portion of the spleen may need to be excised. The remaining spleen segment is then repaired. The splenic artery may be ligated if bleeding is not controlled by sutures and staples alone. The remaining spleen segment may be wrapped in omentum or synthetic mesh and a drain inserted. The abdomen is then closed around the drain.

38120

38120 Laparoscopy, surgical, splenectomy

A laparoscopic splenectomy is performed. Trocars are placed through small incisions and a pneumoperitoneum is created. The laparoscope is inserted and the abdominal cavity is explored. A retractor is inserted and the inferior aspect of the spleen is lifted superiorly. The splenorenal and splenocolic ligaments are divided. Dissection continues in a superior and lateral direction to expose the posterior aspect of the splenic hilum and completely mobilize the spleen. A stapler is inserted and the splenic hilum is transected. Short gastric vessels are divided as needed. The spleen is detached. The most lateral trocar is removed, the incision is enlarged, and a larger trocar is placed. A specimen retrieval bag is inserted through the enlarged trocar site, and the spleen is placed in the bag, which is then brought to the abdominal wall and opened. The spleen is sectioned into smaller pieces and then removed. A drain is placed in the abdomen, surgical instruments are removed, the abdomen is deflated, and trocars removed. Incisions are closed.

38200

38200 Injection procedure for splenoportography

The skin of the abdomen is cleansed and a local anesthetic is injected overlying the spleen and then into deeper tissues. A sheathed needle is inserted into the spleen under fluoroscopic guidance. The needle is passed along the long axis of the spleen toward the splenic hilum. The needle is then removed and the correct sheath position is verified by the presence of free blood return. Splenic pulp pressure is measured using a manometer. A small amount of contrast is then injected to confirm proper sheath placement. Following the test injection, contrast media is injected into the spleen and recorded by cineangiography. The splenic veins are visualized and the contrast is observed as it drains from the splenic vasculature into the portal vein. Separately reportable radiographs are obtained of the splenic vasculature and the portal vein. When the injection procedure is complete, compressed Gelfoam plugs are inserted through the sheath to tamponade the entire needle tract. The sheath is removed and a dressing is applied.

38204

38204 Management of recipient hematopoietic progenitor cell donor search and cell acquisition

The management of locating donor hematopoietic progenitor cells and the physical acquisition of the cells for the recipients transplant.

38205-38206

38205 Blood-derived hematopoietic progenitor cell harvesting for transplantation, per collection; allogeneic
38206 Blood-derived hematopoietic progenitor cell harvesting for transplantation, per collection; autologous

Whole blood is removed from a donor and processed through a machine to separate the hematopoietic progenitor cells from other blood components. The remaining blood components are treated and reinfused into the donor. Code 38205 for each collection of blood-derived donor cells. Code 38206 for each collection of cells removed from the patient's own blood.

38207

38207 Transplant preparation of hematopoietic progenitor cells; cryopreservation and storage

Hematopoietic progenitor cells are harvested for transplantation at a later date. The cells are preserved with a cryoprotectant solution and stored at a low temperature.

38208-38209

38208 Transplant preparation of hematopoietic progenitor cells; thawing of previously frozen harvest, without washing, per donor
38209 Transplant preparation of hematopoietic progenitor cells; thawing of previously frozen harvest, with washing, per donor

Hematopoietic progenitor cells (HPCs), also called hematopoietic stem cells (HSCs), previously harvested for transplantation are thawed and treated for use in a stem cell transplant. HPCs are cells present in the blood and bone marrow that are capable of forming mature blood cells, including red blood cells, platelets, and white blood cells. HPCs are used in the treatment of malignant neoplasms such as leukemia and lymphoma and in the treatment of other conditions such as sickle cell disease. In 38208, the blood-derived HPCs from a single donor that have been preserved with a cryoprotectant solution and stored at a low temperature are thawed in a heated water bath. A sample is obtained following thawing for quality assessment which is performed by a technician. The quality assessment may include nucleated cell count, differential, viability, sterility and/or immunophenotyping. Once the quality assessment has been completed by the technician, the physician reviews the results and determines whether the product can be used in the transplant procedure. In 38209, the cells from a single donor are thawed and washed. Washing of cells is needed when multiple aliquots (bags of harvested cells) are frozen over multiple days. When multiple aliquots are needed, the amount of DMSO used in the preservation process is greater and can reach toxic levels. Some of the DMSO is removed by washing using an automated cell washer. During the wash process the cells are concentrated and resuspended in an infusible solution such as saline or albumin. Quality assessment is then performed on the washed cells to ensure that the product is still suitable for transplant.

38210

38210 Transplant preparation of hematopoietic progenitor cells; specific cell depletion within harvest, T-cell depletion

T-cells are depleted at the time of blood-derived hematopoietic progenitor cell harvesting for future transplantation. T-cell depletion is performed for allogeneic transplant procedures to help reduce the risk of graft-versus-host disease. The harvested cells are passed through an automated device that passively removes T-cells and other unwanted cells. Quality assessment of the T-cell depleted transplant product is performed to ensure that the undesired cells have been sufficiently depleted and that the product is suitable for transplant. Separately reportable cryopreservation and storage is then performed.

Hemic/Lymphatic Systems

38211-38213

38211 Transplant preparation of hematopoietic progenitor cells; tumor cell depletion

38212 Transplant preparation of hematopoietic progenitor cells; red blood cell removal

38213 Transplant preparation of hematopoietic progenitor cells; platelet depletion

Hematopoietic progenitor cells previously harvested for transplantation are treated for use. The cells preserved with a cryoprotectant solution and stored at a low temperature are thawed for infusion. Code 38211 if the specific tumor cells are separated out to prevent reinfusion of the patient's own diseased cells. Code 38212 if red blood cells are specifically removed from the harvested collection . Code 38213 if platelets are specifically removed from the harvested collection.

38214-38215

38214 Transplant preparation of hematopoietic progenitor cells; plasma (volume) depletion

38215 Transplant preparation of hematopoietic progenitor cells; cell concentration in plasma, mononuclear, or buffy coat layer

Hematopoietic progenitor cells previously harvested for transplantation are treated for use. The cells preserved with a cryoprotectant solution and stored at a low temperature are thawed for infusion. Code 38214 if the volume of cells is reduced by removal of plasma from the harvested collection. Code 38215 if the volume of cells is reduced by removing a portion of the concentration of mononuclear cells or buffy coat layer of white blood cells from the plasma.

38220

38220 Bone marrow; aspiration only

A needle is inserted through the skin and advanced until bone is penetrated. Bone marrow is aspirated through the needle and into a syringe.

38221

38221 Bone marrow; biopsy, needle or trocar

A needle is inserted through the skin and advanced until bone is penetrated. A small chip of bone marrow is removed for biopsy by a trocar or needle.

38230-38232

38230 Bone marrow harvesting for transplantation; allogeneic

38232 Bone marrow harvesting for transplantation; autologous

Bone marrow is a thick red liquid that is contained in the inner cavities of bones. It contains hematopoietic progenitor cells (HPCs) , also called hematopoietic stem cells (HSCs), that are capable of forming mature blood cells, including red blood cells, platelets, and white blood cells. With the patient lying prone on the operating table, a general anesthetic is administered. The hip area over the iliac crest is cleansed and a needle is inserted through the skin and into the bone. Bone marrow is extracted from the first bone puncture site using a needle and syringe. The needle is withdrawn from the bone. Without removing the needle completely from the skin, the needle is reinserted at a different site or angle in the bone. Once the available bone marrow has been harvested from this area of the iliac crest, the needle is completely removed from the bone and skin and reinserted at another site in the iliac crest on the same side. This may be repeated several times. The procedure is repeated as needed on the opposite side until approximately 2 quarts of bone marrow have been harvested. Use 38230 when bone marrow is harvested from a donor (allogeneic). Use 38232 when bone marrow is harvested from the patient (autologous).

38240-38241

38240 Hematopoietic progenitor cell (HPC); allogeneic transplantation per donor

38241 Hematopoietic progenitor cell (HPC); autologous transplantation

Hematopoietic progenitor cell (HPC) transplantation, also referred to as hematopoietic stem cell (HSC) transplantation, is a procedure in which progenitor (stem) cells are transplanted, or infused, intravenously into the recipient. Progenitor cells are harvested from bone marrow, peripheral blood, or umbilical cord blood obtained from the patient (i.e., autologous) or from a donor (i.e., allogeneic) in a separately reportable procedure. These cells are then frozen and stored until the time of the transplant procedure. The patient receives pre-transplant myeloablative or immunosuppressive conditioning. The hematopoietic progenitor cells are then thawed and prepared for transplant in a separately reportable procedure. The prepared hematopoietic progenitor cells are then transplanted or infused intravenously. Use 38240 for HPC allogeneic transplantation. If multiple HPC donors are used, report 38240 for each HPC allogeneic transplantation from a new donor. Use 38241 for HPC autologous transplantation.

38242

38242 Allogeneic lymphocyte infusions

Allogeneic (donor) lymphocyte transfusion (infusion) is performed on patients who have had a previous allogeneic hematopoietic progenitor cell (HPC) transplant who develop a hematologic malignancy, such as leukemia or lymphoma, following the HPC transplant. A separately reportable leukopheresis procedure is performed on the original HPC donor to collect lymphocytes. After collection, the donor lymphocytes are infused into the recipient either immediately or after frozen storage. The procedure is performed in an attempt to induce a favorable graft versus leukemia/lymphoma response that will destroy the malignant cells.

38243

38243 Hematopoietic progenitor cell (HPC); HPC boost

Hematopoietic progenitor cell (HPC) transplantation, also referred to as hematopoietic stem cell (HSC) transplantation, is a procedure in which progenitor (stem) cells are transplanted, or infused, intravenously into the recipient. Progenitor cells are harvested from bone marrow, peripheral blood, or umbilical cord blood obtained from the patient (i.e., autologous) or from a donor (i.e., allogeneic) in a separately reportable procedure, usually prior to the initial transplant procedure. An HPC "boost" is an infusion of additional hematopoietic stem cells to a recent HPC transplant patient who has poor graft function, graft failure, or graft rejection with or without immunosuppression. An HPC boost is different from a repeat transplant because the recipient does not require any pre-transplant myeloablative or immunosuppressive conditioning.

38300-38305

38300 Drainage of lymph node abscess or lymphadenitis; simple

38305 Drainage of lymph node abscess or lymphadenitis; extensive

The enlarged lymph node is palpated and the greatest area of fluctuance identified. A local anesthetic is injected. The skin over the lymph node is incised and deeper tissue dissected as needed to expose the abscess site. The lymph node is incised and drained. Cultures may be obtained and sent to the laboratory for separately reportable identification of organisms. The incision may be packed open, a drain placed, or the incision may be closed. Use 38300 for a simple procedure involving superficial lymph nodes and primary closure. Use 38305 for an extensive procedure involving deep tissue dissection, packing or drain placement, and/or secondary closure.

38308

38308 Lymphangiotomy or other operations on lymphatic channels

Surgical treatment of abnormalities or conditions affecting the lymph vessels, also called lymphatics, is uncommon with most abnormalities and conditions being treated medically rather than surgically. Lymphangioma and intestinal lymphangiectasia are examples of two conditions that are treated surgically. Lymphangioma is a congenital abnormality characterized by an abnormal mass of lymphatic vessels. The most common type is lymphangioma circumscriptum which is a cutaneous lymphatic mass composed of multiple vesicular lesions on the skin usually occurring in clusters. These vesicles are actually the dilated ends of lymph vessels and the lesions contain lymphatic fluid. Intestinal lymphangiectasia is a dilatation of the intestinal lymphatics which causes loss of lymphatic fluid into the gastrointestinal tract resulting hypoproteinuria, edema, and lymphocytopenia A condition treated less commonly by surgery is lymphatic obstruction caused by resection of lymph nodes or a mass obstructing the lymphatic vessels. Lymphatic obstruction causes lymphedema. To perform lymphangiotomy or another operation on lymph vessels, an incision is made in the skin over the involved lymph vessel(s). Overlying soft tissues are dissected and the lymph vessel(s) exposed. The affected lymph vessel is incised and explored. If an obstruction is present, the lymph vessel may be excised or the obstructed portion bypassed using a vein graft harvested from the patient. If a lymphangioma is present it is excised taking care to completely excise all abnormal lymph vessels and in the case of lymphangioma circumscriptum the involved dermis. If an intestinal lymphagiectasia is present it is resected. The abdomen is opened and the mass of abnormal intestinal lymphatics exposed and completely excised. Overlying soft tissues are then closed in layers.

Lymphangiotomy or other operations on lymphatic channels

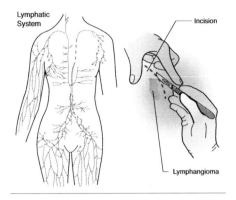

Lymphatic System

Incision

Lymphangioma

38380-38382

38380 Suture and/or ligation of thoracic duct; cervical approach
38381 Suture and/or ligation of thoracic duct; thoracic approach
38382 Suture and/or ligation of thoracic duct; abdominal approach

The physician performs a suture and/or ligation of the thoracic duct. The thoracic duct is the main conduit of the lymphatic system extending from the abdomen through the thoracic cavity and into the neck. While the course of the thoracic duct can vary considerably, it typically begins in the cisterna chyli at the level of the second lumbar vertebral body. It ascends through the abdominal region just anterior to the vertebral bodies. It enters the thoracic cavity on the right through the aortic hiatus and then crosses from the right side to the left at the level of the fourth or fifth thoracic vertebra. It empties into the left jugulosubclavian venous junction. The duct is paper-thin and susceptible to surgical or other traumatic injury causing a lymphatic leak at the site of the injury. The approach depends on the site of the injury. The thoracic duct is exposed and the site of the leak located. Once the leak is located, the injury is repaired with sutures or the duct is tied or ligated a few cm above and below the leak. A dry gauze pad is placed over the repaired or ligated tear and observed for any evidence of continuing leakage. The gauze is removed and the repair is reinforced with a spray or glue type sealant. Use 38380 for a cervical approach. A supraclavicular incision is made on the left side and soft tissues dissected to expose the upper aspect of the thoracic duct. Use 38381 for a thoracic approach. This approach requires a thoracotomy. Chest tubes are placed following repair of the leak. Use 38382 for an abdominal approach. An incision is made in the upper abdomen. The peritoneal cavity is opened and the falciform ligament divided. The liver is mobilized and retracted. Depending on the site of the leak, the diaphragm may be incised and mediastinum entered.

38500-38505

38500 Biopsy or excision of lymph node(s); open, superficial
38505 Biopsy or excision of lymph node(s); by needle, superficial (eg, cervical, inguinal, axillary)

A biopsy or excision of one or more superficial lymph nodes is performed. Superficial cervical, inguinal, and axillary lymph nodes lie close to the surface of the skin and can be accessed with only minimal dissection of overlying tissues. In 38500, an open biopsy or excision is performed. The lymph node to be biopsied is identified by palpation. The skin overlying the node is disinfected and a local anesthetic administered. The skin is incised and the lymph node exposed. If an excisional biopsy is performed, the lymph node is dissected free of surrounding and removed. If an incisional biopsy is performed, a tissue sample is obtained from the lymph node. The lymph node or the tissue sample is then sent for separately reportable laboratory analysis. In 38505, a needle biopsy is obtained. The lymph node is identified by palpation. The skin is cleansed over the planned puncture site and local anesthesia administered. Separately reportable imaging guidance is used as needed. A large bore needle is then advanced into the lymph node, and tissue samples obtained and sent for separately reportable laboratory evaluation.

38510-38520

38510 Biopsy or excision of lymph node(s); open, deep cervical node(s)
38520 Biopsy or excision of lymph node(s); open, deep cervical node(s) with excision scalene fat pad

Open biopsy or excision of deep cervical lymph nodes is performed. Deep cervical lymph nodes include the spinal accessory chain, transverse cervical chain, and Delphian node. An incision is made in the skin of the neck over the involved deep cervical nodes. The platysma muscle is incised. Dissection is carried down through soft tissues taking care to protect surrounding nerves and blood vessels. One or more deep cervical lymph nodes are dissected free of surrounding tissue and removed or tissue samples obtained. Lymph nodes within the scalene fat pad may also be biopsied or excised. The scalene fat pad lies beneath the inferior aspect of the scalene muscle and contains a small number of small lymph nodes. A supraclavicular skin incision is made in the skin and carried down through the platysma muscle. The sternocleidomastoid muscle is divided near its attachment to the clavicle and the scalene fat pad exposed. The scalene fat pad is carefully dissected from surrounding tissues and removed in its entirety. The tissue samples, lymph nodes, and scalene fat pad are sent to the laboratory for separately reportable histological evaluation. Use 38510 when deep cervical lymph node biopsy or excision is performed without scalene fat pad excision and 38520 when scalene fat pad excision is performed.

38525

38525 Biopsy or excision of lymph node(s); open, deep axillary node(s)

Open biopsy or excision of deep axillary lymph nodes is performed. The axillary lymph nodes are divided into five groups including the lateral, subscapular, pectoral, central, and apical (infraclavicular) nodes. The central and apical groups are the deep axillary lymph nodes. An incision is made in the skin of the axilla over the involved deep axillary nodes. Dissection is carried down through soft tissues taking care to protect surrounding nerves and blood vessels. One or more deep axillary lymph nodes are dissected free of surrounding tissue and removed or tissue samples obtained. The nodes or tissue samples are sent to the laboratory for separately reportable pathological evaluation.

38530

38530 Biopsy or excision of lymph node(s); open, internal mammary node(s)

An incision is made in the skin of the chest and overlying breast tissue detached from the pectoralis major fascia. The pectoralis major is divided longitudinally and the sternum, ribs, and the intercostal muscles overlying the internal mammary nodes exposed. The intercostal muscle is divided or a short strip removed to provide access to the subcostal space. The internal mammary vein and artery are identified and the fatty tissue containing the internal mammary nodes dissected free of surrounding tissues and removed or tissue samples of the lymph nodes obtained. The nodes or tissue samples are sent to the laboratory for separately reportable pathological evaluation.

38542

38542 Dissection, deep jugular node(s)

The deep jugular nodes are located along the internal jugular vein. An incision is made along the medial border of the sternocleidomastoid muscle and the plane between the sternocleidomastoid and strap muscles opened. The omohyoid muscle is exposed, dissected free of surrounding tissue, and excised to expose the internal jugular vein and carotid artery. Lymph nodes anterior to the internal jugular vein at the level of the thyroid are excised. The fascia overlying the internal jugular vein is incised laterally and lymph nodes along the lateral border exposed. The internal jugular vein is mobilized, retracted medially and elevated to expose the tissue behind the vein. The phrenic nerve is identified on the anterior scalene muscle and protected. Dissection continues along the posterior aspect of the vein both inferiorly and superiorly until all lymph nodes along the internal jugular vein have been identified and excised. The lymph nodes are sent for pathology for separately reportable evaluation. The neck incision is closed in layers.

38550-38555

38550 Excision of cystic hygroma, axillary or cervical; without deep neurovascular dissection
38555 Excision of cystic hygroma, axillary or cervical; with deep neurovascular dissection

Excision of an axillary or cervical cystic hygroma, also referred to as a cystic lymphangioma, is performed. A cystic hygroma consists of a one or more cysts filled with lymphatic fluid caused by a blockage of the lymphatic system. Cystic hygromas may be present at birth or may develop at any time during a person's life. The skin and subcutaneous

Hemic/Lymphatic Systems

tissue overlying the cystic hygroma is incised. If the cystic hygroma is in the axilla, deeper tissues are opened and the cystic mass exposed by careful dissection around nerves and blood vessels. Once the mass has been dissected free of surrounding tissue it is excised. If the cystic hygroma is in the neck, the platysmal muscle is incised and subplatysmal flaps created. Depending on the depth of the cystic mass, deeper tissues may need to be dissected. This is accomplished by careful dissection and preservation of the carotid sheath which contains the carotid artery, internal jugular vein, and vagus nerve. Dissection continues around all involved blood vessels and nerves until the cystic sac is completely freed from surrounding tissue. The cystic sac is then removed. If multiple cystic sacs are present each is dissected and excised. Use 38550 for excision of a cystic hygroma without deep neurovascular dissection and 38555 if deep neurovascular dissection is required.

38562

38562   Limited lymphadenectomy for staging (separate procedure); pelvic and para-aortic

The abdomen is incised. Before opening the peritoneum, pelvic lymph nodes are explored and removed. Taking care to preserve the genitofemoral nerve and psoas muscle, fatty tissue is stripped from the mid-portion of both common iliac vessels and along the internal and external iliac vessels to the level of the circumflex iliac vein. Iliac, hypogastric and obturator nodes are excised bilaterally. The peritoneal cavity is opened and the abdomen and pelvis explored for evidence of metastatic disease. The para-aortic lymph nodes are exposed and biopsies taken and sent for frozen section. Involved para-aortic lymph nodes are excised. The abdomen is then closed in layers.

38564

38564   Limited lymphadenectomy for staging (separate procedure); retroperitoneal (aortic and/or splenic)

The two most common approaches are transabdominal and thoracoabdominal. Typically the procedure is performed first on the same side as the malignancy. The retroperitoneum is fully exposed. The aortic lymph node dissection begins at the take-off of the renal vessels and then extends laterally to the ureters and inferiorly to the bifurcation of the inferior mesenteric artery. The dissection includes lymph nodes between the aorta and inferior vena cava. Lymph nodes along the splenic artery may also be sampled and positive nodes excised. Frozen section is performed on all lymph node samples to determine the extent of lymph node involvement and the procedure is tailored based on frozen section findings. Depending on the extent of involvement of lymph nodes on the ipsilateral (same) side, lymph nodes on the contralateral (opposite) side may also be sampled and excised.

38570

38570   Laparoscopy, surgical; with retroperitoneal lymph node sampling (biopsy), single or multiple

The physician performs laparoscopic retroperitoneal lymph sampling (biopsy). Using a transperitoneal approach, a trocar is placed off the midline just lateral to the umbilicus on the same side as the malignancy and the laparoscope is inserted. Two additional operating trocars are placed above and below the first just lateral to the rectus muscle. Additional trocars are placed as needed. The colon is mobilized to allow full exposure of the retroperitoneum. The lymph node sampling begins along the aorta at the take-off of the renal vessels and then extends laterally to the ureters and inferiorly to the bifurcation of the inferior mesenteric artery. The sampling includes lymph nodes between the aorta and inferior vena cava. Lymph nodes along the splenic artery may also be sampled and positive nodes excised. Frozen section is performed on all lymph node samples to determine the extent of lymph node involvement and the procedure is tailored based on frozen section findings. Depending on the extent of involvement of lymph nodes on the ipsilateral (same) side, lymph nodes on the contralateral (opposite) side may also be sampled. Upon completion of the procedure, surgical instruments are removed along with the laparoscope and incisions are sutured closed.

38571-38572

38571   Laparoscopy, surgical; with bilateral total pelvic lymphadenectomy
38572   Laparoscopy, surgical; with bilateral total pelvic lymphadenectomy and peri-aortic lymph node sampling (biopsy), single or multiple

The physician performs a laparoscopic bilateral total pelvic lymphadenectomy with or without sampling of the para-aortic lymph nodes. A small incision is made just below the umbilicus, a trocar placed and pneumoperitoneum established. A laparoscope is introduced through the umbilical port and additional portal incisions made and trocars placed for the introduction of surgical instruments. The peritoneal cavity is inspected and the abdomen and pelvis explored for evidence of metastatic disease. Taking care to preserve the genitofemoral nerve and psoas muscle, fatty tissue is stripped from the mid-portion of both common iliac vessels and along the internal and external iliac vessels to the level of the circumflex iliac vein. Iliac, hypogastric and obturator nodes are excised bilaterally. The excised lymph nodes and surrounding tissue are placed in an endobag and removed through an enlarged portal incision. The para-aortic lymph nodes are exposed and biopsies taken and sent for frozen section. Involved para-aortic lymph nodes are excised and removed in an endobag. Use 38571 for bilateral total pelvic lymphadenectomy

performed without para-aortic lymph node sampling and 38572 when para-aortic lymph node sampling is performed. One or more para-aortic nodes may be biopsied and/or excised.

38700

38700   Suprahyoid lymphadenectomy

Lymph nodes of the neck are categorized in six levels with the suprahyoid lymph nodes being in level I, and more specifically in level Ia. The suprahyoid lymph nodes lie beneath the chin between the anterior bellies of the digastric muscles on each side and the hyoid bone below. An incision is made in the skin of the neck below the chin typically in a skin fold. Underlying soft tissues are dissected and the suprahyoid lymph nodes exposed. The lymph nodes are dissected free of surrounding tissue, removed and sent for separately reportable pathological evaluation. A drain is placed in the surgical wound and incisions closed around the drain.

38720-38724

38720   Cervical lymphadenectomy (complete)
38724   Cervical lymphadenectomy (modified radical neck dissection)

The physician performs a complete cervical lymphadenectomy, also referred to as a radical neck dissection (38720) or a modified radical neck dissection (38724). Lymph nodes of the neck are categorized in six levels. Level I includes the submandibular and submental (suprahyoid) lymph nodes; levels II-IV refer the compartments along the jugular lymph node chain with level II extending along the upper third of the jugular vein above the hyoid, level III extending along the middle third of the jugular between the hyoid and the inferior border of the cricoid cartilage, and level IV extending along the lower third of the jugular from the inferior border of the cricoid cartilage to the clavicle. Level V nodes are located in the posterior triangle of the neck and include the spinal accessory, transverse cervical and supraclavicular nodes. Level VI includes nodes lie in the anterior or central compartment of the neck but these nodes are not part of a radical or modified radical neck dissection. The determination of which lymph node levels (I-V) require removal depends on the location of the primary malignancy and the predicted spread from local to regional sites. A curvalinear apron-type incision is used to expose the lymph nodes. The incision begins at one mastoid tip, descends to the lower neck, is carried transversely in one of the skin folds, and ascends to the opposite mastoid tip. Alternatively, a vertical incision anterior to the sternocleidomastoid muscles on the side of the malignancy may be employed. Subcutaneous tissues are dissected and a subplatysmal flap elevated. In 38720, lymph node levels I-V on the side of the malignancy are dissected free of surrounding tissue and excised. The sternocleidomastoid muscle and the internal jugular vein are removed. The submandibular gland is removed. The anterior belly of the digastric muscle as well as the sternohyoid and sternothyroid muscles may also be removed. In 38724, lymph node levels II-VI on the side of the malignancy are removed. The fascia over the sternocleidomastoid muscle is divided. The spinal accessory nerve is identified and skeletonized from the skull base to the sternocleidomastoid. Lymph nodes and surrounding fat are carefully dissected along the entire length of the jugular vein, removed and prepared for pathology examination. The platysma and subcutaneous tissues are closed in a single layer followed by the skin. Several drains are placed deep to the sternocleidomastoid muscle.

38740-38745

38740   Axillary lymphadenectomy; superficial
38745   Axillary lymphadenectomy; complete

An axillary lymphadectomy is performed. There are three levels of axillary lymph nodes with level I lying below the lower edge of the pectoralis minor muscle, level II underneath the muscle, and level III above the muscle. An incision is made in the lowest area of the axilla. The borders of the pectoralis major and latissimus dorsi muscles are identified. The axillary vein is identified and dissected from surrounding tissue. The axillary neural structures are identified and protected. Axillary lymph nodes are excised along with the surrounding fat pad. Usually 15-25 axillary nodes are removed from under the axillary vein and along the nerves and muscles of the axilla. Once all cancerous or suspicious tissue has been excised, a drain is placed and the surgical wound is closed. Use 38740 for excision of superficial lymph nodes which would include those in level I. Use 38745 for complete removal of axillary lymph nodes (levels I-III).

38746

38746   Thoracic lymphadenectomy by thoracotomy, mediastinal and regional lymphadenectomy (List separately in addition to code for primary procedure)

Regional removal of lymph nodes is performed when a malignant neoplasm has spread (metastasized) to the lymph nodes. Thoracic lymph nodes include the intrapulmonary nodes, bronchopulmonary (hilar) nodes, tracheobronchial nodes, peritracheal nodes, intercostal nodes, mediastinal nodes, and parasternal nodes. During a separately reportable thoracic procedure requiring a thoracotomy, the physician locates the involved lymph node chain(s) usually by separately reportable lymph node mapping to identify the sentinel node. The lymph nodes in all involved thoracic lymph node chains are then

● New Code   ▲ Revised Code

carefully dissected from surrounding tissues taking care to protect blood vessels and nerves. The excised lymph nodes are then sent for separately reportable pathological examination.

38747

38747   Abdominal lymphadenectomy, regional, including celiac, gastric, portal, peripancreatic, with or without para-aortic and vena caval nodes (List separately in addition to code for primary procedure)

Regional removal of lymph nodes is performed when a malignant neoplasm has spread (metastasized) to the lymph nodes. The physician locates the involved lymph node chain(s) usually by separately reportable lymph node mapping to identify the sentinel node. The lymph nodes in all involved abdominal lymph node chains are then carefully dissected from surrounding tissues taking care to protect blood vessels and nerves. The excised lymph nodes are then prepared for separately reportable pathology examination.

38760-38765

38760   Inguinofemoral lymphadenectomy, superficial, including Cloquets node (separate procedure)

38765   Inguinofemoral lymphadenectomy, superficial, in continuity with pelvic lymphadenectomy, including external iliac, hypogastric, and obturator nodes (separate procedure)

A superficial inguinofemoral lymphadenectomy is performed in a separate procedure. In 38760, the procedure is performed with excision of Cloquets node. Cloquets node is the deep inguinal lymph node that represents the transitional zone between the inguinal and iliac region. An incision is made parallel to the inguinofemoral ligament and carried down to Camper's fascia. Skin flaps are elevated while simultaneously separating the flaps from the underlying fat pad. Deep tissues at the superior aspect of the inguinal region are dissected. Cloquets node is identified, excised and frozen section performed. The fat pad containing nodal tissue is elevated and mobilized down to the inferior margin of the inguinal ligament. Dissection continues into the femoral triangle. The cribiform fascia is opened. Once the nodal tissue over the common femoral vein has been completely freed the inguinofemoral nodal tissue is removed as a single specimen. In 38765, inguinofemoral lymphadenectomy is performed as described above. If Cloquets node is positive for malignancy, pelvic lymphadenectomy including excision of external iliac, hypogastric, and obturator nodes is also performed. The abdomen is incised and without opening the peritoneum the pelvic lymph nodes on the side of the malignancy are explored. Taking care to preserve the genitofemoral nerve and psoas muscle, fatty tissue is stripped from the mid-portion of the common iliac vessel and along the internal and external iliac vessels to the level of the circumflex iliac vein. Iliac, hypogastric and obturator nodes are excised and sent for separately reportable pathology evaluation. The groin and abdominal incisions are closed in layers.

38770

38770   Pelvic lymphadenectomy, including external iliac, hypogastric, and obturator nodes (separate procedure)

The abdomen is incised and without opening the peritoneum the pelvic lymph nodes on the side of the malignancy are explored. Taking care to preserve the genitofemoral nerve and psoas muscle, fatty tissue is stripped from the mid-portion of both common iliac vessels and along the internal and external iliac vessels to the level of the circumflex iliac vein. Iliac, hypogastric and obturator nodes are excised and sent for separately reportable pathology evaluation. The abdominal incision is closed in layers.

38780

38780   Retroperitoneal transabdominal lymphadenectomy, extensive, including pelvic, aortic, and renal nodes (separate procedure)

Typically the procedure is performed first on the same side as the malignancy. Before opening the retroperitoneum, pelvic lymph nodes are explored and removed. Taking care to preserve the genitofemoral nerve and psoas muscle, fatty tissue is stripped from the mid-portion of both common iliac vessels and along the internal and external iliac vessels to the level of the circumflex iliac vein. Iliac, hypogastric and obturator nodes are excised bilaterally. The retroperitoneum is fully exposed via a transabdominal approach. The retroperitoneum is inspected for evidence of metastatic disease. The aortic lymph node dissection begins at the take-off of the renal vessels and then extends laterally to the ureters and inferiorly to the bifurcation of the inferior mesenteric artery. The dissection includes lymph nodes between the aorta and inferior vena cava. Aortic lymph nodes are excised along with surrounding tissue. Lymph nodes along the renal and splenic arteries may also be excised. Depending on the extent of involvement of lymph nodes on the ipsilateral (same) side, lymph nodes on the contralateral (opposite) side may also be sampled and excised.

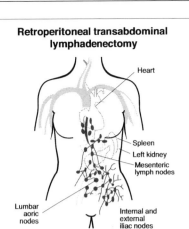

Retroperitoneal transabdominal lymphadenectomy

Heart

Spleen
Left kidney
Mesenteric lymph nodes

Lumbar aoric nodes

Internal and external iliac nodes

Extensive removal of lymph nodes of the retroperitoneal area is performed

38790

38790   Injection procedure; lymphangiography

The skin of the foot is cleansed and blue indicator dye is injected between several toes. The provider waits and observes the dye as it spreads into the small lymph vessels of the foot which takes 15-30 minutes. When there is good delineation of the lymph vessels in the foot, a local anesthetic is injected over one of the larger lymph vessels. The skin is incised and the lymph vessel exposed. A needle or catheter is inserted into the exposed lymph vessel and contrast media injected. Separately reportable lymphangiograms are obtained as the contrast travels through the lymph vessels. Images may be obtained of extremity vessels and/or pelvic and/or abdominal vessels.

38792

38792   Injection procedure; radioactive tracer for identification of sentinel node

An injection procedure is performed for identification of a sentinel node, also referred to as lymph node mapping. Lymph ducts usually drain to one lymph node first, called the sentinel node, which is identified using a combination of weak radioactive dye (technetium-labeled sulfur colloid, technetium-99) measured by a hand held probe, followed by injection of a blue dye (isosulfan blue) that stains the lymph tissue bright blue so it can be seen. The radioactive dye is injected into the tumor site or tumor bed and travels from the tumor site to the sentinel node. This may take as little as 45 minutes or as much as 8 hours. The radioactive dye is followed by an injection of the blue dye. When the radioactive and blue dyes have reached the lymph nodes, a separately reportable lymph node biopsy is performed.

38794

38794   Cannulation, thoracic duct

The thoracic duct is the main conduit of the lymphatic system extending from the abdomen through the thoracic cavity and into the neck. While the course of the thoracic duct can vary considerably, it typically begins in the cisterna chyli at the level of the second lumbar vertebral body. It ascends through the abdominal region just anterior to the vertebral bodies. It enters the thoracic cavity on the right through the aortic hiatus and then crosses from the right side to the left at the level of the fourth or fifth thoracic vertebra. It empties into the left jugulosubclavian venous junction. Cannulation is performed to relieve obstruction of lymph flow due to compression by malignant tumors or in patients with cirrhoisis complicated by ascites and portal hypertension as well as other conditions. An incision is typically made above the clavicle and the thoracic duct is exposed. The duct is punctured and cannulated and advanced as needed. Following cannulation lymphatic fluid is monitored for flow, pressure and composition which can help identify the underlying cause of the obstruction.

38900

38900   Intraoperative identification (eg, mapping) of sentinel lymph node(s) includes injection of non-radioactive dye, when performed (List separately in addition to code for primary procedure)

An injection procedure for identification of the sentinel node(s), also referred to as lymph node mapping, is performed during a separately reportable operative procedure. Lymph ducts usually drain to one lymph node first and this lymph node is called the sentinel node. The sentinel node is identified by injection of a blue dye (isosulfan blue) that stains the lymph tissue bright blue so it can be seen. The dye is injected into the exposed tumor bed. The dye then travels from the tumor bed to the sentinel node. When the dye has reached the sentinel node, one or more separately reportable lymph node biopsies may be performed to determine whether a malignant neoplasm has metastasized to surrounding lymph nodes.

Mediastinum and Diaphragm

39000-39010

39000 Mediastinotomy with exploration, drainage, removal of foreign body, or biopsy; cervical approach

39010 Mediastinotomy with exploration, drainage, removal of foreign body, or biopsy; transthoracic approach, including either transthoracic or median sternotomy

A mediastinotomy is performed using a cervical approach with exploration, drainage, removal of foreign body, or biopsy. A cervical approach is used to explore the superior mediastinum. An incision is made above the suprasternal notch between the borders of the sternocleidomastoid muscle and carried down to pretracheal fascia which is divided. Tissue dissection continues down to the superior mediastinum which is opened and explored. The superior mediastinal space may be drained, foreign bodies removed, and/ or biopsies taken. In 39010, a transthoracic or median sternotomy approach is used. If a transthoracic approach is used, an incision is made over the right or left third costal cartilage. The cartilage bed is incised. Dissection is carried down toward the hilus of the lung. The mediastinal space is explored, drained, any foreign bodies are removed, and/or the lung pleura and lymph nodes biopsied. The pleural space may be entered and biopsies obtained of the lungs. If the pleural space is entered, a chest tube is placed. Incisions are then closed in layers.

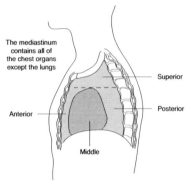

Mediastinotomy

Mediastinum exploration includes the drainage of fluids, removal of a foreign body, or removal of tissue for biopsy

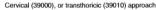

The mediastinum contains all of the chest organs except the lungs

Superior

Posterior

Anterior

Middle

Cervical (39000), or transthoricic (39010) approach

39200-39220

39200 Resection of mediastinal cyst

39220 Resection of mediastinal tumor

The physician resects a mediastinal cyst (39200) or mediastinal tumor (39220). The approach is dictated by the location of the mass. A median sternotomy is typically used for anterior lesions while a posterolateral approach is used for posterior lesions. Dissection is carried down to the mediastinum and the mediastinal space is explored. The mediastinal cyst or tumor is located and exposed. If the lesion is cystic in nature, it is resected and, if possible, the entire cyst wall is removed to prevent recurrence. If the cyst wall is adherent to the tracheobronchial tree, esophagus, or other mediastinal structure and complete resection is not possible, the mucosal lining of the adherent portion of the cyst is removed. If a mediastinal tumor is removed, the tumor is resected in its entirety if possible. Following removal of the cyst or tumor, incisions are closed in layers.

39401-39402

39401 Mediastinoscopy; includes biopsy(ies) of mediastinal mass (eg, lymphoma), when performed

39402 Mediastinoscopy; with lymph node biopsy(ies) (eg, lung cancer staging)

Mediastinoscopy may be performed for evaluation of mediastinal lesions and to assess treatment options for patients with suspected bronchogenic carcinoma. A small skin incision is made above the suprasternal notch between the borders of the sternocleidomastoid muscle and carried down to pretracheal fascia, which is divided. The mediastinoscope is then inserted behind the suprasternal notch and advanced behind the aortic arch into the superior mediastinum. The mediastinoscope is advanced to the level of the carina, which is examined for lesions, tumors, diseased tissue, or any other abnormalities, along with the main bronchi. In 39401, biopsies of a mass or lesion in the mediastinum (eg, lymphoma) may be taken through the endoscope as needed. In 39402,

mediastinal lymph nodes are examined and biopsied as needed (eg, for lung cancer staging). The mediastinoscope is withdrawn and incisions are closed.

39501

39501 Repair, laceration of diaphragm, any approach

The most common cause of diaphragm laceration is blunt trauma due to motor vehicle accident, but laceration may also occur as a result of a fall or penetrating trauma to the abdomen. Even small lacerations of the diaphragm require surgical repair due to the potential for enlargement with herniation of abdominal contents into the chest. The most common approach is abdominal, although a thoracic or combined approach may also be used. The abdomen and/or thorax is opened and explored and the extent of injury determined. The laceration is repaired in layers or a synthetic patch graft applied.

39503

39503 Repair, neonatal diaphragmatic hernia, with or without chest tube insertion and with or without creation of ventral hernia

There are two types of neonatal diaphragmatic hernia. A Bochdalek hernia occurs on the left side of the diaphragm with herniation of stomach and intestines and a Morgagni hernia occurs on the right side with herniation of the liver and intestines. An abdominal, thoracic, or combined approach may be used depending on the size and location of diaphragmatic hernia. Typically, an incision is made below the ribs (subcostal) and the abdominal viscera examined. Herniated abdominal contents are reduced and the hernia sac is excised. The defect in the diaphragm may be suture repaired in a single layer for small defects or a synthetic patch graft may be used for larger defects. If the abdominal cavity is too small to accommodate the abdominal contents, the abdominal wall is repaired with a prosthetic patch that is placed over the abdominal contents. This leaves a ventral hernia in the abdominal wall that will be repaired during a subsequent surgery. One or more chest tubes may be placed at the conclusion of the procedure.

39540-39541

39540 Repair, diaphragmatic hernia (other than neonatal), traumatic; acute

39541 Repair, diaphragmatic hernia (other than neonatal), traumatic; chronic

The physician repairs a traumatic diaphragmatic hernia. This may also be referred to as rupture of the diaphragm with herniation of abdominal contents into the thorax. The most common cause of traumatic diaphragmatic hernia is blunt trauma due to motor vehicle accident, but diaphragmatic hernia may also occur as a result of a fall or penetrating trauma to the abdomen. The most common approach is abdominal, although a thoracic or combined approach may also be used. The abdomen and/or thorax is opened and explored and the extent of injury determined. The edges of the torn diaphragm are freed from surrounding tissue. The herniated abdominal contents are reduced using gentle traction. The hernia defect is repaired primarily with sutures. The suture repair may be reinforced with a fascial graft. Alternatively, a synthetic patch graft may be applied. Use 39540 for repair of an acute (current) traumatic diaphragmatic hernia and 39541 when a chronic traumatic diaphragmatic hernia is repaired. Chronic herniation is often associated with atrophy of the diaphragm requiring repair with a synthetic patch.

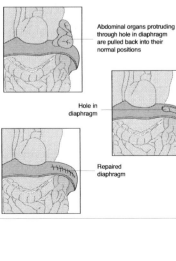

Repair of diaphragmatic hernia

Abdominal organs protruding through hole in diaphragm are pulled back into their normal positions

Hole in diaphragm

Repaired diaphragm

● New Code   ▲ Revised Code

Mediastinum & Diaphragm

39545

39545   Imbrication of diaphragm for eventration, transthoracic or transabdominal, paralytic or nonparalytic

Diaphragmatic eventration refers to relaxation of the diaphragmatic dome. This causes elevation of the diaphragm and protrusion of intestine into the thoracic cavity which can compromise both lung and bowel function. The condition may be present at birth, which is referred to as congenital or nonparalytic eventration, or it may be an acquired condition, also referred to as paralytic eventration. A transthoracic approach is used for severe diaphragmatic elevation, while less severe cases can be treated by a transabdominal approach. Using a thoracic approach, an anterolateral thoracotomy is performed through the intercostal space. The intercostal level depends on the level of elevation of the diaphragm. The anterior portion of the diaphragmatic leaflet is exposed. The dome of the diaphragm is opened taking care to protect the phrenic nerve. Displaced abdominal contents are reduced into the abdominal cavity. The redundant diaphragmatic dome is trimmed and the remaining diaphragm reconstructed by overlapping the edges of the diaphragm muscle.

39560-39561

39560   Resection, diaphragm; with simple repair (eg, primary suture)

39561   Resection, diaphragm; with complex repair (eg, prosthetic material, local muscle flap)

The physician resects the diaphragm which is typically performed to treat metastatic lesions from the lungs or other thoracic structures to the diaphragm. Using a thoracic approach, an anterolateral thoracotomy is performed through an intercostal space. Alternatively, a median sternotomy, abdominal, or other approach may be used. The involved portion of the diaphragm is excised along with a margin of healthy tissue. In 39560, following a limited resection a simple primary suture repair is used to close the diaphragm. In 39561, following an extended resection the diaphragm is repaired using prosthetic replacement (synthetic patch) of the diaphragm. Alternatively, a local muscle or fascial flap may be developed to close the diaphragm.

● New Code   ▲ Revised Code   CPT © 2016 American Medical Association. All Rights Reserved.   © 2017 DecisionHealth

Mediastinum & Diaphragm

40490

40490   Biopsy of lip

A biopsy of the lip is performed to evaluate changes in lip tissue such as scaling, fissuring, plaques, or other lesions. The area to the biopsied is disinfected and a local anesthetic administered. The abnormal area is then incised. A tissue sample is obtained and sent for separately reportable pathology evaluation.

40500

40500   Vermilionectomy (lip shave), with mucosal advancement

The lips are composed of skin, muscle, and mucosa and are divided into three main regions, the cutaneous, vermilion, and mucosal. The cutaneous portion of the upper lip extends from the bottom of the nose to the nasolabial folds laterally to the vermilion border. The lower cutaneous lip extends from the vermilion border to the extension of the nasolabial folds laterally to the mental crease at the chin. The vermilion portion is the pink to red colored portion of the lip which is composed of modified mucosal membrane. The mucosal portion lies inside the mouth and abuts the teeth. Vermilionectomy is performed to treat conditions such as actinic cheilitis, carcinoma in situ, and squamous cell carcinoma of the vermilion. An incision is made along the vermilion border of the affected lip (upper or lower) and the vermilion excised along the submucosal plane. The posterior lip mucosa is then incised and developed to reconstruct the vermilion. The lip mucosa is advanced and meticulously sutured to the skin (cutaneous lip) to reconstruct the vermilion.

40510–40520

40510   Excision of lip; transverse wedge excision with primary closure
40520   Excision of lip; V-excision with primary direct linear closure

The physician performs a transverse wedge excision (40510) or V-excision (40520) of a lesion, scar, or other defect of the lip followed by primary closure. The planned incision lines are marked with a surgical marking pen. If the procedure is performed to excise a lesion, the incision line includes a margin of healthy tissue on all sides of the lesion. The lip is then injected with a local anesthetic and epinephrine to control bleeding. In 40510, a transverse wedge resection of the lip is performed. The lip is incised as planned in a perpendicular fashion through the vermilion on each side of the lesion or defect. Once the white of the lip is reached, the incision on each side converges and a wedge shaped piece of tissue is removed. The edges of the surgical wound are then reapproximated in layers taking care to align the vermilion border. In 40520, a V-excision is performed. V-excisions are used for small lesions, scars or defects. The physician follows the previously marked V-shaped incision lines on the surface of the lip and carries the incision line down through the vermilion to the white of the lip. The lesion is excised. The surgical wound is repaired with sutures in a direct linear fashion.

40525–40527

40525   Excision of lip; full thickness, reconstruction with local flap (eg, Estlander or fan)
40527   Excision of lip; full thickness, reconstruction with cross lip flap (Abbe-Estlander)

A full thickness excision of the lip is performed with reconstruction using a local flap, also referred to as an Estlander or fan flap (40525), or a cross lip flap, also referred to as an Abbe-Estlander flap (40527). The planned incision lines are marked with a surgical marking pen. If the procedure is performed to excise a lesion, the incision line includes a margin of healthy tissue on all sides of the lesion. The lip is then injected with a local anesthetic and epinephrine to control bleeding. A wedge resection of the lip is performed first. The lip is incised as planned in a perpendicular fashion through the cutaneous lip and vermilion on each side of the lesion or defect. Once the white of the lip is reached, the incision on each side converges and a wedge shaped piece of tissue is removed. In 40525, the defect is repaired using a local flap. The incision lines for the flap are marked on the skin using a surgical marker. The flap includes cutaneous lip and vermilion. The incision is carried down through the orbicularis muscle leaving the underlying mucosa intact. The flap is then advanced over the defect and the lip reconstructed. In 40527, the defect is repaired using a cross lip flap which is a type of pedicle flap that is developed and transferred in a two-stage procedure. If the defect is on the lower lip, a full-thickness triangular flap is created using upper lip tissue which includes cutaneous lip and vermilion. If the defect is in the upper lip, the flap is created using lower lip tissue. In the first stage of the procedure, the flap is created. The incision is carried to the vermilion border of the lip and then through the orbicularis muscle leaving underlying labial mucosa intact. The pedicle flap is created maintaining the labial artery for blood supply to the flap. The flap is placed in the defect, but is not severed from its blood supply in the opposite lip. In the second stage of the

procedure performed several weeks later, the flap is divided, the pedicle inserted, and the transfer procedure completed.

40530

40530   Resection of lip, more than one-fourth, without reconstruction

The planned incision lines are marked with a surgical marking pen. If the procedure is performed to excise a lesion, the incision line includes a margin of healthy tissue on all sides of the lesion. The lip is then injected with a local anesthetic and epinephrine to control bleeding. The full-thickness of more than 1/4th of the lip is incised including the cutaneous lip, vermilion, and underlying mucosa. The lip is then excised without plastic reconstruction. The edges of the surgical wound are repaired with sutures.

40650–40654

40650   Repair lip, full thickness; vermilion only
40652   Repair lip, full thickness; up to half vertical height
40654   Repair lip, full thickness; over one-half vertical height, or complex

The lips are composed of skin, muscle, and mucosa and are divided into three main regions, the cutaneous, vermilion, and mucosal. The cutaneous portion of the upper lip extends from the bottom of the nose to the nasolabial folds laterally to the vermilion border. The lower cutaneous lip extends from the vermilion border to the extension of the nasolabial folds laterally to the mental crease at the chin. The vermilion portion is the pink to red colored portion of the lip which is composed of modified mucosal membrane. The mucosal portion lies inside the mouth and abuts the teeth. In 40650, a full thickness repair of the vermilion only is performed. The submucosa is repaired first using small-caliber, soft, nonirritating suture material with the knots buried. The orbicularis oris muscle is repaired next using absorbable suture. The vermilion is repaired last taking care to carefully align the vermilion border. In 40652 and 40654, the vermilion is repaired as described above. The surgeon then closes the dermis and subcutaneous tissue of the cutaneous lip followed by the epidermis which is everted to prevent depression and minimize scarring. If the mucosa is involved, such as when a through-and-through laceration occurs, it may be closed before or after repair of the vermilion and cutaneous lips. Use 40652 for full-thickness repair up to half of the vertical height of the lip and 40654 for lacerations that are over one-half of vertical height or complex. Complex repairs are those that require debridement, extensive undermining, stents, retention sutures or other repair techniques to achieve an acceptable cosmetic appearance.

40700

40700   Plastic repair of cleft lip/nasal deformity; primary, partial or complete, unilateral

The physician performs a primary repair of a unilateral partial or complete cleft lip and associated nasal deformity. Cleft lip is a congenital deformity caused by failure of embryonic connective tissue composed of mesenchymal cells to migrate properly during palate formation resulting in disfigurement of the upper lip and nose. Cleft lip and nasal deformity may be unilateral or bilateral. Each cleft lip deformity is unique requiring individualized procedure planning and surgical technique. In 40700, a unilateral deformity is repaired. The physician identifies the center of Cupid's bow, Cupid's bow peak on the noncleft side, the midline of the columella, and the alar base on both sides of the nose. This information is used to plan reconstruction of the cleft lip. Planned incision lines are marked. The physician then creates a series of flaps to repair the cleft lip and restore continuity of the orbicularis muscle. The nasal deformity is also corrected by undermining the nasal skin on the cleft side and freeing it from the nasal skeleton. The depressed alar cartilage on the cleft side is elevated and the lateral crus and alar base are advanced medially.

40701–40702

40701   Plastic repair of cleft lip/nasal deformity; primary bilateral, 1-stage procedure
40702   Plastic repair of cleft lip/nasal deformity; primary bilateral, 1 of 2 stages

The physician performs a primary repair of a bilateral cleft lip and associated nasal deformity. Cleft lip is a congenital deformity caused by failure of embryonic connective tissue composed of mesenchymal cells to migrate properly during palate formation resulting in disfigurement of the upper lip and nose. Cleft lip and nasal deformity may be unilateral or bilateral. Each cleft lip deformity is unique requiring individualized procedure planning and surgical technique. In 40701, a bilateral deformity is repaired in a single surgical session. The anatomic landmarks are tattooed and incision lines marked. The orbicularis muscle is dissected from overlying skin and muscle bundles divided. The portion

Digestive System

of the muscle that will be used to create the vermillion of Cupid's bow is left attached to the mucosa. A cutaneous labial flap is created along with mucosal flaps that are turned over to create the vermilion and Cupid's bow. The nose is then repaired by freeing overlying tissue from the nasal skeleton. The nasal domes are approximated and the lower lateral cartilage is suspended from the upper lateral cartilage on each side. The muscle bundles of the orbicularis muscle are approximated. All skin incisions are then closed using fine sutures or skin adhesive. In 40702, a bilateral deformity is repaired in two stages. This code reports both stages. Report the first stage and then report the code again for the second stage.

40720

40720   Plastic repair of cleft lip/nasal deformity; secondary, by recreation of defect and reclosure

The physician performs a secondary repair of a cleft lip and associated nasal deformity by recreating the defect, then repairing and reclosing the defect. Cleft lip is a congenital deformity caused by failure of embryonic connective tissue composed of mesenchymal cells to migrate properly during palate formation resulting in disfigurement of the upper lip and nose. Cleft lip and nasal deformity may be unilateral or bilateral. Each cleft lip deformity is unique requiring individualized procedure planning and surgical technique. In this type of secondary repair the physician incises the lip and nose along the original incision lines from the primary repair. Scar tissue is released and excised. Undermining of underlying tissues is performed to allow a tension free closure. The lip and nose are then repaired in the same manner as the primary procedure. The physician identifies the anatomical landmarks. The previously created flaps are then advanced or rotated as needed to repair the cleft lip and restore continuity of the orbicularis muscle. The nasal deformity is also corrected by undermining the nasal skin and freeing it from the nasal skeleton. The physician then repositions the cartilaginous components of the nose and reapproximates the overlying tissues. All skin incisions are closed with fine sutures or skin adhesive.

40761

40761   Plastic repair of cleft lip/nasal deformity; with cross lip pedicle flap (Abbe-Estlander type), including sectioning and inserting of pedicle

Cleft lip is a congenital deformity caused by failure of embryonic connective tissue composed of mesenchymal cells to migrate properly during palate formation resulting in disfigurement of the upper lip and nose. Cleft lip and nasal deformity may be unilateral or bilateral and each cleft lip deformity is unique requiring inidividualized procedure planning and surgical technique. A cross lip pedicle flap, also referred to as an Abbe-Estlander flap, is developed and transferred in a two-stage procedure. The anatomic landmarks are tattooed and incision lines marked. The orbicularis muscle is dissected from overlying skin and muscle bundles divided. The portion of the muscle that will be used to create the vermillion of Cupid's bow is left attached to the mucosa. The defect is repaired using a series of flaps including a cross lip pedicle flap. The cross lip pedicle flap on the lower lip is created by incising the vermilion border of the lip. The incision is carried through the orbicularis muscle leaving underlying labial mucosa intact and protecting the labial artery for blood supply to the flap. The flap is placed in the defect in the upper lip, but is not severed from its blood supply in the lower lip. The nose is then repaired by freeing overlying tissue from the nasal skeleton. The nasal domes are approximated and the lower lateral cartilage is suspended from the upper lateral cartilage on each side. The muscle bundles of the orbicularis muscle are approximated. In the second stage of the procedure performed several weeks later, the flap is divided, the pedicle inserted, and the transfer procedure completed.

40800-40801

40800   Drainage of abscess, cyst, hematoma, vestibule of mouth; simple
40801   Drainage of abscess, cyst, hematoma, vestibule of mouth; complicated

The vestibule of the mouth, also referred to as the buccal or oral cavity includes the mucosa and submucosa of the lips and cheeks but excludes dentoalveolar structures. The abscess, cyst or hematoma is identified and a local anesthetic injected. Mucosal tissue is incised and the abscess pocket, cyst, or hematoma opened and drained. Any loculations in the abscess pocket are broken up. Any blood clots in the hematoma are removed. Use 40800 for a simple procedure in which the incision is closed or left open to heal by secondary intention. Use 40801 for a complicated procedure that requires deeper dissection. Complicated procedures may also require gauze packing or a drain until drainage subsides.

40804-40805

40804   Removal of embedded foreign body, vestibule of mouth; simple
40805   Removal of embedded foreign body, vestibule of mouth; complicated

A straight or elliptical incision is made, the mucosa and submucosa separated, and the foreign body identified. A hemostat or grasping forceps is then used to remove the foreign body. The incision may be closed or left open to heal by secondary intention. Use 40804 for a simple incision and removal. Use 40805 for a complicated incision and removal if

the foreign body is deeply embedded and difficult to localize. The physician may need to dissect underlying tissues to remove the foreign body.

40806

40806   Incision of labial frenum (frenotomy)

A straight or elliptical incision is made, the mucosa and submucosa separated, and the foreign body identified. A hemostat or grasping forceps is then used to remove the foreign body. The incision may be closed or left open to heal by secondary intention. Use 40804 for a simple incision and removal. Use 40805 for a complicated incision and removal if the foreign body is deeply embedded and difficult to localize. The physician may need to dissect underlying tissues to remove the foreign body.

40808

40808   Biopsy, vestibule of mouth

A biopsy of the vestibule of the mouth involving the mucosa and deeper submucosal tissues is performed. The vestibule of the mouth, also referred to as the buccal or oral cavity includes the mucosa and submucosa of the lips and cheeks but excludes dentoalveolar structures. The lesion is identified and a local anesthetic injected. An incision is made in the mucosa and carried down to submucosal tissue. A tissue sample is obtained and sent for separately reportable pathology examination.

40810-40812

40810   Excision of lesion of mucosa and submucosa, vestibule of mouth; without repair
40812   Excision of lesion of mucosa and submucosa, vestibule of mouth; with simple repair

The vestibule of the mouth, also referred to as the buccal or oral cavity includes the mucosa and submucosa of the lips and cheeks but excludes dentoalveolar structures. The lesion is identified and a local anesthetic injected. A margin of healthy tissue is identified and an incision is made through the mucosa and submucosa. The incision is carried around the lesion and the entire lesion is excised. The excised tissue is sent to the laboratory for separately reportable histologic evaluation. Use 40810 when the surgical wound is left open to heal by secondary intention. Use 40812 when the wound is closed by simple single layer suture technique.

40814-40816

40814   Excision of lesion of mucosa and submucosa, vestibule of mouth; with complex repair
40816   Excision of lesion of mucosa and submucosa, vestibule of mouth; complex, with excision of underlying muscle

The vestibule of the mouth, also referred to as the buccal or oral cavity includes the mucosa and submucosa of the lips and cheeks but excludes dentoalveolar structures. The lesion is identified and a local anesthetic injected. A margin of healthy tissue is identified and an incision is made through the mucosa and submucosa. The incision is carried around the lesion and the entire lesion is excised. The surgical wound is inspected to ensure that all abnormal tissue has been removed. The tissue is sent to the laboratory for separately reportable histologic evaluation. A complex repair is performed. Extensive undermining of tissues is performed using a scissors or scalpel to minimize tension on the wound. Bleeding is controlled by chemical or electrocautery. The deepest layers are then closed with absorbable sutures and the knot is buried. Alternatively, stents or retention sutures may be used. The superficial layer is closed taking care to ensure that the wound edges are aligned and everted. Use 40814 when the excision involves only mucosa and submucosa and requires complex repair. Use 40816 when the excision involves muscle in addition to mucosa and submucosa and requires a complex repair.

40818

40818   Excision of mucosa of vestibule of mouth as donor graft

The mucosa of the lips or cheeks may be used. The parotid duct is identified and cannulated as needed to ensure that it is not disturbed. The graft configuration is outlined with a waterproof pen. A local anesthetic is administered. Parallel incisions are made through the mucosa at upper and lower borders of the graft. The incision lines of the upper and lower borders are then sharply angled so that they meet at both ends. The section of mucosa is then harvested using sharp dissection. The defect in the buccal mucosa is then repaired with sutures in a single layer. The mucosal graft is prepared for transfer to the recipient site.

40819

40819   Excision of frenum, labial or buccal (frenumectomy, frenulectomy, frenectomy)

This procedure may also be referred to as a frenumectomy, frenulectomy, or a frenectomy and may be required when the frenum causes displacement of dentures or when it is in close proximity to periodontal implant tissue. A diamond shaped incision is made in the frenum and the frenum is excised. Alternatively, if the frenum is broad, a Z-plasty type incision is made to remove the frenum and lengthen the vestibule.

40820

40820   Destruction of lesion or scar of vestibule of mouth by physical methods (eg, laser, thermal, cryo, chemical)

The lesion is examined and the most appropriate form of destruction determined. Local anesthesia is administered as needed. Cryosurgery using liquid nitrogen to freeze the lesion is one destruction technique. Surgical curettage followed by electrosurgery is another common method of destruction. Other techniques include chemosurgery with a chemotherapeutic agent such as 5-fluorouracil (5-FU) or laser destruction with a carbon dioxide laser.

40830-40831

40830   Closure of laceration, vestibule of mouth; 2.5 cm or less
40831   Closure of laceration, vestibule of mouth; over 2.5 cm or complex

The wound is cleansed and a local anesthetic administered. The wound is inspected and determined to involve the mucosa, submucosa, and deeper connective tissue. Debridement is performed as needed. A layered closure using sutures, staples, and/or tissue adhesive is performed. Tissues are undermined using a scissors or scalpel to minimize tension on the wound. Bleeding is controlled by chemical or electrocautery. The deepest layers are then closed with absorbable sutures and the knot is buried. The superficial layer is closed taking care to ensure that the wound edges are aligned and everted to prevent depression of the scar. Use 40830 for laceration with a length of 2.5 cm or less. Use 40831 when the laceration is over 2.5 cm or when complex repair is required. Complex repair includes extensive debridement and/or undermining of tissue. Stents or retention sutures may be needed to close the wound.

40840

40840   Vestibuloplasty; anterior

The vestibule of the mouth, also referred to as the buccal or oral cavity includes the mucosa and submucosa of the lips and cheeks but excludes dentoalveolar structures. Vestibuloplasty is performed to restore alveolar ridge height. The alveolar ridge is the ridge of bone on the inferior surface of the bodies of the maxilla and mandible that contains the tooth sockets. In patients with cleft lip and/or palate or other facial deformities, the vestibular soft tissue and underlying alveolar ridge bone may require remodeling to achieve the required cosmetic and functional results. This procedure may also be performed in edentulous patients with shallow vestibular sulcus to provide a better fit for dentures. Anterior vestibuloplasty involves reconstruction of tissue between the lips and the front teeth. An incision is made in the mucosa in the sulcus between the lip (labia) and alveolar ridge. Any excess mucosal tissue is excised and a mucosal flap developed. The mucosal flap is then used to cover exposed muscle and alveolar ridge tissue. Alternatively, the tissue may be excised and the underlying tissue allowed to heal by secondary intention.

40842-40843

40842   Vestibuloplasty; posterior, unilateral
40843   Vestibuloplasty; posterior, bilateral

The physician performs a posterior vestibuloplasty. The vestibule of the mouth, also referred to as the buccal or oral cavity includes the mucosa and submucosa of the lips and cheeks but excludes dentoalveolar structures. Vestibuloplasty is performed to restore alveolar ridge height. The alveolar ridge is the ridge of bone on the inferior surface of the bodies of the maxilla and mandible that contains the tooth sockets. In patients with cleft lip and/or palate or other facial deformities, the vestibular soft tissue and underlying alveolar ridge bone may require remodeling to achieve the required cosmetic and functional results. This procedure may also be performed in edentulous patients with shallow vestibular sulcus to provide a better fit for dentures. Posterior vestibuloplasty involves reconstruction of tissue between the cheeks and teeth. An incision is made in the mucosa in the sulcus between the cheek (buccal) and alveolar ridge. Any excess mucosal tissue is excised and a mucosal flap developed. The mucosal flap is then used to cover exposed muscle and alveolar ridge tissue. Alternatively, the tissue may be excised and the underlying tissue allowed to heal by secondary intention. Use 40842 for a unilateral posterior vestibuloplasty and 40843 when a bilateral procedure is performed.

40844

40844   Vestibuloplasty; entire arch

The vestibule of the mouth, also referred to as the buccal or oral cavity includes the mucosa and submucosa of the lips and cheeks but excludes dentoalveolar structures. Vestibuloplasty is performed to restore alveolar ridge height. The alveolar ridge is the ridge of bone on the inferior surface of the bodies of the maxilla and mandible that contains the tooth sockets. In patients with cleft lip and/or palate or other facial deformities, the vestibular soft tissue and underlying alveolar ridge bone may require remodeling to achieve the required cosmetic and functional results. This procedure may also be performed in edentulous patients with shallow vestibular sulcus to provide a better fit for dentures. An

incision is along the crest of the alveolar ridge and the unattached labiobuccal mucosa beginning at one retromolar pad and is carried around the alveolar ridge to the opposite retromolar pad. Any excess mucosal tissue is excised and a mucosal flap developed. If the vestibuloplasty is performed on the mandible, the lingual aspect of the vestibule is may also be incised from one side to the other and excess tissue removed. The previously developed mucosal flap is then used to cover exposed muscle and alveolar ridge tissue. Alternatively, the tissue may be excised and the underlying tissue allowed healing by secondary intention.

40845

40845   Vestibuloplasty; complex (including ridge extension, muscle repositioning)

The vestibule of the mouth, also referred to as the buccal or oral cavity includes the mucosa and submucosa of the lips and cheeks but excludes dentoalveolar structures. Vestibuloplasty is performed to restore alveolar ridge height. The alveolar ridge is the ridge of bone on the inferior surface of the bodies of the maxilla and mandible that contains the tooth sockets. In patients with cleft lip and/or palate or other facial deformities, the vestibular soft tissue and underlying alveolar ridge bone may require remodeling to achieve the required cosmetic and functional results. This procedure may also be performed in edentulous patients with shallow vestibular sulcus to provide a better fit for dentures. An incision is made in the mucosa in the sulcus between the lip (labial incision) and/or cheek (buccal incision) and alveolar ridge. Any excess mucosal tissue is excised and a mucosal flap developed. The incision is then carried down to underlying muscle and the muscles are detached. The muscles may then be reattached in such a way that lengthening of the vestibule occurs. The mucosal flap is used to cover any exposed muscle and alveolar ridge tissue. Alternatively, ridge extension may be performed by dissecting muscle and soft tissue attachments down to supraperiosteal tissue as far as the crest of the maxillary or mandibular alveolus. Excess tissue is excised or repositioned. The surgical incision is closed. A post-surgical stent or denture is placed over the alveolar ridge and secured with screws to allow the overlying tissue to adhere to the periosteum. The stent or denture is removed approximately 2 weeks later.

41000-41006

41000   Intraoral incision and drainage of abscess, cyst, or hematoma of tongue or floor of mouth; lingual
41005   Intraoral incision and drainage of abscess, cyst, or hematoma of tongue or floor of mouth; sublingual, superficial
41006   Intraoral incision and drainage of abscess, cyst, or hematoma of tongue or floor of mouth; sublingual, deep, supramylohyoid

The abscess, cyst or hematoma is identified. Mucosal tissue is incised and the abscess pocket, cyst, or hematoma opened and drained. Any compartments that have formed in the abscess pocket are broken up. Any blood clots in the hematoma are removed. Drains are placed as needed. Use 41000 when the procedure is performed on the lingual (tongue) region. Use 41005 when the abscess, cyst, or hematoma is located in the superficial sublingual (under the tongue) region. Use 41006 when deeper sublingual tissues are involved requiring dissection of the soft tissue lying just above the posterior portion of the lower jaw and hyoid bone (supramylohyoid).

41007-41009

41007   Intraoral incision and drainage of abscess, cyst, or hematoma of tongue or floor of mouth; submental space
41008   Intraoral incision and drainage of abscess, cyst, or hematoma of tongue or floor of mouth; submandibular space
41009   Intraoral incision and drainage of abscess, cyst, or hematoma of tongue or floor of mouth; masticator space

The submental, submandibular, or masticator space in the floor of mouth are deep fascial spaces located around the mandible (lower jaw). The submental space lies in the center of the lower jaw just beneath the chin. The submandibular space extends from the hyoid bone to the mucosal layer in the floor of the mouth. The mandible provides the anterior and lateral boundaries of the space and the superficial layer of the deep cervical fascial provides the inferior boundary. The masticator space is formed by a split in the layer of superficial cervical fascia that encloses the ramus of the mandible, the masseter, the medial pterygoid, and the lower portion of the temporal muscle. Loose connective tissue and fat between the fascia forms these spaces. An incision is made in the mouth over the submental, submandibular, or masticator space and underlying tissues dissected. The abscess, cyst or hematoma is exposed, opened, and drained. Any compartments that have formed in the abscess pocket or cyst are broken up. Any blood clots in the hematoma are removed. Drains are placed as needed. Use 41007 when the procedure is performed on the submental space, 41008 for the submandibular space, and 41009 for the masticator space.

41010

41010   Incision of lingual frenum (frenotomy) The lingual frenum lies in the midline of the tongue and connects the tongue to the floor of the mouth. This procedure is also referred to as lingual frenotomy and is performed to treat tongue-tie

CPT © 2016 American Medical Association. All Rights Reserved.

● New Code   ▲ Revised Code

Digestive System

(ankyloglossia) which occurs when the frenum is too short or too tight. The tongue is lifted up towards the roof of the mouth. The physician then cuts through the frenum parallel to and fairly close to the tongue. Anesthesia is typically not necessary as the cut is made in a single motion that lasts less than a second.

41015-41018

41015   **Extraoral incision and drainage of abscess, cyst, or hematoma of floor of mouth; sublingual**

41016   **Extraoral incision and drainage of abscess, cyst, or hematoma of floor of mouth; submental**

41017   **Extraoral incision and drainage of abscess, cyst, or hematoma of floor of mouth; submandibular**

41018   **Extraoral incision and drainage of abscess, cyst, or hematoma of floor of mouth; masticator space**

The sublingual, submental, submandibular, or masticator space in the floor of mouth are deep fascial spaces located in the floor of the mouth and around the mandible (lower jaw). The sublingual space lies in the floor of the mouth under the tongue. The submental space lies in the center of the lower jaw just beneath the chin. The submandibular space extends from the hyoid bone to the mucosal layer in the floor of the mouth. The mandible provides the anterior and lateral boundaries of the space and the superficial layer of the deep cervical fascia provides the inferior boundary. The masticator space is formed by a split in the layer of superficial cervical fascia that encloses the ramus of the mandible, the masseter, the medial pterygoid, and the lower portion of the temporal muscle. Loose connective tissue and fat between the fascia forms these spaces. A submandibular approach is used. Dissection is carried down through skin and subcutaneous tissue. Regardless of which space is involved the approach is through the submandibular space. The platysma muscle is divided and the submandibular space entered. If the sublingual space is involved, the incision is carried through the submandibular space, the mylohyoid muscle is divided, and the sublingual space entered. If the submental space is involved, the submandibular space is entered and dissection is carried into the submental space below the chin. If the masticator space is involved, the submandibular space is entered; dissection is carried along the lateral surface of the ramus to the masticator space. The abscess, cyst or hematoma is exposed, opened, and drained. Any loculations in the abscess pocket or cyst are broken up. Any blood clots in the hematoma are removed. Drains are placed. Use 41015 for the sublingual space, 41016 for the submental space, 41017 for the submandibular space, and 41018 for the masticator space.

41019

41019   **Placement of needles, catheters, or other device(s) into the head and/ or neck region (percutaneous, transoral, or transnasal) for subsequent interstitial radioelement application**

Needles, catheters, or other devices are placed in the head and/or neck region for interstitial radioelement application, whether percutaneous, transoral, or transnasal. This code reports the placement of the needles or catheters only. The interstitial radioelement application (brachytherapy) is reported separately. Tumor volume to be treated is first assessed and the relationship of the tumor to normal structures is evaluated. Catheter entrance and exit sites are determined and marked on the skin. Needles, catheters, or other devices are selected and prepared for placement. The skin over the first insertion site is punctured with a beveled needle that is advanced to the selected exit site while monitoring the needle's advance around the tumor to the optimal catheter tube placement site. The needle is advanced until it exits the skin at the selected exit site. A wire is inserted through the needle and brought out through the same cavity. The catheter tube, button, and silk tie are threaded over the wire, advanced until they are visible, and the external portion of the catheter tube is secured with a color coded button. The silk tie is brought out through the exit site. This process is repeated until all catheter tubes are in place. The stiff inner catheter ribbons used to stabilize the catheter during insertion are removed. The silk ties are joined and then pulled through a drain that is secured externally with tape.

41100-41105

41100   **Biopsy of tongue; anterior two-thirds**

41105   **Biopsy of tongue; posterior one-third**

Incisional biopsy is done to evaluate abnormal growths, lesions, or suspicious appearing areas of the tongue. A local anesthetic is injected at the planned biopsy site. An incision is then made in the tongue and a slice of tissue removed from the suspicious area. The tissue sample is then sent for separately reportable pathology examination. Use 41100 for biopsy of the anterior two-thirds of the tongue and 41105 for biopsy of the posterior two-thirds.

41108

41108   **Biopsy of floor of mouth**

This procedure is done to evaluate abnormal growths, lesions, or suspicious appearing areas of the floor of the mouth. A local anesthetic is injected at the planned biopsy site. An incision is then made in the floor of the mouth and a slice of tissue removed from the suspicious area. The tissue sample is then sent for separately reportable pathology examination.

41110-41114

41110   **Excision of lesion of tongue without closure**

41112   **Excision of lesion of tongue with closure; anterior two-thirds**

41113   **Excision of lesion of tongue with closure; posterior one-third**

41114   **Excision of lesion of tongue with closure; with local tongue flap**

A local anesthetic is injected around and below the lesion. An incision is made through the epithelium and into the underlying fibrous tissue and muscle. The incision is carried around the lesion and the lesion is excised along with a margin of healthy tissue. The lesion is sent to the laboratory for separately reportable pathology examination. In 41110, a small superficial lesion is excised without closure of surgical site. In 41112, a larger, deeper lesion in the anterior two-thirds of the tongue is excised with suture repair of the surgical site. In 41113, a larger, deeper lesion in the posterior one-third of the tongue is excised with suture repair of the surgical site. In 41114 a lesion is excised and the tongue is repaired with a local tongue flap. Adjacent myomucosal tongue tissue is incised, elevated and rotated over the surgical defect created by excision of the lesion. The flap is sutured over the defect and the donor site closed with sutures.

41115

41115   **Excision of lingual frenum (frenectomy)**

This is also referred to as a lingual frenectomy. The procedure is performed to treat ankyloglossia more commonly referred to as tongue-tie. The frenum is exposed by placement of tension sutures bilaterally through the sides of the tongue. The frenum is then excised beginning at the tip of the tongue moving backward to the mandibular lingual alveolus. Once the frenum is completely excised the mucosa of the tongue and floor of the mouth is undermined and repaired with sutures.

41116

41116   **Excision, lesion of floor of mouth**

A local anesthetic is injected around and below the lesion. An incision is made through the mucosa and submucosal tissue. The incision is carried around the lesion and the lesion is excised along with a margin of healthy tissue. The lesion is sent to the laboratory for separately reportable pathology examination.

41120-41135

41120   **Glossectomy; less than one-half tongue**

41130   **Glossectomy; hemiglossectomy**

41135   **Glossectomy; partial, with unilateral radical neck dissection**

A glossectomy is performed to remove less than one-half of the tongue. Partial glossectomy is usually performed to treat cancer of the tongue, but may also be performed to relieve obstruction of the lower pharynx, to treat an injury to the tongue, as well as other conditions. When performed for cancer of the tongue, an incision is made in the tongue and the tongue lesion is excised along with a margin of healthy surrounding tongue tissue. The tongue defect is repaired by suture. If the excision is more extensive, separately reportable skin graft or a free flap graft may be used to repair the defect. In 41130, a hemiglossectomy is performed. Hemiglossectomy is the removal of one-side or one-half of the tongue. An incision is made in the lower jaw under the mandible on the affected side. The mandible is split to allow access to the floor of the mouth. The side of the tongue with the lesion or tumor is removed along with a margin of healthy tongue tissue. The defect in the tongue is closed by primary suture or a separately reportable skin graft or free flap graft is placed. The mandible is wired together. The incision is closed and drains placed. In 41135, a partial glossectomy is performed with a unilateral radical neck dissection. A partial or hemiglossectomy is performed as described above. A unilateral radical neck dissection (RND) is then performed. Lymph node groups levels I-V are dissected free of surrounding tissue and excised. The sternocleidomastoid muscle and the internal jugular vein are removed. The submandibular gland on the affected side is removed. The anterior belly of the digastric muscle as well as the sternohyoid and sternothyroid muscles may also be removed.

41140-41145

41140   **Glossectomy; complete or total, with or without tracheostomy, without radical neck dissection**

41145   **Glossectomy; complete or total, with or without tracheostomy, with unilateral radical neck dissection**

Complete or total glossectomy is performed to treat cancer of the tongue. Complete or total glossectomy is the removal of more the one-half or one side of the tongue. If a tracheostomy is required, a vertical or horizontal incision is made in the neck over the cricoid cartilage. Subcutaneous fat is removed by electrocautery. Dissection is carried out through the platysma to the raphe between the strap muscles. The strap muscles are separated and the pretracheal fascia and thyroid isthmus exposed. The thyroid isthmus is divided. The trachea is incised and a tracheostomy tube is inserted and secured. Following placement of the tracheostomy tube, an incision is made in the lower jaw under the mandible. The mandible is split to allow access to the floor of the mouth. The entire tongue or a portion involving more than half the tongue is removed along with a margin of

   ● New Code   ▲ Revised Code

Digestive System

healthy tissue. The defect is closed by primary suture. Alternatively, a separately reportable skin graft or free flap graft may be placed or a separately reportable reconstruction of the tongue may be performed. The mandible is wired together. The incision is closed and drains placed. In 41145, a complete or total glossectomy is performed with a unilateral radical neck dissection. A complete or total glossectomy with or without tracheostomy is performed as described above. A unilateral radical neck dissection (RND) is then performed. Lymph node groups levels I-V are dissected free of surrounding tissue and excised. The sternocleidomastoid muscle and the internal jugular vein are removed. The submandibular gland on the affected side is removed. The anterior belly of the digastric muscle as well as the sternohyoid and sternothyroid muscles may also be removed.

41150-41155

41150   Glossectomy; composite procedure with resection floor of mouth and mandibular resection, without radical neck dissection

41153   Glossectomy; composite procedure with resection floor of mouth, with suprahyoid neck dissection

41155   Glossectomy; composite procedure with resection floor of mouth, mandibular resection, and radical neck dissection (Commando type)

A glossectomy is performed in a composite procedure that includes resection of the floor of the mouth and a mandibular resection. This procedure is typically performed to treat cancer of the tongue and oropharynx with involvement of the mandible. The mandible is resected first. A visor flap is employed to gain access to the mandible. This involves incision of the lower gingival buccal sulcus along the mandible. The periosteum of the mandible is undermined and the skin of the chin and lower lip is elevated. The involved mandible is resected. The mucosa of the floor of the mouth is incised and the diseased tissue is removed along with a margin of surrounding healthy tissue. Typically resection of the floor of the mouth includes the soft tissue deep to the sublingual glands with transection of the Wharton duct. The involved portion of the tongue is removed along with a margin of healthy tissue. The defects are typically repaired by separately reportable reconstructive surgeries that may include skin grafts, free flap grafts, and mandibular reconstruction. Code 41150 is used when the procedure described above is performed without radical neck resection. Code 41153 is used when the composite procedure is performed with suprahyoid neck dissection. A suprahyoid neck dissection is a limited neck dissection with excision of the submandibular salivary gland and the lymph nodes of the submandibular triangle only. Code 41155 is used when the composite procedure is performed with a radical neck dissection (RND). The composite procedure that includes glossectomy, resection of the floor of the mouth, and a RND is also called a Commando procedure. In RND, the lymph node groups levels I-V are dissected free of surrounding tissue and excised. The sternocleidomastoid muscle and the internal jugular vein are removed. The submandibular gland on the affected side is removed. The anterior belly of the digastric muscle as well as the sternohyoid and sternothyroid muscles may also be removed.

41250-41252

41250   Repair of laceration 2.5 cm or less; floor of mouth and/or anterior two-thirds of tongue

41251   Repair of laceration 2.5 cm or less; posterior one-third of tongue

41252   Repair of laceration of tongue, floor of mouth, over 2.6 cm or complex

The laceration is irrigated and debridement is performed as needed. A layered closure using sutures is performed. Tissues are undermined using a scissors or scalpel to minimize tension on the wound. Bleeding is controlled by chemical or electrocautery. The deepest layers are then closed with absorbable sutures and the knot is buried. The superficial layer is closed taking care to ensure that the wound edges are aligned and everted to prevent depression of the scar. If there is a deep or through-and -through laceration of the tongue, a three layer closure is performed. The muscular mucosa is closed first followed by the inferior mucosa. Sutures are carried around the side or tip of the tongue to the superior aspect which is the last layer closed. Use 41250 for a laceration of the floor of the mouth and/or anterior 2/3 of the tongue with a length of 2.5 cm or less. Use 41251 when the laceration is 2.5 cm or less and involves the posterior 1/3 of the tongue. Use 41252 for a laceration of the floor of the mouth and/or tongue with a length of 2.6 cm or more or when a complex repair is required. Complex repair includes extensive debridement and/or undermining of tissue. Stents or retention sutures may be needed to close the wound.

41500

41500   Fixation of tongue, mechanical, other than suture (eg, K-wire)

Mechanical fixation of the tongue is used to treat conditions where the tongue falls back and obstructs the airway. K-wire fixation is accomplished by making an incision in the buccal mucosa over the mandibular oblique ridge bilaterally. The mandibular angle is then exposed and a K-wire is passed into the angle of the mandible on one side across the floor of the mouth and through base of the tongue, and through the angle of the mandible on the opposite side.

41510

41510   Suture of tongue to lip for micrognathia (Douglas type procedure)

The tongue is sutured to the lip to treat micrognathia, a congenital anomaly in which the jaw and chin is smaller than normal. This can lead to feeding and breathing problems. An incision is made in the lower lip and a strip of mucosa excised. A second incision is made in the posterior aspect of the tongue and a strip of mucosa excised. The tongue is released from the mandibular symphysis and traction applied. The lip and tongue are then sutured together along the length of the previously excised mucosal strips.

41512

41512   Tongue base suspension, permanent suture technique

Tongue base suspension is performed using permanent suture technique. This procedure is performed to treat obstructive sleep apnea and snoring. This is accomplished by placing a suture at the base of the tongue to provide support and prevent backward prolapse of the posterior tongue base when the patient is in a supine position. A bite block or mouth retractor is placed in the mouth to facilitate exposure of the tongue base. A temporary suture is placed in the tip of the tongue to allow easy manipulation of the tongue during the surgery. The anterior mandible is palpated intraorally and the genioglossal tubercle is identified. A stab incision is made at the base of the frenulum. A screw with attached suture is placed in the mandible at the level of the genioglossal tubercle and below the teeth roots using an inserter device. The tongue is retracted using the previously placed suture at the tip, and the floor of the mouth is exposed. A suture is passed through a previously created insertion hole or incision in the mouth floor and through the tongue to create a looped suture at the base of the tongue. The looped suture is threaded from the anterior portion of the tongue to the posterior base on one side of the tongue. This is repeated on the contralateral side. The screw suture is attached to a needle and passed through the looped suture protruding from the posterior tongue base. The looped suture is tightened to move the screw suture in an anterior direction toward the floor of the mouth. This creates a triangular suture pattern to anchor the tongue base. The suture ends are tied and the posterior tongue base is palpated to ensure that the anchor incision is properly placed. The knot is secured and buried. The incision at the base of the tongue is closed.

41520

41520   Frenoplasty (surgical revision of frenum, eg, with Z-plasty)

A frenoplasty, also referred to as frenuloplasty, is performed. Frenoplasty may be performed to treat recurrent ankyloglossia (tongue-tie) following a previous frenotomy or frenectomy. A four flap Z-plasty or Z-frenoplasty is one method. Four flaps are required rather than two because the scar extends from the floor of the mouth along the posterior aspect of the tongue. Two triangular flaps are created with an angle of approximately 60 degrees in the floor of the mouth. This is repeated in the tongue. The lateral incisions must be the exact length of the central incision with the central incision being placed along the scar from the previous frenotomy or frenectomy. The incision lines are undermined and the flaps in the floor of the mouth are rotated and sutured into place. This is repeated with the tongue flaps.

41530

41530   Submucosal ablation of the tongue base, radiofrequency, 1 or more sites, per session

Submucosal ablation of the tongue base is performed at one or more sites using radiofrequency tissue ablation (RFTA) to reshape and reduce the base of the tongue. This procedure is performed to treat obstructive sleep apnea caused by hypertrophy of the tongue base. Using a percutaneous approach, a radiofrequency electrode is inserted upward through the chin and advanced up into the base of the tongue, taking care not to puncture the mucosa. The electrode is activated, creating a thermal lesion that lies entirely within the muscular portion of the tongue. The electrode may be repositioned and activated at several sites along the tongue base to create a lesion of the desired size and configuration. Tongue base reduction using radiofrequency requires multiple treatment sessions, and each treatment session is reported separately.

41800

41800   Drainage of abscess, cyst, hematoma from dentoalveolar structures

The dentoalveolar structures include the periapical region and dental pulp, the periodontal region comprised of the periodontal ligaments and alveolar bone, and the gum surrounding the teeth. The tooth is extracted as needed. The abscess, cyst or hematoma is exposed, incised, and drained. Any loculations in the abscess pocket or cyst are broken up. Any blood clots in the hematoma are removed. The incision is left open to drain or packed with gauze.

42000

42000   Drainage of abscess of palate, uvula

The palate forms the roof of the mouth and is composed of a bony anterior portion referred to as the hard palate and a muscular posterior portion referred to as the soft palate. The uvula is a conical structure projecting from the soft palate that is composed of connective

Digestive System

tissue, racemose glands, and some muscular fibers. The roof of the mouth is examined and the abscess pocket in the soft palate and/or uvula identified. A needle is used to puncture the abscess pocket and the pus is aspirated. Alternatively, the abscess pocket is incised and as the pus drains from the pocket it is suctioned from the throat. The incision is left open to drain.

42100

42100   Biopsy of palate, uvula

The palate forms the roof of the mouth and is composed of a bony anterior portion referred to as the hard palate and a muscular posterior portion referred to as the soft palate. The uvula is a conical structure projecting from the soft palate that is composed of connective tissue, racemose glands, and some muscular fibers. The roof of the mouth is examined and the lesion in the palate and/or uvula identified. The lesion is incised and a tissue sample obtained. The tissue sample is sent to the laboratory for separately reportable histological evaluation.

42104-42107

42104   Excision, lesion of palate, uvula; without closure
42106   Excision, lesion of palate, uvula; with simple primary closure
42107   Excision, lesion of palate, uvula; with local flap closure

The palate is forms the roof of the mouth and is composed of a bony anterior portion referred to as the hard palate and a muscular posterior portion referred to as the soft palate. The uvula is a conical structure projecting from the soft palate that is composed of connective tissue, racemose glands, and some muscular fibers. The roof of the mouth is examined and the lesion in the palate and/or uvula identified. A margin of healthy tissue is identified and an incision is made through the mucosa and submucosa. The incision is carried around the lesion and the entire lesion is excised. The lesion is sent to the laboratory for separately reportable histologic evaluation. Use 42104 when the surgical wound is left open to heal by secondary intention. Use 42106 when the wound is closed by simple single layer suture technique. Use 42107 when local flap closure is performed which involves elevating a flap of mucosa adjacent to the excision site and suturing it over the surgical wound.

42120

42120   Resection of palate or extensive resection of lesion

This procedure is performed for benign tumors or premalignant or malignant lesions of the hard or soft palate. A mucosal incision is made around the periphery of the lesion or the area of the palate to be resected. If the area is in the soft palate, the incision is carried down through submucosal and connective tissue and the involved region removed with a margin a healthy tissue. If the hard palate is involved, the incision is carried down through the periosteum and the periosteum is elevated. An osteotome or oscillating saw is used to cut through involved bone in the hard palate. The involved region is removed along with a margin of healthy tissue. The tissue is sent to for separately reportable pathology examination. The surgical defect may be closed using lateral relaxing incisions and a local mucosal advancement flap and primary closure of the donor site. Larger defects may require a local palatal flap with the donor site left to heal by secondary intension. Separately reportable extraoral tissue grafts may also be used for reconstruction. Excision of the bone typically requires separately reportable reconstruction with a palatal obturator.

42140

42140   Uvulectomy, excision of uvula

This procedure is typically performed on patients with enlarged or elongated uvulas to reduce snoring or treat obstructive sleep apnea. The back of the throat is treated with a topical anesthetic. A local anesthetic is injected around the uvula. The uvula is then removed using electrocautery. The electrocautery device excises the uvula and controls bleeding.

42145

42145   Palatopharyngoplasty (eg, uvulopalatopharyngoplasty, uvulopharyngoplasty)

This procedure is performed to treat obstructive sleep apnea caused by collapse of the oropharyngeal airway. The uvula, all or part of the soft palate and/or excess tissue in the throat is removed. The area to be excised is marked and the mucosa incised. The incision is carried down through submucosal tissue and the tissue causing the airway obstruction during sleep is excised. Once all excess tissue has been removed, primary suture closure of the surgical wound is performed.

42160

42160   Destruction of lesion, palate or uvula (thermal, cryo or chemical)

The lesion is examined and the most appropriate form of destruction determined. Local anesthesia is administered as needed. Cryosurgery using liquid nitrogen to freeze the lesion is one destruction technique. Surgical curettage followed by electrosurgery is another common method of destruction. Alternatively, chemosurgery with a chemotherapeutic agent such as 5-fluorouracil (5-FU) may be used to destroy the lesion.

42180-42182

42180   Repair, laceration of palate; up to 2 cm
42182   Repair, laceration of palate; over 2 cm or complex

The laceration is irrigated and debridement is performed as needed. A layered closure using sutures is performed. Tissues are undermined using a scissors or scalpel to minimize tension on the wound. Bleeding is controlled by chemical or electrocautery. The deepest layers are then closed with absorbable sutures and the knot is buried. The superficial layer is closed taking care to ensure that the wound edges are aligned and everted to prevent depression of the scar. Use 42180 for a laceration of 2 cm or less. Use 42182 for a laceration over 2 cm or a complex repair. Complex repair includes extensive debridement and/or undermining of tissue. Stents or retention sutures may be needed to close the wound.

42200

42200   Palatoplasty for cleft palate, soft and/or hard palate only

Cleft palate is a congenital deformity in which the roof of the mouth does not develop normally during pregnancy, leaving an opening into the nasal cavity. Cleft palate can occur in the hard palate at the front of the mouth, the soft palate at the back of the mouth, or in both the hard and soft palate. It may occur alone or with other congenital defects of the face and skull with the most common associated defect being cleft lip. The hard and/ or soft palate is repaired by creating bipedicle mucoperiosteal flaps. The lateral edges of the oral aspect of the cleft are incised to a point behind (posterior to) the alveolar ridge. The flaps are elevated and advanced medially taking care to preserve the greater palatine arteries. The flaps are sutured together in layers to cover the defect and separate the oral and nasal cavities. The nasal mucosa is then repaired using a mucoperiosteal flap from the non-cleft side of the vomer. The flap is elevated, advanced over the defect and sutured in layers to close the nasal defect. Open areas are left to heal by secondary intention.

42205-42210

42205   Palatoplasty for cleft palate, with closure of alveolar ridge; soft tissue only
42210   Palatoplasty for cleft palate, with closure of alveolar ridge; with bone graft to alveolar ridge (includes obtaining graft)

A palatoplasty for cleft palate is performed with closure of the alveolar ridge. Cleft palate is a congenital deformity in which the roof of the mouth does not develop normally during pregnancy, leaving an opening into the nasal cavity. Cleft palate can occur in the hard palate at the front of the mouth, the soft palate at the back of the mouth, or in both the hard and soft palate. It may occur alone or with other congenital defects of the face and skull with the most common associated defect being cleft lip. In 42205, closure of soft tissue only is performed. Bipedicle mucoperiosteal flaps are created that extend into to alveolar ridge. The lateral edges of the oral aspect of the cleft are incised to include the alveolar ridge. The flaps are elevated and advanced medially taking care to preserve the greater palatine arteries. The flaps are sutured together in layers to cover the palatal defect including the alveolar ridge and separate the oral and nasal cavities. The nasal mucosa is then repaired using a mucoperiosteal flap from the non-cleft side of the vomer. The flap is elevated, advanced over the defect and sutured in layers to close the nasal defect. Open areas are left to heal by secondary intention. In 42210, a palatoplasty is performed and a bone graft is also used to repair the alveolar ridge. The mucoperiosteum is incised along the defect as described above. The alveolar ridge defect is exposed. A bone graft is harvested, usually from the mandible, and inserted into the alveolar ridge defect. The repair then proceeds as described above.

42215-42225

42215   Palatoplasty for cleft palate; major revision
42220   Palatoplasty for cleft palate; secondary lengthening procedure
42225   Palatoplasty for cleft palate; attachment pharyngeal flap

A secondary palatoplasty is performed for cleft palate which may involve a major revision (42215), secondary lengthening procedure (42220), or attachment of a pharyngeal flap (42225). The primary objectives of cleft palate repair are closure of the defect with good velopharyngeal function that allows normal eating, breathing and intelligible speech. Some patients require a secondary procedure to achieve these objectives. In 42215, a major revision of a previous palatoplasty is performed. The procedure depends on the exact nature of the residual defect. The physician assesses the post-operative deficits following the first procedure and revises the repair. Tissue including mucosa, submucosa, mucoperiosteum, and muscle is rearranged as needed to close the defect. In 42220, a secondary lengthening procedure is performed with the most common procedure being the V-Y pushback procedure. Two posterior unipedicle flaps are created taking care to preserve the greater palatine artery along with one or two anterior pedicle flaps. The anterior flaps are rotated over the anterior aspect of the defect. The anterior flaps are sutured at the midline. The posterior flaps are rotated over the defect to the anterior flaps using V-Y advancement technique to increase the length of the palate. The posterior flaps are then sutured to the anterior flaps and to each other at the midline. In 42225, a pharyngeal flap is attached. The soft palate is incised at the uvula and the incision is extended anteriorly toward the hard palate to create a superiorly based flap. The flap is elevated off the

Digestive System

prevertebral fascia. It is then rotated and inset over the defect. The donor site may be closed with sutures or a separately reportable graft placed.

42226-42227

42226   Lengthening of palate, and pharyngeal flap
42227   Lengthening of palate, with island flap

The palate is lengthened with a pharyngeal flap (42226) or with an island flap (42227). In 42226, a pharyngeal flap is created by incising the soft palate at the uvula. The incision is extended anteriorly toward the hard palate to create a superiorly based flap. The flap is elevated off the prevertebral fascia. It is then rotated and inset over the defect. The donor site is closed with sutures. In 42227, the palate is lengthened using an island flap such as a buccinator sandwich flap. This requires bilateral buccinator flaps. The flaps are outlined on the midpart of each cheek, below the parotid duct opening (papilla). The mucosa on each side is raised along with full-thickness of the buccinator muscle in an anteroposterior direction. The flaps are islanded on a pedicle of the buccinator muscle taking care to preserve blood supply from the buccinator artery. The first flap is sutured with the muscosal surface facing upward into the nasal layer. The second flap from the opposite check is sutured over the first flap with the mucosal surface facing down into the oral layer of the defect. The donor sites are closed with sutures.

42235

42235   Repair of anterior palate, including vomer flap

The anterior palate is repaired which may include use of a vomer flap to close nasal or oral defects in the palate. The defect in the anterior aspect of the palate may be repaired by elevating a full-thickness or split-thickness mucosal flap from the unaffected aspect of the palate. The flap is then rotated and sutured over the defect. The vomer bone forms the inferior and posterior portion of the nasal septum. The palatal tissue is incised over the base of the vomer in an anterior to posterior direction. The mucoperisteum is elevated off the vomer on one or both sides. The vomer flap is then advanced over the defect and secured with sutures. Open areas are left to heal by secondary intention.

42260

42260   Repair of nasolabial fistula

A nasolabial fistula is an abnormal communication or opening located between the upper lip and the nose and is a frequent complication of cleft palate repair. The intraoral aspect of the lip is divided and the nasolabial fistula is exposed. The nasal mucosa is elevated and the mucosal edges of the fistula trimmed and approximated with sutures to close the nasal floor. A flap of mucosa is elevated adjacent to the labial aspect of the fistula and rotated over the defect. The defect is closed with sutures.

42280

42280   Maxillary impression for palatal prosthesis

A maxillary impression is taken for fabrication of a palatal prosthesis. A palatal prosthesis is placed when there is a defect in the palate or maxilla that cannot be immediately repaired using another technique such as tissue flaps or grafts. Pliable impression material is applied to the maxilla including the hard palate and alveolar ridge. The impression material is allowed to harden and is then removed. A palatal prosthesis will be fashioned in a separately reportable procedure using the maxillary impression.

42281

42281   Insertion of pin-retained palatal prosthesis

A previously fabricated palatal prosthesis is inserted and secured with pins to the maxilla. The defect in the palate is exposed. The prosthesis is placed in the defect and the fit evaluated and adjusted as needed. The fixation sites are identified and drill holes placed. Pins are then placed into the drill holes to secure the prosthesis.

42300-42305

42300   Drainage of abscess; parotid, simple
42305   Drainage of abscess; parotid, complicated

Salivary gland abscess is also referred to as sialoadenitis. The parotid glands, which are the largest salivary glands, are located in front of the ears and extend to the area beneath the earlobe along the border of the mandible. An incision is made anterior to the ear and carried under the jaw. Skin flaps are raised and the fat and fascia overlying the parotid gland is exposed. The fat is dissected and the fascia overlying the parotid gland exposed. One or more incisions are made in the parotid gland parallel to the facial nerve branches. Pus is drained from the abscess cavity. The abscess cavity is irrigated with sterile saline or antibiotic solution. Drains are placed as needed and the incision closed. Use 42300 for simple drainage of a small abscess and 42305 for complicated drainage of a more extensive abscess requiring multiple incisions.

42310-42320

42310   Drainage of abscess; submaxillary or sublingual, intraoral
42320   Drainage of abscess; submaxillary, external

Salivary gland abscess is also referred to sialoadentis. The sublingual salivary glands lie below the tongue and open through several ducts into the floor of the mouth. The submaxillary gland, also referred to as the submandibular gland, is the second largest salivary gland and is located in front of the angle of the jaw in the triangle of the neck below the mandible. It drains into a duct (Warthin's duct) in the floor of the mouth lateral to the lingual frenum. The submandibular gland is divided into superficial lobes, which lie superficial to the mylohyoid muscle, and deep lobes that wrap around the posterior aspect of the mylohyoid muscle. In 42310, an intraoral drainage of a submaxillary or sublingual gland is performed. To drain the submaxillary or sublingual glands, the Wharton duct is identified and protected. The mucosa overlying the submaxillary and sublingual glands is incised and the lingual nerve identified and protected. The mylohyoid muscle is retracted and the sublingual gland exposed. If the abcess is in the sublingual gland it is incised and drained. If the abscess is in the submaxillary gland, the soft tissue dissection continues until the submaxillary gland is exposed. It is then incised and drained. In 42320, an external (extraoral) drainage of a submaxillary gland abscess is performed. The neck is incised just below the lower jaw. Overlying soft tissue is dissected and surrounding muscles divided taking care to protect the mandibular branch of the facial nerve. The gland is incised and the abscess drained. Drains are placed and incisions closed around the drains.

42330-42340

42330   Sialolithotomy; submandibular (submaxillary), sublingual or parotid, uncomplicated, intraoral
42335   Sialolithotomy; submandibular (submaxillary), complicated, intraoral
42340   Sialolithotomy; parotid, extraoral or complicated intraoral

A calculus is removed from the submandibular (submaxillary) or parotid salivary gland or duct. This procedure is also referred to as a sialolithomy. In 42330, an uncomplicated, intraoral procedure is performed to remove a calculus from either the sublingual or parotid duct or gland. The papilla of the salivary duct of the involved gland is identified and protected. The mucosa over the duct or gland is incised and the region of the duct or gland containing the calculus is exposed. The salivary gland or duct is incised and the calculus dissected free of the surrounding tissue. The duct or gland is repaired with sutures as is the overlying mucosa. In 42335 and 42340, a complicated intraoral procedure is performed to remove a calculus from the submandibular duct/gland or parotid duct/gland respectively. Complicated removal typically involves a calculus located at a site that is more difficult to access requiring more extensive dissection of surrounding tissue with identification and protection of surrounding nerves and blood vessels. Complicated removal may also be performed if there are multiple calculi or a very large calculus.

42400-42405

42400   Biopsy of salivary gland; needle
42405   Biopsy of salivary gland; incisional

Needle or incisional biopsy of a salivary gland is performed. Biopsy is performed to determine the cause of enlargement of the gland, to evaluate a lump or mass on the gland, or to diagnose Sjogren's disease. Sjogren's disease is an autoimmune disorder characterized by decreased tearing, dry mouth, and dry mucous membranes. In 42400, a core needle biopsy is performed. The skin over the biopsy site is disinfected and a local anesthetic injected. A small incision is made in the skin. The needle is then inserted into the salivary gland and a tissue sample obtained. Separately reportable imaging guidance may be used to help guide the needle to the desired location if a lump or mass is present. The tissue sample is prepared for separately reportable histological evaluation. In 42405, an incision is made in the skin and subcutaneous tissues dissected to expose the salivary gland and/or the suspicious lump or mass. A tissue sample is then obtained and sent for separately reportable histological evaluation.

42408-42409

42408   Excision of sublingual salivary cyst (ranula)
42409   Marsupialization of sublingual salivary cyst (ranula)

Salivary cysts or ranulas are mucoceles that occur in the floor of the mouth due to trauma to the sublingual gland or duct, obstruction of the duct, or infection of the gland. Mucous escapes from the damaged gland or duct and collects in the soft tissues of the floor of the mouth forming a cyst. In 42408, the cyst is excised. Whartun's duct is cannulated prior to dissection of tissue so that it can be identified and protected. An incision is made over the cyst that is carefully dissected from surrounding tissue, taking care not to cause additional injury to the sublingual salivary gland, submandibular duct or lingual nerve. The cyst is removed and the surgical wound is repaired in layers. In 42409, the cyst is marsupialized. The cyst is exposed as described above. The roof of the cyst is excised, the wall is sutured to surrounding mucosa, and the lumen of the cyst is packed with gauze. This allows the cyst to heal from the inside out.

Digestive System

42410-42415

42410 Excision of parotid tumor or parotid gland; lateral lobe, without nerve dissection

42415 Excision of parotid tumor or parotid gland; lateral lobe, with dissection and preservation of facial nerve

The lateral lobe of the parotid gland or a parotid tumor in the lateral aspect of the gland is excised with or without nerve dissection. The parotid gland is the largest of the three major paired salivary glands located below and in front of the ear. An incision is made just in front of the auricle of the ear, carried down around the ear lobe, and extended along the mandible. A skin flap is elevated and the parotid gland exposed. The inferior aspect of the parotid gland is dissected off the sternocleidomastoid muscle. Dissection continues to the digastric muscle. The tissue anterior to the tip and superior to the tragus is carefully dissected and the trunk of the facial nerve exposed. The lateral lobe of the parotid gland or the parotid tumor in the lateral lobe is excised. If deeper dissection is required, a nerve stimulator is used to identify facial nerve branches. The parotid gland is divided and retracted to expose the nerve branches. The parotid gland or tumor is carefully dissected free of the facial nerve and branches which are preserved. Bleeding is controlled with electrocautery. A drain is placed through a separate incision behind the ear. The platysma muscle, subcutaneous tissue and skin are then closed in layers. Use 42410 if the lateral lobe of the parotid gland or a parotid tumor in the lateral lobe is excised without nerve dissection. Use 42415, if nerve dissection is performed with preservation of the facial nerve.

42420-42425

42420 Excision of parotid tumor or parotid gland; total, with dissection and preservation of facial nerve

42425 Excision of parotid tumor or parotid gland; total, en bloc removal with sacrifice of facial nerve

Total excision of the parotid gland or a parotid tumor in is performed with nerve dissection and preservation of the facial nerve (42420) or en bloc removal is performed with sacrifice of the facial nerve (42425). The parotid gland is the largest of the three major paired salivary glands located below and in front of the ear. An incision is made just in front of the auricle of the ear, carried down around the ear lobe, and extended along the mandible. A skin flap is elevated and the parotid gland exposed. The inferior aspect of the parotid gland is dissected off the sternocleidomastoid muscle. Dissection continues to the digastric muscle. The tissue anterior to the tip and superior to the tragus is carefully dissected and the trunk of the facial nerve exposed. A nerve stimulator is used to identify facial nerve branches. The parotid gland is divided and retracted to expose the nerve branches. In 42420, the entire parotid gland or tumor is carefully dissected free of the facial nerve and branches and the facial nerve is preserved. In 42425, the tumor has invaded the facial nerve and an en bloc removal of the entire parotid gland and tumor is performed with sacrifice of the facial nerve. Bleeding is controlled with electrocautery. A drain is placed through a separate incision behind the ear. The platysma muscle, subcutaneous tissue and skin are then closed in layers.

42426

42426 Excision of parotid tumor or parotid gland; total, with unilateral radical neck dissection

The parotid gland is the largest of the three major paired salivary glands located below and in front of the ear. An incision is made just in front of the auricle of the ear, carried down around the ear lobe, and extended along the mandible. A skin flap is elevated and the parotid gland exposed. The inferior aspect of the parotid gland is dissected off the sternocleidomastoid muscle. Dissection continues to the digastric muscle. The tissue anterior to the tip and superior to the tragus is carefully dissected and the trunk of the facial nerve exposed. A nerve stimulator is used to identify facial nerve branches. The parotid gland is divided and retracted to expose the nerve branches. Typically, the tumor has invaded the facial nerve and an en bloc removal of the entire parotid gland and tumor is performed with sacrifice of the facial nerve. Bleeding is controlled with electrocautery. A drain is placed through a separate incision behind the ear. A radical neck dissection is then performed. The lymph node groups levels I-V are dissected free of surrounding tissue and excised. The sternocleidomastoid muscle and the internal jugular vein are removed. The submandibular gland on the affected side is removed. The anterior belly of the digastric muscle as well as the sternohyoid and sternothyroid muscles may also be removed. The surgical wounds are repaired and suction drains placed as needed.

42440

42440 Excision of submandibular (submaxillary) gland

The paired submandibular glands are one or three pairs of major salivary glands. In this procedure one of the submandibular glands is removed. An incision is made in the upper aspect of the neck just below the mandible. The submandibular gland is exposed and dissected free of surrounding tissue taking care to protect the marginal mandibular branch of the facial nerve. The submandibular gland is removed. A drain is placed in the surgical wound and the incision closed around the drain.

42450

42450 Excision of sublingual gland

Wharton's duct is cannulated prior to dissection of tissue so that it can be identified and protected. An incision is made medial to the sublingual salivary gland and the gland is dissected from surrounding tissue taking care to protect the submandibular duct and the lingual nerve. The sublingual gland is removed. The surgical wound is repaired in layers.

42500-42505

42500 Plastic repair of salivary duct, sialodochoplasty; primary or simple

42505 Plastic repair of salivary duct, sialodochoplasty; secondary or complicated

Plastic repair of a salivary duct, also referred to as sialodochoplasty, is performed. Repair of a salivary duct is usually related to penetrating injury to the face with involvement of the salivary duct. The parotid ducts are more commonly injured due to their location, although injury to the submandibular (submaxillary) or sublingual ducts may also occur. The wound is explored, the salivary duct located, and the extent of injury determined. In 42500, a primary or simple repair is performed. The proximal and distal segments are of the duct are located and the edges trimmed as needed. A catheter is placed through the duct papilla (opening) and advanced to the site of injury. The duct is then repaired over the catheter which is left in place while the duct heals. In 42505, a secondary or complicated repair is performed. Secondary repair is performed following a failed primary repair. Complicated repair may be required for an old injury, a heavily contaminated or infected wound, or when the location of the injury requires extensive dissection of overlying tissues. The salivary duct is exposed. The wound is copiously irrigated to remove debris. Surrounding and ductal tissue is debrided as needed. The distal and proximal segments of the duct are mobilized to allow tension free anastomosis. A catheter is placed as described above and the duct is repaired (anastomosed) over the catheter. The catheter is left in place until the duct heals.

42507-42510

42507 Parotid duct diversion, bilateral (Wilke type procedure)

42509 Parotid duct diversion, bilateral (Wilke type procedure); with excision of both submandibular glands

42510 Parotid duct diversion, bilateral (Wilke type procedure); with ligation of both submandibular (Wharton's) ducts

A bilateral parotid duct diversion, also referred to as a Wilke procedure, is performed to treat excessive salivation (sialorrhea) which results in uncontrolled drooling. Sialorrhea is usually caused by a neurological deficit such as cerebral palsy or a head injury. Saliva is produced primarily by the three major paired salivary glands, the parotid, submandibular, and sublingual glands. In 42507, the parotid ducts are individually dissected from surrounding tissue with a cuff of mucosa and removed. Each duct is then transposed to the tonsillar fossae and secured with sutures. In 42509, the parotid duct diversion procedure is performed as described above and both submandibular glands are also excised. Bilateral incisions are made in the upper aspect of the neck just below the mandible. Both submandibular glands are exposed and dissected free of surrounding tissue, taking care to protect the marginal mandibular branch of the facial nerve. The submandibular glands are removed, a drain is placed in the surgical wound, and the incision is closed around the drain. In 42510, the submandibular (Wharton's) ducts are also suture ligated and divided. The Wharton's duct openings (papillae) are identified on the floor of the mouth just lateral to the frenulum of the tongue. An incision is made between the papillae. The first duct is exposed distally for a length of approximately 1 cm. The duct is then tied in two places with sutures. The procedure is repeated on the opposite side. The incision in the floor of the mouth may be closed or left open to heal.

42550

42550 Injection procedure for sialography

An injection procedure for sialography is performed. Separately reportable x-rays are taken of the salivary duct prior to the injection procedure to determine if a stone is present. If no stone is detected, a small catheter is inserted into the salivary duct and contrast media is injected. The flow of contrast is monitored radiographically. A sour liquid such as lemon juice may be given to the patient by mouth to stimulate production of saliva and additional radiographs obtained.

42600

42600 Closure salivary fistula

The physician closes a salivary fistula which is an abnormal communication between the salivary gland and the skin or mucous membrane of the mouth. Fistulas may occur as a postoperative complication of salivary gland or other neck surgery, salivary gland injury, or other condition. The fistulous tract is exposed. The wound is irrigated and tissue debrided as needed. The proximal end of the fistula is closed with sutures or a tissue flap as is the distal end.

● New Code   ▲ Revised Code

42650-42660

42650   Dilation salivary duct
42660   Dilation and catheterization of salivary duct, with or without injection

A narrowing of the salivary duct, also referred to as a stenosis or stricture, is treated with dilation (42650) or dilation and catheterization of salivary duct with or without injection (42660). The mucosa around the salivary duct is injected with local anesthetic. In 42650, a salivary dilator is passed into the duct papilla (opening) and advanced through the narrowed region and into the salivary gland. The duct is sequentially dilated with a series of dilators until the desired diameter of the stenotic region is obtained. In 42660, the dilation procedure is performed using a catheter with or without an injection procedure. A guidewire is inserted into the duct papilla and advanced to area of stenosis. A balloon catheter is passed over the guidewire to the stenotic region and the guidewire is removed. The balloon catheter is then inflated and deflated several times until the desired dilation has been achieved. Contrast material may be injected following the procedure and separately reportable radiographs obtained to ensure that the dilation procedure has been successful.

42665

42665   Ligation salivary duct, intraoral

This procedure may be performed to treat excessive salivation (sialorrhea) which results in uncontrolled drooling. Sialorrhea is usually caused by a neurological deficit such as cerebral palsy or a head injury. Saliva is produced primarily by the three major paired salivary glands, the parotid, submandibular (submaxillary), and sublingual glands. The parotid gland ducts, also referred to as Stenson's ducts, empty near the upper second molar in the cheek (buccal cavity). The submandibular ducts, also referred to as Wharton's ducts, open on the floor of the mouth just lateral to the frenulum of the tongue. The sublingual glands have multiple ducts along the floor of the mouth and some ducts may join with the Wharton's duct. The opening of the duct is identified and the duct may be cannulated for a short distance. An incision is made over the duct and the duct exposed distally for a length of approximately 1 cm. The duct is then tied in two places with sutures. The incision in the mouth may be closed with sutures or left open to heal.

42700-42725

42700   Incision and drainage abscess; peritonsillar
42720   Incision and drainage abscess; retropharyngeal or parapharyngeal, intraoral approach
42725   Incision and drainage abscess; retropharyngeal or parapharyngeal, external approach

Incision and drainage of a peritonsillar, retropharyngeal, or parapharyngeal abscess is performed. Peritonsillar abscess typically occurs near the superior aspect of the palatine tonsils outside the tonsillar capsule in the space between the superior constrictor and palotopharyngeus muscle. Retropharyngeal abscesses are located deep in the neck spaces behind the pharynx and parapharyngeal abscesses are located on both sides of the pharynx in the lateral spaces. In 42700, a peritonillar incision and drainage is performed. A small incision is made in the soft palate, usually superior to the tonsil with a guarded scalpel to prevent deep incision. A Kelly clamp is used to gently dissect tissue inferiorly, posteriorly and slightly laterally over the area of fluctuance until the abscess cavity is located. The abscess cavity is entered and drained. In 42720, an intraoral approach is used to drain a retropharyngeal or parapharyngeal abscess. Intraoral approach is used when the abscess cavity is small and localized. In 42725, an external approach is used to drain a retropharyngeal or parapharyngeal abscess. The external approach used depends on the location and size of the abscess and its proximity to blood vessels as well as other anatomic structures in the neck. One approach commonly used to access the retropharyngeal space involves incising along the anterior border of the sternocleidomastoid muscle. The carotid artery sheath is retracted. The deep spaces behind the pharynx are then opened, the abscess located and drained.

42800

42800   Biopsy; oropharynx

The oropharynx is the middle portion of the throat that is continuous with the mouth lying below the soft palate and above the epiglottis. The oropharynx is visually inspected and the abnormal growth or lesion identified. A local anesthetic is injected to numb the area to be biopsied. One or more tissue samplse are then taken from the abnormal growth or lesion and sent for separately reportable laboratory analysis.

42804-42806

42804   Biopsy; nasopharynx, visible lesion, simple
42806   Biopsy; nasopharynx, survey for unknown primary lesion

The nasopharynx is the upper part of the pharynx that is continuous with the nasal passages. In 42804, a simple biopsy is performed on a visible lesion of the nasopharynx. A local anesthetic is injected. One or more tissue samples are then taken from a visible lesion and sent for separately reportable laboratory analysis. In 42806, a survey for an unknown primary lesion is performed by taking a biopsy of an abnormal growth or lesion in the nasopharynx. Survey for an unknown primary lesion requires a large tissue sample

to ensure that there is enough tissue to identify the origin of the lesion and to classify the neoplasm. A general anesthetic is typically required.

42808

42808   Excision or destruction of lesion of pharynx, any method

The physician excises or destroys a pharyngeal lesion by any method. A local anesthetic is injected or a general anesthetic is administered depending on the lesion's location and size. The lesion is then removed by excising the entire lesion along with a margin of healthy tissue to ensure that it is removed in its entirety. The excision site may be left open to heal by secondary intention or closed with sutures. Alternatively, the lesion may be destroyed by any method including electrosurgery, cryosurgery, or laser or chemical destruction applied directly to the tissue.

42809

42809   Removal of foreign body from pharynx

The physician removes a foreign body from the pharynx that may be located in any part of the pharynx, including the nasopharynx, oropharynx, or hypopharynx. The exact nature of the procedure is determined by the location of the foreign body. The patient is asked to identify the location by sensation. If the foreign body is in the nasopharynx, it is approached through the nose and removed with forceps. If the foreign body sensation is in the oropharynx, the oropharynx is inspected using a tongue depressor. A foreign body in this area is usually visible and can be removed using forceps. If the sensation is in the hypopharynx, the hypopharynx is inspected paying careful attention to the base of the tongue, tonsils, and vallecula. Once the foreign body is localized, it is grasped with forceps and removed.

42810-42815

42810   Excision branchial cleft cyst or vestige, confined to skin and subcutaneous tissues
42815   Excision branchial cleft cyst, vestige, or fistula, extending beneath subcutaneous tissues and/or into pharynx

The physician excises a branchial cleft cyst, vestige, or fistula. A branchial cleft cyst, vestige, or fistula is a congenital anomaly located at the lateral part of the neck and caused by failure of the branchial cleft to close during embryonic development. In 42810, the branchial cleft cyst or vestige is confined to the skin and subcutaneous tissues. A series of horizontal incisions are made in the skin of the neck overlying branchial cyst or vestige to expose the cyst or vestige which often lies in a tortuous path beneath the skin and subcutaneous tissue. Once the cyst or vestige has been exposed, it is dissected out taking care to remove the cyst in its entirety. In 42815, a branchial cleft cyst, vestige, or fistula extending beneath the subcutaneous tissues and/or into the pharynx is removed. The branchial cleft cyst, vestige, or fistula may be exposed as described above with dissection being carried down to deeper tissues to allow complete excision of the cyst, vestige, or fistula. If a branchial cleft cyst or vestige is located close to the pharyngeal wall a peroral route may be used. A branchial cleft fistula may also be removed by a combined approach when the fistula extends from the neck into the pharynx. The cervical end of the fistula is freed from surrounding tissue. The fistulous tract is then approached through the mouth and the freed cervical end of the fistulous tract attached to the stripper. The fistulous tract is removed using steady traction on the oral end. When the entire fistulous tract has been avulsed with the stripper, it is excised by detaching the oral end. The oral and cervical wounds are closed.

42820-42821

42820   Tonsillectomy and adenoidectomy; younger than age 12
42821   Tonsillectomy and adenoidectomy; age 12 or over

A tonsillectomy and adenoidectomy is performed. A mouth prop is used to open and suspend the mouth. Clamps are applied to the tonsils to provide traction during dissection. Dissection of the tonsils may be performed using one of several techniques including scissors and curettes (sharp and blunt dissection), cautery, radiofrequency or laser ablation, harmonic scalpel or other instrument. Using the standard dissection and snare technique, the mucosa is incised with a sickle knife. Dissection begins at the superior pole and is carried inferiorly through the loose connective tissue layer. At the inferior pole, a snare is passed around the tonsil and the tonsil amputated by closing the snare loop. The surgical site is inspected and any tonsil remnants removed. Bleeding is controlled by pressure, suture ties, or cautery. The adenoids are resected using an adenotome, adenoid curette, or microdebrider or vaporized using a laser. To perform resection using an adenoid curette, the physician first retracts the soft palate. An appropriately sized curette is selected and positioned at the posterior edge of the vomer. The curette is then pushed along the vault of the nasopharynx and over the odontoid process. The surgical site is inspected and any adenoid remnants are removed using a small curette or electrocautery. Bleeding is controlled by cautery and/or gauze sponges soaked in epinephrine. Use code 42820 if the patient is younger than age 12 and 42821 if the patient is age 12 or older.

Digestive System

42825-42826

42825   Tonsillectomy, primary or secondary; younger than age 12
42826   Tonsillectomy, primary or secondary; age 12 or over

A primary or secondary tonsillectomy is performed. A primary tonsillectomy refers to the initial removal of the tonsils whereas a secondary tonsillectomy refers to a repeat procedure to remove residual tonsil tissue or regrowth. A mouth prop is used to open and suspend the mouth. Clamps are applied to the tonsils to provide traction during dissection. Dissection of the tonsils may be performed using one of several techniques including scissors and curettes (sharp and blunt dissection), cautery, radiofrequency or laser ablation, harmonic scalpel or other instrument. Using the standard dissection and snare technique, the mucosa is incised with a sickle knife. Dissection begins at the superior pole and is carried inferiorly through the loose connective tissue layer. At the inferior pole, a snare is passed around the tonsil and the tonsil amputated by closing the snare loop. The surgical site is inspected and any tonsil remnants removed. Bleeding is controlled by pressure, suture ties, or cautery. Use code 42825 if the patient is younger than age 12 and 42826 if the patient is age 12 or older.

42830-42836

42830   Adenoidectomy, primary; younger than age 12
42831   Adenoidectomy, primary; age 12 or over
42835   Adenoidectomy, secondary; younger than age 12
42836   Adenoidectomy, secondary; age 12 or over

A primary or secondary adenoidectomy is performed. A primary adenoidectomy refers to the initial removal of the adenoids. A secondary adenoidectomy refers to a repeat procedure for removal of residual adenoid tissue or regrowth. A mouth prop is used to open and suspend the mouth. The adenoids are resected using an adenotome, adenoid curette, or microdebrider or vaporized using a laser. To perform resection using an adenoid curette, the physician first retracts the soft palate. An appropriately sized curette is selected and positioned at the posterior edge of the vomer. The curette is then pushed along the vault of the nasopharynx and over the odontoid process. The surgical site is inspected and any adenoid remnants are removed using a small curette or electrocautery. Bleeding is controlled by cautery and/or gauze sponges soaked in epinephrine. Use code 42830 to report primary adenoidectomy for a patient younger than age 12 and 42831 for primary adenoidectomy for a patient age 12 or older. Use code 42835 to report secondary adenoidectomy for a patient younger than age 12 and 42836 for secondary adenoidectomy for a patient age 12 or older.

42842-42845

42842   Radical resection of tonsil, tonsillar pillars, and/or retromolar trigone; without closure
42844   Radical resection of tonsil, tonsillar pillars, and/or retromolar trigone; closure with local flap (eg, tongue, buccal)
42845   Radical resection of tonsil, tonsillar pillars, and/or retromolar trigone; closure with other flap

The physician performs a radical resection of tonsil, tonsillar pillars, and/or retromolar trigone. The tonsils, tonsillar pillars, and the retromolar trigones are the most common locations of primary malignant neoplasm of the oropharynx. The tonsils, or more specifically the palatine tonsils, are collections of lymphoid tissue situated laterally at the back of the oropharynx or throat and embedded between the tonsillar pillars. The anterior and posterior tonsillar pillars are formed by the palatoglossus muscle (anteriorly) and the palatopharygeus muscle (posteriorly). The retromolar trigone is the small mucosal area behind the wisdom teeth. The extent of the tumor is determined by separately reportable radiographic studies and other diagnostic studies such as biopsies. The area to be resected is identified and may include the tonsil, tonsillar pillars, and/or retromolar trigone. The resection may be performed by an oral approach or through a neck incision. The area of tumor involvement is resected in its entirety along with a margin of healthy tissue. Frozen sections are sent for separately reportable laboratory analysis to ensure that all malignant tissue has been removed. Following frozen section evaluation, additional tissue is excised as needed until all malignant tissue has been removed. In 42842, the area of the resection is left exposed to heal by secondary intention. In 42844, local flap closure is performed. An area of tissue close to the wound, such as tissue from the tongue or cheek, is freed leaving it attached at its base. The flap is then rotated over the resection site and sutured over the surgical wound. The donor site is repaired with sutures. In 42845, closure is performed using another type of flap. Tissue is obtained from another area of the body and configured to cover the surgical wound in the oropharynx. It is then sutured into place using microvascular technique. The donor site is repaired with sutures.

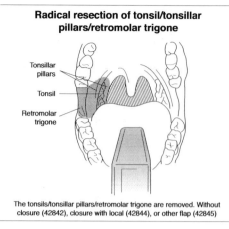

Radical resection of tonsil/tonsillar pillars/retromolar trigone

Tonsillar pillars
Tonsil
Retromolar trigone

The tonsils/tonsillar pillars/retromolar trigone are removed. Without closure (42842), closure with local (42844), or other flap (42845)

42860

42860   Excision of tonsil tags

Tonsil tags are excised. Tonsil tags are small amounts of tonsil tissue that were not removed during a previous tonsillectomy. If the tonsil tags become symptomatic, they are removed. Dissection of the tonsil tags may be performed using scissors and curettes (sharp and blunt dissection), cautery, radiofrequency or laser ablation, harmonic scalpel or other instrument. Bleeding is controlled by pressure, suture ties, or cautery.

42870

42870   Excision or destruction lingual tonsil, any method (separate procedure)

The lingual tonsil is excised or destroyed by any method. The lingual tonsil is a collection of lymphoid tissue located at the posterior (back or base) of the tongue. For a peroral approach, a mouth prop is used to open and suspend the mouth. Dissection of the lingual tonsil may be performed using one of several techniques including scissors and curettes (sharp and blunt dissection), cautery, radiofrequency or laser ablation, or other instrument. Some techniques require a neck incision. Bleeding is controlled by pressure, suture ties, or cautery.

42890

42890   Limited pharyngectomy

This procedure is typically performed for malignant tumors of the pharynx, but may also be performed for benign lesions or strictures. A horizontal incision is made in the neck over the thyrohyoid membrane. The suprahyoid muscles are separated from the hyoid laterally. The valleculae are entered, and the pharynx exposed by retracting the larynx inferiorly and the tongue superiorly. The region of the pharynx to be resected is identified and excised. If a lesion is excised the lesion is removed with a margin of healthy tissue. The surgical defect in the pharynx is closed with sutures or a separately reportable reconstruction with flaps or grafts is performed.

42892-42894

42892   Resection of lateral pharyngeal wall or pyriform sinus, direct closure by advancement of lateral and posterior pharyngeal walls
42894   Resection of pharyngeal wall requiring closure with myocutaneous or fasciocutaneous flap or free muscle, skin, or fascial flap with microvascular anastomosis

The lateral wall of the pharynx or the pyriform sinus is resected. The pyriform sinus, also referred to as the pyriform fossa is a funnel shaped recess in the anterolateral wall of the nasopharynx on each side of the vestibule of the larynx. This procedure is typically performed for malignant tumors of the pharynx or pyriform sinus, but may also be performed for benign lesions or strictures. A horizontal incision is made in the neck over the thyrohyoid membrane. The suprahyoid muscles are separated from the hyoid laterally. The valleculae are entered, and the pharynx exposed by retracting the larynx inferiorly and the tongue superiorly. The lateral pharynx and/or pyriform sinus is exposed and the lesion or defect identified. The lesion or defect is excised along with a margin of healthy tissue. In 42892, the defect is closed by advancement of the lateral and posterior pharyngeal walls. The lateral and posterior walls are mobilized and the edges are approximated and closed with sutures. In 42894, a myocutaneous flap is used to close the defect. Commonly used flaps include latissimus dorsi and pectoralis major. If a pectoralis major flap is used, the size of the defect is measured and the skin over the planned flap site marked. Vessels supplying the flap are identified. The skin and muscle are incised and the flap developed. The myocutaneous flap is rotated into the neck with the skin side facing inward. The flap is sutured to the pharyngeal wall closing the defect. Overlying subcutaneous tissue and skin are then closed over the flap.

Digestive System

42900

42900   **Suture pharynx for wound or injury**

Wounds or injuries to the pharynx are rare. The exact procedure depends on the location of the wound or injury. The pharynx may be approached through the mouth (transoral) or an incision may be made in the neck. The wound or injury is exposed and bleeding controlled. The wound is explored and the extent of injury determined. Any debris is removed and the wound inspected for the presence of foreign bodies. The edges of the wound are trimmed and the wound is repaired with sutures.

42950-42953

42950   **Pharyngoplasty (plastic or reconstructive operation on pharynx)**
42953   **Pharyngoesophageal repair**

A plastic or reconstructive procedure is performed on the pharynx (42950), also referred to as a pharyngoplasty, or the pharynx and esophagus are repaired, also referred to as a pharyngoesophageal repair (42953). The exact procedure depends on the type of pharyngeal defect or malformation. An incision is made in the skin of the neck, usually an apron-type incision in one of the skin folds or vertical incisions anterior to the sternocleidomastoid muscles. The sternocleidomastoids are retracted laterally and the strap muscles and larynx rotated medially to expose the pharynx. The tissue plane behind the pharynx and anterior to the cervical spine is dissected and the posterior aspect of the pharynx exposed. The pharynx is carefully inspected to determine the extent and type of plastic or reconstructive procedure required. The wound is flushed with sterile saline to remove debris. Necrotic tissue is debrided. The edges of the pharyngeal injury are trimmed. In 42950, the pharynx is repaired. Reconstruction of the oropharynx or hypopharynx requires a dynamic, sensate local flap that will preserve swallowing function and prevent aspiration. The physician selects the donor site for the myocutaneous or other tissue flap which is developed in a separately reportable procedure. The flap is then sutured over the pharyngeal defect. In 42953, the pharynx and cervical esophagus are repaired. The esophagus is also exposed and mobilized and the pharyngeal and esophageal injuries or defects evaluated. Depending on the extent of the injury or defect, a direct repair may be performed using a layered closure of the mucosa followed by repair of the overlying muscular layer. Alternatively, a separately reportable myocutaneous or other flap may be used in the repair. Drains are placed in the neck as needed and the overlying tissues and skin repaired in layers.

42955

42955   **Pharyngostomy (fistulization of pharynx, external for feeding)**

Pharyngostomy is performed following injury or surgery at a more proximal point in the pharynx to allow it to heal or following a massive injury or surgical removal of the pharynx without reconstruction to allow drainage of saliva and mucus and/or external feeding. An incision is made in the lateral aspect of the neck. If the pharyngostomy is performed for drainage, the distal segment of the cervical esophagus is closed. The proximal aspect of the pharynx is brought through the lateral incision, everted, and sutured to the skin of the neck. A tube is placed in the stoma and secured with sutures. The tube is attached to a drainage bag or suction pump. If the pharyngostomy is performed for feeding, the proximal segment is attached to some type of drainage device and the distal segment is exteriorized as described above and a feeding tube is placed.

42960-42962

42960   **Control oropharyngeal hemorrhage, primary or secondary (eg, post-tonsillectomy); simple**
42961   **Control oropharyngeal hemorrhage, primary or secondary (eg, post-tonsillectomy); complicated, requiring hospitalization**
42962   **Control oropharyngeal hemorrhage, primary or secondary (eg, post-tonsillectomy); with secondary surgical intervention**

The physician controls a primary or secondary oropharyngeal hemorrhage. Primary oropharyngeal hemorrhage refers to bleeding that was not caused by a surgical procedure while secondary oropharyngeal hemorrhage refers to bleeding resulting from a surgical procedure such as a tonsillectomy. In 42960, a simple outpatient service is performed. The throat is examined and the bleeding site(s) identified. Minor bleeding may be treated with ice water gargling, the application of a topical vasoconstrictor at the bleeding site, and/or the cauterization with silver nitrate. In 42961, control of the oropharyngeal hemorrhage is complicated by the need for hospitalization. The throat is examined and the bleeding site(s) identified. The bleeding may be controlled using the techniques described above. If bleeding continues, the patient is admitted to the hospital for overnight observation and the administration of intravenous fluids. In 42962, the oropharyngeal hemorrhage requires secondary surgical intervention. The throat is examined and any fresh blood clot removed. The bleeding sites are identified and bleeding controlled with cautery or suture tie. If bleeding continues, suture ligature of the bleeding site(s) may be required.

42970-42972

42970   **Control of nasopharyngeal hemorrhage, primary or secondary (eg, postadenoidectomy); simple, with posterior nasal packs, with or without anterior packs and/or cautery**
42971   **Control of nasopharyngeal hemorrhage, primary or secondary (eg, postadenoidectomy); complicated, requiring hospitalization**
42972   **Control of nasopharyngeal hemorrhage, primary or secondary (eg, postadenoidectomy); with secondary surgical intervention**

The physician controls a primary or secondary nasopharyngeal hemorrhage. Primary nasopharyngeal hemorrhage refers to bleeding that was not caused by a surgical procedure while secondary nasopharyngeal hemorrhage refers to bleeding resulting from a surgical procedure such as a adenoidectomy. In 42970, a simple outpatient service is performed with the application of posterior nasal packs with or without anterior nasal packs and cautery. The nasopharyngeal area is examined and the bleeding site(s) identified. Bleeding is treated with cautery of the bleeding sites if needed and the application of posterior nasal packing. If bleeding continues anterior nasal packing may also be used. In 42971, control of the nasopharyngeal hemorrhage is complicated by the need for hospitalization. The nasopharygeal area is examined and the bleeding site(s) identified. The bleeding may be controlled using the techniques described above. If bleeding continues, the patient is admitted to the hospital for overnight observation and the administration of intravenous fluids. In 42972, the nasopharyngeal hemorrhage requires secondary surgical intervention. The nasopharygeal area is examined and any fresh blood clot removed. The bleeding sites are identified and bleeding controlled with cautery or suture tie. If bleeding continues, suture ligature of the bleeding site(s) may be required. Posterior and/or anterior nasal packing is applied as needed.

43020

43020   **Esophagotomy, cervical approach, with removal of foreign body**

An esophagotomy is performed using a cervical approach for removal of an incarcerated or impacted foreign body. An incision is made in the neck, usually on the left side. The internal jugular vein and carotid artery are identified and retracted laterally. The esophagus is exposed. An incision is made in the esophagus at the level of the incarcerated or impacted foreign body. The foreign body is grasped with forceps and carefully removed. The esophagus is inspected for evidence of tearing or other injury and repair performed as needed. The esophageal incision is closed. The neck is closed in a layered fashion.

43030

43030   **Cricopharyngeal myotomy**

Cricopharyngeal myotomy is performed to treat spasm of the cricopharyngeal muscle causing difficulty swallowing (dysphagia). The cricopharyngeal muscle is a sphincter muscle that arises from the lateral borders of the cricoid cartilage. The striated muscle fibers form a sling around the wall of the superior portion of the cervical esophagus. The cricopharyngeal muscle is approached through a left-sided neck incision overlying the cricoid cartilage. Subplastysmal skin flaps are created superiorly and inferiorly to provide wide exposure of the cricopharyngeus. The anterior border of the sternocleidomastoid muscle is identified and reflected posteriorly to expose the carotid sheath. A plane of dissection is created between the carotid sheath and the laryngotracheal complex. If needed, the omohyoid muscle is sectioned to provide better exposure. The larynx is rotated to the right to expose the cervical esophagus. The fan-shaped band of cricopharyngeal muscle fibers is identified. The cricopharyngeus fibers are cut until underlying esophageal mucosa can be seen. The myotomy is extended superiorly and inferiorly until all fibers have been cut. The wound is irrigated and a suction drain placed. The platysma is reapproximated and the skin closed around the drain. To report cricopharyngeal myotomy with diverticulectomy of the hypopharynx or cervical esophagus, see 43130.

43045

43045   **Esophagotomy, thoracic approach, with removal of foreign body**

The esophagus is approached using a right posterior thoracotomy. The skin is incised and the incision extended through the soft tissues. The scapula is retracted and the thorax entered without disrupting the pleura. Retropleural dissection is performed, the lung retracted, and the esophagus is exposed. An incision is made in the esophagus at the level of the incarcerated or impacted foreign body. The foreign body is grasped with forceps and carefully removed. The esophagus is inspected for evidence of tearing or other injury and repaired as needed. The esophageal incision is closed. The thorax is closed in a layered fashion.

43100-43101

43100   **Excision of lesion, esophagus, with primary repair; cervical approach**
43101   **Excision of lesion, esophagus, with primary repair; thoracic or abdominal approach**

The physician performs an open excision of an esophageal lesion with primary closure. The approach depends on the level of the lesion. In 43100, a cervical approach is used. An incision is made in the neck, usually on the left side. The internal jugular vein and carotid

Digestive System

● New Code   ▲ Revised Code

artery are identified and retracted laterally. The esophagus is exposed. An incision is made in the cervical esophagus immediately above or below the level of the lesion. The lesion is exposed and excised along with a margin of healthy tissue and sent to the laboratory for separately reportable histologic evaluation. The esophagus is repaired with sutures. The cervical incision is closed in layers. In 43101, a thoracic or abdominal approach is used. In a thoracic approach, a right posterior thoracotomy is generally used. The skin is incised and the incision extended through the soft tissues. The scapula is retracted and the thorax entered without disrupting the pleura. Retropleural dissection is performed, the lung retracted, and the esophagus is exposed. Using an abdominal approach, also referred to as a transhiatal approach, an incision is made in the upper abdomen and the peritoneal cavity explored. The stomach is mobilized at the gastroesophageal junction and the diaphragmatic hiatus is split to expose the lower posterior mediastinum and esophagus. Once the mid or distal esophagus has been exposed, an incision is made in the esophagus immediately above or below the level of the lesion. The lesion is exposed and excised along with a margin of healthy tissue and sent to the laboratory for separately reportable histologic evaluation. The esophagus is repaired with sutures. The thoracic or abdominal surgical wound is closed in layers.

43107

43107   Total or near total esophagectomy, without thoracotomy; with pharyngogastrostomy or cervical esophagogastrostomy, with or without pyloroplasty (transhiatal)

Using an abdominal approach, also referred to as a transhiatal approach, an incision is made in the upper abdomen and the peritoneal cavity explored. The stomach is mobilized at the gastroesophageal junction and the diaphragmatic hiatus is split to expose the lower posterior mediastinum and esophagus. The esophagus is freed from surrounding tissues using blunt and sharp dissection. The esophagus is transected at the esophagogastric junction. The pharynx or cervical esophagus is also transected through an incision in the neck and the esophagus is removed. A gastric tube is then created from the stomach. The left gastric and gastroepiploic arteries are ligated and divided as are the short splenic vessels. The right gastroepiploic artery is preserved to provide blood supply to the greater curvature of the stomach. The stomach is divided using a linear stapler at a point about 3 cm from the line of the greater curvature. The pyloric sphincter is evaluated. If a pyloroplasty is needed, the pylorus is divided laterally and then sutured longitudinally to provide a wider opening into the duodenum. The seromuscular layer of the stomach is closed with sutures to a point approximately 4 cm from the end. The surgically created gastric tube is mobilized and brought into the neck either behind the sternum (retrosternal) or behind the mediastinum (posterior mediastinal) using a pull-up technique. The gastric tube is prepared for anastomosis as is the pharynx or cervical esophagus and an end-to-end anastomosis is then performed. Esophagectomy is performed without thoracic incision using a pull-up technique to bring the gastric tube into the neck. Thoracic incisions are avoided whenever possible due to the increased risk of developing mediastinitis from an esophageal leak.

43108

43108   Total or near total esophagectomy, without thoracotomy; with colon interposition or small intestine reconstruction, including intestine mobilization, preparation and anastomosis(es)

The procedure includes mobilization and preparation of the colon or small intestine with anastomosis to the pharynx or remaining portion of esophagus. The procedure varies somewhat based on whether the esophagus is reconstructed with a section of small intestine or colon and what portion of the colon or small intestine is used. Using an abdominal approach, also referred to as a transhiatal approach, an incision is made in the upper abdomen and the peritoneal cavity explored. The stomach is mobilized and the diaphragmatic hiatus is split to expose the lower posterior mediastinum and esophagus. The distal esophagus is freed from surrounding tissue. A second incision is made in the neck, the proximal esophagus exposed and mobilized. The esophagus is transected and removed. If a section of colon is used to replace the esophagus, the omentum is dissected off the colon. For a left colon interposition graft, the middle colic artery is ligated and the left and right flexures are mobilized taking care to preserve the arterial and venous collateral circulation for graft perfusion. Alternatively, a section of the left colon may be harvested along with the ascending colon. In this case, the right flexure is taken down. The middle and right colic arteries are ligated and the left colic artery is preserved for graft perfusion. The required length of the colon graft is determined by pulling the colon upward into the neck and measuring the distance between the tethering left colic artery that forms the pedicle for the graft and the planned anastomosis site. The colon transection site is marked. The proximal anastomosis site in the pharynx or cervical esophagus is prepared. Following preparation of the anastomosis site, the colon is transected and the colon graft is placed in a bowel bag to protect it as it is passed through the substernal tunnel to the anastomosis site. The pharynx or remaining cervical esophagus and colon graft are anastomosed. The colon graft is secured with sutures at the diaphragm. The distal end of the colon graft is anastomosed to the stomach. The remaining segments of colon distal and proximal to the harvested segment are then anastomosed to restore continuity of the remaining colon. A jejunostomy tube is placed for feeding and decompression.

Esophagectomy is performed without thoracic incision using a pull-up technique to bring the bowel segment into the neck. Thoracic incisions are avoided whenever possible due to the increased risk of developing mediastinitis from an esophageal leak.

43112

43112   Total or near total esophagectomy, with thoracotomy; with pharyngogastrostomy or cervical esophagogastrostomy, with or without pyloroplasty

A right posterior thoracotomy is generally used. The skin is incised and the incision extended through the soft tissues. The scapula is retracted and the thorax entered without disrupting the pleura. Retropleural dissection is performed, the lung retracted, and the esophagus is exposed. The pneumogastric and recurrent nerves are identified. The azygous vein and bronchial artery are also identified. The esophagus is freed from surrounding tissues using blunt and sharp dissection. The esophagus is transected at the esophagogastric junction. The pharynx or cervical esophagus is also transected through an incision in the neck and the esophagus is removed. A gastric tube is then created from the stomach. The left gastric and gastroepiploic arteries are ligated and divided as are the short splenic vessels. The right gastroepiploic artery is preserved to provide blood supply to the greater curvature of the stomach. The stomach is then divided using a linear stapler at a point about 3 cm from the line of the greater curvature. The pyloric sphincter is evaluated. If a pyloroplasty is needed, the pylorus is divided laterally and then sutured longtitudinally to provide a wider opening into the duodenum. The seromuscular layer of the stomach is closed with sutures to a point approximately 4 cm from the end. The surgically created gastric tube is mobilized and brought into the neck either behind the sternum (retrosternal) or behind the mediastinum (posterior mediastinal). The gastric tube is prepared for anastomosis as is the pharynx or cervical esophagus and an end-to-end anastomosis is then performed.

43113

43113   Total or near total esophagectomy, with thoracotomy; with colon interposition or small intestine reconstruction, including intestine mobilization, preparation, and anastomosis(es)

The procedure includes mobilization and preparation of the colon or small intestine with anastomosis to the pharynx or remaining portion of esophagus. The procedure varies somewhat based on whether the esophagus is reconstructed with a section of intestine or colon and what portion colon or small intestine is used. A right posterior thoracotomy is generally used. The skin is incised and the incision extended through the soft tissues. The scapula is retracted and the thorax entered without disrupting the pleura. Retropleural dissection is performed, the lung retracted, and the esophagus is exposed. The pneumogastric and recurrent nerves are identified. The azygous vein and bronchial artery are also identified. The esophagus is freed from surrounding tissues using blunt and sharp dissection. The esophagus is transected at the esophagogastric junction. The pharynx or cervical esophagus is transected through an incision in the neck and the esophagus is removed. If a section of colon is used to replace the esophagus, the omentum is dissected off the colon. For a left colon interposition graft, the middle colic artery is ligated and the left and right flexures are mobilized taking care to preserve the arterial and venous collateral circulation for graft perfusion. Alternatively, a section of the left colon may be harvested along with the ascending colon. In this case, the right flexure is taken down. The middle and right colic arteries are ligated and the left colic artery is preserved for graft perfusion. The required length of the colon graft is determined by pulling the colon upward into the neck and measuring the distance between the tethering left colic artery that forms the pedicle for the graft and the planned anastomosis site. The colon transection site is marked. The proximal anastomosis site in the pharynx or cervical esophagus is prepared. Following preparation of the anastomosis site, the colon is transected and the colon graft is placed in a bowel bag to protect it as it is passed through the substernal tunnel to the anastomosis site. The pharynx or remaining cervical esophagus and colon graft are anastomosed. The colon graft is secured at the diaphragm with sutures. The distal end of the colon graft is anastomosed to the stomach. The remaining segments of colon distal and proximal to the harvested segment are then anastomosed to restore continuity of the remaining colon. A jejunostomy tube is placed for feeding and decompression.

43116

43116   Partial esophagectomy, cervical, with free intestinal graft, including microvascular anastomosis, obtaining the graft and intestinal reconstruction

The procedure includes obtaining the intestinal graft (flap), microvascular anastomosis of the graft, and reconstruction of the intestines. Cervical esophagectomy is typically performed for malignant neoplasm confined to the cervical region, but may also be performed for benign stricture of the esophagus. An incision is made in the neck, usually on the left side. The internal jugular vein and carotid artery are identified and retracted laterally. The cervical esophagus is exposed and mobilized. A separate incision is made in the abdomen to obtain a free intestinal graft, usually a portion of the jejunum. The jejunum is exposed and the segment to be harvested identified. The distal end of the jejunal segment to be harvested is marked so that the segment will be oriented in the

● New Code   ▲ Revised Code   CPT © 2016 American Medical Association. All Rights Reserved.   © 2017 DecisionHealth

neck to allow for normal peristalsis. The artery supplying the segment of jejunum to be harvested is located. Blood vessels are dissected back to their branching points off the supplying vessels where they are suture ligated and divided. The jejunum is divided and the graft segment removed along with the supplying blood vessels. The remaining small bowel segments are anastomosed. A feeding tube is placed in the jejunum. During the jejunal graft harvest the neck vessels are simultaneously prepared for anastomosis by a second surgeon. The diseased portion of the esophagus is removed and prepared for anastomosis. The jejunal graft is placed in the neck and properly oriented by locating the mark indicating the distal end. The jejunal serosa is first secured to the prevertebral fascia to take tension off the proximal anastomosis and then the proximal and distal ends of the graft are anastomosed to the remaining esophageal segments. Microvascular anastomoses of the jejunal vessels to the neck vessels, typically the thyroid artery and jugular vein, is then performed. Abdominal and neck incisions are closed. This procedure may be performed using a surgical team consisting of a general surgeon for the free jejunal graft (flap) harvest, a head and neck surgeon for the exposure and excision of the cervical esophagus, and a microvascular surgeon for anastomosis of the free jejunal graft (flap). It is performed primarily for malignancy, but also for benign stricture complication of cervical spine surgery with perforation of esophagus.

43117

43117 Partial esophagectomy, distal two-thirds, with thoracotomy and separate abdominal incision, with or without proximal gastrectomy; with thoracic esophagogastrostomy, with or without pyloroplasty (Ivor Lewis)

This procedure may be performed with or without partial gastrectomy and with or without pyloroplasty. The upper abdomen is opened first and the peritoneal cavity inspected. The stomach is mobilized. If the malignancy has invaded the upper aspect of the stomach, the physician excises the involved portion of the stomach. A gastric tube is then created from the stomach. The left gastric and gastroepiploic arteries are ligated and divided as are the short splenic vessels. The right gastroepiploic artery is preserved to provide blood supply to the greater curvature of the stomach. The stomach is divided using a linear stapler at a point about 3 cm from the line of the greater curvature. The pyloric sphincter is evaluated. If a pyloroplasty is needed, the pylorus is divided laterally and then sutured longtitudinally to provide a wider opening into the duodenum. The seromuscular layer of the stomach is closed with sutures to a point approximately 4 cm from the end. A separate incision is then made in the thorax to remove the diseased part of the esophagus. The skin and soft tissues in the right posterior aspect of the thorax are incised. The scapula is retracted and the thorax entered without disrupting the pleura. Retropleural dissection is performed, the lung retracted, and the esophagus is exposed. The pneumogastric and recurrent nerves are identified. The azygous vein and bronchial artery are also identified. The esophagus is freed from surrounding tissues using blunt and sharp dissection. The thoracic esophagus is transected above and below the level of the malignancy and removed. The diaphragmatic hiatus is split to allow the surgically created gastric tube to be brought into the posterior mediastinum. An end-to-end anastomosis of the gastric tube and remaining esophagus is performed.

43118

43118 Partial esophagectomy, distal two-thirds, with thoracotomy and separate abdominal incision, with or without proximal gastrectomy; with colon interposition or small intestine reconstruction, including intestine mobilization, preparation, and anastomosis(es)

The procedure may be performed with or without partial gastrectomy. The procedure includes mobilization and preparation of the colon or small intestine with anastomosis to the pharynx or remaining portion of esophagus. The procedure varies somewhat based on whether the esophagus is reconstructed with a section of intestine or colon and what portion colon or small intestine is used. A right posterior thoracotomy is generally used. The skin is incised and the incision extended through the soft tissues. The scapula is retracted and the thorax entered without disrupting the pleura. Retropleural dissection is performed, the lung retracted, and the esophagus is exposed. The pneumogastric and recurrent nerves are identified. The azygous vein and bronchial artery are also identified. The esophagus is freed from surrounding tissues using blunt and sharp dissection. A separate incision is made in the upper abdomen and the peritoneal cavity explored. The stomach is mobilized and the diaphragmatic hiatus is split to expose the lower posterior mediastinum and esophagus. The esophagus is transected near the esophagogastric junction. Alternatively, it may be necessary to excise a portion of the stomach in order to remove all the malignancy. The thoracic esophagus is also transected, and the esophagus is removed. If a section of colon is used to replace the esophagus, the omentum is dissected off the colon. For a left colon interposition graft, the middle colic artery is ligated and the left and right flexures are mobilized taking care to preserve the arterial and venous collateral circulation for graft perfusion. Alternatively, a section of the left colon may be harvested along with the ascending colon. In this case, the right flexure is taken down. The middle and right colic arteries are ligated and the left colic artery is preserved for graft perfusion. The required length of the colon graft is determined by pulling the colon into the thorax and measuring the distance between the tethering left colic artery that forms the pedicle for the graft and the planned anastomosis site. The colon transection site is marked. Following preparation

of the anastomosis sites, the colon is transected and the colon graft is placed in a bowel bag to protect it as it is passed into the posterior mediastinum to the anastomosis site. The thoracic esophagus and colon graft are anastomosed. The colon graft is secured with sutures at the diaphragm. The distal end of the colon graft is anastomosed to the stomach. The remaining segments of colon distal and proximal to the harvested segment are then anastomosed to restore continuity of the remaining colon. A jejunostomy tube is placed for feeding and decompression.

43121–43122

43121 Partial esophagectomy, distal two-thirds, with thoracotomy only, with or without proximal gastrectomy, with thoracic esophagogastrostomy, with or without pyloroplasty

43122 Partial esophagectomy, thoracoabdominal or abdominal approach, with or without proximal gastrectomy; with esophagogastrostomy, with or without pyloroplasty

The physician performs a partial esophagectomy of the distal two-thirds of the esophagus by thoracotomy only (43121) or by a thoracoabdominal or abdominal approach (43122) with or without partial gastrectomy and with or without pyloroplasty. In 43121, a right posterior thoracotomy is generally used. The skin is incised and the incision extended through the soft tissues. The scapula is retracted and the thorax entered without disrupting the pleura. Retropleural dissection is performed, the lung retracted, and the esophagus is exposed. The pneumogastric and recurrent nerves are identified. The azygous vein and bronchial artery are also identified. The esophagus is freed from surrounding tissues using blunt and sharp dissection. The stomach is exposed by splitting the diaphragmatic hiatus and the stomach is mobilized. The esophagus is transected near the esophagogastric junction. Alternatively, it may be necessary to excise a portion of the stomach in order to remove all the malignancy. The thoracic esophagus is transected, and the esophagus is removed. A gastric tube is created from the stomach. The left gastric and gastroepiploic arteries are ligated and divided as are the short splenic vessels. The right gastroepiploic artery is preserved to provide blood supply to the greater curvature of the stomach. The stomach is then divided using a linear stapler at a point about 3 cm from the line of the greater curvature. The pyloric sphincter is evaluated. If a pyloroplasty is needed, the pylorus is divided laterally and then sutured longtitudinally to provide a wider opening into the duodenum. The seromuscular layer of the stomach is closed with sutures to a point approximately 4 cm from the end. The surgically created gastric tube is mobilized and brought into the mediastinum by a posterior mediastinal approach. The gastric tube is prepared for anastomosis as is the remaining thoracic esophagus and an end-to-end anastomosis is performed. In 43122, the procedure is performed by a thoracoabdominal or abdominal approach. Using a thoracoabdominal approach, a single incision is made over the thorax and carried down into the upper abdomen. Alternatively, an abdominal approach, also referred to as a transhiatal approach is used. The stomach is mobilized and the diaphragmatic hiatus is split to expose the lower posterior mediastinum and the esophagus. The remainder of the procedure is performed as described above.

43123

43123 Partial esophagectomy, thoracoabdominal or abdominal approach, with or without proximal gastrectomy; with colon interposition or small intestine reconstruction, including intestine mobilization, preparation, and anastomosis(es)

The procedure includes mobilization and preparation of the colon or small intestine with anastomosis to the pharynx or remaining portion of esophagus. The procedure varies somewhat based on whether the esophagus is reconstructed with a section of intestine or colon and what portion of colon or small intestine is used. Using a thoracoabdominal approach, a median sternotomy is performed and the incision extended into the upper abdomen. The esophagus is freed from surrounding tissue. Alternatively, an abdominal (transhiatal) approach is used. The stomach is mobilized and the diaphragmatic hiatus is split to expose the lower posterior mediastinum and the esophagus. The esophagus is transected near the esophagogastric junction. Alternatively, it may be necessary to excise a portion of the stomach in order to remove all the malignancy. The thoracic esophagus is also transected, and the esophagus is removed. If a section of colon is used to replace the esophagus, the omentum is dissected off the colon. For a left colon interposition graft, the middle colic artery is ligated and the left and right flexures are mobilized taking care to preserve the arterial and venous collateral circulation for graft perfusion. Alternatively, a section of the left colon may be harvested along with the ascending colon. In this case, the right flexure is taken down. The middle and right colic arteries are ligated and the left colic artery is preserved for graft perfusion. The required length of the colon graft is determined by pulling the colon into the thorax and measuring the distance between the tethering left colic artery that forms the pedicle for the graft and the planned anastomosis site. The colon transection site is marked. Following preparation of the anastomosis sites, the colon is transected and the colon graft is placed in a bowel bag to protect it as it is passed into the posterior mediastinum to the anastomosis site. The thoracic esophagus and colon graft are anastomosed. The colon graft is secured with sutures at the diaphragm. The distal end of the colon graft is anastomosed to the stomach. The remaining segments of colon distal

Digestive System

and proximal to the harvested segment are then anastomosed to restore continuity of the remaining colon. A jejunostomy tube is placed for feeding and decompression.

43124

43124   Total or partial esophagectomy, without reconstruction (any approach), with cervical esophagostomy

If a cervical approach is used, an incision is made in the neck, usually on the left side. The internal jugular vein and carotid artery are identified and retracted laterally. The esophagus is exposed. For a thoracic approach, a right posterior thoracotomy is generally used. The skin is incised and the incision extended through the soft tissues. The scapula is retracted and the thorax entered without disrupting the pleura. Retropleural dissection is performed, the lung retracted, and the esophagus is exposed. If an abdominal (transhiatal) approach is used an incision is made in the upper abdomen and the peritoneal cavity explored. The stomach is mobilized at the gastroesophageal junction and the diaphragmatic hiatus is split to expose the lower posterior mediastinum and esophagus. Once the esophagus has been exposed, the esophagus is mobilized and transected above or below the level of the malignancy or other lesion or defect. The diseased segment of esophagus is removed and the proximal and distal stumps are repaired. A cervical esophagostomy is then created for placement of a feeding tube. The neck is incised if it has not been previously exposed during the esophagectomy. A feeding tube is then passed through the tunnel created by the esophagectomy to the level of the distal esophageal stump. A longitudinal incision is made in the wall of the remaining distal esophageal segment and the feeding tube passed through the incision in the esophagus and into the stomach. The incision in the esophagus is closed around the feeding tube with a purse string suture. The incision in the neck is closed around the feeding tube.

43130-43135

43130   Diverticulectomy of hypopharynx or esophagus, with or without myotomy; cervical approach

43135   Diverticulectomy of hypopharynx or esophagus, with or without myotomy; thoracic approach

A diverticulum is a sac or pouch that arises from a tubular organ and can be either congenital or acquired in origin. One type of acquired diverticulum of the hypharynx is a Zenker diverticulum which is cause by a herniation of mucosa through an area of weakness in the posterior wall of the hypopharynx. Diverticula in the esophagus are relatively rare and usually occur in the middle or lower esophagus. If a cervical approach (43130) is used, an incision is made in the neck, usually on the left side. The internal jugular vein and carotid artery are identified and retracted laterally. The esophagus and/or hypopharynx is exposed. For a thoracic approach (43135), a right posterior thoracotomy is generally used. The skin is incised and the incision extended through the soft tissues. The scapula is retracted and the thorax entered without disrupting the pleura. Retropleural dissection is performed, the lung retracted, and the esophagus is exposed. The esophagus or hypopharynx is mobilized to allow complete exposure of the diverticulum which appears as a muscosal outpouching in the muscular wall. The diverticulum is divided at its neck using a stapler and completely excised. The muscular wall is closed with sutures over the staple line. A myotomy is performed as needed on the side of the hypharynx or esophagus opposite to the diverticulum. The muscular wall of the hypopharynx of esophagus is incised longitudinally using blunt and sharp dissection taking care not to injure the underlying muscosa.

43180

43180   Esophagoscopy, rigid, transoral with diverticulectomy of hypopharynx or cervical esophagus (eg, Zenker's diverticulum), with cricopharyngeal myotomy, includes use of telescope or operating microscope and repair, when performed

Zenker's diverticulum, a pouch that forms in the back of the throat between the cricopharyngeus muscle and the inferior pharyngeal constrictor muscles, usually results from cricopharyngeal muscle spasms. The condition is rare and occurs primarily in the elderly causing food trapping and regurgitation that may lead to aspiration and pneumonia. A transoral endoscopic repair may be performed using a rigid double bladed endoscope and linear stapler and/or a carbon dioxide (CO2) laser or potassium-titanyl-phosphate (KTP) laser. To perform a diverticulectomy using staples, the blades of the endoscope are inserted into the diverticulum and the esophagus. The staple arms are then placed into the diverticulum and the esophagus, locked across the common septum, and fired repeatedly to adhere the mucosal edges together and close off the pouch. To perform a cricopharyngeal myotomy, a laser or needle knife is used to cut the septum between the diverticulum and the esophageal lumen to create a common room. This procedure increases the esophageal lumen and decreases pressure on the cricopharyngeus muscle, which reduces muscle spasms and allows food to travel normally down the esophagus.

43191

43191   Esophagoscopy, rigid, transoral; diagnostic, including collection of specimen(s) by brushing or washing when performed (separate procedure)

A diagnostic esophagoscopy using a rigid endoscope is performed with or without collection of specimens by brushing or washing. The endoscope is introduced through

the mouth and advanced into the esophagus. The velopharyngeal closure, the base of the tongue, and the hypopharynx are examined. Vocal cord motion is observed and the pharyngeal musculature is evaluated. When the scope reaches the cricopharyngeus, the patient is asked to burp or swallow to facilitate passage of the scope which is then advanced along the entire length of the esophagus to the gastroesophageal junction. Any abnormalities are noted. The scope is then withdrawn and the entire circumference of the esophagus is examined. Tissue samples may be obtained by brushing or washing saline fluid into the esophagus and then collecting it.

43192

43192   Esophagoscopy, rigid, transoral; with directed submucosal injection(s), any substance

Esophagoscopy using a rigid endoscope is performed with directed submucosal injection(s) of any substance. Commonly used substances include India ink, botulinum toxin, saline, epinephrine, or corticosteroids. India ink is used to help delineate a lesion prior to separately reportable excision which may also be referred to as tattooing of the lesion. Saline or epinephrine may also be injected prior to separately reportable lesion excision to help separate the mucosal layer from the muscle layer of the esophagus and elevate the lesion. Botulinum toxin is used to treat esophageal achalasia. The endoscope is introduced through the mouth and advanced into the esophagus. The velopharyngeal closure, the base of the tongue, and the hypopharynx are examined. Vocal cord motion is observed and the pharyngeal musculature is evaluated. When the scope reaches the cricopharyngeus, the patient is asked to burp or swallow to facilitate passage of the scope which is then advanced along the entire length of the esophagus to the gastroesophageal junction. Any abnormalities are noted. The scope is then withdrawn and the entire circumference of the esophagus is examined. The lesion is identified and one or more submucosal injections are performed prior to separately reportable lesion excision. Alternatively, if the injection procedure is performed to treat achalasia, the esophageal sphincter is injected with botulinum toxin.

43193

43193   Esophagoscopy, rigid, transoral; with biopsy, single or multiple

Esophagoscopy using a rigid endoscope is performed with biopsy. The endoscope is introduced through the mouth and advanced into the esophagus. The velopharyngeal closure, the base of the tongue, and the hypopharynx are examined. Vocal cord motion is observed and the pharyngeal musculature is evaluated. When the scope reaches the cricopharyngeus, the patient is asked to burp or swallow to facilitate passage of the scope which is then advanced along the entire length of the esophagus to the gastroesophageal junction. Any abnormalities are noted. The scope is then withdrawn and the entire circumference of the esophagus is examined. The site to be biopsied is identified and biopsy forceps are placed through the biopsy channel in the endoscope. The forceps are opened; the tissue is spiked; the forceps are closed; and the tissue sample is removed through the endoscope. One or more tissue samples may be obtained and are sent for separately reportable laboratory analysis.

43194

43194   Esophagoscopy, rigid, transoral; with removal of foreign body(s)

Esophagoscopy using a rigid endoscope is performed to remove a foreign body(s) lodged in the esophagus. The endoscope is introduced through the mouth and advanced into the esophagus. A balloon catheter may be used to remove a smooth-edged foreign body, such as a coin. The catheter tip is passed beyond the level of the foreign body and the balloon is inflated. The catheter is then withdrawn and the foreign body is carefully pulled out of the esophagus. An impacted foreign body, such as a piece of meat, is removed with forceps passed through the endoscope to the impacted foreign body, which is then grasped and removed. Alternatively, impacted food is sometimes nudged into the stomach using the forceps. A rigid endoscope may also be used to remove a sharp foreign body such as a tack or razor blade. The rigid endoscope is introduced and the foreign body is visualized and maneuvered into the lumen of the scope using forceps. The foreign body and scope are removed. Following removal of the foreign body(s), the endoscope is reintroduced and the esophagus is re-examined for evidence of perforation or other injury.

43195

43195   Esophagoscopy, rigid, transoral; with balloon dilation (less than 30 mm diameter)

Esophagoscopy using a rigid endoscope is performed with balloon dilation using a balloon diameter of less than 30 mm. Esophageal dilation is performed to treat a stricture (narrowing) of the esophagus. The stricture may be the result of reflux esophagitis which causes inflammation and scarring of the esophagus, Schatzki's ring which is a ring of benign fibrous tissue in the distal esophagus, congenital esophageal atresia, or malignant disease. The endoscope is introduced through the mouth and advanced into the esophagus to the area of stricture. The deflated balloon catheter is advanced through the instrument channel of the scope to the middle of the stricture. The balloon is inflated while using a pressure gauge to determine the optimal level of inflation. The inflated balloon is left in place for a short period of time (30 seconds to two minutes), deflated, and then removed. Following dilation, the area of stricture is inspected using the scope to ensure that the dilation has been successful and that there are no injuries resulting from the procedure.

43196

43196   Esophagoscopy, rigid, transoral; with insertion of guide wire followed by dilation over guide wire

Esophagoscopy using a rigid endoscope is performed by insertion of guide wire followed by dilation. Esophageal dilation is performed to treat a stricture (narrowing) of the esophagus. The stricture may be the result of reflux esophagitis which causes inflammation and scarring of the esophagus, Schatzki's ring which is a ring of benign fibrous tissue in the distal esophagus, congenital esophageal atresia, or malignant disease. The endoscope is introduced through the mouth and advanced into the esophagus to the area of stricture. A guide wire is inserted through the scope. A series of rigid tubes of increasing diameter are then passed over the guide wire to dilate the stricture. Following dilation, the area of stricture is inspected using the scope to ensure that the dilation has been successful and that there are no injuries resulting from the procedure.

43197

43197   Esophagoscopy, flexible, transnasal; diagnostic, including collection of specimen(s) by brushing or washing, when performed (separate procedure)

A diagnostic transnasal esophagoscopy using a flexible endoscope is performed with or without collection of specimens by brushing or washing. The flexible endoscope is introduced through the nose and advanced into the esophagus. The velopharyngeal closure, the base of the tongue, and the hypopharynx are examined. Vocal cord motion is observed and the pharyngeal musculature is evaluated. When the scope reaches the cricopharyngeus, the patient is asked to burp or swallow to facilitate passage of the scope which is then advanced along the entire length of the esophagus to the gastroesophageal junction. Any abnormalities are noted. The scope is then withdrawn and the entire circumference of the esophagus is examined. Tissue samples may be obtained by brushing or washing saline fluid into the esophagus and then collecting it.

43198

43198   Esophagoscopy, flexible, transnasal; with biopsy, single or multiple

Esophagoscopy using a flexible endoscope is performed with biopsy. The flexible endoscope is introduced through the nose and advanced into the esophagus. The velopharyngeal closure, the base of the tongue, and the hypopharynx are examined. Vocal cord motion is observed and the pharyngeal musculature is evaluated. When the scope reaches the cricopharyngeus, the patient is asked to burp or swallow to facilitate passage of the scope which is then advanced along the entire length of the esophagus to the gastroesophageal junction. Any abnormalities are noted. The scope is then withdrawn and the entire circumference of the esophagus is examined. The site to be biopsied is then identified and biopsy forceps are placed through the biopsy channel in the endoscope. The forceps are opened; the tissue is spiked; the forceps are closed; and the tissue sample is removed through the endoscope. One or more tissue samples may be obtained and are sent for separately reportable laboratory analysis.

43200

43200   Esophagoscopy, flexible, transoral; diagnostic, including collection of specimen(s) by brushing or washing, when performed (separate procedure)

A diagnostic esophagoscopy using a flexible endoscope is performed with or without collection of specimens by brushing or washing. The endoscope is introduced through the mouth and advanced into the esophagus. Velopharyngeal closure, base of the tongue, and the hypopharynx are examined. Vocal cord motion is observed and the pharyngeal musculature is evaluated. When the scope reaches the cricopharyngeus, the patient is asked to burp or swallow to facilitate passage of the scope which is then advanced along the entire length of the esophagus to the gastroesophageal junction. Any abnormalities are noted. The scope is then withdrawn and the entire circumference of the esophagus is examined. Tissue samples may be obtained by brushing or washing saline fluid into the esophagus and then collecting it.

43201

43201   Esophagoscopy, flexible, transoral; with directed submucosal injection(s), any substance

Esophagoscopy using a flexible endoscope is performed with directed submucosal injection(s) of any substance. Commonly used substances include India ink, botulinum toxin, saline, epinephrine, or corticosteroid substances. India ink is used to help delineate a lesion prior to separately reportable excision which may also be referred to as tattooing of the lesion. Saline or epinephrine may also be injected prior to separately reportable lesion excision to help separate the mucosal layer from the muscle layer of the esophagus and elevate the lesion. Botulinum toxin is used to treat esophageal achalasia. The endoscope is introduced through the mouth and advanced into the esophagus. Velopharyngeal closure, base of the tongue, and the hypopharynx are examined. Vocal cord motion is observed and

the pharyngeal musculature is evaluated. When the scope reaches the cricopharyngeus, the patient is asked to burp or swallow to facilitate passage of the scope which is then advanced along the entire length of the esophagus to the gastroesophageal junction. Any abnormalities are noted. The scope is then withdrawn and the entire circumference of the esophagus is examined. The lesion is identified and one or more submucosal injections are performed prior to separately reportable lesion excision. Alternatively, if the injection procedure is performed to treat achalasia, the esophageal sphincter is injected with botulinum toxin.

43202

43202   Esophagoscopy, flexible, transoral; with biopsy, single or multiple

Esophagoscopy using a flexible endoscope is performed with biopsy. The endoscope is introduced through the mouth and advanced into the esophagus. Velopharyngeal closure, base of the tongue, and the hypopharynx are examined. Vocal cord motion is observed and the pharyngeal musculature is evaluated. When the scope reaches the cricopharyngeus, the patient is asked to burp or swallow to facilitate passage of the scope which is then advanced along the entire length of the esophagus to the gastroesophageal junction. Any abnormalities are noted. The scope is then withdrawn and the entire circumference of the esophagus is examined. The site to be biopsied is identified and biopsy forceps are placed through the biopsy channel in the endoscope. The forceps are opened; the tissue is spiked; the forceps are closed; and the tissue sample is removed through the endoscope. One or more tissue samples may be obtained and are sent for separately reportable laboratory analysis.

43204-43205

43204   Esophagoscopy, flexible, transoral; with injection sclerosis of esophageal varices

43205   Esophagoscopy, flexible, transoral; with band ligation of esophageal varices

Esophagoscopy using a flexible endoscope is performed for treatment of esophageal varices by injection sclerosis (43204) or band ligation (43205). Esophageal varices are dilated blood vessels within the wall of the esophagus and are usually associated with portal hypertension caused by cirrhosis of the liver. The endoscope is introduced through the mouth and advanced into the esophagus. Velopharyngeal closure, the base of the tongue, and the hypopharynx are examined. Vocal cord motion is observed and the pharyngeal musculature is evaluated. When the scope reaches the cricopharyngeus, the patient is asked to burp or swallow to facilitate passage of the scope which is then advanced along the entire length of the esophagus to the gastroesophageal junction. Any abnormalities are noted. The scope is then withdrawn and the entire circumference of the esophagus is examined. In 43204, the esophageal varices are injected with sclerosing solution to shrink them. In 43205, a snare is introduced through the endoscope and an elastic band is placed around each varix to tie off (strangle) the vein.

43206

43206   Esophagoscopy, flexible, transoral; with optical endomicroscopy

Optical endomicroscopy provides in vivo visualization and characterization of the esophageal mucosal tissue and pathophysiological processes at the microscopic level. This allows the physician to see histological details during an endoscopy. A flexible endoscope is introduced through the mouth and advanced into the esophagus. The velopharyngeal closure, the base of the tongue, and the hypopharynx are examined. Vocal cord motion is observed and the pharyngeal musculature is evaluated. When the scope reaches the cricopharyngeus, the patient is asked to burp or swallow to facilitate passage of the scope which is then advanced along the entire length of the esophagus to the gastroesophageal junction. Any abnormalities are noted. The scope is then withdrawn while the entire circumference of the esophagus is examined. Any abnormalities are noted. Following the application of a contrast agent, endomicroscopy is performed with a miniaturized endomicroscope integrated into or inserted through the endoscope with a blue laser light that scans the esophageal mucosa from the surface to the deepest mucosal layer. Endomicroscopy allows the physician to obtain separately reportable targeted biopsies from areas with microscopic changes rather than random tissue sampling and provides instant histological information for immediate treatment.

43210

43210   Esophagogastroduodenoscopy, flexible, transoral; with esophagogastric fundoplasty, partial or complete, includes duodenoscopy when performed

Transoral incisionless fundoplication is a procedure that reconstructs a defective gastroesophageal valve, with or without hiatal hernia, and may be used to treat gastroesophageal reflux disease. An endoscope specially outfitted with invaginator, tissue mold and chassis, helical retractor, stylet and fasteners is inserted orally and passed down the esophagus into the stomach. The stomach is inflated and the endoscope is retroflexed to view the gastroesophageal junction. The invaginator provides circumferential tissue retraction, reduces a hernia, if present, and facilitates proper positioning of the fundoplication. The tissue mold and chassis is advanced to rotate the fundus around the esophagus creating a fold and compressing the esophageal and gastric tissue together

Digestive System

along the lesser curvature of the stomach. The helical retractor is then advanced out of the tissue mold, and fasteners are deployed to secure the full thickness serosa tissue above and below the diaphragm at the gastroesophageal junction. The helical retractor is then secured back into the tissue mold and the device is rotated to the opposing side at the greater curvature of the stomach. The steps are repeated to create a tight omega shaped valve. The resulting esophagogastric fundoplasty is 270-310 degrees in circumference and 3-5 cm in length. Endoscopic examination of the duodenum may also be performed. The endoscope is removed after the surgical site has been carefully inspected and no evidence of bleeding is present.

43211

43211   Esophagoscopy, flexible, transoral; with endoscopic mucosal resection

Esophagoscopy using a flexible endoscope is performed with endoscopic mucosal resection. Endoscopic mucosal resection is used to treat dysplastic, or precancerous, lesions and small, early cancerous lesions limited to the mucosa of the esophagus. The endoscope is introduced through the mouth and advanced into the esophagus to the area of the lesion. The borders of the lesion are marked with electrocautery. Diluted adrenaline is then injected into the submucosal layer around the lesion to lift the mucosal layer containing the lesion and separate it from the underlying muscle. A snare with a suction cup is used to lift the lesion which is then excised and captured using the snare. The scope is withdrawn and the entire circumference of the esophagus is examined. The excised tissue is sent for separately reportable pathology examination.

43212

43212   Esophagoscopy, flexible, transoral; with placement of endoscopic stent (includes pre- and post-dilation and guide wire passage, when performed)

Esophagoscopy using a flexible endoscope is performed with stent placement. Indications for stent placement include narrowing or stricture of the esophagus due to esophageal cancer or lung cancer and malignant bronchoesophageal fistula. The endoscope is introduced through the mouth and advanced into the esophagus to the area of the stricture or fistula. If treatment is for a stricture, the stricture is examined and the need for pre-dilation is evaluated. If pre-dilation is needed, a guide wire is inserted through the scope. A series of rigid tubes of increasing diameter are then passed over the guide wire to dilate the stricture. Alternately, a balloon catheter may be advanced to the site of the stricture and inflated to dilate the stricture. Stent placement is then performed. A guide wire is passed through the scope followed by the stent delivery system which is passed over the guide wire and positioned in the narrowed portion of the esophagus or over the fistula. The stent is then deployed. A balloon catheter may again be inserted and inflated to seat the stent. The endoscope is advanced through the stent to check stent position and ensure proper deployment.

43213

43213   Esophagoscopy, flexible, transoral; with dilation of esophagus, by balloon or dilator, retrograde (includes fluoroscopic guidance, when performed)

Esophagoscopy using a flexible endoscope is performed for dilation of the esophagus by balloon or dilator by a retrograde approach. Esophageal dilation is performed to treat a stricture (narrowing) of the esophagus. Retrograde approach is typically used for esophageal strictures that develop after radiation therapy to the head and neck region or in patients who have had an esophagectomy followed by gastric or colonic reconstruction of the esophagus. The stomach is accessed through a previously established jejunostomy or gastrostomy tract. Using fluoroscopic guidance as needed, the endoscope is passed from the stomach to the distal esophagus. A guidewire is advanced in a retrograde fashion from the stomach, into the esophagus, through the stricture, and then pulled into the mouth using a second endoscope that has been introduced through the mouth. The deflated balloon catheter is advanced in a retrograde fashion through the instrument channel of the scope and over the guidewire to the middle of the stricture. The balloon is inflated while using a pressure gauge to determine the optimal level of inflation. The inflated balloon is left in place for a short period of time (30 seconds to two minutes), deflated, and then removed. Alternatively, a guide wire may be introduced followed by a series of rigid tubes of increasing diameter that are passed over the guide wire to dilate the stricture. Upon completion of the procedure, the entire circumference of the esophagus is again inspected as the scopes are withdrawn to ensure adequate dilation of the stricture and to verify that the esophagus has not been damaged during the dilation procedure.

43214

43214   Esophagoscopy, flexible, transoral; with dilation of esophagus with balloon (30 mm diameter or larger) (includes fluoroscopic guidance, when performed)

Esophagoscopy using a flexible endoscope is performed for dilation of the esophagus with a balloon 30 mm or larger in diameter. Esophageal dilation is performed to treat a stricture (narrowing) of the esophagus. The stricture may be the result of reflux esophagitis which causes inflammation and scarring of the esophagus, Schatzki's ring which is a ring of benign fibrous tissue in the distal esophagus, congenital esophageal atresia, or malignant disease. The endoscope is introduced through the mouth. The velopharyngeal closure, the

base of the tongue, and the hypopharynx are examined. Vocal cord motion is observed and the pharyngeal musculature is evaluated. When the scope reaches the cricopharyngeus, the patient is asked to burp or swallow to facilitate passage of the scope which is then advanced along the entire length of the esophagus to the gastroesophageal junction. Any abnormalities are noted. The scope is then withdrawn and the entire circumference of the esophagus is examined noting the area of stricture. Using fluoroscopic guidance as needed, the deflated balloon catheter is advanced through the instrument channel of the scope to the middle of the stricture. The balloon is inflated while using a pressure gauge to determine the optimal level of inflation. The inflated balloon is left in place for a short period of time (30 seconds to two minutes), deflated, and then removed. Following dilation, the area of stricture is inspected using the scope to ensure that the dilation has been successful and that there are no injuries resulting from the procedure.

43215

43215   Esophagoscopy, flexible, transoral; with removal of foreign body(s)

Esophagoscopy using a flexible endoscope is performed to remove a foreign body(s) lodged in the esophagus. The endoscope is introduced through the mouth and advanced into the esophagus. A balloon catheter may be used to remove a smooth-edged foreign body, such as a coin. The catheter tip is passed beyond the level of the foreign body and the balloon is inflated. The catheter is then withdrawn and the foreign body is carefully pulled out of the esophagus. An impacted foreign body, such as a piece of meat, is removed with forceps. The forceps are passed through the endoscope and the impacted foreign body is grasped and removed. Alternatively, impacted food is sometimes nudged into the stomach using the forceps. A flexible endoscope may be used to remove a sharp foreign body such as a tack or razor blade. The endoscope is introduced and the foreign body is visualized and maneuvered into the lumen of the scope using forceps. The foreign body and scope are removed. Following removal of the foreign body(s), the endoscope is reintroduced and the esophagus is re-examined for evidence of perforation or other injury.

43216-43217

43216   Esophagoscopy, flexible, transoral; with removal of tumor(s), polyp(s), or other lesion(s) by hot biopsy forceps

43217   Esophagoscopy, flexible, transoral; with removal of tumor(s), polyp(s), or other lesion(s) by snare technique

Esophagoscopy using a flexible endoscope is performed with removal of tumors, polyps, or other lesions by hot biopsy forceps (43216) or by snare technique (43217). The endoscope is introduced through the mouth and advanced into the esophagus. Velopharyngeal closure, the base of the tongue, and the hypopharynx are examined. Vocal cord motion is observed and the pharyngeal musculature is evaluated. When the scope reaches the cricopharyngeus, the patient is asked to burp or swallow to facilitate passage of the scope which is then advanced along the entire length of the esophagus to the gastroesophageal junction. Any abnormalities are noted. The scope is then withdrawn and the entire circumference of the esophagus is examined. The tumor, polyp, or other lesion is identified. In 43216, hot biopsy forceps are used to remove the lesion. Hot biopsy method uses insulated monopolar forceps to remove and electrocoagulate (cauterize) tissue simultaneously. Hot biopsy forceps are used primarily for removal of small polyps and treatment of vascular ectasias. In 43217, a wire snare loop is placed around the lesion. The loop is heated to shave off and cauterize the lesion. Lesions may be removed en bloc with one placement of the snare or in a piecemeal fashion, which requires multiple snare applications.

43220-43226

43220   Esophagoscopy, flexible, transoral; with transendoscopic balloon dilation (less than 30 mm diameter)

43226   Esophagoscopy, flexible, transoral; with insertion of guide wire followed by passage of dilator(s) over guide wire

Esophagoscopy using a flexible endoscope is performed with transendoscopic balloon dilation using a balloon diameter of less than 30 mm (43220) or insertion of guide wire followed by dilation (43226). Esophageal dilation is performed to treat a stricture (narrowing) of the esophagus. The stricture may be the result of reflux esophagitis which causes inflammation and scarring of the esophagus, Schatzki's ring which is a ring of benign fibrous tissue in the distal esophagus, congenital esophageal atresia, or malignant disease. The endoscope is introduced through the mouth and advanced into the esophagus to the area of stricture. In 43220, the deflated balloon catheter is advanced through the instrument channel of the scope to the middle of the stricture. The balloon is inflated while using a pressure gauge to determine the optimal level of inflation. The inflated balloon is left in place for a short period of time (30 seconds to two minutes), deflated, and then removed. In 43226, a guide wire is inserted through the scope. A series of rigid tubes of increasing diameter are then passed over the guide wire to dilate the stricture. Following dilation, the area of stricture is inspected using the scope to ensure that the dilation has been successful and that there are no injuries resulting from the procedure.

● New Code   ▲ Revised Code   CPT © 2016 American Medical Association. All Rights Reserved.   © 2017 DecisionHealth

43227

43227   Esophagoscopy, flexible, transoral; with control of bleeding, any method

Esophagoscopy using a flexible endoscope is performed with control of bleeding by injection, bipolar/unipolar cautery, laser, heater probe, stapler, plasma coagulator, or other technique. This procedure is performed to treat bleeding due to esophageal injury or conditions such as Mallory-Weiss syndrome. The endoscope is introduced through the mouth and advanced into the esophagus. Velopharyngeal closure, the base of the tongue, and the hypopharynx are examined. Vocal cord motion is observed and the pharyngeal musculature is evaluated. When the scope reaches the cricopharyngeus, the patient is asked to burp or swallow to facilitate passage of the scope which is then advanced along the entire length of the esophagus to the gastroesophageal junction. Any abnormalities are noted. The scope is then withdrawn and the entire circumference of the esophagus is examined. The bleeding site is identified. Bleeding is typically controlled using a contact thermal modality, such as bipolar or unipolar cautery or a heater probe. The cautery device or heater probe is applied to the bleeding point and pressure is applied along with heat to control bleeding. An injection of epinephrine, which works as a vasoconstrictor and tamponade, can also be used to reduce or stop bleeding. YAG laser coagulation and a newer modality, the argon plasma coagulator, are noncontact devices used to coagulate the bleeding site. Staples or hemoclips may be used to approximate the margins of a tear or laceration.

43229

43229   Esophagoscopy, flexible, transoral; with ablation of tumor(s), polyp(s), or other lesion(s) (includes pre- and post-dilation and guide wire passage, when performed)

Esophagoscopy using a flexible endoscope is performed with ablation of one or more tumors, polyps, or other lesions. The endoscope is introduced through the mouth. The velopharyngeal closure, the base of the tongue, and the hypopharynx are examined. Vocal cord motion is observed and the pharyngeal musculature is evaluated. When the scope reaches the cricopharyngeus, the patient is asked to burp or swallow to facilitate passage of the scope which is then advanced along the entire length of the esophagus to the gastroesophageal junction. Any abnormalities are noted. The scope is then withdrawn and the entire circumference of the esophagus is examined noting the site of the lesions to be ablated. If dilation is required prior to the ablation procedure, a guide wire is inserted through the scope. A series of rigid tubes of increasing diameter are then passed over the guide wire and the esophageal lumen is dilated as needed. Alternately, a balloon catheter may be advanced to the site of the stricture and inflated to dilate the esophagus. The laser device is then delivered through the endoscope to the distal margin of the most distal lesion. The lesion is ablated as the endoscope is retracted. The entire lesion is destroyed as the laser traverses the lesion in a distal to proximal direction. This is repeated until all lesions have been destroyed. If dilation is required following destruction of lesions, it is performed again as described above. The esophagus is once again examined using the endoscope to ensure that all lesions have been destroyed and that there are no injuries resulting from the procedure.

43231

43231   Esophagoscopy, flexible, transoral; with endoscopic ultrasound examination

Esophagoscopy using a flexible endoscope is performed with an endoscopic ultrasound examination. The endoscope is introduced through the mouth and advanced into the esophagus. Velopharyngeal closure, the base of the tongue, and the hypopharynx are examined. Vocal cord motion is observed and the pharyngeal musculature is evaluated. When the scope reaches the cricopharyngeus, the patient is asked to burp or swallow to facilitate passage of the scope which is then advanced the entire length of the esophagus to the gastroesophageal junction. Any abnormalities are noted. The scope is then withdrawn and the entire circumference of the esophagus is examined. Following endoscopic examination, an echoendoscope is introduced and advanced to the gastroesophageal junction or to the site of the abnormality or lesion. Ultrasound images are obtained to determine whether the abnormality or lesion is intrinsic (within) or extrinsic (outside) the esophagus. If the lesion is intrinsic to the esophagus, it is evaluated to determine whether it is limited to the mucosa or involves the muscular wall. If it is extrinsic, it is evaluated to determine whether it is in the mediastinal space or has invaded the mediastinal wall, what thoracic organs are involved, and whether there is any lymph node involvement. Hard copies of ultrasound images are made and the abnormalities are again evaluated.

43232

43232   Esophagoscopy, flexible, transoral; with transendoscopic ultrasound-guided intramural or transmural fine needle aspiration/biopsy(s)

Esophagoscopy using a flexible endoscope is performed with transendoscopic ultrasound-guided intramural or transmural fine needle aspiration/biopsy. The endoscope is introduced through the mouth and advanced into the distal esophagus. Velopharyngeal closure, the base of the tongue, and the hypopharynx are examined. Vocal cord motion is observed and the pharyngeal musculature is evaluated. When the scope reaches the cricopharyngeus, the patient is asked to burp or swallow to facilitate passage of the scope which is then advanced the entire length of the esophagus to the gastroesophageal junction. Any abnormalities are noted. A radial scanning echoendoscope is then introduced and advanced under direct endoscopic visualization. Ultrasound imaging is used to evaluate the thoracic region. The mediastinum and adjacent structures are assessed for the presence of enlarged lymph nodes. Other lesions are identified and determination is made whether they arise from the esophagus or other structures and whether the tumor(s) has invaded other vital structures. The lungs are evaluated for the presence of pleural effusion and other abnormalities. Ultrasound images are then sent to a hard copy device and evaluated. Lymph nodes and other lesions that can be biopsied through the esophagus are identified. The radial scanning echoendoscope is removed and replaced with a linear scanning echoendoscope. A needle biopsy catheter is advanced through the biopsy channel of the echoendoscope. Doppler images are obtained to ensure that there are no vascular structures obstructing the planned biopsy route. The needle is then advanced through the esophageal wall into the lesion or lymph node and an aspiration biopsy is obtained and sent for separately reportable cytologic evaluation. Multiple passes are made at each biopsy site. After each pass, the biopsy device is removed, cleaned, and reassembled. Once an adequate specimen has been obtained from the first biopsy site, the next biopsy site is addressed in the same manner.

43233

43233   Esophagogastroduodenoscopy, flexible, transoral; with dilation of esophagus with balloon (30 mm diameter or larger) (includes fluoroscopic guidance, when performed)

Esophagogastroduodenoscopy using a flexible endoscope is performed for dilation of the esophagus with a balloon 30 mm or larger in diameter. Esophageal dilation is performed to treat a stricture (narrowing) of the esophagus. The stricture may be the result of reflux esophagitis which causes inflammation and scarring of the esophagus, Schatzki's ring which is a ring of benign fibrous tissue in the distal esophagus, congenital esophageal atresia, or malignant disease. The endoscope is introduced through the mouth. The velopharyngeal closure, the base of the tongue, and the hypopharynx are examined. Vocal cord motion is observed and the pharyngeal musculature is evaluated. When the scope reaches the cricopharyngeus, the patient is asked to burp or swallow to facilitate passage of the scope which is then advanced along the entire length of the esophagus and any abnormalities are noted. The endoscope is advanced into the stomach, through the pylorus, and into the duodenum. Mucosal surfaces of the duodenum are inspected as the endoscope is withdrawn. The pylorus is examined and the mucosal surfaces of the stomach are also inspected. The entire circumference of the esophagus is examined noting the area of stricture. Using fluoroscopic guidance as needed, the deflated balloon catheter is advanced through the instrument channel of the scope to the middle of the stricture. The balloon is inflated while using a pressure gauge to determine the optimal level of inflation. The inflated balloon is left in place for a short period of time (30 seconds to two minutes), deflated, and then removed. Following dilation, the area of stricture is inspected using the scope to ensure that the dilation has been successful and that there are no injuries resulting from the procedure.

43235

43235   Esophagogastroduodenoscopy, flexible, transoral; diagnostic, including collection of specimen(s) by brushing or washing, when performed (separate procedure)

A diagnostic upper gastrointestinal (UGI) endoscopic examination is performed of the esophagus, stomach, duodenum and/or jejunum with or without collection of specimens by brushing or washing. This procedure may also be referred to as an esophagogastroduodenoscopy (EGD). The mouth and throat are numbed using an anesthetic spray. A hollow mouthpiece is placed in the mouth. The flexible fiberoptic endoscope is then inserted and advanced as it is swallowed by the patient. Once the endoscope has been advanced beyond the cricopharyngeal region, it is guided using direct visualization. The esophagus is inspected and any abnormalities are noted. The endoscope is then advanced beyond the gastroesophageal junction into the stomach and the stomach is insufflated with air. The cardia, fundus, greater and lesser curvature, and antrum of the stomach are inspected and any abnormalities are noted. The tip of the endoscope is then advanced through the pylorus and into the duodenum and/or jejunum. Mucosal surfaces of the duodenum and/or jejunum are inspected and any abnormalities are noted. The endoscope is then withdrawn and mucosal surfaces are again inspected for ulcerations, varices, bleeding sites, lesions, strictures, or other abnormalities. Cytology samples may be obtained by cell brushing or washing.

43236

43236   Esophagogastroduodenoscopy, flexible, transoral; with directed submucosal injection(s), any substance

An upper gastrointestinal (UGI) endoscopic examination, also referred to as an esophagogastroduodenoscopy (EGD) is performed of the esophagus, stomach, duodenum and/or jejunum with directed submucosal injections. Common substances injected include india ink, botulinum toxin, saline, epinephrine, and corticosteroid solutions. The mouth and throat are numbed using an anesthetic spray. A hollow mouthpiece is placed in the mouth.

Digestive System

The flexible fiberoptic endoscope is then inserted and advanced as it is swallowed by the patient. Once the endoscope has been advanced beyond the cricopharyngeal region, it is guided using direct visualization. The esophagus is inspected and any abnormalities noted. The endoscope is then advanced into the stomach and the stomach is insufflated with air. The cardia, fundus, greater and lesser curvature, and antrum of the stomach are inspected and any abnormalities noted. The tip of the endoscope is then advanced through the pylorus and into the duodenum and/or jejunum. Mucosal surfaces of the duodenum and/or jejunum are inspected and any abnormalities are noted. One or more directed submucosal injections are administered. Submucosal injections may be used to mark (tattoo) a lesion for better visualization prior to separately reportable removal of the lesion, or to create a submucosal fluid cushion prior to removal and help separate the mucosal layer from the muscle layer and elevate the lesion. The endoscope is withdrawn and mucosal surfaces are again inspected for ulcerations, varices, bleeding sites, lesions, strictures, or other abnormalities.

43237-43238

43237   **Esophagogastroduodenoscopy, flexible, transoral; with endoscopic ultrasound examination limited to the esophagus, stomach or duodenum, and adjacent structures**

43238   **Esophagogastroduodenoscopy, flexible, transoral; with transendoscopic ultrasound-guided intramural or transmural fine needle aspiration/biopsy(s), (includes endoscopic ultrasound examination limited to the esophagus, stomach or duodenum, and adjacent structures)**

An upper gastrointestinal (UGI) endoscopic examination, also referred to as an esophagogastroduodenoscopy (EGD), is performed of the esophagus, stomach, duodenum and/or jejunum with endoscopic ultrasound (EUS). The mouth and throat are numbed using an anesthetic spray. A hollow mouthpiece is placed in the mouth. The flexible fiberoptic endoscope is then inserted and advanced as it is swallowed by the patient. Once the endoscope has been advanced beyond the cricopharyngeal region, it is guided using direct visualization. The esophagus is inspected and any abnormalities are noted. An endoscopic ultrasound is then advanced for more detailed examination of the wall of the esophagus. EUS allows the esophagus to be imaged as a five-layer structure, the first two layers being the mucosa, the third layer the submusoca, the fourth layer the muscularis propria, and the fifth layer the serosa or adventitia. The endoscope is then advanced into the stomach and the stomach is insufflated with air. The cardia, fundus, greater and lesser curvature, and antrum of the stomach are inspected and any abnormalities are noted. The tip of the endoscope is then advanced through the pylorus and into the duodenum and/or jejunum. Mucosal surfaces of the duodenum and/or jejunum are inspected and any abnormalities are noted. The endoscope is withdrawn and mucosal surfaces are again inspected for ulcerations, varices, bleeding sites, lesions, strictures, or other abnormalities. In 43237, the EGD of the entire UGI tract is performed in conjunction with an endoscopic ultrasound (EUS) examination. Use 43238 when transendoscopic ultrasound-guided intramural or transmural fine needle aspiration or biopsy of one or more sites is also performed. Using endoscopic ultrasound-guidance, a fine needle aspiration device or other biopsy tool is advanced into the (esophageal) wall at the site of the lesion and intramural tissue samples are obtained. If a fine needle biopsy is required from surrounding structures, such as lymph nodes, the needle is passed through the esophageal wall and transmural biopsies are obtained.

43239

43239   **Esophagogastroduodenoscopy, flexible, transoral; with biopsy, single or multiple**

An upper gastrointestinal (UGI) endoscopic examination, also referred to as an esophagogastroduodenoscopy (EGD), is performed on the esophagus, stomach, duodenum and/or jejunum with biopsy(s). The mouth and throat are numbed using an anesthetic spray. A hollow mouthpiece is placed in the mouth. The flexible fiberoptic endoscope is then inserted and advanced as it is swallowed by the patient. Once the endoscope has been advanced beyond the cricopharyngeal region, it is guided using direct visualization. The esophagus is inspected and any abnormalities are noted. The endoscope is then advanced beyond the gastroesophageal junction into the stomach and the stomach is insufflated with air. The cardia, fundus, greater and lesser curvature, and antrum are inspected and any abnormalities are noted. The tip of the endoscope is then advanced through the pylorus and into the duodenum and/or jejunum where mucosal surfaces are inspected for any abnormalities. Single or multiple samples of suspect tissue are taken through the scope. The endoscope is withdrawn and mucosal surfaces are again inspected for ulcerations, varices, bleeding sites, lesions, strictures, or other abnormalities.

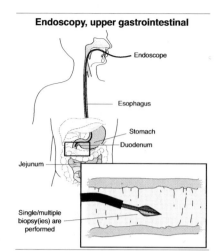

Endoscopy, upper gastrointestinal

Endoscope

Esophagus

Stomach

Duodenum

Jejunum

Single/multiple biopsy(ies) are performed

43240

43240   **Esophagogastroduodenoscopy, flexible, transoral; with transmural drainage of pseudocyst (includes placement of transmural drainage catheter[s]/stent[s], when performed, and endoscopic ultrasound, when performed)**

An upper gastrointestinal (UGI) endoscopic examination, also referred to as an esophagogastroduodenoscopy (EGD), is performed on the esophagus, stomach, duodenum and/or jejunum with transmural drainage of a pseudocyst. The mouth and throat are numbed using an anesthetic spray. A hollow mouthpiece is placed in the mouth. The flexible fiberoptic endoscope is then inserted and advanced as it is swallowed by the patient. Once the endoscope has been advanced beyond the cricopharyngeal region, it is guided using direct visualization. The esophagus is inspected and any abnormalities are noted. The endoscope is then advanced into the stomach and the stomach is insufflated with air. The cardia, fundus, greater and lesser curvature, and antrum are inspected and any abnormalities are noted. The tip of the endoscope is then advanced through the pylorus and into the duodenum and/or jejunum where mucosal surfaces are inspected for any abnormalities. The pseudocyst in the gastrointestinal wall is located. A scanning echoendoscope may be introduced and advanced under direct endoscopic visualization and ultrasound imaging used to locate the pseudocyst. A needle is used to puncture the pseudocyst and the fluid is drained. Diathermic needle cautery may be used to create a fistula between the pseudocyst and the lumen of the gastrointestinal tract or a transmural drainage tube may be inserted to maintain patency of the tract. The endoscope is withdrawn and mucosal surfaces are again inspected for ulcerations, varices, bleeding sites, lesions, strictures, or other abnormalities

43241

43241   **Esophagogastroduodenoscopy, flexible, transoral; with insertion of intraluminal tube or catheter**

An upper gastrointestinal (UGI) endoscopic examination is performed on the esophagus, stomach, duodenum and/or jejunum with transendoscopic tube or catheter placement. The mouth and throat are numbed using an anesthetic spray. A hollow mouthpiece is placed in the mouth. The flexible fiberoptic endoscope is then inserted and advanced as it is swallowed by the patient. Once the endoscope has been advanced beyond the cricopharyngeal region, it is guided using direct visualization. The esophagus is inspected and any abnormalities are noted. The endoscope is then advanced into the stomach and the stomach is insufflated with air. The cardia, fundus, greater and lesser curvature, and antrum of the stomach are inspected and any abnormalities are noted. The tip of the endoscope is then passed through the pylorus into the duodenum and/or jejunum and the mucosal surfaces are inspected. The area of obstruction is identified. The position and length of the obstructed area are determined. An appropriately sized tube or catheter is selected and introduced through the scope. The tube or catheter is then positioned in the obstructed portion of the upper digestive tract. Images are obtained to ensure that the tube is properly placed and opening the lumen of the obstructed area of the upper GI tract.

43242

43242   **Esophagogastroduodenoscopy, flexible, transoral; with transendoscopic ultrasound-guided intramural or transmural fine needle aspiration/biopsy(s) (includes endoscopic ultrasound examination of the esophagus, stomach, and either the duodenum or a surgically altered stomach where the jejunum is examined distal to the anastomosis)**

An upper gastrointestinal (UGI) endoscopic examination is performed on the esophagus, stomach, and either the duodenum, or the jejunum of a surgically altered stomach with ultrasound-guided fine needle aspiration or biopsy(s). The mouth and throat are numbed using an anesthetic spray. A hollow mouthpiece is placed in the mouth. The flexible fiberoptic endoscope is then inserted and advanced as the patient swallows it. Once the endoscope has been advanced beyond the cricopharyngeal region, it is guided using direct visualization. The esophagus is inspected and any abnormalities are noted. The endoscope is then advanced into the stomach and the stomach is insufflated with air. The cardia, fundus, greater and lesser curvature, and antrum of the stomach are inspected and any abnormalities are noted. The tip of the endoscope is then advanced through the pylorus and into the duodenum and/or the jejunum when anastomosed to a surgically altered stomach. Mucosal surfaces of the duodenum and/or jejunum are inspected and any abnormalities are noted. The upper GI EGD is performed in conjunction with an endoscopic ultrasound (EUS) examination. A radial scanning echoendoscope is then introduced and advanced under direct endoscopic visualization. Ultrasound imaging is used to evaluate the UGI tract and the thoracic and upper abdominal region for the presence of enlarged lymph nodes or other lesions adjacent to the upper digestive tract. Lymph nodes and other lesions that can be biopsied are identified. The radial scanning echoendoscope is removed and replaced with a linear scanning echoendoscope. Transendoscopic ultrasound-guided intramural or transmural fine needle aspiration or biopsy is performed. A needle biopsy catheter is then advanced through the biopsy channel of the echoendoscope to the site of the lesion and intramural tissue samples are obtained. If a fine needle biopsy is required from surrounding structures, doppler images are obtained to ensure that there are no vascular structures obstructing the planned biopsy route and the needle is advanced through the wall of the esophagus, stomach, duodenum or jejunum into the lesion or lymph node and the biopsy(s) is obtained.

43243-43244

43243 Esophagogastroduodenoscopy, flexible, transoral; with injection sclerosis of esophageal/gastric varices

43244 Esophagogastroduodenoscopy, flexible, transoral; with band ligation of esophageal/gastric varices

An upper gastrointestinal (UGI) endoscopic examination, also referred to as an esophagogastroduodenoscopy (EGD), is performed on the esophagus, stomach, duodenum and/or jejunum with injection sclerosis (43243) or band ligation (43244) of esophageal and/or gastric varices. Esophageal varices are dilated blood vessels within the wall of the esophagus and are usually associated with portal hypertension caused by cirrhosis of the liver. The mouth and throat are numbed using an anesthetic spray. A hollow mouthpiece is placed in the mouth. The flexible fiberoptic endoscope is then inserted and advanced as it is swallowed by the patient. Once the endoscope has been advanced beyond the cricopharyngeal region, it is guided using direct visualization. The esophagus is inspected and any abnormalities are noted. The endoscope is then advanced beyond the gastroesophageal junction into the stomach and the stomach is insufflated with air. The cardia, fundus, greater and lesser curvature, and antrum of the stomach are inspected and any abnormalities are noted. The tip of the endoscope is then advanced through the pylorus and into the duodenum and/or jejunum. Mucosal surfaces of the duodenum and/or jejunum are inspected and any abnormalities are noted. In 43243, esophageal and/or gastric varices are injected with a sclerosing solution to shrink them. In 43244, a snare is introduced through the endoscope and an elastic band is placed around each varix to tie off (ligate) the vein.

43245

43245 Esophagogastroduodenoscopy, flexible, transoral; with dilation of gastric/duodenal stricture(s) (eg, balloon, bougie)

An upper gastrointestinal (UGI) endoscopic examination, also referred to as an esophagogastroduodenoscopy (EGD), is performed on the esophagus, stomach, duodenum and/or jejunum with dilation of gastric/duodenal stricture(s). The mouth and throat are numbed using an anesthetic spray. A hollow mouthpiece is placed in the mouth. The flexible fiberoptic endoscope is then inserted and advanced as it is swallowed by the patient. Once the endoscope has been advanced beyond the cricopharyngeal region, it is guided using direct visualization. The esophagus is inspected and any abnormalities are noted. The endoscope is then advanced beyond the gastroesophageal junction into the stomach and the stomach is insufflated with air. The cardia, fundus, greater and lesser curvature, and antrum of the stomach are inspected and any abnormalities are noted. The tip of the endoscope is then advanced to the pylorus (gastric outlet) and a dilator such as a balloon or bougie is used to dilate the gastric outlet. If a balloon is used, it is inflated and left in place for a short period of time. The balloon is then deflated. Inflation and deflation may be repeated several times until the outlet is sufficiently dilated. Alternatively, a series of bougie dilators (tubes) of increasing diameter are passed over a guidewire until the obstruction has been relieved. The gastric outlet is inspected for any evidence of tearing or other injury. The endoscope is then passed into the duodenum and/or jejunum and mucosal surfaces are inspected.

43246

43246 Esophagogastroduodenoscopy, flexible, transoral; with directed placement of percutaneous gastrostomy tube

This procedure is also referred to as percutaneous endoscopic gastrostomy (PEG) and is used in patients who are unable to take liquids or food by mouth for an extended period of time. The mouth and throat are numbed using an anesthetic spray. A hollow mouthpiece

is placed in the mouth. The flexible fiberoptic endoscope is then inserted and advanced as it is swallowed by the patient. Once the endoscope has been advanced beyond the cricopharyngeal region, it is guided using direct visualization. The esophagus is inspected and any abnormalities are noted. The endoscope is then advanced into the stomach and the stomach is insufflated with air. The cardia, fundus, greater and lesser curvature, and antrum of the stomach are inspected and any abnormalities are noted. The tip of the endoscope is then passed through the pylorus into the duodenum and/or jejunum and the mucosal surfaces are inspected. The endoscope is then withdrawn into the stomach and the PEG procedure is performed. A small incision is made through the skin and upper abdominal wall on the left side. Using a push technique, a guidewire is inserted through the incision and advanced through the stomach into the gastric cavity under endoscopic visualization. A feeding tube is advanced over the guidewire and into the stomach. The guidewire is removed. Using a pull technique, the feeding tube is advanced endoscopically through the mouth and into the stomach. The feeding tube is advanced through the stomach wall. A snare passed through the abdominal incision is used to capture the feeding tube and pull the tube out through the abdominal incision. The feeding tube is secured internally with a bumper or balloon and externally with a bumper, flange, or other device.

43247

43247 Esophagogastroduodenoscopy, flexible, transoral; with removal of foreign body(s)

An upper gastrointestinal (UGI) endoscopic examination, also referred to as an esophagogastroduodenoscopy (EGD), is performed on the esophagus, stomach, duodenum and/or jejunum with removal of a foreign body(s). The mouth and throat are numbed using an anesthetic spray. A hollow mouthpiece is placed in the mouth. The flexible fiberoptic endoscope is then inserted and advanced as it is swallowed by the patient. Once the endoscope has been advanced beyond the cricopharyngeal region, it is guided using direct visualization. The endoscope is advanced to the site of the foreign body. A balloon catheter may be used to remove a smooth edged foreign body, such as a coin. The catheter tip is passed beyond the level of the foreign body and the balloon is inflated. The catheter is then withdrawn and the foreign body is carefully pulled out of the esophagus. An impacted foreign body such as a piece of meat is removed with forceps. The forceps are passed through the endoscope and the impacted foreign body is grasped and removed. A sharp foreign body such as a tack or razor blade is first maneuvered into the lumen of the scope using forceps and the foreign body and scope are removed. Following removal of the foreign body(s), the endoscope is reintroduced and the esophagus, stomach, duodenum and/or jejunum are examined for evidence of perforation or other injury.

43248-43249

43248 Esophagogastroduodenoscopy, flexible, transoral; with insertion of guide wire followed by passage of dilator(s) through esophagus over guide wire

43249 Esophagogastroduodenoscopy, flexible, transoral; with transendoscopic balloon dilation of esophagus (less than 30 mm diameter)

An upper gastrointestinal (UGI) endoscopic examination is performed on the esophagus, stomach, duodenum and/or jejunum with dilation of the esophagus by insertion of guide wire followed by the passage of dilators (43248) or by balloon dilation using a balloon diameter of less than 30 mm (43249). Esophageal dilation is performed to treat a stricture in the esophagus, which may be the result of reflux esophagitis, causing inflammation and scarring of the esophagus; Schatizki's ring, which is a ring of benign fibrous tissue in the distal esophagus; congenital esophageal atresia; or malignant disease. The mouth and throat are numbed using an anesthetic spray. A hollow mouthpiece is placed in the mouth. The flexible fiberoptic endoscope is then inserted and advanced as it is swallowed by the patient. Once the endoscope has been advanced beyond the cricopharyngeal region, it is guided using direct visualization and advanced into the esophagus to the area of stricture. In 43248, a guide wire is inserted through the scope. A series of rigid tubes of increasing diameter are then passed over the guide wire to dilate the stricture. In 43249, a deflated balloon catheter is advanced through the instrument channel of the scope to the middle of the stricture. The balloon is then inflated while using a pressure gauge to determine the optimal level of inflation. The inflated balloon is left in place for a short period of time (30 seconds to two minutes), deflated, and then removed. Following dilation, the area of stricture is inspected using the scope to ensure that the dilation has been successful and there are no injuries to the esophagus. The endoscope is then advanced into the stomach, duodenum and/or jejunum, which are also examined.

43250-43251

43250 Esophagogastroduodenoscopy, flexible, transoral; with removal of tumor(s), polyp(s), or other lesion(s) by hot biopsy forceps

43251 Esophagogastroduodenoscopy, flexible, transoral; with removal of tumor(s), polyp(s), or other lesion(s) by snare technique

An upper gastrointestinal (UGI) endoscopic examination, also referred to as an esophagogastroduodenoscopy (EGD), is performed on the esophagus, stomach, duodenum and/or jejunum with removal of removal of tumors, polyps, or other lesions by hot biopsy forceps (43250) or by snare technique (43251). The mouth and throat are numbed using

Digestive System

● New Code   ▲ Revised Code

an anesthetic spray. A hollow mouthpiece is placed in the mouth. The flexible fiberoptic endoscope is then inserted and advanced as it is swallowed by the patient. Once the endoscope has been advanced beyond the cricopharyngeal region, it is guided using direct visualization. The esophagus is inspected and any abnormalities are noted. The endoscope is then advanced into the stomach and the stomach is insufflated with air. The cardia, fundus, greater and lesser curvature, and antrum of the stomach are inspected for any abnormalities. The tip of the endoscope is then passed through the pylorus into the duodenum and/or jejunum and mucosal surfaces are inspected. The scope is then withdrawn and tumors, polyps, or other lesions noted are removed. In 43250, hot biopsy forceps are used to remove the lesions. Hot biopsy method uses insulated monopolar forceps to remove and electrocoagulate (cauterize) tissue simultaneously. Hot biopsy forceps are used primarily for removal of small polyps and treatment of vascular ectasias. In 43251, a wire snare loop is placed around the lesion. The loop is heated to shave off and cauterize the lesion. Lesions may be removed in total with one placement of the snare or piecemeal which requires multiple applications of the snare.

Endoscopy, upper gastrointestinal

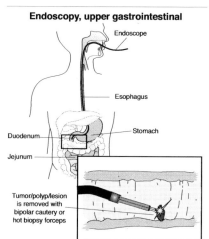

Endoscope

Esophagus

Duodenum

Stomach

Jejunum

Tumor/polyp/lesion is removed with bipolar cautery or hot biopsy forceps

43252

43252   Esophagogastroduodenoscopy, flexible, transoral; with optical endomicroscopy

Esophagogastroduodenoscopy using a flexible endoscope is performed with optical endomicroscopy, which provides in vivo visualization and characterization of the mucosal tissue and pathophysiological processes at the microscopic level. This allows the physician to see histological details during ongoing endoscopy. During an upper gastrointestinal (UGI) endoscopic examination, a small diameter flexible endoscope is inserted through the mouth and advanced into the esophagus, stomach, and duodenum, which are then visualized as the endoscope is slowly withdrawn. Any abnormalities are noted. After the application of contrast agent, endomicroscopy is performed with a miniaturized endomicroscope integrated into the endoscope or inserted through the endoscope that uses a blue laser light to scan the gastrointestinal mucosa from the surface to the deepest mucosal layer. This allows the physician to obtain separately reportable targeted biopsies from areas with microscopic changes rather than random tissue samples and provides instant histological information for immediate treatment. Endomicroscopy can provide histological information in many upper and lower gastrointestinal tract diseases such as Barrett's esophagus, gastric cancer, colorectal neoplasia, celiac disease, Crohn's disease, and ulcerative colitis.

43253

43253   Esophagogastroduodenoscopy, flexible, transoral; with transendoscopic ultrasound-guided transmural injection of diagnostic or therapeutic substance(s) (eg, anesthetic, neurolytic agent) or fiducial marker(s) (includes endoscopic ultrasound examination of the esophagus, stomach, and either the duodenum or a surgically altered stomach where the jejunum is examined distal to the anastomosis)

Esophagogastroduodenoscopy using a flexible endoscope is performed for transmural injection of diagnostic or therapeutic substances or placement of fiducial marker(s) using transendoscopic ultrasound. The most common indications for transmural injections of diagnostic or therapeutic substances through the wall of the stomach or intestines are neurolysis of the celiac plexus in patients with pancreatic cancer or pancreatitis for pain control, as well as injection of chemotherapeutic agents into tumors of the pancreas and liver, and substromal tumors of the gastrointestinal tract. Transmural placement of fiducial markers is most often performed on luminal and extraluminal gastrointestinal tumors, such as pancreatic tumors. The endoscope is introduced through the mouth and structures of the oropharynx and hypopharynx are examined. When the scope reaches the cricopharyngeus, the patient is asked to burp or swallow to facilitate passage of the scope

which is then advanced along the entire length of the esophagus into the stomach, through the pylorus, and into the duodenum. Mucosal surfaces of the duodenum and stomach are inspected as the endoscope is withdrawn. Alternatively, the jejunum is examined in a surgically altered stomach in which the jejunum is anastomosed to the stomach. Next, a radial scanning echoendoscope is introduced and advanced under direct endoscopic visualization. Ultrasound imaging is used to evaluate the wall of the gastrointestinal tract and structures contained in the abdominal and/or thoracic cavity. Ultrasound is used to help determine if a tumor arises from the gastrointestinal tract or surrounding tissues and whether the tumor has invaded other vital structures. Tumors that can be treated through the gastrointestinal tract are identified. The radial scanning echoendoscope is removed and a linear scanning echoendoscope is introduced. A fine needle injection catheter is introduced through the surgical channel of the echoendoscopic. Doppler images are obtained to ensure that there are no vascular structures obstructing the planned injection route. The needle is then advanced through the wall of the stomach or intestine and the tumor is injected with the therapeutic substance, usually a chemotherapeutic agent. Alternatively, the celiac plexus may be identified and a neurolytic substance injected for pain control. If the endoscopic ultrasound is being used to place fiducial markers, the markers are delivered through the wall of the stomach or intestine and placed at strategic sites to mark the tumor borders and critical structures for planned radiotherapy treatments.

43254

43254   Esophagogastroduodenoscopy, flexible, transoral; with endoscopic mucosal resection

Esophagogastroduodenoscopy using a flexible endoscope is performed with endoscopic mucosal resection. Endoscopic mucosal resection is used to treat dysplastic, precancerous lesions and small, early cancerous lesions limited to the mucosa of the esophagus, stomach, or duodenum. The endoscope is introduced through the mouth. The velopharyngeal closure, the base of the tongue, and the hypopharynx are examined. Vocal cord motion is observed and the pharyngeal musculature is evaluated. When the scope reaches the cricopharyngeus, the patient is asked to burp or swallow to facilitate passage of the scope which is then advanced along the entire length of the esophagus and any abnormalities are noted. The endoscope is advanced into the stomach, through the pylorus, and into the duodenum. Mucosal surfaces are inspected as the endoscope is withdrawn. The mucosal lesion is identified. The borders of the lesion are marked with electrocautery. Diluted adrenaline is injected into the submucosal layer around the lesion to separate the mucosal layer containing the lesion from the underlying muscle. A snare with a suction cup is used to further separate the mucosal lesion from underlying tissue. The lesion is then excised and captured using the snare and the scope is withdrawn.

43255

43255   Esophagogastroduodenoscopy, flexible, transoral; with control of bleeding, any method

Esophagogastroduodenoscopy using a flexible endoscope is performed with control of bleeding. The mouth and throat are numbed using an anesthetic spray. A hollow mouthpiece is placed in the mouth. The flexible fiberoptic endoscope is then inserted and advanced as it is swallowed by the patient. Once the endoscope has been advanced beyond the cricopharyngeal region, it is guided using direct visualization. The esophagus is inspected and any abnormalities are noted. The endoscope is then advanced into the stomach and the stomach is insufflated with air. The cardia, fundus, greater and lesser curvature, and antrum of the stomach are inspected and for any abnormalities. The tip of the endoscope is then passed through the pylorus into the duodenum and/or jejunum and the mucosal surfaces are inspected. Any abnormalities are noted. The scope is then withdrawn and the bleeding site is identified. Bleeding is typically controlled using a contact thermal modality, such as bipolar or unipolar cautery, or a heater probe. The cautery device or heater probe is applied to the bleeding point and pressure is applied along with heat to control bleeding. An injection of epinephrine, which works as a vascoconstrictor and tamponade can also be used to reduce or stop bleeding. YAG laser coagulation and a newer modality, the argon plasma coagulator, are noncontact devices used to coagulate the bleeding site. Staples or hemoclips may be used to approximate the margins of a tear or laceration.

43257

43257   Esophagogastroduodenoscopy, flexible, transoral; with delivery of thermal energy to the muscle of lower esophageal sphincter and/or gastric cardia, for treatment of gastroesophageal reflux disease

The mouth and throat are numbed using an anesthetic spray. A hollow mouthpiece is placed in the mouth. The flexible fiberoptic endoscope is then inserted and advanced as it is swallowed by the patient. Once the endoscope has been advanced beyond the cricopharyngeal region, it is guided using direct visualization. The esophagus is inspected and any abnormalities noted. The endoscope is then advanced into the stomach and the stomach is insufflated with air. The cardia, fundus, greater and lesser curvature, and antrum of the stomach are inspected and any abnormalities noted. The tip of the endoscope is then passed through the pylorus into the duodenum and/or jejunum and mucosal surfaces inspected. A guidewire is passed through the endoscope to the duodenum or gastric antrum. The endoscope is withdrawn and a thermal catheter passed over the guidewire to the region to the lower esophageal sphincter. The thermal catheter balloon is inflated, needle electrodes deployed, and radiofrequency energy delivered. This is repeated around the circumference of the sphincter. The thermal catheter is advanced into the stomach, correct positioning verified endoscopically, and thermal energy delivered to the gastric cardia in the same manner as described above. Treatment may require delivery of thermal energy at multiple levels in the esophageal sphincter and gastric cardia. Once thermal lesions have been created at multiple levels the thermal catheter is withdrawn, the endoscope reintroduced, and the region inspected to ensure correct lesion placement.

43259

43259 **Esophagogastroduodenoscopy, flexible, transoral; with endoscopic ultrasound examination, including the esophagus, stomach, and either the duodenum or a surgically altered stomach where the jejunum is examined distal to the anastomosis**

The mouth and throat are numbed using an anesthetic spray. A hollow mouthpiece is placed in the mouth. The flexible fiberoptic endoscope is inserted and advanced as it is swallowed by the patient. Once the endoscope has been advanced beyond the cricopharyngeal region, it is guided using direct visualization. The esophagus is inspected and any abnormalities are noted. The endoscope is then advanced into the stomach and the stomach is insufflated with air. The cardia, fundus, greater and lesser curvature, and antrum of the stomach are inspected and any abnormalities noted. The tip of the endoscope is passed through the pylorus into the duodenum or into the jejunum in the case of a surgically altered stomach where the jejunum is examined distal to the anastomosis. The mucosal surfaces inspected. The scope is then withdrawn and the entire circumference of the duodenum or jejunum (where the stomach has been surgically altered), stomach, and esophagus are again examined. Following endoscopic examination, an echoendoscope is introduced and any abnormalities or lesions are again carefully evaluated. Ultrasound images are obtained to determine whether the abnormality or lesion is intrinsic (within) or extrinsic (outside) the upper gastrointestinal tract. If the lesion is intrinsic, it is evaluated to determine whether it is limited to the mucosa or involves the muscular wall. If it is extrinsic and located in the esophagus, it is evaluated to determine whether it is in the mediastinal space or has invaded the mediastinal wall, what thoracic organs are involved, and whether there is any lymph node involvement. If it is in the stomach or small intestines it is evaluated in the same manner to determine whether invasion is limited the peritoneal cavity or whether other sites and/or structures are involved. Hard copies of ultrasound images are made and the abnormalities are again evaluated.

43260-43261

43260 **Endoscopic retrograde cholangiopancreatography (ERCP); diagnostic, including collection of specimen(s) by brushing or washing, when performed (separate procedure)**
43261 **Endoscopic retrograde cholangiopancreatography (ERCP); with biopsy, single or multiple**

Diagnostic endoscopic retrograde cholangiopancreatography helps to diagnose problems in the liver, gallbladder, bile ducts, and pancreas, particularly conditions of the bile ducts. An endoscope is passed through the esophagus, stomach, and into the duodenum to the point where the pancreatic duct and the common bile duct meet (the Ampulla of Vater), at the major duodenal papilla. A smaller catheter is placed through the scope, the Ampulla of Vater is cannulated, and contrast dye is injected into the ducts. The common bile duct, biliary tract, gallbladder, and pancreas are visualized on x-rays, taken as soon as the dye is injected, to look for any gallstones, strictures, leaks, scarring, or cancer. The catheter may be advanced over a guidewire into the common duct, biliary tract, gallbladder, and/or pancreas to collect cells from one or more of these sites by brushing or injecting saline solution (washing). Use code 43261 when one or more tissue samples (biopsies) are obtained.

43262

43262 **Endoscopic retrograde cholangiopancreatography (ERCP); with sphincterotomy/papillotomy**

Endoscopic retrograde cholangiopancreatography is performed with sphincterotomy or papillotomy. An endoscope is passed through the esophagus, stomach, and into the duodenum to the point where the pancreatic duct and the common bile duct meet (the Ampulla of Vater), at the major duodenal papilla. A smaller catheter is placed through the scope, the Ampulla of Vater is cannulated, and contrast dye is injected into the ducts. The common bile duct, biliary tract, gallbladder, and pancreas are visualized on x-rays, taken as soon as the dye is injected. The catheter is advanced over a guidewire into the common duct, biliary tract, gallbladder, and/or pancreas. The muscle between the bile duct and the pancreatic duct is severed in a sphincterotomy, or a stricture (narrowing) in the bile duct is incised in a papillotomy. A balloon catheter is then inserted to inspect for gallstones or other disease.

43263

43263 **Endoscopic retrograde cholangiopancreatography (ERCP); with pressure measurement of sphincter of Oddi**

Endoscopic retrograde cholangiopancreatography is performed with a pressure measurement of the sphincter of Oddi. An endoscope is passed through the esophagus, stomach, and into the duodenum to the point where the pancreatic duct and the common bile duct meet (the Ampulla of Vater), at the major duodenal papilla. A smaller catheter is placed through the scope, the Ampulla of Vater is cannulated, and contrast dye is injected into the ducts. The common bile duct, biliary tract, gallbladder, and pancreas are visualized on x-rays, taken as soon as the dye is injected. The catheter is advanced over a guidewire into the common bile duct, biliary tract, gallbladder, and/or pancreas and a small tube is inserted into the bile duct or pancreatic duct. A manometer is used to measure the squeeze pressure in the sphincter of Oddi, the muscular valve that controls the opening and closing of the bile duct and the introduction of bile and pancreatic secretions into the duodenal papilla (Ampulla of Vater). The sphincter of Oddi also prevents the contents of the duodenum from entering the Ampulla of Vater.

43264

43264 **Endoscopic retrograde cholangiopancreatography (ERCP); with removal of calculi/debris from biliary/pancreatic duct(s)**

Endoscopic retrograde cholangiopancreatography is performed with removal of stone(s) from the biliary and/or pancreatic ducts. An endoscope is passed through the esophagus, stomach, and into the duodenum to the point where the pancreatic duct and the common bile duct meet, (the Ampulla of Vater), at the major duodenal papilla. A smaller catheter is placed through the scope, the ampulla of Vater is cannulated, and contrast dye is injected into the ducts. The common bile duct, biliary tract, gallbladder, and pancreas are visualized on x-rays, taken as soon as the dye is injected. A balloon catheter is inserted and swept down past the biliary or pancreatic duct calculus (stone). The balloon is inflated and the stone is extracted by slow withdrawal of the balloon catheter. Alternatively, a basket extraction can be performed. The basket extraction device is inserted, the calculus is trapped within the device, and the basket is then slowly withdrawn. One or more calculi may be removed during this procedure.

43265

43265 **Endoscopic retrograde cholangiopancreatography (ERCP); with destruction of calculi, any method (eg, mechanical, electrohydraulic, lithotripsy)**

Endoscopic retrograde cholangiopancreatography is performed with destruction of gallstone(s) (calculi) using any method including mechanical, electrohydraulic, or lithotripsy. An endoscope is passed through the esophagus, stomach, and into the duodenum to the point where the pancreatic duct and the common bile duct meet, (the Ampulla of Vater), at the major duodenal papilla. A smaller catheter is placed through the scope, the Ampulla of Vater is cannulated, and contrast dye is injected into the ducts. The common bile duct, biliary tract, gallbladder, and pancreas are visualized on x-rays, taken as soon as the dye is injected. The catheter is advanced over a guidewire to the site of the gallstone in the biliary tract. Mechanical destruction is performed using a crushing basket device. The crushed gallstone is trapped within the device and the basket is slowly withdrawn. Alternatively an electrohydraulic or laser lithotripsy device may be used. The elecrohydraulic or laser probe is advanced to the stone, activated, and the stone is shattered. One or more stones may be shattered or crushed during this procedure.

43266

43266 **Esophagogastroduodenoscopy, flexible, transoral; with placement of endoscopic stent (includes pre- and post-dilation and guide wire passage, when performed)**

Esophagogastroduodenoscopy using a flexible endoscope is performed with placement of an esophageal stent. Indications for stent placement include narrowing or stricture of the esophagus due to esophageal or lung cancer and malignant bronchoesophageal fistula. The endoscope is introduced through the mouth. The velopharyngeal closure, the base of the tongue, and the hypopharynx are examined. Vocal cord motion is observed and the pharyngeal musculature is evaluated. When the scope reaches the cricopharyngeus, the patient is asked to burp or swallow to facilitate passage of the scope which is then advanced along the entire length of the esophagus and any abnormalities are noted. The endoscope is advanced into the stomach, through the pylorus, and into the duodenum. Mucosal surfaces are inspected as the endoscope is inserted and again as it is withdrawn. Any abnormalities are noted. The scope is then positioned at the site of the narrowing or stricture. The stricture is examined and the need for pre-dilation is evaluated. If pre-dilation is needed, a guide wire is inserted through the scope. A series of rigid tubes of increasing diameter are then passed over the guide wire to dilate the stricture. Alternatively, a balloon catheter may be advanced to the site of the stricture and inflated to dilate the stricture. Stent placement is then performed. A guide wire is passed through the scope followed by the stent delivery system which is passed over the guide wire and positioned in the narrowed portion of the esophagus or over the fistula. The stent is then deployed. A balloon

Digestive System

catheter may again be inserted and inflated to seat the stent. The endoscope is advanced through the stent to check stent position and ensure proper deployment.

43270

43270   Esophagogastroduodenoscopy, flexible, transoral; with ablation of tumor(s), polyp(s), or other lesion(s) (includes pre- and post-dilation and guide wire passage, when performed)

Esophagogastroduodenoscopy using a flexible endoscope is performed with ablation of one or more tumors, polyps, or other lesions. The endoscope is introduced through the mouth. The velopharyngeal closure, the base of the tongue, and the hypopharynx are examined. Vocal cord motion is observed and the pharyngeal musculature is evaluated. When the scope reaches the cricopharyngeus, the patient is asked to burp or swallow to facilitate passage of the scope which is then advanced along the entire length of the esophagus and any abnormalities are noted. The endoscope is advanced into the stomach, through the pylorus, and into the duodenum. Mucosal surfaces are inspected as the endoscope is inserted and again as it is withdrawn, and the site of the lesion is noted. If there is narrowing of the esophageal or gastrointestinal lumen at the site of the lesion, dilation of the lumen may be required prior to the ablation procedure. This is accomplished by inserting a guide wire through the scope. A series of rigid tubes of increasing diameter are then passed over the guide wire and the lumen is dilated as needed. Alternately, a balloon catheter may be advanced to the site of the stricture and inflated to dilate the lumen. The laser device is then delivered through the endoscope to the distal margin of the most distal lesion. The lesion is ablated as the endoscope is retracted. The entire lesion is destroyed as the laser traverses the lesion in a distal to proximal direction. This is repeated until all lesions have been destroyed. If dilation is required following destruction of the lesion(s), it is again performed as described above. The upper gastrointestinal tract is again examined using the endoscope to ensure that all lesions have been destroyed and that there are no injuries resulting from the procedure.

43273

43273   Endoscopic cannulation of papilla with direct visualization of pancreatic/common bile duct(s) (List separately in addition to code(s) for primary procedure)

Endoscopic cannulation of papilla with direct visualization of common bile and/or pancreatic duct(s) is performed. This procedure is performed during a separately reportable endoscopic retrograde cholangiopancreatography (ERCP). Direct visualization of the common bile and/or pancreatic ducts is performed to evaluate the ducts for conditions that may not be evident using radiography procedures alone. The separately reportable ERCP is performed first. A duodenoscope is inserted through the mouth and passed down the esophagus and stomach and into the duodenum to the papilla of Vater. A catheter is inserted through the scope and contrast is injected into the pancreatic and biliary ducts. Fluoroscopic images are obtained and evaluated. Direct visualization is then accomplished by passing a guidewire through the scope until the tip is at the proximal biliary tree. A biliary sphincterotomy is performed. A cholangioscope is then passed through the duodenoscope and into the biliary tree. Common bile ducts and/or pancreatic ducts are examined and any evidence of disease is noted. The cholangioscope is then withdrawn and the physician completes the ERCP procedure.

43274

43274   Endoscopic retrograde cholangiopancreatography (ERCP); with placement of endoscopic stent into biliary or pancreatic duct, including pre- and post-dilation and guide wire passage, when performed, including sphincterotomy, when performed, each stent

An endoscope is passed through the esophagus, stomach, and into the duodenum to the point where the pancreatic duct and the common bile duct meet at the ampulla of Vater, also referred to as the duodenal papilla or papilla of Vater. The muscle between the bile duct and the pancreatic duct is severed as needed to allow passage of the catheter (sphincterotomy). A smaller catheter is then placed through the scope and the ampulla of Vater is cannulated. Contrast is injected to allow visualization of the common bile duct, biliary tract, gallbladder, and pancreas. Images are obtained. A guide wire is placed and a balloon catheter is advanced over the guide wire to the site stricture in the biliary or pancreatic duct. The balloon is inflated and the narrowed region is dilated. The guide wire is removed and a stent delivery catheter is advanced across the narrowed region. The stent is positioned in the narrowed portion of the biliary or pancreatic duct and deployed. A balloon catheter is again delivered and positioned within the stent and inflated to seat the stent. Additional contrast is injected and the biliary system is again visualized to verify correct stent placement.

43275

43275   Endoscopic retrograde cholangiopancreatography (ERCP); with removal of foreign body(s) or stent(s) from biliary/pancreatic duct(s)

An endoscope is passed through the esophagus, stomach, and into the duodenum to the point where the pancreatic duct and the common bile duct meet at the ampulla of Vater, also referred to as the duodenal papilla or papilla of Vater. A smaller catheter is then placed through the scope and the ampulla of Vater is cannulated. Contrast is injected to allow visualization of the common bile duct, biliary tract, gallbladder, and pancreas. Images are obtained. A guide wire is placed and the catheter is advanced over the guide wire to the site of the foreign body or stent. The guide wire is removed and a snare is introduced. The foreign body or stent is captured and removed using the snare. Additional contrast is injected and the biliary system is again visualized to identify any strictures, filling defects, extravasation of contrast, or other abnormalities.

43276

43276   Endoscopic retrograde cholangiopancreatography (ERCP); with removal and exchange of stent(s), biliary or pancreatic duct, including pre- and post-dilation and guide wire passage, when performed, including sphincterotomy, when performed, each stent exchanged

An endoscope is passed through the esophagus, stomach, and into the duodenum to the point where the pancreatic duct and the common bile duct meet at the ampulla of Vater, also referred to as the duodenal papilla or papilla of Vater. A smaller catheter is then placed through the scope and the ampulla of Vater is cannulated. Contrast is injected to allow visualization of the common bile duct, biliary tract, gallbladder, and pancreas. Images are obtained. The sphincter of Oddi is inspected and incised as needed to allow removal of the existing stent and/or placement of the new stent. A guide wire is placed and the catheter is advanced over the guide wire to the site of the existing stent in the biliary or pancreatic duct. The stent is then removed using a snare. Additional contrast is injected and the biliary system is again visualized to identify any strictures, filling defects, extravasation of contrast, or other abnormalities. A balloon catheter is advanced and inflated at the site of the stricture to dilate the narrowed portion as needed. The balloon catheter is removed and the new stent is advanced over the guide wire to the site of the stricture in the biliary or pancreatic duct. Proper positioning is verified and the stent is expanded. The balloon catheter may again be used within the stent to fully expand and seat (secure) the stent at the site of the stricture. Contrast is again injected to ensure that the stent is properly placed and that the narrowed portion of the pancreatic or biliary duct has been opened enough to allow drainage of bile or pancreatic secretions. If more than one stent is exchanged, report code 43276 for each stent that is exchanged.

43277

43277   Endoscopic retrograde cholangiopancreatography (ERCP); with trans-endoscopic balloon dilation of biliary/pancreatic duct(s) or of ampulla (sphincteroplasty), including sphincterotomy, when performed, each duct

An endoscope is passed through the esophagus, stomach, and into the duodenum to the point where the pancreatic duct and the common bile duct meet at the ampulla of Vater, also referred to as the duodenal papilla or papilla of Vater. A smaller catheter is then placed through the scope and the ampulla of Vater is cannulated. Contrast is injected to allow visualization of the ampulla of Vater, common bile duct, biliary tract, gallbladder, and pancreas. Images are obtained. If the ampulla of Vater is narrowed, a balloon catheter may be advanced into the ampulla and inflated. Next, the sphincter of Oddi is inspected and if it is narrowed, an incision may be made to enlarge the opening. If the biliary or pancreatic duct is narrowed, a guide wire is placed and a balloon catheter is advanced and inflated at the site of the stricture in the biliary or pancreatic duct to dilate the narrowed portion. The balloon catheter may be deflated and inflated multiple times until the duct is adequately dilated. The balloon catheter is removed. Contrast is again injected to ensure that the narrowed portion of the pancreatic and/or biliary duct and/or Ampulla of Vater has been opened enough to allow drainage of bile or pancreatic secretions. Report code 43277 for each duct that is dilated.

43278

43278   Endoscopic retrograde cholangiopancreatography (ERCP); with ablation of tumor(s), polyp(s), or other lesion(s), including pre- and post-dilation and guide wire passage, when performed

An endoscope is passed through the esophagus, stomach, and into the duodenum to the point where the pancreatic duct and the common bile duct meet at the ampulla of Vater, also referred to as the duodenal papilla or papilla of Vater. A smaller catheter is then placed through the scope and the ampulla of Vater is cannulated. Contrast is injected to allow visualization of the common bile duct, biliary tract, gallbladder, and pancreas. Images are obtained. The sphincter of Oddi is inspected. A guide wire is placed and the catheter is advanced over the guide wire into the biliary tract. Additional contrast is injected and the biliary system is again visualized to identify any strictures, filling defects, extravasation of contrast, or other abnormalities. The site of the lesion in the biliary or pancreatic duct is noted. A balloon catheter may be advanced and inflated at the site of the lesion to enlarge the biliary or pancreatic duct allowing better access for the ablation procedure. The balloon catheter is removed and the laser device is then delivered through the endoscope to the distal margin of the most distal lesion. The lesion is ablated as the endoscope is retracted. The entire lesion is destroyed as the laser traverses the lesion in a distal to proximal direction. This is repeated until all lesions have been destroyed. If dilation is required following destruction of the lesion(s), it is performed as described above.

● New Code   ▲ Revised Code

43279

43279   Laparoscopy, surgical, esophagomyotomy (Heller type), with fundoplasty, when performed

A laparoscopic Heller-type esophagomyotomy is performed including a fundoplasty when needed. Pneumoperitoneum is established and four to five laparoscopic ports are inserted across the upper abdomen. The laparoscope is inserted and the stomach and esophagus are inspected. The gastric fundus is grasped and pulled down and short gastric vessels are divided. The phrenoesophageal ligament is cut to allow exposure of the anterior gastric cardia and distal esophagus. The area behind the esophagogastric junction is dissected and a drain is placed. The vagus nerves are identified and protected. An endoscope is used to identify the squamocolumnar junction. Traction is applied at the esophagogastric junction and the gastric cardia is incised longitudinally beginning just distal to the squamocolumnar junction and extending into the esophageal muscle approximately 6-8 cm. Longitudinal and circular muscle fibers are divided (myotomy) and the submucosa is exposed. The stomach is insufflated through the endoscope and the incision is inspected to ensure that all muscle fibers along the entire length of the incision have been divided. Any undivided muscle fibers are cut. A manometry catheter is placed in the stomach and pressure recordings are obtained. Areas of positive pressure along the incision site are inspected again, and intact muscle fibers are identified and divided. Following completion of the myotomy, a fundoplasty is performed as needed. To perform a Dor anterior fundoplasty, the fundus is folded over the abdominal side of the myotomy and sutured to the crural diaphragm.

43280

43280   Laparoscopy, surgical, esophagogastric fundoplasty (eg, Nissen, Toupet procedures)

A laparoscopic esophagogastric fundoplasty is performed. There are two common variations of this procedure, the Nissen fundoplication and the Toupet fundoplication. In the Nissen fundoplication, the fundus (top) of the stomach is completely wrapped around the esophagus to produce a short, loose 360 degree wrap. In the Toupet fundoplication, the fundus of the stomach is partially wrapped around the esophagus to produce a shorter, looser, 270 degree wrap. Four small incisions are made in the upper abdomen and trocars are placed. A fifth incision is made just above the umbilicus and the laparoscope is introduced through a port. The liver is retracted and the esophageal hiatus is exposed. A clamp is placed in the esophageal fat pad, which is retracted inferiorly to expose the gastrohepatic ligament and the phrenoesophageal membrane. The gastrohepatic ligament is incised and the right crus of the diaphragm is exposed. Dissection is carried around anteriorly and the left crus of the diaphragm is exposed. Dissection continues to create a window posterior to the esophagus. The hiatal hernia is repaired by closing the hiatus. Once the hiatal hernia is repaired, the short gastric vessels are identified and divided as the spleen is dissected off the stomach. Dissection continues until the fundus of the stomach is completely mobilized. Graspers are used to pull the fundus behind the esophagus and through the previously created window. The fundus is pulled around the esophagus and then either sutured to the muscle layer of the esophagus (270 degree Toupet fundoplication) or to the other side of the fundus with stitches placed through the fundus and then anchored to the muscle layer of the esophagus (360 degree Nissen fundoplication).

43281-43282

43281   Laparoscopy, surgical, repair of paraesophageal hernia, includes fundoplasty, when performed; without implantation of mesh

43282   Laparoscopy, surgical, repair of paraesophageal hernia, includes fundoplasty, when performed; with implantation of mesh

A paraesophageal hernia is characterized by normal position of the gastroesophgeal junction with protrusion of the fundus stomach into the chest cavity alongside the esophagus. Four incisions are made in the upper abdomen and trocars placed. A fifth small incision is made just above the umbilicus and the laparoscope is introduced through a port. The liver is retracted and the esophageal hiatus exposed. The stomach is reduced into the abdomen using endoscopic atraumatic graspers. A clamp is placed in the esophageal fat pad, which is retracted inferiorly to expose the gastrohepatic ligament and the phrenoesophageal membrane. The gastrohepatic ligament is incised and the right crus of the diaphragm exposed. Dissection is carried around anteriorly and the left crus of the diaphragm exposed. Dissection continues to create a window posterior to the esophagus. The hernia sac and gastroesophageal fat pad are mobilized taking care to protect the anterior vagus nerve. The hernia sac is removed. The diaphragm is repaired with sutures in 43281 or reinforced with mesh in 43282. A fundoplication is performed as needed. There are two common variations of this procedure, the Nissen fundoplication and the Toupet fundoplication. In the Nissen fundoplication, the fundus (top) of the stomach is completely wrapped around the esophagus to produce a short, loose 360 degree wrap. In the Toupet fundoplication, the fundus of the stomach is partially wrapped around the esophagus to produce a shorter, looser, 270 degree wrap.

43283

43283   Laparoscopy, surgical, esophageal lengthening procedure (eg, Collis gastroplasty or wedge gastroplasty) (List separately in addition to code for primary procedure)

During a separately reportable laparoscopic procedure on a hiatal hernia, the esophagus is lengthened by Collis or wedge gastroplasty. The gastroesophageal fat pad is removed taking care to preserve the vagal nerves. A dilator (bougie) is passed through the mouth and into the esophagus and stomach. A laparoscopic stapling device is inserted into the abdominal cavity through one of the existing ports. Axial traction is applied to esophagus. The greater curvature of the stomach is grasped and rotated into an anteroposterior position. The endostapler is placed parallel to the distal esophagus at the angle of His. The stapler is fired to create a 2-4 cm neoesophagus and a new angle of His. The primary laparoscopic procedure is completed which typically involves fundoplication with placement of anchoring sutures from the esophagus to the fundoplication and then to the diaphragm. The fundoplication is then reduced through the diaphragm into the abdomen and anchoring sutures tied. The dilator is removed.

43284-43285

● 43284   Laparoscopy, surgical, esophageal sphincter augmentation procedure, placement of sphincter augmentation device (ie, magnetic band), including cruroplasty when performed

● 43285   Removal of esophageal sphincter augmentation device

A laparoscopic procedure is performed to implant or remove a sphincter augmentation device (magnetic band) around the lower esophageal sphincter (LES) to treat gastroesophageal reflux. Using a standard laparoscopy approach, the gastroesophageal junction (GEJ) is visualized and the area where the device is to be implanted is minimally dissected. The peritoneal reflection is divided and the mediastinal cavity and phrenoesophageal ligament are preserved. The posterior vagus nerve is identified and exposed, followed by creation of a small opening between the posterior vagus nerve and the esophageal body. The circumferential diameter of the esophagus at the GEJ is measured using a sizing instrument and the appropriate band is selected. The band consists of a string of interlinked titanium beads with magnetic cores that fit snugly together to keep the LES closed, but expand to open the LES in response to swallowing. The band is inserted through the opening between the vagus nerve and the esophagus, encircling the esophagus at the LES with the ends of the band positioned and secured anteriorly. Cruroplasty for esophageal hernia repair may also be performed as well. An enlarged hiatal (esophageal) opening in the diaphragm allows the stomach to protrude upwards into the chest. The crura are tendinous/muscular extensions tethering the diaphragm to the spine and surrounding the esophagus at the esophageal opening where the fibers of the right crus part to allow the esophagus to pass. The contents of the hernia sac are first reduced and the opening adjusted to the right size by reapproximating the diaphragmatic crura with permanent interrupted sutures. To remove the implanted device (43285), the GEJ is visualized, the device is identified, dissected free of the esophagus, and removed from the abdomen. The laparoscope and other instruments are removed from the abdominal cavity, the carbon dioxide is released, and the incisions are closed with sutures, staples, or steristrips.

43300-43305

43300   Esophagoplasty (plastic repair or reconstruction), cervical approach; without repair of tracheoesophageal fistula

43305   Esophagoplasty (plastic repair or reconstruction), cervical approach; with repair of tracheoesophageal fistula

Esophagoplasty involves plastic repair or reconstruction of the esophagus, which may be performed for a variety of reasons including blunt trauma, an avulsion type injury, or an acquired or traumatic tracheoesophageal fistula. An incision is made in the neck, usually on the left side. The internal jugular vein and carotid artery are identified and retracted laterally. The trachea and esophagus are exposed. An incision is made in the cervical esophagus immediately above or below the level of the lesion. In 43300, the esophageal defect does not include a tracheoesophageal fistula. The esophagus is dissected free of surrounding tissue to allow inspection and repair of the defect. Any ragged or necrotic tissue in the muscular wall of the esophagus is debrided and the mucosal defect is exposed. Mucosal tissue is trimmed back until healthy tissue is encountered. The mucosal tissue is inverted and suture repaired. A second layer of sutures is placed in the muscular wall of the esophagus. The repair may be reinforced using separately reportable microvascular anastomosis of an intercostal muscle flap. In 43305, the esophagoplasty is performed with repair of a tracheoesophageal fistula. The fistula is identified and divided. The trachea is repaired with sutures. The esophageal defect is closed in layers. Pedicle flaps are created from the sternohyoid or sternothyroid muscles. The pedicle flaps are positioned between the trachea and esophagus to reinforce the closure.

Digestive System

              ● New Code   ▲ Revised Code

43310-43312

43310 Esophagoplasty (plastic repair or reconstruction), thoracic approach; without repair of tracheoesophageal fistula

43312 Esophagoplasty (plastic repair or reconstruction), thoracic approach; with repair of tracheoesophageal fistula

Esophagoplasty involves plastic repair or reconstruction of the esophagus, which may be performed for a variety of reasons including blunt trauma, an avulsion type injury, or an acquired or traumatic tracheoesophageal fistula. In a thoracic approach, a right posterolateral thoracotomy is generally used. The skin is incised and the incision extended through the soft tissues. The scapula is retracted and the thorax entered without disrupting the pleura. Retropleural dissection is performed, the lung retracted, and the esophagus is exposed. The mediastinal pleura are opened as needed to fully expose the defect. In 43310, the esophageal defect does not include a tracheoesophageal fistula. The esophagus is dissected free of surrounding tissue to allow inspection and repair of the defect. Any ragged or necrotic tissue in the muscular wall of the esophagus is debrided and the mucosal defect is exposed. Mucosal tissue is trimmed back until healthy tissue is encountered. The mucosal tissue is inverted and suture repaired. A second layer of sutures is placed in the muscular wall of the esophagus. The repair may be reinforced using microvascular anastomosis of an intercostal muscle flap. In 43312, the esophagoplasty is performed with repair of a tracheoesophageal fistula. The fistula is divided. The trachea is repaired with sutures. The esophagus is then repaired in two layers. The suture line is reinforced with a flap of mediastinal pleura, intercostal muscle, and rib periosteum as needed.

43313-43314

43313 Esophagoplasty for congenital defect (plastic repair or reconstruction), thoracic approach; without repair of congenital tracheoesophageal fistula

43314 Esophagoplasty for congenital defect (plastic repair or reconstruction), thoracic approach; with repair of congenital tracheoesophageal fistula

Esophagoplasty involves plastic repair or reconstruction of the esophagus. In a thoracic approach, a right posterolateral thoracotomy is generally used. The skin is incised and the incision extended through the soft tissues. The scapula is retracted and the thorax entered without disrupting the pleura. Retropleural dissection is performed, the lung retracted, and the esophagus is exposed. The mediastinal pleura are opened as needed to fully expose the defect. In 43313, the esophageal defect does not include a tracheoesophageal fistula. The esophagus is dissected free of surrounding tissue to allow inspection and repair of the defect. The muscular wall of the esophagus at the site of the defect is inspected and debrided as needed. The mucosal defect is exposed. Mucosal tissue is trimmed back until healthy tissue is encountered. The mucosal tissue is inverted and suture repaired. A second layer of sutures is placed in the muscular wall of the esophagus. The repair may be reinforced using microvascular anastomosis of an intercostal muscle flap. A nasogastric feeding tube is placed prior to closure of the chest. A chest tube is placed in the retropleural space and the thoracic incision is closed. In 43314, the esophagoplasty is performed with repair of a tracheoesophageal fistula. The fistula is divided. The trachea is repaired with sutures. The esophagus is then repaired in two layers. The suture line is reinforced with a flap of mediastinal pleura, intercostal muscle, and rib periosteum as needed.

43320

43320 Esophagogastrostomy (cardioplasty), with or without vagotomy and pyloroplasty, transabdominal or transthoracic approach

In a thoracic approach, a right posterior thoracotomy is generally used. The skin is incised and the incision extended through the soft tissues. The scapula is retracted and the thorax entered without disrupting the pleura. Retropleural dissection is performed, the lung retracted, and the distal esophagus is exposed. Using an abdominal approach, also referred to as a transhiatal approach, an incision is made in the upper abdomen and the peritoneal cavity explored. The stomach is mobilized at the gastroesophageal junction and the diaphragmatic hiatus is split to expose the lower posterior mediastinum and distal esophagus. A gastric tube is created from the stomach. The left gastric and gastroepiploic arteries are ligated and divided as are the short splenic vessels. The right gastroepiploic artery is preserved to provide blood supply to the greater curvature of the stomach. The stomach is divided using a linear stapler at a point about 3 cm from the line of the greater curvature. The pyloric sphincter is evaluated. If a pyloroplasty is needed, the pylorus is divided laterally and then sutured longtitudinally to provide a wider opening into the duodenum. The seromuscular layer of the stomach is closed with sutures to a point approximately 4 cm from the end. The esophagus is freed from surrounding tissues using blunt and sharp dissection. The esophagus is transected above the esophagogastric junction. The surgically created gastric tube is mobilized and an end-to-end anastomosis to the distal esophagus is performed. If a vagotomy is performed, the vagus nerve or nerve branches that supply the stomach are cut or severed by electrocautery.

43325

43325 Esophagogastric fundoplasty; with fundic patch (Thal-Nissen procedure)

Fundoplasty is performed to treat hiatal hernia with gastroesophageal reflux. Using a transpleural approach, the esophagus is mobilized. A radial incision is made through the diaphragm; the stomach is exposed; and the greater curvature is mobilized. The fundus of the stomach is allowed to prolapse into the chest. The lower aspect of the esophagus is incised longitudinally to the fundus of the stomach. The gastric inlet is widened by approximating the edges of the incision transversely. A split thickness skin graft is harvested and tacked to the fundus. A dilator is then passed through the mouth into the esophagus and stomach to maintain the desired width of the lumen at the esophagogastric junction. The fundus is wrapped around the esophagus and sutured to the right side of the esophagus to create pressure distally and prevent gastroesophageal reflux. Anchoring sutures are placed from the esophagus to the fundus and then to the diaphragm. The fundus is reduced through the diaphragm into the abdomen and anchoring sutures are tied. The dilator is removed; chest tubes are placed; and incisions are closed.

43327-43328

43327 Esophagogastric fundoplasty partial or complete; laparotomy

43328 Esophagogastric fundoplasty partial or complete; thoracotomy

A partial or complete esophagogastric fundoplasty is performed to treat a sliding hiatal hernia. In 43327, the procedure is performed by an abdominal approach using a complete (360 degree) wrap such as a Nissen fundoplication, or a partial (270 degree) wrap such as a Toupet fundoplication. In a complete fundoplasty, the fundus (top) of the stomach is completely wrapped around the esophagus. In a partial fundoplasty, the fundus of the stomach is partially wrapped around the esophagus to produce a shorter, looser wrap. A midline incision is made in the abdomen and the liver is retracted. The esophageal hiatus is exposed. The gastroesophageal fat pad is retracted inferiorly to expose the gastrohepatic ligament and the phrenoesophageal membrane. The gastrohepatic ligament is incised and the right crus of the diaphragm is exposed. Dissection is carried around the anterior aspect of the diaphragm and the left crus is exposed. A window is then created posterior to the esophagus. The hiatal hernia is repaired. Once the hiatal hernia has been repaired, the short gastric vessels are identified and divided as the spleen is dissected off the stomach. The fundus of the stomach is completely mobilized. The fundus is pulled behind the esophagus through the previously created window and around to the front of the esophagus where it is sutured to itself and then to the esophageal muscle layer. In 43328, the procedure is performed by a transthoracic approach using a technique such as a Belsey IV or Belsey Mark IV (BMIV). In this technique example, the fundus is partially wrapped around the esophagus. This may also be referred to as a 270 degree wrap. An incision is made through the chest just above the diaphragm. The stomach is mobilized and pulled into the chest cavity. A window is created behind the esophagus. The stomach is partially wrapped around the esophagus and sutured to the muscle layer of the esophagus. The stomach is returned to the abdomen and the hiatal hernia is repaired. Another technique is the Hill procedure which involves anchoring the stomach to the diaphragm to prevent recurrent herniation and suturing the right and left crura of the diaphragm to narrow the hiatus.

43330-43331

43330 Esophagomyotomy (Heller type); abdominal approach

43331 Esophagomyotomy (Heller type); thoracic approach

This procedure is performed to treat esophageal achalasia which is a failure of the esophageal sphincter to relax causing uncoordinated contraction in the thoracic esophagus which in turn causes difficulty swallowing and functional obstruction of the esophagus. In 43330, and abdominal approach also referred to as a transhiatal approach is used. An incision is made in the upper abdomen and the peritoneal cavity explored. The stomach is mobilized at the gastroesophageal junction and the diaphragmatic hiatus is split to expose the lower posterior mediastinum and distal esophagus. In 43331, a thoracic approach, usually a right posterior thoracotomy is used. The skin is incised and the incision extended through the soft tissues. The scapula is retracted and the thorax entered without disrupting the pleura. Retropleural dissection is performed, the lung retracted, and the distal esophagus is exposed. The diaphragmatic hiatus is split and the gastroesophageal junction exposed. A longitudinal incision is then made in the muscular wall of the distal esophagus and carried down onto the gastric cardia (stomach). All muscle fibers are severed down to the submucosal layer of the esophagus and stomach. A nasogastric tube is placed. If a thoracic approach is used, a chest tube may be placed. Abdominal or thoracic incisions are then closed in layers.

● New Code   ▲ Revised Code   CPT © 2016 American Medical Association. All Rights Reserved.   © 2017 DecisionHealth

43332-43333

43332 Repair, paraesophageal hiatal hernia (including fundoplication), via laparotomy, except neonatal; without implantation of mesh or other prosthesis

43333 Repair, paraesophageal hiatal hernia (including fundoplication), via laparotomy, except neonatal; with implantation of mesh or other prosthesis

A paraesophageal hernia is characterized by normal position of the gastroesophageal junction with protrusion of the fundus (top) of the stomach into the chest cavity alongside the esophagus. A midline incision is made in the abdomen. The liver is retracted and the esophageal hiatus is exposed. The herniated portion of the stomach is reduced back into the abdomen using atraumatic graspers. The gastroesophageal fat pad is retracted inferiorly to expose the gastrohepatic ligament and the phrenoesophageal membrane. The gastrohepatic ligament is incised and the right crus of the diaphragm is exposed. Dissection is carried around the anterior aspect of the diaphragm and the left crus is exposed. A window is then created posterior to the esophagus. The hernia sac is mobilized taking care to protect the anterior vagus nerve. The hernia sac is excised. The diaphragm is repaired with sutures in 43332 or reinforced with mesh or other prosthetic material in 43333. A fundoplication is performed as needed. There are two common variations of this procedure--the Nissen fundoplication and the Toupet fundoplication. In the Nissen fundoplication, the fundus (top) of the stomach is completely wrapped around the esophagus to produce a short, loose 360 degree wrap. In the Toupet fundoplication, the fundus of the stomach is partially wrapped around the esophagus to produce a shorter, looser, 270 degree wrap.

43334-43335

43334 Repair, paraesophageal hiatal hernia (including fundoplication), via thoracotomy, except neonatal; without implantation of mesh or other prosthesis

43335 Repair, paraesophageal hiatal hernia (including fundoplication), via thoracotomy, except neonatal; with implantation of mesh or other prosthesis

A paraesophageal hernia is characterized by normal position of the gastroesophageal junction with protrusion of the fundus (top) of the stomach into the chest cavity alongside the esophagus. An incision is made through the chest just above the diaphragm. The stomach is mobilized and pulled into the chest cavity. A window is created behind the esophagus. If a fundoplication is performed, the stomach is partially or completely wrapped around the esophagus and sutured to the muscle layer of the fundus and/or esophagus. Common techniques performed via a thoracic approach include Belsey IV or Belsey Mark IV (BMIV) which employ a partial 270 degree wrap. The stomach is returned to the abdomen and the paraesophageal hernia is repaired. The hernia sac is mobilized taking care to protect the anterior vagus nerve. The hernia sac is excised. The diaphragm is repaired with sutures in 43334 or reinforced with mesh or other prosthetic material in 43335. The thorax is closed and chest tubes are placed as needed.

43336-43337

43336 Repair, paraesophageal hiatal hernia, (including fundoplication), via thoracoabdominal incision, except neonatal; without implantation of mesh or other prosthesis

43337 Repair, paraesophageal hiatal hernia, (including fundoplication), via thoracoabdominal incision, except neonatal; with implantation of mesh or other prosthesis

A paraesophageal hernia is characterized by normal position of the gastroesophageal junction with protrusion of the fundus (top) of the stomach into the chest cavity alongside the esophagus. A combined thoracoabdominal approach for repair is typically used in patients who have had previous diaphragmatic hernia surgery or those who have an irreducible hernia. A left posterolateral thoracotomy is used to expose the esophagus and an upper abdominal incision is used to expose the diaphragm and stomach. Simultaneous dissection in the upper abdomen and left chest is performed and adhesions are divided. The paraesophageal hernia sac, muscular origins (crura) of the diaphragm and esophageal hiatus are identified. If a previous fundoplication has been performed, it is taken down. The herniated portion of the stomach is mobilized and returned to the abdomen. The hernia sac is mobilized taking care to protect the anterior vagus nerve. The hernia sac is excised. If a fundoplication is performed, the fundus (top) of the stomach is partially or completely wrapped around the esophagus and sutured to the muscle layer of the stomach and/or esophagus. Common fundoplication techniques include Nissen or Toupet procedures which employ a complete 360 degree wrap or Belsey IV or Belsey Mark IV (BMIV) which employ a partial 270 degree wrap. The diaphragm is repaired with sutures in 43336 or reinforced with mesh or other prosthetic material in 43337. The abdomen and thorax are closed and chest tubes are placed as needed.

43338

43338 Esophageal lengthening procedure (eg, Collis gastroplasty or wedge gastroplasty) (List separately in addition to code for primary procedure)

During a separately reportable open procedure on a hiatal hernia, the esophagus is lengthened by Collis or wedge gastroplasty. The gastroesophageal fat pad is removed taking care to preserve the vagal nerves. A dilator (bougie) is passed through the mouth and into the esophagus and stomach. A stapling device is inserted into the abdominal cavity through the existing abdominal incision. Axial traction is applied to the esophagus. The greater curvature of the stomach is mobilized and rotated into an anteroposterior position. The stapler is placed parallel to the distal esophagus at the angle of His. The stapler is fired to create a 2-4 cm neoesophagus and a new angle of His. The primary open procedure is completed which typically involves fundoplication with placement of anchoring sutures from the esophagus to the fundoplication and then to the diaphragm. The fundoplication is then reduced through the diaphragm into the abdomen and anchoring sutures are tied. The dilator is removed.

43340-43341

43340 Esophagojejunostomy (without total gastrectomy); abdominal approach

43341 Esophagojejunostomy (without total gastrectomy); thoracic approach

This procedure may be performed when the stomach has been removed in a previous procedure, such as when a previous esophagogastrojejunostomy has failed requiring excision of the ischemic segment of jejunum with reanastomosis to the esophagus. In 43340, an abdominal approach also referred to as a transhiatal approach is used. An incision is made in the upper abdomen and the peritoneal cavity explored. The diaphragmatic hiatus is split to expose the lower posterior mediastinum and distal esophagus. In 43341, a thoracic approach, usually a right posterior thoracotomy is used. The skin is incised and the incision extended through the soft tissues. The scapula is retracted and the thorax entered without disrupting the pleura. Retropleural dissection is performed, the lung retracted, and the distal esophagus is exposed. The diaphragmatic hiatus is split and to access abdominal contents. The remaining stump of the esophagus is grasped with forceps. The esophageal stump may be opened or the ischemic segment of esophagus or jejunum excised. A 10-15 cm segment of jejunum is dissected free of mesentery taking care to preserve the jejunal vascular arcade. The freed segment of jejunum is pulled up to the esophageal stump. The esophagus and jejunum are then anastomosed in an end-to-end or end-to side fashion. If an end-to-side anastomosis is performed, the side of the jejunum is incised and the esophagus sutured to the side of the jejunum. The proximal jejunal stump is then closed. If a thoracic approach is used, a chest tube may be placed. Abdominal or thoracic incisions are then closed in layers.

43351-43352

43351 Esophagostomy, fistulization of esophagus, external; thoracic approach

43352 Esophagostomy, fistulization of esophagus, external; cervical approach

Fistulization of the esophagus is performed to allow the patient to eat normally. The proximal (upper) aspect of the esophagus is exteriorized creating a stoma and the distal (lower) aspect is closed. The stoma is allowed to heal for two weeks and then an esophageal tube with a flange is inserted. The flange is positioned within the esophagus completely under the skin. Part of the esophageal tube lies exterior to the skin. The exterior portion is connected to a gastrostomy tube. In 43351, the thoracic esophagus is exteriorized. A right posterior thoracotomy is generally used. The skin is incised and the incision is extended through the soft tissues. The scapula is retracted and the thorax is entered without disrupting the pleura. Retropleural dissection is performed; the lung is retracted; and the esophagus is exposed. Once the esophagus has been exposed, the esophagus is mobilized and divided. The distal segment is closed. The proximal esophageal segment is brought out through the left posterior chest wall. The muscular wall is sutured to the fascia. The full thickness of the esophagus is anastomosed to the skin. In 43352, the cervical esophagus is exteriorized. The esophagus is usually exteriorized on the left side of the neck. An incision is made anterior to the sternocleidomastoid muscle, between the thyroid gland and the trachea medially, and the carotid sheath laterally. The esophagus is mobilized below the cricopharynx taking care to protect the recurrent laryngeal nerves. The esophagus is divided and the distal end is sutured closed. The proximal stump is exteriorized. The muscular layers of the esophagus are sutured to the cervical fascia. The full thickness of the esophagus is anastomosed to the skin.

43360

43360 Gastrointestinal reconstruction for previous esophagectomy, for obstructing esophageal lesion or fistula, or for previous esophageal exclusion; with stomach, with or without pyloroplasty

Prior to the gastrointestinal reconstruction, the gastroepiploic vessels are ligated along the greater curvature of the stomach approximately four cm proximal to the pylorus, the tail of the pancreas is freed from its bed, and the spleen is resected. The blood supply to the greater curvature of the stomach is enhanced and vessels are lengthened so that the gastric tube will have an adequate blood supply. Next, a pedicle tube approximately one foot long and one inch in diameter is constructed from the greater curvature of the

Digestive System

stomach. An incision is made in the greater curvature of the stomach approximately four cm from the pylorus. A double row of staples is then inserted parallel to the greater curvature of the stomach about one inch from the edge. The stomach is incised between the two rows of staples creating the first six-inch portion of the gastric tube. A second double row of staples is inserted proximal to the first row in the stomach. The stomach is again incised between the second double row of staples to create the second six inch portion of the gastric tube. The completed tube is one foot long and will be used to replace the esophagus. The staples in the tube and the residual stomach are then inverted using a continuous suture. The gastric tube remains attached to the fundus of the stomach. The gastric tube is reversed in direction and the antral end of the tube is anastomosed to the remaining portion of the cervical esophagus, or if the cervical esophagus has been completely obliterated, to the pharynx. If the distal esophagus has not been completely removed during a previous surgery, the distal portion is closed. The tube can be routed subcutaneously, retrosternally, or intrathoracically. Pyloroplasty is performed as needed to widen the pyloric canal and relieve any stricture in the duodenum. This is accomplished by a longitudinal incision through the duodenum and pylorus that is closed transversely.

43361

43361   **Gastrointestinal reconstruction for previous esophagectomy, for obstructing esophageal lesion or fistula, or for previous esophageal exclusion; with colon interposition or small intestine reconstruction, including intestine mobilization, preparation, and anastomosis(es)**

The procedure varies somewhat based on whether the esophagus is reconstructed with a section of intestine or colon and what portion colon or small intestine is used. If a section of colon is used, the omentum is dissected off the colon. For a left colon interposition graft, the middle colic artery is ligated and the left and right flexures are mobilized taking care to preserve the arterial and venous collateral circulation for graft perfusion. Alternatively, a section of the left colon may be harvested along with the ascending colon. In this case, the right flexure is taken down, The middle and right colic arteries are ligated and the left colic artery is preserved for graft perfusion. The required length of the colon graft is determined by tethering the colon upward into the chest or neck area and measuring the distance between the tethering left colic artery that forms the pedicle for the graft and the planned anastomosis site. The planned transection site is marked. The proximal anastomosis site in the chest or neck is prepared. If the anastomisis is in the distal esophagus enlargement of the thoracic inlet may be required. This is accomplished by removal of the left half of the manubrium, the medial end of the first rib, and the sternal head of the left clavicle. If the anastomosis is in the middle third of the esophagus, a median sternotomy is performed to access the anastomosis site. Following preparation of the anastomosis site, the colon is transected and the colon graft is placed in a bowel bag to protect it as it is passed through the substernal tunnel to the anastomosis site. The esophagus is divided. The esophagus and colon graft are anastomosed. The colon graft is sutured to the left crus of the diaphragm or at the opening of the diaphragm into the substernal tunnel. The distal end of the colon graft is anastomosed to the posterior surface of the stomach. The remaining segments of colon distal and proximal to the harvested segment are then anastomosed to restore continuity of the remaining colon. A jejunostomy tube is placed for feeding and decompression.

43400-43401

43400   **Ligation, direct, esophageal varices**
43401   **Transection of esophagus with repair, for esophageal varices**

Open procedures are rarely used to treat esophageal varices except in patients who have variceal bleeding that cannot be controlled using pharmacologic or endoscopic interventions. The esophagus is exposed by a right posterolateral thoracotomy. The skin is incised and the incision extended through the soft tissues. The scapula is retracted and the thorax entered without disrupting the pleura. Retropleural dissection is performed, the lung retracted, and the distal third of the esophagus is exposed. Alternatively, a transhiatal abdominal approach may be used. In 43400, the esophagus is dissected free of surrounding tissue and incised to allow inspection of the varices. The varices are then tied off (ligated) under direct vision using sutures or bands. In 43401, the distal aspect of the esophagus is exposed and transected using a staple gun to devascularize the esophageal varices. When bleeding from varices has been controlled, the esophagus is repaired and the surgical incisions closed.

43405

43405   **Ligation or stapling at gastroesophageal junction for pre-existing esophageal perforation**

The esophagus is exposed by a right posterolateral thoracotomy. The skin is incised and the incision extended through the soft tissues. The scapula is retracted and the thorax entered without disrupting the pleura. Retropleural dissection is performed, the lung retracted, and the perforation at the gastroesophageal junction exposed. Alternatively, a transhiatal abdominal approach may be used. The esophagus and stomach are dissected free of surrounding tissue to allow inspection and repair of the defect. Any ragged or necrotic tissue is debrided. The perforation is then repaired by ligation or stapling of the defect and the thoracic or abdominal incision is closed.

43410-43415

43410   **Suture of esophageal wound or injury; cervical approach**
43415   **Suture of esophageal wound or injury; transthoracic or transabdominal approach**

In 43410, the injury is in the cervical esophagus. An incision is made in the neck, anterior to the sternocleidomastoid muscle, between the thyroid gland and trachea medially, and the carotid sheath laterally. The internal jugular vein and carotid artery are identified and retracted laterally. In 43415, the wound or injury is repaired using either a thoracic or abdominal approach. For a thoracic approach, a right posterior thoracotomy is generally used. The skin is incised and the incision extended through the soft tissues. The scapula is retracted and the thorax entered without disrupting the pleura. Retropleural dissection is performed, the lung retracted, and the esophagus is exposed. If an abdominal approach, also referred to as a transhiatal approach, is used an incision is made in the upper abdomen and the peritoneal cavity explored. The stomach is mobilized at the gastroesophageal junction and the diaphragmatic hiatus is split to expose the lower posterior mediastinum and esophagus. Once the esophagus has been exposed, the wound or injury is inspected and debrided as needed. Any ragged edges are trimmed. The wound or injury is then suture repaired.

43420-43425

43420   **Closure of esophagostomy or fistula; cervical approach**
43425   **Closure of esophagostomy or fistula; transthoracic or transabdominal approach**

In 43420, the esophagostomy or fistula site is in the cervical esophagus. An incision is made in the neck anterior to the sternocleidomastoid muscle, between the thyroid gland and trachea medially, and the carotid sheath laterally. The internal jugular vein and carotid artery are identified and retracted laterally. In 43425, the esophagostomy or fistula site is in the thorax or abdomen. For a thoracic approach, a right posterior thoracotomy is generally used. The skin is incised and the incision extended through the soft tissues. The scapula is retracted and the thorax entered without disrupting the pleura. Retropleural dissection is performed, the lung retracted, and the esophagus is exposed. If an abdominal approach, also referred to as a transhiatal approach, is used an incision is made in the upper abdomen and the peritoneal cavity explored. The stomach is mobilized at the gastroesophageal junction and the diaphragmatic hiatus is split to expose the esophagus. The exteriorized segment of the esophagus is dissected free of the skin and fascia. The interior stump is located dissected free of surrounding tissue and opened. The interior and exterior segments are reanastomosed or prepared for another surgical procedure. The stoma or fistula site is closed in layers and the surgical incision to expose the internal segment closed.

43450-43453

43450   **Dilation of esophagus, by unguided sound or bougie, single or multiple passes**
43453   **Dilation of esophagus, over guide wire**

The physician dilates the esophagus by unguided sound or bougie (43450) or over a guide wire (43453). These procedures are performed without direct visualization of the esophagus. Dilation is performed to treat esophageal stricture caused by esophageal reflux, benign or malignant lesions, or other injury/disease. Separately reportable esophagram is performed to identify the site and extent of the stricture. Separately reportable fluoroscopy may be used during the dilation procedure. A series of progressively larger rigid rubber tubes, also referred to as sounds or bougies, are passed through the mouth and down into the esophagus to dilate the stricture. In 43450, no guide is used to pass the sounds or bougies. In 43453, the sounds or bougies are passed over a guide wire.

43460

43460   **Esophagogastric tamponade, with balloon (Sengstaken type)**

Esophagogastric tamponade, also called balloon tamponade, is a procedure used to temporarily treat bleeding veins from gastric or esophageal varices, by applying pressure with the balloon against the bleeding vessels, compressing them, and stopping the bleeding. The patient is intubated to protect the airway. The tube is advanced into the stomach; air is injected into the balloon; and the tube is clamped. X-rays are taken to confirm placement. Additional air is placed in the rounded gastric balloon, and the tube is clamped. A type of helmet for traction is placed on the patient's head. The tube is pulled out until tension is achieved and the balloon is compressing the vessels, applying pressure to stop the bleeding. Traction is maintained by securing the tube to the helmet's facemask. For varices in the esophagus, an elongated, esophageal balloon is inflated after intubation and insertion. A pressure manometer and stopcock are securely inserted within the esophageal balloon lumen. Air is slowly injected into the elongated balloon until optimal pressure is reached and the lumen is clamped. Both gastric and esophageal aspiration is monitored for continued bleeding.

● New Code   ▲ Revised Code

Digestive System

43496

43496   Free jejunum transfer with microvascular anastomosis

This may also be referred to as a free jejunal graft or flap. An incision is made in the abdomen to obtain the free jejunal graft. The jejunum is exposed and the segment to be harvested identified. The distal end of the graft segment is marked so that it will be oriented to allow for normal peristalsis. The artery supplying the segment of jejunum to be harvested is located. Blood vessels are dissected back to their branching points off the supplying vessels where they are suture ligated and divided. The jejunum is divided and the graft segment removed along with the supplying blood vessels. The remaining distal and proximal jejunal segments are anastomosed to maintain small bowel continuity. The free segment of jejunum is then transferred to the site where the jejunal graft will be placed. The transfer site is prepared in a separately reportable procedure. The jejunal graft is properly oriented by locating the mark indicating the distal end. The jejunal serosa is first secured to surrounding tissue to take tension off the anastomosis sites and then the proximal and distal ends of the graft are anastomosed to the remaining esophageal or bowel segments. Microvascular anastomosis of the jejunal vessels to vessels at the anastomosis site is then performed.

43500

43500   Gastrotomy; with exploration or foreign body removal

The physician performs a gastrotomy for exploration of the stomach or removal of foreign body. An incision is made in the abdomen and the stomach exposed. The stomach wall is incised and the inner lumen of the stomach is visually inspected. Any abnormalities are noted. If a foreign body is present, it is removed and the stomach again inspected for the presence of injury or disease. The stomach is closed, the surgical wound irrigated, and the overlying muscle and skin closed in a layered fashion.

43501-43502

43501   Gastrotomy; with suture repair of bleeding ulcer
43502   Gastrotomy; with suture repair of pre-existing esophagogastric laceration (eg, Mallory-Weiss)

The physician performs a gastrotomy for suture repair of a bleeding ulcer (43501) or suture repair of a pre-existing esophagogastric laceration (43502). An esophagogastric laceration may also be referred to as a Mallory-Weiss tear. An incision is made in the abdomen and the stomach exposed. To repair a bleeding ulcer, the stomach is palpated and the site of the ulcer located. The stomach is incised and blood evacuated. The ulcer is located and bleeding controlled by applying pressure to the ulcer using a finger inserted into the ulcer crater. Once the bleeding has stopped, the blood vessels are suture ligated. In 43502, the esophagogastric laceration is identified, bleeding controlled, and the bleeding vessels are suture ligated.

43510

43510   Gastrotomy; with esophageal dilation and insertion of permanent intraluminal tube (eg, Celestin or Mousseaux-Barbin)

This procedure is typically performed as a palliative measure in patients with advanced esophageal cancer when a tube cannot be passed using a transoral endoscopic approach. An incision is made in the abdomen. The stomach is incised. A balloon catheter is advanced to the site of the stenosis and inflated. The inflated balloon remains in place for a short period of time and is then deflated. Inflation and deflation may be repeated several times until the narrowed segment of esophagus has been dilated to the desired diameter. Alternatively, a series of tubes of increasing diameter may be inserted through the stomach to the narrowed segment of esophagus and the stricture dilated. When the desired diameter is attained, a permanent intraluminal tube is placed at the site of the esophageal stenosis to maintain patency of the esophagus. The stomach incision is closed. The abdominal incision is closed in layers.

43520

43520   Pyloromyotomy, cutting of pyloric muscle (Fredet-Ramstedt type operation)

This procedure is typically performed during the neonatal period to treat congenital hypertrophic pyloric stenosis. A right upper abdominal incision is made just below the costal margin and above the inferior aspect of the liver. Dissection is carried down through subcutaneous tissue and the muscle layer of the abdomen is exposed and divided. The omentum and transverse colon are exposed. The transverse colon is mobilized and the stomach is exposed. The pylorus is identified and incised longitudinally through the serosal and muscle layers while taking care not to incise the mucosa. The muscle layer is gently spread allowing the mucosa to protrude up to the level of the serosa which increases the internal opening (lumen) at the pyloric junction. The incision in the pylorus is left open. The abdominal incision is closed in layers.

43605

43605   Biopsy of stomach, by laparotomy

The stomach is biopsied using an open approach. An incision is made in the abdomen. The stomach is exposed and incised. Biopsy forceps are used to obtain tissue samples from the stomach mucosa. Alternatively, a larger wedge of tissue may be excised. The abdominal incision is closed in layers and the tissue samples are sent for separately reportable pathological evaluation.

43610-43611

43610   Excision, local; ulcer or benign tumor of stomach
43611   Excision, local; malignant tumor of stomach

Local excision of an ulcer or tumor is performed. An incision is made in the abdomen and the stomach exposed. The stomach is palpated to identify the location of the ulcer or tumor. Depending on the location of the ulcer or tumor, the stomach may be mobilized to provide better access to the site of the lesion. Gastric arteries are identified and the vascular pedicle clamped. The stomach is incised and blood evacuated from the stomach. The ulcer or tumor is located and excised. Report 43610 for local excision of an ulcer or benign tumor and 43611 for local excision of a malignant tumor.

43620-43622

43620   Gastrectomy, total; with esophagoenterostomy
43621   Gastrectomy, total; with Roux-en-Y reconstruction
43622   Gastrectomy, total; with formation of intestinal pouch, any type

An upper midline abdominal incision is used to access the stomach. The abdominal cavity is explored. The stomach is mobilized and clamps placed just above the gastroesophageal junction and just below the gastroduodenal junction. The esophagus is transected just distal to the clamp and the duodenum transected proximal to the clamp. The stomach is removed. In 43620, an esophagogastroenterostomy is performed. The small intestine is mobilized, usually the duodenum, and brought up to the esophageal stump. The esophagus and duodenum are sutured together in an end-to-end fashion. In 43621, a Roux-en-Y reconstruction is performed. The proximal stump of the duodenum is closed. A section of jejunum is mobilized. The jejunum is divided and a Roux-en-Y limb is constructed. The side of the distal end of the jejunum is anastomosed to the side of the esophagus and the proximal end is anastomosed to the side of the jejunum. In 43622, an intestinal pouch is created. A long segment of small bowel is mobilized. The segment is folded back on itself in an S or J configuration and then incised and sutured in such a manner as to create a reservoir or pouch. The pouch is then anastomosed to the esophagus and to the remaining segment of small bowel.

43631-43632

43631   Gastrectomy, partial, distal; with gastroduodenostomy
43632   Gastrectomy, partial, distal; with gastrojejunostomy

A partial gastrectomy is performed to remove the lower (distal) portion of the stomach. An incision is made in the abdomen and the stomach exposed. The stomach is divided at the pylorus and mobilized to expose the left gastric artery. The vascular pedicle is clamped, the stomach contents evacuated, and the stomach decompressed. Branches of the left gastric artery are identified, divided, and suture ligated distal to the vascular clamp. The clamp is released and hemostasis verified. The proximal resection site is identified and marked with a suture. The distal point of the resection is identified and marked with noncrushing clamps. The stomach is divided and staples applied. The staple line is oversewn with sutures and hemostasis secured. The remaining stomach segment is aligned with the remaining segment of intestine and temporary stay sutures placed. The temporary sutures are replaced with running sutures and the stomach serosa approximated to the intestinal serosa. Report 43631 if the stomach is sutured (anastomosed) to the duodenum and 43632 if the stomach is anastomosed to the jejunum.

43633-43634

43633   Gastrectomy, partial, distal; with Roux-en-Y reconstruction
43634   Gastrectomy, partial, distal; with formation of intestinal pouch

An upper midline abdominal incision is used to access the stomach. The abdominal cavity is explored. The stomach is mobilized and clamps placed across the stomach just above the planned transection site and just below the gastroduodenal junction. The stomach is transected just distal to the clamp and the duodenum transected proximal to the clamp. The distal aspect of the stomach is removed. In 43633, a Roux-en-Y reconstruction is performed. The proximal stump of the duodenum is closed. A section of jejunum is mobilized. The jejunum is divided and a Roux-en-Y limb is constructed. The side of the distal end of the jejunum is anastomosed to the side of the stomach and the proximal end is anastomosed to the side of the jejunum. In 43634, an intestinal pouch is created. A long segment of small bowel is mobilized. The segment is folded back on itself in an S or J configuration and then incised and sutured in such a manner as to create a reservoir or pouch. The pouch is then anastomosed to the remaining portion of the stomach and the remaining segment of small bowel.

Digestive System

● New Code   ▲ Revised Code

43635

43635   Vagotomy when performed with partial distal gastrectomy (List separately in addition to code[s] for primary procedure)

The vagus nerve is the tenth cranial nerve. It arises from the brainstem and travels through the neck, thorax, and abdomen giving rise to multiple branches along its path. At the stomach, the vagus nerve divides into branches that innervate different parts of the stomach and upper digestive tract. Cutting of the vagus nerve is performed to decrease excessive acid production in the stomach to help prevent peptic ulcers. Vagotomy used to be a common procedure but is now performed rarely due to the success of pharmacologic treatments for ulcers. The vagus nerve is identified and freed from surrounding structures. The main vagal nerve trunks are divided.

43640-43641

43640   Vagotomy including pyloroplasty, with or without gastrostomy; truncal or selective

43641   Vagotomy including pyloroplasty, with or without gastrostomy; parietal cell (highly selective)

The vagus nerve is the tenth cranial nerve. It arises from the brainstem and travels through the neck, thorax, and abdomen, giving rise to multiple branches along its path. At the stomach, the vagus nerve divides into branches that innervate different parts of the stomach and upper digestive tract. Cutting of the vagus nerve is performed to decrease excessive acid production in the stomach to help prevent peptic ulcers. A midline upper abdominal incision is used to expose the stomach and vagus nerve. In 43640, a truncal or selective vagotomy is performed. The vagus nerve is identified and freed from surrounding structures. To perform a truncal vagotomy, the main vagal trunks are located and divided. To perform a selective vagotomy, the main vagal trunks are identified and dissected up to the branch leading to the biliary tree. This branch is followed to the hepatic branch and the nerve is transected as close to the hepatic branch as possible. In 43641, a highly selective vagotomy is performed. The vagal nerve is identified and followed to the Latarjet's nerve branches, also referred to as the parietal cell branches. These branches are divided beginning at the esophagogastric junction and continuing along the lesser curvature of the stomach. Because vagotomy also affects gastric motility, which may delay gastric emptying, a pyloroplasty is performed to enlarge the opening from the stomach to the duodenum. The gastroduodenal junction is exposed and the pyloric sphincter is incised longitudinally and the incision repaired transversely to relax the sphincter and enlarge the opening. A gastrostomy may also be performed. Two concentric pursestring sutures are placed in the stomach around the planned incision site. The serosa of the stomach is incised in the center of the pursestring sutures, the inner mucosal layer is grasped and a small portion excised. The hole in the mucosa is dilated to allow placement of a balloon catheter. The balloon catheter is inserted into the stomach, the balloon inflated, and traction applied to the external catheter to position the balloon against the wall of the stomach. The pursestring sutures are securely tied around the catheter. The stomach is positioned against the abdominal wall and the site of the abdominal incision determined. A stab incision is made in the abdomen, a forceps inserted through the skin into the abdominal cavity, the catheter grasped, and exteriorized. Anchoring sutures are placed on the internal abdominal wall. The abdominal incision is closed in layers.

43644-43645

43644   Laparoscopy, surgical, gastric restrictive procedure; with gastric bypass and Roux-en-Y gastroenterostomy (roux limb 150 cm or less)

43645   Laparoscopy, surgical, gastric restrictive procedure; with gastric bypass and small intestine reconstruction to limit absorption

These procedures are performed to treat morbid obesity. A small portal incision is made and a trocar placed in the upper abdomen and pneumoperitoneum established. The laparoscope is then introduced. Several more portal incisions are made in the upper abdomen for introduction of surgical instruments. The liver is retracted and the upper aspect of the stomach exposed. The gastroesophageal junction is identified. The gastrohepatic ligament is incised at the edge of the lesser curvature of the stomach and a tunnel is created behind the upper aspect of the stomach. An endoscopic linear stapler is used to transect the stomach and create a small gastric pouch in the proximal aspect of the stomach. The ligament of Trietz is identified and the jejunum is transected a few cm distal to this point. In 43644, a Roux-en-Y gastroenterostomy is then performed. The distal Roux-en-Y limb is mobilized and brought up to the gastric pouch through a tunnel in the transverse mesocolon. The mesenteric defect is closed around the distal Roux limb. The jejunum is anastomosed to the small gastric pouch using a side-to-side technique. The proximal Roux limb is measured to ensure that it does not exceed 150 cm and it is then anastomosed to the jejunum. In 43645, small intestine reconstruction is performed to limit absorption. This procedure combines gastric restriction with bypass of a large segment of small bowel to promote fat malabsorption. This also involves creation of a Roux limb of greater than 150 cm. The physician may either create a short biliopancreatic limb (20-90 cm) with a very long Roux limb (>150 cm) or a very long limb (>150 cm) that is anastomosed distal to the ileocecal valve.

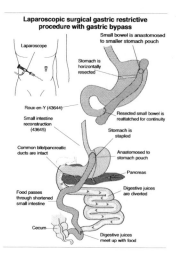

Laparoscopic surgical gastric restrictive procedure with gastric bypass

43647-43648

43647   Laparoscopy, surgical; implantation or replacement of gastric neurostimulator electrodes, antrum

43648   Laparoscopy, surgical; revision or removal of gastric neurostimulator electrodes, antrum

Laparoscopic implantation or replacement of gastric neurostimulator electrodes within the antrum of the stomach is done for cases of medically refractory gastroparesis. This is also known as a gastric pacemaker. The neurostimulator or generator portion of the device is implanted into a subcutaneous pocket created in the abdominal wall beneath the rib cage. Two intramuscular lead wires with electrodes are implanted in the muscle wall of the stomach antrum. The electrodes provide continuous high frequency, low energy electrical stimulation to the nerves of the lower stomach. The electrical stimulation encourages the stomach to contract and this helps relieve accompanying symptoms of severe vomiting, nausea, and related gastrointestinal problems of gastroparesis. Code 43647 for initial implantation or replacement of gastric neurostimulator electrodes via laparascope. Code 43648 for revision or removal of previously placed gastric neurostimulator electrodes via laparoscope.

43651-43652

43651   Laparoscopy, surgical; transection of vagus nerves, truncal

43652   Laparoscopy, surgical; transection of vagus nerves, selective or highly selective

A surgical laparoscopy is performed with transection of the vagus nerves, also referred to as vagotomy. The vagus nerve is the tenth cranial nerve. It arises from the brainstem and travels through the neck, thorax, and abdomen giving rise to multiple branches along its path. At the stomach, the vagus nerve divides into branches that innervate different parts of the stomach and upper digestive tract. Cutting of the vagus nerve is performed to decrease excessive acid production in the stomach to help prevent peptic ulcers. Vagotomy used to be a common procedure but is now performed rarely due to the success of pharmacologic treatments for ulcers. A small incision is made in the upper abdomen, a trocar placed and pneumoperitoneum established. The laparoscope is introduced. Additional portal incisions are made to allow introduction of surgical instruments. The vagus nerve is identified and freed from surrounding structures. In 43651, a truncal vagotomy is performed. The main vagal trunks are divided. In 43652, a selective or highly selective vagotomy is performed. To perform selective vagotomy, the main vagal trunks are identified and dissected up to the branch leading to the biliary tree. This branch is followed to the hepatic branch and the nerve is transected as close to the hepatic branch as possible. To perform highly selective vagotomy, dissection continues to the Latarjet's nerve branches which are divided beginning at the esophagogastric junction and continuing along the lesser curvature of the stomach. Upon completion of the procedure, surgical instruments and the laparoscope are removed. Air is released from the abdomen and the portal incisions are closed.

43653

43653   Laparoscopy, surgical; gastrostomy, without construction of gastric tube (eg, Stamm procedure) (separate procedure)

A small portal incision is made and a trocar is placed in the upper abdomen. Pneumoperitoneum is established. The laparoscope is then introduced. Several more portal incisions are made for introduction of surgical instruments. The stomach is exposed and mobilized. Two concentric pursestring sutures are placed in the stomach around the planned incision site. The serosa of the stomach is incised in the center of the pursestring sutures, the inner mucosal layer is grasped, and a small portion is excised. The hole in the mucosa is dilated to allow placement of a balloon catheter. The balloon catheter is inserted into the stomach, inflated, and traction applied to the external catheter to position the balloon against the wall of the stomach. The pursestring sutures are securely tied around the catheter. The stomach is positioned against the abdominal wall and the site of the abdominal incision is determined. An existing trocar site may be used or a separate stab incision may be made in the abdomen. Forceps are inserted through the skin into the abdominal cavity and the catheter is grasped and exteriorized. Anchoring sutures are placed on the internal abdominal wall. The surgical instruments and laparoscope are removed, air is released from the peritoneum, and portal incisions are closed with sutures.

43752

43752 Naso- or oro-gastric tube placement, requiring physician's skill and fluoroscopic guidance (includes fluoroscopy, image documentation and report)

The length of tube to be inserted is determined and the tube marked. If a nasogastric tube is being inserted, the nostrils are inspected for patency. The tube is lubricated and inserted into the largest patent nostril. If an orogastric tube is used, it is inserted through the mouth. If alert and able, the patient is instructed to swallow as the tube is passed under fluoroscopic guidance through the pharynx, esophagus, and into the stomach. Placement may be verified radiographically, by aspiration of stomach contents, or by using a stethoscope to listen for the sound of air entering the stomach when an air bolus is instilled using an irrigation syringe.

43753

43753 Gastric intubation and aspiration(s) therapeutic, necessitating physician's skill (eg, for gastrointestinal hemorrhage), including lavage if performed

A gastric tube is inserted through the nose or mouth. If the tube is inserted through the nose, the nostrils are examined and the more patent nostril is selected for tube insertion. The patient's head is tipped backward and viscous lidocaine is instilled into the nostril to provide local anesthesia. The length of tube needed for insertion into the stomach is estimated and the tube is marked. The tube is inserted into the nose and advanced to the nasopharynx. The patient may sip water to assist in advancing the tube through the oropharynx, esophagus, and then into the stomach. Proper placement is verified by instilling air into the stomach and auscultating for a rush of air or by aspirating gastric content. The physician performs a therapeutic aspiration procedure. The physician may also wash out the stomach by instilling liquid and then aspirating the instilled liquid along with gastric contents. The gastric tube may be left in place or removed following the aspiration procedure.

43754-43755

43754 Gastric intubation and aspiration, diagnostic; single specimen (eg, acid analysis)

43755 Gastric intubation and aspiration, diagnostic; collection of multiple fractional specimens with gastric stimulation, single or double lumen tube (gastric secretory study) (eg, histamine, insulin, pentagastrin, calcium, secretin), includes drug administration

A gastric tube is inserted through the nose or mouth. If the tube is inserted through the nose, the nostrils are examined and the more patent nostril is selected for tube insertion. The patient's head is tipped backward and viscous lidocaine is instilled into the nostril to provide local anesthesia. The length of tube needed for insertion into the stomach is estimated and the tube is marked. The tube is inserted into the nose and advanced to the nasopharynx. The patient may sip water to assist in advancing the tube through the oropharynx, esophagus, and then into the stomach. Proper placement is verified by instilling air into the stomach and auscultating for a rush of air or by aspirating gastric content. The physician performs a diagnostic aspiration procedure. In 43754, a single specimen of gastric content is obtained for analysis. In 43755, multiple fractional specimens are obtained to evaluate gastric secretions. The test includes administration of drugs such as histamine, insulin, pentagastrin, calcium, and secretin that stimulate gastric secretion.

43756-43757

43756 Duodenal intubation and aspiration, diagnostic, includes image guidance; single specimen (eg, bile study for crystals or afferent loop culture)

43757 Duodenal intubation and aspiration, diagnostic, includes image guidance; collection of multiple fractional specimens with pancreatic or gallbladder stimulation, single or double lumen tube, includes drug administration

A gastric tube is inserted through the nose or mouth. If the tube is inserted through the nose, the nostrils are examined and the more patent nostril is selected for tube insertion. The patient's head is tipped backward and viscous lidocaine is instilled into the nostril to provide local anesthesia. The length of tube needed for insertion into the dudenum is estimated and the tube is marked. The tube is inserted into the nose and advanced to the nasopharynx. The patient may sip water to assist in advancement through the oropharynx, esophagus and then into the stomach and duodenum. Image guidance is used to ensure that the tube is successfully advanced into the duodenum. Once the tube has been successfully advanced into the duodenum one or more specimens are obtained for analysis.¬† In 43756, a single specimen of duodenal content is obtained for analysis. In 43757, multiple fractional specimens are obtained to evaluate duodenal content and

pancreatic and gallbladder secretions. The test includes administration of drugs that stimulate pancreatic and gallbladder secretion of bile salts.

43760

43760 Change of gastrostomy tube, percutaneous, without imaging or endoscopic guidance

A percutaneous change of a gastrostomy tube is performed without imaging or endoscopic guidance. The existing gastrostomy tube site is examined. If the gastrostomy tube is a balloon catheter type, the balloon is deflated and the gastrostomy tube is removed. If it is a retention dome type, the gastrostomy tube may be cut, allowing the dome to pass through the digestive tract or the dome may be removed along with the gastrostomy tube using external traction. A new gastrostomy tube is inserted. If the gastrostomy tube is a balloon catheter type, the balloon is filled. The tube is pulled back and secured, and patency is verified.

43761

43761 Repositioning of a naso- or oro-gastric feeding tube, through the duodenum for enteric nutrition

An existing nasogastric or orogastric tube is repositioned from the stomach to the duodenum to provide enteric nutrition. The exposed tube is lubricated. If alert and able, the patient is instructed to swallow as the tube is advanced under separately reportable fluoroscopic guidance from the stomach into the duodenum. Fluoroscopy may also be used to verify correct positioning of the gastric feeding tube in the duodenum.

43770

43770 Laparoscopy, surgical, gastric restrictive procedure; placement of adjustable gastric restrictive device (eg, gastric band and subcutaneous port components)

A laparoscopic gastric restrictive procedure is performed with placement of an adjustable gastric restrictive device, including a gastric band and subcutaneous port components. A Verres needle is introduced and the abdomen is insufflated. Five trocars are placed, one below the xiphoid with the camera and optical system; one in the midline below the first trocar for the liver retractor; one in the right upper quadrant for the grasping forceps and gastric band tool; one in the left upper quadrant for the cautery hook, needle holder and grasping forceps; and one on the left anterior axillary line for the grasping forceps. A nasogastric tube is placed and inflated to identify the location of the stomach. The lesser curvature is dissected. One set of grasping forceps are placed on the gastrohepatic ligament and another on the gastric wall placing the lesser curvature under tension. A small opening is created between the gastrohepatic ligament and lesser curvature to allow placement of the band. The phrenogastric ligament is put under tension and a small window is created using the coagulation hook. An endograsp is introduced, passed through the retrogastric tunnel until it is visible in the phrenogastric window, and advanced until it emerges above the spleen and grasps the diaphragm. The gastric band is introduced and grasped using the endograsp, looped around the stomach, and tightened. The position of the band is checked, adjusted as needed, and then locked. Saline solution is injected into the inflatable balloon and tension is calibrated. The tube is clamped and any redundant portion is cut and removed. The band is secured with sutures. The access port is placed in the subcutaneous tissue of the abdomen and connected to the injection reservoir. The reservoir is fixed to the abdominal fascia in the left hypochondrium. Gastric band adjustment is performed postoperatively in the radiology department.

43771-43774

43771 Laparoscopy, surgical, gastric restrictive procedure; revision of adjustable gastric restrictive device component only

43772 Laparoscopy, surgical, gastric restrictive procedure; removal of adjustable gastric restrictive device component only

43773 Laparoscopy, surgical, gastric restrictive procedure; removal and replacement of adjustable gastric restrictive device component only

43774 Laparoscopy, surgical, gastric restrictive procedure; removal of adjustable gastric restrictive device and subcutaneous port components

A laparoscopic revision of an adjustable gastric restrictive device, gastric band component only, is performed in 43771. A revision procedure of the gastric band component is typically performed when slippage occurs. The gastric band component is equipped with a locking mechanism that can be opened when slippage occurs so the band can be repositioned. A Verres needle is inserted and the abdomen is insufflated. Trocars are introduced for placing laparoscopic tools. A nasogastric tube is placed for decompression. The gastric band is dissected free, unlocked, and repositioned. Use 43772 when the gastric band is dissected free, unlocked, and removed laparoscopically without the removal of other components. In 43773, the defective gastric band is dissected free, unlocked, and removed, then replaced. An endograsp is introduced, passed through the retrogastric tunnel until it is visible in the phrenogastric window, and advanced until it emerges above the spleen and grasps the diaphragm. The replacement gastric band is then introduced and grasped using the endograsp, looped around the stomach, and tightened. The position of the band is checked, adjusted as needed, and then locked. Saline solution is injected into the inflatable

Digestive System

balloon and tension is calibrated. The tube is clamped and any redundant portion is cut and removed. The band is secured with sutures and connected to the existing reservoir. Gastric band adjustment is performed postoperatively in the radiology department. Use 43774 when both the gastric band and subcutaneous port components are removed laparoscopically. The subcutaneous port components are dissected and removed first to allow traction on the band. After trocars and laparoscopic instruments are placed, the gastric band is dissected free, unlocked, and removed.

43775

43775   Laparoscopy, surgical, gastric restrictive procedure; longitudinal gastrectomy (ie, sleeve gastrectomy)

Sleeve gastrectomy is a bariatric (weight loss) procedure that involves removing more than 85% of the stomach leaving only a very narrow vertical segment intact. A small incision is made and pneumoperitoneum established. Additional incisions are made in the upper abdomen and trocars placed. A fifth small incision is made just above the umbilicus and the laparoscope is introduced through a port. The liver is retracted. The greater curvature of the stomach is mobilized. Gastric vessels along the greater curvature are divided. The short gastric vessels are mobilized. Once the greater curvature of the stomach is completely mobilized a bougie is inserted endoscopically through the esophagus and passed into the stomach. The bougie is used to size the portion of the stomach that will remain after the gastrectomy. A gastric stapler is used to divide the stomach vertically. The staple line is checked for bleeding which is controlled by electrocautery. The severed portion of the stomach is removed through one of the ports. Surgical tools and the laparoscope are removed. The portal incisions are closed with sutures.

43800

43800   Pyloroplasty

The pyloric sphincter is a band of muscle at the lower aspect of the stomach that acts as a valve between the stomach and duodenum. The pyloric sphincter prevents regurgitation of duodenal contents back into the stomach. When the sphincter is too tight, a condition referred to as pyloric stenosis, the sphincter slows the passage of food from the stomach to the duodenum which can cause gastroesophageal reflux or peptic ulcer disease. Pyloroplasty is performed to relax the sphincter and increase the diameter of pylorus. A midline incision is made in the abdomen and the stomach and duodenum exposed. The pylorus is divided laterally and then sutured longtitudinally to create a wider opening into the duodenum. The abdominal incision is closed in layers.

43810

43810   Gastroduodenostomy

This procedure is performed without resecting (removing) a portion of the stomach or duodenum. The abdomen is opened in the midline and the stomach and duodenum exposed. Any adhesions are lysed and the stomach and duodenum are mobilized. An incision is made in the stomach, usually the greater curvature. The stomach and duodenum are divided at the gastroduodenal junction and the opening in the stomach closed with sutures. An incision is then made in the stomach usually along the greater curvature and the duodenum is sutured to the stomach in an end-to-side fashion. Alternatively, the duodenum may be rotated up to meet the stomach. The stomach and duodenum are incised longitudinally and sutured together in a side-to-side fashion. The surgical wound is irrigated, drains placed as needed, and the abdominal incision closed in layers.

43820-43825

43820   Gastrojejunostomy; without vagotomy
43825   Gastrojejunostomy; with vagotomy, any type

This procedure is performed without resecting (removing) a portion of the stomach, duodenum or jejunum. There are several techniques including retrocolic and antecolic. The abdomen is opened in the midline and the stomach and jejunum exposed. Any adhesions are lysed and the stomach and jejunum are mobilized. Using a retrocolic technique, the stoma is located as close to the pylorus as possible at the most dependent (lowest) portion or greater curvature of the stomach. Clamps are placed along the greater and lesser curvatures. The transverse colon is lifted, the mesocolon inspected, and the middle colic artery identified and protected. An avascular segment of mesentery is identified and incised. The stomach protrudes through the incision in the mesocolon with the lesser curvature located at the lowest corner of the mesenteric opening. The lesser curvature is sutured to the mesocolon. A jejunal loop distal to the ligament of Trietz is selected and clamped and incised. The greater curvature of the stomach is also incised and the jejunum is then sutured (anastomosed) to the opening in the stomach in a side-to-side fashion. Using an antecolic technique, an incision is made in the gastrocolic ligament instead of the mesocolon and the stomach and jejunum are then anastomosed using the same technique described above. The surgical wound is irrigated, drains placed as needed, and the abdominal incision closed in layers. In 43820 the procedure is performed without vagotomy. In 43825, a vagotomy is also performed. The vagus nerve innervates the stomach and causes the stomach to secrete acid. Patients with peptic ulcer disease sometimes

require severing of the vagus nerve to reduce acid production. The vagus nerve is located and either the trunk or branches are cut.

43830-43832

43830   Gastrostomy, open; without construction of gastric tube (eg, Stamm procedure) (separate procedure)
43831   Gastrostomy, open; neonatal, for feeding
43832   Gastrostomy, open; with construction of gastric tube (eg, Janeway procedure)

In 43830, the procedure is performed without construction of a gastric tube (Stamm procedure). A small incision is made in the midline of the upper abdomen. The peritoneum is grasped with forceps and incised. The abdominal cavity is opened and any adhesions along the inner abdominal wall lysed. The anterior aspect of the stomach is grasped. Two concentric pursestring sutures are placed in the stomach around the planned incision site. The serosa of the stomach is incised in the center of the pursestring sutures, the inner mucosal layer grasped and a small portion excised. The hole in the mucosa is dilated to allow placement of a balloon catheter. The balloon catheter is inserted into the stomach, the balloon inflated, and traction applied to the external catheter to position the balloon against the wall of the stomach. The pursestring sutures are securely tied around the catheter. The stomach is positioned against the abdominal wall and the site of the abdominal incision determined. A stab incision is made in the abdomen, a forceps inserted through the skin into the abdominal cavity, the catheter grasped, and exteriorized. Anchoring sutures are placed on the internal abdominal wall. The abdominal incision is closed in layers. In 43831, an open gastrostomy is performed to place a neonatal feeding tube. This procedure is performed as described in 43830 with the only exception being that the procedure is for placement of a feeding tube in a neonate. In 43832, an open gastrostomy is performed with construction of a gastric tube. The stomach is exposed as described above and incised to create a stomach flap. The stomach flap is then advanced to the abdominal wall taking care to ensure that there is no undo tension on the stomach. A stab incision is made in the abdomen and the stoma site prepared. The flap of stomach is then pulled through the stab incision, everted, and sutured to the abdominal wall. A gastrostomy tube is inserted into the abdomen.

43840

43840   Gastrorrhaphy, suture of perforated duodenal or gastric ulcer, wound, or injury

The abdomen is opened in the midline and the abdominal cavity explored. Any adhesions are lysed and the stomach and duodenum are exposed. The perforation is identified. The hole in the stomach and/or duodenum is closed in a layered fashion with sutures. If the perforation is due to a penetrating wound or injury, the abdomen is thoroughly explored to ensure that there is no injury to other organs, blood vessels, or nerves. The abdomen is copiously flushed with sterile saline to remove gastric fluids that have escaped into the abdominal cavity as well as blood or other debris. Drains are placed as needed and the abdomen closed in layers.

43842-43843

43842   Gastric restrictive procedure, without gastric bypass, for morbid obesity; vertical-banded gastroplasty
43843   Gastric restrictive procedure, without gastric bypass, for morbid obesity; other than vertical-banded gastroplasty

A midline abdominal incision is used to expose the stomach. In 43842, vertical banded gastroplasty is performed. A small window is created in both the anterior and posterior walls of the stomach at the upper aspect of. A line of staples is then placed from the window to the esophagus to create a small pouch at the upper aspect of the stomach along the lesser curvature. The edges of the windows in the anterior and posterior walls are sutured together to create a through and through hole through which a plastic band is inserted. The vertical band is wrapped around the lesser curvature just below the small gastric pouch to create a small outlet from the pouch. The band keeps food in the pouch longer and makes the patient feel full. Vertical banded gastroplasty is not commonly used today. In 43843, a technique other than vertical banded gastroplasty is used. This procedure involves any other technique used to create a gastric pouch and restrict the passage of food through the stomach without the use of a bypass procedure.

43845

43845   Gastric restrictive procedure with partial gastrectomy, pylorus-preserving duodenoileostomy and ileoileostomy (50 to 100 cm common channel) to limit absorption (biliopancreatic diversion with duodenal switch)

This procedure may also be referred to as biliopancreatic diversion with duodenal switch. A midline abdominal incision is made to expose the stomach. The stomach is mobilized. A longitudinal pouch is then created by staple division of the stomach beginning at the top of the gastric fundus and continuing laterally to the gastroesophageal juncation at the angle of His. The lateral aspect of the stomach is removed. The pyloric sphincter and a small portion of the proximal duodenum are preserved. The first portion of the duodenum is mobilized and transected approximately 3-5 cm from the pylorus. The small bowel is

● New Code   ▲ Revised Code

transected approximately 250 cm from the ileocecal valve. The distal limb is sutured to the remaining duodenal segment using and end-to-end technique. The proximal biliopancreatic limb is sutured to the small bowel approximately 50-100 cm proximal to the ileocecal valve. Drains are placed and abdominal incisions are closed.

43846-43847

43846 Gastric restrictive procedure, with gastric bypass for morbid obesity; with short limb (150 cm or less) Roux-en-Y gastroenterostomy

43847 Gastric restrictive procedure, with gastric bypass for morbid obesity; with small intestine reconstruction to limit absorption

These procedures are performed to treat morbid obesity. An upper abdominal midline incision is made to access the stomach. The liver is retracted and the upper aspect of the stomach exposed. The gastroesophageal junction is identified. The gastrohepatic ligament is incised at the edge of the lesser curvature of the stomach and a tunnel is created behind the upper aspect of the stomach. A linear stapler is used to transect the stomach and create a small gastric pouch in the proximal aspect of the stomach. The ligament of Trietz is identified and the jejunum is transected a few cm distal to this point. In 43846, a Roux-en-Y gastroenterostomy is then performed. The distal Roux-en-Y limb is mobilized and brought up to the gastric pouch through a tunnel in the transverse mesocolon. The mesenteric defect is closed around the distal Roux limb. The jejunum is anastomosed to the small gastric pouch using a side-to-side technique. The proximal Roux limb is measured to ensure that it does not exceed 150 cm and it is then anastomosed to the jejunum. In 43847, small intestine reconstruction is performed to limit absorption. This procedure combines gastric restriction with bypass of a large segment of small bowel to promote fat malabsorption. This also involves creation of a Roux limb of greater than 150 cm. The physician may either create a short biliopancreatic limb (20-90 cm) with a very long Roux limb (>150 cm) or a very long limb (>150 cm) that is anastomosed distal to the ileocecal valve. Once all anastomoses have been completed, drains are placed and the abdominal incision is closed.

43848

43848 Revision, open, of gastric restrictive procedure for morbid obesity, other than adjustable gastric restrictive device (separate procedure)

An open revision of a gastric restrictive procedure other than an adjustable gastric band is performed for morbid obesity. Revision is done when the previously performed gastric procedure fails, which may be due to weight regain, mechanical complications, or intolerance to the restriction. The revision performed is dependent on the nature of the original gastric restrictive procedure and the reason for the failure. Possible revision procedures include mini-gastric bypass or Roux-en-Y gastric bypass procedure. An incision is made in the abdomen. The stomach is exposed and dissected free. Any previous gastric restrictive devices are removed, such as a vertical gastric band. The revision procedure is then performed. If a mini-gastric bypass procedure is performed, the stomach is stapled to create a narrow long tube on one side and a larger section of stomach on the other side that is partitioned off. The smaller section of the stomach is anastomosed (attached) to the lower portion of the small intestine just in front of the large intestine. Bypassing the upper portion of the small intestine excludes approximately six feet of highly absorptive tissue where the majority of calories are absorbed. The larger portion of stomach is sealed off and left unattached to the small intestine. If a Roux-en-Y gastric bypass is performed, a portion of the stomach is stapled to create a small pouch about the size of the thumb. The small intestine is bisected and the lower portion of the small intestine is anastomosed to the stomach pouch. Food now bypasses the lower stomach and upper portion of small intestine where the majority of calories are absorbed. Because the top section of small intestine is where bile and pancreatic juices enter the digestive system, the bisected end of small bowel is anastomosed to the lower small intestine. This creates the Y-shaped connection that gives this procedure its name (Roux-en-Y gastric bypass).

43850-43855

43850 Revision of gastroduodenal anastomosis (gastroduodenostomy) with reconstruction; without vagotomy

43855 Revision of gastroduodenal anastomosis (gastroduodenostomy) with reconstruction; with vagotomy

The abdomen is opened the site of the previous anastomosis inspected. The exact procedure depends on the indication for the revision. A stricture at the anastomosis site may be released by incising the muscular wall longitudinally and repairing the stricture transversely. A perforation at the anastomosis site may be repaired with sutures. In 43850, the procedure is performed without vagotomy. In 43855, a vagotomy is performed. The vagus nerve is the tenth cranial nerve. It arises from the brainstem and travels through the neck, thorax, and abdomen, giving rise to multiple branches along its path. At the stomach, the vagus nerve divides into branches that innervate different parts of the stomach and upper digestive tract. Cutting of the vagus nerve is performed to decrease excessive acid production in the stomach to help prevent peptic ulcers. Following revision of the gastroduodenostomy, the vagus nerve is identified and freed from surrounding structures. The main vagal trunks are located and divided. Drains are then placed in the abdomen as needed and the abdominal incision closed.

43860-43865

43860 Revision of gastrojejunal anastomosis (gastrojejunostomy) with reconstruction, with or without partial gastrectomy or intestine resection; without vagotomy

43865 Revision of gastrojejunal anastomosis (gastrojejunostomy) with reconstruction, with or without partial gastrectomy or intestine resection; with vagotomy

The abdomen is opened and the site of the previous anastomosis inspected. The exact procedure depends on the indication for the revision. A stricture at the anastomosis site may be released by incising the muscular wall longitudinally and repairing the stricture transversely. A perforation at the anastomosis site may be repaired with sutures. In 43860, the procedure is performed without vagotomy. A portion of the stomach and/or jejunum may be excised and the stomach and jejunum reanastomosed. In 43860, the procedure is performed without a vagotomy. In 43865, a vagotomy is performed. The vagus nerve is the tenth cranial nerve. It arises from the brainstem and travels through the neck, thorax, and abdomen, giving rise to multiple branches along its path. At the stomach, the vagus nerve divides into branches that innervate different parts of the stomach and upper digestive tract. Cutting of the vagus nerve is performed to decrease excessive acid production in the stomach to help prevent peptic ulcers. Following revision of the gastroduodenostomy, the vagus nerve is identified and freed from surrounding structures. The main vagal trunks are located and divided. Drains are then placed in the abdomen as needed and the abdominal incision closed.

43870

43870 Closure of gastrostomy, surgical

The gastrostomy tube is removed. A small incision is made in the abdomen near the site of the gastrostomy. The stomach is released from the abdominal wall and the opening in the stomach exposed. The edges of the opening are debrided and the opening is closed with sutures. The gastrostomy site in the abdomen is then closed as is the abdominal wall incision.

43880

43880 Closure of gastrocolic fistula

Gastrocolic fistulas are typically a complication malignant ulceration caused by cancer of the stomach or colon but may also occur due to benign ulcers of the stomach. The abdomen is opened and the fistula between the stomach and colon identified. The fistulous tract is severed at its connection to the colon and the opening in the colon closed. The tract is then severed at the opening in the stomach and the stomach opening is closed. Drains are placed in the abdomen as needed and the abdominal incision is closed.

43881-43882

43881 Implantation or replacement of gastric neurostimulator electrodes, antrum, open

43882 Revision or removal of gastric neurostimulator electrodes, antrum, open

Implantation or replacement of gastric neurostimulator electrodes within the antrum of the stomach is done for cases of medically refractory gastroparesis. This is also known as a gastric pacemaker. The neurostimulator or generator portion of the device is implanted into a subcutaneous pocket created in the abdominal wall beneath the rib cage. Two intramuscular lead wires with electrodes are implanted in the muscle wall of the stomach antrum. The electrodes provide continuous high frequency, low energy electrical stimulation to the nerves of the lower stomach. The electrical stimulation encourages the stomach to contract and this helps relieve accompanying symptoms of severe vomiting, nausea, and related gastrointestinal problems of gastroparesis. Code 43881 for initial implantation or replacement of gastric neurostimulator electrodes by open surgery. Code 43882 for open revision or removal of previously placed gastric neurostimulator electrodes.

43886-43888

43886 Gastric restrictive procedure, open; revision of subcutaneous port component only

43887 Gastric restrictive procedure, open; removal of subcutaneous port component only

43888 Gastric restrictive procedure, open; removal and replacement of subcutaneous port component only

An incision is made over the access port and the subcutaneous fat and capsule around the port are divided. The port is exposed and inspected. In 43886, the port is revised which may be required due to a malfunctioning component or when the port becomes malpositioned. The malfunctioning component is repaired or replaced or the port is returned to the proper position. The port is then secured with sutures to the abdominal fascia. In 43887, the port is removed without replacement which may be performed due to infection at the port site. The port is released from the abdominal wall. The access tubing to the band is severed and the port is removed. The remaining tubing is tied off and placed in the peritoneal cavity. The band component is left in place. The port site is irrigated, packed with gauze and left open to heal by secondary intention. In 43888, the port is removed and

Digestive System

replaced. This procedure is performed for a malfunctioning port that cannot be repaired. The port is released from the abdominal wall, the access tubing to the band is severed and the port is removed. The new access port is connected to the tubing and the port is secured with sutures to the abdominal wall fascia. The port is tested by injecting saline into the band to tighten it. Once the band has been tightened to the desired level, the surgical incisions are closed.

44005

44005   Enterolysis (freeing of intestinal adhesion) (separate procedure)

Enterolysis refers to the severing of intestinal adhesions which is performed when adhesions cause the bowel to stick together and twist or kink causing bowel obstruction. A midline abdominal incision is used to expose the intestines. The abdominal cavity is inspected. Intestinal adhesions are lysed using blunt and sharp dissection. Once all adhesions have been released, the incision is closed in layers.

44010

44010   Duodenotomy, for exploration, biopsy(s), or foreign body removal

A duodenotomy is performed for exploration, biopsy, or foreign body removal. An incision is made in the abdomen and the duodenum is exposed. The duodenal segment to be explored is removed from the abdominal cavity and placed on the operating table. Pressure is applied to the duodenal segment to express intestinal contents. The intestine is clamped distal and proximal to the operative site. An incision is made in the intestine and the internal lumen is explored. Tissue samples are taken and sent to the laboratory for pathology. If a foreign body is present, it is removed. The duodenal incision is closed; the distal and proximal clamps are removed; the duodenal segment is returned to the abdomen; and the abdominal incision is closed.

44015

44015   Tube or needle catheter jejunostomy for enteral alimentation, intraoperative, any method (List separately in addition to primary procedure)

Following major abdominal surgery, physiological changes occur, including cellular and morphological changes. Enteral feeding following surgery helps maintain digestive tract integrity and function. Upon completion of the operative procedure, a segment of jejunum is selected that can reach the abdominal wall without tension. For tube jejunostomy placement, a small incision is made through the skin and upper abdominal wall on the left side. A guidewire is inserted through the incision and advanced into the jejunum. A tube for enteral alimentation is then advanced over the guidewire and into the jejunum. The guidewire is removed. The tube is secured internally with a bumper or balloon and externally with a bumper, flange, or other device. For NCJ placement a commercial kit is used consisting of a 90 cm French catheter with a flexible stainless steel stylet; two thin walled needles, a blunt adaptor needle, and catheter sleeve retainer. A pursestring suture is placed in the antimesenteric border of the jejunum at the planned puncture site. One of the two thin walled needles is introduced with the bevel point up, advanced through the pursestring suture and a submucosal tunnel is created. The needle is advanced for its full length along the submucosal layer and then passed through the mucosa into the jejunal lumen. The flexible stylet is attached to the catheter and the stylet and catheter are advanced through the needle into the jejunal lumen. The thin walled needle is removed and the catheter advanced approximately 25 cm within the jejunum. The stylet is removed. The pursestring suture is closed around the catheter. An exit site is selected in abdomen and the second thin walled catheter advanced through the skin and abdominal wall into the peritoneum. The catheter is threaded through the needle. The jejunum is sutured to the abdominal wall. The external segment of catheter is shortened to the desired length and anchored to the skin. A needle is inserted into the catheter and a bolus of normal saline injected to confirm patency.

44020-44021

44020   Enterotomy, small intestine, other than duodenum; for exploration, biopsy(s), or foreign body removal
44021   Enterotomy, small intestine, other than duodenum; for decompression (eg, Baker tube)

An enterotomy is performed on a segment of small intestine other than the duodenum for exploration, biopsy, or foreign body removal. An incision is made in the abdomen and the intestinal segment exposed. The segment to be explored is removed from the abdominal cavity and placed on the operating table. Pressure is applied to the intestinal segment to express its contents. The intestine is clamped distal and proximal to the operative site. An incision is made in the intestine and the internal lumen explored. Tissue samples are taken and sent to the laboratory for pathology. If a foreign body is present it is removed. The intestinal incision is closed, the distal and proximal clamps removed, the intestinal segment returned to the abdomen, and the abdominal incision closed. In 44021, an enterotomy is performed on a segment of small intestine other than the duodenum for decompression. The segment of bowel to be incised is isolated as described above. A purse string suture is placed in the intestine and a small nick incision made through the wall of the intestine. A trocar and cannula connected to suction tubing are inserted through the

incision. The suction tubing is advanced up and down the distended loops of intestine and the intestine is decompressed. Following completion of the decompression, the suction tubing is removed, the pursestring suture tied around the incision, and a second pursestring suture placed around the wound.

44025

44025   Colotomy, for exploration, biopsy(s), or foreign body removal

A colotomy is performed for exploration, biopsy, or foreign body removal. An incision is made in the abdomen and the colon segment is exposed; removed from the abdominal cavity; and placed on the operating table. Pressure is applied to the colon segment to express its contents. The colon is clamped distal and proximal to the operative site. An incision is made in the colon and the internal lumen is then explored. Tissue samples are taken and sent to the laboratory for pathology. Any foreign body is removed. The colon incision is closed; the distal and proximal clamps are removed; the colon segment is returned to the abdomen; and the abdominal incision is closed.

44050

44050   Reduction of volvulus, intussusception, internal hernia, by laparotomy

A laparotomy is performed to reduce a case of volvulus, intussusception, or internal hernia. Volvulus is a twisting of the intestines. Intussusception is a condition where one segment of intestine slides or telescopes into another segment. Internal hernia occurs when part of the intestine protrudes out of its normal location. An incision is made in the abdomen and the volvulus, intussusception, or internal hernia site of intestine is located. To correct a volvulus, the physician manipulates the twisted segment of colon into the correct position. To correct an intussusception, the physician starts at the top of the mass and gently squeezes the telescoped section of intestine back into its normal position. To reduce an internal hernia, the physician manipulates the protruding segment of bowel back into its normal position.

44055

44055   Correction of malrotation by lysis of duodenal bands and/or reduction of midgut volvulus (eg, Ladd procedure)

Malrotation of the intestines is a congenital anomaly that results from failure of the intestines to rotate to the left of the superior mesenteric artery (SMA) at the ligament of Trietz, which normally occurs between the 4th through 12th weeks of fetal development. The intestines are exposed through a midline abdominal incision. If a midgut volvulus is present, the entire small bowel and transverse colon are delivered out of the abdomen. Malrotation usually results in a clockwise twisting of the intestine, so the surgeon reduces the volvulus by twisting the intestine in a counterclockwise direction. The bowel is inspected to ensure that it is viable. The cecum is placed in the left upper quadrant and the duodenum exposed along its entire length. The duodenum is inspected for any external sites of obstruction caused by bands of tissue between the duodenum and peritoneum. Any bands are lysed. Bands may also occur at the ileum or jejunum and these sometimes are attached to the gallbladder and liver. These bands are also lysed. An NG tube is then passed through the duodenum to ensure that there are no internal sites of obstruction. An incidental appendectomy is also performed prior to closing the abdomen due to the possibility of damage to the appendiceal vessels during band lysis.

44100

44100   Biopsy of intestine by capsule, tube, peroral (1 or more specimens)

The physician may obtain one or more specimens. Using fluoroscopic guidance, a capsule attached to a flexible tube is inserted into the mouth and the patient is instructed to swallow the capsule and tube. Once the capsule and tube has reached the stomach, the patient then drinks water and changes position as instructed until the capsule and tube have passed into the desired location in the jejunum. Alternatively, a flexible tube is passed through the mouth and into the stomach. It is then advanced through the pylorus and into the duodenum. The tube is manipulated to the duodenojejunal junction and into the first loop of jejunum where the first set of specimens is usually obtained, although the physician may advance the tube beyond this point if needed. The biopsy capsule is fired and biopsies are taken from the jejunum and the tube is withdrawn into the duodenum. Biopsies are then taken from the duodenum. The tube is completely withdrawn and the specimens are prepared and sent to the laboratory for separately reportable evaluation.

44110-44111

44110   Excision of 1 or more lesions of small or large intestine not requiring anastomosis, exteriorization, or fistulization; single enterotomy
44111   Excision of 1 or more lesions of small or large intestine not requiring anastomosis, exteriorization, or fistulization; multiple enterotomies

A midline incision is made in the abdomen and the diseased segment of small or large intestine exposed. The antimesenteric side of the intestine is incised and the mucosa inspected. The lesion is identified and excised along with a margin of healthy tissue and sent to the laboratory for separately reportable histological analysis. One or more lesions are removed. Lesion removal does not involve removal of an entire segment of bowel so anastomosis, exteriorization, or fistulization are not required. The intestinal incision is

Digestive System

closed in layers as is the abdominal incision. In 44110, a single enterotomy is performed with excision of one of more lesions. In 44111, multiple enterotomies are required and one or more lesions are removed from each enterotomy site.

44120-44121

44120   Enterectomy, resection of small intestine; single resection and anastomosis

44121   Enterectomy, resection of small intestine; each additional resection and anastomosis (List separately in addition to code for primary procedure)

The physician performs an enterectomy, also referred to as a resection of the small intestine, with anastomosis. The abdominal cavity is exposed through a midline incision. Adhesions are lysed using blunt and sharp dissection. The abdominal contents including the liver, gallbladder, and other organs are exposed and inspected. The diseased section of the small intestine is identified and dissected free of surrounding tissue. Blood vessels are clamped and suture ligated as needed. The small intestine is divided using staples or noncrushing clamps. The diseased section of intestine is removed and the residual proximal and distal small intestine segments are sutured together (anastomosed). There are a number of different anastomosis configurations that can be used including end-to-end, end-to-side, or side-to-side. Following repair of the intestine, the abdomen is closed in layers. Use 44120 to report a single resection and anastomosis and 44121 for each additional resection and anastomosis.

44125

44125   Enterectomy, resection of small intestine; with enterostomy

The physician performs an enterectomy, also referred to as a resection of the small intestine, with enterostomy. The abdominal cavity is exposed through a midline incision. Adhesions are lysed using blunt and sharp dissection. The abdominal contents including the liver, gallbladder, and other organs are exposed and inspected. The diseased section of the small intestine is identified and dissected free of surrounding tissue. Blood vessels are clamped and suture ligated as needed. The small intestine is divided using staples or noncrushing clamps. The diseased section of intestine is removed. The remaining distal segment of intestine is closed off and the proximal segment is prepared for exteriorization. A small incision is made over the planned enterostomy site and carried down through subcutaneous tissue. Fat is excised and the anterior rectus fascia is exposed and opened. The rectus muscle fibers are separated using blunt dissection. The peritoneum is entered. An opening of sufficient diameter is created for the stoma. The segment of small bowel to be exteriorized is brought through the peritoneum and abdominal wall and everted (turned back on itself) and then sutured to the skin.

44126-44128

44126   Enterectomy, resection of small intestine for congenital atresia, single resection and anastomosis of proximal segment of intestine; without tapering

44127   Enterectomy, resection of small intestine for congenital atresia, single resection and anastomosis of proximal segment of intestine; with tapering

44128   Enterectomy, resection of small intestine for congenital atresia, single resection and anastomosis of proximal segment of intestine; each additional resection and anastomosis (List separately in addition to code for primary procedure)

The physician performs an enterectomy, also referred to as a resection of the small intestine, for congenital atresia with anastomosis of the proximal segment of intestine. Congenital atresia is a condition in which the small intestine is completely obstructed resulting in dilation of the segment of intestine proximal to the site of obstruction. The stomach may also be dilated and the pylorus hypertrophied and distended. The abdominal cavity is exposed through a midline incision. The abdominal contents including the liver, gallbladder, and other organs are exposed and inspected. The dilated section of the small intestine is identified and dissected free of surrounding tissue. Blood vessels are clamped and suture ligated as needed. The small intestine is divided using staples or noncrushing clamps. The dilated section of intestine is removed. The residual proximal and distal small intestine segments are sutured together (anastomosed). Because the proximal segment of small intestine is usually dilated and the distal segment thin-walled and flattened, a diamond-shaped anastomosis may be created. This involves making a longitudinal incision in the distal, collapsed segment and a transverse incision in the inferior aspect of the dilated proximal segment. The two segments are then sutured together. In 44126, the residual proximal and distal small intestine segments are sutured together (anastomosed) without tapering the dilated proximal segment. In 44127, the dilated proximal segment is tapered by plicating (creating folds) on the lateral antimesenteric side. Use 44126 or 44127 for a single resection and anastomosis and 44128 for each additional small intestine segment requiring resection and anastomosis.

44130

44130   Enteroenterostomy, anastomosis of intestine, with or without cutaneous enterostomy (separate procedure)

The physician performs an enteroenterostomy with or without cutaneous enterostomy. This procedure is typically performed to reconnect a previously resected or bypassed segment

of small intestine. The abdominal cavity is exposed through a midline incision. Adhesions are lysed using blunt and sharp dissection. The abdominal contents including the liver, gallbladder, and other organs are exposed and inspected. The previously divided segments of the small intestine are identified and dissected free of surrounding tissue. Blood vessels are clamped and suture ligated as needed. The previously divided segments are incised at the planned anastomosis sites and the proximal and distal segments are sutured together (anastomosed). There are a number of different anastomosis configurations that can be used including end-to-end, end-to-side, or side-to-side. Following repair of the intestine, the abdomen may be closed in layers or a cutaneous enterostomy may be created prior to closure by making a small skin incision over the planned enterostomy site and carrying the incision down through subcutaneous tissue. Fat is excised and the anterior rectus fascia is exposed and opened. The rectus muscle fibers are separated using blunt dissection. The peritoneum is entered. An opening of sufficient diameter is created for the stoma. The segment of small bowel to be exteriorized is brought through the peritoneum and abdominal wall and everted (turned back on itself), then sutured to the skin.

44132-44133

44132   Donor enterectomy (including cold preservation), open; from cadaver donor

44133   Donor enterectomy (including cold preservation), open; partial, from living donor

An open donor enterectomy is performed including cold preservation from a cadaver donor (44132) or a living donor (44133). Intestinal transplantation is performed in patients with irreversible intestinal failure with life-threatening complications due to long-term total parenteral nutrition. In 44132, the abdomen of the cadaver donor is incised and the organs to be harvested are exposed. The donor organs are dissected from surrounding tissue. To procure the intestine, it is first dissected from the pancreas by separating the superior mesenteric artery and vein. The intestine is then removed, perfused with cold preservation solution and placed on ice. In 44133, the abdomen of the living donor is incised in the midline and the intestines are exposed. The small intestine is inspected and its length is measured from the ligament of Trietz to the ileocecal valve. The terminal ileum is identified and a marker is placed approximately 15-20 cm from the ileocecal valve to identify the proximal aspect of the segment to be harvested. The length of the small bowel segment to be harvested is determined based on the anatomic characteristics of the transplant recipient and donor's total intestinal length. The distal aspect of the transplant segment is then marked. The terminal branches of the superior mesenteric artery and vein are dissected from surrounding tissue and marked with vessel loops. The origin of the right colic artery is identified and marked with a vessel loop. Mesenteric tissue is dissected. Vascular arcades are ligated and divided. The segment of intestine is then transected and transferred to the recipient surgical suite. The living donor intestine is re-anastomosed.

44135-44136

44135   Intestinal allotransplantation; from cadaver donor

44136   Intestinal allotransplantation; from living donor

The physician performs intestinal allotransplantation with or without enterectomy. The abdominal cavity is entered and inspected. Any adhesions are lysed. The falciform ligament is taken down and the liver is inspected. The incision is then extended subcostally to the right. The gallbladder is exposed and resected as needed. The cecum is mobilized. The mesentery is dissected from the retroperitoneal structures. The inferior vena cava is identified and dissected to the level of the renal vein. The superior mesenteric and renal veins are dissected followed by dissection of the infrarenal aorta. Arterial and venous grafts are placed on the aorta and inferior vena cava respectively. The donor intestine is then brought into the operative field, anastomosed to the aortic and inferior vena cava grafts, and perfused. The recipient native jejunum is resected and the donor intestine is anastomosed proximally and distally. Bleeding is controlled. A gastrostomy tube is placed and the stomach is anchored to the abdominal wall. A jejunostomy tube is inserted. The donor intestine is exteriorized in the right lower quadrant in a chimney ileostomy. Drains are placed as needed and incisions are closed. The gastrostomy and jejunostomy tubes are secured with sutures. Use 44135 for intestine allotransplantation using a cadaver donor and 44136 when the intestine is harvested from a living donor.

44137

44137   Removal of transplanted intestinal allograft, complete

The physician performs complete removal of a transplanted intestinal allograft. Removal is performed for graft failure due to chronic rejection or for other complications such as thrombosis of major arteries. The abdominal cavity is exposed through a midline incision. Adhesions are lysed using blunt and sharp dissection. The intestine is retracted and the aorta is exposed. The aortic and venous grafts constructed at the time of the transplant are dissected and controlled with vessel loops, then clamped and transected. The anastomosis sites of the transplanted intestine are identified and the transplanted intestine is divided from native intestine and removed en bloc. The aortic and venous graft remnants are sutured closed. The distal stump of native bowel is oversewn. The proximal end of native intestine is exteriorized. A small incision is made over the planned enterostomy site and carried down through subcutaneous tissue. Fat is excised and the anterior rectus fascia is exposed and opened. The rectus muscle fibers are separated using blunt dissection.

Digestive System

The peritoneum is entered. An opening of sufficient diameter is created for the stoma. The segment of small bowel to be exteriorized is brought out through the peritoneum and abdominal wall and everted (turned back on itself), then sutured to the skin. A gastrostomy tube is inserted and anchored to the abdominal wall. Abdominal drains are placed and the surgical wound is closed.

44139

44139   Mobilization (take-down) of splenic flexure performed in conjunction with partial colectomy (List separately in addition to primary procedure)

A mobilization (take-down) of the splenic flexure is performed in conjunction with a separately reportable partial colectomy. The splenic flexure, also referred to as the left colic flexure, is the second bend in the large intestine at the junction of the transverse and descending colon. The splenic flexure has multiple attachments to surrounding tissue including the splenocolic ligament, the renocolic ligament (the region of fusion between the Toldt's retroperitoneal fascia and the mesentery of the left colon), and the omentum. Take-down is performed to allow a tension-free anastomosis between the splenic flexure and the remaining colon or a tension-free externalization of the remaining intestine. An inferior approach is used to access the splenic flexure. The sigmoid colon is retracted anteriorly and superiorly revealing the renocolic ligament. Retroperitoneal fascia overlying the left kidney is dissected free of the posterior mesentery of the left colon. When the upper pole of the left kidney is visible, the splenic flexure is approached and the splenocolic ligament is divided by electrocautery. The omentum is then dissected off the splenic flexure and away from the transverse colon as the splenic flexure is retracted inferiorly. All remaining attachments are divided. Following mobilization of the splenic flexure, the surgeon completes the separately reportable partial colectomy by anastomosis of the distal and proximal segments of colon or externalization of the intestine.

44140

44140   Colectomy, partial; with anastomosis

A segment of the colon (large intestine) is removed. This procedure may also be referred to as a right or left hemicolectomy. The procedure differs slightly depending on the location and length of the segment being removed. In a left colectomy, the proximal bowel is lifted out of the abdomen and held in place using a retractor. The attachments between the left gutter and the colon are incised and the colon is mobilized and moved to the center and down. The left ureter is identified and protected. The distal resection site is identified and prepared and the mesenteric peritoneum is divided. The retroperitoneal tissues are spread and the right ureter is identified and protected. The mesenteric vessels are then clamped, divided, and suture ligated and the mesentery is divided. The colon is divided using staples or noncrushing clamps. The diseased section of bowel is removed and the residual proximal and distal bowel segments are sutured or stapled together (anastomosed). In a right colectomy, the sigmoid colon is identified and the resection site is identified and marked. The left retroperitoneum is entered and the left ureter is identified and protected. The mesentery is incised. The retroperitoneum on the right is entered and the right ureter is identified and protected. The proximal colon is divided using staples or noncrushing clamps. Attention then turns to the segment of bowel to be removed. Vascular structures attached to the bowel segment are dissected. Vessels are clamped, divided, and suture ligated. The distal resection site is identified and the colon is divided. The diseased section of bowel is removed. The residual proximal and distal bowel segments are sutured together (anastomosed).

44141

44141   Colectomy, partial; with skin level cecostomy or colostomy

A segment of the colon (large intestine) is removed and a colostomy or skin level cecostomy is created. The segment of colon to be removed is mobilized by dividing the embryonic fusion planes and the peritoneum, taking care to preserve blood supply. The mesentery is divided. The colon is divided and the diseased or damaged segment is removed. Next, a colostomy or skin level cecostomy is created. A small incision is made in the skin over the planned colostomy or cecostomy site and carried down through subcutaneous space. Fat is excised down to the anterior rectus fascia. The fascia is opened, taking care to protect the underlying rectus muscle and its blood supply. The rectus fibers are separated by blunt dissection. The peritoneum is entered and an opening of sufficient diameter is created for the stoma. Ideally, the proximal segment of cecum or colon should be brought through a peritoneal tunnel to prevent postoperative obstruction of the stoma. The colon or cecum is brought through the abdominal wall and everted (folded back on itself). The segment of colon or cecum is then sutured to the skin.

44143

44143   Colectomy, partial; with end colostomy and closure of distal segment (Hartmann type procedure)

A segment of the colon (large intestine) is removed through a midline incision, the distal (end-segment) of bowel is closed and an end colostomy is created. End colostomies are created when the lower segment of bowel, the sigmoid colon, is used to create the colostomy. A Hartmann type procedure is used when the distal segment of bowel and the

rectum are not removed, but are sutured closed instead, creating a Hartmann pouch. The segment of colon to be removed is mobilized by dividing the embryonic fusion planes and the peritoneum, taking care to preserve blood supply. The mesentery is divided. The colon is divided and the diseased or damaged segment is removed. The distal segment of colon is sutured closed. Next, an end colostomy is created. A small incision is made in the skin over the planned colostomy site and carried down through subcutaneous space. Fat is excised down to the anterior rectus fascia. The fascia is opened taking care to protect the underlying rectus muscle and its blood supply. The rectus fibers are separated by blunt dissection. The peritoneum is entered and an opening of sufficient diameter is created for the stoma. Ideally, the colon should be brought through a peritoneal tunnel to prevent postoperative obstruction of the stoma. The colon is brought through the abdominal wall and everted (folded back on itself). The segment of colon is then sutured to the skin.

44144

44144   Colectomy, partial; with resection, with colostomy or ileostomy and creation of mucofistula

A segment of the colon (large intestine) is removed and two openings (stomas) are created. The first stoma is a colostomy or ileostomy connected to the functioning bowel that drains stool. The second stoma is a mucofistula connected to the rectum that drains mucous. This procedure is also referred to as a double-barrel colostomy. The segment of colon to be removed is mobilized by dividing the embryonic fusion planes and the peritoneum, taking care to preserve blood supply. The mesentery is divided. The colon is divided and the diseased or damaged segment is removed. Next, the colostomy or ileostomy is created. A small incision is made in the skin over the planned colostomy or ileostomy site and carried down through the subcutaneous space. Fat is excised down to the anterior rectus fascia. The fascia is opened, taking care to protect the underlying rectus muscle and its blood supply. The rectus fibers are separated by blunt dissection. The peritoneum is entered and an opening of sufficient diameter is created for the stoma. Ideally, the proximal segment of colon or ileum should be brought through a peritoneal tunnel to prevent postoperative obstruction of the stoma. The colon or cecum is brought through the abdominal wall and everted (folded back on itself). The segment of colon or ileum is then sutured to the skin. The site of the second stoma for the mucofistula is opened and prepared in the same fashion. The distal segment of colon attached to the rectum is used to create the mucofistula.

44145-44146

44145   Colectomy, partial; with coloproctostomy (low pelvic anastomosis)
44146   Colectomy, partial; with coloproctostomy (low pelvic anastomosis), with colostomy

A midline incision is made in the abdomen and the abdominal cavity is inspected. The superior rectal vessels are located, dissected from the sacral promontory, ligated, and divided. The rectum is mobilized from the proximal aspect to the mid to distal aspect as needed. The segment of colon to be resected is also mobilized. The colon is clamped above and below the planned transection sites, the colon is transected and the diseased segment removed. The remaining distal and proximal segments are sutured together (anastomosed). Use 44145 when the procedure is performed without a colostomy. Use 44146 when a colostomy is performed. The resection and anastomosis is performed as described above. A diverting colostomy is then created. An incision is made in the lower abdomen, usually on the right side. The colon is transected and the distal segment closed with sutures. The stoma site is prepared and the proximal segment brought through the abdominal wall, folded back on itself (everted), and sutured to the skin and subcutaneous tissue. A colostomy appliance is placed at the stoma site. Drains are placed and the abdominal incision is closed in layers.

44147

44147   Colectomy, partial; abdominal and transanal approach

A midline incision is made in the abdomen and the abdominal cavity is inspected. The segment of colon to be resected is identified and mobilized. The superior rectal vessels are located, dissected from the sacral promontory, ligated, and divided. The ureters are identified and protected and the peritoneum incised. The presacral space is entered and dissection is carried down to the pelvic floor. An elliptical incision is made around the anus and the rectum is freed from surrounding tissue. The colon is clamped above and below the planned transection sites, the colon is transected and the diseased segment removed. The anal incision is closed. The remaining distal and proximal segments of bowel are sutured together (anastomosed). Drains are placed and the abdominal incision is closed in layers.

44150-44151

44150   Colectomy, total, abdominal, without proctectomy; with ileostomy or ileoproctostomy
44151   Colectomy, total, abdominal, without proctectomy; with continent ileostomy

A midline abdominal incision is made and the abdominal cavity is inspected. The entire colon is mobilized beginning with division of the lateral peritoneal attachments and separation of the omentum from the transverse colon. The mesentery of the colon is divided

Digestive System

beginning at the left colon and continuing proximally. The bowel is divided distally at the rectosigmoid junction and proximally just above the ileocecal valve. The diseased colon is removed. In 44150, an ileostomy is created or a low pelvic anastomosis (ileoproctostomy) is performed. If an ileostomy is performed, the distal transection site at the rectosigmoid junction is closed with sutures. The terminal ileum is brought through a separate incision, usually in the right lower quadrant. The exteriorized segment of ileum is folded back on itself (everted), and sutured to the skin and subcutaneous tissue. If an ileoproctostomy is performed, the terminal ileum is sutured to the rectum in an end-to-end fashion. In 44151, a continent ileostomy is created to allow collection of stool in a surgically created internal pouch. A 45-60 cm segment of ileum is mobilized. This segment of ileum is folded back on itself, opened and the sutured back together to create a reservoir or pouch (S or J) leaving a distal segment of approximately 15 to create the ileal valve. Electrocautery is used to scarify the segment of ileum immediately distal to the reservoir. Adjacent mesentery is excised. The scarified segment of ileum is pushed (telescoped) into the reservoir to create an ileal valve. The telescoped portion is secured to the pouch with staples or sutures. The pouch is then sutured closed. The distal-most end of ileum is brought through the abdominal wall at the prepared stoma site and sutured flush with the skin. The ileal pouch is sutured to the abdominal wall. A large diameter plastic tube is placed in the stoma. The tube remains in place for several weeks and is occluded for increasingly longer periods of time to expand the pouch. When the patient can tolerate occlusion for up to 8 hours, the tube is removed. The patient then intubates the pouch through the ileal stoma several times a day to drain of fecal matter from the reservoir.

44155-44156

44155   Colectomy, total, abdominal, with proctectomy; with ileostomy
44156   Colectomy, total, abdominal, with proctectomy; with continent ileostomy

A midline abdominal incision is made and the abdominal cavity is inspected. The entire colon is mobilized beginning with division of the lateral peritoneal attachments and separation of the omentum from the transverse colon. The mesentery of the colon is divided beginning at the left colon and continuing proximally. The bowel is divided in the ileum just proximal to the ileocecal valve. Attention then turns to the rectum. The superior rectal vessels are located, dissected from the sacral promontory, ligated, and divided. The ureters are identified and protected and the peritoneum incised. The presacral space is entered and dissection is carried down to the pelvic floor. An elliptical incision is made around the anus and the rectum is freed from surrounding tissue. The entire colon and rectum are removed. The perineal incision is closed in layers. In 44155, an ileostomy is created. An incision is made in the lower abdomen, usually in the right lower quadrant. The terminal end of ileum is brought through the abdominal wall, folded back on itself (everted), and sutured to the skin and subcutaneous tissue. In 44156, a continent ileostomy is created to allow collection of stool in a surgically created internal pouch. A 45-60 cm segment of ileum is mobilized. This segment of ileum is folded back on itself, opened and the sutured back together to create a reservoir or pouch (S or J) leaving a distal segment of approximately 15 to create the ileal valve. Electrocautery is used to scarify the remaining 15 cm segment of ileum immediately distal to the reservoir. Adjacent mesentery is excised. The scarified segment of ileum is pushed (telescoped) into the reservoir to create an ileal valve, which is secured to the pouch with staples or sutures. The pouch is then sutured closed. The distal-most end of ileum is brought through the abdominal wall at the prepared stoma site and sutured flush with the skin. The ileal pouch is sutured to the abdominal wall. A large diameter plastic tube is placed in the stoma and remains in place for several weeks. The tube is occluded for increasingly longer periods of time to expand the pouch. When the patient can tolerate occlusion for up to 8 hours, the tube is removed. The patient then intubates the pouch through the ileal stoma several times a day to drain of fecal matter from the reservoir.

44157

44157   Colectomy, total, abdominal, with proctectomy; with ileoanal anastomosis, includes loop ileostomy, and rectal mucosectomy, when performed

The physician performs a total colectomy, abdominal, with proctectomy; with ileoanal anastomosis, including a loop ileostomy and rectal mucosectomy, when performed. Through an abdominal incision, the entire colon and rectum are mobilized. The colon between the terminal portion of the ileum and the distal rectum is divided and removed. The remaining portion of the distal rectum may have the mucosa stripped. The end of the terminal ileum is then brought out through the remaining cuff of the distal rectum and anastomosed to the anus with sutures. Another loop of the ileum above the newly created ileoanal anastomosis may be brought out through an opening made in the abdominal wall and sutured onto the skin for an artificial opening through which the ileum can empty while the anal anastomosis heals.

44158

44158   Colectomy, total, abdominal, with proctectomy; with ileoanal anastomosis, creation of ileal reservoir (S or J), includes loop ileostomy, and rectal mucosectomy, when performed

The physician performs a total colectomy, abdominal, with proctectomy; with ileoanal anastomosis, creation of ileal reservoir (S or J), including a loop ileostomy and rectal

mucosectomy, when performed. Through an abdominal incision, the entire colon and rectum are mobilized. The colon between the terminal portion of the ileum and the distal rectum is divided and removed. The remaining portion of the distal rectum may have the mucosal lining stripped, but the muscle is left intact. A portion of the terminal ileum is then folded on itself and formed into a pouch or ileal reservoir, which is then brought out through the remaining cuff of muscle in the distal rectum and anastomosed to the anus with sutures. This pouch of small intestine will provide a storage place for stool in the absence of the large intestine and the rectal muscles will allow for holding and passing stool normally. Another loop of the ileum above the newly created ileoanal anastomosis may be brought out through an opening made in the abdominal wall and sutured onto the skin for an artificial opening through which the ileum can empty temporarily while the anal anastomosis heals.

44160

44160   Colectomy, partial, with removal of terminal ileum with ileocolostomy

A midline abdominal incision is made and the abdominal cavity is inspected. The diseased segment of colon is mobilized along with a portion of the terminal ileum. The colon and terminal ileum are clamped above and below the planned transection sites, the diseased segment colon and terminal ileum is divided and removed. An ileocolostomy is then performed. The remaining segment of terminal ileum is sutured to the remaining segment of colon in an end-to-end fashion. Drains are placed and abdominal incisions are closed.

44180

44180   Laparoscopy, surgical, enterolysis (freeing of intestinal adhesion) (separate procedure)

Enterolysis refers to the severing of intestinal adhesions which is performed when adhesions cause the bowel to stick together and twist or kink causing bowel obstruction. A small portal incision is made near the umbilicus, a trocar inserted, and pneumoperitoneum established. Additional portal incisions are made and trocars placed in the upper and lower quadrants of the abdomen. The abdominal cavity is inspected. Intestinal adhesions are lysed using blunt and sharp dissection. Once all adhesions have been released, the laparoscope and trocars are removed, and the portal incisions closed.

44186-44187

44186   Laparoscopy, surgical; jejunostomy (eg, for decompression or feeding)
44187   Laparoscopy, surgical; ileostomy or jejunostomy, non-tube

A small portal incision is made near the umbilicus, a trocar inserted, and pneumoperitoneum established. Additional portal incisions are made and trocars placed in the upper and lower quadrants of the abdomen. The abdominal cavity is inspected. Any adhesions are lysed using blunt and sharp dissection. In 44186, a jejunostomy tube is placed for decompression or feeding. A small incision is made through the skin and upper abdominal wall on the left side. Using a push technique, a guidewire is inserted through the incision and using laparoscopic guidance it is advanced into the jejunum. A tube for feeding or decompression is then advanced over the guidewire and into the jejunum. The guidewire is removed. The tube is secured internally with a bumper or balloon and externally with a bumper, flange, or other device. In 44187, a non-tube ileostomy or jejunostomy is performed. The segment of ileum or jejunum to be exteriorized is identified and mobilized. A trocar is placed in the planned stoma site. The jejunum or ileum is clamped above and below the planned transection site. The stoma site is prepared around the previously placed trocar. Gas is released from the abdomen and the jejunum or ileum exteriorized through the stoma incision. The jejunum or ileum is transected. The distal segment is closed with sutures, the clamp removed, and the distal segment returned to the abdomen. The proximal clamp is removed. The proximal segment of jejunum or ileum is folded back on itself (everted) and sutured to the skin and subcutaneous tissue. Pneumoperitoneum is reestablished. The abdomen and the segment of exteriorized intestine are inspected to ensure that there is no tension on the stoma. The laparoscope and trocars are removed, and the portal incisions closed. A stoma appliance is placed.

44188

44188   Laparoscopy, surgical, colostomy or skin level cecostomy

A small portal incision is made near the umbilicus, a trocar inserted, and pneumoperitoneum established. Additional portal incisions are made and trocars placed in the upper and lower quadrants of the abdomen. The abdominal cavity is inspected. Any adhesions are lysed using blunt and sharp dissection. The segment of colon or cecum to be exteriorized is identified and mobilized. A trocar is placed in the planned stoma site. The colon or cecum is clamped above and below the planned transection site. The stoma site is prepared around the previously placed trocar. Gas is released from the abdomen and the colon or cecum exteriorized through the stoma incision. The colon or cecum is transected. The distal segment is closed with sutures, the clamp removed, and the distal segment returned to the abdomen. The proximal clamp is removed. The proximal segment of colon or cecum is folded back on itself (everted) and sutured to the skin and subcutaneous tissue. Pneumoperitoneum is reestablished. The abdomen and the segment of exteriorized

Digestive System

bowel are inspected to ensure that there is no tension on the stoma. The laparoscope and trocars are removed, and the portal incisions closed. A stoma appliance is placed.

44202-44203

44202 Laparoscopy, surgical; enterectomy, resection of small intestine, single resection and anastomosis

44203 Laparoscopy, surgical; each additional small intestine resection and anastomosis (List separately in addition to code for primary procedure)

A small portal incision is made near the umbilicus, a trocar inserted, and pneumoperitoneum established. Additional portal incisions are made and trocars placed in the upper and lower quadrants of the abdomen. The abdominal cavity is inspected. The segment of small intestine to be resected is identified and mobilized to allow for exteriorization of the bowel. The distal resection site in the small intestine is identified and the intestine clamped and divided. The incision at one of the abdominal trocar sites is enlarged. The proximal segment of small intestine is brought though the incision in the abdominal wall and the small intestine exteriorized to a point beyond the proximal resection site. The proximal resection site is identified and resected using clips and harmonic scalpel. The remaining segment of exteriorized small intestine is returned to the abdomen and the exteriorization incision closed. The distal and proximal segments of small intestine are sutured or stapled together (anastomosed). The small bowel is clamped above and below the segment to be removed. The proximal and distal resection sites are identified and the small intestine is divided at these sites. The proximal and distal segments are sutured together (anastomosed) with sutures or staples and the clamps released. Use 44202 for a single resection and anastomosis and 44203 for each additional segment that is resected and anastomosed.

44204-44205

44204 Laparoscopy, surgical; colectomy, partial, with anastomosis

44205 Laparoscopy, surgical; colectomy, partial, with removal of terminal ileum with ileocolostomy

A small portal incision is made near the umbilicus, a trocar inserted, and pneumoperitoneum established. Additional portal incisions are made and trocars placed in the upper and lower quadrants of the abdomen. The abdominal cavity is inspected. In 44204, the segment of colon to be resected is mobilized to allow for exteriorization of the bowel. The distal resection site in the colon is identified and the colon is divided. The incision at one of the lower abdominal trocar sites is enlarged. The proximal segment of colon is brought though the incision in the abdominal wall and the bowel exteriorized to a point beyond the proximal resection site. The proximal resection site is identified and resected using clips and harmonic scalpel. The remaining segment of exteriorized bowel is returned to the abdomen and the exteriorization incision closed. The distal and proximal segments of colon are sutured or stapled together (anastomosed). In 44205, the segment of colon to be resected is mobilized along with the terminal ileum to allow for exteriorization of the bowel. The distal resection site in the colon is identified and the colon is divided. The incision at one of the lower abdominal trocar sites is enlarged. The proximal segment of colon is brought though the incision in the abdominal wall and the bowel exteriorized to a point beyond the proximal resection site. The proximal resection site in the ileum is identified and resected using clips and harmonic scalpel. The exteriorized bowel is returned to the abdomen and the exteriorization incision closed. The distal segment of colon and the proximal segment of ileum are sutured or stapled together (anastomosed).

44206

44206 Laparoscopy, surgical; colectomy, partial, with end colostomy and closure of distal segment (Hartmann type procedure)

A small portal incision is made near the umbilicus, a trocar inserted, and pneumoperitoneum established. Additional portal incisions are made and trocars placed in the upper and lower quadrants of the abdomen. The abdominal cavity is inspected. The segment of bowel to be resected is identified and mobilized. The distal resection is performed with a linear cutter and the distal segment of bowel is closed with sutures. The incision at one of the lower abdominal trocar sites is enlarged. The proximal segment of colon is brought though the incision in the abdominal wall and the bowel exteriorized to a point beyond the proximal resection site. The proximal resection site is identified and resected using clips and harmonic scalpel. The stoma site is prepared and the remaining proximal segment of colon folded back on itself (everted), and sutured to the skin and subcutaneous tissue. Trocars are removed and portal incisions closed. A colostomy appliance is placed at the stoma site.

44207-44208

44207 Laparoscopy, surgical; colectomy, partial, with anastomosis, with coloproctostomy (low pelvic anastomosis)

44208 Laparoscopy, surgical; colectomy, partial, with anastomosis, with coloproctostomy (low pelvic anastomosis) with colostomy

A small portal incision is made near the umbilicus, a trocar inserted, and pneumoperitoneum established. Additional portal incisions are made and trocars placed in the upper and lower quadrants of the abdomen. The abdominal cavity is inspected. The

superior rectal vessels are located, dissected from the sacral promontory, ligated, and divided. The rectum is mobilized from the proximal aspect to the mid to distal aspect. The distal resection is performed with an endoscopic linear stapler/cutter. The mesorectum is divided. The segment of colon to be resected is mobilized to allow for exteriorization of the bowel. The incision at one of the lower abdominal trocar site is enlarged. In 44207, the divided end of the rectosigmoid colon is brought though the incision in the abdominal wall and the bowel exteriorized to a point beyond the proximal resection site. The proximal resection site is identified and resected using clips and harmonic scalpel. After placing a pursestring suture and anvil around the end of the remaining portion of bowel, the exteriorized bowel is returned to the abdomen and the exteriorization incision closed. A stapler is passed through the anus and the spike advanced out through the rectal stump. The stapler and anvil are mated and the stapler fired to create an end-to-end anastomosis of the rectal stump and colon. In 44208, the resection and anastomosis is performed as described above. A diverting colostomy is then created. An incision is made in the lower abdomen, usually the on the right side. The stoma site is prepared and a loop of colon brought through the abdominal wall, folded back on itself (everted), and sutured to the skin and subcutaneous tissue. Trocars are removed and portal incisions closed. A colostomy appliance is placed at the stoma site.

44210

44210 Laparoscopy, surgical; colectomy, total, abdominal, without proctectomy, with ileostomy or ileoproctostomy

A small portal incision is made near the umbilicus, a trocar inserted, and pneumoperitoneum established. Additional portal incisions are made and trocars placed in the upper and lower quadrants of the abdomen. The abdominal cavity is inspected. The entire colon is mobilized beginning with division of the lateral peritoneal attachments and separation of the omentum from the transverse colon. The mesentery of the colon is divided beginning at the left colon and continuing proximally. The bowel is divided distally at the rectosigmoid junction. The incision at one of the lower abdominal trocar sites is enlarged. The divided end of the rectosigmoid colon is brought though the incision in the abdominal wall and the bowel exteriorized to a point proximal to the ileocecal valve. The terminal ileum is divided and the entire colon removed. If an ileoproctostomy is to be created, a pursestring suture and anvil are placed around the end of the terminal ileum. The exteriorized bowel is returned to the abdomen and the exteriorization incision closed. A stapler is passed through the anus and the spike advanced out through the rectum. The stapler and anvil are mated and the stapler fired to create and end-to-end anastomosis of the rectum and colon. Alternatively, an ileostomy may be performed. The distal transection site in the rectum is closed with sutures. The exteriorized segment of ileum is folded back on itself (everted), and sutured to the skin and subcutaneous tissue. Trocars are removed and portal incisions closed. An ileostomy appliance is placed at the stoma site.

44211

44211 Laparoscopy, surgical; colectomy, total, abdominal, with proctectomy, with ileoanal anastomosis, creation of ileal reservoir (S or J), with loop ileostomy, includes rectal mucosectomy, when performed

The physician does a laparoscopic total abdominal colectomy with proctectomy and ileoanal anastomosis, creation of ileal reservoir (S or J), with a loop ileostomy, and including rectal mucosectomy, when performed. Carbon dioxide gas is used to insufflate the abdomen through the umbilicus. Through small abdominal incisions, the laparoscopic instruments are then inserted into the abdominal cavity in the right and left midquadrant and suprapubic area. The entire colon and rectum are mobilized. The colon between the terminal portion of the ileum and the distal rectum is divided and removed. The remaining portion of the distal rectum may have the mucosal lining stripped, but the muscle is left intact. A portion of the terminal ileum is then folded on itself and formed into a pouch or ileal reservoir, which is then brought out through the remaining cuff of muscle in the distal rectum and anastomosed to the anus with sutures. This pouch of small intestine will provide a storage place for stool in the absence of the large intestine and the rectal muscles will allow for holding and passing stool normally. Another loop of the ileum above the newly created ileoanal anastomosis may be brought out through an opening made in the abdominal wall and sutured onto the skin for an artificial opening through which the ileum can empty temporarily while the anal anastomosis heals.

44212

44212 Laparoscopy, surgical; colectomy, total, abdominal, with proctectomy, with ileostomy

The physician performs a laparoscopic total abdominal colectomy with proctectomy with ileostomy. A small portal incision is made near the umbilicus, a trocar inserted, and pneumoperitoneum established. Additional portal incisions are made and trocars placed in the upper and lower quadrants of the abdomen. The abdominal cavity is inspected. The entire colon is mobilized beginning with division of the lateral peritoneal attachments and separation of the omentum from the transverse colon. The mesentery of the colon is divided beginning at the left colon and continuing proximally. The bowel is divided in the ileum just proximal to the ileocecal valve.¬† Attention then turns to the rectum. The superior rectal vessels are located, dissected from the sacral promontory, ligated, and divided. The

● New Code   ▲ Revised Code

Digestive System

ureters are identified and protected and the peritoneum incised and air released from the abdominal cavity. The presacral space is entered and dissection is carried down to the pelvic floor. An elliptical incision is made around the anus and the rectum is freed from surrounding tissue. The entire colon and rectum are removed through the perineal incision which is then closed in layers. Pneumoperitoneum is reestablished. An ileostomy is then performed. An incision is made in the lower abdomen, usually in the right lower quadrant. The stoma site is prepared and the terminal end of ileum brought through the abdominal wall, folded back on itself (everted), and sutured to the skin and subcutaneous tissue. Trocars are removed and portal incisions closed. An ileostomy appliance is placed at the stoma site.

44213

44213 **Laparoscopy, surgical, mobilization (take-down) of splenic flexure performed in conjunction with partial colectomy (List separately in addition to primary procedure)**

Laparoscopic mobilization (take-down) of the splenic flexure is performed in conjunction with a separately reportable partial colectomy procedure. Take-down is performed to allow exteriorization of the segment of colon to be resected and tension-free anastomosis of the remaining segments of colon. The inferior mesenteric vein is divided and the mesentery of the left colon is dissected free of Gerota's fascia. A hole is made in the mesentery of the transverse colon to allow gas to enter and distend the lesser sac for better visualization. The mesentery of the splenic flexure is then detached from the pancreas. The colon is detached from the omentum and the left abdominal gutter to complete the mobilization.

44227

44227 **Laparoscopy, surgical, closure of enterostomy, large or small intestine, with resection and anastomosis**

Laparoscopic closure of an enterostomy of the small or large intestine is performed with resection and anastomosis. A small portal incision is made near the umbilicus, a trocar inserted, and pneumoperitoneum established. The laparoscope is inserted. Additional trocars are placed in the upper and lower abdomen. The abdominal viscera are inspected. Adhesions are lysed. The distal intestinal or rectal stump is identified and mobilized. The stoma is dissected from the abdominal wall and the proximal segment of intestine mobilized. The intestine is freed from the skin at the stoma site which releases gas from the abdomen. During the temporary loss of pneumoperitoneum, the enterostomy is resected and anvil of a circular stapler is placed in the proximal segment of intestine and secured with a purse-string suture. The exteriorized intestinal segment is returned to the abdomen and pneumoperitoneum is re-established. The proximal and distal segments of intestine are sutured together (anastomosed) using the stapler device. Bleeding is controlled and the trocars removed. The small portal incisions are then closed in a layered fashion.

44300

44300 **Placement, enterostomy or cecostomy, tube open (eg, for feeding or decompression) (separate procedure)**

Open placement of a tube into the small intestine for feeding or into the large intestine for decompression is performed. For placement of a feeding tube, an incision is made in the abdomen. A loop of small intestine, usually jejunum, is exposed. Two concentric purse-string sutures are placed into the seromuscular layer. An incision is made in the bowel at the center of the previously placed purse-string sutures. A catheter is inserted and threaded distally several centimeters. The sutures are secured around the catheter and the catheter is brought to the abdominal wall at a site separate from the initial incision site. A stab incision is made. The catheter (feeding tube) is advanced through the stab incision and secured with sutures. For placement of a cecostomy tube for decompression, the cecum is exposed and incised. A catheter is threaded into the cecum and secured with sutures. A separate stab incision is made through the abdominal wall and the catheter is advanced through the stab incision and secured with sutures.

44310

44310 **Ileostomy or jejunostomy, non-tube**

A jejunostomy or ileostomy is made without tube insertion. An incision is made in the abdomen at the intended stoma site. A loop of jejunum or ileum is brought to the incision site. The loop may be passed through an intraperitoneal tunnel to the abdominal wall or taken directly to the anterior abdominal wall. The loop of jejunum or ileum is then divided and a 5-6 cm segment is brought out through the abdominal wall. The distal 2-3 cm are folded back over the exposed segment of small bowel and sutured to the abdominal wall to create an artificial opening.

44312-44314

44312 **Revision of ileostomy; simple (release of superficial scar) (separate procedure)**

44314 **Revision of ileostomy; complicated (reconstruction in-depth) (separate procedure)**

Revision may be necessary if the stoma becomes constricted or obstructed, the intestine prolapses through the stoma, the intestine retracts causing the stoma to sink below the level of the skin, the intestine detaches from the skin, or necrosis occurs. In 44312, a simple revision is performed such as release of a superficial scar. A skin incision is made around the entire circumference of the ileostomy. Local release of scar tissue (adhesions) around the stoma may be performed. Alternatively, dissection may continue down through fascia and peritoneum and the distal tip of the ileum may be resected. Resection is performed by elevating the ileum above the abdominal wall for a length of 3-5 cm. Retention sutures are placed in the fascia and the distal tip resected. The ileum is everted and sutured to skin and subcutaneous tissue. In 44314, a complicated revision is performed which may involve excision of necrotic bowel and reconstruction of the stoma or relocation the stoma. The abdomen is opened in the midline and the abdomen explored. Adhesions are lysed and the exteriorized segment mobilized. If necrotic ileum is present, an incision is made around the stoma and the incision is carried down through fascia and peritoneum. The necrotic segment of ileum is excised. The terminal end of the remaining segment of ileum is brought through the abdominal wall, folded back on itself (everted), and sutured to the skin and subcutaneous tissue. If the ileostomy requires relocation, it is taken down in the same manner as described above. The abdomen is incised at the new stoma site. The stoma site is prepared and the stoma fashioned as described above. The abdomen is closed and an ileostomy appliance is placed at the stoma site.

44316

44316 **Continent ileostomy (Kock procedure) (separate procedure)**

A continent ileostomy, also referred to as a Kock procedure, is performed as a separate procedure on a patient who has had a previously performed coloproctectomy. A continent ileostomy allows collection of stool in a surgically created internal pouch which means that the patient does not have to use external stoma bags or devices to collect fecal matter. A midline incision is made in the abdomen and the ileum exposed. A 45-60 cm segment of ileum is mobilized. This segment of ileum is folded back on itself, opened and the sutured back together to create a reservoir or pouch (S or J) leaving a distal segment of approximately 15 to create the ileal valve. Electrocautery is used to scarify the 15 cm segment of ileum immediately distal to the reservoir. Adjacent mesentery is excised. The scarified segment of ileum is pushed into the reservoir, which is referred to as telescoping or intussusception of the bowel, to create an ileal valve. The telescoped portion is secured to the pouch with staples or sutures. The pouch is then sutured closed. A separate incision is made, usually in the right lower quadrant, and the distal-most end of ileum is brought through the abdominal wall and sutured flush with the skin. The ileal pouch is sutured to the abdominal wall. A large diameter plastic tube is placed in the stoma. The tube will remain in place for several weeks and will be occluded for increasingly longer periods of time to expand the pouch. When the patient can tolerate occlusion for up to 8 hours, the tube is removed. The patient will then intubate the pouch through the ileal stoma several times a day to allow drainage of fecal matter from the reservoir.

44320-44322

44320 **Colostomy or skin level cecostomy**

44322 **Colostomy or skin level cecostomy; with multiple biopsies (eg, for congenital megacolon) (separate procedure)**

A midline abdominal incision is made and the peritoneum entered. The abdomen is carefully explored. Any adhesions are lysed using blunt and sharp dissection. The segment of colon or cecum to be exteriorized is identified and mobilized. A separate incision is made in the lower abdomen, usually on the right side and a stoma site prepared. The colon or cecum is clamped above and below the planned transection site. The colon or cecum is transected and the distal segment closed with sutures and the distal clamp removed. The proximal segment of the colon or cecum is exteriorized, the clamp removed, the colon or cecum folded back on itself (everted) and sutured to the skin and subcutaneous tissue. The abdominal incision is closed and a stomal appliance is placed. Use 44320 when the procedure is performed without multiple biopsies and 44322 when multiple biopsies of the intestinal mucosa are obtained for a condition such as congenital megacolon. Following transection of the intestine, multiple biopsies are obtained and sent to the laboratory for separately reportable pathological evaluation.

Digestive System

44340-44346

44340 Revision of colostomy; simple (release of superficial scar) (separate procedure)

44345 Revision of colostomy; complicated (reconstruction in-depth) (separate procedure)

44346 Revision of colostomy; with repair of paracolostomy hernia (separate procedure)

Revision may be necessary if the stoma becomes constricted or obstructed, the intestine prolapses through the stoma, the intestine retracts causing the stoma to sink below the level of the skin, the intestine detaches from the skin, necrosis occurs or the patient develops a parastomal hernia. In 44340, a simple revision is performed such as release of a superficial scar. A skin incision is made around the entire circumference of the colostomy. Local release of scar tissue (adhesions) around the stoma may be performed. Alternatively, dissection may continue down through fascia and peritoneum and the distal tip of the colon may be resected. Resection is performed by elevating the colon above the abdominal wall for a length of 3-5 cm. Retention sutures are placed in the fascia and the distal tip resected. The colon is everted and sutured to skin and subcutaneous tissue. In 44345, a complicated revision is performed which may involve excision of necrotic bowel and reconstruction of the stoma or relocating the stoma. The abdomen is opened in the midline and the abdomen inspected. Adhesions are lysed and the exteriorized segment of bowel mobilized. If necrotic bowel is present, an incision is made around the stoma and the incision is carried down through fascia and peritoneum. The necrotic segment of bowel is excised. The terminal end of the remaining segment of bowel is brought through the abdominal wall, folded back on itself (everted), and sutured to the skin and subcutaneous tissue. If the colostomy requires relocation, it is taken down in the same manner as described above. The abdomen is incised at the new stoma site. The new stoma site is fashioned as described above. In 44346, a paracolostomy hernia is repaired. An incision is made over the hernia and the hernia is reduced. Overlying fascia is then repaired with sutures or fascial repair with a mesh implant is performed.

44360-44361

44360 Small intestinal endoscopy, enteroscopy beyond second portion of duodenum, not including ileum; diagnostic, including collection of specimen(s) by brushing or washing, when performed (separate procedure)

44361 Small intestinal endoscopy, enteroscopy beyond second portion of duodenum, not including ileum; with biopsy, single or multiple

An endoscopic examination is performed on the small intestine beyond the second portion of the duodenum and may include collection of specimens by brushing or washing (44360) or single or multiple biopsies (44361). The duodenum is divided into four portions: the duodenal bulb or cap, the descending portion, the transverse portion, and the ascending portion. The mouth and throat are numbed using an anesthetic spray. A hollow mouthpiece is placed in the mouth. The flexible fiberoptic endoscope is then inserted and advanced as it is swallowed by the patient. Once the endoscope has been advanced beyond the cricopharyngeal region, it is guided using direct visualization into the duodenum. The mucosal surfaces are inspected to a point beyond the second portion of the duodenum and any abnormalities are noted. The examination may include the entire jejunum as well but does not include the ileum. The scope is then withdrawn and the entire circumference of the duodenum and jejunum are inspected again. In 44360, cell samples may be obtained by brushing or washing saline fluid into the small intestine and then collecting it. In 44361, the site(s) to be biopsied is identified and biopsy forceps are placed through the biopsy channel of the endoscope. The forceps are opened, the tissue is spiked, and the forceps are closed. The biopsied tissue is removed through the endoscope. One or more tissue samples may be obtained. The cell or tissue samples are sent for separately reportable laboratory analysis.

44363

44363 Small intestinal endoscopy, enteroscopy beyond second portion of duodenum, not including ileum; with removal of foreign body(s)

An endoscopic examination is performed on the small intestine beyond the second portion of the duodenum with removal of foreign body(s). The duodenum is divided into four portions: the duodenal bulb or cap, the descending portion, the transverse portion, and the ascending portion. The mouth and throat are numbed using an anesthetic spray. A hollow mouthpiece is placed in the mouth. The flexible fiberoptic endoscope is then inserted and advanced as it is swallowed by the patient. Once the endoscope has been advanced beyond the cricopharyngeal region, it is guided using direct visualization into the duodenum and advanced to the foreign body. The foreign body may lie within the duodenum or the jejunum. A balloon catheter may be used to remove a smooth edged foreign body, such as a coin. The catheter tip is passed beyond the level of the foreign body and the balloon is inflated. The catheter is then withdrawn and the foreign body is carefully pulled out. An impacted foreign body such as a piece of meat is removed with forceps. The forceps are passed through the endoscope and the impacted foreign body is grasped and removed. A sharp foreign body such as a tack or razor blade is first maneuvered into the lumen of the scope using forceps and then the foreign body and scope are removed. Following removal of the foreign body(s), the endoscope is reintroduced and the small

intestine is examined to a point beyond the second portion of the duodenum for evidence of perforation or other injury.

44364-44365

44364 Small intestinal endoscopy, enteroscopy beyond second portion of duodenum, not including ileum; with removal of tumor(s), polyp(s), or other lesion(s) by snare technique

44365 Small intestinal endoscopy, enteroscopy beyond second portion of duodenum, not including ileum; with removal of tumor(s), polyp(s), or other lesion(s) by hot biopsy forceps or bipolar cautery

An endoscopic examination is performed on the small intestine beyond the second portion of the duodenum with removal of tumors, polys, or other lesions by snare technique (44364) or by hot biopsy forceps or biopsy cautery (44365). The duodenum is divided into four portions: the duodenal bulb or cap, the descending portion, the transverse portion, and the ascending portion. The mouth and throat are numbed using an anesthetic spray. A hollow mouthpiece is placed in the mouth. The flexible fiberoptic endoscope is then inserted and advanced as it is swallowed by the patient. Once the endoscope has been advanced beyond the cricopharyngeal region, it is guided using direct visualization into the duodenum. The mucosal surfaces are inspected to a point beyond the second portion of the duodenum and any abnormalities are noted. The examination may include the entire jejunum as well, but not the ileum. The scope is then withdrawn and the entire circumference of the duodenum and jejunum are inspected again. In 44364, a wire snare loop is placed around the lesion. The loop is heated to shave off and cauterize the lesion. Lesions may be removed in total with one placement of the snare or in a piecemeal fashion, which requires multiple applications of the snare. In 44365, hot biopsy forceps or bipolar cautery is used to remove the lesion. Hot biopsy forceps use insulated monopolar forceps to remove and electrocoagulate (cauterize) tissue simultaneously. Bipolar cautery also uses electrical current to remove and cauterize the lesion; however, in this case the current runs from one part of the tip of the forceps to another portion of the forceps. Both hot biopsy forceps and bipolar cautery are used primarily for removal of small polyps and treatment of vascular ectasias.

44366

44366 Small intestinal endoscopy, enteroscopy beyond second portion of duodenum, not including ileum; with control of bleeding (eg, injection, bipolar cautery, unipolar cautery, laser, heater probe, stapler, plasma coagulator)

An endoscopic examination is performed on the small intestine beyond the second portion of the duodenum with control of bleeding. The duodenum is divided into four portions: the duodenal bulb or cap, the descending portion, the transverse portion, and the ascending portion. The mouth and throat are numbed using an anesthetic spray. A hollow mouthpiece is placed in the mouth. The flexible fiberoptic endoscope is then inserted and advanced as it is swallowed by the patient. Once the endoscope has been advanced beyond the cricopharyngeal region, it is guided using direct visualization into the duodenum. The mucosal surfaces are inspected to a point beyond the second portion of the duodenum and any abnormalities are noted. The examination may include the entire jejunum as well, but not the ileum. The scope is then withdrawn and the entire circumference of the duodenum and jejunum are inspected again. The bleeding site is identified. Bleeding is typically controlled using a contact thermal modality, such as bipolar or unipolar cautery or a heater probe. The cautery device or heater probe is applied to the bleeding point and pressure is applied along with heat to control bleeding. An injection of epinephrine, which works as a vasoconstrictor and tamponade, can also be used to reduce or stop bleeding. YAG laser coagulation and a newer modality, the argon plasma coagulator, are noncontact devices used to coagulate the bleeding site. Staples or hemoclips may be used to approximate the margins of a tear or laceration.

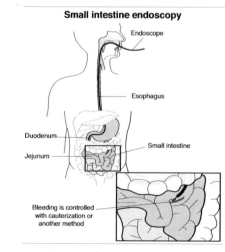

Small intestine endoscopy

Endoscope

Esophagus

Duodenum

Jejunum

Small intestine

Bleeding is controlled with cauterization or another method

● New Code   ▲ Revised Code

44369

44369 Small intestinal endoscopy, enteroscopy beyond second portion of duodenum, not including ileum; with ablation of tumor(s), polyp(s), or other lesion(s) not amenable to removal by hot biopsy forceps, bipolar cautery or snare technique

An endoscopic examination is performed on the small intestine beyond the second portion of the duodenum with removal of tumors, polys, or other lesions that are not suited to removal by snare technique, hot biopsy forceps, or biopsy cautery. The duodenum is divided into four portions: the duodenal bulb or cap, the descending portion, the transverse portion, and the ascending portion. The mouth and throat are numbed using an anesthetic spray. A hollow mouthpiece is placed in the mouth. The flexible fiberoptic endoscope is then inserted and advanced as it is swallowed by the patient. Once the endoscope has been advanced beyond the cricopharyngeal region, it is guided using direct visualization into the duodenum. The mucosal surfaces are inspected to a point beyond the second portion of the duodenum and any abnormalities are noted. The examination may include the entire jejunum as well but not the ieum. The scope is then withdrawn and tumors, polyps, or other lesions are ablated using a technique such as laser ablation. The laser device is delivered through the endoscope to the distal margin of the lesion. Beginning at the distal margin, the lesion is ablated as the endoscope is retracted until the laser device has traversed the entire lesion and destroyed it.

44370

44370 Small intestinal endoscopy, enteroscopy beyond second portion of duodenum, not including ileum; with transendoscopic stent placement (includes predilation)

An endoscopic examination is performed on the small intestine beyond the second portion of the duodenum with stent placement. The duodenum is divided into four portions: the duodenal bulb or cap, the descending portion, the transverse portion, and the ascending portion. The mouth and throat are numbed using an anesthetic spray. A hollow mouthpiece is placed in the mouth. The flexible fiberoptic endoscope is then inserted and advanced as it is swallowed by the patient. Once the endoscope has been advanced beyond the cricopharyngeal region, it is guided using direct visualization into the duodenum. The mucosal surfaces are inspected to a point beyond the second portion of the duodenum, which may include the jejunum but not the ileum, and any abnormalities are noted. The area of stenosis is identified and predilated as needed before the stent is placed. The position and length of the stenosis are determined. An appropriately sized stent is selected and introduced through the scope. The stent is positioned in the narrowed portion of the small intestine and deployed (expanded). Separately reportable radiographs are obtained to evaluate expansion of the stent and ensure that it is properly positioned.

44372-44373

44372 Small intestinal endoscopy, enteroscopy beyond second portion of duodenum, not including ileum; with placement of percutaneous jejunostomy tube

44373 Small intestinal endoscopy, enteroscopy beyond second portion of duodenum, not including ileum; with conversion of percutaneous gastrostomy tube to percutaneous jejunostomy tube

An endoscopic examination is performed on the small intestine beyond the second portion of the duodenum with placement of percutaneous feeding tube in the jejunum. A percutaneous endoscopic jejunostomy tube (PEJ-tube) is used to provide nutrients to individuals who are unable to take liquids or food by mouth. The duodenum is divided into four portions. The first is the duodenal bulb or cap, the second is the descending portion, the third is the transverse portion, and the fourth is the ascending portion. The mouth and throat are numbed using an anesthetic spray. A hollow mouthpiece is placed in the mouth. The flexible fiberoptic endoscope is then inserted and advanced as it is swallowed by the patient. Once the endoscope has been advanced beyond the cricopharyngeal region, it is guided using direct visualization into the duodenum. The mucosal surfaces are inspected to a point beyond the second portion of the duodenum and any abnormalities are noted. The inspection includes the entire jejunum as well but does not include the ileum. In 44372, a (PEJ-tube) is inserted. A small incision is made through the skin and abdominal wall over the jejunum. Using a pull technique, the feeding tube is advanced endoscopically through the mouth and into the jejunum. The jejunum is punctured and the feeding tube is advanced through the jejunal wall. A snare is passed through the abdominal incision to capture the feeding tube and pull the tube out through the abdominal incision. The feeding tube is secured internally with a bumper or balloon and externally with a bumper, flange, or other device. In 44373, a gastrostomy is converted to a PEJ-tube, usually due to repeat aspiration of stomach contents into the lungs. The gastrostomy tube is removed. An angiocatheter and guidewire are inserted through the existing gastrostomy incision and using endoscopic control, guided through the pylorus, into the duodenum, and advanced beyond the ligament of Trietz into the jejunum. The angiocatheter is removed and a G-J tube advanced over the guidewire into the jejunum. The G-J tube is secured internally with a bumper or balloon and externally with a bumper, flange, or other device.

44376-44377

44376 Small intestinal endoscopy, enteroscopy beyond second portion of duodenum, including ileum; diagnostic, with or without collection of specimen(s) by brushing or washing (separate procedure)

44377 Small intestinal endoscopy, enteroscopy beyond second portion of duodenum, including ileum; with biopsy, single or multiple

A small intestine endoscopic examination is performed beyond the second portion of the duodenum including the ileum with or without collection of specimens by brushing or washing (44376) or with single or multiple biopsy (44377). The mouth and throat are numbed using an anesthetic spray. A hollow mouthpiece is placed in the mouth. The flexible fiberoptic endoscope is then inserted and advanced as it is swallowed by the patient. Once the endoscope has been advanced beyond the cricopharyngeal region, it is guided using direct visualization into the duodenum. The mucosal surfaces of the duodenum, jejunum, and ileum are inspected and any abnormalities are noted. The scope is then withdrawn and the entire circumference of the intestinal mucosa is inspected again. In 44376, cell samples may be obtained by brushing or washing saline fluid into the small intestine and then collecting it. In 44377, the site to be biopsied is identified and biopsy forceps are placed through the biopsy channel in the endoscope. The forceps are opened, the tissue is spiked, and the forceps are closed. The biopsied tissue sample is removed through the endoscope. One or more tissue samples may be obtained. The cell or tissue samples are sent for separately reportable laboratory analysis.

44378

44378 Small intestinal endoscopy, enteroscopy beyond second portion of duodenum, including ileum; with control of bleeding (eg, injection, bipolar cautery, unipolar cautery, laser, heater probe, stapler, plasma coagulator)

A small intestine endoscopic examination is performed beyond the second portion of the duodenum including the ileum with control of bleeding. The mouth and throat are numbed using an anesthetic spray. A hollow mouthpiece is placed in the mouth. The flexible fiberoptic endoscope is then inserted and advanced as it is swallowed by the patient. Once the endoscope has been advanced beyond the cricopharyngeal region, it is guided using direct visualization into the duodenum. The mucosal surfaces of the duodenum, jejunum, and ileum are inspected and any abnormalities are noted. The scope is then withdrawn and the entire circumference of the intestinal mucosa is inspected again. The bleeding site is identified. Bleeding is typically controlled using a contact thermal modality, such as bipolar or unipolar cautery or a heater probe. The cautery device or heater probe is applied to the bleeding point and pressure applied along with heat to control bleeding. An injection of epinephrine, which works as a vasoconstrictor and tamponade, can also be used to reduce or stop bleeding. YAG laser coagulation and a newer modality, the argon plasma coagulator, are noncontact devices used to coagulate the bleeding site. Staples or hemoclips may be used to approximate the margins of a tear or laceration.

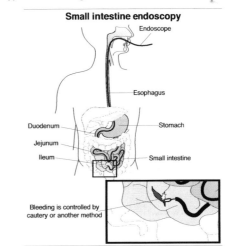

Small intestine endoscopy

Endoscope

Esophagus

Duodenum

Stomach

Jejunum

Ileum

Small intestine

Bleeding is controlled by cautery or another method

44379

44379 Small intestinal endoscopy, enteroscopy beyond second portion of duodenum, including ileum; with transendoscopic stent placement (includes predilation)

A small intestine endoscopic examination is performed beyond the second portion of the duodenum including the ileum with stent placement. The mouth and throat are numbed using an anesthetic spray. A hollow mouthpiece is placed in the mouth. The flexible fiberoptic endoscope is then inserted and advanced as it is swallowed by the patient. Once the endoscope has been advanced beyond the cricopharyngeal region, it is guided using direct visualization into the duodenum. The mucosal surfaces of the duodenum, jejunum, and ileum are inspected and any abnormalities are noted. The area of stenosis is identified and predilated as needed before the stent is placed. The position and length of the stenosis are determined. An appropriately sized stent is selected and introduced through the scope. The stent is positioned in the narrowed portion of the small intestine and deployed (expanded). Separately reportable radiographs are obtained to evaluate expansion of the stent and ensure that it is properly positioned.

44380-44382

44380   Ileoscopy, through stoma; diagnostic, including collection of specimen(s) by brushing or washing, when performed (separate procedure)

44381   Ileoscopy, through stoma; with transendoscopic balloon dilation

44382   Ileoscopy, through stoma; with biopsy, single or multiple

Ileoscopy is performed through an existing stoma with biopsy(s) (44382), collection of brushing or washing cell samples (44380), and transendoscopic balloon dilation (44381). The endoscope is inserted into the ileum through the ileostomy opening. The ileum is inflated with a small amount of air to expand the mucosal folds and allow better visualization of the mucosa. The scope is advanced along the ileum and the mucosa is carefully inspected. In 44380, cell samples may be obtained by brushing or washing saline fluid into the small intestine and then collecting it. In 44382, the site(s) to be biopsied is identified and biopsy forceps are placed through the biopsy channel in the endoscope. The forceps are opened, the tissue is spiked, and the forceps are closed. The biopsied tissue is then removed through the endoscope. One or more tissue samples may be obtained. The cell and tissue samples are sent for separately reportable laboratory analysis. In 44381, a narrowed area of the ileum is identified and dilated with a balloon device through the scope. The deflated balloon catheter is advanced through the instrument channel of the scope to the middle of the stricture. The balloon is then inflated while using a pressure gauge to determine the optimal level of inflation. The inflated balloon is left in place for a short period of time (30 seconds to two minutes), deflated, and then removed. Following dilation, the area of stricture is inspected using the scope to ensure that the dilation has been successful and there are no injuries to the ileum.

44384

44384   Ileoscopy, through stoma; with placement of endoscopic stent (includes pre- and post-dilation and guide wire passage, when performed)

An ileoscopy is performed through an existing stoma with endoscopic stent placement including pre- and post-dilation of the narrowed segment of ileum over a guidewire. The endoscope is inserted into the ileum through the ileostomy opening. The ileum is inflated with a small amount of air to expand the mucosal folds and allow better visualization of the mucosa. The scope is advanced along the ileum and the mucosa is carefully inspected. The scope is then positioned at the area of stenosis and the position and length of the stenosis are determined. The stricture is examined and the need for pre-dilation is evaluated. If pre-dilation is needed, a guide wire is inserted through the scope and a series of rigid tubes of increasing diameter are passed over the guide wire to dilate the stricture. Alternatively, a balloon catheter may be advanced to the site of the stricture and inflated to dilate the stricture. Stent placement is then performed. A guide wire is passed through the scope followed by the stent delivery system which is passed over the guide wire and positioned in the narrowed portion of the ileum. An appropriately sized stent is selected and introduced through the scope. The stent is then positioned in the narrowed portion of the small intestine and deployed (expanded). A balloon catheter may again be inserted and inflated to seat the stent. The endoscope is advanced through the stent to verify correct stent position and ensure proper deployment and the scope is withdrawn.

44385-44386

44385   Endoscopic evaluation of small intestinal pouch (eg, Kock pouch, ileal reservoir [S or J]); diagnostic, including collection of specimen(s) by brushing or washing, when performed (separate procedure)

44386   Endoscopic evaluation of small intestinal pouch (eg, Kock pouch, ileal reservoir [S or J]); with biopsy, single or multiple

A Kock pouch is a continent ileostomy made from the terminal ileum after a colectomy. It consists of a reservoir and a nipple type valve exiting to the skin. The bowel contents remain inside the body in this pouch until the patient decides to empty it by inserting a simple, hollow tube or catheter through the valve. An S or J pouch is another type of ileoanal reservoir performed after total colectomy in which the small intestine is used to construct an internal pouch that is connected to the top of the anal canal. The S or J type is the manner in which the surgeon loops the intestine for pouch creation. S and J pouches are usually performed in a 2-stage procedure in which a loop ileostomy is first brought out to the skin surface for a few weeks until the internal pouch is healthy enough for internal continuity of the bowel to be re-established. Endoscopic evaluation is done to monitor the condition of the small intestinal pouch. An endoscope is inserted into the pouch through the stoma or valve. The mucosa of the pouch is carefully inspected. In 44385, cell samples may be obtained by brushing or washing saline fluid into the pouch and then collecting it. In 44386, any suspect site(s) to be biopsied is identified and biopsy forceps are placed through the biopsy channel in the endoscope. The forceps are opened, the tissue is spiked, and the forceps are closed. The biopsied tissue is removed through the endoscope. One or more tissue samples may be obtained. The cell or tissue samples are sent for separately reportable laboratory analysis.

44388-44389

44388   Colonoscopy through stoma; diagnostic, including collection of specimen(s) by brushing or washing, when performed (separate procedure)

44389   Colonoscopy through stoma; with biopsy, single or multiple

A colonoscopy is performed through an existing stoma with or without collection of specimens by brushing or washing in 44388 and with single or multiple biopsies in 44389. A colonoscope is introduced through the colostomy opening and advanced through the colon. Mucosal surfaces of the colon are inspected and any abnormalities are noted. The endoscope is then withdrawn and mucosal surfaces are again inspected for ulcerations, varices, bleeding sites, lesions, strictures, or other abnormalities. A brush is introduced through the endoscope and cell (cytology) samples are obtained. Alternatively, sterile water may be introduced to wash the mucosal lining and the fluid aspirated to obtain cell samples. In 44389, any suspect site(s) to be biopsied is identified and biopsy forceps are placed through the biopsy channel in the endoscope. The forceps are opened, the tissue is spiked, and the forceps are closed. The biopsied tissue is then removed through the endoscope. One or more tissue samples may be obtained. The cell or tissue samples are sent for separately reportable laboratory analysis.

44390

44390   Colonoscopy through stoma; with removal of foreign body(s)

A colonoscopy is performed through an existing stoma with removal of a foreign body(s). A colonoscope is introduced through the colostomy opening and advanced through the colon to the site of the foreign body. A balloon catheter may be used to remove a smooth edged foreign body. The catheter tip is passed beyond the level of the foreign body and the balloon is inflated. The catheter is then withdrawn and the foreign body is carefully pulled out of the colon. An impacted foreign body is removed with forceps, which are passed through the endoscope. The impacted foreign body is then grasped in the forceps and removed. Following removal of the foreign body(s), the endoscope is reintroduced and the colon is examined for evidence of perforation or other injury.

44391

44391   Colonoscopy through stoma; with control of bleeding, any method

A colonoscopy is performed through an existing stoma with control of bleeding by any method, which may include injection, bipolar/unipolar cautery, laser, heater probe, stapler, plasma coagulator, or other technique. The endoscope is introduced through the colostomy opening. Mucosal surfaces of the colon are inspected and any abnormalities are noted. The bleeding site is identified. Bleeding is typically controlled using a contact thermal modality, such as bipolar or unipolar cautery or a heater probe. The cautery device or heater probe is applied to the bleeding point and pressure is applied along with heat to control the bleeding. An injection of epinephrine, which works as a vasoconstrictor and tamponade, can also be used to reduce or stop bleeding. YAG laser coagulation and a newer modality, the argon plasma coagulator, are noncontact devices used to coagulate the bleeding site. Staples or hemoclips may be used to approximate the margins of a tear or laceration.

44392-44394

44392   Colonoscopy through stoma; with removal of tumor(s), polyp(s), or other lesion(s) by hot biopsy forceps

44394   Colonoscopy through stoma; with removal of tumor(s), polyp(s), or other lesion(s) by snare technique

A colonoscopy is performed through an existing stoma with removal of tumors, polyps, or lesions. The endoscope is introduced through the colostomy opening. Mucosal surfaces of the colon from the stoma to the cecum or a small intestine anastomosis are inspected and abnormalities are noted. The scope is then withdrawn as the entire circumference of the colon is examined. Any tumor, polyp, or other lesion is identified. In 44392, hot biopsy forceps are used to remove the lesion(s). The hot biopsy method uses insulated monopolar forceps to remove and electrocoagulate (cauterize) tissue simultaneously. Hot biopsy forceps are used primarily for removal of small polyps and treatment of vascular ectasias. In 44394, a wire snare loop is placed around the lesion. The loop is heated to shave off and cauterize the lesion(s), which may be removed en bloc with one placement of the snare or in a piecemeal fashion, which requires multiple applications of the snare.

44401

44401   Colonoscopy through stoma; with ablation of tumor(s), polyp(s), or other lesion(s) (includes pre-and post-dilation and guide wire passage, when performed)

A colonoscopy is performed through an existing stoma with tumor, polyp, or lesion ablation. The endoscope is introduced through the colostomy opening. Mucosal surfaces of the colon from the stoma to the cecum or a small intestine anastomosis are inspected and abnormalities are noted. The scope is then withdrawn as the entire circumference of the colon is examined. The site of the tumor(s), polyp(s), or other lesion(s) to be ablated is identified. If dilation is required to allow better access for the ablation procedure, a guide wire is inserted through the scope. A series of rigid tubes of increasing diameter are then passed over the guide wire and the lumen of the large intestine is dilated as needed.

Digestive System

Alternately, a balloon catheter may be advanced to the site of the stricture and inflated to dilate the narrowed area. The balloon catheter is removed and the laser device is then delivered through the endoscope to the distal margin of the most distal lesion. The lesion is ablated as the endoscope is retracted. The entire lesion is destroyed as the laser traverses the lesion in a distal to proximal direction. This is repeated until all lesions have been destroyed. If dilation is required following destruction of lesions, it is performed again. The colon is once again examined using the endoscope to ensure that all lesions have been destroyed and that there are no injuries resulting from the procedure.

44402

44402   Colonoscopy through stoma; with endoscopic stent placement (including pre- and post-dilation and guide wire passage, when performed)

A colonoscopy is performed through an existing stoma with endoscopic stent placement including pre- and post-dilation of the narrowed segment of colon and any necessary guide wire passage. A colonoscope is introduced through the colostomy opening and mucosal surfaces of the colon from the stoma to the cecum or small intestine proximal to an anastomosis are inspected. Any abnormalities are noted. The scope is then withdrawn as the entire circumference of the colon is examined. The scope is then advanced to the area of stenosis. Under separately reportable fluoroscopic guidance, a biliary catheter is advanced through the stricture and contrast is injected through the catheter to determine the length of the stricture. If pre-dilation is needed, a guide wire is inserted through the scope and a series of rigid tubes of increasing diameter are passed over the guide wire to dilate the stricture. Alternatively, a balloon catheter may be advanced to the site of the stricture and inflated to dilate the stricture. Stent placement is then performed. A guide wire is passed through the scope followed by the stent delivery system which is passed over the guide wire and positioned in the narrowed portion of the colon. An appropriately sized stent is selected and introduced through the scope. The stent is then positioned in the stenosed area and deployed (expanded). A balloon catheter may again be inserted and inflated to seat the stent. The endoscope is advanced through the stent to verify correct stent position and ensure proper deployment and the scope is withdrawn..

44403-44404

44403   Colonoscopy through stoma; with endoscopic mucosal resection
44404   Colonoscopy through stoma; with directed submucosal injection(s), any substance

A colonoscopy is performed through an existing stoma with mucosal resection (44403) or submucosal injection(s) (44404). The endoscope is introduced through the colostomy opening. Mucosal surfaces of the colon from the stoma to the cecum or a small intestine anastomosis are inspected and abnormalities are noted. The scope is then withdrawn as the entire circumference of the colon is examined. The mucosal lesion is identified. In 44403, the borders of the lesion are marked with electrocautery. Diluted adrenaline is injected into the submucosal layer around the lesion to separate the mucosal layer containing the lesion from the underlying muscle. A snare with a suction cup is used to further separate the mucosal lesion from underlying tissue. The lesion is then excised and captured using the snare and the scope is withdrawn. In 44404, one or more directed submucosal injections are administered. Submucosal injections may be used to mark (tattoo) a lesion for better visualization prior to separately reportable excision or to create a submucosal fluid cushion prior to removal. This helps separate the mucosal layer from the muscle layer and elevate the lesion. Commonly used substances include India ink, botulinum toxin, saline, epinephrine, or corticosteroids.The endoscope is withdrawn and mucosal surfaces are again inspected for ulcerations, bleeding sites, lesions, strictures, or other abnormalities.

44405

44405   Colonoscopy through stoma; with transendoscopic balloon dilation

A colonoscopy is performed through an existing stoma with balloon dilation of a stricture. The endoscope is introduced through the colostomy opening. Mucosal surfaces of the colon from the stoma to the cecum or a small intestine anastomosis are inspected and abnormalities are noted. The scope is then withdrawn as the entire circumference of the colon is examined. The narrowed area of the colon is identified and dilated with a balloon device through the scope. The deflated balloon catheter is advanced through the instrument channel of the scope to the middle of the stricture. The balloon is then inflated while using a pressure gauge to determine the optimal level of inflation. The inflated balloon is left in place for a short period of time (30 seconds to two minutes), deflated, and then removed. Following dilation, the area of stricture is inspected using the scope to ensure that the dilation has been successful and there are no injuries to the colon.

44406

44406   Colonoscopy through stoma; with endoscopic ultrasound examination, limited to the sigmoid, descending, transverse, or ascending colon and cecum and adjacent structures

A colonoscopy is performed through an existing stoma with endoscopic ultrasound examination. The endoscope is introduced through the colostomy opening. Mucosal surfaces of the colon from the stoma to the cecum or a small intestine anastomosis

are inspected and abnormalities are noted. The scope is then withdrawn as the entire circumference of the colon is examined. An echoendoscope is introduced and advanced under direct visualization to the area of concern. The balloon which covers the transducer housing is filled with water to facilitate acoustic coupling. Continuous ultrasound imaging is performed. Ultrasound allows visualization of the lesion or other area of concern along with the walls of the colon and pericolonic structures such as lymph nodes. Upon completion of the ultrasound examination, the echoendoscope is withdrawn followed by removal of the colonoscope.

44407

44407   Colonoscopy through stoma; with transendoscopic ultrasound guided intramural or transmural fine needle aspiration/biopsy(s), includes endoscopic ultrasound examination limited to the sigmoid, descending, transverse, or ascending colon and cecum and adjacent structures

A colonoscopy is performed through an existing stoma with transendoscopic ultrasound guided intramural or transmural fine needle aspiration/biopsy(s). The endoscope is introduced through the colostomy opening. Mucosal surfaces of the colon from the stoma to the cecum or a small intestine anastomosis are inspected and abnormalities are noted. The scope is then withdrawn as the entire circumference of the colon is examined. A radial scanning echoendoscope is introduced and advanced under direct visualization to an area of compression in the colon that is exterior to the colonic mucosa and continuous ultrasound imaging is performed. The mass exterior to the colon is identified. Ultrasound images are obtained and evaluated. Lymph nodes and other lesions that can be biopsied through the colon are identified. The radial scanning echoendoscope is removed and replaced with a linear scanning echoendoscope. A fine needle aspiration/biopsy catheter is advanced through the biopsy channel of the echoendoscope. Doppler images are obtained to ensure that there are no vascular structures obstructing the planned biopsy route. The needle is then advanced through the colon wall into the lesion or lymph node and a needle biopsy is obtained. Multiple passes are made at each biopsy site. After each pass, the biopsy device is removed, cleaned, and reassembled. Once an adequate specimen has been obtained from the first biopsy site, the next biopsy site is addressed in the same manner.

44408

44408   Colonoscopy through stoma; with decompression (for pathologic distention) (eg, volvulus, megacolon), including placement of decompression tube, when performed

A colonoscopy is performed through an existing stoma with decompression of pathologic distention, such as volvulus, and tube placement, if performed. Volvulus is a twisting of the intestine on its mesenteric pedicle, causing obstruction and leaving a loop of intestine distended with feces and gas. Volvulus tends to occur particularly in the sigmoid segment of the colon from long standing constipation when an elongated and atonic colon develops. This is also known as acquired megacolon and can lead to tissue infarction from disruption of the blood supply, and perforation with peritonitis. The endoscope is introduced through the colostomy opening. Mucosal surfaces of the colon from the stoma to the cecum are inspected as far as possible to the point of the volvulus using air insufflation to separate the musocal folds. The mucosa is carefully inspected for evidence of ischemia or necrosis. If the mucosa appears healthy, a flatus tube is passed alongside the scope and gently passed through the twisted segment of intestine to a site just proximal to the obstruction. As rapid decompression occurs, the backed up liquid feces and gas evacuate with relief of the obstruction. Or, a suction device may be attached to the scope and fluid, stool, and debris are evacuated from the colon. After decompression of the distended colon, the tube is left in place for 24-48 hours to maintain the decompression and allow time for oxygenation of the previously twisted bowel wall. The scope is then withdrawn.

44500

44500   Introduction of long gastrointestinal tube (eg, Miller-Abbott) (separate procedure)

Types of long GI tubes include: Miller-Abbot, used for aspiration; Harris, used for suction and irrigation; and Cantor with a balloon at the distal end. The nostrils are inspected for patency. The patient is placed in Fowler's position with the head slightly hyperextended. The tube is lubricated and inserted into the largest patent nostril. If alert and able, the patient is instructed to swallow as the tube is passed through the pharynx, esophagus, and into the stomach. The patient is turned to the right side to allow the GI tube to pass spontaneously into the duodenum. Positioning of the tube is confirmed radiographically. If the GI tube has not passed into the duodenum spontaneously within 24 hours, separately reportable fluoroscopic guidance may be used to help manipulate the tube to the desired position in the small bowel.

Digestive System

44602-44603

44602 Suture of small intestine (enterorrhaphy) for perforated ulcer, diverticulum, wound, injury or rupture; single perforation

44603 Suture of small intestine (enterorrhaphy) for perforated ulcer, diverticulum, wound, injury or rupture; multiple perforations

Suture repair of the small intestine (enterorrhaphy) is performed to treat a perforated ulcer, diverticulum, wound, injury or rupture. An incision is made in the abdomen and the segment of small intestine requiring repair is removed from the abdomen and placed on the operating table. Intestinal contents are expressed from the intestinal segment. The intestine is clamped above and below the perforation. Bleeding is controlled by suture ligation of involved blood vessels. The opening in the intestine is closed by suturing the mucous membranes followed by the serous coat and then the muscular wall. The abdominal cavity is cleansed using gauze and irrigation fluid as needed. Drains are placed as needed, and the abdominal incision closed. Report 44602 for suture of a single perforation and 44603 when multiple perforations are repaired.

44604-44605

44604 Suture of large intestine (colorrhaphy) for perforated ulcer, diverticulum, wound, injury or rupture (single or multiple perforations); without colostomy

44605 Suture of large intestine (colorrhaphy) for perforated ulcer, diverticulum, wound, injury or rupture (single or multiple perforations); with colostomy

Suture repair of the large intestine (colorrhaphy) is performed to treat a perforated ulcer, diverticulum, wound, injury or rupture. An incision is made in the abdomen and the segment of large intestine requiring repair is removed from the abdomen and placed on the operating table. Intestinal contents are expressed from the intestinal segment. The intestine is clamped above and below the perforation. Bleeding is controlled by suture ligation of involved blood vessels. The opening in the intestine is closed by suturing the mucous membranes followed by the serous coat and then the muscular wall. The abdominal cavity is cleansed using gauze and irrigation fluid as needed. Drains are placed as needed and the abdominal incision closed. Report 44604 for suture repair without colostomy. Report 44605 when a colostomy is also performed. The colon is divided above the site of the colorrhaphy. The colostomy is created by making a small incision over the planned colostomy site. Fat is excised down to the anterior rectus fascia. The fascia is opened taking care to protect the underlying rectus muscle and its blood supply. The rectus fibers are separated by blunt dissection. The peritoneum is entered and an opening created for the stoma. A peritoneal tunnel may be created to prevent postoperative obstruction of the stoma. The colon is then brought through the abdominal wall and everted (folded back on itself). The segment of colon is sutured to the skin.

44615

44615 Intestinal stricturoplasty (enterotomy and enterorrhaphy) with or without dilation, for intestinal obstruction

Stricturoplasty is performed primarily for treatment of short strictures in patients with long-standing Crohn's disease. The abdomen is incised and the narrowed segment of small bowel exposed. For stricutres, usually less than 10 cm, a Heineke-Mikulicz stricutorplasty is performed. A longitudinal incision (enterotomy) is made in the narrowed segment of intestine along the anti-mesenteric border and extended 1-2 cm into normal diameter intestine on each side. The intestinal mucosa is carefully examined along the entire length of the stricture to ensure that there is no evidence of malignancy or other disease. Biopsies are obtained as needed. The longitudinal enterotomy is then closed with sutures or staples (enterorrhaphy) in a transverse fashion which increases the diameter stricutred segment. For strictures 10-20 cm in length, a Finney stricturoplasty is performed. The strictured segment is folded into a U-shape. Seromuscular sutures are placed between the two sides of the U. A longitudinal U-shaped incision is made around the suture line. The mucosa is inspected and biopsies obtained as needed. The incision in the posterior wall of the intestine is repaired with sutures and the suture line carried around to the anterior aspect of the intestine and the incision in the anterior bowel closed.

44620-44626

44620 Closure of enterostomy, large or small intestine

44625 Closure of enterostomy, large or small intestine; with resection and anastomosis other than colorectal

44626 Closure of enterostomy, large or small intestine; with resection and colorectal anastomosis (eg, closure of Hartmann type procedure)

The physician closes an enterostomy of the large or small intestine. If a duodenostomy or jejunostomy is present it is removed. In 44620, a small incision is made in the abdomen near the site of the enterostomy. The intestine is released from the abdominal wall and the opening in the intestine exposed. The edges of the intestinal opening are debrided and trimmed and the opening is closed with sutures. The enterostomy site in the abdominal wall is then closed as is the abdominal incision. In 44625, the enterostomy is closed and the remaining segments of intestine resected and anastomosed. This excludes a colorectal anastomosis. The abdomen is opened and adhesions lysed. The distal intestinal stump is

located and mobilized. The proximal segment that was used to create the enterostomy is freed from the abdominal wall. The proximal and distal stumps are resected as needed and the two segments are then sutured together to restore the integrity of the bowel. In 44626, the enterostomy is closed the remaining segments of colon and rectum resected and anastomosed. This may also be referred to as a take-down or closure of a Hartmann procedure. The procedure is performed as described in 44625, except that the physician must locate the rectal segment which may lie low in the sacrum. Once the rectal segment has been located and mobilized, the proximal segment of colon is freed from the abdominal wall the colon and rectal segments are resected as needed and anastomosed. Drains are placed in the abdomen as needed and the abdominal incision is closed.

44640

44640 Closure of intestinal cutaneous fistula

The physician closes an intestinal cutaneous fistula which is an abnormal communication or passage between the intestine and the skin. The abdomen is incised and fistulous tract located. The tract is severed at the intestinal opening and the opening closed with sutures. The tract in the abdominal wall is excised and the abdominal wall closed in layers. The surgical incision is also closed.

44650

44650 Closure of enteroenteric or enterocolic fistula

The physician closes an enteroenteric or enterocolic fistula, which are abnormal communications or passages between two segments of small intestine or between a segment of small intestine and a segment of colon (large intestine). The abdomen is incised and the fistulous tract located. The tract is severed at both intestinal openings and excised. The openings in the intestines are closed with sutures. The surgical incision is closed.

44660-44661

44660 Closure of enterovesical fistula; without intestinal or bladder resection

44661 Closure of enterovesical fistula; with intestine and/or bladder resection

An enterovesical fistula is an abnormal communication between a segment of intestine and the urinary bladder. The most common cause of enterovesical fistula is diverticular disease of the colon with other common causes being colon cancer, inflammatory bowel diseases such as Crohn's disease, complications of radiation therapy, or trauma. The abdomen is opened and the fistulous tract located. The fistulous tract is divided and bladder and bowel separated. The tract is examined to determine whether the bowel and bladder can be repaired by primary closure or whether resection is required. In 44660, primary closure is performed. The fistulous tract is excised. The openings in the bowel and bladder are each repaired separately with sutures. In 44661, resection of the bladder and/or intestine is required. The fistulous tract between the bowel and bladder is severed. The bowel is clamped above and below the fistulous tract, transected, and the portion containing the fistulous tract removed. An end-to-end anastomosis is then used to reapproximate the bowel. If the bladder requires resection, the fistulous tract is excised along with a portion of the surrounding bladder. The remaining bladder wall is then reapproximated with sutures. A separately reportable omental flap may be developed and placed between the bowel and bladder to prevent recurrence. Drains are placed in the abdomen and the abdominal incision is closed.

44680

44680 Intestinal plication (separate procedure)

This procedure may be performed on patients who have had multiple bowel surgeries or those with peritonitis in an effort to prevent bowel obstruction. Plication creates folds in loops of bowel in an orderly fashion rather than the disorderly fashion that occurs when adhesions form. The abdomen is opened and the segments of intestine to be plicated identified. The intestine is mobilized and arranged in loops approximately 8 inches in length. A long needle carrying the suture material is passed through the mesentery of each bowel loop approximately 3 mm from the bowel wall. The suture is then threaded through the mesentery. The needle is then passed back in the opposite direction approximately 3 cm from the first suture line and the suture passed through the mesentery in the same manner. The suture is tied loosely to avoid strangulating the bowel. Upon completion of the plication procedure the abdomen is closed in layers.

44700

44700 Exclusion of small intestine from pelvis by mesh or other prosthesis, or native tissue (eg, bladder or omentum)

The physician performs a procedure to exclude the small intestine from the pelvis using mesh or other prosthetic tissue or native tissue such as bladder or omentum. This procedure is performed prior to radiation therapy to prevent radiation injury to the small intestine. The abdomen is opened and the small intestine mobilized and elevated out of the pelvic cavity. A piece of mesh is then trimmed to the appropriate dimensions, placed under the intestines, and sutured to surrounding structures to keep the small intestines elevated out of the radiation field. Alternatively, another prosthetic device such as soft

Digestive System

silicone plastic that conforms to the pelvis may be used. This device is filled with saline and contrast material so that it can be visualized on radiographs. Radiographs are obtained prior to each radiation session to ensure that the bowel is outside the radiation field. The device remains in place throughout the radiation therapy sessions and is then is removed through a small incision following drainage of the device. Another alternative is the creation of an omental sling. An omental flap is created, positioned under the intestines, and secured with sutures to keep the intestines elevated and out of the radiation field.

44701

44701   Intraoperative colonic lavage (List separately in addition to code for primary procedure)

Intraoperative colonic lavage is performed to cleanse the colon of fecal matter prior to a separately reportable colectomy or colon repair. Following mobilization of the splenic flexure, the colon contents are milked into the descending colon by manual massage. A drain is inserted in the descending colon for evacuation of the fecal matter. An incision is made in the cecum and a catheter is inserted. Irrigating solution is flushed through the catheter into the colon while the colon is massaged to break up solid stool. Stool and irrigating solution empty from the descending colon through the previously placed drain. Upon completion of the lavage procedure, the catheter and drain are removed and the incision in the cecum closed. The physician then proceeds with the definitive procedure.

44705

44705   Preparation of fecal microbiota for instillation, including assessment of donor specimen

Fecal microbiota transplantation (FMT), also called fecal bacteriotherapy, is an effective treatment for recurrent Clostridium difficile infection in which a feces sample is taken from a donor for transplantation into the infected patient's gastrointestinal tract to restore normal bacterial flora. Administration is usually done via enema or nasogastric tube. Code 44705 reports the physician work provided for donor assessment and oversight of fecal microbiota preparation. Material preparation includes obtaining the stool sample before the procedure. The donor must be free of infectious diseases (hepatitis A, B, and C viruses; HIV-1 and HIV-2), parasitic diseases, yeast overgrowth, and other digestive tract conditions. All donor stool samples are cultured for enteric bacterial pathogens, and screened by light microscopy for presence of ova and parasites in accordance with standard laboratory protocols. Donor sample preparation includes the choice of diluent (e.g., sterile saline), homogenization, and filtration of stool sample.

44715

44715   Backbench standard preparation of cadaver or living donor intestine allograft prior to transplantation, including mobilization and fashioning of the superior mesenteric artery and vein

Backbench standard preparation of cadaver or live donor intestine allograft is performed prior to transplantation including mobilization and fashioning of the superior mesenteric artery and vein. The allograft is removed from the sterile container, placed on ice, and maintained in a cold preservation bath. The graft is inspected to ensure that it is intact and healthy enough for transplant. Surrounding soft tissues are dissected off the graft. The mesenteric artery and vein are identified and inspected to ensure that they are intact and of adequate length to perform the anastomosis. If the mesenteric artery and vein are not of sufficient length, they are reconstructed in separately reportable procedures. The graft is maintained in cold preservation until the recipient is ready for the transplant procedure.

44720-44721

44720   Backbench reconstruction of cadaver or living donor intestine allograft prior to transplantation; venous anastomosis, each

44721   Backbench reconstruction of cadaver or living donor intestine allograft prior to transplantation; arterial anastomosis, each

Backbench reconstruction of a cadaver or live donor intestinal allograft is performed prior to transplantation including venous anastomosis (44720) and/or arterial anastomosis (44721). In 44720, a vein graft that has been procured from the cadaver donor or from a live compatible donor is received on ice and bathed in cold preservation solution. The superior mesenteric vein attached to the intestinal allograft and the extension venous graft are sutured together in an end-to-end fashion. If additional venous extension grafts are required, each is reported separately. In 44721, an arterial graft that has been procured from the cadaver donor or from a live compatible donor is received on ice and bathed in cold preservation solution. The superior mesenteric artery attached to the intestinal allograft and the extension arterial graft are sutured together in an end-to-end fashion. If additional arterial extension grafts are required, each is reported separately.

44800

44800   Excision of Meckel's diverticulum (diverticulectomy) or omphalomesenteric duct

Meckel's diverticulum is a congenital anomaly caused by incomplete obliteration of the omphalomesenteric (vitelline) duct which results in a vestigial pouch or connection

between the intestine and umbilicus. A midline incision is made in the abdomen and carried down to the Meckel's diverticulum. If the diverticulum has a mesentery, the mesentery is isolated, clamped, divided, and ligated. The Meckel's diverticulum is then clamed and excised in the transverse axis of the ileum. The artery on the ileal mesentery that supplies the Meckel's diverticulum is divided and the distal artery segment excised. The operative site is irrigated and incisions are closed.

44820

44820   Excision of lesion of mesentery (separate procedure)

The mesentery of the gastrointestinal tract is a contiguous fanlike structure composed of fibrous and fatty tissues that contain arterial, venous, lymphatic, and neural structures supplying the intestinal tract. Tumors or lesions of the mesentery may be cystic or solid and may be malignant or benign. The abdomen is incised and the region of the mesentery containing the lesion is exposed. The abdomen is explored and the mesentery carefully examined prior to excision of the lesion to determine if there are any other masses or abnormalities. The lesion is excised along with a margin of healthy tissue and sent to the laboratory for separately reportable pathological evaluation. The operative site is irrigated, bleeding controlled, and incisions closed.

44850

44850   Suture of mesentery (separate procedure)

The mesentery of the gastrointestinal tract is a contiguous fanlike structure composed of fibrous and fatty tissues that contain arterial, venous, lymphatic, and neural structures supplying the gastrointestinal tract. A midline incision is made in the abdomen and the peritoneum opened. Blood and fluid is aspirated and the abdomen explored to determine the extent of injury. The injury to the mesentery is located and bleeding controlled. Blood and blood clots are aspirated. The mesentery is inspected to determine whether any major blood vessels, lymphatic structures, or nerves have been damaged. The mesentery is repaired with sutures. The operative site is irrigated and the abdomen again inspected for evidence of injury to other organs or structures. The operative wound is then closed in a layered fashion.

44900

44900   Incision and drainage of appendiceal abscess, open

The appendix is a short blind-end tubular structure arising from the cecum. An appendiceal abscess results when the appendix ruptures due to acute appendicitis and an abscess pocket forms. In 44900, open incision and drainage is performed. An incision is made in the right lower quadrant. The external and oblique muscles are split and the peritoneum divided. Dissection is carried down to the site of the abscess. The abscess pocket is incised and purulent material drained. Blunt finger dissection is used to break of loculations. The abscess pocket is irrigated with saline or antibiotic solution. A drain placed and the surgical wound closed around the drain.

44950-44955

44950   Appendectomy

44955   Appendectomy; when done for indicated purpose at time of other major procedure (not as separate procedure) (List separately in addition to code for primary procedure)

An incision is made in the right lower quadrant overlying the appendix for its removal. The external and internal oblique muscles are split and the peritoneum is divided. Blunt dissection is used to mobilize the appendix, which is grasped and delivered into the operative wound. The base of the appendix is clamped and suture ligated. Purse string sutures are placed in the cecum. The appendix is divided; the appendiceal stump is folded (invaginated) beneath the purse string sutures in the cecum; and The incision is closed with sutures. Use 44955 when an appendectomy is performed for a documented medical reason at the time of another major abdominal procedure.

44960

44960   Appendectomy; for ruptured appendix with abscess or generalized peritonitis

A ruptured appendix that has caused peritonitis or that has an abscess is removed. An incision is made in the right lower quadrant overlying the appendix. The external and internal oblique muscles are split and the peritoneum is divided. Peritoneal fluid is inspected and purulent fluid is cultured. The opening in the peritoneum is widened and the appendix is manually and visually inspected to the level of the cecum and terminal ileum. Blunt dissection is used to mobilize the appendix, which is grasped and delivered into the operative wound. The extent of rupture is determined, taking care to note any extension into the base of the appendix. If the base is not involved, the appendix is isolated from the mesoappendix and crushed using a straight clamp placed proximal to the rupture. Purse string sutures are placed in the cecum. The appendix is resected off the stump and removed. The appendiceal stump is folded (invaginated) beneath the purse string sutures in the cecum. The surgical area is inspected for bleeding and pockets of infection. The abdominal cavity is irrigated with saline and antibiotics. Drains are placed. The incision is

Digestive System

closed around the drains. Alternatively, the skin and subcutaneous tissue may be left open to heal by secondary intention (from the inside out).

44970

44970   Laparoscopy, surgical, appendectomy

An appendix is removed laparoscopically. Three small incisions are made in the abdomen: one at the umbilical level, one in the suprapubic region, and one in the right upper quadrant. Trocars are inserted. A pneumoperitoneum is created by pumping air into the abdominal cavity to separate the abdominal wall from the internal organs. The laparoscope is inserted through the umbilical trocar. A grasper inserted into the right upper quadrant is used to retract the cecum, elevating the appendix into the operative field. The appendix is grasped and inserted into the suprapubic trocar. A mesenteric window is created under the base of the appendix, which is then transected and its base inspected for bleeding. Once bleeding subsides, the appendix is amputated from the gastrointestinal tract, delivered into the specimen bag, and removed from the intra-abdominal cavity. The abdominal cavity is irrigated, instruments are removed, and incisions are closed.

45000

45000   Transrectal drainage of pelvic abscess

Transrectal drainage of a pelvic abscess is performed. A digital rectal exam is performed and the abscess is palpated. With the tip of the index finger placed at the intended incision site, closed thin-curved scissors are inserted along the index finger and a stab incision is made with the tip of the scissors into the abscess. The scissors are opened slightly to enlarge the incision and the abscess is drained. A drain may be placed.

45005-45020

45005   Incision and drainage of submucosal abscess, rectum
45020   Incision and drainage of deep supralevator, pelvirectal, or retrorectal abscess

Incision and drainage of a submucosal abscess of the rectum (45005) or a deep supralevator, pelvirectal, or rectorectal abscess (45020) is performed. A proctoscope or sigmoidoscope may be used to locate the abscess. In 45005, the submucosal rectal abscess is opened using one of several techniques. A radial or cross-shaped (cruciate) incision is made over the area of fluctuance as close to the anal verge as possible. The edges of the incision are excised to expose the abscess cavity and permit wide drainage. The incisions may be left open to drain, packed with iodophor gauze for 24 hours, or a drain placed. In 45020, the approach depends on the location of the abscess and the site where the abscess originated. Radial or cruciate incisions are used to permit wide drainage. To drain a supralevator abscess that originated in the intersphincteric region, an incision is made through the rectal mucosa. A pelvirectal abscess is approached through the rectum just above the anorectal line. A retrorectal abscess may be approached through the posterior anal canal with tissue dissection from the intersphincteric plane through the puborectalis sling and into the space posterior to (behind) the anus and rectum. The supralevator, pelvirectal, or retrorectal abscess is then probed using a gloved finger and any loculations broken up. The abscess cavity is inspected to ensure that there are no fistulous tracts. Incisions may be left open to drain, packed with iodophor gauze, or a drain placed.

45100

45100   Biopsy of anorectal wall, anal approach (eg, congenital megacolon)

A biopsy of the anorectal wall is performed for a condition such as congenital megacolon, also referred to as Hirschprung's disease. Congenital megacolon is a dilation or enlargement (hypertrophy) of the colon due to the absence or a greatly reduced number of ganglion cells normally found in the muscular wall of the rectum and colon. The area to be biopsied is identified, cleansed, and a local anesthetic injected. The anorectal wall is incised and a tissue sample obtained. The tissue sample is prepared and sent for separately reportable laboratory evaluation.

45108

45108   Anorectal myomectomy

This procedure is typically performed to treat Hirschprung disease, a developmental disorder of the nervous system in which there is an absence of ganglion cells in the distal colon that causes functional bowel obstruction. The anus is dilated using narrow retractors. A transverse incision is made in the posterior wall of the anal mucosa just above the mucocutaneous junction. The mucosa is elevated and a 6-10 cm strip of the muscularis is excised along with a portion of the internal sphincter. The overlying mucosa is closed over a small drain.

45110

45110   Proctectomy; complete, combined abdominoperineal, with colostomy

A midline incision is made in the abdomen and the abdomen explored. The proximal transection site is identified which may include the sigmoid colon. The sigmoid colon and rectum are mobilized and a clamp placed above the planned transection site. The

perineum is incised and the outer layer of the rectal wall divided in a circular fashion. The rectum and surrounding mesentery are then freed from pelvic and abdominal attachments and delivered en bloc through the perineal incision. The perineal incision is closed. The anal mucosa is closed. A separate incision is made for creation of a stoma. The proximal segment of colon is exteriorized through the stoma incision. The colon is folded back on itself (everted) and sutured to the skin and subcutaneous tissue. Drains are placed in the abdomen and the abdominal incision closed. A stoma appliance is placed.

45111

45111   Proctectomy; partial resection of rectum, transabdominal approach

Transabdominal approach is typically used for resection of the proximal aspect of the rectum. A midline incision is made in the lower abdomen and the abdomen explored. The proximal transection site is identified which may include a portion of the sigmoid colon. The sigmoid colon and rectum are mobilized and a clamp placed above the planned proximal transection site. A second clamp is placed below the planned distal resection site in the rectum. The rectum is divided and the diseased or injured segment removed. The distal and proximal segments are then anastomosed in an end-to-end fashion. Drains are placed in the abdomen and the midline abdominal incision is closed.

45112

45112   Proctectomy, combined abdominoperineal, pull-through procedure (eg, colo-anal anastomosis)

A midline incision is made in the abdomen and the abdomen explored. The proximal transection site is identified which may include a portion of the sigmoid colon. The sigmoid colon and rectum are mobilized and a clamp placed above the planned transection site. The perineum is incised and the outer layer of the rectal wall divided in a circular fashion. The rectum and surrounding mesentery are then freed from pelvic and abdominal attachments. The rectum and mesentery are separated and removed en bloc leaving the anal mucosa intact. The anastomosis site in the anus is prepared by placing sutures around the circumference of the anus. The anal mucosa and the colon are sutured together (anastomosed). Drains are placed in the abdomen and the midline abdominal incision is closed.

45113

45113   Proctectomy, partial, with rectal mucosectomy, ileoanal anastomosis, creation of ileal reservoir (S or J), with or without loop ileostomy

A midline incision is made in the abdomen and the abdomen explored. The proximal transection site is identified which may include the sigmoid colon. The sigmoid colon and rectum are mobilized and a clamp placed above the planned transection site. A second clamp is placed below the planned distal resection site in the rectum. The rectum is divided and the diseased or injured segment removed. The remaining proximal segment of rectum or sigmoid colon is then closed with sutures. The remaining segment of distal rectum may have the mucosa stripped but the muscular wall is left intact. The terminal ileum is divided just above the cecum and the distal segment sutured closed. An ileal reservoir is then created. A portion of the terminal ileum is folded on itself in an S or J configuration and then sutured in such a manner as to form a pouch. The distal segment of terminal ileum just below the pouch is sutured to the anal mucosa. The pouch provides a storage place for stool in the absence of the proximal rectum and the muscular wall of the distal rectum allows for holding and passing of stool normally. A loop ileostomy may also be created to provide passage of stool until the pouch and ileoanal anastomosis have healed. A small incision is made in the abdominal wall at the planned ileostomy site. A loop of ileum above the pouch is mobilized and brought out of the abdominal wall at the stoma site. The loop is incised longitudinally and the edges folded back to expose the mucosa which is sutured to the abdomen. This creates two stomas. The one from above eliminates stool and the one from below, also called a mucous fistula, eliminates mucus from the bowel above the pouch. Drains are placed and the abdomen is closed in layers.

45114-45116

45114   Proctectomy, partial, with anastomosis; abdominal and transsacral approach
45116   Proctectomy, partial, with anastomosis; transsacral approach only (Kraske type)

The transsacral approach is rarely performed. In 45114, the patient is placed prone in a jack-knife position. An incision is made at the midline of the back beginning 2 cm proximal to the anal verge and extending up the back approximately 8-10 cm. The coccyx is excised and the two lower sacral segments resected to allow exposure of the distal segment of the rectum. The rectum is mobilized and divided distally. The incision in the back is closed. The patient is placed in the supine position and a midline incision is made in the abdomen and the abdomen explored. The proximal transection site is identified which may include the sigmoid colon. The sigmoid colon and proximal rectum are mobilized and the sigmoid colon or rectum is divided above the diseased segment. The remaining proximal and distal segments are anastomosed in an end-to-end fashion. Drains are placed and the abdominal incision is closed. In 45116, only a transsacral approach is used. An incision is made at the midline of the back beginning 2 cm proximal to the anal verge and extending up the back

Digestive System

approximately 8-10 cm. The coccyx is excised and the two lower sacral segments resected to allow exposure of the distal segment of the rectum. The rectum is mobilized and divided above and below the diseased or injured segment which is removed. The remaining proximal and distal segments are anastomosed in an end-to-end fashion. Drains are placed and the transsacral incision is closed.

45119

45119   Proctectomy, combined abdominoperineal pull-through procedure (eg, colo-anal anastomosis), with creation of colonic reservoir (eg, J-pouch), with diverting enterostomy when performed

A midline incision is made in the abdomen and the abdomen explored. The segment of colon to be used as the reservoir is identified and the colon is mobilized. The proximal transection site is identified which may include the sigmoid colon. The sigmoid colon and rectum are mobilized and a clamp placed above the planned transection site. The perineum is incised and the outer layer of the rectal wall divided in a circular fashion. The rectum and surrounding mesentery are then freed from pelvic and abdominal attachments. The rectum and mesentery are separated and removed en bloc leaving the anal mucosa intact. A colonic reservoir is created by folding the colon back on itself. The colon is then sutured together and the antimesenteric border incised parallel to the suture line to open the pouch and expose the mucosa. The previously placed suture lines in the colon wall are reinforced by suturing the mucosal layer to create a two layer closure. The pouch is closed and positioned in the pelvis. The anastomosis site in the anus is prepared by placing sutures around the circumference of the anus. The anal mucosa and the colon are sutured together (anastomosed). If a diverting enterostomy is required, the enterostomy site is selected and the abdomen incised. The segment of colon or ileum is mobilized and transected. The distal segment is closed and the proximal segment brought out through the stoma incision. The intestine is folded back on itself (everted) and sutured to the skin and subcutaneous tissue. Drains are placed in the abdomen and the midline abdominal incision is closed. A stoma appliance is placed.

45120-45121

45120   Proctectomy, complete (for congenital megacolon), abdominal and perineal approach; with pull-through procedure and anastomosis (eg, Swenson, Duhamel, or Soave type operation)

45121   Proctectomy, complete (for congenital megacolon), abdominal and perineal approach; with subtotal or total colectomy, with multiple biopsies

This procedure may also be referred to as a Swenson, Duhamel, or Soave operation. A midline incision is made in the abdomen and the abdomen explored. Congenital megacolon, also known as Hirschsprung's disease, is characterized by the absence of ganglion cells, a type of specialized nerve cell, in the rectum and for variable lengths of the colon. The condition is caused by failure of ganglion cells to migrate along the entire length of the bowel during fetal development. The result is abnormal intestinal function that can range from complete obstruction to severe constipation. Treatment involves removing the abnormal bowel segments and replacing those segments with bowel that has normal nerve cells by pulling normal bowel down and connecting it with anal mucosa. In 45120, only the rectum and possibly a small segment of sigmoid colon are removed. The proximal transection site is identified which may include a small portion of the sigmoid colon. The sigmoid colon and rectum are mobilized and a clamp placed above the planned transection site. The perineum is incised and the outer layer of the rectal wall divided in a circular fashion. The rectum and surrounding mesentery are then freed from pelvic and abdominal attachments. The rectum and mesentery are separated and removed en bloc leaving the anal mucosa intact. The anastomosis site in the anus is prepared by placing sutures around the circumference of the anus. The anal mucosa and the remaining segment of rectum or sigmoid colon are sutured together (anastomosed). Drains are placed in the abdomen and the midline abdominal incision is closed. In 45121, the rectum and part or all of the colon are removed and multiple biopsies of the bowel are obtained. The procedure is the same as in 45120 except that prior to the resection, biopsies are obtained to determine the location in the bowel of normal nerve tissue. The transection site in the colon is identified and the colon is mobilized and resected along with the entire rectum.

45123

45123   Proctectomy, partial, without anastomosis, perineal approach

This procedure is performed to treat malignant neoplasm of the rectum. The lower bowel is cleansed by rectal irrigation. Lateral incisions are made on either side of the anus and carried anteriorly and posteriorly. Closure of the anus is accomplished with a pursestring suture. Pudendal vessels are clamped and ligated as they are encountered. Posteriorly, the incision is carried proximally through the anococcygeal ligament and anterior to the pre-sacral fascia. Anteriorly, the incision is carried proximally posterior to the prostatic or vaginal fascia. The rectum is then closed below the planned transection site with pursestring suture. The rectum is transected above the level of the neoplasm. The levator muscles are divided. The diseased portion of the colon is delivered through the perineal incision. The rectum is divided above the level of the pursestring sutures placed around

the anus and the diseased section of rectum removed. Bleeding is controlled and incisions closed.

45126

45126   Pelvic exenteration for colorectal malignancy, with proctectomy (with or without colostomy), with removal of bladder and ureteral transplantations, and/or hysterectomy, or cervicectomy, with or without removal of tube(s), with or without removal of ovary(s), or any combination thereof

This procedure is performed to treat bulky, locally advanced primary or recurrent colorectal cancer with metastases to adjacent organs. All of the large bowel and rectum and the bladder are removed. The ureters are transplanted and a colostomy may be performed. In women, the uterus and/or cervix, fallopian tubes, and ovaries may also be removed. Wide exposure of the abdomen is achieved by a midline abdominal incision. The abdomen is explored to determine the extent of involvement of adjacent organs. The pelvic dissection begins at the level of the aortic bifurcation. The inferior mesenteric artery is transected at its origin and a wide lymphadenectomy is performed. The sigmoid colon is mobilized and transected. The plane between the fascia of the mesorectum and the endopelvic fascia is dissected as far distally as possible. The ureters are located and traced proximally and distally. The bladder is mobilized and the superior and inferior pedicles of the bladder are ligated and transected. In men, the puboprostatic ligaments, the dorsal vein of the penis, and the urethra are divided. In women, the ovaries and ureters are mobilized. Once the abdomen dissection is complete, perineal dissection is performed. The entire sphincter musculature and the urogenital diaphragm are dissected and the dissection is carried up to the abdominal dissection. When the abdominal plane is met, all the mobilized contents of the perineum, pelvis, and abdomen are removed en bloc. A segment of distal ileum is isolated and the ureters are anastomosed directly into the isolated segment which is then exteriorized and sutured to the skin to create an incontinent ileal conduit. Alternatively, a colonic reservoir may be fashioned and a continent urinary conduit created. If a colostomy is required, a separate incision is made for creation of a stoma. The proximal segment of colon exteriorized through the stoma incision. The colon is folded back on itself (everted) and sutured to the skin and subcutaneous tissue. The pelvic floor is reconstructed using mesh, Alloderm, omentum or other tissue from the patient. Once reconstructive procedures have been completed the pelvic dead space is filled using myocutaneous flaps. Drains are placed and the perineal and abdominal incisions are closed.

45130-45135

45130   Excision of rectal procidentia, with anastomosis; perineal approach

45135   Excision of rectal procidentia, with anastomosis; abdominal and perineal approach

Rectal proccidentia is a complete prolapse of the entire thickness of the rectum. In 45130, an excision of the prolapsed rectum is performed via a perineal approach. This procedure may also be referred to as an Altemeier procedure or a proctosigmoidectomy. The patient is placed in lithotomy position and the perineum exposed. The perineum is incised and the outer layer of the bowel wall divided in a circular fashion. The rectum is then freed from pelvic and abdominal attachments to a point just above (proximal to) the dentate line by dividing the fat and mesentery. The rectum is then separated and removed leaving the anal mucosa intact along with a short proximal rectal segment. The anal mucosa and rectal stump are then anastomosed. In 45135, a combined abdominal and perineal approach is used. The perineum and the rectum are divided as described above. An abdominal incision is made and the sigmoid colon and rectum are mobilized up to the level of the levator ligaments. The lateral ligaments are divided and sutured to the presacral fascia. The fat and mesentery surrounding the sigmoid colon is divided taking care to preserve the inferior mesenteric artery. A portion of the sigmoid colon and the entire rectum are removed. The anal musoca is then anastomosed to the remaining segment of sigmoid colon. Abdominal incisions are closed in a layered fashion.

45136

45136   Excision of ileoanal reservoir with ileostomy

An ileoanal reservoir also referred to as an intestinal pouch or J-pouch, is created out of small intestine to collect stool following removal of the entire large bowel and lining of the rectum. Removal of an ileoanal pouch is performed when complications occur, such as functional problems or sepsis. A midline abdominal incision is made. Intra-abdominal and small bowel adhesion are lysed. The ileoanal pouch is dissected free of surrounding tissue. The pouch is severed from the anal mucosa using a perineal approach. The pouch is removed from the abdomen. A second incision is made, usually in the right side of the lower abdomen for creation of an ileostomy. The distal ileal segment is brought through the abdominal wall and sutured to the skin.

45150

45150   Division of stricture of rectum

A rectal stricture is a narrowing of a segment of the rectum. Rectal strictures may caused by inflammation, trauma or injury to the rectum including trauma from a previous surgical procedure or radiation therapy. Scar tissue from the trauma can contract causing the narrowing. Using a transanal approach, the narrowed segment of the rectum is located.

Digestive System

● New Code   ▲ Revised Code

The rectum is incised and the contracted tissue divided. The wound is left open to heal by secondary intention.

45160-45172

45160 Excision of rectal tumor by proctotomy, transsacral or transcoccygeal approach

45171 Excision of rectal tumor, transanal approach; not including muscularis propria (ie, partial thickness)

45172 Excision of rectal tumor, transanal approach; including muscularis propria (ie, full thickness)

In 45160, a transacral or transcoccygeal approach is used to remove a rectal tumor. An incision is made at the midline of the back beginning 2 cm proximal to the anal verge and extending up the back approximately 8-10 cm. The coccyx is excised and the two lower sacral segments resected as needed to allow exposure of the rectum. The rectum is incised at the site of the tumor or mass. The tumor is excised along with a margin of healthy tissue. Separately reportable frozen sections are obtained to ensure that the margins are clear. The specimen is then sent to the laboratory for separately reportable pathology evaluation. The rectum is then repaired with sutures and the transsacral or transscoccygeal incision is closed. In 45171 and 45172, a transanal approach is used. An anoscope may be used to locate the tumor. Once the tumor is located, the rectal mucosa is incised. The incision is carried through deeper tissues and the tumor excised along with a margin of healthy tissue. Frozen sections are obtained to ensure that margins are clear and the specimen is sent to the laboratory for pathology evaluation. The incision in the rectum is closed. Use 45171 for a partial thickness excision. Partial thickness excision may include the first three layers of the rectum, the inner lining or mucosa, the thin muscle layer called the muscularis mucosa, and the fibrous tissue or submucosa beneath the mucularis mucosa. Partial thickness excision does not include the muscularis propria. Use 45172 for a full thickness excision that includes the first three layers described above as well as the mucularis propria which is the thick muscle layer that contracts to expel stool.

45190

45190 Destruction of rectal tumor (eg, electrodesiccation, electrosurgery, laser ablation, laser resection, cryosurgery) transanal approach

The sphincter is stretched and anal retractors applied to expose the tumor. The lesion is examined and the most appropriate form of destruction determined. Saline or epinephrine may be injected into the submucosa beneath the tumor to elevate it and help control bleeding. The area to be destroyed is marked which includes the tumor along with a surrounding margin of health tissue. Electrodessication uses a monopolar high-frequency electric current to destroy the mass and control bleeding. Electrosurgery is a common method of destruction that uses heat applied with a high frequency current using a metal probe or needle. Laser ablation involves the use of a non-contact Nd-YAG laser or a contact laser probe with coaxial water to vaporize the tumor. Laser resection is performed with a CO_2 laser that is used to sharply excise the tumor which is then removed. Cryosurgery using liquid nitrogen to freeze the lesion is another destruction technique. A series of freeze-thaw cycles may be required to completely destroy the tumor.

45300

45300 Proctosigmoidoscopy, rigid; diagnostic, with or without collection of specimen(s) by brushing or washing (separate procedure)

A diagnostic rigid proctosigmoidoscopy is performed with or without collection of specimens by brushing or washing. An obturator is inserted into the scope which is introduced into the anus and advanced approximately 5 cm. The obturator is removed and the eyepiece is attached. The scope is advanced into the rectum using air insufflation to separate the mucosal folds. The scope is advanced to the rectosigmoid junction and, if possible, a short distance into the sigmoid colon. The scope is then withdrawn and the mucosa carefully inspected. Cytology (cell) samples may be obtained using a brush. Alternatively, water may be introduced to wash the mucosal lining, and the fluid aspirated to obtain cell samples. Cytology samples are sent for separately reportable laboratory analysis.

45303

45303 Proctosigmoidoscopy, rigid; with dilation (eg, balloon, guide wire, bougie)

A rigid proctosigmoidoscopy is performed with dilation to treat a stricture of the rectum or sigmoid colon. Strictures are usually a complication of surgery, radiation, or inflammatory disease of the intestine. An obturator is inserted into the scope which is introduced into the anus and advanced approximately 5 cm. The obturator is removed and the eyepiece is attached. The scope is advanced into the rectum to the point of the stricture using air insufflation to separate the mucosal folds. A guide wire is advanced under direct visualization to a point just proximal to the stricture. A balloon catheter is then passed over the guide wire and positioned in the middle of the stricture. The balloon is inflated and left in place for a short period of time, deflated, and then removed. Alternatively, a flexible cylindrical instrument called a bougie may be used to dilate the stricture. The bougie is passed through the stricture to stretch it. Following dilation, the area is inspected using the

scope to ensure that the dilation has been successful and that there are no injuries to the rectum or sigmoid colon resulting from the procedure.

45305

45305 Proctosigmoidoscopy, rigid; with biopsy, single or multiple

The physician inserts an endoscope into the rectal cavity to visualize the rectum and the last section of the large intestine. One or more tissue samples are taken for examination and diagnosis.

45307

45307 Proctosigmoidoscopy, rigid; with removal of foreign body

A rigid proctosigmoidoscopy is performed with removal of a foreign body. An obturator is inserted into the scope which is introduced into the anus and advanced approximately 5 cm. The obturator is removed and the eyepiece is attached. The scope is advanced into the rectum to the site of the foreign body. A balloon catheter may be used to remove a smooth edged foreign body. The catheter tip is passed beyond the level of the foreign body and the balloon is inflated. The catheter is then withdrawn and the foreign body carefully pulled out of the rectum. An impacted foreign body is removed with forceps passed through the endoscope. The impacted foreign body is then grasped and removed. Following removal of the foreign body, the endoscope is reintroduced and the rectum is examined for evidence of perforation or other injury.

45308-45315

45308 Proctosigmoidoscopy, rigid; with removal of single tumor, polyp, or other lesion by hot biopsy forceps or bipolar cautery

45309 Proctosigmoidoscopy, rigid; with removal of single tumor, polyp, or other lesion by snare technique

45315 Proctosigmoidoscopy, rigid; with removal of multiple tumors, polyps, or other lesions by hot biopsy forceps, bipolar cautery or snare technique

A rigid proctosigmoidoscopy is performed with removal of a single tumor, polyp, or other lesion by hot biopsy forceps or bipolar cautery (45308) or snare technique (45309), or multiple tumors, polyps, or other lesions by these techniques (45315). An obturator is inserted into the scope which is introduced into the anus and advanced approximately 5 cm. The obturator is removed and the eyepiece is attached. The scope is advanced into the rectum using air insufflation to separate the mucosal folds. The scope is advanced to the rectosigmoid junction and, if possible, a short distance into the sigmoid colon. The scope is then withdrawn and the mucosa is carefully inspected. The tumor, polyp, or other lesion is identified. In 45308, hot biopsy forceps or bipolar cautery is used to remove the lesion. The hot biopsy method use insulated monopolar forceps to remove and electrocoagulate (cauterize) tissue simultaneously. Bipolar cautery also uses electrical current to remove and cauterize the lesion; however, the current runs from one part of the tip of the forceps to another portion of the forceps. Both hot biopsy forceps and bipolar cautery are used primarily for removal of small polyps and treatment of vascular ectasias. In 45309, a wire loop is placed around the lesion. The loop is heated to shave off and cauterize the lesion. Lesions may be removed en bloc with one placement of the snare or in a piecemeal fashion, which requires multiple applications of the snare. In 45315, one or more of the techniques described above are used to remove multiple tumors, polyps, or other lesions.

45317

45317 Proctosigmoidoscopy, rigid; with control of bleeding (eg, injection, bipolar cautery, unipolar cautery, laser, heater probe, stapler, plasma coagulator)

A rigid proctosigmoidoscopy is performed with control of bleeding by injection, bipolar/unipolar cautery, laser, heater probe, stapler, plasma coagulator, or other technique. An obturator is inserted into the scope which is introduced into the anus and advanced approximately 5 cm. The obturator is removed and the eyepiece is attached. The scope is advanced into the rectum using air insufflation to separate the mucosal folds. The scope is advanced to the rectosigmoid junction and, if possible, a short distance into the sigmoid colon. The scope is then withdrawn and the mucosa is carefully inspected. The bleeding site is identified. Bleeding is typically controlled using a contact thermal modality, such as bipolar or unipolar cautery, or a heater probe. The cautery device or heater probe is applied to the bleeding point and pressure is applied along with heat to control bleeding. An injection of epinephrine, which works as a vasoconstrictor and tamponade, can also be used to reduce or stop bleeding. YAG laser coagulation and a newer modality, the argon plasma coagulator, are noncontact devices used to coagulate the bleeding site. Staples or hemoclips may be used to approximate the margins of a tear or laceration.

45320

45320 Proctosigmoidoscopy, rigid; with ablation of tumor(s), polyp(s), or other lesion(s) not amenable to removal by hot biopsy forceps, bipolar cautery or snare technique (eg, laser)

A rigid proctosigmoidoscopy is performed with ablation of tumors, polyps, or lesions by a technique other than hot biopsy forceps, bipolar cautery, or snare technique. An obturator is inserted into the scope which is introduced into the anus and advanced approximately

Digestive System

5 cm. The obturator is removed and the eyepiece is attached. The scope is advanced into the rectum using air insufflation to separate the mucosal folds. The scope is advanced to the rectosigmoid junction and, if possible, a short distance into the sigmoid colon. The scope is then withdrawn and the mucosa is carefully inspected. The tumor, polyp, or other lesion is identified and ablated using a technique such as laser ablation. The laser device is delivered through the endoscope to the proximal margin of the lesion. Beginning at the proximal margin, the lesion is ablated as the endoscope is retracted. The laser device traverses the entire lesion and destroys it.

45321

45321   Proctosigmoidoscopy, rigid; with decompression of volvulus

A rigid proctosigmoidoscopy is performed with decompression of volvulus. Volvulus is a twisting of the intestines causing obstruction. An obturator is inserted into the scope which is introduced into the anus and advanced approximately 5 cm. The obturator is removed and the eyepiece is attached. The scope is advanced into the rectum to the point of the volvulus using air insufflation to separate the mucosal folds. The mucosa is carefully inspected for evidence of ischemia or necrosis. If the mucosa appears healthy, a rectal tube is passed beyond the twisted segment of intestine until gas and stool is released. The scope is removed and the rectal tube is secured to the perianal region and left in place for 48 hours.

45327

45327   Proctosigmoidoscopy, rigid; with transendoscopic stent placement (includes predilation)

A rigid proctosigmoidoscopy is performed with transendoscopic stent placement including predilation. Stenting is performed to treat intestinal obstruction due to malignant neoplasm. An obturator is inserted into the scope which is introduced into the anus and advanced approximately 5 cm. The obturator is removed and the eyepiece is attached. The scope is advanced to the point of the obstruction using air insufflation to separate the mucosal folds. The scope is then withdrawn and the mucosa is carefully inspected for evidence of ischemia or necrosis. If the mucosa appears healthy, a guide wire is introduced through the scope and advanced across the lesion. If predilation is required, a balloon catheter is passed over the guide wire and positioned in the middle of the stricture. The balloon is inflated and left in place for a short period of time, deflated, and then removed. An appropriately sized stent is selected and passed over the guide wire and across the area of obstruction. The stent is deployed under endoscopic vision and the scope is removed.

45330-45331

45330   Sigmoidoscopy, flexible; diagnostic, including collection of specimen(s) by brushing or washing, when performed (separate procedure)
45331   Sigmoidoscopy, flexible; with biopsy, single or multiple

A flexible sigmoidoscopy is performed with or without collection of specimens by brushing or washing in 45330 and with single or multiple biopsies in 45331. A standard flexible sigmoidoscope is introduced into the anus and advanced through the rectum and into the sigmoid colon while using air insufflation to separate the mucosal folds. Mucosal surfaces of the colon are inspected and any abnormalities are noted. The endoscope is then withdrawn and mucosal surfaces are again inspected for ulcerations, varices, bleeding sites, lesions, strictures, or other abnormalities. A brush is introduced through the endoscope and cell (cytology) samples are obtained. Alternatively, sterile water may be introduced to wash the mucosal lining and the fluid aspirated to obtain cell samples. In 45331, any suspect site to be biopsied is identified and biopsy forceps are placed through the biopsy channel in the endoscope. The forceps are opened, the tissue is spiked, and the forceps are closed. The biopsied tissue is then removed through the endoscope. One or more tissue samples may be obtained. The cell or tissue samples are sent for separately reportable laboratory analysis.

45332

45332   Sigmoidoscopy, flexible; with removal of foreign body(s)

A flexible sigmoidoscopy is performed with removal of foreign body(s). A standard flexible sigmoidoscope is introduced into the anus and advanced through the rectum and into the sigmoid colon while using air insufflation to separate the mucosal folds. Mucosal surfaces of the colon are inspected and any abnormalities are noted. The scope is advanced to the site of the foreign body. A balloon catheter may be used to remove a smooth-edged foreign body. The catheter tip is passed beyond the level of the foreign body and the balloon is inflated. The catheter is then withdrawn and the foreign body is carefully pulled out of the sigmoid colon and rectum. An impacted foreign body is removed with forceps passed through the endoscope. The impacted foreign body is grasped and removed. Following removal of the foreign body(s), the endoscope is reintroduced and the rectum and sigmoid colon are examined for evidence of perforation or other injury.

45333

45333   Sigmoidoscopy, flexible; with removal of tumor(s), polyp(s), or other lesion(s) by hot biopsy forceps

A flexible sigmoidoscopy is performed with removal of tumors, polyps, or other lesions by hot biopsy forceps. A standard flexible sigmoidoscope is introduced into the anus and advanced through the rectum into the sigmoid colon while using air insufflation to separate the mucosal folds. The scope is then withdrawn and the mucosa is carefully inspected. The tumor, polyp, or other lesion is identified and hot biopsy forceps are used to remove the lesion. Hot biopsy method uses insulated monopolar forceps to remove and electrocoagulate (cauterize) tissue simultaneously. Hot biopsy forceps are used primarily for removal of small polyps and treatment of vascular ectasias. The endoscope is then withdrawn and mucosal surfaces are again inspected for ulcerations, varices, bleeding sites, lesions, strictures, or other abnormalities.

45334

45334   Sigmoidoscopy, flexible; with control of bleeding, any method

A flexible sigmoidoscopy is performed with control of bleeding by any method. Some methods used for controlling bleeding include injection, bipolar/unipolar cautery, laser, heater probe, stapler, plasma coagulator, or other technique. A standard flexible sigmoidoscope is introduced into the anus and advanced through the rectum into the sigmoid colon while using air insufflation to separate the mucosal folds. The scope is then withdrawn and the mucosa is carefully inspected. The bleeding site is identified. Bleeding is typically controlled using a contact thermal modality, such as bipolar or unipolar cautery, or a heater probe. The cautery device or heater probe is applied to the bleeding point and pressure is applied along with heat to control bleeding. An injection of epinephrine, which works as a vasoconstrictor and tamponade, can also be used to reduce or stop bleeding. YAG laser coagulation and a newer modality, the argon plasma coagulator, are noncontact devices used to coagulate the bleeding site. Staples or hemoclips may be used to approximate the margins of a tear or laceration. The endoscope is then withdrawn and mucosal surfaces are again inspected for ulcerations, varices, other bleeding sites, lesions, strictures, or other abnormalities.

45335

45335   Sigmoidoscopy, flexible; with directed submucosal injection(s), any substance

A flexible sigmoidoscopy is performed with directed submucosal injection(s) of any substance. Commonly used substances include India ink, saline, epinephrine, or corticosteroids. India ink is used to help mark or delineate a lesion for better visualization prior to separately reportable excision, also referred to as tattooing. Saline or epinephrine may also be injected prior to removal to create a submucosal fluid cushion and help separate the mucosal layer from the muscle layer of the colon and elevate the lesion. A standard flexible sigmoidoscope is introduced into the anus and advanced through the rectum into the sigmoid colon while using air insufflation to separate the mucosal folds. The scope is then withdrawn and the mucosa is carefully inspected. The lesion is identified and one or more submucosal injections are administered. The endoscope is withdrawn and mucosal surfaces are again inspected for ulcerations, varices, bleeding sites, lesions, strictures, or other abnormalities.

45337

45337   Sigmoidoscopy, flexible; with decompression (for pathologic distention) (eg, volvulus, megacolon), including placement of decompression tube, when performed

A flexible sigmoidoscopy is performed with decompression of pathologic distention such as volvulus and tube placement, if performed. Volvulus is a twisting of the intestine on its mesenteric pedicle, causing obstruction and leaving a loop of intestine distended with feces and gas. Volvulus tends to occur particularly in the sigmoid segment of the colon from long standing constipation when an elongated and atonic colon develops. This is also known as acquired megacolon and can lead to tissue infarction from disruption of the blood supply and perforation with peritonitis. A standard flexible sigmoidoscope is introduced into the anus and advanced through the rectum as far as possible to the point of the volvulus using air insufflation to separate the musocal folds. The mucosa is carefully inspected for evidence of ischemia or necrosis. If the mucosa appears healthy, a flatus tube is passed alongside the scope and gently passed through the twisted segment of intestine to a site just proximal to the obstruction. As rapid decompression occurs, the backed up liquid feces and gas evacuate with relief of the obstruction. Or, a suction device may be attached to the scope and fluid, stool, and debris evacuated from the colon. After decompression of the distended colon, the tube is left in place for 24-48 hours to maintain the decompression and allow time for oxygenation of the previously twisted bowel wall. The scope is then withdrawn.

45338

45338   Sigmoidoscopy, flexible; with removal of tumor(s), polyp(s), or other lesion(s) by snare technique

A flexible sigmoidoscopy is performed with removal of tumors, polyps, or other lesions by snare technique. A standard flexible sigmoidoscope is introduced into the anus and advanced through the rectum into the sigmoid colon while using air insufflation to separate the mucosal folds. The scope is then withdrawn and the mucosa is carefully inspected. The tumor, polyp, or other lesion is identified and a wire snare loop is placed around the lesion. The loop is heated to shave off and cauterize the lesion. Lesions may be removed en bloc with one placement of the snare or in a piecemeal fashion which requires multiple applications of the snare. The endoscope is then withdrawn and mucosal surfaces are again inspected for ulcerations, varices, bleeding sites, lesions, strictures, or other abnormalities.

45340

45340   Sigmoidoscopy, flexible; with transendoscopic balloon dilation

A flexible sigmoidoscopy is performed with transendoscopic balloon dilation. Strictures are usually a complication of surgery, radiation, or inflammatory disease of the intestine. A standard flexible sigmoidoscope is introduced into the anus and advanced through the rectum into the sigmoid colon. The narrowed area of the colon is identified and dilated with a balloon device through the scope. The deflated balloon catheter is advanced through the instrument channel of the scope to the middle of the stricture. The balloon is then inflated while using a pressure gauge to determine the optimal level of inflation. The inflated balloon is left in place for a short period of time (30 seconds to two minutes), deflated, and then removed. Following dilation, the area of stricture is inspected using the scope to ensure that the dilation has been successful and there are no injuries to the colon.

45341

45341   Sigmoidoscopy, flexible; with endoscopic ultrasound examination

A flexible sigmoidoscopy is performed with an endoscopic ultrasound examination. A standard flexible sigmoidoscope is introduced into the anus and advanced through the rectum into the sigmoid colon while using air insufflation to separate the mucosal folds. The scope is then withdrawn and the mucosa is carefully inspected. Any abnormalities are noted. Following endoscopic examination, an echoendoscope is introduced and may be advanced as far as a part of the descending colon. The balloon which covers the transducer housing is filled with water to facilitate acoustic coupling. Continuous ultrasound imaging is performed. Ultrasound images are obtained to help evaluate abnormalities. Typically, echoendoscopy is performed to evaluate the depth of a tumor or lesion and to determine whether it has advanced beyond the mucosa into the submucosa or muscular wall of the colon and whether there is transmural or adjacent organ involvement. Once the tumor or lesion has been fully evaluated, the echoendoscope is then removed.

45342

45342   Sigmoidoscopy, flexible; with transendoscopic ultrasound guided intramural or transmural fine needle aspiration/biopsy(s)

A flexible sigmoidoscopy is performed with transendoscopic ultrasound-guided intramural or transmural fine needle aspiration/biopsy. A standard flexible sigmoidoscope is introduced into the anus and advanced through the rectum into the sigmoid colon while using air insufflation to separate the mucosal folds. The mucosa is carefully inspected. Any abnormalities are noted. A radial scanning echoendoscope is then introduced and advanced under direct endoscopic visualization. Ultrasound imaging is used to evaluate the structures exterior to the rectum and sigmoid colon. Adjacent structures are assessed for the presence of enlarged lymph nodes. Other lesions are identified and determination is made whether they arise from the sigmoid colon or rectum or other structures and whether the tumor(s) has invaded other vital structures. Ultrasound images are then sent to a hard copy device and evaluated. Lymph nodes and other lesions that can be biopsied through the sigmoid colon or rectum are identified. The radial scanning echoendoscope is removed and replaced with a linear scanning echoendoscope. A needle biopsy catheter is advanced through the biopsy channel of the echoendoscope. Doppler images are obtained to ensure that there are no vascular structures obstructing the planned biopsy route. The needle is then advanced through the intestinal wall into the lesion or lymph node and an aspiration biopsy is obtained and sent for separately reportable cytologic evaluation. Multiple passes are made at each biopsy site. After each pass, the biopsy device is removed, cleaned, and reassembled. Once an adequate specimen has been obtained from the first biopsy site, the next biopsy site is addressed in the same manner.

45346

45346   Sigmoidoscopy, flexible; with ablation of tumor(s), polyp(s), or other lesion(s) (includes pre- and post-dilation and guide wire passage, when performed)

A flexible sigmoidoscopy is performed with tumor, polyp, or lesion ablation. A standard flexible sigmoidoscope is introduced into the anus and advanced through the rectum into the sigmoid colon while using air insufflation to separate the mucosal folds. The scope is

then withdrawn and the mucosa is carefully inspected. The site of the tumor(s), polyp(s), or other lesion(s) to be ablated is identified. If dilation is required to allow better access for the ablation procedure, a guide wire is inserted through the scope. A series of rigid tubes of increasing diameter are then passed over the guide wire and the lumen of the large intestine is dilated as needed. Alternately, a balloon catheter may be advanced to the site of the stricture and inflated to dilate the narrowed area. The balloon catheter is removed and the laser device is then delivered through the endoscope to the distal margin of the most distal lesion. The lesion is ablated as the endoscope is retracted. The entire lesion is destroyed as the laser traverses the lesion in a distal to proximal direction. This is repeated until all lesions have been destroyed. If dilation is required following destruction of lesions, it is performed again. The colon is once again examined using the endoscope to ensure that all lesions have been destroyed and that there are no injuries resulting from the procedure.

45347

45347   Sigmoidoscopy, flexible; with placement of endoscopic stent (includes pre- and post-dilation and guide wire passage, when performed)

A flexible sigmoidoscopy is performed with endoscopic stent placement including pre- and post-dilation of the narrowed segment of colon over a guidewire. A standard flexible sigmoidoscope is introduced into the anus and advanced through the rectum into the sigmoid colon while using air insufflation to separate the mucosal folds and allow better visualization of the mucosa. The scope is then positioned at the area of stenosis and the position and length of the stenosis are determined. The stricture is examined and the need for pre-dilation is evaluated. If pre-dilation is needed, a guide wire is inserted through the scope and a series of rigid tubes of increasing diameter are passed over the guide wire to dilate the stricture. Alternatively, a balloon catheter may be advanced to the site of the stricture and inflated to dilate the stricture. Stent placement is then performed. A guide wire is passed through the scope followed by the stent delivery system which is passed over the guide wire and positioned in the narrowed portion of the colon. An appropriately sized stent is selected and introduced through the scope. The stent is then positioned in the narrowed portion of the colon and deployed (expanded). A balloon catheter may again be inserted and inflated to seat the stent. The endoscope is advanced through the stent to verify correct stent position and ensure proper deployment and the scope is withdrawn.

45349

45349   Sigmoidoscopy, flexible; with endoscopic mucosal resection

A flexible sigmoidoscopy is performed with endoscopic mucosal resection. A standard flexible sigmoidoscope is introduced into the anus and advanced through the rectum into the sigmoid colon or a portion of the descending colon while using air insufflation to separate the mucosal folds for better visualization. The scope is then withdrawn as the entire circumference of the colon is examined. The mucosal lesion is identified. The borders of the lesion are marked with electrocautery. Diluted adrenaline is injected into the submucosal layer around the lesion to separate the mucosal layer containing the lesion from the underlying muscle. A snare with a suction cup is used to further separate the mucosal lesion from underlying tissue. The lesion is then excised and captured using the snare and the scope is withdrawn.

45350

45350   Sigmoidoscopy, flexible; with band ligation(s) (eg, hemorrhoids)

A flexible sigmoidoscopy is performed with band ligation of hemorrhoids. A standard flexible sigmoidoscope is introduced into the anus and advanced through the rectum into the sigmoid colon or a portion of the descending colon while using air insufflation to separate the mucosal folds for better visualization. The scope is then withdrawn as the entire circumference of the colon is examined. Band ligation, or rubber band ligature, is then used to treat one or more internal hemorrhoids. The hemorrhoid(s) is located, grasped with forceps, and pulled through the barrel of the ligature device. The physician takes care to ensure that the entire hemorrhoid is contained in the barrel. The rubber band is then applied to the hemorrhoid by squeezing the handle of the ligator. A second rubber band is placed in the same manner to ensure that blood supply to the hemorrhoid is interrupted even if one of the bands breaks. After all hemorrhoids are ligated, the instruments are removed.

45378

45378   Colonoscopy, flexible; diagnostic, including collection of specimen(s) by brushing or washing, when performed (separate procedure)

A flexible colonoscopy is performed with or without collection of specimens by brushing or washing. The colonoscope is inserted into the rectum and advanced through the colon to the cecum or a point within the terminal ileum, using air insufflation to separate the mucosal folds for better visualization. Mucosal surfaces of the colon are inspected and any abnormalities are noted. The endoscope is then withdrawn as mucosal surfaces are again inspected for ulcerations, varices, bleeding sites, lesions, strictures, or other abnormalities. Cytology (cell) samples may be obtained using a brush introduced through the endoscope. Alternatively, sterile water may be introduced to wash the mucosal lining and the fluid aspirated to obtain cell samples. Cytology samples are sent for separately reportable laboratory analysis.

Colonoscopy

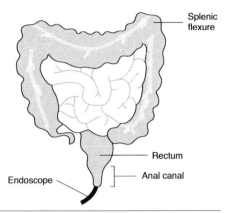

Splenic flexure

Rectum

Anal canal

Endoscope

45379

45379   Colonoscopy, flexible; with removal of foreign body(s)

A flexible colonoscopy is performed with removal of foreign body(s). The colonoscope is inserted into the rectum and advanced through the colon to the cecum or a point within the terminal ileum, using air insufflation to separate the mucosal folds for better visualization. Mucosal surfaces of the colon are inspected and the foreign body is located. A balloon catheter may be used to remove a smooth-edged foreign body. The catheter tip is passed beyond the level of the foreign body and the balloon is inflated. The catheter is then withdrawn and the foreign body is carefully pulled out of the sigmoid colon and rectum. An impacted foreign body is removed with forceps passed through the endoscope. The impacted foreign body is grasped and removed. Following removal of the foreign body(s), the endoscope is reintroduced and the colon is examined for evidence of perforation or other injury.

45380

45380   Colonoscopy, flexible; with biopsy, single or multiple

A flexible colonoscopy is performed with with single or multiple biopsies. The colonoscope is inserted into the rectum and advanced through the colon to the cecum or a point within the terminal ileum, using air insufflation to separate the mucosal folds for better visualization. Mucosal surfaces of the colon are inspected and any abnormalities are noted. The endoscope is then withdrawn and mucosal surfaces are again inspected for ulcerations, varices, bleeding sites, lesions, strictures, or other abnormalities. Any suspect site(s) to be biopsied is identified and biopsy forceps are placed through the biopsy channel in the endoscope. The forceps are opened, the tissue is spiked, and the forceps are closed. The biopsied tissue is then removed through the endoscope. One or more tissue samples may be obtained and are sent for separately reportable laboratory analysis.

Colonoscopy

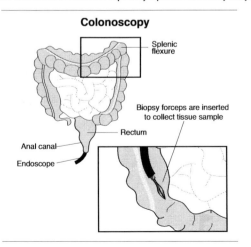

Splenic flexure

Biopsy forceps are inserted to collect tissue sample

Rectum

Anal canal

Endoscope

45381

45381   Colonoscopy, flexible; with directed submucosal injection(s), any substance

A flexible colonoscopy is performed with directed submucosal injection(s) of any substance. Commonly used substances include India ink, saline, epinephrine, or corticosteroid

substances. India ink is used to help delineate a lesion prior to separately reportable excision which may also be referred to as tattooing of the lesion. Saline or epinephrine may also be injected prior to separately reportable lesion excision to help separate the mucosal layer from the muscle layer of the colon and elevate the lesion. The colonoscope is inserted into the rectum and advanced through the colon to the cecum or a point within the terminal ileum, using air insufflation to separate the mucosal folds for better visualization. Mucosal surfaces of the colon are inspected and any abnormalities are noted. The lesion is identified and one or more submucosal injections are administered. The endoscope is withdrawn and mucosal surfaces are again inspected for ulcerations, bleeding sites, lesions, strictures, or other abnormalities.

45382

45382   Colonoscopy, flexible; with control of bleeding, any method

A flexible colonoscopy is performed beyond with control of bleeding by any method. Some methods used for controlling bleeding include injection, bipolar/unipolar cautery, laser, heater probe, stapler, plasma coagulator, or other technique. The colonoscope is inserted into the rectum and advanced through the colon to the cecum or a point within the terminal ileum, using air insufflation to separate the mucosal folds for better visualization. Mucosal surfaces of the colon are inspected and any abnormalities are noted. The bleeding site is identified. Bleeding is typically controlled using a contact thermal modality, such as bipolar or unipolar cautery or a heater probe. The cautery device or heater probe is applied to the bleeding point and pressure is applied along with heat to control bleeding. An injection of epinephrine, which works as a vascoconstrictor and tamponade, can also be used to reduce or stop bleeding. YAG laser coagulation and a newer modality, the argon plasma coagulator, are noncontact devices used to coagulate the bleeding site. Staples or hemoclips may be used to approximate the margins of a tear or laceration. The endoscope is then withdrawn and mucosal surfaces are again inspected for ulcerations, varices, other bleeding sites, lesions, strictures, or other abnormalities.

45384–45385

45384   Colonoscopy, flexible; with removal of tumor(s), polyp(s), or other lesion(s) by hot biopsy forceps

45385   Colonoscopy, flexible; with removal of tumor(s), polyp(s), or other lesion(s) by snare technique

A flexible colonoscopy is performed with removal of tumors, polyps, or other lesions by hot biopsy forceps (45384) or snare technique (45385). The colonoscope is inserted into the rectum and advanced through the colon to the cecum or a point within the terminal ileum, using air insufflation to separate the mucosal folds for better visualization. Mucosal surfaces of the colon are inspected and any abnormalities are noted. The tumor, polyp, or other lesion is identified. In 45384, hot biopsy forceps are used to remove the lesion. Hot biopsy method uses insulated monopolar forceps to remove and electrocoagulate (cauterize) tissue simultaneously. Hot biopsy forceps are used primarily for removal of small polyps and treatment of vascular ectasias. In 45385, a wire snare loop is placed around the lesion. The loop is heated to shave off and cauterize the lesion. Lesions may be removed en bloc with one placement of the snare or in a piecemeal fashion which requires multiple applications of the snare. The endoscope is withdrawn and mucosal surfaces are again inspected for ulcerations, bleeding sites, lesions, strictures, or other abnormalities.

45386

45386   Colonoscopy, flexible; with transendoscopic balloon dilation

A flexible colonoscopy is performed with transendoscopic balloon dilation of one or more strictures. Strictures are usually a complication of surgery, radiation, or inflammatory disease of the intestine. The flexible colonoscope is inserted into the rectum and advanced through the colon. The narrowed area of the colon is identified and dilated with a balloon device through the scope. The deflated balloon catheter is advanced through the instrument channel of the scope to the middle of the stricture. The balloon is then inflated while using a pressure gauge to determine the optimal level of inflation. The inflated balloon is left in place for a short period of time, deflated, and then removed. If multiple strictures are present, the scope and balloon catheter are advanced to the next stricture and the dilation procedure is repeated until all areas of stricture have been addressed. Following dilation, each area of stricture is inspected to ensure that the dilation has been successful and there are no injuries to the colon.

45388

45388   Colonoscopy, flexible; with ablation of tumor(s), polyp(s), or other lesion(s) (includes pre- and post-dilation and guide wire passage, when performed)

A flexible colonoscopy is performed with tumor, polyp, or lesion ablation. A standard flexible colonoscope is introduced into the rectum and advanced through the colon to the cecum or a point within the terminal ileum while using air insufflation to separate the mucosal folds for better visualization. The scope is then withdrawn and the mucosa is carefully inspected. The site of the tumor(s), polyp(s), or other lesion(s) to be ablated is identified. If dilation is required to allow better access for the ablation procedure, a guide wire is inserted through the scope. A series of rigid tubes of increasing diameter are

Digestive System

then passed over the guide wire and the lumen of the large intestine is dilated as needed. Alternately, a balloon catheter may be advanced to the site of the stricture and inflated to dilate the narrowed area. The balloon catheter is removed and the laser device is then delivered through the endoscope to the distal margin of the most distal lesion. The lesion is ablated as the endoscope is retracted. The entire lesion is destroyed as the laser traverses the lesion in a distal to proximal direction. This is repeated until all lesions have been destroyed. If dilation is required following destruction of lesions, it is performed again. The colon is once again examined using the endoscope to ensure that all lesions have been destroyed and that there are no injuries resulting from the procedure.

45389

45389　Colonoscopy, flexible; with endoscopic stent placement (includes pre- and post-dilation and guide wire passage, when performed)

A flexible colonoscopy is performed with endoscopic stent placement including pre- and post-dilation of the narrowed segment of colon over a guidewire. A standard flexible colonoscope is introduced into the anus and advanced through the rectum into the colon while using air insufflation to separate the mucosal folds and allow better visualization of the mucosa. The scope is then positioned at the area of stenosis and the position and length of the stenosis are determined. The stricture is examined and the need for pre-dilation is evaluated. If pre-dilation is needed, a guide wire is inserted through the scope and a series of rigid tubes of increasing diameter are passed over the guide wire to dilate the stricture. Alternatively, a balloon catheter may be advanced to the site of the stricture and inflated to dilate the stricture. Stent placement is then performed. A guide wire is passed through the scope followed by the stent delivery system which is passed over the guide wire and positioned in the narrowed portion of the colon. An appropriately sized stent is selected and introduced through the scope. The stent is then positioned in the narrowed portion of the colon and deployed (expanded). A balloon catheter may again be inserted and inflated to seat the stent. The endoscope is advanced through the stent to verify correct stent position and ensure proper deployment and the scope is withdrawn.

45390

45390　Colonoscopy, flexible; with endoscopic mucosal resection

A flexible colonoscopy is performed with endoscopic mucosal resection. A standard flexible colonoscope is introduced into the rectum and advanced through the colon to the cecum or a point within the terminal ileum while using air insufflation to separate the mucosal folds for better visualization. The scope is then withdrawn as the entire circumference of the colon is examined. The mucosal lesion is identified. The borders of the lesion are marked with electrocautery. Diluted adrenaline is injected into the submucosal layer around the lesion to separate the mucosal layer containing the lesion from the underlying muscle. A snare with a suction cup is used to further separate the mucosal lesion from underlying tissue. The lesion is then excised and captured using the snare and the scope is withdrawn.

45391-45392

45391　Colonoscopy, flexible; with endoscopic ultrasound examination limited to the rectum, sigmoid, descending, transverse, or ascending colon and cecum, and adjacent structures

45392　Colonoscopy, flexible; with transendoscopic ultrasound guided intramural or transmural fine needle aspiration/biopsy(s), includes endoscopic ultrasound examination limited to the rectum, sigmoid, descending, transverse, or ascending colon and cecum, and adjacent structures

A flexible colonoscopy is performed with endoscopic ultrasound examination. A standard flexible colonoscope is introduced into the rectum and advanced through the colon to the cecum or a point within the terminal ileum while using air insufflation to separate the mucosal folds for better visualization. The scope is then withdrawn as the entire circumference of the colon is examined for any evidence of disease or injury. An echoendoscope is then inserted into the rectum for ultrasound examination of the rectum, the entire colon, cecum, and adjacent structures. The balloon which covers the transducer housing is filled with water to facilitate acoustic coupling. Continuous ultrasound imaging is performed. Ultrasound allows visualization of a lesion, mass, compression, or other area of concern along with the walls of the colon and pericolonic structures such as lymph nodes. In 45392, the echoendoscope is advanced under direct visualization to an area of compression in the colon that is exterior to the colon mucosa. The mass exterior to the colon or within the muscular wall of the colon is identified. Ultrasound images are obtained and lymph nodes and other lesions that can be biopsied through the colon are identified. A fine needle aspiration/biopsy catheter is advanced through the biopsy channel of the echoendoscope. Doppler images are obtained to ensure that there are no vascular structures obstructing the planned biopsy route. The needle is then advanced through the colon wall into the lesion or lymph node and a needle biopsy is obtained. Multiple passes are made at each biopsy site. After each pass, the biopsy device is removed, cleaned, and reassembled. Once an adequate specimen has been obtained from the first biopsy site, the next biopsy site is addressed in the same manner. All biopsy specimens are sent to the laboratory for separately reportable cytologic examination.

45393

45393　Colonoscopy, flexible; with decompression (for pathologic distention) (eg, volvulus, megacolon), including placement of decompression tube, when performed

A flexible colonoscopy is performed with decompression of pathologic distention, such as volvulus, and tube placement, if performed. Volvulus is a twisting of the intestine on its mesenteric pedicle, causing obstruction and leaving a loop of intestine distended with feces and gas. Volvulus tends to occur particularly in the sigmoid segment of the colon from long standing constipation when an elongated and atonic colon develops. This is also known as acquired megacolon and can lead to tissue infarction from disruption of the blood supply, and perforation with peritonitis. A standard flexible colonoscope is introduced into the rectum and advanced through the colon. Mucosal surfaces of the colon from the rectum to the cecum are inspected as far as possible to the point of the volvulus using air insufflation to separate the musocal folds. The mucosa is carefully inspected for evidence of ischemia or necrosis. If the mucosa appears healthy, a flatus tube is passed alongside the scope and gently passed through the twisted segment of intestine to a site just proximal to the obstruction. As rapid decompression occurs, the backed up liquid feces and gas evacuate with relief of the obstruction. Or, a suction device may be attached to the scope and fluid, stool, and debris are evacuated from the colon. After decompression of the distended colon, the tube is left in place for 24-48 hours to maintain the decompression and allow time for oxygenation of the previously twisted bowel wall. The scope is then withdrawn.

45395-45397

45395　Laparoscopy, surgical; proctectomy, complete, combined abdominoperineal, with colostomy

45397　Laparoscopy, surgical; proctectomy, combined abdominoperineal pull-through procedure (eg, colo-anal anastomosis), with creation of colonic reservoir (eg, J-pouch), with diverting enterostomy, when performed

A small portal incision is made near the umbilicus, a trocar inserted, and pneumoperitoneum established. Additional portal incisions are made and trocars placed in the upper and lower quadrants of the abdomen. The abdominal cavity is inspected. In 45395, a complete proctectomy with colostomy is performed. The sigmoid colon is retracted medially and mobilized along the line of Toldt to the splenic flexure. The sigmoid colon is then retracted laterally. The left ureter is identified and protected. The sigmoid mesentery is incised at the pelvic brim and dissected and the inferior mesenteric artery and vein are isolated, ligated, and transected. The rectum and surrounding mesentery are freed from pelvic and abdominal attachments. The colon is clamped and divided at the level of the sigmoid junction. The perineum is incised in a circular fashion around the rectum. The rectum and surrounding mesentery are delivered en bloc through the perineal incision. The perineal incision is closed. The stoma site is prepared around one of the previously placed trocars. Gas is released from the abdomen and the proximal segment of colon exteriorized through the stoma incision. The colon is folded back on itself (everted) and sutured to the skin and subcutaneous tissue. Drains are placed in the abdomen and the portal incisions closed. A stoma appliance is placed. In 45397, a proctectomy is performed using pull-through procedure with creation of a colonic reservoir such as a J-pouch with a diverting enterostomy when performed. The proctectomy is performed as described above. The segment of colon to be used as the reservoir is identified and the colon is mobilized. Folding the colon back on itself creates a colonic reservoir. The colon is then sutured together and the antimesenteric border incised parallel to the suture line to open the pouch and expose the mucosa. The previously placed suture lines in the colon wall are reinforced by suturing the mucosal layer to create a two-layer closure. The pouch is closed and positioned in the pelvis. The anastomosis site in the anus is prepared by placing sutures around the circumference of the anus. The anal mucosa and the colon are sutured together (anastomosed). If a diverting enterostomy is required, the enterostomy site is selected and the abdomen incised. The intestinal segment is mobilized and transected. The distal segment is closed and the proximal segment brought out through the stoma incision. The intestine is folded back on itself (everted) and sutured to the skin and subcutaneous tissue. The procedure is completed as described above.

45398

45398　Colonoscopy, flexible; with band ligation(s) (eg, hemorrhoids)

A flexible colonoscopy is performed with band ligation of hemorrhoids. A standard flexible colonoscope is introduced into the rectum and advanced through the colon to the cecum or a point within the terminal ileum while using air insufflation to separate the mucosal folds for better visualization. The scope is then withdrawn as the entire circumference of the colon is examined for any evidence of disease or injury. Band ligation, or rubber band ligature, is then used to treat one or more internal hemorrhoids. The hemorrhoid(s) is located, grasped with forceps, and pulled through the barrel of the ligature device. The physician takes care to ensure that the entire hemorrhoid is contained in the barrel. The rubber band is then applied to the hemorrhoid by squeezing the handle of the ligator. A second rubber band is placed in the same manner to ensure that blood supply to the hemorrhoid is interrupted even if one of the bands breaks. After all hemorrhoids are ligated, the instruments are removed.

Digestive System

45400-45402

45400 Laparoscopy, surgical; proctopexy (for prolapse)
45402 Laparoscopy, surgical; proctopexy (for prolapse), with sigmoid resection

A small portal incision is made near the umbilicus, a trocar inserted, and pneumoperitoneum established. Additional portal incisions are made and trocars placed in the upper and lower quadrants of the abdomen. The abdominal cavity is inspected. The sigmoid colon and rectum are dissected off the presacral fascia and mobilized. The presacral space is entered, the rectum mobilized distally. The rectal prolapse is reduced and the segment of colon that is to be attached to the sacrum identified. The sigmoid colon may be resected along with a portion of the upper rectum to allow adequate reduction of the prolapse. The vascular supply is interrupted by ligating and dividing the inferior mesenteric artery or the individual sigmoid arteries. The transection sites are identified and clamps placed above and below the proximal and distal transection sites. The sigmoid colon is transected distally. A small muscle splitting incision is made in the abdomen and the proximal segment is exteriorized and transected. The anvil of the stapler device is inserted in the remaining proximal segment and secured with a pursestring suture. The proximal segment is returned to the abdomen and the remaining sigmoid colon and rectum anastomosed by a transanal approach. The clamps are removed. The rectum is fixed to the sacrum or sacral promontory with sutures. The laparoscope and trocars are removed and the portal incisions closed. Use 45400, when the procedure is performed without sigmoid colon resection and 45402 when sigmoid colon resection is performed.

45500-45505

45500 Proctoplasty; for stenosis
45505 Proctoplasty; for prolapse of mucous membrane

These proctoplasty procedures are not specific as to technique. Any procedure that effectively rearranges the tissue to relieve the stenosis or relieve the prolapse may be used. In 45500, proctoplasty for stenosis is performed. The narrowed segment of the rectum is inspected. The physician then makes a series of incisions to relieve the stenosis. Tissue is rearranged as needed or local flaps created to widen the stenotic region. In 45505, proctoplasty is performed for prolapse of the mucous membrane of the rectum. One method is to excise the excess mucosal tissue from the rectum. The muscular wall is then arranged in folds to narrow and tighten the wall of the rectum. The remaining rectal mucosa is then sutured to the anal mucosa.

45520

45520 Perirectal injection of sclerosing solution for prolapse

Rectal prolapse may be partial or complete. Partial prolapse involves protrusion of only the rectal mucosa through the anus while complete prolapse involves protrusion of a portion of the entire thickness of the rectum. Injection of sclerosing solution is used primarily to treat partial prolapse. Sclerosing solution such as saline, alcohol, or phenol is prepared. A gloved finger may be inserted into the rectum to help position the needle tip appropriately. The sclerosing solution is infiltrated into perirectal tissue laterally and posteriorly.

45540-45550

45540 Proctopexy (eg, for prolapse); abdominal approach
45541 Proctopexy (eg, for prolapse); perineal approach
45550 Proctopexy (eg, for prolapse); with sigmoid resection, abdominal approach

These procedures are performed to treat prolapse of the rectum. In 45540, a midline abdominal incision is made. The sigmoid colon and rectum are dissected off the presacral fascia and mobilized. The presacral space is entered and the rectum mobilized distally. The rectal prolapse is reduced and the segment of colon that is to be attached to the sacrum identified. The rectum is fixed to the sacrum or sacral promontory with sutures. In 45541, the perineum is incised circumferentially at the rectoanal junction. The rectum is mobilized and rectal prolapse reduced. The rectum is fixed to the sacrum or sacral promontory with sutures. The perineum is repaired in layers. In 45550, the sigmoid colon is resected along with a portion of the upper rectum to allow adequate reduction of the prolapse. The procedure is performed as described in 45540 with the resection performed prior to fixing the rectum to the sacrum or sacral promontory. The vascular supply is interrupted by ligating and dividing the inferior mesenteric artery or the individual sigmoid arteries. Clamps placed above and below the planned proximal and distal transection sites. The sigmoid colon is transected and the segment of sigmoid colon removed. The remaining segments are sutured together (anastomosed) and the clamps are removed.

45560

45560 Repair of rectocele (separate procedure)

A rectocele, also called a proctocele, is a prolapse or herniation of the anterior wall of the rectum into the back wall of the vagina. While rectoceles do occur in men, this is rare. There are a number of different approaches that can be used including transanal, transvaginal, perineal, abdominal or a combined approach. Using a transvaginal approach, the posterior vaginal mucosa is opened up to the vaginal apex. An ellipse of skin at the junction of the vagina and perineum is excised. Perirectal fascia is dissected free of the posterior vaginal mucosa to expose the rectocele. The rectocele is reduced and the margins of the

levator ani muscles located. Sutures are placed from the apical margin of the levator ani to the posterior fourchette and then tied. Excessive vaginal mucosa is trimmed exposing the surgically created triangular defect in the perineal body and the insertion of the bulbocavernosus muscle. The perirectal fascia is closed followed by closure of the posterior vaginal wall. The hymenal ring is reconstructed. The vaginal mucosa is then sutured to the perirectal fascia. The pelvic floor is reinforced by placing sutures in the insertions of the bulbocavernosus muscle. The surgically created defect in the perineal body is closed. Subcutaneous tissues and skin are closed.

45562-45563

45562 Exploration, repair, and presacral drainage for rectal injury
45563 Exploration, repair, and presacral drainage for rectal injury; with colostomy

A penetrating injury to the rectum is explored and repaired and presacral drains are placed. The abdomen is opened and explored. The rectal injury is identified and bleeding controlled. The rectal wound is repaired with sutures. Depending on the nature of the injury a colostomy may be performed to temporarily divert stool from the rectum. If possible the colostomy is performed in the sigmoid colon. The physician may create any type of colostomy with more commonly employed methods being loop colostomy, loop with distal closure, or an end colostomy with mucous fistula. Following the abdominal procedure and stoma creation presacral drains are placed. A curvilinear incision is made between the coccyx and the posterior margin of the anus. The incision is extended through the endopelvic fascia. Blunt dissection is used to open the presacral space. Dissection continues to the site of the rectal injury. A drain is then inserted to the level of the injury and secured to the perianal skin. Use 45562 when the procedure is performed without a colostomy and 45563 when a colostomy is performed.

45800-45805

45800 Closure of rectovesical fistula
45805 Closure of rectovesical fistula; with colostomy

A rectovesical fistula is an abnormal communication or passage between the rectum and urinary bladder. This type of fistula can occur postoperatively or result from chronic infection or inflammation of pelvic structures. The abdomen is opened and the rectovesical fistula located. Adhesions between the rectum and bladder are lysed and the two structures are separated. The opening in the bladder is located and repaired with sutures. The opening in the rectum is inspected and the rectum is closed with sutures. Omentum may be interposed between the bladder and rectum to help prevent recurrence of the fistula. A colostomy may be performed to temporarily divert stool from the rectum. If possible the colostomy is performed in the sigmoid colon. The physician may create any type of colostomy with more commonly employed methods being loop colostomy, loop with distal closure, or an end colostomy with mucous fistula. Drains are placed in the abdomen as needed and the abdominal incision is closed. Use 45800 for closure of rectovesical fistula without colostomy and 45805 if a colostomy is performed.

45820-45825

45820 Closure of rectourethral fistula
45825 Closure of rectourethral fistula; with colostomy

A rectourethral fistula is an abnormal communication or passage between the rectum and urethra. This type of fistula can occur postoperatively or result from chronic infection or inflammation of bowel, malignant neoplasm, or trauma. There are a number of different approaches including abdominal, perineal, and parasacrococcygeal (trans-sphincteric). Prior to the procedure a suprapubic cystostomy may be performed to temporarily divert urine from the urethra. Alternatively, a catheter may be placed in the urethra. Using a trans-sphincteric approach, a curvilinear incision is made between the coccyx and the posterior margin of the anus. The internal sphincter mechanism and posterior rectal wall are divided and the fistula exposed. An incision is made around the fistula and the incision is extended to the opening in the urethra. The rectal wall is undermined and mobilized. The opening in the urethra is closed. Rectal wall flaps are created and sutured over the opening in the rectum. The incision in the posterior rectal wall is closed and the internal sphincter reapproximated. A colostomy may be performed to temporarily divert stool from the rectum. If the closure of the rectourethral fistula has been performed by other than an abdominal approach, the abdomen is opened and a length of sigmoid or other segment of colon mobilized and brought to the abdominal wall. A separate incision may be made for the stoma. The physician may create any type of colostomy with more commonly employed methods being loop colostomy, loop with distal closure, or an end colostomy with mucous fistula. If a loop colostomy is performed, the loop is brought out of the abdominal wall at the stoma site. The loop is incised longitudinally and the edges folded back to expose the mucosa, which is sutured to the abdomen. This creates two stomas. The one from above eliminates stool and the one below, also called a mucous fistula, eliminates mucus. Use 45820 for closure of rectourethral fistula without colostomy and 45825 if a colostomy is performed.

Digestive System

45900

45900   Reduction of procidentia (separate procedure) under anesthesia

The physician reduces procidentia under anesthesia in a separate procedure. Procidentia is complete prolapse of the full-thickness of the rectum through the anus. Following induction of anesthesia, the physician manually manipulates the rectum back through the anus and into normal position. The buttocks are tightly taped together to prevent repeat prolapse. Reduction is usually a temporary measure as most patients require surgical fixation of the rectum to prevent repeat prolapse.

45905-45910

45905   Dilation of anal sphincter (separate procedure) under anesthesia other than local

45910   Dilation of rectal stricture (separate procedure) under anesthesia other than local

In 45905, following induction of anesthesia, manual dilation of the anal sphincter is performed. Using gloved hands, the anus is lubricated. The physician then inserts two gloved fingers of the left hand into the anus. While lifting up with the left hand the physician inserts the gloved index finger of the right hand and presses downward to locate the constricting band in the sphincter. The physician then uses gentle pressure along the band to release it and dilate the sphincter. As the band releases, additional gloved fingers are inserted until the desired dilation has been achieved. In 45910, a rectal stricture is dilated. This may be accomplished manually as described in 45905 or using a balloon or other type of dilator for a rectal stricture. Balloon dilation is accomplished using separately reportable fluoroscopic guidance. A feeding catheter is introduced into the rectum. A contrast agent may be injected into the catheter to outline the stricture. The catheter is positioned at the stricture or across the stricture orifice. A guidewire is advanced through the catheter and beyond the stricture. The catheter is removed and a balloon catheter advanced over the guidewire and positioned within the stricture. The guidewire is removed. The balloon is inflated using contrast media for 3-5 minutes. The balloon is deflated. Inflation and deflation is repeated until the desired amount of dilation of the stricture has been achieved. The balloon catheter is then removed.

45915

45915   Removal of fecal impaction or foreign body (separate procedure) under anesthesia

Fecal impaction results from extreme constipation where a large, hard mass of stool accumulates in the rectum and sometimes extends into the sigmoid colon. The impacted stool cannot be passed by the patient. Foreign bodies in the rectum are usually inserted during sexual activity. Another reason for insertion is an attempt to conceal a weapon or contraband substance. General anesthesia is administered. A gloved finger is inserted into the rectum and the mass of stool is broken up into smaller pieces that are then dislodged and removed from the rectum. Low-lying foreign bodies are able to be palpated during a rectal exam. Once located, a forcep or snare is used to grasp and remove the foreign body. Alternatively, if a vacuum has formed around the object, a foley catheter may be inserted beyond the proximal aspect of the foreign body and the balloon inflated to break the vacuum after which the foreign body is removed.

45990

45990   Anorectal exam, surgical, requiring anesthesia (general, spinal, or epidural), diagnostic

Anesthesia is rarely required for anorectal examination but may be used in patients experiencing significant pain or those who are extremely apprehensive. This procedure is typically used to diagnose the cause of pain in the anorectal region. General, spinal, or epidural anesthesia is administered. The patient is positioned in left lateral or Sim's (lateral) position. The perineal region is inspected visually for lesions, fissures, hemorrhoids, drainage or other abnormalities. The physician performs a digital exam to determine if there are any masses or areas of fluctuance that might indicate an abscess. An anoscope or proctoscope with a good light source may also be used to visualize the anal canal and distal rectum for evidence of lesions, masses, fistulas, or other abnormalities.

46020-46030

46020   Placement of seton

46030   Removal of anal seton, other marker

An anal seton is placed in a fistula tract. A fistula is an abnormal tunnel or passage that connects one body surface to another. Anal fistulas usually result from a rectal abscess that opens and drains into the anal canal. Anal setons are used to promote drainage or fibrosis of the tract or to cut the fistula. The fistula tract identified. A length of non-absorbable suture material inserted into the external opening of the fistula tract using a fine buttonhole probe. The suture material is passed through the internal opening of the fistula and then pulled back out of the anal canal. If the seton is placed for drainage and/or fibrosis, it is left loose. If a cutting type seton is placed, the two ends of the suture material are tied together to create a loop. The diameter of the loop is tightened over a period of

weeks which causes it to slowly cut through and open the fistula tract so that it can heal. Use 46020 for placement of the seton and 46030 for removal.

46040

46040   Incision and drainage of ischiorectal and/or perirectal abscess (separate procedure)

Incision and drainage of an ischiorectal and/or perirectal abscess is performed. Ischiorectal and perirectal abscesses lie in the deeper tissues surrounding the rectum. An ischiorectal abscess is contained in a wedge-shaped space between the tuberosity of the ischium and the obturator internus muscle laterally and the external anal sphincter and the levator ani muscle medially. An ischiorectal abscess may be present only on one side or may spread posteriorly around to the other side forming a horseshoe abscess. A perirectal abscess is located in the connective tissue adjacent to the rectum. A digital rectal examination is performed and the location of abscess identified. A radial or cross-shaped (cruciate) incision is made over the most prominent aspect of the abscess mass or the area of greatest fluctuance. The edges of the incision are excised to expose the abscess cavity and permit wide drainage. The abscess cavity is inspected manually with the fingers and any loculations (pockets) broken up. The incisions may be left open to drain, packed with iodophor gauze for 24 hours, or a drain placed.

46045

46045   Incision and drainage of intramural, intramuscular, or submucosal abscess, transanal, under anesthesia

An intramural abscess is located within the substance of the anal wall. An intramuscular abscess lies within the muscle tissue of the anal sphincter or levator ani muscles. A submucosal abscess lies just below the mucosa of the anus within the submucosal tissue. A digital examination is performed and the location of the abscess identified. A radial or cross-shaped (cruciate) incision is made over the most prominent aspect of the abscess mass or the area of greatest fluctuance. The edges of the incision are excised to expose the abscess cavity and permit wide drainage. The abscess cavity is inspected manually with the fingers and any loculations (pockets) broken up. The incisions may be left open to drain, packed with iodophor gauze for 24 hours, or a drain placed.

46050

46050   Incision and drainage, perianal abscess, superficial

A superficial perianal abscess is located in the connective tissue adjacent to the anus. A digital examination is performed and the location of abscess identified. A radial or cross-shaped (cruciate) incision is made over the most prominent aspect of the abscess mass or the area of greatest fluctuance. The edges of the incision are excised to expose the abscess cavity and permit wide drainage. The abscess cavity is inspected manually with the fingers and any loculations (pockets) broken up. The incisions may be left open to drain, packed with iodophor gauze for 24 hours, or a drain placed.

46060

46060   Incision and drainage of ischiorectal or intramural abscess, with fistulectomy or fistulotomy, submuscular, with or without placement of seton

An ischiorectal abscess is contained in a wedge-shaped space between the tuberosity of the ischium and the obturator internus muscle laterally and the external anal sphincter and the levator ani muscle medially. An ischiorectal abscess may be present only on one side or may spread posteriorly around to the other side forming a horseshoe abscess. An intramural abscess is located within the substance of the anal or rectal wall. A fistula, which is an abnormal passage connecting one epithelial surface to another, forms when the abscess ruptures. A digital rectal examination is performed and the location of abscess identified. The location of the fistula tract is also located. A radial or cross-shaped (cruciate) incision is made over the most prominent aspect of the abscess mass or the area of greatest fluctuance. The edges of the incision are excised to expose the abscess cavity and permit wide drainage. The abscess cavity is inspected manually with the fingers and any loculations (pockets) broken up. The incisions may be left open to drain, packed with iodophor gauze for 24 hours, or a drain placed. The fistula tract is then opened (fistulotomy) or excised (fistulectomy). If an anal seton is placed, a length of non-absorbable suture material inserted into the external opening of the fistula tract using a fine buttonhole probe. The suture material is passed through the internal opening of the fistula and then pulled back out of the anal canal. If the seton is placed for drainage and/or fibrosis, it is left loose. Alternatively, a cutting type seton may be placed to gradually open the fistulous tract, which is another means of fistulotomy. For a cutting seton, the two ends of the suture material are tied together to create a loop. The diameter of the loop is tightened over a period of weeks which causes it to slowly cut through and open the fistula tract so that it can heal.

● New Code   ▲ Revised Code   © 2017 DecisionHealth

Digestive System

46070

46070   Incision, anal septum (infant)

A congenital anal septum is divided in an infant. A congenital anal septum is an abnormal wall or membrane that divides the anus into two cavities instead of the normal single tubular canal. The anus is inspected and the extent of the septum identified. The septum is then sharply incised to create a single tubular anal canal.

46080

46080   Sphincterotomy, anal, division of sphincter (separate procedure)

The internal and external anal sphincters are rings of muscle that form the opening of the anus. These rings of muscle keep the anus closed while stool collects in the rectum. To pass stool, the anal sphincters relax and open. The internal sphincter is not under conscious control. If the resting pressure of the internal sphincter is too high, it may spasm. The spasms can prevent healing of fissures. Anal fissures are painful cracks in the mucous membrane of the anus. By incising the internal anal sphincter, muscle tension is relaxed which allows stool to pass more easily and the fissures to heal. A lateral incision is made in the internal sphincter to divide the muscle tissue without completing cutting through the entire ring of muscle.

46083

46083   Incision of thrombosed hemorrhoid, external

An external thrombosed hemorrhoid is incised to remove the clotted blood. External hemorrhoids are enlarged blood vessels (varices) that are on the outside (external to) the anal canal. External hemorrhoids that develop blood clots can become very tender making it difficult to sit, walk, or pass stool. An incision is made in the hemorrhoid and pressure applied over the hemorrhoid to remove one or more large blood clots.

46200

46200   Fissurectomy, including sphincterotomy, when performed

Anal fissures are painful cracks in the mucous membrane of the anus. The internal and external anal sphincters are rings of muscle that form the opening of the anus. These rings of muscle keep the anus closed while stool collects in the rectum. To pass stool, the anal sphincters relax and open. The internal sphincter is not under conscious control. If the resting pressure of the internal sphincter is too high, it may spasm. The spasms can reduce blood supply to the internal sphincter which can cause fissures to develop and prevent existing fissures from healing. By incising the internal anal sphincter, muscle tension is relaxed which allows stool to pass more easily and the fissures to heal. An incision is made adjacent to the fissure and carried around the entire aspect of the fissure which is then completely excised. The surgical wound is closed with sutures. If a sphincterotomy is performed, a lateral incision is made in the internal sphincter to divide the muscle tissue without completing cutting through the entire ring of muscle.

46220

46220   Excision of single external papilla or tag, anus

Anal papillae are normal projections in the epithelium at the upper end of the anal canal. Papillae sometimes become inflamed or enlarged requiring removal. Anal tags are flaps of skin at the anal verge. The anal verge is the transitional zone between the mucous membrane of the anal canal and the perianal skin. These tags are sometimes referred to as hemorrhoidal tags because external hemorrhoids that have resolved often result in a tag. The area is cleansed and a local anesthetic injected. The enlarged papilla or tag is excised and the mucous membrane closed as needed with sutures.

46221

46221   Hemorrhoidectomy, internal, by rubber band ligation(s)

This procedure is also referred to as rubber band ligature and may be used to treat one or more hemorrhoids. An anoscope or proctoscope may be used to locate the hemorrhoid. The hemorrhoid is grasped with forceps and pulled through the barrel of the ligature device. The physician takes care to ensure that the entire hemorrhoid is contained in the barrel. The rubber band is then applied to the hemorrhoid by squeezing the handle of the ligator. A second rubber band is placed in the same manner to ensure that blood supply to the hemorrhoid is interrupted even if one of the bands breaks.

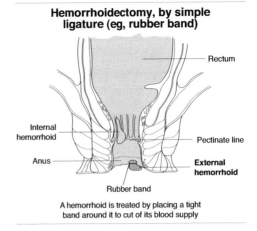

Hemorrhoidectomy, by simple ligature (eg, rubber band)

A hemorrhoid is treated by placing a tight band around it to cut of its blood supply

46230

46230   Excision of multiple external papillae or tags, anus

Anal tags are flaps of skin at the anal verge. The anal verge is the transitional zone between the mucous membrane of the anal canal and the perianal skin. These tags are sometimes referred to as hemorrhoidal tags because external hemorrhoids that have resolved often result in a tag. Anal papillae are normal projections in the epithelium at the upper end of the anal canal. Papillae sometimes become inflamed or enlarged requiring removal. The area is cleansed. The enlarged papillae or external hemorrhoid tags are excised and the mucous membrane closed as needed with sutures.

46250

46250   Hemorrhoidectomy, external, 2 or more columns/groups

Hemorrhoids are enlarged blood vessels (varices) in the anal region. External hemorrhoids are external to the anal canal. In this procedure two or more columns or groups of hemorrhoids are excised. The perianal tissue is examined and the extent of hemorrhoidal disease evaluated using an anoscope. The perianal skin and anal canal are cleansed and a local anesthetic injected at the base of the hemorrhoid. A clamp may be placed to provide traction to the skin and allow better exposure of the hemorrhoid. A radial or circumferential incision is made over the hemorrhoid to remove blood clots. The entire hemorrhoid is then sharply excised. Once the hemorrhoidal plexus and blood clots have been removed, the base of the wound is examined and any residual hemorrhoidal tissue or clots excised. Bleeding is controlled by pressure or electrocautery. The surgical wound may be sutured closed or left open to heal. This is repeated for each column or group of hemorrhoids.

46255-46258

46255   Hemorrhoidectomy, internal and external, single column/group
46257   Hemorrhoidectomy, internal and external, single column/group; with fissurectomy
46258   Hemorrhoidectomy, internal and external, single column/group; with fistulectomy, including fissurectomy, when performed

Hemorrhoids are enlarged blood vessels (varices) in the anal region. Internal hemorrhoids are on the inside of the anal canal while external hemorrhoids are on the outside. In these procedures excision of the internal or external hemorrhoids is limited to a single column or group. In 46255, the physician makes an elliptical incision that encompasses the entire external hemorrhoid. Dissection is carried down to muscle tissue. The entire hemorrhoidal mass is excised. Bleeding is controlled by electrocautery. The surgical wound may be closed with sutures or left open to granulate. This is repeated for each hemorrhoidal mass excised. The same technique is used to excise the internal hemorrhoids. In 46257, hemorrhoidectomy is performed with fissurectomy. Anal fissures are painful cracks in the mucous membrane of the anus. Following the hemorrhoidectomy procedure, an incision is made adjacent to the fissure and carried around the entire aspect of the fissure which is then completely excised. In 46258, hemorrhoidectomy is performed with fistulectomy. A fissurectomy may also be performed. A fistula is an abnormal passage connecting one epithelial surface to another. The hemorrhoidectomy is performed as described above. The fistula tract is located. A probe or suture may be passed through the external opening of the tract to determine the location of the internal opening. The fistula tract is then excised. If an anal fissure is present, the fissure is excised as described above.

Digestive System

46260-46262

46260 Hemorrhoidectomy, internal and external, 2 or more columns/groups

46261 Hemorrhoidectomy, internal and external, 2 or more columns/groups; with fissurectomy

46262 Hemorrhoidectomy, internal and external, 2 or more columns/groups; with fistulectomy, including fissurectomy, when performed

Hemorrhoids are enlarged blood vessels (varices) in the anal region. Internal hemorrhoids are on the inside of the anal canal while external hemorrhoids are on the outside. In these procedures excision of the internal or external hemorrhoids is performed on two or more columns or groups. In 46260, the physician makes an elliptical incision that encompasses the entire external hemorrhoid. Dissection is carried down to muscle tissue. The entire hemorrhoidal mass is excised. Bleeding is controlled by electrocautery. The surgical wound may be closed with sutures or left open to granulate. This is repeated for each hemorrhoidal mass excised. The same technique is used to excise the internal hemorrhoids. In 46261, hemorrhoidectomy is performed with fissurectomy. Anal fissures are painful cracks in the mucous membrane of the anus. Following the hemorrhoidectomy procedure, an incision is made adjacent to the fissure and carried around the entire aspect of the fissure which is then completely excised. In 46262, hemorrhoidectomy is performed with fistulectomy. A fissurectomy may also be performed. A fistula is an abnormal passage connecting one epithelial surface to another. The hemorrhoidectomy is performed as described above. The fistula tract is located. A probe or suture may be passed through the external opening of the tract to determine the location of the internal opening. The fistula tract is then excised. If an anal fissure is present, the fissure is excised as described above.

46270-46285

46270 Surgical treatment of anal fistula (fistulectomy/fistulotomy); subcutaneous

46275 Surgical treatment of anal fistula (fistulectomy/fistulotomy); intersphincteric

46280 Surgical treatment of anal fistula (fistulectomy/fistulotomy); transsphincteric, suprasphincteric, extrasphincteric or multiple, including placement of seton, when performed

46285 Surgical treatment of anal fistula (fistulectomy/fistulotomy); second stage

A fistula is an abnormal passage connecting one epithelial surface to another. The fistula tract is located. A probe or suture may be passed through the external opening of the tract to determine the location of the internal opening. The fistula tract is then incised and opened (fistulotomy) to allow healing from the inside out or the fistula tract is excised (fistulectomy). Use 46270 for a subcutaneous anal fistula and 46275 if the fistula is intersphincteric. Use 46280 for a transsphincteric, suprasphincteric, or extrasphincteric fistula or multiple anal fistulas. Transsphincteric, suprasphincteric, and extrasphincteric fistulas are in deeper tissues and require more extensive dissection to locate. If an anal seton is placed, a length of non-absorbable suture material inserted into the external opening of the fistula tract using a fine buttonhole probe. The suture material is passed through the internal opening of the fistula and then pulled back out of the anal canal. If the seton is placed for drainage and/or fibrosis, it is left loose. Alternatively, a cutting type seton may be placed to gradually open the fistulous tract, which is another means of fistulotomy. For a cutting seton, the two ends of the suture material are tied together to create a loop. The diameter of the loop is tightened over a period of weeks which causes it to slowly cut through and open the fistula tract so that it can heal. Use 46285 for second stage fistulectomy or fistulotomy. In order to decrease the risk of incontinence when the fistula tract traverses the anal sphincter, a two-stage procedure may be performed. A portion of the fistula is opened or excised and allowed to heal during the primary procedure. Then, the remainder of the fistula is opened or excised at a second surgical session.

46288

46288 Closure of anal fistula with rectal advancement flap

Repair with an advancement flap is used for high perianal fistulas that are located in the upper two-thirds of the external anal sphincter. High perianal fistulas cannot be opened or excised because disruption of the external anal sphincter is associated with a high risk of incontinence. The external opening of the fistula is identified and a probe inserted to locate the internal opening. The internal opening is excised. The mucosa and submucosa along with a small amount of muscle fibers are mobilized from the internal sphincter taking care to keep the base of the flap wide enough to ensure adequate vascularization. The fistula tract is curetted. The internal opening is left open. The flap is then sutured over the internal fistula opening. Following placement of the flap, fibrin glue is sometimes instilled through the external opening taking care not to disrupt the flap.

46320

46320 Excision of thrombosed hemorrhoid, external

External hemorrhoids are enlarged blood vessels (varices) that are on the outside (external to) the anal canal. Thrombotic external hemorrhoids develop blood clots and can become very tender making it difficult to sit, walk, or pass stool. The perianal tissue is examined and the extent of hemorrhoidal disease evaluated using an anoscope. The perianal skin

and anal canal are cleansed and a local anesthetic injected at the base of the hemorrhoid. A clamp may be placed to provide traction to the skin and allow better exposure of the hemorrhoid. A radial or circumferential incision is made over the hemorrhoid to remove blood clots. Excision is performed using an elliptical incision that encompasses the entire external hemorrhoid. Once the hemorrhoidal plexus and blood clots have been removed, the base of the wound is examined and any residual hemorrhoidal tissue or clots excised. Bleeding is controlled by pressure or electrocautery. The surgical wound may be sutured closed or left open to heal.

46500

46500 Injection of sclerosing solution, hemorrhoids

One or more hemorrhoids are treated by injection of sclerosing solution, also referred to as sclerotherapy. The sclerosing solution causes the hemorrhoid to become inflamed, the vein walls to stick together and then close permanently. Injection of sclerosing solution causes the hemorrhoid to disappear or become smaller over time as the hemorrhoidal mass is reabsorbed by the body.

46505

46505 Chemodenervation of internal anal sphincter

Chemodenervation of the internal anal sphincter is performed to treat chronic anal fissure. This procedure uses an injection of botulinum toxin or other denervation agent to relax the internal anal sphincter muscle which reduces tension at the anal opening and allows the fissure to heal. The location of the fissure is noted and the area to be denervated is identified. The physician then injects the denervation agent in divided amounts around the internal anal sphincter area. The denervation agent acts rapidly with paralysis occurring in a few hours.

46600-46601

46600 Anoscopy; diagnostic, including collection of specimen(s) by brushing or washing, when performed (separate procedure)

46601 Anoscopy; diagnostic, with high-resolution magnification (HRA) (eg, colposcope, operating microscope) and chemical agent enhancement, including collection of specimen(s) by brushing or washing, when performed

In diagnostic anoscopy, the anus is visually inspected and a digital rectal exam is performed as needed. A blunt tip obturator is inserted into the scope which is introduced into the anus using an advancing twisting motion while the patient bears down. Once the anoscope is completely inserted, the obturator is withdrawn and an eye piece is attached. In 46601, the diagnostic anoscopy is performed with high-resolution magnification (HRA) and chemical enhancement. After the anoscope is inserted approximately two inches into the anal canal, a standard colposcope or operating microscope is used to magnify the area for visual examination. A chemical agent such as 3% acetic acid is applied to any suspicious areas to be examined. The anal mucosa is carefully inspected and cytology (cell) samples may be obtained via brushing the mucosal lining. Alternatively, water may be introduced, the mucosal lining washed, and the fluid aspirated to obtain cell samples. Cytology samples are sent for separately reportable laboratory analysis.

46604

46604 Anoscopy; with dilation (eg, balloon, guide wire, bougie)

Dilation is performed to treat a stricture of the anus. Strictures are usually a complication of surgery, radiation, or inflammatory disease. The anus is visually inspected and a digital rectal exam is performed as needed. The obturator is inserted into the scope which is introduced into the anus and advanced to the point of the stricture using a twisting motion while the patient bears down. The obturator is removed and the eyepiece attached. A guide wire is advanced under direct visualization to a point just proximal to the stricture. A balloon catheter is passed over the guide wire and positioned in the middle of the stricture. The balloon is inflated and left in place for a short period of time, deflated, and then removed. Alternatively, a flexible cylindrical instrument called a bougie may be used to dilate the stricture. The bougie is passed through the stricture to stretch it. Following dilation, the area is inspected using the scope to ensure that the dilation has been successful and that there are no injuries to the anus resulting from the procedure.

46606

46606 Anoscopy; with biopsy, single or multiple

The anus is visually inspected and a digital rectal exam is performed as needed. The obturator is inserted into the scope which is introduced into the anus and advanced using a twisting motion while the patient bears down. The obturator is removed and the eyepiece attached. The scope is then withdrawn and the mucosa carefully inspected. A biopsy forceps is passed through the biopsy channel in the endoscope. The biopsy forceps is opened and a tissue sample captured. The forceps is closed and then removed from the anoscope with the tissue sample. One or more tissue samples (biopsies) are obtained and sent for separately reportable laboratory analysis.

● New Code ▲ Revised Code CPT © 2016 American Medical Association. All Rights Reserved. © 2017 DecisionHealth

Digestive System

46607

46607 Anoscopy; with high-resolution magnification (HRA) (eg, colposcope, operating microscope) and chemical agent enhancement, with biopsy, single or multiple

Anoscopy with high-resolution magnification and chemical agent enhancement is performed with biopsy(s). An anoscope is introduced into the anus using an advancing twisting motion while the patient bears down. After the anoscope is inserted approximately two inches into the anal canal, a standard colposcope or operating microscope is used to magnify the area for visual examination. The entire circumference of the anal mucosa is then carefully inspected and any abnormalities are noted. A chemical agent such as 3% acetic acid is applied to enhance visualization of any suspicious areas being examined. If lesions or other areas of concern are identified, single or multiple biopsies are taken of the suspect site(s) through the scope and removed. The tissue specimens are sent for separate laboratory analysis. The anal mucosa is again inspected and instruments are removed.

46608

46608 Anoscopy; with removal of foreign body

The anus is visually inspected and a digital rectal exam is performed as needed. The obturator is inserted into the scope which is introduced into the anus and advanced to the site of the foreign body. The obturator is removed and the eyepiece attached. A balloon catheter may be used to remove a smooth edged foreign body. The catheter tip is passed beyond the level of the foreign body and the balloon inflated. The catheter is then withdrawn and the foreign body carefully pulled out of the rectum. An impacted foreign body is removed with a forceps. The forceps is passed through the endoscope, the impacted foreign body grasped and removed. Following removal of the foreign body, the endoscope is reintroduced and the rectum examined for evidence of perforation or other injury.

46610-46612

46610 Anoscopy; with removal of single tumor, polyp, or other lesion by hot biopsy forceps or bipolar cautery
46611 Anoscopy; with removal of single tumor, polyp, or other lesion by snare technique
46612 Anoscopy; with removal of multiple tumors, polyps, or other lesions by hot biopsy forceps, bipolar cautery or snare technique

The obturator is inserted into the scope which is introduced into the anus and advanced using a twisting motion while the patient bears down. The obturator is removed and the eyepiece attached. The scope is then withdrawn and the mucosa carefully inspected. The tumor, polyp or other lesion is identified. In 46610, hot biopsy forceps or bipolar cautery is used to remove the lesion. Hot biopsy forceps use an insulated monopolar forceps to simultaneously remove and electrocoagulate (cauterize) tissue. Bipolar cautery also uses electrical current to remove and cauterize the lesion however in this case the current runs from one part of the tip of the forceps to another portion of the forceps. Both hot biopsy forceps and bipolar cautery are used primarily for removal of small polyps and treatment of vascular ectasias. In 46611, a wire loop is placed around the lesion. The loop is heated to shave off and cauterize the lesion. Lesions may be removed in total with one placement of the snare or piecemeal which requires multiple applications of the snare. In 46612, one or more of the techniques described above are used to remove multiple tumors, polyps, or other lesions.

46614

46614 Anoscopy; with control of bleeding (eg, injection, bipolar cautery, unipolar cautery, laser, heater probe, stapler, plasma coagulator)

The obturator is inserted into the scope which is introduced into the anus and advanced using a twisting motion while the patient bears down. The obturator is removed and the eyepiece attached. The scope is then withdrawn and the mucosa carefully inspected. The bleeding site is identified. Bleeding is typically controlled using a contact thermal modality, such as bipolar or unipolar cautery or a heater probe. The cautery device or heater probe is applied to the bleeding point and pressure applied along with heat to control bleeding. An injection of epinephrine which works as a vascoconstrictor and tamponade can also be used to reduce or stop bleeding. YAG laser coagulation and a newer modality, the argon plasma coagulator, are noncontact devices used to coagulate the bleeding site. Staples or hemoclips may be used to approximate the margins of a tear or laceration.

46615

46615 Anoscopy; with ablation of tumor(s), polyp(s), or other lesion(s) not amenable to removal by hot biopsy forceps, bipolar cautery or snare technique

The obturator is inserted into the scope which is introduced into the anus and advanced using a twisting motion while the patient bears down. The obturator is removed and the eyepiece attached. The scope is then withdrawn and the mucosa carefully inspected. The tumor, polyp or other lesion is identified. The tumor, polyp or other lesion is identified and ablated using a technique such as laser ablation. The laser device is delivered through

the endoscope to the proximal margin of the lesion. Beginning at the proximal margin, the lesion is ablated as the endoscope is retracted. The laser device traverses the entire lesion and destroys it. The procedure is repeated if there are multiple tumors, polyps, or lesions until all have been ablated.

46700-46705

46700 Anoplasty, plastic operation for stricture; adult
46705 Anoplasty, plastic operation for stricture; infant

Anal strictures may be acquired or congenital. An acquired anal stricture results from scar tissue that constricts the anal canal causing difficulty in passing stool. The stricture may be the result of scarring due to a tear, radiation therapy for cancers in the perianal region, trauma from a previous surgical procedure, or other trauma. A congenital anal stricture, also called anal stenosis, is present at birth. The anal muscosa is incised and the scar tissue exposed. The scar tissue is then incised in the anal canal or anal sphincter to release the stricture and widen the anal canal. Overlying tissues are repaired in layers. Use 46700 for repair of anal stricture in an adult and 46705 for an infant.

46706

46706 Repair of anal fistula with fibrin glue

The perineum is prepped and draped and a digital rectal exam performed. An anoscope is used to examine the anus and identify the site of the fistula. A probe is introduced into the internal opening of the fistula and passed through the fistula to the external opening. A curette is used to remove granulation tissue from the fistula tract. A flexible catheter is inserted at the internal opening of the fistula and the entire fistulous tract is filled with fibrin glue.

46707

46707 Repair of anorectal fistula with plug (eg, porcine small intestine submucosa [SIS])

Placement of a plug, such as a porcine small intestine submucosa (SIS), to repair an anorectal fistula is a minimally invasive procedure with few complications. The internal and external openings of the fistula tract are identified. The fistula is curetted and irrigated with antibiotic solution. If a porcine SIS plug is used, it is prepared by taking a 4-ply sheet of SIS, rolling it tightly, and securing the edge with sutures. Suture ligatures are then placed at the ends of the plug and used to pull and position the plug within the fistula tract. The plug is then trimmed flush with the internal opening and the opening is closed with sutures. Alternatively, a sliding mucosal flap may be used to close the internal opening. The fistula usually closes in about 5 weeks.

46710-46712

46710 Repair of ileoanal pouch fistula/sinus (eg, perineal or vaginal), pouch advancement; transperineal approach
46712 Repair of ileoanal pouch fistula/sinus (eg, perineal or vaginal), pouch advancement; combined transperineal and transabdominal approach

In 46710, an incision is made in the perineum around the anus. Any residual anal mucosa is excised. An anoscope is inserted into the anus and the distal anastomosis site identified. Epinephrine is injected below the distal anastomosis site. The distal aspect of the pouch is mobilized taking care to protect the internal sphincter. Dissection continues proximally until the entire pouch is mobilized and the proximal anastomosis site is identified. The process of dissecting the pouch also divides the fistula or sinus. Dissection is then extended approximaly 6-10 cm beyond the proximal anastomosis site. The vaginal or perineal end of the fistula or sinus is located, excised, and debrided. The fistula or sinus tract is then closed in layers. The distal end of the pouch is trimmed and the anal transitional zone or fistula site excised. The new distal aspect of the pouch is sutured to the anus at the dentate line. In 46712, the lower abdomen is incised and the proximal aspect of the ileoanal pouch mobilized. The perineum is then incised and the distal aspect of the pouch mobilized as described above up to the level of the abdominal dissection which also divides the fistula or sinus tract. The pouch is transected at the distal anastomosis site and brought into the abdomen and inspected. The distal aspect of the pouch is trimmed, returned to the pelvis, and sutured to the anal canal. Abdominal and perineal incisions are closed in layers.

46715-46716

46715 Repair of low imperforate anus; with anoperineal fistula (cut-back procedure)
46716 Repair of low imperforate anus; with transposition of anoperineal or anovestibular fistula

An imperforate anus is a congenital anomaly in which the anal opening fails to form at all or in which the only opening is a small malpositioned fistulous tract. The term low imperforate anus is outdated but generally describes a malformation at or below the levator ani muscles. Current anorectal malformations are now classified based on anatomic characteristics. An anoperineal fistula occurs in both sexes. The anus is closed but there is an opening in the perineal body or in boys there may not be an opening in

Digestive System

the perineum, but there may be a fistula extending into the scrotum and evidence of a mucus or meconium in the scrotal tissues. An anovestibular fistula occurs in girls as a small opening in the posterior vestibule of the vagina. In 46715, an imperforate anus characterized by an anoperineal fistula is repaired using a cut-back procedure. The perineal region is prepped and a muscle stimulator used to identify the anorectal muscle complex so that the cut-back can be positioned properly within the external anal sphinter. The fistula is cannulated and a scissors is then used to cut the tissue back (posteriorly) so that the fistula opens within the external anal sphincter. The exposed mucosa may be repaired with sutures or local skin flaps developed to close the defect. This provides a larger outlet for stool and prevents bowel obstruction and hypertrophy of the colon. In 46716, the imperforate anus is characterized by an anoperineal or anovestibular fistula and is treated using a transposition anoplasty. Following identification of the anorectal muscle complex using a muscle stimulating device, the anoperineal or anovestibular fistula is dissected from surrounding tissue. The skin over the anal sphincter is opened and the fistula is transposed so that it opens within the anal sphincter. The skin around the anus is sutured to the fistula. The perineum or vestibule of the vagina where the fistula had previously terminated is also repaired.

46730-46735

46730 **Repair of high imperforate anus without fistula; perineal or sacroperineal approach**
46735 **Repair of high imperforate anus without fistula; combined transabdominal and sacroperineal approaches**

An imperforate anus is a congenital anomaly in which the anal opening fails to form or in which the opening is a small malpositioned fistulous tract. The term high imperforate anus is outdated but generally describes a malformation above the levator ani muscles. Anorectal malformations are now classified based on anatomic characteristics. In 46730, the anorectal muscle complex is identified using a muscle stimulating device. An incision is made anterior to the anorectal muscles in the perineum or posterior to the anorectal muscles where dissection is carried up to the presacral space (sacroperineal approach). Dissection continues until the rectal pouch is identified. The rectal pouch is mobilized taking care to completely separate the rectum from all attachments to the genitorurinary tract. The muscle stimulator device is again used to identify and mark the anterior and posterior limits of the muscle complex. The rectum is sutured to the anorectal muscle complex. The perineal or sacroperineal incision is closed. The skin over the anal sphincter is incised. The rectal pouch is opened and rectal mucosa sutured circumferentially to the skin to create the anal opening. In 46735, an incision is made posterior to the anorectal muscles in the perineum. Dissection is carried up to the presacral space and continues until the rectal pouch is identified. The rectal pouch is mobilized taking care to completely separate the rectum from all attachments to the genitorurinary tract. The abdomen is incised and the abdominal cavity inspected. The proximal aspect of the rectum is exposed and the superior rectal vessels are located and protected. The ureters are identified and protected. The peritoneum is incised and the presacral space is entered. Dissection continues through these two incisions until the rectum is completely mobilized and can be pulled-through to the area of the anal sphincter. The abdominal incision is closed. The anoplasty is then completed as described above.

46740-46742

46740 **Repair of high imperforate anus with rectourethral or rectovaginal fistula; perineal or sacroperineal approach**
46742 **Repair of high imperforate anus with rectourethral or rectovaginal fistula; combined transabdominal and sacroperineal approaches**

An imperforate anus is a congenital anomaly in which the anal opening fails to form or in which the only opening is a small fistulous tract. The term high imperforate anus is outdated but generally describes a malformation above the levator ani muscles. Anorectal malformations are now classified based on anatomic characteristics. In 46740, the anorectal muscle complex is identified using a muscle stimulating device. An incision is made anterior to the anorectal muscles in the perineum or posterior to the anorectal muscles where dissection is carried up to the presacral space (sacroperineal approach). Dissection continues until the rectal pouch is identified. The rectal pouch is mobilized taking care to completely separate the rectum from all attachments to the genitorurinary tract. As the rectal pouch is dissected the rectourethral or rectovaginal fistula is identified and the fistulous opening in the rectum severed. The fistulous tract is excised and the wound closed. The muscle stimulator device is again used to identify and mark the anterior and posterior limits of the anorectal muscle complex. The rectum is sutured to the anorectal muscle complex. The perineal or sacroperineal incision is closed. The skin over the anal sphincter is incised. The rectal pouch is opened and rectal mucosa sutured circumferentially to the skin to create the anal opening. In 46742, an incision is made posterior to the anorectal muscles in the perineum. Dissection is carried up to the presacral space and continues until the rectal pouch is identified. The rectal pouch is mobilized taking care to completely separate the rectum from all attachments to the genitorurinary tract. The abdomen is incised and the abdominal cavity inspected. The proximal aspect of the rectum is exposed and the superior rectal vessels are located and protected. The ureters are identified and protected. The peritoneum is incised and

the presacral space is entered. Dissection continues through these two incisions until the rectum is completely mobilized and can be pulled-through to the area of the anal sphincter. The fistulous tract is identified, the opening severed, the tract excised, and the wound closed. The abdominal incision is closed. The anoplasty is then completed as described above.

46744-46748

46744 **Repair of cloacal anomaly by anorectovaginoplasty and urethroplasty, sacroperineal approach**
46746 **Repair of cloacal anomaly by anorectovaginoplasty and urethroplasty, combined abdominal and sacroperineal approach**
46748 **Repair of cloacal anomaly by anorectovaginoplasty and urethroplasty, combined abdominal and sacroperineal approach; with vaginal lengthening by intestinal graft or pedicle flaps**

Cloacal anomalies occur only in girls and are characterized by merging of the rectum, vagina, and urethra into a single common channel. The approach and surgical repair depends on the exact nature of the cloaca and exactly where the rectum, vagina, and urethra merge. In 46744, a low cloacal anomaly is repaired by a sacroperineal approach. An incision is made in the posterior aspect of the perineum and dissection is carried up to the presacral space (sacroperineal approach). Dissection continues until the rectal pouch is identified. The rectal pouch is mobilized. The vagina and urethra are then mobilized together as one unit. The muscle stimulator device is used to identify and mark the anterior and posterior limits of the anorectal muscle complex. The rectum is pulled down and sutured to the anorectal muscle complex. The vagina and urethra are also pulled down to the perineum and sutured into place. A vaginoplasty and urethroplasty are performed to construct functional openings in the perineum. The sacroperineal incision is closed. The skin over the anal sphincter is incised. The rectal pouch is opened and rectal mucosa sutured circumferentially to the skin to create the anal opening. In 46746, a high cloaca is repaired using a combined abdominal and sacroperineal approach. An incision is made in the lower abdomen and carried down to the bladder and rectum. The rectum is mobilized and repaired as described above. In high cloaca the vagina and urinary tract usually require separation to gain the length needed to pull these structures down to the perineum. This is accomplished by careful dissection of urogenital structures. When the vagina and urethra have been separated, they are pulled down and vaginoplasty and urethroplasty performed to construct functional openings in the perineum. In 46748, a high cloaca is repaired using a combined abdominal and sacroperineal approach with vaginal lengthening by intestinal graft or pedicle flaps. Rectal, vaginal and urethral mobilization is performed as described above. A segment of small intestine or colon is harvested and prepared for grafting. The intestinal graft is configured to the size and shape required to achieve the necessary lengthening of the vagina and is sutured to the vaginal remnant and perineum. Alternatively, the physician may use pedicle flaps from surrounding tissue to lengthen the vagina.

46750-46751

46750 **Sphincteroplasty, anal, for incontinence or prolapse; adult**
46751 **Sphincteroplasty, anal, for incontinence or prolapse; child**

Anal or fecal incontinence caused by muscle damage or weakening of the external and/ or internal anal sphincters or by rectal prolapse is treated by sphincteroplasty. Anal incontinence is the inability to store and hold stool in the rectum and is typically caused by a tear or laceration in adults. In children the anal incontinence is more often the result of a congenital anomaly. The perineum is cleansed and local anesthetic and vasoconstrictor injected at the surgical site. A curvalinear incision is made parallel to the external sphincter. The anal mucosa is dissected free of scar tissue and the underlying external and internal sphincters. Dissection continues up the levator ani. Scar tissue is excised. Muscle ends may be overlapped to reduce anal diameter. The internal and external sphincters are repaired with sutures. Overlying mucosa and skin is repaired with sutures. Use 46750 for sphincteroplasty on an adult and 46751 if the procedure is performed on a child.

46753-46754

46753 **Graft (Thiersch operation) for rectal incontinence and/or prolapse**
46754 **Removal of Thiersch wire or suture, anal canal**

A Thiersch operation, also referred to as anal encirclement, is performed for rectal incontinence or prolapse. The procedure involves placing a thin band of non-absorbable material such as a wire or suture under the skin at the anus. The wire, suture, or other material is then advanced around the entire circumference of the anus. The foreign material eventually results in formation of a fibrous ring that helps prevents prolapse of the rectum and resulting incontinence. Use 46753 for placement of the wire or suture and 46754 for removal of the Thiersch wire or suture.

● New Code   ▲ Revised Code   CPT © 2016 American Medical Association. All Rights Reserved.   © 2017 DecisionHealth

Digestive System

46760-46762

46760 Sphincteroplasty, anal, for incontinence, adult; muscle transplant
46761 Sphincteroplasty, anal, for incontinence, adult; levator muscle imbrication (Park posterior anal repair)
46762 Sphincteroplasty, anal, for incontinence, adult; implantation artificial sphincter

An anal sphincteroplasty is performed for adult incontinence using a muscle transplant (46760), levator muscle imbrication, also referred to as a Park posterior anal repair (46761), or implantation of an artificial sphincter (46762). In 46760, sphincteroplasty is performed using a muscle transplant, usually the gracilis or gluteus maximus muscle is used. If the repair is performed using the gracilis muscle, the gracilis muscle is detached from the tibia, and mobilized. A subcutaneous tunnel is created from the pubic tubercle to the anal canal. The gracilis muscle is then wrapped around the anal sphincter to restore muscle tone to the sphincter. In 46761, the levator muscle is imbricated. The levator ani muscles are exposed using a posterior approach. A series of folds are then created and secured with sutures to recreate the normal anorectal angle and lengthen the anal canal. In 46762, an artificial bowel (anal) sphincter is inserted. The skin and muscosa around the anal canal are incised and a cuff is placed around the canal. A reservoir and pump are then placed in the scrotum or labium. The reservoir, pump, and cuff are connected by a thin tube that is tunneled subcutaneously. The skin incisions are closed over the reservoir, pump, and cuff. Once the tissue has healed, fluid is transferred from the reservoir to the cuff which inflates the cuff and closes the anal canal. To deflate the cuff and allow passage of stool, the patient presses on the pump which moves the fluid into the reservoir allowing the anal canal to open. Fluid automatically moves back into the cuff after several minutes.

46900-46924

46900 Destruction of lesion(s), anus (eg, condyloma, papilloma, molluscum contagiosum, herpetic vesicle), simple; chemical
46910 Destruction of lesion(s), anus (eg, condyloma, papilloma, molluscum contagiosum, herpetic vesicle), simple; electrodesiccation
46916 Destruction of lesion(s), anus (eg, condyloma, papilloma, molluscum contagiosum, herpetic vesicle), simple; cryosurgery
46917 Destruction of lesion(s), anus (eg, condyloma, papilloma, molluscum contagiosum, herpetic vesicle), simple; laser surgery
46922 Destruction of lesion(s), anus (eg, condyloma, papilloma, molluscum contagiosum, herpetic vesicle), simple; surgical excision
46924 Destruction of lesion(s), anus (eg, condyloma, papilloma, molluscum contagiosum, herpetic vesicle), extensive (eg, laser surgery, electrosurgery, cryosurgery, chemosurgery)

The physician destroys one or more anal lesions using a method such as chemical destruction, electrodessication, cryosurgery, laser surgery, electrosurgery, or surgical excision. Common types of lesions treated include condylomata, papillomata, molluscum contagiosum, and herpetic vesicles. The lesion is examined and the most appropriate form of destruction determined. Local anesthesia is administered as needed. In 46900, a simple chemical destruction is performed with silver nitrate or other chemical compound. In 46910, a simple electrodessication is performed using a monopolar high-frequency electric current to destroy the lesion and control bleeding. In 46916, cryosurgery is performed using liquid nitrogen to freeze the lesion. A series of freeze-thaw cycles may be required to completely destroy the lesion. In 46917, a simple laser ablation is performed using a non-contact Nd-YAG laser or a contact laser probe with coaxial water to vaporize the lesion. In 46922, a simple excision is performed. A narrow margin of healthy tissue is identified and a full-thickness incision is made through the mucous and submucous tissue. The incision is carried around the lesion and the entire lesion is excised. The lesion is sent to the laboratory for separately reportable histologic evaluation. Bleeding is controlled by electrocautery or chemical cautery. The wound may be closed using simple single layer suture technique or left open to granulate. In 46924, extensive destruction of a large lesion or multiple lesions is performed using laser surgery, electrosurgery, cryosurgery, or chemosurgery. Laser surgery, cryosurgery, or chemosurgery is performed as described above over an extensive area. Alternatively, electrosurgery may be performed. Electrosurgery uses heat applied to the lesion(s) with a high frequency current that passes through a metal probe or needle.

46930

46930 Destruction of internal hemorrhoid(s) by thermal energy (eg, infrared coagulation, cautery, radiofrequency)

Internal hemorrhoids are destroyed using thermal energy such as infrared coagulation, cautery, or radiofrequency. Internal hemorrhoids are sac-like protrusions of blood vessels in the rectum that may prolapse through the anus and become thrombosed. The anal canal is gently dilated by inserting one or two gloved fingers. The hemorrhoid is grasped with forceps, traction is applied, and the internal hemorrhoid is drawn out of the anal canal. Infrared coagulation, cautery, or radiofrequency is then applied to tissue just proximal to the hemorrhoid. Infrared coagulation uses an infrared light, cautery uses an electrocautery probe, and radiofrequency uses an electrode. When any of these thermal energy sources

are directed at the tissue proximal to the hemorrhoid, they create a thermal lesion (burn) that disrupts the blood supply, causing the hemorrhoid to shrink.

46940-46942

46940 Curettage or cautery of anal fissure, including dilation of anal sphincter (separate procedure); initial
46942 Curettage or cautery of anal fissure, including dilation of anal sphincter (separate procedure); subsequent

Curettage or cautery of an anal fissure including dilation of anal sphincter is performed in a separate procedure. Anal fissures are painful cracks in the mucous membrane of the anus. When the fissures are chronic, a stricture of the anal sphincter may result requiring dilation. The fissure is treated using curettage which involves scraping the lesion to expose healthy underlying mucosa. Surgical curettage may be followed by chemical cautery or electrocautery. Chemical cautery is performed using silver nitrate or phenol in glycerine. Electrocautery uses heat applied to the fissure with a high frequency current that passes through a metal probe or needle. If a stricture is present it is dilated using a flexible cylindrical instrument called a bougie. The bougie is passed through the stricture to stretch it. Use 46940 for the initial procedure and 46942 for subsequent procedures.

46945-46946

46945 Hemorrhoidectomy, internal, by ligation other than rubber band; single hemorrhoid column/group
46946 Hemorrhoidectomy, internal, by ligation other than rubber band; 2 or more hemorrhoid columns/groups

Hemorrhoids are enlarged blood vessels (varices) in the anal region. Internal hemorrhoids are on the inside of the anal canal. The perianal tissue is examined and the extent of hemorrhoidal disease evaluated using an anoscope or proctoscope. The perianal skin and anal canal are cleansed and a local anesthetic injected at the base of the hemorrhoid. A clamp may be placed to provide traction to the skin and allow better exposure of the hemorrhoid. The hemorrhoid is grasped with forceps and, and a ligature device other than a rubber band is placed around the hemorrhoid. The physician takes care to ensure that the ligature is placed at the base of the hemorrhoid. A second ligature is then applied just below the first to ensure that blood supply to the hemorrhoid is interrupted even if one of the bands breaks. Use 46945 when a single hemorrhoid column or group is treated by ligation other than rubber band; use 46946 for 2 or more hemorrhoid columns or groups.

46947

46947 Hemorrhoidopexy (eg, for prolapsing internal hemorrhoids) by stapling

A circular hollow tube is inserted into the anal canal. A long suture is placed in the anal canal above the internal hemorrhoids. The ends of the suture are passed out of the anus through the hollow tube. A stapler is placed in the hollow tube and the ends of the suture are pulled which pulls the tissue supporting the hemorrhoids into the stapler jaws. At the same time, the hemorrhoidal cushions are pulled into their normal position higher up in the anal canal. The stapler is fired which divides the circumferential ring of hemorrhoidal tissue and at the same time staples closed the upper and lower edges of the divided tissue. As the cut tissues heal, scar tissue forms which anchors the hemorrhoidal cushions into their normal position higher in the anal canal. When the tissue has healed, the staples fall off and are expelled in the stool.

47000-47001

47000 Biopsy of liver, needle; percutaneous
47001 Biopsy of liver, needle; when done for indicated purpose at time of other major procedure (List separately in addition to code for primary procedure)

The skin is cleansed and a local anesthetic is injected before a tissue sample (biopsy) of the liver is obtained using percutaneous needle technique. Separately reportable ultrasound, fluoroscopy, CT, or MRI imaging guidance may be used to help identify the abnormal tissue location. A large bore needle or spring loaded biopsy gun is inserted through the skin into the liver and a tissue sample is withdrawn. Use 47001 when a needle biopsy of the liver is obtained during another major procedure, most often through an existing abdominal incision.

47010

47010 Hepatotomy, for open drainage of abscess or cyst, 1 or 2 stages

In 47010, one of two open approaches is used. The more common approach is through a right subcostal incision that may extend up to the xiphoid process or into the left subcostal region. The right rectus muscle is transected and the oblique muscles are split. The liver is visualized and the abscess or cyst located, incised, and drained. The abdomen is explored for signs of peritonitis and other abscess sites. If a one stage procedure is performed, a drain is placed in the abscess or cyst and the abdomen is closed around the drain. If two stages are required, the wound is left open to drain and closed later during a separate surgical session after the infection has resolved. If the abscess or cyst is in the upper posterior aspect of the liver, a transpleural approach may be used, but is less common as it does not allow for abdominal exploration.

Digestive System

47015

47015 **Laparotomy, with aspiration and/or injection of hepatic parasitic (eg, amoebic or echinococcal) cyst(s) or abscess(es)**

The abdomen is opened (laparotomy) and a parasitic abscess or cyst on the liver is aspirated and/or injected with a solution containing an agent destructive to the parasite. An incision is made in the right subcostal area over the liver and may be extended into the left subcostal region or craniad over the xiphoid process. The right rectus muscle is transected and the oblique muscles are split. The abdomen is inspected and the site of the parasitic abscess or cyst on the liver is identified and punctured. A needle or catheter is placed and fluid and debris are suctioned (aspirated) from the abscess or cyst pocket. For an amebic cyst or abscess, aspiration is typically not followed by injection, but the infection is treated with oral antibiotics. For echinococcal infection, also referred to as hydatid liver cyst, a protosclocidal agent such as hypertonic saline or ethanol is injected and left in the cyst pocket for approximately 15 minutes before being reaspirated.

47100

47100 **Biopsy of liver, wedge**

A small triangular section of the liver is removed for examination and diagnosis. An incision is made in the right subcostal region. The right rectus muscle is transected and the oblique muscles are split. The sternum is retracted. The biopsy site is identified and a wedge of liver is excised. Bleeding is controlled, the wound is irrigated, and the incision site is closed.

47120

47120 **Hepatectomy, resection of liver; partial lobectomy**

The physician resects a portion of the right or left lobe of the liver. An incision is made in the right subcostal region and extended into the left subcostal region or into the craniad over the xiphoid process. The right rectus muscle is transected, the oblique muscles are split, and the medial portion of the left rectus muscle is transected. Ligaments attached to the segment of the liver to be removed are severed and the liver is mobilized. The inferior vena cava and the hepatic veins above the liver are dissected. Arteries to the segment of liver being removed are identified and ligated and veins are dissected and divided. A line of transection for the liver segment is marked with electrocautery. The liver parenchyma is divided using scissors and blunt clamp dissection and the liver segment is then removed. Vascular and biliary structures are ligated and the raw surface of the liver is examined for bleeding and bile leaks. Bleeding is controlled by coagulation. Biliary leaks are controlled with clipping and suture ligation. The wound is irrigated, drains are placed as needed, and The incision is closed with sutures.

47122

47122 **Hepatectomy, resection of liver; trisegmentectomy**

The physician resects the entire right lobe of the liver, the medial segment of the left lobe, and the hepatic parenchyma to the right of the falciform ligament and the ligamentum teres. This is referred to as a right extended lobectomy or a trisegmentectomy. An incision is made in the right subcostal region, extending into the left subcostal region or into the craniad over the xiphoid process. The right rectus muscle is transected, the oblique muscles are split, and the medial portion of the left rectus muscle is transected. The right lobe of the liver is mobilized toward the left. The cystic artery and duct are ligated and divided. The peritoneum is incised and the right main hepatic artery is identified and protected. Dissection is continued superiorly and posteriorly taking care to protect the portal vein. The right main hepatic duct is dissected free. The hepatic vein is located and transected. The liver capsule is incised and the parenchyma transected. Alternatively, the hepatic parenchyma in the interlobar plane is transected. An incision is made to the right of the falciform ligament and the parenchyma is crushed to permit access to the umbilical fissure. Vessels and ducts passing to the medial segment of the left lobe are divided, preserving vessels and ducts to the lateral segment of the left lobe. The three segments are devascularized and excised. The incision is closed over drains after bleeding is controlled and the wound is irrigated.

47125

47125 **Hepatectomy, resection of liver; total left lobectomy**

The physician resects the entire left lobe of the liver. An incision is made in the right subcostal region and extended into the left subcostal region or into the craniad over the xiphoid process. The right rectus muscle is transected and the oblique muscles are split. The medial portion of the left rectus muscle is transected. Ligaments on the left lobe of the liver are severed and the left lobe is mobilized. The inferior vena cava and the hepatic veins above the liver are dissected. The left hepatic artery is divided and the left branch of the portal vein is identified and ligated. The left lobe is retracted to the right and the lesser omentum is transected. The ligamentum venosum is identified and divided near its attachment to the left hepatic vein. The middle and left hepatic veins are then located and ligated. Vessels supplying the right liver are temporary occluded with clamps. The liver is divided by first marking the line of transection with electrocautery and dividing the parenchyma with scissors and blunt clamp dissection. The left lobe is removed. Vascular and biliary structures are ligated. Blood supply is restored to the right lobe. The raw surface

of the right lobe is examined for bleeding and bile leaks. Any bleeding is controlled by coagulation and biliary leaks are controlled with clipping and suture ligation. The wound is irrigated, drains are placed as needed, and the incision is closed with sutures.

47130

47130 **Hepatectomy, resection of liver; total right lobectomy**

The physician resects the right lobe of the liver. An incision is made in the right subcostal region, extending into the left subcostal region or into the craniad over the xiphoid process. The right rectus muscle is transected, the oblique muscles are split, and the medial portion of the left rectus muscle is transected. The right lobe of the liver is mobilized toward the left. The cystic artery and duct are ligated and divided. The peritoneum is incised and the right main hepatic artery is identified and protected. Dissection is continued superiorly and posteriorly taking care to protect the portal vein. The right main hepatic duct is dissected free. The hepatic vein is located and transected. The liver capsule is incised, the parenchyma transected, and the right lobe is excised. Alternatively, the hepatic parenchyma in the interlobar plane is transected and the right lobe is excised. The incision is closed over drains after bleeding is controlled and the wound is irrigated.

47133

47133 **Donor hepatectomy (including cold preservation), from cadaver donor**

The liver is removed from a cadaver donor and cold preserved for transplant. A midline incision is made from the substernal notch to the pubis. The round and falciform ligaments are divided. The liver is exposed and inspected. The gastrohepatic ligament is inspected, and the left hepatic artery is identified and preserved. The common hepatic and right hepatic arteries are identified and preserved. The common bile duct is divided and the gallbladder is flushed with normal saline. The distal aorta and inferior mesenteric vein are isolated. The right gastric artery and gastroduodenal arteries are ligated. The main hepatic artery is dissected back to the aorta. The splenic and left gastric arteries are located and ligated unless there is an anatomic variance that requires a modified approach. The portal vein is isolated and dissected back to the superior mesenteric and splenic veins. When dissection is complete, the aorta is cross clamped below the diaphragm and preservation solution is instilled into the aortic and portal vein. The liver is removed and packed in ice for transport.

47135

47135 **Liver allotransplantation; orthotopic, partial or whole, from cadaver or living donor, any age**

The liver is exposed using a bilateral subcostal incision with upper midline extension. The falciform ligament is taken down and the porta hepatis is dissected. The hepatic artery is ligated. The bile duct is transected as close to the liver as possible. The portal vein is isolated and venovenous bypass is initiated. The hepatic triangular ligaments are taken down. The inferior vena cava is located and cross clamped above and below the liver and the diseased liver is removed. The donor graft is placed in the usual anatomic position (orthotopic placement) and flushed to remove the preservation solution. Blood vessels are anastomosed beginning with the portal vein followed by arterial anastomosis. The bile duct in the donor liver is then anastomosed to the recipient bile duct. Alternatively, the donor bile duct may be implanted in the recipient jejunum. A T-tube is placed in the bile duct for external drainage. Additional drains are placed as needed in the abdomen and the abdominal incision is closed.

47140-47142

47140 **Donor hepatectomy (including cold preservation), from living donor; left lateral segment only (segments II and III)**

47141 **Donor hepatectomy (including cold preservation), from living donor; total left lobectomy (segments II, III and IV)**

47142 **Donor hepatectomy (including cold preservation), from living donor; total right lobectomy (segments V, VI, VII and VIII)**

The left lateral segment (segments II and III) is removed from a living donor and cold preserved for liver transplant. A midline incision is made from the substernal notch to the pubis. Alternatively, an upper midline approach may be used. The liver is exposed and inspected. The left lateral segment is mobilized by dividing the left triangular, the left coronary, and the falciform ligaments. The left lateral segment is then displaced downward and the porta hepatis is exposed. The tributaries of the left branch of the portal vein, the left hepatic duct, and the left branch of the hepatic artery are dissected and occluded. The liver parenchyma is separated to the level of the hepatic vein, which is double ligated and transected. The liver segment is removed, perfused with cold preservation solution, and prepared for transplant by another member of the transplant team. In the donor, bleeding is controlled and the wound is irrigated and closed around drains. In 47142, segments V, VI, VII, and VIII are removed for a total right lobectomy.

● New Code ▲ Revised Code

Digestive System

47143-47145

47143 Backbench standard preparation of cadaver donor whole liver graft prior to allotransplantation, including cholecystectomy, if necessary, and dissection and removal of surrounding soft tissues to prepare the vena cava, portal vein, hepatic artery, and common bile duct for implantation; without trisegment or lobe split

47144 Backbench standard preparation of cadaver donor whole liver graft prior to allotransplantation, including cholecystectomy, if necessary, and dissection and removal of surrounding soft tissues to prepare the vena cava, portal vein, hepatic artery, and common bile duct for implantation; with trisegment split of whole liver graft into 2 partial liver grafts (ie, left lateral segment [segments II and III] and right trisegment [segments I and IV through VIII])

47145 Backbench standard preparation of cadaver donor whole liver graft prior to allotransplantation, including cholecystectomy, if necessary, and dissection and removal of surrounding soft tissues to prepare the vena cava, portal vein, hepatic artery, and common bile duct for implantation; with lobe split of whole liver graft into 2 partial liver grafts (ie, left lobe [segments II, III, and IV] and right lobe [segments I and V through VIII])

A liver that has been removed from a cadaver is prepared for transplant. This is referred to as backbench or back table preparation. The liver may be received with or without the gallbladder intact. If the gallbladder is intact, it is removed (cholecystectomy). Surrounding soft tissue on the liver is dissected free. The vena cava is prepared and suspended by suture material. The suprahepatic vena cava is closed and the infrahepatic vena cava is cannulated and inflated with preservation solution to identify any caval leaks. Caval tributaries are suture ligated to prevent hemorrhage following transplant. The portal vein and hepatic artery are dissected free of surrounding tissue and isolated. Anomalous vessels are identified and dissected free of surrounding tissue in preparation for reconstructive venous and arterial procedures that are reported separately. The common bile duct is dissected free from surrounding tissue in preparation for transplant. The entire liver may be implanted or it may be split into two partial grafts for transplant into two patients. Use 47143 if the entire liver is transplanted into a single patient. Use 47144 if a trisegment split is performed in which the liver is divided into a left lateral segment containing segments II and III and a right trisegment containing the remainder of the liver segments I, IV, V, VI, VII, and VIII. Use 47145 if the liver is split into two partial grafts of right and left lobes. The left lobe contains segments II, III, and IV, and the right lobe contains segment I, V, VI, VII, and VIII.

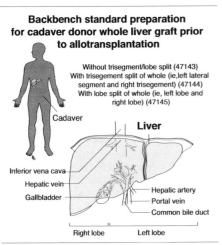

Backbench standard preparation for cadaver donor whole liver graft prior to allotransplantation

Without trisegment/lobe split (47143)
With trisegement split of whole (ie,left lateral segment) and right trisegement) (47144)
With lobe split of whole (ie, left lobe and right lobe) (47145)

Cadaver

Liver

Inferior vena cava
Hepatic vein
Gallbladder

Hepatic artery
Portal vein
Common bile duct

Right lobe   Left lobe

47146-47147

47146 Backbench reconstruction of cadaver or living donor liver graft prior to allotransplantation; venous anastomosis, each

47147 Backbench reconstruction of cadaver or living donor liver graft prior to allotransplantation; arterial anastomosis, each

Any anatomic variations in venous or arterial blood supply to a donor liver are identified and reconstructed in a back table procedure prior to transplant. The hepatic venous drainage is inspected and anatomic variations are corrected by reconstructing and anastomosing anomalous vessels to the hepatic venous drainage. The common hepatic artery, one of the three branches of the celiac artery, typically provides the blood supply to the liver. However, the liver may receive some or all of its blood supply from the other two celiac branches comprised of the splenic and gastric arteries or from the superior mesenteric artery. These arteries are preserved and revascularized by attaching them to the main hepatic circulation. Use 47146 for each venous anastomosis and 47147 for each arterial anastomosis.

47300

47300 Marsupialization of cyst or abscess of liver

A cyst or abscess in the liver is treated by exteriorization and creation of a pouch so that fluid and debris can drain. An incision is made in the right subcostal region and extended into the left subcostal region or into the craniad over the xiphoid process. The right rectus muscle is transected and the oblique muscles are split. The medial portion of the left rectus muscle is transected. The cyst or abscess is opened and drained. The anterior wall of the cyst is then resected and the remaining wall is inspected for biliary orifices which are sutured to prevent bile leakage. Any biliary vessels draining into the cyst or abscess are suture ligated. The cut edges of the remaining wall are then sutured back to the adjacent edges of the skin creating a pouch that remains open.

47350-47362

47350 Management of liver hemorrhage; simple suture of liver wound or injury

47360 Management of liver hemorrhage; complex suture of liver wound or injury, with or without hepatic artery ligation

47361 Management of liver hemorrhage; exploration of hepatic wound, extensive debridement, coagulation and/or suture, with or without packing of liver

47362 Management of liver hemorrhage; re-exploration of hepatic wound for removal of packing

A midline abdominal incision is used to expose the liver. The abdominal cavity is explored to determine the extent of injury and whether or not there are injuries to other organs, blood vessels or nerves. The falciform ligament is divided. Overlying bowel is retracted. Packs are placed above the liver. The right and left peritoneal ligaments are incised and the right and left triangular ligaments excised to expose and mobilize the liver and expose the hepatic artery and inferior vena cava. The liver wound is explored. In 47350, simple suture of a liver wound or injury is performed. Sutures are used to repair the liver parenchyma and capsule. In 47360, complex suture of liver wound or injury is performed. Intrahepatic blood vessels and bile ducts are ligated. If bleeding continues following repair of the intrahepatic blood vessels, a selective hepatic artery ligation (SHAL) is performed. The liver is carefully inspected for any signs of continued bleeding. In 47361, the liver wound is treated with extensive debridement, coagulation and/or suture with or without packing of liver. Devitalized tissue is removed (debrided) using finger dissection and cautery. Resectional debriment is performed using clips or a stapler device. Other hemostatic agents are used as needed including thrombin, fibrin sealant, collagen, electrocautery, laser or radiofrequency coagulation, packing and sutures. The abdomen is copiously irrigated to remove blood clots and debris. If bleeding cannot be controlled without packing, the packing is left in place. The abdomen is then closed in layers. In 47362, the abdomen is re-opened and packing removed. One to two days following liver repair, the abdomen is re-opened along the previous incision. Overlying tissues are dissected and the packing removed. The liver is inspected for evidence of bleeding or necrosis. Additional debriment is performed as needed. The abdomen is then closed in layers.

47370-47371

47370 Laparoscopy, surgical, ablation of 1 or more liver tumor(s); radiofrequency

47371 Laparoscopy, surgical, ablation of 1 or more liver tumor(s); cryosurgical

A small portal incision is made near the umbilicus, a trocar inserted, and pneumoperitoneum established. Additional portal incisions are made and trocars placed in the upper and lower quadrants of the abdomen. The abdominal cavity is inspected for extrahepatic tumors and other abnormalities. Any adhesions are lysed using blunt and sharp dissection. The liver is mobilized, all eight hepatic segments inspected, and liver tumors located. In 47370, using separately reportable ultrasound imaging, the radiofrequency needle electrode is placed in the center of the tumor and radiofrequency energy used to heat the tumor to the desired temperature. The temperature is maintained at the desired level for the planned period of time. Following the heating cycle the tissue is cooled while monitoring the site to ensure that the entire tumor has been destroyed along with a margin of health tissue. The electrode needle may be removed and reinserted at a different angle or location in the tumor to ensure necrosis of the entire tumor. This is repeated for separate tumors until all tumors have been destroyed. This is repeated for separate tumors until all tumors have been destroyed. In 47371, cryosurgical ablation of the liver tumors is performed. Using separately reportable ultrasound guidance, one or more cryoprobes are inserted into the tumor and the freeze cycle initiated. The tumor is frozen creating an iceball. Following the freeze cycle, the tissue is thawed while monitoring the site to ensure that the entire tumor has been destroyed along with a margin of healthy tissue. Several freeze-thaw cycles may be required to completely destroy the tumor. This is repeated for separate tumors until all tumors have been destroyed. Following completion of the procedure, gas is released from the abdomen, the laparoscope and surgical tools removed, and the portal incisions are closed.

Digestive System

47380-47381

47380 Ablation, open, of 1 or more liver tumor(s); radiofrequency
47381 Ablation, open, of 1 or more liver tumor(s); cryosurgical

An open ablation of one or more liver tumors is performed. A midline incision is made in the abdomen. Any adhesions are lysed using blunt and sharp dissection. The abdominal cavity is inspected for extrahepatic tumors and other abnormalities. The liver is mobilized, all eight hepatic segments inspected, and liver tumors located. In 47380, radiofrequency ablation is performed. Using separately reportable ultrasound guidance, the radiofrequency electrode needle is placed in the center of the tumor and radiofrequency energy used to heat the tumor to the desired temperature. The temperature is maintained at the desired level for the planned period of time. Following the heating cycle the tissue is cooled while monitoring the site to ensure that the entire tumor has been destroyed along with a margin of healthy tissue. The electrode needle may be removed and reinserted at a different angle or location in the tumor to ensure necrosis of the entire tumor. This is repeated for separate tumors until all tumors have been destroyed. In 47381, cryosurgical ablation of the liver tumors is performed. Using separately reportable ultrasound guidance, one or more cryoprobes are inserted into the tumor and the freeze cycle initiated. The tumor is frozen creating an iceball. Following the freeze cycle, the tissue is thawed while monitoring the site to ensure that the entire tumor has been destroyed along with a margin of health tissue. Several freeze-thaw cycles may be required to completely destroy the tumor. This is repeated for separate tumors until all tumors have been destroyed. Following completion of the procedure, gas is released from the abdomen, the laparoscope and surgical tools removed, and the portal incisions are closed.

47382

47382 Ablation, 1 or more liver tumor(s), percutaneous, radiofrequency

Using continuous separately reportable ultrasound, CT, or MRI guidance, a stab incision is made in the upper abdomen to allow insertion of the radiofrequency thermal ablation device. The radiofrequency electrode needle inserted through the skin incision and advanced into the liver. Using radiographic guidance, the needle is placed in the center of the tumor and radiofrequency energy used to heat the tumor to the desired temperature. The temperature is maintained at the desired level for the planned period of time. Following the heating cycle the tissue is cooled while monitoring the site to ensure that the entire tumor has been destroyed along with a margin of healthy tissue. The electrode needle may be removed and reinserted at a different angle or location in the tumor to ensure necrosis of the entire tumor. This is repeated for separate tumors until all tumors have been destroyed. Following completion of the ablation procedure, the stab incision is closed in layers.

47383

47383 Ablation, 1 or more liver tumor(s), percutaneous, cryoablation

Cryoablation involves the use of extreme cold to destroy abnormal cells. Percutaneous liver ablation is a minimally invasive technique performed under the guidance of ultrasound (US), computerized tomography (CT), or magnetic resonance imaging (MRI) to identify the liver tumor(s) and then a thin, hollow cryoprobe is inserted percutaneously through the skin to the targeted area. Liquid nitrogen or argon gas is injected though the probe to freeze the tumor tissue. The destroyed tissue will be absorbed by the body, mechanical removal is not necessary. Cryoablation is suitable for large or small tumors and is often performed when open resection is contraindicated due to patient age, a preexisting disease or condition, or when palliative treatment is desired for systemic disseminated disease.

47400

47400 Hepaticotomy or hepaticostomy with exploration, drainage, or removal of calculus

A midline abdominal incision is used to expose the liver. The falciform ligament is divided. Overlying bowel is retracted and the liver exposed. The right and left peritoneal ligaments are incised and the right and left triangular ligaments excised to mobilize the liver. The liver is inspected for evidence of disease. The obstructed extrahepatic or intrahepatic duct is exposed. The duct is incised and bile drained. If an intrahepatic calculus is present, it is removed. The incision in the duct may be closed or a drain placed. The abdominal incision is then closed in layers.

47420-47425

47420 Choledochotomy or choledochostomy with exploration, drainage, or removal of calculus, with or without cholecystotomy; without transduodenal sphincterotomy or sphincteroplasty
47425 Choledochotomy or choledochostomy with exploration, drainage, or removal of calculus, with or without cholecystotomy; with transduodenal sphincterotomy or sphincteroplasty

An open choledochotomy or choledochostomy with or without cholecystotomy is performed for exploration, drainage, or removal of calculus. Choledochotomy and choledochostomy are typically performed on patients with acute cholecystitis who are critically ill and unable to undergo more definitive surgical treatment, such as cholecystectomy. An incision is made

in the common bile duct and any stones are removed using forceps, scoops, or irrigation as needed. The main and segmental intrahepatic ducts are explored. Any stones in the right and left hepatic ducts are removed in the same fashion. The segmental ducts are explored and any stones are removed by basket extraction or balloon catheter. Cholecystotomy is performed, if needed: an incision is made in the gallbladder which is decompressed. Any stones present are removed. The gallbladder is inspected for free flow of bile; the cystic duct is explored; and any obstructing stones are manually milked back into the gallbladder. If many stones are present or continuous drainage is required, a choledochostomy tube (T-tube) is placed. The gallbladder is closed around the T-tube and drains are placed in the abdomen before closure. Use 47425 if transduodenal sphincterotomy or sphincteroplasty is also performed, in which the second part of the duodenum is exposed and incised, and the sphincter of Oddi is identified and divided. The division is extended to the dilated portion of the bile duct and any stones are removed. The common bile duct and duodenum are then sutured together.

47460

47460 Transduodenal sphincterotomy or sphincteroplasty, with or without transduodenal extraction of calculus (separate procedure)

Open transduodenal sphincterotomy or sphincteroplasty is performed with or without extraction of calculus. Sphincterotomy or sphincteroplasty is typically performed for sphincter of Oddi dysfunction (SOD). The sphincter of Oddi is the site where the pancreatic and bile ducts enter the duodenum. This sphincter acts as a one-way valve that allows bile to enter the duodenum while preventing the contents of the bowel from entering the bile ducts. When a stricture or stone is present, adequate bile drainage into the duodenum is compromised, resulting in pancreatitis or biliary dilatation and pain. Open transduodenal sphincterotomy or sphincteroplasty may be performed by extraperitoneal approach through a flank incision or intraperitoneally through an abdominal incision. The second part of the duodenum is exposed and incised. The sphincter of Oddi is identified and divided. The division is extended to the dilated portion of the bile duct and any stones are removed. The common bile duct and duodenum are then sutured together.

47480

47480 Cholecystotomy or cholecystostomy, open, with exploration, drainage, or removal of calculus (separate procedure)

An open cholecystotomy or cholecystostomy is performed for exploration, drainage, or removal of calculus. Cholecystotomy and cholecystostomy are typically performed on patients with acute cholecystitis who are critically ill and unable to undergo more definitive surgical treatment, such as cholecystectomy. An incision is made in the gallbladder. If any stones (calculi) are present, they are removed. The gallbladder is inspected for free flow of bile. If free flow of bile is not present, the cystic duct is explored and any obstructing stones are manually milked back into the gallbladder. If many stones are present, a cholecystostomy tube is placed. The gallbladder is closed around the tube and drains are placed in the abdomen before closure.

47490

47490 Cholecystostomy, percutaneous, complete procedure, including imaging guidance, catheter placement, cholecystogram when performed, and radiological supervision and interpretation

Cholecystostomy is typically performed on patients with acute cholecystitis who are critically ill and unable to undergo more definitive surgical treatment, such as cholecystectomy. The skin is prepped and a local anesthetic is administered. A small incision is made in the skin. Using Seldinger technique, a needle is advanced into the abdomen and then into the gallbladder using ultrasonic, fluoroscopic, or CT guidance. A guidewire is threaded through the needle and into the gallbladder and the needle is withdrawn. A catheter is threaded over the guidewire and situated in the gallbladder. The guidewire is withdrawn. Alternatively, direct trocar technique may be used to obtain access to the gallbladder, followed by catheter insertion. The gallbladder is decompressed. Contrast media may be injected into the cystic duct to allow visualization and evaluation of bile ducts. Following injection of contrast media, radiographic images are obtained. These images are reviewed and interpreted by the physician. The gallbladder catheter may be removed or left in place for prolonged drainage.

47531-47532

47531 Injection procedure for cholangiography, percutaneous, complete diagnostic procedure including imaging guidance (eg, ultrasound and/or fluoroscopy) and all associated radiological supervision and interpretation; existing access
47532 Injection procedure for cholangiography, percutaneous, complete diagnostic procedure including imaging guidance (eg, ultrasound and/or fluoroscopy) and all associated radiological supervision and interpretation; new access (eg, percutaneous transhepatic cholangiogram)

In 47532, a percutaneous transhepatic cholangiogram is performed to diagnose the cause of a blockage in the bile duct. The skin is prepped and an incision is made over the intended catheter insertion site, typically over the right midaxillary line below the

Digestive System

tenth rib for access to the right hepatic lobe, or over the epigastrium for access to the left hepatic lobe. A long, thin, flexible, small diameter needle is inserted through the skin into the liver, and advanced into the bile duct. A small amount of contrast medium is injected to confirm the location of the needle. A guidewire is threaded through the needle into the bile duct and the needle is removed. An angiography catheter is then passed over the guidewire and the guidewire is removed. Dye is injected into the bile ducts, which are visualized. More radiographic images are taken as the contrast continues to flow through the bile ducts into the small intestine. In 47531, contrast medium for percutaneous diagnostic cholangiography is injected through an existing access that is already secured in place, such as a transhepatic drainage catheter or T-tube, and then the bile ducts are visualized. These codes include ultrasonic or fluoroscopic guidance supervision and image interpretation of the cholangiogram.

47533-47534

47533 **Placement of biliary drainage catheter, percutaneous, including diagnostic cholangiography when performed, imaging guidance (eg, ultrasound and/or fluoroscopy), and all associated radiological supervision and interpretation; external**

47534 **Placement of biliary drainage catheter, percutaneous, including diagnostic cholangiography when performed, imaging guidance (eg, ultrasound and/or fluoroscopy), and all associated radiological supervision and interpretation; internal-external**

A transhepatic biliary drainage catheter is introduced through the skin for external drainage (47533) or internal-external drainage (47534) when the bile ducts are blocked from stenosis, impacted stones, or tumors. The skin is prepped and an incision is made over the insertion site. Typically this is either over the right midaxillary line below the tenth rib for access to the right hepatic lobe or over the epigastrium for access to the left hepatic lobe. A long, thin, flexible needle is inserted through the skin into the liver, and advanced into the bile duct. A small amount of contrast medium is injected to confirm needle location. A guidewire is passed through the needle into the bile duct and the needle is removed. If cholangiography is performed, an angiography catheter is passed over the guidewire. Dye is injected into the bile ducts, which are visualized on x-ray. More radiographic images are taken as the contrast continues to flow through the bile ducts into the small intestine. The bile duct may be probed and any strictures dilated before the transhepatic biliary drainage catheter is inserted over the guidewire. In 47534, an internal-external biliary drainage tube is placed across the narrowed portion of the bile duct with its curled end in the small intestine. The side drainage holes along the tube's length allow bile to drain past the narrowing into the small intestine. The other end of the tube exits the skin to allow external drainage. Alternatively, if the drain cannot be manipulated past the obstructed site, an external transhepatic biliary drainage tube is placed proximal to the obstruction (47533). Additional contrast is injected following placement of the catheter or tube to ensure that the bile duct is patent. The end of the tube exiting the skin is then attached to a bag for bile collection. These codes report the insertion of the biliary drainage catheter or tube, ultrasonic or fluoroscopic guidance for placement, contrast injection for bile duct visualization, and all radiographic supervision and interpretation of the images.

47535

47535 **Conversion of external biliary drainage catheter to internal-external biliary drainage catheter, percutaneous, including diagnostic cholangiography when performed, imaging guidance (eg, fluoroscopy), and all associated radiological supervision and interpretation**

A procedure is performed to convert an existing external biliary drainage catheter to an internal-external biliary drainage catheter for treating obstruction, which may be caused by gall stones, tumors, infection, inflammation, or trauma. When obstruction is present, an external biliary drainage catheter is usually placed first for decompression. The initial external catheter is inserted through the skin with the tip located above the blockage. The bile is collected in a drainage bag. After successful decompression has been accomplished, the external biliary drainage system is converted to an internal-external system. Under fluoroscopic guidance, a guidewire is advanced via the existing percutaneous catheter through the obstructed area and into the duodenum. The existing catheter is removed and a new catheter is inserted over the guidewire. Dye may be injected though the catheter to view the biliary system (cholangiography) and confirm catheter placement past the obstruction into the duodenum, after which the guidewire is removed. The catheter is secured to the skin and a drainage bag is connected to the external portion of the catheter. An external-internal biliary drainage system allows bile to flow in two directions. Code 47535 includes all imaging guidance, supervision, and interpretation of images for converting an external biliary drainage catheter to an internal-external drainage system.

47536

47536 **Exchange of biliary drainage catheter (eg, external, internal-external, or conversion of internal-external to external only), percutaneous, including diagnostic cholangiography when performed, imaging guidance (eg, fluoroscopy), and all associated radiological supervision and interpretation**

A procedure is performed to exchange a percutaneous biliary drainage catheter (external only, internal-external) or to convert an internal-external catheter to an external only catheter. A biliary drainage catheter is used to treat obstruction, which may be caused by gallstones, tumor, infection, inflammation, or trauma. A catheter may need to be exchanged when sediment collects in the lumen and impedes the drainage of bile or when decompression is successful and the patient can move on to the next level of treatment. The catheter exchange or conversion is performed under fluoroscopic guidance. A guidewire is advanced through the existing catheter to the area just above the obstruction (external only) or past the obstruction into the duodenum (internal-external), and the old catheter is removed. A new catheter is then inserted over the guidewire with the tip above the obstruction (external only) or into the duodenum, (internal-external) and the guidewire is removed. The exchange of an internal-external biliary drainage catheter to an external only catheter is also performed over a guidewire placed through the existing catheter followed by removal of the old catheter. Stents may be placed in the area of obstruction to maintain patency of the bile duct. The new external catheter is advanced over the guidewire to the area of obstruction or stent(s) placement, and the guidewire is removed. Dye may be injected though the catheter to view the biliary system (cholangiography) and confirm catheter placement and patency of the bile duct. The catheter is secured to the skin and a drainage bag is connected to the external portion of the catheter. Code 47536 includes all imaging guidance, supervision, and interpretation of images for exchange of an external or internal-external biliary drainage catheter or conversion of an internal-external biliary drainage catheter to external only.

47537

47537 **Removal of biliary drainage catheter, percutaneous, requiring fluoroscopic guidance (eg, with concurrent indwelling biliary stents), including diagnostic cholangiography when performed, imaging guidance (eg, fluoroscopy), and all associated radiological supervision and interpretation**

A procedure is performed to remove a percutaneous biliary drainage catheter following successful decompression of the biliary system and placement of internal biliary stent(s). Obstruction of the biliary system may be caused by gallstones, tumor, infection, inflammation, or trauma. Staged procedures are often necessary to treat an obstruction. The initial external catheter may be changed to an internal-external system, followed by stent placement, and then removal of the catheter. The external catheter remains in place for 1-2 days following stent placement and the patient returns for fluoroscopic imaging of the biliary system (cholangiography) to confirm that the stent is functional and bile is flowing into the duodenum. The percutaneous biliary catheter is then removed and the skin incision is closed. Code 47537 includes all imaging guidance, supervision, and interpretation of images for removal of the percutaneous biliary catheter.

47538-47540

▲ **47538** **Placement of stent(s) into a bile duct, percutaneous, including diagnostic cholangiography, imaging guidance (eg, fluoroscopy and/or ultrasound), balloon dilation, catheter exchange(s) and catheter removal(s) when performed, and all associated radiological supervision and interpretation; existing access**

▲ **47539** **Placement of stent(s) into a bile duct, percutaneous, including diagnostic cholangiography, imaging guidance (eg, fluoroscopy and/or ultrasound), balloon dilation, catheter exchange(s) and catheter removal(s) when performed, and all associated radiological supervision and interpretation; new access, without placement of separate biliary drainage catheter**

▲ **47540** **Placement of stent(s) into a bile duct, percutaneous, including diagnostic cholangiography, imaging guidance (eg, fluoroscopy and/or ultrasound), balloon dilation, catheter exchange(s) and catheter removal(s) when performed, and all associated radiological supervision and interpretation; new access, with placement of separate biliary drainage catheter (eg, external or internal-external)**

A stent(s) is placed through the skin into a bile duct to hold a blocked area open and allow bile to flow through to the small intestine. In 47539 and 47540, the skin is prepped and an incision is made over the insertion site, usually over the right midaxillary line below the tenth rib for access to the right hepatic lobe, or over the epigastrium for access to the left hepatic lobe. A long, thin, flexible needle is inserted through the skin into the liver, and advanced into the bile duct. For 47538, the needle is inserted into the bile duct through an existing access already secured in place, such as through a previously placed transhepatic drainage catheter or T-tube. A small amount of contrast medium is injected to confirm needle location. A guidewire is passed through the needle into the bile duct and the needle is removed. If cholangiography is performed, an angiography catheter is passed over the guidewire. Dye is injected into the bile ducts, which are visualized on x-ray. More radiographic images are taken as the contrast continues to flow through the bile ducts

Digestive System

into the small intestine. A balloon catheter may then be inserted over the guidewire to the site of the stricture and inflated to dilate the narrowed portion of the duct. A stent(s) is advanced to the site of the stricture over the guidewire and placed within the bile duct to maintain the narrowed portion open and allow the blocked bile to flow into the small intestine. In 47539, internal biliary stent(s) only are placed through a newly created access. In 47538, the stent(s) is placed into the duct through a previously existing access. In 47540, a separate drainage tube or catheter is also placed in addition to the stent. An internal-external biliary drainage tube is placed across the narrowed portion with its curled end in the small intestine and the other end exiting the skin. An external transhepatic biliary drainage tube may be placed proximal to the obstructed area and exiting through the skin. Additional contrast is injected following placement of the stent(s) and drainage catheter to ensure patency of the bile duct. The end of the drainage tube exiting the skin is then attached to a bag for bile collection.

47541

47541   Placement of access through the biliary tree and into small bowel to assist with an endoscopic biliary procedure (eg, rendezvous procedure), percutaneous, including diagnostic cholangiography when performed, imaging guidance (eg, ultrasound and/or fluoroscopy), and all associated radiological supervision and interpretation, new access

A procedure is performed to assist with endoscopic retrograde cholangiography (ERC) or endoscopic ultrasound guided rendezvous procedure (EUS-RV). During ERC or EUS-RV, an endoscope is inserted through the nose or mouth into the stomach and small intestine to locate the opening of the biliary duct in the papilla of the duodenum. A catheter containing contrast dye is passed down the working channel of the endoscope into the biliary and pancreatic duct openings into the small intestine. The dye is injected and x-rays are obtained to study the system. When the biliary duct opening cannot be visualized through the endoscope, an ultrasound transducer may be inserted over the endoscope or through the working channel to assist in locating the opening. If EUS fails to locate the biliary opening, a new, percutaneous access to the biliary tree may be necessary. In these cases, a small gauge needle is advanced through the skin into the liver. Dye may be injected and the biliary system visualized (cholangiography). Under fluoroscopic or ultrasonic guidance, a guide wire protected by a catheter is advanced transhepatically over the needle and manipulated to the opening of the bile duct in the major papilla of the duodenum. With the tip of the guide wire exposed in the duodenum, the endoscopic biliary procedure can be resumed with location of the biliary duct opening marked by the exposed guide wire. Code 47541 includes all imaging guidance, supervision, and interpretation of the ultrasound and/or fluoroscopic films or video for placing the new biliary access.

47542

47542   Balloon dilation of biliary duct(s) or of ampulla (sphincteroplasty), percutaneous, including imaging guidance (eg, fluoroscopy), and all associated radiological supervision and interpretation, each duct (List separately in addition to code for primary procedure)

A procedure is performed to open a stricture in the biliary duct or ampulla. Strictures may result from stones, tumors, infection or inflammation, surgery, radiation, trauma, alcohol or drug abuse. Using fluoroscopic or ultrasonic (US) guidance, a small gauge needle is advanced through the skin and into the liver. A guide wire is advanced transhepatically through the needle and manipulated into the appropriate biliary duct area with the stricture. Placement is confirmed by fluoroscopic visualization and mapping. A stricture will appear as a narrowing or blockage in a branch of the biliary tree. A balloon tipped catheter is then passed over the guide wire to the stricture or blockage site and the balloon is inflated to widen the lumen of the duct. Code 47542 includes guidance and all associated supervision and interpretation of images for each duct dilated.

47543

47543   Endoluminal biopsy(ies) of biliary tree, percutaneous, any method(s) (eg, brush, forceps, and/or needle), including imaging guidance (eg, fluoroscopy), and all associated radiological supervision and interpretation, single or multiple (List separately in addition to code for primary procedure)

A procedure is performed to obtain cell or tissue samples from the lumen of a biliary duct. Endoluminal biopsy is usually performed pre-operatively when imaging alone fails to differentiate benign and malignant lesions in patients with biliary stenosis. If a percutaneous transhepatic drainage catheter is already in place, access to the biliary tree can be gained through the existing catheter. To establish access in the absence of an existing catheter, a small gauge needle is advanced through the skin and into the liver under fluoroscopic guidance. A guide wire and catheter are then advanced transhepatically over the needle and manipulated to the target area in the biliary duct. To obtain cell samples using brush method, a sheath and a flexible brush-tipped probe are introduced through the catheter and advanced to a point beyond the stricture. The sheath is then pulled back to expose the brush which is rotated back and forth across the stricture. The brush is then pulled back into the sheath and both brush and sheath are removed. To obtain tissue samples using needle or forceps method, a sheath is introduced through the

catheter and a cholangioscope is inserted and advanced to the stricture. A flexible needle unit or flexible forceps are passed through the working channel of the cholangioscope. The needle or forceps are advanced into the area of the stricture and tissue samples are collected within the needle or grasped and cut by the forceps. Once an adequate tissue sample has been obtained, the cholangioscope and sheath are removed. An existing percutaneous transhepatic drainage catheter is usually replaced at the end of the procedure. Code 47543 includes all associated guidance, supervision and interpretation of images necessary for single or multiple endolumical biopsy(ies) withing the biliary tree.

47544

47544   Removal of calculi/debris from biliary duct(s) and/or gallbladder, percutaneous, including destruction of calculi by any method (eg, mechanical, electrohydraulic, lithotripsy) when performed, imaging guidance (eg, fluoroscopy), and all associated radiological supervision and interpretation (List separately in addition to code for primary procedure)

A procedure is performed to remove calculi/debris from the biliary ducts and/or gallbladder. The percutaneous approach provides minimally invasive management of biliary stones when endoscopic extraction fails or is refused by the patient. If a percutaneous transhepatic drainage catheter is already in place, access to the biliary tree/gallbladder can be gained through the existing catheter. To establish access in the absence of an existing catheter, a small gauge needle is advanced through the skin and into the liver under fluoroscopic guidance. A guide wire and catheter are then advanced transhepatically over the needle and manipulated to the target area in the biliary duct. Small stones within a duct may be mechanically removed using a balloon catheter. A stiff guide wire is inserted through the catheter and advanced into the duodenum. A sheath is introduced over the guide wire and a balloon tipped catheter is inserted through the sheath. The balloon is inflated distal to the stone(s) and the bile duct is dilated to the size of the largest stone. The balloon is deflated and the catheter is withdrawn with the tip placed proximal to the stone(s). The balloon is then re-inflated and used to push the stone(s) through the duct into the duodenum. Stones may also be removed mechanically using a basket with or without destruction using electrohydraulic lithotripsy (EHL). A sheath is introduced through the catheter over the guide wire and a cholangioscope is inserted and advanced to the stone. The basket is passed through the working channel of the cholangioscope to grasp the stones, which are then removed through the scope. For stones that are too large for the diameter of the scope, the lithotripsy probe is inserted through the working channel and the stone(s) are first fragmented. The fragments may then be removed using irrigation and suction or the basket may be reinserted through the working channel and the fragments grasped and removed. After careful examination of the duct(s) to ensure that all stones have been removed and there is no bleeding, the cholangioscope is removed. An existing percutaneous transhepatic drainage catheter is usually replaced at the end of the procedure. Code 47544 includes guidance and all associated supervision and interpretation of images during removal of calculi.

47550

47550   Biliary endoscopy, intraoperative (choledochoscopy) (List separately in addition to code for primary procedure)

During a separate operative procedure, a biliary endoscopy (choledochoscopy) is performed. A flexible biliary endoscope attached to an irrigation system is inserted through an incision in the common duct. The entire length of the common bile duct is inspected down to the papilla and any abnormalities are noted. The scope is then withdrawn and reinserted proximally and the hepatic ducts inspected.

47552-47553

47552   Biliary endoscopy, percutaneous via T-tube or other tract; diagnostic, with collection of specimen(s) by brushing and/or washing, when performed (separate procedure)
47553   Biliary endoscopy, percutaneous via T-tube or other tract; with biopsy, single or multiple

A flexible fiberoptic endoscope is inserted percutaneously through a T-tube or other external biliary drainage tract. The endoscope is advanced into the bile ducts which are inspected for evidence of disease or other abnormalities. In 47552, cell samples may be obtained by brushing or washing saline fluid into bile duct and then collecting it. The cell samples are sent to the laboratory for separately reportable cytology evaluation. In 47553, the site to be biopsied is identified and a biopsy forceps is placed through the biopsy channel in the endoscope. The forceps is opened, the tissue spiked, the forceps closed, and the tissue sample removed through the endoscope. One or more tissue samples may be obtained. The tissue samples are sent for separately reportable laboratory analysis.

47554

47554   Biliary endoscopy, percutaneous via T-tube or other tract; with removal of calculus/calculi

A flexible fiberoptic endoscope is inserted through the T-tube or other tract. The bile ducts are inspected for evidence of disease or other abnormalities. The endoscope is advanced to the site of the calculus. A snare or basket is placed through a separate channel in the endoscope. The collapsed basket or snare is manipulated to a point beyond the calculus, opened and the calculus captured and extracted through the endoscope. Alternatively, a balloon catheter may be advanced beyond the calculus, the balloon inflated and the calculus removed. This is repeated until all calculi have been removed. The endoscope is then withdrawn and the biliary ducts inspected for any signs of injury resulting from removal of the calculi.

47555-47556

47555   Biliary endoscopy, percutaneous via T-tube or other tract; with dilation of biliary duct stricture(s) without stent
47556   Biliary endoscopy, percutaneous via T-tube or other tract; with dilation of biliary duct stricture(s) with stent

A flexible fiberoptic endoscope is inserted through the T-tube or other tract. The bile ducts are inspected for evidence of disease or other abnormalities. The endoscope is advanced to the site of the stricture. A balloon catheter is placed through a separate channel in the endoscope. The balloon is positioned within the narrowed segment of the duct and inflated for short period of time. The balloon is then deflated and the narrowed segment re-evaluated. The balloon may be inflated and deflated several times to achieve the desired result. The procedure is repeated at a separate site if multiple strictures are present. In 47555, no stent is placed. The endoscope is withdrawn and the bile ducts inspected for any signs of injury dilation procedure. In 47556, following the dilation procedure, a collapsed stent is advanced through the endoscope to the site of the stricture. Once properly positioned in the duct, the stent is deployed (expanded). The bile duct is examined at the site of the stent to ensure proper positioning. The physician may then evaluate the bile ducts beyond the narrowed segment. Following completions of the endoscopic exam, the scope is withdrawn and the bile ducts again inspected for any signs of injury or disease.

47562-47563

47562   Laparoscopy, surgical; cholecystectomy
47563   Laparoscopy, surgical; cholecystectomy with cholangiography

The gallbladder is removed by laparoscopic technique. A small portal incision is made at the navel and a trocar is inserted. The scope and video camera are then inserted at this site. The abdomen is inflated with carbon dioxide. Two to three additional abdominal portal incisions are made and trocars are inserted for placing surgical instruments. The gallbladder is identified. If the gallbladder is distended, a needle may be used to drain bile from the gallbladder. Grasper clamps are applied. The Hartmann's pouch is identified and retracted, exposing the triangle of Calot. The cystic artery and cystic duct are identified. The cystic duct is dissected free and transected. The cystic artery is dissected free, ligated, and doubly divided. Electrocautery is used to dissect the gallbladder off the liver bed. The gallbladder is placed in an extraction sac and removed from the abdomen through one of the small incisions. Use 47563 if intraoperative cholangiography is also performed by placing a small catheter in the cystic duct, instilling 10-20 ml of dye, and then visualizing the ducts using fluoroscopy.

47564

47564   Laparoscopy, surgical; cholecystectomy with exploration of common duct

The gallbladder is removed by laparoscopic technique and the common duct is explored. A small portal incision is made at the navel and a trocar is inserted. The scope and video camera are then inserted at this site. The abdomen is inflated with carbon dioxide. Two to three additional abdominal portal incisions are made and trocars are inserted for placing surgical instruments. The gallbladder is identified. If the gallbladder is distended, a needle may be used to drain bile from the gallbladder. Grasper clamps are applied. The Hartmann's pouch is identified and retracted, exposing the triangle of Calot. The cystic artery and cystic duct are identified. The cystic duct is dissected free and transected. The common bile duct is explored by making a small incision in the duct's anterior superior aspect and advancing a catheter for visualization. If calculi are encountered, a basket extraction catheter is used to remove the stones. Once all calculi are removed, the biliary tract is flushed and filled with saline. A drainage catheter may be placed. Following exploration of the common duct, the cystic artery is dissected free, ligated, and doubly divided. Electrocautery is used to dissect the gallbladder off the liver bed. The gallbladder is placed in an extraction sac and removed from the abdomen through one of the small incisions.

47570

47570   Laparoscopy, surgical; cholecystoenterostomy

A laparoscopic cholecystoenterostomy, also referred to as a laparoscopic biliary bypass procedure, is performed. A small portal incision is made at the navel and a trocar is inserted. The scope and video camera are then inserted at this site. The abdomen is inflated with carbon dioxide. Two to three additional abdominal portal incisions are made and trocars are inserted for placing surgical instruments. The gallbladder is visualized. A laparoscopic intracorporeal linear stapling device is inserted. The gallbladder is exposed as well as a loop of small bowel, usually from the jejunum. The gallbladder and small bowel are then anastomosed using intracorporeal stapler insertion. The stapler insertion sites

are sutured closed. The laparoscopic and surgical instruments are removed and the portal incisions are closed.

47600-47605

47600   Cholecystectomy
47605   Cholecystectomy; with cholangiography

The gallbladder is removed by open surgical technique. An incision is made in the upper abdomen, typically in the right subcostal region. Retractors are inserted and the hepatoduodenal ligament, gallbladder, and triangle of Calot are visualized. Tissue is carefully dissected down to the level of the cystic duct at its junction with the common duct. Dissection continues to the level of the cystic artery. The gallbladder is then dissected from the hepatic bed and the cystic duct ligated. The cystic artery is dissected, doubly ligated, and divided. The gallbladder is removed. Drains may be placed and the incision closed. Use 47605 if intraoperative cholangiography is also performed by placing a small catheter into the cystic duct, instilling 10-20 ml of contrast, and then visualizing the ducts using fluoroscopy.

47610

47610   Cholecystectomy with exploration of common duct

The gallbladder is removed by open surgical technique and the common duct is explored. An incision is made in the upper abdomen, typically in the right subcostal region. Retractors are inserted and the hepatoduodenal ligament, gallbladder, and triangle of Calot are visualized. Tissue is carefully dissected down to the level of the cystic duct at its junction with the common duct. Dissection continues to the level of the cystic artery. The gallbladder is dissected free from the hepatic bed and the cystic duct is ligated. The common bile duct is then explored. The lesser omentum is first exposed and the right lobe of the liver is retracted upward with the duodenum downward, and the stomach is moved to the left. The peritoneum over the common bile duct is divided and the common duct is exposed and opened longitudinally. Any calculi are extracted by inserting a biliary balloon catheter into the common duct. The catheter is passed into the right and then the left hepatic ducts. The balloon is inflated in each duct and the catheter is withdrawn to extract any stones. The catheter is then passed into the lower choledochal sphincter, the balloon is inflated, and the catheter is withdrawn to extract any stones there. A T-tube is placed in the common duct, which is closed around it. The cystic artery is dissected, doubly ligated, and divided. The gallbladder is then removed. The incision is closed around the T-tube and drains.

47612

47612   Cholecystectomy with exploration of common duct; with choledochoenterostomy

The gallbladder is removed by open surgical technique with common duct exploration and a choledochoenterostomy. An incision is made in the upper abdomen, typically in the right subcostal region. Retractors are inserted and the hepatoduodenal ligament, gallbladder, and triangle of Calot are visualized. Tissue is carefully dissected down to the level of the cystic duct at its junction with the common duct. Dissection continues to the level of the cystic artery. The gallbladder is dissected free from the hepatic bed and the cystic duct is ligated. The common bile duct is then explored. The lesser omentum is first exposed and the right lobe of the liver is retracted upward with the duodenum downward, and the stomach is moved to the left. The peritoneum over the common bile duct is divided and the common duct is exposed and opened longitudinally. Any calculi are extracted by inserting a biliary balloon catheter into the common duct. The catheter is passed into the right and then the left hepatic ducts. The balloon is inflated in each duct and the catheter is withdrawn to extract any stones. The catheter is then passed into the lower choledochal sphincter, the balloon is inflated, and the catheter is withdrawn to extract any stones there. A choledochoenterostomy is then performed. This can be performed in a side-to-side or end-to-end anastomosis. The end-to-side configuration is also referred to as a transaction choledochoenterostomy and is the preferred type. In an end-to-side anastomosis, the lower end of the common bile duct is mobilized above the duodenum and the head of the pancreas. The duct is then completely transected and the distal (pancreatic) end is closed. The proximal end is anastomosed end-to-side to the duodenum. The cystic artery is dissected, doubly ligated, and divided. The gallbladder is then removed. The incision is closed around drains.

47620

47620   Cholecystectomy with exploration of common duct; with transduodenal sphincterotomy or sphincteroplasty, with or without cholangiography

The gallbladder is removed by open surgical technique with common duct exploration and a sphincterotomy or sphincteroplasty. An incision is made in the upper abdomen, typically in the right subcostal region. Retractors are inserted and the hepatoduodenal ligament, gallbladder, and triangle of Calot are visualized. Tissue is carefully dissected down to the level of the cystic duct at its junction with the common duct. Dissection continues to the level of the cystic artery. The gallbladder is dissected free from the hepatic bed and the cystic duct is ligated. Intraoperative cholangiography is performed if indicated by placing a

Digestive System

small catheter in the cystic duct, instilling 10-20 ml of dye, and then visualizing the ducts using fluoroscopy. The common bile duct is then explored. The lesser omentum is first exposed and the right lobe of the liver is retracted upward with the duodenum downward, and the stomach is moved to the left. The peritoneum over the common bile duct is divided and the common duct is exposed and opened longitudinally. Any calculi are extracted by inserting a biliary balloon catheter into the common duct. The catheter is passed into the right and then the left hepatic ducts. The balloon is inflated in each duct and the catheter is withdrawn to extract any stones. The catheter is then passed into the lower choledochal sphincter, the balloon is inflated, and the catheter is withdrawn to extract any stones there. A sphincterotomy or sphincteroplasty is then performed. The entire length of the musculature of the lower, middle, and upper choledochal sphincters surrounding the lower end of the common bile duct are divided. The musoca is then approximated at the cut edges and repaired with interrupted sutures. The cystic artery is dissected, doubly ligated, and divided. The gallbladder is removed and the incision is closed around drains.

47700

47700   Exploration for congenital atresia of bile ducts, without repair, with or without liver biopsy, with or without cholangiography

Congenital biliary atresia is a condition in which there is obliteration or discontinuity of the extrahepatic bile ducts which causes obstruction of the flow of bile from the liver. Untreated biliary atresia eventually causes cirrhosis and destruction of the liver. An abdominal incision is made in the upper midline and the gallbladder and liver are exposed. The extrahepatic bile ducts or biliary tract remnant is identified and the patency evaluated. Intraoperative cholangiography may be performed by placing a small catheter in the cystic duct and instilling contast media. The anatomy of the biliary tree from the liver to the small intestine is evaluated radiographically. Failure of contrast media to reach the gastrointestinal tract is indicative of biliary atresia. Tissue samples are taken from the liver as needed and histologic evaluation performed to determine whether there is histologic evidence of bile duct proliferation or obstruction.

47701

47701   Portoenterostomy (eg, Kasai procedure)

Portoenterostomy is performed to treat congenital biliary atresia, a condition in which there is obliteration or discontinuity of the extrahepatic bile ducts which causes obstruction of the flow of bile from the liver. Untreated biliary atresia eventually causes cirrhosis and destruction of the liver. An abdominal incision is made in the upper midline and the gallbladder and liver are exposed. The hilum of the liver is dissected and the biliary tract remnant identified. The jejunum is mobilized and divided. A Roux-en-Y limb is constructed. The distal end of the divided jejunum is anastomosed to the liver hilum and the proximal end is anastomosed to the side of the jejunum. Drains are placed as needed and the abdomen is closed.

47711-47712

47711   Excision of bile duct tumor, with or without primary repair of bile duct; extrahepatic

47712   Excision of bile duct tumor, with or without primary repair of bile duct; intrahepatic

Bile duct tumors are rare. Lesions may be benign or malignant, although malignant tumors are more common. Extrahepatic bile duct tumors occur outside the liver while intrahepatic bile duct tumors occur in the portion of the bile duct inside the liver. Local excision of an intrahepatic bile duct tumor is not commonly performed as these tumors are more likely to be malignant and prone to metastasis. When local excision is performed, an abdominal incision is made in the midline, the gallbladder and liver are exposed, and the bile duct tumor identified. The bile duct is transected above and below the tumor and both the duct and tumor are excised. The bile duct may be repaired by suturing the remaining portions together or by separately reportable Roux-en-Y hepaticojejunuostomy or other reconstruction technique. Use 47711 for excision of an extrahepatic bile duct tumor and 47712 for excision of intrahepatic bile duct tumor.

47715

47715   Excision of choledochal cyst

The physician excises a choledochal cyst which is a congenital bile duct anomaly characterized by cystic dilation of the biliary duct(s). An abdominal incision is made in the midline, the gallbladder and liver are exposed, and the choledochal cyst identified. The bile duct is transected above and below the cyst and dilated portion of the duct is excised. The bile duct may be repaired by suturing the remaining portions together or by separately reportable Roux-en-Y hepaticojejunuostomy or other reconstruction technique.

47720-47721

47720   Cholecystoenterostomy; direct
47721   Cholecystoenterostomy; with gastroenterostomy

A cholecystoenterostomy, also referred to as a biliary bypass procedure, is performed to treat biliary obstruction. In 47720, a direct choledochoenterostomy is performed.

An abdominal incision is made in the midline. The gallbladder and a segment of small intestine are exposed and mobilized. The gallbladder is dissected and asegment of small intestine rotated up to the gallbladder and incised longitudinally. The gallbladder is then anastomosed to the small intestine. This allows bile to drain directly from the gallbladder into the small intestine. In 47721, a cholecystoenterostomy is performed with gastroenterostomy. The cholecystoenterostomy is performed as described above. If a gastroduodenostomy is performed, the stomach and duodenum are divided at the gastroduodenal junction and the opening in the stomach closed with sutures. An incision is then made in the stomach usually along the greater curvature and the duodenum is sutured to the stomach in an end-to-side fashion. Alternatively, a segment of duodenum or jejunum may be rotated up to meet the stomach. The stomach and duodenum or jejunum are incised longitudinally and sutured together in a side-to-side fashion. The surgical wound is irrigated, drains placed as needed, and the abdominal incision closed in layers.

47740-47741

47740   Cholecystoenterostomy; Roux-en-Y
47741   Cholecystoenterostomy; Roux-en-Y with gastroenterostomy

A Roux-en-Y cholecystoenterostomy, also referred to as a biliary bypass procedure, is performed to treat biliary obstruction. In 47740, a Roux-en-Y choledochoenterostomy is performed without gastroenterostomy. An abdominal incision is made in the midline and the gallbladder and a segment of small intestine are exposed. The gallbladder is dissected. The jejunum is mobilized and divided. A Roux-en-Y limb is constructed. The distal end of the divided jejunum is anastomosed to the gallbladder and the proximal end is anastomosed to the side of the jejunum. This allows bile to drain directly from the gallbladder into the small intestine. In 47741, a Roux-en-Y cholecystoenterostomy is performed with gastroenterostomy. The cholecystoenterostomy is performed as described above. If a gastroduodenostomy is performed, the stomach and duodenum are divided at the gastroduodenal junction and the opening in the stomach closed with sutures. An incision is then made in the stomach usually along the greater curvature and the duodenum is sutured to the stomach in an end-to-side fashion. Alternatively, a segment of duodenum or jejunum may be rotated up to meet the stomach. The stomach and duodenum or jejunum are incised longitudinally and sutured together in a side-to-side fashion. The surgical wound is irrigated, drains placed as needed, and the abdominal incision closed in layers.

47760-47765

47760   Anastomosis, of extrahepatic biliary ducts and gastrointestinal tract
47765   Anastomosis, of intrahepatic ducts and gastrointestinal tract

An anastomosis of extrahepatic or intrahepatic bile ducts to the gastrointestinal tract is performed, also referred to as a biliary bypass procedure. This procedure is performed to treat biliary obstruction. In 47760, anastomosis of extrahepatic bile ducts is performed. An abdominal incision is made in the midline and the liver, gallbladder and a segment of small intestine and/or stomach are exposed. The obstructed bile duct is divided above the obstruction and the ends closed with sutures. The stomach, or a segment of small intestine, usually the jejunum, is mobilized and brought up to the bile duct. The bile duct is incised longitudinally. The stomach or small intestine is incised and the bile duct anastomosed to the stomach or small intestine. This allows bile to drain directly from the bile duct into the small intestine. The surgical wound is irrigated, drains placed as needed, and the abdominal incision closed in layers. In 47765, anastomosis of intrahepatic bile ducts is performed. The procedure is performed as described above, except that the liver hilum is dissected and the intrahepatic bile ducts are exposed and divided. The intrahepatic bile duct is then anastomosed to the gastrointestinal tract as described above.

47780-47785

47780   Anastomosis, Roux-en-Y, of extrahepatic biliary ducts and gastrointestinal tract

47785   Anastomosis, Roux-en-Y, of intrahepatic biliary ducts and gastrointestinal tract

A Roux-en-Y anastomosis of extrahepatic or intrahepatic bile ducts to the gastrointestinal tract is performed, also referred to as a biliary bypass procedure. This procedure is performed to treat biliary obstruction. In 47780, a Roux-en-Y anastomosis of extrahepatic bile ducts is performed. An abdominal incision is made in the midline and the liver, gallbladder, obstructed bile duct and a segment of small intestine are exposed. A segment of small intestine, usually the jejunum, is mobilized and divided. A Roux-en-Y limb is constructed. The extrahepatic bile duct is divided above the obstruction and the ends closed. A longitudinal incision is then made in the bile duct. The distal end of the divided small intestine is closed and a small incision is made near the distal end intestine. The small intestine is anastomosed to the extrahepatic bile duct and the proximal end is anastomosed to the side of the small intestine. This allows bile to drain directly from the liver into the small intestine. The surgical wound is irrigated, drains placed as needed, and the abdominal incision closed in layers. In 47785, a Roux-en-Y anastomosis of intrahepatic bile ducts is performed. The procedure is performed as described above, except that the liver hilum is dissected and the intrahepatic bile ducts are exposed. The distal end of the small intestine is then anastomosed to the intrahepatic bile ducts.

Digestive System

47800

47800 Reconstruction, plastic, of extrahepatic biliary ducts with end-to-end anastomosis

An abdominal incision is made in the midline and the liver, gallbladder and extrahepatic bile ducts exposed. The diseased or injured extrahepatic bile duct is identified and the injury evaluated. The injured or diseased segment is excised and the ends of the remaining segments are sutured together. The surgical wound is irrigated, drains placed as needed, and the abdominal incision closed in layers.

47801

47801 Placement of choledochal stent

This procedure is performed for chronic obstruction of the common bile duct, especially that due to malignancy. An abdominal incision is made in the midline and the liver, gallbladder and common bile duct exposed. The common bile duct is incised and a biliary plastic or metal tube or stent placed into the narrowed segment of the duct. The common bile duct incision is closed and patency verified by separately reportable cholangiogram. The surgical wound is irrigated, drains placed as needed, and the abdominal incision closed in layers.

47802

47802 U-tube hepaticoenterostomy

An abdominal incision is made in the midline and the liver, gallbladder and bile ducts exposed. The hilum of the liver is dissected and the U-tube placed into the proximal aspect of the intrahepatic bile duct. One end of the U-tube is then threaded through the liver into the small intestine, usually to a jejunal Roux-en-Y limb. A separate enterotomy is performed and the U-tube brought out through the intestine. Stab incisions are then made in the abdomen and both ends of the U-tube, the one exiting the liver and the one exiting the intestine, are then brought out through the stab incisions and secured to the abdominal wall.

47900

47900 Suture of extrahepatic biliary duct for pre-existing injury (separate procedure)

An abdominal incision is made in the midline and the liver, gallbladder and extrahepatic bile ducts exposed. The injured bile duct is identified and the injury evaluated. The injury is repaired with sutures. The surgical wound is irrigated, drains placed as needed, and the abdominal incision closed in layers.

48000-48001

48000 Placement of drains, peripancreatic, for acute pancreatitis
48001 Placement of drains, peripancreatic, for acute pancreatitis; with cholecystostomy, gastrostomy, and jejunostomy

In 48000, a small stab wound is made in the abdomen over the site of the fluid collection. A catheter is inserted over a guidewire and into the fluid collection. The catheter is secured and left in place until the pancreatitis subsides. One or more drains may be placed. In 48001, drains are placed as described above. Drainage catheters are then also placed in the gallbladder (cholecystostomy), stomach (gastrostomy), and small intestine (jejunostomy). Cholecystostomy is performed by inserting a catheter over a guidewire and passing it thought the abdominal wall, the liver, and into the gallbladder. Gastrostomy and jejunostomy are performed by making a small incision in the abdominal wall and passing a tube into the stomach or small intestine. All catheters are secured and left in place until the pancreatitis subsides.

48020

48020 Removal of pancreatic calculus

A calculus (stone) is removed from the pancreas. A subcostal or midline incision is made in the abdomen. The pancreas is inspected and the stone is identified. An incision is made in the pancreas overlying the stone contained in one of the pancreatic ducts. The stone is removed. The incision in the pancreatic duct and pancreas are closed. The surgical wound is irrigated, drains are placed, and the wound is closed over the drains.

48100-48102

48100 Biopsy of pancreas, open (eg, fine needle aspiration, needle core biopsy, wedge biopsy)
48102 Biopsy of pancreas, percutaneous needle

In 48100, an incision is made in the abdomen over the pancreas and the pancreas is exposed. The lesion is identified. If a fine needle aspiration (FNA) is performed, a thin needle is inserted into the pancreatic lesion and cells are extracted for cytopathology examination. The needle may need to be inserted into the lesion multiple times to obtain an adequate cell specimen. If needle core biopsy (NCB) is performed, a large bore needle is inserted into the pancreatic lesion and a tissue sample is obtained. The tissue sample is visually inspected and additional samples obtained as needed. If a wedge biopsy is

performed, a small wedge-shaped section of the pancreas containing the lesion is excised. In 48102, a percutaneous needle biopsy is performed. The skin is prepped and a local anesthetic administered. A small incision is made overlying the previously identified pancreatic lesion. Using separately reportable fluoroscopic, ultrasound, CT or MR guidance, a thin walled needle is advanced through the incision and positioned adjacent to the lesion. A second needle is advanced into the lesion and tissue samples are obtained usually by making multiple passes with the needle.

48105

48105 Resection or debridement of pancreas and peripancreatic tissue for acute necrotizing pancreatitis

Resection or debridement is done on the pancreas and peripancreatic tissue for acute necrotizing pancreatitis. This condition happens when extensive inflammation caused by autodigestion of the gland by its own enzymes involves parenchymal abscesses and hemorrhaging from enzymes being walled off in granulation and bacteria seeding throughout the tissue. Aggressive surgical debridement is delayed as long as possible for better survival, and only done on patients with necrosis positive for bacteria or fungi on Gram stain or culture of aspirate. An abdominal incision is made and tissue is dissected and retracted to reach the pancreas. Peripancreatic fat is predominantly involved as it is the first to necrotize while the gland may be less involved. The surrounding diseased tissue is removed and areas of necrosis in the pancreas are resected and debrided. Drains are put into place and the wound is closed.

48120

48120 Excision of lesion of pancreas (eg, cyst, adenoma)

A lesion such as a cyst or adenoma is excised from the pancreas. A subcostal or midline incision is made in the abdomen. The pancreas is inspected and the lesion is identified. Depending on the nature and site of the lesion, several different techniques may be used. One technique for cystic lesions that are connected to the pancreas by a tubular structure is to suture ligate and divide the lesion. Another technique is to dissect the lesion from ductal and vascular structures and then resect the lesion.

48140-48145

48140 Pancreatectomy, distal subtotal, with or without splenectomy; without pancreaticojejunostomy
48145 Pancreatectomy, distal subtotal, with or without splenectomy; with pancreaticojejunostomy

A subcostal or midline incision is made in the abdomen. The gastrocolic and colosplenic ligaments are divided. The duodenum and head of the pancreas are mobilized. The peritoneum is incised along the inferior border of the body and tail of the pancreas. Blunt dissection is used to free the body and tail from the posterior abdominal wall. If the spleen is removed, the dissection is extended from the superior mesenteric vein to the hilum of the spleen. The splenic artery is identified, divided, and doubly ligated. The spleen is then freed from the diaphragm. The spleen and distal pancreas are retracted so that the inferior mesenteric vein can be seen. The splenic vein is identified and preserved. The mesentery of the uncinate process is ligated and divided. The freed pancreas and spleen are temporarily returned to their normal position. The body of the pancreas is incised and a portion of the body and entire tail are removed. If the spleen is removed it is excised in conjunction with the distal pancreas. In 48140, the procedure is performed without pancreaticojejunuostomy. The pancreatic duct is identified and drainage to the duodenum is verified. In 48145, a pancreaticojejunostomy is also performed. A Roux-en-Y jejunal segment is constructed. The head of the pancreas is anastomosed to the defunctionalized (distal) jejunal segment. Gastrointestinal continuity is restored by anastomosis of the proximal jejunal segment to the distal segment in a Y configuration. The pancreas is closed with interrupted mattress sutures. The wound is flushed with normal saline and drains placed. The abdomen is closed around the drains.

48146

48146 Pancreatectomy, distal, near-total with preservation of duodenum (Child-type procedure)

A distal near-total pancreatectomy to remove the entire body of the pancreas along with the tail of the pancreas is performed with preservation of the duodenum. This procedure is also referred to as a ninety-five percent distal pancreatectomy. A subcostal or midline incision is made in the abdomen. The gastrocolic and colosplenic ligaments are divided. The duodenum and head of the pancreas are mobilized. The peritoneum is incised along the inferior border of the body and tail of the pancreas. Blunt dissection is used to free the body and tail from the posterior abdominal wall. The spleen is dissected free. The spleen and distal pancreas are retracted so that the inferior mesenteric vein can be seen. The mesentery of the uncinate process is ligated and divided. The pancreas and spleen are temporarily returned to their normal position. The pancreas is incised between the head and the body, and the body and tail are excised, taking care to preserve the vessels that provide adequate blood supply to the duodenum. The pancreatic duct is identified and drainage to the duodenum is verified. The pancreas is closed with interrupted mattress

Digestive System

● New Code   ▲ Revised Code

sutures. The wound is flushed with normal saline and drains are placed. The abdomen is closed around the drains.

48148

48148   Excision of ampulla of Vater

The ampulla of Vater is excised. This procedure is also referred to as an ampullectomy. A subcostal or midline incision is made in the abdomen. The second part of the duodenum is mobilized. Stay sutures are placed in the duodenal wall. The bile and pancreatic ducts are cannulated using a catheter. The duodenal mucosa is resected around the ampulla of Vater. The biliary and pancreatic ducts are transected and the ampulla of Vater is excised. The biliary and pancreatic ducts are reconstructed by approximating the common walls of these ducts and suturing them together on the duodenal wall. The ducts are probed with biliary dilators to ensure adequate size. Drainage of the ducts into the duodenum is verified and the duodenum is closed. The surgical wound is flushed with normal saline and drains may be placed. The abdomen is closed around the drains.

48150-48152

48150   Pancreatectomy, proximal subtotal with total duodenectomy, partial gastrectomy, choledochoenterostomy and gastrojejunostomy (Whipple-type procedure); with pancreatojejunostomy

48152   Pancreatectomy, proximal subtotal with total duodenectomy, partial gastrectomy, choledochoenterostomy and gastrojejunostomy (Whipple-type procedure); without pancreatojejunostomy

A subcostal or midline incision is made in the abdomen. The duodenum and head of the pancreas are mobilized. The superior mesenteric vein is identified. The common bile duct and portal vein are mobilized. The neck of the pancreas is elevated. The stomach is divided. The common bile duct and neck of the pancreas are divided. The pancreas is dissected from mesenteric vessels. The proximal jejunum is mobilized and divided. The distal duodenum is dissected from the posterior abdominal wall. The transected portion of jejunum is passed under the mesenteric vessels and delivered to the anastomosis site. The mesoduodenum and mesentery of the uncinate process are divided. The head of the pancreas, the portion of the bile duct, the duodenum, and the portion of the stomach are now free from all attachments and are removed. In 48150, the pancreas and jejunum are anastomosed (pancreatojejunostomy) using either an end-to-side or end-to-end technique. Next, the bile duct is anastomosed to the jejunum (choledochojejunostomy). In 48152, the pancreatic duct is identified and drainage to the small bowel verified, and the procedure is performed without pancreatojejunostomy. The pancreas is closed with mattress sutures. A T-tube may be placed in the bile duct to ensure that it remains open. The remaining portion of the stomach is then anastomosed to the jejunum (gastrojejunostomy). The abdomen is irrigated with normal saline, drains are placed, and the abdomen is closed.

48153-48154

48153   Pancreatectomy, proximal subtotal with near-total duodenectomy, choledochoenterostomy and duodenojejunostomy (pylorus-sparing, Whipple-type procedure); with pancreatojejunostomy

48154   Pancreatectomy, proximal subtotal with near-total duodenectomy, choledochoenterostomy and duodenojejunostomy (pylorus-sparing, Whipple-type procedure); without pancreatojejunostomy

The head (proximal portion) of the pancreas is removed along with a portion of the bile duct and nearly the entire duodenum, preserving only the proximal 3-4 cm of the duodenum. A pancreatojejunostomy may also be performed. A subcostal or midline incision is made in the abdomen. The duodenum and head of the pancreas are mobilized. The superior mesenteric vein is identified. The common bile duct and portal vein are mobilized. The neck of the pancreas is elevated. The duodenum is divided 3-4 cm distal to the pylorus. The common bile duct and neck of the pancreas are divided. The pancreas is dissected from mesenteric vessels. The proximal jejunum is mobilized and divided. The distal duodenum is dissected from the posterior abdominal wall. The transected portion of jejunum is passed under the mesenteric vessels and delivered to the anastomosis site. The mesoduodenum and mesentery of the uncinate process are divided. The head of the pancreas, a portion of the bile duct, and a section of duodenum are now free from all attachments and are removed. In 48153, the pancreas and jejunum are anastomosed (pancreatojejunostomy) using either an end-to-side or end-to-end technique. Next, the bile duct is anastomosed to the jejunum (choledochojejunostomy). In 48154, the pancreatic duct is identified, drainage to the small bowel verified, and the procedure is performed without pancreatojejunostomy. The pancreas is closed with mattress sutures. A T-tube may be placed in the bile duct to ensure that it remains open. The remaining portion of the duodenum is then anastomosed to the jejunum (gastrojejunostomy). The abdomen is irrigated with normal saline, drains are placed, and the abdomen is closed.

48155

48155   Pancreatectomy, total

A subcostal or midline incision is made in the abdomen. The gastrocolic omentum is divided and the lesser sac is entered. The splenic and hepatic flexures are mobilized. Attachments between the posterior stomach and pancreas are divided. The stomach is

elevated and the anterior surface of the pancreas is exposed. The peritoneum along the inferior border of the pancreas is incised and the body and tail are mobilized. Mobilization of the tail of the pancreas also requires division of the splenic ligaments and short gastric arteries (vasa brevia). The pancreas is dissected from the mesenteric vessels and the entire pancreas is removed. The abdomen is irrigated with normal saline and drains are placed. The abdomen is closed around the drains.

48160

48160   Pancreatectomy, total or subtotal, with autologous transplantation of pancreas or pancreatic islet cells

All or part of the pancreas is removed. Following removal of the pancreas, a portion of the pancreas or the islet cells are harvested from the resected pancreas and transferred to a different site in the same patient (autologous transplant). A subcostal or midline incision is made in the abdomen. The gastrocolic omentum is divided and the lesser sac is entered. The splenic and hepatic flexures are mobilized. Attachments between the posterior stomach and pancreas are divided. The stomach is elevated and the anterior surface of the pancreas is exposed. The peritoneum along the inferior border of the pancreas is incised and the body and tail are mobilized. Mobilization of the tail of the pancreas also requires division of the splenic ligaments and short gastric arteries (vasa brevia). The pancreas is dissected from the mesenteric vessels. All or part of the pancreas is removed. If an islet cell transplant is performed, the cells must first be extracted from the resected pancreas by injecting a collagenase solution into the pancreas. This separates the cells from the acinar tissue (secretory portion of the pancreas). The islet cell tissue is then collected, washed, and diluted in plasma. The plasma is injected into the portal vein of the liver (portal embolization). Alternatively, the islet cells may be transplanted beneath the kidneys.

48400

48400   Injection procedure for intraoperative pancreatography (List separately in addition to code for primary procedure)

The pancreatic ducts are visualized following injection of contrast (dye) during a separately reportable operative procedure. The distal pancreatic duct is identified. A catheter is inserted and contrast is injected in a retrograde fashion. The pancreatic ducts are visualized and evaluated for possible injury or obstruction. This code reports the injection procedure only. The radiological component is reported separately.

48500

48500   Marsupialization of pancreatic cyst

A pancreatic cyst is opened and a pouch is created (marsupialization) to allow exterior drainage of the cyst. The approach is either by a subcostal or a midline incision. The pancreas is visualized and the cyst is inspected. Fluid is aspirated from the cyst to verify that it is a fluid-filled type. The anterior wall of the cyst is incised and fluid and debris is extracted. A biopsy is taken to rule out malignancy. The anterior wall of the cyst is resected and a pouch is then fashioned. The cut edges of the pouch are sutured to the skin to allow exterior drainage of the cyst.

48510

48510   External drainage, pseudocyst of pancreas, open

External drainage of a pancreatic pseudocyst is performed by open approach. The pancreas is exposed by a subcostal or midline abdominal incision. The pseudocyst is located. The cyst is aspirated to verify that it is a fluid-filled type. A small incision is made in the cyst and the wall is biopsied to rule-out malignancy. One or more drains are placed and secured in the cyst cavity to drain fluid. The drains are left in place and the abdomen is closed around the drains.

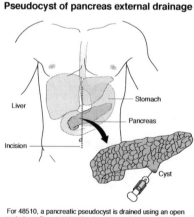

Pseudocyst of pancreas external drainage

Liver | Stomach | Pancreas | Incision | Cyst

For 48510, a pancreatic pseudocyst is drained using an open technique. Report 48511 if using using radiological guidance.

   ● New Code   ▲ Revised Code

Digestive System

48520-48540

48520   Internal anastomosis of pancreatic cyst to gastrointestinal tract; direct
48540   Internal anastomosis of pancreatic cyst to gastrointestinal tract; Roux-en-Y

A pancreatic cyst is connected by internal anastomosis to the gastrointestinal tract for drainage. The approach may be either by bilateral subcostal incisions or a midline abdominal incision. The cyst is exposed and fluid is aspirated from the cyst to verify that it is a fluid-filled type. Aspiration also allows the thickness of the cyst wall to be evaluated. A biopsy of the cyst wall is performed to rule-out malignancy. In 48520, the anastomosis is performed directly to the posterior wall of the stomach or the duodenum. If the anastomosis is to the stomach (cystgastrostomy), the stomach is opened and stay sutures are placed directly above the pancreatic cyst, which is typically already adherent to the posterior wall of the stomach. An incision is then made through the cystic and the gastric wall tissue. Fluid and debris are evaluated from the cyst. The incised posterior gastric wall and the anterior cyst wall are then sutured together. Less commonly a cyst in the head of the pancreas will be anastomosed to the duodenum (cystduodenostomy). The head of the pancreas is mobilized. An incision is made in the wall of the duodenum and the adjacent cyst wall and the incised edges sutured together. In 48540, a Roux-en-Y limb is constructed and the cyst is anastomosed to the jejunum (cystjejunostomy). The jejunum is mobilized and divided. A Roux-en-Y limb is constructed and brought to the cyst wall. The cyst is incised and fluid and debris evacuated. The distal end of the divided jejunum is anastomosed to the cyst wall. The proximal end of the jejunum is anastomosed to the side of the jejunum approximately 40 cm from the distal anastomosis in a Y-shaped configuration. Drains are placed in the abdomen and the abdominal incision is closed.

48545

48545   Pancreatorrhaphy for injury

Following traumatic injury to the pancreas, lacerations are repaired. A subcostal or midline incision is made in the abdomen. The entire pancreas is exposed and inspected. The lesser sac is mobilized, opened, and inspected. Attachments to the transverse colon and stomach are severed and the transverse colon is retracted downward and the stomach upward for better visualization of the body of the pancreas. The hepatic flexure of the colon is mobilized for better visualization of the pancreatic head and neck. To visualize the tail of the pancreas, the splenic hilum is exposed. The peritoneal attachments lateral to the spleen and colon are divided. The colon, spleen, and pancreas are then mobilized to allow palpation and visual inspection of the posterior pancreas. Bleeding from small lacerations is controlled. Large lacerations are repaired with mattress sutures, or less frequently, with staples. The operative wound is irrigated and drains are placed. The abdomen is closed around the drains.

48547

48547   Duodenal exclusion with gastrojejunostomy for pancreatic injury

Following traumatic injury to the pancreas with involvement of the pancreatic duct and duodenum, a duodenal exclusion, also referred to as a pyloric exclusion, is performed to divert gastric contents away from the duodenum until the duodenal and pancreatic duct injuries heal. A subcostal or midline incision is made in the abdomen. The pancreas and duodenum are exposed and inspected. An incision is made in the stomach (gastrotomy) and the pylorus is grasped, clamped, and sutured closed. A loop gastrojejunostomy is constructed by dividing the jejunum, which is then anastomosed to the stomach. This diverts gastric flow away from the duodenum for several weeks or months to allow the duodenum and pancreatic duct to heal. The abdomen is irrigated, drains are placed, and the abdomen is closed around the drains. The exclusion suture in the pylorus will open and the gastrojejunostomy will functionally close without further surgical intervention.

48548

48548   Pancreaticojejunostomy, side-to-side anastomosis (Puestow-type operation)

A pancreaticojejunostomy, side-to-side anastomosis, or Puestow-type operation is done in cases of severe pain from chronic pancreatitis. An abdominal incision is made from under the breastbone to the navel. The pancreas is exposed and the main duct of the pancreas is opened from the head to the tail. A loop of jejunum is brought up to create a connecting fistula and the entire open pancreatic duct is then sutured into the defunctionalized jejunal loop to allow pancreatic secretions to drain directly into the intestine through the formation of a longitudinal pancreaticojejunostomy in a side-to-side anastomosis.

48550

48550   Donor pancreatectomy (including cold preservation), with or without duodenal segment for transplantation

A pancreatectomy is performed from a cadaver (brain-dead) patient for transplantation, including cold preservation. The pancreas is removed with or without a duodenal segment. Typically, the pancreas is harvested along with other organs such as the heart, lung, liver, and kidneys. An incision is made from the sternal notch to the pubis and from the right to the left flank to expose the thoracic and abdominal contents. The pancreas and liver are mobilized together. The portal vein, hepatic artery, and bile duct are dissected and the gastro-duodenal artery is ligated. The origin of the hepatic artery is dissected from

the pancreas at the celiac axis. The origin of the splenic artery is located. The left gastric artery is ligated. The origins of the celiac and superior mesenteric arteries are isolated at the aorta. The duodenum is mobilized. As the thoracic organs are removed, the aorta and inferior mesenteric vein are infused with preservative solution. The duodenum is divided at the pylorus and the ligament of Treitz. The liver is removed first to provide access to the pancreas. The superior mesenteric artery is divided at its origin and the pancreas is removed. The pancreas is flushed again with preservative solution and transferred to the back table for backbench preparation prior to transplantation.

48551

48551   Backbench standard preparation of cadaver donor pancreas allograft prior to transplantation, including dissection of allograft from surrounding soft tissues, splenectomy, duodenotomy, ligation of bile duct, ligation of mesenteric vessels, and Y-graft arterial anastomoses from iliac artery to superior mesenteric artery and to splenic artery

Standard backbench preparation of a cadaver donor pancreas is performed prior to transplantation. The pancreas is removed from the sterile container, placed on ice, and bathed in cold preservation solution. The pancreas is inspected to ensure that it is intact and healthy enough for transplant. The attached spleen is removed by carefully ligating and dividing splenic vessels. The duodenum is opened and the Sphincter of Oddi is located. A catheter is inserted into the common bile duct and passed through the sphincter to confirm sphincter location. The duodenum is shortened both proximally and distally. The mesenteric vessels are ligated and divided as the duodenum is separated from the distal pancreas. Both ends of the remaining duodenum are stapled and oversewn. The common bile duct is ligated. The middle colic vessels are ligated at the base of the transverse mesocolon. The superior mesenteric vessels are ligated at the root of the small bowel mesentery. A Y-graft is constructed between the external and internal iliac arteries by suturing each of these iliac limbs to the superior mesenteric artery. The pancreas is maintained on ice and bathed in cold preservation solution until the recipient has been prepared for transplant.

48552

48552   Backbench reconstruction of cadaver donor pancreas allograft prior to transplantation, venous anastomosis, each

Venous anastomosis is performed on a cadaver donor pancreas in a backbench reconstruction procedure prior to transplantation. Venous extension graft is sometimes needed when the portal vein is too short or there is an unusual anatomic configuration. A segment of donor vein that matches the diameter of portal vein is procured usually from the cadaver donor. Typically either the common or external iliac vein is used. The donor vein is anastomosed in an end-to-end fashion to the portal vein using loupe magnification. Report 48552 for each venous anastomosis performed.

48554

48554   Transplantation of pancreatic allograft

The physician transplants a pancreas allograft. There are two different surgical techniques for pancreas transplantation. One places the pancreas in the lower abdomen with the digestive enzymes draining into the urinary bladder. The other places the pancreas in the abdomen and uses anastomosis of the attached segment of duodenum to the jejunum to drain digestive enzymes into the intestine. In addition, pancreas transplant is frequently performed with concurrent kidney transplant. The recipient procedure is performed using a midline intraperitoneal approach. If kidney transplant is performed at the same surgical session, it is performed first. Next, the pancreas is transplanted. To perform abdominal placement of the donor pancreas with digestive enzymes draining to the intestine, attention is first directed to the portal vein. The portal vein in the donor pancreas is anastomosed end-to-side to a major tributary of the superior mesenteric vein of the recipient. The donor iliac artery is brought through a window in the distal mesentery and anastomosed end-to-side to the right common iliac artery. The segment of duodenum attached to the donor pancreas is anastomosed to a diverting Roux-en-Y in the recipient jejunum. The pancreas is revascularized and the tail of the pancreas is anchored to the anterior abdominal wall with interrupted sutures to permit subsequent allograft biopsy using percutaneous ultrasound-guided technique. A nasogastric tube is placed. Drains are placed as needed in the abdomen and the surgical wound is closed.

48556

48556   Removal of transplanted pancreatic allograft

The physician removes a transplanted pancreatic allograft. Removal is performed due to complications including graft rejection, infection, or malignancy. The abdomen is opened and the pancreatic allograft is exposed and evaluated. Once it has been determined that the transplanted pancreas is not functioning properly and must be removed, the donor portal vein and donor iliac artery are clamped and transected, and vascular anastomosis sites in the recipient vessels are repaired. The pancreas allograft is severed at the anastomosis sites in the jejunum or urinary bladder. The jejunum or urinary bladder graft sites are repaired. Drains are placed and the abdomen is closed.

Digestive System

49000-49002

49000 Exploratory laparotomy, exploratory celiotomy with or without biopsy(s) (separate procedure)

49002 Reopening of recent laparotomy

The physician performs an exploratory laparotomy or celiotomy with or without biopsies in a separate procedure. The abdomen is incised. Abdominal organs are visually examined for evidence of infection, inflammation, perforations, lesions, or other injuries or diseased conditions. Any abnormalities are noted, including the presence of blood, bile, or other fluids in the abdominal cavity. Fluid or tissue samples may be obtained and sent for separately reportable laboratory analysis. Following examination, abdominal organs are returned to their normal positions and the abdominal incision is closed in layers. In 49002, a laparotomy site is opened and re-explored, as above.

49010

49010 Exploration, retroperitoneal area with or without biopsy(s) (separate procedure)

An exploration of the retroperitoneal area with or without biopsies is performed. The retroperitoneal area lies behind the peritoneum, the sac that lines the abdominopelvic cavity. Organs that lie within the retroperitoneal cavity include the adrenal glands, kidneys, ureters, bladder, aorta, inferior vena cava, and part of the esophagus, rectum, and uterus. The retroperitoneum may be approached anteriorly through a transverse, subcostal, midline rectus or paramedial lateral rectus incision or posteriorly through a flank incision just below the 11th or 12th rib. The retroperitoneal area and organs are visually examined for evidence of infection, inflammation, perforations, lesions, injuries, abnormalities, or other diseased condition. Any abnormalities are noted, including the presence of blood or other fluids in the retroperitoneal space. Fluid or tissue samples may be obtained and sent for separately reportable laboratory analysis. Following examination, the incision is closed in layers.

49020

49020 Drainage of peritoneal abscess or localized peritonitis, exclusive of appendiceal abscess, open

An abscess is a localized collection of pus. A peritoneal abscess is one contained within the peritoneum and may also be referred to as an intraperitoneal abscess. Localized peritonitis is an inflammation of the peritoneal tissue in a circumscribed region. An incision is made in the abdomen. The entire peritoneal cavity is explored and the abscess is located. Loculations are separated and all debris, which may include pus, blood, and necrotic tissue, is evacuated. The abscess site is vigorously irrigated with sterile saline or antibiotic solution until all debris has been removed. A drain is placed in the abscess cavity and the abdomen is closed around the drain.

49040

49040 Drainage of subdiaphragmatic or subphrenic abscess, open

A subdiaphragmatic abscess is a collection of pus that is located in the abdominal cavity below the diaphragm. A subphrenic abscess is located above the diaphragm in the space that separates the chest cavities from the abdominal cavity. The subdiaphragmatic or subphrenic abscess is accessed by a transpleural, extrapleural, retroperitoneal (extraperitoneal), or transperitoneal open approach. The entire subdiaphragmatic or subphrenic cavity is explored and the abscess located. Loculations are separated and all debris, which may include pus, blood, and necrotic tissue, is evacuated. The abscess site is vigorously irrigated with sterile saline or antibiotic solution until all debris has been removed. A drain is placed in the abscess cavity and the incision is closed around the drain.

49060

49060 Drainage of retroperitoneal abscess, open

A retroperitoneal abscess is a collection of pus that is located in the abdominal cavity behind the peritoneum and may also be referred to as an extraperitoneal abscess. The retroperitoneum is accessed using an open approach through an anterior or posterior subcostal incision, a midline abdominal incision, or a flank incision. The entire retroperitoneal cavity is explored and the abscess located. Loculations are separated and all debris, which may include pus, blood, and necrotic tissue, is evacuated. The abscess site is vigorously irrigated with sterile saline or antibiotic solution until all debris has been removed. A drain is placed in the abscess cavity and the incision is closed around the drain.

49062

49062 Drainage of extraperitoneal lymphocele to peritoneal cavity, open

An extraperitoneal lymphocele is a fluid collection composed of lymph that is contained behind the peritoneum in the retroperitoneal space. Lymphoceles typically occur due to surgical or other trauma to lymphatic vessels in the retroperitoneum. An incision is made in the abdomen and the posterior aspect of the peritoneum exposed. The posterior

peritoneum is incised and a small window (fenestration) created to allow lymphatic fluid to drain from the retroperitoneum into the peritoneal cavity. The window is left open and the abdomen is closed.

49082-49083

49082 Abdominal paracentesis (diagnostic or therapeutic); without imaging guidance

49083 Abdominal paracentesis (diagnostic or therapeutic); with imaging guidance

An abdominal paracentesis may be performed as a diagnostic procedure to help determine the cause of fluid buildup in the abdominal cavity. It may also be performed therapeutically when fluid buildup causes pain or impairs breathing. The skin over the planned puncture site is cleansed and a local anesthetic is injected. A paracentesis needle attached to a syringe is inserted into the abdominal cavity using imaging guidance as needed. Fluid is aspirated. The fluid is visually examined for evidence of bleeding or other conditions. If the procedure is performed for diagnostic purposes, only a small amount of fluid is withdrawn and the fluid is then sent to the laboratory for separately reportable analysis. If the procedure is performed for therapeutic purposes, fluid continues to be aspirated until as much fluid as possible has been removed from the abdominal cavity. Use 49082 when the procedure is performed without imaging guidance. Use 49083 when imaging guidance is used.

49084

49084 Peritoneal lavage, including imaging guidance, when performed

The abdomen is cleansed and a local anesthetic is injected. A small incision is made in the skin and carried down through the abdominal wall. Using imaging guidance as needed, a dialysis-type catheter is inserted into the peritoneal cavity. Fluid is drained from the peritoneal cavity and visually examined for evidence of bleeding or other conditions. The fluid is then sent to a laboratory for separately reportable analysis. A saline solution is instilled into the cavity and withdrawn to flush the cavity of blood clots or debris.

49180

49180 Biopsy, abdominal or retroperitoneal mass, percutaneous needle

This procedure is typically performed using separately reportable imaging guidance to identify the mass and to facilitate accurate placement of the needle within the mass. Using continuous imaging guidance, the core biopsy needle is inserted through the abdomen into the mass. A tissue sample is obtained. The physician may make multiple passes through the same puncture site or may approach the lesion through a different puncture site until an adequate tissue sample is obtained. The tissue sample is then sent to the laboratory for separately reportable histologic evaluation.

49185

49185 Sclerotherapy of a fluid collection (eg, lymphocele, cyst, or seroma), percutaneous, including contrast injection(s), sclerosant injection(s), diagnostic study, imaging guidance (eg, ultrasound, fluoroscopy) and radiological supervision and interpretation when performed

A procedure is performed to remove a collection of fluid such as from a lymphocele, cyst, or seroma, and instill a chemical sclerosant into the cavity. Sclerotherapy induces inflammatory fibrosis of the cyst or lesion wall to prevent re-accumulation of fluid. A small bore needle is inserted through the skin into the lesion. A pigtail catheter is inserted over the needle and fluid is aspirated and measured. A sample is sent for laboratory analysis (Gram stain, culture, cytology). Dilute contrast dye is injected through the catheter and observed using fluoroscopy to rule out fistula communication and/or leakage into the peritoneum, blood vessels, biliary system, or renal collecting system. Communication of the cyst or fluid cavity to any of these structures contraindicates injection of a sclerosant. After determining that no leakage is present, approximately 50% of the aspirated volume is replaced with the sclerosant. Ethanol is the most commonly used sclerosant. Other chemicals that may be used include bismuth, providone-iodine, tetracycline, bleomycin, hypertonic saline, ethanolamine oleate, and acetic acid. The patient's position is rotated to ensure that the entire cyst wall has contact with the sclerosant. After a prescribed period of time, minimally 20 minutes, the sclerosant is removed via aspiration. The catheter is connected to bulb suction and US or CT is performed to insure complete evacuation of the sclerosant. The catheter may be removed immediately or be left in place if subsequent treatments are anticipated or planned. Code 49185 includes all imaging guidance and associated supervision and interpretation during sclerotherapy.

49203-49205

49203 Excision or destruction, open, intra-abdominal tumors, cysts or endometriomas, 1 or more peritoneal, mesenteric, or retroperitoneal primary or secondary tumors; largest tumor 5 cm diameter or less

49204 Excision or destruction, open, intra-abdominal tumors, cysts or endometriomas, 1 or more peritoneal, mesenteric, or retroperitoneal primary or secondary tumors; largest tumor 5.1-10.0 cm diameter

49205 Excision or destruction, open, intra-abdominal tumors, cysts or endometriomas, 1 or more peritoneal, mesenteric, or retroperitoneal primary or secondary tumors; largest tumor greater than 10.0 cm diameter

Open excision or destruction of intra-abdominal or retroperitoneal tumors, cysts, or endometriomas is performed. Tumors may be benign, such as endometrioma or benign cystic mesothelioma, or malignant, such as adenocarcinoma, malignant mesothelioma, desmoplastic small cell tumors, or liposarcoma. Malignant tumors may be primary or secondary. Tumors may be completely excised or they may be destroyed by electrocautery or laser. Destruction is also referred to as surgical ablation. An incision is made in the abdomen to the level of the peritoneum, which is grasped, elevated, and incised taking care to avoid injury to the bowel and other internal organs. The peritoneal cavity is opened. Any adhesions are dissected and the abdominal viscera is exposed. The entire abdominal cavity is explored visually and by palpation and all masses and other abnormalities are noted. The location, size, and extent of the first tumor are noted. The tumor is either excised or destroyed by electrocautery or laser. This is repeated until all tumors have been excised or destroyed. Retroperitoneal tumors are treated in the same fashion taking care to avoid injury to the kidneys, ureters, and renal vessels. Use 49203 if the diameter of the largest tumor is 5.0 cm or less in diameter, 49204 if the largest tumor is 5.1 to 10.0 cm in diameter, and 49205 if the largest tumor is greater than 10.0 cm in diameter.

49215

49215 Excision of presacral or sacrococcygeal tumor

Tumors arising in the presacral space or sacrococcygeal region are rare. The abdomen is incised and dissection carried down to the posterior peritoneum. The posterior peritoneum is incised and the tumor in the presacral or sacrococcygeal region exposed. The ureters are identified and protected. The tumor is mobilized which may require ligation and division of sacral blood vessels. The tumor is dissected free of the rectum and removed. The peritoneum is closed. Drains are placed a needed in the presacral space or sacrococcygeal area. The abdominal incision is closed in layers.

49220

49220 Staging laparotomy for Hodgkins disease or lymphoma (includes splenectomy, needle or open biopsies of both liver lobes, possibly also removal of abdominal nodes, abdominal node and/or bone marrow biopsies, ovarian repositioning)

Staging laparotomy was standard procedure in the evaluation of patients with early Hodgkin's disease to distinguish patients with disease confined to above the diaphragm and those with more extensive disease. The procedure is used less frequently today due to the emergence of new imaging techniques. A midline incision is made in the abdomen. The spleen is exposed, mobilized, and displaced medially to expose the splenorenal, splenocolic, and gastrosplenic ligaments which are ligated and divided. The splenic artery and vein are then visualized, ligated and divided. The spleen is removed and the surgery site inspected for bleeding with particular attention being paid to the splenic pedicle and retroperitoneal space. Any bleeding is controlled by electrocautery or by suture ligation of blood vessels. The liver is exposed and tissue samples obtained from both lobes. Abdominal lymph nodes are exposed and inspected. Tissue samples are obtained from multiple nodes and any enlarged nodes are excised. If radiation therapy is planned for treatment of Hodgkin's disease, the ovaries may be surgically repositioned outside of the radiation field in women of child-bearing age. Bone marrow biopsies may also be obtained with common biopsy sites being the sternum or iliac crest. Following completion of all staging procedures, the abdominal wound is irrigated and the abdomen closed.

49250

49250 Umbilectomy, omphalectomy, excision of umbilicus (separate procedure)

Umbilical structures may be approached through the umbilicus or an infraumbilical incision. The umbilicus is explored and all structures identified, including the umbilical vein and arteries, median umbilical ligament (urachus). The physician then excises the urachus and any omphalomesenteric remnants. The umbilical ring is closed and the skin is closed over the umbilicus taking care to maintain a normal appearing umbilicus.

49255

49255 Omentectomy, epiploectomy, resection of omentum (separate procedure)

The omentum is a sheet of fat covered by peritoneum that extends from the stomach to other organs in the abdominal cavity. The greater omentum extends from the bottom edge of the stomach to the transverse colon and overlies the small intestine. An upper midline abdominal incision is used to expose the omentum. The omentum is explored to identify

masses, lesions, or other evidence of disease or injury. The omentum is lifted off the colon and the posterior aspect explored. The segment of omentum to be resected is identified. Blood vessels are individually clamped and ligated as the omentum is dissected free of surrounding tissues and removed. Drains are placed as needed and the abdominal incision closed.

49320

49320 Laparoscopy, abdomen, peritoneum, and omentum, diagnostic, with or without collection of specimen(s) by brushing or washing (separate procedure)

A periumbilical port is placed and pneumoperitoneum established by the insufflation of air. The laparoscope is inserted and the entire abdominal cavity, peritoneum, and/or omentum inspected for signs of malignancy, disease, or injury using a video camera. A biopsy brush may be inserted through the laparoscope and cell samples obtained. Alternatively, cells may be obtained by washing which involves instilling a small amount of sterile saline through the laparoscopic and then aspirating the fluid. Brushings or washings are sent to the laboratory for separately reportable cytology evaluation. Following completion of the procedure, the instruments are withdrawn and pressure applied to the abdomen to express any remaining air in the peritoneum. The portal incisions are closed.

49321

49321 Laparoscopy, surgical; with biopsy (single or multiple)

A periumbilical port is placed and pneumoperitoneum established by the insufflation of air. The laparoscope is inserted and the entire abdominal cavity, peritoneum, and/or omentum inspected for signs of malignancy, disease, or injury using a video camera. Biopsy forceps are inserted through the laparoscope and a tissue sample obtained. One or more tissue samples may be obtained from a single or multiple sites. Tissue samples are sent to the laboratory for separately reportable histologic evaluation. Following completion of the procedure, the biopsy sites are inspected for bleeding and any bleeding controlled by laser or electrocautery. The instruments are withdrawn and pressure applied to the abdomen to express any remaining air in the peritoneum. The portal incisions are closed.

49322

49322 Laparoscopy, surgical; with aspiration of cavity or cyst (eg, ovarian cyst) (single or multiple)

A periumbilical port is placed and pneumoperitoneum established by the insufflation of air. The laparoscope is inserted and the entire abdominal cavity, peritoneum, and/or omentum inspected for signs of malignancy, disease, or injury using a video camera. The cavity or cyst is located and an aspiration needle inserted through the laparoscope. The cavity or cyst is punctured, and fluid aspirated. Fluid from one or more cavities or cysts may be aspirated. Following completion of the procedure, the puncture sites are inspected for bleeding and any bleeding controlled by laser or electrocautery. The instruments are withdrawn and pressure applied to the abdomen to express any remaining air in the peritoneum. The portal incisions are closed.

49323

49323 Laparoscopy, surgical; with drainage of lymphocele to peritoneal cavity

An extraperitoneal lymphocele is a fluid collection composed of lymph that is contained behind the peritoneum in the retroperitoneal space. Lymphoceles typically occur due to surgical or other trauma to lymphatic vessels in the retroperitoneum. A small incision is made in the area of the umbilicus and the laparoscope is inserted. The abdomen is inflated with gas. Two or three additional small incisions are made in the abdomen and trocars are inserted. Surgical instruments are inserted through the trocars. The posterior peritoneum exposed, incised and a small window (fenestration) created to allow lymphatic fluid to drain from the retroperitoneum into the peritoneal cavity. The window is left open. Surgical tools are removed from the abdomen and the gas (pneumoperitoneum) is released. The laparoscope and trocars are removed and portal incisions closed with sutures.

49324-49325

49324 Laparoscopy, surgical; with insertion of tunneled intraperitoneal catheter

49325 Laparoscopy, surgical; with revision of previously placed intraperitoneal cannula or catheter, with removal of intraluminal obstructive material if performed

An intraperitoneal catheter is inserted (49324) or revised (49325). A small incision is made in the area of the umbilicus and the laparoscope is inserted. The abdomen is inflated with gas. Two or three additional small incisions are made in the abdomen and trocars are inserted. Surgical instruments are inserted through the trocars. The abdomen is inspected for adhesions and the site of entry for the catheter into the peritoneum is identified. In 49324, the catheter is attached to the tunneler, and the tunneler and catheter are passed into the subcutaneous tissue deep to Scarpa's fascia and through the subcutaneous tissue to the site where the catheter will enter the peritoneum. The tunneler and catheter are passed out through the skin and the tunneler is removed. An introducer needle is placed into the peritoneum adjacent to the catheter under laparoscopic guidance. A guidewire is placed through the introducer into the peritoneum and the introducer is removed. A combined catheter introducer and dilator are advanced over the guidewire into the peritoneum. The guidewire and dilator are removed. The intraperitoneal catheter is then passed into the abdomen through the introducer. Proper positioning of the catheter is verified laparoscopically. The introducer is removed from the abdomen and the gas (pneumoperitoneum) is released. The laparoscope and trocars are removed and portal incisions are closed with sutures. In 49325, a previously placed intraperitoneal catheter is inspected using the laparoscope. The tip of the catheter may be repositioned or obstructive debris that has collected in the catheter may be flushed out of the lumen.

49326

49326   Laparoscopy, surgical; with omentopexy (omental tacking procedure) (List separately in addition to code for primary procedure)

A laparoscopic omentopexy, also referred to as an omental tacking procedure, is performed during a separately reportable laparoscopic procedure to insert or revise an intraperitoneal catheter or cannula. The omentum is a sheet of fat covered by peritoneum that extends from the stomach to other organs in the abdominal cavity. The greater omentum extends from the bottom edge of the stomach to the transverse colon and overlies the small intestine. A forceps is inserted into the abdominal cavity through a previously established laparoscopic port. The greater omentum is grasped, lifted into the upper abdomen, and attached to the upper abdominal wall, falciform ligament, or other structure using sutures or laparoscopic tacks.

49327

49327   Laparoscopy, surgical; with placement of interstitial device(s) for radiation therapy guidance (eg, fiducial markers, dosimeter), intra-abdominal, intrapelvic, and/or retroperitoneum, including imaging guidance, if performed, single or multiple (List separately in addition to code for primary procedure)

Interstitial devices, such as fiducial markers and dosimeters, are placed prior to radiation therapy and are used to locate the tumor or mass and/or measure the radiation dose precisely. Placement of interstitial fiducial markers allows radiation to be directed at the malignant tissue while preventing extensive radiation damage to surrounding tissues and structures. Fiducial markers are gold seeds that are implanted in or around the malignant tumor. Implantable dosimeters measure the amount of radiation at the site of the tumor. During a separately reportable laparoscopic procedure, the planned placement sites in the abdomen, pelvis, or retroperitoneum are identified and measured using imaging guidance. One or more markers are passed through one of the operating ports into the tumor, tumor bed, and/or the tissue surrounding the tumor. The positions of the markers are checked radiographically to ensure that they are properly placed. The same technique is used for placement of an interstitial dosimeter. The laparoscopic procedure is completed; the laparoscope and trocars are removed and portal incisions are closed with sutures.

49400

49400   Injection of air or contrast into peritoneal cavity (separate procedure)

Using separately reportable radiographic guidance, a needle is inserted through the abdomen into the peritoneal cavity. The peritoneal cavity is then filled with air to create a pneumoperitoneum or contrast is injected and separately reportable radiographs are obtained.

49402

49402   Removal of peritoneal foreign body from peritoneal cavity

A peritoneal foreign body is removed from the peritoneal cavity. The abdominal wall is incised and the peritoneum is entered to allow the physician to explore the cavity and locate the foreign body, which is removed and The incision is closed with sutures.

49405-49407

49405   Image-guided fluid collection drainage by catheter (eg, abscess, hematoma, seroma, lymphocele, cyst); visceral (eg, kidney, liver, spleen, lung/mediastinum), percutaneous

49406   Image-guided fluid collection drainage by catheter (eg, abscess, hematoma, seroma, lymphocele, cyst); peritoneal or retroperitoneal, percutaneous

49407   Image-guided fluid collection drainage by catheter (eg, abscess, hematoma, seroma, lymphocele, cyst); peritoneal or retroperitoneal, transvaginal or transrectal

The physician performs image-guided drainage of a fluid collection such as an abscess, hematoma, seroma, lymphocele, or cyst of the digestive, respiratory, urogenital, or endocrine system or in the spleen, heart, or great vessels. Using fluoroscopic, ultrasonic, or CT guidance, the fluid collection is identified. A catheter with a sheath is introduced into the mediastinal, pleural, peritoneal, or retroperitoneal cavity. The catheter and sheath is passed through the organ that contains the fluid collection and into the fluid filled cavity. The fluid collection is then drained. The fluid filled cavity may be flushed with sterile saline or antibiotic solution to clear all pus, blood, and other fluid from the site. The catheter may

be removed or left in place to provide continuous drainage. For code 49405, access is gained using a needle, and localization is confirmed by imaging. Then a wire is advanced into the cavity, and a dilator is used to perform a fascial dilatation to accommodate the drainage catheter. A catheter is advanced over the wire into the fluid collection, the wire removed and the catheter is locked. Use code 49406 for a percutaneous approach to a fluid collection contained in the peritoneal and retroperitoneal cavity and located in the digestive system, urogenital system, or endocrine system including the kidney, liver, or spleen. Use 49407 for a transvaginal or transrectal approach to a fluid collection contained in the peritoneal or retroperitoneal cavity. Transvaginal or transrectal approach is most commonly performed for drainage of fluid collections of urogenital organs such as the ovary or a pericolic fluid collection. Transvaginal approach uses an ultrasound probe with a drainage catheter mounted in the transducer groove that is placed in the vagina. The catheter tip is positioned over the fluid collection site. The stylet is inserted through the catheter tip and advanced through the vaginal wall into the fluid collection. A trocar is then advanced into the center of the fluid collection and it is drained. The catheter may be removed once the fluid is completely drained or it may be left in place to provide continuous drainage. If it is left in place, the stylet is removed and the catheter is attached to a drainage bag or to wall suction. Transrectal approach is performed in the same manner except that the catheter is introduced through the rectum using radiological guidance.

49411-49412

49411   Placement of interstitial device(s) for radiation therapy guidance (eg, fiducial markers, dosimeter), percutaneous, intra-abdominal, intra-pelvic (except prostate), and/or retroperitoneum, single or multiple

49412   Placement of interstitial device(s) for radiation therapy guidance (eg, fiducial markers, dosimeter), open, intra-abdominal, intrapelvic, and/or retroperitoneum, including image guidance, if performed, single or multiple (List separately in addition to code for primary procedure)

Interstitial devices, such as fiducial markers and dosimeters, are placed prior to radiation therapy and are used to locate the tumor or mass and/or measure the radiation dose precisely. Placement of interstitial fiducial markers allows radiation to be directed at the malignant tissue while preventing extensive radiation damage to surrounding tissues and structures. Fiducial markers are gold seeds that are implanted in or around the malignant tumor. Implantable dosimeters measure the amount of radiation at the site of the tumor. In 49411, the planned placement sites in the abdomen, pelvis, or retroperitoneum are identified and measured using separately reportable imaging guidance. A local anesthetic is administered to numb tissue along the planned insertion sites. Using radiologic guidance, one or more markers are passed through an introducer needle into the tumor and/or the tissue surrounding the tumor. The positions of the markers are checked radiographically to ensure that they are properly placed. The same technique is used for placement of an interstitial dosimeter. In 49412, the interstitial devices are placed during a separately reportable open procedure. The sites for placement of fiducial markers and/or a dosimeter are selected. The markers and/or dosimeter are advanced into any remaining tumor tissue, the tumor bed, and/or surrounding tissues. Imaging guidance is used as needed to ensure proper placement of the devices. The open procedure is completed and the operative wound is closed.

49418

49418   Insertion of tunneled intraperitoneal catheter (eg, dialysis, intraperitoneal chemotherapy instillation, management of ascites), complete procedure, including imaging guidance, catheter placement, contrast injection when performed, and radiological supervision and interpretation, percutaneous

A tunneled intraperitoneal catheter is inserted using percutaneous technique. Using imaging guidance, the sites for the catheter insertion into the skin and the puncture site for insertion into the peritoneum are selected and marked on the skin. The catheter is attached to the tunneler, and the tunneler and catheter are passed into the subcutaneous tissue deep to Scarpa's fascia at the skin insertion site. The tunneler and catheter are then passed through the subcutaneous tissue to the site where the catheter will enter the peritoneum, and the tunneler and catheter are passed out through the skin. The tunneler is removed. An introducer needle is placed into the peritoneum adjacent to the catheter using imaging guidance. A guidewire is placed through the introducer into the peritoneum and the introducer is removed. A combined catheter introducer and dilator are advanced over the guidewire and into the peritoneum. The guidewire and dilator are removed. The catheter is passed into the abdomen through the introducer. A small amount of contrast may be injected through the catheter and observed radiographically to ensure proper positioning of the catheter. The introducer is removed from the abdomen.

Digestive System

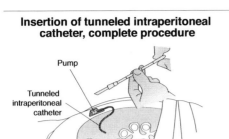

Insertion of tunneled intraperitoneal catheter, complete procedure

A complete catheter procedure (e.g., dialysis, chemotherapy, management of ascites)

49419

49419   Insertion of tunneled intraperitoneal catheter, with subcutaneous port (ie, totally implantable)

A tunneled intraperitoneal catheter with a subcutaneous port is completely indwelling without any external access ports. An incision is made in the upper abdomen and carried down through the peritoneum. Any adhesions are lysed and bowel is dissected as needed to provide a cavity in the peritoneum that is not obstructed by other structures. The skin and subcutaneous tissue over the rectus fascia is incised and a subcutaneous pocket is created. The port is then sutured to the fascia and filled with heparinized saline. A catheter or cannula is tunneled through the subcutaneous tissue and to the site where the catheter will enter the peritoneal cavity. The peritoneum is punctured and the catheter is advanced into the peritoneum. The port and catheter are checked to ensure that medication or other fluid flows freely into the cavity. The upper abdominal incision is closed and the skin pocket is closed over the reservoir.

49421-49422

49421   Insertion of tunneled intraperitoneal catheter for dialysis, open
49422   Removal of tunneled intraperitoneal catheter

A tunneled intraperitoneal catheter is inserted (49421) or removed (49422). Open insertion of a cannula or catheter is performed by making an incision in the upper abdomen carried down through the peritoneum. Any adhesions are lysed and bowel is dissected as needed to provide a cavity in the peritoneum that is not obstructed by other structures. The catheter or cannula is inserted and clamped or connected to an external port. The upper abdominal incision is closed. In 49422, a tunneled intraperitoneal catheter is removed. The area around the insertion site is cleansed and a local anesthetic is injected. Using blunt dissection as needed, the catheter is freed from the tunnel and removed. Bleeding is controlled with pressure; the insertion site is closed as needed; and a pressure dressing is applied.

49423

49423   Exchange of previously placed abscess or cyst drainage catheter under radiological guidance (separate procedure)

Using continuous radiological guidance throughout the procedure, a guidewire is placed into the existing catheter which is removed over the guidewire. A replacement catheter is then placed over the guidewire and advanced through the existing tract into the abscess pocket or cyst. The guidewire is removed.

49424

49424   Contrast injection for assessment of abscess or cyst via previously placed drainage catheter or tube (separate procedure)

A contrast injection is performed through a previously placed drainage catheter to assess an abscess or cyst. The draining abscess or cyst is evaluated to determine the size and location of the abscess pocket or cyst. Contrast media is injected through the existing catheter and distribution of the contrast material is observed radiographically. Separately reportable radiographic supervision and interpretation is performed during the injection procedure.

49425-49426

49425   Insertion of peritoneal-venous shunt
49426   Revision of peritoneal-venous shunt

The physician inserts or revises a peritoneal venous shunt. A peritoneal venous shunt is used to treat ascites which is an accumulation of fluid in the peritoneal cavity. In 49425, the peritoneal-venous shunt is inserted. The shunt is typically inserted into the subclavian

vein although the internal jugular vein may also be used. A small incision is made over the subclavian or internal jugular vein. The vein is exposed and an introducer sheath inserted. The venous catheter portion of the shunt is inserted through introducer sheath and advanced into the superior vena cava. A tunnel is created in the subcutaneous tissue from the upper abdomen traversing the chest wall to the site of the venous catheter. The shunt tubing is advanced through the tunnel and inserted into the peritoneal cavity. A pressure sensitive one-way valve is then connected to both the venous catheter and shunt which allows fluid to move from the peritoneal cavity into the vein while prevents backflow of blood. In 49426, the peritoneal-venous shunt is revised. The exact nature of the procedure depends on which portion of the shunt is malfunctioning. If the peritoneal shunt is malfunctioning it may be repositioned or replaced. If the valve is malfunctioning it is removed and replaced. If the venous catheter is malfunctioning, it may be repositioned or replaced.

49427

49427   Injection procedure (eg, contrast media) for evaluation of previously placed peritoneal-venous shunt

A peritoneal venous shunt is used to treat ascites which is an accumulation of fluid in the peritoneal cavity. A local anesthetic is injected into the peritoneal cavity. Contrast media or a radiotracer, such as TC99m-SC or TC99m-MAA, is injected into the left lower quadrant. If the patient has a LeVeen shunt, the abdomen is massaged to distribute the radiotracer. If the patient has a Denver shunt, the patient is instructed to pump the system. Following the injection procedure, separately reportable radiographs are obtained to evaluate patency of the peritoneal venous shunt.

49428-49429

49428   Ligation of peritoneal-venous shunt
49429   Removal of peritoneal-venous shunt

The physician performs a ligation or removal of a peritoneal venous shunt. A peritoneal venous shunt is used to treat ascites which is an accumulation of fluid in the peritoneal cavity. In 49428, the peritoneal-venous shunt is ligated. Shunt tubing traverses the subcutaneous tissue of the chest wall and is easily exposed by incising the skin and subcutaneous tissue over the shunt. A segment of shunt tubing is dissected free of surrounding tissue and a ligature, such as a flexible cord, placed around the tubing to tie it off. In 49429, the peritoneal-venous shunt is removed. An incision is made in skin and subcutaneous tissue of the upper chest at the point where the tubing enters the jugular vein and in the abdomen at the point where the shunt enters the peritoneal cavity. The shunt tubing is dissected free of surrounding tissue and is removed. Incisions in the upper chest and abdomen are closed with sutures.

49435

49435   Insertion of subcutaneous extension to intraperitoneal cannula or catheter with remote chest exit site (List separately in addition to code for primary procedure)

As an add-on procedure, the physician inserts an additional extension to an abdominal cannula/catheter subcutaneously, beginning in the peritoneum. The external site is threaded through, exiting through a remote site in the chest.

49436

49436   Delayed creation of exit site from embedded subcutaneous segment of intraperitoneal cannula or catheter

After another procedure, the physician creates an embedded portion of an abdominal cannula/catheter subcutaneously, beginning in the peritoneum. The external site is threaded through, exiting through a remote site in the chest.

49440-49441

49440   Insertion of gastrostomy tube, percutaneous, under fluoroscopic guidance including contrast injection(s), image documentation and report
49441   Insertion of duodenostomy or jejunostomy tube, percutaneous, under fluoroscopic guidance including contrast injection(s), image documentation and report

A percutaneous insertion of a gastrostomy tube is performed under fluoroscopic guidance. Percutaneous gastrostomy tube placement can be performed using either a push (Sacks-Vine) technique or pull (Ponsky-Gauderer) technique. Glucagon is administered and a nasogastric tube is placed. The stomach is insufflated, the skin over the insertion site is cleansed, and a local anesthetic is administered. Under fluoroscopic guidance, the needle is passed through the skin and into the stomach. This is confirmed radiographically. Fasteners are used to secure the stomach to the abdominal wall. A guidewire is then passed through the needle into the stomach and the needle is withdrawn. The abdominal wall and gastric wall are dilated using serial dilators or an angioplasty balloon. The gastrostomy tube is then inserted over the guidewire and anchored in the stomach. The guidewire is withdrawn. If a pull technique is used, a feeding tube is advanced through the patient's mouth and into the stomach. A needle is passed into the stomach and a snare is

Digestive System

introduced under fluoroscopic guidance. The gastrostomy tube is then captured and pulled through the gastric and abdominal wall and out through the skin. Radiographic imaging guidance is performed continuously during the entire procedure, also using contrast injections, to monitor placement of the tube and verify correct positioning. Contrast injection(s), image documentation, and a written report is provided in the code. Use 49441 for percutaneous insertion of a duodenostomy or jejunostomy tube by the same technique into the duodenum or jejunum, instead of the stomach.

49442

49442   Insertion of cecostomy or other colonic tube, percutaneous, under fluoroscopic guidance including contrast injection(s), image documentation and report

Percutaneous insertion of a cecostomy or other colonic tube is performed under fluoroscopic guidance. The cecostomy tube example described here is usually performed for fecal incontinence. Prior to the cecostomy tube insertion, a standard bowel prep is done. Only clear liquids are allowed for one to two days and an oral laxative is given the evening before the procedure. The colon is inflated with air until the bowel is distended. The skin is cleansed and a local anesthetic is administered. The bowel is paralyzed and a needle is inserted into the cecum or other colon segment under fluoroscopic guidance. The cecum or other colon segment is secured to the abdominal wall using one to three fasteners. A guidewire is inserted into the cecum or other part of the colon and the tract is dilated. A sheath is introduced and the tube is inserted through the abdominal wall and into the cecum or other colon section. The tube is flushed with normal saline and capped. The patient then uses this tube to administer a small volume phosphate enema followed by a saline enema that completely evacuates the bowel, avoiding fecal incontinence. Radiographic imaging guidance is performed continuously during the entire procedure, also using contrast injections, to monitor placement of the tube and verify correct positioning. Contrast injection(s), image documentation, and a written report are provided in the code.

49446

49446   Conversion of gastrostomy tube to gastro-jejunostomy tube, percutaneous, under fluoroscopic guidance including contrast injection(s), image documentation and report

A gastrostomy tube is converted to a gastrojejunostomy tube using percutaneous technique under fluoroscopic guidance. The skin is cleansed at the gastroscopy tube site and a topical anesthetic is applied. A stiff guidewire is placed under fluoroscopic guidance and the gastrostomy tube is removed. A gastrojejunostomy tube is advanced over the guidewire. The tube is advanced through the stomach, across the pylorus, and into the jejunum just beyond the ligament of Trietz. The stiff wire is removed and the tube is secured by inflating the balloon. Radiographic imaging guidance is performed continuously during the entire procedure, also using contrast injections, to monitor placement of the tube and verify correct positioning. Contrast injection(s), image documentation, and a written report are provided in the code.

49450-49452

49450   Replacement of gastrostomy or cecostomy (or other colonic) tube, percutaneous, under fluoroscopic guidance including contrast injection(s), image documentation and report

49451   Replacement of duodenostomy or jejunostomy tube, percutaneous, under fluoroscopic guidance including contrast injection(s), image documentation and report

49452   Replacement of gastro-jejunostomy tube, percutaneous, under fluoroscopic guidance including contrast injection(s), image documentation and report

A percutaneous replacement of a gastrostomy, cecostomy or other colonic tube is performed under fluoroscopic guidance. Replacement is required particularly in the case of a tube being accidentally pulled out. The gastrostomy, cecostomy, or other colonic tube tract is inspected and cleansed. Contrast media is injected into the tract, which is then assessed. A guidewire is inserted. The replacement tube is then pushed through the tract over the guidewire and into the stomach, cecum, or other segment of colon. The replacement tube is secured both internally with retention devices and externally to the skin. Radiographic imaging guidance is performed continuously during the entire procedure, also using contrast injections, to monitor placement of the tube and verify correct positioning. Contrast injection(s), image documentation, and a written report are provided in the code. Use 49451 to report percutaneous replacement of a duodenostomy or jejunostomy tube. Use 49452 to report replacement of a gastrojejunostomy tube.

49460

49460   Mechanical removal of obstructive material from gastrostomy, duodenostomy, jejunostomy, gastro-jejunostomy, or cecostomy (or other colonic) tube, any method, under fluoroscopic guidance including contrast injection(s), if performed, image documentation and report

Obstructive material is removed mechanically from a gastrostomy, duodenostomy, jejunostomy, gastrojejunostomy, cecostomy, or other colonic tube. This may be performed by any method under fluoroscopic guidance. The position of the tube is first checked.

An attempt is made to break up the obstructive material using various wires and/or guidewires. If this is unsuccessful, a mechanical device may be used, followed by reinsertion of a wire through the catheter to dislodge material that has been broken up or softened by the mechanical device. Multiple passes of the wire may be necessary to completely dislodge all obstructive material and push it into the stomach or intestine. When the obstruction is completely cleared, the catheter is flushed, and contrast media is injected to verify that the tube is functioning properly. Radiographic imaging guidance is performed continuously during the entire procedure, also using contrast injections, to monitor the procedure. Contrast injection(s), image documentation, and a written report are provided in the code.

49465

49465   Contrast injection(s) for radiological evaluation of existing gastrostomy, duodenostomy, jejunostomy, gastro-jejunostomy, or cecostomy (or other colonic) tube, from a percutaneous approach including image documentation and report

An existing gastrostomy, duodenostomy, jejunostomy, gastrojejunostomy, cecostomy, or other colonic tube is injected with contrast to verify that the tubing is still is the correct position and functioning properly. After contrast is injected, fluoroscopic imaging is used to check the tube's position and that it is still patent and functioning. Image documentation and a written report of the procedure is provided in the code.

49491-49492

49491   Repair, initial inguinal hernia, preterm infant (younger than 37 weeks gestation at birth), performed from birth up to 50 weeks postconception age, with or without hydrocelectomy; reducible

49492   Repair, initial inguinal hernia, preterm infant (younger than 37 weeks gestation at birth), performed from birth up to 50 weeks postconception age, with or without hydrocelectomy; incarcerated or strangulated

An initial inguinal hernia repair is performed on a preterm infant (younger than 37 weeks gestation at birth) from birth up to 50 post-conceptual weeks of age. An inguinal hernia is a condition where structures protrude through a weakness in the abdominal wall in the groin area. In 49491, a reducible hernia in which the contents of the hernia sac can be pushed back into normal position, is repaired. In 49492, an incarcerated or strangulated hernia is repaired. Incarcerated hernia tissue cannot be pushed back into its normal position. Strangulated hernias are those in which circulation is compromised. This procedure may be performed with or without a hydrocelectomy. A hydrocele is an accumulation of excess fluid in a sac or cavity. In this case, the hydrocele is typically in the tunica vaginalis of the testis. In males, a small incision is made over the external ring. Scarpa's fascia is elevated and incised. The cord is isolated and dissected free of fat and the external ring is exposed. The cord is elevated, overlying fascia is opened distal to the external ring, and the hernia sac is exposed. The sac is dissected free of surrounding tissue, opened, and the contents are inspected. Loops of bowel proximal and distal to the obstruction are extracted and examined. If the bowel is healthy and peristalsis is present, the hernia is repaired. The distal end of the sac is transected. The proximal stump of the sac is freed up through the internal ring to the level of the extraperitoneal fat. The sac is rotated to ensure that it is emptied of all hernia contents before it is ligated and the excess stump excised. The cord structures are returned to the peritoneal cavity and the opening in the cord covering is sutured closed. Scarpa's fascia is closed and the skin is reapproximated. If a hydrocele is present, it is drained and a partial excision of the tunica vaginalis may also be performed. In females, the procedure is the same, except that the hernia sac must be explored for the presence of the ovary. If the ovary is not contained in the sac, the round ligament is ligated together with the sac. If the ovary is present and healthy, it is returned to the abdomen, taking care to avoid damage to the fallopian tube. Once the ovary is returned to the abdomen, the sac is then clamped and transected.

49495-49496

49495   Repair, initial inguinal hernia, full term infant younger than age 6 months, or preterm infant older than 50 weeks postconception age and younger than age 6 months at the time of surgery, with or without hydrocelectomy; reducible

49496   Repair, initial inguinal hernia, full term infant younger than age 6 months, or preterm infant older than 50 weeks postconception age and younger than age 6 months at the time of surgery, with or without hydrocelectomy; incarcerated or strangulated

An initial inguinal hernia repair is performed on a full-term infant younger than six months or a preterm infant (less than 37 weeks gestation at birth) older than 50 weeks post-conception age, but still younger than six months. An inguinal hernia is a protrusion of tissues through a weakness in the abdominal wall in the groin area. In 49495, a reducible hernia in which the contents of the hernia sac can be pushed back into normal position, is repaired. In 49496, an incarcerated or strangulated hernia is repaired. Incarcerated hernia tissue cannot be pushed back into its normal position. Strangulated hernias are those in which circulation is compromised. The repair may be performed with or without a hydrocelectomy. A hydrocele is an accumulation of excess fluid in a sac or cavity. In this case, the hydrocele is typically in the tunica vaginalis of the testis. In males, a small incision is made over the external ring. Scarpa's fascia is elevated and incised. The cord is isolated and dissected free of fat and the external ring is exposed. The cord is elevated, overlying fascia is opened distal to the external ring, and the hernia sac is exposed. The sac is dissected free of surrounding tissue, opened, and the contents are inspected. Loops of bowel proximal and distal to the obstruction are extracted and examined. If the bowel is healthy and peristalsis is present, the hernia is repaired. The distal end of the sac is transected. The proximal stump of the sac is freed up through the internal ring to the level of the extraperitoneal fat. The sac is rotated to ensure that it is emptied of all hernia contents before it is ligated and the excess stump excised. The cord structures are returned to the peritoneal cavity and the opening in the cord covering is sutured closed. Scarpa's fascia is closed and the skin is reapproximated. If a hydrocele is present, it is drained and a partial excision of the tunica vaginalis may also be performed. In females, the procedure is the same, except that the hernia sac must be explored for the presence of the ovary. If the ovary is not contained in the sac, the round ligament is ligated together with the sac. If the ovary is present and healthy, it is returned to the abdomen, taking care to avoid damage to the fallopian tube. Once the ovary is returned to the abdomen, the sac is then clamped and transected.

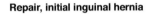

Repair, initial inguinal hernia

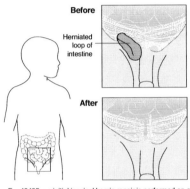

Before

Herniated loop of intestine

After

For 49495, an initial inguinal hernia repair is performed on a full-term infant younger than six months or a preterm infant. Report 49577 if hernia is incarcerated or strangulated

49500-49501

49500 Repair initial inguinal hernia, age 6 months to younger than 5 years, with or without hydrocelectomy; reducible

49501 Repair initial inguinal hernia, age 6 months to younger than 5 years, with or without hydrocelectomy; incarcerated or strangulated

An initial inguinal hernia repair is performed on a child between six months and under five years of age. An inguinal hernia is a protrusion of tissues through a weakness in the abdominal wall in the groin area. In 49500, a reducible hernia in which the contents of the hernia sac can be pushed back into normal position, is repaired. In 49501, an incarcerated or strangulated hernia is repaired. Incarcerated hernia tissue cannot be pushed back into its normal position. Strangulated hernias are those in which circulation is compromised. The repair may be performed with or without a hydrocelectomy. A hydrocele is an accumulation of excess fluid in a sac or cavity. In this case, the hydrocele is typically in the tunica vaginalis of the testis. In males, a small incision is made over the external ring. Scarpa's fascia is elevated and incised. The cord is isolated and dissected free of fat and the external ring is exposed. The cord is elevated, overlying fascia is opened distal to the external ring, and the hernia sac is exposed. The sac is dissected free of surrounding tissue, opened, and the contents are inspected. Loops of bowel proximal and distal to the obstruction are extracted and examined. If the bowel is healthy and peristalsis is present, the hernia is repaired. The distal end of the sac is transected. The proximal stump of the sac is freed up through the internal ring to the level of the extraperitoneal fat. The sac is rotated to ensure that it is emptied of all hernia contents before it is ligated and the excess stump excised. The cord structures are returned to the peritoneal cavity and the opening in the cord covering is sutured closed. Scarpa's fascia is closed and the skin is reapproximated. If a hydrocele is present, it is drained and a partial excision of the tunica vaginalis may also be performed. In females, the procedure is the same, except that the hernia sac must be explored for the presence of the ovary. If the ovary is not contained in the sac, the round ligament is ligated together with the sac. If the ovary is present and healthy, it is returned to the abdomen, taking care to avoid damage to the fallopian tube. Once the ovary is returned to the abdomen, the sac is then clamped and transected.

49505-49507

49505 Repair initial inguinal hernia, age 5 years or older; reducible

49507 Repair initial inguinal hernia, age 5 years or older; incarcerated or strangulated

An initial inguinal hernia repair is performed on a patient who is five years or older. An inguinal hernia is a condition where structures protrude through a weakness in the abdominal wall in the groin area. In 49505, a reducible hernia in which the contents of the hernia sac can be pushed back into normal position, is repaired. In 49507, an incarcerated or strangulated hernia is repaired. Incarcerated hernia tissue cannot be pushed back into its normal position. Strangulated hernias are those in which circulation is compromised. An incision is made over the internal ring. The skin, fat, and subcutaneous fascia are incised down to the aponeurosis of the external oblique muscle. The external ring is identified and the external oblique aponeurosis is slit. The internal ring is opened and the inguinal canal is exposed. In males, the spermatic cord and its covering are mobilized and the covering is removed. The hernia sac is dissected free into the retroperitoneum, opened, and inspected for the presence of bowel or bladder wall. Any bowel or bladder content is reduced (pushed back into the abdominal cavity) and the hernia sac is transected and inverted into the abdominal cavity. A mesh plug may be placed to reinforce the repair. In women, the sac is inspected for the ovary. If the ovary is present, it is returned to the abdomen. The sac is then resected together with the round ligament. The internal ring is closed and the posterior wall of the inguinal canal is repaired.

49520-49521

49520 Repair recurrent inguinal hernia, any age; reducible

49521 Repair recurrent inguinal hernia, any age; incarcerated or strangulated

A recurrent inguinal hernia is repaired on a patient of any age. An inguinal hernia is a condition where structures protrude through a weakness in the abdominal wall in the groin area. In 49520, a reducible hernia in which the contents of the hernia sac can be pushed back into normal position, is repaired. In 49521, an incarcerated or strangulated hernia is repaired. Incarcerated hernia tissue cannot be pushed back into its normal position. Strangulated hernias are those in which circulation is compromised. Recurrent hernia repairs vary in complexity depending on the extent of the defect and the amount of scarring and tissue damage resulting from the initial repair. An incision is made over the internal ring. As the previous repair is taken apart, care is taken to preserve healthy tissue. Meticulous dissection of the anatomic layers is required. The skin, fat, and subcutaneous fascia are incised down to the aponeurosis of the external oblique muscle. The external ring is identified and the external oblique aponeurosis is slit. The internal ring is opened and the inguinal canal exposed. In males, the spermatic cord and its covering are mobilized and the covering is removed. The hernia sac is dissected free into the retroperitoneum, opened, and inspected for the presence of bowel or bladder wall. Any bowel or bladder content is reduced (pushed back into the abdominal cavity) and the sac is transected and inverted into the abdominal cavity. A mesh plug may be placed to reinforce the repair. In women, the sac is inspected for the ovary. If the ovary is present, it is inspected and returned to the abdomen when healthy. The sac is then resected together with the round ligament. The internal ring is closed and the posterior wall of the inguinal canal is repaired.

49525

49525 Repair inguinal hernia, sliding, any age

A sliding inguinal hernia repair is performed on a patient of any age. A sliding inguinal hernia is one in which structures protrude through a weakness in the abdominal wall in the groin area and the condition is complicated by a hernia sac that is partially comprised of the abdominal viscus. An incision is made over the internal ring. The skin, fat, and subcutaneous fascia are incised down to the aponeurosis of the external oblique muscle. The external ring is identified and the external oblique aponeurosis is slit. The internal ring is opened and the inguinal canal exposed. In males, the spermatic cord and its covering are mobilized and the covering is removed. The hernia sac is identified and opened, revealing visceral peritoneum continuous with a portion of the sac wall. Any bowel or bladder content is reduced (pushed back into the abdominal cavity). The sac is then transected, taking care to protect the viscera and avoid damage to the mesenteric vessels. The sac is inverted into the abdominal cavity. A mesh plug may be placed to reinforce the repair. In women, the sac is inspected for the ovary. If the ovary is present, it is inspected and returned to the abdomen when healthy. The sac is then resected together with the round ligament. The internal ring is closed and the posterior wall of the inguinal canal is repaired.

49540

49540 Repair lumbar hernia

A lumbar hernia is repaired. Lumbar hernias occur between the erector spinae muscles posteriorly and a vertical line from the twelfth rib to the iliac crest anteriorly. The most common site is herniation through the inferior lumbar triangle (of Petit). This is the region above the iliac crest behind the posterior edge of the external oblique muscle and in front of the anterior border of the latissimus dorsi muscle. Lumbar hernias also occur in the superior lumbar triangle, the region below the twelfth rib and above the serratus

           ● New Code   ▲ Revised Code

Digestive System

posterior inferior muscle, behind the border of the internal oblique muscle and in front of the quadratus lumborum and erector spinae muscles. An incision is made over the hernia defect. The sac is dissected down to its neck, opened, and its contents inspected. If the bowel is healthy, it is reduced into the abdomen. The empty sac is excised or inverted. If the defect is small, it is sutured closed. Larger defects may require reinforcement with a mesh plug. The mesh is fixed between the peritoneum and abdominal wall muscles.

49550-49553

49550   Repair initial femoral hernia, any age; reducible
49553   Repair initial femoral hernia, any age; incarcerated or strangulated

An initial femoral hernia repair is performed on a patient of any age. A femoral hernia is a condition in which tissues protrude through a weakness in the groin area into the top of the thigh. Code 49550 reports repair of a reducible hernia, in which the contents of the hernia sac can be pushed back into their normal position. An incision is made in the thigh below the inguinal ligament over the femoral canal. The subcutaneous fat is split, exposing the extraperitoneal fat enveloping the hernia sac. The mass of peritoneal fat is freed by blunt dissection. The inguinal ligament, overlying fascia, and neck of the hernia are exposed. The fat mass is split and the sac is also exposed, then dissected up to and beyond the neck, and opened so the contents can be inspected. The bowel and omentum are returned to the abdominal cavity. The sac is ligated at the neck and transected. The stump is returned to the abdominal cavity and the inguinal ligament is sutured to Cooper's ligament. A mesh plug may be applied. Use 49553 if the hernia was strangulated or incarcerated. Incarcerated hernias are those in which the contents of the hernia sac cannot be pushed back to their normal position. Strangulated hernias are those in which circulation is compromised.

49555-49557

49555   Repair recurrent femoral hernia; reducible
49557   Repair recurrent femoral hernia; incarcerated or strangulated

A recurrent femoral hernia repair is performed on a person of any age. A femoral hernia is a condition in which structures protrude through a weakness in the groin area into the top of the thigh. Code 49555 reports repair of a reducible hernia, in which the contents of the hernia sac can be pushed back into their normal position. Recurrent hernia repairs vary in complexity depending on the extent of the defect and the amount of scarring and tissue damage from the initial repair. An incision is made in the thigh below the inguinal ligament over the femoral canal. The subcutaneous fat is split, exposing the extraperitoneal fat enveloping the hernia sac. The mass of peritoneal fat is freed by blunt dissection. As the previous repair is taken apart, care is taken to preserve healthy tissue. The inguinal ligament, overlying fascia, and neck of the hernia are exposed. The fat mass is split and the sac is also exposed, then dissected up to and beyond the neck, and opened so the contents can be inspected. Adhesions between the bowel, omentum, and sac wall are severed. The bowel and omentum are returned to the abdominal cavity. The sac is ligated at the neck and transected. The stump is returned to the abdominal cavity and the inguinal ligament is sutured to Cooper's ligament. A mesh plug may be applied. Use 49557 if the hernia was strangulated or incarcerated. Incarcerated hernias are those in which the contents of the hernia sac cannot be pushed back to their normal position. Strangulated hernias are those in which circulation is compromised.

49560-49561

49560   Repair initial incisional or ventral hernia; reducible
49561   Repair initial incisional or ventral hernia; incarcerated or strangulated

An initial repair of an incisional or ventral hernia is performed. An incisional hernia, also referred to as a ventral hernia, occurs at the site of an old abdominal wall (laparotomy) incision that has not closed properly. Tissues in the abdominal wall separate at the site of the old incision and the abdominal organs bulge through the opening. Code 49560 reports repair of a reducible hernia, in which the contents of the hernia sac can be pushed back into their normal position in the abdomen. A small incisional hernia is repaired by resuturing the tissue. The old scar is excised and separated from the hernia sac. The skin on each side of the incision is freed and the entire sac is exposed and opened. Adherent omentum and bowel are dissected off the inner surface of the hernia sac and freed from the inner surface of the abdominal wall. The sac and its peritoneal lining, scar tissue, and suture material are excised. Normal tissue of the linea alba, a band of fibrous tissue in the midline of the abdomen, is exposed and the abdominal wall is sutured closed. Excess skin is removed before being sutured closed. A large defect may be repaired by either shoelace technique or reinforced with a mesh implant. If shoelace technique is used, the old scar is excised and skin and fat are dissected off the hernia sac. The anterior rectus muscle sheaths are exposed. The unopened hernia sac and its contents are returned to the abdominal cavity. Following reduction of the hernia, an incision is made in each anterior rectus sheath about one cm from the medial edge and the rectus muscle is exposed. The incision is extended superiorly and inferiorly along the entire length of the hernia. The linea alba is reconstructed by suturing the two strips of anterior rectus muscle together. The lateral cut edges of the rectus sheaths meet at the midline and are anchored to the new linea alba. Larger defects may require mesh reinforcement. Use code 49561 if the hernia is strangulated or incarcerated. Incarcerated hernias are those in which the contents of the

hernia sac cannot be pushed back to their normal position. Strangulated hernias are those in which circulation is compromised.

49565-49566

49565   Repair recurrent incisional or ventral hernia; reducible
49566   Repair recurrent incisional or ventral hernia; incarcerated or strangulated

A recurrent incisional or ventral hernia is repaired. An incisional hernia, also referred to as a ventral hernia, occurs at the site of an old abdominal wall (laparotomy) incision that has not closed properly. Tissues in the abdominal wall separate at the site of the old incision and the abdominal organs bulge through the opening. Code 49565 reports repair of a reducible hernia, in which the contents of the hernia sac can be pushed back into their normal position in the abdomen. Recurrent hernia repairs vary in complexity depending on the extent of the defect and the amount of scarring and tissue damage resulting from the initial repair. A small incisional hernia is repaired by resuturing the tissue. The old scar is excised and separated from the hernia sac. The skin on each side of the incision is freed and the entire sac is exposed and opened. Adherent omentum and bowel are dissected off the inner surface of the hernia sac and freed from the inner surface of the abdominal wall. The sac and its peritoneal lining, scar tissue, and suture material are excised. Normal tissue of the linea alba, a band of fibrous tissue in the midline of the abdomen, is exposed and the abdominal wall is sutured closed. Excess skin is removed before being sutured closed. A large defect may be repaired, either by shoelace technique or reinforced with a mesh implant. If shoelace technique is used, the old scar is excised and skin and fat are dissected off the hernia sac. The anterior rectus muscle sheaths are exposed. The unopened hernia sac and its contents are returned to the abdominal cavity. Following reduction of the hernia, an incision is made in each anterior rectus sheath about one cm from the medial edge and the rectus muscle is exposed. The incision is extended superiorly and inferiorly along the entire length of the hernia. The linea alba is reconstructed by suturing the two strips of anterior rectus muscle together. The lateral cut edges of the rectus sheaths meet at the midline and are anchored to the new linea alba. Larger defects may require mesh reinforcement. Use code 49566 if the hernia is strangulated or incarcerated. Incarcerated hernias are those in which the contents of the hernia sac cannot be pushed back to their normal position. Strangulated hernias are those in which circulation is compromised.

49568

49568   Implantation of mesh or other prosthesis for open incisional or ventral hernia repair or mesh for closure of debridement for necrotizing soft tissue infection (List separately in addition to code for the incisional or ventral hernia repair)

Mesh or other prosthesis is implanted to provide reinforcement during a separately reportable incisional or ventral hernia repair or for closure following a separately reportable debridement for necrotizing soft tissue infection (NSTI). Placement of mesh or prosthetic implant may be performed using a variety of techniques including underlay, onlay, inlay, wrap-around, or a combination of these techniques. Mesh or other implant material is cut to the desired shape to reinforce the hernia or support the NSTI debridement defect. In an underlay technique, a large piece of mesh extending beyond the edges of the defect is sutured deep to the peritoneum or between the peritoneum and the abdominal wall. The edges of the mesh are fixed using mattress sutures passing through the entire thickness of the abdominal wall taking care to place omentum between the bowel and the prosthesis. In an inlay technique, the mesh is cut to the size and shape of the defect and sutured to the edges of the defect. In an onlay technique, a large piece of mesh is sutured to the outer surface of the abdominal wall over the external oblique muscles. In a wrap-around technique, two sheets of mesh are wrapped around the abdominal wall and sutured first to each side of the defect using vertical sutures. The mesh on each side of the defect is then sutured together bringing the opposing medial edges together.

49570-49572

49570   Repair epigastric hernia (eg, preperitoneal fat); reducible (separate procedure)
49572   Repair epigastric hernia (eg, preperitoneal fat); incarcerated or strangulated

An epigastric hernia is repaired. Epigastric hernias are those where abdominal contents protrude through the linea alba, a sheet of muscle fiber in the midline of the abdomen. Epigastric hernias occur in the midline in the region between the umbilicus and the xiphoid process. Code 49570 reports repair of a reducible hernia, in which the contents of the hernia sac can be pushed back to their normal position. An incision is made over the hernia defect and herniated fat is excised, exposing the linea alba. The hernia sac is opened and the contents inspected. If the contents are healthy, they are returned to the abdomen. Omentum adherent to the sac and the sac are excised. The opening in the fascia is closed. In rare cases, a more complex repair is required with reconstruction of the linea alba. An incision is made in each anterior rectus sheath about one cm from the medial edge and the rectus muscle is identified. The incision is extended up and down the entire length of the hernia opening. The two strips of anterior rectus muscle are approximated in the midline to create a new linea alba. The lateral cut edges of the rectus sheaths are anchored in the midline to the new linea alba. Use code 49572 if the hernia is

Digestive System

strangulated or incarcerated. Incarcerated hernias are those in which the contents of the hernia sac cannot be pushed back to their normal position. Strangulated hernias are those in which circulation is compromised.

49580-49582

49580 Repair umbilical hernia, younger than age 5 years; reducible
49582 Repair umbilical hernia, younger than age 5 years; incarcerated or strangulated

An umbilical hernia in a child younger than age five is repaired. Umbilical hernias are protrusions of omentum and bowel through the abdominal wall at the umbilicus. Code 49580 reports repair of a reducible hernia, in which the contents of the hernia sac can be pushed back into their normal position. A curved incision is made in the skin below the umbilicus. The skin is raised and the subcutaneous fat is dissected off the aponeurosis of the external oblique muscle to the level of the hernia sac. The distal end of the sac is freed from the skin. The sac may be opened and the contents inspected. If the bowel is healthy, the sac is inverted into the abdominal cavity and then snipped off at its base. The hernia defect in the abdominal wall is closed and the skin is tacked down over the aponeurosis and closed. A pressure dressing may be applied. Use code 49582 if the hernia is strangulated or incarcerated. Incarcerated hernias are those in which the contents of the hernia sac cannot be pushed back to their normal position. Strangulated hernias are those in which circulation is compromised.

49585-49587

49585 Repair umbilical hernia, age 5 years or older; reducible
49587 Repair umbilical hernia, age 5 years or older; incarcerated or strangulated

An umbilical hernia in a patient aged five years or older is repaired. Umbilical hernias are protrusions of omentum and bowel through the abdominal wall at the umbilicus. Code 49585 reports repair of a reducible hernia, in which the contents of the hernia sac can be pushed back into their normal position. A curved incision is made in the skin below the umbilicus. The skin is raised by dissecting it free of the subcutaneous fat. The fascial edge of the hernia defect and the neck of the sac are exposed. The anterior rectus muscle sheath is exposed. The neck of the sac is incised along the edge of the hernia defect and lifted away from the abdominal wall. The hernia contents are extracted and inspected. Any adhesions are severed. If the bowel is healthy, it is returned to the abdomen. The omentum and hernia sac are excised. The hernia defect in the abdominal wall is closed. If the defect is large, a mesh plug may be applied. The skin is tacked down over the aponeurosis and the skin is closed. A pressure dressing may be applied. Use code 49587 if the hernia is strangulated or incarcerated. Incarcerated hernias are those in which the contents of the hernia sac cannot be pushed back to their normal position. Strangulated hernias are those in which circulation is compromised.

49590

49590 Repair spigelian hernia

A Spigelian hernia is repaired. Spigelian hernias, also referred to as lateral ventral hernias, are protrusions of abdominal contents through the semilunar line. The semilunar line is at the lateral (outer) border of the rectus sheath and extends from the tip of the ninth rib to the pubic tubercle. The most common site for a Spigelian hernia is in the lower abdomen. Low spigelian hernias pass through the conjoined tendon of the transversus abdominis and the internal oblique muscles. A skin incision is made over the defect. If the hernia sac protrudes into subcutaneous tissue, the skin incision will immediately reveal the hernia sac. If the hernia sac is interstitial, the incision is extended into the external oblique muscle. The hernia sac is dissected free of surrounding tissue down to the hernia neck. The sac is then opened and the contents are inspected. If the bowel is healthy, it is returned to the abdomen. Any adhesions present are severed and the sac is then excised or inverted. The defects in the fascia of the transversus abdominis muscle and the internal oblique muscle are closed. The external oblique muscle incision is closed.

49600

49600 Repair of small omphalocele, with primary closure

The physician repairs a small umbilical ring defect (omphalocele) present at birth. Small defects are usually 1-2 cm in diameter and contain only one or two loops of small bowel. The unopened omphalocele sac or the remaining ruptured sac is excised. The bowel is examined to rule out other problems that need to be addressed. If no other problems exist, the abdominal wall is stretched by inserting the fingers of both hands and pushing out on the abdominal wall. Once sufficient space has been achieved, the bowel is pushed into the abdomen. The defect in the abdominal wall is then closed and covered with skin.

49605-49606

49605 Repair of large omphalocele or gastroschisis; with or without prosthesis
49606 Repair of large omphalocele or gastroschisis; with removal of prosthesis, final reduction and closure, in operating room

The physician repairs a large umbilical ring defect (omphalocele) or a defect lateral to the umbilicus (gastroschisis) containing bowel and other internal organs present at birth. The

physician may use one of two techniques. In the first technique, the large defect is closed without a prosthesis. The abdominal wall is stretched by inserting the fingers of both hands and pushing out on the abdominal wall. If the physician is able to stretch the abdominal wall enough to allow the bowel and other internal organs to be replaced in the abdomen without causing excessive tension, the abdominal wall may be closed and covered with skin. The second technique is to construct a prosthetic silo or pouch to enclose the bowel. The skin is dissected off the edge of the defect. One edge of the prosthesis is sutured to the abdominal wall defect. The other two edges of the prosthesis are sutured together and a silo or pouch is constructed that contains the bowel and internal organs. Tension is then used to slowly stretch the abdominal wall. As the abdominal wall is stretched, the silo or pouch is closed to force more of the bowel and internal organs into the abdomen. This may take several days or a week or more to accomplish. Once all the bowel and internal organs are contained in the abdomen, a second procedure (49606) is performed to remove the prosthesis. The abdominal wall is then closed and covered with skin.

49610-49611

49610 Repair of omphalocele (Gross type operation); first stage
49611 Repair of omphalocele (Gross type operation); second stage

An omphalocele is a congenital defect of the ventral abdominal wall in which there is an absence of abdominal muscles, fascia and skin. Intra-abdominal structures protrude from the abdominal region and are covered by a membrane consisting of peritoneum and amnion. The classic omphalocele occurs at the umbilical ring and the umbilical cord is attached to the omphalocele. During the first stage of the repair, umbilical vessels are ligated and the umbilical cord is amputated. The skin is incised at the edge of the defect. The skin is dissected from the fascia and elevated. The amnion remains intact. Skin flaps are developed and closed over the omphalocele, leaving a large ventral hernia. During the second stage which is typically performed 6 months to two years later, the skin flaps are opened and the large ventral hernia is repaired. Use 49610 for the first stage of the Gross operation and 49611 for the second stage.

49650-49651

49650 Laparoscopy, surgical; repair initial inguinal hernia
49651 Laparoscopy, surgical; repair recurrent inguinal hernia

A small incision is made in the area of the umbilicus and the laparoscope is inserted. The abdomen is inflated with gas. Two or three additional small incisions are made in the abdomen and trocars are inserted. Surgical instruments are inserted through the trocars. The hernia is identified and a peritoneal incision made from the lateral aspect of the inguinal canal to the lateral umbilical ligament. Cooper's ligament is exposed along with the inferior epigastric vessels and in males the spermatic cord. Iliac vessels are identified and protected. The abdominal wall is exposed and surrounding fatty tissue excised. The hernia sac is dissected from surrounding tissues. The hernia sac is pushed back into the abdominal cavity and the defect in the abdominal wall exposed. A mesh patch is anchored to Cooper's ligament and tacked to the abdominal wall over the abdominal wall defect. The peritoneum is closed over the abdominal wall completely covering the mesh. The laparoscope, surgical instruments, and trocars are removed and the portal incisions closed. Use 49650 for the initial repair of an inguinal hernia and 49651 for repair of a recurrent inguinal hernia.

49652-49653

49652 Laparoscopy, surgical, repair, ventral, umbilical, spigelian or epigastric hernia (includes mesh insertion, when performed); reducible
49653 Laparoscopy, surgical, repair, ventral, umbilical, spigelian or epigastric hernia (includes mesh insertion, when performed); incarcerated or strangulated

Laparoscopic repair of a ventral, umbilical, spigelian, or epigastric hernia is performed, including mesh insertion if needed. A ventral hernia is a type that occurs at the site of an old, weakened abdominal-wall incision. An umbilical hernia is a protrusion of omentum and bowel through the abdominal wall at the umbilicus. A spigelian hernia is a protrusion of abdominal contents through the semilunar line through the lateral border of the rectus sheath. An epigastric hernia is a protrusion of abdominal contents through the linea alba, a sheet of muscle fiber in the midline of the abdomen. In 49652, a small incision is made at a site distant from any prior abdominal incisions and the hernia defect. A trocar is placed and pneumoperitoneum is established. The laparoscope is introduced and additional portal incisions are made under direct vision for insertion of surgical instruments. Adhesions are lysed. The abdominal wall is examined and the extent of the hernia is evaluated. The edges of the defect are cleared of peritoneum and fat. The location of the hernia defects are drawn on the overlying skin. The hernia contents are reduced. The hernia defect may be closed by primary suture, or a mesh insert may need to be placed. If mesh is required, the hernia defect is measured and the mesh is cut to size, inserted, and positioned over the reduced hernia defect. Tacks or sutures are used to affix the mesh to the abdominal wall. The laparoscope and surgical instruments are removed, the pneumoperitoneum is released, and the portal incisions are closed. In 49653, an incarcerated or strangulated hernia is repaired. After lysing adhesions and evaluating the extent of the hernia, the hernia sac is opened and the incarcerated loop of bowel is inspected, released, and returned to

● New Code ▲ Revised Code

Digestive System

the abdominal cavity. For a strangulated hernia, the necrotic tissue (which may include omentum, bowel or other contents) is resected, placed in a retrieval bag, and removed. The hernia repair is then performed as described above.

49654-49655

49654   Laparoscopy, surgical, repair, incisional hernia (includes mesh insertion, when performed); reducible

49655   Laparoscopy, surgical, repair, incisional hernia (includes mesh insertion, when performed); incarcerated or strangulated

Laparoscopic repair of an incisional hernia is performed, including mesh insertion if needed. An incisional hernia occurs as a protrusion defect at the site of an incompletely healed abdominal surgical wound or incision. In 49654, a small incision is made at a site distant from the prior abdominal incision and the hernia defect. A trocar is placed and pneumoperitoneum is established. The laparoscope is introduced and additional portal incisions are made under direct vision for insertion of surgical instruments. Adhesions are lysed. The abdominal wall is examined and the extent of the hernia is evaluated. The edges of the defect are cleared of peritoneum and fat. The location of the hernia defects are drawn on the overlying skin. The hernia contents are reduced. The hernia defect may be closed by primary suture, or a mesh insert may need to be placed. If mesh is required, the hernia defect is measured and the mesh is cut to size, inserted, and positioned over the reduced hernia defect. Tacks or sutures are used to affix the mesh to the abdominal wall. The laparoscope and surgical instruments are removed, the pneumoperitoneum is released, and the portal incisions are closed. In 49655, an incarcerated or strangulated hernia is repaired. After lysing adhesions and evaluating the extent of the hernia, the hernia sac is opened and the incarcerated loop of bowel is inspected, released, and returned to the abdominal cavity. For a strangulated hernia, the necrotic tissue (which may include omentum, bowel, or other abdominal contents) is resected, placed in a retrieval bag, and removed. The hernia repair is then performed as described above.

49656-49657

49656   Laparoscopy, surgical, repair, recurrent incisional hernia (includes mesh insertion, when performed); reducible

49657   Laparoscopy, surgical, repair, recurrent incisional hernia (includes mesh insertion, when performed); incarcerated or strangulated

Laparoscopic repair of a recurrent incisional hernia is performed, including mesh insertion if needed. An incisional hernia occurs as a protrusion defect at the site of an incompletely healed abdominal surgical wound or incision. These can be frustrating and difficult hernias to treat as the tissue of the abdominal wall is already weakened, thin, and stretched. In 49656, a small incision is made at a site distant from the prior abdominal incision and the hernia defect. A trocar is placed and pneumoperitoneum is established. The laparoscope is introduced and additional portal incisions are made under direct vision for insertion of surgical instruments. Adhesions are lysed. The abdominal wall is examined and the extent of the hernia is evaluated. The edges of the defect are cleared of peritoneum and fat. The location of the hernia defects are drawn on the overlying skin. The hernia contents are reduced. The hernia defect may be closed by primary suture or a mesh insert may need to be placed. If mesh is required, the hernia defect is measured and the mesh is cut to size, inserted, and positioned over the hernia defect. Tacks or sutures are used to affix the mesh to the abdominal wall. The laparoscope and surgical instruments are removed; the pneumoperitoneum is released; and the portal incisions are closed. In 49657, an incarcerated or strangulated recurrent hernia is repaired. After lysing adhesions and evaluating the extent of the hernia, the hernia sac is opened and the incarcerated loop of bowel is inspected, released, and returned to the abdominal cavity. For a strangulated hernia, the necrotic tissue (which may include omentum, bowel, or other abdominal contents) is resected, placed in a retrieval bag, and removed. The hernia repair is then performed as described above.

49900

49900   Suture, secondary, of abdominal wall for evisceration or dehiscence

Dehiscence refers to opening of an abdominal wound or surgical incision that was closed with sutures during a previous surgery. Evisceration is protrusion of intra-abdominal contents through the open wound. The suture line and abdominal wall are inspected for evidence of infection. Old sutures are removed. Any abdominal contents that have eviscerated are also inspected and returned to the abdominal cavity. The edges the wound, including peritoneum, fascia, subcutaneous tissue, and skin are trimmed. Running sutures are loosely placed along the entire aspect of the surgical wound through peritoneum, fascia, and muscle. Once all sutures have been placed, they are tightened and the knot is tied. Subcutaneous tissue and skin is then closed over the abdominal wall.

49904-49906

49904   Omental flap, extra-abdominal (eg, for reconstruction of sternal and chest wall defects)

49906   Free omental flap with microvascular anastomosis

49905   Omental flap, intra-abdominal (List separately in addition to code for primary procedure)

Omental flaps are used in reconstruction procedures when there are large defects in soft and/or connective tissues caused by injury, disease, or surgical removal of tissue. In 49904, an extra-abdominal omental flap is used to reconstruct a defect in the sternum or chest. An upper midline abdominal incision is used to expose the omentum. The omentum is evaluated to determine which vessels are dominant and which vessel pedicle would provide adequate flap length and vascular supply for the extra-abdominal reconstruction. The omentum is lifted off the colon and carefully dissected free of the transverse colon. Blood vessels are individually clamped and ligated. The omentum is then lifted and rotated over the chest to ensure that it has been sufficiently mobilized to cover the entire defect. The anterior diaphragm is incised and the omental flap passed into the chest. It is placed over the defect and evaluated to ensure that there is no tension on the vessel pedicle and that blood flow to the flap is unobstructed. The omental flap is then secured with sutures to the surrounding structures. Drains are placed as needed and the abdominal incision closed. In 49905, an intra-abdominal omental flap is used during a separately reportable abdominal procedure to repair a defect in the abdomen. The omentum is exposed and evaluated as described above. The omental flap is created as described above, rotated over the abdominal defect, and secured with sutures. In 49906, a free omental flap is used to repair a defect. The segment of omentum to be used in the free flap is identified. The vascular pedicle is isolated and the amount of omentum needed to fill the defect is dissected from surrounding omentum. The recipient site is prepared and the recipient vessels isolated and prepared for microvascular anastomosis. The omental vessels are divided and the free omental flap is transferred to the recipient site. Microvascular anastomosis of omental and recipient vessels is performed. The omentum is secured to the edges of the defect with sutures. Overlying subcutaneous tissue and skin may be closed over the free omental flap or a separately reportable skin graft may be used to cover the flap. The abdominal incision is closed.

Omental flap, intra/extra-abdominal

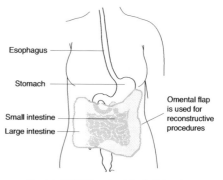

Esophagus

Stomach

Small intestine

Large intestine

Omental flap is used for reconstructive procedures

Use code (49904) for extra-abdominal (sternal or chest wall); use code (49905) for intra-abdominal; use code (49906) for free vascularized repair flap

50010

50010   **Renal exploration, not necessitating other specific procedures**

Renal exploration may be performed following blunt or penetrating renal trauma, particularly when there is evidence of persistent hemorrhage, the presence of devitalized renal tissue, or persistent urinary leakage. The approach depends on whether there are other intra-abdominal injuries that require exploration. The renal artery is exposed and a loop is placed around the artery to prevent hemorrhage. Gerota's fascia is incised and perirenal fat is dissected. The kidney is exposed and visually examined to determine the extent of injury. The surgical wound is irrigated and perioperative drains are placed as needed. No additional surgical interventions are required in this procedure. Once the kidney and surrounding tissue have been thoroughly explored, Gerota's fascia is closed, vessel loops are removed, and the incision is closed in layers. Perirenal drains may be left in place.

50020

50020   **Drainage of perirenal or renal abscess, open**

Perirenal abscess, renal abscesss, or infected urinoma resulting from blunt or penetrating trauma or other cause is treated with open drainage. The skin is incised and underlying soft tissues are dissected. Gerota's fascia is incised and perirenal fat is dissected. The abscess is located and incised. Loculations are separated and all debris, which may include pus, blood, and necrotic tissue is evacuated. The abscess site is vigorously irrigated with sterile saline or antibiotic solution until all debris has been cleared from the abscess pocket. A drain is placed in the abscess cavity and incisions are closed in layers around the drain.

50040-50045

50040   **Nephrostomy, nephrotomy with drainage**
50045   **Nephrotomy, with exploration**

Open nephrostomy or nephrotomy may be performed to drain urine from the kidney when the ureter is blocked due to a kidney stone or tumor, when the ureter or bladder has been injured causing urine to leak into the retroperitoneal or peritoneal cavity, or as a diagnostic procedure to assess kidney anatomy and function. A skin incision is made over the kidney and soft tissues are dissected. Gerota's fascia is incised and perirenal fat is dissected. Blood vessels are identified and controlled by placing a loop around each vessel. The kidney is exposed and visually examined. In 50040, a small incision is made in the kidney and a drainage catheter or tube is placed in the renal pelvis to drain urine from the kidney. The catheter or tube is secured with sutures and overlying tissues are closed around the drainage device. In 50045, the kidney is incised and visually examined. Once the kidney and surrounding tissue have been thoroughly explored, drains are placed as needed, Gerota's fascia is closed, vessel loops are removed, and the incision is closed in layers.

50060-50065

50060   **Nephrolithotomy; removal of calculus**
50065   **Nephrolithotomy; secondary surgical operation for calculus**

Open nephrolithotomy is performed to remove a renal calculus. A skin incision is made over the kidney and soft tissues are dissected. Gerota's fascia is incised and perirenal fat is dissected. Blood vessels are identified and controlled by placing a loop around each vessel. The kidney is exposed and visually examined. An incision is made in the kidney over the site of the renal calculus. The calculus is located and removed and sent to the laboratory for separately reportable analysis. Drains are placed as needed, Gerota's fascia is closed, vessel loops are removed, and the incision is closed in layers. Use 50060 for the primary surgical procedure to remove the renal calculus. Use 50065 if this is a secondary surgical operation to remove the calculus.

50070-50075

50075   **Nephrolithotomy; removal of large staghorn calculus filling renal pelvis and calyces (including anatrophic pyelolithotomy)**
50070   **Nephrolithotomy; complicated by congenital kidney abnormality**

Open nephrolithotomy is performed to remove a renal calculus in a procedure complicated by congenital kidney abnormality or by removal of a large staghorn calculus. A skin incision is made over the kidney and soft tissues are dissected. Gerota's fascia is incised and perirenal fat is dissected. Blood vessels are identified and controlled by placing a loop around each vessel. The kidney is exposed and visually examined. An incision is made in the kidney over the site of the renal calculus. Use 50070 for open removal of a renal calculus when the patient has a congenital kidney abnormality such as parenchymal disease, congenital obstruction of the ureteropelvic junction with or without hydronephrosis, or polycystic kidneys. The calculus is located and removed and sent to the laboratory for

separately reportable analysis. Drains are placed as needed, Gerota's fascia is closed, vessel loops are removed, and the incision is closed in layers. Use 50075 if the patient has a large staghorn calculus, which may also be referred to as a struvite calculus. To be classified as a staghorn calculus, the stone must involve the renal pelvis and extend into at least two calyces. In order to completely expose and excise the stone, the kidney is bivalved along the lateral aspect, which is also referred to as anatrophic nephrolithotomy, or the renal pelvis is opened, which is also referred to as anatrophic pyelolithotomy. The staghorn calculus is then carefully dissected free of the renal parenchyma and removed. The renal pelvis and calyces are carefully inspected to ensure that all stone fragments are removed.

50080-50081

50080   **Percutaneous nephrostolithotomy or pyelostolithotomy, with or without dilation, endoscopy, lithotripsy, stenting, or basket extraction; up to 2 cm**
50081   **Percutaneous nephrostolithotomy or pyelostolithotomy, with or without dilation, endoscopy, lithotripsy, stenting, or basket extraction; over 2 cm**

A renal calculus is removed by percutaneous technique. The skin over the planned puncture site is cleansed and a local anesthetic is injected. The skin is punctured and a needle is advanced into the kidney to the site of the calculus using separately reportable fluoroscopic guidance. A guidewire is then advanced through the needle and the needle is removed. A rigid and/or flexible nephroscope is introduced over the guidewire and the guidewire is removed. The calculus is visualized. If the calculus is large, a series of dilators may be passed through the nephroscope to widen the tract and provide better access to the calculus. A permanent indwelling stent may be placed to maintain the opening. Lithotripsy is performed as needed using ultrasound, an electrohydraulic device, pneumatic lithotrites, and/or laser to fragment the stone. A basket extraction device may be used to remove the calculus. Once the calculus and any fragments have been completely removed, a nephrostomy tube is placed to ensure good post-procedural drainage of the kidney. A large branched staghorn calculus may require multiple percutaneous nephrolithotomy or pyelolithotomy tracts for complete removal of the calculus. Use 50080 for a calculus up to 2 cm. Use 50081 if the calculus is over 2 cm.

50100

50100   **Transection or repositioning of aberrant renal vessels (separate procedure)**

Aberrant renal blood vessels are one cause of ureteropelvic junction (UPJ) obstruction. This occurs when the renal arteries and/or veins at the inferior pole of the kidney cross anterior to the ureter causing obstruction and hydronephrosis. An anterior approach is used to expose the aberrant blood vessels, ureter, and kidney. The aberrant blood vessels are dissected free of surrounding tissue. If the kidney has adequate blood supply from other renal vessels, the aberrant vessels are ligated and transected. If the aberrant blood vessels must be preserved, vessel loops are placed superior and inferior to the planned transection site. The vessels are transected between the vessel loops and repositioned so that they no longer obstruct the UPJ. The vessels are anastomosed. The vessel loops are removed and the operative wound is closed in layers.

50120-50135

50120   **Pyelotomy; with exploration**
50125   **Pyelotomy; with drainage, pyelostomy**
50130   **Pyelotomy; with removal of calculus (pyelolithotomy, pelviolithotomy, including coagulum pyelolithotomy)**
50135   **Pyelotomy; complicated (eg, secondary operation, congenital kidney abnormality)**

A pyelotomy is an incision into the renal pelvis, the large cavity in the center of the kidney where urine is collected. The renal pelvis collects urine from the calyces. Urine drains from the renal pelvis into the ureter. A skin incision is made over the kidney. Gerota's fascia is incised and perirenal fat is dissected. Blood vessels are identified and controlled by placing a loop around each vessel. The kidney and ureter are exposed and visually examined. The ureter is traced upwards to the ureteropelvic junction (UPJ) and the renal pelvis is located. The posterior aspect of the renal pelvis is exposed and incised. In 50120, the renal pelvis is carefully explored for signs of disease or injury. In 50125, the renal pelvis is incised and a pyelostomy tube is placed into the pelvis to drain urine. A pursestring suture is placed around the pyelostomy tube to secure it to the renal pelvis. The surgical wound is closed in layers around the tube and a pyelostomy bag is attached to the tube to collect urine. In 50130, a calculus is removed from the renal pelvis. A single stone is removed using stone forceps. A coagulum pyelolithotomy may be used to remove multiple small stones. This involves creating a coagulum (clot) that envelops the small stones. For coagulum pyelolithotomy, a noncrushing clamp is placed around the ureter at the UPJ. Prior to incising the renal pelvis, thrombin and calcium chloride solution are injected into the renal pelvis to precipitate clot formation. Once the clot has formed, the renal pelvis is incised and the clot containing the small stones is removed. In 50135, a complicated pyelotomy is performed on a patient who has had previous surgery on the kidney or a patient who has a congenital kidney abnormality such as parenchymal disease, congenital obstruction of the ureteropelvic junction with or without hydronephrosis, or polycystic kidneys. The physician may explore the renal pelvis, place a pyelostomy tube, or remove a calculus. Upon completion of the procedure, drains are placed as needed and the surgical wound is closed in layers.

50200-50205

50200   **Renal biopsy; percutaneous, by trocar or needle**
50205   **Renal biopsy; by surgical exposure of kidney**

In 50200, a percutaneous, trocar or needle biopsy is performed using separately reportable radiological guidance. The patient is sedated and a local anesthetic administered. The patient is placed prone on top of pillows or folded sheets to compress the abdomen and upper ribs allowing better access to the kidney. The kidneys are visualized using ultrasound, fluoroscopy, CT, or MRI with the most common modality being ultrasound. The trocar or needle is then placed through the skin over the kidney and advanced under direct vision to the renal capsule. A tissue sample is obtained. In 50205, an open biopsy is performed by surgical exposure of the kidney. A small incision is made in the back over the kidney and the renal capsule exposed. A tissue sample is obtained and sent for separately reportable pathological evaluation.

50220-50225

50220   **Nephrectomy, including partial ureterectomy, any open approach including rib resection**
50225   **Nephrectomy, including partial ureterectomy, any open approach including rib resection; complicated because of previous surgery on same kidney**

An open nephrectomy is performed including partial ureterectomy and rib resection when needed. A wide flank incision is made immediately below the lower border of the ribs or near the 11th or 12th rib. The 11th and/or 12th ribs are removed as needed to allow surgical access to the kidney. Alternatively, an anterior subcostal approach may be utilized. The kidney and ureter are exposed. The renal artery and vein are isolated, ligated and divided. The kidney is dissected free from surrounding tissue. A section of ureter is removed by first dissecting the involved section of ureter free of surrounding tissue. The ureter is then divided and the diseased section removed along with the kidney. Bleeding is controlled, drains placed as needed, and the incisions closed. Report 50220 when no previous surgery on the kidney has been performed and 50225 when the procedure is complicated by previous surgery on the same kidney.

50230

50230   **Nephrectomy, including partial ureterectomy, any open approach including rib resection; radical, with regional lymphadenectomy and/or vena caval thrombectomy**

An open radical nephrectomy is performed including partial ureterectomy, regional lymph node excision, vena caval thrombectomy, and rib resection, when needed. A wide flank incision is made immediately below the lower border of the ribs or near the 11th or 12th rib. The 11th and/or 12th ribs are removed as needed to allow surgical access to the kidney. Alternatively, an anterior subcostal approach may be utilized. The kidney and ureter are exposed. The aortocaval space is entered and regional lymph nodes are excised. The renal artery is isolated, ligated, and divided and the renal vein is palpated to identify any evidence of tumor thrombus. If tumor thrombus is present, the thrombus is milked back toward the kidney and the renal vein is ligated near the vena cava. If this is not possible, the renal vein is divided, the vena cava is incised, and the thrombus is resected. The Gerota's fascia is dissected free from surrounding structures and the lymphatic vessels are ligated. The gonadal vein is mobilized, clamped, and ligated. The ureter is dissected free of surrounding tissue and divided. The kidney is then mobilized and retracted to expose the adrenal gland. The adrenal gland is dissected free of surrounding tissue and removed along with the kidney. Bleeding is controlled, drains are placed as needed, and The incision is closed with sutures.

50234-50236

50234   **Nephrectomy with total ureterectomy and bladder cuff; through same incision**
50236   **Nephrectomy with total ureterectomy and bladder cuff; through separate incision**

An open nephrectomy with total ureterectomy and excision of the bladder cuff is performed. A Foley catheter is placed and the bladder is drained. A wide flank incision is made immediately below the lower border of the ribs or near the 11th or 12th rib. Alternatively, an anterior subcostal approach may be utilized. The kidney and ureter are exposed. The renal artery and vein are isolated, ligated and divided. The kidney is dissected free from surrounding tissue and removed. The entire ureter along with a section of bladder at the ureterovesical junction (UVJ) is removed by first dissecting the ureter free from surrounding

tissue. The bladder is then incised just below the UVJ and the bladder cuff removed. The bladder incision is closed. Bleeding is controlled, drains placed as needed, and the incisions closed. Report 50234 when the procedure is performed through a single incision; report 50236 when the kidney is removed through a subcostal or flank incision and a separate incision is used to remove the ureter and bladder cuff.

50240

50240   **Nephrectomy, partial**

An open partial nephrectomy is performed. A wide flank incision is made immediately below the lower border of the ribs. Alternatively, an anterior subcostal approach may be utilized. The kidney and ureter are exposed taking care to preserve the kidney vasculature. The renal artery is isolated and a vascular loop placed. Perirenal fat is dissected free of the kidney. The kidney lesion is located. Small lesions are enucleated and excised using blunt and sharp dissection. Large lesions require diuresis, temporary occlusion of the renal artery supplying the tumor site, and renal hypothermia. The renal mass is then resected by blunt and sharp dissection. Bleeding is controlled by suture-ligation of bleeding arteries and veins. The parenchymal defect in the kidney is closed.

50250

50250   **Ablation, open, 1 or more renal mass lesion(s), cryosurgical, including intraoperative ultrasound guidance and monitoring, if performed**

The physician performs an open procedure to destroy (ablate) one or more lesions in the kidney using cryosurgery with intraoperative ultrasound guidance as needed. A wide flank incision is made over the affected kidney. The kidney is exposed and the lesion is identified. One or more cryosurgical probes are then inserted into the lesion and the first freeze-thaw cycle is initiated. The ice ball created during the freeze cycle is monitored using ultrasound to ensure adequate extension of the ice ball beyond the lesion margins. A second freeze-thaw cycle is performed in the same manner. Additional lesions are treated in the same manner. The probes are removed, bleeding is controlled, drains are placed, and the incision is closed around the drains.

50280

50280   **Excision or unroofing of cyst(s) of kidney**

One or more cysts of the kidney are treated by open surgical excision or unroofing of the cyst(s). A wide flank incision is made over the affected kidney and the kidney is exposed. The cyst is then opened and the fluid is drained. The redundant cyst wall is excised in its entirety using blunt and sharp dissection. The base of the cyst is fulgurated to prevent recurrence and the defect is filled with perirenal fat. Alternatively, an unroofing procedure may be performed, which involves creating a window in the cyst wall or partially resecting the cyst wall and then marsupializing the cyst-creating an open pocket of the remaining cyst wall. Drains may be placed in the window to facilitate drainage and the remaining cyst wall I closed around the drains. Bleeding is controlled and incisions are closed.

50290

50290   **Excision of perinephric cyst**

The physician performs an excision of a perinephric cyst. Perinephric cysts, also referred to as perirenal cysts, occur on the exterior surface of the kidney in the space surrounding it. A wide flank incision is made over the affected kidney. Gerota's fascia is dissected off the surface of the cyst and excised along with perinephric fat overlying the cyst. The cyst is exposed and may be decompressed by aspirating the fluid or it may be left intact and dissected free from the surface of the kidney to facilitate identification of the margins. If the cyst has been decompressed, the redundant cyst wall is then excised in its entirety using blunt and sharp dissection. Depending on the location of the cyst, the base may be fulgurated to prevent recurrence. If the base of the cyst is in close proximity to the renal pelvis or hilum, fulguration may not be performed due to the risk of damage to surrounding vasculature. The defect is filled with perirenal fat. Bleeding is controlled and incisions are closed.

50300

50300   **Donor nephrectomy (including cold preservation); from cadaver donor, unilateral or bilateral**

One or both kidneys are harvested from a deceased (cadaver) donor that has been maintained medically until the surgical transplant team arrives. The inferior vena cava, aorta, and both renal pedicles are dissected free of surrounding structures. The gonadal, lumbar, and adrenal veins are clipped and divided. The renal artery is identified and dissected free of surrounding tissue. Lateral, posterior, and inferior kidney attachments are left intact to prevent torsion of the kidney and damage to its vascular pedicle. The ureter is dissected free of surrounding tissue to the level of the iliac vessels and divided. The kidney is dissected free from the remaining lateral and inferior attachments. The lower pole of the kidney is elevated and dissected free of posterior attachments. The vascular pedicle containing the renal artery and vein is divided. If cardiocirculatory arrest is initiated, retrograde cannulation of the aorta above the renal arteries is performed and the kidneys are cooled in situ by perfusing them with cold preservation solution. The kidneys and ureters are then removed and packed in ice and delivered to the recipient transplant team(s).

50320

50320   Donor nephrectomy (including cold preservation); open, from living donor

A living donor nephrectomy inclusive of cold preservation of the donor kidney is performed via an open approach. The lateral line of Toldt is identified and incised. The peritoneum over the kidney is mobilized and the anterior surface of the kidney is visualized. The colon is mobilized and rolled medially. The colorenal ligaments are divided and Gerota's fascia is exposed. The ureter and surrounding vascular structures are identified and retracted to expose the lower pole of the kidney and the renal hilum. The lower pole is partially mobilized. The kidney is retracted laterally and superiorly to allow access to the renal hilum. The renal hilum is dissected free of the surrounding structures. The renal vein is exposed. The gonadal, lumbar, and adrenal veins are clipped and divided. The renal artery is identified and dissected free of surrounding tissue. Lateral, posterior, and inferior kidney attachments are left intact to prevent torsion of the kidney and damage to its vascular pedicle. The ureter is dissected free of surrounding tissue to the level of the iliac vessels and divided. The kidney is dissected free from the remaining lateral and inferior attachments. The lower pole of the kidney is elevated and dissected free of posterior attachments. The vascular pedicle containing the renal artery and vein is divided. The kidney and ureter are then removed. The kidney may be perfused with cold preservation solution and/or placed on ice and delivered to the recipient surgical team.

50323-50325

50323   Backbench standard preparation of cadaver donor renal allograft prior to transplantation, including dissection and removal of perinephric fat, diaphragmatic and retroperitoneal attachments, excision of adrenal gland, and preparation of ureter(s), renal vein(s), and renal artery(s), ligating branches, as necessary

50325   Backbench standard preparation of living donor renal allograft (open or laparoscopic) prior to transplantation, including dissection and removal of perinephric fat and preparation of ureter(s), renal vein(s), and renal artery(s), ligating branches, as necessary

Standard backbench (backtable) preparation of a kidney harvested from a cadaver or living donor is performed prior to transplant. The kidney is unpackaged and transferred to a backtable basin and placed in iced Ringers lactate solution. Cultures are taken of the preservation fluid and sent to the laboratory. Fat and surrounding tissue is dissected off the external surface of the kidney. The adrenal gland is excised. The kidney is inspected and all open ends of small blood vessels are suture ligated to prevent post transplant bleeding. Lymphatic vessels are also suture ligated to prevent post transplant lymphocele formation. Large blood vessels are then addressed. The gonadal, adrenal, and any lumbar vein branches are divided and ligated. The renal vein is trimmed. If any reconstruction of the renal vein is required it is reported separately. The renal arteries are evaluated. Some donors have only a single renal artery and others have multiple renal arteries. The renal arteries are trimmed and branches ligated as needed. If any reconstruction is required on the renal arteries, it is reported separately. The ureter is then prepared leaving as much surrounding tissue as possible undisturbed to prevent damage to the vascular structures. The renal vessels are then flushed with Ringers lactate to identify any vascular defects or leaks that may require additional preparation or repair. Report 50323 for backbench preparation on a cadaver donor kidney and 50325 for backbench preparation on a living donor kidney.

50327-50328

50327   Backbench reconstruction of cadaver or living donor renal allograft prior to transplantation; venous anastomosis, each

50328   Backbench reconstruction of cadaver or living donor renal allograft prior to transplantation; arterial anastomosis, each

Backbench venous or arterial reconstruction is performed on a cadaver or living donor kidney. In 50327 the renal vein is reconstructed using a section of the vena cava or a vein graft. The renal vein is trimmed. The section of vena cava or vein graft is then fashioned to the correct length and width and anastomosed to the renal vein. If multiple renal vein branches are present, these may be anastomosed to form single vein or each may be prepared separately. Report 50327 for each venous anastomosis performed. In 50328, a one or more renal arteries are reconstructed using the gonadal vein obtained from the harvested kidney. The donor gonadal vein is used to create a patch or graft when a single renal artery requires repair or lengthening. When multiple renal artery branches are present, the renal arteries may be anastomosed to each other in a side-to-side fashion to create a single renal artery or each artery may be prepared separately with a venous graft. Report 50328 for each arterial anastomosis performed.

50329

50329   Backbench reconstruction of cadaver or living donor renal allograft prior to transplantation; ureteral anastomosis, each

Backbench reconstruction of the ureter is performed on a cadaver or living donor renal allograft prior to transplant. This may be required when the donor kidney has an anomaly, such as the presence of double ureters. The ureter is carefully dissected free of surrounding tissue, taking care not to compromise the vascular supply. A patch or graft is then prepared, usually with a section of ureter from the transplant recipient, and anastomosed to the ureter. When double ureters are present, they may be anastomosed to each other or each ureter may require separate preparation with graft anastomosis. Report 50329 for each ureteral anastomosis performed.

50340

50340   Recipient nephrectomy (separate procedure)

A kidney is removed from the donor recipient prior to transplantation in a separate procedure. A wide flank incision is made immediately below the lower border of the ribs or near the 11th or 12th rib. Alternatively, an anterior subcostal approach may be utilized. The peritoneum over the kidney is mobilized and the anterior surface of the kidney is visualized. The colon is mobilized and rolled medially. The colorenal ligaments are divided and Gerota's fascia is exposed. The ureter and surrounding vascular structures are identified and retracted to expose the lower pole of the kidney and the renal hilum. The lower pole is partially mobilized. The kidney is retracted laterally and superiorly to allow access to the renal hilum. The renal hilum is dissected free of the surrounding structures. The renal vein is exposed. The gonadal, lumbar, and adrenal veins are clipped and divided. The renal artery is identified and dissected free of surrounding tissue. Lateral, posterior, and inferior kidney attachments are left intact to prevent torsion of the kidney and damage to its vascular pedicle. The ureter is dissected free of surrounding tissue to the level of the iliac vessels and divided. The kidney is dissected free from the remaining lateral and inferior attachments. The lower pole of the kidney is elevated and dissected free of posterior attachments. The vascular pedicle containing the renal artery and vein is divided. The kidney is removed and the intact segment of ureter is closed. Bleeding is controlled, drains placed as needed, and the incisions closed.

50360-50365

50360   Renal allotransplantation, implantation of graft; without recipient nephrectomy

50365   Renal allotransplantation, implantation of graft; with recipient nephrectomy

The physician transplants the prepared kidney obtained from a cadaver or living donor in the transplant recipient. An incision is made in the lower abdomen. The transversalis fascia is incised and the retroperitoneal space entered. The peritoneum is retracted medially to allow exposure of the iliac blood vessels. Lymphatic vessels surrounding the iliac blood vessels are ligated and divided. The iliac blood vessels are dissected free of surrounding tissue from the region immediately above of the iliac lymph nodes to the bifurcation of the external and internal iliac artery. Vascular clamps are applied. The external iliac vein is incised and the prepared renal vein in the renal allograft is anastomosed to the external iliac vein. If more than one renal vein is present in the allograft, these are anastomosed separately to the external iliac vein. The prepared renal artery is then anastomosed to the internal or external iliac artery. If more than one renal artery is present, separate incisions are made and each artery is anastomosed to a separate site in the internal or external iliac artery. Vascular clamps are released, the anastomosis sites inspected, and any bleeding controlled. The ureter in the donor kidney is now prepared for anastomosis. The dome of the bladder is exposed and incised. The ureter is trimmed to the correct length and the end spatulated to match the opening in the bladder. The mucosa of the bladder and ureter are anastomosed followed by closure of the destrusor muscle layer over the ureter. A temporary stent may be placed to ensure patency at the anastomosis site. The kidney is then placed in the parapsoas fossa taking care to avoid any kinking of the blood vessels or ureter. Incisions are closed. Report 50360 when the kidney transplant is performed as described above leaving the recipient kidney intact. Report 50365 when the recipient kidney is removed at the time of the transplant procedure. A wide flank incision is made immediately below the lower border of the ribs or near the 11th or 12th rib. Alternatively, an anterior subcostal approach may be utilized. The kidney and ureter are exposed. The renal artery and vein are isolated, ligated and divided. The kidney is dissected free from surrounding tissue. The ureter is divided and the intact segment of ureter closed. Bleeding is controlled, drains placed as needed, and the incisions closed. The physician then proceeds with the transplant procedure as described above.

50370

50370   Removal of transplanted renal allograft

The physician removes a previously transplanted donor kidney. An incision is made in the lower abdomen. The transversalis fascia is incised and the retroperitoneal space is entered. The peritoneum is retracted medially and the transplanted kidney is exposed, then dissected free of surrounding tissue. The anastomosis sites of the transplanted ureter and renal vessels are exposed. The ureter is dissected free of surrounding tissue, ligated, and

Urinary System

divided. The renal vessels are dissected free of surrounding tissues, ligated, and divided. The transplanted kidney is removed, bleeding is controlled, and incisions are closed.

50380

50380   Renal autotransplantation, reimplantation of kidney

The physician removes the patient's kidney from the normal anatomic location and reimplants it in the parapsoas fossa or other site. The lateral line of Toldt is identified and incised. The peritoneum over the kidney is mobilized and the anterior surface of the kidney is visualized. The colon is mobilized and rolled medially. The colorenal ligaments are divided and Gerota's fascia is exposed. The ureter and surrounding vascular structures are identified and retracted to expose the lower pole of the kidney and the renal hilum. The lower pole is partially mobilized. The kidney is retracted laterally and superiorly to allow access to the renal hilum, which is dissected free of the surrounding structures. The renal vein is exposed. The gonadal, lumbar, and adrenal veins are clipped and divided. The renal artery is identified and dissected free of surrounding tissue. Lateral, posterior, and inferior kidney attachments are left intact to prevent torsion of the kidney and damage to its vascular pedicle. The ureter is dissected free of surrounding tissue to the level of the iliac vessels and divided. The kidney is dissected free from the remaining lateral and inferior attachments. The lower pole of the kidney is elevated and dissected free of posterior attachments. The vascular pedicle containing the renal artery and vein is divided. The kidney and ureter are removed. The kidney is prepared for reimplantation into the parapsoas fossa or other site. For implantation into the parapsoas fossa, an incision is made in the lower abdomen. The transversalis fascia is incised and the retroperitoneal space is entered. The peritoneum is retracted medially to allow exposure of the iliac vessels. Surrounding lymphatic vessels are ligated and divided. The iliac vessels are dissected free of surrounding tissue from the region immediately above the iliac lymph nodes to the bifurcation of the external and internal iliac artery. Vascular clamps are applied. The external iliac vein is incised and the prepared renal vein in the renal autograft is anastomosed to the external iliac vein. If more than one renal vein is present, they are anastomosed separately to the external iliac vein. The prepared renal artery is then anastomosed to the internal or external iliac artery. If more than one renal artery is present, separate incisions are made and each artery is anastomosed to a separate site in the internal or external iliac artery. Vascular clamps are released and the anastomosis sites are inspected. The ureter is prepared for anastomosis. The dome of the bladder is exposed and incised. The ureter is trimmed to the correct length and the end is spatulated to match the opening in the bladder. The mucosa of the bladder and ureter are anastomosed, followed by closure of the destrusor muscle layer over the ureter. A temporary stent may be placed to ensure patency at the anastomosis site. The kidney is then placed in the parapsoas fossa taking care to avoid any kinking of the blood vessels or ureter. Drains placed as needed and incisions are closed.

Renal autotransplantation, reimplantation of kidney

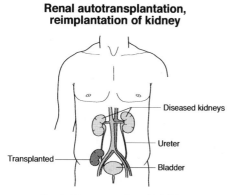

Diseased kidneys

Ureter

Transplanted

Bladder

The physician removes the patient's kidney from the normal anatomic location and reimplants it in the parapsoas fossa or other site.

50382-50384

50382   Removal (via snare/capture) and replacement of internally dwelling ureteral stent via percutaneous approach, including radiological supervision and interpretation

50384   Removal (via snare/capture) of internally dwelling ureteral stent via percutaneous approach, including radiological supervision and interpretation

The physician removes and replaces an indwelling ureteral stent via a percutaneous approach using radiographic guidance. A small skin incision is made over the selected entry site in the kidney. A needle is inserted into the renal calyx and positioned using radiographic guidance. Contrast media is injected and fluoroscopy performed. The kidney and ureter are visualized. A guidewire is introduced into the renal pelvis, the needle is removed, and the tract is dilated. A sheath is placed over the guidewire and into the renal

pelvis. A snare device is then passed through the renal pelvis and into the ureter to capture the indwelling stent. The stent is retracted until the proximal end is exposed. A guidewire is placed through the partially externalized stent and positioned in the ureter. The stent is then removed leaving the guidewire in place. The replacement stent is advanced over the guidewire and the distal end of the stent positioned in the bladder. Correct positioning of the replacement stent is verified radiographically. All surgical instruments are removed. A final set of radiographs are obtained to document correct positioning of the stent. Use 50382 to report removal and replacement of an indwelling ureteral stent. Use 50384 to report removal only.

50385-50386

50385   Removal (via snare/capture) and replacement of internally dwelling ureteral stent via transurethral approach, without use of cystoscopy, including radiological supervision and interpretation

50386   Removal (via snare/capture) of internally dwelling ureteral stent via transurethral approach, without use of cystoscopy, including radiological supervision and interpretation

An internally dwelling ureteral stent is removed via snare or other capture device and replaced using a transurethral catheter approach under fluoroscopic guidance without the use of cystoscopy. This procedure includes radiological supervision and interpretation. A ureteral stent is a soft, hollow tube about the size of a strand of spaghetti that holds the ureter open to allow urine to drain from the kidney to the bladder in cases of obstruction or blockage. Most stents are left in place only until the obstruction has been relieved, which typically takes from a few weeks to a few months. A catheter is advanced into the bladder and contrast is injected for visualization. A guidewire is advanced into the bladder, the first catheter is replaced with a larger catheter, the snare or other capture device is introduced and advanced to the distal pigtail portion of the ureteral stent in the bladder. The stent is grasped and pulled into the bladder and urethra until it is exposed. A guidewire is then introduced through the stent and advanced into the renal pelvis using fluoroscopic guidance. The stent is then removed and a catheter is advanced over the guidewire. Additional contrast is injected, the catheter is removed, and a new stent is passed over the guidewire and positioned with the proximal pigtail in the renal pelvis and the distal pigtail in the bladder. The guidewire is then removed. Stent position is confirmed by fluoroscopy and X-ray images are obtained to document correct placement. Use 50386 if the ureteral stent is removed without being replaced.

50387

▲ 50387   Removal and replacement of externally accessible nephroureteral catheter (eg, external/internal stent) requiring fluoroscopic guidance, including radiological supervision and interpretation

An externally accessible transnephric stent is a thin flexible tube that extends from the kidney through the ureter and into the bladder with a hub exiting the skin over the kidney. For removal and replacement of the transnephric stent, contrast is injected as needed through the existing external/internal stent to enhance fluoroscopic visualization of the kidney, ureter, bladder, and the existing stent. Using continuous fluoroscopic guidance, the proximal suture fixing the stent to the kidney is cut. A guidewire is inserted through the stent and advanced into the bladder. The existing stent is removed over the guidewire. A new stent is advanced over the guidewire into the bladder. Once the stent is properly positioned in the bladder, the guidewire is partially removed and the stent is visualized to ensure that the stent has coiled in the bladder. The coil, which is referred to as a pigtail, is necessary to prevent accidental dislodgement of the stent from the bladder. The remaining length of stent is assessed to ensure that it is long enough to coil properly in the renal pelvis. The guidewire is removed. A suture is placed to secure the proximal aspect of the stent in the kidney. Contrast is injected as needed to ensure that the stent is patent and functioning properly. The stent hub is secured to the skin with sutures and capped or a drainage device is attached to allow external drainage of urine. Final radiographic images are obtained to ensure that the stent is properly positioned.

50389

50389   Removal of nephrostomy tube, requiring fluoroscopic guidance (eg, with concurrent indwelling ureteral stent)

A nephrostomy tube, also referred to as a stent or catheter, is a tube that passes through the skin into the renal pelvis or a calyx of the kidney. It may be used alone or with a concurrent indwelling ureteral stent. For removal of the tube, contrast is injected as needed into the nephrostomy tube to enhance fluoroscopic visualization of the kidney, ureter, bladder, and any existing stent. Using continuous fluoroscopic guidance, the suture fixing the tube to the kidney is cut. A guidewire is inserted through the tube into the renal pelvis, taking care to avoid accidentally hooking any existing indwelling ureteral stent or the stent retention suture. The nephrostomy tube is removed over the guidewire and the guidewire is then removed. Final radiographic images are obtained to ensure that any existing stent remains properly positioned.

● New Code   ▲ Revised Code

50390

50390   Aspiration and/or injection of renal cyst or pelvis by needle, percutaneous

Aspiration and/or injection is performed to treat a renal cyst or to remove fluid from the renal pelvis. Kidney cysts are fluid filled sacs that form in the kidneys. Simple cysts are typically benign and asymptomatic. When a kidney cyst causes flank pain, frequent urination, or blood in the urine, aspiration is performed followed by injection of a sclerotic solution. The skin in the flank region over the kidney is cleansed. A local anesthetic is infiltrated as a needle is passed under separately reportable radiologic supervision to the site of the planned aspiration and/or injection. If the procedure is a simple aspiration of urine from the renal pelvis, a needle is advanced into the renal pelvis and urine is removed. If the procedure is for treatment of a real cyst, the needle is advanced into the renal cyst. Cystic fluid is aspirated and sent for separately reportable laboratory evaluation. Contrast is then injected into the cystic lesion to determine if there is any communication (opening) between the cyst and the collecting system. If there is no communication, a sclerosing solution, usually 95% ethanol, is injected into the cyst. The sclerosing solution is left in the cyst for several minutes and then removed.

50391

50391   Instillation(s) of therapeutic agent into renal pelvis and/or ureter through established nephrostomy, pyelostomy or ureterostomy tube (eg, anticarcinogenic or antifungal agent)

A therapeutic agent, such as an anticarcinogenic or antifungal agent, is instilled into the renal pelvis and/or ureter through an established nephrostomy, pyelostomy, or ureterostomy tube. This procedure is usually performed to treat malignancy of the epithelial lining of the urinary tract. It may also be used to treat fungal infection of the renal pelvis caused by Candida albicans. Using separately reportable fluoroscopic guidance, the position of the previously placed nephrostomy, pyelostomy, or ureterostomy tube is checked. The anticarcinogenic, antifungal, or other agent is prepared and placed in a syringe, which is connected to the ostomy tube and instilled into the kidney or ureter. The agent is left in the kidney or ureter for the appropriate amount of time and then drained and disposed of properly. The ostomy tube is then reconnected to the drainage system.

50395

50395   Introduction of guide into renal pelvis and/or ureter with dilation to establish nephrostomy tract, percutaneous

The skin in the flank region over the kidney is cleansed. A local anesthetic is infiltrated as a needle is passed. A guidewire is advanced through the skin to the renal pelvis of the kidney and/or ureter under separately reportable radiologic supervision. A series of dilators are advanced over the guidewire to establish a nephrostomy tract. Once the required tract diameter is established, the dilator is removed.

50396

50396   Manometric studies through nephrostomy or pyelostomy tube, or indwelling ureteral catheter

Manometric studies of the renal pelvis and/or ureter are also referred to as a Whitaker test. The procedure may be performed to evaluate persistent upper urinary tract dilatation, particularly in patients who have undergone previous operative intervention to relieve obstruction of the upper urinary tract. The procedure may also be performed to evaluate patency of an indwelling ureteral catheter. A bladder catheter is inserted through the urethra. The skin around an existing nephrostomy or pyelostomy tube insertion site and the external tube components are cleansed with antibacterial solution. The drainage bag is disconnected from the nephrostomy tube. The nephrostomy tube and bladder catheter are connected to a pressure transducer and baseline pressures are obtained. Saline or a contrast dilution is slowly perfused into the kidney and serial pressures in the kidney and bladder are obtained. Upon completion of the manometric studies, the manometer is disconnected from the nephrostomy tube and bladder catheter; the external drainage bag is connected to the tube; and the bladder catheter is removed. The physician reviews the manometry recording and provides a written interpretation of the studies.

50400-50405

50400   Pyeloplasty (Foley Y-pyeloplasty), plastic operation on renal pelvis, with or without plastic operation on ureter, nephropexy, nephrostomy, pyelostomy, or ureteral splinting; simple

50405   Pyeloplasty (Foley Y-pyeloplasty), plastic operation on renal pelvis, with or without plastic operation on ureter, nephropexy, nephrostomy, pyelostomy, or ureteral splinting; complicated (congenital kidney abnormality, secondary pyeloplasty, solitary kidney, calicoplasty)

Pyeloplasty is a plastic operation on the kidney typically performed to treat congenital high insertion of the ureter into the renal pelvis with obstruction. Foley Y-pyeloplasty, one of the more common surgical techniques, is described here. A skin incision is made over the kidney. Gerota's fascia is incised and perirenal fat is dissected. Blood vessels are identified and controlled by placing a loop around each vessel. The kidney and ureter are exposed and visually examined. Because of the upper urinary tract obstruction, the renal

pelvis is typically extremely dilated. A Y-shaped incision is made in the dilated renal pelvis beginning with an anterior incision at the ureteropelvic junction that is extended laterally and downward toward the hilum of the kidney, creating the first arm of the Y incision. A posterior incision is then made in the renal pelvis in the same fashion, creating the second arm of the Y. Next, the ureter is incised longitudinally in the lateral aspect, which is the side facing the renal pelvis. The renal pelvis flap is trimmed as needed. Prior to repositioning and anastomosis of the ureter, a nephrostomy or pyelostomy tube may be placed and/or a ureteral splint (stent) may be introduced to maintain the diameter of the ureter. The ureter is then positioned along the incision lines in the renal pelvis and anastomosed. Drains are placed as needed and the operative wound is closed around the drains. Use 50400 for a simple pyeloplasty. Use 50405 when the procedure is complicated by other congenital kidney abnormalities, or previous surgery on the kidney or ureter such as a previous pyeloplasty or repair of the renal calyces (calicoplasty).

50430-50431

50430   Injection procedure for antegrade nephrostogram and/or ureterogram, complete diagnostic procedure including imaging guidance (eg, ultrasound and fluoroscopy) and all associated radiological supervision and interpretation; new access

50431   Injection procedure for antegrade nephrostogram and/or ureterogram, complete diagnostic procedure including imaging guidance (eg, ultrasound and fluoroscopy) and all associated radiological supervision and interpretation; existing access

Antegrade nephrostogram and/or ureterogram is performed to visualize the kidney and/or ureter and detect urinary tract obstruction caused by strictures, stones, blood clots, or tumors, or to assess kidney and ureter function prior to or following surgical treatment. When a nephrostomy or pyelostomy tube is already in place, this procedure may be performed to check for tube patency, blockage, or leakage. To establish a new access, the patient is positioned prone, a local anesthetic is injected, and a needle is inserted and advanced into the ureter/renal pelvis under ultrasound and/or fluoroscopic guidance. Contrast dye is injected and a series of x-rays are taken to visualize movement through the tube and urinary tract. A thin wire may be threaded through the needle to facilitate placement of a catheter or nephrostomy tube. The needle and wire are then removed. If placement of a catheter/tube is not indicated, the needle is simply removed after completion of the procedure. To perform the nephrostogram/ureterogram through an existing access, the tube and surrounding skin are first washed with an antibacterial solution and contrast is injected through the catheter/tube. A series of x-rays are taken to monitor and record the movement of contrast through the tube and the urinary tract. At the conclusion of the study, the catheter/tube may be plugged or connected to drainage. These codes include the injection, imaging guidance, and associated radiologic supervision and interpretation for new access in 50430 or an existing access in 50431.

50432-50433

50432   Placement of nephrostomy catheter, percutaneous, including diagnostic nephrostogram and/or ureterogram when performed, imaging guidance (eg, ultrasound and/or fluoroscopy) and all associated radiological supervision and interpretation

50433   Placement of nephroureteral catheter, percutaneous, including diagnostic nephrostogram and/or ureterogram when performed, imaging guidance (eg, ultrasound and/or fluoroscopy) and all associated radiological supervision and interpretation, new access

Percutaneous placement of a nephrostomy catheter (50432) or nephroureteral catheter (50433) is performed to treat urinary obstruction caused by stones, tumors, or strictures; to diagnose urinary conditions; provide access for therapeutic interventions; or divert urine in the presence of traumatic injury, leaks, fistulas, or hemorrhagic cystitis. A single or double needle technique may be employed. Under ultrasound and/or fluoroscopic guidance, a single trocar or Chiba needle is inserted below the 12th rib to minimize the risk of puncturing the pleura. The needle is advanced into the posterior mid or lower pole calyx and urine is aspirated to verify location and decompress the system. Contrast dye is injected and a series of x-rays are taken to visualize movement of dye through the urinary tract. Once satisfactory placement of the needle has been established, a thin wire is threaded through the needle into the proximal ureter (nephroureteral) or upper pole of the calyx (nephrostomy). A self-restraining nephrostomy or nephroureteral catheter is inserted over the wire and the wire is then removed. For double needle technique, the first needle is inserted directly into the renal pelvis and contrast dye is injected to obtain a series of x-rays. A small amount of air or CO2 may be injected after the contrast to enhance visualization of the posterior calyces. A clamp applied to the skin is used to mark the entry site of the second needle placed under the 12th rib in the posterior axillary line. The insertion of the second needle and placement of the catheter is identical to the single needle technique. The first needle is removed at the end of the procedure. These codes include the percutaneous placement of the catheter, any diagnostic nephrostogram and/or ureterogram, the imaging guidance, and all associated radiologic supervision and interpretation.

Urinary System

50434-50435

50434 Convert nephrostomy catheter to nephroureteral catheter, percutaneous, including diagnostic nephrostogram and/or ureterogram when performed, imaging guidance (eg, ultrasound and/or fluoroscopy) and all associated radiological supervision and interpretation, via pre-existing nephrostomy tract

50435 Exchange nephrostomy catheter, percutaneous, including diagnostic nephrostogram and/or ureterogram when performed, imaging guidance (eg, ultrasound and/or fluoroscopy) and all associated radiological supervision and interpretation

A procedure is performed to convert an existing percutaneous nephrostomy catheter to a nephroureteral catheter (50434) or to exchange an existing nephrostomy catheter with a new catheter (50435). A nephrostomy or nephroureteral catheter may be used to restore or maintain the flow of urine through the kidney/ureter when strictures, leaks, or fistulas are present. With the patient positioned prone, contrast dye may be injected through the existing catheter and a series of x-rays taken to monitor contrast movement through the tube and urinary tract. For conversion to a nephroureteral catheter, a guide wire is inserted through the exiting nephrostomy catheter into the kidney and advanced into the proximal ureter. The catheter is then removed and a new catheter is inserted over the guide wire and advanced to the new position. Once placement has been confirmed with fluoroscopy, the guide wire is removed. For nephrostomy catheter exchange, a guidewire is advanced through the catheter into the renal pelvis. The old catheter is removed over the guide wire and replaced with a new catheter. Once the position has been confirmed with fluoroscopy, the guide wire is removed. These codes include any diagnostic nephrostogram and/or ureterogram, imaging guidance, and associated radiologic supervision and interpretation.

50500

50500 Nephrorrhaphy, suture of kidney wound or injury

The physician performs an open procedure to suture repair a wound or injury to the kidney. A flank incision is made, the injured kidney is exposed, and the area of the lesion is identified. The wound or injury is repaired with sutures. The operative site is irrigated and inspected for any additional injuries which are also repaired. Any bleeding is controlled. Drains may be placed in the operative site and the surgical wound is closed around the drains.

50520

50520 Closure of nephrocutaneous or pyelocutaneous fistula

A fistulous (sinus) tract from the kidney or ureteropelvic junction (UPJ) leading out to the skin is surgically closed. Fistulous tracts are most often caused by kidney stones or tuberculosis, but may also be caused by injury during percutaneous procedures or lithotripsy. The termination site of the fistulous tract in the abdomen is identified by injecting the fistula with a radiopaque substance. Suture ligation is then used to close the open sinus tract, along with fulguration or injection of fibrin glue.

50525-50526

50525 Closure of nephrovisceral fistula (eg, renocolic), including visceral repair; abdominal approach

50526 Closure of nephrovisceral fistula (eg, renocolic), including visceral repair; thoracic approach

A fistulous (sinus) tract from the kidney to another internal organ is closed and the involved organ is repaired as needed. Fistulous tracts are most often caused by renal stones or tuberculosis, but may also be caused by injury during percutaneous procedures or lithotripsy. An abdominal or thoracic surgical approach may be employed depending on the location of the fistulous tract. The kidney and ureter are exposed. A catheter is inserted into the ureter and a radiopaque substance injected to identify the fistulous tract. The fistula is followed down to where it enters the involved organ, such as the colon, and is suture ligated and divided. The involved organ is repaired. The origin of the fistula in the kidney is closed. Use 50525 for an abdominal approach and 50526 for a thoracic approach.

50540

50540 Symphysiotomy for horseshoe kidney with or without pyeloplasty and/or other plastic procedure, unilateral or bilateral (1 operation)

The physician performs an open procedure to divide the isthmus (symphysiotomy) connecting the lower poles of a horseshoe kidney. A unilateral or bilateral pyeloplasty or other plastic repair of the kidney may also be performed. A horseshoe kidney is a type of renal fusion anomaly consisting of two distinct functioning kidneys connected at the lower poles by an isthmus of functioning renal or fibrous tissue at the midline. A midline abdominal incision is typically employed to allow access to both sides of the horseshoe kidney and its anomalous vasculature. The isthmus is dissected free of surrounding tissue and divided, taking care to preserve the vasculature to both sides of the horseshoe kidney. If the ureter is obstructed at the ureteropelvic junction (UPJ), a pyeloplasty or other plastic

procedure is performed to treat the blockage or narrowing. The ureter and surrounding vascular structures are identified and retracted to expose the lower poles of the horseshoe kidney and the UPJ. The UPJ defect is repaired. One or both ureters may be repaired. A stent is then placed in the ureter bridging the repair to facilitate healing and allow drainage of urine. Drains are placed in the surgical wound. The site is irrigated and inspected, bleeding is controlled, surgical instruments are removed, and incisions are closed.

50541-50542

50541 Laparoscopy, surgical; ablation of renal cysts

50542 Laparoscopy, surgical; ablation of renal mass lesion(s), including intraoperative ultrasound guidance and monitoring, when performed

The physician performs a laparoscopic procedure to destroy (ablate) cysts or mass lesions in the kidney. The lesion(s) may be destroyed using any of a number of techniques including cryoablation, radiofrequency ablation (RFA), high-intensity focused ultrasound (HIFU), laser thermal ablation, or other method. Pneumoperitoneum is achieved and trocars are placed. The laparoscope is inserted through the umbilical port. The peritoneum over the kidney is mobilized and the anterior surface of the kidney is visualized. The kidney lesion is identified. One or more cryosurgical probes or other ablation instruments are inserted into the lesion. If cryoablation is the technique used, the first freeze-thaw cycle is initiated. The ice ball created during the freeze cycle is monitored using ultrasound to ensure adequate extension of the ice ball beyond the margins of the lesion. A second freeze-thaw cycle is performed in the same manner. Additional lesions are treated in the same manner. RFA is a thermal technique that heats the lesion and surrounding tissue. If RFA is performed, the appropriate electrode needle or array is selected based on the size and shape of the cyst or lesion. The RFA device is activated and the lesion is ablated. Laser thermal ablation uses a laser to produce heat and destroy the lesion. HIFU uses focused sound waves to produce heat and cavitation. Following ablation of all lesions, the surgical instruments are removed, bleeding is controlled, drains are placed, and portal incisions are closed around the drains. Report 50541 for ablation of renal cysts and 50542 for ablation of other renal mass lesions.

50543

50543 Laparoscopy, surgical; partial nephrectomy

The physician performs a partial nephrectomy via a laparoscopic approach. Small portal incisions are made and pneumoperitoneum is achieved by insufflating the abdomen with air. Trocars are placed and the laparoscope is inserted through an umbilical port. The lateral line of Toldt is identified and incised. The peritoneum over the kidney is mobilized and the anterior surface of the kidney is visualized. The colon is mobilized and rolled medially. The ureter and surrounding vascular structures are identified and retracted to expose the lower pole of the kidney and the renal hilum. The kidney mass is identified and dissected free from surrounding healthy kidney tissue. The defect left after removal is repaired using sutures and sealant glue. The laparoscope is removed from the umbilical port and inserted into the lateral port. A bag is inserted through the umbilical port and the excised kidney mass is placed in the bag. The umbilical incision is extended and the bag containing the kidney mass is removed. The surgical site is inspected, bleeding is controlled, surgical instruments are removed, and incisions are closed.

50544

50544 Laparoscopy, surgical; pyeloplasty

The physician performs a pyeloplasty via a laparoscopic approach. Pyeloplasty is a reconstructive operation performed to treat blockage or narrowing of the ureter at the ureteropelvic junction (UPJ). Small portal incisions are made and pneumoperitoneum is achieved by insufflating the abdomen with air. Trocars are placed and the laparoscope is inserted through an umbilical port. The lateral line of Toldt is identified and incised. The peritoneum over the kidney is mobilized and the anterior surface of the kidney is visualized. The colon is mobilized and rolled medially. The ureter and surrounding vascular structures are identified. The ureter is dissected free of surrounding tissue, taking care to ensure adequate fat is maintained around the ureter. The ureteropelvic junction (UPJ) is exposed and the lower pole of the kidney is mobilized. The UPJ is isolated and any aberrant blood vessels impinging on the UPJ are identified and dissected free. The obstructed segment of the UPJ is then dissected free and excised. The renal pelvis is trimmed as needed and the ureteral stump is examined and spatulated. A stent is placed through the ureter into the bladder. The posterior wall of the UPJ is anastomosed, followed by closure of the renal pelvis. The proximal end of the ureteral stent is then placed in the renal pelvis and the anterior UPJ incision is closed. A drain may be placed. The surgical site is inspected, bleeding is controlled, surgical instruments are removed, and incisions are closed.

50545

50545 Laparoscopy, surgical; radical nephrectomy (includes removal of Gerota's fascia and surrounding fatty tissue, removal of regional lymph nodes, and adrenalectomy)

The physician performs a radical nephrectomy including removal of Gerota's fascia, surrounding fatty tissue, regional lymph nodes, and adrenal glands via a laparoscopic

Urinary System

approach. Small portal incisions are made and pneumoperitoneum is achieved by insufflating the abdomen with air. Trocars are placed and the laparoscope is inserted through an umbilical port. The lateral line of Toldt is identified and incised. The peritoneum over the kidney is mobilized and the anterior surface of the kidney visualized. The colon is mobilized and rolled medially. The colorenal ligaments are divided and Gerota's fascia is exposed. Regional lymph nodes are excised, the Gerota's fascia is dissected free from surrounding structures, and the lymphatic vessels are ligated. The ureter and surrounding vascular structures are identified and retracted to expose the lower pole of the kidney and the renal hilum. The lower pole is dissected free of surrounding structures. The kidney is retracted laterally and superiorly to allow access to the renal hilum, which is dissected free of surrounding structures. The renal artery and vein are identified, divided, and ligated. Dissection continues medially along the inferior vena cava to the adrenal vein which is divided and ligated. The adrenal gland is dissected free of surrounding tissue and the adrenal arteries are divided. The kidney is dissected free from any remaining lateral and superior attachments and the ureter is divided. The laparoscope is removed from the umbilical port and inserted into the lateral port. A bag is inserted through the umbilical port and the kidney, Gerota's fascia, surrounding fatty tissue, regional lymph nodes and the adrenal gland are placed in the bag for removal. The umbilical incision is extended and the bag containing the kidney and surrounding structures is removed. The surgical site is inspected, bleeding is controlled, surgical instruments are removed, and incisions are closed.

50546

50546   Laparoscopy, surgical; nephrectomy, including partial ureterectomy

The physician performs a nephrectomy with partial ureterectomy via a laparoscopic approach. Small portal incisions are made and pneumoperitoneum is achieved by insufflating the abdomen with air. Trocars are placed and the laparoscope is inserted through an umbilical port. The lateral line of Toldt is identified and incised. The peritoneum over the kidney is mobilized and the anterior surface of the kidney is visualized. The colon is mobilized and rolled medially. The ureter and surrounding vascular structures are identified and retracted to expose the lower pole of the kidney and the renal hilum. The lower pole is then dissected free of surrounding structures. The kidney is retracted laterally and superiorly to allow access to the renal hilum, which is dissected free of surrounding structures. The renal artery and vein are identified and divided. The diseased section of ureter is also dissected and divided. The kidney is mobilized from any remaining lateral and superior attachments. The laparoscope is removed from the umbilical port and inserted into the lateral port. A bag is inserted through the umbilical port. The kidney, along with the section of diseased ureter, is placed in the bag. The umbilical incision is extended and the bag containing the kidney and ureter is removed. The surgical site is inspected, bleeding is controlled, surgical instruments are removed, and incisions are closed.

50547

50547   Laparoscopy, surgical; donor nephrectomy (including cold preservation), from living donor

A living donor nephrectomy inclusive of cold preservation of the donor kidney is performed via a laparoscopic approach. Small portal incisions are made and pneumoperitoneum is achieved by insufflating the abdomen with air. Trocars are placed and the laparoscope is inserted through an umbilical port. The lateral line of Toldt is identified and incised. The peritoneum over the kidney is mobilized and the anterior surface of the kidney is visualized. The colon is mobilized and rolled medially. The colorenal ligaments are divided and Gerota's fascia is exposed. The ureter and surrounding vascular structures are identified and retracted to expose the lower pole of the kidney and the renal hilum. The lower pole is partially mobilized. The kidney is retracted laterally and superiorly to allow access to the renal hilum, which is dissected free of surrounding structures. The renal vein is exposed. The gonadal, lumbar, and adrenal veins are clipped and divided. The renal artery is identified and dissected free of surrounding tissue. Lateral, posterior, and inferior kidney attachments are left intact to prevent torsion of the kidney and damage to its vascular pedicle. The ureter is dissected free of surrounding tissue to the level of the iliac vessels and divided. The kidney is dissected free from the remaining lateral and inferior attachments. The lower pole of the kidney is elevated and dissected free of the remaining posterior attachments. The periumbilical incision is extended taking care to keep the peritoneum intact and preserve the pneumoperitoneum. The vascular pedicle containing the renal artery and vein is divided. The laparoscope is removed from the umbilical port and inserted into the lateral port. A bag is inserted through the umbilical port and the kidney is placed in the bag. The peritoneum is opened and the kidney is delivered. The kidney may be perfused with cold preservation solution and/or placed on ice and is then delivered to the recipient surgical team.

50548

50548   Laparoscopy, surgical; nephrectomy with total ureterectomy

The physician performs a nephrectomy with total ureterectomy via a laparoscopic approach. Small portal incisions are made and pneumoperitoneum is achieved by insufflating the abdomen with air. Trocars are placed and the laparoscope is inserted through an umbilical port. The lateral line of Toldt is identified and incised. The peritoneum

over the kidney is mobilized and the anterior surface of the kidney is visualized. The colon is mobilized and rolled medially. The ureter and surrounding vascular structures are identified and retracted to expose the lower pole of the kidney and the renal hilum. The lower pole is dissected free of surrounding structures. The kidney is retracted laterally and superiorly to allow access to the renal hilum, which is dissected free of surrounding structures. The renal artery and vein are identified and divided. The entire ureter is dissected free of surrounding tissue and divided just above the ureterovesical junction (UVJ). The kidney is dissected free from any remaining lateral and superior attachments. The laparoscope is removed from the umbilical port and inserted into the lateral port. A bag is inserted through the umbilical port and the kidney and ureter are placed in the bag. The umbilical incision is extended and the bag containing the kidney and ureter is removed. The surgical site is inspected, bleeding is controlled, surgical instruments are removed, and incisions are closed.

50551-50553

50551   Renal endoscopy through established nephrostomy or pyelostomy, with or without irrigation, instillation, or ureteropyelography, exclusive of radiologic service

50553   Renal endoscopy through established nephrostomy or pyelostomy, with or without irrigation, instillation, or ureteropyelography, exclusive of radiologic service; with ureteral catheterization, with or without dilation of ureter

To perform endoscopy through an existing nephrostomy, the external drainage bag is removed from the nephrostomy or pyelostomy tube. A guidewire is advanced through the tube and the nephrostomy tube is removed over the guidewire. A series of dilators are then advanced over the guidewire and the tract is dilated to allow insertion of the endoscope. The renal endoscope is inserted into the kidney through the established nephrostomy or pyelostomy tract. The kidney is carefully examined. In 50551, sterile saline or other solution may be used to irrigate the kidney; a diagnostic or therapeutic solution may be instilled into the kidney; or contrast may be instilled for separately reportable radiopyelography. In 50553, ureteral catheterization is performed in addition to the procedures described above. A ureteral catheter is advanced through the endoscope and into the ureter, which is carefully examined for obstruction or stenosis. If stenosis is present, a balloon tipped catheter is introduced to the site of the stenosis and inflated. The balloon may be deflated and inflated several times until the stenotic region is adequately dilated. All instruments are then removed, the nephrostomy tube is replaced, and the external drainage bag is reattached to the nephrostomy tube.

50555-50557

50555   Renal endoscopy through established nephrostomy or pyelostomy, with or without irrigation, instillation, or ureteropyelography, exclusive of radiologic service; with biopsy

50557   Renal endoscopy through established nephrostomy or pyelostomy, with or without irrigation, instillation, or ureteropyelography, exclusive of radiologic service; with fulguration and/or incision, with or without biopsy

To obtain a biopsy or fulgurate lesions of the kidney endoscopically through an existing nephrostomy, the external drainage bag is first removed from the nephrostomy or pyelostomy tube. A guidewire is advanced through the tube and the nephrostomy tube is removed over the guidewire. A series of dilators are then advanced over the guidewire and the tract is dilated to allow insertion of the endoscope. A renal endoscope is inserted into the kidney through the established nephrostomy or pyelostomy tract. The kidney is carefully examined. Sterile saline or other solution may be used to irrigate the kidney; a diagnostic or therapeutic solution may be instilled into the kidney; or contrast may be instilled for separately reportable radiopyelography. In 50555, following the endoscopic examination of the kidney, biopsy forceps are introduced through the endoscope and one or more tissue samples are obtained. In 50557, following endoscopic examination, an electrocautery tool is introduced through the endoscope and lesions or tissue in the kidney is destroyed and/or the renal pelvis or calyces may be incised. Tissue samples may also be obtained. All instruments are then removed; the nephrostomy tube is replaced; and the external drainage bag is reattached to the nephrostomy tube.

50561

50561   Renal endoscopy through established nephrostomy or pyelostomy, with or without irrigation, instillation, or ureteropyelography, exclusive of radiologic service; with removal of foreign body or calculus

To remove a foreign body or stone endoscopically through an existing nephrostomy, the external drainage bag is first removed from the nephrostomy or pyelostomy tube. A guidewire is advanced through the tube and the nephrostomy tube is removed over the guidewire. A series of dilators are then advanced over the guidewire and the tract is dilated to allow insertion of the endoscope. A renal endoscope (nephroscope) is inserted into the kidney through the established nephrostomy or pyelostomy tract. The kidney is carefully examined and the foreign body or calculus is located. Sterile saline or other solution may be used to irrigate the kidney; a diagnostic or therapeutic solution may be instilled into the kidney; or contrast may be instilled for separately reportable radiopyelography. An endograsper is introduced through the nephroscope and the foreign body or calculus

Urinary System

is grasped and removed through the endoscope. The renal pelvis and calyces are again inspected to ensure that all foreign body or calculus fragments have been removed. All instruments are removed; the nephrostomy tube is replaced; and the external drainage bag is reattached to the nephrostomy tube.

50562

50562   **Renal endoscopy through established nephrostomy or pyelostomy, with or without irrigation, instillation, or ureteropyelography, exclusive of radiologic service; with resection of tumor**

The external drainage bag is removed from the existing nephrostomy or pyelostomy tube. A guidewire is advanced through the nephrostomy tube and the tube is removed. A series of dilators are then advanced over the guidewire and the tract is dilated to allow insertion of the endoscope. A renal endoscope is inserted into the kidney through the established nephrostomy or pyelostomy tract. The kidney is carefully examined and the tumor is located. Sterile saline or other solution may be used to irrigate the kidney; a diagnostic or therapeutic solution may be instilled into the kidney; or contrast may be instilled for separately reportable radiopyelography. The nephroscope is exchanged for a resectoscope and the renal tumor is resected and removed using irrigation and an endoscopic evacuation device. The kidney is then re-examined to ensure that all of the tumor has been removed. Bleeding is controlled by fulguration. The resectoscope is removed. The nephrostomy tube is replaced and the external drainage bag is reattached to the nephrostomy tube.

50570-50572

50570   **Renal endoscopy through nephrotomy or pyelotomy, with or without irrigation, instillation, or ureteropyelography, exclusive of radiologic service**

50572   **Renal endoscopy through nephrotomy or pyelotomy, with or without irrigation, instillation, or ureteropyelography, exclusive of radiologic service; with ureteral catheterization, with or without dilation of ureter**

A small incision is made in the kidney. A renal endoscope is inserted into the kidney through the incision and the kidney is carefully examined. In 50570, sterile saline or other solution may be used to irrigate the kidney; a diagnostic or therapeutic solution may be instilled into the kidney; or contrast may be instilled for separately reportable radiopyelography. In 50572, a ureteral catheterization is also performed in addition to the endoscopic examination with or without irrigation, instillation, or ureteropyelography. Following renal endoscopy, a ureteral catheter is advanced through the endoscope and into the ureter. The ureter is carefully examined for obstruction or stenosis. If stenosis is present, a balloon tipped catheter is introduced to the site of the stenosis and inflated. This balloon may be deflated and inflated several times until the stenotic region is adequately dilated. All instruments are then removed. A nephrostomy tube is placed as needed and the incision is closed.

50574

50574   **Renal endoscopy through nephrotomy or pyelotomy, with or without irrigation, instillation, or ureteropyelography, exclusive of radiologic service; with biopsy**

A small incision is made in the kidney. A renal endoscope is inserted into the kidney through the incision and the kidney is carefully examined. Sterile saline or other solution may be used to irrigate the kidney, a diagnostic or therapeutic solution may be instilled into the kidney; or contrast may be instilled for separately reportable radiopyelography. Biopsy forceps are introduced through the endoscope and one or more tissue samples are obtained from the kidney. All instruments are then removed. A nephrostomy tube is placed as needed and the incision is closed.

50575

50575   **Renal endoscopy through nephrotomy or pyelotomy, with or without irrigation, instillation, or ureteropyelography, exclusive of radiologic service; with endopyelotomy (includes cystoscopy, ureteroscopy, dilation of ureter and ureteral pelvic junction, incision of ureteral pelvic junction and insertion of endopyelotomy stent)**

A small incision is made in the kidney. A renal endoscope is inserted into the kidney through the incision and the kidney is carefully examined. Sterile saline or other solution may be used to irrigate the kidney, a diagnostic or therapeutic solution may be instilled into the kidney; or contrast may be instilled for separately reportable radiopyelography to assess a narrowed ureteropelvic junction. A cystoscope is introduced through the urethra and the bladder is examined. A guidewire is passed through the ureter and obstructed region of the renal pelvis in a retrograde fashion. A ureteroscope is advanced into the ureter over the guidewire and the ureter is examined. A second guidewire may be passed from the renal pelvis into the ureter in an antegrade fashion. Using endoscopic surgical tools such as an electrode device or laser, an endopyelotomy incision is made in the inner (tunica mucosa) and middle layers (tunica muscularis) of the ureteral pelvic junction. The outer fibrous layer (tunica adventia) is left intact. A balloon dilator may then be used to increase the diameter of the tunica adventia at the site of the stricture. An endopyelotomy stent is placed to maintain patency while the incision heals. Guidewires and surgical

instruments are removed. A nephrostomy tube is placed as needed and the kidney incision is closed.

50576

50576   **Renal endoscopy through nephrotomy or pyelotomy, with or without irrigation, instillation, or ureteropyelography, exclusive of radiologic service; with fulguration and/or incision, with or without biopsy**

A small incision is made in the kidney. A renal endoscope is inserted into the kidney through the incision and the kidney is carefully examined. Sterile saline or other solution may be used to irrigate the kidney; a diagnostic or therapeutic solution may be instilled into the kidney; or contrast may be instilled for separately reportable radiopyelography. Following endoscopic examination, an electrocautery tool is introduced through the endoscope and lesions or tissue in the kidney are destroyed and/or the renal pelvis or calyces may be incised. Biopsy forceps may also be introduced and one or more tissue samples obtained. All instruments are then removed. A nephrostomy tube is placed as needed and the incision is closed.

50580

50580   **Renal endoscopy through nephrotomy or pyelotomy, with or without irrigation, instillation, or ureteropyelography, exclusive of radiologic service; with removal of foreign body or calculus**

A small incision is made in the kidney. A renal endoscope is inserted into the kidney through the incision and the kidney is carefully examined. The foreign body or calculus is located. Sterile saline or other solution may be used to irrigate the kidney; a diagnostic or therapeutic solution may be instilled into the kidney; or contrast may be instilled for separately reportable radiopyelography. An endograsper is introduced through the nephroscope and the foreign body or calculus is grasped and removed through the endoscope. The renal pelvis and calyces are again inspected to ensure that all foreign body or calculus fragments have been removed. All instruments are then removed. A nephrostomy tube is placed as needed and the incision is closed.

50590

50590   **Lithotripsy, extracorporeal shock wave**

Extracorporeal shock wave lithotripsy (ESWL) is the preferred method of treatment for renal and ureteral stones (calculi). Lithotripsy machines have four basic components: a shockwave generator, a focusing system, a coupling mechanism, and an imaging unit that localizes the stone and monitors fragmentation. Most lithotripter machines are powered with an electromagnetic shockwave generator. The focusing system is used to concentrate the shockwaves on the target, which is the stone. The coupling mechanism consists of water contained in a silicone membrane. These small water filled drums, or cushions on the shock tube, provide air-free contact between the patient's skin and the tube. The imaging unit is required for localizing the stone and monitoring the fragmentation. Depending on the location of the stone, the patient is placed either on the back or abdomen on the treatment table. Using fluoroscopic or ultrasound imaging, the stone is positioned in the focus of the shock wave. Coupling gel is applied on the skin at the site where the shock tube is to be placed. The shock tube is pressed against the skin and shock waves are then delivered through the tube at rates of up to 120 per minute. Stone fragmentation is monitored radiographically as the ESWL treatment is delivered. Once the stone fragments are small enough to allow them to pass through the kidney and ureter, ESWL is terminated.

50592

50592   **Ablation, 1 or more renal tumor(s), percutaneous, unilateral, radiofrequency**

One or more renal tumors of the right or left kidney are destroyed (ablated) by radiofrequency using percutaneous technique. Radiofrequency uses electrical currents in the range of radiofrequency waves. The electrical currents produce heat around the needle to destroy tumor tissue. The heat also cauterizes blood vessels which reduces the risk of bleeding. Grounding pads are placed on the back and thighs. Using separately reportable ultrasound, CT, or MRI guidance, the tumor is located. The optimal track and placement of the electrode needle is determined. The electrode needle is inserted through the skin and into the tumor using continuous imaging guidance, taking care to avoid other organs and major blood vessels. The location of the needle tip is confirmed and the electrode needle is connected to the radiofrequency generator which is activated. Imaging guidance is used to monitor and assess tumor destruction. For multiple or very large tumors, more than one needle may be used. Alternatively, the needle may be partially withdrawn and repositioned following each radiofrequency application. When treatment is complete, the needle is withdrawn and pressure is applied to prevent bleeding along the needle track.

50593

50593   **Ablation, renal tumor(s), unilateral, percutaneous, cryotherapy**

One or more renal tumors are destroyed (ablated) by cryotherapy using percutaneous technique. Cryotherapy uses extreme cold to freeze and destroy tissue. The tumor(s) is identified using separately reportable ultrasound, CT, or MRI guidance. Most tumors require placement of multiple probes to ensure complete tumor destruction and allow sufficient

● New Code   ▲ Revised Code   CPT © 2016 American Medical Association. All Rights Reserved.   © 2017 DecisionHealth

Urinary System

margins. The entry sites for cryotherapy probe placement are determined and small incisions are made to facilitate placement. The probes are inserted into the center of the tumor(s) using imaging guidance and taking care to avoid other organs and major blood vessels. The location of the probe tips is confirmed and the cryoablation unit is activated. The probes are filled with argon gas, resulting in rapid freezing at temperatures as low as -100 degrees centigrade. This is followed by a thawing cycle that is initiated by replacing the argon with helium. Imaging guidance is used to monitor the creation of the cryoablation sphere (ice ball) and assess tumor destruction (necrosis). Complete destruction typically requires two freeze/thaw cycles. When treatment is complete, the probes are withdrawn, the skin incisions are cleansed, and a dressing is applied.

50600

50600   Ureterotomy with exploration or drainage (separate procedure)

Ureterotomy with exploration or drainage is performed. An incision is made in the abdomen over the upper, middle, or lower ureter depending on the nature of the exploration or drainage procedure. Muscles of the abdominal wall are divided and the peritoneum is pushed aside. The ureter is identified and dissected free of the serosa and periureteral fat and then incised. Exploration is done to identify any disease or abnormalities. A soft Penrose drainage or suction tube is placed and the ureter is drained and flushed with irrigation solution. The drainage tube is left in place and incisions are closed around the drain.

50605

50605   Ureterotomy for insertion of indwelling stent, all types

Ureterotomy with stent placement is performed. An incision is made in the abdomen over the upper, middle, or lower ureter depending on the location of the stricture or other abnormality. Muscles of the abdominal wall are divided and the peritoneum is pushed aside. The ureter is identified and dissected free of the serosa and periureteral fat. The ureter is then incised and explored. A soft Penrose drainage or suction tube is placed above the site of the stricture or other abnormality and the ureter is drained and flushed with irrigation solution. A double J stent is placed in the ureter at the stricture site. The ureterotomy site may be left open with a drainage tube in place. Abdominal and skin incisions are closed around the drain.

50610-50630

50610   Ureterolithotomy; upper one-third of ureter
50620   Ureterolithotomy; middle one-third of ureter
50630   Ureterolithotomy; lower one-third of ureter

An ureterolithotomy is performed to remove a calculus or stone from the ureter. An incision is made in the abdomen over the upper, middle, or lower ureter depending on the location of the stone. Muscles of the abdominal wall are divided and the peritoneum is pushed aside. The ureter is identified and dissected free of the serosa and periureteral fat. The site of the stone is identified visually by noting a bulge in the ureter or manually by palpating the ureter. The stone is immobilized by placement of vascular loops above and below the stone. The ureter is incised over the stone and the stone is removed. A catheter is placed in the ureter, the ureter is irrigated and any stone fragments are removed. A soft Penrose drainage tube or suction tube is placed and the ureter drained. The incision in the ureter is closed taking care not to constrict the ureter. A drainage tube is placed and the abdomen is closed around the drain. Report 50610 for removal of a stone from the upper one-third of the ureter, 50620 for removal from the middle one-third of the ureter, and 50630 for removal from the lower one-third of the ureter.

50650

50650   Ureterectomy, with bladder cuff (separate procedure)

The distal ureter is excised along with a section of bladder at the site of the ureteral orifice. A Foley catheter is placed and the bladder is drained. An incision is made in the abdomen over the affected ureter and bladder, which are exposed and inspected. The distal ureter and bladder cuff are then excised by first transecting the ureter above the site of the abnormality or lesion and then incising the bladder just below the ureterovesical junction (UVJ) and removing the bladder cuff. The opening in the bladder is repaired and a drainage tube is placed. The incisions are closed around the drain.

50660

50660   Ureterectomy, total, ectopic ureter, combination abdominal, vaginal and/or perineal approach

An ectopic ureter is excised by a combined abdominal, vaginal, and/or perineal approach. An ectopic ureter is one that terminates in an abnormal location. An ectopic ureter may terminate in the epididymus, vas deferens, ejaculatory duct, seminal vesicle, urethra or utriculus in males or in the Gartner's duct, upper vagina, cervix, uterus, or urethra in females. Less commonly it may terminate in the rectum in both sexes. A Foley catheter is placed and the bladder is drained. An incision is made in the abdomen over the ureter. The ureter is exposed and inspected. A second incision may be made in the vagina or perineum at the site where the ureter terminates. The ureter is excised.

50684

50684   Injection procedure for ureterography or ureteropyelography through ureterostomy or indwelling ureteral catheter

An injection procedure is performed through a previously created ureterostomy or a previously placed indwelling ureteral catheter to visualize the ureter and/or renal pelvis. A catheter is placed through the stoma in the skin into the ureter or through the indwelling ureteral catheter. Radiographic contrast media is injected through the catheter into the ureter and renal pelvis. Following the injection procedure, separately reportable radiographs of the ureter and renal pelvis are obtained.

50686

50686   Manometric studies through ureterostomy or indwelling ureteral catheter

Manometric studies are performed through a previously created ureterostomy or previously placed indwelling ureteral catheter to evaluate ureteral function and diagnose ureteral reflux. Ureteral eflux occurs when the direction of the flow of urine is reversed and travels back into the kidneys. This may occur when the muscular attachments of the ureter to the bladder that create the valve-like mechanism which closes the ureteric opening when urine is stored and voided fails of function. The reasons may be anatomical or functional. Manometry measures the strength of an organ's muscles. A catheter with a specialized manometer sensor is placed within the ureter, either through the stoma opening or the indwelling ureteral catheter. The pressure sensor in the catheter transmits muscle impulses to a computer and pressure recordings are obtained and analyzed.

50688

50688   Change of ureterostomy tube or externally accessible ureteral stent via ileal conduit

The physician changes a ureterostomy tube or an externally accessible ureteral stent via a previously created ileal conduit. Under separately reportable radiographic guidance, a guidewire and sheath are introduced through the previously created the ileal conduit. The ureterostomy tube or externally accessible stent is grasped and removed through the sheath. The replacement tube or stent is then loaded and advanced over the guidewire to into the ureter. Correct positioning is verified radiographically before the guidewire is removed.

50690

50690   Injection procedure for visualization of ileal conduit and/or ureteropyelography, exclusive of radiologic service

An injection procedure is performed to visualize a previously created ileal conduit and/or for ureteropyelography. A catheter is placed in the ileal conduit. Radiographic contrast media is injected through the catheter into the ileal conduit, ureter, and renal pelvis. Following the injection, separately reportable radiographs of the ileal conduit, ureter, and renal pelvis are obtained.

50700

50700   Ureteroplasty, plastic operation on ureter (eg, stricture)

The ureter is exposed and the narrowed, injured, or diseased portion is isolated. Plastic repair of the ureter depends on the exact nature of the ureteral abnormality. One type of repair involves the use of a Z-plasty. Horizontal and oblique incisions are made over the narrowed or injured portion of the ureter. The flaps are then rotated and re-anastomosed.

50693

50693   Placement of ureteral stent, percutaneous, including diagnostic nephrostogram and/or ureterogram when performed, imaging guidance (eg, ultrasound and/or fluoroscopy), and all associated radiological supervision and interpretation; pre-existing nephrostomy tract

A procedure is performed to place a ureteral stent through a pre-existing nephrostomy tract. A ureteral stent may be required to facilitate the flow of urine from the kidney to the bladder through the ureter in the presence of strictures, leaks, or fistulas. With the patient positioned prone, contract dye is injected through the pre-existing nephrostomy catheter and the urinary system is visualized using ultrasound and/or fluoroscopy. A guide wire is inserted through the catheter into the renal collecting system, coiled through the renal pelvis, and advanced down the ureter and into the bladder. The old nephrostomy catheter is removed and the stent is inserted over the guide wire and advanced into position. The proximal end remains outside the body with the distal pigtail threaded through the kidney, down the ureter, and into the bladder. This includes any diagnostic nephrostogram and/or ureterogram done, imaging guidance, and all associated radiologic supervision and interpretation.

Urinary System

50694-50695

50694 Placement of ureteral stent, percutaneous, including diagnostic nephrostogram and/or ureterogram when performed, imaging guidance (eg, ultrasound and/or fluoroscopy), and all associated radiological supervision and interpretation; new access, without separate nephrostomy catheter

50695 Placement of ureteral stent, percutaneous, including diagnostic nephrostogram and/or ureterogram when performed, imaging guidance (eg, ultrasound and/or fluoroscopy), and all associated radiological supervision and interpretation; new access, with separate nephrostomy catheter

Percutaneous placement of a ureteral stent with or without placement of a separate nephrostomy catheter may be performed to treat urinary obstruction caused by stones, tumors, or strictures; to diagnose urinary conditions; provide access for therapeutic interventions; or divert urine in the presence of traumatic injury, leaks, fistulas, or hemorrhagic cystitis. A single or double needle technique may be employed. Under ultrasound and/or fluoroscopic guidance, a single trocar or Chiba needle is inserted below the 12th rib to minimize the risk of puncturing the pleura. The needle is advanced into the renal pelvis, and urine is aspirated to verify location and decompress the system. Contrast dye is then injected and a series of x-rays are taken to visualize movement of dye through the urinary tract. Once satisfactory needle placement has been established, a thin wire is threaded through the needle into the renal pelvis and advanced down the ureter into the bladder. The stent is inserted over the guide wire and advanced into position. The proximal end is coiled within the renal pelvis with the distal pigtail in the bladder. If a separate nephrostomy catheter is not inserted (50694), the proximal end of the stent may remain outside the body or lie entirely inside the renal system. When a separate nephrostomy catheter is inserted (50695), the catheter is threaded over the guide wire into the upper pole of the calyx with the end outside the body. For double needle technique, the first needle is inserted directly into the renal pelvis and contrast dye is injected to obtain a series of x-rays. A small amount of air or CO2 may be injected to enhance visualization of the posterior calyces. A clamp applied to the skin is used to mark the entry site of the second needle placed under the 12th rib in the posterior axillary line. Insertion of the second needle and placement of the stent/catheter is identical to the single needle technique. These codes include any diagnostic nephrostogram and/or ureterogram, imaging guidance, and all associated radiologic supervision and interpretation.

50705

50705 Ureteral embolization or occlusion, including imaging guidance (eg, ultrasound and/or fluoroscopy) and all associated radiological supervision and interpretation (List separately in addition to code for primary procedure)

Ureteral embolization or occlusion may be used to interrupt the flow of urine from the kidney(s) to the bladder when chronic or refractory lower urinary tract fistulas are present. The development of fistulas can be due to trauma, malignancy, or radiation. If percutaneous access is first required, a trocar or Chiba needle is inserted below the 12th rib under ultrasound and/or fluoroscopic guidance to minimize the risk of puncturing the pleura. The needle is advanced into the renal pelvis and urine is aspirated to verify location and decompress the system. After satisfactory placement of the needle, a thin wire is threaded through the needle into the distal ureter. A guidewire may also be placed through an existing percutaneous tube or catheter into the ureter. A delivery catheter or access sheath is inserted over the wire; and the wire is removed. The delivery catheter or access sheath may also be introduced through a cystoscope/ureteroscope. Stainless steel coils and gelatin sponge pledgets are inserted through the catheter/sheath to occlude the ureter. Additional images are obtained to confirm ureteral occlusion. This includes imaging guidance and associated radiologic supervision and interpretation for ureteral embolization or occlusion done in conjunction with a separate primary procedure.

50706

50706 Balloon dilation, ureteral stricture, including imaging guidance (eg, ultrasound and/or fluoroscopy) and all associated radiological supervision and interpretation (List separately in addition to code for primary procedure)

Balloon dilation of a ureteral stricture may be performed through a percutaneously placed catheter or through the bladder and ureteroscope. Radiologic guidance is required for either approach to ensure that the balloon is centered directly over the stricture. Strictures are narrowed segments of the ureteral lumen that obstruct urine flow. Common causes include tumors and fibrosis. If percutaneous access is first required, a trocar or Chiba needle is inserted below the 12th rib under ultrasound and/or fluoroscopic guidance to minimize the risk of puncturing the pleura. The needle is advanced into the renal pelvis and urine is aspirated to verify location and decompress the system. After satisfactory placement of the needle has been established, a thin wire is threaded through the needle to the location of the ureteral stricture. A guidewire may also be placed through an existing percutaneous tube or catheter to the stricture. The balloon catheter is placed over the guide wire and the guide wire is removed. Once the balloon is positioned directly over

the stricture, the balloon is serially dilated until the narrowed area is open. A stent may be inserted following dilation to maintain patency of the ureter. Additional imaging may confirm that the ureter is patent. The balloon catheter may also be introduced through a cystoscope/ureteroscope and placed directly over the stricture, confirmed by fluoroscopy. The balloon is serially dilated until the narrowed ureteral lumen is open. A stent may be inserted following the balloon dilation to maintain patency of the ureter. Uretogram images confirm that the ureter is patent. The balloon catheter is removed. Code 50706 includes imaging guidance and associated radiologic supervision and interpretation for balloon dilation of a ureteral stricture done in conjunction with a separate primary procedure. This type of repair increases the lumen diameter at the site of the narrowing or injury.

50715

50715 Ureterolysis, with or without repositioning of ureter for retroperitoneal fibrosis

An open ureterolysis is performed on an obstructed ureter that is entrapped by fibrous tissue in the retroperitoneum. This condition is referred to as retroperitoneal fibrosis (RPF). RPF is a rare condition characterized by chronic inflammation of the retroperitoneal structures, including the ureters. The ureter is approached using a flank incision. The colon is mobilized medially to the level of the vena cava and iliac vessels and the retroperitoneum and ureter are exposed. The extent of fibrosis is evaluated and the ureter is then dissected free of the fibrotic mass, which is biopsied for analysis. The ureter may be divided and the normal distal segment repositioned and reattached to the kidney, or the ureter may be left intact and wrapped in omentum.

50722-50725

50722 Ureterolysis for ovarian vein syndrome

50725 Ureterolysis for retrocaval ureter, with reanastomosis of upper urinary tract or vena cava

An open ureterolysis is performed on an obstructed ureter that has become entrapped due to ovarian vein syndrome or retrocaval ureter. In 50722, the ureteral obstruction is due to ovarian vein syndrome. Ovarian vein syndrome occurs when an enlarged or tortuous ovarian vein compresses the ureter. An incision is made in the abdomen and the enlarged ovarian vein exposed. Adhesions between the ureter, ovarian vein, or other structures are severed. The ovarian vein may be divided and the enlarged section excised to release the entrapped ureter. In 50725, the ureteral obstruction is due to a retrocaval ureter. Retrocaval ureter, also referred to as circumcaval ureter, is a rare congenital anomaly resulting from persistence of the posterior cardinal veins. This causes malposition of the ureter behind the inferior vena cava where it can become compressed and obstructed between the inferior vena cava and aorta. The retrocaval ureter is exposed by a subcostal incision. The ureter is dissected free of surrounding tissues and mobilized. The compressed segment of ureter is excised. The distal and proximal ends of ureter are spatulated and continuity of the ureter restored by anastomosis. A temporary double J stent is placed to maintain patency and facilitate healing of the ureter. External drainage tubes may be placed in the operative wound. Bleeding is controlled and incisions closed. Alternatively, the vena cava may be divided, the ureter repositioned, and the vena cava reanastomosed.

50727-50728

50727 Revision of urinary-cutaneous anastomosis (any type urostomy)

50728 Revision of urinary-cutaneous anastomosis (any type urostomy); with repair of fascial defect and hernia

A previously created urostomy is revised. The exact nature of the procedure depends on the type of urostomy which may be a cutaneous ureterostomy, cystostomy, or nephrostomy. Revision may be necessary if the stoma becomes constricted or obstructed; if the urinary tract tissue prolapses through the stoma or if it retracts, causing the stoma to sink below the level of the skin, or even detaches from the skin; if necrosis occurs; or if the patient develops a parastomal hernia. In 50727, a skin incision is made around the entire circumference of the urostomy. Local release of scar tissue (adhesions) around the stoma may be performed. Alternatively, dissection may continue down through fascia and peritoneum and the distal portion of the urinary tissue may be resected, then everted, and sutured back to the skin and subcutaneous tissue. If the stoma needs to be relocated, the abdomen is opened at the new stoma site. Adhesions are lysed and the exteriorized urinary tissue is mobilized. Any necrotic tissue is excised. The terminal end of the urinary tissue is brought through the abdominal wall, folded back on itself (everted), and sutured to the skin and subcutaneous tissue. In 50728, a urostomy fascial defect and hernia is repaired. An incision is made over the hernia and the hernia is reduced. Overlying fascia is then repaired with sutures or a mesh implant.

50740-50750

50740 Ureteropyelostomy, anastomosis of ureter and renal pelvis

50750 Ureterocalycostomy, anastomosis of ureter to renal calyx

Ureteropyelostomy is a procedure that joins the upper aspect of the ureter to the lower aspect of the renal pelvis while ureterocalycostomy joins the ureter to the calyces at a point above the lower aspect of the renal pelvis. These procedures are performed

● New Code   ▲ Revised Code   CPT © 2016 American Medical Association. All Rights Reserved.   © 2017 DecisionHealth

Urinary System

to treat ureteropelvic junction (UPJ) obstruction or a long proximal ureteral stricture. Ureterocalycostomy is performed when the renal pelvis is severely fibrosed or scarred. The ureter is exposed and mobilized taking care to preserve periureteral tissue. The ureter is divided just distal to the narrowed region. The proximal ureteral stump is ligated. The kidney is exposed and mobilized. In 50740, the lower aspect of the renal pelvis is excised at a point above the narrowed or obstructed portion. The proximal aspect of the remaining segment of healthy ureter is spatulated. A stent is placed and the ureteropelvic anastomosis is performed over the stent. The repair is reinforced with perinephric fat or omentum. In 50750, the procedure is performed as described above except that the lower pole calyx is exposed and the parenchyma over the lower pole is resected. Any remaining fibrotic or diseased tissue is excised. The proximal ureter is spatulated. A stent is placed and the ureterocalyceal anastosmosis is performed over the stent.

50760-50770

50760   Ureteroureterostomy
50770   Transureteroureterostomy, anastomosis of ureter to contralateral ureter

Ureteroureterostomy is a procedure that joins two segments of the same ureter while transureteroureterostomy joins one ureter to the contralateral ureter. These procedures are performed to treat ureteral stenosis, obstruction, or injury. In 50760, the ureter is exposed and the narrowed or injured portion is identified. The ureter is dissected free of surrounding tissues and mobilized between soft rubber loops. Care is taken to preserve periureteral tissues and blood supply. The narrowed or damaged portion is excised. A ureteral catheter is inserted extending from the renal pelvis to the bladder. The two segments of ureter are anastomosed over the ureteral catheter. A drain is placed in the abdomen adjacent to the anastomosis. The surgical wound is closed in layers. In 50770, both ureters are exposed and mobility and length are evaluated. The diseased ureter is mobilized above the area of the diseased portion up to the ureteropelvic junction (UPJ) taking care to preserve periureteral tissue and blood supply. A retroperitoneal tunnel is created. The diseased ureter is transected above the diseased segment. The proximal healthy segment of the ureter is brought across the midline through the tunnel to the opposite ureter. The recipient ureter is mobilized. The transposed ureter is spatulated. An incision is made in the recipient ureter and the transposed ureter is sutured to the recipient ureter. Ureteral stenting is performed as needed. A drain is placed in the abdomen and the surgical wound is closed.

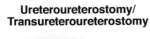

Ureteroureterostomy/ Transureteroureterostomy

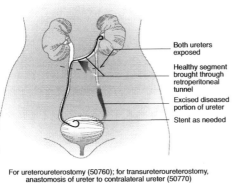

Both ureters exposed

Healthy segment brought through retroperitoneal tunnel

Excised diseased portion of ureter

Stent as needed

For ureteroureterostomy (50760); for transureteroureterostomy, anastomosis of ureter to contralateral ureter (50770)

50780-50785

50780   Ureteroneocystostomy; anastomosis of single ureter to bladder
50782   Ureteroneocystostomy; anastomosis of duplicated ureter to bladder
50783   Ureteroneocystostomy; with extensive ureteral tailoring
50785   Ureteroneocystostomy; with vesico-psoas hitch or bladder flap

An open ureteroneocystostomy is performed. The distal ureter is divided at or near the ureterovescical junction (UVJ). An incision is then made in the dome of the bladder wall to the level of the mucosa. A smaller incision is made in the bladder mucosa. The detached segment of ureter is trimmed and the end spatulated. The full thickness of the ureter is anastomosed to the bladder mucosa. The bladder wall is then closed over a 2-3 cm segment of ureter to create a tunnel for the ureter to help prevent reflux. The opening at the UVJ is closed. A temporary ureteral stent may be placed to ensure patency and facilitate healing. Report 50780 when the procedure is performed on a single ureter. Report 50782 when the procedure is performed on a duplicated (double) ureter. Duplicated ureters are the result of a duplicated collecting system in a single kidney with two ureters that may be fused into a single ureter or may each empty separately into the bladder. Report 50783 when extensive ureteral tailoring or reconstruction is required prior to implantation into the bladder. Report 50785 when the procedure is performed with a vesico-psoas hitch or bladder flap. The procedure is performed as described above; however prior to implantation of the ureter, the bladder is mobilized and sutured (fixed) to the psoas muscle. The bladder

is then incised at the point of fixation to the psoas muscle and the ureter implanted in the immobile bladder portion along the line of fixation using a long submucosal tunnel. Alternatively, a bladder flap, also referred to as a Boari flap, may be used when the distal ureteral segment is too short to reach the bladder.

50800

50800   Ureteroenterostomy, direct anastomosis of ureter to intestine

A diseased or injured segment of the middle or distal ureter is excised and the healthy proximal ureteral segment is anastomosed to the intestine. The abdomen is incised in the midline and the peritoneum is opened. The small bowel is isolated and packed out of the surgical field. The ureter is exposed and mobilized taking care to preserve perirenal tissue and blood supply. The diseased segment of ureter is excised and the distal ureteral stump is ligated at the ureterovesical junction. A segment of intestine, usually ileum, is selected and mobilized as needed. The ureter is spatulated, stented, and anastomosed to the intestine in an end-to-side fashion. A nephrostomy tube is placed as needed. The surgical wound is closed in layers.

50810

50810   Ureterosigmoidostomy, with creation of sigmoid bladder and establishment of abdominal or perineal colostomy, including intestine anastomosis

Ureterosigmoidostomy is one type of urinary diversion that may be performed on patients with bladder cancer, neurogenic bladder, radiation injury to the bladder, intractable incontinence, as well as other conditions. The abdomen is incised in the midline and the peritoneum is opened. The small bowel is isolated and packed out of the surgical field. The ureters are exposed, mobilized, and divided distally near the ureterovesical junction. The ureteral stumps are ligated. A segment of sigmoid colon is selected and mobilized. The segment from which the sigmoid bladder is to be constructed is isolated. The sigmoid colon is divided and an appropriately sized segment is isolated. The remaining distal and proximal portions of the sigmoid colon are then anastomosed and bowel continuity is restored. The sigmoid bladder is fashioned. A tunnel is created from the sigmoid bladder to the ureters. The ureters are pulled through the tunnel to the sigmoid bladder and into the lumen of the sigmoid. The ends of the ureters are spatulated along the anterior aspect. Stents are placed in both ureters. The ureters are anastomosed to the sigmoid colon approximately 3 cm apart. A separate abdominal or perineal incision is made for creation of the stoma through which urine will be expelled. The sigmoid bladder is exteriorized through the stoma, folded back on itself (everted), and sutured to the skin or subcutaneous tissue, creating either an abdominal or perineal colostomy. An ostomy bag is secured over the sigmoidostomy site or a catheter is placed in the stoma. Drains are placed as needed and surgical incisions are closed in layers.

50815-50820

50815   Ureterocolon conduit, including intestine anastomosis
50820   Ureteroileal conduit (ileal bladder), including intestine anastomosis (Bricker operation)

Ureterocolon and ureteroileal conduits are types of urinary diversions that may be performed on patients with bladder cancer, neurogenic bladder, radiation injury to the bladder, and intractable incontinence as well as other conditions. The abdomen is incised in the midline and the peritoneum is opened. The small bowel is isolated and packed out of the surgical field. The ureters are exposed and mobilized. The ureters are divided distally near the ureterovesical junction and the ureteral stumps are ligated. The portion of colon or ileum to be used for the conduit is identified and isolated. The remaining segments of bowel distal and proximal to the isolated segment are anastamosed and bowel continuity is restored. A stoma site is selected and the skin is incised. Dissection is carried down to the anterior rectus fascia which is incised. The rectus muscle is divided using blunt dissection. The distal end of the conduit is pulled through the abdominal wall, everted, and sutured to skin or subcutaneous tissues to create the stoma. The proximal end of the conduit is closed with sutures. A tunnel is created from the conduit to the ureters. The ureters are pulled through the tunnel to the conduit. The ends of the ureters are spatulated. Stents are placed in both ureters. Small incisions are made in the conduit and the ureters are anastomosed to the conduit approximately 3 cm apart. Drains are placed as needed and surgical incisions are closed in layers. An ostomy bag is placed over the ostomy site to collect urine. Use 50815 when the conduit is created using a portion of the colon; use 50820 when a portion of the ileum is used.

50825

50825   Continent diversion, including intestine anastomosis using any segment of small and/or large intestine (Kock pouch or Camey enterocystoplasty)

A continent urinary diversion procedure is performed. Continent urinary diversion differs from other urinary diversion procedures in that the patient may void normally through the urethra. Alternatively, a stoma may be created with a valve mechanism using intussuscepted colon that prevents leakage of urine. With this type of stoma, the patient removes urine by periodically catheterizing the pouch. The abdomen in incised in the midline. The small bowel is isolated and packed out of the surgical field. The ureters are

Urinary System

exposed, mobilized, and divided distally near the ureterovesical junction. The ureteral stumps are ligated. A segment of small or large intestine is selected and mobilized. The segment, usually 30-35 cm of intestine from which the pouch is to be constructed, is isolated. The intestine is divided, leaving the isolated segment attached to the mesenteric pedicle keeping blood supply intact. The remaining distal and proximal portions of the intestine are then anastomosed and bowel continuity is restored. The intestinal pouch is fashioned by arranging the isolated segment in a U or W configuration. The segment is incised longitudinally along the mesenteric border to detubularize it. The intestine is fashioned into a pouch. A tunnel is created from the pouch to the ureters. The ureters are pulled through the tunnel to the pouch. The ends of the ureters are spatulated along the anterior aspect. The ureters are anastomosed to the pouch approximately 3 cm apart. The distal aspect of the pouch may be incised and anastomosed to the bladder neck in females or the proximal urethra in males. Alternatively, a stoma may be created through a separate incision. When a stoma is created, the pouch is configured and detubularized as described above except for the portion of intestine that will be used to form the valve. The remaining tubular segment is scarified using electrocautery and adjacent mesentery is excised. The scarified segment is telescoped (intussuscepted) into the pouch and secured with sutures, creating the valve. The valve component is then sutured to the previously prepared stoma site in the abdominal wall. A catheter is placed through the valve into the stoma. Drains are placed as needed and surgical incisions are closed in layers.

50830

50830   Urinary undiversion (eg, taking down of ureteroileal conduit, ureterosigmoidostomy or ureteroenterostomy with ureteroureterostomy or ureteroneocystostomy)

Urinary undiversion or take-down procedure is performed to restore the continuity of the urinary tract. This procedure is done primarily on patients with previous injury to the ureter or bladder that required temporary diversion, and children with urologic conditions that require temporary diversion until the condition can be surgically corrected or until it resolves. The exact procedure performed depends on the type of urinary diversion and the patient's anatomy. The abdomen is incised in the midline and the peritoneum is opened. The small bowel is isolated and packed out of the surgical field. Adhesions are lysed and the previously reconfigured anatomy is evaluated, including the remaining proximal ureteral segments, ureteral anastomosis sites, any distal ureteral segments, urinary bladder, and the ileal conduit, if present. The proximal ureters are exposed and dissected free of surrounding tissue taking care to preserve surrounding periureteral tissue and blood supply. If ureterosigmoidostomy or ureteroenterostomy has been performed, the ureters are disconnected from the bowel, stents are removed, and the anastomosis sites in the bowel are repaired. The proximal ureteral segments are then reconnected to the distal ureteral segments, if present, or to the bladder. Reconnecting the ureters may require mobilization of the renal pelvis in order to achieve reimplantation of the ureters in the bladder. Stents are placed in the ureters as needed. If an ileal conduit has been used, the cutaneous connection is severed. The ileal conduit is mobilized taking care to preserve blood supply. The bladder is incised and a submucosal tunnel is created in the internal bladder wall. The distal aspect of the ileal conduit is passed through the tunnel and anchored to the bladder muscle. The conduit exits the bladder musosa near the bladder trigone. Stents are placed in the ureters as needed. The cutaneous stoma is closed. Drains are placed and the abdominal incision is closed in layers.

50840

50840   Replacement of all or part of ureter by intestine segment, including intestine anastomosis

A diseased or injured segment of the ureter is excised and any remaining healthy proximal ureteral segment is anastomosed to the intestine as a ureteral replacement. The abdomen is incised in the midline and the peritoneum is opened. The small bowel is isolated and packed out of the surgical field. The ureter is exposed and mobilized. The diseased segment of ureter is excised and the distal ureteral stump is ligated at the ureterovesical junction. A segment of intestine, usually ileum, is selected and mobilized. The length of intestine required for ureteral replacement is determined. The intestine is divided and a segment of the required length is isolated. The intestinal segments proximal and distal to the isolated segment are then anastomosed and bowel continuity is restored. The isolated segment of intestine is prepared for anastomosis to the ureter and bladder. The proximal end of the isolated segment of intestine is closed with sutures. The ureter is spatulated, stented, and anastomosed to the proximal end of the isolated segment of intestine in an end-to-side fashion. The distal end of isolated intestine is anastomosed to the bladder. An incision is made in the bladder wall usually 1-2 cm posterolateral to the native ureteral orifice. A full-thickness segment of bladder wall matching the diameter of the distal segment of intestine is excised. The distal segment of intestine is anastomosed to the bladder. A nephrostomy tube is placed as needed. The surgical wound is closed in layers.

50845

50845   Cutaneous appendico-vesicostomy

Appendicovesicostomy is performed primarily in children and young adults to treat conditions such as neuropathic bladder due to myelomeningocele, extrophy-epispadias,

cloacal anomalies, prune belly syndrome, and posterior urethral valves. The procedure involves creation of an appendiceal channel, referred to as a Mitrofanoff channel, within the bladder. The appendiceal channel extends from the bladder to the skin. This type of channel is easy to catheterize and durable enough to last a lifetime. The right colon is mobilized beyond the hepatic flexure. The appendix and bladder are mobilized. The appendix is detached from the cecum and the cecum is closed. The terminal aspect of the appendix is incised and dilated as needed to increase the size of the lumen. The bladder is incised. A submucosal bladder tunnel is created. The terminal aspect of the appendix is passed into the bladder, through the submucosal tunnel, spatulated, and sutured to the bladder making sure that the sutures pass through the detrusor muscle and mucosa at the distal aspect of the bladder tunnel. The appendix is also secured at the proximal aspect where it enters the bladder. The appendiceal channel is catheterized to ensure that a catheter can pass easily into the bladder. A stoma site is selected, usually at the umbilicus or in the right lower quadrant. The skin is incised and underlying soft tissues are dissected to the level of the fascia. The fascia is incised and widened until the opening is large enough to allow passage of the index finger. The appendix is brought through the opening to the skin until the bladder is positioned against the posterior fascial wall. The appendix and bladder are sutured to the fascia. The cecal end of the appendix is spatulated and any redundant appendix is trimmed. The spatulated appendix is then sutured to the skin or subcutaneous tissues at the stoma site. A temporary indwelling catheter is placed until the surgical wounds have healed sufficiently to allow intermittent catheterization through the stoma. Abdominal drains are placed as needed and the abdominal incision is closed in layers.

50860

50860   Ureterostomy, transplantation of ureter to skin

A cutaneous ureterostomy is performed. A lateral incision is made in the abdomen, overlying muscle is divided, and the peritoneum is retracted to expose the ureter, which is divided as close to the ureterovesical junction (UVJ) as possible. The distal stump of the ureter is ligated. The proximal ureter is then dissected free of surrounding tissue and brought up into the surgical wound. A catheter is passed through the ureter into the renal pelvis to drain the kidney. The catheter may be left in place and sutured to the abdominal wall. Alternatively, an artificial opening, or stoma, may be created on the surface of the abdomen with the ureter sutured to the stoma to divert the passage of urine from the bladder out through the abdomen. A drain is inserted into the abdominal wound and the wound is closed around the drain.

50900

50900   Ureterorrhaphy, suture of ureter (separate procedure)

Suture repair of a ureter is performed in a separate procedure. The damaged ureter is exposed. The injury is located, inspected, and determined to be minor and suitable for suture repair alone. The edges of the ureteral laceration are approximated and fine sutures are placed. Drains are placed as needed and the surgical wound is closed in layers.

50920-50930

50920   Closure of ureterocutaneous fistula
50930   Closure of ureterovisceral fistula (including visceral repair)

A ureterocutaneous fistula is an abnormal communication between a ureter and the skin while a ureterovisceral fistula is an abnormal communication between a ureter and a hollow multilayered walled organ. The ureter is exposed and the abnormal communication is located. The fistula tract is followed from the ureter to the skin or the visceral organ and excised. The fistulous opening in the ureter is debrided as needed and closed with sutures. In 50920, the skin and subcutaneous tissues in the skin are also debrided and closed with sutures. In 50930, the opening in the visceral organ is debrided and closed with sutures or repaired by another technique. The operative wound is closed in layers.

50940

50940   Deligation of ureter

The physician performs deligation of the ureter. Deligation is performed to remove a ligature from a ureter that has been unintentionally tied off during an abdominal or retroperitoneal procedure. This can happen when blood vessels around the ureter are ligated and the ureter is inadvertently caught in the ligature. Inadvertent ligation of the ureter causes complete or partial obstruction. The ureter is exposed by a retroperitoneal or transperitoneal approach. The health of the ureter is evaluated to determine whether blood supply to the ureter is intact. If the ureter is healthy, the ligature is removed to relieve the obstruction.

50945

50945   Laparoscopy, surgical; ureterolithotomy

Ureterolithotomy is performed to remove a ureteral stone (calculus) from the ureter. The laparoscopic procedure can be performed using a retroperitoneal or transperitoneal approach. Using a retroperitoneal approach, the laparoscope is introduced either through an incision below the tip of the twelfth rib if the ureteral stone is in the upper ureter or through an incision medial to the anterosuperior iliac spine if the stone is in the lower ureter. Muscles are split and the peritoneum separated from the abdominal wall with blunt dissection. Additional portal incisions are made for the introduction of surgical instruments. The ureter is identified and the stone, which is seen as a bulge in the ureter, located. Forceps are used to grasp the ureter at the site of the stone to prevent it from moving. The ureter is dissected and incised. The stone is extracted from the ureter using forceps and carefully removed through one of the portal incisions. A double J-stent may be placed if needed through the ureteral incision. The ureter is repaired, the laparoscopic and surgical instruments removed, and the abdomen closed.

50947-50948

50947 Laparoscopy, surgical; ureteroneocystostomy with cystoscopy and ureteral stent placement

50948 Laparoscopy, surgical; ureteroneocystostomy without cystoscopy and ureteral stent placement

Ureteroneocystostomy is performed by laparoscopic approach. In 50948, a small incision is made inferior to the umbilicus. A trocar is placed into the peritoneal cavity; the laparoscope is introduced through the trocar; and the abdomen is insufflated. Several additional portal incisions are made for the introduction of surgical instruments. Dissection is then performed under laparoscopic control to mobilize the ureter, beginning proximal to the broad ligament and carried down to the ureterovesical junction. An incision is made in the muscular wall of the bladder (detrusor muscle) to create a trough at the planned ureteral transplant site along the lateral aspect of the bladder. An incision is made in the bladder and the ureter is inserted into the detrusor trough. The ureter is anastomosed to the detrusor edges and the trough is closed around the ureter. In 50947, ureteroneocystostomy is performed as described above followed by cystoscopy and ureteral stent placement. A cystoscope is inserted through the urethra and into the urinary bladder. The opening in the ureter is identified. A guide wire is advanced into the ureter and a stent is then advanced over the guide wire and positioned in the ureter under laparoscopic visualization. Following completion of the procedure, a urethral catheter is placed; the cystoscope and laparoscope are removed; and the abdominal incisions are closed.

50951-50953

50951 Ureteral endoscopy through established ureterostomy, with or without irrigation, instillation, or ureteropyelography, exclusive of radiologic service

50953 Ureteral endoscopy through established ureterostomy, with or without irrigation, instillation, or ureteropyelography, exclusive of radiologic service; with ureteral catheterization, with or without dilation of ureter

Ureteral endoscopy is performed through an existing ureteral stoma or ureteral catheter exiting the skin. The ureteroscope is introduced through the ureterostomy. In 50951, the ureter is inspected and any obstruction, stenosis, stricture, or other abnormal condition is noted. The ureter may be irrigated with normal saline, or diagnostic or therapeutic solution may be instilled. Contrast material may be injected and separately reportable ureteropyelography performed. In 50953, following visual examination, a ureteral catheter is advanced through the ureteroscope. If stenosis is present, a balloon tipped catheter is introduced to the site of the stenosis and inflated. This balloon may be deflated and inflated several times until the stenotic region is adequately dilated. The ureter may be irrigated with normal saline or diagnostic or therapeutic solution may be instilled. Contrast material may be injected and separately reportable ureteropyelography performed. All instruments are then removed.

50955-50961

50955 Ureteral endoscopy through established ureterostomy, with or without irrigation, instillation, or ureteropyelography, exclusive of radiologic service; with biopsy

50957 Ureteral endoscopy through established ureterostomy, with or without irrigation, instillation, or ureteropyelography, exclusive of radiologic service; with fulguration and/or incision, with or without biopsy

50961 Ureteral endoscopy through established ureterostomy, with or without irrigation, instillation, or ureteropyelography, exclusive of radiologic service; with removal of foreign body or calculus

Ureteral endoscopy is performed through an existing ureteral stoma or ureteral catheter exiting the skin. The ureteroscope is introduced through the ureterostomy. The ureter is inspected for abnormal tissue, foreign body, or calculus. The ureter may be irrigated with normal saline or diagnostic or therapeutic solution may be instilled. Contrast material may be injected and separately reportable ureteropyelography performed. In 50955, a biopsy is performed. Biopsy forceps are inserted through the ureteroscope and one or more tissue samples are obtained. In 50957, fulguration and/or incision of abnormal tissue is performed. A biopsy may be performed prior to the fulguration procedure as described above. To destroy abnormal tissue, an electrocautery device is advanced through the ureteroscope to the site of the lesion. The device is activated and the abnormal tissue is destroyed. Alternatively, a laser or cryoprobe may be used to destroy the abnormal tissue. The physician may introduce a blade and incise the abnormal tissue instead of, or in addition to, the fulguration procedure. In 50961, the ureter is inspected and a foreign body,

such as a stent or calculus, is located. A grasping device or basket is advanced through the working channel of the ureteroscope and the foreign body or calculus is captured and removed. The ureter is re-inspected to ensure that there has not been any injury to the ureter during the procedure.

50970-50972

50970 Ureteral endoscopy through ureterotomy, with or without irrigation, instillation, or ureteropyelography, exclusive of radiologic service

50972 Ureteral endoscopy through ureterotomy, with or without irrigation, instillation, or ureteropyelography, exclusive of radiologic service; with ureteral catheterization, with or without dilation of ureter

Ureteral endoscopy is performed through an incision in the ureter. An incision is made to expose the ureter. A small incision is made in the ureter and the ureteroscope is introduced. In 50970, the ureter is inspected and any obstruction, stenosis, stricture, or other abnormal condition is noted. The ureter may be irrigated with normal saline, or diagnostic or therapeutic solution may be instilled. Contrast material may be injected and separately reportable ureteropyelography performed. In 50972, following visual examination, a ureteral catheter is advanced through the ureteroscope. If stenosis is present, a balloon tipped catheter is introduced to the site of the stenosis and inflated. This balloon may be deflated and inflated several times until the stenotic region is adequately dilated. The ureter may be irrigated with normal saline or diagnostic or therapeutic solution may be instilled. Contrast material may be injected and separately reportable ureteropyelography performed. All instruments are removed and the ureterotomy is closed with sutures.

50974-50980

50974 Ureteral endoscopy through ureterotomy, with or without irrigation, instillation, or ureteropyelography, exclusive of radiologic service; with biopsy

50976 Ureteral endoscopy through ureterotomy, with or without irrigation, instillation, or ureteropyelography, exclusive of radiologic service; with fulguration and/or incision, with or without biopsy

50980 Ureteral endoscopy through ureterotomy, with or without irrigation, instillation, or ureteropyelography, exclusive of radiologic service; with removal of foreign body or calculus

Ureteral endoscopy is performed through an incision in the ureter. An incision is made to expose the ureter. A small incision is made in the ureter and the ureteroscope is introduced. The ureter is inspected for abnormal tissue, foreign body, or calculus. The ureter may be irrigated with normal saline, or diagnostic or therapeutic solution may be instilled. Contrast material may be injected and separately reportable ureteropyelography performed. In 50974, a biopsy is performed. Biopsy forceps are inserted through the ureteroscope and one or more tissue samples are obtained. In 50976, fulguration and/or incision of abnormal tissue is performed. A biopsy may be performed prior to the fulguration procedure as described above. To destroy abnormal tissue, an electrocautery device is advanced through the ureteroscope to the site of the lesion. The device is activated and the abnormal tissue is destroyed. Alternatively, a laser or cryoprobe may be used to destroy the abnormal tissue. The physician may introduce a blade and incise the abnormal tissue instead of, or in addition to, the fulguration procedure. In 50980, the ureter is inspected and a foreign body, such as a stent or calculus, is located. A grasping device or basket is advanced through the working channel of the ureteroscope and the foreign body or calculus is captured and removed. The ureter is re-inspected to ensure that there has not been any injury to the ureter during the procedure.

51020-51030

51020 Cystotomy or cystostomy; with fulguration and/or insertion of radioactive material

51030 Cystotomy or cystostomy; with cryosurgical destruction of intravesical lesion

The urinary bladder is exposed and incised. Alternatively, a small incision is made over the bladder and the bladder wall is punctured to provide surgical access to the internal lumen. In 51020, abnormal tissue is destroyed by fulguration or radioactive material is inserted into a lesion. To destroy abnormal tissue, an electrocautery device is advanced through the incision to the site where the abnormal tissue is located. The device is activated and the lesion is destroyed. Alternatively, a laser may be used to destroy the abnormal tissue. If a radioactive material is used to treat a lesion, the delivery device is inserted into the bladder and positioned at the site of the lesion or abnormal tissue. The radioactive pellet is then embedded in the mucosa or bladder wall at the site of the lesion or abnormal tissue. In 51030, a cryoprobe is introduced through the incision and abnormal tissue is frozen. Several freeze-thaw cycles may be required to completely destroy all abnormal tissue.

51040

51040 Cystostomy, cystotomy with drainage

A cystostomy or cystotomy with drainage is performed. The skin over the lower abdomen is cleansed. An incision is made in the abdominal wall and into the bladder. A drainage tube (catheter) is inserted and secured to the abdomen to facilitate drainage, and a sterile dressing is applied.

51045

51045   Cystotomy, with insertion of ureteral catheter or stent (separate procedure)

The urinary bladder is exposed and a small incision is made in the bladder wall. A guidewire is introduced through the incision and advanced through the ureter to the renal pelvis. A catheter is advanced over the guidewire to the renal pelvis. The guidewire is removed. The ureter may be irrigated with normal saline, or diagnostic or therapeutic solution may be instilled. Alternatively, a ureteral stent may be placed over the guidewire. The stent is advanced over the guidewire and the proximal end is positioned in the renal pelvis. The guidewire is slowly withdrawn taking care not to dislodge the stent. The distal end of the stent is positioned in the urinary bladder.

51050

51050   Cystolithotomy, cystotomy with removal of calculus, without vesical neck resection

A skin incision is made in the lower abdomen over the urinary bladder. Tissues are dissected down to the anterior rectus muscle sheath. The rectus abdominus and pyramidalis muscles are separated and retracted. The peritoneum is reflected. The urinary bladder is exposed and an incision is made in the bladder wall to perform a cystotomy and remove a calculus from the bladder. Two stay sutures are placed in the bladder wall lateral to the planned incision site. The stay sutures are pulled to tent the bladder. A stab incision is made between the stay sutures in the tented portion of the bladder. The incision is enlarged until it is wide enough to accommodate extraction of the calculus. Grasping forceps are introduced and the calculus is captured and removed. The bladder incision is closed followed by layered closure of the abdominal incision.

51060

51060   Transvesical ureterolithotomy

A skin incision is made in the lower abdomen over the urinary bladder. Tissues are dissected down to the anterior rectus muscle sheath. The rectus abdominus and pyramidalis muscles are separated and retracted. The peritoneum is reflected. The urinary bladder is exposed and an incision is made in the bladder wall. Two stay sutures are placed in the bladder wall lateral to the planned incision site. The stay sutures are pulled to tent the bladder. A stab incision is made between the stay sutures in the tented portion of the bladder. The incision is enlarged until the ureteral orifice is visible. A second incision is made through the bladder wall near the ureter. The calculus in the distal aspect of the ureter is located. The ureter is incised and the calculus extracted through the bladder. The ureteral incision is closed, followed by the proximal bladder incision. The anterior wall of the bladder is closed, followed by layered closure of the abdominal incision.

51065

51065   Cystotomy, with calculus basket extraction and/or ultrasonic or electrohydraulic fragmentation of ureteral calculus

A skin incision is made in the lower abdomen over the urinary bladder. Tissues are dissected down to the anterior rectus muscle sheath. The rectus abdominus and pyramidalis muscles are separated and retracted. The peritoneum is reflected. The urinary bladder is then exposed and an incision is made in the bladder wall to perform a cystotomy for basket extraction and/or fragmentation of a ureteral calculus. Two stay sutures are placed in the bladder wall lateral to the planned incision site. The stay sutures are pulled to tent the bladder. A stab incision is made between the stay sutures in the tented portion of the bladder. The incision is enlarged until the ureteral orifice is visible. The basket extraction device is advanced through the bladder and into the ureter. The calculus is captured and removed. Lithotripsy may be performed using ultrasound or an electrohydraulic device to fragment the ureteral calculus prior to, or instead of, basket extraction. Once all stone fragments have been removed, the bladder incision is closed, followed by the abdominal incision which is closed in layers.

51080

51080   Drainage of perivesical or prevesical space abscess

The physician drains fluid from an abscess located in the tissue around the bladder. A skin incision is made in the lower abdomen over the urinary bladder. Tissues are dissected down to the anterior rectus muscle sheath. The rectus abdominus and pyramidalis muscles are separated and retracted. The peritoneum is reflected. An abscess in the perivesical or prevesical space is located. The abscess cavity is opened and drained. Blunt dissection is used to break up loculations. The cavity is flushed with sterile saline or antibiotic solution, and a drain is placed. The incision is closed over the drain.

51100-51102

51100   Aspiration of bladder; by needle
51101   Aspiration of bladder; by trocar or intracatheter
51102   Aspiration of bladder; with insertion of suprapubic catheter

A needle aspiration of the bladder is performed in 51100. A needle is inserted through the skin in the suprapubic region and advanced into the bladder. A small amount of urine is aspirated. This procedure is usually performed for urinalysis and culture for suspected urinary tract infection and requires a minimum of 2 ml of urine. Use 51101 for bladder aspiration using a trocar or intracatheter. A small incision is made in the skin over the suprapubic region. A trocar or intracatheter is inserted into the bladder and urine is aspirated. Use 51102 for bladder aspiration with insertion of a suprapubic catheter. A needle aspiration is performed as described above prior to insertion of the suprapubic catheter. The syringe is then removed and a guidewire is placed through the needle. The needle is removed and a small incision is made adjacent to the guidewire. A peel-away sheath introducer is placed over the guidewire and the guidewire is removed. A Foley catheter is advanced through the sheath introducer into the bladder and the balloon is deployed. The sheath introducer is removed and the catheter pulled back until resistance is met. The catheter tubing is secured on the abdominal wall and a drainage bag is attached.

51500

51500   Excision of urachal cyst or sinus, with or without umbilical hernia repair

The urachus is a duct present in the fetus that is usually obliterated between the 2nd and 4th month of gestation, becoming the median umbilical ligament. However, in some individuals this duct persists as a sinus that communicates with the umbilicus and bladder, or as a cyst. A persistent urachal sinus or cyst is usually asymptomatic and is not surgically excised unless infection occurs. A catheter is placed through the urethra and into the bladder. The skin is incised over the midline of the abdomen beginning just below the umbilicus and extending over the bladder. Underlying tissues are dissected; the anterior rectus abdominus muscle is divided; and the sinus or cyst is exposed. Usually a portion of the median umbilical ligament has begun to form and this is detached from the umbilicus. The sinus or cyst is mobilized using sharp dissection down towards the bladder. The bladder is filled with sterile saline. The peritoneum is incised and mobilization of the sinus or cyst continues down to the bladder dome. All connections between the sinus or cyst and the bladder dome are severed. This may require resection of the bladder cuff which is then repaired with sutures. The sinus or cyst is completely excised. If an umbilical hernia is present, it is repaired. The hernia sac is exposed. The neck of the sac is incised and lifted away from the abdominal wall. The hernia contents are extracted and inspected. Any adhesions are severed. The bowel is returned to the abdomen. The hernia sac is excised. The defect in the abdominal wall is closed with sutures and/or a mesh implant is applied. Skin and subcutaneous tissues are closed is layers.

51520-51530

51520   Cystotomy; for simple excision of vesical neck (separate procedure)
51525   Cystotomy; for excision of bladder diverticulum, single or multiple (separate procedure)
51530   Cystotomy; for excision of bladder tumor

A midline extraperitoneal abdominal approach is used to expose the bladder. The rectus and transversalis fascia are divided and the incision is carried down through the space of Retzius. The anterior bladder wall and vesical neck are identified. The bladder dome is incised and the bladder wall is inspected including the trigone, ureteral orifices, and bladder neck. In 51520, the bladder (vesical) neck is excised. The bladder neck is mobilized and resected. Visceral bladder fascia is used to reconstruct the neck. In 51525, one or more bladder diverticula are excised. A bladder diverticulum is a protrusion of mucosal tissue through the detrusor muscles of the bladder and into the abdominal cavity. Intravesical excision involves pulling the diverticulum into the bladder. Tension is then applied to the everted diverticulum and it is excised or divided at its base using electrocautery. If the diverticulum cannot be pulled into the bladder due to adhesions, the mucosa around the diverticular orifice is divided. Adhesions are lysed and the diverticulum is then pulled into the bladder and removed. The defect in the bladder wall is repaired. In 51530, a bladder tumor is excised. The tumor is excised along with a margin of health tissue using sharp dissection. The defect in the bladder is repaired with sutures. The bladder incision is closed. The abdominal incision is closed in layers.

51535

51535   Cystotomy for excision, incision, or repair of ureterocele

A ureterocele is a congenital cystic dilation of the submucosa of the ureter occurring in the distal aspect near the ureterovesical junction and protruding into the bladder. A midline extraperitoneal abdominal approach is used to expose the bladder. The rectus and transversalis fascia are divided and the incision is carried down through the space of Retzius. The anterior bladder wall and vesical neck are identified. The bladder dome is incised and the bladder wall is inspected including the trigone, ureteral orifices, and bladder neck. The ureterocele is identified. One of three surgical interventions is then used to treat the ureterocele -excision, incision, or repair. Excision involves making a

Urinary System

circumferential incision around the ureterocele using electrocautery and removing the dilated submucosal tissue. Incision is used to deflate the ureterocele. The full-thickness incision begins at the roof of the ureterocele. The incision is extended to the base of the defect. Repair involves excision of the ureterocele using electrocautery and then repairing any defects in the ureteral or bladder wall associated with the ureterocele.

51550-51565

51550   **Cystectomy, partial; simple**

51555   **Cystectomy, partial; complicated (eg, postradiation, previous surgery, difficult location)**

51565   **Cystectomy, partial, with reimplantation of ureter(s) into bladder (ureteroneocystostomy)**

Partial cystectomy is typically performed for localized malignant neoplasm of the bladder. The bladder is exposed using a low midline or transverse suprapubic incision. Lesions in the posterior bladder are typically approached intraperitoneally while lesions in the dome or anterior bladder are approached extraperitoneally. Separately reportable pelvic lymph node dissection is performed as needed. The bladder is then mobilized. Stay sutures are strategically placed at a site distant from the lesion. The bladder is incised between the stay sutures and enlarged to allow good visualization of the lesion. The portion of the bladder containing the lesion is then excised along with overlying perivesical fat and peritoneum, taking care to remove a margin of healthy tissue as well. The submucosa and muscle of the bladder wall are closed in layers. Use 51550, a simple partial cystectomy is done, which includes initial bladder procedures and/or those where the lesion is easily accessible. Use 51555, a complicated procedure is done, which includes those where a previous bladder surgery has been performed, the patient has received radiation treatment affecting the lower abdomen or bladder, or lesions are difficult to access. Use 51565, ureteral re-implantation is also performed. Ureteral re-implantation is required when the ureteral orifice must be sacrificed in order to ensure complete removal of the lesion. The site for the re-implantation is selected and incised. A submucosal tunnel is created from the incision site to the desired exit site of the ureter. The ureter is passed through the tunnel and secured with sutures.

51570-51575

51570   **Cystectomy, complete; (separate procedure)**

51575   **Cystectomy, complete; with bilateral pelvic lymphadenectomy, including external iliac, hypogastric, and obturator nodes**

Complete cystectomy is performed for conditions such as malignant neoplasm, severe radiation or chemical cystitis, refractory interstitial cystitis, hemorrhagic cystitis, neurogenic bladder disease, severe incontinence, trauma, fistula, upper urinary tract obstruction, or refractory urethral stricture. When urinary diversion has been performed during a previous surgical encounter, an extraperitoneal approach is typically used. The bladder is exposed using a low midline or transverse suprapubic incision. Overlying fascia is divided and the space of Retzius is entered. Pelvic lymph node dissection is performed as needed. Fatty tissue is stripped from the mid-portion of the common iliac vessels bilaterally and from the internal and external iliac vessels to the level of the circumflex iliac vein. Iliac, hypogastric, and obturator nodes are excised bilaterally. Following pelvic lymphadenectomy, blunt and sharp dissection is used to separate the parietal peritoneum from the dome and posterior wall of the bladder. The superior bladder (vesical) pedicles are clamped and divided. Any remaining portions of the distal ureters are freed from surrounding structures. Dissection of the posterior bladder, bladder neck, and base of the bladder continues until the entire bladder is completely freed from all surrounding structures. The lateral vascular pedicles are ligated and divided. The urethra is divided and the bladder is removed. If complete cystectomy is performed without pelvic lymphadenectomy, use code 51570; if pelvic lymphadenectomy is performed, use code 51575.

51580-51585

51580   **Cystectomy, complete, with ureterosigmoidostomy or ureterocutaneous transplantations**

51585   **Cystectomy, complete, with ureterosigmoidostomy or ureterocutaneous transplantations; with bilateral pelvic lymphadenectomy, including external iliac, hypogastric, and obturator nodes**

The entire bladder is removed, and the ureters are connected to the large intestine or the skin surface to drain urine. When urinary diversion is performed in conjunction with complete cystectomy, an intraperitoneal approach is used. The abdomen is incised in the midline. Prior to opening the peritoneum, pelvic lymph nodes are dissected as needed. Fatty tissue is stripped from the mid-portion of the common iliac vessels bilaterally and from the internal and external iliac vessels to the level of the circumflex iliac vein. Iliac, hypogastric, and obturator nodes are excised bilaterally. The peritoneum opened. The small bowel is isolated and packed out of the surgical field. The ureters are exposed and mobilized taking care to preserve perirenal tissue and blood supply. The ureters are divided as close to the ureterovesical junction as possible. A segment of the sigmoid colon is selected and mobilized. A tunnel is created from the sigmoid colon to the ureters. The ureters are pulled through the tunnel and into the lumen of the sigmoid colon. The ends of the ureters are spatulated along the anterior aspect. Stents are placed in both ureters.

The ureters are anastomosed to the sigmoid colon. The stents are then pulled through the colon exiting through the anus. Alternatively, the ureters may be transplanted to the skin. Following mobilization of the ureters, a catheter is passed through each ureter and into the renal pelvis. The catheters may be left in place and attached to the skin or a stoma may be created the ureters sutured to the stoma. Following completion of the urinary diversion procedure, blunt and sharp dissection is used to mobilize the bladder. The superior bladder (vesical) pedicles are clamped and divided. Any remaining portions of the distal ureters are freed from surrounding structures. Dissection continues until the entire bladder is completely freed from all surrounding structures. The lateral vascular pedicles are ligated and divided. The urethra is divided and the bladder is removed. Drains are placed as needed and surgical incisions are closed in layers. If the procedure is performed without pelvic lymphadenectomy, use code 51580; if pelvic lymphadenectomy is performed, use code 51585.

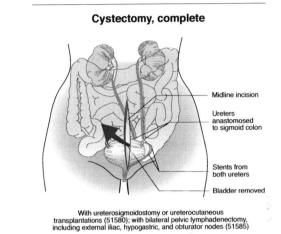

Cystectomy, complete

Midline incision

Ureters anastomosed to sigmoid colon

Stents from both ureters

Bladder removed

With ureterosigmoidostomy or ureterocutaneous transplantations (51580); with bilateral pelvic lymphadenectomy, including external iliac, hypogastric, and obturator nodes (51585)

51590-51595

51590   **Cystectomy, complete, with ureteroileal conduit or sigmoid bladder, including intestine anastomosis**

51595   **Cystectomy, complete, with ureteroileal conduit or sigmoid bladder, including intestine anastomosis; with bilateral pelvic lymphadenectomy, including external iliac, hypogastric, and obturator nodes**

When urinary diversion is performed in conjunction with complete cystectomy, an intraperitoneal approach is used. The abdomen is incised in the midline. Prior to opening the peritoneum, pelvic lymph nodes are dissected as needed. Fatty tissue is stripped from the mid-portion of the common iliac vessels bilaterally and from the internal and external iliac vessels to the level of the circumflex iliac vein. Iliac, hypogastric, and obturator nodes are excised bilaterally. The peritoneum is opened. The small bowel is isolated and packed out of the surgical field. The ureters are exposed and mobilized taking care to preserve perirenal tissue and blood supply. The ureters are divided as close to the ureterovesical junction as possible. Either a segment of ileum or sigmoid colon is isolated depending on whether a ureteroileal conduit or sigmoid bladder is constructed. The remaining bowel segments distal and proximal to the isolated segment are anastomosed and bowel continuity is resorted. A separate abdominal or perineal incision is made for creation of the stoma through which urine will be expelled. Dissection is carried down to the anterior rectus fascia which is incised. The rectus muscle is divided using blunt dissection. If an ileal conduit is constructed, the distal end of the conduit is pulled through the abdominal wall, everted, and sutured to skin or subcutaneous tissues to create the stoma. The proximal end of the conduit is closed with sutures. A tunnel is created from the conduit to the ureters. The ureters are pulled through the tunnel to the conduit. The ends of the ureters are spatulated. Stents are placed in both ureters. Small incisions are made in the conduit and the ureters are anastomosed to the conduit approximately 3 cm apart. If a sigmoid bladder is constructed, the sigmoid bladder is fashioned. A tunnel is created from the sigmoid bladder to the ureters. The ureters are pulled through the tunnel to the sigmoid bladder and into the lumen of the sigmoid. The ends of the ureters are spatulated along the anterior aspect. Stents are placed in both ureters. The ureters are anastomosed to the sigmoid bladder approximately 3 cm apart. The sigmoid bladder is exteriorized through the stomal incision, folded back on itself (everted), and sutured to the skin or subcutaneous tissue, creating either an abdominal or perineal colostomy. An ostomy bag is secured over the ostomy site. Following completion of the urinary diversion procedure, blunt and sharp dissection is used to mobilize the bladder. The superior bladder (vesical) pedicles are clamped and divided. Any remaining portions of the distal ureters are freed from surrounding structures. Dissection continues until the entire bladder is completely freed from all surrounding structures. The lateral vascular pedicles are ligated and divided. The urethra is divided and the bladder is removed. Drains are placed as needed and surgical incisions are closed in layers. If the procedure is performed without pelvic

Urinary System

lymphadenectomy, use code 51590; if pelvic lymphadenectomy is performed, use code 51595.

51596

51596   Cystectomy, complete, with continent diversion, any open technique, using any segment of small and/or large intestine to construct neobladder

Bladder resection is performed in conjunction with continent urinary diversion. Continent urinary diversion differs from other urinary diversion procedures in that the patient may void normally through the urethra. Alternatively, a stoma may be created with a valve mechanism using intussuscepted colon that prevents leakage of urine. With this type of stoma, the patient removes urine by periodically catheterizing the pouch. The abdomen is incised in the midline. The small bowel is isolated and packed out of the surgical field. The ureters are exposed, mobilized, and divided distally near the ureterovesical junction and the ureteral stumps are ligated. Blunt and sharp dissection is used to mobilize the bladder. The superior bladder (vesical) pedicles are clamped and divided. Any remaining portions of the distal ureters are freed from surrounding structures. Dissection continues until the entire bladder is completely freed from all surrounding structures. The lateral vascular pedicles are ligated and divided. The urethra is divided and the bladder is removed. A segment of small or large intestine is selected and mobilized. The segment, usually 30-35 cm of intestine, from which the pouch is to be constructed, is isolated. The intestine is divided leaving the isolated segment attached to the mesenteric pedicle keeping blood supply intact. The remaining distal and proximal portions of the intestine are then anastomosed and bowel continuity is restored. The intestinal pouch is fashioned by arranging the isolated segment in a U or W configuration. The segment is incised longitudinally along the mesenteric border to detubularize it. The intestine is fashioned into a pouch. A tunnel is created from the pouch to the ureters. The ureters are pulled through the tunnel to the pouch. The ends of the ureters are spatulated along the anterior aspect and anastomosed to the pouch approximately 3 cm apart. The distal aspect of the pouch may be incised and anastomosed to the bladder neck in females or the proximal urethra in males. Alternatively, a stoma may be created through a separate incision. When a stoma is created, the pouch is configured and detubularized as described above except for the portion of intestine that will be used to form the valve. The remaining tubular segment is scarified using electrocautery and adjacent mesentery is excised. The scarified segment is telescoped (intussuscepted) into the pouch and secured with sutures, creating the valve. The valve component is then sutured to the previously prepared stoma site in the abdominal wall. A catheter is placed through the valve into the stoma. Drains are placed as needed and surgical incisions are closed in layers.

51597

51597   Pelvic exenteration, complete, for vesical, prostatic or urethral malignancy, with removal of bladder and ureteral transplantations, with or without hysterectomy and/or abdominoperineal resection of rectum and colon and colostomy, or any combination thereof

Pelvic exenteration is performed to treat a primary bladder, prostatic, and/or urethral malignancy that has spread to other pelvic tissues or organs. The extent of the procedure depends on which organs have metastatic disease. The procedure includes removal of the bladder with urinary diversion and resection of the rectum and colon with colostomy as needed. Reproductive organs may also be removed if they have not been removed during a previous surgery. Females will have the uterus, ovaries, fallopian tubes, and cervix removed. Males will have the prostate removed. The abdomen is opened and explored. The liver, peritoneum, bowel, and aortic and pelvic lymph nodes are inspected. Biopsies are taken as needed. The pararectal, paravesical, and Retzius spaces are opened. If a total hysterectomy is needed, the round ligaments are cut and tied. The broad ligaments are opened. The infundibulopelvic ligaments are clamped, cut, and tied along with the ovarian vessels. If a prostatectomy is needed, the prostate is dissected free of surrounding tissues and removed. The retroperitoneal space is opened and the ureters are exposed. The hypogastric artery is identified and divided. The cardinal ligaments are divided. The ureters are dissected free of surrounding tissue, ligated, and divided. The rectal space between the rectosigmoid colon and the sacrum/coccyx is developed. The sigmoid arcade and superior vessels are ligated. The rectosigmoid colon is divided. The rectum is elevated and freed from surrounding tissues. The bladder is freed from the pubic symphysis. The urethra, rectum, and vagina are divided below the level of the malignancy. All involved pelvic organs are removed, including some or all of the following: ovaries, tubes, uterus, cervix, bladder, distal ureters, rectum, and colon. Following removal of involved organs, the rectum and colon are anastomosed or a colostomy is performed. The proximal ureters are then transplanted to provide urinary diversion. If noncontinent diversion is employed, a ureteroileal conduit may be created by implanting the ureters in a segment of ileum which is then brought out in a cutaneous stoma. Alternatively, a continent pouch using the right colon may be developed. The exenterated pelvis is reconstructed using omental, myocutaneous and/or muscle flaps.

51600

51600   Injection procedure for cystography or voiding urethrocystography

Contrast media is instilled into the bladder using a technique other than retrograde injection of contrast. For example, if the patient has a suprapubic catheter, contrast is injected through the existing catheter. For cystography, separately reportable radiographs are taken of the bladder as it is filled with contrast. Any filling abnormalities are noted. For voiding cystourethrography, separately reportable radiographs are taken as the bladder is filled and additional radiographs are obtained of the bladder and urethra as the bladder is emptied.

51605

51605   Injection procedure and placement of chain for contrast and/or chain urethrocystography

A tube containing a beaded chain and catheter are introduced through the urethra. Contrast is injected. Separately reportable radiographs are obtained. Chain cystourethrography is an outdated diagnostic procedure that was used to evaluate stress incontinence in women. The chain allowed assessment of urethral hypermobility and the degree of bladder descent. This procedure has largely been replaced by video urodynamic studies.

51610

51610   Injection procedure for retrograde urethrocystography

Retrograde cystourethrography is performed to evaluate the size, shape, and capacity of the bladder and urethra. The physician also evaluates whether there is any vesicoureteral reflux, which is reverse flow of urine back into the ureters and kidneys. The urethral orifice is cleansed with antiseptic. A sterile catheter is inserted through the urethra into the bladder. Contrast media is then instilled into the bladder. Separately reportable radiographs are taken of the bladder as it is filled with contrast. Any filling abnormalities are noted. The patient may be asked to strain, or pressure may be applied to the abdomen to see if there is any reflux into the ureters and kidneys. The head of the x-ray table may be lowered and additional radiographs taken. The catheter is then removed and additional radiographs are obtained of the bladder and urethra as the bladder is emptied.

51700

51700   Bladder irrigation, simple, lavage and/or instillation

A lavage procedure which involves instillation and removal of fluid or only an instillation procedure may be performed. A catheter is inserted into the bladder. If a lavage is being performed for bladder irrigation, normal saline is instilled and then removed from the bladder. Lavage is performed to help prevent or treat blood clots in bladder. Instillation may be performed with normal saline or a medication such as an antibiotic. Antibiotic instillation may be done over a period of time as a continuous drip into the bladder. Once the lavage and/or instillation procedure is completed, the catheter may be removed from the bladder or left in place to drain urine.

51701

51701   Insertion of non-indwelling bladder catheter (eg, straight catheterization for residual urine)

A non-indwelling catheter is inserted into the bladder. This may be referred to as straight catheterization. Straight catheterization is performed to empty the bladder of urine or to test for residual urine following urination which indicates incomplete emptying of the bladder. If the patient is being checked for residual urine, the patient first empties the bladder into a container and the amount is measured. A catheter kit is prepared. The urethra is cleansed with antiseptic solution. A sterile catheter is then inserted through the urethra into the bladder. Urine is drained from the bladder and the amount of residual urine is measured.

51702-51703

51702   Insertion of temporary indwelling bladder catheter; simple (eg, Foley)
51703   Insertion of temporary indwelling bladder catheter; complicated (eg, altered anatomy, fractured catheter/balloon)

A temporary indwelling catheter is inserted into the bladder. This may be referred to as Foley catheterization. A catheter kit is prepared. The urethra is cleansed with antiseptic solution. A sterile Foley catheter is inserted through the urethra into the bladder. The balloon is then inflated with about 10 cc of water to keep it in place. The catheter is attached to a sterile drainage bag and urine is continuously drained from the bladder. Use 51702 for a simple catheterization procedure and 51703 for a procedure complicated by altered anatomy or a fractured catheter or balloon.

51705-51710

51705   Change of cystostomy tube; simple
51710   Change of cystostomy tube; complicated

The physician changes a previously placed cystostomy tube. The cystostomy tube is changed periodically to prevent encrustation of the tube. Separately reportable imaging guidance may be used. A guidewire is inserted through the existing cystostomy tube. The pursestring suture securing the existing catheter is removed. The existing tube is removed. A new cystostomy tube is passed over the guidewire and into the bladder. The new tube is secured with a pursestring suture. Use 51705 if the tube change is simple and 51710 if it is complicated, such as a procedure performed on a patient with altered anatomy or when the tube has adhered to the cystostomy tunnel.

51715

51715   Endoscopic injection of implant material into the submucosal tissues of the urethra and/or bladder neck

This procedure is performed to treat mild incontinence due to thinning of tissues at the bladder outlet. A cystourethroscope is placed at the bladder outlet so that the outlet can be visualized while the injection procedure is performed. The physician then injects implant material, usually collagen or a newer material composed of water based gel containing carbon coated beads. The implant material is injected into the submucosal tissues surrounding the urethra and/or bladder neck. Once the bladder outlet tissues have been plumped up and any floppiness of the bladder outlet valve relieved, the cystourethroscope is removed. The injection procedure may need to be repeated two to three times over the course of several weeks to achieve the desired level of valve closure and prevent incontinence.

51720

51720   Bladder instillation of anticarcinogenic agent (including retention time)

An anticarcinogenic agent is prepared per the manufacturer's instructions. The urethral orifice is cleansed and a catheter is inserted through the urethra into the bladder. The bladder is drained of urine. The anticarcinogenic agent is instilled into the bladder through the catheter and the catheter is removed. The patient is then repositioned, periodically rotating from the right side, back, left side, and stomach to ensure that the anticarcinogenic agent comes in contact with all bladder surfaces over the course of the treatment period which may be as long as two hours. Upon completion of the treatment, the patient empties the bladder into the toilet.

51725

51725   Simple cystometrogram (CMG) (eg, spinal manometer)

A cystometrogram (CMG) is performed to measure bladder capacity and bladder storage pressures. CMG is used to evaluate conditions such as urinary incontinence, difficulty with urination, and neurogenic bladder. Prior to the CMG, the patient empties the bladder and the amount is measured. The urethra is cleansed with antiseptic solution. A sterile catheter with a sensor is then inserted through the urethra into the bladder. The bladder is then filled with sterile saline and the physician queries the patient about the sensations experienced during the filling process including fullness, pain, urgency, and leakage. Simple CMG (51725) measures bladder capacity and storage pressures using a spinal manometer or by simply observing the column of fluid entering the bladder. The patient may be asked to cough or strain to increase abdominal pressure which allows the physician to evaluate any stress incontinence. Complex CMG (51726) uses calibrated electronic equipment and measures intra-abdominal, total bladder, and true detrusor pressures simultaneously. The detrusor is the muscular wall of the bladder. Complex CMG can differentiate between involuntary detrusor contraction or reversed bladder compliance due to increased intra-abdominal pressure. Emptying pressures are not measured during simple or complex CMG. Only bladder capacity and storage pressures are measured.

51726-51729

51726   Complex cystometrogram (ie, calibrated electronic equipment)
51727   Complex cystometrogram (ie, calibrated electronic equipment); with urethral pressure profile studies (ie, urethral closure pressure profile), any technique
51728   Complex cystometrogram (ie, calibrated electronic equipment); with voiding pressure studies (ie, bladder voiding pressure), any technique
51729   Complex cystometrogram (ie, calibrated electronic equipment); with voiding pressure studies (ie, bladder voiding pressure) and urethral pressure profile studies (ie, urethral closure pressure profile), any technique

A cystometrogram (CMG) is performed to measure bladder capacity and bladder storage pressures. CMG is used to evaluate conditions such as urinary incontinence, difficulty with urination, and neurogenic bladder. Prior to the CMG, the patient empties the bladder and the amount is measured. The urethra is cleansed with antiseptic solution. A sterile catheter with a sensor is then inserted through the urethra into the bladder. The bladder is then filled with sterile saline and the physician queries the patient about the sensations experienced during the filling process including fullness, pain, urgency, and leakage. In

51726, a complex CMG is performed using calibrated electronic equipment that measures intra-abdominal, total bladder and true detrusor pressures simultaneously. The detrusor is the muscular wall of the bladder. Complex CMG can differentiate between involuntary detrusor contraction and reversed bladder compliance due to increased intra-abdominal pressure. In 51727, a complex CMG is performed as described above with urethral pressure profile studies that provide information on the ability of the urethra to prevent leakage of urine. A fluid-filled catheter with multiple radial lumen openings is advanced into the bladder. The catheter is continuously perfused with saline solution as the catheter is pulled through the urethra at a slow continuous rate. The catheter contains a sensor that is connected to recording device. As the catheter is removed urethral pressures are recorded and a tracing of the pressures provided. In 51728, a complex CMG is performed voiding pressure studies (VP) are performed using any technique. A catheter is inserted into the bladder and the bladder filled with fluid. A device is used to measure the amount of pressure the bladder can generate and the flow of urine. After filling the bladder with fluid, the patient is asked to void. Sensors record pressures prior to voiding, sphincter opening pressure and opening time, maximum voiding pressure, pressure at maximum flow, and flow during and after bladder contractions. Multiple bladder fills may be necessary to accurately evaluate bladder voiding pressure. In 51729, a complex CMG is performed with urethral pressure profile and voiding pressure studies as described above. Following completion of the complex CMG and additional studies, the physician interprets the studies and provides a written report.

51736-51741

51736   Simple uroflowmetry (UFR) (eg, stop-watch flow rate, mechanical uroflowmeter)
51741   Complex uroflowmetry (eg, calibrated electronic equipment)

Simple (51736) or complex (51741) uroflowmetry (UFR) is performed to measure urine flow rate. This test evaluates detrusor muscle contraction and bladder neck and urethral function. The detrusor muscle is the muscular wall of the bladder that contracts during urination. Contraction of the detrusor works in conjunction with gravity and increased intra-abdominal pressure to facilitate emptying of the bladder. Decreased flow rate may be caused by poor detrusor function due to neurological lesions, obstruction due to benign prostatic hypertrophy, or bladder prolapse (cystocele). Increased flow rate may be due to urethral sphincter dysfunction. In 51736, the flow of urine is visually observed to gauge the flow and a stop watch may be used to determine how long it takes to empty the bladder. In 51741, calibrated electronic equipment is used to measure the flow of urine.

51784-51785

51784   Electromyography studies (EMG) of anal or urethral sphincter, other than needle, any technique
51785   Needle electromyography studies (EMG) of anal or urethral sphincter, any technique

Electromyography (EMG) measures the electrical activity in the anal or urethral sphincter muscles. Muscles and nerves generate electrical impulses that facilitate sphincter contraction and relaxation. If electrical impulses are impaired, the sphincter will not open and close properly. In 51784, an EMG electrode patch is placed around the urethral sphincter or anal sphincter and muscle impulses recorded. EMG of the anal or urethral sphincter using an electrode patch is performed at the time of separately reportable complex cystometrogram (CMG) or voiding pressure (VP) studies. Electrical activity is recorded during filling and emptying of the bladder. In 51785, needles are placed in the urethral or anal sphincter to obtain information on pelvic floor muscle activity. This test is performed during separately reportable complex CMG in patients with neurological disease to record electrical impulses during filling and emptying of the bladder.

51792

51792   Stimulus evoked response (eg, measurement of bulbocavernosus reflex latency time)

Stimulus evoked response is performed to measure bulbocavernosus reflex latency time. In men, the bulbocavernosus muscle constricts the bulbous urethra during urination allowing the last drops of urine to be expelled. In women, the bulbocavernosus muscle helps support the pelvic floor. Stimulus evoked response is used to help evaluate cauda equina syndrome. The glans penis or clitoris is stimulated, which in turn stimulates the sacral reflex arch (S2-S4). As the sacral reflex arch is stimulated, motor activity of the urethral sphincter in men or the pelvic floor in women is evaluated.

51797

51797   Voiding pressure studies, intra-abdominal (ie, rectal, gastric, intraperitoneal) (List separately in addition to code for primary procedure)

Abdominal voiding pressure measures how much the patient must strain to void. A catheter is inserted into the rectum and a device used to measure intra-abdominal pressure. The bladder is filled with fluid. Intra-abdominal pressure is recorded as the patient voids. Multiple bladder fills may be necessary to accurately evaluate intra-abdominal pressure. The physician then interprets the intra-abdominal voiding pressure and compares it to the total bladder (intravesical) voiding pressure to obtain the true intravesical pressure during

Urinary System

voiding. Intra-abdominal voiding pressure (AP) (rectal, gastric, intraperitoneal) is evaluated at the time of a separately reportable bladder voiding pressure study.

51798

51798   Measurement of post-voiding residual urine and/or bladder capacity by ultrasound, non-imaging

Post-voiding residual urine and/or bladder capacity is measured using nonimaging ultrasound. An ultrasound probe which may be part of a hand-held unit or a larger conventional ultrasound unit is placed on the patient's abdomen over the bladder. Sound waves are transmitted from the transducer to the bladder and reflected back from the bladder to the transducer. Data from multiple cross-sectional scans are then transmitted to a computer within the ultrasound unit and the computer calculates bladder capacity including bladder volume measurements. When post-voiding residual is measured, the patient is asked to urinate and the amount of urine remaining in the bladder after urination is then measured using the ultrasound device and computer calculations.

51800-51820

51800   Cystoplasty or cystourethroplasty, plastic operation on bladder and/or vesical neck (anterior Y-plasty, vesical fundus resection), any procedure, with or without wedge resection of posterior vesical neck

51820   Cystourethroplasty with unilateral or bilateral ureteroneocystostomy

Plastic reconstruction of the bladder, which may also include reconstruction of the vesical neck and urethra, is performed. Plastic reconstruction may be performed for congential anamolies, scarring or acquired deformities due to previous surgery, or traumatic injuries. There are a number of different reconstruction techniques that may be employed depending on the condition being treated. The bladder is exposed using a low midline or transverse suprapubic incision. A defect in the posterior bladder is typically approached intraperitoneally while defects in the dome, anterior bladder, vesical neck, and/or urethra are approached extraperitoneally. In 51800, the bladder is incised and the bladder defect is inspected. Portions of the bladder, bladder neck, or urethra may be excised. The bladder wall is reconfigured as needed. For example, to reconfigure an enlarged bladder trigone, the wall of the bladder neck may be plicated or a Y-plasty may be performed. In 51820, the bladder defect is located near one or both ureteral orifices, and a ureteroneocystostomy is performed in conjunction with the cystourethroplasty. One or both ureters are ligated and transected at the ureterovesical junction. The bladder defect is then repaired and the ureters are transplanted to a new site in the bladder. An incision is made in the muscular wall of the bladder and a trough is created. The ureter(s) is placed in the trough in the detrusor muscle. An incision is made in the bladder mucosa at the distal aspect of the trough. The ureter(s) is secured to the interior aspect of the bladder with sutures. The trough is closed over the proximal aspect of the ureter(s).

51840-51841

51840   Anterior vesicourethropexy, or urethropexy (eg, Marshall-Marchetti-Krantz, Burch); simple

51841   Anterior vesicourethropexy, or urethropexy (eg, Marshall-Marchetti-Krantz, Burch); complicated (eg, secondary repair)

The physician performs an anterior vesicourethropexy or urethropexy, also referred to as a Marshall-Marchetti-Kranz or Burch procedure or an abdominal bladder suspension. This procedure is performed to treat incontinence in women caused by stretching of the pelvic ligaments with vaginal wall prolapse. An incision is made in the abdomen and the bladder neck and urethra are exposed. The prolapsed vaginal wall and urethra are then suspended. Two sutures are placed through the paravaginal fascia, one on each side of the urethrovesical junction and oriented perpendicular to the vaginal axis. The sutures are then passed through the Cooper's ligament, pelvic fascia, or pubic bone, and tied to provide suspension and support to the bladder and urethra. If additional suspension is required, a second set of sutures may be placed along the base of the bladder. Use 51840 for simple bladder suspension in patients who have not been operated on previously (primary bladder suspension or repair). Use code 51841 for a complex procedure in patients with a failed suspension procedure requiring secondary repair.

51845

51845   Abdomino-vaginal vesical neck suspension, with or without endoscopic control (eg, Stamey, Raz, modified Pereyra)

The physician performs an abdomino-vaginal vesical neck suspension, also referred to as a Stamey, Raz, or modified Pereyra procedure, or as a transvaginal needle bladder suspension, which may be performed with or without endoscopic control. This procedure is performed to treat anatomical incontinence in women caused by vaginal wall prolapse. Modified Pereyra procedure begins with a small transverse incision made at the distal urethra. A second vertical incision is made in the vagina and extended until it transects the incision at the distal urethra. The vaginal epithelium is dissected to the pubic rami. The endopelvic fascia is perforated and the puborethral ligaments are exposed. Heavy, nonabsorbable suture material is used to secure the puborethral ligaments to the endopelvic fascia. A small incision is made above the pubic bone (suprapubic incision). A ligature carrier is then passed through the suprapubic incision and advanced through

the vaginal incision. The sutures on each side of the urethra are threaded through the eye of the ligature carrier and then transferred to the abdominal wall. This may be performed using cystoscopic control to prevent bladder injury. Vaginal incisions are closed. The left and right sutures are then approached via the suprapubic incision and tied to suspend the bladder. The suprapubic incision is closed. The Raz procedure differs in that the retropubic space is entered to facilitate passage of the needle. The vaginal wall, excluding the vaginal musosa, is then anchored to the endopelvic fascia. The Stamey procedure uses two transverse suprapubic incisions, one on each side of the symphysis pubis. The rectus fascia is exposed. A T-shaped vaginal incision is made below the urethral meatus. The Stamey needle is introduced through one of the suprapubic incisions and passed through the vaginal incision at the level of the bladder neck. A suture is placed through the needle which is then withdrawn through the suprapubic incision. The needle is passed through the same suprapubic incision just lateral to the original needle entry site and carried into the vagina at a point just distal to the original entry site in the vagina. The suture is passed through a small synthetic tube which acts as a buttress for the vaginal loop. After capturing a large loop of vaginal tissue, the suture is again passed through the vaginal incision and pulled through the suprapubic incision. This is repeated on the opposite side. The vaginal incision is closed. Using cystoscopic control, tension is applied to the sutures via the suprapubic incisions to suspend the bladder and the sutures are tied. The suprapubic incisions are closed.

51860-51865

51860   Cystorrhaphy, suture of bladder wound, injury or rupture; simple

51865   Cystorrhaphy, suture of bladder wound, injury or rupture; complicated

A cystorrhaphy is performed for suture repair of bladder wound, injury or rupture. Types of bladder injuries include contusion with tear of the bladder mucosa, intraperitoneal laceration or rupture, interstitial injury, extraperitoneal laceration or rupture or a combination of these types of injuries. A Foley catheter is inserted and the bladder drained. A vertical midline incision is made in the abdomen. The pelvic viscera, ureters, bowel, and blood vessels, are inspected. The exterior of the bladder is inspected. The dome of the bladder is opened and the interior of the bladder inspected. Any foreign bodies are removed. The ureteral orifices are inspected to ensure that they are intact. The bladder injury is localized and any nonviable tissue debrided. The bladder injury is closed in layers in a watertight fashion. Omental fat may be interposed on the closure to cushion the bladder from associated pelvic fractures. Following closure, water or saline is instilled through the Foley catheter to ensure that no leakage occurs at the repair site. A suprapubic catheter may be placed through a separate incision along with a drain in the perivesical space. The abdomen is then closed in layers. Use code 51860 for a simple suture repair and code 51865 for a complicated repair. Complicated repairs include bladder injuries with foreign body, debris, extensive nonviable tissue, and pelvic fracture or other injury that complicates the

51880

51880   Closure of cystostomy (separate procedure)

The physician closes a cystostomy, a surgically created opening through the abdomen into the bladder through which a catheter is inserted for drainage. The drainage catheter is removed and the surgically created opening in the bladder is closed in a layered fashion. The opening in the abdominal wall and skin are also closed.

51900

51900   Closure of vesicovaginal fistula, abdominal approach

A vesicovaginal fistula is closed using an abdominal approach. A vesicovaginal fistula is an abnormal passage between the bladder and vagina through which urine is passing into the vaginal vault. The abdomen is incised and the bladder is exposed. An incision is made in the bladder, the ureters are catheterized, and the fistula tract is located. Stay sutures are placed around the fistula tract, which is then excised along with any scar tissue or necrotic tissue. The bladder wall is dissected free of the endopelvic fascia and vaginal wall. The vaginal wall defect is closed. The bladder wall defect is closed. The ureteral catheters are removed and the cystotomy is closed.

51920-51925

51920   Closure of vesicouterine fistula

51925   Closure of vesicouterine fistula; with hysterectomy

The physician closes a vesicouterine fistula. An incision is made in the lower abdomen and the abdomen and pelvis inspected. The vesicouterine space is dissected using sharp and blunt dissection. The fistulous tract is located and excised. The fistulous opening in the bladder is closed. The fistulous opening in the uterus is closed and omentum interposed between the bladder and uterus. The bladder is filled in a retrograde fashion and watertight repair of the bladder wall verified. The abdominal wall and skin are closed in a layered fashion. In 51925, the vesicouterine fistula is closed and a hysterectomy is performed. The fistula is excised and the bladder wall defect is closed as described above. The abdominal hysterectomy is then performed. The infundibulopelvic and round ligaments are identified, suture ligated, and divided. The bladder is reflected away from the cervix. Uterine and

● New Code   ▲ Revised Code   © 2017 DecisionHealth

Urinary System

cervical vessels are cross clamped, divided, and ligated. The vagina is incised and the cervix separated from the vagina. The vaginal cuff is closed. The uterus and cervix are removed, bleeding controlled, and the abdominal incision closed in a layered fashion.

51940

51940   Closure, exstrophy of bladder

Bladder exstophy is a congenital defect in which the bladder is flat instead of round and exposed outside the body. The defect also affects the abdominal wall, pelvic bones, bladder neck, perineum, urethra, and external genitalia. The abdominal wall is open. The symphysis pubis is widely separated at the midline with bony deficits at the anterior pubic rami as well as anterior rotation of the posterior and anterior aspects of the pelvis. There is also a shortening of the distance between the umbilicus and the anus due to shortening and broadening of the perineum. The musculature at the bladder neck does not form properly, affecting bladder control. There is shortening and broadening of the perineum. In girls, the urethra and vagina are shorter than normal and the labia are widely separated with a bifid clitoris. In boys, the penis appears shorter than normal because the base of the penis remains attached to the pubic bones internally. The failure of the pubic bones to fuse causes the base of the penis to spread apart internally. The procedure begins by bringing the pelvic bones together. Minor pelvic bone separation may be treated by medial rotation of the greater trochanters which will bring the pubic bones together at the midline. If the pelvic bones are widely separated, osteotomy may be required. Bilateral transverse anterior innominate bone and anterior vertical iliac bone osteotomies are performed with pin placement to close the separation at the symphysis pubis. Next, the bladder, posterior urethra, and abdominal wall are closed. An incision is made around the umbilicus and bladder and carried down to the urethral plate. The umbilical vessels are doubly ligated and transected. The bladder dome is separated from the peritoneum. The retropubic space is developed and the bladder is separated from the rectus sheath and muscle. In males, the prostrate is freed from the rectus muscle. The upper border of the urogenital diaphragm fibers between the bladder neck, posterior urethra, and pubic bone are sharply incised and separated down to the pelvic floor. In males, the prostate and anterior corpus are freed from the pubis by deep incision. Ureteral stents are placed; the bladder neck and urethra are reconstructed as needed; and the bladder wall is closed. The pubic bones are approximated using nylon sutures placed between the fibrous cartilages of the pubic rami. A drain is placed near the umbilicus and the abdominal wall is closed in layers.

51960

51960   Enterocystoplasty, including intestinal anastomosis

Enterocystoplasty, also referred to as bladder augmentation, uses a segment of intestine to enlarge the bladder and reduce intravesical pressure in patients with bladder neuropathy and high pressure detrusor contractions. Cystoscopic examination of the bladder is performed. Internal ureteral stents or external ureteral catheters are placed. The cystoscope is removed and a Foley catheter is placed. The abdomen is incised in the midline and the peritoneum is opened. The small bowel is isolated and packed out of the surgical field. The ureters are identified and protected. The portion of colon or ileum to be used for the augmentation is isolated and harvested. The remaining segments of bowel distal and proximal to the isolated segment are anastamosed and bowel continuity is restored. The harvested segment of bowel is detubularized and reconfigured into a U, S, or W shaped graft. The bladder is bivalved. A large caliber suprapubic catheter is placed in addition to the Foley catheter. The intestinal graft is sutured to the bladder. Drains are placed as needed and the abdomen is closed around the drains.

51980

51980   Cutaneous vesicostomy

Cutaneous vesicostomy, also referred to as cutaneous cystostomy, involves incising the bladder and creating a stoma on the skin to allow drainage of urine. The abdomen is incised and the rectus fascia is exposed. A triangular segment of fascia is excised. The rectus muscle is divided and the space of Retzius is entered. The dome of the bladder is exposed. The bladder is incised. The bladder wall is sutured to the rectus fascia. The bladder epithelium is sutured to the skin. An ostomy bag is placed over the stoma.

51990

51990   Laparoscopy, surgical; urethral suspension for stress incontinence

A urethral suspension procedure for stress incontinence is performed via a laparoscopic approach. A small incision is made just below the umbilicus and the laparoscope is introduced. Two or three additional small incisions are made in the abdomen to allow introduction of surgical instruments. The intraperitoneal cavity is inspected. The space of Retzius is dissected and the paravaginal fascia is identified and elevated. Two endoscopic sutures are then placed through the paravaginal fascia-one on each side of the urethrovesical junction and oriented perpendicular to the vaginal axis. The sutures are passed through Cooper's ligament and tied. This elevates the urethrovesical angle and provides a platform on which the bladder neck rests. The suspension is then checked visually, manually, or by cystoscopy to ensure that it is adequate. If additional suspension

is required, a second set of sutures may be placed along the base of the bladder. The laparoscope and surgical instruments are removed and the abdominal incisions are closed.

51992

51992   Laparoscopy, surgical; sling operation for stress incontinence (eg, fascia or synthetic)

A sling operation is performed to treat stress incontinence using a fascial or synthetic graft via a laparoscopic approach. If a fascial autograft is being used, a small incision is made over the lower abdomen or thigh and a strip of fascia is removed. Four small incisions are then made in the abdomen and trocars are placed. The laparoscope is introduced and the retropubic space is dissected out. The fascial or synthetic graft is introduced laparoscopically. An incision is made in the anterior vaginal wall over the bladder neck. A small tunnel is created on one side of the bladder neck and a long clamp is advanced through the vaginal incision into the retropubic space. One end of the fascial or synthetic sling is grasped and pulled into the vagina. The sling is then placed under the urethra and around the bladder neck and returned to the retropubic space through a second small tunnel on the other side of the bladder neck. The ends of the sling are sutured to the Cooper's ligament, pelvic fascia, or the abdominal wall. The laparoscope and surgical instruments are removed. The incisions in the abdomen and vaginal wall are closed.

52000

52000   Cystourethroscopy (separate procedure)

A cystourethroscopy is performed to visualize the inside of the bladder and urethra in a separate procedure. The urethra is cleansed with antiseptic solution. A rigid or flexible cystoscope consisting of a thin, telescope-like tube with a light and camera is introduced through the urethra into the bladder. The camera allows images of the urethra and bladder to be viewed on a computer or television monitor. The bladder may be filled with sterile saline or water to improve visualization of the bladder wall. Once the procedure is complete, the saline or water is drained from the bladder and the cystoscope is removed.

52001

52001   Cystourethroscopy with irrigation and evacuation of multiple obstructing clots

Cystourethroscopy is performed to visualize the inside of the bladder and urethra and remove obstructing blood clots. The urethra is cleansed with antiseptic solution. A rigid or flexible cystoscope is introduced through the urethra into the bladder. The bladder is inspected and obstructing blood clots are noted. The cystoscope is removed and a resectoscope is introduced into the bladder. The clots are broken up and evacuated. The bladder is flushed with sterile saline and inspected for any residual blood clots or bleeding. The resectoscope is removed. A catheter is inserted as needed for continuous bladder irrigation and/or drainage.

52005-52007

52005   Cystourethroscopy, with ureteral catheterization, with or without irrigation, instillation, or ureteropyelography, exclusive of radiologic service

52007   Cystourethroscopy, with ureteral catheterization, with or without irrigation, instillation, or ureteropyelography, exclusive of radiologic service; with brush biopsy of ureter and/or renal pelvis

Cystourethroscopy is performed to visualize the inside of the bladder and urethra with catheterization of the ureters. The urethra is cleansed with antiseptic solution. A rigid or flexible cystoscope is introduced through the urethra into the bladder. The bladder may be filled with sterile saline to allow better visualization of the bladder wall. In 52005, following inspection of the bladder, the ureters are catheterized. A guidewire is introduced through the cystoscope and advanced into the first ureter and through the ureter to the renal pelvis. A catheter is advanced over the guidewire to the renal pelvis. The ureter may be irrigated with normal saline, or diagnostic or therapeutic solution may be instilled. Contrast material may be injected and separately reportable ureteropyelography performed. The procedure may be repeated on the opposite ureter. Upon completion of the procedure, the catheter and guidewire are removed. In 52007, the ureters are catheterized as described above and tissue samples are obtained using a nylon or steel brush.

52010

52010   Cystourethroscopy, with ejaculatory duct catheterization, with or without irrigation, instillation, or duct radiography, exclusive of radiologic service

Cystourethroscopy is performed to visualize the inside of the bladder and urethra with catheterization of the ejaculatory ducts. The urethra is cleansed with antiseptic solution. A rigid or flexible cystoscope is introduced through the urethra into the bladder. The bladder may be filled with sterile saline to allow better visualization of the bladder wall. The bladder is inspected and the ureteral orifices are identified and examined. The cystoscope is pulled back into the proximal urethra, which is inspected and the ejaculatory ducts are located. Guidewires are advanced through the urethra and into the ejaculatory ducts. A catheter is threaded through each ejaculatory duct and the guidewires are removed. The ducts may be flushed with sterile saline or contrast injected for separately reportable ejaculatory duct

Urinary System

radiography. Upon completion of the procedure, the catheters are removed. The bladder, urethra, and ejaculatory duct orifices are re-inspected with the cystoscope, which is then removed.

52204

52204   Cystourethroscopy, with biopsy(s)

Cystourethroscopy is performed to visualize the inside of the bladder and urethra and tissue samples are obtained. The urethra is cleansed with antiseptic solution. A rigid or flexible cystoscope is introduced through the urethra into the bladder. The bladder may be filled with sterile saline to allow better visualization of the bladder wall. The bladder is inspected and the ureteral orifices are identified and examined. Biopsy forceps are introduced through the cystoscope and tissue samples are obtained. The bladder and urethra are re-inspected following biopsy and any bleeding is controlled. The cystoscope is removed.

52214

52214   Cystourethroscopy, with fulguration (including cryosurgery or laser surgery) of trigone, bladder neck, prostatic fossa, urethra, or periurethral glands

Cystourethroscopy is performed to visualize the inside of the bladder and urethra. Abnormal tissue in the distal aspect of the bladder (bladder trigone), bladder neck, prostatic fossa, urethra, or periurethral glands is destroyed using a high-frequency electrical current. The urethral orifice is cleansed with antiseptic solution. A rigid or flexible cystoscope is introduced through the urethra into the bladder. The bladder may be filled with sterile saline to allow better visualization of the bladder wall. The bladder is inspected and the ureteral orifices are identified and examined. The cystoscope is withdrawn and the prostatic fossa, urethra, and periurethral glands are examined and any abnormal tissue is noted. An electrocautery device is then advanced through the urethroscope to the site where the abnormal tissue is located. The device is activated and the lesion is destroyed. Alternatively, a laser or cryoprobe may be used to destroy the abnormal tissue. Upon completion of the procedure, the bladder trigone and neck, prostatic fossa, urethra, and periurethral glands are re-inspected to ensure that all abnormal tissue has been destroyed. The cystoscope is then removed.

52224-52240

52224   Cystourethroscopy, with fulguration (including cryosurgery or laser surgery) or treatment of MINOR (less than 0.5 cm) lesion(s) with or without biopsy
52234   Cystourethroscopy, with fulguration (including cryosurgery or laser surgery) and/or resection of; SMALL bladder tumor(s) (0.5 up to 2.0 cm)
52235   Cystourethroscopy, with fulguration (including cryosurgery or laser surgery) and/or resection of; MEDIUM bladder tumor(s) (2.0 to 5.0 cm)
52240   Cystourethroscopy, with fulguration (including cryosurgery or laser surgery) and/or resection of; LARGE bladder tumor(s)

Cystourethroscopy is performed to visualize the inside of the bladder and urethra and bladder tumors are destroyed using a high-frequency electrical current. The urethral orifice is cleansed with antiseptic solution. A rigid or flexible cystoscope is introduced through the urethra into the bladder. The bladder may be filled with sterile saline to allow better visualization of the bladder wall. The bladder is inspected and the ureteral orifices are identified and examined. Bladder tumors are located. An electrocautery device is then advanced through the urethroscope to the site where the tumors are located. The device is activated and the tumors are destroyed. Alternatively, a laser or cryoprobe may be used to destroy the tumors. Upon completion of the procedure, the bladder is re-inspected to ensure that all tumors have been destroyed. The cystoscope is then removed. In 52224, a minor lesion less than 0.5 cm is destroyed. In 52234, 52235, or 52240, larger bladder tumors are destroyed as described above, or resected. If resection is performed, the tumors are located as described above. The cystoscope is removed, a resectoscope is advanced to the site of the tumor and the tumor is resected. The tumor is removed using irrigation and a cystoscopic evacuation device. This is repeated until all tumors have been removed. Bleeding is controlled as needed using electrocoagulation or laser coagulation. Use 52234 for one or more small bladder tumors measuring 0.5 up to 2.0 cm in greatest diameter; use 52235 for medium bladder tumors measuring 2 to 5 cm, or 52240 for large bladder tumors measuring greater than 5 cm.

52250

52250   Cystourethroscopy with insertion of radioactive substance, with or without biopsy or fulguration

Cystourethroscopy is performed to visualize the inside of the bladder and urethra and bladder tumors are destroyed using a radioactive substance inserted at the tumor site. The urethral orifice is cleansed with antiseptic solution. A rigid or flexible cystoscope is introduced through the urethra into the bladder. The bladder may be filled with sterile saline to allow better visualization of the bladder wall. The bladder is inspected and the ureteral orifices are identified and examined. The bladder tumors are located. A tissue sample may be obtained using biopsy forceps. Tissue may also be destroyed by

electrocautery, laser, or other technique. If electrocautery is used, an electrocautery device is advanced through the urethroscope to the site where the tumor is located. The device is activated and the tumor is destroyed. The radioactive substance is then loaded into a delivery device and implanted into the bladder at the site of the malignancy. All surgical tools are removed along with the cystoscope. The radioactive implant may be left in the bladder for several days. When the internal radiation treatment is completed, the implant is removed using the cystoscope.

52260-52265

52260   Cystourethroscopy, with dilation of bladder for interstitial cystitis; general or conduction (spinal) anesthesia
52265   Cystourethroscopy, with dilation of bladder for interstitial cystitis; local anesthesia

Interstitial cystitis (IC), also referred to as painful bladder syndrome, is characterized by recurring bladder and pelvic pain that may be accompanied by frequent urination. Cystourethroscopy is performed to visualize the inside of the bladder and urethra. The urethral orifice is cleansed with antiseptic solution. A rigid or flexible cystoscope is introduced through the urethra into the bladder. The bladder is inspected and the ureteral orifices are identified and examined. Areas of inflammation, scarring, and fibrosis are noted. Any ulcerations in the bladder wall are also noted. Bladder distention is then performed to dilate the urinary bladder. This is accomplished by inserting a catheter and filling the bladder with normal saline or gas. If normal saline is used, it may be mixed with a local anesthetic agent. The saline or gas is left in the bladder for 10-15 minutes and then removed. The catheter is removed. The bladder and urethra may be re-examined using the cystoscope, which is then removed. Use 52260 when the procedure is performed using general or conduction (spinal anesthesia); use 52265 when local anesthesia is used.

52270-52276

52270   Cystourethroscopy, with internal urethrotomy; female
52275   Cystourethroscopy, with internal urethrotomy; male
52276   Cystourethroscopy with direct vision internal urethrotomy

Internal urethrotomy is performed to treat internal urethral stricture. Cystourethroscopy is performed to visualize the inside of the bladder and urethra and identify the area of urethral stricture. The urethral orifice is cleansed with antiseptic solution. A rigid or flexible cystoscope is introduced through the urethra into the bladder. The bladder is inspected and the ureteral orifices are identified and examined. The cystoscope is slowly removed and the area of stricture is identified. A cold knife incision is made at 12 o'clock or multiple radial incisions are made at the site of the stricture. If multiple areas of stricture are noted, the procedure is repeated until all narrowed portions of the urethra have been incised. The urethra is then re-examined using the cystoscope. The cystoscope is removed and a Foley catheter is placed through the urethra and into the bladder to help maintain the diameter of the treated areas. Use 52270 for incision of a female urethral stricture; use 52275 for a male; and use 52276 for direct vision urethrotomy. Direct vision urethrotomy is performed by inserting a special telescope which allows the physician to see the stricture and make incisions while visualizing the stricture.

52277

52277   Cystourethroscopy, with resection of external sphincter (sphincterotomy)

The external urethral sphincter is a ring-like muscle in the urethra that controls emptying of the bladder. Cystourethroscopy is performed to visualize the inside of the bladder and urethra and identify the area of the external sphincter. The urethral orifice is cleansed with antiseptic solution. A rigid or flexible cystoscope is introduced through the urethra into the bladder. The bladder is inspected and the ureteral orifices are identified and examined. The cystoscope is slowly removed and the area of the urethral sphincter is identified. Multiple radial incisions are made in the external urethral sphincter to help relax it and allow urine to pass more easily. The urethra is then re-examined using the cystoscope and any bleeding is controlled. The cystoscope is removed and a Foley catheter is placed through the urethra and into the bladder to help maintain the diameter of the urethral sphincter.

52281

52281   Cystourethroscopy, with calibration and/or dilation of urethral stricture or stenosis, with or without meatotomy, with or without injection procedure for cystography, male or female

Urethral calibration involves measuring the diameter of the narrowed portion of the urethra. Calibration and/or dilation of a urethral stricture or stenosis is typically performed only when the narrowed portion is at the distal aspect of the urethra or the urethral opening, called the urethral meatus. A series of cone-shaped instruments of increasing diameter called Bougies are advanced into the tip of the urethra and then withdrawn. The physician begins with the smallest size, usually an 8 French Bougie. If this size can be easily inserted and withdrawn, progressively larger diameter Bougies are inserted until resistance is felt. The largest size Bougie that can be inserted determines the diameter of the distal urethra. Once the diameter of the narrowed distal segment has been determined, the physician then examines the urethra using a cystourethroscope. Following visualization through the urethroscope, the physician determines the best treatment method. The stricture may be dilated using progressively larger sounds, a filiform and progressively larger followers, or a balloon catheter that is inflated and deflated at the site of the stricture. The urethral meatus may be incised in a radial fashion to open the narrowed portion. Contrast material may also be injected through the urethra and into the bladder and separately reportable cystography performed.

52282

52282   Cystourethroscopy, with insertion of permanent urethral stent

A permanent urethral stent is used to treat a persistent stricture or narrowing of the urethra. The urethral orifice is cleansed with antiseptic solution. A rigid or flexible cystoscope consisting of a thin, telescope-like tube with a light and camera is introduced through the urethra into the bladder. The camera allows images of the urethra and bladder to be viewed on a computer or television monitor. The bladder may be filled with sterile saline or water to improve visualization of the bladder wall. The saline or water is drained from the bladder and the narrowed portion of the urethra evaluated. An appropriately sized permanent urethral stent is selected and introduced into the urethra through the working channel of the cystoscope. The stent is positioned in the narrowed segment and deployed. The cystoscope is then removed.

52283

52283   Cystourethroscopy, with steroid injection into stricture

Steroid injection is performed to treat urethral stricture. Steroid injection is typically reserved for strictures of the distal urethra or meatus, strictures that occur following radical prostatectomy, or for patients who have had multiple urethroplasties. Cystourethroscopy is performed to visualize the urethra and identify the area of stricture. The urethral orifice is cleansed with antiseptic solution. A rigid or flexible cystoscope is introduced through the urethra and advanced to the area of the stricture. The narrowed portion of the urethra is injected with a steroid medication, and the cystoscope is removed.

52285

52285   Cystourethroscopy for treatment of the female urethral syndrome with any or all of the following: urethral meatotomy, urethral dilation, internal urethrotomy, lysis of urethrovaginal septal fibrosis, lateral incisions of the bladder neck, and fulguration of polyp(s) of urethra, bladder neck, and/or trigone

Female urethral syndrome is characterized by urinary frequency and pain on urination without the presence of a urinary tract infection or other urinary tract abnormality. The urethral orifice is cleansed with antiseptic solution. A rigid or flexible cystoscope is introduced through the urethra into the bladder. The bladder may be filled with sterile saline to allow better visualization of the bladder wall. The bladder is inspected and the ureteral orifices are identified and examined. The cystoscope is slowly withdrawn and the urethra is inspected. The physician may perform one or more therapeutic procedures depending on the cystoscopic findings, including urethral meatotomy or dilation, internal urethrotomy, lysis of urethrovaginal septum fibrosis, lateral incisions of the bladder neck, and/or fulguration of polyps. If the meatus is stenosed, a meatotomy may be performed by incising the urethral meatus. A urethral stricture may be dilated using progressively larger sounds, a filiform and progressively larger followers, or a balloon catheter. Polyps of the urethra, bladder neck, and/or trigone may be treated using an electrocautery device that is advanced through the urethroscope to the site where the polyps are located. The device is activated and the polyps are destroyed. Alternatively, a laser or cryoprobe may be used to destroy the polyps. Fibrotic adhesions at the urethrovaginal septum are severed as needed. Transurethral relaxing incisions are made at the bladder neck as needed. Upon completion of the procedure, the bladder trigone, neck, and urethra are re-inspected with the cystoscope and any bleeding is controlled. The cystoscope is then removed.

52287

52287   Cystourethroscopy, with injection(s) for chemodenervation of the bladder

Chemodenervation involves the injection of a toxin (type A botulinum) directly into a muscle to produce temporary muscle paralysis by blocking the release of acetylcholine. Multiple injections are often required to achieve denervation. Chemical denervation begins within 2 to 3 days of the injection and lasts approximately 3 to 6 months. After anesthetizing the urethra and bladder, the physician places the cystoscope and begins injecting Botox across the back of the trigone and in a radial fashion from the trigone up the posterior wall, and toward the dome of the bladder. Treatment of urinary incontinence due to detrusor overactivity involves Botox injected cystoscopically into the detrusor muscle at 30 different locations. Intravesical or sphincteric injections of Botox A are used to treat overactive bladder and functional outlet obstruction.

52290

52290   Cystourethroscopy; with ureteral meatotomy, unilateral or bilateral

Cystourethroscopy is performed to visualize the inside of the bladder, ureteral orifices, and urethra and incise restricted ureteral opening(s). The urethral orifice is cleansed with

antiseptic solution. A rigid or flexible cystoscope is introduced through the urethra into the bladder. The bladder is inspected and the ureteral orifices are identified and examined. A retractable blade is introduced through the cystoscope and advanced to the ureteral orifice. The blade is exposed and the intravesical ureteral orifice is incised. The procedure is repeated on the opposite side as needed. The incisions are inspected with the cystoscope and bleeding is controlled. The cystoscope is removed.

52300-52301

52300   Cystourethroscopy; with resection or fulguration of orthotopic ureterocele(s), unilateral or bilateral

52301   Cystourethroscopy; with resection or fulguration of ectopic ureterocele(s), unilateral or bilateral

This procedure may also be referred to as endoscopic or transurethral resection or fulguration of ureterocele. An ureterocele is a saccular out-pouching of the distal ureter that protrudes into the urinary bladder. An orthotopic ureterocele has its orifice located in the normal anatomic position in the bladder. An ectopic ureterocele has its orifice located in an abnormal position, often in the bladder neck or urethra. Cystourethroscopy is performed to visualize the inside of the bladder and ureteral orifices. The urethral orifice is cleansed with antiseptic solution. A rigid or flexible cystoscope is introduced through the urethra into the bladder. The bladder may be filled with sterile saline to allow better visualization of the bladder wall. The bladder is inspected and the ureterocele is identified and examined. If the ureterocele is fulgurated, an electrocautery device is then advanced through the urethroscope to the ureterocele. The device is activated and the out-pouching is destroyed. Alternatively, a laser or cryoprobe may be used to destroy the ureterocele. If resection is performed, the cystoscope is removed and a resectoscope is advanced to the site of the ureterocele, which is resected. Tissue is removed using irrigation and a cystoscopic evacuation device. Bleeding is controlled as needed using electrocoagulation or laser coagulation. The procedure is repeated on the contralateral ureter as needed. Upon completion of the procedure, the bladder and ureteral orifices are re-inspected to ensure that the abnormal portion of the ureter has been completed resected or destroyed. Use 52300 for unilateral or bilateral orthotopic ureteroceles; use 52301 for unilateral or bilateral ectopic ureteroceles.

52305

52305   Cystourethroscopy; with incision or resection of orifice of bladder diverticulum, single or multiple

A bladder diverticulum is a pouch in the bladder wall that may be congenital or acquired. Diverticula may cause ureteral obstruction or vesicoureteral reflux, recurrent urinary tract infections, or stone formation in the bladder. Cystourethroscopy is performed to visualize the inside of the bladder, ureteral orifices, or urethra. The urethral orifice is cleansed with antiseptic solution. A rigid or flexible cystoscope is introduced through the urethra into the bladder. The bladder may be filled with sterile saline to allow better visualization of the bladder wall. The bladder is inspected and the diverticulum is identified and examined. If the diverticulum is incised, a retractable blade is introduced through the cystoscope, the blade is exposed, and the diverticulum is incised. If resection is performed, the cystoscope is removed and a resectoscope is advanced to the site of the diverticulum, which is resected. Tissue is removed using irrigation and a cystoscopic evacuation device. Bleeding is controlled as needed using electrocoagulation or laser coagulation. If multiple diverticula are present, the procedure is repeated until all diverticula have been treated.

52310-52315

52310   Cystourethroscopy, with removal of foreign body, calculus, or ureteral stent from urethra or bladder (separate procedure); simple

52315   Cystourethroscopy, with removal of foreign body, calculus, or ureteral stent from urethra or bladder (separate procedure); complicated

Cystourethroscopy is performed to visualize the inside of the bladder, ureteral orifices, and urethra. The urethral orifice is cleansed with antiseptic solution. A rigid or flexible cystoscope is introduced through the urethra into the bladder. The bladder is inspected and a foreign body or calculus, or a ureteral stent is located. A grasping device is advanced through the working channel of the cystoscope and the foreign body, calculus, or ureteral stent is captured and removed from the bladder. The bladder and ureteral orifices are re-inspected to ensure that there has not been any injury to the bladder or ureters. The cystoscope is removed. Use 52310 for a simple removal; use 52315 for a complicated removal.

52317-52318

52317   Litholapaxy: crushing or fragmentation of calculus by any means in bladder and removal of fragments; simple or small (less than 2.5 cm)

52318   Litholapaxy: crushing or fragmentation of calculus by any means in bladder and removal of fragments; complicated or large (over 2.5 cm)

A scope is inserted into the bladder and the stone is visualized. To remove the stone by litholapaxy, a crushing instrument or mechanical disintegration probe or laser is inserted through the urethra into the bladder. The stone is then fragmented into smaller and smaller pieces until the remaining fragments are small enough to pass through an evacuation

Urinary System

catheter, which is then inserted through the urethra and into the bladder. The bladder is irrigated with sterile saline or other solution and the stone fragments are flushed out of the bladder through the catheter. The bladder is re-inspected with the scope to ensure that all stones have been pulverized and that all fragments have been flushed from the bladder. Use 52317 for simple litholaplaxy or small stones less than 2.5 cm; use 52318 for complicated litholaplaxy or large stones over 2.5 cm.

52320-52325

52320 **Cystourethroscopy (including ureteral catheterization); with removal of ureteral calculus**

52325 **Cystourethroscopy (including ureteral catheterization); with fragmentation of ureteral calculus (eg, ultrasonic or electro-hydraulic technique)**

The urethra is cleansed with antiseptic solution. A rigid or flexible cystoscope is introduced through the urethra into the bladder for cystourethroscopy to remove a stone from the ureter. The bladder may be filled with sterile saline to allow better visualization of the bladder wall. Following inspection of the bladder, the ureters are catheterized. A guidewire is introduced through the cystoscope and advanced through the ureter into the renal pelvis. In 52320, a grasping or retrieval device is advanced through the cystoscope over the guidewire to the calculus in the ureter, and the calculus is captured and removed. In 52325, the calculus is first fragmented using an ultrasonic or electrohydraulic technique. The ultrasonic or electrohydraulic probe is advanced through the cystoscope to the ureteral stone. The probe is activated and shockwaves are generated, causing fragmentation of the calculus. Following retrieval or fragmentation of the calculus, a catheter may be advanced over the guidewire to the renal pelvis and the ureter may be irrigated to remove calculus fragments. Diagnostic or therapeutic solution may also be instilled into the ureter through the catheter. Upon completion of the procedure, the catheter, guidewire, and cystoscope are removed.

52327

52327 **Cystourethroscopy (including ureteral catheterization); with subureteric injection of implant material**

The physician performs cystourethroscopy with subureteric injection of implant material including any required ureteral catheterization. This procedure may also be referred to as a subureteral transurethral injection or STING procedure. A modification of the STING procedure is the hydrodistention-implantation technique also referred to as a HIT procedure. A catheter is used to drain urine from the bladder. A cystourethroscope is inserted into the urethra and advanced into the bladder. The bladder is then partially filled with fluid in a retrograde fashion to allow better visualization of the ureteral orifice. The scope is advanced to the ureteral orifice. The ureter may be distended using a pressurized stream of irrigation fluid directed into the ureter. If ureteral catheterization is required, a couple of techniques may be employed. If guidewires are used, two are required. A safety guidewire is passed into the ureter first. A semirigid or flexible ureteroscope is then passed alongside the safety guidewire over a working guidewire and the ureter is catheterized by passing a temporary ureteral catheter over the working guidewire and positioning it in the ureter. Alternatively, a wireless or "no touch" technique may be used to position the catheter in the ureter. The ureteroscope is removed and a needle is passed through the cystourethroscope into the submucosa below the ureteral orifice. Implant material is then injected to elevate and narrow the ureteral orifice and support the ureter. The scope is withdrawn to the level of the bladder neck and the implant site is visualized to ensure that the implant material has been properly placed. The bladder is then emptied and the scope is withdrawn.

52330

52330 **Cystourethroscopy (including ureteral catheterization); with manipulation, without removal of ureteral calculus**

The urethra is cleansed with antiseptic solution. A rigid or flexible cystoscope is introduced through the urethra into the bladder. The bladder may be filled with sterile saline to allow better visualization of the bladder wall. Following inspection of the bladder, the ureter is catheterized. A guidewire is introduced through the cystoscope and advanced into the ureter and through the ureter to the renal pelvis. A grasping device is advanced through the cystoscope and the calculus is grasped and manipulated into a different location without removal. The ureter may be irrigated with normal saline. Upon completion of the procedure the catheter, guidewire, and cystoscope are removed.

52332

52332 **Cystourethroscopy, with insertion of indwelling ureteral stent (eg, Gibbons or double-J type)**

The urethra is cleansed with antiseptic solution. A rigid or flexible cystoscope is introduced through the urethra into the bladder. The bladder may be filled with sterile saline to allow better visualization of the bladder wall. Following inspection of the bladder, the ureter is catheterized. A guidewire is introduced through the cystoscope and advanced into the ureter and through the ureter to the renal pelvis. A stent is then advanced through the cystoscope, over the guidewire, and positioned within the ureter. The guidewire is removed, leaving the stent in place. The bladder is re-inspected and the position of the distal tail

of the stent is inspected to ensure that it is properly positioned in the bladder. Upon completion of the procedure, the cystoscope is removed.

52334

52334 **Cystourethroscopy with insertion of ureteral guide wire through kidney to establish a percutaneous nephrostomy, retrograde**

A nephrostomy is created endoscopically by means of a controlled, retrograde fine wire puncture from within the renal pelvis or calyx to provide percutaneous access to the kidney. The urethra is cleansed with antiseptic solution. A rigid or flexible cystoscope is introduced through the urethra into the bladder. The bladder may be filled with sterile saline to allow better visualization of the bladder wall. Following inspection of the bladder, the ureter is catheterized. A guidewire is introduced through the cystoscope and advanced into the ureter and through the ureter to the renal pelvis or desired calyx. A nephrostomy catheter is then advanced over the guidewire into the renal pelvis and then into the desired calix. The guidewire is removed, leaving the nephrostomy catheter in place. A sheathed needle is then advanced through the catheter. The needle is exposed and advanced through the calyx until it exits the skin. The nephrostomy tract is dilated over the needle. Once the desired diameter has been achieved, a nephrostomy tube is placed and secured with sutures. The needle, cystoscope, and other surgical devices are removed.

52341-52343

52341 **Cystourethroscopy; with treatment of ureteral stricture (eg, balloon dilation, laser, electrocautery, and incision)**

52342 **Cystourethroscopy; with treatment of ureteropelvic junction stricture (eg, balloon dilation, laser, electrocautery, and incision)**

52343 **Cystourethroscopy; with treatment of intra-renal stricture (eg, balloon dilation, laser, electrocautery, and incision)**

The physician performs cystourethroscopy to treat a ureteral, ureteropelvic junction (UPJ), or intra-renal stricture using balloon dilation, laser, electrocautery and/or incision. A cystourethroscope is inserted into the urethra, and advanced through the bladder and into the ureter. A guidewire is passed under ureteroscopic control through the area of the stricture. A semi-rigid or flexible ureteroscope is then passed alongside the guidewire to the area of the stricture. A balloon dilator may be advanced and inflated to dilate the stricture. This may be followed by incision of the stricture using an endoincision technique with a laser fiber, electrocautery, or other endoscopic surgical tool. Incisions are made through the full-thickness of the ureter or UPJ until periureteric or perirenal fat is encountered. Dilation and/or incisions are made along the length of the srtricture until the ureteroscope can be passed through the area of stricture. A temporary indwelling stent is then placed across the surgical site and surgical instruments are removed. Report 52341 for treatment of a ureteral stricture, 52342 for treatment of a UPJ stricture, and 52343 for treatment of an intra-renal stricture.

52344-52346

52344 **Cystourethroscopy with ureteroscopy; with treatment of ureteral stricture (eg, balloon dilation, laser, electrocautery, and incision)**

52345 **Cystourethroscopy with ureteroscopy; with treatment of ureteropelvic junction stricture (eg, balloon dilation, laser, electrocautery, and incision)**

52346 **Cystourethroscopy with ureteroscopy; with treatment of intra-renal stricture (eg, balloon dilation, laser, electrocautery, and incision)**

Cystourethroscopy with ureteroscopy is performed to treat a ureteral stricture (52344), ureteropelvic junction stricture (52345), or intra-renal stricture (52346) using balloon dilation, laser, electrocautery, and/or incision. Cystoscopy with ureteroscopy uses an ureteroscope that is passed through the urethra into the bladder and then into the ureter. The ureteroscope is used to directly visualize the ureter, pass guidewires, and direct the use of laser, balloons, or incisional or electrocautery devices. In 52344, the ureteroscope is passed from the bladder into the ureter to the site of the stricture. The stricture is visualized. A guide wire is then passed through the stricture. If a balloon catheter is used, it is advanced over the guidewire, inflated at the site of the narrowing, deflated, and removed. If a laser is used, the laser fiber is passed to the site of the stricture and fired to incise the narrowed area. Electrocautery and/or incision may also be performed via the ureteroscope to open the narrowed area. In 52345, the ureteroscope is advanced into the upper ureter. The ureteropelvic junction is visualized. A guidewire is passed through the stricture at the ureteropelvic junction and the stricture is treated as described above. In 52346, the ureteroscope is passed further up into the renal pelvis; a guidewire is passed through the stricture; and the narrowing is treated as described above.

52351

52351 **Cystourethroscopy, with ureteroscopy and/or pyeloscopy; diagnostic**

The urethra is cleansed with antiseptic solution. A rigid or flexible cystoscope is introduced through the urethra into the bladder. The bladder may be filled with sterile saline to allow better visualization of the bladder wall. Following inspection of the bladder, a guidewire is introduced through the cystoscope and advanced into the first ureter and through the ureter to the renal pelvis. The cystoscope is removed. A ureteroscope is then advanced over the guidewire and into the renal pelvis. The guidewire is removed. The renal pelvis is inspected and any abnormalities are noted. The ureteroscope is slowly withdrawn and the entire length of the ureter is inspected. The diagnostic ureteroscopy and/or pyeloscopy is repeated on the opposite ureter as needed. Upon completion of the procedure, the ureteroscope is removed.

52352-52353

52352   **Cystourethroscopy, with ureteroscopy and/or pyeloscopy; with removal or manipulation of calculus (ureteral catheterization is included)**
52353   **Cystourethroscopy, with ureteroscopy and/or pyeloscopy; with lithotripsy (ureteral catheterization is included)**

The urethra is cleansed with antiseptic solution. A rigid or flexible cystoscope is introduced through the urethra into the bladder. The bladder may be filled with sterile saline to allow better visualization of the bladder wall. Following inspection of the bladder, the ureters are catheterized. A guidewire is introduced through the cystoscope and advanced into the ureter and through the ureter to the site of the calculus within the ureter or renal pelvis. The cystoscope is removed. A ureteroscope is then advanced over the guidewire to the site of the calculus. In 52352, the calculus is manipulated or removed. A grasping or retrieval device is advanced through the cystoscope over the guidewire to the calculus, which is captured and extracted. Alternatively, the calculus may be grasped and manipulated into a different location without removal. In 52353, the calculus is fragmented with lithotripsy, using an ultrasonic or electrohydraulic technique. The ultrasonic or electrohydraulic probe is advanced through the ureteroscope to the ureter. The probe is activated and shockwaves are generated, causing fragmentation of the calculus. Following retrieval, manipulation, or fragmentation of the calculus, a catheter may be advanced over the guidewire to the renal pelvis and the ureter may be irrigated to remove the calculus fragments. Diagnostic or therapeutic solution may also be instilled into the ureter through the catheter. The ureteroscope may be advanced into the renal pelvis and the renal pelvis and ureter examined again as the ureteroscope is slowly withdrawn.

52354-52355

52354   **Cystourethroscopy, with ureteroscopy and/or pyeloscopy; with biopsy and/or fulguration of ureteral or renal pelvic lesion**
52355   **Cystourethroscopy, with ureteroscopy and/or pyeloscopy; with resection of ureteral or renal pelvic tumor**

The urethra is cleansed with antiseptic solution. A rigid or flexible cystoscope is introduced through the urethra into the bladder. The bladder may be filled with sterile saline to allow better visualization of the bladder wall. Following inspection of the bladder, the ureters are catheterized. A guidewire is introduced through the cystoscope and advanced into the ureter or renal pelvis to the site of the lesion or abnormal tissue. The cystoscope is removed. A ureteroscope is then advanced over the guidewire to the site of the tumor or lesion. In 52354, biopsy forceps are introduced through the ureteroscope and tissue samples are obtained. The renal pelvis and/or ureter are re-inspected following biopsy and any bleeding is controlled. Alternatively, an electrocautery device, laser, or cryoprobe is advanced through the ureteroscope to the site of the lesion. The device is activated and the abnormal tissue is destroyed by fulguration. In 52355, the renal pelvis and/or ureteral tumor is located and a resectoscope is advanced to the site of the tumor, which is then resected. The tumor is removed using irrigation and an endoscopic evacuation device. Bleeding is controlled as needed using electrocoagulation or laser coagulation. Following biopsy, fulguration, or tumor resection, a catheter may be advanced over the guidewire to the renal pelvis and the ureter and renal pelvis may be irrigated. Diagnostic or therapeutic solution may also be instilled through the catheter. The ureteroscope may be advanced into the renal pelvis and the renal pelvis and ureter examined as the ureteroscope is slowly withdrawn.

52356

52356   **Cystourethroscopy, with ureteroscopy and/or pyeloscopy; with lithotripsy including insertion of indwelling ureteral stent (eg, Gibbons or double-J type)**

The urethra is cleansed with antiseptic solution. A rigid or flexible cystoscope is introduced through the urethra and into the bladder. The bladder may be filled with sterile saline to allow better visualization of the bladder wall. Following inspection of the bladder, the ureters are catheterized. A guide wire is introduced through the cystoscope and advanced into and through the ureter to the site of the calculus in the ureter or renal pelvis. A ureteroscope is then advanced over the guide wire to the site of the calculus, which is fragmented using lithotripsy by either ultrasonic or electrohydraulic technique. The ultrasonic or electrohydraulic probe is advanced through the ureteroscope to the calculus. The probe is activated and shockwaves are generated to fragment the calculus. The probe is withdrawn and a catheter is advanced over the guide wire. The ureter and/or renal pelvis are irrigated to help flush out the calculus fragments. The catheter is removed and the ureteroscope is again advanced through the ureter to the renal pelvis. The renal pelvis and ureter are examined prior to stent placement as the ureteroscope is slowly withdrawn. A stent is advanced over the guide wire and positioned in the ureter. The guide wire is removed leaving the stent in place. The bladder is inspected again using the cystoscope

and the position of the distal tail of the stent in the bladder is noted. Upon completion of the procedure, the cystoscope is removed.

52400

52400   **Cystourethroscopy with incision, fulguration, or resection of congenital posterior urethral valves, or congenital obstructive hypertrophic mucosal folds**

Cystourethroscopy is performed with incision, fulguration, or resection of posterior urethral valves or obstructive hypertrophic mucosal folds. Both posterior urethral valves and obstructive hypertrophic mucosal folds are congenital anomalies of the urethra characterized by an obstructing membrane in the posterior segment of the male urethra causing bladder outlet obstruction. A cystourethroscope is inserted into the urethra and advanced into the bladder. The valves or mucosal folds are then incised, ablated (fulgurated), or resected through the cystourethroscope using cold knife, electrocautery, or laser energy.

52402

52402   **Cystourethroscopy with transurethral resection or incision of ejaculatory ducts**

The physician performs a cystourethroscopy with transurethral resection or incision of ejaculatory ducts to treat an obstruction caused by scar tissue, prostatic cysts, or stones. This procedure may also be referred to as a TURED (transurethral resection of ejaculatory ducts), TUIED (transurethral incision of ejaculatory ducts), or a resection of the verumontanum. The verumontanum is a small protuberance in the distal end of the prostatic urethra where the ejaculatory ducts enter the urethra. A cystourethroscope is inserted into the urethra and the urethra and bladder are examined endoscopically with careful attention to the region of the prostatic urethra and the ejaculatory duct orifices at the verumontanum. A resectoscope is then inserted and a hook electrode is used to incise one or both ejaculatory ducts. Alternatively, a loop electrode may be used to perform a resection of the verumontanum. This may require several passes of the cutting loop. Adequate incision or resection of the ejaculatory ducts is verified endoscopically by visualization of fluid refluxing from the opened ducts. Bleeding is controlled by cauterization of blood vessels taking care to avoid damage to the duct openings. The surgical instruments are then removed along with the cystourethroscope and a Foley catheter is placed in the bladder for 24-48 hours.

52441-52442

52441   **Cystourethroscopy, with insertion of permanent adjustable transprostatic implant; single implant**
52442   **Cystourethroscopy, with insertion of permanent adjustable transprostatic implant; each additional permanent adjustable transprostatic implant (List separately in addition to code for primary procedure)**

A permanent adjustable transprostatic implant is inserted via cystourethroscopy to retract obstructing lateral lobes of an enlarged prostate and expand the urethral lumen. This minimally invasive procedure can provide rapid relief of lower urinary symptoms associated with benign prostatic hypertrophy. A rigid cystoscope is inserted into the urethra and under visualization the implant delivery device is advanced into the sheath and angled anterolaterally to compress the obstructive lobe. A needle loaded with a monofilament and metallic tab is deployed through the prostate lobe and the needle is retracted, leaving the tab engaged and the monofilament tensioned. The implant is delivered by attaching the urethral end-piece to the monofilament which is then cut. The urethral end-piece invaginates into the urethral wall causing focal injury and epithelialization. Code 52441 is reported for a single implant and code 52442 is reported for each additional implant.

52450

52450   **Transurethral incision of prostate**

The physician performs a transurethral incision of the prostate (TUIP). An incision is made through the urethra using electrocautery or a laser beam at the site where the prostate meets the bladder. The incision is carried down through the muscle tissue and into the prostate where one or two small incisions or grooves are made in the prostate. No tissue is removed. This is done to release the tension on the urethra allowing urine to flow out of the bladder more easily.

52500

52500   **Transurethral resection of bladder neck (separate procedure)**

The physician performs transurethral resection of the bladder neck. A cystourethroscope is inserted into the urethra and the urethra and bladder are examined endoscopically with careful attention to the region of the prostatic urethra and bladder neck. Meatotomy or urethrotomy are performed as needed prior to insertion of the resectoscope. An irrigating resectoscope is then introduced and the prostate is resected at four and eight o'clock to the level of the prostate capsule. The prostate is incised using a diathermy loop and the incision is carried down to the level of the extracapsular fat. The incision is then extended from the verumontanum to the level immediately below the bladder trigone. Bleeding is

Urinary System

controlled, surgical instruments and the cystourethroscope are removed, and the resected prostate chips are submitted for pathological examination.

52601

52601   Transurethral electrosurgical resection of prostate, including control of postoperative bleeding, complete (vasectomy, meatotomy, cystourethroscopy, urethral calibration and/or dilation, and internal urethrotomy are included)

The physician performs a complete transurethral electrosurgical resection of the prostate (TURP). The following procedures may also be performed and are included: vasectomy, meatotomy, cystourethroscopy, urethral calibration, urethral dilation, internal urethrotomy, and control of postoperative bleeding. A cystourethroscope is inserted into the urethra and the urethra and bladder are examined endoscopically with careful attention to the region of the prostatic urethra and prostate. The physician may need to incise the urethral meatus (meatotomy), dilate and/or calibrate the urethra, or incise the internal urethra (internal urethrotomy) for better surgical access prior to insertion of the resectoscope. An irrigating resectoscope is introduced and the prostate is completely resected using an electrical loop that simultaneously cuts or vaporizes the obstructive tissue and cauterizes the blood vessels. The prostate is irrigated and the chips of prostate tissue are flushed from the prostate and into the bladder. A vasectomy may also be done by resecting the vas deferens along with the prostate. Following completion of the procedure, the irrigation fluid, prostatic tissue, and surgical debris are flushed from the bladder. Bleeding is controlled, surgical instruments and cystourethroscope are removed, and the resected prostate chips are submitted for pathological examination. Postoperative bleeding is monitored and any excessive bleeding may require a return to the operating room for cystourethroscopy and cauterization of blood vessels.

52630

52630   Transurethral resection; residual or regrowth of obstructive prostate tissue including control of postoperative bleeding, complete (vasectomy, meatotomy, cystourethroscopy, urethral calibration and/or dilation, and internal urethrotomy are included)

The physician performs a transurethral resection of residual obstructive tissue or regrowth following a previous resection of the prostate. A cystourethroscope is inserted into the urethra, and the urethra and bladder are examined endoscopically with careful attention to the region of the prostatic urethra and prostate. The physician may need to incise the urethral meatus (meatotomy), dilate and/or calibrate the urethra, and incise the internal urethra (internal urethrotomy) for better surgical access prior to insertion of the resectoscope. An irrigating resectoscope is introduced, and the obstructive regrowth of prostatic tissue is resected using an electrical loop that simultaneously cuts or vaporizes the obstructive tissue and cauterizes the blood vessels. The prostate is irrigated and the chips of prostatic tissue are flushed from the prostate into the bladder. Following completion of the procedure, the irrigation fluid, prostatic tissue, and surgical debris are flushed from the bladder. Bleeding is controlled, surgical instruments and the cystourethroscope are removed, surgical instruments are submitted for pathological examination.

52640

52640   Transurethral resection; of postoperative bladder neck contracture

The physician performs transurethral resection of a postoperative contracture of the bladder neck. A cystourethroscope is inserted into the urethra and both the urethra and bladder are examined endoscopically with careful attention to the bladder neck regions. Meatotomy or urethrotomy are performed as needed prior to insertion of the resectoscope. An irrigating resectoscope is then introduced into the bladder neck region and scar tissue is incised and resected. Bleeding is controlled and the surgical instruments and cystourethroscope are removed.

52647

52647   Laser coagulation of prostate, including control of postoperative bleeding, complete (vasectomy, meatotomy, cystourethroscopy, urethral calibration and/or dilation, and internal urethrotomy are included if performed)

A complete laser coagulation of the prostate is performed including control of postoperative bleeding. This procedure is also referred to as transurethral ultrasound-guided laser prostatectomy (TULIP) using a free fiber or free-fiber visually guided laser ablation of the prostate (VLAP). TULIP and VLAP result in gradual sloughing of necrotic prostate tissue. The following procedures may also be performed and are included: vasectomy, meatotomy, cystourethroscopy, urethral calibration, urethral dilation, internal urethrotomy, and control of postoperative bleeding. A cystourethroscope is inserted into the urethra and both the urethra and bladder are examined endoscopically with careful attention to the prostatic region. The physician may need to incise the urethral meatus (meatotomy), dilate and/or calibrate the urethra, and/or incise the internal urethra (internal urethrotomy) for better surgical access. The laser probe is advanced through the endoscope to the base of the middle lobe of the prostate. The laser is activated, the temperature is increased to 85 degrees centigrade, and the middle lobe is coagulated.

The probe is held in position for up to 3 minutes using direct visualization or fluoroscopic video guidance. An irrigation tube is used to continuously flush blood and debris from the surgical site into the bladder. The bladder is drained and irrigated as needed to maintain good visibility. The probe is then retracted and placed in each lateral lobe and the laser coagulation procedure is repeated. When all lobes of the prostate have been treated, bleeding is controlled, the surgical tools and cystourethroscope are removed, and a Foley catheter is inserted.

52648

52648   Laser vaporization of prostate, including control of postoperative bleeding, complete (vasectomy, meatotomy, cystourethroscopy, urethral calibration and/or dilation, internal urethrotomy and transurethral resection of prostate are included if performed)

A complete laser vaporization of the prostate is performed including control of postoperative bleeding. This procedure may also be referred to as interstitial laser coagulation of the prostate (ILCP) or contact laser ablation of the prostate (CLAP). ILCP and CLAP result in immediate laser destruction and vaporization of prostate tissue. The following procedures may also be performed and are included: vasectomy, meatotomy, cystourethroscopy, urethral calibration, urethral dilation, internal urethrotomy, and control of postoperative bleeding. A cystourethroscope is inserted into the urethra and both the urethra and bladder are examined endoscopically with careful attention to anatomy of the urethral sphincter and prostate. The position of the ureters and bladder neck are also noted. The physician may need to incise the urethral meatus (meatotomy), dilate and/or calibrate the urethra, and/or incise the internal urethra (internal urethrotomy) for better surgical access. The laser fiber is introduced and positioned taking care to avoid direct contact with the prostate tissue. The laser is fired perpendicularly using slow side-to-side sweeping movements. Effective vaporization of prostate tissue results in formation of bubbles. When all lobes of the prostate have been treated, the bladder is emptied and the surgical cavity is inspected to verify that sufficient tissue has been removed. The bladder neck should be visible from the verumontanum. The integrity of the ureters is also verified. Any bleeding is controlled. The surgical tools and cystourethroscope are removed. Generally, little postoperative bleeding occurs following laser vaporization and a Foley catheter is not typically required.

52649

52649   Laser enucleation of the prostate with morcellation, including control of postoperative bleeding, complete (vasectomy, meatotomy, cystourethroscopy, urethral calibration and/or dilation, internal urethrotomy and transurethral resection of prostate are included if performed)

A complete laser enucleation of the prostrate is performed with morcellation including control of postoperative bleeding. Morcellation of the prostate involves dividing it into smaller pieces so that it can be more easily removed. Also included in this procedure are a vasectomy, meatotomy, cystourethroscopy (cystoscopy), urethral calibration and/or dilation, internal urethrotomy, and transurethral resection of the prostate, if performed. Prior to the laser enucleation procedure, a cystoscopy is performed to examine the bladder for the presence of any tumors or masses. The urethra is then calibrated and dilated using a series of sounds. If the meatus is narrowed, it is incised (meatotomy). A continuous flow resectoscope sheath is placed, followed by a laser fiber stabilizing catheter, video system, and lastly the laser fiber. Normal saline irrigant is then run through the resection tubing into the resectoscope. The resectoscope is then used to visualize the anatomy and determine the extent of each lobe's enlargement. Each lobe of the prostrate is then sequentially enucleated and resected, usually beginning with the median lobe. This process begins by first cutting a groove with the laser along the sulcus just lateral to the verumontanum (seminal colliculus). The groove is then deepened, undermined, and widened to separate it from the lateral lobe. A second groove may be created by repeating this process. All attachments in the median lobe are divided and the median lobe is enucleated. Dissection of the right lateral lobe is then performed freeing it from the capsular floor by moving the laser in a side-to-side, transverse fashion. When the floor of the right lobe is dissected free of all attachments, an anterior groove is created along the anterior commisure to separate the right lateral lobe from the roof of the capsule. The remaining lateral attachments at the apex of the right lateral lobe are identified and cut with the laser. Enucleation of the right lobe is completed by dividing any remaining attachments at the bladder neck. Attention is then directed to the left lateral lobe and the left lateral lobe is enucleated in the same fashion as the right. Once all three lobes of the prostate have been enucleated and pushed into the bladder, bleeding is controlled by laser coagulation. The inner sheath of the resectoscope, the laser fiber, and the stabilizing catheter are removed. A morcellator is introduced. Inflow tubing with normal saline is used to distend the bladder. Prostate tissue from one of the lobes that has been pushed into the bladder is isolated and the morcellator blades activated. The prostrate tissue is cut into smaller pieces by the morcellator and these smaller pieces of prostate tissue are removed by suction. This is repeated until the bladder is cleared of all prostate tissue.

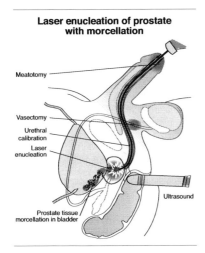

Laser enucleation of prostate with morcellation

Meatotomy

Vasectomy

Urethral calibration

Laser enucleation

Ultrasound

Prostate tissue morcellation in bladder

52700

52700   Transurethral drainage of prostatic abscess

The physician performs transurethral drainage of a prostatic abscess. The abscess is located using digital rectal exam (DRE) and/or separately reportable transrectal ultrasound (TRUS) guidance. A cystourethroscope is inserted into the urethra and both the urethra and bladder are examined. A needle is used to puncture the abscess and a small amount of fluid is aspirated and sent to the laboratory for culture. An incision is then made in the abscess wall and the abscess is drained.

53000-53010

53000   Urethrotomy or urethrostomy, external (separate procedure); pendulous urethra

53010   Urethrotomy or urethrostomy, external (separate procedure); perineal urethra, external

Urethrotomy or urethrostomy is performed to allow access to the penile or perineal urethra, bladder neck, and/or bladder. In males, the urethra is divided into anterior and posterior segments. The anterior urethra includes the meatus, fossa navicularis, penile or pendulous urethra, and bulbar urethra. The posterior urethra includes the membranous and prostatic urethra which may also be referred to as the perineal urethra. In 53000, the spongiosum is incised and the pendulous urethra is exposed and incised. A catheter is placed into the bladder through the incision in the pendulous urethra to provide drainage of urine. In 53010, the perineum is incised and the perineal urethra is exposed. A catheter is placed into the bladder through the incision in the perineal urethra to provide drainage of urine.

53020-53025

53020   Meatotomy, cutting of meatus (separate procedure); except infant

53025   Meatotomy, cutting of meatus (separate procedure); infant

The external urethral meatus is the most distal aspect of the urethra, also referred to as the external urethral orifice. Meatotomy is performed to enlarge the orifice. The urethral meatus is cleansed. A local anesthetic is administered. The meatus is incised. Use 53020 when meatotomy is performed on a child older than an infant, and adolescent, or adult. Use 53025 when meatotomy is performed on an infant.

53040

53040   Drainage of deep periurethral abscess

A deep periurethral abscess is an infection that frequently occurs as a complication of gonococcal infection, urethral stricture, or urethral catheterization. The perineum is incised over the abscess site. The abscess pocket is opened and pus is drained. Loculations are broken up using finger dissection. The abscess pocket is flushed with sterile saline or antibiotic solution. The abscess pocket may be packed with gauze or a drain may be placed.

53060

53060   Drainage of Skene's gland abscess or cyst

Skene's glands are small mucus glands located adjacent to the distal urethra, also known as periurethral glands, which deliver secretions into the female urethra near the urethral meatus. Cysts form when the Skene's ducts become obstructed. The cysts can become infected and turn into abcesses. The cyst or abscess is located by palpation. The cyst or abscess is then incised and drained.

53080-53085

53080   Drainage of perineal urinary extravasation; uncomplicated (separate procedure)

53085   Drainage of perineal urinary extravasation; complicated

Perineal urinary extravasation occurs when there is a disruption in the continuity of the perineal urethra and urine leaks out into the perineal tissue, which causes it to become red, tender, and edematous. The disruption may be caused by rupture of the urethra due to a stricture in the distal end, or traumatic injury. The urethra cannot be repaired until the urine has been drained from the perineal tissue. In 53080, uncomplicated drainage is performed using multiple incisions in the superficial perineal tissue to allow drainage of the urine. In 53085, complicated drainage is performed, which may be required when there is a traumatic injury to the urethra or when dissection of deeper tissues is required to allow drainage of urine.

53200

53200   Biopsy of urethra

The lesion on the external aspect of the urethra is visually inspected. The surgical site is cleansed and a local anesthetic administered as needed. One or more tissue samples are obtained. The tissue samples are then prepared and examined by a pathologist in a separately reportable procedure to determine if cancer or other abnormal cells are present.

53210

53210   Urethrectomy, total, including cystostomy; female

The urethra in women is located in the pelvic floor (perineum), in front of and above the vagina. A total urethrectomy is the complete removal of the urethra from the bladder to the perineum. A urethral catheter is inserted. An incision is made around the external urethra and the urethra is dissected free of surrounding tissue. The pubourethral ligament is exposed and transected. The posterior aspect of the urethra is dissected free of the vaginal septum. The right and left urethropelvic ligaments are exposed, isolated, and transected. Once the urethra is completely free of all surrounding tissue from the external meatus to the bladder neck, an incision is made just above the pubis. The completely isolated urethra is pulled into the pelvis and the bladder neck is dissected from surrounding tissue. The urethra is excised at the level of the bladder neck and removed along with the urethral catheter. The bladder is neck is closed with sutures. An opening called a cystostomy, also referred to as an epicystostomy or vesicostomy, is surgically created in the lower abdomen to facilitate urine drainage from the bladder. This is accomplished by making an incision in the lower abdomen to the level of the rectus fascia. A triangular section of the rectus fascia is completely excised. The rectus muscle is incised and the dome of the bladder is exposed. The bladder is opened and the bladder wall secured to the opening in the rectus fascia with sutures. The bladder epithelium is then secured to the skin. A catheter or tube is inserted and secured to the abdominal wall with sutures.

53215

53215   Urethrectomy, total, including cystostomy; male

The urethra in men is located centrally down the shaft of the penis. A total urethrectomy is performed by making an incision in the perineum and removing the urethra from the prostate area to the tip of the penis. A Foley catheter or urethral sound is inserted into the urethra. An incision is made in the lower abdomen and the bladder neck exposed. The bulbocavernosus muscle is exposed and incised in the midline. The bulbar urethra is dissected free of surrounding tissue. Buck's fascia is incised and a window created between Buck's fascia and the corpora cavernosa to allow mobilization of the cavernous urethra. The cavernous urethra is dissected from surrounding tissue as tension is applied to the urethra drawing the urethra into the pelvic incision. Dissection continues distally. Tension is applied and the glans penis is inverted. The urethra is mobilized to the level of the coronal sulcus in the glans penis. The glans penis is returned to its normal orientation and a traction suture placed in the glans. An incision is made over the frenulum and the mobilized portion of the urethra captured using umbilical tape or a vessel loop. An incision is made around the external urethral meatus and carried up to the incision over the frenulum. The urethra is dissected free of the glans penis. Once the distal aspect of the urethra has been completely mobilized, the urethra is brought into the pelvis and excised at the level of the bladder neck. The urethra and catheter are removed and the bladder neck is closed. Incisions in the penis are closed in layers. A drain or catheter may be left in place to facilitate drainage from the area. An opening called a cystostomy, also referred to as an epicystostomy or vesicostomy, is surgically created in the lower abdomen to facilitate urine drainage from the bladder. This is accomplished by making an incision in the lower abdomen to the level of the rectus fascia. A triangular section of the rectus fascia is completely excised. The rectus muscle is incised and the dome of the bladder is exposed. The bladder is opened and the bladder wall secured to the opening in the rectus fascia with sutures. The bladder epithelium is then secured to the skin. A catheter or tube is inserted and secured to the abdominal wall with sutures.

● New Code   ▲ Revised Code

Urinary System

53220

53220   Excision or fulguration of carcinoma of urethra

Treatment of external urethral cancers in both men and women may be performed by excision or fulguration, also referred to as electrocautery, electroresection, or laser destruction. The lesion on the external urethra may have been previously diagnosed or biopsied and diagnosed during the same surgical session. If excision is performed, the lesion along with a margin of healthy tissue is sharply excised. The specimen is evaluated in a separately reportable procedure by a pathologist to ensure that the margins are free of malignant tissue. If any malignant tissue is identified the margins are widened until they are completely free of malignancy. Fulguration may be performed using an electrocautery device or laser. The electrocautery device or laser is activated and the abnormal tissue is destroyed.

53230

53230   Excision of urethral diverticulum (separate procedure); female

Partial ablation and total excision are the most effective treatment when urethral divertuclum are in the middle or proximal area of the female urethra. A percutaneous suprapubic catheter is inserted as needed. The vagina is prepped and draped, a Foley catheter placed transurethrally. A vaginal incision is made via midline vertical, transverse or U-shape with the apex distal to the diverticulum. In partial ablation the periurethral fascia is exposed and dissected into proximal and distal flaps exposing the diverticular sac. The body of the diverticular sac is then entered and the sac excised from the periurethral fascia. A metal probe is placed through the ostia to identify the opening and the bulk of the sac excised leaving attenuated tissue around the ostia. The probe is removed and the attenuated tissue is sewn closed in multiple layers. Total excision or urethral diverticulectomy removes the diverticular sac and the surrounding mucosal lining. The vaginal flap is dissected using scissors preserving the periurethral fascia. The periurethral fascia is opened in proximal and distal flaps exposing the diverticular sac. The sac is not entered. The diverticulum is dissected circumferentially to the ostia. Attenuated tissue at the ostia is excised and the entire sac removed. The muscular and mucosal layers of the urethral defect are closed vertically over the catheter. In both procedures, the periurethral fascia is closed transversely and the anterior vaginal wall is also sutured. The urethral catheter is left in place. The suprapubic catheter, if used, may be removed or left in place.

53235

53235   Excision of urethral diverticulum (separate procedure); male

Male urethral diverticula are quite rare but can be found in the proximal part of the penile urethra and distal part of the bulbous urethra. With the patient prepped and the penis and scrotum draped a catheter is placed transurethrally. An incision is made in the skin exposing the corpus spongiosum. The diverticular sac is dissected free of the corpus spongiosum including the attenuated tissue at the ostia. The muscular and mucosal layers of the urethral defect are closed vertically over the catheter. Drains may be placed and the corpus spongiosum closed with sutures followed by closure of the skin. The urethral catheter is left in place.

53240

53240   Marsupialization of urethral diverticulum, male or female

Marsupialization or Spence procedure is performed on women when the diverticulum is located in the distal urethra, away from the bladder neck. A transurethral catheter is placed and the bladder emptied. The catheter is then withdrawn. Using straight Mayo scissors, one blade in the urethra and the second along the anterior wall of the vagina an incision is made midline beneath the posterior wall of the urethra and the diverticular sac entered. The incision is enlarged as needed. The diverticulum is inspected for suspicious appearing tissue. If a biopsy is performed to rule out malignancy, tissue samples are prepared and examined by a pathologist in a separately reportable procedure. The urethral and diverticular epithelial lining is then sutured to the incised vaginal epithelial lining exteriorizing the urinary tract epithelium and creating a large posterior meatotomy. A similar meatotomy is performed in men with distal diverticulum close to the penile tip. The diverticulum and meatus are opened together with scalpel or scissors to form a single, large meatal opening. Spontaneous voiding can be expected following either procedure and a urinary catheter is not usually necessary.

53250

53250   Excision of bulbourethral gland (Cowper's gland)

The bulbourethral or Cowper's gland is located at the base of the penis, posterior and lateral to the membranous portion of the urethra. A horizontal curved incision is made in the skin of the perineum above the anal opening and carried down through the superficial Camper's fascia and then the deep Colles' fascia. The rectus urethralis muscular band is then transected allowing entry into the urogenital diaphragm. The perirectal fascia which makes up the posterior layer of Denonvillier's fascia is identified and opened and the bulbourethral gland is located and dissected free. The ductal opening of the gland into the urethra is identified and ligated. The gland and surrounding tissue is removed and inspected. Tissue samples may be prepared and examined by a pathologist in a separately

reportable procedure. The incision is closed in layers with absorbable sutures, skin edges are approximated with interrupted sutures. A Penrose drain may be left in place.

53260

53260   Excision or fulguration; urethral polyp(s), distal urethra

Open excision to remove polyps in the distal urethra is most often performed when the polyp is large or has reoccurred. With the female patient in dorsal lithotomy position the vulva, vagina and perineum is prepped and draped. The male patient is positioned supine and the penis prepped and draped. The urinary meatus and urethra may be dilated using a catheter or balloon to aid with visualization of the polyp. The polyp is grasped using a clamp or forceps and pulled out to elongate the stalk and expose the base of the polyp where it attaches to the urethra. The polyp is completely excised from the urethra by fulguration at the base using an electrocautery device or laser. The polyp is removed and inspected. Tissue samples are prepared and examined by a pathologist in a separately reportable procedure. The patient may have a Foley catheter placed following the procedure.

53265

53265   Excision or fulguration; urethral caruncle

Removal of external urethral caruncle in both men and women may be performed by excision or fulguration, also referred to as electrocautery, electroresection, or laser destruction. With the female in dorsal lithotomy position the vulva and perineum are prepped and draped. The male is positioned supine and the penis is prepped and draped. Using an Allis clamp, the caruncle is grasped and retracted with slight pressure forward. A scalpel is then used to excise part of the vestibular epithelium and the urethra is transected proximally to the caruncle. The urethral mucosa and vestibular epithelium are now exposed. The two layers are closed using interrupted absorbable sutures, sewing the urethral mucosa to the vestibular epithelium. Fulguration may be performed using an electrocautery device or laser. The electrocautery device or laser is activated and the abnormal tissue is destroyed. A Foley catheter may be placed transurethrally following the procedures.

53270

53270   Excision or fulguration; Skene's glands

Skene's glands, also referred to as lesser vestibular glands, periurethral glands or paraurethral glands are located along the sides of the female urethra. Glands that are enlarged due to cysts or infection may be excised by marsupialization or electrocoagulation technique. The glands are located by visualization and/or palpation and an incision made using straight Mayo scissors, one blade in the urethra and the second in the sac of the periurethral gland. The incision is enlarged as needed. The gland is dissected free of surrounding tissue. Tissue samples are prepared and examined by a pathologist as needed in a separately reportable procedure. The incision is closed in layers. The urethral lining and the epithelial lining of the gland are repaired with sutures. Exteriorization of the urinary tract epithelium may result in an enlarged urethral meatus. Fulguration may be performed using an electrocautery device or laser. The electrocautery device or laser is activated and the abnormal tissue is destroyed.

53275

53275   Excision or fulguration; urethral prolapse

Several surgical procedures are acceptable to correct a urethral prolapse or urethrocele. Using the Lowe technique, a meatotomy is performed to release constriction of the meatal ring and the prolapsed mucosa is manually reduced. The mucosa and urethra are then tied to the periurethral vestibule using multiple mattress sutures. With the Kelly-Burnham technique a Foley catheter is placed transurethrally and the prolapsed mucosa is excised circumferentially around it. The edges of the urethral mucosa and introital mucosa are approximated and the incision is closed with interrupted sutures. This technique may be modified by placing holding sutures in the prolapsed mucosa to form quadrants around the urethra. The mucosa is then excised in sections. Prolapsed urethral mucosa may also be removed by fulguration, also referred to as electrocautery, electroresection, or laser destruction. Using an electrocautery device or laser, the device or laser is activated and the abnormal tissue destroyed.

53400-53405

53400   Urethroplasty; first stage, for fistula, diverticulum, or stricture (eg, Johannsen type)

53405   Urethroplasty; second stage (formation of urethra), including urinary diversion

Urethroplasty is performed in two stages. In 53400, the first stage is performed. A skin graft is harvested. In an uncircumcised male, the foreskin can be used. The coronal ridge is marked with ink circumferentially. The prepuce is retracted and adhesions between the glans and prepuce epithelium are lysed. A clamp may be placed with one blade inside the preputial sac and the second on the outer skin creating a crush area at the dorsal midline of the prepuce. The clamp is removed after a few minutes and the crush line is incised

● New Code   ▲ Revised Code   CPT © 2016 American Medical Association. All Rights Reserved.   © 2017 DecisionHealth

Urinary System

using scissors. The prepuce tissue is dissected free of the penis circumferentially along the coronal ridge. Hemostasis is maintained with electrocautery and absorbable sutures are placed to join the skin and preputial epithelium. Alternatively, skin from the inside thigh, groin above the hairline, buttocks or buccal mucosa is harvested. After the graft has been harvested and prepared, the skin on the penile shaft is incised with a scalpel to expose the urethra. The urethra in incised along the length of the stricture, diverticulum, or fistula until healthy tissue has been exposed proximally and distally. The ostia are calibrated at each end. The prepared graft tissue is laid around the marsupialized urethra and sewn medially to the urethral margin and laterally to the edge of the penile skin with interrupted absorbable sutures. A catheter is placed transurethrally. A percutaneous suprapubic catheter may also be placed into the bladder to divert urine during the postoperative period. In 53405, the second stage is performed once the graft has healed and the epithelium has vascularized. The vascularized epithelial tissue is excised using longitudinal incisions on each side. The proximal and distal ostia are calibrated. If narrowing has occurred, revision of the graft may be performed. The vascularized epithelial tissue is formed into a tubular neourethral structure over a transurethral catheter or stent. The tubular graft is secured using midline anastomosis with a running suture, interspersed with interlocking sutures and the wound is closed in layers. The catheter or stent is left in place.

53410

53410   Urethroplasty, 1-stage reconstruction of male anterior urethra

A single stage urethroplasty on the male anterior urethra is most often indicated following trauma or injury. The anterior urethra extends distally from the membranous urethra in three segments. The bulbar segment extends through the proximal corpus spongiosum, ischeal cavernosus and bulbospongiosum until it reaches the penile plane. The penile segment runs the length of the pendulous penis into the third segment, the fossa navicularis in the glans penis. A catheter or urethral sound is used to locate the level of the stricture. A Foley catheter is placed transurethrally into the bladder. A midline incision is made along the ventral penile plane and dissection extended through Buck's fascia until the urethra is identified and adequately exposed. An incision is made along the urethral stricture over the catheter and extended at least 1 cm distally and proximally into healthy urethral tissue is encountered. Using an onlay flap technique, one skin margin is excised to a width not exceeding 25 mm and carried down into the subcutaneous connective tissue. The flap is tapered at each end with the length corresponding to the size of the urethral deficit. At this point the skin edges are checked for approximation to ensure that minimal tension will occur during wound closure. The medial border of the flap is sutured to the incised urethra creating an anchor and then beginning at the distal margin, the flap and the urethral epithelium are sutured together with a running stitch to form a lateral suture line. The free edge of the flap is then rolled and secured to the contralateral margin creating a urethral lumen and a running stitch is made along that margin. Drains may be placed. The subcutaneous connective tissue is closed over the urethral suture lines without injuring the pedicle of the flap. The skin is approximated with minimal tension and closed with a running stitch. The transurethral catheter remains in place.

53415

53415   Urethroplasty, transpubic or perineal, 1-stage, for reconstruction or repair of prostatic or membranous urethra

A single stage repair or reconstruction of the posterior urethra can be accomplished through a transpubic and perineal approach. It is most often indicated following injury or trauma such as pelvic fracture. The posterior urethra is comprised of the prostatic and membranous segments and extends from the bladder neck through the prostate gland, between the prostatic apex and perineal membrane until it connects to the anterior urethra at the bulbar segment. A midline incision is made in the perineum, bifurcating at the posterior end. Dissection continues through the bulbospongiosum muscle, exposing the corpus spongiosum until the urethra is located and mobilized. Proceeding in the direction of the bulbar urethra, the proximal point of obliteration is identified using a catheter and the distal point as far as the suspensory ligament to the penis is assessed. A sound is passed via a previously created suprapubic cystotomy tract through the bladder neck and into the prostatic urethra. Beginning at the level of the crus and working distally, the right and left corporal bodies are separated in the midline for a distance of 4-5 cm allowing the urethra to move upwards and shortening the distance between the urethral ends. If urethral tension remains after separating the corporal bodies, dissection continues by displacing or ligating the penile vessels laterally. Then using bone rongeurs or an osteotome, a wedge of bone is removed from the pubis at the inferior aspect creating a groove for the urethra to settle into and adding 1-2 cm of urethral length. If anastomosis is still not possible due to urethral tension, the urethra is rerouted around the corporal body through a larger resection of the pubic bone by circumferentially mobilizing one of the corporal bodies proximal to the suspensory penile ligament. The distal urethral stump is spatulated and brought down from a 12-o'clock position and the proximal urethral stump is also spatulated and lifted from the 6-o'clock position, healthy tissue is identified along with the seminal ducts in the verumontanum of the prostatic urethra. Anastomosis of the two ends of the urethra is accomplished by placing 8-10 sutures through the urethral mucosa. A fenestrated French catheter is placed transurethrally. The incision is closed in layers and the suprapubic catheter is replaced.

53420-53425

53420   Urethroplasty, 2-stage reconstruction or repair of prostatic or membranous urethra; first stage

53425   Urethroplasty, 2-stage reconstruction or repair of prostatic or membranous urethra; second stage

A 2-stage repair of the prostatic or membranous urethra is typically indicated following injury or trauma such as pelvic fracture, prostate surgery or radiation therapy. In 53420, the first stage is performed using a perineal approach. The prostatic and membranous urethral segments extend from the bladder neck through the prostate gland, between the prostatic apex and perineal membrane, and terminate at the bulbar segment. A previously placed suprapubic catheter is not usually left in place. A midline perineal incision is made. Dissection continues through the bulbospongiosum muscle, exposing the corpus spongiosum until the urethra is located. In the instance of a stricture, the urethra is opened and resected to expose healthy urethral tissue at the distal and proximal ends. If complete transection of the urethra has occurred, the distal and proximal ends are identified and brought to the midline. A previously prepared buccal mucosal graft is used to line the urethral deficit or encase the urethral stumps. The graft is sutured to the perineal skin edges and around the urethral stumps. Urine remains diverted by the suprapubic catheter. In 53425, the second stage of a 2-stage repair is carried out after the graft has vascularized and adequate epithelial tissue is visualized at the perineum. A previously placed suprapubic catheter is left in place. The graft is incised circumferentially from the perineal edge and mobilized laterally. A Foley catheter is placed transurethrally into the bladder and the graft is rolled into a tubular structure around the catheter to form a neourethra. The graft is fixed with sutures at the proximal and distal edges of the stricture opening or the urethral stumps. Drains may be placed and the corpus spongiosum is closed over the newly formed urethra followed by closure of the bulbospongiosum muscle and finally, closure of the skin. The suprapubic catheter is left in place along with the transurethral catheter.

53430

53430   Urethroplasty, reconstruction of female urethra

There are a number of accepted techniques for reconstruction of the female urethra. A Foley catheter is inserted transurethrally. A suprapubic catheter may also be inserted. Using an inverted U-shaped incision on the anterior wall of the vagina, the urethral defect is identified. An incision is made over one of the labia forming a flap that includes the labial fat pad. The urethra is repaired using a Martius flap which includes the labial flap and the fat pad. The flap is sutured under the urethral repair to provide support. If there is limited periurethral or vaginal tissue, a technique that allows for rotation of the flap may be used. Using a U-shaped anterior vaginal incision, the flap is mobilized from the vaginal wall, rotated distally and sutured as a dorsal onlay flap creating a tubular neourethra over the foley catheter. The vaginal wall harvest site is closed with sutures. In both procedures, drains may be placed and the vaginal mucosa is then closed in layers with absorbable sutures. A less used technique involves a dorsal approach and a buccal mucosal graft. The dorsal area of the urethral meatus is exposed using a U-shaped incision. The vulvar mucosa is dissected from the urethral channel to develop a plane between the urethra and the cavernous tissue of the clitoris. The anterior portion of the urethral sphincter is identified and carefully moved upward. The bladder neck is located and identified with a stitch and an incision made lengthwise in the urethra. The prepared buccal mucosal graft is sutured to the right and left sides of the urethral opening. The reinforced dorsal urethra is sutured to the clitoral body forming the new urethral roof. The graft tissue is tailored to make a normal meatal opening. The vulvar incision is closed with absorbable sutures. The Foley catheter remains in place.

53431

53431   Urethroplasty with tubularization of posterior urethra and/or lower bladder for incontinence (eg, Tenago, Leadbetter procedure)

The physician lengthens the urethra or the lower part of the bladder with muscle tissue from the bladder. This procedure is done to relieve a condition in which the patient cannot control the release of urine.

53440

53440   Sling operation for correction of male urinary incontinence (eg, fascia or synthetic)

The sling procedure to correct male urinary incontinence is accomplished by using an allograft, xenograft or synthetic mesh graft. A Foley catheter is inserted transurethrally. A transverse suprapubic incision is made and the rectus fascia exposed. The rectus fascia is incised allowing access to the retropubic space. A U-shaped perineal incision is made in the skin and carried down through the bulbospongiosum muscle to the corpus spongiosum. Dissection continues until the urethra is identified. The urethra is dissected and the retropubic space entered on both sides of the urethra. A ligature passer is inserted into the retropubic space through the suprapubic incision, the endopelvic fascia is perforated and the ligature passer then exits through the perineal incision on one side of the urethra. A sling graft is placed under the urethra and one end attached to the ligature passer. The

Urinary System

graft is then pulled through the endopelvic fascia into the retropubic space. The graft is detached from the ligature passer and the ligature passer is again passed through the suprapubic incision and endopelvic fascia exiting on the opposite side of the urethra. The other end of the sling graft is attached to the ligature passer and pulled into the retropubic space. The sling is now seated under the urethra. Tension of the sling is adjusted to provide adequate support without obstructing the urethra. The perineal wound is closed. The sling sutures are tunneled through the rectus fascia. The rectus fascia is closed and the sling sutures are tied down over the closed fascia. The suprapubic fascia is closed. Alternatively, the graft may be secured to the pubic rami. Using a bone drill, three screws with sutures are driven into each side of the pubic rami proximally at the level of the bulbar urethra and distally just below the pubic symphysis. The graft material is secured to the bone on one side with sutures and on the other it is secured with temporary pass through sutures. The tension on the sling is adjusted. The sutures are then securely tied down. The incision is closed in layers.

Sling operation for correction of male urinary incontinence

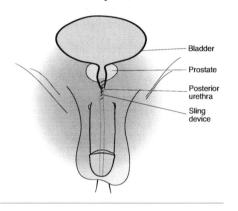

Bladder

Prostate

Posterior urethra

Sling device

53442

53442   Removal or revision of sling for male urinary incontinence (eg, fascia or synthetic)

Removal or revision of the urethral sling in males is rarely necessary, but may be performed for failure of the sling, pain, or infection. A transurethral catheter is inserted into the bladder. The perineum is incised under the scrotum. Dissection is carried down to the bulbospoongiosus muscles and continues until the urethra and sling are exposed. If the sling is revised, it is freed from surrounding tissue and tension readjusted as needed. If the sling is removed, the sling is freed from the surrounding tissue taking care not to cause further injury to the urethra or surrounding blood vessels. The sling is mobilized up to the endopelvic fascia on both sides of the pelvis. The abdomen is incised just above the pubic bone and the abdominal ends of the sling identified. The rectus fascia is incised and the sling mobilized within the retropubic space down to the endopelvic fascia. Alternatively if the sling has been secured to the pubic rami, the bone screws are removed. When the sling is completely mobilized it is removed through the perineal incision. Eroded urethral tissue is debrided and the urethra closed. The abdominal and perineal wounds are irrigated with antibiotic solution. Drains are placed as needed. The abdominal and perineal incisions are individually closed around the drains.

53444

53444   Insertion of tandem cuff (dual cuff)

Insertion of a tandem or dual cuff following insertion of an artificial urinary sphincter (AUS) system is performed when there is failure with the originally placed cuff. An incision is made at the level of the bulbous urethra where the cuff is located. The cuff is exposed and mobilized. The cuff and tubing are freed from the urethra. The tubing is clamped and the existing cuff removed. The urethral diameter is sized. Two appropriately sized cuffs are then placed around the urethra and connected to the existing tubing. The AUS system is activated. The bladder is filled and the cuffs evaluated for leakage. Once it has been determined that the AUS system is functioning properly without leakage, the surgical wound is closed.

53445

53445   Insertion of inflatable urethral/bladder neck sphincter, including placement of pump, reservoir, and cuff

An artificial urinary sphincter (AUS) is used to control the flow of urine from the bladder through the urethra and can be implanted in both men and women A catheter is placed transurethrally. In male patients, a midline incision is made in the perineum just below the scrotum, carried down through the Colles' fascia and the bulbocavernosus muscle. The urethra is freed circumferentially from surrounding tissue. The catheter is removed so that

an accurate circumference of the urethra can be measured. The urethra is measured and an appropriately sized urethral sphincter cuff is chosen. The cuff is prepared and filled with an iso-osmotic solution and passed tab first around the urethra, snapped in place and the tab rotated dorsally. The cuff tubing is then routed through a subcutaneous tunnel to the abdomen. The perineal incision is closed in layers and the surgeon begins the next phase of the surgery through the abdomen. A midline or transverse suprapubic incision is made in the skin and carried down to divide the rectus fascia. The linea alba is opened and the prevesical space is accessed creating a pocket large enough to accommodate the balloon. The balloon is prepared and filled with the iso-osmotic solution and the tubing clamped. The balloon is positioned in the prevesical space and the tubing routed through the rectus fascia to the abdominal incision. The pump is prepared with the iso-osmotic solution. From the abdominal incision, dissection is carried down to the chosen hemiscrotum creating a dependent subdartos pouch. The pump is placed in the pouch with the locking button facing out. The pump tubing should remain above the rectus muscle and fascia in the abdominal incision. After the components are in place the connecting tubing is trimmed and ends sealed with sutureless connectors. The device is cycled 2 or 3 times to check for fluid leaks and functionality and the cuff is then locked in open position. The abdominal incision is closed in layers and a catheter is again inserted transurethrally. Implantation an AUS in women is accomplished through a transverse midline incision in the lower abdomen with or without a U-shaped anterior wall incision in the vagina. The abdomen is incised and the rectus muscle separated to enter the retropubic space. The bladder is separated from the pubic symphysis. Bilateral tunnels are created through the endopelvic fascia extending below the urethra and exiting in the anterior wall of the vagina. If the procedure is performed with an anterior vaginal wall incision, the retro pubic space is entered laterally from the undersurface of the pubic bone. The bladder neck and urethra are mobilized. The cuff, tubing and balloon are placed as described above and the pump is placed in the labia majora. The device is tested as described above and the incisions are closed.

53446-53448

53446   Removal of inflatable urethral/bladder neck sphincter, including pump, reservoir, and cuff

53447   Removal and replacement of inflatable urethral/bladder neck sphincter including pump, reservoir, and cuff at the same operative session

53448   Removal and replacement of inflatable urethral/bladder neck sphincter including pump, reservoir, and cuff through an infected field at the same operative session including irrigation and debridement of infected tissue

The artificial urinary sphincter or AUS is removed through the same incision site(s) used to implant the device. In, 53446, the AUS is removed without replacement. A catheter is placed transurethrally. In male patients a midline incision is made in the perineum just below the scrotum, carried down through the Colles' fascia and the bulbocavernosus muscle. The tubing is clamped and the cuff is freed from the urethra and surrounding tissue. The tubing is tracked through the subcutaneous tunnel to the abdomen and dissected free from surrounding tissue. A midline or transverse suprapubic incision is made in the skin and carried down to divide the rectus fascia. The linea alba is opened and the balloon and tubing dissected free from the tissue in the prevesical space. The tubing is then tracked to the subdartos pouch in the hemiscrotum and the pump and tubing are dissected free from the surrounding tissue. In women, removal is accomplished through an incision in the lower abdomen with or without a separate anterior wall incision in the vagina. The abdomen is incised and the rectus muscle separated to enter the retropubic space. The balloon is located and dissected free from surrounding tissue, tubing is tracked and dissected to the endopelvic fascia and the anterior wall of the vagina. In a transvaginal approach, tubing is tracked and dissected upwards to the retropubic space. The cuff is located and dissected free from the urethra followed by tracking of tubing and dissection to the pump in the labia majora. In both men and women, the tubing is then clamped to avoid fluid leakage into the surgical wound and the device is removed though the incisions. Drains may be placed and the abdominal and perineal/vaginal incisions are closed in layers. In 53447, the removal is performed as described above and replaced with a new AUS system. A flexible cuff is placed around the bladder neck or urethra. A reservoir of liquid is placed next to the cuff and attached to the cuff with tubing. A pump is placed in the scrotum in males or the labia majora in females. The AUS system is tested for functionality and the incisions are closed. Use 53448 if the removal and replacement is performed on a patient with an infection due to the device. The procedure is performed as described above except that the wound is copiously irrigated with an antibiotic solution and extra care must be taken to ensure that all infected and necrotic tissue has been debrided.

53449

53449   Repair of inflatable urethral/bladder neck sphincter, including pump, reservoir, and cuff

Mechanical failure of the artificial urinary sphincter (AUS) is most often due to depressurization such as loss of fluid or disconnection but may also result from obstruction caused by tubing kinks or inadequate position of the pump. Physical examination, radiologic or urodynamic studies are employed first to try and diagnose the problem. If surgical intervention is necessary small incisions are made in the lower abdomen to access the balloon and tubing that connects the balloon to the cuff and pump. The tubing is disconnected and using a syringe, iso-osmotic fluid is injected into the balloon to visually inspect for leaks. Next a syringe is used to inject 1-2 ml of solution into the cuff to check for leaks. After a minute has elapsed, the same amount of fluid should be drawn back out if no leak is present. Pump function is assessed by attaching syringes to the tubing coming from the cuff and balloon and with external manipulation of the pump, fluid is observed shifting between the two syringes. This manipulation may remove air bubbles or debris which could be the cause of pump malfunction. If any component of the device is found to defective it is replaced. Tubing that is kinked is shortened or rerouted in a straighter pathway. Tubing is reconnected and the device is cycled a few times before the small surgical incisions are closed in layers.

53450-53460

53450   Urethromeatoplasty, with mucosal advancement
53460   Urethromeatoplasty, with partial excision of distal urethral segment (Richardson type procedure)

The physician widens the opening of the urethra to improve urination. The physician removes some tissue from the penis, so it will not constrict the urethra.

53500

53500   Urethrolysis, transvaginal, secondary, open, including cystourethroscopy (eg, postsurgical obstruction, scarring)

To identify postoperative obstruction or scarring and determine if urethrolysis is necessary, cystourethroscopy is performed first. The cystourethroscope is inserted through the urethral meatus and advanced toward the bladder as the surgeon searches for areas of tissue erosion, scarring, stenosis, obstruction or fistula formation. The scope is removed and the procedure continues by making a midline or U-shaped incision in the anterior wall of the vagina. Dissection continues along the surface of the periurethral fascia to the pubic bone. Retracting the endopelvic fascia, periurethral fascia and vaginal wall laterally exposes the retropubic space which is entered between the attachment of the endopelvic fascia to the obturator fascia. The urethra is then dissected free of the proximal bladder at the underside of the pubic bone. Any adhesions are lysed. Previously placed sutures may be cut to allow mobility of the bladder and urethra. Once the urethra is completely freed of adhesions and scar tissue, the wound is closed in layers. A catheter may be placed transurethrally following the procedure.

53502

53502   Urethrorrhaphy, suture of urethral wound or injury, female

Surgical repair of a urethral wound or injury in a female is performed. With the patient in dorsal lithotomy position, the vagina, vulva and perineum are prepped and draped. A midline or U-shaped incision is made in the anterior vaginal wall. The periurethral fascia is dissected and the urethra identified. The mucosal and muscular layers of the urethral defect are closed over a previously placed transurethral catheter. The periurethral fascia is closed with absorbable sutures followed by the vaginal wall. The urethral catheter is left in place.

53505-53510

53505   Urethrorrhaphy, suture of urethral wound or injury; penile
53510   Urethrorrhaphy, suture of urethral wound or injury; perineal

Surgical repair of an injury to the male urethra is performed. In 53505, surgical repair of the penile urethra is accomplished with the patient supine or in low lithotomy position. The penis, scrotum and perineal area are prepped and draped. For a penetrating injury, the wound it cleaned, corpus spongiosum or corpus cavernosum debrided and the area is examined for associated injuries. The urethral wound is repaired with sutures over a catheter previously placed transurethrally into the bladder. Drains may be placed if the wound is large or contaminated. The corpus spongiosum or corpus cavernosum is closed with absorbable sutures followed by closure of the skin. In 53510, surgical repair of an injury to the bulbar urethra is approached through a midline perineal incision. The bulbocavernosus muscle is divided and corpus spongiosum entered at the site of the injury. The wound is cleaned and corpus spongiosum debrided if necessary. The urethra is exposed and examined. The technique for repair is similar to a urethroplasty for strictures. For a urethral defect of <25 mm, the repair is accomplished by anastomosis. To repair a longer defect, the urethra is dissected distally from the corpus spongiosum to maximize the length. The distal end is spatulated dorsally, the proximal end ventrally. Anastomosis of the urethral ends is accomplished with a single layer suture through the urethral mucosa and spongiosal adventitia on the dorsal surface and two layers of sutures on the ventral surface. Drains may be placed if the wound is large or contaminated. The corpus spongiosum is closed followed by the bulbocavernosus muscle and the skin. A catheter may be placed transurethrally into the bladder at the end of the procedure.

53515

53515   Urethrorrhaphy, suture of urethral wound or injury; prostatomembranous

Surgical repair of an injury to the prostatomembranous urethra may be attempted immediately if the patient requires exploratory surgery to identify rectal or vascular injuries but is most often delayed as long as 6-12 weeks to allow for absorption of a hematoma. In either case a suprapubic catheter is necessary and can be placed percutaneously or with open cystotomy. The surgical technique for immediate repair will vary depending on other injuries sustained by the patient. For delayed repair, a midline perineal incision is made and the bulbospongiosum muscle divided. Dissection continues through the corpus spongiosum until the urethra is located. Proceeding in the direction of the bulbar urethra, the proximal point of obliteration is identified using a catheter and the distal point as far as the suspensory ligament to the penis is assessed. A sound is then passed via the suprapubic cystotomy tract through the bladder neck and into the prostatic urethra. Beginning at the level of the crus and working distally, the right and left corporal bodies are separated in the midline for a distance of 4-5 cm allowing the urethra to move upwards and shortening the distance between the urethral ends. If urethral tension remains after separating the corporal bodies, dissection continues by displacing or ligating the penile vessels laterally. Then using bone rongeurs or an osteotome, a wedge of bone is removed from the pubis at the inferior aspect creating a groove for the urethra to settle into and adding 1-2 cm of urethral length. If anastomosis is still not possible due to urethral tension, the urethra is rerouted around the corporal body through a larger resection of the pubic bone by circumferentially mobilizing one of the corporal bodies proximal to the suspensory penile ligament and dissecting away from the surface to avoid injury to neurovascular tissue. The distal urethral stump is spatulated and brought down from a 12-o'clock position and the proximal urethral stump is also spatulated and lifted from the 6-o'clock position, healthy tissue is identified along with the seminal ducts in the verumontanum of the prostatic urethra. Anastomosis of the two ends of the urethra is accomplished by placing sutures through the urethral mucosa and tying them after all have been placed. A fenestrated catheter is placed transurethrally. The corpus spongiosum is closed followed by the bulbospongiosum muscle. The perineal skin is sutured and the suprapubic catheter is replaced.

53520

53520   Closure of urethrostomy or urethrocutaneous fistula, male (separate procedure)

To close an urethrostomy or urethrocutaneous fistula as a separate procedure in males, a catheter is placed transurethrally. A midline incision is made along the urethral opening in the penile skin and the epithelialized fistula/urethrostomy is excised, inverting the urethral mucosa and closing the defect over the catheter. Next, the skin layer of the penile incision is extended proximally toward the scrotum until the subcutaneous dartos muscle is visualized. The scrotal skin is undermined and a flap marked in the dartos muscle. The flap is excised along the marks, elevated and flipped over the fistula/urethrostomy. Needle point cautery is used to control bleeding. The edges of the flap are sutured over the urethral repair. The dartos muscle is approximated in the scrotum and sutured. A drain may be placed. The scrotal skin is closed. The penile skin is closed without tension over the dartos flap and the foley catheter is left in place.

53600-53601

53600   Dilation of urethral stricture by passage of sound or urethral dilator, male; initial
53601   Dilation of urethral stricture by passage of sound or urethral dilator, male; subsequent

A urethral stricture in a male is dilated by passage of a sound or urethral dilator. A urethral stricture is a narrowing of the urethra typically due to infection or trauma. A series of increasingly larger sounds are inserted. Sounds are rods with rounded ends. Alternatively, a special balloon catheter may be used to dilate the stricture. Some balloon dilators have an integral urinary drainage catheter that can be left in the bladder. If sounds are used to dilate the stricture, a urinary catheter may be inserted following dilation to maintain the opening. Use 53600 for the initial dilation using a sound or urethral dilator and 53601 for subsequent procedures.

53605

53605   Dilation of urethral stricture or vesical neck by passage of sound or urethral dilator, male, general or conduction (spinal) anesthesia

After satisfactory induction of general or regional anesthesia, the male patient is placed in dorsal lithotomy position and the penis and scrotum are prepped and draped. Serial dilatation of the urethral stricture or vesical neck is accomplished using urethral sounds or S-curve urethral dilators of increasing size and thickness until the narrowed area of the urethra or vesical neck has widened. A catheter is placed transurethrally following the procedure.

Urinary System

53620-53621

53620 Dilation of urethral stricture by passage of filiform and follower, male; initial

53621 Dilation of urethral stricture by passage of filiform and follower, male; subsequent

A urethral stricture in a male is dilated by passage of a filiform and follower. A urethral stricture is a narrowing of the urethra typically due to infection or trauma. There are two types of filiform dilators available. One type uses a filiform wire guide with a series of followers, which are threadlike instruments. The wire guide is inserted into the urethra. Followers of increasing diameter are then inserted over the wire guide to expand the narrowed portion of the urethra. A second type is an integral filiform urethral dilator that eliminates the need for followers. Use 53620 for the initial dilation using a filiform and follower and 53621 for subsequent procedures.

53660-53665

53660 Dilation of female urethra including suppository and/or instillation; initial

53661 Dilation of female urethra including suppository and/or instillation; subsequent

53665 Dilation of female urethra, general or conduction (spinal) anesthesia

Dilation of the female urethra is performed. This procedure is done to treat a narrowing or stricture of the urethra caused by injury, scarring, congenital anomaly, or other conditions. The urethral opening is cleansed. A local anesthetic is applied in the form of a suppository, jelly, or liquid to numb the urethra. Alternatively, general or conduction (spinal) anesthesia may be used. A series of tubes or dilators are then passed through the urethral opening to the urethrovesical junction to increase the diameter of the narrowed segment of urethra. A urethroscope may be used to guide the dilators. Following the dilation procedure, a catheter may be inserted and left in place to drain the bladder. Use 53660 for initial dilation or 53661 for subsequent dilation performed under local anesthesia. Use 53665 for dilation (initial or subsequent) performed under general or conduction (spinal) anesthesia.

53850

53850 Transurethral destruction of prostate tissue; by microwave thermotherapy

Transurethral microwave thermotherapy (TUMT) is used to treat benign prostatic hypertrophy (BPH). With the patient awake and positioned supine, the penis is prepped with an antiseptic solution and 10-20 ml of 1-2 % Lidocaine gel is instilled into the urethra for local anesthesia. A special catheter is inserted through the urethra to the bladder and anchored in place with a balloon tip. The catheter contains a microwave antenna which is positioned within the prostatic urethra. Position of the catheter may be verified using separately reportable transrectal ultrasound. A probe is then placed in the rectum to monitor temperature during the procedure. The machine is activated and treatment begins. Microwave currents raise the temperature to above 45 degrees centigrade in the prostate gland, destroying excess tissue. At the same time, water flows through the catheter and cools the urethra to prevent damage to surrounding tissue. The patient is monitored throughout the 30-60 minute procedure for pain or discomfort. At the end of the procedure the treatment catheter is removed and replaced by a Foley catheter inserted transurethrally.

53852

53852 Transurethral destruction of prostate tissue; by radiofrequency thermotherapy

Transurethral radiofrequency thermotherapy also known as transurethral needle ablation (TUNA) is used to treat benign prostatic hypertrophy (BPH). With the patient awake and in a dorsal lithotomy position, the penis is prepped with an antiseptic solution and 10-20 ml of 1-2 % Lidocaine gel is instilled into the urethra for local anesthesia. A rectal probe may be placed to monitor temperature during the procedure. A special catheter is inserted to the level of the prostatic urethra and an interstitial radiofrequency needle is deployed through the urethral wall into the prostatic tissue. Bipolar electrodes in the needle are activated by a machine. The low wave radiofrequency energy produces heat to between 60-100 degrees centigrade destroying excess prostatic tissue within minutes. At the same time, water flows through the catheter and cools the urethra to prevent damage to surrounding tissue. The needle is withdrawn and repositioned a few centimeters away and the machine is activated again until all lobes of the prostate have been treated. At the end of the procedure the treatment catheter is removed and may be replaced by a Foley catheter inserted transurethrally.

53855

53855 Insertion of a temporary prostatic urethral stent, including urethral measurement

A temporary urethral stent is used to treat obstruction of the prostatic urethra due to benign prostatic hyperplasia (BPH) or following surgical treatment for BPH, prostatic cancer, or radiation therapy. Temporary stenting of the prostatic urethra is used as an alternative to placement of a Foley catheter and allows the patient to urinate normally. One type of stent is consists of a proximal balloon to prevent migration or displacement of the stent, a urine port is situated above the balloon, a stent that spans the prostatic urethra, an anchor in the distal meatus, and a retrieval string for removal of the temporary stent. The urethral orifice is cleansed with antiseptic solution. An introducer is inserted into the urethra and the stent device advanced until the tip is in the bladder and the stent positioned in the prostatic urethra above the urethral sphincter. The balloon is inflated with sterile water to secure the soft tip in the bladder. The introducer is removed. The stent holds the prostatic urethra open so that urine can be passed normally.

53860

53860 Transurethral radiofrequency micro-remodeling of the female bladder neck and proximal urethra for stress urinary incontinence

The physician performs transurethral radiofrequency micro-remodeling of the female bladder neck and proximal urethra for urinary stress incontinence due to hypermobility. Low temperature radiofrequency energy is used to remodel the submucosal tissue of the bladder neck and urethra and change the luminal function without causing narrowing or thickening of the lumen. A local anesthetic is administered. The transurethral probe is inserted into the urethra, and controlled radiofrequency energy is applied to heat the submucosal tissue at target sites in the lower urinary tract. This results in collagen denaturation at the multiple small treatment sites. When the tissue heals, the treated sites have increased resistance to intra-abdominal pressure, which reduces or eliminates involuntary leakage of urine.

54000-54001

54000   Slitting of prepuce, dorsal or lateral (separate procedure); newborn

54001   Slitting of prepuce, dorsal or lateral (separate procedure); except newborn

The physician makes a dorsal or lateral slit in the prepuce. The prepuce, also referred to as the foreskin, is the free fold of skin that covers the glans penis in uncircumcised males. If the prepuce is too tight, it is incised (slit) on the back (dorsum) or sides (lateral). Use 54000 when the procedure is performed on a newborn and 54001 when it is performed on a patient other than a newborn.

54015

54015   Incision and drainage of penis, deep

The patient is positioned supine and the penis is prepped with an antiseptic solution. The area is infiltrated with local anesthetic and an incision made through the skin and carried down to the corpus cavernosum and/or the corpus spongiosum until the infected area is opened and pus/fluid starts to drain. Infected or devitalized tissue is debrided including the epithelial cell lining. The wound is cleaned and irrigated with saline and/or antibacterial solution. A drain is placed and the wound closed with simple sutures. A sterile dressing is applied immediately following the procedure. The dressing and drain are removed 2-3 days later.

54050-54065

54050   Destruction of lesion(s), penis (eg, condyloma, papilloma, molluscum contagiosum, herpetic vesicle), simple; chemical

54055   Destruction of lesion(s), penis (eg, condyloma, papilloma, molluscum contagiosum, herpetic vesicle), simple; electrodesiccation

54056   Destruction of lesion(s), penis (eg, condyloma, papilloma, molluscum contagiosum, herpetic vesicle), simple; cryosurgery

54057   Destruction of lesion(s), penis (eg, condyloma, papilloma, molluscum contagiosum, herpetic vesicle), simple; laser surgery

54060   Destruction of lesion(s), penis (eg, condyloma, papilloma, molluscum contagiosum, herpetic vesicle), simple; surgical excision

54065   Destruction of lesion(s), penis (eg, condyloma, papilloma, molluscum contagiosum, herpetic vesicle), extensive (eg, laser surgery, electrosurgery, cryosurgery, chemosurgery)

The physician destroys one or more lesions on the penis using a method such as chemical destruction, electrodessication, cryosurgery, laser surgery, electrosurgery, or surgical excision. Common types of lesions treated include condylomata, papillomata, molluscum contagiosum, and herpetic vesicles. The lesion is examined and the most appropriate form of destruction determined. Local anesthesia is administered as needed. In 54050, a simple chemical destruction is performed with silver nitrate or other chemical compound. In 54055, a simple electrodessication is performed using a monopolar high-frequency electric current to destroy the lesion and control bleeding. In 54056, cryosurgery is performed using liquid nitrogen to freeze the lesion. A series of freeze-thaw cycles may be required to completely destroy the lesion. In 54057, a simple laser ablation is performed using a non-contact Nd-YAG laser or a contact laser probe with coaxial water to vaporize the lesion. In, 54060 a simple excision is performed. A narrow margin of healthy tissue is identified and a full-thickness incision is made through the mucous and submucous tissue. The incision is carried around the lesion and the entire lesion is excised. The lesion is sent to the laboratory for separately reportable histologic evaluation. Bleeding is controlled by electrocautery or chemical cautery. The wound may be closed using simple single layer suture technique or left open to granulate. In 54065, extensive destruction of a large lesion or multiple lesions is performed using laser surgery, electrosurgery, cryosurgery, or chemosurgery. Laser surgery, cryosurgery, or chemosurgery is performed as described above over an extensive area. Alternatively, electrosurgery may be performed. Electrosurgery uses heat applied to the lesion(s) with a high frequency current that passes through a metal probe or needle.

54100-54105

54100   Biopsy of penis; (separate procedure)

54105   Biopsy of penis; deep structures

A biopsy of the penis is performed. In 54100, a simple biopsy is performed. The area to be biopsied is disinfected and a local anesthetic administered. An incision is in the skin overlying the lesion. A tissue sample is obtained. The tissue is sent to the laboratory for separately reportable histological evaluation. In 54105, a biopsy of deeper tissue is performed which may require use of a general anesthetic. Overlying tissues are dissected

until the suspicious mass or lump is exposed. A tissue sample is obtained and sent for separately reportable histological evaluation.

54110-54112

54110   Excision of penile plaque (Peyronie disease)

54111   Excision of penile plaque (Peyronie disease); with graft to 5 cm in length

54112   Excision of penile plaque (Peyronie disease); with graft greater than 5 cm in length

Excision of penile plaque associated with Peyronie's disease is performed with or without graft repair. Peyronie's disease is characterized by the development of a hard, fibrous layer of scar tissue (plaque) under the skin in the spongy erectile tissue on the upper or lower side of the penis. The plaque causes the penis to curve when erect. The overlying tissue is incised and the plaque exposed. The plaque is then expanded by making several linear cuts in the plaque or excised. The areas of excision or expansion are covered as needed using a graft of skin, vein, or synthetic material. Use 54110, if the procedure is performed without a graft, 54111 if a graft of 5 cm or less is used, and 54112 if a graft of greater than 5 cm is required.

54115

54115   Removal foreign body from deep penile tissue (eg, plastic implant)

To remove a foreign body, such as an implant, from deep penile tissue, the patient is positioned supine and the penis is prepped and draped. An incision is made along the shaft of the penis overlying the foreign body and carried down to the corpus cavernosum and/or corpus spongiosum until the object is visualized. Tissue surrounding the object is dissected free including devitalized or infected tissue and the wound irrigated with saline and/or antibacterial solution. A drain is placed and the wound closed with simple sutures. A sterile dressing is applied immediately following the procedure. The dressing and drain are removed 2-3 days later.

54120

54120   Amputation of penis; partial

Partial amputation of the penis or penectomy is performed with the patient in supine position under local, regional or general anesthesia. The penis is prepped and draped and the tumor or lesion may be isolated by suturing a sterile condom or glove to the penile tip. A tourniquet is placed around the base of the penis and a circumferential incision is made in the skin 1.5 to 2.0 cm proximal to the tumor or lesion. Superficial and deep dorsal veins are identified, cut and tied with sutures. Dissection continues through Buck's fascia and the tunica albuginea of the corpora. The corpora cavernosa is divided down to the urethra to identify the central cavernosal arteries which are tied off with sutures. The urethra is now dissected free from the corpus spongiosum, leaving a 1 cm urethral stump distally to the transected corpora cavernosa and the specimen is removed. Tissue samples from the amputated penis are then prepared and examined by a pathologist in a separately reportable procedure to determine if margins are clear of cancer or other abnormal cells. The remaining urethral stump and transected corpora are washed off with an antiseptic or antibiotic solution and the closure begins by placing horizontal mattress sutures using through the corpora, incorporating Buck's fascia, tunica albuginea and intercavernous septum. The tourniquet is released from the base of the penis and bleeding controlled by fulguration. The urethra is spatulated and sutured to the skin. The skin is closed or if a dorsal skin flap has been left, a button-hole incision is made in the flap, the flap is rotated ventrally anastomosing the dorsally spatulated urethra to the button-hole opening, and finally closing the skin flaps. One other option is to leave a slightly longer urethral stump, 1.5 to 2 cm and spatulate ventrally, the dorsal flap is then rotated and sutured to the tunica albuginea of the corpora cavernosa and skin. A catheter is inserted transurethrally at the conclusion of the procedure.

54125

54125   Amputation of penis; complete

Complete amputation of penis may be necessary when a tumor or lesion is large or infiltrating. With the patient in dorsal lithotomy position the penis, scrotum and perineum are prepped and draped. The tumor or lesion is isolated with a sterile condom or glove sheathing the entire penis and sutured at the base. An elliptical skin incision is made at the base of the penis and carried through the subcutaneous tissue to the pubis. Blood vessels and lymphatic tissue are ligated or fulgurated. Penile suspensory ligaments are identified and isolated. The dorsal vein and penile arteries are identified, clamped and ligated. Positioning the penis upward, Buck's fascia is opened and the urethra is dissected free from the corpora cavernosa. The urethra is divided at the distal bulbar region with adequate length to route to the perineuem. Dissection of the corpora cavernosa continues to the ischiopubic rami where it is ligated and transected and the amputation is complete. Tissue samples from the amputated penis are then prepared and examined by a pathologist in a separately reportable procedure to determine if margins are clear of cancer or other abnormal cells. Dissection continues around the urethra to the urogenital diaphragm attempting a straight course to the perineal urethostomy site. A 1 cm wedge of skin and subcutaneous tissue is removed from the perineum midline between the scrotum and the rectum. Using a curved clamp, a tunnel is created in the perineal subcutaneous tissue and the urethra is pulled through the perineal incision. After spatulating the urethra dorsally, a V-shaped skin inlay is created and anastomosed to the lining of the urethra. A catheter is inserted transurethrally. Penrose drains are placed on either side of the scrotum and the wound is closed transversely allowing elevation of the scrotum away from the perineal urethrostomy site.

54130-54135

54130   Amputation of penis, radical; with bilateral inguinofemoral lymphadenectomy

54135   Amputation of penis, radical; in continuity with bilateral pelvic lymphadenectomy, including external iliac, hypogastric and obturator nodes

The tumor or lesion in the penis is isolated with a sterile condom or glove sheathing the entire penis and sutured at the base. An elliptical skin incision is made at the base of the penis and carried through the subcutaneous tissue to the pubis. Blood vessels and lymphatic tissue are ligated or fulgurated. Penile suspensory ligaments are identified and isolated. The dorsal vein and penile arteries are identified, clamped and ligated. Positioning the penis upward, Buck's fascia is opened and the urethra is dissected free from the corpora cavernosa. The urethra is divided at the distal bulbar region leaving adequate length to route to the perineum. The corpora cavernosa is dissected to the ischiopubic rami where it is ligated and transected and the amputation is complete. Dissection continues around the urethra to the urogenital diaphragm attempting a straight course to the perineal urethostomy site. A wedge of skin and subcutaneous tissue is removed from the perineum midline between the scrotum and the rectum. Using a curved clamp, a tunnel is created in the perineal subcutaneous tissue and the urethra is pulled through the perineal incision. After spatulating the urethra dorsally, a V-shaped skin inlay is created and anastomosed to the lining of the urethra. A catheter is inserted. Penrose drains are placed on either side of the scrotum and the wound is closed transversely to elevate the scrotum away from the perineal urethrostomy site. In 54130, amputation of the penis is performed with bilateral inguinofemoral lymphadenectomy. An incision is made parallel to the inguinofemoral ligament and carried down to Camper's fascia. Skin flaps are elevated and separated from the underlying fat pad. Deep tissues at the superior aspect of the inguinal region are dissected. Cloquets node is identified, excised and frozen section performed. The fat pad containing nodal tissue is elevated and mobilized down to the inferior margin of the inguinal ligament. Dissection continues into the femoral triangle. The cribiform fascia is opened. Once the nodal tissue over the common femoral vein has been completely freed the inguinofemoral nodal tissue is removed as a single specimen. In 54135, the amputation of the penis and inguinofemoral lymphadenectomy is performed as described above. If Cloquets node is positive for malignancy, bilateral pelvic lymphadenectomy including excision of external iliac, hypogastric, and obturator nodes is performed. The abdomen is incised without opening the peritoneum, and the pelvic lymph nodes are explored. Fatty tissue is stripped from the mid-portion of the common iliac vessel and along the internal and external iliac vessels to the level of the circumflex iliac vein. Iliac, hypogastric and obturator nodes are excised. The groin and abdominal incisions are closed in layers.

54150

54150   Circumcision, using clamp or other device with regional dorsal penile or ring block

The foreskin on the head of the penis of a newborn is removed. The physician places a clamp or other device over the head of the penis to expose the foreskin, which is then removed. The clamp stays in place for a few days until all of the foreskin is gone. A regional block is included.

54160-54161

54160   Circumcision, surgical excision other than clamp, device, or dorsal slit; neonate (28 days of age or less)

54161   Circumcision, surgical excision other than clamp, device, or dorsal slit; older than 28 days of age

A male circumcision is performed using a method other than a clamp, device, or dorsal slit technique. Circumcision involves excision or removal of the prepuce, also referred to as the foreskin, which is the free fold of skin that covers the glans penis in uncircumcised males. A local anesthetic is injected. Alternatively, for older children and adults, a general anesthetic may be used. The physician then uses a free hand technique to excise of the prepuce. Use 54160 for a neonate defined as a patient aged 28 days or less. Use 54161 for a patient older than 28 days of age.

54162

54162   Lysis or excision of penile post-circumcision adhesions

Adhesions sometimes form between the remaining prepuce (foreskin) and the glans penis following circumcision. While most adhesions resolve without surgical intervention, persistent adhesions may be cut (lysed) or excised. A general, regional, or local anesthetic is administered. A scalpel is then used to lyse or excise the adhesions.

54163

54163   Repair incomplete circumcision

This procedure is performed when there is excessive residual prepuce (foreskin) remaining following a previously performed circumcision. A general, regional, or local anesthetic is administered. If the head of the penis can be exposed, residual prepuce is the excised. If the head of the penis cannot be exposed due to the formation of adhesions between the glans penis and residual prepuce, the adhesions are first cut (lysed) and then the residual prepuce is excised.

54164

54164   Frenulotomy of penis

A frenulotomy of the penis may also be referred to as a frenuloplasty. With the patient positioned supine after a local anesthetic has been applied topically or injected, the penis is prepped and draped. A Z-shaped superficial skin incision is made with a slanting cut in the glans, followed by a vertical cut along the preputial fold and a second slanting cut in the prepuce. The incision is then straightened allowing the penis to elongate. Fine absorbable sutures are used to close the incision. A variation of this procedure may be performed using vascular clips. One clip is placed under the glans and the second parallel to the foreskin. A vertical incision is made between the two clips and they are pulled apart to stretch and elongate the frenulum. Sutures are not usually necessary and the clips fall off in a few days.

54200-54205

54200   Injection procedure for Peyronie disease

54205   Injection procedure for Peyronie disease; with surgical exposure of plaque

Peyronie's disease is treated with an injection procedure with or without surgical exposure of plaque. Peyronie's disease is characterized by the development of a hard, fibrous layer of scar tissue (plaque) under the skin in the spongy erectile tissue on the upper or lower side of the penis. The plaque causes the penis to curve when erect. In 54200, the physician injects a drug that breaks down scar tissue and allows normal tissues to regenerate. Common drugs used include collagenase, calcium channel blockers such as verapimil, or interferons. The drugs are injected through the skin and into the plaque at multiple sites on the affected side of the penis. In 54205, the skin is incised and tissue dissected to expose the plaque. The drug is then injected at multiple sites directly into the plaque.

54220

54220   Irrigation of corpora cavernosa for priapism

Irrigation of the corpora cavernosa for priapism is accomplished with the patient awake. A penile ring block or local infiltration of anesthetic into the skin and tunica albuginea may be used for pain control. A 16 or 18 gauge needle is used to enter the lateral aspect of the corpus cavernosa. A 10 cc syringe is attached and an attempt made to aspirate blood from the tissue. If aspiration is unsuccessful, the syringe is removed from the needle and a 3-way stopcock attached. A liter of saline solution is connected via intravenous tubing to the stopcock opposite the needle and the syringe placed into the top port. Saline is drawn into the syringe and injected through the needle into the corpus cavernosa. The syringe is then used to aspirate thinned blood and the irrigation fluid back out of the tissue. The cycle continues until detumescence occurs. The needle can then be removed and firm pressure applied to the site for 5 minutes. Unilateral irrigation is usually successful in draining both sides of the corpora cavernosa. If saline alone does not relieve the priapism, epinephrine or phenylephrine may be added to the irrigation fluid.

54230

54230   Injection procedure for corpora cavernosography

Cavernosography involves the injection of contrast medium into the corpora cavernosa to examine radiographically the structure of the corpora cavernosa and the veins that drain blood from it. A 19-22 gauge needle is inserted into the tissue of the corpora cavernosa on the dorsal lateral aspect proximal to the glans penis. Contrast medium is injected and separately radiographic images are taken immediately from two angles, anterior/posterior and lateral/oblique. In less than a minute, the contrast medium should begin to flow through the channels between the two sides of the corpora cavernosa and drain down into the deep dorsal or crural veins. The needle is removed at the end of the procedure and pressure applied to the site. This code reports only the injection procedure. The radiologist's supervision and interpretation is reported separately.

● New Code   ▲ Revised Code   CPT © 2016 American Medical Association. All Rights Reserved.   © 2017 DecisionHealth

54231

54231	**Dynamic cavernosometry, including intracavernosal injection of vasoactive drugs (eg, papaverine, phentolamine)**

Dynamic cavernosometry measures the vascular pressure in the corpus cavernosum during an erection. Using a 27-30 gauge needle, a vasodilatory drug such as Caverject or papaverine is injected into the corpora to produce arterial and sinusoidal relaxation. Following local injection of an anesthetic, a 19 gauge Butterfly needle is inserted into the corpus cavernosum at a vertical angle to the penile axis to allow for movement during the erection. A perfusion pump with normal saline is attached to the needle and the fluid is pumped into the tissue until an erection is achieved. The pressure continues to be monitored and erectile activity observed until it reaches about 150 mm/Hg. The infusion is then stopped and the cavernosum pressure measured. Rapid fall in pressure and loss of an erection may indicate leakage into the vessels.

54235

54235	**Injection of corpora cavernosa with pharmacologic agent(s) (eg, papaverine, phentolamine)**

The penis is laid across the thigh to stabilize and stretch it and the foreskin is retracted if the penis is uncircumcised. The injection site is selected and skin cleansed with alcohol. The site may be on either side of the penis, anywhere from the base to the glans. Care must be taken not to inject in the midline or underside of the penis or through visible veins. A needle is inserted at a 90 degree angle up to the needle hub and medication is injected over 1-2 minutes. The needle is removed and pressure applied to control bleeding. The corpora cavernosa is squeezed along one side and then the other and then pinched transversely at intervals to evenly distribute the medication along the entire length of the penis.

54240

54240	**Penile plethysmography**

A plethysmograph is a device that meaures blood flow in the various parts of the body. Penile plethysmography, also referred to as penile pulse volume recording, is used to diagnose erectile dysfunction. Either a volumetric air chamber type or a circumferential transducer type may be used. The volumetric air chamber type is placed over the patient's penis. As the penis becomes erect, air is displaced and the amount of air displacement is measured. The circumferential transducer type uses a rubber ring filled with mercury or indium/gallium that is placed around the shaft of the patient's penis. As the penis becomes erect, changes in diameter are measured. The physician reviews the results of the plethysmography and provides a written interpretation of the results.

54250

54250	**Nocturnal penile tumescence and/or rigidity test**

This test is performed to determine whether the patient is having normal erections during sleep. The results are used to evaluate the cause of and/or level of erectile dysfunction. The test may be done at home or in a sleep lab. An electronic monitoring device is used to record how many erections occur during sleep, how long the erections last, and how rigid the penis becomes during each erection. The physician reviews the recording and provides a written interpretation of the results.

54300

54300	**Plastic operation of penis for straightening of chordee (eg, hypospadias), with or without mobilization of urethra**

There are several accepted techniques to straighten a penile curve or chordee. A longitudinal incision is made through the circumcision scar along the shaft of the penis, carried down to the superficial layer of Buck's fascia and the penile skin is degloved. A needle is inserted into the corpus cavernosum at a vertical angle to the penile axis to allow for movement during the erection. A perfusion pump with normal saline is attached to the needle and fluid pumped into the tissue until an erection is achieved and the location and degree of curvature observed. For a ventral curvature, the fibrous tissue in dartos fascia is mobilized for removal and the fibrous tissue in Buck's fascia is opened using scissors allowing mobilization of the urethra and corpus spongiosum between the glans and the penoscrotal junction. An erection is again induced with saline and if the penis is straight, the degloved skin is repositioned and the wound closed. An alternative approach when penile length does not need to be considered is excision and plication of the tunica albuginea. A circumferential skin incision is made at the glans and the penis degloved allowing the urethra to be mobilized by resection from the dartos and Buck's fascia. Erection is induced as described previously and if curvature remains, an ellipse of tissue opposite the concave curve is marked and excised from the tunica albuginea. The edges of the ellipse are sutured closed. If a penile curve remains, additional elliptical incisions are made until the penis is straight. The degloved skin is then mobilized back up the shaft of the penis and sutured around the glans. When only a lateral curve requires correction, erection is induced as previously described and a small vertical incision is made through Buck's fascia at the point of maximal curvature. A horizontal ellipse of tissue is removed from the tunica albuginea as previously described and the edges sutured. An erection

is again induced and if the penis is straight Buck's fascia is sutured closed followed by closure of the skin.

54304

54304	**Plastic operation on penis for correction of chordee or for first stage hypospadias repair with or without transplantation of prepuce and/or skin flaps**

The penis may have a normal glans and urethral meatus but thin and poorly developed urethral mucosa and spongiosum tissue causing penile curvature. A staged repair is undertaken to correct the chordee and augment the urethra with an onlay island graft. The patient is positioned supine and the penis is prepped and draped. The repair begins with identification of the flat ventral glans surface as it begins to curve around the meatus. A vertical incision is made at the midline and widened along the glanular groove until an adequate meatal opening is formed. This incision will be left open to epithelialize. Next an incision is made in the subcoronal tissue around the glans with extensions on either side of the urethral plate where it joins normal skin and on the side of the glandular groove to the apex of the glansplasty. The penile skin is then degloved exposing Buck's fascia but preserving the vascular connection to the preputial flap. The vascular pedicle is separated from the outer preputial skin maintaining blood supply to both layers. An onlay flap is created from the inner prepuce and running sutures are placed beginning under the pedicle to draw the glans together. The wing flaps are rotated medially around the neo-urethra and approximated in the midline with mattress sutures.

54308-54316

54308	**Urethroplasty for second stage hypospadias repair (including urinary diversion); less than 3 cm**

54312	**Urethroplasty for second stage hypospadias repair (including urinary diversion); greater than 3 cm**

54316	**Urethroplasty for second stage hypospadias repair (including urinary diversion) with free skin graft obtained from site other than genitalia**

The physician performs the second stage of a procedure to fix a birth defect in which the urethral opening is somewhere other than the tip of the penis. The urethra is moved less than 3 cm. Code 54312 if the urethra is moved more than 3 cm. Code 54316 if the physician uses a skin graft to complete the procedure. The graft is taken from somewhere other than the genitals.

54318

54318	**Urethroplasty for third stage hypospadias repair to release penis from scrotum (eg, third stage Cecil repair)**

The 3rd stage of a hypospadius repair to release the penis from the scrotum is performed a minimum of six weeks following the 2nd stage to allow for adequate epithelialization of the neo-urethra. The patient is positioned supine and the penis and scrotum are prepped and draped. A Foley catheter is placed transurethrally into the bladder. The approximated skin edges of the penis and scrotum are carefully excised to prevent any transfer of scrotal skin to the penile shaft. The soft tissue of the penile shaft is preserved and the edges of the penile skin from glans to scrotum are approximated and closed in the midline with absorbable sutures. The scrotal skin is then approximated and closed in the same fashion. The Foley catheter may be removed or left in place following the procedure.

54322-54326

54322	**1-stage distal hypospadias repair (with or without chordee or circumcision); with simple meatal advancement (eg, Magpi, V-flap)**

54324	**1-stage distal hypospadias repair (with or without chordee or circumcision); with urethroplasty by local skin flaps (eg, flip-flap, prepucial flap)**

54326	**1-stage distal hypospadias repair (with or without chordee or circumcision); with urethroplasty by local skin flaps and mobilization of urethra**

Hypospadius is a condition in which the urethral meatus is displaced from its normal position at the tip of the penis to the underside of the penis in males. Hypospadius is classified as distal or mild when the meatal opening is small and located in or near the glans. In 54322, mild hypospadias is repaired using simple meatal advancement, also referred to as a meatal advancement and glanduloplasty (MAGPI), inverted Y-meatoglanduloplasty, or V-flap. To perform a MAGPI, a longitudinal circumcising incision is made in the glans followed by dorsal meatotomy to advance the edge of the meatus distally. The ventral edge of the meatus is elevated and brought forward. The flattened wings of the glans are rotated upwards and ventrally to form a cone shape after detaching the glans from the corpus spongiosum at the lateral margin and the corpora cavernosa at the side. The edges of the glans tissue are reapproximated in the midline around the excised urethral meatus in two layers, first incorporating the mesenchyme of the glans and finally the superficial glans epithelium. To perform an inverted Y-meatoglanuloplasty, a longitudinal incision is made midline from the meatus to the edge of the glans. Diverging limb incisions are made along the upper edge of the meatus creating space for the new urethra. The Y-incision is sutured as an inverted V and the glans flaps are wrapped around the urethra and sutured in the midline. In 54324, a single stage repair with urethroplasty using local skin flaps is performed, such as a Mathieu or tubularized incised plate (TIP)

● New Code   ▲ Revised Code

urethroplasty, also known as a Snodgrass procedure. A U-shaped incision along the urethral plate is made and the penis is degloved. Longitudinal incisions are made along the urethral plate to create the glans wings. In the Mathieu procedure, a skin flap is developed proximal to the urethral meatus with sufficient length to reach the tip of the glans. The flap is elevated and sutured to each side of the distal urethra. In the Snodgrass procedure, a midline incision is made from the tip of the glans to the urethral meatus and carried down through the mucosal and submucosal tissue to the corporal bodies creating a tube over a catheter. Both procedures continue with dissection of dorsal subcutaneous tissue from the prepucial and penile shaft skin which is then rotated ventrally covering the neo-urethra. The wings of the glans form a second layer of support for the neo-urethra and are closed symmetrically in 2 layers. A urethral stent or catheter remains in place following the procedure. In 54326, a procedure similar to the Mathieu or Snodgrass procedure is performed except that the urethra is also mobilized. This involves detaching the entire urethra from the anterior aspect of the corpora cavernosa to increase ureteral length, also referred to as Koff technique. If more length is required, the urethra is also freed proximally. This may be referred to as a Turner-Warwick procedure.

54328

54328　　1-stage distal hypospadias repair (with or without chordee or circumcision); with extensive dissection to correct chordee and urethroplasty with local skin flaps, skin graft patch, and/or island flap

Hypospadius is a condition in which the urethral meatus is displaced from its normal position at the tip of the penis to the underside of the penis in males. Hypospadius is classified as distal or mild when the meatal opening is small and located in or near the glans. This procedure involves creation of a distal neourethra using grafts and/or flaps so that the urethral metaus can be relocated to the tip of the penis and also corrects chordee which refers to curvature of the erect penis. An example of this type of hypospadias repair is a transverse preputial island flap (TPIF). A stent or catheter is placed in the urethra. A Y-shaped incision is made in the glans. The short limbs are approximately 0.5 cm long and the vertical limb extends to the coronal sulcus. Fibrotic tissue is identified and excised from the midline and laterally and the glans flaps elevated to allow the meatus to be enlarged and a core space made for the neourethra. A circumferential incision is made in the subcoronal tissue below the glans extending laterally to the area of excised fibrous tissue. The penile and preputial skin is degloved exposing Buck's fascia but preserving the vascular connection to the preputial flap. Once the penis has been degloved an erection is induced and the degree of curvature evaluated. Due to the severity of the chordee, tissues are extensively dissected and the chordee corrected. The neourethra is then constructed. A rectangular flap is created and if necessary extended by using a horseshoe incision incorporating penile skin on either side. The flap is tubularized around a catheter with interrupted sutures beginning at the meatus under the vascular pedicle. The pedicle is separated from the preputial skin below the vascular bed of the outer prepuce. Next the small upper median flap formed by the Y incision is anchored with sutures to the upper dorsal aspect of the tube. To create an aesthetic appearing meatus, a small V shaped wedge of tissue is excised from the tip of the glans. The mobilized glans wings are then rotated medially around the neo urethra and anchored with 3 mattress sutures placed transversely to approximate the wings in the midline which completes construction of the neourethra. Alternatively, a local skin flap or skin patch graft may be used to construct the neourethra. Following completion of the procedure, the urethral stent or catheter remains in place.

54332

54332　　1-stage proximal penile or penoscrotal hypospadias repair requiring extensive dissection to correct chordee and urethroplasty by use of skin graft tube and/or island flap

Hypospadius is a condition in which the urethral meatus is displaced from its normal position at the tip of the penis to the underside of the penis in males. In proximal hypospadias, the meatal opening is typically in the penoscrotal region and may range from a normal sized meatus to a long opening extending from the penoscrotal region to the midshaft. A lateral based flap can be used for proximal and penoscrotal hypospadias in a single stage repair. A Y-shaped incision is made in the glans with the long vertical segment extending to the coronary sulcus. Fibrotic tissue is identified and excised from the midline and laterally to correct chordee followed by elevation of the three glans flaps to allow space for the neourethra. A long rectangular skin flap is created including a small cuff of skin containing the urethral meatus by incising proximally in the midline of the scrotum with distal and lateral extension to the prepuce if necessary. The penile skin is elevated and mobilized dorsally down to the root, carefully avoiding rotation of the flap. The flap is then tubularized over a catheter or stent, suturing distal to proximal using a continuous subcuticular stitch reinforced at intervals with interrupted sutures. The neomeatus is created by suturing the terminal end of the neourethra to the ventral V-shaped incision in the glans. A slit like opening and a conical glans can be accomplished by excising a small V-shaped tip in the neo-urethra. Next the glanular wings wrap around the neourethra distally and are approximated in the midline. A layer of vascular areolar subcutaneous tissue is placed as reinforcement over the tubularized graft. The skin is approximated in

the midline to simulate the normal penile raphae and closed with a continuous transverse mattress stitch.

54336

54336　　1-stage perineal hypospadias repair requiring extensive dissection to correct chordee and urethroplasty by use of skin graft tube and/or island flap

Perineal hypospadius is a condition in which the urethral meatus is displaced from its normal position at the tip of the penis to the perineal region near the anus in males. Often there is a cleft deformity of the scrotum as well. A single stage repair of perineal hypospadias and chordee can be accomplished using a Koyanagi-Nonomura bucket release technique or a modified/augmented version of this repair. A catheter is placed transurethrally into the bladder. A circumferential incision is made just proximal to the coronal sulcus and carried down between dartos and Buck's fascia on the dorsal side. The urethral plate is exposed and fibrous bands on the ventral aspect proximal to the hypospadias meatus are excised down to the corpus spongiosum inside the scrotum to correct chordee. A U-shaped incision is made around the hypospadias meatus with extensions lateral and dorsal into the prepuce. The incisions in the prepuce are joined at the 12 o'clock position. The portion between the prepuce and dartos is dissected free on the dorsal side. The prepuce is fixed to the dartos as the neourethra without vascular compromise. A buttonhole incision is made through the pedicle of the dartos and the glans penis is passed through the hole. The parameatal skin flap and vascular pedicle are then mobilized to the ventral side maintaining a loop shape. The internal side of the loop is closed over the catheter with a running stitch beginning at the front wall and incorporating the full thickness. The external side of the loop is closed with a running subcuticular stitch beginning at the back wall of the neourethra. The neomeatus is created by making a slit like midline incision in the glans penis extending from the tip to the coronal sulcus and dissecting bilaterally to create a plane between the glans cap and the corpora. The neourethra fits into the created groove and the length is adjusted with the end of the neourethra finally sutured to the tip of the glans to complete the neomeatus. The catheter now extends out the tip of the penis. The wings of the created flap are mobilized over the neourethra and sutured in the midline and Byer's flaps created from the dorsal foreskin are divided and sutured to cover the remaining ventral skin defects. The circumferential incision is closed around the corona creating the appearance of a circumcision. The catheter is left in place.

54340-54348

54340　　Repair of hypospadias complications (ie, fistula, stricture, diverticula); by closure, incision, or excision, simple

54344　　Repair of hypospadias complications (ie, fistula, stricture, diverticula); requiring mobilization of skin flaps and urethroplasty with flap or patch graft

54348　　Repair of hypospadias complications (ie, fistula, stricture, diverticula); requiring extensive dissection and urethroplasty with flap, patch or tubed graft (includes urinary diversion)

The physician repairs any complications to a procedure in which birth defect in which the urethra opens somewhere besides the tip of the penis is fixed. The complications which may be fixed include any abnormal passages, any tissue that is sticking together, or any abnormal sacs or pouches. The physician may fix these defects by closing them, cutting them, or removing them. Code 54344 if in order to fix these defects, the physician must use skin flaps. Additionally, the urethra must be repaired with flaps or patches of skin. Code 54348 if the physician must perform extensive procedures to fix the defects, including repairing the urethra with a patch, flap, or tube of skin.

54352

54352　　Repair of hypospadias cripple requiring extensive dissection and excision of previously constructed structures including re-release of chordee and reconstruction of urethra and penis by use of local skin as grafts and island flaps and skin brought in as flaps or grafts

The physician fixes an extensive deformity of the penis that is the result of surgery to repair a birth defect in which the urethra opens somewhere besides the tip of the penis. Some of the repairs that were done during the original surgery must be reversed. The physician must perform extensive procedures to fix the defects, including repairing the urethra with a patch, flap, or tube of skin.

54380-54390

54380　　Plastic operation on penis for epispadias distal to external sphincter

54385　　Plastic operation on penis for epispadias distal to external sphincter; with incontinence

54390　　Plastic operation on penis for epispadias distal to external sphincter; with exstrophy of bladder

Epispadias is a congenital defect of the urinary tract in which the urethra does not fully develop causing urine to exit the body in an abnormal location. In males, the urethral opening is generally on the top or side of the penis rather than at the tip. The condition can be complicated by bladder neck and sphincter malformation and/or exstrophy of the bladder. These malformations may be treated in a single procedure or in a staged

　　● New Code　　▲ Revised Code　　CPT © 2016 American Medical Association. All Rights Reserved.　　© 2016 DecisionHealth

fashion. In 54380, surgical correction of penile epispadias is performed. A circumferential incision is made below the glans and the penile skin is degloved exposing Buck's fascia. The urethral meatus is resected to the distal edge of the hypoplastic urethral tissue. An island flap is harvested from the penile preputial skin. A neourethra is then developed over a stent or catheter. The glans is split and flaps elevated to cover the distal neourethra, foreskin is trimmed and excess tissue removed. The degloved penile skin is mobilized back up the penile shaft and the incision is sutured. In 54385, epispadias is complicated by absence of the bladder neck and sphincter resulting in incontinence. Epispadias repair and bladder neck reconstruction are typically performed in a staged fashion with the epispadias repair being performed around age 2 and bladder neck reconstruction at around age 4. To accomplish the bladder neck reconstruction, triangular lateral bladder mucosal wedges about 15 mm wide and 30 mm long are marked, developed and demucosalized. The flaps are brought over the neourethra using a "vest-over-pants" technique to form the bladder neck. Suspension sutures are placed to suspend to the bladder neck. In 54390, bladder exstrophy, a condition where the bladder is turned inside out and protrudes through the abdominal wall, is also repaired. A skin incision is made above the umbilicus, carried around the sides of the bladder mucosa to approximately 1 cm from the midline, and continued parallel along the distal urethral plate to the lateral region of the male verumontanum. The incision is deepened around the umbilicus and a plane developed between the rectus muscle and the bladder wall. The peritoneum is dissected off the bladder and developed laterally until the trigone and the urogenital diaphragm are encountered. Ureteral stents are placed. The urogenital diaphragm is dissected completely off of the pubic bone parallel to the bladder and posterior urethra. Traction is placed on the pubic bone to bring the bladder neck deep into the pelvis. The bladder neck and posterior urethra are closed. An osteotomy is performed by bringing the pubic bone together in the midline with suture or wire and the abdominal wall defect is closed in layers. The pelvis may be immobilized with traction, cast or external fixator.

Plastic operation on penis for epispadias distal to external sphincter

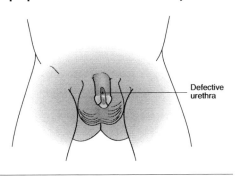

Defective urethra

54400-54401

54400   Insertion of penile prosthesis; non-inflatable (semi-rigid)
54401   Insertion of penile prosthesis; inflatable (self-contained)

Placement of a penile prosthesis is performed to treat erectile dysfunction. In 54400, a non-inflatable/semi-rigid penile prosthesis is inserted. A catheter is placed transurethrally. A 180 degree skin incision is made along the subcoronal area of the penis and carried down to Buck's fascia. Stay sutures are then placed through the tunica albuginea lateral to the penile nerves securing each corpora cavernosa. Longitudinal incisions are made along the dorsal surface of the corpora cavernosa between the stay sutures. The incisions are extended and a space created on each side in the corporal tissue. The spaces are enlarged using a dilator. The tip of the dilator is positioned under the dorsolateral surface of the tunica albuginea and dilation proceeds at an angle away from the urethra and the penile septum. The spaces are measured and appropriately sized prosthetic cylinders are loaded into an inserter and placed into each of the corporal spaces. The inserting instrument is removed and the corporal incision is closed followed by closure of the tunica albuginea and skin. In 54401, an inflatable, self- contained penile prosthesis is inserted. A penoscrotal approach is most often used. A skin incision is made in the mid-raphe area of the penoscrotal junction and carried down to the dartos fascia. The fascia is carefully divided and a circular self-retaining hook retractor used as needed to facilitate exposure of the operative field. The corpus spongiosum is identified and dissection continues lateral to the urethra and spongiosum tissue until the corpora cavernosa is encountered. Stay sutures are placed through the tunica albuginea to secure each corpora cavernosa. A corporotomy is made between the sutures. The incisions are extended, spaces created, and the inflatable prosthesis placed as described above. A pouch is then created in the sub-dartos tissue of the scrotum. The pump is inserted and connected to the cylinders. The device is cycled to ensure that it is functioning properly and to check for leaks. Incisions are closed.

54405

54405   Insertion of multi-component, inflatable penile prosthesis, including placement of pump, cylinders, and reservoir

A multi-component inflatable device is installed in the penis, allowing the patient to increase penile rigidity for intercourse. The device consists of an two inflatable cylinders in the penis, a liquid reservoir, and a pump located in the scrotum.

54406

54406   Removal of all components of a multi-component, inflatable penile prosthesis without replacement of prosthesis

A catheter is passed transurethrally. A midline skin incision is made in the lower abdomen and carried down through the subcutaneous tissue to the fascia. The dorsal venous complex and corporal bodies are identified and the incision is explored until tubing to the reservoir is encountered and tracked to its position under the rectus muscle. Using sharp and blunt dissection, the reservoir is freed. Tubing is tracked to the pump in the dartos pouch in the scrotum, dissected free, and brought out through the abdominal incision. Tubing is tracked to the two lateral cylinders in the corporal bodies and the cylinders are dissected free. All components are removed. Corporotomy incisions are closed. The tunica albuginea is closed followed by scrotal/dartos fascia. A drain may be placed in the abdominal incision. The rectus muscle, subcutaneous tissue and skin are closed.

54408

54408   Repair of component(s) of a multi-component, inflatable penile prosthesis

A catheter is inserted transurethrally. A midline skin incision is made in the lower abdomen and carried down through the subcutaneous tissue to the fascia. The dorsal venous complex and corporal bodies are identified and the incision is explored until tubing to the reservoir is encountered and tracked to its position under the rectus muscle. The tubing is checked for kinks and the reservoir for kinks/leaks. Tubing is then tracked to the pump in the dartos pouch in the scrotum which is also examined for kinks/leaks. Finally tubing is tracked to the cylinders in the corporal bodies and examined for kinks/leaks. Repair may include shortening of tubing if kinks are present, replacement of tubing, or replacement of connecters if leaks are occurring at the connection sites. The penile prosthesis is cycled to ensure that it is working properly and that there are no leaks. The tunica albuginea is closed followed by scrotal/dartos fascia. A drain may be placed in the abdominal incision. The rectus muscle, subcutaneous tissue and skin are closed.

54410-54411

54410   Removal and replacement of all component(s) of a multi-component, inflatable penile prosthesis at the same operative session
54411   Removal and replacement of all components of a multi-component inflatable penile prosthesis through an infected field at the same operative session, including irrigation and debridement of infected tissue

A catheter is passed transurethrally. A midline skin incision is made in the lower abdomen and carried down through the subcutaneous tissue to the fascia. The dorsal venous complex and corporal bodies are identified and the incision is explored until tubing to the reservoir is encountered and tracked to its position under the rectus muscle. Using sharp and blunt dissection, the reservoir is freed. Tubing is tracked to the pump in the dartos pouch in the scrotum, dissected free, and brought out through the abdominal incision. Tubing is tracked to the two lateral cylinders in the corporal bodies and the cylinders are dissected free. All components are removed. If the removal is performed for infection, the wounds are copiously irrigated with antibiotic solution and any infected or necrotic tissue is debrided. The corporal bodies are resized and an appropriately sized replacement prosthetic device selected. The cylinders are filled with saline and cycled to check for leaks. The cylinders are then loaded into an inserter and placed into each of the corporal spaces. The inserting instrument is removed. The corporotomy incisions are closed. The pump is placed into the dartos pouch in the scrotum. The reservoir is placed in the rectus space in the lower abdomen. Tubing length is adjusted and connections secured. The device is cycled to ensure that it is functioning properly and to check for leaks. The tunica albuginea is closed followed by scrotal/dartos fascia. A drain may be placed in the abdominal incision. The rectus muscle, subcutaneous tissue and skin are closed. Use 54410 for removal and replacement of all components for a reason other than infection. Use 54411 for removal and replacement through an infected field.

54415

54415   Removal of non-inflatable (semi-rigid) or inflatable (self-contained) penile prosthesis, without replacement of prosthesis

Removal of a penile prosthesis is typically performed through the same incision used for placement. A catheter is placed transurethrally. To remove a non-inflatable, semi-rigid penile prosthesis, a 180 degree skin incision is made along the subcoronal area of the penis and carried down to Buck's fascia. Stay sutures are then placed through the tunica albuginea lateral to the penile nerves securing each corpora cavernosa. Longitudinal incisions are made along the dorsal surface of the corpora cavernosa between the stay sutures. The cylinder implants are identified within the corporal bodies. Each implant (right and left) is dissected free of surrounding tissue. Hemostasis is achieved with electrocautery and the wound is irrigated with antibiotic solution. If infection is present the wound may be left open to drain or a drain inserted. The incision is closed in layers. To remove an inflatable, self-contained penile prosthesis placed through a penoscrotal approach, a skin incision is made in the mid-raphe area of the penoscrotal junction and carried down to the dartos fascia. The fascia is divided and a self-retaining hook retractor placed to facilitate exposure of the operative field. The corpus spongiosum is identified. Dissection is performed lateral to the urethra and spongiosum tissue until the corpora cavernosa is encountered. Stay sutures are placed through the tunica albuginea to secure each corpora cavernosa. A corporotomy is made between the sutures. The cylinder implants are identified in the corporal bodies. The cylinder implants are identified within the corporal bodies. Each implant (right and left) is dissected free of surrounding tissue. Tubing is tracked to the pump in the sub-dartos pouch and the tubing and pump are dissected from surrounding tissue and removed. Incisions are closed as described above.

54416-54417

54416 **Removal and replacement of non-inflatable (semi-rigid) or inflatable (self-contained) penile prosthesis at the same operative session**

54417 **Removal and replacement of non-inflatable (semi-rigid) or inflatable (self-contained) penile prosthesis through an infected field at the same operative session, including irrigation and debridement of infected tissue**

A penile prosthesis is removed and replaced at the same operative session. A catheter is placed transurethrally. The incision used for the insertion is reopened. The corpora cavernosa is exposed. Longitudinal incisions are made along the dorsal surface of the corpora cavernosa and the cylinder implants identified. Each prosthesis (right and left) is dissected free of surrounding tissue and removed. If the prosthesis is an inflatable semi-contained type, the tubing is tracked to the pump in the sub-dartos pouch and the tubing and pump are dissected from surrounding tissue and removed. Hemostasis is achieved with electrocautery and the wound is irrigated with antibiotic solution. If the procedure is performed through an infected surgical field, the wound is copiously irrigated and tissue debrided as needed. The penile prosthesis is then replaced. To replace a non-inflatable semi-rigid prosthesis, the length is measured and appropriately sized prosthetic cylinders are loaded into the insertion device. The cylinders are placed into each of the corporal spaces (right and left). The insertion device is removed and the incision is closed in layers. To replace a self-contained inflatable penile prosthesis, the cylinders are replaced as described above. The pump is inserted into the dartos pouch and connected to the cylinders. The device is cycled to evaluate function and to check for leaks. The corporal incisions are closed in layers. Use 54416 for removal and replacement for a reason other than infection. Use 54417 for removal and replacement through an infected field.

54420-54430

54420 **Corpora cavernosa-saphenous vein shunt (priapism operation), unilateral or bilateral**

54430 **Corpora cavernosa-corpus spongiosum shunt (priapism operation), unilateral or bilateral**

A shunt procedure is performed to treat priapism. A Foley catheter is placed transurethrally. In 54420, a Grayhack procedure is performed which creates a shunt between the corpora cavernosa and saphenous. The first incision is made below the inguinal ligament at the saphenofemoral junction on either the right or left side and carried down until the saphenous vein is identified. An 8-10 cm length of vein is mobilized from surrounding tissue for harvesting. A lateral second incision is made in the skin at the base of the penis on the same side as the first incision and carried down to the corpora cavernosa/corpus spongiosum. An elliptical incision is then made in the tunica albuginea. The penis and glans may be irrigated using heparinized saline solution to remove accumulated blood and clots. A tunnel is created between the two incisions. The ligated saphenous vein is brought through to the penile incision. The end of the vein is spatulated open and sewn to the elliptical incision in the tunica albuginea. The skin of the penile incision is closed and then the inguinal/thigh incision is closed in layers. If a unilateral procedure fails to relieve pressure in the corpora cavernosa an identical procedure may be performed on the opposite side. In 54430, a Quackles procedure procedure is performed which creates a shunt between the corpora cavernosa and corpus spongiosum. A vertical skin incision is made in the perineum posterior to the scrotum. The incision is carried down to the bulbocavernous muscle which is reflected off the urethra. The junction of the cavernosa and spongiosum is identified and longitudinal or elliptical incisions are made through the tunica albuginea into one of corpora cavernosa bodies and the tissue of the corpus spongiosum. The blood is evacuated from the corpora cavernosa by milking the penis. The posterior walls of the corpora cavernosa and corpus spongiosum are sutured together followed by the anterior walls. Pressure is measured for 10 minutes and if the intercavernosal pressure remains less than 40 mm Hg, the skin is closed. If the pressure is higher than 40 mm Hg an identical procedure is performed on the opposite side.

54435

54435 **Corpora cavernosa-glans penis fistulization (eg, biopsy needle, Winter procedure, rongeur, or punch) for priapism**

Creation of a fistula in the corpora cavernosa-glans penis to relieve priapism may also be referred to as an Ebbehof or Winter procedure. These are minimally invasive surgical procedures and can often be performed using only a local anesthetic for pain control. With the patient positioned supine, the penis is prepped and draped. A large bore biopsy needle or scalpel tip is inserted through the glans penis into the corpora cavernosa and a core of tissue is removed, which allows accumulated blood to drain. Gentle pressure may be applied from the base of the penis toward the glans to milk blood out of the corporal tissue. The fistula is allowed to close spontaneously.

54437

54437 **Repair of traumatic corporeal tear(s)**

A procedure is performed to repair traumatic corporeal tear(s). The corpora cavernosa and corpus spongiosum are surrounded by a tough fibroelastic tissue called the tunica albuginea that stretches and thins during an erection. Traumatic corporeal injury occurs most often when the erect penile head strikes the pubic symphysis or perineum. Symptoms include a "popping" sound, rapid detumescence, pain, swelling, and abnormal penile curvature. Rarely, corporeal tears occur in the flaccid penis usually from sports injuries or other trauma. Tearing of the tunica albuginea and/or the corpora cavernosa causes a hematoma deep in Buck's fascia. Repair may be accomplished through a distal circumferential degloving incision or a lateral incision over the hematoma. For circumferential degloving, an incision is made in the skin between the glans and penile shaft, carried down to dartos fascia and Buck's fascia and then de-gloved to the base of the penis. The right and left corpora cavernosa and the corpus spongiosum surrounding the urethra are carefully inspected. If a corporeal hematoma is present, Buck's fascia is incised and the hematoma is evacuated. The tunica albuginea is then inspected and lacerations are repaired. The fascia is closed with sutures; the skin is brought back up to cover the penile shaft (re-gloved); and the circumferential incision is closed. For a lateral incision over the hematoma, the skin is incised, carried down to dartos fascia and Buck's fascia, and the hematoma is evacuated. The tunica albuginea laceration is repaired with sutures and the incision is then closed in layers.

54438

54438 **Replantation, penis, complete amputation including urethral repair**

A procedure is performed to replant the penis following complete amputation. Bleeding from the penile stump may be controlled with a penrose drain placed circumferentially and tightened with a hemostat. Necrotic tissue is debrided from the stump and penile remnant. Using a microscope, the skin is undermined from the stump and shaft to expose the dorsal veins, artery, and nerves and the urethra is spatulated. A foley catheter is inserted into the urethra to bridge and stabilize the segments. The urethral mucosa is approximated and sutured 360° followed by a second layer of sutures through the corpus spongiosum. The deep cavernosal arteries may be reanastomosed if the amputation is proximal. The corporeal bodies are reattached and the tunica albuginea is approximated and sutured. Microvascular identification of the dorsal neurovascular bundles is performed and the dorsal arteries, vein, and nerves are reanastomosed. The dartos fascia is approximated and closed, followed by closure of the skin. Penrose drains may be placed as well as a suprapubic catheter.

54440

54440 **Plastic operation of penis for injury**

A plastic operation for penis injury called a phalloplasty is accomplished in stages. The first stage involves harvesting tissue from a donor site to create a neo-phallus with attachment of the neo-phallus to the genital area. The most common harvest site is a free transfer flap from the musculocutaneous latissimus dorsi (MLD). A skin incision is made and carried down to deep fascia to develop a plane between the latissimus dorsi and serratus cutaneous muscles. The flap is divided inferiorly and medially and then lifted to expose the neurovascular pedicle. After isolating a small strip of muscle to preserve the blood supply, dissection of the pedicle and subcutaneous fat continues proximally to the axillary vessels. The thoracodorsal nerve is identified and isolated, including the vascular blood supply for 3-4 cm proximally. Next the neo-phallus is created while the graft is still attached to the blood supply of the vascular pedicle. The harvested flap is tubularized and a neo-glans is created by folding what will be the distal edge over and attaching it to the shaft. While the MLD is being harvested, a second surgical team is preparing the groin site. An inguinal skin incision is made and tissue gently dissected to locate and mobilize the superficial femoral artery, saphenous vein and ilioinguinal nerve. A Y-incision is then made over the pubis and a tunnel created between the inguinal and Y incisions for the pedicle of the transfer graft. The neo-phallus is removed from the chest and transferred to the pubis. Using microsurgical technique, a lateral-to-terminal anastomosis is made between the subscapular and femoral arteries and a terminal-to-terminal anastomosis is made between the subscapular and saphenous veins. An epineural microneuorrhaphy is then completed between the ilioinguinal and thoracodorsal nerves. The next stage is a separately reportable urethroplasty which may be combined with the first stage if a buccal mucosa graft is used or performed on its own after the neo-phallus has been implanted and is viable. The final stage is separately reportable penile prosthesis insertion. The penile implants are inserted 3-6 months after a successful urethroplasty has been accomplished.

54450

54450   Foreskin manipulation including lysis of preputial adhesions and stretching

This procedure may be performed for tight foreskin (phimosis) or adhesions in an uncircumcised male or adhesions between the remaining foreskin and glans pens in a circumcised male. In a circumscribed male the remaining foreskin is manually manipulated by the physician to break up adhesions. In an uncircumcised male, the foreskin is pulled back to expose the glans penis and stretched which also breaks up any adhesions.

54500-54505

54500   Biopsy of testis, needle (separate procedure)
54505   Biopsy of testis, incisional (separate procedure)

A biopsy of the testis is performed. In 54500, a needle biopsy is performed. The skin over the planned puncture site is cleansed and a local anesthetic is administered as needed. A large bore needle is then inserted into the testis and a tissue sample obtained. In 54505, an incisional biopsy is performed. The skin is cleansed and a local anesthetic administered. If the biopsy is performed to evaluate a mass, the mass is exposed and a tissue sample obtained. The tissue sample is sent to the laboratory for separately reportable histological evaluation. If the biopsy is performed to evaluate the absence of living sperm in a semen sample (azoospermia), a sample of testis tissue is obtained. The tissue is placed in Bouin's fluid and sent to the infertility laboratory to determine whether sperm are present.

54512

54512   Excision of extraparenchymal lesion of testis

An extraparenchymal lesion of the testis is excised. This type of lesion is located beneath the membranous covering (tunica vaginalis) of the testis and within the testicular capsule (tunica albuginea). Excision is performed for benign lesions such as fibroma, calcified pseudotumor, adenomatoid tumor, or testicular appendages. The scrotum is explored through a groin incision. The external oblique fascia is opened, taking care to protect the ilioinguinal nerve. The spermatic cord is mobilized and a tourniquet is placed around the cord. The testicle is delivered through the incision with the cord attached. The tunica vaginalis is incised and the testis and epididymis are inspected. The lesion is identified. Biopsies are obtained prior to excision and sent for separately reportable frozen section to confirm that the lesion is benign. The lesion is excised. The testis is replaced in the scrotal sac; the tourniquet around the cord is removed; the surgical wound irrigated; and the wound is closed.

54520

54520   Orchiectomy, simple (including subcapsular), with or without testicular prosthesis, scrotal or inguinal approach

A simple orchiectomy or orchidectomy involves the removal of the testis. The surgical approach may be through the scrotum or inguinal area and testicular prosthesis may be implanted in the same operative session. In a scrotal approach the skin incision is made at the median raphe and carried down through the subcutaneous tissue to the dartos fascia and cremasteric fibers to expose the tunica vaginalis. The gubernacular attachments are ligated and divided. The testis is removed through the scrotal incision. If an inguinal approach is used a 4-6 cm skin incision is made superior to the pubic bone and parallel to the inguinal ligament on either the right or left side. The incision is carried down through the subcutaneous tissue to the aponeurosis of the external oblique muscle. Using a scalpel, an incision is made in the muscle between the internal and external rings following the direction of the fibers. The incision is widened preserving the ilioinguinal nerve and opening the inguinal canal to expose the spermatic cord. Using gentle pressure and traction on the spermatic cord, the testis is manipulated out of the scrotum through the open external inguinal ring and inguinal canal and delivered through the surgical wound to the operative field. If a gubernaculum is present at the inferior aspect of the testis it is clamped, cut and tied with absorbable suture. The surgical steps are the same at this point for scrotal and inguinal approach. The spermatic cord is clamped and divided above the epididymis, the vas deferens and vascular sections are ligated with sutures and then divided to facilitate removal of the testis. The scrotal structures are visually inspected, the wound is irrigated with saline solution and hemostasis is achieved using electrocautery. A prosthetic testicular implant may be placed at this time into the empty scrotal sac. The hemiscrotum is closed. The surgical wound is closed in layers.

54522

54522   Orchiectomy, partial

A partial orchiectomy is performed as a conservative intervention for benign intratesticular tumor or cyst, such as benign epidermoid cyst, hamartoma, or squamous epithelial cyst. Partial orchiectomy preserves the healthy testicular tissue. The scrotum is explored through a groin incision. The external oblique fascia is opened, taking care to protect the

ilioinguinal nerve. The spermatic cord is mobilized and a tourniquet is placed around the cord. The testicle is delivered through the incision with the cord attached. The tunica vaginalis is incised and the testis and epididymis are inspected. The lesion is identified. Biopsies are obtained prior to excision and sent for separately reportable frozen section to confirm that the lesion is benign. The mass is carefully excised from the surrounding germinal testicular tissue. The testicular capsule (tunica albuginea) is closed. The testis is replaced in the scrotal sac; the tourniquet around the cord is removed; the surgical wound is irrigated; and the wound is closed.

54530-54535

54530   Orchiectomy, radical, for tumor; inguinal approach
54535   Orchiectomy, radical, for tumor; with abdominal exploration

Radical orchiectomy or orchidectomy for known or suspected testicular tumor is performed through an inguinal incision. In 54530, a 4-6 cm skin incision is made superior to the pubic bone and parallel to the inguinal ligament on the side correlating to the tumor. The incision is carried down through the subcutaneous tissue to the aponeurosis of the external oblique muscle. An incision is made in the muscle between the internal and external rings following the direction of the fibers. The incision is widened preserving the ilioinguinal nerve and opening the inguinal canal to expose the spermatic cord. The spermatic cord is bluntly dissected from the floor of the inguinal canal along its length to the pubic tubercle. A drain is then wrapped tightly around the spermatic cord and secured forming a tourniquet. With pressure and gentle traction on the spermatic cord, the testis is manipulated out of the scrotum through the open external inguinal ring and inguinal canal and delivered through the surgical wound to the operative field. If a gubernaculum is present at the inferior aspect of the testis it is clamped, cut and tied with absorbable suture. The vas deferens and vascular section of spermatic cord are then clamped, ligated and divided as close to the inguinal ring as possible. A long silk or polypropylene suture is placed through the stump of the spermatic cord as a marker should later retroperitoneal lymph node dissection be necessary. Hemostasis is achieved using electrocautery and the wound irrigated. Closure begins at the inguinal floor, reinforcing with interrupted sutures if the area appears weak. Next the ilioinguinal nerve is released and the external oblique muscle is closed with sutures beginning at the internal ring and terminating at the pubic tubercle. The wound may be irrigated again and the skin is the n closed with skin sutures, staples or clips. In 54535, following excision of the testis as described above, the abdomen is also explored. The incision is then extended cephalad and the peritoneum opened and explored for tumor. A separately reportable radical lymphadenectomy is performed as needed. Hemostasis is achieved using electrocautery and the wound irrigated. The peritoneum is closed with absorbable suture.

54550-54560

54550   Exploration for undescended testis (inguinal or scrotal area)
54560   Exploration for undescended testis with abdominal exploration

Undescended testicle or cryptorchism occurs when one or both testes fail to descend into the scrotum before birth. Testes that have not descended by age 1 are typically treated surgically. The inguinal or scrotal area is explored for the undescended testis. Using an inguinal approach, the skin incision is made superior to the pubic bone and parallel to the inguinal ligament on either the right or left side. The incision is carried down through the subcutaneous tissue to the aponeurosis of the external oblique muscle. Using a scalpel, an incision is made in the muscle between the internal and external rings following the direction of the fibers. The incision is widened preserving the ilioinguinal nerve and opening the inguinal canal. If a spermatic cord is present, it is elevated and freed from the cremaster muscle with careful dissection and the undescended testis is repositioned in the scrotum. If spermatic cord structures and/or testicular remnants are present, they are removed and the surgery terminated at this point. If no cord structures or testicle can be identified, dissection moves to inside the internal ring and if the results are still negative for cord structure or testis an abdominal exploration may be performed. Abdominal exploration is performed through an incision in the lower abdomen. The abdominal muscles are separated and the peritoneum is entered and explored for spermatic cord and/or testis. If only remnants of spermatic cord structures and/or testis are present, they are removed and the surgery terminated at this point, closing the surgical incision in layers. If spermatic structures and testis are present, the spermatic vessels are dissected free from attachments and a broad flap shaped from the peritoneum with attachment to the vas deferens is brought down through a newly created external ring lateral to the pubic tubercle. The length of the spermatic cord is assessed and if there is sufficient length the testis is brought down into the scrotum. If there is not sufficient length or blood supply is compromised, a staged procedure may be required. Use 54550 for an inguinal or scrotal exploration. Use 54560 when abdominal exploration is required in addition to or instead of the inguinal or scrotal exploration.

54600-54620

54600 **Reduction of torsion of testis, surgical, with or without fixation of contralateral testis**
54620 **Fixation of contralateral testis (separate procedure)**

Testicular torsion is a condition in which the spermatic cord that is attached to the testicle becomes twisted, cutting off the blood supply to the testicle. The testis may be approached through single vertical midline incision in the scrotum, two separate hemiscrotal incisions or a transverse incision. The incision is down to the dartos muscle. The testis is identified and the layers of the tunica albuginea are gently opened to expose the testis. The testis is inspected and gently manipulated to relieve the torsion. The testis may then be wrapped in warm moist gauze to recover while exploration of the contralateral testis is made. If the contralateral testis is normal it may be fixed in place by everting the tunica vaginalis creating contact between the tunica albuginea and the dartos muscle and placing the testis in an extravaginal position. Two to three sutures are used to attach the peritesticular tissue to the dartos muscle anchoring the testis in place. The wrapped testis is then reexamined for viability. A dusty rose or pink color signifies adequate blood perfusion and the testis is fixed in the same manner as for the contralateral testis. The dartos layer is closed with sutures followed by closure of the skin. Use 54600 for reduction of torsion of testis with or without fixation of contralateral testis. Use 54620 for fixation of contralateral testiso only, when performed as a separate procedure.

54640

54640 **Orchiopexy, inguinal approach, with or without hernia repair**

Orchiopexy is performed to reposition an undescended testis in the scrotum. A transverse inguinal incision is made in the skin and then carried down through the subcutaneous tissue to the external oblique aponeurosis. The inguinal canal is opened and the ilioinguinal nerve is identified and isolated. The spermatic cord and testicle are identified. If fibrous cord called a gubernaculum is present, it is divided at the proximal end using a hemostat to allow for manipulation of the spermatic cord. Once the spermatic cord is free it is elevated and blunt dissection continues off the anterior cremaster muscle fibers to the internal ring. If a hernia sac is present, it is dissected from the spermatic fascia and the cord structures are separated from the hernia sac. The sac can then be transected and dissected up to the internal inguinal ring where is it ligated with sutures. The testis and spermatic cord along with the distal hernia sac if present are delivered out of the inguinal incision. The hernia sac may be repositioned with absorbable suture behind the spermatic cord or testis to prevent formation of a hydrocele. A tunnel is made from the groin to the scrotum. A second transverse incision is made in the hemiscrotum on the same side as the inguinal incision and a pouch created by dissecting the scrotal skin from the underlying dartos muscle. A suture can be placed through the testicle and used to deliver the testis through the tunnel or a clamp can be passed from the scrotum to the inguinal incision grasping the testis and pulling it through to the dartos pouch. The spermatic cord is carefully examined for torsion. To prevent the testis from migrating back to the inguinal area, the inlet to the pouch may be narrowed to a diameter smaller than the testis by placing a non suture through the dartos muscle and incorporating the parietal tunica vaginalis in the stitch. Alternatively, the testis may be sutured to the scrotal septum to anchor it in the new location. The scrotal incision is closed. If a hernia sac was present the transversalis fascia may require approximation to close the internal inguinal ring followed by closure of the external oblique aponeurosis and subcutaneous tissue and finally the skin edges.

54650

54650 **Orchiopexy, abdominal approach, for intra-abdominal testis (eg, Fowler-Stephens)**

An orchiopexy performed through an open abdominal incision may be accomplished in a single stage or a two stage Fowler-Stephens technique. A midline skin incision is made from pubis to just below the umbilicus, carried down through the rectus muscle and the peritoneum opened. The intestines are moved aside to visualize the peritoneal cavity and the testis and spermatic cord located and inspected. The spermatic vessels are dissected free and vascular clips applied. The peritoneum is excised around the internal inguinal ring and the gubernaculum is transected distally leaving some testicular tissue attached. Grasping the freed gubernaculum, the peritoneum is incised laterally and medially over the spermatic vessels with the incisions joined proximally. Dissection continues until adequate length is obtained in the spermatic cord to allow mobilization of the testis to the scrotum. In a single stage procedure, the spermatic vessels are divided between the previously applied vascular clips and the peritoneum incised lateral to the distal vessels with extension distally to the internal inguinal ring, superiorly to the vas deferens and medially to the bladder. A skin incision is made in the scrotum on the same side as the testis. A pouch is developed in the dartos tissue and a neo-inguinal ring created using a clamp or forceps to open a tunnel from the dartos pouch, over the pubic tubercle, and through the peritoneum. The forceps are used to grasp the testis and gently mobilize it through the tunnel to the scrotum. The spermatic cord is inspected for tension or torsion. To prevent the testis from migrating back to the abdomen it may be anchored to the scrotal septum with sutures. The scrotal incision is closed. The abdominal incision is checked for bleeding and

hemostasis obtained with electrocautery. The intestines are moved back to their original position in the abdominal cavity. The incision is closed in layers. If a two stage procedure is performed, the incision is closed following mobilization of the testis. The testes are given approximately 6 months to develop collateral vascular circulation from the cremasteric and vasal arteries. The abdomen is then reopened and the testis mobilized to the scrotum as described above.

54660

54660 **Insertion of testicular prosthesis (separate procedure)**

Insertion of a testicular prosthesis in a procedure separate from removal of testis can be accomplished through either an inguinal or a suprascrotal incision. Using an inguinal approach, the skin is incised over and carried down to the oblique muscle. The muscle is incised and the surgeon's finger used to probe and locate the scrotal neck and previous tunnel. Forceps are then used to dissect adhesions along the tunnel to the scrotum. The wound is irrigated and the prosthesis inserted through the incision. Using pressure on the outside skin, the prosthesis is gently manipulated through the tunnel into the scrotal space. Alternatively, Hegar dilators of increasing size may be used to expand the tunnel to the scrotum. Once the correct size dilator has been passed into the scrotum an identical Hegar is placed on the outside of the scrotum and pushed up to invaginate the base of the scrotum through the inguinal incision. The prosthesis is placed into the invaginated scrotum, anchored with a suture and manipulated back through the incision and tunnel to its original position. The wound is checked for bleeding and the incision closed in layers. Using a suprascrotal approach, the skin incision is made above the scrotum lateral to the penis and blunt dissection is used to form a pouch in the intrascrotal space. The prosthesis is inserted through the incision into the space and the incision is closed with absorbable suture.

54670

54670 **Suture or repair of testicular injury**

If the injury is closed, the scrotum is incised. The tunica vaginalis is opened and the testis is exposed. If there is an open wound to the testis, the wound is explored and enlarged as needed to allow evaluation of the injury. The testis, spermatic cord, and tunical vaginalis are irrigated. Any foreign bodies are removed. The spermatic cord and testis are inspected for evidence of injury. If vascular injury is suspected, the tunica albuginea is incised and the blood flow to the testis evaluated. If the injury has resulted in extrusion of testicular contents, the contaminated seminiferous tubules are removed using sharp dissection and debridement. Following evaluation and repair of the testicular injury, the tunica albuginea is closed. The tunica vaginalis may be closed or left open and a drain placed. If the tunica vaginalis is closed, the scrotal fascia and skin are also closed.

54680

54680 **Transplantation of testis(es) to thigh (because of scrotal destruction)**

One or both testes can be preserved after scrotal destruction by surgical transplantation to the thigh. Small skin incisions are made in the thigh at the level of the scrotum. The skin is elevated with blunt dissection and a superficial subcutaneous pouch created. The dissection is extended to create a tunnel to the perineum to allow the spermatic cord to descend into the pouch without traction or torsion. The testis is gently manipulated through the tunnel to the subcutaneous pouch in the thigh and secured with absorbable suture. The skin incision in the thigh is closed. The procedure is repeated on the contralateral side as needed. The scrotal injury may be treated in a separately reportable procedure.

54690

54690 **Laparoscopy, surgical; orchiectomy**

Laparoscopic orchiectomy is performed with the patient in supine, Trendelenburg position. A Foley catheter is placed transurethrally. A small U-shaped skin incision is made at the umbilicus, and a clamp used to dissect down to the anterior rectus fascia which is then opened a few millimeters to allow a Veress needle to be introduced into the peritoneal cavity. A pneumoperitoneum is created with insufflation of CO_2. Using upward traction on the abdominal wall, the laparoscope is inserted through the umbilical incision and trocars placed into the abdomen along the mid-clavicular line. Abdominal organs are identified and inspected. The testis is grasped and dissected free from surrounding tissue, spermatic cord including the spermatic vessels and vas deferens are clipped and cut and the testis is sealed and removed from the abdominal cavity through the ports. The laparoscopic instruments are withdrawn and CO_2 removed from the cavity. The fascia is closed with suture followed by closure of the skin.

54692

54692 **Laparoscopy, surgical; orchiopexy for intra-abdominal testis**

Laparoscopic orchiopexy is performed with the patient in supine, Trendelenburg position. A Foley catheter is placed transurethrally. A small U-shaped skin incision is made at the umbilicus, and a clamp is used to dissect down to the anterior rectus fascia which is then opened a few millimeters to allow a Veress needle to be introduced into the peritoneal cavity. A pneumoperitoneum is created with insufflation of CO_2. With upward traction on the abdominal wall, the laparoscope is inserted through the umbilical incision and trocars are placed into the abdomen along the mid-clavicular line. Abdominal organs are identified and inspected. To free the testis and spermatic cord, dissection begins lateral to the structures at the gubernaculum near the internal inguinal ring. After dividing the gubernaculum the peritoneum is incised and elevated off the spermatic vessels. The spermatic vessels are mobilized. The testis is grasped and stretched toward the contralateral inguinal ring to evaluate length. If necessary, additional mobility is achieved by incising a triangular section of peritoneum between the spermatic vessels and the vas deferens. Once adequate length of the spermatic cord has been obtained, a small transverse incision is made in the hemiscrotum ipsilateral to the testis and a subdartos pouch created by dissecting the scrotal skin from the underlying dartos muscle. A trocar is introduced through the scrotal incision and manipulated through the external inguinal ring lateral to the bladder and into the abdomen. The testis is grasped and delivered to the subdartos pouch where it is sutured to the scrotal septum anchoring it in the new location. The scrotal incision is closed. The laparoscopic instruments are withdrawn and CO2 removed from the cavity. The fascia is closed followed by closure of the skin.

54700

54700   **Incision and drainage of epididymis, testis and/or scrotal space (eg, abscess or hematoma)**

The scrotum is examined and the location of the fluid collection determined. The scrotum is incised. If the abscess or hematoma is located in the scrotal space, the abscess pocket or hematoma is located and opened. If there is an abscess pocket any loculations are broken up using blunt dissection and the pus drained. The abscess cavity is irrigated with sterile saline or antibiotic solution. If there is a hematoma, any blood clots are removed. If the abscess or hematoma is in the testis, the tunica vaginalis is opened, and the abscess or hematoma drained as described above. If the abscess involves the epididymus, the epididymis is exposed and the abscess or hematoma drained. The incisions may be left open and packed with gauze or a drain placed. Alternatively, the incision may be closed.

54800

54800   **Biopsy of epididymis, needle**

A needle biopsy of the epididymis is performed under local anesthetic with the patient positioned supine and the scrotum prepped and draped. The testis is palpated in the scrotal sac and the epididymis located and stabilized between the surgeon's index finger and thumb. The scrotal skin is stretched tightly and a small skin incision made with the point of a scalpel. A spring loaded needle is fired through the incision into the epididymal tissue to obtain tissue samples. The tissue samples are then prepared and examined by a pathologist in a separately reportable procedure to determine if cancer or other abnormal cells are present.

54830

54830   **Excision of local lesion of epididymis**

To excise a local lesion from the epididymis the patient is positioned supine and the scrotum prepped and draped. The surgical approach may be through a vertical median raphe or a transverse hemiscrotal incision which is then carried down to the tunica vaginalis. The testis and epididymis are brought out of the dartos fascia using blunt dissection or alternatively brought out through a completely incised tunica vaginalis. The lesion is then excised from the epididymal tissue. Bleeding is controlled with electrocautery. Tissue samples are prepared and examined by a pathologist in a separately reportable procedure to determine if cancer or other abnormal cells are present. If the lesion was large, the tunica vaginalis may be suture plicated in a radial fashion. The testis is returned to the scrotum and the tunica vaginalis or dartos layer closed followed by closure of the skin.

54840

54840   **Excision of spermatocele, with or without epididymectomy**

Excision of a spermatocele, with or without epididymectomy is accomplished with the patient positioned supine and the scrotum prepped and draped. The surgical approach may be through a vertical median raphe or a transverse hemiscrotal incision which is then carried down to the tunica vaginalis. The testis with epididymis are brought out of the dartos fascia using blunt dissection or alternatively brought out through a completely incised tunica vaginalis. Using sharp and blunt dissection, the spermatocele is isolated from the epididymis and the area explored for the connecting neck of the spermatocele to the epididymis. If located, the neck is suture ligated and divided. If the connecting neck cannot be located or the spermatocele is multiloculated, a partial epididymectomy is performed by excising a plane of normal epididymal tissue adjacent to the spermatocele. Bleeding in the epididymal bed is controlled by electrocautery. If the spermatocele was large in size, the tunica vaginalis may be suture plicated in a radial fashion. The testis is returned to the scrotum. The tunica vaginalis or dartos layer is closed followed by closure of the skin.

54860-54861

54860   **Epididymectomy; unilateral**
54861   **Epididymectomy; bilateral**

Epididymectomy is performed with the patient positioned supine and the penis and scrotum prepped and draped. A transverse incision is made in the skin of the hemiscrotum and carried down to the tunica vaginalis. Using sharp and blunt dissection in a plane between the tunica vaginalis and dartos fascia, the testis, epididymis and vas deferens are freed and delivered to the operative field. If a vasectomy was previously performed, dissection of the epididymis and vas deferens continues to a level above the vasectomy site. In the absence of a vasectomy, the vas deferens may be divided and ligated with absorbable suture at the junction of convoluted and straight vas deferens. After dividing the vas deferens, dissection continues to the vaso-epididymal junction creating a plane between the epididymis and testis. The epididymis is then grasped and lifted off the testis as the surgeon continues to dissect in an inferior to superior line, ligating the epididymal artery if encountered. When dissection reaches the testicular efferent ducts, they are ligated with absorbable suture or cauterized and the entire specimen is removed intact. The surgical site is irrigated and bleeding in the epididymal bed is controlled with electrocautery or fine absorbable sutures. The testis is then returned to the scrotal sac and the edges of the tunica vaginalis closed followed by layered closure of the dartos fascia and skin. Use 54860 for a unilateral epididymectomy. Use 54861 if the procedure is performed bilaterally.

54865

54865   **Exploration of epididymis, with or without biopsy**

Epididymal exploration, with or without biopsy, is done in cases of infertility in which the patient is suspected of having an obstructed epididymis with azoospermia. Exploration is done through a midline scrotal incision. The testis is delivered from the scrotal sac and the tunica vaginalis is opened to access the epididymis. The operating microscope is used to examine the epididymis under magnification. An obstructed epididymis will have a characteristic appearance as the tail end will have dilated tubules of a yellowish color due to the presence of macrophages that phagocytize sperm remnants of degenerating and necrotic sperm which has been blocked in its passage. The epididymal tunic may be punctured or opened to access the tubules and biopsies may be taken. Puncture sites or tunic incisions are closed, the tunica vaginalis is closed in a watertight way to avoid inflammation and later adhesions, the testicle is then returned to its position, and the incision is closed with sutures.

54900-54901

54900   **Epididymovasostomy, anastomosis of epididymis to vas deferens; unilateral**
54901   **Epididymovasostomy, anastomosis of epididymis to vas deferens; bilateral**

The physician bypasses a blockage between the small organ that sits next to the testicle and stores sperm and the tube that carries sperm to the penis. The organ is reconnected to the tube at a different point, bypassing the blockage. Code 54900 if this procedure is only performed on one of the two sperm-storing organs. Code 54901 if this procedure is performing on both of the sperm-storing organs.

55000

55000   **Puncture aspiration of hydrocele, tunica vaginalis, with or without injection of medication**

The tunica vaginalis is the serous sheath covering the testis and epididymis that consists of an outer parietal and inner visceral layer. A hydrocele is a collection of fluid between the parietal and visceral layers. The skin over the hydrocele is disinfected and a local anesthetic administered as needed. The skin is then punctured and the needle advanced into the fluid collection which is aspirated. Following aspiration, a sclerosing medication may be injected to help prevent recurrence of the hydrocele.

55040-55041

55040   **Excision of hydrocele; unilateral**
55041   **Excision of hydrocele; bilateral**

The physician excises a hydrocele, also referred to as hydrocelectomy. The tunica vaginalis is the serous sheath covering the testis and epididymis that consists of an outer parietal and inner visceral layer. A hydrocele is a collection of fluid between the parietal and visceral layers. The scrotum is examined and the location of the fluid collection determined. An incision is made in the groin for children or in the scrotum for adults. The parietal layer of the tunica vaginalis is incised and the fluid drained. The wall of the hydrocele sac is closed or partially excised to prevent recurrence. Overlying tissues are closed in layers. Use 55040 for a unilateral procedure and 55041 for a bilateral hydrocele.

55060

55060   **Repair of tunica vaginalis hydrocele (Bottle type)**

A tunica vaginalis hydrocele is a collection of fluid within the tunica vaginalis of the scrotum. In a Bottle-type procedure, a transverse incision is made in the skin of the anterior scrotum and carried down through the dartos fascia to the tunica vaginalis exposing the fluid filled sac surrounding the testis. The sac is incised vertically along the anterior border at the upper edge of the cord and the fluid drained. The hydrocele is everted around the testicle and secured with sutures. The scrotal incision is then closed in layers with absorbable suture starting with the dartos fascia followed by the skin.

55100

55100   Drainage of scrotal wall abscess

The scrotum is the sac that contains the testes. The scrotum is composed of skin that contains a network of nonstriated muscle fibers referred to as the dartos or scrotal fascia. An abscess of the scrotal wall involves the superficial layers of the scrotum. The skin of the scrotum is incised over the area of greatest fluctuance and the abscess pocket identified and opened. Any loculations are broken up using blunt dissection and the pus drained. The abscess cavity is irrigated with sterile saline or antibiotic solution. The incisions may be left open and packed with gauze or a drain placed. Alternatively, the incision may be closed.

55110

55110   Scrotal exploration

A scrotal exploration may be performed after an injury, for acute symptoms indicating testicular pathology or as part of a male infertility workup. The scrotal skin is incised transversely over the affected hemiscrotum or vertically along the median raphe and carried down through the dartos fascia to the tunica vaginalis and the testis/testes delivered out of the scrotum to the operative field. The structures are examined and any abnormalities noted. The incision is closed in layers starting with the dartos fascia and then the skin.

55120

55120   Removal of foreign body in scrotum

The physician removes a foreign body from the scrotum following traumatic injury. The scrotum is the sac that contains the testes. The scrotum is composed of skin that contains a network of nonstriated muscle fibers referred to as the dartos or scrotal fascia. If there is a puncture wound, a straight or elliptical incision is made, the skin separated and the scrotum explored. The foreign body is located. A hemostat or grasping forceps is then used to remove the foreign body. Alternatively, an open wound to the scrotum is explored and enlarged as needed to allow evaluation of the injury. The foreign body is located and removed. The wound is irrigated to remove any debris. The incision may be closed or packed open and a drain placed.

55150

55150   Resection of scrotum

Scrotal resection may be necessary when skin lesions, soft tissue tumors or excessive lymphatic tissue is present. An incision is made along the margin of healthy and affected skin and carried down to the dartos fascia in the inguinal, perineal and crural areas. The testes and spermatic cords are dissected free and isolated. The abnormal skin and tissue are excised completely and sent to pathology where they may be prepared and examined by a pathologist in a separately reportable procedure. The tunica vaginalis is then inverted and the skin edges brought together to cover the scrotal structures. Bleeding is controlled with electrocautery, a drain is placed, and the edges of the incision are approximated and sutured in layers at the midline to simulate the scrotal raphe, starting with the dartos fascia followed by the skin.

55200

55200   Vasotomy, cannulization with or without incision of vas, unilateral or bilateral (separate procedure)

For a vasotomy with incision of the vas deferens, the scrotum is palpated to identify the vas, a small incision is made in the skin and the vas is pulled up and delivered to the operative field. A straight clamp is placed under the vas and a hemi-vasotomy incision created utilizing an operative microscope and a micro-knife, with the clamp serving as a platform. Fluid is obtained from the opening of the vas and may be examined under a microscope in the operating room or sent to the laboratory for a separately reportable procedure. The vas deferens is then cannulized using an angiocath inserted into the distal end of the vasotomy and more fluid samples are obtained, examined or sent to the laboratory for a separately reportable procedure. The angiocath is removed and the hemi-vasotomy closed in layers followed by closure of the skin. If both the right and left vas deferens are to be examined, the procedure is repeated on the opposite side. For a vasotomy without incision of the vas deferens, the scrotum is palpated to locate a straight portion of the structure. An angiocath or lymphangiogram needle with silastic tubing and a syringe attached is carefully threaded into the vasal lumen and fluid is aspirated and examined under a microscope in the operating room or sent to the laboratory for a separately reportable procedure. The needle is withdrawn from the vas deferens and removed from the scrotum. Firm pressure is applied to the puncture area to minimize bleeding. If both the right and left vas deferens are to be examined, the procedure is repeated on the opposite side.

55250

55250   Vasectomy, unilateral or bilateral (separate procedure), including postoperative semen examination(s)

Vasectomy is considered a permanent form of birth control which involves interrupting the duct (vas deferens) that carries sperm from the testicles to the seminal vesicles. The vas deferens is located by palpation. A local anesthetic is injected. An incision is made in the scrotum and the vas deferens exposed. The vas deferens is cut and the ends tied, sutured, or closed using electrocautery. Scar tissue will develop over the cut ends to seal the duct and prevent release of sperm into the seminal vesicles. The vas deferens is replaced in the scrotum which is closed with absorbable suture material. The procedure is repeated on the opposite side. Some physicians use a single incision of the scrotum to expose both vas deferens while others two separate incisions, one on each side. It usually takes several months for all remaining sperm in the remaining vas deferens and seminal vesicles to be ejaculated or reabsorbed so the patient must use an alternative form of birth control. The patient returns as instructed by the physician and postoperative semen examination is performed to ensure that the vas deferens has closed and that there are no sperm in the semen.

55300

55300   Vasotomy for vasograms, seminal vesiculograms, or epididymograms, unilateral or bilateral

A vasotomy is performed for injection of contrast for a unilateral or bilateral vasogram, seminal vesiculogram or epididymogram. This code reports the vasotomy and injection procedure only. For vasotomy with incision of the vas, the scrotum is palpated to identify the vas, a small incision is made in the skin and the vas is pulled up and delivered to the operative field. A straight clamp is placed under the vas and a hemi-vasotomy incision created utilizing an operative microscope and a micro-knife and the clamp serving as a platform. Fluid may be obtained from the opening of the vas and examined under a microscope in the operating room or sent to the laboratory for a separately reportable procedure. The vas deferens is then cannulized using an angiocath inserted into the distal end of the vasotomy and more fluid samples are obtained and examined or sent to the laboratory. A syringe containing 5-10 ml of contrast media is attached to the angiocath and the fluid is injected to examine the distal seminal duct under fluoroscopy. Proximal patency of the vas deferens and epididymal tubule may also be examined using the same technique by allowing passive flow contrast media into these structures. The angiocath is then removed and the hemi-vasotomy closed in layers followed by closure of the skin. If bilateral studies are performed, the procedure is repeated on the opposite side. For a procedure without incision of the vas, the scrotum is palpated to locate a straight portion of the structure. An angiocath or lymphangiogram needle with silastic tubing and a syringe attached is carefully threaded into the vasal lumen and the procedure continues as described for a vasotomy with incision. Upon completion of the procedure, the needle is removed from the scrotum and firm pressure applied to the puncture area to minimize bleeding. If bilateral studies are performed, the procedure is repeated on the opposite side.

55400

55400   Vasovasostomy, vasovasorrhaphy

A vasovasostomy or vasovasorrhaphy is a performed to reconnect the ends of the vas deferens following a vasectomy or to repair an iatrogenic vasal injury that occurred during another surgical procedure. The scrotal skin is incised over the previous surgical scar and the vas deferens pulled up and delivered to the operative field. The ends of the vas deferens are incised and dilated using fine forceps, an angiocath is introduced into the vasal lumen and the vas deferens is irrigated with saline to assess patency. The irrigation fluid is examined microscopically for spermatozoa or sperm fragments. The ends of the vas deferens are anastomosed using a single layer or multiple layer technique. The reconnected/repaired vas deferens is returned to the scrotum and the skin is then closed with absorbable suture.

55450

55450   Ligation (percutaneous) of vas deferens, unilateral or bilateral (separate procedure)

Percutaneous ligation of the vas deferens, unilateral or bilateral, may be accomplished using a needle and diathermy wire or with conventional vasectomy technique of cutting the vas and sealing the ends. The scrotum is palpated to locate the vas deferens. With the scrotal skin pulled taut to stabilize the vas, a sharp needle with removable cannula is inserted through the skin and threaded into the vasal lumen. The cannula is then removed and a diathermy snare wire inserted through the needle. The vas deferens is cauterized by the diathermy wire. The needle and wire are then removed from the scrotum and firm pressure applied to the site to minimize bleeding. If a bilateral ligation is desired an identical procedure is performed on the opposite side. For conventional vasectomy technique a hemostat is used to make a puncture in the scrotal skin over the vas deferens and a ring clamp passed through the puncture to encompass the vas and pull it through to the operative field. The vas deferens is then clamped in two places and cut. In an open end vasectomy, the vas section leading to the testis is left open and the section to the prostate is closed using cautery or sutures. In a closed end vasectomy, both the vas sections are closed using cautery or sutures. The vas ends are then returned to the scrotum and the skin puncture is closed with a suture or steri-strip. If a bilateral ligation is desired an identical procedure is performed on the opposite side.

55500

55500   Excision of hydrocele of spermatic cord, unilateral (separate procedure)

Excision of a spermatic hydrocele is most often performed through an inguinal incision. A transverse inguinal incision is made in the skin and then carried down through the subcutaneous tissue to the external oblique aponeurosis. The inguinal canal is opened and the ilioinguinal nerve is identified and isolated. Next the surgical wound is explored until the spermatic cord is identified and bluntly dissected off the anterior cremaster muscle fibers to the internal ring. After placement of a ligature suture near the base of the hydrocele sac, the sac is then carefully elevated off the spermatic cord, preserving the spermatic vessels and the vas deferens and the sac dissected free from the spermatic fascia. The sac is then transected and dissected up to the internal inguinal ring where is it ligated with suture and bleeding controlled with electrocautery. The spermatic fascia is closed around the cord structures, and the external oblique muscle is closed followed by the skin.

55520

55520   Excision of lesion of spermatic cord (separate procedure)

The excision of a lesion from the spermatic cord is most often performed through an inguinal incision. A transverse inguinal incision is made in the skin and carried down through the subcutaneous tissue, Camper's fascia and Scarpa's fascia to the external oblique aponeurosis. The inguinal canal is opened and the ilioinguinal nerve is identified and isolated. The surgical wound is explored until the spermatic cord is identified and bluntly dissected off the anterior cremaster muscle fibers to the internal ring. The cord is then stabilized using non-crushing clamps and ligated at the gubernaculum. The lesion is identified and excised. Bleeding is controlled with electrocautery and the spermatic fascia is closed with fine suture. The external oblique muscle , Scarpa's fascia and Camper's fascia are closed in layers followed by the skin.

55530-55535

55530   Excision of varicocele or ligation of spermatic veins for varicocele; (separate procedure)

55535   Excision of varicocele or ligation of spermatic veins for varicocele; abdominal approach

A varicocele is an enlargement of the veins in the scrotum. A varicocele may be treated by excision or ligation of the spermatic veins. In 55530, an inguinal or subinguinal approach is used. Using an inguinal approach, the external inguinal ring is located by invaginating the scrotal skin upwards. A transverse incision is made in the skin starting at the external inguinal ring and extending laterally along the line of Langer. The incision is carried down through the subcutaneous tissue, Camper's fascia and Scarpa's fascia to the external oblique aponeurosis. The muscle fibers are incised and the ilioinguinal nerve identified and isolated. Alternatively, using a subinguinal approach, a skin incision is made in the groin above and to the side of the penis and then carried down through the subcutaneous tissue and fascia. Using blunt dissection the spermatic cord is exposed to the level of the pubic tubercle. A ring clamp or Penrose drain is passed around the cord and the testis is delivered to the operative field. The external spermatic perforator, scrotal and gubernacular collateral veins are identified, clamped, divided and ligated and the testis is returned to the scrotal sac. The spermatic cord is elevated with a Penrose drain and the external and internal spermatic fascia opened to expose the varicocele. A solution of 1% Papaverine may be used to irrigate and induce dilation and pulsation of the arteries to facilitate identification. The testicular artery and lymphatic channels are identified and preserved. The spermatic veins are clamped, divided and suture ligated. Alternatively, the varicocele may be excised. The vas deferens is examined and one set of vasal vessels may be ligated if enlarged. The Penrose drain is removed and the spermatic cord placed back into the incision. The incision is closed in layers. In 55535, a retroperitoneal approach is used. A skin incision is made along the line of Langer in the lower abdomen and carried down through the subcutaneous tissue to the external oblique aponeurosis. The muscle fibers are incised and the ilioinguinal nerve identified and isolated. The internal oblique muscle is exposed and blunt dissection used to expose the transverse abdominis muscle which is then transected. The retroperitoneal space is entered just above the inguinal ligament. The peritoneum is displaced medially to expose the testicular artery and vein near the ureter and the femoral artery and inferior epigastric artery and vein near the vas deferens. The vessels are elevated using a loop and a solution of 1% Papaverine may be used for irrigation to induce dilation and pulsation to facilitate identification of the arteries. The veins, arteries and lymphatic vessels are identified and the veins ligated using vascular clips or intracorporeal sutures. Alternatively the varicocele may be excised. Hemostasis is obtained with electrocautery. The incision is closed in layers.

55540

55540   Excision of varicocele or ligation of spermatic veins for varicocele; with hernia repair

A varicocele is an enlargement of the veins in the scrotum. A varicocele may be treated by excision or ligation of the spermatic veins. A varicocelectomy or ligation of spermatic veins with concurrent hernia repair may be performed through a retroperitoneal incision in the lower abdomen. A skin incision is made along the line of Langer in the lower abdomen and carried down through the subcutaneous tissue to the external oblique aponeurosis. The muscle fibers are incised and the ilioinguinal nerve identified and isolated. The internal oblique muscle is exposed and blunt dissection used to expose the transverse abdominis muscle which is then transected. The retroperitoneal space is entered just above the inguinal ligament. The peritoneum is displaced medially to expose the testicular artery and vein near the ureter and the femoral artery and inferior epigastric artery and vein near the vas deferens. The vessels are elevated using a loop and a solution of 1% Papaverine may be used for irrigation to induce dilation and pulsation to facilitate identification of the arteries. The veins, arteries and lymphatic vessels are identified and the veins ligated using vascular clips or intracorporeal sutures. Alternatively the varicocele may be excised. To repair an inguinal hernia from this approach a mesh patch is most often used. The hernia sac is identified and dissected free of the surrounding tissue. The sac and contents are pulled into the abdominal cavity. The patch is laid over the opening in the inguinal canal and sutured in place. Hemostasis is obtained with electrocautery and the incision then closed in layers.

55550

55550   Laparoscopy, surgical, with ligation of spermatic veins for varicocele

A varicocele is an enlargement of the veins in the scrotum. Using a laparoscopic approach the spermatic veins are ligated. A small U-shaped skin incision is made at the umbilicus, and a clamp used to dissect down to the anterior rectus fascia which is then opened a few millimeters to allow a Veress needle to be introduced into the peritoneal cavity. A pneumoperitoneum is created with insufflation of CO_2. Using upward traction on the abdominal wall the laproscope is inserted through the umbilical incision and 3 ports are placed in a baseball diamond configuration in the lower abdomen. The intra-abdominal vas deferens is identified at the junction of the spermatic cord above the internal inguinal ring along with the gonadal vessels. The posterior peritoneum is then excised using cautery, laser or endoscopic scissors. The gonadal artery is identified and preserved. The gonadal vein is isolated by blunt dissection using atraumatic graspers and ligated with vascular clips or intracorporeal sutures. The laparoscopic instruments are withdrawn and CO_2 removed from the cavity. The fascia is closed with absorbable suture followed by closure of the skin with suture, skin clips or surgical glue.

55650

55650   Vesiculectomy, any approach

Vesiculectomy, removal the seminal vesicle, is performed by any approach. Open surgical approaches to the seminal vesicles include: transperineal, transvesical through the posterior bladder wall, paravesical, retrovesical, or transcoccygeal. The procedure may also be performed laparoscopically. Using a transperineal approach, an inverted-U incision is made in the perineum and the central tendon is divided. A retractor is used to expose the anterior rectal fascial fibers. The rectourethralis is divided near the apex of the prostate. A weighted speculum is then used to expose the seminal vesicle. The rectum is dissected off the prostate and Denonvilliers fascia is incised. The seminal vesicle is dissected off the prostate, suture ligated at the base, and divided. Dissection is carried to the apex of the gland. The vascular pedicle is clamp ligated and the seminal vesicle is excised. To perform the procedure laparoscopically, a small U-shaped skin incision is made at the umbilicus, and a clamp used to dissect down to the anterior rectus fascia which is then opened a few millimeters to allow a Veress needle to be introduced into the peritoneal cavity. A pneumoperitoneum is created with insufflation of CO_2. Using upward traction on the abdominal wall the laproscope is inserted through the umbilical incision and 3-4 ports are placed in the lower abdomen. A transverse opening is made in the retrovesical peritoneum and the vas deferens is identified. The seminal vesicle is dissected from the vas deferens and the seminal artery is identified, ligated with vascular clips and cut. Dissection of the seminal vesicle continues along the posterior trigone of the bladder and around the urethra. The seminal vesicle is then excised and removed from the abdomen. The laparoscopic instruments are withdrawn and CO_2 removed from the cavity. The fascia is closed with absorbable suture followed by closure of the skin with suture, skin clips or surgical glue.

55680

55680   Excision of Mullerian duct cyst

A Mullerian duct cyst is a rare congenital anomaly in males that is a remnant of the caudal ends of the fused Mullerian duct, that usually regresses before birth. These cysts are typically located in the midline, behind the bladder. They originate in the region of the vermontanum and are attached to the vermontanum with a stalk. They do not communicate with the urethra. Using a suprapubic approach, the abdomen is incised and the peritoneum is opened behind the bladder. The prostate gland and prostatic utricle are identified. The area is until the Mullerian duct and cyst are identified. The neck of the cyst is ligated and the cyst is excised. The peritoneum is closed and the abdominal incision is closed in layers.

55700-55705

55700 Biopsy, prostate; needle or punch, single or multiple, any approach
55705 Biopsy, prostate; incisional, any approach

A biopsy of the prostate is performed. Biopsy is performed when there is an enlargement or palpable mass of the prostate or when the patient has an elevated prostatic-specific antigen (PSA) blood test. In 55700, a needle or punch biopsy is performed by any approach. A large bore needle or spring-loaded (punch) needle is inserted through the rectum (transrectal biopsy) or through the urethra (transurethral biopsy), using a needle guide. The needle may be passed into a single site or multiple sites in the prostate may be punctured to obtain a tissue sample. If a transrectal approach is used a separately reportable transrectal ultrasound (TRUS) may be used to guide placement of the needle. If a transurethral approach is used, the physician uses a cystoscope to visualize the prostate gland and obtain the biopsy. The tissue sample is sent to the laboratory for separately reportable histological evaluation. In 55705, an incisional biopsy is performed by any approach. Incisional biopsy is typically performed using a transperineal approach. The perineum between the anus and scrotum is incised and the prostate exposed. A tissue sample is obtained from one or more sites in the prostate.

55706

55706 Biopsies, prostate, needle, transperineal, stereotactic template guided saturation sampling, including imaging guidance

A transperineal needle biopsy of the prostate is performed by stereotactic template-guided saturation sampling, including imaging guidance. Using transrectal ultrasound (TRUS), a stereotactic template, and a stabilizing device, the prostate is positioned on the implant grid. The implant grid is divided into six or more sections. A linear probe with an attachment for needle guidance is used to obtain the tissue samples. Tissue cores are then obtained from each section and placed in separate specimen jars corresponding to the sections. As many as 60 tissue cores may be obtained and are sent to the laboratory for separately reportable pathology analysis.

55720-55725

55720 Prostatotomy, external drainage of prostatic abscess, any approach; simple
55725 Prostatotomy, external drainage of prostatic abscess, any approach; complicated

A prostatotomy by any approach is performed to drain an abscess in the prostate gland. In 55720, a simple prostatotomy with drainage is performed. The procedure may be performed using separately reportable transrectal ultrasound (TRUS) guidance. If TRUS guidance is used, the TRUS probe is inserted into the rectum. A small incision is made in the perineum and a biopsy needle and guide inserted and advanced under TRUS guidance into the abscess pocket in the prostate. Pus is aspirated. The needle is removed and a pigtail catheter is inserted into the abscess pocket to allow continued drainage. The catheter is secured and the perineum is dressed. In 55725, a complicated prostatotomy is performed. Using a perineal approach, an inverted-U incision is made in the mid-perineum above the anal opening. The incision is carried down to the ischiorectal fossa incising each side of the central tendon which is then divided and cut. The fibrous confluence is exposed and dissected posterior to the raphe of the bulbospongiosus muscle which is divided to expose the rectourethralis and levator ani muscles. With careful dissection around the rectum, the rectourethralis muscle is divided and the fibrous confluence elevated with forceps to expose the rectum and urethra at the apex of the prostate. The prostate is exposed and an incision is made in the prostate over the abscess pocket. The abscess pocket is opened and drained. Any loculations are broken up using blunt dissection. The abscess pocket is flushed with antibiotic solution, a drain is placed, and the incision is closed around the drain.

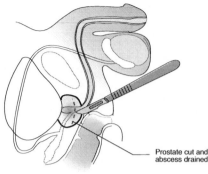

Prostatotomy, external drainage of prostatic abscess

Prostate cut and abscess drained

Any approach, simple (55720); any approach, complicated (55725)

55801

55801 Prostatectomy, perineal, subtotal (including control of postoperative bleeding, vasectomy, meatotomy, urethral calibration and/or dilation, and internal urethrotomy)

The physician enters the pubic cavity from the area between the rectum and the genitals and removes the prostate gland. The physician leaves in the seminal vesicles. During the procedure, the physician may control bleeding tissue, remove a section of the vas deferens, enlarge the opening of the urethra in the penis, increase or reduce the diameter of the urethra, and remove a section of the urethra.

55810-55815

55810 Prostatectomy, perineal radical
55812 Prostatectomy, perineal radical; with lymph node biopsy(s) (limited pelvic lymphadenectomy)
55815 Prostatectomy, perineal radical; with bilateral pelvic lymphadenectomy, including external iliac, hypogastric and obturator nodes

The prostate gland and seminal vesicles are removed through an incision in the perineum. If lymphadenectomy is needed, it is performed first. The lower abdomen is incised and without opening the peritoneum the pelvic lymph nodes on one side are explored. Taking care to preserve the genitofemoral nerve and psoas muscle, fatty tissue is stripped from the mid-portion of the common iliac vessel and along the external iliac vessel. Iliac, hypogastric and obturator nodes are biopsied and sent for separately reportable frozen section. If the malignancy has spread to these lymph nodes, they are excised. The procedure may be repeated on the opposite side. Radical perineal prostatectomy is then performed. An inverted-U incision is made in the perineum above the anal opening. The incision is carried down to the ischiorectal fossa and each side of the central tendon divided. The fibrous confluence is exposed and dissected posterior to the raphe of the bulbospongiosus muscle which is divided to expose the rectourethralis and levator ani muscles. The rectourethralis muscle is divided and the rectum and urethra exposed. The rectum is mobilized posteriorly from the prostatic apex the Denonvilliers fascia is exposed. The prostate gland is mobilized toward the perineum. The rectum is mobilized away from the prostate. A transverse incision is made through the Denonvilliers fascia between the medial aspects of the vas deferens and seminal vesicles. Each vas deferens is freed from surrounding tissue, ligated and divided. The seminal vesicles are retracted medially and the lateral aspects exposed, ligated and divided. The base of the prostate is exposed. In a nerve sparing approach, the Denonvilliers aponeurosis is incised and the cavernosal nerve bundles separated from the prostate. In a non-nerve sparing approach, the periprostataic tissue is dissected from the levator muscles and excised with the prostate. For both nerve sparing and non-nerve sparing procedure, the puboprostatic ligaments anterior to the prostate are divided. Prostate attachments anterior to the bladder neck are exposed and divided. A plane of dissection is created between the bladder neck and the base of the prostate. The urethra is exposed at its junction with the prostate. The urethra is dissected from the surrounding tissue and divided 1 cm below the bladder neck. The prostate is removed. The urethral ends are anastomosed. If the bladder neck cannot be preserved, it is excised and the bladder opening reduced in size to allow anastomosis of the urethra. A catheter is placed transurethrally into the bladder and the bladder is irrigated to remove clots. The perineal incision is closed. Use 55810 for radical perineal prostatectomy without lymph node biopsy or excision. Use 55812 when the procedure is performed with lymph node biopsy or limited pelvic lymphadenectomy. Use 55815 when the procedure is performed with bilateral excision of pelvic lymph nodes, including excision of the external iliac, hypogastric, and obturator nodes.

● New Code ▲ Revised Code

55821

55821   Prostatectomy (including control of postoperative bleeding, vasectomy, meatotomy, urethral calibration and/or dilation, and internal urethrotomy); suprapubic, subtotal, 1 or 2 stages

The physician enters the pubic cavity from above the lower abdomen and removes the prostate gland. The physician leaves in the seminal vesicles. During the procedure, the physician may control bleeding tissue, remove a section of the vas deferens, enlarge the opening of the urethra in the penis, increase or reduce the diameter of the urethra, and remove a section of the urethra. The procedure can be performed in one or two stages.

55831

55831   Prostatectomy (including control of postoperative bleeding, vasectomy, meatotomy, urethral calibration and/or dilation, and internal urethrotomy); retropubic, subtotal

The physician enters the pubic cavity from the lower abdomen and removes the prostate gland. The physician leaves in the seminal vesicles. During the procedure, the physician may control bleeding tissue, remove a section of the vas deferens, enlarge the opening of the urethra in the penis, increase or reduce the diameter of the urethra, and remove a section of the urethra.

55840-55845

55840   Prostatectomy, retropubic radical, with or without nerve sparing
55842   Prostatectomy, retropubic radical, with or without nerve sparing; with lymph node biopsy(s) (limited pelvic lymphadenectomy)
55845   Prostatectomy, retropubic radical, with or without nerve sparing; with bilateral pelvic lymphadenectomy, including external iliac, hypogastric, and obturator nodes

The lower abdomen is incised in the midline. If lymphadenectomy is needed, it is performed first. Without opening the peritoneum the pelvic lymph nodes on one side are explored. Taking care to preserve the genitofemoral nerve and psoas muscle, fatty tissue is stripped from the mid-portion of the common iliac vessel and along the external iliac vessel. Iliac, hypogastric and obturator nodes are biopsied and sent for separately reportable pathology frozen section. If the malignancy has spread to these lymph nodes, they are excised. The procedure may be repeated on the opposite side. The prostate is approached by first removing retropubic fat. The superficial branch of the dorsal venous complex is isolated and cauterized. The prostatic fascia and dorsal venous complex are exposed. The dorsal venous complex is ligated and divided. The prostatic fascia is incised and the neurovascular bundles on either side of the prostate are identified, mobilized posteriorly and protected. Alternatively, if the malignancy has spread to surrounding tissues, the neurovascular complex is excised. Using finger dissection the Denonvilliers fascia covering the posterior prostate and anterior rectum is separated. Finger dissection continues to the prostato-apical junction bilaterally. The lateral prostatic fascia on one side is incised. The membranous urethra is exposed and divided. The prostate is then completely mobilized while ligating vascular pedicles close to the prostate. The anterior layer of Denonvilliers fascia is divided and the ampullae of the vas deferens located, dissected off the medial aspect of the seminal vesicles and divided. The seminal vesicles are dissected free of the bladder base and posterior aspect of the bladder. The prostate is now free from all surrounding tissue and is removed en bloc. The bladder neck is repaired as needed. A sound is placed in the urethra and the bladder is anastomosed to the urethra. The surgical wound is closed in layers. Use 55840 for radical retropubic prostatectomy without lymph node biopsy or excision. Use 55842 when the procedure is peformed with lymph node biopsy or limited pelvic lymphadenectomy. Use 55845 when the procedure is performed with bilateral pelvic lymphadenectomy, including the external iliac, hypogastric, and obturator nodes.

55866

55866   Laparoscopy, surgical prostatectomy, retropubic radical, including nerve sparing, includes robotic assistance, when performed

Laparoscopic prostatectomy may be performed using either a transperitoneal or extraperitoneal approach. If a transperitoneal approach is used, a periumbilical incision is made for the initial laparoscopic port. Pneumoperitoneum is established. A conventional or robotic laparoscope is then inserted through the infraumbilical port into the peritoneum and the abdomen is inspected. Additional portal incisions are made for introduction of surgical instruments. An incision is made in the peritoneal fold between the rectum and bladder and the seminal vesicles are dissected and then retracted to allow exposure of Denonvilliers aponeurosis. The aponeurosis is incised and dissection continues to the rectourethral muscle, separating the prostate from the rectum. The peritoneum is incised and the space of Retzius is entered, resulting in the bladder falling posteriorly. The endopelvic fascia is incised and the levator muscle is pushed out of the way so that the prostate gland can be resected. The dorsal vein is ligated. The bladder neck is incised. The lateral pedicles are dissected. The urethra is transected and the prostate is removed along with the seminal vesicles. The urethra is re-anastomosed to the bladder neck. A drain is placed; the laparoscope and surgical intruments are removed; and portal incisions are

closed. If an extraperitoneal approach is used, a small incision is made, the preperitoneum is insufflated, and the space of Retzius is developed using blunt dissection until the pubic symphysis is reached. The retropubic space is then further developed by placing a port in the midline above the symphysis and extraperitoneal robotic instruments through additional right and left ports. The procedure then continues as described above.

55873

55873   Cryosurgical ablation of the prostate (includes ultrasonic guidance and monitoring)

Cryosurgical ablation of the prostate is performed which includes ultrasonic guidance for interstitial cryosurgical probe placement. Cryosurgical ablation may be performed as an initial procedure to treat prostate cancer or it may be performed subsequent to a failed intervention such as failed radiation therapy. An ultrasound probe is placed in the rectum. Cryosurgical probes are then placed through the perineum into the prostate using real-time ultrasound imaging to monitor probe placement. The cryoprobes are then cooled to the appropriate temperature to create an iceball. The growth of the iceball is monitored with ultrasound. When it has reached the appropriate size, the cryoprobes are thawed. A second freeze/thaw cycle may be required. On occasion a third freeze/thaw cycle is performed on a selected region such as the urethral diaphragm. This is accomplished by first removing posterior probes and then repeating the freeze/thaw cycle on the target region. The cryoprobes are thawed and removed. The cryoprobe sheath sites in the perineum are closed with sutures.

55875

55875   Transperineal placement of needles or catheters into prostate for interstitial radioelement application, with or without cystoscopy

Transperineal placement of needles or catheters into the prostate is done for interstitial radioelement application, a form of brachytherapy. Radioactive isotopes are used for the slow delivery of internal radiation to the target tissue. Using fluoroscopy or ultrasonic guidance, encapsulated radioactive seeds are placed directly into prostate tissue through the perineum using applicators in the form of needles or tiny catheter tubes. The prostate will have been mapped out in a previous procedure to determine the exact locations and number of seeds to be placed. The tiny radioactive seeds contain isotopes such as Iodine-125 or Palladium-103, and are left in the prostate to deliver their dose of radiation steadily over a period of a few months before becoming inert. They do not need to be removed and cause no harm after becoming inert. By this method, the targeted tissue receives the radiation with minimal exposure to any surrounding tissue.

55876

55876   Placement of interstitial device(s) for radiation therapy guidance (eg, fiducial markers, dosimeter), prostate (via needle, any approach), single or multiple

Single or multiple interstitial devices for radiation therapy guidance, such as fiducial markers or dosimeter, are placed into the prostate using a needle by any approach. The protate lies between the bladder and the rectum and its position changes in relation to the amount of rectal or bladder fullness. Since the rectum becomes less distended during a pelvic radiotherapy course, the prostate generally moves in a posterior, inferior direction. The change in position cannot be assessed with external landmarks. Since target motion is the major source of error in radiation treatment delivery, a safety margin is applied to ensure accurate, daily target localization for correct radiation. Radiopaque fiducial markers are one type of interstitial device placed in the prostate prior to starting therapy to be used with X-ray imaging to monitor and guide accuracy of the beam isocenter before delivery. Interstitial devices, such as fiducial markers, are placed prior to radiation therapy and are used to precisely locate the tumor or mass in the prostate. This allows radiation to be directed at the malignant tissue and helps prevent extensive radiation damage to surrounding tissues and structures. Fiducial markers are gold seeds that are implanted in or around a malignant tumor or the prostate. The procedure is performed using separately reportable ultrasound, fluoroscopic, CT, or MR guidance. A digital rectal exam is performed. If ultrasound guidance is used, the anus is dilated and a transrectal ultrasound probe inserted. The prostate is visualized and measured. A local anesthetic is administered to numb tissue along the planned insertion sites. Using radiological guidance, one or more gold seeds are passed through a needle that is passed through the ultrasound probe. The gold seeds are placed at strategic locations in and around the prostate or the prostate tumor. The positions of the gold seeds are checked radiographically to ensure that they are properly placed. The transrectal ultrasound probe is removed.

55920

55920   Placement of needles or catheters into pelvic organs and/or genitalia (except prostate) for subsequent interstitial radioelement application

Needles or catheters are placed in the pelvic organs and/or genitalia, excluding the prostate, for interstitial radioelement application. This code reports the placement of the needles or catheters only. The interstitial radioelement application (brachytherapy) is reported separately. This procedure varies depending on the exact site of the malignant neoplasm and male or female anatomy. A radiopaque urinary tract catheter with a steel ring to mark the urethral meatus may be inserted into the bladder. Tumor volume is assessed. The relationship of the tumor to normal structures is evaluated. A template device may be selected and prepared to orient the brachytherapy needles or catheters, and then sutured into place. Needles, catheters, and other devices, such as guide probes, guide wires, or a vaginal cylinder in females, are selected and prepared for placement. The number of needles or catheters and depth of insertion are adjusted depending on the extent and anatomic distribution of the tumor. The skin over the first insertion site is punctured and the brachytherapy needle or catheter is advanced to the selected site. Digital rectal palpation may be used to guide placement of needles and catheters in the posterior aspect of the genital region. This is repeated until all catheter tubes are in place.

56405

56405   Incision and drainage of vulva or perineal abscess

The physician performs incision and drainage of an abscess of the vulva or perineum. A small incision is made in the skin over the vulvar or perineal abscess to drain it. Laboratory specimens are sent for culture. Pressure is applied to control bleeding. The abscess site is packed with gauze which is removed approximately 24 hours later.

56420

56420   Incision and drainage of Bartholin's gland abscess

The physician performs incision and drainage of a Bartholin's gland abscess. The Bartholin's glands are located on both sides of the posterior introitus and drain through ducts that empty into the vestibule. The wall of the abscess is grasped with small forceps and the abscess is opened using stab incision. The abscess is drained and laboratory specimens are obtained for culture. A small balloon tipped catheter may be inserted into the Bartholin's duct and the balloon inflated. The inflated balloon catheter is left in the abscess cavity for three to four weeks to allow epithelialization of the surgically created tract.

56440

56440   Marsupialization of Bartholin's gland cyst

The physician performs marsupialization of a Bartholin's gland cyst. The Bartholin's glands are located on both sides of the posterior introitus and drain through ducts that empty into the vestibule. The wall of the cyst is grasped with two small hemostats. The cyst is incised vertically over the center of the cyst at a point outside the hymenal ring and the cyst is drained. Cultures are taken and sent for separately reportable laboratory analysis. The cyst wall is everted and sutured to the edge of the vestibular musoca.

56441

56441   Lysis of labial adhesions

The physician performs lysis of labial adhesions, also referred to as vaginal synechiae. Labial adhesions occur in children and appear as thin, pale, semitranslucent membranes between the labia minora that cover or completely close the vaginal opening. A local anesthetic cream is applied to the labia minora and the adhesions are separated using blunt dissection. Estrogen cream is applied to the labia for several weeks to prevent recurrence.

56442

56442   Hymenotomy, simple incision

Hymenotomy is done by simple incision. The hymen is the membrane that either partly or completely covers the opening of the vagina. This is a minor procedure to open the membrane covering to allow for the normal flow of menstrual products and normal intercourse in cases of an unusually thick or rigid hymen. The tissue is incised in a star-shaped pattern under local anesthesia.

56501-56515

56501   Destruction of lesion(s), vulva; simple (eg, laser surgery, electrosurgery, cryosurgery, chemosurgery)
56515   Destruction of lesion(s), vulva; extensive (eg, laser surgery, electrosurgery, cryosurgery, chemosurgery)

Vulvar lesions are destroyed using laser surgery, electrosurgery, cryosurgery, or chemosurgery. A local anesthetic may be administered. The type of destruction technique depends on the type of lesion and physician preference. Destruction may be used in conjunction with scraping (curettement) of the lesion. The physician uses laser energy, heat, cold, or a chemical to destroy one or more lesions. Use code 56501 for simple destruction or 56515 for extensive destruction.

56605-56606

56605   Biopsy of vulva or perineum (separate procedure); 1 lesion
56606   Biopsy of vulva or perineum (separate procedure); each separate additional lesion (List separately in addition to code for primary procedure)

The skin is cleansed and a local anesthetic injected. A tissue sample is obtained and sent to the laboratory for separately reportable pathology examination. Use code 56605 for biopsy of one lesion and 56606 for each separate additional lesion biopsied.

56620-56625

56620   Vulvectomy simple; partial
56625   Vulvectomy simple; complete

A partial or complete simple vulvectomy is performed. The vulva includes the following structures of the external genitalia: mons pubis, labia major and minora, clitoris, vaginal vestibule and glands, opening of urethra, and opening of vagina. Simple vulvectomy is typically performed to treat a severe leukoplakia or a confirmed malignancy of the vulva, such as extensive carcinoma in situ, microinvasive carcinoma, or Paget's disease. Simple vulvectomy is differentiated from radical vulvectomy in that excision does not extend into the perineal fascia. In 56620, the malignancy or disease involves only part of the vulva and only the involved portion is removed. The exact nature of the procedure will depend on the location and extent of the disease. Excision margins are marked taking care to include an adequate margin of healthy tissue and the skin is incised down to the level of subcutaneous fat. The involved portion of the vulva is excised. In 56625, all vulvar structures are removed. The incision begins above the labial folds in the mons pubis. The incision is extended down the lateral fold of the labia majora and across the posterior fourchette. The pudendal arteries and veins are clamped and tied bilaterally as they are encountered. The urethral orifice is protected and the incision extended from the meatus around the vaginal introitus. The rectum is protected as the incision is carried inferiorly. The last regions to be transected are the fat pad in the mons pubis and the vascular plexus surrounding the clitoris which is clamped and tied prior to transection to control bleeding. The surgical defect is repaired taking care to undermine and mobilize the vaginal mucosa to prevent contracture of the introitus. Following placement of a catheter in the urethral meatus, the periurethral mucosa is sutured to the skin.

56630-56632

56630   Vulvectomy, radical, partial
56631   Vulvectomy, radical, partial; with unilateral inguinofemoral lymphadenectomy
56632   Vulvectomy, radical, partial; with bilateral inguinofemoral lymphadenectomy

The vulva includes the following structures of the external genitalia: mons pubis, labia major and minora, clitoris, vaginal vestibule and glands, opening of urethra, and opening of vagina. Radical vulvectomy is typically performed to treat invasive carcinoma. Radical vulvectomy is differentiated from simple vulvectomy in that excision extends into the perineal fascia. In 56630-56632, the malignancy involves only part of the vulva and only the involved portion is removed. The exact nature of the procedure will depend on the location and extent of the disease. Excision margins are marked taking care to include an adequate margin of healthy tissue. The skin is incised down to the level of subcutaneous fat and with deep dissection continuing down to the perineal fascia and even into the periosteum of the pubic symphysis if needed. The involved portion of the vulva along with deep fascia and involved periosteum is excised. Examples of structures excised in a partial vulvectomy include the right or left side (labia majora and minora, vaginal ventibule and glands on the involved side), the upper portion (mons pubis, upper portion of labia majora and minora, clitoris, upper aspect of vaginal vestibule and involved glands), or the lower portion (lower portion of labia major and minora, lower aspect of vaginal vestibule and involved glands). Partial radical vulvectomy may be performed with unilateral (56631) or bilateral (56632) inguinofemoral lymphadenectomy. Inguinofemoral lymphadenectomy is typically performed only on the side with the malignancy. If the cancer is in the middle of the vulva, a bilateral lymphadenectomy is performed. When lymphadenectomy is indicated, this is typically performed first. A skin incision is made just below and parallel to the groin crease. The incision is carried through the membranes that cover the inguinal vein and artery to expose the inguinofemoral lymph nodes which are then removed. The procedure is repeated on the contralateral side when a bilateral lymphadenectomy is indicated. The physician then proceeds with the radical partial vulvectomy.

56633-56640

56633   Vulvectomy, radical, complete
56634   Vulvectomy, radical, complete; with unilateral inguinofemoral lymphadenectomy
56637   Vulvectomy, radical, complete; with bilateral inguinofemoral lymphadenectomy
56640   Vulvectomy, radical, complete, with inguinofemoral, iliac, and pelvic lymphadenectomy

The vulva includes the following structures of the external genitalia: mons pubis, labia major and minora, clitoris, vaginal vestibule and glands, opening of urethra, and opening of vagina. Radical vulvectomy is typically performed to treat invasive carcinoma. Radical vulvectomy is differentiated from simple vulvectomy in that excision extends into the perineal fascia and may also extend into the periosteum of the pubic symphysis. In 56633-56640, the invasive malignancy requires that all vulvar structures be removed. Excision margins are marked taking care to include an adequate margin of healthy tissue. The incision begins above the labial folds in the mons pubis. The skin is incised down to the level of subcutaneous fat and with deep dissection continuing down to the perineal fascia and even into the periosteum of the pubic symphysis if needed. The incision is extended down the lateral fold of the labia majora and across the posterior fourchette. The pudendal arteries and veins are clamped and tied bilaterally as they are encountered. The urethral orifice is protected and the incision extended from the meatus around the vaginal introitus. The rectum is protected as the incision is carried inferiorly. The last regions to be transected are the fat pad in the mons pubis and the vascular plexus surrounding the clitoris which is clamped and tied prior to transection to control bleeding. The surgical defect is repaired taking care to undermine and mobilize the vaginal mucosa to prevent contracture of the introitus. Following placement of a catheter in the urethral meatus, the periurethral mucosa is sutured to the skin. Complete radical vulvectomy may be performed with unilateral (56634) or bilateral (56637) inguinofemoral lymphadenectomy. When lymphadenectomy is indicated, this is typically performed first. A skin incision is made just below and parallel to the groin crease. The incision is carried through the membranes that cover the inguinal vein and artery to expose the inguinofemoral lymph nodes which are then removed. The procedure is repeated on the contralateral side when a bilateral lymphadenectomy is indicated. In 56640, radical vulvectomy is performed with inguinofemoral, iliac and pelvic lymphadenectomy. The inguinofemoral lymphadenectomy and radical vulvectomy are completed as described above. An incision is then made in the abdomen to expose the iliac and pelvic lymph nodes. Involved lymph nodes, which may include external and common iliac nodes, hypogastric nodes, and/or obturator nodes, are dissected free of surrounding tissues and removed.

56700

56700   Partial hymenectomy or revision of hymenal ring

The physician performs a partial hymenectomy or revision of hymenal ring. The procedure is performed to enlarge the hymenal orifice. A circular incision is made that follows the normal line of the hymenal ring (annulus) and the excess hymenal tissue is excised. The hymenal ring is then repaired by suturing it to the vaginal epithelium.

56740

56740   Excision of Bartholin's gland or cyst

The physician performs excision of a Bartholin's gland or cyst. The Bartholin's glands are located on both sides of the posterior introitus and drain through ducts that empty into the vestibule. An incision is made in the skin overlying the opening of the Bartholin's gland and the wall of the gland is exposed. Adhesions between the wall of the gland or cyst and the overlying vaginal mucosa are lysed. The wall of the cyst is grasped with forceps and retracted to allow identification of blood vessels. The entire Bartholin's gland and cyst, duct, and surrounding tissue are excised. Bleeding is controlled using electrocoagulation and suture ligation of blood vessels. The bed of the gland is closed and a drain placed in the surgical wound.

56800

56800   Plastic repair of introitus

The physician performs a plastic repair of the vaginal introitus (outlet). This procedure is performed to treat vaginal outlet stenosis that may occur as a complication of an episiotomy or following posterior repair. An incision is made at the posterior fold of the labia minora (posterior fourchette). The posterior vaginal wall is dissected free of the perineal body. A triangular section of skin is removed from the perineum beginning at the posterior fourchette and continuing posteriorly toward the anus. The superficial transverse perineal muscle is exposed and a series of small incisions are made in this muscle to open the vaginal outlet. The posterior vaginal mucosa is mobilized and used to cover the triangular surgical defect in the perineum by suturing it to the skin of the perineum.

56805

56805   Clitoroplasty for intersex state

The physician performs a clitoroplasty for intersex state. Intersex state is a condition where the genitalia have characteristics of both sexes making gender identification impossible from the outward appearance of the genitalia alone. Intersex states include: true hermaphrodite and female or male pseudohermaphrodite. A true hermaphrodite has mixed male and female sex organs with both ovaries and testicles. A female pseudohermaphrodite is a genetic female with external genitalia that appears male, including a penis. A male pseudohermaphrodite is a genetic male with external genitalia that has failed to develop normally. Clitoroplasty is typically performed on a true hermaphrodite with female gender identification or a female pseudohermaphrodite and involves plastic surgery to reconstruct what may appear to be a large clitoris or small penis into a more normal appearing clitoris.

The clitoris is reduced in size while the physician takes care to preserve the neurovascular function.

56810

56810   Perineoplasty, repair of perineum, nonobstetrical (separate procedure)

The physician performs a nonobstetrical repair of the perineum (perineoplasty) in a separate procedure. This procedure is performed to treat an enlarged or gaping vaginal introitus (opening). The perineum is the region between the vagina and rectum. An incision is made over the perineal body and a triangular section of skin is excised. The perineum is rebuilt in layers. First the underlying musculature is inspected and suture repaired as needed. Subcutaneous tissues are closed and any perineal bulging is eliminated. The triangular surgical defect in the skin is then closed by pulling the posterior vaginal mucosa over the defect and suturing it to the skin of the perineum.

56820-56821

56820   Colposcopy of the vulva
56821   Colposcopy of the vulva; with biopsy(s)

The physician performs a colposcopy of the vulva. A colposcope is an instrument that looks like a pair of binoculars mounted on a pedestal with a light attached. The colposcope lenses magnify the tissue of the vulva allowing better visualization of abnormal tissue. The colposcope is placed at the vulva. The vulva is inspected in its entirety. The vulva is examined under two or three different magnifications. Acetic acid is then applied to allow better visualization of abnormal cells. Following the application of acetic acid, different colored filters are used to visualize blood vessels and any abnormal blood vessel patterns noted. Next, the vulva is painted with an iodine solution that stains the glycogen in the cells. Normal cells stain a dark-brown color. Any areas that do not stain are biopsied as are previously identified areas showing abnormal blood vessel patterns. Use code 56820 for colposcopy of the vulva without biopsy and code 56821 when the procedure is performed with one or more biopsies of the vulva.

57000-57010

57000   Colpotomy; with exploration
57010   Colpotomy; with drainage of pelvic abscess

The posterior cervical lip is grasped with a tenaculum and the cervix elevated to expose the posterior vagina. A stab incision is made in the posterior vaginal wall and widened as needed. In 57000, the physician explores the posterior cul-de-sac for evidence of infection, disease, or other abnormalities. In 57010, the physician drains an abscess in the posterior cul-de-sac. The physician inserts blunt forceps or a finger to break up loculi in the abscess cavity. The abscess cavity is drained. The drainage is sent for separately reportable laboratory cultures. The abscess site may be catheterized and flushed with sterile saline or antibiotic solution. A drain may be placed to allow continued drainage of the abscess site. The incision is closed around the drain.

57020

57020   Colpocentesis (separate procedure)

The physician performs a colpocentesis, also referred to as a culdocentesis, in a separate procedure. The posterior cervical lip is grasped with a tenaculum and the cervix is elevated to expose the posterior vagina. A needle and syringe are inserted into the vagina. With the needle tip postioned just below the posterior lip of the cervix, the vaginal wall is punctured and fluid is aspirated from the posterior cul-de-sac. The fluid is sent to the laboratory for separately reported culture or analysis.

57022-57023

57022   Incision and drainage of vaginal hematoma; obstetrical/postpartum
57023   Incision and drainage of vaginal hematoma; non-obstetrical (eg, post-trauma, spontaneous bleeding)

The physician performs an incision and drainage of a vaginal hematoma. The vaginal hematoma is identified and evaluated as to location and size. An incision is made in the skin overlying the hematoma and the hematoma is drained and all blood clots evacuated. The hematoma site is evaluated for active bleeding and any bleeding vessels are ligated. The incision may be closed or left open to heal. Vaginal packing is applied as needed. Use code 57022 for an obstetrical or postpartum vaginal hematoma. Use code 57023 for a non-obstetrical vaginal hematoma, such as one occurring spontaneously or following trauma.

57061-57065

57061   Destruction of vaginal lesion(s); simple (eg, laser surgery, electrosurgery, cryosurgery, chemosurgery)
57065   Destruction of vaginal lesion(s); extensive (eg, laser surgery, electrosurgery, cryosurgery, chemosurgery)

Vaginal lesions are destroyed using laser surgery, electrosurgery, cryosurgery, or chemosurgery. A local anesthetic may be administered. The type of destruction technique depends on the type of lesion and physician preference. Destruction may be used in conjunction with scraping (curettement) of the lesion. The physician uses laser energy, heat, cold, or a chemical to destroy one or more lesions. Use code 57061 for simple destruction or 57065 for extensive destruction.

57100-57105

57100 Biopsy of vaginal mucosa; simple (separate procedure)

57105 Biopsy of vaginal mucosa; extensive, requiring suture (including cysts)

The physician performs a biopsy of the vaginal mucosa. The skin is cleansed and a local anesthetic injected. In 57100, a simple biopsy of the vaginal mucosa is performed in a separate procedure. A tissue sample is obtained from the vaginal lesion and sent to the laboratory for separately reportable pathology examination. The biopsy site does not require suture repair. In 57105, an extensive biopsy requiring suture closure including biopsy of cystic lesions is performed. Cystic lesions of the vaginal mucosa include inclusion cysts caused by trauma to the vaginal wall, Gartner's duct cysts, or benign cystic tumors. An incision is made in the vaginal mucosa at the site of the cystic or other vaginal lesion. A large section of abnormal tissue is removed and sent to the laboratory for pathology examination. The incision is closed with sutures.

57106-57109

57106 Vaginectomy, partial removal of vaginal wall

57107 Vaginectomy, partial removal of vaginal wall; with removal of paravaginal tissue (radical vaginectomy)

57109 Vaginectomy, partial removal of vaginal wall; with removal of paravaginal tissue (radical vaginectomy) with bilateral total pelvic lymphadenectomy and para-aortic lymph node sampling (biopsy)

The physician removes part of the vaginal wall (partial vaginectomy). In 57106, the vaginal epithelium is removed without removing the paravaginal tissue (paracolpium) surrounding the vagina. The vaginal wall is excised along with a two cm margin of healthy tissue distal to the lesion and the entire vaginal wall proximal to the lesion. An incision is made across the top of the vaginal vault. Two longitudinal full-thickness incisions are then made, one along the ventral (anterior) aspect and a second along the dorsal (posterior) aspect of the vaginal wall. These incisions extend from the top of the vaginal vault to a point two cm distal to the lesion. The upper vaginal wall containing the lesion is excised. Separately reportable vaginal reconstruction with skin grafts may be performed at the same or a subsequent surgical session. In 57107, a partial radical vaginectomy is performed which involves removal of the upper portion of vaginal wall and removal of paravaginal tissue. The vaginal wall is incised as described above. The bladder and rectal pillars are transected at their attachment sites on the bladder and rectum. The anterior and posterior vaginal walls along with the two lateral paravaginal spaces are resected to a point two cm distal to the lesion. In 57109 a partial radical vaginectomy is performed with bilateral total pelvic lymphadenectomy and para-aortic lymph node sampling. This procedure requires a combined approach and the procedure may be performed by two surgeons. A midline incision is made in the abdomen extending from the symphysis pubis to a point just above the umbilicus. The abdomen is explored to ascertain whether pelvic metastases are present. The pelvic lymph nodes are exposed. Involved lymph nodes, which may include external and common iliac nodes, hypogastric nodes, and/or obturator nodes, are dissected free of surrounding tissues and removed. The para-aortic lymph nodes are exposed and frozen sections sent for pathology exam. The vaginal wall and paravaginal tissue are removed as described above.

Vaginectomy, partial removal of vaginal wall

Pelvic lymph nodes removed
Bladder wall
Paravaginal tissue
Vaginal wall

Partial (57106); with removal of paravaginal tissue (57107);
with removal of paravaginal tissue, with bilateral
total pelvic lympadenectomy and biopsy (57109)

57110-57112

57110 Vaginectomy, complete removal of vaginal wall

57111 Vaginectomy, complete removal of vaginal wall; with removal of paravaginal tissue (radical vaginectomy)

57112 Vaginectomy, complete removal of vaginal wall; with removal of paravaginal tissue (radical vaginectomy) with bilateral total pelvic lymphadenectomy and para-aortic lymph node sampling (biopsy)

In 57110, the vaginal epithelium is removed without removing the paravaginal tissue (paracolpium) surrounding the vagina. An incision is made across the top of the vaginal vault. Two longitudinal full-thickness incisions are then made, one along the ventral (anterior) aspect and a second along the dorsal (posterior) aspect of the vaginal wall. These incisions extend from the top of the vaginal vault to the introitus (vaginal opening). An incision is then made around the introitus. The right and left halves of the vaginal wall are excised. Separately reportable vaginal reconstruction with skin grafts may be performed at the same or a subsequent surgical session. In 57111, a complete radical vaginectomy is performed which involves removal of the entire vaginal wall and removal of paravaginal tissue. The vaginal wall is incised as described above. The bladder and rectal pillars are transected at their attachment sites on the bladder and rectum. The anterior and posterior vaginal walls along with the two lateral paravaginal spaces are resected. In 57112 a complete radical vaginectomy is performed with bilateral total pelvic lymphadenectomy and para-aortic lymph node sampling. This procedure requires a combined approach and the procedure may be performed by two surgeons. A midline incision is made in the abdomen extending from the symphysis pubis to a point just above the umbilicus. The abdomen is explored to ascertain whether pelvic metastases are present. The pelvic lymph nodes are exposed. Involved lymph nodes, which may include external and common iliac nodes, hypogastric nodes, and/or obturator nodes, are dissected free of surrounding tissues and removed. The para-aortic lymph nodes are exposed and frozen sections sent for pathology exam. The vaginal wall and paravaginal tissue are removed as described above.

57120

57120 Colpocleisis (Le Fort type)

The physician performs a Le Fort type colpocleisis, also referred to as a partial colpocleisis. This procedure is performed to treat a medically fragile patient with an intact uterus and cervix and symptomatic pelvic organ prolapse (POP). Anterior and posterior segments of the vaginal wall are removed. The segments may be rectangular or triangular in shape. The uterus and cervix are then pushed back into the pelvic cavity and the raw edges of the vagina are sutured together leaving a channel through which uterine and cervical secretions can flow. Imbricating sutures are used to secure the raw vaginal surfaces, providing a corset-like support structure to prevent prolapse of the pelvic organs.

57130

57130 Excision of vaginal septum

The physician excises the vaginal septum. A transverse vaginal septum results from failure of the vaginal plate to regress completely during fetal development. The vaginal septum may completely obstruct the vagina or may contain small perforations that allow the flow of secretions and menstrual blood. The vaginal walls are retracted and the septum is exposed. A vertical incision is made through the center of the septum dividing it in half. Traction is applied to the septum with tissue forceps while the septum is separated from the vaginal mucosa using sharp excision on first one side and then the other. The vaginal mucosa at the site of the septal attachment is repaired with sutures.

57135

57135 Excision of vaginal cyst or tumor

The physician excises a vaginal cyst or tumor. Cystic lesions of the vaginal mucosa may be inclusion cysts caused by trauma to the vaginal wall, Gartner's duct cysts, or benign cystic tumors. Tumors include both benign and malignant neoplasms. An incision is made in the vaginal mucosa over the cystic lesion. The cyst is excised and sent to the laboratory for pathology examination. If the physician is removing a tumor, the tumor is removed along with a margin of healthy tissue. The incision is closed with sutures.

57150

57150 Irrigation of vagina and/or application of medicament for treatment of bacterial, parasitic, or fungoid disease

The physician irrigates the vagina or applies a medicament for treatment of bacterial, parasitic, or fungoid disease. A tube or catheter is inserted into the vagina and attached to a syringe containing an anti-bacterial, anti-parasitic, or anti-fungoid irrigation solution, which is instilled into the vagina. Alternatively, a vaginal film, gel, or pessary containing anti-bacterial, anti-parasitic, or anti-fungoid medication is inserted into the vaginal vault to treat a local vaginal infection.

57155

57155   Insertion of uterine tandem and/or vaginal ovoids for clinical brachytherapy

A uterine tandem and/or vaginal ovoids are inserted for separately reportable delivery of clinical brachytherapy. Uterine tandem and vaginal ovoids are empty radiation applicator devices that are loaded with a radiation source after being placed by the surgeon. Intracavitary radiation of the uterus or vagina using a tandem or ovoids delivers high dose radiation to a malignant neoplasm while limiting the volume of tissue affected by the radiation. A uterine tandem is used for treatment of neoplasms of the lower uterus and uterine cervix. Vaginal ovoids are used primarily for vaginal cuff neoplasms and neoplasms in the upper third of the vagina. Often both a uterine tandem and vaginal ovoids are placed simultaneously. The physician determines the appropriate number and location of the tandem and/or ovoids to be placed in the lower uterus and/or vagina. The tandem is inserted at the site of a tumor in the lower uterus or uterine cervix. The vaginal ovoids are placed laterally on each side of the fornix. Once the empty radiation applicator shells are placed, separately reportable afterloading of the radiation source is performed.

57156

57156   Insertion of a vaginal radiation afterloading apparatus for clinical brachytherapy

Vaginal brachytherapy is typically performed following a hysterectomy for uterine cancer. Brachytherapy is delivered to the upper vaginal region using a cylinder apparatus placed within the vagina when there is a high risk for cancer recurrence. The bowel is prepped with a Fleet enema the night before the procedure. With the patient supine and the feet in stirrups, the perineal and genital area is cleansed. Catheters are inserted into the bladder and rectum. The physician inserts the vaginal cylinder and secures it in the vagina. Contrast is injected into the bladder and rectal catheters and images are obtained so the physician can evaluate the cylinder in relation to surrounding organs. In separately reportable procedures, the physician evaluates the images, creates a treatment plan, and tailors the radiation doses and exposure amounts to treat sites at risk for cancer recurrence while minimizing radiation exposure to other areas. Following the treatment planning, the physician then delivers the prescribed radiation dose through the channels in the cylinder. Upon completion of the brachytherapy procedure, the vaginal cylinder and bladder and rectal catheters are removed.

57160

57160   Fitting and insertion of pessary or other intravaginal support device

The physician fits and inserts a pessary or other intravaginal support device. These devices provide a nonsurgical method of treating pelvic organ prolapse. Pessaries and intravaginal support devices come in a variety of shapes and sizes. The physician selects the device based on the severity of the prolapse and the patient's anatomy and fits the patient with a properly sized device. The physician inserts the selected device and positions it properly in the vagina to reduce the pelvic organ prolapse.

57170

57170   Diaphragm or cervical cap fitting with instructions

The physician fits a diaphragm or cervical cap and instructs the patient on the use of the device. These devices are barrier type birth control devices. A diaphragm is a dome shaped soft rubber disc with a flexible rim. A cervical cap is a thimble shaped device that fits snugly over the cervix. When inserted into the vagina, both devices cover the cervix preventing sperm from entering the uterus. Both devices are used with spermicidal jellies or creams to kill sperm and to prevent pregnancy. The physician selects the proper size of diaphragm or cap and positions it over the cervix to verify that the fit is correct. If the patient has not used a barrier device before, the patient is instructed on how to insert and position the device. The patient then inserts the diaphragm or cap without assistance from the physician. When the patient has inserted the device, the physician checks the device to verify that it is properly positioned over the cervix.

57180

57180   Introduction of any hemostatic agent or pack for spontaneous or traumatic nonobstetrical vaginal hemorrhage (separate procedure)

A hemostatic agent or pack is placed in the vagina to control spontaneous or traumatic nonobstetrical hemorrhage. Packing provides a tamponade effect on the bleeding site. Packing techniques vary, but most physicians use a long continuous segment of sterile gauze. The gauze may be placed directly in the vagina or inserted into a sterile plastic bag or glove to allow easy removal. The patient is carefully monitored while the pack is in place to ensure that the hemostatic agent or pack has controlled the bleeding and that there is no undetected bleeding proximal to the pack or internally.

57200-57210

57200   Colporrhaphy, suture of injury of vagina (nonobstetrical)
57210   Colpoperineorrhaphy, suture of injury of vagina and/or perineum (nonobstetrical)

The physician repairs a nonobstetrical injury (open wound or laceration) to the vagina and/or perineum. This procedure may also be referred to as a colporrhaphy, colpoperineorrhaphy, or perineorrhaphy. In 57200, a vaginal laceration is repaired. The apex of the vaginal laceration is identified and an anchor suture placed approximately one cm above the apex. The vaginal mucosa and rectovaginal fascia are sutured closed from the apex down to the level of the hymenal ring. In 57210, the vaginal laceration is repaired as described above then the perineal laceration is addressed. The transverse muscles of the perineal body are identified on each side of the perineal laceration and reapproximated followed by repair of the bulbocavernosus muscle. If the laceration has caused separation of the rectovaginal fascia from the perineal body, the fascia is reattached. Anatomical repair of the perineal muscles provides good approximation of the overlying skin and skin sutures are not generally required. If skin suture is required, running subcuticular sutures are used.

57220

57220   Plastic operation on urethral sphincter, vaginal approach (eg, Kelly urethral plication)

The physician performs a plastic operation on the urethral sphincter via a vaginal approach, such as a Kelly plication or urethral plication. This procedure is performed to treat stress incontinence and is accomplished using a plication procedure to reduce the diameter of the urethra. Using a vaginal approach, a tenaculum is placed on the cervix and a transverse incision made at the junction of the vaginal mucosa and cervix and carried down to the pubovesical cervical fascia. The vaginal mucosa is dissected off the pubovesical cervical fascia. The vaginal mucosa is opened in the midline to approximately one cm from the urethral meatus. Dissection continues until the bladder and urethra are separated from the vaginal mucosa and the urethral vesical angle has been identified. A mattress suture is placed in the wall of the urethra along the lateral margin approximately one cm below the urethral meatus. The urethral tissue is then inverted and plicated, and the suture tied. Additional plication sutures are placed along the urethra to a point approximately two cm beyond the urethral vesical angle. Overlying tissues are reapproximated and a Foley or suprapubic catheter placed.

57230

57230   Plastic repair of urethrocele

The physician performs a plastic repair of a prolapsed urethra. Using a vaginal approach, a tenaculum is placed on the cervix and a transverse incision is made at the junction of the vaginal mucosa and cervix and carried down to the cervical fascia. The vaginal mucosa is dissected off the cervical fascia down to the level of the pubic bone and bladder. The vaginal mucosa is opened in the midline to approximately 1 cm from the urethral opening (meatus). Dissection continues until the urethra is separated from the vaginal mucosa and the junction between the urethra and bladder (urethrovesical angle) has been identified. Beginning immediately below the urethral meatus, plication sutures are placed in the fascia. By folding (plicating) the fascia, the prolapsed urethra is returned to normal position (reduced). The vaginal mucosa is then closed. A Foley or suprapubic catheter is placed.

57240

57240   Anterior colporrhaphy, repair of cystocele with or without repair of urethrocele

This procedure is performed on the anterior aspect (front) of vaginal wall to treat prolapse of the bladder (cystocele) with prolapse of the urethra (urethrocele), if present. Using a vaginal approach, a tenaculum is placed on the cervix and a transverse incision is made at the junction of the vaginal mucosa and cervix and carried down to the cervical fascia. The vaginal mucosa is dissected off underlying fascia. Dissection continues until the urethra is separated from the vaginal mucosa and the junction between the urethra and bladder (urethrovesical angle) has been exposed. The defect in the underlying fascia is repaired using plication sutures. By folding (plicating) the fascia, the prolapsed bladder and urethra are returned to normal position (reduced). Excessive vaginal mucosa is excised. The vaginal mucosa is then closed in the midline and the vaginal cuff is repaired with sutures. A Foley or suprapubic catheter is placed.

57250

57250   Posterior colporrhaphy, repair of rectocele with or without perineorrhaphy

The physician performs a posterior colporrhaphy for repair of rectocele with or without perineorrhaphy. A rectocele occurs when the rectum prolapses (herniates) through the levator sling due to a weakness in the anterior perirectal fascia. A transverse incision is made in the vaginal mucosa at the posterior fold of the labia minora (posterior fourchette). The posterior vaginal mucosa is dissected off the perirectal fascia. If a perineorrhaphy is performed, a second incision is made in the perineal body and a triangular section is removed to expose the bulbocavernosus muscle. The rectocele is exposed and reduced to expose the margins of the levator ani muscles. Sutures are placed from the apical margin of the levator ani to the posterior fourchette and then tied. Excessive vaginal musoca is trimmed, exposing the surgically created triangular defect in the perineal body and the insertion of the bulbocavernosus muscle. The perirectal fascia is closed, followed by closure of the posterior vaginal wall. The hymenal ring is reconstructed. The vaginal mucosa is then approximated to the perirectal fascia and the surgically created defect in the perineal body is closed. Sutures are also placed in the insertions of the bulbocavernosus muscle as part of the perineal body reconstruction. Subcutaneous tissues and skin are closed in a layered fashion.

57260-57265

57260   Combined anteroposterior colporrhaphy
57265   Combined anteroposterior colporrhaphy; with enterocele repair

A combined anterior and posterior colporrhaphy is performed with or without enterocele repair. An enterocele is a herniation of the peritoneal sac with protrusion of a portion of small bowel into the rectovaginal space between the posterior surface of the vagina and the anterior surface of the rectum. To perform the anterior repair using a vaginal approach, a tenaculum is placed on the cervix and a transverse incision made at the junction of the vaginal mucosa and cervix and carried down to the pubovesical cervical fascia. The vaginal mucosa is dissected off the pubovesical cervical fascia which is then opened using scissor dissection in the midline. The vaginal mucosa is opened in the midline to approximately one cm from the urethral meatus. Dissection continues until the bladder and urethra are separated from the vaginal mucosa and the urethral vesical angle has been identified. Beginning immediately below the urethral meatus, plication sutures are placed in the pubovesical cervical fascia until the entire cystocele and urethrocele have been reduced. Excess vaginal mucosa is excised. The vaginal mucosa is then closed in the midline and the vaginal cuff suture repaired. If an enterocele is present, it is repaired prior to the posterior repair. The posterior vaginal mucosa overlying the enterocele is opened up to the vaginal apex. An ellipse of skin at the junction of the vagina and perineum is excised. Perirectal fascia is dissected free of the posterior vaginal mucosa to expose the enterocele sac. The sac is incised and the small bowel pushed back into the abdomen. The sac is closed with two pursestring sutures placed around the neck of the enterocele. The redundant sac is excised. The physician now performs a posterior repair. The rectocele is exposed and reduced. Sutures are placed from the apical margin of the levator ani to the posterior fourchette and then tied. Excessive vaginal musoca is trimmed exposing the surgically created elliptical defect in the perineal body and the insertion of the bulbocavernosus muscle. The perirectal fascia is closed followed by closure of the posterior vaginal wall. The hymenal ring is reconstructed. The vaginal mucosa is then approximated to the perirectal fascia and the surgically created defect in the perineal body closed. Sutures are also placed in the insertions of the bulbocavernosus muscle as part of the perineal body reconstruction. Subcutaneous tissues and skin are closed in a layered fashion. Use code 57260, for combined repair of prolapsed bladder, urethra, and rectum. Use code 57265, for repair of prolapsed bladder, urethra, and rectum treated in conjunction with an enterocele.

57267

57267   Insertion of mesh or other prosthesis for repair of pelvic floor defect, each site (anterior, posterior compartment), vaginal approach (List separately in addition to code for primary procedure)

The physician inserts mesh or other prosthetic material for repair of a pelvic floor defect via a vaginal approach at the time of a separately reportable anterior and/or posterior colporrhaphy and/or rectocele repair. An incision is made in the vagina to access deep supportive muscle, fascia, and ligaments. The mesh or other prosthetic material is cut to the desired size and configuration to accomplish the repair. Alternatively, a preconfigured prosthetic (mesh) implant may be used. The mesh or prosthetic material is then placed over the anterior or posterior fascia and secured to underlying musculature along the pelvic floor defect in the compartment being repaired (anterior, posterior). Report 57267 for each compartment repaired with mesh.

57268-57270

57268   Repair of enterocele, vaginal approach (separate procedure)
57270   Repair of enterocele, abdominal approach (separate procedure)

An enterocele is repaired in a separate procedure. An enterocele is a herniation of the peritoneal sac and a portion of small bowel into the rectovaginal space between the posterior surface of the vagina and the anterior surface of the rectum. In 57268, the enterocele is repaired via a vaginal approach. The posterior vaginal mucosa overlying the enterocele is opened up to the vaginal apex. Perirectal fascia is dissected free of the posterior vaginal mucosa to expose the enterocele sac. The sac is incised and the small bowel pushed back into the abdomen. The enterocele sac is closed with two pursestring sutures placed around the neck of the enterocele. The redundant sac is excised. Sutures are then placed between the anterior rectal wall, the stump of the enterocele sac, and the uterosacral ligaments to reinforce the repair and prevent future enterocele formation. Excessive vaginal mucosa is trimmed and the incisions closed in layers. In 57270, the enterocele is repaired via an abdominal approach. An incision is made in the

lower abdomen. The peritoneum is incised at the vaginal cuff and the endopelvic fascia identified. The enterocele sac is exposed, incised, and the small bowel pushed back into the abdomen. The sac is ligated and resected. The endopelvic fascia is suture repaired using one of several techniques. In a Halban repair, permanent sutures are placed just below the peritoneum from the posterior wall of the vagina to the cul-de-sac and then to the anterior wall of the rectum. In a Moschcowitz repair, the cul-de-sac is obliterated by placing horizontal purse-string sutures distally deep in the cul-de-sac and carrying them proximally.

57280

57280   Colpopexy, abdominal approach

The physician performs a suspension of the vaginal apex, also referred to as a colpopexy, via an abdominal approach. An obturator is first placed in the vaginal vault to elevate the vaginal apex. An incision is made in the lower abdomen and the bowel is exposed. The sigmoid colon is retracted laterally to the left pelvic sidewall. The peritoneum is incised at the right paracolic gutter from the sacral promontory to the cul-de-sac. The anterior longitudinal ligament is exposed. Two to four sutures are placed in the anterior longitudinal ligament at the S2-S3 level. The vesicovaginal space is entered. A previously prepared Y-shaped piece of mesh is sutured to the anterior and posterior vaginal apex and then attached to the sacral sutures to suspend the vaginal apex. The peritoneum is closed over the mesh and the incision in the abdomen is closed.

57282-57283

57282   Colpopexy, vaginal; extra-peritoneal approach (sacrospinous, iliococcygeus)
57283   Colpopexy, vaginal; intra-peritoneal approach (uterosacral, levator myorrhaphy)

The physician performs a suspension of the vaginal apex, also referred to as a colpopexy, via a vaginal approach using either an extraperitoneal (57282) or intraperitoneal (57283) technique. In 57282, the vaginal apex is suspended by attaching it to the sacrospinous or iliococcygeus ligaments. An incision is made in the perineum and posterior vaginal mucosa to open the rectovaginal space. The right rectal pillar overlying the right pararectal space is penetrated. The rectum is then displaced to the left and the right ischial spine palpated. A window is created through the descending rectal septum over the ischial spine. The sacrospinous ligament -coccygeus muscle complex is visualized, grasped with the long tip of a clamp, and then penetrated with the blunt tip of a ligature carrier and sutures placed in the sacrospinous ligament. Alternatively, the vaginal apex may be suspended to the iliococcygeus fascia bilaterally. The colpopexy sutures are grasped and held while sutures are then placed in the vaginal submucosa and buried in the fibromuscular wall. The colpopexy sutures are then tied to suspend the vaginal apex. In 57283, the vaginal apex is suspended by attaching it to the uterosacral ligaments or levator muscle. The vaginal mucosa is incised at the vaginal apex. The endopelvic fascia is dissected away from the muscosa. The peritoneum is exposed and incised. The bowel is retracted. The ureters and uterosacral ligaments are identified bilaterally. The uterosacral ligaments are grasped with clamps and traction applied. Sutures are then placed through the uterosacral ligaments bilaterally. Alernatively, sutures may be placed in the levator ani muscle. The sutures are then tied to the vaginal apex and the vaginal apex suspended. The incision in the vagina is closed.

57284

57284   Paravaginal defect repair (including repair of cystocele, if performed); open abdominal approach

A paravaginal defect is repaired using an open abdominal approach. Any repair of cystocele is included. A paravaginal defect results from loss of support of the arcus tendineus fascia pelvis (ATFP) which forms the lateral attachments of the vagina. Without the support of the ATFP, the bladder and urethra drop from their normal position (prolapse), resulting in a cystocele or cystourethrocele. The defect may affect only one side(unilateral) or both sides (bilateral) of the ATFP. Using an open abdominal approach, the retropubic space of Retzius is accessed, taking care to protect vascular structures. The bladder is mobilized and the lateral retropubic spaces are exposed. The ischial spine is identified by palpation. The entire length of the ATFP is visualized as a white ligamentus band extending from the ischial spine toward the ipsilateral posterior pubic symphysis. The paravaginal defect is visualized, which may present as a unilateral or bilateral defect with avulsion of the vagina off the ATFP or as avulsion of the ATFP off the obturator internus muscle. The bladder is deflected. A few fingers of the nondominant hand are inserted into the vagina and the ipsilateral anterolateral vaginal sulcus is elevated. A suture is placed through the fibromuscular tissue of the lateral vaginal apex and into the ATFP or obturator internus fascia just distal to the ischial spine. Additional sutures are placed in a similar fashion with the last suture placed into the pubourethral ligament as close as possible to the pubic ramus. The sutures are tied sequentially and the defect is obliterated. If a bilateral defect is present, the procedure is repeated on the contralateral side.

57285

57285 **Paravaginal defect repair (including repair of cystocele, if performed); vaginal approach**

A paravaginal defect is repaired using a vaginal approach. Any cystocele repair is included, when performed. A paravaginal defect results from loss of support of the arcus tendineus fascia pelvis (ATFP) which forms the lateral attachments of the vagina. Without the support of the ATFP, the bladder and urethra drop out of their normal position (prolapse), resulting in a cystocele or cystourethrocele. Using a vaginal approach, the anterior vaginal wall is incised and the bladder is dissected free of the vaginal epithelium to gain access to the retropubic space (space of Retzius). The ATFP is exposed. Sutures are placed along the anterior lateral vaginal sulcus at the site of the defect, which may be either unilateral or bilateral, and carried through the pubocervical fascia. The sutures are then brought through the internal obturator muscle immediately above the ATFP and placed from the underside along the full length of the pubic synthesis to the ischial spine. The sutures are tied sequentially and the defect is obliterated. The incisions in the vaginal wall are repaired.

57287

57287 **Removal or revision of sling for stress incontinence (eg, fascia or synthetic)**

A previously placed fascial or synthetic sling used to treat stress incontinence is removed or revised. Removal of the sling is usually performed for complications such as urethral erosion and may also be performed for vaginal extrusion of the sling. Revision may be performed for recurrent stress incontinence or vaginal extrusion of the sling. A Foley catheter is placed through the urethra and into the bladder. Removal is performed using a vaginal approach. The sling is dissected free of surrounding tissue and removed along with any permanent suture material. If urethral erosion is present, the urethral defect is repaired over the catheter by suture repair of the periurethral fascia. A labial fat graft may be used to strengthen the repair. If the sling has extruded through the vagina, the sling may be removed or revised. Removal is performed as described above and the vaginal defect is then repaired. Revision following vaginal extrusion of the sling consists of trimming the mesh, excising granulation tissue, and a two-layer repair of the vaginal defect. If revision is performed for recurrent stress incontinence, the sling may be shortened. An incision is made in the vagina and the sling is dissected free of surrounding tissue, then shortened and reattached to the pelvic fascia or abdominal wall.

57288

57288 **Sling operation for stress incontinence (eg, fascia or synthetic)**

A sling operation is done to treat stress incontinence using a fascial or synthetic graft. If a fascial autograft is being used, an incision is made in the lower abdomen and a strip of abdominal fascia is removed. A second incision is then made in the vaginal wall just below the urethra. Two small tunnels are created on either side of the urethra and extended into the space below the pubic bone. The fascial or synthetic sling is placed under the urethra and around the bladder neck. The ends of the sling are then brought up through the tunnels and sutured to the pelvic fascia or the abdominal wall. The incisions in the abdomen and vaginal wall are closed.

57289

57289 **Pereyra procedure, including anterior colporrhaphy**

The physician performs an operation to fix a condition in which the patient is unable to control the release of urine. The physician makes incisions in the pubic area and the lower abdominal area to run thin cords to tie the urethrovesical junction to the muscles by the rectum. The physician also repairs a condition in which the bladder protrudes through the vaginal wall.

57291-57292

57291 **Construction of artificial vagina; without graft**
57292 **Construction of artificial vagina; with graft**

Construction of an artificial vagina is performed to treat congenital absence of the vagina. The procedure varies depending on whether a functioning uterus is present and whether or not a tissue graft is used. In 57291, the procedure is performed without a graft. An H-shaped incision is made between the urethra and rectum. Using blunt dissection, a cavity is created. If a functioning uterus is present, the cavity is created up to the lowest pole of the uterine cavity. A sound is inserted into the uterus. If the uterus is absent, the cavity is created up to the peritoneum. Bleeding is controlled by electrocoagulation. A vaginal stent is then placed in the newly created cavity. A Foley catheter may also be inserted into the uterus to maintain patency of the cervical canal. Sutures are placed in the labial musculature to temporarily secure the vaginal stent until healing of the surgical wound occurs. In 57292, a tissue graft is applied following creation of the cavity between the urethra and rectum. A full or split thickness skin graft is harvested from the buttocks or upper thigh. The graft is applied to an obturator that is then inserted into the vaginal vault. The graft edges are sutured to the introitus. The obturator is retained until the graft has healed sufficiently to permit removal. The patient is then fitted with a polyfoam dilator which must be inserted daily and remain in place for 10-12 hours each day.

57295

57295 **Revision (including removal) of prosthetic vaginal graft; vaginal approach**

A prosthetic vaginal graft is revised or removed using a vaginal approach. Deep vaginal retractors are placed to expose the vaginal apex. An assessment is made of the prosthetically reinforced vaginal apex to determine whether the mesh should be excised in its entirety, only the eroded portions removed, or the mesh removed and replaced. Tissue around the outside edges of the mesh is incised and the vaginal epithelium is dissected off the endopelvic fascia. The mesh is grasped and tension is applied as all or part of the mesh is excised. If vaginal apical support is not adequate without the mesh, a new prosthetic mesh graft is configured and sutured in place. The endopelvic fascia is closed with sutures and the vaginal epithelium is closed over the fascia. The vagina is irrigated to remove blood and debris and vaginal packing is applied.

57296

57296 **Revision (including removal) of prosthetic vaginal graft; open abdominal approach**

A previously placed prosthetic vaginal graft is revised or removed by open abdominal approach. An incision is made in the lower abdomen to access the newly formed vagina and reach the affected graft material. An assessment of the complication necessitating revision, such as a stricture or infection, will determine if portions of eroded mesh material must be excised and removed; if graft material needs to be replaced; or if the existing graft and surrounding tissue can be revised. The appropriate vaginal incisions to access the graft for revision or removal are made. Graft material and vaginal tissue are rearranged and re-approximated so as to form a functioning neovagina again and all layers of tissue are closed with vaginal packing put in place.

57300

57300 **Closure of rectovaginal fistula; vaginal or transanal approach**

The physician closes a rectovaginal fistula using a vaginal or transanal approach. A rectovaginal fistula is an abnormal passage between the rectum and vagina that may be congenital or acquired. Acquired fistulas may be caused by infection, an injury to the perineum while giving birth, a complication of vaginal or rectal surgical procedures, or a complication of radiation therapy for malignancy. For transvaginal repair, the vaginal mucosa is elevated around the fistula and the fistula is exposed. Pursestring sutures are placed around the fistula and it is inverted into the rectal lumen. The vaginal mucosa is closed. For a transanal approach, an anoscope is used to identify the fistula. An advancement flap is outlined. The flap of mucosal and submucosal tissue is elevated. Sometimes muscle tissue is also required. The fistula tract is debrided and the muscle tissue over the fistula is sutured closed. The tip of the fistula in the rectum above the closed muscle tissue is excised. The flap is advanced and sutured over the closed fistula tract. The vaginal side of the fistula is left open.

57305-57307

57305 **Closure of rectovaginal fistula; abdominal approach**
57307 **Closure of rectovaginal fistula; abdominal approach, with concomitant colostomy**

An abdominal approach is used when the fistula is located high in the rectum. These types of fistulas result most often from malignant neoplasm or radiation therapy. In 57305, an incision is made in the lower abdomen. The rectovaginal septum is dissected and the fistula identified. The fistula is divided and the openings in the rectum and vagina closed with sutures. In 57307, the fistula is closed as described above and a concomitant colostomy is performed. A second incision is made in the abdomen for the colostomy opening. The section of intestine to be diverted is transected and the distal segment closed. The proximal segment is brought out through the skin. The intestine is sutured to the skin creating the stoma. A colostomy bag is placed over the stoma.

57308

57308 **Closure of rectovaginal fistula; transperineal approach, with perineal body reconstruction, with or without levator plication**

A rectovaginal fistula is closed using a transperineal approach with perineal body reconstruction with or without levator plication. A rectovaginal fistula is an abnormal passage between the rectum and vagina that may be congenital or acquired. Acquired fistulas may be caused by infection, an injury to the perineum while giving birth, a complication of vaginal or rectal surgical procedures, or a complication of radiation therapy for malignancy. The perineum is incised; the anal sphincter and superficial transverse peritoneal muscles are transected; and the rectovaginal space is developed. The posterior vaginal mucosa is incised around the fistula. The fistula tract is excised down to the rectal mucosa. The surrounding vaginal tissue is elevated and mobilized. The rectum is repaired by inverting the mucosa into the rectal lumen. Suture repair continues down to the anal mucosa. The bulbocavernosus muscle along with the fat pad is sutured over the repaired rectum to provide blood supply to the region. If the levator ani muscles require plication, this is done. The anal sphincter and superficial transverse peritoneal muscles are repaired. The vaginal mucosa is closed and the perineal incision is suture repaired.

● New Code   ▲ Revised Code

57310-57311

57310 Closure of urethrovaginal fistula
57311 Closure of urethrovaginal fistula; with bulbocavernosus transplant

A urethrovaginal fistula is closed. Urethrovaginal fistula is typically a complication of surgical trauma following anterior vaginal repair or obstetrical trauma during vaginal delivery. In 57310, the fistula is exposed and the vaginal mucosa incised from the urethral meatus to the fistula site. Fascial flaps are developed and mobilized on each side of the urethra. The fistula is closed by suturing the urethral mucosa. The fascial flap on one side is sutured to the base of the flap on the opposite side. The flap on the opposite side is then closed over the first flap in a double breasted fashion. The vaginal mucosa is closed. In 57311, the fistula is repaired as described above and a bulbocavernosus flap developed to provide vascularization to tissues that have been damaged by a previous surgical procedure or radiation. The labia majora is incised and the bulbocavernosus muscle and fat pad mobilized. The muscle is transected and tunneled under the vaginal mucosa, labia minora and labia majora. The muscle flap is sutured over the repaired fistula and the fascia then closed over the flap in a double breasted fashion. The labia majora and vaginal mucosa are repaired. A suprapubic catheter is placed to allow the urethra to heal.

57320-57330

57320 Closure of vesicovaginal fistula; vaginal approach
57330 Closure of vesicovaginal fistula; transvesical and vaginal approach

A vesicovaginal fistula (VVF) is closed using a vaginal approach (57320) or a combined transvesical and vaginal approach (57330). A vesicovaginal fistula is an abnormal passage between the bladder and vagina through which urine is discharged from the bladder into the vaginal vault. In 57320, a deep vaginoperineal incision is made and the fistula tract exposed. The fistula tract is may be catheterized with a balloon catheter and traction applied to draw the fistula into the surgical field. Traction sutures are placed around the fistula tract. The vaginal mucosa is denuded and the incision extended to the bladder wall. The fistula tract is resected. Defects in the bladder wall, fascia, and vaginal wall are closed sequentially. In 57330, a combined transvesical and vaginal approach are employed. An incision is made in the abdomen and the bladder exposed. The bladder is opened (cystotomy) and the ureters catheterized. The fistula is identified and excised along with surrounding scar tissue. A second incision is made in the vagina and any remaining fistula dissected free of surrounding tissue and excised. The vaginal defect is closed by either the abdominal or vaginal route depending on its location. The fascia and bladder wall defect are closed by an abdominal approach. The ureteral catheters are removed and the cystotomy closed.

57335

57335 Vaginoplasty for intersex state

The physician performs a vaginoplasty for intersex state. Intersex state is a condition where the genitalia have characteristics of both sexes making gender identification impossible from the outward appearance of the genitalia alone. Intersex states include: true hermaphrodite and female or male pseudohermaphrodite. A true hermaphrodite has mixed male and female sex organs with both ovaries and testicles. A female pseudohermaphrodite is a genetic female with external genitalia that appears male, including a penis. A male pseudohermaphrodite is a genetic male with external genitalia that has failed to develop normally. There are a number of techniques for vaginoplasty that depend on what genitalia is present. The existing genitalia may be used to create a vagina. If a penis or testes are present, they may be inverted to create the vagina. If existing genitalia is not sufficient for inversion technique, grafts may be taken from existing labia, penile tissue, or scrotal skin. Other skin or tissue grafts or flaps from the oral mucosa, buttocks, lower abdomen, or intestinal mucosa may also be used.

57400

57400 Dilation of vagina under anesthesia (other than local)

Vaginal dilation under anesthesia may be done in cases of vaginal genetic anomaly, such as incomplete transverse vaginal septa or vaginal agenesis (absent or underdeveloped vaginal vault). It may also be performed to maintain established patency or depth and prevent stenosis following surgery, or to treat scarring or stenosis of the vagina due to injury or radiation. Dilation of the vagina under anesthesia may be performed as an initial procedure to increase the diameter of the vaginal vault sufficiently enough to allow subsequent home dilation by the patient. The patient is placed under anesthesia, other than local type, and vaginal obturators or dilators, of increasingly larger size are inserted and held with firm, gentle pressure for several minutes to stretch and lengthen the tissue of the vaginal walls and enlarge the vaginal canal.

57410

57410 Pelvic examination under anesthesia (other than local)

The physician carries out a manual pelvic examination with the patient under anesthesia, other than local. The pelvic exam is used to check the vulva, vagina, cervix, uterus, fallopian tubes, and ovaries. The patient is positioned on the exam table. External genitalia are visually examined first to check for swelling, sores, or abnormalities. A speculum is inserted into the vagina and opened so the vaginal canal and cervix can be viewed. A small sample of cells or fluid may be taken from the cervix or vagina for testing. The speculum is removed and the physician conducts a bimanual exam to check the organs that cannot be viewed, even with the speculum. The physician places fingers inside the vagina and presses down on the lower abdomen to feel that the uterus and ovaries are the right size and shape and to check for cysts or other irregular growths. Sometimes, a rectal exam is also done.

57415

57415 Removal of impacted vaginal foreign body (separate procedure) under anesthesia (other than local)

A foreign body impacted in the vaginal tissue is removed under anesthesia, other than local. With the patient positioned on the exam table, a speculum is inserted into the vagina and opened so the vaginal canal can be viewed. The physician may shine a light to help locate the foreign body, which is extracted as carefully as possible while the patient is under anesthesia, due to the patient's young age or the size or depth of the imbedded foreign object.

57420-57421

57420 Colposcopy of the entire vagina, with cervix if present
57421 Colposcopy of the entire vagina, with cervix if present; with biopsy(s) of vagina/cervix

The physician performs a colposcopy of the entire vagina and cervix if the cervix has not been surgically removed. A colposcope is an instrument that looks like a pair of binoculars mounted on a pedestal with a light attached. The colposcope lenses magnify the tissue of the vagina and cervix, if present, allowing better visualization of abnormal tissue. The colposcope is placed at the vaginal opening. A speculum is then placed into the vagina to separate the vaginal wall. The vaginal wall is inspected in its entirety by rotating the speculum so that the entire vagina can be examined. If the cervix is present, the speculum is then placed to allow visualization of the entire cervix. The vagina and cervix are examined under two or three different magnifications. Acetic acid is then applied to allow better visualization of abnormal cells. Following the application of acetic acid, different colored filters are used to visualize blood vessels and any abnormal blood vessel patterns noted. Next, the vagina and cervix are painted with an iodine solution that stains the glycogen in the cells. Normal cells stain a dark-brown color. Any areas that do not stain are biopsied as are previously identified areas showing abnormal blood vessel patterns. Use code 57420 for colposcopy of the entire vagina and cervix without biopsy and code 57421 when the procedure is performed with one or more biopsies of the vagina and/or cervix.

57423

57423 Paravaginal defect repair (including repair of cystocele, if performed), laparoscopic approach

A paravaginal defect is repaired using a laparoscopic approach. Any repair of a cystocele is included, when performed. A paravaginal defect results from loss of support of the arcus tendineus fascia pelvis (ATFP) which forms the lateral attachments of the vagina. Without the support of the ATFP, the bladder and urethra drop out of their normal position (prolapse), resulting in a cystocele or cystourethrocele. Using a laparoscopic approach, a small incision is made below the umbilicus and the laparoscope is inserted. Additional small incisions are made and trocars are placed, including a small incision into the peritoneum above the bladder and behind the pubic bone. The retropubic space (space of Retzius) is entered and dissected. Using the laparoscope, the paravaginal defect is identified and the location is confirmed with digital vaginal exam. Sutures are placed along the anterior lateral vaginal sulcus at the site of the defect, which may be either unilateral or bilateral, and carried through the pubocervical fascia. The sutures are then brought through the internal obturator muscle immediately above the ATFP and placed from the underside along the full length of the pubic synthesis to the ischial spine. A retractor is placed in the vaginal vault and the sutures are tied sequentially using intracorporeal or extracorporeal knot tying technique. Repair of the defect is confirmed by digital vaginal exam and direct laparascopic view.

57425

57425 Laparoscopy, surgical, colpopexy (suspension of vaginal apex)

The physician performs a suspension of the vaginal apex, also referred to as a colpopexy, via a laparoscopic approach. Four small incisions are made in the abdomen and trocars are placed. The laparoscope is introduced and the bowel is mobilized to allow access to the sacrum. The peritoneum over the sacrum is elevated and incised. A vaginal probe is introduced into the vaginal vault to elevate the apex. The peritoneum over the vaginal apex is incised. The bladder and rectum are dissected free from the vagina and a piece of prepared mesh configured into a Y-shape is sutured to the posterior and anterior aspects of the vaginal apex. Sutures are then placed in the sacrum and the long arm of the mesh is attached to the sacrum to form a bridge suspending the vaginal apex. Alternatively, the long arm of the mesh can be sutured to the anterior longitudinal sacral ligament. The peritoneum is closed over the mesh. The laparoscope and surgical instruments are removed from the abdomen and the incisions are closed.

57426

57426   Revision (including removal) of prosthetic vaginal graft, laparoscopic approach

A prosthetic vaginal graft may need to be revised due to infection, stricture, or erosion of the mesh through overlying tissues. Using a laparoscopic approach, a small incision is made below the umbilicus and the laparoscope inserted. Additional small incisions are made and trocars placed. An instrument is placed within the vaginal cavity to elevate the vagina. Using the laparoscope, the peritoneum over the prosthetic vaginal graft is opened and the graft is inspected. Tissue surrounding the area of the graft attachment is dissected. All or part of the prosthetic graft material may be removed. Any remaining graft material is rearranged along with endopelvic fascia and vaginal tissue to allow coverage the vaginal apex. The endopelvic fascia is reapproximated with sutures and the vaginal epithelium closed in layers. The vaginal mucosa is repaired. The peritoneum overlying the vaginal apex is closed laparoscopically, the laparoscope and surgical tools removed and the portal incisions closed.

57452-57456

57452   Colposcopy of the cervix including upper/adjacent vagina

57454   Colposcopy of the cervix including upper/adjacent vagina; with biopsy(s) of the cervix and endocervical curettage

57455   Colposcopy of the cervix including upper/adjacent vagina; with biopsy(s) of the cervix

57456   Colposcopy of the cervix including upper/adjacent vagina; with endocervical curettage

The physician performs a colposcopy of the cervix and upper adjacent vagina. A colposcope is an instrument that looks like a pair of binoculars mounted on a pedestal with a light attached. The colposcope lenses magnify the tissue of the cervix and upper adjacent vagina allowing better visualization of abnormal tissue. The colposcope is placed at the vaginal opening. A speculum is then placed into the vagina to separate the vaginal wall and allow visualization of the cervix and upper adjacent vaginal wall. The cervix and upper adjacent vagina are examined under two or three different magnifications. Acetic acid is then applied to allow better visualization of abnormal cells. Following the application of acetic acid, different colored filters are used to visualize blood vessels and any abnormal blood vessel patterns noted. Next, the cervix and upper adjacent vagina are painted with an iodine solution that stains the glycogen in the cells. Normal cells stain a dark-brown color. Any areas that do not stain are biopsied as are previously identified areas showing abnormal blood vessel patterns. An endocervical curettage (ECC) is performed as needed. ECC is accomplished by scraping the cervical canal using a curet inserted into the cervix. Use code 57452 for colposcopy only, 57454 for colposcopy with biopsy and ECC, 57455 for colposcopy with biopsy, and 57456 for colposcopy with ECC.

57460-57461

57460   Colposcopy of the cervix including upper/adjacent vagina; with loop electrode biopsy(s) of the cervix

57461   Colposcopy of the cervix including upper/adjacent vagina; with loop electrode conization of the cervix

The physician performs a colposcopy of the cervix and upper adjacent vagina with a loop electrode biopsy of the cervix. A colposcope is an instrument that looks like a pair of binoculars mounted on a pedestal with a light attached. The colposcope lenses magnify the tissue of the vagina and cervix, if present, allowing better visualization of abnormal tissue. The colposcope is placed at the vaginal opening. A speculum is then placed into the vagina to separate the vaginal wall and allow visualization of the cervix and upper adjacent vaginal wall. The cervix and upper adjacent vagina are examined under two or three different magnifications. Acetic acid is then applied to allow better visualization of abnormal cells. Following the application of acetic acid, different colored filters are used to visualize blood vessels and any abnormal blood vessel patterns noted. Next, the cervix and upper adjacent vagina are painted with an iodine solution that stains the glycogen in the cells. Normal cells stain a dark-brown color. Any areas that do not stain are biopsied as are previously identified areas showing abnormal blood vessel patterns using a thin wire loop that conducts an electrical current to remove the piece of tissue (57460). This may be referred to as a loop electrical excision procedure (LEEP). Following the colposcopy procedure, the patient is placed on a grounding pad and an insulated speculum connected to smoke-evacuator tubing is inserted into the vagina. The cervix is visualized and a local anesthetic with epinephrine is injected beneath the surface of the cervical epithelium. Abnormal tissue is biopsied using the thin wire loop that conducts the electrical current. Alternatively, a loop electrode conization of the cervix may be performed (57461). Conization refers to the removal of a cone-shaped section of tissue from the cervix. Conization is accomplished using a thin wire loop for deep excision of the entire transformation zone. This may be accomplished in a single pass of the loop or using a two pass technique. Bleeding is controlled by painting the cervix with Monsel solution or by electrocautery.

57500

57500   Biopsy of cervix, single or multiple, or local excision of lesion, with or without fulguration (separate procedure)

Single or multiple biopsies of the cervix are obtained or local excision of a lesion of the cervix is performed with or without fulguration of the biopsy/excision site. A speculum is inserted into the vagina and the cervix is exposed. The cervix is cleansed and then soaked with acetic acid to enhance visibility of the lesion(s). A local anesthetic may be administered. A tenaculum may be inserted to hold the cervix during the biopsy/excision. One or more tissue samples are obtained or the lesion is excised. Bleeding is controlled using topical medication or electrocautery (fulguration). The tissue samples are sent to the laboratory for evaluation.

57505

57505   Endocervical curettage (not done as part of a dilation and curettage)

The physician performs endocervical curettage that is not part of a dilation and curettage procedure. A speculum is placed in the vaginal vault and the cervix is visualized. A curette is inserted into the cervical canal and a tissue sample is obtained by scraping a small amount of tissue from high inside the cervical canal. The tissue sample is sent to the laboratory for separately reportable microscopic exam.

57510-57513

57510   Cautery of cervix; electro or thermal

57511   Cautery of cervix; cryocautery, initial or repeat

57513   Cautery of cervix; laser ablation

The physician cauterizes the cervix. A speculum is inserted into the vaginal vault and the cervix visualized. In 57510, cervical cautery is performed using thermal or electrocautery. Heat or an electric current is used to destroy abnormal cervical tissue. This is accomplished by inserting a cautery probe and touching the heated tip of the probe to the abnormal cervical tissue. This burns away the abnormal tissue. In 57511, cryocautery is used to ablate abnormal cervical tissue. Cyrocautery uses extreme cold in the form of compressed nitrous oxide (liquid nitrogen) or carbon dioxide gas to freeze the abnormal cervical tissue. The cold source is delivered through a hand-held instrument inserted into the vaginal vault. This may be performed as an initial or repeat procedure. In 57513, cervical cautery is performed by laser ablation. A focused beam of light is used to evaporate eroded or abnormal cervical tissue. The laser delivery device is inserted into the vagina, directed at the area of abnormal tissue, and activated to destroy the tissue.

57520-57522

57520   Conization of cervix, with or without fulguration, with or without dilation and curettage, with or without repair; cold knife or laser

57522   Conization of cervix, with or without fulguration, with or without dilation and curettage, with or without repair; loop electrode excision

A conization of the cervix is performed with or without fulguration, with or without dilation and curettage, and with or without repair using cold knife or laser (57520) or loop electrode excision (57522). In 57520, following placement of a weighted speculum, cervical cerclage may be performed to control bleeding. The cervix is sounded to determine cervical length and the position of the internal os. The cervix is painted with Lugol solution and lateral traction applied to the cerclage sutures. A cone or wedge shaped section of cervical tissue is removed using blade excision (cold knife) including the entire transformation zone and a 2-3 mm margin of healthy tissue. Alternatively, laser conization may be used. For laser conization, bleeding is controlled by placing a cervical cerclage or by local injection of a vasoconstrictor. The exocervical margin is outlined with small dots produced by the laser. Laser incision is accomplished by connecting the dots and extending the depth of the incision. The cone or wedge excision may be completed using the laser, a scalpel or scissors. If the laser is used, the stromal edge of the incision is grasped and lifted with a hook to allow penetration of the laser beam toward the apex. The cone specimen is removed in one piece if possible. The endocervical canal is dilated and cervical tissue is removed by curettage as needed. Excessive bleeding is controlled by coagulation (cautery, fulguration). Suture repair using figure-eight or U sutures is performed as needed. In 57522, a loop electrode excision is performed, also referred to as loop electrosurgical excision procedure (LEEP) or large loop excision of transformation zone (LLETZ). The patient is attached to a grounding pad. An insulated speculum is placed in the vagina and connected to smoke evacuator tubing. A local anesthetic with a vasoconstrictor is injected into the cervical epithelium. The appropriate sized electrical loop is selected to perform the excision. Cervical tissue is then excised to a depth of approximately one cm on the first pass. Additional passes are made until the entire transformation zone and a margin of healthy tissue have been excised. Fulguration, dilation and curettage, and cervical repair are performed if needed as described above.

57530

57530   Trachelectomy (cervicectomy), amputation of cervix (separate procedure)

The physician performs an amputation of the cervix, also referred to as a trachelectomy or cervicectomy. Using a vaginal approach, the paravesical, rectovaginal, and vesicovaginal

● New Code   ▲ Revised Code

spaces are dissected. The cardinal and uterosacral ligaments are clamped and divided. The uterovesical ligament distal to the ureter is transected. The vaginal branch of the uterine artery is ligated. The cervix is transected at its junction with the uterine isthmus. In younger patients wishing to preserve fertility, a new cervical os may be created. A catheter is inserted and sutured to the new cervical os to maintain uterine patency. A suture is placed around the lower uterine segment to prevent cervical incompetence. The diseased cervix is removed along with the upper third of the vagina. The proximal vaginal cuff is sutured to the new cervical os or the remaining uterine body. If an abdominal approach is used, the abdomen is incised and the uterine vessels are ligated at their origins. The uterus is transected at the level of the internal os and the cervix is removed along with the parametria and upper third of the vagina. The proximal vaginal margins are sutured to uterine body.

57531

57531   Radical trachelectomy, with bilateral total pelvic lymphadenectomy and para-aortic lymph node sampling biopsy, with or without removal of tube(s), with or without removal of ovary(s)

The physician performs a radical trachelectomy (cervicectomy) with bilateral total pelvic lymphadenectomy and para-aortic lymph node sampling with or without removal of tubes and/or ovaries. The pelvic lymphadenectomy and para-aortic lymph node sampling is performed first using a laparoscopic, transperitoneal, or retroperitoneal approach. The pelvic lymph nodes including the external and common iliac nodes, hypogastric nodes, and obturator nodes, are dissected free of surrounding tissues, removed, and sent for frozen section. The para-aortic lymph nodes are then exposed; biopsies are taken; and they are sent for frozen section. Following removal of the pelvic lymph nodes, the fallopian tubes and ovaries are inspected and may be removed if needed. To remove the tubes and/or ovaries, the round ligament is transected and the posterior leaf of the broad ligament is opened. The infundibulopelvic ligament is undermined using blunt dissection. The ureter is identified and protected. The infundibulopelvic ligament is clamped, incised, and suture ligated. The fallopian tube, suspensory ligament, and mesosalpinx are clamped and transected near the opening into the uterus. The tube and ovary are removed. The procedure is repeated on the opposite side as needed. The uterine cervix is then resected. This may be performed via an abdominal, vaginal, or combined approach. Uterine vessels are ligated at their origins. The body of the uterus (uterine corpus) is transected just above the internal cervical os. The cervix is removed along with parametrial tissue and a portion of the vagina. The tissue is sent for frozen section. Further resection of the uterus is performed as needed until all of the tumor and an adequate margin of healthy tissue has been removed. In younger patients wishing to preserve fertility, a catheter is placed in the uterine opening (neocervix) to maintain patency, a cerclage is placed around the uterus and the proximal vaginal margins are sutured to the body of the uterus.

57540-57545

57540   Excision of cervical stump, abdominal approach
57545   Excision of cervical stump, abdominal approach; with pelvic floor repair

The physician excises the cervical stump via an abdominal approach. Excision of cervical stump may be performed in patients with a previous subtotal abdominal hysterectomy who develop cervical neoplasm or myoma. The lower abdomen is incised and the incision carried down to the rectus abdominus muscles which are separated in the midline. The peritoneum is elevated and opened. The round ligaments are identified, elevated and suture ligated. The bladder is freed from the cervix. The cervical stump is elevated and the broad ligament identified. The bladder peritoneum, posterior leaf of the broad ligament, and the peritoneum overlying the cul-de-sac and rectum are incised. Any attachment of the bladder to the cervix is taken down using blunt and sharp dissection. The infundibulopelvic ligament is clamped and transected. The cervical stump is freed from the round and infundibulopelvic ligaments. The peritoneum is opened around the cervical stump and traction is applied to the cervical stump. The cardinal and uterosacral ligaments are ligated and divided and the cervical stump is removed. The vaginal cuff is suspended. The space between the rectum and vagina is closed with sutures. The edge of the vagina is repaired with sutures and the angle of the vagina is attached to the uterosacral and cardinal liagments. The abdominal incision is closed in layers.

57550-57556

57550   Excision of cervical stump, vaginal approach
57555   Excision of cervical stump, vaginal approach; with anterior and/or posterior repair
57556   Excision of cervical stump, vaginal approach; with repair of enterocele

The physician excises the cervical stump via a vaginal approach. Cervical stump excision is performed on patients who have had a previous sub-total hysterectomy and subsequently develop a malignancy of the cervix. In 57550, a tenaculum is placed on the cervix. An incision is made in the upper aspect of the vaginal mucosa around the entire cervix stump. Tension is placed on the tenaculum and sharp and blunt dissection used to free the bladder from the cervix and lyse adhesions. The cervical stump is removed along with parametrial tissue and a portion of the vagina and sent for frozen section. In 57555, the cervical stump is removed as described above followed by an anterior and/

or posterior repair. The pubovesical fascia is exposed. The vaginal mucosa is dissected off the pubovesical fascia which is then opened using scissor dissection in the midline. The vaginal mucosa is opened in the midline to approximately one cm from the urethral meatus. Dissection continues until the bladder and urethra are separated from the vaginal mucosa and the urethral vesical angle has been identified. Beginning immediately below the urethral meatus, plication sutures are placed in the pubovesical cervical fascia until the entire cystocele and urethrocele have been reduced. Excess vaginal mucosa is excised. The vaginal mucosa is then closed in the midline and the vaginal cuff suture repaired. If a posterior repair is performed, a transverse incision is made in the vaginal mucosa at the posterior fold of the labia minora (posterior fourchette). The posterior vaginal mucosa is dissected off the perirectal fascia. If a perineorrhaphy is required a second incision is made in the perineal body and a triangular section removed to expose the bulbocavernosus muscle. The rectocele is exposed and reduced to expose the margins of the levator ani muscles. Sutures are placed from the apical margin of the levator ani to the posterior fourchette and then tied. Excessive vaginal musoca is trimmed exposing the surgically created triangular defect in the perineal body and the insertion of the bulbocavernosus muscle. The perirectal fascia is closed followed by closure of the posterior vaginal wall. The hymenal ring is reconstructed. The vaginal mucosa is then approximated to the perirectal fascia and the surgically created defect in the perineal body closed. Sutures are also placed in the insertions of the bulbocavernosus muscle as part of the perineal body reconstruction. Subcutaneous tissues and skin are closed in a layered fashion. In 57556, the cervical stump is removed as described above and an enterocele is repaired. The posterior vaginal mucosa overlying the enterocele is opened up to the vaginal apex. An ellipse of skin at the junction of the vagina and perineum is excised. Perirectal fascia is dissected free of the posterior vaginal mucosa to expose the enterocele sac. The sac is incised and the small bowel pushed back into the abdomen. The sac is closed with two pursestring sutures placed around the neck of the enterocele. The redundant sac is excised.

57558

57558   Dilation and curettage of cervical stump

Dilation and curettage of the cervical stump is performed for surgical scraping of the part of the uterus that is left after hysterectomy. A speculum is inserted vaginally to facilitate viewing the cervix, which is then enlarged with a dilator. The physician scrapes tissue from the cervical stump and removes the speculum.

57700

57700   Cerclage of uterine cervix, nonobstetrical

Using a vaginal approach, the physician may perform a McDonald type cerclage by weaving a pursestring suture in and out of the skin around the cervix and then tightening it to cinch the cervix together; or in a Shirodkar type procedure, the pursestring suture is tunneled subcutaneously around the cervix and then cinched together. Alternatively, an abdominal approach may be used through an incision in the lower abdomen. A stitch is then placed through the lower part of the uterus to cinch the lower uterus and upper cervix together.

57720

57720   Trachelorrhaphy, plastic repair of uterine cervix, vaginal approach

A plastic repair of the uterine cervix, also referred to as a trachelorrhaphy, is performed via a vaginal approach. The cervix is exposed and the laceration is identified. The cervix is cleansed and infiltrated with local anesthetic. The first suture is placed above the apex of the cervical laceration to control bleeding. Sutures are then carried distally along the entire length of the laceration.

57800

57800   Dilation of cervical canal, instrumental (separate procedure)

An instrumental dilation of the cervical canal is performed in a separate procedure. The cervix is exposed and cleansed with antiseptic solution. The cervix is numbed and dilated by passing a series of metal rods of increasing diameter into the cervical canal.

58100-58110

58100   Endometrial sampling (biopsy) with or without endocervical sampling (biopsy), without cervical dilation, any method (separate procedure)
58110   Endometrial sampling (biopsy) performed in conjunction with colposcopy (List separately in addition to code for primary procedure)

A speculum is placed in the vagina. The cervix is exposed and cleansed with antiseptic solution. The anterior cervical lip is grasped with a tenaculum and the uterus is sounded. An endometrial curette is passed through the cervix and biopsies are taken from multiple sites in the uterus. Biopsies may also be taken of the endocervical canal. The curette is withdrawn and the tissue sent to pathology. The tenaculum is removed and bleeding from the cervix controlled with pressure. The speculum is removed. Use code 58100 if endometrial biopsy is performed alone as a separate procedure. Use code 58110 if it is performed as an add-on service in conjunction with a separately reportable colposcopy procedure.

58120

58120   Dilation and curettage, diagnostic and/or therapeutic (nonobstetrical)

A speculum is placed in the vagina. The cervix is exposed and cleansed with antiseptic solution. The anterior cervical lip is grasped with a tenaculum. A sound is passed to determine the depth and angle of the uterus. The cervix is numbed and dilated by passing a series of metal rods of increasing diameter into the cervical canal. Alternatively, a laminaria tent may be inserted into the cervix 8-20 hours prior to the procedure. The laminaria absorbs water and swells, slowly dilating the cervical canal. Biopsies may be taken of the endocervical canal. A curette is then inserted through the cervix and the uterine wall is scraped or suctioned. Endocervical and endometrial tissue is sent for pathology exam. Following the procedure, the tenaculum is removed and bleeding from the cervix is controlled with pressure.

58140-58146

58140   Myomectomy, excision of fibroid tumor(s) of uterus, 1 to 4 intramural myoma(s) with total weight of 250 g or less and/or removal of surface myomas; abdominal approach

58145   Myomectomy, excision of fibroid tumor(s) of uterus, 1 to 4 intramural myoma(s) with total weight of 250 g or less and/or removal of surface myomas; vaginal approach

58146   Myomectomy, excision of fibroid tumor(s) of uterus, 5 or more intramural myomas and/or intramural myomas with total weight greater than 250 g, abdominal approach

Uterine fibroids are benign tumors of the muscle tissue (myometrium) of the uterus. Fibroid tumors may be submucous, intramural, subserous, or pedunculated. Submucous fibroids protrude into the uterine cavity and are typically removed by hysteroscopy. Intramural fibroids are contained within the uterine muscle. Subserous fibroids occur on the exterior of the uterus and may be pedunculated, that is attached by a thin stalk to the exterior of the uterine muscle. In 58140 and 58146, an incision is made in the abdomen and uterus is exposed. The uterus is visually inspected and palpated to determine the location of the fibroid(s). If the fibroid is subserous or pedunculated it is removed from the exterior surface of the uterus. For an intramural fibroid, the uterus is incised down to the level of the fibroid. The fibroid tumor is peeled off of the uterine wall (myometrium). Bleeding is controlled by electrocautery. The uterus is suture repaired in layers. Use code 58140 for one to four intramural myoma(s) with a total weight of 250 grams or less or for surface (subserous or pedunculated) myomas. Use code 58146 for removal of five or more intramural myomas or for myomas with a total weight greater than 250 grams. In 58145, a vaginal myomectomy is performed to remove one to four intramural myomas with a total weight of 250 grams or less or to remove surface (subserous or pedunculated) myomas. The procedure may be performed by an anterior or posterior vaginal approach. The vaginal mucosa is incised and the incision is carried down through the fascia to expose the peritoneum. The peritoneum is opened. If a posterior approach is used a long narrow retractor is placed in the Douglas pouch and a second retractor placed on the posterior wall of the cervix to allow exposure of the posterior uterine wall. If an anterior approach is used, the ureters must be identified and the pillars clamped and cut. A stitch is then placed in the stump of each pillar so that they can be easily identified and reconstructed following the myomectomy. The vesicouterine space is then dissected and the anterior uterine wall exposed. The location, number, and size of the fibroids are determined by digital palpation of the uterus. If the fibroid is subserous or pedunculated it is removed from the exterior surface of the uterus. For an intramural fibroid, the first fibroid is grasped and the uterine wall incised to the level of the fibroid. The fibroid capsule is exposed and dissected. The fibroid is enucleated and removed. This is repeated until all fibroids have been removed. The uterine wall and serosa are then reconstructed in layers.

58150-58152

58150   Total abdominal hysterectomy (corpus and cervix), with or without removal of tube(s), with or without removal of ovary(s)

58152   Total abdominal hysterectomy (corpus and cervix), with or without removal of tube(s), with or without removal of ovary(s); with colpo-urethrocystopexy (eg, Marshall-Marchetti-Krantz, Burch)

The physician performs a total abdominal hysterectomy with or without removal of the fallopian tubes and/or ovaries. An incision is made in the abdomen and the anterior uterine surface exposed. The peritoneum at the cervicovesical fold is incised. Blunt dissection is used to expose the broad ligament, round ligament and fallopian tubes. If the fallopian tubes and/or ovaries are removed, an incision is made in the exposed broad ligament. The ovarian vessels are visualized and suture ligated. The cut edges of the broad ligament are plicated with mattress sutures. The fallopian tubes and ovaries are dissected free of surrounding tissue. The round ligaments are clamped, divided, and blood vessels suture ligated bilaterally. The cervix is palpated and the position of the bladder ascertained. The bladder is then dissected off the uterus and the dissection carried down to the vaginal wall. The posterior aspect of the uterus is visualized and inspected to verify that it is not adhered to the rectum. The uterine vessels are exposed, clamped, divided and suture ligated. The posterior cervical peritoneum is incised and the incision is extended around the cervix. The vaginal wall is incised and the cervix separated from the vagina. The uterus

and cervix with or without the ovaries and tubes are removed. The vaginal opening is closed. The surgical site is inspected, bleeding controlled, and the abdominal incision closed. In 58152, a total abdominal hysterectomy is performed with a colpo-urethrocystopexy with or without removal of tubes and/or ovaries. The hysterectomy is performed as described above. The prolapsed vaginal wall and urethra are then suspended. Two sutures are placed through the paravaginal fascia, one on each side of the urethrovesical junction, oriented perpendicular to the vaginal axis. The sutures are then passed through the Cooper's ligament, pelvic fascia, or pubic bone and tied to provide suspension and support to the bladder and urethra. If additional suspension is required, a second set of sutures may be placed along the base of the bladder.

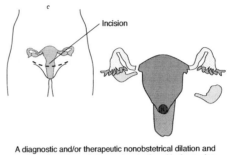

Total abdominal hysterectomy with or without removal of tube

Incision

A diagnostic and/or therapeutic nonobstetrical dilation and curettage is performed. A speculum is placed in the vagina.

58180

58180   Supracervical abdominal hysterectomy (subtotal hysterectomy), with or without removal of tube(s), with or without removal of ovary(s)

The physician performs a supracervical (subtotal) abdominal hysterectomy with or without removal of the fallopian tubes and/or ovaries. An incision is made in the abdomen and the anterior uterine surface is exposed. The peritoneum is incised. Blunt dissection is used to expose the broad ligament, round ligament, and fallopian tubes. If the fallopian tubes and/or ovaries are to be removed, an incision is made in the exposed broad ligament. The ovarian vessels are visualized and suture ligated. The cut edges of the broad ligament are plicated with mattress sutures. The fallopian tubes and ovaries are dissected free of surrounding tissue. The round ligaments are clamped and divided, and blood vessels are ligated bilaterally. The cervix is palpated and the position of the bladder ascertained before it is dissected off the uterus. The posterior aspect of the uterus is visualized and inspected to verify that it has not adhered to the rectum. The uterine vessels are exposed, clamped, divided, and suture ligated. The uterus is separated from the cervix and removed, with or without the tube(s)/ovary(ies) leaving the cervix intact. Sutures are placed to suspend the cervix, which is coagulated and covered with peritoneum. The surgical site is inspected and the abdominal incision is closed.

58200

58200   Total abdominal hysterectomy, including partial vaginectomy, with para-aortic and pelvic lymph node sampling, with or without removal of tube(s), with or without removal of ovary(s)

The physician performs a total abdominal hysterectomy including partial vaginectomy with para-aortic and pelvic lymph node sampling biopsy, with or without removal of tubes and/or ovaries. The abdomen is incised. Before opening the peritoneum, pelvic lymph node sampling biopsies are taken and sent for frozen section. The peritoneal cavity is then opened. The abdomen and pelvis are explored for evidence of metastatic disease. The para-aortic lymph nodes are exposed and biopsies are taken and sent for frozen section. Blunt dissection is used to expose the broad ligament, round ligament, and fallopian tubes. If the fallopian tubes and/or ovaries are removed, an incision is made in the exposed broad ligament. The ovarian vessels are visualized and suture ligated. The cut edges of the broad ligament are plicated with mattress sutures. The fallopian tubes and ovaries are dissected free of surrounding tissue. The round ligaments are clamped and divided, and blood vessels are suture ligated bilaterally. The bladder is mobilized and the uterus is exposed. The uterine artery and vein are ligated. The ureters are dissected from the parametrium and from the tunnel of the cardinal ligament. The posterior peritoneum and rectovaginal space are opened. The uterosacral ligaments are freed and divided as are the cardinal ligaments. The parametria is freed from inferior attachments to the level of the vagina. The uterus and cervix are removed with or without removal of the ovaries and/or tubes. The partial vaginectomy is then performed. The proximal portion of the vagina is excised along with a margin of healthy tissue distal to the lesion and the entire vaginal wall proximal to the lesion. An incision is made across the top of the vaginal vault. Two longitudinal full-

● New Code   ▲ Revised Code

thickness incisions are then made, one along the ventral (anterior) aspect and a second along the dorsal (posterior) aspect of the vaginal wall. These incisions extend from the top of the vaginal vault to a point 2 cm distal to the lesion. The bladder and rectal pillars are transected at their attachment sites on the bladder and rectum. The anterior and posterior vaginal walls along with the two lateral paravaginal spaces are resected to a point 2 cm distal to the lesion. The upper portion of the vagina is then removed. Separately reportable vaginal reconstruction with skin grafts may be performed at the same or a subsequent surgical session.

58210

58210 **Radical abdominal hysterectomy, with bilateral total pelvic lymphadenectomy and para-aortic lymph node sampling (biopsy), with or without removal of tube(s), with or without removal of ovary(s)**

The physician performs a radical abdominal hysterectomy with bilateral total pelvic lymphadenectomy and para-aortic lymph node sampling biopsy, with or without removal of tubes and/or ovaries. A radical hysterectomy is most commonly performed for cervical cancer and involves more extensive surgery than a total hysterectomy. Tissue surrounding the uterus and the upper vagina are also removed. The abdomen is incised. Before opening the peritoneum, pelvic lymph nodes are explored and removed. Taking care to preserve the genitofemoral nerve and psoas muscle, fatty tissue is stripped from the mid-portion of both common iliac vessels along the internal and external iliac vessels to the level of the circumflex iliac vein. Iliac, hypogastric, and obturator nodes are excised bilaterally and sent for separately reportable frozen section exam. The peritoneal cavity is opened and the abdomen and pelvis are explored for evidence of metastatic disease. The para-aortic lymph nodes are exposed and biopsies are taken and sent for frozen section. Blunt dissection is used to expose the broad ligament, round ligament, and fallopian tubes. If the fallopian tubes and/or ovaries are removed, an incision is made in the exposed broad ligament. The ovarian vessels are visualized and suture ligated. The cut edges of the broad ligament are plicated with mattress sutures. The fallopian tubes and ovaries are dissected free of surrounding tissue. The round ligaments are clamped and divided and blood vessels are suture ligated bilaterally. The bladder is mobilized and the uterus is exposed. The uterine artery and vein are ligated. The ureters are dissected from the parametrium and from the tunnel of the cardinal ligament. The posterior peritoneum and rectovaginal space are opened. The uterosacral ligaments are freed and divided as are the cardinal ligaments. The parametria is freed from inferior attachments to the level of the vagina. The uterus, cervix, and pelvic tissue around the uterus are removed with or without removal of the ovaries and/or tubes. The proximal portion of the vagina is also excised. An incision is made across the top of the vaginal vault. Two longitudinal full-thickness incisions are then made, one along the ventral (anterior) aspect and a second along the dorsal (posterior) aspect of the vaginal wall. The bladder and rectal pillars are transected at their attachment sites on the bladder and rectum. The anterior and posterior vaginal walls along with the two lateral paravaginal spaces are resected. The upper portion of the vagina is then removed. Separately reportable vaginal reconstruction with skin grafts may be performed at the same or a subsequent surgical session.

58240

58240 **Pelvic exenteration for gynecologic malignancy, with total abdominal hysterectomy or cervicectomy, with or without removal of tube(s), with or without removal of ovary(s), with removal of bladder and ureteral transplantations, and/or abdominoperineal resection of rectum and colon and colostomy, or any combination thereof**

The physician performs pelvic exenteration for gynecologic malignancy. This procedure includes a total abdominal hysterectomy or cervicectomy with or without removal of tubes and/or ovaries, removal of the bladder with ureteral transplantations, and/or abdominoperineal resection of the rectum and colon with colostomy. The abdomen is opened and explored. The liver, peritoneum, bowel, and aortic and pelvic lymph nodes are carefully inspected. Biopsies are taken as needed. The pararectal, paravesical, and Retzius spaces are opened and the cardinal ligaments are exposed. The round ligaments are cut and tied and the broad ligaments are opened. The infundibulopelvic ligaments, in conjunction with the ovarian vessels, are clamped, cut, and tied. The retroperitoneal space is opened and the ureters are exposed. The hypogastric artery is identified and divided. The cardinal ligaments are divided. The ureters are dissected free of surrounding tissue, ligated, and divided. The rectal space between the rectosigmoid colon and the sacrum/coccyx is developed. The sigmoid arcade and the superior vessels are ligated. The rectosigmoid colon is divided. The rectum is elevated and freed from surrounding tissues. The bladder is freed from the pubic symphysis. The urethra, rectum, and vagina are divided below the level of the malignancy, leaving adequate margins of healthy tissue. All involved pelvic organs are removed, including some or all of the following: ovaries, tubes, uterus, cervix, bladder, distal ureters, rectum, and colon. Following removal of involved organs, the rectum/colon is anastomosed or a colostomy is performed. The proximal ureters are then transplanted to provide urinary diversion. If noncontinent diversion is employed, an ileal urinary conduit may be created by implanting the ureters into a segment of small bowel which is then brought out in a cutaneous stoma. Alternatively, a continent pouch using the

right colon may be developed. The exenterated pelvis is then reconstructed using omental, myocutaneous, and/or muscle flaps.

58260-58263

58260 **Vaginal hysterectomy, for uterus 250 g or less**
58262 **Vaginal hysterectomy, for uterus 250 g or less; with removal of tube(s), and/or ovary(s)**
58263 **Vaginal hysterectomy, for uterus 250 g or less; with removal of tube(s), and/or ovary(s), with repair of enterocele**

The physician performs a vaginal hysterectomy on a uterus weighing 250 grams or less. Tenacula are placed on the cervix. The vaginal mucosa is incised around the entire cervix. Traction is applied to the tenacula, and the bladder is separated from the uterus using blunt and sharp dissection. The bladder is elevated to expose the peritoneal vesicouterine fold which is then incised. The cul-de-sac is exposed and the peritoneum incised. The broad ligament is exposed. The uterosacral ligaments are clamped and divided. The cardinal ligaments are clamped at the lower uterine segment, incised, and suture ligated. The lower portion of the broad ligament is clamped and divided at its attachment to the lower uterine segment. The posterior uterine wall is grasped and the uterus delivered into the vagina. The tubo-ovarian round ligaments are exposed, clamped, and incised close to the uterine fundus bilaterally. The fallopian tubes are transected. The tubo-ovarian round ligaments are doubly ligated. The uterus is removed. The fallopian tubes are returned to the abdomen. Alternatively, if the tubes and ovaries are to be removed, the round ligament is cut and tied bilaterally. Tension is then applied to the infundibulopelvic ligament which is cut allowing delivery of the tubes and ovaries along with the uterus into the vagina and all of these structures are removed. The anterior vaginal wall is elevated. The entire length of the broad ligament is exposed and bleeding controlled. The peritoneum is closed. The vaginal cuff is left open to drainage of the pelvis. Use code 58260 when only the uterus is removed. Use code 58262 when the uterus is removed along with the tubes and ovaries. Use code 58263 when the uterus, tubes and ovaries are removed and an enterocele is repaired. To repair the enterocele, the vaginal mucosa overlying the enterocele is opened. The perirectal fascia is dissected free of the posterior vaginal mucosa to expose the enterocele sac. The sac is incised and the small bowel pushed back into the abdomen. The sac is closed with two pursestring sutures placed around the neck of the enterocele. The redundant sac is excised.

58267

58267 **Vaginal hysterectomy, for uterus 250 g or less; with colpo-urethrocystopexy (Marshall-Marchetti-Krantz type, Pereyra type) with or without endoscopic control**

Tenacula are placed on the cervix. The vaginal mucosa is incised around the entire cervix. Traction is applied to the tenacula and the bladder is separated from the uterus using blunt and sharp dissection. The bladder is elevated to expose the peritoneal vesicouterine fold which is then incised. The cul-de-sac is exposed and the peritoneum is incised. The broad ligament is exposed. The uterosacral ligaments are clamped and divided. The cardinal ligaments are clamped at the lower uterine segment, incised, and suture ligated. The lower portion of the broad ligament is clamped and divided at its attachment to the lower uterine segment. The posterior uterine wall is grasped and the uterus is delivered into the vagina. The tubo-ovarian round ligaments are exposed, clamped, and incised close to the uterine fundus bilaterally. The fallopian tubes are transected. The tubo-ovarian ligaments are doubly ligated. The uterus is removed. The fallopian tubes are returned to the abdomen. Next, the colpourethrocystopexy is performed to suspend the prolapsed vaginal wall and urethra. Two sutures are placed through the paravaginal fascia, one on each side of the urethrovesical junction, oriented perpendicular to the vaginal axis. The sutures are then passed through the Cooper's ligament, pelvic fascia, or pubic bone and tied to provide suspension and support to the bladder and urethra. If additional suspension is required, a second set of sutures may be placed along the base of the bladder. The surgical site is inspected and bleeding is controlled. The peritoneum is closed. The vaginal cuff is left open to allow drainage of the pelvis.

58270

58270 **Vaginal hysterectomy, for uterus 250 g or less; with repair of enterocele**

Tenacula are placed on the cervix. The vaginal mucosa is incised around the entire cervix. Traction is applied to the tenacula and the bladder is separated from the uterus using blunt and sharp dissection. The bladder is elevated to expose the peritoneal vesicouterine fold which is then incised. The cul-de-sac is exposed and the peritoneum is incised. The broad ligament is exposed. The uterosacral ligaments are clamped and divided. The cardinal ligaments are clamped at the lower uterine segment, incised, and suture ligated. The lower portion of the broad ligament is clamped and divided at its attachment to the lower uterine segment. The posterior uterine wall is grasped and the uterus is delivered into the vagina. The tubo-ovarian round ligaments are exposed, clamped, and incised close to the uterine fundus bilaterally. The fallopian tubes are transected. The tubo-ovarian ligaments are doubly ligated. The uterus is removed. The fallopian tubes are returned to the abdomen. The surgical site is inspected and bleeding is controlled. The peritoneum is closed. The vaginal cuff is left open to allow drainage of the pelvis. To repair the enterocele, the vaginal mucosa overlying the enterocele is opened. The perirectal fascia is dissected free of the posterior vaginal mucosa to expose the enterocele sac. The sac is incised and the small bowel is pushed back into the abdomen. The sac is closed with two pursestring sutures placed around the neck of the enterocele. The redundant sac is excised

58275-58280

58275   **Vaginal hysterectomy, with total or partial vaginectomy**
58280   **Vaginal hysterectomy, with total or partial vaginectomy; with repair of enterocele**

Tenacula are placed on the cervix. The vaginal mucosa is incised around the entire cervix. Traction is applied to the tenacula, and the bladder is separated from the uterus using blunt and sharp dissection. The bladder is elevated to expose the peritoneal vesicouterine fold which is then incised. The cul-de-sac is exposed and the peritoneum incised. The broad ligament is exposed. The uterosacral ligaments are clamped and divided. The cardinal ligaments are clamped at the lower uterine segment, incised, and suture ligated. The lower portion of the broad ligament is clamped and divided at its attachment to the lower uterine segment. The posterior uterine wall is grasped and the uterus delivered into the vagina. The tubo-ovarian round ligaments are exposed, clamped, and incised close to the uterine fundus bilaterally. The fallopian tubes are transected. The tubo-ovarian ligaments are doubly ligated. The uterus is removed. The fallopian tubes are returned to the abdomen. The surgical site is inspected and bleeding controlled. The peritoneum is closed. Following the hysterectomy part or all of vaginal wall is removed. Two longitudinal full-thickness incisions are then made, one along the ventral (anterior) aspect and a second along the dorsal (posterior) aspect of the vaginal wall. These incisions extend from the top of the vaginal vault to a point approximately two cm distal to the neoplasm for a partial vaginectomy or to the introitus (vaginal opening) for a total vaginectomy. An incision is then made around the vaginal wall two cm distal to the neoplasm or at the introitus. The right and left halves of the vaginal wall are excised. Separately reportable vaginal reconstruction with skin grafts may be performed at the same or a subsequent surgical session. Use code 58275 when vaginal hysterectomy and total or partial vaginectomy is performed without enterocele repair. Use code 58280 when an enterocele is also repaired. To repair the enterocele, the vaginal mucosa overlying the enterocele is opened. The perirectal fascia is dissected free of the posterior vaginal mucosa to expose the enterocele sac. The sac is incised and the small bowel pushed back into the abdomen. The sac is closed with two pursestring sutures placed around the neck of the enterocele. The redundant sac is excised.

58285

58285   **Vaginal hysterectomy, radical (Schauta type operation)**

A radical hysterectomy by definition includes removal of the uterus, cervix, pelvic lymph nodes, and upper third of the vagina. The tubes and ovaries are also typically removed as is parametrial tissue. Para-aortic lymph node sampling may also be performed. The physician uses a vaginal approach for the hysterectomy but must also open the abdomen to access the pelvic and para-aortic lymph nodes. Para-aortic lymph node sampling and pelvic lymph node excision is performed first. The abdomen is incised; para-aortic lymph nodes are isolated bilaterally; and sampling biopsies areobtained and sent for frozen section. The common iliac nodes may be approached retroperitoneally by extending the incision from the para-aortic node dissection site. Other pelvic lymph nodes are approached through pelvic incisions. Taking care to preserve the genitofemoral nerve and psoas muscle, fatty tissue is stripped from the mid-portion of both common iliac vessels and along the internal and external iliac vessels to the level of the circumflex iliac vein. Iliac, hypogastric, and obturator nodes are excised bilaterally and sent for separately reportable frozen section exam. The radical vaginal hysterectomy is now performed. An incision is made in the upper vaginal wall and the paravesical and pararectal spaces are opened. The uterine artery is identified, isolated, and divided. The uterine vein is clipped and mobilized. The cardinal ligament is detached from the pelvic sidewall and all lateral cardinal ligament tissue is removed. The peritoneum is divided. The uterosacral ligament is dissected to allow mobilization of the rectum. The vesicouterine ligament is divided. The prevesical space is developed and the bladder pillar is isolated from the cardinal ligaments. The cardinal ligament attachments to the vagina are clamped, divided, and ligated. The uterus is mobilized and the ureters are dissected free of surrounding tissues pushed out of the way. Any additional peritoneal attachments are severed; the posterior uterine wall is grasped; and the uterus is delivered through the vagina. The tubo-ovarian round ligaments are exposed, clamped, and incised close to the uterine fundus bilaterally. The fallopian tubes are transected. The tubo-ovarian round ligaments are doubly ligated. The uterus is removed and the fallopian tubes are returned to the abdomen. Alternatively, if the tubes and ovaries are to be removed, the round ligament is cut and tied bilaterally. Tension is then applied to the infundibulopelvic ligament which is cut, allowing delivery of the tubes and ovaries along with the uterus into the vagina and all of these structures are removed. The anterior vaginal wall is elevated. The entire length of the broad ligament is exposed and bleeding is controlled. The peritoneum is closed. Following the hysterectomy, the upper third of the vaginal wall is removed. Two longitudinal full-thickness incisions are made, one along the ventral (anterior) aspect and a second along the dorsal (posterior) aspect of the vaginal wall. An incision is then made around the vaginal wall. The right and left halves of the upper

vaginal wall are excised. Separately reportable vaginal reconstruction with skin grafts may be performed at the same or a subsequent surgical session.

58290-58292

58290   **Vaginal hysterectomy, for uterus greater than 250 g**
58291   **Vaginal hysterectomy, for uterus greater than 250 g; with removal of tube(s) and/or ovary(s)**
58292   **Vaginal hysterectomy, for uterus greater than 250 g; with removal of tube(s) and/or ovary(s), with repair of enterocele**

Removal of an enlarged uterus often requires that the uterus be removed in multiple pieces which may also be referred to as morcellization. This may be performed by hemisection which involves cutting the uterus into two halves, intramyometrial coring which reduces the diameter of the uterus by removing a core of tissue from the interior aspect of the uterus, or wedge resection which involves cutting the uterus into multiple pieces. Tenacula are placed on the cervix. The vaginal mucosa is incised around the entire cervix. Traction is applied to the tenacula, and the bladder is separated from the uterus using blunt and sharp dissection. The bladder is elevated to expose the peritoneal vesicouterine fold which is then incised. The cul-de-sac is exposed and the peritoneum incised. Uterine vessels are ligated. One of the morcellization techniques described above is employed to remove the uterus as uterine attachments are severed. As portions of the uterus are exteriorized and removed, the broad ligament is exposed. The uterosacral ligaments are clamped and divided. The cardinal ligaments are clamped at the lower uterine segment, incised, and suture ligated. The lower portion of the broad ligament is clamped and divided at its attachment to the lower uterine segment. The tubo-ovarian round ligaments are exposed, clamped, and incised close to the uterine fundus bilaterally. The fallopian tubes are transected. The tubo-ovarian round ligaments are doubly ligated. The entire uterus is removed. The fallopian tubes are returned to the abdomen. Alternatively, if the tubes and ovaries are to be removed, the round ligament is cut and tied bilaterally. Tension is then applied to the infundibulopelvic ligament which is cut allowing delivery of the tubes and ovaries along with the morcellized uterus into the vagina and all of these structures are removed. The anterior vaginal wall is elevated. The entire length of the broad ligament is exposed and bleeding controlled. The peritoneum is closed. The vaginal cuff is left open to allow drainage of the pelvis. Use code 58290 when only the uterus is removed. Use code 58291 when the uterus is removed along with the tubes and ovaries. Use code 58292 when the uterus, tubes and ovaries are removed and an enterocele is repaired. To repair the enterocele, the vaginal mucosa overlying the enterocele is opened. The perirectal fascia is dissected free of the posterior vaginal mucosa to expose the enterocele sac. The sac is incised and the small bowel pushed back into the abdomen. The sac is closed with two pursestring sutures placed around the neck of the enterocele. The redundant sac is excised.

58293

58293   **Vaginal hysterectomy, for uterus greater than 250 g; with colpo-urethrocystopexy (Marshall-Marchetti-Krantz type, Pereyra type) with or without endoscopic control**

The physician performs a vaginal hysterectomy on a uterus weighing more than 250 grams with a colpo-urethrocystopexy with or without endoscopic control. Removal of an enlarged uterus often requires that it be removed in multiple pieces, referred to as morcellization. This may be performed by hemisection which involves cutting the uterus into two halves, intramyometrial coring which reduces the diameter of the uterus by removing a core of tissue from the interior aspect, or wedge resection which involves cutting the uterus into multiple pieces. Tenacula are placed on the cervix. The vaginal mucosa is incised around the entire cervix. Traction is applied to the tenacula and the bladder is separated from the uterus using blunt and sharp dissection. The bladder is elevated to expose the peritoneal vesicouterine fold which is then incised. The cul-de-sac is exposed and the peritoneum is incised. Uterine vessels are ligated. One of the morcellization techniques described above is employed to remove the uterus as uterine attachments are severed. As portions of the uterus are exteriorized and removed, the broad ligament is exposed. The uterosacral ligaments are clamped and divided. The cardinal ligaments are clamped at the lower uterine segment, incised, and suture ligated. The lower portion of the broad ligament is clamped and divided at its attachment to the lower uterine segment. The tubo-ovarian round ligaments are exposed, clamped, and incised close to the uterine fundus bilaterally. The fallopian tubes are transected. The tubo-ovarian round ligaments are doubly ligated. The entire morcellized uterus is removed. The fallopian tubes are returned to the abdomen. Alternatively, if the tubes and ovaries are to be removed, the round ligament is cut and tied bilaterally. Tension is then applied to the infundibulopelvic ligament which is cut, allowing delivery of the tubes and ovaries along with the morcellized uterus into the vagina and all of these structures are removed. The anterior vaginal wall is elevated. The entire length of the broad ligament is exposed and bleeding is controlled. Next, the colpourethrocystopexy is performed to suspend the prolapsed vaginal wall and urethra. Two sutures are placed through the paravaginal fascia, one on each side of the urethrovesical junction, oriented perpendicular to the vaginal axis. The sutures are then passed through the Cooper's ligament, pelvic fascia, or pubic bone and tied to provide suspension and support to the bladder and urethra. If additional suspension is required, a second set of sutures may be placed along the base of the bladder. The surgical site is inspected and bleeding is controlled. The peritoneum is closed. The vaginal cuff is left open to allow drainage of the pelvis.

58294

58294 Vaginal hysterectomy, for uterus greater than 250 g; with repair of enterocele

The physician performs a vaginal hysterectomy on a uterus weighing more than 250 grams with repair of an enterocele. Removal of an enlarged uterus often requires that it be removed in multiple pieces, referred to as morcellization. This may be performed by hemisection which involves cutting the uterus into two halves, intramyometrial coring which reduces the diameter of the uterus by removing a core of tissue from the interior aspect, or wedge resection which involves cutting the uterus into multiple pieces. Tenacula are placed on the cervix. The vaginal mucosa is incised around the entire cervix. Traction is applied to the tenacula, and the bladder is separated from the uterus using blunt and sharp dissection. The bladder is elevated to expose the peritoneal vesicouterine fold which is then incised. The cul-de-sac is exposed and the peritoneum is incised. Uterine vessels are ligated. One of the morcellization techniques described above is employed to remove the uterus as uterine attachments are severed. As portions of the uterus are exteriorized and removed, the broad ligament is exposed. The uterosacral ligaments are clamped and divided. The cardinal ligaments are clamped at the lower uterine segment, incised, and suture ligated. The lower portion of the broad ligament is clamped and divided at its attachment to the lower uterine segment. The tubo-ovarian round ligaments are exposed, clamped, and incised close to the uterine fundus bilaterally. The fallopian tubes are transected. The tubo-ovarian round ligaments are doubly ligated. The entire morcellized uterus is removed. The fallopian tubes are returned to the abdomen. Alternatively, if the tubes and ovaries are to be removed, the round ligament is cut and tied bilaterally. Tension is then applied to the infundibulopelvic ligament which is cut, allowing delivery of the tubes and ovaries along with the morcellized uterus into the vagina and all of these structures are removed. The anterior vaginal wall is elevated. The entire length of the broad ligament is exposed and bleeding is controlled. The peritoneum is closed. The vaginal cuff is left open to allow drainage of the pelvis. To repair the enterocele, the vaginal mucosa overlying the enterocele is opened. The perirectal fascia is dissected free of the posterior vaginal mucosa to expose the enterocele sac. The sac is incised and the small bowel is pushed back into the abdomen. The sac is closed with two pursestring sutures placed around the neck of the enterocele. The redundant sac is excised.

58300-58301

58300 Insertion of intrauterine device (IUD)
58301 Removal of intrauterine device (IUD)

Two types of IUDs are available for contraception, a copper-releasing device and a hormone releasing devise. Prior to insertion of the IUD (58300), a bimanual examination is performed to assess the position of the uterus. The cervix is cleansed and then stabilized using a tenaculum. A uterine sound is passed into the uterus and the depth of the uterine cavity ascertained. The IUD is positioned in the insertion tube and the insertion rod is attached. The IUD is inserted and the tube pulled back slightly to allow expansion of the IUD. When the IUD is properly positioned, the insertion rod is removed followed by removal of the insertion tube. The threads are released automatically and extend through the cervical os. The tenaculum is removed from the cervix and the threads are cut to approximately three cm in length. To remove the IUD (58301), the threads are identified extending through the cervical os. The threads are grasped with ring forceps and traction applied away from the cervix to remove the IUD.

Insertion of intrauterine device

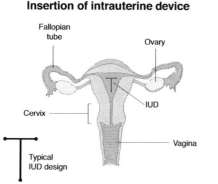

The physician inserts (58300), or removes (58301) a contraceptive device in the uterus.

58321-58322

58321 Artificial insemination; intra-cervical
58322 Artificial insemination; intra-uterine

Intra-cervical (58321) or intra-uterine (58322) artificial insemination is performed. Artificial insemination may be performed for male infertility caused by the absence of sperm or low sperm count or retrograde ejaculation, female infertility caused by a cervical injury or deformity that prevents sperm from passing through the cervix, the absence of a male partner, or other reasons. In 58321, a thin flexible catheter is inserted into the cervical os and attached to a syringe containing washed and concentrated sperm. The sperm are injected into the cervical os. In 58322, the catheter is inserted into the uterine cavity and the sperm injected.

58323

58323 Sperm washing for artificial insemination

Sperm washing is performed prior to artificial insemination. Sperm washing separates sperm cells from semen, gets rid of dead or slow moving sperm, and removes chemicals that may impair fertilization. There are three commonly used sperm washing techniques which include simple wash, density gradient wash, and swim up technique. Semen is collected following masturbation or in the case of retrograde ejaculation, a separately reportable collection procedure is performed. In a simple sperm wash, the semen is diluted in a test tube solution containing antibiotics and protein supplements. It is then centrifuged, causing sperm cells to fall to the bottom of the test tube and concentrating the highly active sperm together in a dense mass. The density gradient sperm wash separates dead sperm cells, white blood cells, and waste products. The test tube is filled with multiple layers of liquids of different densities. Semen is placed on the top layer and the test tube is centrifuged. Debris and dead sperm are caught in the top layers while active healthy sperm are concentrated at the bottom of the test tube. Following either simple or density gradient sperm wash, the mass of sperm is removed from the test tube and used in a separately reportable artificial insemination procedure. Swim up technique involves placing semen in a culture dish with a layer of media culture that attracts the sperm. Sperm are collected as they swim up to the media culture. When a sufficient number of sperm have been collected, they are used in a separately reportable artificial insemination procedure.

58340

58340 Catheterization and introduction of saline or contrast material for saline infusion sonohysterography (SIS) or hysterosalpingography

The physician inserts a catheter into the uterus and injects saline or contrast material for saline infusion sonohysterography (SIS) or hysterosalpingography. For SIS, the physician first performs a baseline transvaginal ultrasound. The vaginal probe is removed and a speculum is inserted. The cervical os is cleansed through the speculum. A small diameter flexible catheter is then placed through the cervix and into the uterine cavity. The speculum is removed and the vaginal probe is reinserted. Using separately reportable ultrasound to visualize the uterus, sterile saline or contrast media is instilled into the uterine cavity through the tube until the uterine cavity is adequately expanded. For hysterosalpingography, the catheter is inserted in the same manner as for SIS. Following removal of the speculum, separately reportable fluoroscopy is used to visualize the uterus and Fallopian tubes as contrast media is instilled.

58345

58345 Transcervical introduction of fallopian tube catheter for diagnosis and/or re-establishing patency (any method), with or without hysterosalpingography

The physician performs transcervical introduction of a fallopian tube catheter for diagnosis and/or reestablishing patency by any method with or without hysterosalpingography. A baseline transvaginal ultrasound is performed. The vaginal probe is removed and a speculum is placed in the vagina. The cervical os is cleansed. Using separately reportable fluoroscopic guidance, a small diameter flexible catheter is placed through the cervix into the uterine cavity and advanced into the proximal tubal ostium. Contrast media is instilled into the fallopian tube and patency is evaluated. If the proximal tube is obstructed, it may be recanalized using a guidewire with or without a coaxial catheter. This is repeated on the opposite side as needed. This procedure may be performed with or without hysterosalpingography. Contrast is instilled into the uterine cavity if both the uterus and fallopian tubes are evaluated.

58346

58346 Insertion of Heyman capsules for clinical brachytherapy

Heyman capsules are inserted into the uterus for separately reportable delivery of clinical brachytherapy. Heyman capsules are small metallic or plastic capsules containing 5-10 mg of radium. Intracavity radiation of the uterus using Heyman capsules delivers low dose radiation to a malignant neoplasm while limiting the volume of healthy tissue affected by the radiation. Heyman capsules are used for treatment of neoplasms of the uterine fundus.

The physician determines the appropriate number and location of Heyman capsules to be placed in the uterus and the capsules are inserted in and around the tumor in the uterus.

58350

58350   Chromotubation of oviduct, including materials

Chromotubation of the oviduct is performed, including the supply of materials. This procedure is used to evaluate tubal patency and allows evaluation of the pelvic cavity. It may also be used to identify peritubal adhesions and endometriosis. Dye is introduced into the uterine cavity and observed as it flows into the fallopian tubes and spills over into the peritoneal cavity. Tubal motility is evaluated as the dye flows through the tubes and any obstruction of the tubes is noted.

58353

58353   Endometrial ablation, thermal, without hysteroscopic guidance

Thermal endometrial ablation is performed without hysteroscopic guidance. This procedure is used to treat menorrhagia due to benign conditions such as dysfunctional uterine bleeding. Thermal ablation destroys the tissue lining the uterus using heat. A baseline transvaginal ultrasound is performed. The vaginal probe is removed and a speculum is placed in the vagina. The cervical os is cleansed. A balloon catheter is placed through the cervix into the uterine cavity. The balloon is inflated against the tissue by filling it with water heated to a high temperature and the uterine lining is ablated.

58356

58356   Endometrial cryoablation with ultrasonic guidance, including endometrial curettage, when performed

A single-toothed tenaculum is placed on the anterior cervical lip and traction is applied. The uterus is sounded. The cervical canal diameter is checked and dilated as needed. A suction curettage is performed as needed to thin the endometrial lining of the uterus. Using ultrasound guidance, the cryoprobe is inserted through the cervix and into the uterus with the tip directed towards the right or left uterine horn (area where the fallopian tube enters the uterus). Sterile saline is injected to remove air from the uterus and improve ultrasound visualization. The cryoprobe is activated and the first freezing cycle is initiated. One or two freeze-thaw cycles may be performed in each freezing zone. When adequate freezing has been achieved in the first freezing zone, the cryoprobe tip is repositioned adjacent to the contralateral horn and the freeze-thaw cycles are repeated. Some physicians perform the procedure using three freeze zones with the third freeze zone in the lower uterine segment. Upon completion of the freezing procedure, the cryoprobe and tenaculum are removed and any bleeding from the cervix is controlled.

58400-58410

58400   Uterine suspension, with or without shortening of round ligaments, with or without shortening of sacrouterine ligaments; (separate procedure)

58410   Uterine suspension, with or without shortening of round ligaments, with or without shortening of sacrouterine ligaments; with presacral sympathectomy

The physician performs uterine suspension with or without shortening of the round and/or sacrouterine ligaments in a separate procedure (58400) or with presacral sympathectomy (58410). Open uterine suspension is rarely performed having largely been replaced by laparoscopic procedures. The abdomen is incised and the uterus, round ligaments, and sacrouterine ligaments are exposed. Using one of several techniques, the round and/or sacrouterine ligaments are shortened. One technique for shortening the round ligaments is to plicate the peritoneum on each side along the length of the round ligaments using mattress sutures. Sacrouterine ligaments may also be plicated. Another technique is to suture the round ligaments to pelvic musculature. In 58410 a presacral sympathectomy is also performed to alleviate pain. The posterior parietal peritoneum is incised in the midline just above the sacral promontory. The incision is carried upward to the bifurcation of the aorta and then downward over the promontory. The flaps of peritoneum are elevated to the level of the common iliac arteries and the sheet of fibrous tissue containing the fibers of the presacral nerve is exposed. The fibrous tissue and nerve fibers are separated beginning at the right common iliac artery near the bifurcation of the aorta. Gentle dissection is continued over the left iliac vein to the left common iliac artery. The freed sheet of tissue is elevated and dissection is carried downward to the division of the hypogastric nerves. The upper and lower attachments are ligated and divided completing the sympathectomy. The posterior parietal peritoneum is closed followed by the layered closure of the abdominal incision.

58520

58520   Hysterorrhaphy, repair of ruptured uterus (nonobstetrical)

The physician performs a hysterorrhaphy of a ruptured uterus caused by a nonobstetrical injury. The abdomen is opened and explored. Any blood clots are removed. The uterus is lifted out of the abdomen to identify the site and extent of injury and determine the exact nature of the required repair. The bladder is separated from the lower edge of the uterine segment. Uterine vessels are located and ligated as needed. If the rupture has

created a broad ligament hematoma, the round ligament is clamped, cut, and tied off, and the anterior leaf of the broad ligament is opened. The hematoma is drained. Any bleeding vessels are ligated. If the rupture extends into the cervix and vagina, the bladder is mobilized. The upper portion of the cervical injury is sutured first and then carried down distally until the entire cervical/vaginal injury is repaired. The ureters are identified and protected. The uterine tear is then repaired in one or two layers. Bleeding is controlled by suture ligation of bleeding vessels. An abdominal drain may be placed. Prior to closing the abdomen, the bladder is also inspected to ensure that it is free of injury. The abdomen is then closed in layers around the drain.

58540

58540   Hysteroplasty, repair of uterine anomaly (Strassman type)

The physician performs a hysteroplasty to repair a uterine anomaly. Mullerian uterine anomalies are the most common type. During fetal development, the mullerian duct system differentiates to form the fallopian tubes, uterus, uterine cervix, and the superior aspect of the vagina. A variety of anomalies can occur when development of this tissue is disrupted. Types of uterine anomalies that may be corrected by hysteroplasty include unicornuate uterus, didelphys (complete or partial duplication of the uterus, cervix, and/or vagina), complete or partial bicornuate uterus, complete or partial septate uterus, and arcuate uterus. The exact nature of the surgical repair is dependent on the type of uterine anomaly. One of the more commonly performed procedures is a Strassman metroplasty used to treat didelphic and bicornuate uterine anomalies. A transverse incision is made in the fundus of the dideplphic uterus between the round ligaments. The myometrial partition between the two uterine cavities is incised and a single uterine cavity is formed. The incision is closed in an anterior to posterior direction. A modification of the Strassman procedure for treatment of bicornuate or septate uterus involves wedge resection of the uterine horns or septum. For repair of a bicornuate uterus, a wedge-shaped incision is made in the uterine fundus on the medial aspect of each uterine horn. The incision extends into the endometrial cavity from the superior aspect of each horn to the inferior aspect of the uterus. The wedge is removed and the uterine fundus is repaired. Another type of hysterorrhaphy procedure is done for a septate uterus, in which a wedge-shaped incision incorporating the septum is made in the uterine fundus in an anteroposterior direction. The wedge of tissue is excised and the uterine fundus is suture repaired.

58541-58542

58541   Laparoscopy, surgical, supracervical hysterectomy, for uterus 250 g or less

58542   Laparoscopy, surgical, supracervical hysterectomy, for uterus 250 g or less; with removal of tube(s) and/or ovary(s)

Laparoscopic supracervical hysterectomy (LSH) is performed to remove a uterus 250g or less. LSH is a minimally invasive way to remove the uterus as an alternative to total abdominal hysterectomy. LSH maintains better pelvic support because the ligaments that hold up the vagina and cervix are left intact. This procedure also preserves sexual function by maintaining the cervix and its secretory glands. LSH is not done on cancer patients or those with history of precancerous cervical pathology. A retractor is placed vaginally into the cervix to aid in moving the uterus for visualization. A small belly button incision and two small hip bone area incisions are made for placing the laparoscopic instruments and the abdomen is inflated with carbon dioxide gas. The scope is inserted in the belly button incision and the cutting/grasping instrument and retractor are operated through the other two incisions. The uterus alone (58541) or the uterus along with the fallopian tubes and/or ovaries (58542) is separated from the blood supply and released from its attachment to the cervix. Permanent sutures are placed in the ligaments that hold up the cervix for greater support against later prolapse. The center of the cervix is coagulated to prevent bleeding problems, and then the cervix is covered with peritoneum, the lining of the abdomen. Instruments are then changed to a morcellator, a rounded blade on the end of a tube, and a small camera. The uterus with or without tubes and/or ovaries are delivered out of the abdomen in strips and sent to pathology. Bleeders are coagulated, instruments are removed, and the gas is emptied from the abdomen before closing the incisions.

58543-58544

58543   Laparoscopy, surgical, supracervical hysterectomy, for uterus greater than 250 g

58544   Laparoscopy, surgical, supracervical hysterectomy, for uterus greater than 250 g; with removal of tube(s) and/or ovary(s)

LSH is a minimally invasive way to remove the uterus as an alternative to total abdominal hysterectomy. LSH maintains better pelvic support because the ligaments that hold up the vagina and cervix are left intact. This procedure also preserves sexual function by maintaining the cervix and its secretory glands. LSH is not done on cancer patients or those with history of precancerous cervical pathology. A retractor is placed vaginally into the cervix to aid in moving the uterus for visualization. A small belly button incision and two small hip bone area incisions are made for placing the laparoscopic instruments and the abdomen is inflated with carbon dioxide gas. The scope is inserted in the belly button incision and the cutting/grasping instrument and retractor are operated through the other two incisions. The uterus alone (58543) or the uterus along with the fallopian tubes and/or ovaries (58544) is separated from the blood supply and released from its attachment to the cervix. Permanent sutures are placed in the ligaments that hold up the cervix for greater support against later prolapse. The center of the cervix is coagulated to prevent bleeding problems, and then the cervix is covered with peritoneum, the lining of the abdomen. Instruments are then changed to a morcellator, a rounded blade on the end of a tube, and a small camera. The uterus with or without tubes and/or ovaries is delivered out of the abdomen in strips and sent to pathology. Bleeders are coagulated, instruments are removed, and the gas is emptied from the abdomen before closing the incisions.

58545-58546

58545   Laparoscopy, surgical, myomectomy, excision; 1 to 4 intramural myomas with total weight of 250 g or less and/or removal of surface myomas

58546   Laparoscopy, surgical, myomectomy, excision; 5 or more intramural myomas and/or intramural myomas with total weight greater than 250 g

The physician performs a laparoscopic myomectomy with excision of intramural fibroid tumor(s) and/or removal of surface myomas. Uterine fibroids are benign tumors of the muscle tissue (myometrium) of the uterus. Fibroid tumors may be submucous, intramural, subserous, or pedunculated. Submucous fibroids protrude into the uterine cavity and are typically removed by hysteroscopy. Intramural fibroids are contained within the uterine muscle. Subserous fibroids occur on the exterior of the uterus and may be pedunculated, that is attached by a thin stalk to the exterior of the uterine muscle. An incision is made just below the umbilicus and a trocar placed, and the laparoscopic is inserted. The uterus is visually inspected to determine the location of the fibroid(s). Two or three portal incisions are made in the lower abdomen for introduction of surgical instruments. For removal of a surface fibroid, an incision is made over the fibroid and the fibroid is freed from its attachments to the exterior uterine wall. For an intramural fibroid, the uterus is incised down to the level of the fibroid. The fibroid tumor is peeled off of the uterine wall (myometrium). Depending on the size of the fibroid it may be removed whole or cut into pieces (morcellized) and the pieces removed. Bleeding is controlled by electrocautery. The uterus is suture repaired in layers. Use code 58545 when one to four intramural myoma(s) with a total weight of 250 grams and/or surface (subserous or pedunculated) myomas are removed laparoscopically. Use code 58546 for laparoscopic removal of five or more intramural myomas or for myomas with a total weight greater than 250 grams.

58548

58548   Laparoscopy, surgical, with radical hysterectomy, with bilateral total pelvic lymphadenectomy and para-aortic lymph node sampling (biopsy), with removal of tube(s) and ovary(s), if performed

Laparoscopic radical hysterectomy, with bilateral total pelvic lymphadenectomy and para-aortic lymph node sampling (biopsy) is performed, including the removal of tube(s) and ovary(s), if done. After inflation with carbon dioxide gas, trocars are inserted in the umbilical and suprapubical region and both lower quadrants and a manipulator is placed in the uterus. The peritoneum between the uterosacral ligaments is incised and careful dissection is done in the rectovaginal space, facilitated by a sponge placed in the posterior vaginal fornix. The left round ligament is divided. The left uterovarian ligament and portion of the fallopian tube is divided. The broad ligament is dissected with the incision carried to the bladder. The vesicovaginal space is created with blunt and sharp dissection, aided by placing a sponge in the anterior vaginal fornix. The bladder pillars are isolated and the left ureter is dissected from surrounding tissue. The left uterine artery is coagulated. The left lymph node packets overlying the external iliac vessels are then separated for left pelvic lymphadenectomy. The perivesical space is opened and the left obturator space is entered. Lymphatic tissue around arteries and nerves is carefully removed and lymph node packets are delivered through the suprapubic port. The left ureteral tunnel is dissected, the bladder pillar divided, and the ureter is rolled laterally. The right uterovarian ligament, the fallopian tube, and then the broad ligament are divided. The pelvic sidewall is entered and the right uterine artery and vein are isolated and coagulated. The right ureter is isolated and dissected from its tunnel and the bladder pillar is divided. The uterosacral ligaments are divided. Right pelvic lymphadenectomy is also done. The uterus is free of all supporting tissues and can be delivered in a vaginal manner to ensure adequate vaginal margins with direct visualization. The vaginal cuff is closed, and vessels, ureters, and nerves are checked before ending the procedure.

58550-58552

58550   Laparoscopy, surgical, with vaginal hysterectomy, for uterus 250 g or less

58552   Laparoscopy, surgical, with vaginal hysterectomy, for uterus 250 g or less; with removal of tube(s) and/or ovary(s)

The physician performs a laparoscopically assisted vaginal hysterectomy (LAVH) for a uterus weighing 250 grams or less with or without removal of tubes and/or ovaries. An incision is made just below the umbilicus and a trocar placed, and the laparoscopic is inserted. The abdominal cavity and uterus are visually inspected. Two or three portal incisions are made in the lower abdomen for introduction of surgical instruments. Using bipolar coagulation to control bleeding, the round ligaments are transected followed by transection of the broad ligament. Ring forceps are placed in the vagina to elevate the vaginal apex while the bladder flap is developed using blunt and sharp dissection. The bladder pillars are coagulated and transected. The perivesical and perivaginal spaces are

developed using blunt and sharp dissection. A linear stapler is used to transect either the infundibulopelvic or utero-ovarian ligaments depending on whether the tubes and/or ovaries are being removed. The ascending branch of the uterine artery is transected. The upper aspect of the vaginal wall is incised. The cardinal ligament is approached vaginally cross-clamped, divided and suture ligated. The uterus is delivered through the vaginal incision and removed. The vaginal cuff is closed. Following closure of the vaginal cuff, the abdomen is inspected laparoscopically and any bleeding controlled by laser cautery. The abdomen is irrigated, instruments removed and portal incisions closed. Use code 58550 for LAVH without removal of tubes and/or ovaries or code 58552 when the tubes and/or ovaries are removed.

58553-58554

58553   Laparoscopy, surgical, with vaginal hysterectomy, for uterus greater than 250 g

58554   Laparoscopy, surgical, with vaginal hysterectomy, for uterus greater than 250 g; with removal of tube(s) and/or ovary(s)

An incision is made just below the umbilicus and a trocar placed, and the laparoscopic is inserted. The abdominal cavity and uterus are visually inspected. Two or three portal incisions are made in the lower abdomen for introduction of surgical instruments. Using bipolar coagulation to control bleeding, the round ligaments are transected followed by transection of the broad ligament. Ring forceps are placed in the vagina to elevate the vaginal apex while the bladder flap is developed using blunt and sharp dissection. The bladder pillars are coagulated and transected. The perivesical and perivaginal spaces are developed using blunt and sharp dissection. A linear stapler is used to transect either the infundibulopelvic or utero-ovarian ligaments depending on whether the tubes and/or ovaries are being removed. The ascending branch of the uterine artery is transected. A circular incision is made upper aspect of the vaginal wall. The cardinal ligament is approached vaginally cross-clamped, divided and suture ligated. The uterus is delivered through the vaginal incision and removed. If necessary, wedge morcellation, coring, or bivalving of the uterus is performed to facilitate removal. The peritoneum and vaginal cuff are closed. Following closure of the vaginal cuff, the abdomen is inspected laparoscopically and any bleeding controlled by laser cautery. The abdomen is irrigated, instruments removed and portal incisions closed. Use code 58553 for LAVH without removal of tubes and/or ovaries or code 58554 when the tubes and/or ovaries are removed.

58555

58555   Hysteroscopy, diagnostic (separate procedure)

A diagnostic hysteroscopy is performed. A bimanual pelvic exam is done prior to hysteroscope insertion. A single-tooth tenaculum is placed on the anterior cervical lip. The cervix is then numbed and dilated using metal dilators to allow insertion of the hysteroscope, which is placed into the endocervical canal and advanced into the uterine cavity under direct vision while simultaneously expanding the uterus with saline or carbon dioxide. The uterus is then examined for polyps, fibroids, or other abnormalities. When the procedure is complete, the hysteroscope and tenaculum are removed and any bleeding from the cervix is controlled.

58558

58558   Hysteroscopy, surgical; with sampling (biopsy) of endometrium and/or polypectomy, with or without D & C

A surgical hysteroscopy with sampling (biopsy) of endometrium and/or polypectomy is performed with or without dilation and curettage (D&C). A bimanual pelvic exam is done prior to hysteroscope insertion. A single-tooth tenaculum is placed on the anterior cervical lip and a sound is passed to determine the depth and angle of the uterus. The cervix is numbed and dilated using metal dilators to allow insertion of the hysteroscope, which is placed into the endocervical canal and advanced into the uterine cavity under direct vision while simultaneously expanding the uterus with saline or carbon dioxide. The uterus is examined for polyps, fibroids, or other abnormalities. An endometrial curette or thin wire biopsy forceps are passed through the cervix and biopsies are taken from multiple sites in the uterus. Any polyps are removed. If a D&C is needed, a curette is inserted through the cervix and the uterine wall is scraped or suctioned. The tissue is sent for pathology exam. All instruments are removed and bleeding from the cervix is controlled with pressure.

58559-58560

58559   Hysteroscopy, surgical; with lysis of intrauterine adhesions (any method)

58560   Hysteroscopy, surgical; with division or resection of intrauterine septum (any method)

Prior to insertion of the hysteroscope, a bimanual pelvic exam is performed. A single-tooth tenaculum is placed on the anterior cervical lip. A sound is then passed to determine the depth and angle of the uterus. The cervix is numbed and dilated using metal dilators to allow insertion of the hysteroscope. The hysterscope is inserted into the endocervical canal and advanced into the uterine cavity under direct vision while simultaneously expanding the uterus with saline or carbon dioxide. The uterus is examined and the presence of adhesions or an intrauterine septum noted. In 58559, intrauterine adhesions, also referred to as synechiae or scar tissue, are lysed. This may be performed using blunt dissection, scissors, laser, or other method. All adhesions are removed and the tubal openings (ostia) visualized. In 58560, a resectoscope, scissors, or a vaporizing electrode is used to divide, resect, or remove the intrauterine septum. All instruments along with the hysterscope are removed. The tenaculum is removed from the cervical lip and bleeding from the cervix controlled with pressure.

58561

58561   Hysteroscopy, surgical; with removal of leiomyomata

A surgical hysteroscopy is done to remove leiomyomatas, also referred to as uterine fibroids, which are benign tumors of the muscle tissue (myometrium) of the uterus. Fibroid tumors may be submucous, intramural, subserous, or pedunculated. Submucous fibroids grow within the endometrial lining of the uterus and protrude into the uterine cavity. These are typically removed by hysteroscopy. Intramural fibroids are contained within the muscle of the uterine wall. Subserous fibroids occur on the exterior of the uterus and may become pedunculated, or attached by a thin stalk as they grow, and can become very large. A bimanual pelvic exam is done prior to hysteroscope insertion. A single-tooth tenaculum is placed on the anterior cervical lip and a sound is passed to determine the depth and angle of the uterus. The cervix is numbed and dilated using metal dilators to allow insertion of the hysteroscope, which is placed into the endocervical canal and advanced into the uterine cavity under direct vision while simultaneously expanding the uterine cavity with saline or carbon dioxide. The uterus is examined and the size, number, and location of leiomyomata are noted and all are removed using a resectoscope, scissors, or laser. Surgical instruments are removed and any bleeding from the cervix is controlled.

58562

58562   Hysteroscopy, surgical; with removal of impacted foreign body

A surgical hysteroscopy is done to remove an impacted foreign body, such as an impacted intrauterine device (IUD). A bimanual pelvic exam is done prior to hysteroscope insertion. A single-tooth tenaculum is placed on the anterior cervical lip and a sound is passed to determine the depth and angle of the uterus. The cervix is numbed and dilated using metal dilators to allow insertion of the hysteroscope, which is placed into the endocervical canal and advanced into the uterine cavity under direct vision while simultaneously expanding the uterine cavity with saline or carbon dioxide. The uterus is examined. The foreign body is located and grasped with a toothed grasper and pulled toward the hysteroscope sheath. The hysteroscope and grasper are removed simultaneously from the uterus. The tenaculum is then removed from the cervical lip and bleeding is controlled with pressure.

58563

58563   Hysteroscopy, surgical; with endometrial ablation (eg, endometrial resection, electrosurgical ablation, thermoablation)

A surgical hysteroscopy with endometrial ablation is performed using any of the different techniques available, such as endometrial resection, electrosurgical ablation, or thermoablation. Endometrial ablation permanently removes a thin layer of tissue lining the uterus to stop or reduce excessive, abnormal bleeding (menorrhagia). A bimanual pelvic exam is done prior to hysteroscope insertion. A single-tooth tenaculum is placed on the anterior cervical lip and a sound is passed to determine the depth and angle of the uterus. The cervix is numbed and dilated using metal dilators to allow insertion of the hysteroscope, which is placed into the endocervical canal and advanced into the uterine cavity under direct vision while simultaneously expanding the uterine cavity with saline or carbon dioxide. The uterine cavity is examined. Using an electrosurgial roller-ball and starting at the uterine horns (cornua), the cornua and tubal angles are ablated first, followed by the lateral and anterior walls, and then the posterior wall. Electric current travels through the roller ball as it is applied around the endometrium and cauterizes the tissue. Thermoablation may be done using a balloon on the end of a catheter inserted into the uterus, then filled with fluid heated to a high temperature against the endometrial lining. A resectoscope may be used, which has a built-in wire in the end of the device through which electrical current flows. Endometrial tissue is resected in strips and removed with polyp forceps. Upon completion of the procedure, instruments are removed and bleeding from the cervical lip is controlled with pressure.

58565

58565   Hysteroscopy, surgical; with bilateral fallopian tube cannulation to induce occlusion by placement of permanent implants

The physician performs a surgical hysteroscopy with bilateral fallopian tube cannulation and placement of permanent implants to occlude the fallopian tubes in an elective sterilization procedure. Following a pelvic examination, a speculum is placed in the vagina and a single-toothed tenaculum is placed on the anterior cervical lip. The cervix is dilated and the hysteroscope is introduced. The uterine cavity is examined and the fallopian tube openings are evaluated. The first tube is cannulated and a small insert is placed to occlude the tube. This is repeated on the contralateral side. The hysteroscope and tenaculum are removed and any bleeding from the cervix is controlled.

58570-58571

58570   Laparoscopy, surgical, with total hysterectomy, for uterus 250 g or less
58571   Laparoscopy, surgical, with total hysterectomy, for uterus 250 g or less; with removal of tube(s) and/or ovary(s)

A total laparoscopic hysterectomy (TLH) is performed to remove a uterus weighing 250 grams or less, typically through the vagina and still intact, in 58570. A urinary catheter is inserted into the bladder through the urethra, the cervix is dilated, and a uterine sound is inserted to measure the uterine length. A uterine manipulator is placed transvaginally through the cervix. A vaginal extender (cervical cup) is placed and an occlusion device is inserted to prevent loss of air from the peritoneum. An incision is made below the umbilicus, the laparoscope is inserted, and the abdomen is insufflated. An additional suprapubic incision and bilateral incisions near the hip bones are made for other surgical instruments. The ureters are identified and protected. The peritoneum overlying the bladder is incised. The bladder is dissected off the lower uterine segment and the anterior vagina is exposed. An incision is made into the anterior aspect of the vagina and extended laterally and posteriorly, while preserving the uterosacral ligament. The utero-ovarian ligament, uterine attachments, and blood vessels are divided. The patient is placed in high lithotomy position and the pneumoperitoneum is allowed to escape. The uterus and cervix are then delivered into the vagina and removed. The occlusion device is replaced and the abdomen is reinflated. The vagina is closed by laparoscopic suturing of the apex, which is supported with sutures in the uterosacral ligaments to prevent vaginal prolapse. Use 58571 when the tube(s) and/or ovary(s) are also delivered into the vagina and removed with the uterus.

58572-58573

58572   Laparoscopy, surgical, with total hysterectomy, for uterus greater than 250 g
58573   Laparoscopy, surgical, with total hysterectomy, for uterus greater than 250 g; with removal of tube(s) and/or ovary(s)

A total laparoscopic hysterectomy (TLH) is performed to remove a uterus weighing more than 250 grams (58572), typically removed through the vagina unless the uterus is too large, in which case it may be morcellized into smaller pieces first. A urinary catheter is first inserted into the bladder through the urethra. The cervix is dilated and a uterine sound is inserted to measure the uterine length. A uterine manipulator is placed transvaginally through the cervix. A vaginal extender (cervical cup) is placed and an occlusion device is inserted to prevent loss of air from the peritoneum. An incision is made below the umbilicus, the laparoscope is inserted, and the abdomen is insufflated. An additional suprapubic incision and bilateral incisions near the hip bones are made for other surgical instruments. The ureters are identified and protected. The peritoneum overlying the bladder is incised. The bladder is dissected off the lower uterine segment and the anterior vagina is exposed. An incision is made into the anterior aspect of the vagina and extended laterally and posteriorly, while preserving the uterosacral ligament. The utero-ovarian ligament, uterine attachments, and blood vessels are divided. Uterine fibroids may be morcellized and removed through the umbilical incision. The patient is placed in high lithotomy position and the pneumoperitoneum is allowed to escape. The uterus and cervix are delivered into the vagina and removed. If the uterus is too large to deliver intact, it is morcellized transvaginally, delivered into the vagina, and then removed. The occlusion device is replaced and the abdomen is reinflated. The vagina is closed by laparoscopic suturing of the apex, which is supported with sutures in the uterosacral ligaments to prevent vaginal prolapse. Use 58573 when the tube(s) and/or ovary(s) are also delivered into the vagina and removed with the uterus.

58600-58611

58600   Ligation or transection of fallopian tube(s), abdominal or vaginal approach, unilateral or bilateral
58605   Ligation or transection of fallopian tube(s), abdominal or vaginal approach, postpartum, unilateral or bilateral, during same hospitalization (separate procedure)
58611   Ligation or transection of fallopian tube(s) when done at the time of cesarean delivery or intra-abdominal surgery (not a separate procedure) (List separately in addition to code for primary procedure)

Using an abdominal approach, an incision is made in the lower abdomen and the fallopian tube exposed. If a mini-laparotomy is utilized, the fallopian tube is identified by first locating the fimbriated end where the round ligament can be identified as a separate structure. The fallopian tube is then grasped in the mid-portion using forceps and the loop of fallopian tube suture ligated. The mesosalpinx of the loop is perforated with sutures and the tube transected. The procedure is repeated on the opposite side as needed. The procedure may be performed using a vaginal approach, although this approach is rarely used. The posterior fornix of the vagina is incised to access the posterior cul-de sac . The fallopian tube is located and grasped in its midportion using forceps. The tube is suture ligated. The mesosalpinx of the loop is perforated with sutures and the tube transected. The procedure is repeated on the opposite side as needed. Use code 58600 when the tubal ligation/transection is performed alone. Use code 58605 when the procedure is performed as a postpartum procedure during the same hospitalization. Use code 58611 when the procedure is performed as an add-on service at the time of a cesarean delivery or other intra-abdominal surgical procedure.

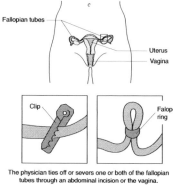

Ligation or transection of fallopian tube(s) when done at the time of cesarean delivery or intra-abdominal surgery

Fallopian tubes

Uterus
Vagina

Clip

Falope ring

The physician ties off or severs one or both of the fallopian tubes through an abdominal incision or the vagina.

58615

58615   Occlusion of fallopian tube(s) by device (eg, band, clip, Falope ring) vaginal or suprapubic approach

The fallopian tubes are occluded using a device such as a band, clip, or Falope ring via a vaginal or suprapubic approach. If a vaginal approach is used, the posterior fornix of the vagina is incised to access the posterior cul-de sac. The fallopian tube is located and grasped in its midportion using forceps. A band, clip or Falope ring is then placed around the loop of fallopian tube. This is repeated on the opposite side as needed. If a suprapubic approach is used, a small incision is made just above the pubic bone. The fallopian tube is identified by first locating the fimbriated end where the round ligament can be identified as a separate structure. The fallopian tube is then grasped in the mid-portion using forceps and the loop of fallopian tube is occluded by placing a band, clip or Falope ring around it. The procedure is repeated on the opposite side as needed.

58660

58660   Laparoscopy, surgical; with lysis of adhesions (salpingolysis, ovariolysis) (separate procedure)

A laparoscopy with lysis of adhesions of the fallopian tubes (salpingolysis) or ovaries (ovariolysis) is performed. A tenaculum is inserted into the vagina, the cervix is grasped, and the uterus is anteflexed. A periumbilical port is placed and pneumoperitoneum is established by insufflating with air. The laparoscope is inserted and the abdominal cavity is inspected. Scar tissue around the tubes and ovaries is meticulously divided. Adhesiolysis may be performed by blunt or sharp dissection, laser, or electrocautery. The procedure continues until all adhesions have been severed and the mobility and function of the tubes and ovaries are restored. A synthetic protective material that breaks down over time may be placed in the pelvic cavity to help prevent formation of new adhesions. The pelvic area is inspected for bleeding, the instruments are withdrawn, and pressure is applied to the abdomen to express any remaining air in the peritoneum. The portal incisions are closed.

58661

58661   Laparoscopy, surgical; with removal of adnexal structures (partial or total oophorectomy and/or salpingectomy)

The physician may remove part or all of one or both fallopian tubes and/or ovaries. A tenaculum is inserted into the vagina, the cervix is grasped, and the uterus is anteflexed. A periumbilical port is placed and pneumoperitoneum is established by insufflating with air. The laparoscope is inserted and the abdominal cavity is inspected. The fimbrial end of the fallopian tube and ovary are elevated. A window is created in the peritoneum of the broad ligament and the infundibulopelvic ligament is grasped, ligated, and transected. The posterior leaf of the broad ligament is severed up to its attachment to the uterus. The fallopian and ovarian ligament is coagulated or ligated with an endoloop at the uterus and severed. A clip is placed across the superior portion of the broad ligament and across the base of the tube at its junction with the uterus. The tube is then severed and removed with or without the ovary through the endoscopic port, or placed in an endobag and removed. The pelvic area is inspected for bleeding, the instruments are withdrawn, and pressure is applied to the abdomen to express any remaining air in the peritoneum. The portal incisions are closed.

58662

58662   Laparoscopy, surgical; with fulguration or excision of lesions of the ovary, pelvic viscera, or peritoneal surface by any method

A laparoscopy with fulguration or excision of lesions of the ovary, pelvic viscera, or peritoneal surface is performed. A tenaculum is inserted into the vagina, the cervix is grasped, and the uterus is anteflexed. A periumbilical port is placed and pneumoperitoneum is established by insufflating with air. The laparoscope is inserted and the abdominal cavity is inspected. Lesions in the ovary, pelvic viscera, or peritoneal surface

are excised using a clip or scissors, or destroyed using a laser or electrocautery. The pelvic area is inspected for bleeding, the instruments are withdrawn, and pressure is applied to the abdomen to express any remaining air in the peritoneum. The portal incisions are closed.

58670-58671

58670   Laparoscopy, surgical; with fulguration of oviducts (with or without transection)

58671   Laparoscopy, surgical; with occlusion of oviducts by device (eg, band, clip, or Falope ring)

A laparoscopy with tubal ligation by fulguration or occlusion of the oviducts is performed. A tenaculum is inserted into the vagina, the cervix grasped, and the uterus anteflexed. A periumbilical port is placed and pneumoperitoneum established by the insufflation of air. The laparoscope is inserted and the abdominal cavity inspected. In 58670, a cautery device is introduced and a section of the fallopian tube is destroyed. The fallopian tube may also be severed (transected). In 58671, the tongs of the band instrument are loaded with the occlusion device (band, clip, or Falope ring) and inserted into the abdomen. The fallopian tube is pulled into the band applicator and the occlusion device is pushed off the applicator around the fallopian tube. The procedure is repeated on the opposite side. The pelvic area is inspected for bleeding, the instruments are withdrawn, and pressure applied to the abdomen to express any remaining air in the peritoneum. The portal incisions are closed.

58672

58672   Laparoscopy, surgical; with fimbrioplasty

A laparoscopic fimbrioplasty is performed. This procedure is used to treat conditions such as agglutination or clubbing of the fimbriae, filmy adhesions, or hydrosalpinx without complete closure of the ostium. An incision is made just below the umbilicus; a trocar is placed, and the laparoscope is inserted. Pneumoperitoneum is established by inflating the abdominal cavity with air. The abdominal cavity, uterus, fallopian tubes, and ovaries are visually inspected. Two or three additional portal incisions are made in the lower abdomen for the introduction of surgical instruments. The fallopian tube may be distended by injecting indigo carbine solution into the tube through a cannula placed vaginally into the uterus. Adhesions around the fallopian tube, ovary, and round ligament are lysed. The clubbed end of the fallopian tube is opened using electrocautery. Microforceps are used to elevate the serosal layer lying over the end of the tube. At this point, the tube should be opened sufficiently to allow the indigo carbine solution to spill out. Microforceps are used to pick up the scarred serosal tissue which is transected to expose the fimbriae. The scarred serosal tissue is then folded back allowing the fimbriae to prolapse out of the tube. The fimbriae are separated by irrigation with warm saline solution. The scarred serosal tissue is sutured to the exterior serosal layer of the tube. Other techniques used to repair the fimbriae include: ostial stretching, deagglutination, and/or lysis of perifimbrial adhesions. Additional indigo carbine dye is injected into the uterus to verify patency of the tube.

58673

58673   Laparoscopy, surgical; with salpingostomy (salpingoneostomy)

A laparoscopic salpingostomy (salpingoneostomy, neosalpingostomy) is performed. This procedure is used primarily to treat hydrosalpinx although it may be used for other conditions causing obstruction of the tube. Hydrosalpinx is an accumulation of fluid in the fallopian tube that occurs as a result of an injury to the end of the tube, causing it to close and preventing tubal secretions from being expelled. The secretions then collect in the tube and cause it to swell. An incision is made just below the umbilicus; a trocar is placed, and the laparoscope is inserted. Pneumoperitoneum is established by inflating the abdominal cavity with air. The abdominal cavity, uterus, fallopian tubes, and ovaries are visually inspected. Two or three additional portal incisions are made in the lower abdomen for the introduction of surgical instruments. Adhesions around the fallopian tube, ovary, and round ligament are lysed. The tube is distended by transcervical injection of saline or dye. The hydrosalpinx is opened using scissors, micro-needle, or laser. The incision runs from the tube outward toward the ovary and will form a new tubal os. The edge of the tubal incision is grasped and everted to allow inspection of the tubal mucosa. Additional radial incisions are made as needed to further open the tube. Additional dye may be injected into the uterus to verify patency of the tube.

58674

● 58674   Laparoscopy, surgical, ablation of uterine fibroid(s) including intraoperative ultrasound guidance and monitoring, radiofrequency

Uterine fibroids are benign tumors of the muscle tissue (myometrium) of the uterus. Fibroid tumors may be submucous, intramural, or subserous. Submucous fibroids protrude into the uterine cavity; intramural fibroids are contained within the uterine muscle; and subserous fibroids occur on the exterior of the uterus. Radiofrequency ablation (RFA) may be used to treat all sizes and locations of fibroid tumors. Two ports are placed, one in the infraumbilical region and a second in the suprapubic region. Pneumoperitoneum is established. A laparoscopic examination is performed which includes uterine ultrasound to identify all fibroid tumors. A small skin incision is made and the RFA device is advanced

● New Code   ▲ Revised Code

percutaneously into the peritoneal cavity to the site of the fibroid. The RFA tip is advanced into the fibroid and the electrode array is deployed. Laparoscopic visualization and ultrasound guidance are used to ensure proper placement and deployment of the electrode array before it is activated. The temperature of the array increases until the target temperature is reached. Target temperature is then maintained for a prescribed period in order to accomplish complete ablation. The electrode array is then deactivated and retracted into the RFA device. Additional fibroids are treated in the same manner. When all fibroid tumors have been ablated, the RFA device is removed, CO2 gas is allowed to empty from the peritoneal cavity, and skin incisions are closed.

58700-58720

58700 **Salpingectomy, complete or partial, unilateral or bilateral (separate procedure)**

58720 **Salpingo-oophorectomy, complete or partial, unilateral or bilateral (separate procedure)**

The physician performs a unilateral or bilateral, complete or partial salpingectomy
. An incision is made in the abdomen. A clamp is applied to the fallopian tube at the tubouterine junction, and the fallopian tube is mobilized. The broad ligament is exposed, clamped in the superior aspect, and incised to free the superior portion of the fallopian tube. The broad ligament is repaired with mattress sutures. An elliptical incision is made around the base of the fallopian tube at its insertion into the uterus. Dissection is carried down through the muscle plane of the uterus. The fallopian tube is severed from the uterus and removed. The incision in the uterus is repaired. The procedure is repeated on the opposite side if a bilateral salpingectomy is required. In 58720, a unilateral or bilateral, complete or partial salpingectomy with oophorectomy is performed. The uterus is pulled forward to allow access to the infundibulopelvic ligament. The infundibulopelvic ligament which contains the ovarian vessels is clamped. The fallopian tube and ovary are mobilized to expose the broad ligament which is incised. The ovarian vessels are identified and suture ligated. An elliptical incision is made around the base of the fallopian tube at its insertion into the uterus. Dissection is carried down through the muscle plane of the uterus. The fallopian tube is severed from the uterus and removed along with the ovary. The incision in the uterus is repaired. The procedure is repeated on the opposite side if a bilateral salpingectomy and oophorectomy is required.

58740

58740 **Lysis of adhesions (salpingolysis, ovariolysis)**

Lysis of adhesions of the fallopian tubes (salpingolysis) or ovaries (ovariolysis) is performed via an incision made in the lower abdomen. The abdominal cavity, uterus, fallopian tubes, and ovaries are visually inspected. Scar tissue around the tubes and ovaries is meticulously divided. Adhesiolysis may be performed by blunt or sharp dissection, laser, or electrocautery. The procedure continues until all adhesions have been severed and the mobility and function of the tubes and ovaries has been restored. A synthetic protective material that breaks down over time may be placed in the pelvic cavity to help prevent formation of new adhesions. The pelvic area is inspected to ensure hemostasis and the abdominal incision is closed.

58750

58750 **Tubotubal anastomosis**

A tubotubal anastomosis is performed via an abdominal incision. This procedure is performed to reverse a previous tubal ligation. Tubotubal anastomosis may also be used following excision of a diseased or damaged portion of the fallopian tube. An incision is made in the lower abdomen. The abdominal cavity, uterus, fallopian tubes, and ovaries are visually inspected. Adhesions around the fallopian tube, ovary, and round ligament are lysed. The blocked tubal segments are opened and a narrow flexible stent is threaded from the fimbriated end through the tube lumen and into the uterine cavity to ensure that the tube is not obstructed at a point distant from the segment involved in the previously performed ligation procedure. The two tubal segments are then brought together by placing a retention suture in the connective tissue beneath the tube. Microsurgical technique is used to anastomose the middle muscular layer of the tube and the outer serosal layer while taking care not to disrupt the inner mucosal layer. Following anastomosis, the stent is withdrawn from the fimbriated end of the tube.

58752

58752 **Tubouterine implantation**

A tubouterine implantation is performed via an abdominal incision. This procedure is performed to reverse a previous tubal ligation in which only the distal portion of the fallopian tube remains. Tubouterine implanation may also be used following excision of the proximal portion of a diseased or damaged tube. An incision is made lower abdomen. The abdominal cavity, uterus, fallopian tubes, and ovaries are visually inspected. Adhesions around the fallopian tube, ovary, and round ligament are lysed. The distal portion of the tube is mobilized and a new opening is created through the uterine wall. The tubal segment is inserted through the new opening into the uterine cavity. Microsurgical technique is used to suture the tube to the uterine wall and reimplant the fallopian tube.

58760

58760 **Fimbrioplasty**

A fimbrioplasty is performed via an abdominal incision. This procedure is used to treat conditions such as agglutination or clubbing of the fimbriae, filmy adhesions, or hydrosalpinx without complete closure of the ostium. An incision is made in the lower abdomen. The abdominal cavity, uterus, fallopian tubes, and ovaries are visually inspected. The fallopian tube may be distended by injecting indigo carbine solution into the tube through a cannula placed vaginally into the uterus. Adhesions around the fallopian tube, ovary, and round ligament are lysed. The clubbed end of the fallopian tube is opened using electrocautery. Microforceps are used to elevate the serosal layer lying over the end of the tube. At this point, the tube should be opened sufficiently to allow the indigo carbine solution to spill out. Microforceps are used to pick up the scarred serosal tissue which is transected to expose the fimbriae. The scarred serosal tissue is then folded back allowing the fimbriae to prolapse out of the tube. The fimbriae are separated by irrigation with warm saline solution. The scarred serosal tissue is sutured to the exterior serosal layer of the tube. Other techniques used to repair the fimbriae include: ostial stretching, deagglutination, and/or lysis of perifimbrial adhesions. Additional indigo carbine dye is injected into the uterus to verify patency of the tube before the abdominal incision is closed.

58770

58770 **Salpingostomy (salpingoneostomy)**

A salpingostomy (salpingoneostomy, neosalpingostomy) is performed via an abdominal incision. This procedure is used primarily to treat hydrosalpinx although it may be used for other conditions causing obstruction of the tube. Hydrosalpinx is an accumulation of fluid in the fallopian tube that occurs as a result of an injury to the end of the tube, causing it to close and preventing tubal secretions from being expelled. The secretions then collect in the tube and cause it to swell. An incision is made in the lower abdomen. The abdominal cavity, uterus, fallopian tubes, and ovaries are visually inspected. Adhesions around the fallopian tube, ovary, and round ligament are lysed. The tube is distended by transcervical injection of saline or dye. The hydrosalpinx is opened using scissors, micro-needle, or laser. The incision runs from the tube outward toward the ovary and will form a new tubal os. The edge of the tubal incision is grasped and everted to allow inspection of the tubal mucosa. Additional radial incisions are made as needed to further open the tube. Additional dye may be injected into the uterus to verify patency of the tube before the abdominal incision is closed.

58800-58805

58800 **Drainage of ovarian cyst(s), unilateral or bilateral (separate procedure); vaginal approach**

58805 **Drainage of ovarian cyst(s), unilateral or bilateral (separate procedure); abdominal approach**

An ovarian cyst is a sac or pouch arising from the ovary. The cyst may be fluid-filled or contain semi-solid or solid material. Using a transvaginal approach, a vaginal ultrasound probe is used to identify internal structures and aid in localization of the cyst. A small incision may be made in the vagina. Alternatively, the needle may be advanced directly through the posterior vaginal fornix and into the ovarian cyst. The cyst is then aspirated and drained until all of the cyst contents have been removed. The transvaginal approach is typically reserved for medically fragile patients who are not good candidates for an open abdominal procedure. Using an abdominal approach, a suprapubic incision is made through the skin and subcutaneous tissue. Subcutaneous fat is cleared and the anterior rectus fascia incised. The rectus muscles are retracted and the underlying transversalis fascia and peritoneum exposed and incised. The ovary and cyst are exposed and inspected along with the uterus, fallopian tubes and the contralateral ovary. The cyst is punctured and drained taking care to prevent spillage of cyst contents. The cyst contents are sent for separately reportable laboratory analysis.

Drainage of ovarian cyst(s), unilateral or bilateral (separate procedure) vaginal/abdominal approach

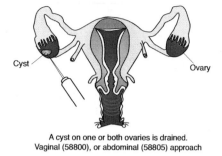

A cyst on one or both ovaries is drained.
Vaginal (58800), or abdominal (58805) approach

58820-58822

58820 **Drainage of ovarian abscess; vaginal approach, open**
58822 **Drainage of ovarian abscess; abdominal approach**

Using a transvaginal approach, an incision is made in the vaginal wall through the posterior vaginal fornix. The ovary is approached through the posterior cul-de-sac. The abscess is incised and the incision carried down into the abscess cavities. The septa within the abscess are opened and the abscess drained. Transvaginal ovarian abscess drainage is typically limited to patients with an unruptured abscess. Using an abdominal approach, an incision is made through the skin and subcutaneous tissue. Subcutaneous fat is cleared and the anterior rectus fascia incised. The rectus muscles are retracted and the underlying transversalis fascia and peritoneum exposed and incised. The abdominal cavity is inspected to ensure that there are no abscesses in the subdiaphragmatic spaces or along the colonic guttars. The bowel is also carefully inspected for the presence of infection. The bowel is then packed into the upper abdomen. The ovarian abscess is incised and the incision carried down into the abscess cavities. The septa within the abscess cavities are opened and the abscess drained. The abdomen is irrigated with antibiotic solution and drains placed. The abdomen is closed around the drains.

58825

58825 **Transposition, ovary(s)**

Transposition of the ovaries is performed. This procedure is done on women of child-bearing age wishing to preserve fertility while receiving radiation treatment for malignant neoplasms of gynecological structures or other malignancies such as colorectal cancer or Hodgkin's lymphoma. An incision is made through the skin and subcutaneous tissue of the abdomen and the anterior rectus fascia is incised. The rectus muscles are retracted and the underlying transversalis fascia and peritoneum are exposed and incised. The peritoneal cavity is inspected. The peritoneum of the both pelvic sidewalls is incised and the retroperitoneal space is developed. Ovarian vessels and the ureters are identified and protected. The utero-ovarian ligaments are separated and the peritoneum is incised to the area outside the true pelvis. The ovarian vessels are then turned laterally taking care not to disrupt the blood supply to the ovaries and tubes. The ovaries and tubes are then transposed and placed high in the paracolic gutters just below the spleen on one side and the liver on the other. The upper and lower poles are marked with hemoclips to ensure that their location can be easily identified on radiographic examination and to ensure that they lie outside the radiation portals.

58900

58900 **Biopsy of ovary, unilateral or bilateral (separate procedure)**

The physician performs a unilateral or bilateral biopsy of the ovary. An incision is made through the skin and subcutaneous tissue of the abdomen. Subcutaneous fat is cleared and the anterior rectus fascia is incised. The rectus muscles are retracted and the underlying transversalis fascia and peritoneum are exposed and incised. The peritoneal cavity is inspected. The ovaries are exposed and inspected along with the uterus and fallopian tubes. The ovarian lesion is identified and tissue samples are obtained and sent for laboratory analysis. The abdomen is then closed in layers.

58920

58920 **Wedge resection or bisection of ovary, unilateral or bilateral**

A unilateral or bilateral wedge resection or bisection of the ovary is performed. An incision is made through the skin and subcutaneous tissue of the abdomen. Subcutaneous fat is cleared and the anterior rectus fascia is incised. The rectus muscles are retracted and the underlying transversalis fascia and peritoneum are exposed and incised. The peritoneal cavity is inspected. The ovaries are exposed and inspected along with the uterus and

fallopian tubes. The ovarian lesion is identified and a wedge of tissue containing the lesion is excised. Alternatively, the ovary may be bisected (cut in half) with the section containing the lesion removed. The ovarian tissue is sent for separately reportable laboratory analysis. The abdomen is then closed in layers.

58925

58925 **Ovarian cystectomy, unilateral or bilateral**

The physician performs a unilateral or bilateral ovarian cystectomy. An ovarian cyst is a sac or pouch arising from the ovary that may be filled with fluid or contain semi-solid or solid material. Using an abdominal approach, a suprapubic incision is made through the skin and subcutaneous tissue. Subcutaneous fat is cleared and the anterior rectus fascia is incised. The rectus muscles are retracted and the underlying transversalis fascia and peritoneum are exposed and incised. The ovary and cyst are exposed and inspected along with the uterus, fallopian tubes, and contralateral ovary. If the cyst is large, the physician may first decompress the cyst by puncturing and draining the contents, taking care to prevent spillage. The cystic pouch is then dissected off the ovary. Alternatively, the cyst may be removed whole by dissecting it off the ovary, taking care not to puncture the cyst wall. The cyst and its contents are sent for separately reportable laboratory analysis. The abdomen is then closed in layers.

58940-58943

58940 **Oophorectomy, partial or total, unilateral or bilateral**
58943 **Oophorectomy, partial or total, unilateral or bilateral; for ovarian, tubal or primary peritoneal malignancy, with para-aortic and pelvic lymph node biopsies, peritoneal washings, peritoneal biopsies, diaphragmatic assessments, with or without salpingectomy(s), with or without omentectomy**

Oophorectomy may be performed due to disease or ovarian malignancy or as a prophylactic measure in patients with breast cancer or at high risk for developing ovarian cancer. In 58940, the skin and subcutaneous tissue of the abdomen are incised. Subcutaneous fat is cleared and the anterior rectus fascia incised. The rectus muscles are retracted and the underlying transversalis fascia and peritoneum exposed and incised. The ovary is exposed and inspected along with the uterus, fallopian tubes and the contralateral ovary. The ovarian ligament is identified, ligated and divided. Part or all of the ovary is dissected free of surrounding tissue and excised. The procedure is repeated on the opposite side as needed. In 58943, one or both ovaries are removed for ovarian, tubal, or primary peritoneal malignancy. In addition, para-aortic and pelvic lymph node biopsies are performed along with peritoneal washings and/or biopsies, the diaphragm is inspected for metatastatic disease, the fallopian tubes may be excised (salpingectomy), and the omentum may be excised (omentectomy). Before opening the peritoneum, pelvic lymph node sampling biopsies are taken and sent for frozen section. The peritoneal cavity is opened and the abdomen and pelvis explored for evidence of metastatic disease. The peritoneal cavity is irrigated with saline solution and the solution aspirated. The washings are sent for laboratory analysis. Tissue samples of the peritoneum may also be obtained and sent for laboratory analysis. The para-aortic lymph nodes are exposed and biopsies taken and sent for frozen section. Blunt dissection is used to expose the broad ligament, round ligament, ovaries, and fallopian tubes. If the fallopian tubes are removed with the ovaries, an incision is made in the exposed broad ligament. The ovarian vessels are visualized and suture ligated. The cut edges of the broad ligament are plicated with mattress sutures. The fallopian tubes and ovaries are dissected free of surrounding tissue. The round ligaments are clamped, divided, and blood vessels suture ligated bilaterally. The fallopian tube is transected near the junction with the uterus. The ovaries and fallopian tube are removed. Alternatively, the ovaries may be separated from surrounding tissues and removed while the fallopian tubes are left intact. The omentum may also be removed. Beginning at the greater curvature of the stomach and taking care to control bleeding from the omental branches of the right gastric artery the omentum is dissected free of the stomach. The left gastroepiploic artery is isolated, ligated and divided, and the remaining omentum removed from the transverse colon. The abdomen is then closed in layers.

58950

58950 **Resection (initial) of ovarian, tubal or primary peritoneal malignancy with bilateral salpingo-oophorectomy and omentectomy**

The abdomen is opened from the symphysis pubis to the xiphoid and the abdominal and pelvic cavities are explored to determine the extent of the malignancy. Blunt dissection is used to expose the broad ligament, round ligament, ovaries, and fallopian tubes. An incision is made in the exposed broad ligament. The ovarian vessels are visualized and suture ligated. The cut edges of the broad ligament are plicated with mattress sutures. The fallopian tubes and ovaries are dissected free of surrounding tissue. The round ligaments are clamped and divided, and blood vessels are suture ligated bilaterally. The fallopian tube is transected near the junction with the uterus. The ovaries and fallopian tubes are removed. If the resection is for a primary peritoneal malignancy, the peritoneal tumor is resected. If the resection is for an ovarian or tubal malignancy, the metastatic disease is resected as much as possible. The omentum is removed. Beginning at the greater curvature of the stomach and taking care to control bleeding from the omental branches of the right gastric artery, the omentum is dissected free of the stomach. The left gastroepiploic artery is isolated, ligated, and divided, and the remaining omentum is removed from the transverse colon. The abdomen is then closed in layers.

58951-58952

58951 Resection (initial) of ovarian, tubal or primary peritoneal malignancy with bilateral salpingo-oophorectomy and omentectomy; with total abdominal hysterectomy, pelvic and limited para-aortic lymphadenectomy

58952 Resection (initial) of ovarian, tubal or primary peritoneal malignancy with bilateral salpingo-oophorectomy and omentectomy; with radical dissection for debulking (ie, radical excision or destruction, intra-abdominal or retroperitoneal tumors)

The abdomen is opened from the symphysis pubis to the xiphoid and the abdominal and pelvic cavities explored to determine the extent of the malignancy. Blunt dissection is used to expose the broad ligament, round ligament, ovaries, and fallopian tubes. An incision is made in the exposed broad ligament. The ovarian vessels are visualized and suture ligated. The cut edges of the broad ligament are plicated with mattress sutures. The fallopian tubes and ovaries are dissected free of surrounding tissue. The round ligaments are clamped, divided, and blood vessels suture ligated bilaterally. The fallopian tube is transected near the junction with the uterus. The ovaries and fallopian tubes are removed. If the resection is for a primary peritoneal malignancy, the peritoneal tumor is resected. If the resection is for an ovarian or tubal malignancy as much metastatic disease as possible is resected. The omentum is removed. Beginning at the greater curvature of the stomach and taking care to control bleeding from the omental branches of the right gastric artery the omentum is dissected free of the stomach. The left gastroepiploic artery is isolated, ligated and divided, and the remaining omentum removed from the transverse colon. The abdomen is then closed in layers. In 58951, the physician performs a total hysterectomy with pelvic and limited para-aortic lymphadenectomy, in addition to resecting the ovarian, tubal or primary peritoneal malignancy and removing the fallopian tubes, ovaries and omentum. The abdomen is incised. Before opening the peritoneum, pelvic lymph nodes are explored and removed. Taking care to preserve the genitofemoral nerve and psoas muscle, fatty tissue is stripped from the mid-portion of the both common iliac vessels and along the internal and external iliac vessels to the level of the circumflex iliac vein. Iliac, hypogastric and obturator nodes are excised bilaterally and sent for separately reportable frozen section exam. The peritoneal cavity is opened and the abdomen and pelvis explored for evidence of metastatic disease. The para-aortic lymph nodes are exposed and biopsies taken and sent for frozen section. Involved para-aortic lymph nodes are excised. The physician then performs the total abdominal hysterectomy with removal of tubes and ovaries. Blunt dissection is used to expose the broad ligament, round ligament and fallopian tubes. An incision is made in the exposed broad ligament. The ovarian vessels are visualized and suture ligated. The cut edges of the broad ligament are plicated with mattress sutures. The fallopian tubes and ovaries are dissected free of surrounding tissue. The round ligaments are clamped, divided, and blood vessels suture ligated bilaterally. The bladder is mobilized and the uterus exposed. The uterine artery and vein are ligated. The ureters are dissected from the parametrium and from the tunnel of the cardinal ligament. The posterior peritoneum is opened and the rectovaginal space opened. The uterosacral ligaments are freed and divided as are the cardinal ligaments. The parametria is freed from inferior attachments to the level of the vagina. The uterus, cervix, fallopian tubes and ovaries are removed. The omentum is also removed as described above. In 58952, the ovarian, tubal, or primary peritoneal malignancy is resected and the tube, ovaries, and omentum removed as described in 58951. The physician also performs a radical dissection for debulking of the tumor which includes radical excision or destruction of intra-abdominal or retroperitoneal tumors. The intra-abdominal and retroperitoneal tumors are approached through the abdominal incision. Each tumor is then addressed individually. Tumor nodules are resected from organ surfaces and/or organ resections performed as needed. Peritoneal stripping is performed to remove all gross tumor nodules from the peritoneum. As much tumor mass as possible is excised or destroyed while taking to protect and preserve function of vital organs.

58953-58954

58953 Bilateral salpingo-oophorectomy with omentectomy, total abdominal hysterectomy and radical dissection for debulking

58954 Bilateral salpingo-oophorectomy with omentectomy, total abdominal hysterectomy and radical dissection for debulking; with pelvic lymphadenectomy and limited para-aortic lymphadenectomy

The physician performs a bilateral salpingo-oophorectomy with total omentectomy and total abdominal hysterectomy with radical dissection for debulking of metastases with or without pelvic lymphadenectomy and limited para-aortic lymphadenectomy. An incision is made in the abdomen and the anterior uterine surface exposed. The peritoneum at the cervicovesical fold is incised. Blunt dissection is used to expose the broad ligament, round ligament and fallopian tubes. An incision is made in the exposed broad ligament. The ovarian vessels are visualized and suture ligated. The cut edges of the broad ligament are plicated with mattress sutures. The fallopian tubes and ovaries are dissected free of surrounding tissue. The round ligaments are clamped, divided, and blood vessels suture

ligated bilaterally. The cervix is palpated and the position of the bladder ascertained. The bladder is then dissected off the uterus and the dissection carried down to the vaginal wall. The posterior aspect of the uterus is visualized and inspected to verify that it is not adhered to the rectum. The uterine vessels are exposed, clamped, divided and suture ligated. The posterior cervical peritoneum is incised and the incision is extended around the cervix. The vaginal wall is incised and the cervix separated from the vagina. The uterus and cervix are removed along with the ovaries and tubes. The vaginal opening is closed. The omentum is freed first from the transverse colon and then from the greater curvature of the stomach up to the splenic hilum. The omentum is removed. The physician then resects (debulks) as much of the tumor as possible. Pelvic and para-aortic lymph nodes are palpated and enlarged nodes are sampled. In 58953, the pelvic and para-aortic lymph nodes are not removed. In 58954, pelvic lymphadenectomy and limited para-aortic lymphadenectomy are also performed. All pelvic lymph nodes are removed and positive para-aortic nodes are also removed. The surgical site is carefully inspected to verify that as much metastatic disease as possible has been removed. Bleeding is controlled, the abdominal wound irrigated, and the abdominal incision closed.

58956

58956 Bilateral salpingo-oophorectomy with total omentectomy, total abdominal hysterectomy for malignancy

The physician performs a bilateral salpingo-oophorectomy with total omentectomy and total abdominal hysterectomy for malignancy. An incision is made in the abdomen and the anterior uterine surface is exposed. The peritoneum at the cervicovesical fold is incised. Blunt dissection is used to expose the broad ligament, round ligament, and fallopian tubes. An incision is made in the exposed broad ligament. The ovarian vessels are visualized and suture ligated. The cut edges of the broad ligament are plicated with mattress sutures. The fallopian tubes and ovaries are dissected free of surrounding tissue. The round ligaments are clamped and divided, and the blood vessels are suture ligated bilaterally. The cervix is palpated and the position of the bladder is ascertained. The bladder is then dissected off the uterus and the dissection is carried down to the vaginal wall. The posterior aspect of the uterus is visualized and inspected to verify that it is not adhered to the rectum. The uterine vessels are exposed, clamped, divided, and suture ligated. The posterior cervical peritoneum is incised and the incision is extended around the cervix. The vaginal wall is incised and the cervix is separated from the vagina. The uterus and cervix are removed along with the ovaries and tubes. The vaginal opening is closed. The omentum is freed first from the transverse colon and then from the greater curvature of the stomach up to the splenic hilum and removed. The surgical site is carefully inspected to verify that all visible metatastic disease has been removed. Bleeding is controlled; the abdominal wound is irrigated; and The incision is closed with sutures.

58957-58958

58957 Resection (tumor debulking) of recurrent ovarian, tubal, primary peritoneal, uterine malignancy (intra-abdominal, retroperitoneal tumors), with omentectomy, if performed

58958 Resection (tumor debulking) of recurrent ovarian, tubal, primary peritoneal, uterine malignancy (intra-abdominal, retroperitoneal tumors), with omentectomy, if performed; with pelvic lymphadenectomy and limited para-aortic lymphadenectomy

Resection or tumor debulking of intra-abdominal or retroperitoneal tumors is done on recurrent ovarian, tubal, primary peritoneal, or uterine malignancies. Tumor debulking is surgically removing as much of the tumor as possible. Through an abdominal incision, the surgeon openly accesses the tumor site, whether on the uterus, the uterine adnexa, such as the ovary or fallopian tube, or the peritoneum, and resects or removes the recurring tumor tissue. Tumor debulking, or incomplete resection, is done when it may not be possible to remove the entire tumor or when attempting to create immunological memory for long-term antitumor immunity, in which case the surgical debulking is followed by combination chemo and immunotherapy. The surgeon may also remove the omentum, a sheet of fat covered by peritoneum that extends from the stomach to other organs, such as the liver (lesser omentum), and covers the small intestines to the transverse colon (greater omentum). Code 58958 when the lymph nodes within the pelvis are also removed along with a portion of the nodes that surround the lower aorta.

58960

58960 Laparotomy, for staging or restaging of ovarian, tubal, or primary peritoneal malignancy (second look), with or without omentectomy, peritoneal washing, biopsy of abdominal and pelvic peritoneum, diaphragmatic assessment with pelvic and limited para-aortic lymphadenectomy

Prior to opening the abdomen, pelvic lymph nodes are explored and removed. Taking care to preserve the genitofemoral nerve and psoas muscle, fatty tissue is stripped from the mid-portion of both common iliac vessels and along the internal and external iliac vessels to the level of the circumflex iliac vein. Iliac, hypogastric and obturator nodes are excised bilaterally. A long midline abdominal incision is made from the xiphoid process to the pubis. The peritoneal cavity is opened and the abdomen and pelvis explored for evidence of metastatic disease. Sterile saline is instilled into the peritoneal cavity and removed by suction to obtain peritoneal washings. The washings are prepared and sent to the laboratory for cytopathology examination. Multiple tissue samples are obtained from the abdominal and pelvic peritoneum. The diaphragm is inspected and scrapings obtained for cytopathology examination. The para-aortic lymph nodes are exposed and biopsies taken and sent for frozen section. Involved para-aortic lymph nodes are excised. If the omentum has not been excised in an earlier procedure it may be removed. The anterior aspect of the omentum is explored to identify masses, lesions, or other evidence of disease or injury. The omentum is lifted off the colon and the posterior aspect explored. The segment of omentum to be resected is identified. Blood vessels are individually clamped and ligated as the omentum is dissected free of surrounding tissues and removed. Drains are placed as needed and the abdominal incision is closed.

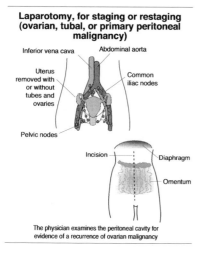

Laparotomy, for staging or restaging (ovarian, tubal, or primary peritoneal malignancy)

Inferior vena cava

Abdominal aorta

Uterus removed with or without tubes and ovaries

Common iliac nodes

Pelvic nodes

Incision

Diaphragm

Omentum

The physician examines the peritoneal cavity for evidence of a recurrence of ovarian malignancy

58970

58970   Follicle puncture for oocyte retrieval, any method

The physician retrieves an egg via follicle puncture for in vitro fertilization. The physician may access the follicle via one of several methods, including laparoscopically, transabdominally, or transvaginally. Ultrasonic guidance or laparoscopic guidance are used to visualize the follicle and a needle is inserted directly into the follicle, which then aspirates the egg and surrounding fluid. The needle and other medical equipment are withdrawn. Closure with Steri-Strips may be necessary.

58974

58974   Embryo transfer, intrauterine

Embryos which have been maintained in a laboratory culture dish for 48 to 72 hours are placed into the uterus of the patient. The physician aspirates the embryos into a catheter, which is then placed through the vagina and cervix. The embryos are evacuated into the uterus and the catheter is withdrawn.

58976

58976   Gamete, zygote, or embryo intrafallopian transfer, any method

The physician transfers a gamete, zygote, or embryo into the patient's fallopian tube via any method (usually GIFT or ZIFT). Gamete intrafallopian transfer (GIFT) occurs when an egg and sperm are aspirated in the laboratory setting and injected into the fallopian tube via a catheter. Zygote intrafallopian transfer (ZIFT) occurs when the physician aspirates a previously fertilized egg into a catheter and injects it into the fallopian tube. Either procedure may be performed laparoscopically or hysteroscopically.

59000

59000   Amniocentesis; diagnostic

The physician performs amniocentesis. Using ultrasonic guidance, the physician inserts a needle through the abdominal wall and uterus, directly into the amniotic sac. Amniotic fluid is aspirated for diagnostic purposes. This procedure often occurs between the 12th and 18th week of pregnancy. The needle is withdrawn.

59001

59001   Amniocentesis; therapeutic amniotic fluid reduction (includes ultrasound guidance)

The physician performs amniotic fluid reduction. Using ultrasonic guidance, the physician inserts a needle through the abdominal wall and uterus, directly into the amniotic sac. Amniotic fluid is aspirated for therapeutic purposes and as much as seven liters may be drained. The needle is withdrawn. This procedure is a common treatment for twin-twin transfusion syndrome.

59012

59012   Cordocentesis (intrauterine), any method

The physician performs cordocentesis, also known as percutaneous umbilical blood sampling (PUBS). Using ultrasonic guidance, the physician inserts a needle through the abdominal wall and into the umbilical artery or vein. Fetal blood is aspirated. The physician may utilize a transamniotic or transplacental approach. The needle is removed.

59015

59015   Chorionic villus sampling, any method

The physician obtains a tissue sample of the chorionic villus (CVS). The chorionic villus is commonly known as the placenta. There are three main approaches used in CVS. After the vagina and cervix have been cleansed with antiseptic, the physician uses ultrasonic guidance to insert a catheter through the cervix. Placental cells are aspirated into the catheter and the catheter is removed. If CVS is performed via the transvaginal or transabdominal approaches, the physician inserts a needle through the abdomen wall or vagina to reach the placenta. Ultrasonic guidance is also used during these approaches. The needle is used to aspirate placental cells, and then removed. This procedure is usually performed 9 to 12 weeks into the pregnancy.

59020

59020   Fetal contraction stress test

The physician performs a fetal contraction stress test, also known as an oxytocin challenge test. Two belts with sensors attached are placed around the patient's abdomen. One belt holds the sensor that detects the fetus's heart rate; the other measures the timing and duration of the uterine contractions. The sensors are attached with wires to a recording device that can indicate or print out a record of the fetal heart rate as well as the strength and duration of uterine contractions. The heart rate monitor may be moved if the fetus changes position. The fetus's heart rate and spontaneous contractions of the uterus are recorded on the external fetal monitor for 10 minutes. If spontaneous contractions do not occur during this 10-minute period, the patient is given an intravenous infusion of oxytocin (Pitocin), and the contractions are recorded on the monitor. The infusion begins with a low dose, which is gradually increased until three contractions occur within 10 minutes, each one lasting longer than 45 seconds. Breast massage, or nipple stimulation, may be utilized instead of an oxytocin infusion. Nipple stimulation prompts the body to produce the hormone oxytocin naturally. The patient massages her nipple by hand until contractions start. If a second contraction does not occur within 2 minutes of the first, the nipple is massaged again. If contractions do not occur within 15 minutes, both nipples are stimulated. This procedure may be repeated for up to a maximum of 10 minutes on one breast. Because nipple stimulation can cause long, uncontrolled contractions, an oxytocin infusion is preferred by some physicians.

59025

59025   Fetal non-stress test

During a non-stress test, the patient is hooked up to a fetal monitor. No medication is given to stimulate or cause movement of the fetus or contractions of the uterus. The fetus may be moving spontaneously, and the test will work without any further stimulation. The patient may encourage the fetus to move by rubbing her hand over her abdomen. Additionally, the clinician may make a loud noise with a special device above the abdomen. When the fetus moves, a recording is made of its heart rate. This procedure is non-invasive and lasts approximately 30 minutes.

59030

59030   Fetal scalp blood sampling

Fetal Blood Sampling (FBS) is a procedure performed for the diagnosis of fetal distress. The fetal scalp is first visualized with an amnioscope inserted vaginally. The fetal scalp is cleaned. The physician creates a small cut made in the scalp from which blood is collected in a microtube. The incision penetrates no farther than 2 mm into the fetal scalp and is closely observed for clotting and closure.

59050-59051

59050   Fetal monitoring during labor by consulting physician (ie, non-attending physician) with written report; supervision and interpretation

59051   Fetal monitoring during labor by consulting physician (ie, non-attending physician) with written report; interpretation only

A non-attending physician or other consultant inserts a catheter into the amniotic sac, via the cervix, in order to monitor and record contraction intervals. An electrode is also placed directly onto the fetus's scalp to record the fetus's electrocardiographic data. Code 59050 if the consultant supervises the labor and interprets the finding of the fetal monitoring in a written report. Code 59051 if the consultant only interprets the data and writes a report. No supervision during labor is associated with code 59051.

59070

59070   Transabdominal amnioinfusion, including ultrasound guidance

The physician performs transabdominal amnioinfusion including ultrasound guidance. Amnioinfusion is performed when amniotic fluid is low so that fetal anatomy can be better visualized and evaluated. The procedure may also be performed in conjunction with invasive procedures such as fetoscopy or placement of fetal shunts. Using continuous ultrasound guidance, a needle is guided into the uterus, taking care to avoid the fetus, and an amniocentesis is performed. Sterile saline is then instilled until optimum visualization of fetal anatomy is obtained. The needle is removed and a detailed ultrasound of the fetus is performed. Following completion of the procedure, the patient is monitored as needed. The physician discusses the findings with the patient and prepares a written report.

59072

59072   Fetal umbilical cord occlusion, including ultrasound guidance

The physician performs fetal umbilical cord occlusion, including ultrasound guidance, on monochorionic twins sharing the same placenta. Fetal umbilical cord occlusion is indicated when one monochorionic twin has a fetal anomaly (discordant anomalous twins) that is not consistent with survival or has suffered a fetal demise, and the second twin's chance for survival is compromised. Occluding the umbilical cord of the anomalous or already demised twin severs the vascular link between the fetuses, causing death of the anomalous twin while improving the chances for survival of the healthy twin. Umbilical cord occlusion may also be performed for twin-twin transfusion syndrome (TTTS), a complication of monochorionic twin pregnancy in which there is an exchange of blood between the two fetuses, resulting in polyhydramnios in one sac and oligohydramnios in the other. Using continuous ultrasound guidance, the umbilical cord of the affected fetus is identified along with a placental free area for access to the umbilical cord. A scope is introduced into the uterus followed by small coagulation forceps. The umbilical cord of the affected fetus is grasped, and the cord is occluded using laser, suture, or bipolar coagulation. The cord is completely occluded in the case of an anomaly or demise or occluded at the level where blood exchange is occurring in the case of TTTS. Color Doppler ultrasound is used to verify occlusion of the cord, indicated by the absence of blood flow. The scope is removed and the patient is monitored as needed. The physician discusses the results of the procedure with the patient and prepares a written report.

59074

59074   Fetal fluid drainage (eg, vesicocentesis, thoracocentesis, paracentesis), including ultrasound guidance

The physician performs fetal fluid drainage, such as vesicocentesis, thoracocentesis, or paracentesis, including ultrasound guidance. Fluid aspiration from the fetal bladder, thorax, abdominal cavity, or other sites is performed to help evaluate or treat fetal congenital abnormalities. Using continuous ultrasound guidance, a needle is directed into the fetal bladder, thorax, abdominal cavity, or other site and fluid is aspirated. The needle is then removed. The patient is monitored and repeat ultrasound is performed to evaluate the site

● New Code   ▲ Revised Code   **407**

of the fetal puncture and aspiration. The physician discusses the findings with the patient and prepares a written report.

59076

59076   Fetal shunt placement, including ultrasound guidance

The physician places a fetal shunt using ultrasound guidance. A shunt may be placed in the fetal thorax or bladder for treatment of pleural effusion or bladder obstruction. The shunt drains fluid from the thorax or bladder into the amniotic cavity. A shunt is selected and sterilized along with the insertion instruments. A local anesthetic is administered to the maternal abdominal wall and fascia. Using continuous ultrasound guidance, a trocar is placed into the maternal abdomen and uterus and into the fetal thorax or bladder. A catheter is passed through the trocar and the proximal end is advanced into the fetus' thorax or bladder. The trocar is then withdrawn slightly to allow placement of the distal portion of the catheter in the amniotic cavity. Correct placement of the conduit is confirmed using ultrasound imaging. The trocar is removed and the patient and fetus are monitored as needed. Additional imaging is obtained to verify that the thorax or bladder is draining properly. The physician discusses the results of the procedure with the patient and prepares a written report.

59100

59100   Hysterotomy, abdominal (eg, for hydatidiform mole, abortion)

The physician performs an abdominal hysterotomy, which may be done to remove a hydatidiform mole (molar pregnancy), complete a failed abortion, or for another indication. A hydatidiform mole is a rare mass or growth formed by abnormally proliferating cells that are supposed to develop into the placenta. A complete molar pregnancy results in only a grapelike mass of placental tissue arising from the chorionic villi. A partial molar pregnancy contains both grapelike mass of abnormal placental tissue and some sign of nonviable embryonic or fetal development. The lower abdomen is incised and the uterus is exposed. The uterus is entered through the lower portion, as for a cesarean section, and the physician removes the hydatidiform mole or the nonviable fetus and placenta. If the procedure is performed for hydatidiform mole, the uterus is inspected to ensure that the entire mass and surrounding abnormal tissue have been removed and the tissue is sent to pathology as hydatidiform moles have a potential of developing into choriocarcinoma. If the procedure is for abortion, the placenta is examined and the uterus is inspected to ensure that all products of conception have been removed. Curettage may be done on the uterine cavity before The incision is closed with sutures. The abdomen is closed in layers.

59120-59121

59120   Surgical treatment of ectopic pregnancy; tubal or ovarian, requiring salpingectomy and/or oophorectomy, abdominal or vaginal approach

59121   Surgical treatment of ectopic pregnancy; tubal or ovarian, without salpingectomy and/or oophorectomy

An incision is made in the abdomen or through the vagina and the fallopian tube and/or ovary exposed. In 59120, the ectopic pregnancy is treated by excising the tube and/or ovary. For ovarian ectopic pregnancy treated by oophorectomy, the ovary is dissected fee of surrounding tissue and removed. For tubal ectopic pregnancy, the fallopian tube is clamped between the uterus and the ectopic pregnancy. The pedicle is divided and suture ligated. The tuboovarian artery is clamped, cut, and ligated. All or part of the fallopian tube is then dissected free of surrounding tissue and removed. In 59121, the ectopic pregnancy is treated without removing the tube or ovary. For an ovarian ectopic pregnancy, the ovary is grasped and the ectopic pregnancy dissected from the ovary using blunt and sharp dissection and removed. Bleeding is controlled with electrocautery. For tubal ectopic pregnancy, an incision is made in the antimesenteric side of the tube. The ectopic pregnancy is then dissected and dislodged by injecting saline deep into the fallopian tube using an aquadissector or syringe. The tube is irrigated at the site of the ectopic pregnancy and the products of conception are removed. Bleeding is controlled using electrocautery or suture ligation of vessels. The incision in the fallopian tube is left open to heal by secondary intention. Alternatively, a tubal pregnancy may be evacuated from the fimbriated end without an incision by milking the tube and expressing the pregnancy or grasping the fimbria, injecting saline, and irrigating and removing the products of conception.

59130

59130   Surgical treatment of ectopic pregnancy; abdominal pregnancy

An abdominal ectopic pregnancy is treated using an abdominal approach. Abdominal pregnancies are those involving extrauterine implantation of the fertilized ovum in the omentum, vital organs, or large vessels. The exact nature of the procedure depends on the location of the implantation and the gestational age. An incision is made in the abdomen and the site of the abdominal pregnancy is exposed. The placental blood supply is interrupted by ligating the umbilical cord and blood vessels. The embryo or fetus and membranes are surgically removed from the abdomen. If the placenta is attached to the fallopian tube, ovary, or other extra-uterine structure, it is also removed. The abdomen is irrigated and blood clots are removed. The abdomen is closed in layers.

59135-59136

59135   Surgical treatment of ectopic pregnancy; interstitial, uterine pregnancy requiring total hysterectomy

59136   Surgical treatment of ectopic pregnancy; interstitial, uterine pregnancy with partial resection of uterus

An interstitial pregnancy is a form of ectopic pregnancy in which the pregnancy is implanted in the interstitial segment of the fallopian tube. The interstitial segment of the fallopian tube lies within the muscular wall (myometrium) of the uterus. An interstitial pregnancy grows into and is surrounded by myometrial tissue. Another term used for interstitial pregnancy is cornual pregnancy. A cornual pregnancy is one that occurs in the interstitial segment of a unicornuate or bicornuate uterus. A unicornuate uterus is an anomaly in which the uterus is incompletely developed comprised of only one lateral half. A bicornuate uterus is another type of anomaly in which the uterus is divided into two lateral horns due to imperfect union of the paramesonephritic ducts. In 59135, the interstitial pregnancy is treated by total hysterectomy. An incision is made in the abdomen and the anterior uterine surface exposed. The peritoneum at the cervicovesical fold is incised. Blunt dissection is used to expose the broad ligament, round ligament and fallopian tubes. The cervix is palpated and the position of the bladder ascertained. The bladder is then dissected off the uterus and the dissection carried down to the vaginal wall. The posterior aspect of the uterus is visualized and inspected to verify that it is not adhered to the rectum. The uterine vessels are exposed, clamped, divided and suture ligated. The posterior cervical peritoneum is incised and the incision is extended around the cervix. The vaginal wall is incised and the cervix separated from the vagina. The fallopian tubes are transected above the level of the interstitial pregnancy. The uterus and cervix are removed. The vaginal opening is closed. The surgical site is inspected, bleeding controlled, and the abdominal incision closed. In 59136, a partial resection of the uterus is performed at the site of the interstitial pregnancy. The part of the uterus containing the interstitial pregnancy is dissected free from surrounding tissue and then excised. The surgical wound in the uterus is closed.

59140

59140   Surgical treatment of ectopic pregnancy; cervical, with evacuation

A cervical ectopic pregnancy is treated surgically by evacuation. Cervical pregnancy involves implantation of the fertilized ovum within the cervical stricture below the internal os. As the ovum grows, the trophoblast invades the endocervix and the pregnancy develops in the fibrous cervical canal. Patients typically present with vaginal bleeding. Conservative treatment is not often possible due to life threatening hemorrhage and hysterectomy is performed. When conservative treatment is possible, it is typically a combination of systemic chemotherapy and cervical evacuation and curettage, although evacuation and curettage is sometimes performed alone. The patient is first given multiple doses of methotrexate and leucovorin over a four day period. If the cervical pregnancy is complicated by hemorrhage, the cervical arteries are ligated. The products of conception are then evacuated from the cervical canal by sharp curettage or using a suction curette. Bleeding is controlled by cervical tamponade using a balloon catheter in the cervical canal or by cervical stay sutures. Another technique involves local injection of vasoconstrictors and cervical cerclage followed by cervical curettage and evacuation.

59150-59151

59150   Laparoscopic treatment of ectopic pregnancy; without salpingectomy and/or oophorectomy

59151   Laparoscopic treatment of ectopic pregnancy; with salpingectomy and/or oophorectomy

Three small incisions are made in the abdomen and ports placed. Pneumoperitoneum is established. The laparoscope is introduced and the presence and location of the ectopic pregnancy confirmed. In 59151, the ectopic pregnancy is treated by excising the tube and/or ovary. For ovarian ectopic pregnancy treated by oophorectomy, the ovary is dissected free of surrounding tissue using laser, electrocautery, clips, or scissors and the ovary is removed. For tubal ectopic pregnancy, the fallopian tube is removed by progressive coagulation and cutting of the mesosalpinx starting at the fimbriated end and progressing to the isthmus. The tuboovarian artery is compressed and dessicated. The tube is separated from the uterus using bipolar coagulation or loop-type ligation and division with scissors and removed. In 59150, the ectopic pregnancy is treated without removing the tube or ovary. For an ovarian ectopic pregnancy, the ovary is grasped and the ectopic pregnancy is removed from the ovary using blunt and sharp dissection. Bleeding is controlled with electrocautery. For tubal ectopic pregnancy, an incision is made in the antimesenteric side of the tube over the site of the tubal swelling. The ectopic pregnancy is then removed with forceps or dissected and dislodged by injecting saline deep into the fallopian tube using an aquadissector. The tube is irrigated. Bleeding is controlled using bipolar diathermy. The incision in the fallopian tube is left open to heal by secondary intention. Alternatively, a tubal pregnancy may be evacuated from the fimbriated end without an incision by milking the tube and expressing the pregnancy or by grasping the fimbria, injecting saline, and irrigating and removing the products of conception. Following completion of the procedure, the pneumoperitoneum is released and the abdomen is checked for bleeding. The abdomen is irrigated and all blood clots are evacuated. The laparoscope is removed.

59160

59160   Curettage, postpartum

Postpartum curettage is performed. A speculum is placed in the vagina. The cervix is exposed and cleansed with antiseptic solution. The anterior cervical lip is grasped with a tenaculum. A sound is then passed to determine the depth and angle of the uterus. A curette is inserted through the cervix and the uterine wall is scraped or suctioned. The tissue is sent for pathology exam. The tenaculum is removed and bleeding from the cervix is controlled with pressure.

59200

59200   Insertion of cervical dilator (eg, laminaria, prostaglandin) (separate procedure)

A cervical dilator such as a laminaria tent or prostaglandin is inserted into the cervix in a separate procedure. Prior to delivery, the cervix normally thins, softens, relaxes, and opens in response to uterine contractions. This is called cervical ripening. When cervical ripening is not rapid enough to facilitate delivery, a cervical dilator may be used. There are several commonly used types, including laminaria tents, prostaglandin gel, and prostaglandin mesh. Laminaria is a type of seaweed. A tube shaped piece of laminaria, called a laminaria tent is placed in the cervix. The laminaria absorbs water and swells, slowly dilating the cervical canal. Alternatively, a prostaglandin gel is placed in the cervix or prostaglandin mesh is placed in the vaginal vault. Prostaglandin is a potent, hormone-like substance used to induce natural labor that softens the cervix and causes uterine muscles to contract.

59300

59300   Episiotomy or vaginal repair, by other than attending

An episiotomy or vaginal tear occurring during vaginal delivery is repaired by a physician or other qualified health care professional other than the attending one that performed the delivery. Perineal lacerations are classified by depth from first to fourth degree and the required repair will depend on the depth of the laceration. Deep laceration (fourth degree) requires approximation of the rectal mucosa and internal and external anal sphincters. The rectal mucosa and anal sphincters are exposed by retracting the vaginal sidewalls. The apex of the rectal mucosal injury is identified and suture repaired carrying the repair to the level of the anal verge. The internal sphincter is identified and suture repaired. The external anal sphincter is then repaired using an end-to-end technique. The physician then begins repair of the vaginal laceration, or in the case of a second degree laceration, the physician begins the procedure by identifying the apex of the vaginal laceration and placing an anchoring suture approximately one cm above the apex. The vaginal mucosa and rectovaginal fascia are sutured closed down to the level of the hymenal ring. The transverse muscles of the perineal body are then identified on each side of the perineal laceration and reapproximated, followed by repair of the bulbocavernosus muscle. If the laceration has caused separation of the rectovaginal fascia from the perineal body, the fascia is reattached. Anatomical repair of the perineal muscles provides good approximation of the overlying skin and skin sutures are not generally required. If skin suture is required, running subcuticular sutures are used.

59320-59325

59320   Cerclage of cervix, during pregnancy; vaginal
59325   Cerclage of cervix, during pregnancy; abdominal

The physician performs cerclage of the cervix during pregnancy. This procedure is performed to treat an incompetent cervix. Other indications include: history of second trimester miscarriage, previous LEEP or cone biopsy of the cervix, other injury to the cervix. Cervical cerclage prevents the cervix from opening too soon and helps prevent premature labor and delivery. The procedure is typically performed at 12-14 weeks gestation, but may also be performed as an emergent procedure later in pregnancy if opening of the cervix is noted. In 59320, the cervical cerclage is placed using a vaginal approach. The physician may perform a McDonald type cerclage by weaving a pursestring suture in and out of the skin around the cervix and then tightening it to cinch the cervix together. Alternatively, using a Shirodkar type procedure, the pursestring suture is tunneled subcutaneously around the cervix and then cinched together. In 59325, an abdominal approach is used. An incision is made in the lower abdomen. A stitch is then placed through the lower part of the uterus to cinch the lower uterus and upper cervix together.

59350

59350   Hysterorrhaphy of ruptured uterus

The physician performs hysterorrhaphy to repair a rupture of the uterus occurring during childbirth. The abdomen is opened and explored and blood clots are removed. The uterus is lifted out of the abdomen to identify the site and extent of injury and determine the exact nature of the required repair. The bladder is separated from the lower edge of the uterine segment. Uterine vessels are located and ligated as needed. If the rupture has created a broad ligament hematoma, the round ligament is clamped, cut, and tied off, and the anterior leaf of the broad ligament is opened. The hematoma is drained. Any bleeding vessels are ligated. If the rupture extends into the cervix and vagina, the bladder is mobilized. The upper portion of the cervical injury is sutured first and then carried down

distally until the entire cervical/vaginal injury is repaired. The ureters are identified and protected. The uterine tear is then repaired in one or two layers. Bleeding is controlled by suture ligation of bleeding vessels. An abdominal drain is placed. Prior to closure, the bladder is inspected to ensure that it is free of injury. The abdomen is then closed in layers around the drain.

59400-59410

59400   Routine obstetric care including antepartum care, vaginal delivery (with or without episiotomy, and/or forceps) and postpartum care
59409   Vaginal delivery only (with or without episiotomy and/or forceps)
59410   Vaginal delivery only (with or without episiotomy and/or forceps); including postpartum care

Routine obstetric care including antepartum and postpartum care with vaginal delivery is performed. The physician provides routine prenatal office care including an initial maternal history and evaluation of the health status of the mother and fetus, monthly office visits for the first 28 weeks of gestation, biweekly visits to 36 weeks, and weekly visits thereafter. The patient is admitted to the hospital when labor begins. Depending on the stage of labor and following an initial assessment by hospital staff, the patient may be allowed to walk or engage in other activities. When active labor begins, the physician monitors the mother and fetus using fetal heart monitoring which will alert him/her to signs of fetal distress. If no contraindications arise, the physician delivers the baby vaginally. An episiotomy is performed if needed. The physician may also use forceps or vacuum extraction to assist the birth process. Following delivery of the baby, the umbilical cord is clamped and cut, the baby is evaluated, airways suctioned, and the baby is given to the parents to hold or to another physician/assistant if the baby requires additional monitoring or care. The physician delivers the placenta and examines the placenta and attached umbilical cord. The uterus is also checked to ensure that all placental tissue has been delivered. If an episiotomy has been performed or significant vaginal tearing has occurred, the episiotomy or tear is sutured. The physician attends the patient in the hospital and provides postpartum office follow-up. Use code 59400 when all of the above services are provided (antepartum care, vaginal delivery, and postpartum care). Use code 59409 when only the vaginal delivery is performed. Use code 59410 when the vaginal delivery and postpartum care are provided.

59412

59412   External cephalic version, with or without tocolysis

External cephalic version with or without tocolysis is performed. External cephalic version is used to rotate the fetus from a breech to a vertex (head down) presentation. Breech presentation includes frank breech with hips flexed and knees extended, complete breech with both hips and knees flexed, and footling breech with one or both hips extended and a foot presenting. The procedure is typically not performed until the mother has reached 37 weeks gestation or term. A separately reportable ultrasound is performed prior to the version to confirm the breech presentation of the fetus, evaluate the degree of engagement of the breech, evaluate amniotic fluid, identify the placental location, rule out congenital anomalies, and rule out a nuchal cord. A separately reportable nonstress test is performed to check for fetal heart rate abnormalities. If no contraindications exist, the physician proceeds with the planned version procedure. An intravenous line is placed. A tocolytic agent is administered as needed to suppress uterine contractions during the procedure. The mother is placed supine or in slight Trendelenberg position. The presenting part (buttocks, foot) is disengaged from the pelvis and the fetus is gently manipulated into a vertex (head down) position using a forward roll or back flip. Typically a forward roll is first attempted and if unsuccessful a back flip is performed. The non-stress test is repeated to check for fetal distress/bradycardia. A second ultrasound is obtained to verify the success or failure of the version procedure.

59414

59414   Delivery of placenta (separate procedure)

The physician delivers the placenta only in a separate procedure. Following vaginal delivery performed in another setting or by another physician, the placenta is delivered from the uterus. The placenta and attached umbilical cord are inspected for anomalies. The uterus is inspected to ensure that all placental tissue has been delivered.

59425-59426

59425   Antepartum care only; 4-6 visits
59426   Antepartum care only; 7 or more visits

The physician provides antepartum care only. The physician may provide antepartum care only due to termination of the pregnancy by miscarriage or abortion or the patient may be transferred to the care of another physician. An initial maternal history and evaluation of the health status of the mother and fetus is performed. On the initial and subsequent visits the mother is weighed, blood pressures and fetal heart tones are checked, and routine chemical urinalysis is performed. Use code 59425 when routine antepartum care is provided for four to six visits or code 59426 for seven or more visits.

59430

59430   Postpartum care only (separate procedure)

The physician performs postpartum care only in a separate procedure. The physician attends the patient in the hospital following a vaginal or cesarean delivery performed in another setting or by another provider. The physician also provides routine office follow-up of the patient following the delivery. For a cesarean delivery this includes a visit for suture removal and a subsequent visit for postpartum pelvic examination. For a vaginal delivery this includes the six week postpartum pelvic examination.

59510-59515

59510   Routine obstetric care including antepartum care, cesarean delivery, and postpartum care

59514   Cesarean delivery only

59515   Cesarean delivery only; including postpartum care

Routine obstetric care including antepartum and postpartum care with cesarean delivery is performed. The physician provides routine prenatal office care including an initial maternal history and evaluation of the health status of the mother and fetus, monthly office visits for the first 28 weeks of gestation, biweekly visits to 36 weeks, and weekly visits thereafter. The cesarean delivery may be planned and performed prior to the onset of labor or it may be performed due to maternal or fetal complications following the onset of labor. An epidural or other anesthetic is administered. An incision is made in the abdomen. The uterus is incised and amniotic fluid removed by suctioning. If the head of the baby is engaged in the pelvis, the physician first disengages the baby's head from the pelvis, delivers the head through the uterine incision, and then suctions the baby's airways. The baby is then completely removed from the uterus while the physician checks for and addresses any umbilical cord entanglement or other complications. The baby is shown to the parents and then placed in a warmer where it will be examined and attended by other physicians/assistants. The placenta is removed from the uterus and examined by the physician. The uterine incision is closed. The abdomen is closed in layers. The physician attends the patient in the hospital and provides post-cesarean office follow-up. Use code 59510 when all of the above services are provided (antepartum care, cesarean delivery, and postpartum care). Use code 59514 when only the cesarean delivery is performed. Use code 59515 when the cesarean delivery and postpartum care is provided.

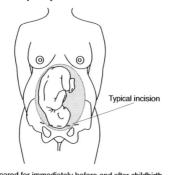

Routine obstetric care including antepartum care, cesarean delivery, and postpartum care

Typical incision

The patient is cared for immediately before and after childbirth, and is attended to during a childbirth by cesarean section

59525

59525   Subtotal or total hysterectomy after cesarean delivery (List separately in addition to code for primary procedure)

A subtotal or total hysterectomy is performed following a separately reportable cesarean delivery. The hysterectomy may be performed as a planned procedure for a medical indication discovered during the pregnancy such as cervical dysplasia or leiomyoma. The hysterectomy may also be performed as an emergent procedure after the cesarean. Total hysterectomy is removal of the entire uterus with the cervix, with or without including the ovaries. Subtotal hysterectomy is removal of the uterus, leaving the cervix. Following the cesarean delivery, the peritoneum at the cervicovesical fold is incised. Blunt dissection is used to expose the broad ligament, round ligament, and fallopian tubes. If the ovaries are to be removed, an incision is made in the exposed broad ligament. The ovarian vessels are visualized and suture ligated. The cut edges of the broad ligament are plicated with mattress sutures. The ovaries are dissected free of surrounding tissue if they are to be removed. The round ligaments are clamped and divided and blood vessels are suture ligated bilaterally. The cervix is palpated and the position of the bladder is ascertained. The bladder is then dissected off the uterus and the dissection is carried down to the vaginal wall. The posterior aspect of the uterus is visualized and inspected to verify that it is not adhered to the rectum. The uterine vessels are exposed, clamped, divided, and suture ligated. The posterior cervical peritoneum is incised and the incision is extended

around the cervix. The vaginal wall is incised and the cervix is separated from the vagina. The uterus and cervix are removed in a total hysterectomy. The cervix is left for a subtotal hysterectomy. The vaginal opening is closed. The surgical site is inspected; bleeding is controlled; and the abdominal incision is closed.

59610-59614

59610   Routine obstetric care including antepartum care, vaginal delivery (with or without episiotomy, and/or forceps) and postpartum care, after previous cesarean delivery

59612   Vaginal delivery only, after previous cesarean delivery (with or without episiotomy and/or forceps)

59614   Vaginal delivery only, after previous cesarean delivery (with or without episiotomy and/or forceps); including postpartum care

Routine obstetric care including antepartum and postpartum care with vaginal delivery is performed following a previous cesarean section. This may be referred to as a vaginal birth after cesarean (VBAC). The physician provides routine prenatal office care including an initial maternal history and evaluation of the health status of the mother and fetus, monthly office visits for the first 28 weeks of gestation, biweekly visits to 36 weeks, and weekly visits thereafter. The patient is admitted to the hospital when labor begins. Depending on the stage of labor and following an initial assessment by hospital staff, the patient may be allowed to walk or engage in other activities. When active labor begins, the physician closely monitors the mother and fetus using continuous fetal heart monitoring which will alert him/her to early signs of fetal distress or uterine rupture. If no contraindications arise, the physician delivers the baby vaginally. An episiotomy is performed if needed. The physician may also use forceps or vacuum extraction to assist the birth process. Following delivery of the baby, the umbilical cord is clamped and cut, the baby is evaluated, airways suctioned, and the baby is given to the parents to hold or to another physician/assistant if the baby requires additional monitoring or care. The physician delivers the placenta and examines the placenta and attached umbilical cord. The uterus is also checked to ensure that all placental tissue has been delivered. If an episiotomy has been performed or significant vaginal tearing has occurred, the episiotomy or tear is sutured. The physician attends the patient in the hospital and provides postpartum office follow-up. Use code 59610 when all of the above services are provided (antepartum care, VBAC delivery, and postpartum care). Use code 59612 when only the VBAC delivery is performed. Use code 59614 when the VBAC delivery and postpartum care is provided.

59618-59622

59618   Routine obstetric care including antepartum care, cesarean delivery, and postpartum care, following attempted vaginal delivery after previous cesarean delivery

59620   Cesarean delivery only, following attempted vaginal delivery after previous cesarean delivery

59622   Cesarean delivery only, following attempted vaginal delivery after previous cesarean delivery; including postpartum care

Routine obstetric care including antepartum and postpartum care with cesarean delivery is performed following attempted vaginal delivery after a previous cesarean section. This may be referred to as a cesarean delivery following failed trial of labor or a failed vaginal birth after cesarean (failed VBAC). The physician provides routine prenatal office care including an initial maternal history and evaluation of the health status of the mother and fetus, monthly office visits for the first 28 weeks of gestation, biweekly visits to 36 weeks, and weekly visits thereafter. Following a failed trial of labor the patient is transferred to the surgical suite and an epidural or other anesthetic administered. An incision is made in the abdomen. The uterus is incised and amniotic fluid removed by suctioning. Because of the attempted vaginal delivery, the head of the baby is likely engaged in the pelvis. The physician first disengages the baby's head from the pelvis, delivers the head through the uterine incision, and then suctions the baby's airways. The baby is then removed from the uterus while the physician checks for and addresses any umbilical cord entanglement or other complications. The baby is shown to the parents and then placed in a warmer where it will be examined and attended by other physicians/assistants. The placenta is removed from the uterus and examined by the physician. The uterine incision is closed. The abdomen is closed in layers. The physician attends the patient in the hospital and provides post-cesarean office follow-up. Use code 59618 when all of the above services are provided (antepartum care, cesarean delivery following failed VBAC, and postpartum care). Use code 59620 when only the cesarean delivery following the failed VBAC is performed. Use code 59622 when the cesarean delivery following failed VBAC and postpartum care are provided.

59812

59812   Treatment of incomplete abortion, any trimester, completed surgically

An incomplete abortion, also referred to as a spontaneous incomplete abortion, occurring during any trimester is completed surgically. An incomplete abortion exists when some of the products of conception have been expelled but some, typically the placenta, are still contained in the uterus. A speculum is placed in the vagina. The cervix is exposed and cleansed with antiseptic solution. The anterior cervical lip is grasped with a tenaculum. A sound is then passed to determine the depth and angle of the uterus. The cervix is numbed and dilated by passing a series of metal rods of increasing diameter into the cervical canal. Alternatively, a laminaria tent may be inserted into the cervix 8-20 hours prior to the procedure. The laminaria absorbs water and swells, slowly dilating the cervical canal. A curette is then inserted through the cervix and the uterine wall is scraped or suctioned to remove the retained products of conception. This tissue is sent for pathology exam. The tenaculum is removed and bleeding from the cervix is controlled with pressure.

59820-59821

59820 Treatment of missed abortion, completed surgically; first trimester
59821 Treatment of missed abortion, completed surgically; second trimester

A missed abortion is completed surgically. A missed abortion exists when the fetus dies in utero or is no longer developing but is not expelled from the uterus. Other terms for a missed abortion include anembryonic gestation, empty sac, and blighted ovum. Suction curettage is the most common surgical method used to treat a missed abortion. A speculum is placed in the vagina. The cervix is exposed and cleansed with antiseptic solution. The anterior cervical lip is grasped with a tenaculum. The cervix is numbed and dilated by passing a series of metal rods of increasing diameter into the cervical canal. Alternatively, a laminaria tent may be inserted into the cervix 8-20 hours prior to the procedure. The laminaria absorbs water and swells, slowly dilating the cervical canal. A suction curette is then inserted through the cervix and suction initiated while the curette is rotated in a full circle several times. When tissue and blood stop passing through the curette, the suction evacuation is complete. It is sometimes necessary to follow the suction curettage with sharp curettage and scraping of the uterus to ensure that all products of conception have been removed. The tissue is then sent for pathology exam. Following the procedure, the tenaculum is removed and bleeding from the cervix controlled with pressure. Use 59820 for a first trimester missed abortion completed by surgical evacuation and 59821 for a second trimester missed abortion.

59830

59830 Treatment of septic abortion, completed surgically

A septic abortion exists when the fetus dies in utero, and the mother develops an infection of the uterus or uterine contents before, during, or after the abortion. A separately reportable culture and sensitivity is performed on the vaginal discharge. An intravenous line is placed and antibiotics are administered. Suction curettage is the most common surgical method used to remove any retained products of conception. A speculum is placed in the vagina. The cervix is exposed and cleansed with antiseptic solution. The anterior cervical lip is grasped with a tenaculum. The cervix is numbed and dilated by passing a series of metal rods of increasing diameter into the cervical canal. A suction curette is then inserted through the cervix and suction initiated while the curette is rotated in a full circle several times. When tissue and blood stop passing through the curette, the suction evacuation is complete. It is sometimes necessary to follow the suction curettage with sharp curettage and scraping of the uterus to ensure that all products of conception have been removed. The tissue is then sent for pathology exam. Following the procedure, the tenaculum is removed and bleeding from the cervix controlled with pressure. The patient remains on intravenous or oral antibiotic therapy following the procedure.

59840-59841

59840 Induced abortion, by dilation and curettage
59841 Induced abortion, by dilation and evacuation

An induced abortion is performed by dilation and curettage (D&C) or dilation and evacuation. An induced abortion, also referred to as a therapeutic abortion, is one that is brought on intentionally. In 59840, the abortion is performed by D&C. A speculum is placed in the vagina. The cervix is exposed and cleansed with antiseptic solution. The anterior cervical lip is grasped with a tenaculum. A sound is then passed to determine the depth and angle of the uterus. The cervix is numbed and dilated by passing a series of metal rods of increasing diameter into the cervical canal. Alternatively, a laminaria tent may be inserted into the cervix 8-20 hours prior to the procedure. The laminaria absorbs water and swells, slowly dilating the cervical canal. A curette is then inserted through the cervix and the uterine wall is scraped. This tissue is sent for pathology exam. Following the procedure, the tenaculum is removed and bleeding from the cervix controlled with pressure. In 59841, the abortion is performed by dilation and evacuation, also referred to as suction curettage. The cervix is cleansed and dilated as described above. Following dilation of the cervix, a suction curette is inserted through the cervix and suction initiated while the curette is rotated in a full circle several times. When tissue and blood stop passing through the curette, the suction evacuation is complete. The tenaculum is removed and bleeding from the cervix controlled with pressure.

59850-59851

59850 Induced abortion, by 1 or more intra-amniotic injections (amniocentesis-injections), including hospital admission and visits, delivery of fetus and secundines
59851 Induced abortion, by 1 or more intra-amniotic injections (amniocentesis-injections), including hospital admission and visits, delivery of fetus and secundines; with dilation and curettage and/or evacuation

An induced abortion, also referred to as a therapeutic abortion, is performed using one or more intra-amniotic injections (amniocentesis injections). Agents injected or instilled include hypertonic saline, hypertonic urea, or prostaglandin F2a. Induced abortion by instillation technique is reserved for patients in the second trimester of pregnancy. The procedure includes hospital admission and physician visits and the delivery of the fetus and secundines with or without dilation and curettage or evacuation. Eight to 24 hours prior to the planned induced abortion, laminaria, prostaglandin, or other cervical dilator, is inserted into the cervix. Following confirmation of cervical dilation, the abdomen is cleansed, a pocket of amniotic fluid identified by ultrasound, and a needle placed in the amniotic fluid pocket. Alternatively, a local anesthetic is administered at the planned amniocentesis puncture site and a spinal needle introduced into the amniotic sac and free flow of amniotic fluid confirmed. A cannula is then inserted through the needle. The needle is withdrawn. The first intra-amniotic injection is performed which causes fetal demise and induces labor. Uterine and fetal activity are monitored along with vital signs of the mother. Additional intra-amniotic injections are performed as needed. The fetus and placenta are delivered vaginally. The products of conception are inspected to verify that the abortion is complete. If an incomplete abortion occurs, a dilation and curettage or evacuation is performed. A speculum is placed in the vagina. The cervix is exposed and cleansed with antiseptic solution. The anterior cervical lip is grasped with a tenaculum. A sound is then passed to determine the depth and angle of the uterus. A curette is inserted through the cervix and the uterine wall is scraped or suctioned. This tissue is sent for pathology exam. Following the procedure, the tenaculum is removed and bleeding from the cervix controlled with pressure. Use code 59850 when the procedure is performed without dilation and curettage or evacuation. Use code 59851 for an incomplete induced abortion requiring dilation and curettage or evacuation.

59852

59852 Induced abortion, by 1 or more intra-amniotic injections (amniocentesis-injections), including hospital admission and visits, delivery of fetus and secundines; with hysterotomy (failed intra-amniotic injection)

An induced abortion, also referred to as a therapeutic abortion, is attempted using one or more intra-amniotic injections (amniocentesis injections) followed by hysterotomy for failed intra-amniotic injection. The procedure includes hospital admission and physician visits. A local anesthetic is administered at the planned amniocentesis puncture site. A needle is introduced into the amniotic sac followed by a cannula inserted through the needle. The needle is withdrawn. The first intra-amniotic injection is performed which causes fetal demise and induces labor. Uterine and fetal activity are monitored along with vital signs of the mother. Additional intra-amniotic injections may be performed in an attempt to stimulate uterine contractions and abort the fetus. When it is evident that the intra-amniotic injections have failed, a hysterotomy is performed. The abdomen is incised and the uterus is exposed and incised. The physician removes the fetus and placenta. The placenta is examined and the uterus is inspected to ensure that all products of conception have been removed. The uterine incision is closed and the abdomen is closed in layers.

59855-59856

59855 Induced abortion, by 1 or more vaginal suppositories (eg, prostaglandin) with or without cervical dilation (eg, laminaria), including hospital admission and visits, delivery of fetus and secundines
59856 Induced abortion, by 1 or more vaginal suppositories (eg, prostaglandin) with or without cervical dilation (eg, laminaria), including hospital admission and visits, delivery of fetus and secundines; with dilation and curettage and/or evacuation

An induced abortion, also referred to as a therapeutic abortion, is performed using one or more vaginal suppositories with or without cervical dilation. Medical abortion agents used include mifepristone with misoprostol, methotrexate with misoprostol, or misoprostol used alone. The procedure includes hospital admission and physician visits and the delivery of the fetus and secundines with or without dilation and curettage or evacuation. For a second trimester abortion, passive dilators, such as laminaria or a balloon catheter are inserted into the cervix. A suppository is inserted into the vaginal fornix. Uterine and fetal activity are monitored along with vital signs of the mother. Additional vaginal suppositories are inserted as needed at six to 12 hour intervals. The fetus and placenta are delivered vaginally. The products of conception are inspected to verify that the abortion is complete. Following delivery of the fetus, intravenous oxytocin is administered. If an incomplete abortion occurs, a dilation and curettage or evacuation is performed. A speculum is placed in the vagina. The cervix is exposed and cleansed with antiseptic solution. The anterior cervical lip is grasped with a tenaculum. A sound is then passed to determine the depth and angle of the uterus. A curette is inserted through the cervix and the uterine wall is scraped or

● New Code   ▲ Revised Code

Maternity Care/Endocrine System

suctioned. This tissue is sent for pathology exam. Following the procedure, the tenaculum is removed and bleeding from the cervix controlled with pressure. Use code 59855 when the procedure is performed without dilation and curettage or evacuation. Use code 59856 for an incomplete induced abortion requiring dilation and curettage or evacuation.

59857

59857   Induced abortion, by 1 or more vaginal suppositories (eg, prostaglandin) with or without cervical dilation (eg, laminaria), including hospital admission and visits, delivery of fetus and secundines; with hysterotomy (failed medical evacuation)

An induced abortion, also referred to as a therapeutic abortion, is attempted using one or more vaginal suppositories with or without cervical dilation followed by hysterotomy for failed medical evacuation. Medical abortion agents used include mifepristone with misoprostol, methotrexate with misoprostol, or misoprostol used alone. The procedure includes hospital admission, physician visits, and the delivery of the fetus and secundines. For a second trimester abortion, passive cervical dilators, such as laminaria or a balloon catheter are inserted into the cervix. A suppository such as prostaglandin is inserted into the vaginal fornix. Prostaglandin is a potent, hormone-like substance used to induce natural labor that softens the cervix and causes uterine muscles to contract. Uterine and fetal activity are monitored along with vital signs of the mother. Additional vaginal suppositories are inserted as needed at 6-12 hour intervals. When it is evident that the attempted medical evacuation has failed, a hysterotomy is performed. The abdomen is incised and the uterus is exposed and incised. The physician removes the fetus and placenta. The placenta is examined and the uterus is inspected to insure that all products of conception have been removed. The uterine incision is closed and the abdomen is closed in layers.

59866

59866   Multifetal pregnancy reduction(s) (MPR)

Multifetal pregnancy reduction (MPR, MFPR) is performed to induce fetal demise of one or more of the fetuses in order to allow the pregnancy to continue with improved chances that one or more healthy fetuses can be carried to term and to reduce the risk of complications associated with preterm delivery. Following patient counseling, confirmation of gestational age at 9-12 weeks, and fetal genetic testing, the physician prepares the patient for MPR. The abdomen is cleansed and a local anesthetic is administered. Using ultrasound guidance, a needle is inserted through the abdomen and into the uterus. The needle is then advanced into the thorax or other site of the selected fetus and potassium chloride solution is injected which stops the fetal heart. The procedure is repeated until the desired number of remaining viable fetuses is reached. The fetuses that have been injected are no longer viable and will be reabsorbed by the mother.

59870

59870   Uterine evacuation and curettage for hydatidiform mole

Uterine evacuation and curettage is performed for hydatidiform mole, also referred to as a molar pregnancy. A hydatidiform mole is a rare mass or growth formed by abnormally proliferating cells that are supposed to develop into the placenta. A complete molar pregnancy results in only a grapelike mass of placental tissue arising from the chorionic villi. A partial molar pregnancy contains both grapelike mass of abnormal placental tissue and some sign of nonviable embryonic or fetal development. The cervix is exposed and cleansed with antiseptic solution. The anterior cervical lip is grasped with a tenaculum. A sound is then passed to determine the depth and angle of the uterus. The cervix is numbed and dilated by passing a series of metal rods of increasing diameter into the cervical canal. Alternatively, a laminaria tent may be inserted into the cervix 8-20 hours prior to the procedure. The laminaria absorbs water and swells, slowly dilating the cervical canal. A curette is then inserted through the cervix and the uterine wall is scraped. Alternatively, a suction curette is inserted and suction is initiated while the curette is rotated in a full circle several times. When tissue and blood stop passing through the curette, the suction evacuation is complete. This tissue is sent for pathology exam. The tenaculum is removed and bleeding from the cervix is controlled with pressure.

59871

59871   Removal of cerclage suture under anesthesia (other than local)

A cervical cerclage suture is removed under regional or general anesthesia either prior to the onset of labor or after the global period for placement of the cerclage. If the patient is planning to deliver vaginally, the cerclage is typically removed around 36-37 weeks gestation in an office procedure using only a local anesthetic. If the patient is scheduled for a cesarean delivery, the cerclage is removed at the time of the cesarean. However, when complications arise, especially if the cerclage was placed through an abdominal incision, it is sometimes necessary to remove the cerclage under regional or general anesthesia at a time other than the delivery. To remove a transabdominally placed cerclage, the lower abdomen is incised. Dissection is carried down to the cervix and the cerclage sutures are exposed and removed.

60000

60000   Incision and drainage of thyroglossal duct cyst, infected

The thyroglossal duct is present during fetal development and allows the thyroid gland to move from the base of the tongue to its final position in the neck. It normally disappears once the thyroid gland reaches its final position. However, in some individuals, remnants of the duct remain leaving cavities in the neck that can fill with fluid or mucus and become infected. The enlarged area of the neck is palpated and the skin incised over the area of greatest fluctuance. The cyst cavity is opened and the cyst drained. Blunt finger dissection is used to break up any loculations. The cyst may be packed with gauze or a drain placed. Incision and drainage is rarely performed because it can lead to scarring that can make future infections difficult to treat. Preferred treatment is antibiotic therapy and excision of the cyst.

60100

60100   Biopsy thyroid, percutaneous core needle

Separately reportable imaging guidance may be used. The skin over the thyroid gland is cleansed and a local anesthetic administered. A large bore needle is introduced into the thyroid and a tissue sample obtained. The needle may be passed multiple times into different sites in the thyroid to obtain an adequate tissue sample. The tissue sample is sent to the laboratory for separately reportable histological evaluation.

60200

60200   Excision of cyst or adenoma of thyroid, or transection of isthmus

The thyroid is composed of two lobes and a central isthmus that connects the two lobes. Thyroid cysts or fluid filled nodules are typically benign lesions. Thyroid adenomas are benign tumors that originate in the cell layer that lines the inner surface of the thyroid gland. Thyroid adenomas secrete thyroid hormone which may cause hyperthyroidism. The neck is extended and a transverse skin incision made over the thyroid in one of the neck creases. The incision is carried down through skin subcutaneous tissue and the platysma taking care to protect the laryngeal nerve and the parathyroid glands. The thyroid gland is exposed and the cyst or adenoma identified. The cyst or adenoma is dissected from surrounding tissue, removed, and sent to the laboratory for separately reportable pathological evaluation. An incision is made in the isthmus and the cross-section containing the cyst or adenoma removed. The neck incision is closed in layers.

Excision of cyst or adenoma of thyroid

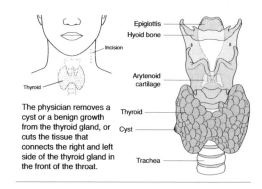

The physician removes a cyst or a benign growth from the thyroid gland, or cuts the tissue that connects the right and left side of the thyroid gland in the front of the throat.

60210-60212

60210   Partial thyroid lobectomy, unilateral; with or without isthmusectomy

60212   Partial thyroid lobectomy, unilateral; with contralateral subtotal lobectomy, including isthmusectomy

The thyroid is composed of two lobes and a central isthmus that connects the two lobes. Partial thyroid lobectomy is not commonly performed. One indication is a hot nodule in the upper or lower portion of one of the lobes that is causing hyperthyroidism. The neck is extended and a transverse skin incision made over the thyroid in one of the neck creases. The incision is carried down through subcutaneous tissue and the platysma taking care to protect the laryngeal nerve and the parathyroid glands. The thyroid gland is exposed. In 60210, part of one of the lobes is excised. If a wider margin is required to ensure that all diseased tissue has been removed, part of or the entire isthmus is also excised. In 60212, part of one of the lobes, part or all of the isthmus and, part of the opposite (contralateral) lobe is removed and sent to the laboratory for separately reportable pathological evaluation. The neck incision is closed in layers.

● New Code   ▲ Revised Code

60220-60225

60220 Total thyroid lobectomy, unilateral; with or without isthmusectomy
60225 Total thyroid lobectomy, unilateral; with contralateral subtotal lobectomy, including isthmusectomy

The thyroid is composed of two lobes and a central isthmus that connects the two lobes. Total thyroid lobectomy is performed for solitary nodules confined to a single lobe that have a high probability of malignancy or are indeterminate following biopsy, follicular adenomas, solitary hot or cold nodules, or goiters contained in one lobe. A transverse skin incision made over the thyroid in one of the neck creases. The incision is carried down through subcutaneous tissue and the platysma taking care to protect the laryngeal nerve and the parathyroid glands. The thyroid gland is exposed. In 60220, the entire lobe on one side is excised. If a wider margin is required to ensure that all diseased tissue has been removed, part or the entire isthmus is also excised. In 60225, the entire on one side, part or all of the isthmus and, part of the opposite (contralateral) lobe is removed and sent to the laboratory for separately reportable pathological evaluation. The neck incision is closed in layers.

60240

60240 Thyroidectomy, total or complete

The thyroid is composed of two lobes and a central isthmus that connects the two lobes. The neck is extended and a transverse skin incision made over the thyroid in one of the neck creases. The incision is carried down through subcutaneous tissue and the platysma. The middle thyroid vein is identified and ligated. The recurrent laryngeal nerve and parathyroid glands are identified and preserved. Blood vessels in the superior pole of the thyroid are identified and ligated followed by ligation of the terminal branches of the inferior thyroid artery. The Berry ligament is divided and the isthmus elevated off the trachea. The thyroid is then removed. The surgical wounds are repaired and suction drains placed as needed.

60252-60254

60252 Thyroidectomy, total or subtotal for malignancy; with limited neck dissection
60254 Thyroidectomy, total or subtotal for malignancy; with radical neck dissection

The thyroid is composed of two lobes and a central isthmus that connects the two lobes. A total thyroidectomy removes entire thyroid while a subtotal thyroidectomy removes one entire lobe, the isthmus, and the majority of the opposite (contralateral) lobe. The neck is extended and a transverse skin incision made over the thyroid in one of the neck creases. The incision is carried down through subcutaneous tissue and the platysma. The middle thyroid vein is identified and ligated. The recurrent laryngeal nerve and parathyroid glands are identified and preserved. Blood vessels in the superior pole of the thyroid are identified and ligated followed by ligation of the terminal branches of the inferior thyroid artery. The Berry ligament is divided and the isthmus elevated off the trachea. The entire thyroid or the majority of the thyroid is then removed. In 60252, a limited neck dissection is then performed. The lymph nodes of the perithyroid region are carefully inspected. Involved lymph node groups are dissected free of surrounding tissues and excised. The sternocleidomastoid and jugular vein are preserved. In 60254, a radical neck dissection (RND) is then performed. The surgical wounds are repaired and suction drains placed as needed. The lymph node groups levels I-V are dissected free of surrounding tissue and excised. The sternocleidomastoid muscle and the internal jugular vein are removed. The submandibular gland on the affected side is removed. The anterior belly of the digastric muscle as well as the sternohyoid and sternothyroid muscles may also be removed. The surgical wounds are repaired and suction drains placed as needed.

60260

60260 Thyroidectomy, removal of all remaining thyroid tissue following previous removal of a portion of thyroid

The neck is extended and a transverse skin incision made over the thyroid in one of the neck creases. The incision is carried down through subcutaneous tissue and the platysma and the remaining thyroid tissue is exposed. The exact procedure depends on the amount of remaining thyroid tissue. The middle thyroid vein is identified and ligated. The recurrent laryngeal nerve and parathyroid glands are identified and preserved. Blood vessels in the superior pole of the thyroid are identified and ligated followed by ligation of the terminal branches of the inferior thyroid artery. The Berry ligament is divided and the isthmus elevated off the trachea. The remaining thyroid tissue is then removed. The surgical wounds are repaired and suction drains placed as needed.

60270-60271

60270 Thyroidectomy, including substernal thyroid; sternal split or transthoracic approach
60271 Thyroidectomy, including substernal thyroid; cervical approach

A thyroidectomy including substernal thyroid is performed using a sternal split or transthoracic approach (60270) or cervical approach (60271). The normal thyroid gland

is located in the neck and has two lobes that wrap around the trachea. Enlargement of the thyroid sometimes causes the thyroid to grow down the neck and into the chest resulting in a substernal thyroid. Excision of the substernal thyroid is performed first. In 60270, a sternotomy or thoracotomy is performed to expose the substernal thyroid. The substernal thyroid is separated from fibrous attachments and lifted into the neck. In 60271, the thyroid is approached using a supraclavicular incision. The portion of the thyroid extending into the mediastinum is dissected using finger dissection to separate the thyroid from fibrous attachments. Once all attachments have been severed, the substernal thyroid is lifted from the mediastinum and delivered into the neck. The physician then proceeds with the thyroidectomy. The middle thyroid vein is identified and ligated. The recurrent laryngeal nerve and parathyroid glands are identified and preserved. Blood vessels in the superior pole of the thyroid are identified and ligated followed by ligation of the terminal branches of the inferior thyroid artery. The Berry ligament is divided and the isthmus elevated off the trachea. The thyroid is then removed. The surgical wounds are repaired and suction drains placed as needed.

60280-60281

60280 Excision of thyroglossal duct cyst or sinus
60281 Excision of thyroglossal duct cyst or sinus; recurrent

The formation of a thyroglossal duct cyst is one of the most common congenital malformations in the neck midline. The cysts appear as small lumps in the center of the neck. When the thyroid gland is developing, the embryonic cells travel the thryoglossal duct from the base of the tongue to the gland's location in the neck. Once there, the duct disappears, or involutes. When the duct fails involution, remnants create pockets, or cysts, that can fill up with fluid or mucus. A sinus occurs when the tube remains and opens out onto the skin. With the Sistrunk procedure, the recurrence rate for duct remnants becoming fluid-filled cysts has dropped significantly. A midline incision is made in the neck with careful dissection up to the hyoid bone in the upper neck. Careful attention not to deviate from the midline is given in order to protect the hypoglossal nerve from damage. The small hyoid bone is in close connection with the thyroglossal duct tract as it runs into the deeper tissue of the tongue. The central portion of the hyoid bone is therefore removed along with a cuff of tongue tissue along the tract of the cyst or sinus. The wound is closed with absorbable sutures and the skin is closed with Derma-Bond, or Steri-Strips, so there are no sutures to be removed for the child. A light pressure dressing is wrapped around the neck. Report 60281 if the excision is done for a recurrent thyroglossal duct cyst or sinus.

60300

60300 Aspiration and/or injection, thyroid cyst

The thyroid is a butterfly shaped gland located in the anterior aspect of the neck. A thyroid cyst is a fluid filled sac occurring in the thyroid gland that may be small or large and may appear suddenly or develop gradually. Some cysts are entirely filled with fluid while others contain both fluid and solid components. The thyroid is palpated and the cyst is located. The skin is cleansed and a needle is inserted into the cyst. The fluid is aspirated (drained), and the aspiration may be followed by injection of medication, such as ethanol, to destroy the cyst.

60500-60512

60500 Parathyroidectomy or exploration of parathyroid(s)
60502 Parathyroidectomy or exploration of parathyroid(s); re-exploration
60505 Parathyroidectomy or exploration of parathyroid(s); with mediastinal exploration, sternal split or transthoracic approach
60512 Parathyroid autotransplantation (List separately in addition to code for primary procedure)

If all parathyroid glands must be removed, the physician will also perform a parathyroid autotransplantation of parathyroid tissue. There are four parathyroid glands that are located behind the thyroid, two in each lobe at the lateral upper and lower aspects of the lobes. The parathyroid glands monitor and regulate calcium levels in the blood by secreting parathyroid hormone when blood calcium levels fall and stopping secretion when blood calcium levels return to normal. Exploration with excision of one or more parathyroids is performed for enlargement of one or more glands which is usually indicative of a parathyroid adenoma. Parathyroid adenomas cause overproduction of parathyroid hormone (hyperparathyroidism). A transverse skin incision is made in the neck over the thyroid in one of the skin creases. The incision is carried down through subcutaneous tissue and the platysma. The thyroid is elevated. The enlarged parathyroid gland is exposed, dissected from surrounding tissue and removed. The physician may expose the remaining parathyroid glands to confirm that they are of normal size. If other glands are found to be enlarged, they are also removed. If all four glands must be removed, the physician will perform a separately reportable parathyroid autotransplantation. One or two parathyroid glands are sliced into small (1x3 mm) pieces. Normal parathyroid tissue is dissected from the slices. The sternocleidomastoid muscle or a muscle in the forearm is opened and a pocket created. Three to four pieces of normal parathyroid tissue are then implanted into the muscle. Use 60500 for the initial surgical procedure to explore and/or excise one or more parathyroids and 60502 for a re-exploration procedure. Use 60505 when a sternal split or transthoracic approach is required to expose the enlarged parathyroid gland. The mediastinum is dissected and explored. The enlarged parathyroid gland is located and explored or excised as described above. Use 60512 when parathyroid autotransplantation is performed.

60520

60520 Thymectomy, partial or total; transcervical approach (separate procedure)

The thymus is a small organ in the upper chest, under the sternum and extending from the base of the throat to the front of the heart. During fetal development and childhood, the thymus produces and aides in the maturation of T-lymphocytes. It reaches its maximum size during puberty and then decreases in size and is replaced by fatty tissue in adulthood. Thymectomy may be done to treat non-metastatic thymoma, thymic carcinoid, thymic carcinoma, or myasthenia gravis. An incision is made above the sternal notch between the sterncleidomastoid muscle. Subplatysmal skin flaps are raised superiorly to the thyroid cartilage and inferiorly to the sternal notch. The strap muscles are dissected in the midline and the upper poles of the thymus are exposed. The upper poles are dissected off surrounding tissue. The thyrothymic ligaments at the superior aspect of the thymus are suture ligated and divided. Dissection of the thymus continues into the superior mediastinum. The thymic veins are isolated and suture ligated. The posterior aspect of the thymus is dissected to a level behind and inferior to the innominate vein. The anterior thymus is dissected from the chest wall. The left lung is deflated and the mediastinal pleura is opened from the diaphragm to the innominate vein. Care is taken to protect the phrenic nerve and internal mammary vessels. The thymus is grasped, retracted, and dissected medially off the anterior surface of the pericardium. Dissection continues as far right of the midline as possible. The left lung is re-inflated; the right lung is deflated; and the right pleura is opened. The phrenic nerve is identified and protected. The thymus is then dissected off the pericardium on the right side and dissection continues until the thymus is free of the mediastinum. The thymus is then removed through the cervical incision as is any remaining mediastinal or pericardial fat. A drain is placed and the right lung is reinflated. The cervical incisions are closed in layered fashion.

60521-60522

60521 Thymectomy, partial or total; sternal split or transthoracic approach, without radical mediastinal dissection (separate procedure)

60522 Thymectomy, partial or total; sternal split or transthoracic approach, with radical mediastinal dissection (separate procedure)

A partial or total thymectomy is performed by sternal split or transthoracic approach. The thymus is a small organ situated in the upper chest under the sternum and extending from the base of the throat to the front of the heart. During fetal development and childhood the thymus produces and aides in the maturation of T-lymphocytes, a white blood cell important in immune response. The thymus reaches its maximum size during puberty and then decreases in size and is replaced by fat tissue in adulthood. Thymectomy may be performed for treatment of non-metastatic thymoma, thymic carcinoid, thymic carcinoma, or myasthenia gravis. If a sternal split is used, the skin is incised over the sternum, the manubrium exposed and completely divided, and the sternal split carried down to the third or fourth intercostal space. The sternum is retracted, both pleural spaces are opened, and the phrenic nerves identified. The overlying mediastinal pleura is divided and the anterior thymus and innominate vein exposed. The thymus along with fat overlying the pericardium is mobilized off the pericardium beginning at the right inferior horn. Once the lower horn is completely free of the pericardium, the right superior horn is mobilized. The thyrothymic ligament is exposed and the right superior horn is divided from the thyroid gland. The thyrothymic ligament is ligated. The thymus is retracted toward the left and the lateral arterial blood supply from the internal mammary artery is isolated, ligated and divided. The left lower and left upper horns of the thymus are freed in the same manner. Following mobilization of all four horns, the innominate vein is clamped, divided, and suture ligated. The thymus is then removed. If a thymic mass is present, frozen sections are taken and sent to pathology. Adjacent anatomic structures are inspected for possible metastatic lesions. If metastatic lesions are identified, the involved structures are removed along with the thymus. A chest tube is placed, the sternum is closed with wire sutures, and the soft tissue and skin closed with absorbable stitches. Use code 60521 for partial or total thymectomy without radical mediastinal dissection. Use 60522 when metastatic lesions necessitate radical mediastinal dissection with removal of involved tissue and mediastinal structures.

60540-60545

60540 Adrenalectomy, partial or complete, or exploration of adrenal gland with or without biopsy, transabdominal, lumbar or dorsal (separate procedure)

60545 Adrenalectomy, partial or complete, or exploration of adrenal gland with or without biopsy, transabdominal, lumbar or dorsal (separate procedure); with excision of adjacent retroperitoneal tumor

The adrenal glands are paired endocrine glands located above each kidney. The adrenal glands excrete hormones including epinephrine, norepinephrine, androgens, estrogens, aldosterone, and cortisol. Exploration, biopsy, and/or excision is typically performed for enlargement or tumors of these glands. Tumors often excrete excessive amounts of hormones causing severe hormonal imbalances. The adrenal gland is typically approached through an anterior or posterior subcostal incision, a midline abdominal incision, or a

flank incision. Overlying tissues are dissected and the adrenal gland exposed. If exploration and biopsy is performed, the adrenal gland is carefully inspected and a tissue sample obtained. If the adrenal gland is excised, blood vessels supplying the adrenal gland are ligated and divided. The adrenal gland is dissected free of surrounding tissue and removed. The wound is irrigated with sterile saline and the wound closed in layers. Use 60540 when exploration and excision of the adrenal gland is performed without excision of an adjacent retroperitoneal tumor and 60545 when an adjacent retroperitoneal tumor is also excised. The most common approach is an abdominal transperitoneal route. The tumor is typically excised along with a wide margin of normal tissue to ensure that all tumor tissue is removed.

60600-60605

60600 Excision of carotid body tumor; without excision of carotid artery

60605 Excision of carotid body tumor; with excision of carotid artery

The physician excises a carotid body tumor. The carotid bodies are a collection of paraganglionic cells called glomus tissue located at the bifurcation of the common carotid arteries into the internal and external carotid arteries. The carotid bodies detect changes in arterial blood, such as high levels of carbon dioxide or low levels of oxygen, and then initiate an autonomic response that leads to changes in respiratory and heart rate in response to these changes to counteract the changes. Carotid body tumors, also referred to as glomus tumors or paragangliomas, are benign tumors. An incision is made in the neck over the bifurcation of the common carotid artery. Vessel loops are used to control proximal and distal blood vessels. The tumor is carefully dissected from the common carotid artery and surrounding tissues. The dissection is extended in a superior direction taking care to protect the internal carotid artery. The tumor is dissected from the internal and external carotid arteries. Once the tumor is freed from all attachments it is removed. Use 60600 for excision of carotid body tumor without excision of the carotid artery. Use 60605 when a portion of the carotid artery must be excised to accomplish the tumor excision.

Excision of carotid body tumor

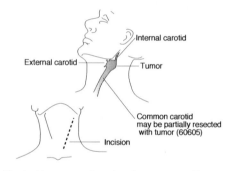

The physician removes a tumor from the common carotid artery

60650

60650 Laparoscopy, surgical, with adrenalectomy, partial or complete, or exploration of adrenal gland with or without biopsy, transabdominal, lumbar or dorsal

The adrenal glands are paired endocrine glands located above each kidney. The adrenal glands excrete hormones including epinephrine, norepinephrine, androgens, estrogens, aldosterone, and cortisol. Exploration, biopsy, and/or excision is typically performed for enlargement or tumors of these glands. Tumors often excrete excessive amounts of hormones causing severe hormonal imbalances. Laparoscopic surgery is typically performed using an abdominal transperitoneal approach, although a retroperitoneal approach is sometimes used instead. A small incision is made in the upper abdomen on the affected side. A trocar is placed and the laparoscope introduced into the abdomen. Pneumoperitoneum is established. If the affected adrenal gland is on the right, the right lobe of the liver is mobilized. The triangular ligament is incised up to the diaphragm. The retroperitoneum is opened. The inferior vena cava is identified and a plane of dissection developed between the vena cava and the adrenal gland. If the affected adrenal gland is on the left, the splenic flexure and pancreas are mobilized and the retroperitoneum opened. Surrounding tissues are dissected and the adrenal gland exposed. If exploration and biopsy is performed, the adrenal gland is carefully inspected and a tissue sample obtained. If the adrenal gland is excised, the adrenal vein and other blood vessels supplying the adrenal gland are ligated and divided. The adrenal gland is dissected free of surrounding tissue, placed in an endobag, and removed. The surgical instruments are removed, gas released from the abdomen, and the laparoscope and trocars are removed. Portal incisions are closed.

61000-61001

61000 Subdural tap through fontanelle, or suture, infant, unilateral or bilateral; initial

61001 Subdural tap through fontanelle, or suture, infant, unilateral or bilateral; subsequent taps

A unilateral or bilateral subdural tap through a fontanelle or suture is performed on an infant. The procedure is typically performed through the lateral aspect of the anterior fontanelle. The scalp is shaved over the planned tap site. Using Z-track insertion technique with the skin displaced laterally over the anterior fontanelle, a subdural or spinal needle is advanced at a 90 degree angle through the skin at the lateral aspect of the coronal suture of the anterior fontanelle. The subdural or spinal needle is then advanced through the dura into the subdural space. The stylet is removed and cerebrospinal fluid and blood is drained. The stylet is then replaced, the needle removed, and a dressing applied. The procedure is repeated as needed on the opposite side. Use code 61000 for the initial unilateral or bilateral subdural tap and code 61001 for a subsequent unilateral or bilateral tap.

61020-61026

61020 Ventricular puncture through previous burr hole, fontanelle, suture, or implanted ventricular catheter/reservoir; without injection

61026 Ventricular puncture through previous burr hole, fontanelle, suture, or implanted ventricular catheter/reservoir; with injection of medication or other substance for diagnosis or treatment

A ventricular puncture through a previous burr hole, fontanelle, suture, or an implanted ventricular catheter/reservoir is performed without injection. The hair is cut or the scalp is shaved over the planned puncture site. If the procedure is performed through a previous burr hole, fontanelle or suture, a spinal needle is advanced through the skin and into the ventricle. The stylet is removed and cerebrospinal fluid and blood is drained. The stylet is then replaced, the needle removed, and a dressing applied. If the procedure is performed through an implanted ventricular catheter/reservoir, the needle is inserted at a 30 to 45 degree angle through the skin into the reservoir bladder. Cerebrospinal fluid and blood is drained. As the intracranial pressure reduces, the flow rate will slow. When the pressure has been reduced sufficiently, the needle is removed and firm pressure is applied to the puncture site until drainage has stopped. Use code 61026 when ventricular puncture is performed through a previous burr hole, fontanelle, suture, or an implanted ventricular catheter/reservoir with injection of medication or other substance for diagnosis or treatment. The puncture procedure is performed as described above. As cerebrospinal fluid is withdrawn from the ventricle an equal amount of medication or other substance, such as gas, contrast media, dye, or radioactive material, is instilled. The head is then rotated to disperse the medication or other substance. If the injection is performed for ventriculography, separately reportable radiographs are obtained.

61050-61055

61050 Cisternal or lateral cervical (C1-C2) puncture; without injection (separate procedure)

61055 Cisternal or lateral cervical (C1-C2) puncture; with injection of medication or other substance for diagnosis or treatment

A cisternal or lateral cervical (C1-C2) puncture is performed without injection. A cisternal puncture uses a spinal needle placed below the occipital bone at the back of the skull. Alternatively, the subarachnoid space in the posterior aspect of the spinal canal can be approached from a lateral direction. The needle shaft is held in place by the muscles in the lateral neck. After insertion of the needle, the stylet is removed and cerebrospinal fluid and blood is drained. The stylet is then replaced and a dressing applied. Use code 61055 for a cisternal or lateral cervical puncture performed with injection of medication or other substance for diagnosis or treatment. The puncture procedure is performed as described above. As cerebrospinal fluid is withdrawn from the subarachnoid space, an equal amount of medication or other substance, such as gas, contrast media, dye, or radioactive material, is instilled. If the injection is performed for gas myelography or other radiologic procedure, separately reportable radiographs are obtained.

61070

61070 Puncture of shunt tubing or reservoir for aspiration or injection procedure

The physician punctures shunt tubing or a reservoir in the skull, meninges, or brain and aspirates fluid or injects medication or another substance. The puncture site is disinfected. A needle with a syringe is advanced into the shunt tubing or reservoir. Cerebrospinal fluid and blood are aspirated, or a medication or other substance is injected through the shunt tubing or into the reservoir.

61105-61107

61105 Twist drill hole for subdural or ventricular puncture

61107 Twist drill hole(s) for subdural, intracerebral, or ventricular puncture; for implanting ventricular catheter, pressure recording device, or other intracerebral monitoring device

A twist drill hole is created in the skull for subdural or ventricular puncture. A twist drill hole is created using a hand twist drill with the safety stop set to the expected thickness of the skull at the drill hole site. The drill is advanced through the outer and inner table of the skull until a change in resistance indicates that the inner table of the skull has been penetrated and the dura punctured. A needle is then inserted through the drill hole into the subdural space or one of the brain ventricles and cerebrospinal fluid is aspirated. Use code 61107 when a twist drill hole is created in the skull for subdural, intracerebral or ventricular puncture with implantation of intraventricular catheter, pressure recording device, or other intracerebral monitoring device. Intracerebral monitoring devices measure diverse physiological parameters including intracerebral oxygenation, blood flow, and temperature. The twist drill hole is created as described above. A catheter is advanced into the space between the dural and arachnoid membranes (subdural space), cerebrum, or one of the ventricles. The catheter is attached to drainage tubing, a pressure transducer, or other intracerebral monitoring device. Catheter patency is tested and/or the monitoring system is tested and calibrated.

61108

61108 Twist drill hole(s) for subdural, intracerebral, or ventricular puncture; for evacuation and/or drainage of subdural hematoma

A twist drill hole is created in the skull for evacuation of a subdural hematoma. A twist drill hole is created using a hand twist drill with the safety stop set to the expected thickness of the skull at the drill site. The drill is advanced through the outer and inner table of the skull until a change in resistance indicates that the inner table of the skull has been penetrated and the dura punctured. A syringe is then inserted through the drill hole into the subdural space and the subdural hematoma is flushed out.

61120

61120 Burr hole(s) for ventricular puncture (including injection of gas, contrast media, dye, or radioactive material)

A burr hole is created for ventricular puncture including injection of gas, contrast media, dye, or radioactive material. The skin of the scalp is incised and flapped forward. A burr hole is created with a surgical drill or perforator. The dura is incised or perforated using pinhole cautery. A needle is then inserted and cerebrospinal fluid is aspirated. An injection procedure for separately reportable ventriculography may also be performed. As cerebrospinal fluid is withdrawn from the ventricle, an equal amount of gas, contrast media, dye, or radioactive material is instilled. The head is then rotated to disperse the contrast material within the ventricles. Separately reportable radiographs are obtained.

61140

61140 Burr hole(s) or trephine; with biopsy of brain or intracranial lesion

A burr or trephine is used to make a small opening in the skull and obtain a biopsy of the brain or an intracranial lesion. The scalp is incised and flapped forward. A burr hole is created with a surgical drill or perforator. Alternatively, a small disc of bone may be removed using a trephine. The dura is incised. Bleeding is controlled by electrocautery. A biopsy needle is inserted and a tissue sample is obtained from the brain or intracranial lesion. The needle is withdrawn; the dura is closed; and the skull defect is repaired by replacing the bone disc or applying bone wax.

61150-61151

61150 Burr hole(s) or trephine; with drainage of brain abscess or cyst

61151 Burr hole(s) or trephine; with subsequent tapping (aspiration) of intracranial abscess or cyst

A burr or trephine is used to make a small opening in the skull followed by drainage of a brain abscess or cyst. The scalp is incised and flapped forward. A burr hole is created with a surgical drill or perforator. Alternatively, a small disc of bone may be removed using a trephine. The dura is incised. Bleeding is controlled by electrocautery. A needle is inserted and advanced to the abscess or cyst site. The abscess or cyst capsule is perforated. The obturator in the needle is removed and a syringe attached to the needle. The cyst or abscess is drained. The needle is withdrawn, the dura closed, and the skull defect repaired by replacing the bone disc or applying bone wax. Use code 61150 for the initial drainage

● New Code   ▲ Revised Code   **415**

Nervous System

of the brain abscess or cyst and 61151 when a subsequent tapping with aspiration of the intracranial abscess or cyst is performed.

61154-61156

61154 Burr hole(s) with evacuation and/or drainage of hematoma, extradural or subdural

61156 Burr hole(s); with aspiration of hematoma or cyst, intracerebral

A burr hole craniotomy is performed for drainage of a subdural or extradural hematoma. The scalp is incised and flapped forward. A burr hole is created with a surgical drill or perforator through the outer and inner table of the skull. For an extradural hematoma, the collection of blood is located between the inner table of the skull and the dural membrane. A cannula with a stylet is inserted through a guide. A syringe is inserted and the collection of blood flushed from the hematoma site. For a subdural hematoma, the dura is incised and the collection of blood between the dura and arachnoid membranes located. A cannula with stylet is inserted. A syringe is inserted and the collection of blood flushed from the hematoma site. The syringe is withdrawn, the dura closed, and the skull defect repaired using bone wax. Use 61156 for aspiration of an intracerebral hematoma or cyst. An intracerebral hematoma or cyst, also referred to as a cerebral hematoma or cyst, is a collection of blood or fluid within the brain in the substance of the cerebrum. The cannula is advanced into the intracerebral hematoma or cyst and blood or fluid removed using gentle suction.

61210

61210 Burr hole(s); for implanting ventricular catheter, reservoir, EEG electrode(s), pressure recording device, or other cerebral monitoring device (separate procedure)

One or more cranial burr holes are created to allow for implantation of a ventricular catheter, reservoir, EEG electrode(s), pressure recording device, or other cerebral monitoring device. The area over the burr hole site(s) is shaved. A small incision is made through the skin and fascia. Overlying muscle is separated and the periosteum is incised. A drill cutter is used to create a small hole through the entire thickness of the skull. The opening is enlarged using a conical or cylindrical burr. If a larger opening is required, a ronguer may be used.

61215

61215 Insertion of subcutaneous reservoir, pump or continuous infusion system for connection to ventricular catheter

The physician inserts a subcutaneous reservoir, pump, or continuous infusion system for connection to a ventricular catheter. An implantable reservoir, pump or continuous infusion system may be used to deliver medication directly into the brain or to drain excess cerebrospinal fluid from the ventricles. An incision is made in the skin under the infraclavicular fossa and a subcutaneous pocket is created. The reservoir, pump, or continuous infusion system is placed within the subcutaneous pocket and connected to a previously placed ventricular catheter. The skin is closed over the reservoir, pump, or continuous infusion system.

61250-61253

61250 Burr hole(s) or trephine, supratentorial, exploratory, not followed by other surgery

61253 Burr hole(s) or trephine, infratentorial, unilateral or bilateral

A burr or trephine is used to make one or more small openings in the skull to access the supratentorial region of the brain for exploration not followed by definitive surgery. The supratentorial region is the part of the brain that lies above the tentorium cerebelli, a fold of dura mater that separates the frontal and occipital lobes of the cerebrum from the cerebellum. The scalp is incised and flapped forward. A burr hole is created with a surgical drill or perforator. Alternatively, a small disc of bone may be removed using a trephine. The dura is incised. Bleeding is controlled by electrocautery. A suspected defect or injury in the supratentorial region is explored through the small opening. The dura is closed and the skull defect repaired by replacing the bone disc or applying bone wax. Use code 61253 when unilateral or bilateral burr holes or trepanation is performed to access the infratentorial region of the brain for exploration not followed by definitive surgery. The infratentorial region is the part of the brain that lies below the tentorium cerebelli.

61304-61305

61304 Craniectomy or craniotomy, exploratory; supratentorial

61305 Craniectomy or craniotomy, exploratory; infratentorial (posterior fossa)

An exploratory supratentorial craniectomy or craniotomy is performed. The supratentorial region is the part of the brain that lies above the tentorium cerebelli, a fold of dura mater that separates the frontal and occipital lobes of the cerebrum from the cerebellum. A craniectomy is performed by creating scalp flaps, followed by several burr holes. The bone between the burr holes is then cut with a saw or craniotome and a large bone flap raised for temporary or permanent removal. A craniotomy is performed by incising the scalp and then raising scalp, bone, and dural flaps to expose the cerebrum. A suspected defect or

injury to the supratentorial region of the brain is explored and any abnormalities noted. No definitive surgery is performed. When the exploratory procedure is complete, the dural flap is placed over the exposed brain and approximated with sutures taking care to tightly close the dura to prevent leakage of cerebrospinal fluid. The bone flap is then placed over the dura and anchored with steel sutures. Alternatively, a craniectomy defect may be plugged with bone wax or silicone. The fascia and muscle are closed followed by the scalp in a layered fashion. Use code 61305 for an exploratory infratentorial craniectomy or craniotomy of the cerebellar region. The infratentorial region is the part of the brain that lies below the tentorium cerebelli.

61312-61313

61312 Craniectomy or craniotomy for evacuation of hematoma, supratentorial; extradural or subdural

61313 Craniectomy or craniotomy for evacuation of hematoma, supratentorial; intracerebral

A supratentorial craniectomy or craniotomy is performed for evacuation of an extradural or subdural hematoma. The supratentorial region is the part of the brain that lies above the tentorium cerebelli, a fold of dura mater that separates the frontal and occipital lobes of the cerebrum from the cerebellum. An extradural hematoma is a collection of blood between the inner table of the skull and the dural membrane. A subdural hematoma is a collection of blood between the dural and arachnoid membranes. A craniectomy is performed by creating scalp flaps, followed by several burr holes. The bone between the burr holes is then cut with a saw or craniotome and a bone flap raised for temporary or permanent removal. A craniotomy is performed by incising the scalp and then raising scalp and bone flaps to expose an extradural hematoma. If a subdural hematoma is present, dural flaps are raised. The collection of blood is removed using biopsy forceps, gentle suction and irrigation. When the procedure is complete, the dural flap is placed over the exposed brain and approximated with sutures taking care to tightly close the dura to prevent leakage of cerebrospinal fluid. Alternatively, a temporary drain may be placed in the subdural space to drain residual fluid. The bone flap is then placed over the dura and anchored with steel sutures. Alternatively, a craniectomy defect may be plugged with bone wax or silicone. The fascia and muscle are closed and then the scalp in a layered fashion. Use code 61313 for a supratentorial craniectomy or craniotomy for evacuation of an intracerebral hematoma. An intracerebral hematoma, also referred to as a cerebral hematoma, is a collection of blood within the brain in the substance of the cerebrum usually caused by rupture of an artery.

61314-61315

61314 Craniectomy or craniotomy for evacuation of hematoma, infratentorial; extradural or subdural

61315 Craniectomy or craniotomy for evacuation of hematoma, infratentorial; intracerebellar

An infratentorial craniectomy or craniotomy is performed for evacuation of an extradural or subdural hematoma. The infratentorial region is the part of the brain that lies below the tentorium cerebelli, a fold of dura mater that separates the frontal and occipital lobes of the cerebrum from the cerebellum. An extradural hematoma is a collection of blood between the inner table of the skull and the dural membrane. A subdural hematoma is a collection of blood between the dural and arachnoid membranes. A craniectomy is performed by creating scalp flaps, followed by several burr holes. The bone between the burr holes is then cut with a saw or craniotome and a bone flap raised for temporary or permanent removal. A craniotomy is performed by incising the scalp and then raising scalp and bone flaps to expose an extradural hematoma. If a subdural hematoma is present, dural flaps are raised. The collection of blood is removed using biopsy forceps, gentle suction and irrigation. When the procedure is complete, the dural flap is placed over the exposed brain and approximated with sutures taking care to tightly close the dura to prevent leakage of cerebrospinal fluid. Alternatively, a temporary drain may be placed in subdural space to drain residual fluid. The bone flap is then placed over the dura and anchored with steel sutures. Alternatively, a craniectomy defect may be plugged with bone wax or silicone. The fascia and muscle are closed and then the scalp in a layered fashion. Use code 61315 for an infratentorial craniectomy or craniotomy for evacuation of an intracerebellar hematoma. An intracerebellar hematoma, also referred to as a cerebellar hematoma, is a collection of blood within the brain in the substance of the cerebellum usually caused by rupture of an artery.

61316

61316 Incision and subcutaneous placement of cranial bone graft (List separately in addition to code for primary procedure)

A cranial bone graft removed at the time of a separately reportable craniectomy procedure is placed in a subcutaneous pocket to be used for future reconstruction of the skull defect. Subcutaneous storage, also referred to as subcutaneous banking, of the removed cranial bone flap preserves the viability of the bone for future use as an autogenous bone graft. An incision is made in the skin of the abdomen and a subcutaneous pocket is fashioned. The cranial bone flap removed during the craniectomy procedure is placed in the subcutaneous pocket and the skin and subcutaneous tissue is closed over the bone flap.

● New Code   ▲ Revised Code

61320-61321

61320   Craniectomy or craniotomy, drainage of intracranial abscess; supratentorial
61321   Craniectomy or craniotomy, drainage of intracranial abscess; infratentorial

A supratentorial craniectomy or craniotomy is performed for drainage of intracranial abscess. The supratentorial region is the part of the brain that lies above the tentorium cerebelli, a fold of dura mater that separates the frontal and occipital lobes of the cerebrum from the cerebellum. An intracranial abscess in the supratentorial region is a collection of pus in the cerebrum, the subdural space or the extradural space. A craniectomy is performed by creating scalp flaps, followed by several burr holes. The bone between the burr holes is then cut with a saw or craniotome and a bone flap raised for temporary or permanent removal. A craniotomy is performed by incising the scalp and then raising scalp and bone flaps to expose an extradural abscess. If a subdural abscess is present, dural flaps are raised. Several approaches and techniques are employed depending on the location of the abscess and whether or not abscess resides in an eloquent or non-eloquent region of the brain. The eloquent brain includes the sensorimotor, language, and visual cortex; the hypothalamus and thalamus, the internal capsule, brainstem; and deep cerebellar nuclei and peduncles. If the abscess is in a non-eloquent region, the abscess wall is dissected from the surrounding brain to allow enucleation of the lesion. If the abscess is in an eloquent region, an operative microscope is used to visualize and preserve cortical vessels within the sulcus. The abscess wall is located and opened widely to create a pouch (marsupialization) and pus is aspirated. The cavity is then irrigated with saline solution. When the procedure is complete, the dural flap is placed over the exposed brain and approximated with sutures taking care to tightly close the dura to prevent leakage of cerebrospinal fluid. The bone flap is then placed over the dura and anchored with steel sutures. Alternatively, a craniectomy defect may be plugged with bone wax or silicone. The fascia and muscle are closed and then the scalp in a layered fashion. Use code 61321 for drainage of an intracranial abscess in the infratentorial region of the brain, the region below the tentorium cerebelli that includes the cerebellum and brainstem.

61322-61323

61322   Craniectomy or craniotomy, decompressive, with or without duraplasty, for treatment of intracranial hypertension, without evacuation of associated intraparenchymal hematoma; without lobectomy
61323   Craniectomy or craniotomy, decompressive, with or without duraplasty, for treatment of intracranial hypertension, without evacuation of associated intraparenchymal hematoma; with lobectomy

A decompressive craniectomy or craniotomy is performed with or without duraplasty to treat intracranial hypertension without evacuation of intraparenchymal hematoma and without lobectomy. A craniectomy is performed by creating scalp flaps, followed by several burr holes. The bone between the burr holes is then cut with a saw or craniotome and a bone flap raised for temporary or permanent removal. A craniotomy is performed by incising the scalp and then raising scalp and bone flaps. The dura is opened. A duraplasty may be performed using an autologous galeal flap graft, a cultured dermal graft, or a synthetic patch graft to enlarge the dura allowing decompression of the brain. The dura and/or dural graft is tightly sutured to prevent leakage of cerebrospinal fluid. A drain is placed. The bone flap is then placed over the dura and anchored with steel sutures. Alternatively, the bone flap may be excised and stored in an abdominal pocket or bone bank until cerebral swelling has resolved. In 61323, the procedure is performed with a lobectomy. The procedure is performed as described above, and then swollen brain tissue is removed to control intracranial pressure.

61330

61330   Decompression of orbit only, transcranial approach

Transcranial approach to the orbit may be performed either by removal of the frontal bone with preservation of the orbital rim or removal of the frontal bone along with the supraorbital arch. This approach is typically used to access the superomedial aspect of the orbit for lesions or defects at the orbital apex, optic canal, and/or involving both the orbit and intracranial structures. A bicoronal incision is made and the scalp reflected. Medial and frontal burr holes are placed above the orbital rims. A bone saw is then used to connect the burr holes and frontal bone is removed. The dura is carefully reflected away from the floor of the frontal fossa. The frontal lobe is retracted and the floor of the frontal fossa exposed. An osteotomy of the orbital rim or frontal bar is created by drilling inferomedial and inferolateral burr holes that are connected using a reciprocating saw. The inferolateral burr hole is connected to the lateral orbital rim. A burr hole is centered in the anterior floor of the frontal fossa and a transverse osteotomy is performed to complete release the orbital rim. The orbit is exposed. Bony defects or other structures impinging on ocular structures are located and removed or reconfigured to relieve pressure on the eye, optic nerve, and other ocular structures. Upon completion of the procedure the orbital bony structures are replaced and the orbit is reconstructed. The dura is inspected for injury. The frontal bone is replaced and secured with mini-plate and screws. The overlying soft tissues and skin are repaired.

61332-61333

61332   Exploration of orbit (transcranial approach); with biopsy
61333   Exploration of orbit (transcranial approach); with removal of lesion

Transcranial approach to the orbit may be performed either by removal of the frontal bone with preservation of the orbital rim or removal of the frontal bone along with the supraorbital arch. This approach is typically used access to the superomedial aspect of the orbit for lesions or defects at the orbital apex, optic canal, and/or involving both the orbit and intracranial structures. A bicoronal incision is made and the scalp reflected. Medial and frontal burr holes are placed above the orbital rims. A bone saw is used to connect the burr holes and frontal bone is removed. The dura is carefully reflected away from the floor of the frontal fossa. The frontal lobe is retracted and the floor of the frontal fossa is exposed. An osteotomy of the orbital rim or frontal bar is created by drilling inferomedial and inferolateral burr holes that are connected using a reciprocating saw. The inferolateral burr hole is connected to the lateral orbital rim. A burr hole is centered in the anterior floor of the frontal fossa and a transverse osteotomy is performed to complete release of the orbital rim. The orbit is exposed. In 61332, the area of abnormal tissue is located and a tissue sample is obtained. In 61333, the lesion is located and carefully dissected free of surrounding tissue along with a margin of healthy tissue. Upon completion of the procedure, the orbital bony structures are replaced and the orbit is reconstructed. The dura is inspected for injury. The frontal bone is replaced and secured with miniplate and screws. The overlying soft tissues and skin are repaired.

61340

61340   Subtemporal cranial decompression (pseudotumor cerebri, slit ventricle syndrome)

Subtemporal cranial decompression involves removing the lateral wall of the middle cranial fossa to relieve pressure in the temporal lobe of the brain due to slit ventricle syndrome or pseudotumor cerebrii. This procedure is rarely performed today to treat these conditions, having been largely replaced by other treatment modalities. Slit ventricle syndrome is characterized by very small slit-like ventricles and is generally a complication of hydrocephalus that has been treated with shunting of cerebrospinal fluid (CSF). Pseudotumor cerebrii, also referred to as idiopathic intracranial hypertension, is a disorder of unknown cause that is characterized by elevated intracranial pressure complicated by swelling of the optic disc (papilledema). Papilledema can lead to optic nerve compression and blindness. An incision is made over the temporal bone and scalp flaps created and raised to expose the underlying temporal bone. Several burr holes are drilled and then a bone saw or craniotome is used to create a bone flap. The bone flap is elevated and the dura opened. The dura is enlarged using a portion of the epicranial aponeurosis, which is the flat tendon joining the epicranial muscles covering the skull. Alternatively, a cultured dermal graft or synthetic patch graft may be used to enlarge the dura. The dura and dural graft are tightly sutured to prevent cerebrospinal fluid leakage. A drain may be placed. The bone flap is then replaced and anchored with steel sutures.

61343

61343   Craniectomy, suboccipital with cervical laminectomy for decompression of medulla and spinal cord, with or without dural graft (eg, Arnold-Chiari malformation)

This procedure is performed to decompress the medulla and spinal cord when compression is caused by bony defects in the suboccipital region of the skull and the C1-C2 region of the spine. This condition is referred to as an Arnold-Chiari malformation. The bony defects put pressure on the medulla oblongata which is the most inferior aspect of the brain stem and also forms the upper portion of the spinal cord. Pressure on the medulla can cause dizziness, muscle weakness, numbness, vision problems, headache, and problems with balance and coordination. The head is fixed in a neutral position using tongs or a Mayfield head holder. A midline incision is made over the lower aspect of the skull, and the occiput and C1 and C2 vertebrae are exposed. A pericranial graft is harvested as needed. Laminectomy retractors are placed at the superior and inferior wound margins. At C1 and C2, the spinous processes are removed with a cutting rongeur and the laminae with a punch rongeur. The ligamentum flavum is incised as needed. Burr holes are created in the suboccipital region and a saw is then used to connect the burr holes and create a bone flap that extends to the posterior margin of the foramen magnum. The posterior margin of the foramen magnum is removed using a high-speed drill. The bone flap is elevated. Decompression of the medulla and spinal cord may require opening the dura. The dura is then enlarged using the previously harvested pericranial graft. Alternatively a cultured dermal graft or synthetic patch graft may be used to enlarge the dura. The dura and dural graft are tightly sutured to prevent cerebrospinal fluid leakage. A drain may be placed. The bone flap is then replaced and anchored with steel sutures.

61345

61345   Other cranial decompression, posterior fossa

A posterior fossa cranial decompression is often done in symptomatic cases of Arnold Chiari malformation with tonsillar herniation causing headache, hydrocephalus, or syringomyelia. The cerebellum is located low down in the back of the head near the

Nervous System

brainstem and has two small areas at the bottom called the cerebellar tonsils. Normally, these structures sit entirely within the skull. In Arnold-Chiari malformation, the cerebellar tonsils, sometimes with the brainstem, herniate through the foramen magnum, down into the spinal canal. Posterior fossa decompression removes the bone at the back of the skull to relieve pressure on the brain and spinal cord, make more room for the herniated cerebellum, and restore normal CSF flow. After the patient is prepped with the head in a skull-fixation device, an incision is made approximately 3 inches down the midline at the base of the head to the upper neck. The muscles attached to the back of the skull and upper vertebrae are elevated and lifted back. A small section of skull at the back of the head is removed to relieve compression of the cerebellar tonsils and expose the dura. Sometimes, bony removal alone restores normal CSF flow and relieves compression. The surgeon may open the dura to observe the tonsils. Electrocautery may be used to shrink the herniated tonsils and unblock CSF flow. If duraplasty is required to expand the opening and space around the tonsils, a patch of synthetic material or a piece of the patient's own pericranium is used and sutured into place in a watertight fashion. Dural sealant is used around the suture line to prevent leakage of CSF. The neck muscles and skin are replaced and sutured together.

61450

61450   Craniectomy, subtemporal, for section, compression, or decompression of sensory root of gasserian ganglion

The gasserian ganglion is a sensory ganglion of the trigeminal nerve (cranial nerve V) (CN V), and is more commonly referred to as the trigeminal ganglion. It is located in a cavity in the dura mater called Meckel's cave near the apex of the petrous portion of the temporal bone. Section, compression, or decompression is performed to treat pain symptoms caused by compression of the gasserian ganglion. A small curvilinear incision is made behind the ear. The temporal muscle is divided and muscle fibers are separated from the bone to expose the temporal fossa. A small piece of the temporal bone is excised to allow access to the sensory root of the gasserian ganglion. Nerve fibers may be divided, a balloon used to temporarily compress the nerve root freeing it from surrounding structures, or the vascular structures compressing the trigeminal nerve may be dissected away from the nerve. That latter procedure, also referred to as microvascular decompression, is the most common procedure. Blood vessels are dissected away from the nerve and a Teflon pad placed between the nerve and blood vessels. The excised portion of temporal bone is replaced and secured with wire sutures. Overlying tissues are closed in layers.

61458-61460

61458   Craniectomy, suboccipital; for exploration or decompression of cranial nerves
61460   Craniectomy, suboccipital; for section of 1 or more cranial nerves

Cranial nerves become compressed when blood vessels cross the nerves putting pressure on them. This compression can cause a variety of symptoms depending on which nerves are affected including vertigo (dizziness) when the vestibular nerve is compressed or tinnitus (ringing or other noise in the ears) when the cochlear nerve is compressed. The patient is placed supine and the head fixed in a Mayfield clamp. The head is rotated to the side and flexed to allow access to the surgical site. A curvilinear skin incision is made behind the ear (retroauricle, retromastoid) taking care to avoid the greater and lesser occipital nerves. A small section of bone is removed using a cutting bur. The dura is incised, the posterior fossa decompressed, and the cerebellopontine angle exposed. In 61458, cranial nerves are explored and/or decompressed with the aid of an operating microscope. Microvascular decompression is accomplished by placing small synthetic sponges between the compressing blood vessels and the affected cranial nerves. In 61460, one or more cranial nerves are sectioned (cut). Cranial nerve section is performed to treat conditions such as severe vertigo caused by Meniere's disease or vestibular neuritis. Following completion of the cranial nerve decompression or cranial nerve section, the dura is reapproximated and exposed mastoid air cells sealed with bone wax. Gelfoam is placed over the dura followed by Gelfilm and muscle, fascia, and skin are closed in layers.

61480

61480   Craniectomy, suboccipital; for mesencephalic tractotomy or pedunculotomy

Tractotomy is a division or cutting of a nerve tract in the brain or spinal cord performed to treat intractable pain such as that caused by head and neck cancer (nociceptive pain). Open tractotomy procedures have largely been replaced by less invasive stereotactic tractotomy procedures. The open surgical technique is accompanied by high morbidity rates that include deafness, gaze palsy, and dysaesthesia. A mesencephalic tractotomy or pedunculotomy is performed to relieve unilateral intractable pain. The mesencephalon, or midbrain, is part of the brainstem, and is approached via a suboccipital craniotomy. The patient is placed in a sitting position to facilitate access to the midbrain. The head is fixed in a neutral position using tongs or a Mayfield head holder. A midline incision is made over the lower aspect of the skull and the occiput is exposed. Burr holes are created in the suboccipital region and a saw is then used to connect the burr holes and create a bone flap that extends to the posterior margin of the foramen magnum. The bone flap is elevated and the mesencephalon is exposed. The spinothalamic tract in the midbrain is then sectioned unilaterally to produce hemi-analgesia. The spinothalamic tract

is the major ascending central pain pathway sending information from the spinal cord up to the brainstem and thalamus. Following completion of the tractotomy, the dura is reapproximated. Gelfoam is placed over the dura followed by Gelfilm and muscle, fascia, and skin are closed in layers.

61500

61500   Craniectomy; with excision of tumor or other bone lesion of skull

Skull tumors or lesions may originate in the bone, cartilage, blood or blood vessels, or other connective tissue, neuroepithelial cells, squamous cells, or they may be metastatic in nature. Incision is made in the skin and carried down through the soft tissue overlying the site of the tumor or bone lesion in the skull. The periosteum is incised and elevated. The tumor or lesion and a margin is healthy tissue is excised. If the periosteum is healthy it is closed over the defect. If the periosteum is not healthy and must be excised, the defect may be plugged with bone wax or silicone. The fascia and muscle are closed over the defect and the scalp is closed in a layered fashion.

61501

61501   Craniectomy; for osteomyelitis

A craniectomy is performed for osteomyelitis of the skull. This procedure may also be referred to as a sequestrectomy of the skull. A sequestrum is a piece of necrotic bone that has become separated from healthy surrounding bone. An incision is made in the skin and carried down through the soft tissue overlying the site of the osteomyelitis. If the periosteum is soft and viable, it is elevated off the necrotic sequestrum. The necrotic bone is excised and the ribbon of elevated periosteum is then approximated over the cortical bone defect. If the periosteum is not viable and an involucrum has formed around the sequestrum, the necrotic bone is removed leaving the involucrum which will form new bone in the cortical bone defect. The incisions in the soft tissue and skin are closed and a dressing is applied.

61510-61512

61510   Craniectomy, trephination, bone flap craniotomy; for excision of brain tumor, supratentorial, except meningioma
61512   Craniectomy, trephination, bone flap craniotomy; for excision of meningioma, supratentorial

The supratentorial region is the part of the brain that lies above the tentorium cerebelli, a fold in the dura mater that separates the frontal and occipital lobes of the cerebrum from the cerebellum. A craniectomy is performed by creating scalp flaps, followed by burr holes. The bone between the burr holes is then cut with a saw or craniotome and a bone flap elevated and removed either temporarily or permanently. Trephination involves removing a circular button of the skull. Craniotomy involves creating scalp and bone flaps which are then elevated to expose the region of the brain with the brain tumor. In 61510, a brain tumor or lesion other than a meningioma is excised. The dura is incised and a dural flap is created. An operative microscope is used to visualize and preserve cortical blood vessels and other critical structures. The brain tumor is located and carefully dissected from the surrounding brain tissue. The physician attempts to resect the tumor in its entirety. If critical structures are involved, as much of the tumor as can safely be removed is excised. The dura is repaired. Bone flaps are placed over the dura and secured with steel sutures. Alternatively the skull defect may be plugged with bone wax or silicone. The scalp flap is reapproximated and the skin incision closed. In 61512 a meningioma is excised. A meningioma is a tumor of the meninges which are the membranes that cover the brain and spinal cord. Meningiomas are usually slow-growing benign tumors. Malignant meningiomas do occur although they are quite rare. The meningioma is exposed. The arterial feeders to the meningioma are identified and coagulated. The meningioma is completely resected including any involved dura and any involved or hyperostotic bone. The dura is then repaired using an autograft of pericranium or fascia lata. Alternatively a synthetic dural substitute may be used. The skull defect, scalp flap, and skin are repaired as described above.

61514-61516

61514   Craniectomy, trephination, bone flap craniotomy; for excision of brain abscess, supratentorial
61516   Craniectomy, trephination, bone flap craniotomy; for excision or fenestration of cyst, supratentorial

The supratentorial region is the part of the brain that lies above the tentorium cerebelli, a fold in the dura mater that separates the frontal and occipital lobes of the cerebrum from the cerebellum. A craniectomy is performed by creating scalp flaps, followed by burr holes. The bone between the burr holes is then cut with a saw or craniotome and a bone flap elevated and removed either temporarily or permanently. Trephination involves removing a circular button of the skull. Craniotomy involves creating scalp and bone flaps which are then elevated to expose the region of the brain with the brain abscess or cyst. In 61514, a brain abscess is excised. The abscess wall is dissected from surrounding brain tissue and the entire abscess pocket removed without rupturing the abscess wall. In 61516, a cyst is excised or fenestrated. If the cyst is excised, it is carefully dissected from surrounding brain

Nervous System

tissue and removed in its entirety without rupturing the cyst wall. If it is fenestrated, the cyst is incised and an opening created so that the cyst can drain into the cerebrospinal fluid pathway. The dura is repaired. Bone flaps are placed over the dura and secured with steel sutures. Alternatively the skull defect may be plugged with bone wax or silicone. The scalp flap is reapproximated and the skin incision closed.

61517

61517   Implantation of brain intracavitary chemotherapy agent (List separately in addition to code for primary procedure)

Following resection of a malignant neoplasm of the brain an intracavity chemotherapy agent is implanted. The chemotherapy agent is removed from the packaging and handled as instructed in the manufacturer's guidelines. The chemotherapy agent is then placed in the resection cavity and secured per the manufacturer's guidelines taking care to avoid covering the ventricles and large vascular structures. Following placement of the chemotherapy agent the cavity may be irrigated. The dura is then tightly closed to prevent cerebrospinal fluid leakage.

61518-61519

61518   Craniectomy for excision of brain tumor, infratentorial or posterior fossa; except meningioma, cerebellopontine angle tumor, or midline tumor at base of skull
61519   Craniectomy for excision of brain tumor, infratentorial or posterior fossa; meningioma

The infratentorial region of the brain is the region below the tentorium cerebelli and includes the cerebellum and brainstem. A craniectomy is performed by creating scalp flaps, followed by burr holes. The bone between the burr holes is then cut with a saw or craniotome and a bone flap elevated and removed either temporarily or permanently. In 61518, a brain tumor or lesion other than a meningioma, cerebellopontine angle tumor, or midline tumor at the base of the skull is excised. The dura is incised and a dural flap is created. An operative microscope is used to visualize and preserve cortical blood vessels and other critical structures. The brain tumor is located and carefully dissected from the surrounding brain tissue. The physician attempts to resect the tumor in its entirety. If critical structures are involved as much of the tumor as can safely be removed is excised. In 61519, a meningioma is excised. A meningioma is a tumor of the meninges which are the membranes that cover the brain and spinal cord. Meningiomas are usually slow-growing benign tumors. Malignant meningiomas do occur although they are quite rare. The meningioma is located and exposed. The arterial feeders to the meningioma are identified and coagulated. The meningioma is completely resected, including any involved dura and any involved or hyperostotic bone. The dura is repaired using an autograft of pericranium or fascia lata, or a synthetic dural substitute. Care is taken to seal the dura from cerebrospinal fluid leakage. Bone flaps are placed over the dura and secured with steel sutures. Alternatively, the skull defect may be plugged with bone wax or silicone. The scalp flap is reapproximated and the skin incision closed.

61520

61520   Craniectomy for excision of brain tumor, infratentorial or posterior fossa; cerebellopontine angle tumor

Cerebellopontine angle tumors are the most common site of intracranial posterior fossa tumors. The cerebellopontine angle is a bilateral space that is filled with cerebrospinal fluid. The medial boundary is the brain stem, the cerebellum lies just above the space, and the temporal bone forms the lateral boundary. The floor of the cerebellopontine angle is formed by the lower cranial nerves (IX, X, XI). The most common type of cerebellopontine angel tumor is an acoustic neuroma which may also be referred to as a vestibular schwannoma. Acoustic neuromas are slow-growing tumors of the acoustic nerve which is located behind the ear and below the cerebellum. Other less common types of tumors in this region include other types of benign tumors and primary or metatastatic malignant tumors. Using a retrosigmoid approach, an occipital craniotomy is performed. The dura is opened and the arachnoid is incised. The tumor is exposed and carefully debulked. The posterior wall of the internal auditory canal is removed so that tumor within the auditory canal can be excised. The dura is opened and the tumor debulking in the auditory canal continues until only the tumor capsule remains. Adherent portions of the tumor capsule are carefully dissected from the brain stem and from the facial nerve (cranial nerve VII). The skull defect, scalp flap and skin are repaired as described above. Following complete removal of the tumor, the dura is closed and the craniotomy repaired.

61521

61521   Craniectomy for excision of brain tumor, infratentorial or posterior fossa; midline tumor at base of skull

The infratentorial region lies below the tentorium cerebelli and includes the cerebellum and the brainstem. The tentorium cerebelli is the second largest fold in the dura mater that provides a strong, arched, membranous covering over the cerebellum, supports the occipital lobes, and separates the two structures. A craniectomy for the infratentorial or posterior fossa region is performed by making a midline incision at the base of the skull down to the upper vertebrae, creating scalp flaps and elevating the muscles, followed

by burr holes. The bone between the burr holes is then cut with a saw or craniotome and the piece of bone is elevated and removed, either temporarily or permanently. The dura is incised and a dural flap is created. An operative microscope is used to visualize and preserve cortical blood vessels and other critical structures. The midline brain tumor at the base of the skull is located and carefully dissected from the surrounding brain tissue. The physician attempts to resect the tumor in its entirety. If critical structures are involved, as much of the tumor as can safely be removed is excised. The dura is repaired using an autograft of pericranium or fascia lata, or a synthetic dural substitute. Care is taken to seal the dura from cerebrospinal fluid leakage. Bone flaps are replaced over the dura and secured with steel sutures. Alternatively, the skull defect may be plugged with bone wax or silicone. The muscles and scalp flap are re-approximated and the skin incision is closed.

61522-61524

61522   Craniectomy, infratentorial or posterior fossa; for excision of brain abscess
61524   Craniectomy, infratentorial or posterior fossa; for excision or fenestration of cyst

The infratentorial region of the brain is the region below the tentorium cerebelli and includes the cerebellum and brainstem. A craniectomy is performed by creating scalp flaps, followed by burr holes. The bone between the burr holes is then cut with a saw or craniotome and a bone flap elevated and removed either temporarily or permanently. Trephination involves removing a circular button of the skull. Craniotomy involves creating scalp and bone flaps which are then elevated to expose the region of the brain with the brain abscess or cyst. In 61522, a brain abscess is excised. The abscess wall is dissected from surrounding brain tissue and the entire abscess pocket removed without rupturing the abscess wall. In 61524, a cyst is excised or fenestrated. If the cyst is excised, it is carefully dissected from surrounding brain tissue and removed in its entirety without rupturing the cyst wall. If it is fenestrated, the cyst is incised and an opening created so that the cyst can drain into the cerebrospinal fluid pathway. The dura is repaired. Bone flaps are placed over the dura and secured with steel sutures. Alternatively the skull defect may be plugged with bone wax or silicone. The scalp flap is reapproximated and the skin incision closed.

61526-61530

61526   Craniectomy, bone flap craniotomy, transtemporal (mastoid) for excision of cerebellopontine angle tumor
61530   Craniectomy, bone flap craniotomy, transtemporal (mastoid) for excision of cerebellopontine angle tumor; combined with middle/posterior fossa craniotomy/craniectomy

Cerebellopontine angle tumors are the most common site of intracranial posterior fossa tumors. The cerebellopontine angle is a bilateral space that is filled with cerebrospinal fluid. The medial boundary is the brain stem, the cerebellum lies just above the space, and the temporal bone forms the lateral boundary. The floor of the cerebellopontine angle is formed by the lower cranial nerves (IX, X, XI). The most common type of cerebellopontine angel tumor is an acoustic neuroma which may also be referred to as a vestibular schwannoma. Acoustic neuromas are slow-growing tumors of the acoustic nerve which is located behind the ear and below the cerebellum. Other less common types of tumors in this region include other types of benign tumors and primary or metatastatic malignant tumors. In 61526, a transtemporal approach is used. A postauricular skin flap is developed and the temporalis muscle and mastoid periosteum exposed. The mastoid periosteum is incised and elevated off the mastoid bone. A mastoidectomy is performed. The middle and posterior fossa dura are exposed. Bone is removed and the temporal lobe dura and the sigmoid sinus exposed and retracted. The antrum, lateral semicircular canal and vertical facial nerve are identified. The incus is removed, the tensor tympani tendon sectioned and the Eustachian tube packed with oxidized cellulose packing. The middle ear space is packed with temporalis muscle. A labyrinthectomy is performed. The jugular bulb is identified. The internal auditory canal is exposed and inferior and superior troughs developed so that the bone of the internal auditory canal can be removed. The facial nerve is identified. The superior vestibular nerve is followed to the ampullated end of the superior semicircular canal. The superior vestibular nerve is reflected inferiorly from the ampullated end of the superior semicircular canal. The facial nerve is located and integrity confirmed using a facial nerve stimulator. The tumor is debulked and dissected free of the facial nerve. The tumor is completely removed. The posterior fossa dura is reapproximated. Fat is packed into the surgical defect. The periosteum is closed followed by layered closure of overlying soft tissue and skin. In 61530, the transtemporal approach is combined with a middle/posterior fossa craniectomy to provide better exposure of the tumor. A skin incision is made either anterior or posterior to the external auditory meatus. The temporalis muscle is incised or reflected inferiorly. A temporal craniotomy is performed. The dura is elevated from the floor of the middle cranial fossa. The temporal lobe dura is elevated off the surface of the temporal bone. The petrosal sinus is identified and protected. Dissection continues until the lateral posterior end of the internal auditory canal is exposed. The greater superficial petrosal nerve is identified and followed retrograde to the geniculate ganglion. The geniculate ganglion is completely exposed. The labyrinthine portion of the nerve is identified and followed medially and inferiorly into the internal auditory canal. Once the medial end of the internal auditory canal is identified overlying bone is removed until adequate exposure has been attained, including exposure of the superior vestibular

Nervous System

nerve where it penetrates the labyrinthine bone to innervate the ampulla. The tumor is then completely removed as described above. Bone is used to fill air cells to prevent leakage of cerebrospinal fluid. Fat is packed into the internal auditory canal. The dura is repaired. The skull is replaced and secured with miniplates. The soft tissues are closed in layers.

61531

61531   Subdural implantation of strip electrodes through 1 or more burr or trephine hole(s) for long-term seizure monitoring

Strip electrodes used for long term seizure monitoring consist of a single row of electrodes that can be placed into the subdural region through burr or trephine holes. The scalp is incised and flapped forward. A burr hole is created with a surgical drill or perforator. Alternatively, a small disc of bone may be removed using a trephine. The dura is incised. Bleeding is controlled by electrocautery. A strip electrode is inserted into the subdural region. The strip electrode is tested to ensure that it is functioning properly. The dura is closed and the skull defect is repaired by replacing the bone disc or applying bone wax. The procedure is repeated at each strip electrode implantation site.

61533

61533   Craniotomy with elevation of bone flap; for subdural implantation of an electrode array, for long-term seizure monitoring

An electrode array used for long term seizure monitoring contains multiple rows of electrodes on a square grid. The skin is incised and scalp flaps created followed by burr holes. The bone between the burr holes is cut with a saw or craniotome and a bone flap elevated. The dura is opened and retracted. The electrode array is placed at the desired site in the subdural region and tested to ensure that it is functioning properly. The electrode array is secured with sutures and the dura closed over the array. The bone flap is replaced and secured with sutures, wires, or miniplate and screws. The overlying muscle is repaired and the galea and skin closed in layers.

61534

61534   Craniotomy with elevation of bone flap; for excision of epileptogenic focus without electrocorticography during surgery

In some patients with epilepsy, a lesional or localized epileptogenic focus can be identified. The site of the lesion is located and confirmed using separately reportable electroencephalography studies and MRI as needed. If the lesion is not in an eloquent region of the brain, the lesion may be excised without the use of intraoperative electrocorticography. The skin is incised and scalp flaps created followed by burr holes. The bone between the burr holes is cut with a saw or craniotome and a bone flap elevated. The dura is opened and retracted. The region of the lesional or localized epileptogenic focus is identified and the abnormal brain tissue is excised. Following removal of all abnormal brain tissue, the dura is closed. The bone flap is replaced and secured with sutures, wires, or miniplate and screws. The overlying muscle is repaired and the galea and skin closed in layers.

61535-61536

61535   Craniotomy with elevation of bone flap; for removal of epidural or subdural electrode array, without excision of cerebral tissue (separate procedure)

61536   Craniotomy with elevation of bone flap; for excision of cerebral epileptogenic focus, with electrocorticography during surgery (includes removal of electrode array)

Following a previous surgery in which an epidural or subdural electrode array is placed to allow identification of epileptogenic focus, the craniotomy site is reopened and the array removed and/or the epileptogenic focus is excised. In 61535, the electrode array is removed without excision of any brain tissue. A skin incision is made along the previous incision lines. Scalp flaps are raised and a bone flap elevated. If an epidural electrode array is present, it is removed from the surface of the dura. If a subdural electrode array is present, the dura is opened and the subdural array removed. In 61536, the electrode array is removed as described above and then the epileptogenic focus is also excised with the help of intraoperative electrocorticography. To perform electrocorticography electrodes are placed on the surface of the cerebral cortex and additional electrodes are inserted into deeper regions of the brain as needed. Brain waves are recorded with and without stimuli. The boundaries of the epileptogenic focus are identified. The region of the lesional or localized epileptogenic focus is identified and the abnormal brain tissue is excised. Following removal of all abnormal brain tissue, the electrocorticography electrodes are removed and the dura is closed. The bone flap is replaced and secured with sutures, wires, or miniplate and screws. The overlying muscle is repaired and the galea and skin closed in layers.

61537-61538

61537   Craniotomy with elevation of bone flap; for lobectomy, temporal lobe, without electrocorticography during surgery

61538   Craniotomy with elevation of bone flap; for lobectomy, temporal lobe, with electrocorticography during surgery

One of the temporal lobes is excised usually for control of epileptic seizures. Temporal lobectomy is may be performed with or without intraoperative electrocorticography, also referred to as brain mapping. This involves recording electrical potentials directly from the cerebral cortex and/or adjacent structures to help identify the boundaries of the epileptogenic zone and to help identify the extent of the required resection of the temporal lobe. The skin is incised and scalp flaps created followed by burr holes. The bone between the burr holes is cut with a saw or craniotome and a bone flap elevated. The dura is opened and retracted. The anterior aspect of the temporal lobe is measured and the location of cortical incisions determined. If electrocorticography is used, electrodes are placed on the surface of the cerebral cortex and additional electrodes are inserted into deeper regions of the brain. Brain waves are recorded with and without stimuli. The boundaries of the epileptogenic zone are identified. The cortex is incised and dissection carried deep to the cortex using an ultrasonic aspirator. Dissection continues along the coronal plane to the temporal horn of the lateral ventricle and hippocampus. Attention then turns to the pia mater of the medial cortex. A subpial dissection is performed and the pia is opened. The anterior and lateral portion of the temporal lobe is removed. Attention is then directed to the hippocampus, amygdala, and uncus which are carefully dissected while taking care to coagulate and divide perforating arteries from the posterior cerebral artery without damaging it. As dissection continues care is taken to preserve the anterior choroidal artery and the pia arachnoid overlying the ambient cistern which contains the internal carotid artery, posterior cerebral artery, CN III, CN IV, CN V, and CN VI, the basilar vein of Rosenthal, the optic tract, the lateral geniculate and the brainstem. The hippocampus, amygdala and uncus are excised which completes the excision of the temporal lobe. The dura is repaired and the bone flap replaced and secured with sutures, wires, or miniplate and screws. The temporalis muscle is repaired and the galea and skin closed in layers. Use 61537 if the procedure is performed without electrocorticography. Use 61538 if electrocorticography is used.

61539

61539   Craniotomy with elevation of bone flap; for lobectomy, other than temporal lobe, partial or total, with electrocorticography during surgery

The physician removes a piece of the skull from over the frontal, parietal, or occipital lobe of the brain. The physician then removes all or part of one lobe of the brain to control seizures. The physician uses a device to monitor the electrical signals in the brain during the procedure.

61540

61540   Craniotomy with elevation of bone flap; for lobectomy, other than temporal lobe, partial or total, without electrocorticography during surgery

Craniotomy with elevation of bone flap (i.e. removing part of the skull to expose the brain) for a partial or complete lobectomy (not including the temporal lobe). Does not include electrocorticography (monitoring of the brain's nervous/electrical activity) during surgery.

61541

61541   Craniotomy with elevation of bone flap; for transection of corpus callosum

The brain is divided into right and left cerebral hemispheres. Each hemisphere has an outer layer of grey matter called the cerebral cortex and an inner layer of white matter. The two hemispheres are separated by the corpus callosum. Transection of the corpus callosum is performed to treat generalized seizure disorders. These types of seizures begin in the cerebral cortex and then spread through the commissural pathways. Transection of the corpus callosum interrupts the generalized or bilateral pathway and can reduce or eliminate certain types of seizures. A long skin incision is made beginning anterior to the coronal suture on the left side of the skull and carried across the midline to the right side. A scalp flap is created. Burr holes are drilled slightly to the left of midline, the bone between the burr holes is cut with a saw or craniotome and a bone flap elevated. The dura is opened in a curvilinear fashion beginning at the sagittal sinus and retracted. Using a surgical microscope, dissection is carried down the interhemispheric fissure. A self-retaining retractor is used to retract the right frontal lobe and a second retractor is used on the falx or contralateral cingulate gyrus to allow adequate exposure of the corpus callosum. The callosal margin and pericallosal arteries are identified passing over the callosum. Callosal fibers are initially divided using suction aspiration and bipolar coagulation through the genu and anterior callosum while taking care to protect the pericallosal arteries. The midline raphe, which is the septum between the lateral ventricles, is identified and a ball dissector is then used to divide the perpendicular fibers in the posterior aspect of the corpus callosum. Once the transection is complete, the dura is closed. The bone flap is replaced and secured with sutures, wires, or miniplate and screws. The overlying muscle is repaired and the galea and skin closed in layers.

● New Code   ▲ Revised Code   CPT © 2016 American Medical Association. All Rights Reserved.   © 2017 DecisionHealth

61543

61543   Craniotomy with elevation of bone flap; for partial or subtotal (functional) hemispherectomy

The brain is divided into right and left cerebral hemispheres. Each hemisphere has an outer layer of grey matter called the cerebral cortex and an inner layer of white matter. The two hemispheres are separated by the corpus callosum. In 61543, a functional hemispherectomy, also referred to as a partial or subtotal hemispherectomy, is performed. This involves removing a portion of the affected hemisphere and then transecting the remaining connecting nerve fibers as well as the corpus callosum between the remaining portion of the affected hemisphere and the contralateral hemisphere. The deeper structures including the basal ganglia, thalamus, and brain stem are left in place. A long skin incision is made beginning anterior to the coronal suture on the left side of the skull and carried across the midline to the right side. A scalp flap is created. Burr holes are drilled slightly to the left of midline; the bone between the burr holes is cut with a saw or craniotome; and a bone flap is elevated. The dura is opened in a curvilinear fashion beginning at the sagittal sinus and retracted. Following exposure of the affected hemisphere, the portion to be removed is identified, which usually includes the frontal lobe and central portion of the cortex on the affected side. Using a surgical microscope, dissection is carried down to the interhemispheric fissure. Callosal fibers are initially divided using suction aspiration and bipolar coagulation and the affected portion of the cerebral hemisphere is mobilized and removed. Any remaining nerve fibers between the two hemispheres are severed. The corpus callosum between the remaining cerebral cortex on the affected side and the contralateral hemisphere is transected. Once the transection is complete, the dura is closed. The bone flap is replaced and secured with sutures, wires, or miniplate and screws. The overlying muscle is repaired and the galea and skin are closed in layers.

61544

61544   Craniotomy with elevation of bone flap; for excision or coagulation of choroid plexus

The choroid plexus is found in each of the four ventricles of the brain. Its function is to produce cerebrospinal fluid (CSF). The choroid plexus consists of capillaries separated from the ventricles by choroid epithelial cells. These cells filter liquid from the blood and this filtered liquid then becomes CSF which circulates through the ventricles and within the subarachnoid space around the brain and spinal canal. Excision or coagulation of the choroid plexus is performed to treat some types of hydrocephalus. The skin is incised and scalp flaps created followed by burr holes. The bone between the burr holes is cut with a saw or craniotome and a bone flap elevated. The dura is opened and retracted. Brain tissue is dissected taking care to preserve critical structures. The ventricular system is entered and a portion of the choroid plexus excised. Alternatively, a portion of the choroid plexus may be destroyed by coagulation using electrocautery or laser. Once the desired region of the choroid plexus has been excised or coagulated, the dura is closed. The bone flap is replaced and secured with sutures, wires, or miniplate and screws. The overlying muscle is repaired and the galea and skin closed in layers.

61545

61545   Craniotomy with elevation of bone flap; for excision of craniopharyngioma

A craniopharyngioma is a benign tumor with both cystic and solid components that arises from the remnants of the craniopharyngeal duct near the base of the pituitary gland. The skin is incised above the eyebrows and the tumor approached via a supraorbital craniotomy. Scalp flaps created followed by burr holes in the supraorbital region. The bone between the burr holes is cut with a saw or craniotome and a bone flap elevated. The dura is opened and retracted. Brain tissue is dissected taking care to preserve critical structures, and the tumor is exposed. The tumor is carefully dissected from surrounding tissue and excised. Separately reportable intraoperative evaluation by a pathologist is performed to assess the margins. If the margins are not free of abnormal tissue, additional tissue is excised if critical structures can be spared. Excision of tissue continues until the margins are clear or until the neurosurgeon determines that he/she has removed as much of the tumor as can be safely removed. The dura is closed. The bone flap is replaced and secured with sutures, wires, or miniplate and screws. The overlying muscle is repaired and the skin closed in layers.

61546-61548

61546   Craniotomy for hypophysectomy or excision of pituitary tumor, intracranial approach

61548   Hypophysectomy or excision of pituitary tumor, transnasal or transseptal approach, nonstereotactic

The pituitary gland or a pituitary tumor is surgically removed. The pituitary gland is a small pea-sized endocrine gland that is located at the center and base of the skull immediately behind the bridge of the nose in a small depression in the skull called the sella turcica. The pituitary gland can be accessed via an intracranial, transnasal or transseptal approach. In 61546, an intracranial approach is used usually to access a tumor that extends beyond the sella turcica. The skin is incised above the eyebrows and the tumor approached via a supraorbital craniotomy. Scalp flaps created followed by burr holes in the supraorbital

region. The bone between the burr holes is cut with a saw or craniotome and a bone flap elevated. The dura is opened and retracted. The frontal lobe is elevated and the pituitary gland or tumor exposed. The pituitary gland or tumor is carefully dissected from surrounding tissue and excised. Separately reportable intraoperative evaluation by a pathologist is performed to assess the margins. If the margins are not free of abnormal tissue, additional tissue is excised if critical structures can be spared. Excision of tissue continues until the margins are clear or until the neurosurgeon determines that he/she has removed as much of the tumor as can be safely removed. The dura is closed. The bone flap is replaced and secured with sutures, wires, or miniplate and screws. The overlying muscle is repaired and the skin closed in layers. In 61548, a transnasal or transseptal approach is used. Stents are placed in the nose, secured with sutures to the nasal septum, and the nose is packed with gauze or sponges to absorb drainage from the operative site. An incision is made in the mouth just below the upper lip at the junction with the upper gum. Soft tissue is dissected and the nasal cavity is entered. A speculum is inserted and the pituitary gland or tumor located. The dura is incised. The pituitary gland may be grasped with forceps and removed or the gland or tumor may be carefully dissected from surrounding tissue and excised. Once the gland or tumor has been completely excised, the dura is closed. This may require a fat graft which is usually harvested from the inner thigh. The speculum is removed and the surgical wound closed in layers.

61550-61552

61550   Craniectomy for craniosynostosis; single cranial suture

61552   Craniectomy for craniosynostosis; multiple cranial sutures

Craniosynostosis is a congenital disorder that causes one or more of the cranial sutures to close prematurely in infants. Early closure of cranial sutures puts pressure on the brain and impairs brain development and also causes abnormalities in the shape of the head. Craniosynostosis may occur alone or be part of a syndrome, such as Crouzon, Apert, Carpenter, Chotzen, or Pfieffer syndrome, which occurs with other abnormalities. Craniosynostosis is classified as simple, when only one cranial suture closes prematurely, or complex, when multiple sutures close prematurely. It is treated with excision of one or more pieces or wedges of bone from the skull. A skin incision is made over the affected cranial suture and a scalp flap elevated. The skull is exposed and burr holes drilled along the planned craniectomy lines. A wedge of bone is removed. For metopic craniosynostosis, the bone wedge removed extends from the soft spot in the crown of the head to the top of the nose. In coronal synostosis, a bone wedge is removed from the soft spot to the ear on the affected side. In sagittal synostosis bone cuts are made in midline across the top of the skull and a second cut is made over the back of the skull near the open suture area. These bone cuts are joined on each side and a rectangular section of the skull removed. The bone is then cut diagonally at the top of the skull and extended to the soft spot where a V-shaped section of the skull is removed. Two side cuts are also made on each side of the skull and the bone wedges removed to allow side expansion of the narrowed skull. The incisions are closed in layers and the infant is placed in a custom-made helmet that helps to reshape the skull as bone growth occurs. Use 61550 for surgical treatment of synostosis involving a single suture. Use 61552 when multiple sutures are involved.

61556-61557

61556   Craniotomy for craniosynostosis; frontal or parietal bone flap

61557   Craniotomy for craniosynostosis; bifrontal bone flap

Craniosynostosis is a congenital disorder that causes one or more of the cranial sutures to close prematurely in infants. Early closure of cranial sutures puts pressure on the brain and impairs brain development and also causes abnormalities in the shape of the head. Craniosynostosis may occur alone or be part of a syndrome, such as Crouzon, Apert, Carpenter, Chotzen, or Pfieffer syndrome, which occurs with other abnormalities. Craniosynostosis is classified as simple, when only one cranial suture closes prematurely, or complex, when multiple sutures close prematurely. In 61556, craniosyntosis is treated by developing a bone flap of the frontal or parietal bone. A skin incision is made over the frontal or parietal bone and a scalp flap elevated. The skull is exposed and bone cuts marked. Burr holes are drilled along the lines of the planned bone cuts. Bone cuts are made using a craniotome or saw to join the burr holes. The bone flap is elevated. The bone is then repositioned as needed to allow normal brain growth and remodeling of the skull. The bone flap is secured with miniplate and screws as needed. The incisions are closed in layers and the infant is placed in a custom-made helmet that helps reshape the skull as bone growth occurs. In 61557, the same procedure is performed except that a bifrontal bone flap is created and elevated.

61558-61559

61558   Extensive craniectomy for multiple cranial suture craniosynostosis (eg, cloverleaf skull); not requiring bone grafts

61559   Extensive craniectomy for multiple cranial suture craniosynostosis (eg, cloverleaf skull); recontouring with multiple osteotomies and bone autografts (eg, barrel-stave procedure) (includes obtaining grafts)

Craniosynostosis is a congenital disorder that causes one or more of the cranial sutures to close prematurely in infants. Early closure of cranial sutures puts pressure on the brain and impairs brain development and also causes abnormalities in the shape of

Nervous System

● New Code   ▲ Revised Code

the head. Craniosynostosis may occur alone or be part of a syndrome, such as Crouzon, Apert, Carpenter, Chotzen, or Pfieffer syndrome, which occurs with other abnormalities. Craniosynostosis is classified as simple, when only one cranial suture closes prematurely, or complex, when multiple sutures close prematurely. Craniosyntosis is treated with excision of multiple pieces or wedges of bone from the skull. Incision lines are marked on the skin, the skin is incised and scalp flaps created that allow complete exposure of the entire surface of the skull. Bone cuts are marked on the skull. Burr holes are drilled along the planned craniectomy lines. The burr holes are connected using a craniotome or saw. The wedges or pieces of bone are removed. The bone pieces or wedges are reshaped and then reoriented in the skull to provide the best cosmetic result. In 61558, the reconfigured bones are then secured using miniplates and screws. In 61559, bone autografts are harvested, configured to the desired size and shape and used to reshape the skull. The bones and bone grafts are then secured with internal fixation. The incisions are closed in layers.

61580-61581

61580 Craniofacial approach to anterior cranial fossa; extradural, including lateral rhinotomy, ethmoidectomy, sphenoidectomy, without maxillectomy or orbital exenteration
61581 Craniofacial approach to anterior cranial fossa; extradural, including lateral rhinotomy, orbital exenteration, ethmoidectomy, sphenoidectomy and/or maxillectomy

An extradural lesion is exposed using a craniofacial approach to the anterior cranial fossa. In 61580, an incision is made beginning at the medial edge of the eyebrow and extends down the side of the nose (lateral rhinotomy) around the nasal ala and down the center of the lip. A second incision line is made from the upper aspect of the side of the nose to the inner canthus and carried below the eye to the outer canthus and aong the maxilla into the temporal region. The facial nerve is mobilized and transected using a technique that will allow reanastomosis of the nerve at the end of the procedure. Subperiosteal dissection is then carried down to the intraorbital nerve which is transected and tagged. A flap is created composed of the upper lip, cheek, lower eyelid and parotid gland. Mucosa and bone of the ethmoid and sphenoid sinuses are completely resected (ethmoidectomy, sphenoidectomy) to provide access to the extradural lesion. In 61581, the exposure is performed as described above but an orbital exenteration is performed which typically requires a maxillectomy. This type of approach is typically performed for malignant tumors that have invaded the maxillarysinus. Orbital structures are removed when the tumor has invaded the periorbital region. The maxillary sinus is exposed. Mucosa and bone of the maxillary sinus are completely resected. Traction sutures are placed posterior to the margins of the closed lids. An incision is made in the superior aspect through the skin of the eyelid behind the eye lashes. The full-thickness skin incision is carried around the entire circumference of the eye and includes the skin around the outer and inner canthi. The incision is carried through the subcutaneous tissues and into the periosteum around the oribital rim. Periorbital elevators are used to free the periosteum from underlying bone. The eyeball and the entire contents of the orbit are removed en bloc. The lesion is now exposed. Once all neurovascular structures are identified and preserved, lesion dissection begins and is reported separately

61582

61582 Craniofacial approach to anterior cranial fossa; extradural, including unilateral or bifrontal craniotomy, elevation of frontal lobe(s), osteotomy of base of anterior cranial fossa

The physician accesses a lesion or defect inside of the front of the skull and outside of the membrane that lines the skull. The lesion is accessed through the face. The physician may pull back bone from one or two sites on the face. The physician will raise the frontal lobes of the brain to access the lesion. The physician may also have to remove bone tissue from the front of the face.

61583

61583 Craniofacial approach to anterior cranial fossa; intradural, including unilateral or bifrontal craniotomy, elevation or resection of frontal lobe, osteotomy of base of anterior cranial fossa

The physician accesses a lesion or defect inside of the front of the skull and outside of the membrane that lines the skull. The lesion is accessed through the face. The physician may pull back bone from one or two sites on the face. The physician will raise or remove frontal lobes of the brain to access the lesion. The physician may also have to remove bone tissue from the front of the face.

61584

61584 Orbitocranial approach to anterior cranial fossa, extradural, including supraorbital ridge osteotomy and elevation of frontal and/or temporal lobe(s); without orbital exenteration

The physician accesses a lesion or defect inside of the front of the skull and outside of the membrane that lines the skull. The lesion is accessed through the face. The physician removes a section of bone over the eyes going across the forehead. The physician will elevate the frontal lobes of the brain during the procedure.

61585

61585 Orbitocranial approach to anterior cranial fossa, extradural, including supraorbital ridge osteotomy and elevation of frontal and/or temporal lobe(s); with orbital exenteration

The physician accesses a lesion or defect inside of the front of the skull and outside of the membrane that lines the skull. The lesion is accessed through the face. The physician removes a section of bone over the eyes going across the forehead. The physician will elevate the frontal lobes of the brain during the procedure. The physician also removes the eyeball, and all other tissue, from the eye socket.

61586

61586 Bicoronal, transzygomatic and/or LeFort I osteotomy approach to anterior cranial fossa with or without internal fixation, without bone graft

The physician accesses a lesion or defect inside of the front of the skull and outside of the membrane that lines the skull. The lesion is accessed through the face. The physician removes the cheekbone, and may remove the section of bone adjacent to the cheekbone that includes the nose. The physician may use, pins, screws, and other materials to reconstruct the face.

61590

61590 Infratemporal pre-auricular approach to middle cranial fossa (parapharyngeal space, infratemporal and midline skull base, nasopharynx), with or without disarticulation of the mandible, including parotidectomy, craniotomy, decompression and/or mobilization of the facial nerve and/or petrous carotid artery

An extradural or intradural lesion is exposed using an infratemporal pre-auricular approach to the middle cranial fossa. This approach provides access to lesions in the parapharyngeal space, infratemporal and midline skull base, and the nasopharynx. The incision begins near the midline at the top of the skull, extends laterally over the temporal region, and is then carried down in front of the ear along the pre-auricular crease to the level of the tragus. The incision is then extended down into the neck to provide access to and control of the internal carotid artery. The scalp flap is elevated. The temporalis muscle is elevated off the temporal fossa. The fascia of the masseter muscle is dissected and the parotid gland is exposed and removed (parotidectomy). For wider exposure, the mandible may be exposed and severed from its attachments to the temporal bone (mandibular disarticulation). A temporal craniotomy is performed with the exact placement of the osteotomies determined by the location of the lesion. Once the cranium is opened, the orbital soft tissues are protected. The frontal lobe is retracted. Soft tissues are then dissected off the infratemporal skull base. The facial nerve is identified and decompressed or mobilized as needed. The petrous carotid artery is also identified and decompressed or mobilized. Once all neurovascular structures are identified and preserved, lesion dissection begins and is reported separately

61591

61591 Infratemporal post-auricular approach to middle cranial fossa (internal auditory meatus, petrous apex, tentorium, cavernous sinus, parasellar area, infratemporal fossa) including mastoidectomy, resection of sigmoid sinus, with or without decompression and/or mobilization of contents of auditory canal or petrous carotid artery

An extradural or intradural lesion is exposed using an infratemporal post-auricular approach to the middle cranial fossa. This approach allows access to lesions in the internal auditory meatus, petrous apex, tentorium, cavernous sinus, parasellar area, and infratemporal fossa. The incision begins in the temporal area and extends behind the ear over the mastoid bone and down into the neck to provide access to and control of the internal carotid artery. The scalp flap is elevated. The temporalis muscle is elevated off the temporal fossa. A mastoidectomy is performed along with resection of the sigmoid sinus to allow exposure of the middle cranial fossa. The middle ear may be sacrificed during the approach. The facial nerve is skeletonized and protected if possible but it may be resected if the tumor has invaded the facial nerve. A temporal craniotomy is performed with the exact placement of the osteotomies determined by the location of the lesion. The frontal lobe is retracted. Soft tissues are then dissected off the infratemporal skull base. If the middle ear has not been sacrificed, the auditory canal is decompressed and mobilized. The petrous carotid artery is also decompressed or mobilized. Once all neurovascular structures are identified and preserved, lesion dissection begins.

61592

61592 Orbitocranial zygomatic approach to middle cranial fossa (cavernous sinus and carotid artery, clivus, basilar artery or petrous apex) including osteotomy of zygoma, craniotomy, extra- or intradural elevation of temporal lobe

The physician removes the small skull bone behind the eye socket, giving the physician access to the middle of the skull. The physician will make incisions in this area and will elevate the part of the brain in the temple.

61595

61595 **Transtemporal approach to posterior cranial fossa, jugular foramen or midline skull base, including mastoidectomy, decompression of sigmoid sinus and/or facial nerve, with or without mobilization**

A C-shaped incision is made beginning above the ear over the temporal bone, extending in a wide arc around the ear and down the neck. A flap is elevated to expose the temporal muscle, mastoid and neck structures. A complete mastoidectomy along with removal of the mastoid tip is performed. The sigmoid sinus, a small S-shaped cavity behind the mastoid bone, is denuded of bone except for a small rectangle of bone called Bill's island. The internal carotid artery is exposed and protected. The internal jugular vein is exposed and ligated. The facial nerve is identified and protected. A transtemporal craniotomy is performed with the exact placement of the osteotomies determined by the location of the lesion. Once all neurovascular structures are identified and preserved, lesion dissection begins and is reported separately.

61596

61596 **Transcochlear approach to posterior cranial fossa, jugular foramen or midline skull base, including labyrinthectomy, decompression, with or without mobilization of facial nerve and/or petrous carotid artery**

The external ear canal is sutured closed. The cochlea is approached using a transmastoid approach. A C-shaped incision is made beginning above the ear over the temporal bone, extending in a wide arc around the ear and down the neck. A flap is elevated to expose the temporal muscle, mastoid and neck structures. The middle ear is approached through the mastoid bone. The middle ear canal including the tympanic membrane and ossicles are removed. The descending portion of the facial nerve is identified and decompressed. The fallopian canal is opened and the epineurium of the facial nerve is freed from surrounding bone. The chochlea is excavated. The horizontal segment of the facial nerve is skeletonized. The facial nerve is elevated from its bony channel. Mobilization and decompression of facial nerve continues into the labyrinthine region. The dura of the internal auditory canal is opened and the facial nerve dissected free of the remaining remnants of the cochlea. The labyrinth is opened. The bony and membranous labyrinth is then completely excised (labyrinthectomy). The petrous carotid artery is mobilized and decompressed as needed. Extradural lesion dissection now begins in a separately reportable procedure. If the lesion is intradural, the posterior fossa dura is incised and separately reportable lesion excision begins.

61623

61623 **Endovascular temporary balloon arterial occlusion, head or neck (extracranial/intracranial) including selective catheterization of vessel to be occluded, positioning and inflation of occlusion balloon, concomitant neurological monitoring, and radiologic supervision and interpretation of all angiography required for balloon occlusion and to exclude vascular injury post occlusion**

Temporary balloon occlusion is performed prior to permanent occlusion to determine whether permanent occlusion of the artery can be performed without causing neurovascular compromise or injury such as a stroke. An access artery is selected and punctured. An introducer sheath is placed over the needle and the needle withdrawn. A guidewire is inserted and advanced to the target vessel in the head and neck under fluoroscopic guidance. A neuroangiography catheter is advanced over the guidewire and the guidewire removed. Diagnostic angiography is performed to confirm the vascular anomaly and to evaluate the vasculature prior to balloon occlusion. Following completion of the diagnostic angiography, the angiography catheter is positioned in the artery to be occluded. A guidewire is reintroduced through the catheter and advanced to the target vessel. The angiography catheter is removed and the temporary balloon occlusion catheter advanced over the guidewire. A neurological examination is performed prior to deployment of the balloon. Intra-arterial pressure measurements are obtained within the target vessel. The balloon is inflated and the artery occluded. Contrast is injected to confirm vessel occlusion. Arterial pressures are again obtained and a neurological examination performed to confirm neurological stability. Timed neurological evaluation and arterial pressure measurements are performed over the next 30 minutes to ensure that there is no change in neurological status. The temporary occlusion balloon is then deflated and removed. A completion angiogram is performed to exclude any vascular injury following the temporary occlusion procedure.

61624-61626

61624 **Transcatheter permanent occlusion or embolization (eg, for tumor destruction, to achieve hemostasis, to occlude a vascular malformation), percutaneous, any method; central nervous system (intracranial, spinal cord)**

61626 **Transcatheter permanent occlusion or embolization (eg, for tumor destruction, to achieve hemostasis, to occlude a vascular malformation), percutaneous, any method; non-central nervous system, head or neck (extracranial, brachiocephalic branch)**

The physician performs a permanent percutaneous transcatheter occlusion or embolization procedure on a central nervous system (CNS) artery (61624) or non-central nervous system head or neck artery (61626). Occlusion or embolization procedures are performed for tumor destruction, to achieve hemostasis, or to occlude a vascular malformation. CNS arteries include intracranial and spinal cord arteries. Non-CNS arteries include extracranial arteries and arterial branches off the brachiocephalic arteries. An access artery is selected and punctured. An introducer sheath is placed over the needle and the needle withdrawn. A guidewire is inserted and advanced to the target vessel using separately reportable imaging guidance. An angiography catheter is advanced over the guidewire and the guidewire removed. Diagnostic angiography is performed to confirm the vascular anomaly and to evaluate the vasculature prior to the permanent occlusion or embolization procedure. Following completion of the diagnostic angiography, the angiography catheter is positioned in the artery to be occluded. A guidewire is reintroduced through the catheter and advanced to the target vessel. The angiography catheter is removed and the embolization or occlusion catheter advanced over the guidewire. A neurological examination is performed prior to placing the occlusion device or injecting the embolizing agent. The occlusion device is then inserted through the catheter and deployed or the embolizing agent is injected. Contrast is injected to confirm vessel occlusion. A post-procedure neurological examination is performed to confirm neurological stability.

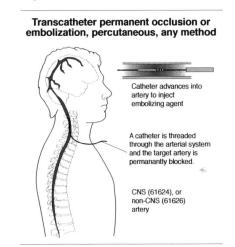

Transcatheter permanent occlusion or embolization, percutaneous, any method

Catheter advances into artery to inject embolizing agent

A catheter is threaded through the arterial system and the target artery is permanantly blocked.

CNS (61624), or non-CNS (61626) artery

61630-61635

61630 **Balloon angioplasty, intracranial (eg, atherosclerotic stenosis), percutaneous**

61635 **Transcatheter placement of intravascular stent(s), intracranial (eg, atherosclerotic stenosis), including balloon angioplasty, if performed**

An intracranial arterial stenosis is treated by percutaneous balloon angioplasty and/or stent placement. The skin is cleansed over the catheter access site. A local anesthetic is injected. A small stab incision is made in the skin and a needle is inserted into the blood vessel followed by a sheath. A microcatheter or neurointerventional guidewire is threaded from the access artery to the carotid circulation. The intracranial artery to be treated is then selectively catheterized by advancing an arteriography catheter over the guide catheter wire. A diagnostic arteriography is performed to evaluate the anatomy and determine whether balloon angioplasty is indicated. In 61630, a balloon angioplasty is performed. Additional angiograms are obtained evaluate the stenotic artery and determine the proper placement and diameter of the angioplasty balloon. The angioplasty balloon catheter is then prepared. A steerable micro-guidewire and microcatheter are advanced through the guide catheter into the intracranial arteries and across the stenosed artery. The micro-guidewire is removed and replaced with an exchange wire. The microcatheter is removed and the angioplasty balloon catheter is advanced over the exchange wire and situated across the stentic region. The balloon is inflated and the stenotic region dilated under fluoroscopic control. Once adequate dilation has been achieved, the balloon catheter is withdrawn into the access artery but not removed. The guidewire is left in place while post-procedure angiograms are obtained to evaluate for hyperacute thrombosis or rebound stenosis. Additional interventional measures are initiated if these conditions occur. Once the stenotic lesion has been successfully dilated and any complications addressed,

● New Code   ▲ Revised Code

Nervous System

the catheters and guidewires are removed. In 61635, an intracranial intravascular stent is placed. If indicated, a balloon angioplasty is performed as described above. Following completion of arteriography studies and balloon angioplasty, the exchange wire or catheter is left in place. The stent delivery system is then advanced over the wire or catheter until it is positioned across the area of stenosis. The stent is deployed and the delivery system withdrawn into the access artery leaving the exchange catheter or wire in place. Angiograms are obtained and the position of the stent evaluated. After a 15-minute interval additional angiograms are obtained to rule-out complications. All catheters and wires are removed.

61640-61642

61640	**Balloon dilatation of intracranial vasospasm, percutaneous; initial vessel**
61641	**Balloon dilatation of intracranial vasospasm, percutaneous; each additional vessel in same vascular family (List separately in addition to code for primary procedure)**
61642	**Balloon dilatation of intracranial vasospasm, percutaneous; each additional vessel in different vascular family (List separately in addition to code for primary procedure)**

Intracranial endovascular balloon dilatation is performed to treat vasospasm of the smooth muscle lining. Vasospasm may occur following subarachnoid hemorrhage which causes changes in the intima that can result in luminal narrowing and rigidity of the vessel wall. The skin is cleansed over the catheter access site. A local anesthetic is injected. A small stab incision is made in the skin and a needle is inserted into the blood vessel followed by a sheath. A microcatheter or neurointerventional guidewire is threaded from the access artery to the carotid circulation. The intracranial artery to be treated is then selectively catheterized by advancing an arteriography catheter over the guidewire. A diagnostic arteriography is performed to evaluate the anatomy and determine whether balloon dilatation is indicated. In 61640, a balloon dilatation of the initial vessel is performed. Additional angiograms are obtained evaluate the arterial lesion and determine the proper placement and diameter of the balloon. The balloon catheter is then prepared. A steerable micro-guidewire and microcatheter are advanced through the guide catheter into the intracranial arteries and across the arterial lesion. The micro-guidewire is removed and replaced with an exchange wire. The microcatheter is removed and the angioplasty balloon catheter is advanced over the exchange wire and situated across the lesion. The balloon is inflated and the arterial lesion dilated under fluoroscopic control. Once adequate dilatation has been achieved, the balloon catheter is withdrawn into the access artery but not removed. The guidewire is left in place while post-procedure angiograms are obtained to evaluate for hyperacute thrombosis or rebound stenosis. Additional interventional measures are initiated if these conditions occur. Once the arterial lesion has been successfully dilated and any complications addressed, the catheters and guidewires are removed. Use 61641 for each additional vessel in the same vascular family that is treated with balloon dilatation. Use 61642 for each additional vessel in a different vascular family that is treated with balloon dilatation.

61645

61645	**Percutaneous arterial transluminal mechanical thrombectomy and/or infusion for thrombolysis, intracranial, any method, including diagnostic angiography, fluoroscopic guidance, catheter placement, and intraprocedural pharmacological thrombolytic injection(s)**

A procedure is performed to remove mechanically and/or dissolve with thrombolytic drugs an intracranial blood clot. Percutaneous access to the intracranial blood vessel(s) is established through a peripheral artery. A needle is introduced into the artery under fluoroscopic guidance and a thin wire is threaded through the needle and advanced to the occluded area. If diagnostic angiography is performed, a catheter is introduced over the guidewire and advanced to the occlusion. The guidewire is removed and dye is injected to obtain detailed images of the intracranial blood vessels. The guidewire is then reinserted and advanced as far as possible through the clot. A mechanical device such as an aspiration catheter, micro-guidewire, micro-snare, or retriever is advanced over the guidewire and the clot is evacuated. An infusion of a thrombolytic agent such as tissue plasminogen activator, urokinase, streptokinase, Acteplase, Reteplase, and Tenacteplase may be used to assists with clot degradation. An infusion catheter is introduced over the guidewire to the clot area and medication is delivered as bolus injection(s) or continuous infusion while clot lysis is monitored with periodic angiograms. The catheter is removed at the end of the treatment period. Code 61645 includes diagnostic angiography and fluoroscopic guidance, catheter placement, and intraprocedural pharmacological thrombolytic injection(s).

61650-61651

61650	**Endovascular intracranial prolonged administration of pharmacologic agent(s) other than for thrombolysis, arterial, including catheter placement, diagnostic angiography, and imaging guidance; initial vascular territory**
61651	**Endovascular intracranial prolonged administration of pharmacologic agent(s) other than for thrombolysis, arterial, including catheter placement, diagnostic angiography, and imaging guidance; each additional vascular territory (List separately in addition to code for primary procedure)**

A procedure is performed to administer endovascular intracranial pharmacologic agent(s) other than for thrombolysis. These agents may include papaverine, nicardipine, and verapamil used to treat arterial vasospasm following stroke. Access to intracranial blood vessels is established through a peripheral artery. A needle is introduced into the artery under fluoroscopic guidance; a thin wire is threaded through the needle and advanced to the targeted vascular area. If diagnostic angiography is performed, a catheter is introduced over the guidewire and the guidewire is removed. Dye is injected to obtain detailed images of the intracranial blood vessels. The guidewire is then reinserted and the angiography catheter is removed. An infusion catheter is introduced over the guidewire to the targeted vascular territory and the pharmacologic agent is delivered as prolonged continuous infusion. The catheter may be moved to access additional vascular territories (61651) with subsequent delivery of pharmacologic agents before being removed at the end of the treatment period. These codes include diagnostic angiography and imaging guidance.

61680-61682

61680	**Surgery of intracranial arteriovenous malformation; supratentorial, simple**
61682	**Surgery of intracranial arteriovenous malformation; supratentorial, complex**

An arteriovenous malformation (AVM) is an abnormal connection between the arterial and venous systems in which one or more arteries and veins connect directly with each other without blood first passing through capillary system. Intracranial AVMs are congenital malformations. The direct connection between the arterial and venous systems results in shunting of blood into the venous system at high pressure. This can result in rupture of the blood vessels and hemorrhage as well as other complications. These surgeries are performed on an AVM in the supratentorial region which is the part of the brain that lies above the tentorium cerebelli, a fold in the dura mater that separates the frontal and occipital lobes of the cerebrum from the cerebellum. A craniotomy is performed by creating scalp flaps, followed by burr holes. The bone between the burr holes is then cut with a saw or craniotome and a bone flap elevated. The dura is opened. The AVM is exposed. Separately reportable angiography may be performed intraoperatively to identify which blood vessels are involved. Using microsurgical technique, the arterial feeders are located, suture ligated and divided. The mass of involved blood vessels is then dissected from surrounding tissue and the draining vein or veins isolated, suture ligated and divided. The AVM is completely excised. Additional angiograms are obtained to ensure that the entire AVM has been removed. Once the AVM has been completely excised, the dura is closed, the bone flap replaced and secured with sutures, wire, or miniplate and screws, and the overlying skin flap closed with sutures. Use 61680 for a simple supratentorial AVM. A simple AVM is a smaller mass of vessels that typically does not have normal vessels incorporated in the mass and is typically not located in a critical region of the brain. Use 61682 for a complex supratentorial AVM. A complex AVM is a larger mass of vessels that may have normal vessels incorporated in the mass or be located in a critical region of the brain.

61684-61686

61684	**Surgery of intracranial arteriovenous malformation; infratentorial, simple**
61686	**Surgery of intracranial arteriovenous malformation; infratentorial, complex**

An arteriovenous malformation (AVM) is an abnormal connection between the arterial and venous systems in which one or more arteries and veins connect directly with each other without blood first passing through the capillary system. Intracranial AVMs are congenital malformations. The direct connection between the arterial and venous systems results in shunting of blood into the venous system at high pressure. This can result in rupture of the blood vessels and hemorrhage as well as other complications. These surgeries are performed on an AVM in the infratentorial region which is the part of the brain that lies below the tentorium cerebelli, a fold in the dura mater that separates the frontal and occipital lobes of the cerebrum from the cerebellum. A craniotomy is performed by creating scalp flaps, followed by burr holes. The bone between the burr holes is then cut with a saw or craniotome and a bone flap elevated. The dura is opened. The AVM is exposed. Separately reportable angiography may be performed intraoperatively to identify which blood vessels are involved. Using microsurgical technique, the arterial feeders are located, suture ligated and divided. The mass of involved blood vessels is then dissected from surrounding tissue and the draining vein or veins isolated, suture ligated and divided. The AVM is completely excised. Additional angiograms are obtained to ensure that the entire AVM has been removed. Once the AVM has been completely excised, the dura is closed, the bone flap replaced and secured with sutures, wire, or miniplate and screws, and the overlying skin flap closed with sutures. Use 61684 for a simple infratentorial AVM. A simple AVM is a smaller mass of vessels that typically does not have normal vessels incorporated in the mass and is typically not located in a critical region of the brain. Use 61686 for

Nervous System

a complex infratentorial AVM. A complex AVM is a larger mass of vessels that may have normal vessels incorporated in the mass or be located in a critical region of the brain.

61690-61692

61690 Surgery of intracranial arteriovenous malformation; dural, simple

61692 Surgery of intracranial arteriovenous malformation; dural, complex

An arteriovenous malformation (AVM) is an abnormal connection between the arterial and venous systems in which one or more arteries and veins connect directly with each other without blood first passing through capillary system. Intracranial AVMs are congenital malformations. The direct connection between the arterial and venous systems results in shunting of blood into the venous system at high pressure. This can result in rupture of the blood vessels and hemorrhage as well as other complications. These surgeries are performed on an AVM in the dura which is the tough fibrous outer membrane that covers the central nervous system. A craniotomy is performed by creating scalp flaps, followed by burr holes. The bone between the burr holes is then cut with a saw or craniotome and a bone flap elevated taking care to carefully dissect the periosteal layer of the dura from the overlying bone. The AVM is exposed. Separately reportable angiography may be performed intraoperatively to identify which blood vessels are involved. Using microsurgical technique, the arterial feeders are located, suture ligated and divided. The mass of involved blood vessels is then dissected from surrounding tissue and the draining vein or veins isolated, suture ligated and divided. The AVM is completely excised. Additional angiograms are obtained to ensure that the entire AVM has been removed. Once the AVM has been completely excised, the dura is repaired, the bone flap replaced and secured with sutures, wire, or miniplate and screws, and the overlying skin flap closed with sutures. Use 61690 for a simple dural AVM. A simple AVM is a smaller mass of vessels that typically does not have normal vessels incorporated in the mass and is typically not located in a critical region of the brain. Use 61692 for a complex dural AVM. A complex AVM is a larger mass of vessels that may have normal vessels incorporated in the mass or be located in a critical region of the brain.

61697-61698

61697 Surgery of complex intracranial aneurysm, intracranial approach; carotid circulation

61698 Surgery of complex intracranial aneurysm, intracranial approach; vertebrobasilar circulation

Surgery is performed on a complex intracranial aneurysm of the carotid (61697) or vertebrobasilar (61698) circulation via an intracranial approach. Complex intracranial aneurysms are those that are larger than 15 mm, have calcification of the aneurysm neck, and/or have normal vessels incorporated into the aneurysm neck. If the surgery requires temporary vessel occlusion, trapping, or cardiopulmonary bypass for successfully treatment, the aneurysm is also classified as complex. The approach depends on the exact location of the aneurysm. An approach through the interhemispheric fissure or pterion may be used. After the skin and subcutaneous tissue have been incised and overlying bone removed (craniectomy), the dura mater is opened. The arachnoid is nicked and cerebrospinal fluid is drained as needed to allow maximal exposure of the internal carotid or vertebrobasilar artery. The artery is located and separated from the arachnoid membrane and the aneurysm is exposed. The aneurysm may treated by clipping and resecting the mass lesion. Vessel reconstruction is then performed using direct repair with bypass graft. Alternatively, if collateral circulation is adequate, the aneurysm may be trapped and clips applied above and below the lesion to become completely occluded.

61700-61702

61700 Surgery of simple intracranial aneurysm, intracranial approach; carotid circulation

61702 Surgery of simple intracranial aneurysm, intracranial approach; vertebrobasilar circulation

Surgery is performed on a simple intracranial aneurysm of the carotid (61700) or vertebrobasilar (61702) artery via an intracranial approach. Simple intracranial aneurysms are those that are 15 mm or less, do not have calcification of the aneurysm neck, and do not have normal vessels incorporated into the aneurysm neck. Simple aneurysm repair does not require temporary vessel occlusion, trapping, or cardiopulmonary bypass for successful treatment. The approach depends on the exact location of the aneurysm. An approach through the interhemispheric fissure or pterion may be used. After the skin and subcutaneous tissue have been incised and overlying bone removed (craniectomy), the dura mater is opened. The arachnoid is nicked and cerebrospinal fluid is drained as needed to allow maximal exposure of the internal carotid or vertebrobasilar artery. The artery is located and separated from the arachnoid membrane and the aneurysm is exposed. Simple aneurysms are typically treated by applying a clip to permanently exclude the aneurysm from the intracranial circulation.

61703

61703 Surgery of intracranial aneurysm, cervical approach by application of occluding clamp to cervical carotid artery (Selverstone-Crutchfield type)

An intracranial aneurysm, also called a cerebral or intracerebral aneurysm is a weakened area in a blood vessel that expands and fills with blood. Depending on the size and location it can put pressure on surrounding brain tissue causing pain and neurological deficits. It can also rupture causing an intracranial hemorrhage. Intracranial aneurysms may be congenital or acquired. In 61703, an intracranial aneurysm that is fed by the cervical carotid artery is occluded by application of a Selverstone-Crutchfield type clamp via a cervical approach. An incision is made on the side of the neck over the proximal aspect of the internal carotid artery that feeds the aneurysm. The artery is dissected from surrounding tissue and an adjustable clamp placed around the artery to partially occlude it. Partial occlusion of the artery allows the artery walls to thicken and clotting to occur within the aneurysmal sac thereby reducing the risk of enlargement or rupture of the aneurysm. This type of clamp can be adjusted postoperatively because a tightening device that is part of the clamp extends to the skin surface. Once the desired amount of occlusion has been achieved, overlying tissues are closed in layers around the tightening device.

61705

61705 Surgery of aneurysm, vascular malformation or carotid-cavernous fistula; by intracranial and cervical occlusion of carotid artery

Blood flow to an intracranial aneurysm, vascular malformation or carotid-cavernous fistula is interrupted using a combined intracranial and cervical approach to clamp the internal or external artery. An intracranial aneurysm, also called a cerebral or intracerebral aneurysm is a weakened area in a blood vessel that expands and fills with blood. Depending on the size and location it can put pressure on surrounding brain tissue causing pain and neurological deficits. It can also rupture causing an intracranial hemorrhage. Intracranial aneurysms may be congenital or acquired. A vascular malformation refers to any type of abnormality of the blood vessels. A carotid-cavernous fistula is an abnormal communication between the external or internal carotid artery and the venous cavernous sinus located behind the eyes. An incision is made on the side of the neck over the proximal aspect of the internal carotid artery that feeds the aneurysm. The artery is dissected from surrounding tissue and an adjustable clamp placed around the artery to partially occlude it. Next, a craniotomy is performed by creating scalp flaps, followed by burr holes. The bone between the burr holes is then cut with a saw or craniotome and a bone flap elevated. The dura is opened. The portion of the internal or external carotid artery that supplies the aneurysm, vascular malformation, or carotid-cavernous fistula is exposed and using microsurgical technique dissected free of surrounding tissue. A clamp is then placed around the carotid artery and slowly closed. Once the artery has been partially or completely occluded, the dura is closed, the bone flap replaced and secured with sutures, wire, or miniplate and screws, and the overlying skin flap closed with sutures.

61708

61708 Surgery of aneurysm, vascular malformation or carotid-cavernous fistula; by intracranial electrothrombosis

TBlood flow to an intracranial aneurysm, vascular malformation or carotid-cavernous fistula is interrupted using intracranial electrothrombosis. An intracranial aneurysm, also called a cerebral or intracerebral aneurysm is a weakened area in a blood vessel that expands and fills with blood. Depending on the size and location it can put pressure on surrounding brain tissue causing pain and neurological deficits. It can also rupture causing an intracranial hemorrhage. Intracranial aneurysms may be congenital or acquired. A vascular malformation refers to any type of abnormality of the blood vessels. A carotid-cavernous fistula is an abnormal communication between the external or internal carotid artery and the venous cavernous sinus located behind the eyes. A craniotomy is performed by creating scalp flaps, followed by burr holes. The bone between the burr holes is then cut with a saw or craniotome and a bone flap elevated. The dura is opened. A catheter is inserted into the carotid artery that supplies the aneurysm, vascular malformation, or carotid-cavernous fistula. A microcatheter is advanced and positioned in the sac of the aneurysm, vascular malformation or in the carotid cavernous fistula. A coil is introduced via a delivery wire. A positive electrical current is applied to the proximal end of the delivery wire. This attracts negatively charged red and white blood cells, platelets, and fibrinogen to the positively charged coil. A thrombus develops in the aneurysmal sac, vascular malformation or fistula. The positive current is applied for several minutes until the coils have dissolved in the thrombus. Once the aneurysmal sac, vascular malformation or fistula has been completely occluded, the microcatheter is removed, the dura is closed, the bone flap replaced and secured with sutures, wire or miniplate and screws, and the overlying skin flap closed with sutures.

61710

61710 Surgery of aneurysm, vascular malformation or carotid-cavernous fistula; by intra-arterial embolization, injection procedure, or balloon catheter

Blood flow to an intracranial aneurysm, vascular malformation or carotid-cavernous fistula is interrupted using intra-arterial embolization, injection or balloon catheter placement.

Nervous System

An intracranial aneurysm, also called a cerebral or intracerebral aneurysm is a weakened area in a blood vessel that expands and fills with blood. Depending on the size and location it can put pressure on surrounding brain tissue causing pain and neurological deficits. It can also rupture causing an intracranial hemorrhage. Intracranial aneurysms may be congenital or acquired. A vascular malformation refers to any type of abnormality of the blood vessels. A carotid-cavernous fistula is an abnormal communication between the external or internal carotid artery and the venous cavernous sinus located behind the eyes. A catheter is inserted through the skin into the access artery and maneuvered into the carotid artery that supplies the aneurysm, vascular malformation, or carotid-cavernous fistula. A microcatheter is advanced and positioned in the sac of the aneurysm, vascular malformation or in the carotid cavernous fistula. One or more coils or a balloon catheter with detachable balloons is introduced via the microcatheter. The coil or balloon is deployed and secured at the site of the aneurysm, malformation or fistula. The balloon immediately occludes the aneurysm, malformation or fistula. In the case of the coils, blood clots will form around the coils and block the flow of blood. Alternatively, an injection procedure may be performed. Angiograms are obtained to ensure that the devices are properly placed. Once the aneurysmal sac, vascular malformation or fistula has been completely occluded or the coils are in place, the catheter is removed.

61711

61711   Anastomosis, arterial, extracranial-intracranial (eg, middle cerebral/cortical) arteries

An extracranial to intracranial (EC-IC) anastomosis is a bypass procedure performed to augment cerebral blood flow. It typically involves connection of the superficial temporal artery to a branch of the middle cerebral or cortical arteries although it can be performed on other arteries as well. A craniotomy is performed by creating scalp flaps, followed by burr holes. The bone between the burr holes is then cut with a saw or craniotome and a bone flap elevated. The dura is opened and the affected intracranial artery exposed. The donor artery is also exposed. If needed, a vein bypass graft may be harvested, usually the saphenous vein in the leg. Using microscopic technique, the obstructed portion of the middle cerebral branch or cortical artery is bypassed either by direct bypass or using a bypass graft. If direct bypass is used, the donor artery is mobilized and transected. The obstructed artery is incised at a point beyond the obstruction and the donor artery is sutured to the obstructed artery. If a vein graft is used, the donor and obstructed arteries are incised and the vein graft sutured to these arteries to provide a conduit that bypasses the obstructed region. Intraoperative angiograms are obtained to verify patency at the anastomosis site and to evaluate blood flow in the brain. The dura is closed, the bone flap replaced and secured with sutures, wire or miniplate and screws, and the overlying skin flap closed with sutures

61720-61735

61720   Creation of lesion by stereotactic method, including burr hole(s) and localizing and recording techniques, single or multiple stages; globus pallidus or thalamus

61735   Creation of lesion by stereotactic method, including burr hole(s) and localizing and recording techniques, single or multiple stages; subcortical structure(s) other than globus pallidus or thalamus

The globus pallidus and thalamus are subcortical structures in the brain which means that they lie below the cerebral cortex. These two structures are located in the forebrain. The globus pallidus is a pale-appearing spherical area that is part of the lentiform nucleus which is a component of the basal ganglia. The basal ganglia are the large masses of gray matter at the base of the cerebral hemisphere of the brain. The thalamus is a large oval structure immediately above the midbrain. Other subcortical structures of the forebrain include the limbic system which contains the hippocampus, amygdala, cingulate gyrus and others, and the hypothalamus. The midbrain and hindbrain are also subcortical structures. The midbrain contains the tectum and tegmentum, and the hindbrain contains the cerebellum, reticular formation, pons, and medulla. Stereotactic lesion creation of the subcortical structures is a type of psychosurgical procedure and is considered investigational or experimental by many payers. A special frame is attached to the skull. MRI or CT scans are used to map out the procedure and determine where the lesions will be created. Surgical apparatus attached to the head frame are adjusted to the MRI or CT coordinates of the target region. Alternatively frameless stereotactic surgery may be performed using fiduciary markers. One or more small incisions are made over the lateral aspect of the skull and the skull is exposed. Burr holes are created to access the subcortical region of the brain. Electrocautery probes are inserted through the burr holes and using the stereotactic coordinates the probes are advanced to the region where the lesion is to be created. A radiofrequency current is then generated and the desired tissue is ablated. If the desired result is not attained during the first surgical session, the procedure is repeated during a subsequent surgery on another day. Use 61720 for creation of a lesion in the globus pallidus or thalamus. Use 61735 for creation of a lesion in other subcortical structures.

61750-61751

61750   Stereotactic biopsy, aspiration, or excision, including burr hole(s), for intracranial lesion

61751   Stereotactic biopsy, aspiration, or excision, including burr hole(s), for intracranial lesion; with computed tomography and/or magnetic resonance guidance

Stereotactic biopsy, aspiration or excision is performed on a deep mass, tumor or lesion that cannot be approached using an open technique. A special frame is attached to the skull. MRI or CT scans are used to map out the location of the mass, tumor or lesion and determine where the lesions will be created. Alternatively angiography may be used. To obtain a biopsy, a stereotactic biopsy apparatus is attached to the head frame and adjusted to the MRI, CT or angiogram coordinates of the target region. Alternatively frameless stereotactic surgery may be performed using fiduciary markers. An incision is made in the skin overlying the site where the burr hole will be created. The burr hole is drilled and the biopsy probe is inserted through the burr hole. Using the stereotactic coordinates the biopsy probe is advanced to the site of the mass, tumor or lesion. Tissue samples are obtained. The same technique is used for an aspiration procedure except that a stereotactic aspiration device is used. To excise a mass, tumor, or lesion, stereotactic surgical instruments are passed through one or more burr holes and the tumor is removed in a piecemeal fashion. Once the procedure is complete, the burr hole is filled with bone wax and the skin incision is closed. The stereotactic frame is removed. Use 61750 when the procedure is performed without CT or MRI guidance. Use 61751 when CT or MRI guidance is used.

61760

61760   Stereotactic implantation of depth electrodes into the cerebrum for long-term seizure monitoring

Stereotactic implantation of depth electrodes in the deep tissues of the cerebrum for long-term seizure monitoring is performed. A special frame is attached to the skull. MRI or CT scans are used to map out the site where the depth electrodes will be placed. An insertion apparatus containing the depth electrodes is attached to the head frame and adjusted to the MRI or CT coordinates. Alternatively frameless stereotactic surgery may be performed using fiduciary markers. An incision is made in the skin overlying the site where the burr hole will be created. The burr hole is drilled and the depth electrodes are inserted through the burr hole. Using the stereotactic coordinates the depth electrodes are advanced to the desired site in the deep tissues of the cerebrum. The electrodes are tested to ensure they are functioning properly. The burr hole is filled with bone wax and the skin incision is closed. The stereotactic frame is removed.

61770

61770   Stereotactic localization, including burr hole(s), with insertion of catheter(s) or probe(s) for placement of radiation source

Stereotactic localization including burr holes is performed with insertion of catheters or probes for placement of a radiation source. This procedure is performed to treat brain tumors. A stereotactic head frame is applied. Stereotactic CT with contrast enhancement is performed to determine the lesion location and dimension, and optimal placement of the catheters or probes. The skin is incised and the skull is exposed. A drill is used to create one or more burr holes. One or more tracks are then created in the brain tissue for placement of the probes or catheters by using a needle followed by dilation until each of these tracks is large enough to accommodate the probe or catheter tips. The housing for the radiation source delivery system is mounted on the head frame. The probe or catheter tips are positioned using the previously acquired target requirements. Radiation monitors are inserted into the carrier ring of the frame to monitor radiation dosing. The device is activated and the prescribed radiation dose is delivered for the calculated time interval. On completion of the radiation delivery service, the probes or catheters are removed and the incision is closed.

61781-61782

61781   Stereotactic computer-assisted (navigational) procedure; cranial, intradural (List separately in addition to code for primary procedure)

61782   Stereotactic computer-assisted (navigational) procedure; cranial, extradural (List separately in addition to code for primary procedure)

Stereotactic procedures are those that are done in a defined three-dimensional space using a computer system. The use of computer-assisted stereotaxis in conjunction with a definitive procedure on the brain allows the physician to perform the procedure without general anesthesia, through much smaller skin incisions and bone openings, and to locate the surgical site more precisely. A local anesthetic is injected into the planned pin sites on the skull. The stereotactic ring is positioned over the skull and pins are placed through the skin and into the skull to immobilize the head. A second localizing ring is then temporarily placed on the stereotactic ring and a CT scan is performed. The information obtained from the CT scan is then analyzed using navigational computer software that provides a set of coordinates to identify the precise optimal location for the skin incision and bone cuts, and to locate the lesion or region of the brain precisely on which the definitive procedure will be performed. The physician then uses the stereotactic equipment and the coordinates obtained from the CT scan to perform the separately reportable definitive procedure. Use 61781 for a procedure within or beneath the dura mater (intradural); use 61782 for a procedure outside the dura mater (extradural).

61783

61783 **Stereotactic computer-assisted (navigational) procedure; spinal (List separately in addition to code for primary procedure)**

Stereotactic procedures are those that are done in a defined three-dimensional space using a computer system. The use of computer-assisted stereotaxis in conjunction with a definitive procedure on the spine allows the physician to perform the procedure without general anesthesia, through much smaller incisions, and to locate the surgical site more precisely. The patient is immobilized and a CT scan is performed on the region of the spine where the definitive procedure will be performed. The information obtained from the CT scan is then analyzed using navigational computer software that provides a set of coordinates to identify the precise optimal location for the skin incision and bone cuts, and to locate precisely the lesion or region of the spine on which the definitive procedure will be performed. The physician then uses the stereotactic equipment and the coordinates obtained from the CT scan to perform the separately reportable definitive procedure.

61790-61791

61790 **Creation of lesion by stereotactic method, percutaneous, by neurolytic agent (eg, alcohol, thermal, electrical, radiofrequency); gasserian ganglion**

61791 **Creation of lesion by stereotactic method, percutaneous, by neurolytic agent (eg, alcohol, thermal, electrical, radiofrequency); trigeminal medullary tract**

A special frame is attached to the skull. MRI or CT scans are used to map out the procedure and determine where the lesions in the gasserian ganglion or trigeminal medullary tract will be created. Depending on the type of destruction procedure performed, a needle or probe apparatus is attached to the head frame and adjusted to the MRI or CT coordinates of the target region. Alternatively frameless stereotactic surgery may be performed using fiduciary markers. The needle or probe is then advanced through the skin to the region where the lesion will be created using the stereotactic coordinates. If an injection procedure is performed, a neurolytic agent such as alcohol is injected. If an electric or radiofrequency probe is used, the probe is activated and the desired tissue is ablated. Use 61790 for creation of a lesion in the gasserian ganglion. Use 61791 for creation of a lesion in the trigeminal medullary tract.

61796-61797

61796 **Stereotactic radiosurgery (particle beam, gamma ray, or linear accelerator); 1 simple cranial lesion**

61797 **Stereotactic radiosurgery (particle beam, gamma ray, or linear accelerator); each additional cranial lesion, simple (List separately in addition to code for primary procedure)**

Stereotactic radiosurgery using a particle beam, gamma ray, or linear accelerator is performed on a single, simple cranial lesion in 61796. Stereotactic radiosurgery delivers a very high radiation dose to a precise location using multiple intersecting beams of radiation. Particle beam or cyclotron technology has limited use in the United States. Gamma ray technology uses a gamma knife composed of 201 beams of highly focused gamma rays to treat small to medium-sized cranial lesions. Linear accelerator (LINAC) technology uses high energy X-ray photons or electrons in curving paths around the head and can be used to treat larger cranial lesions. A rigid stereotactic frame is attached to the head in a separately reportable procedure to secure the head in a fixed position and ensure that the radiation beams are directed at the lesion with the necessary precision. During a separately reportable planning procedure, the lesion is visualized using three-dimensional MRI or CT scans. The required treatment is defined and includes determination of lesion location and volume, identification of surrounding structures and assessment of risk of damage to these structures, and dose computation. If a gamma knife is used, the patient is placed on the gamma bed. A helmet with several hundred holes is attached to the head frame. The gamma bed moves backward into the treatment area. The helmet locks into the radiation source and the radiation dose is delivered. If a linear accelerator is used, a computer is used in conjunction with a micro-multileaf collimator attached to the linear accelerator which arranges and shapes high-energy radiation beams in the exact configuration of the lesion. The gantry rotates around the patient and delivers the planned radiation dose to the lesion. Use code 61796 for a single, simple cranial lesion and code 61797 for each additional simple cranial lesion.

61798-61799

61798 **Stereotactic radiosurgery (particle beam, gamma ray, or linear accelerator); 1 complex cranial lesion**

61799 **Stereotactic radiosurgery (particle beam, gamma ray, or linear accelerator); each additional cranial lesion, complex (List separately in addition to code for primary procedure)**

Stereotactic radiosurgery using a particle beam, gamma ray, or linear accelerator is performed on a single, complex cranial lesion in 61798. Stereotactic radiosurgery delivers a very high radiation dose to a precise location using multiple intersecting beams of radiation. Particle beam or cyclotron technology has limited use in the United States. Gamma ray technology uses a gamma knife composed of 201 beams of highly focused gamma rays to treat small to medium-sized cranial lesions. Linear accelerator (LINAC) technology uses high energy X-ray photons or electrons in curving paths around the head and can be used to treat larger cranial lesions. A rigid stereotactic frame is attached to the head in a separately reportable procedure to secure the head in a fixed position and ensure that the radiation beams are directed at the lesion with the necessary precision. During a separately reportable planning procedure, the lesion is visualized using three-dimensional MRI or CT scans. The required treatment is defined and includes determination of lesion location and volume, identification of surrounding structures and assessment of risk of damage to these structures, and dose computation. If a gamma knife is used, the patient is placed on the gamma bed. A helmet with several hundred holes is attached to the head frame. The gamma bed moves backward into the treatment area. The helmet locks into the radiation source and the radiation dose is delivered. If a linear accelerator is used, a computer is used in conjunction with a micro-multileaf collimator attached to the linear accelerator, which arranges and shapes high-energy radiation beams in the exact configuration of the lesion. The gantry rotates around the patient and delivers the planned radiation dose to the lesion. Use code 61798 for a single, complex cranial lesion and code 61799 for each additional complex cranial lesion.

61800

61800 **Application of stereotactic headframe for stereotactic radiosurgery (List separately in addition to code for primary procedure)**

A stereotactic head frame is applied for a separately reportable stereotactic radiosurgery procedure. A local anesthetic is injected at each of the stabilization sites in the skull. The frame is then fitted to the patient's head and attached to the skull using metal screws.

61863-61864

61863 **Twist drill, burr hole, craniotomy, or craniectomy with stereotactic implantation of neurostimulator electrode array in subcortical site (eg, thalamus, globus pallidus, subthalamic nucleus, periventricular, periaqueductal gray), without use of intraoperative microelectrode recording; first array**

61864 **Twist drill, burr hole, craniotomy, or craniectomy with stereotactic implantation of neurostimulator electrode array in subcortical site (eg, thalamus, globus pallidus, subthalamic nucleus, periventricular, periaqueductal gray), without use of intraoperative microelectrode recording; each additional array (List separately in addition to primary procedure)**

Implantation of a neurostimulator array in the subcortical region of the brain is performed to treat functional disorders due to Parkinson's disease, various types of tremors, multiple sclerosis, medically intractable primary dystonias and those due to psychotropic medications, bradykinesia, dyskinesia, rigidity and severe pain from cancer or other causes. A stereotactic frame is attached to the skull. MRI or CT scans are used to map out the procedure and determine how many electrode arrays will be placed and where they will be placed. The trajectories for the array placements in the target regions are also determined. The components required to implant the arrays are attached to the stereotactic head frame. If twist holes or burr holes are used to access the implantation sites, the entry points are localized, marked on the skin and the skin is incised. The twist holes or burr holes are then created. The dura is coagulated and punctured. Alternatively, a craniotomy or craniectomy is performed. Scalp flaps are developed. Burr holes are drilled and the bone between the burr holes is then cut with a saw or craniotome. A bone flap is elevated or a portion of the skull is removed. The dura is opened and the surface of the brain exposed. The entry site for the guide cannula is inspected to ensure there are no large vessels and the brain surface is coagulated. The guide cannula is inserted into the brain. The deep brain stimulation array is introduced and positioned in the target area. Test stimulation is performed and the adjustment made in the position of the array until the desired functional results are achieved. The guide cannula is then removed leaving the electrode array in place. An anchoring device is used to maintain the array in the desired position. The lead is coiled in a subgaleal pocket. The procedure is repeated if more than one array is implanted. The galea is closed with sutures followed by the skin. The stereotactic frame is removed. Use 61863 for implantation of the first array without the use of intraoperative microelectrode recording (MER) and 61864 for each additional array placed without MER.

Nervous System

61867-61868

61867 Twist drill, burr hole, craniotomy, or craniectomy with stereotactic implantation of neurostimulator electrode array in subcortical site (eg, thalamus, globus pallidus, subthalamic nucleus, periventricular, periaqueductal gray), with use of intraoperative microelectrode recording; first array

61868 Twist drill, burr hole, craniotomy, or craniectomy with stereotactic implantation of neurostimulator electrode array in subcortical site (eg, thalamus, globus pallidus, subthalamic nucleus, periventricular, periaqueductal gray), with use of intraoperative microelectrode recording; each additional array (List separately in addition to primary procedure)

Implantation of a neurostimulator array in the subcortical region of the brain is performed to treat functional disorders due to Parkinson's disease, various types of tremors, multiple sclerosis, medically intractable primary dystonias and those due to psychotropic medications, bradykinesia, dyskinesia, rigidity and severe pain from cancer or other causes. A stereotactic frame is attached to the skull. MRI or CT scans are used to map out the procedure and determine how many electrode arrays will be placed and where they will be placed. The trajectories for the array placements in the target regions are also determined. The components required to implant the arrays are attached to stereotactic head frame. If twist holes or burr holes are used to access the implantation sites, the entry points are localized, marked on the skin and the skin is incised. The twist holes or burr holes are then created. The dura is coagulated and punctured. Alternatively, a craniotomy or craniectomy is performed. Scalp flaps are developed. Burr holes are drilled and the bone between the burr holes is then cut with a saw or craniotome. A bone flap is elevated or a portion of the skull is removed. The dura is opened and the surface of the brain exposed. The entry site for the guide cannula is inspected to ensure there are no large vessels, and the brain surface is coagulated. The guide cannula is inserted into the brain. A microdrive/electrode assembly component is attached to the stereotactic frame and a microelectrode inserted into the guide cannula. As the microelectrode is advanced into the brain tissue, recordings from individual neurons are obtained and response of these neurons to light touch, passive joint movement, and other stimuli is evaluated. Multiple microelectrode tracks may be required to identify the optimal target region for electrode array placement. Once optimal placement of the electrode array is determined, the microelectrode is removed. The deep brain stimulation array is introduced and positioned in the target area. Test stimulation is performed and the adjustment made in the position of the array until the desired functional results are achieved. The guide cannula is then removed leaving the electrode array in place. An anchoring device is used to maintain the array in the desired position. The lead is coiled in a subgaleal pocket. The procedure is repeated if more than one array is implanted. The galea is closed with sutures followed by the skin. The stereotactic frame is removed. Use 61867 for implantation of the first array with the use of intraoperative microelectrode recording (MER) and 61868 for each additional array placed with MER.

62000-62010

62000 Elevation of depressed skull fracture; simple, extradural

62005 Elevation of depressed skull fracture; compound or comminuted, extradural

62010 Elevation of depressed skull fracture; with repair of dura and/or debridement of brain

A depressed skull fracture results from a high-energy, direct blow to a small surface area of the skull from a blunt object. Depressed skull fractures may be open or closed and may result in loss of consciousness. Depressed skull fracture may also be associated with intracranial injuries such epidural or subdural hematoma and dural tearing. In 62000, elevation of a closed fracture without a dural tear is performed. A closed skull fracture is one in which the skin is intact at the site of the fracture. A lazy-S or horseshoe incision is made over the depressed region and the bone exposed. The bone is elevated. The depressed area is inspected to insure that the dura is intact. In 62005, elevation of an open fracture or a fracture in which there is fragmentation of the bone is performed. The skin is inspected and debrided as needed. The skin laceration may be extended to allow inspection of the skull. Fracture fragments are detached using a pneumatic drill. The dura is inspected and found to be intact. The bone fragments are washed in antiseptic solution. The skull is reconstructed and the fracture fragments secured with sutures, wire, or miniplates and screws. In 62010, a depressed skull fracture complicated by a dural tear and/or contamination or damage to brain tissue is performed. Fracture fragments are detached and cleansed as described above. Debris including fracture fragments is removed from the brain. Any damaged or contaminated tissue is carefully debrided. The dura is then repaired with sutures, fibrin glue or a patch graft. The skull is reconstructed as described above. Overlying soft tissues and skin are closed in layers.

62100

62100 Craniotomy for repair of dural/cerebrospinal fluid leak, including surgery for rhinorrhea/otorrhea

A cerebrospinal fluid (CSF) leak may occur from the nose (rhinorrhea), external auditory canal (otorrhea), or other tear in the dura as a result of trauma or a complication of surgery. Separately reportable radiological studies are performed to identify the site of the cerebrospinal fluid leak. An incision is made over the skull at the site of the CSF leak and the skull is exposed. Burr holes are created in the skull and a saw is then used to connect the burr holes and create a bone flap. The bone flap is elevated and the dura exposed. The dural tear is located and repaired with sutures, fibrin glue or a dural patch. The bone flap is replaced and secured with sutures, wire, or miniplates and screws. Overlying soft tissue and skin are closed in layers.

62120-62121

62120 Repair of encephalocele, skull vault, including cranioplasty

62121 Craniotomy for repair of encephalocele, skull base

An encephalocele is a congenital anomaly in which intracranial contents protrude through a skull defect. An encephalocele may contain only cerebral spinal fluid or it may contain brain tissue as well. Encephaloceles are divided into two broad categories, those that protrude from the skull vault and those that protrude at the skull base. Cranial vault encephaloceles occur in the outer aspect of the skull, usually along the suture lines in the frontal, parietal or occipital regions or less commonly at the pterion, and result in a visible external bulge. Skull base encephaloceles are subclassified into two types based on site. Skull base frontoethmoidal encephaloceles project forward causing a mass in the face while basal encephaloceles project downward producing a mass in the nasopharynx. The exact procedure depends on the site and the contents of the encephalocele. A skin flap is created to allow exposure of the encephalocele. Burr holes are created in the skull and a saw is then used to connect the burr holes to create a bone flap around the skull defect. The bone flap is elevated around the encephalocele and the stalk identified. If there is no brain or other tissue in the encephalocele, the stalk is suture ligated and the encephalocele excised. If brain or other tissue is present in the encephalocele, it is reduced back into the skull vault and the encephocele is then excised. The dura is repaired with a sutures or a patch graft. Bone flaps are replaced and the defect in the skull is then repaired using a bone graft, bone wax or other techniques. Bone flaps are secured with sutures, wire, or miniplates and screws. Use 62120 for repair of an encephalocele of the skull vault and 62121 for repair of an encephalocele located in the skull base.

62140-62141

62140 Cranioplasty for skull defect; up to 5 cm diameter

62141 Cranioplasty for skull defect; larger than 5 cm diameter

A cranioplasty to repair a skull defect may be performed using a cranial bone graft or other materials. The site of the skull defect is exposed. If a previously removed cranial bone is used, it is retrieved from the subcutaneous pocket in a separately reportable procedure. The cranial bone graft is returned to the site of the skull defect and secured with sutures, wires, or miniplate and screws. Alternatively, a prosthetic plate may be used to repair the defect. Use 62140 for repair of a skull defect up to 5 cm in diameter. Use 62141 for repair of a skull defect larger than 5 cm.

62142

62142 Removal of bone flap or prosthetic plate of skull

The physician removes a flap of bone or a prosthetic plate that was implanted in a previous procedure to cover a defect. A U-incision is made over the site of the bone flap or prosthetic plate. A skin flap is elevated and the bone flap or prosthetic plate exposed. Any external fixation such as wire or miniplates and screws is removed. The bone flap or prosthetic plate is separated from skull using drill, saw or other device. The bone flap or prosthetic plate is then removed. The dura is inspected to ensure that it is intact. A separately reportable procedure may then be used to repair the skull defect.

62143

62143 Replacement of bone flap or prosthetic plate of skull

The site of the skull injury or defect is exposed. If a previously removed cranial bone is used, it is retrieved from the subcutaneous pocket in a separately reportable procedure. The cranial bone graft is returned to the site of the skull defect and secured with sutures, wires, or miniplate and screws. Alternatively, a prosthetic plate may be used to repair the defect. An appropriately sized plate is selected and secured with wires or a miniplate and screws. Overlying soft tissue and skin is repaired in layers.

62145

62145 Cranioplasty for skull defect with reparative brain surgery

A cranioplasty to repair a skull injury or defect is performed at the time of reparative brain surgery. The site of the skull injury or defect is exposed. If a temporary prosthetic plate has been placed over the defect, it is removed. The reparative procedure performed is dependent on the type of brain injury. Following the reparative procedure the skull is repaired. If a previously removed cranial bone is used, it is retrieved from the subcutaneous pocket in a separately reportable procedure. The cranial bone graft is returned to the site of the skull defect and secured with sutures, wires, or miniplate and screws. Use of a local bone graft is accomplished by taking a large bone graft from another site in the skull, splitting the bone with a chisel, replacing the cortical bone at the donor site and then repairing the skull defect with the inner plate of the donor bone. Both sites are repaired with sutures or wires. Alternatively, the bone graft may be harvested from tibia, scapula, ribs, or iliac crest. The bone graft is configured to the size and shape of the defect. The bone graft is then secured as described above. Another option is the use of a prosthetic plate which is secured with wires or miniplate and screws. The overlying soft tissue and skin is then closed in layers.

62146-62147

62146 **Cranioplasty with autograft (includes obtaining bone grafts); up to 5 cm diameter**

62147 **Cranioplasty with autograft (includes obtaining bone grafts); larger than 5 cm diameter**

A cranioplasty to repair a skull defect may be performed using a bone graft. The site of the skull injury or defect is exposed. If a previously removed cranial bone is used, it is retrieved from the subcutaneous pocket in a separately reportable procedure. The cranial bone graft is returned to the site of the skull defect and secured with sutures, wires, or miniplate and screws. Use of a local bone graft is accomplished by taking a large bone graft from another site in the skull, splitting the bone with a chisel, replacing the cortical bone at the donor site and then repairing the skull defect with the inner plate of the donor bone. Both sites are repaired with sutures or wires. Alternatively, the bone graft may be harvested from tibia, scapula, ribs, or iliac crest. The bone graft is configured to the size and shape of the defect. The bone graft is then secured as described above. Use 62146 for repair of a skull defect up to 5 cm in diameter. Use 62147 for repair of a skull defect larger than 5 cm.

62148

62148 **Incision and retrieval of subcutaneous cranial bone graft for cranioplasty (List separately in addition to code for primary procedure)**

A previously placed cranial bone graft is removed from the subcutaneous pocket and used to repair the skull defect. The subcutaneous pocket is opened along the previous incision. The bone graft is located, freed from surrounding tissue, and placed in an antibiotic solution until it is needed for the separately reportable cranioplasty. The subcutaneous pocket is irrigated, hemostasis obtained by electrocautery, and the skin pocket is closed.

62160

62160 **Neuroendoscopy, intracranial, for placement or replacement of ventricular catheter and attachment to shunt system or external drainage (List separately in addition to code for primary procedure)**

An intracranial neuroendoscopy is performed during a separately reportable ventricular catheter placement or replacement. A small incision is made in the scalp and the skull exposed. The periosteum is incised and a burr hole strategically created to allow visualization of the ventricular catheter. A neuroendoscope is inserted through the burr hole and advanced into the ventricle and surrounding intracranial structures identified and inspected. If the ventricular catheter is being replaced, the existing catheter is located using the neuroendoscope and removed under direct visualization. In a placement or replacement procedure, a ventricular catheter is then advanced into the ventricle using the neuroendoscope to ensure the catheter is properly positioned. The neuroendoscope is removed and the burr hole filled with bone graft or bone wax. The periosteum is closed followed by soft tissues and skin.

62161-62162

62161 **Neuroendoscopy, intracranial; with dissection of adhesions, fenestration of septum pellucidum or intraventricular cysts (including placement, replacement, or removal of ventricular catheter)**

62162 **Neuroendoscopy, intracranial; with fenestration or excision of colloid cyst, including placement of external ventricular catheter for drainage**

A small incision is made in the scalp and the skull exposed. A burr hole is strategically created to allow visualization of the site where the adhesions or cyst is located or to allow visualization of the septum pellucidum. The dura is incised and a neuroendoscope is inserted through the burr hole. The brain cortex is inspected to ensure that large blood vessels are not in the path of the planned trocar insertion site. A trocar is then introduced into the ventricle. The inner stylet is removed from the trocar and the neuroendoscope inserted and advanced to the site of the adhesions, cyst or septum pellucidum. In 62161, any adhesions obstructing the flow of cerebrospinal fluid are dissected. If an intraventricular cyst is present, the cyst wall is opened. The neuroendoscope is advanced into the cyst and a second opening created in the opposite side (back) of the cyst wall. The openings are enlarged. The neuroendoscope is advanced within the ventricular system which is inspected to ensure that there is good communication of cerebrospinal fluid throughout the system. The septum pellucidum may be opened to allow better circulation of cerebrospinal fluid. The septum pellucidum is a thin plate of brain tissue dividing the column and body of the fornix below and the corpus callosum above and anteriorly. It is usually fused in the middle forming a partition between the left and right frontal horn of the lateral ventricles. The neuroendoscope is removed. If a ventricular catheter is needed, it is advanced into the ventricle through the trocar and positioned in the ventricle. The trocar is removed. The catheter is cut to the desired length, attached to a one-way, flow-controlled valve proximally. Shunt tubing distal to the valve is then tunneled through the scalp to the neck and into the jugular vein or other shunt termination site in a separately reportable

procedure. All incisions are closed. In 62162, a colloid cyst is opened or excised. The neuroendoscope is advanced toward the colloid cyst. The cyst is opened and the contents of the cyst evacuated using a suction catheter. The suction catheter is removed and a cautery device advanced through the working channel of the neuroendoscope. The site of attachment of the cyst wall is located and coagulated. The cautery device is removed and a cutting device inserted. The attachment cut. The cutting device is removed and a grasping device inserted. The cyst is then removed, the area inspected for bleeding, and the neuroendoscope removed. A ventricular catheter is inserted as described above but instead of being tunneled to the internal shunt system it is attached to an external drainage system.

62163

62163 **Neuroendoscopy, intracranial; with retrieval of foreign body**

A foreign body, such as a ventricular catheter, is retrieved from the ventricular system using neuroendoscopy. A small incision is made in the scalp and the skull exposed. A burr hole is strategically placed to allow insertion of the neuroendoscope into the ventricular system. The dura is incised and a neuroendoscope is inserted through the burr hole. The brain cortex is inspected to ensure that large blood vessels are not in the path of the planned trocar insertion site. A trocar is then introduced into the ventricle. The ventricular system is inspected and the foreign body located. The foreign body is freed from adhesions or scar tissue. A grasping device is inserted through the working channel and the foreign body is captured and removed. The ventricular system is then reinspected to ensure that there is no bleeding and no obstruction to the flow of cerebrospinal fluid. The neuroendoscope is removed. The dura is repaired, the burr hole closed with bone wax, and the overlying soft tissue and skin closed in layers.

62164

62164 **Neuroendoscopy, intracranial; with excision of brain tumor, including placement of external ventricular catheter for drainage**

A brain tumor is excised using neuroendoscopy. A small incision is made in the scalp and the skull exposed. A burr hole is strategically placed to allow insertion of the neuroendoscope into the ventricular system. The dura is incised and a neuroendoscope is inserted through the burr hole. The brain cortex is inspected to ensure that large blood vessels are not in the path of the planned trocar insertion site. A trocar is then introduced into the ventricle. The ventricular system is inspected as the neuroendoscope is advanced to the tumor site. A tissue sample may be obtained and sent for separately reportable pathological examination. The tumor is then excised. A large tumor may require multiple passes and the use of a variety of instruments such as forceps, currettes, and suction devices. Following removal of the tumor, a cautery device is advanced through the working channel of the neuroendoscope to control bleeding. The neuroendoscope is removed. If a ventricular catheter is needed, it is advanced into the ventricle through the trocar and positioned in the ventricle. The trocar is removed. The catheter is cut to the desired length and attached to an external drainage system.

62165

62165 **Neuroendoscopy, intracranial; with excision of pituitary tumor, transnasal or trans-sphenoidal approach**

A pituitary tumor is excised using neuroendoscopy via a transnasal or transsphenoidal approach. The neuroendoscope is inserted into one of the nostrils to the sphenoid ostium. The sphenoid ostium is opened using a rongeur. The sphenoid muscosa is stripped and bleeding controlled with electrocautery. The sinus is irrigated with antibiotic solution. Using endoscopic guidance a small osteotome is used to remove the floor of the sella and expose the dura. The dura is incised. The pituitary tumor is visualized through the endoscope. A tissue sample may be obtained and sent for separately reportable pathological examination. The tumor is then excised. A large tumor may require multiple passes and the use of a variety of instruments such as forceps, currettes, and suction devices. Following removal of the tumor, a cautery device is advanced through the working channel of the endoscope to control bleeding. The endoscope is retracted into the nasal sinus so that the dural repair and sella reconstruction can be performed under direct visualization. The dural defect is packed with Gelfoam and the sella floor repaired. The sphenoid sinus is packed with Vaseline-impregnated gauze. The endoscope is withdrawn.

62180

62180 **Ventriculocisternostomy (Torkildsen type operation)**

In this procedure, a shunt is placed in the lateral ventricle terminating in the cisterna magna (cerebellomedullary cistern) to bypass an obstruction in the cerebral aqueduct. A curved skin incision is made in the scalp to create a skin flap. The scalp is flapped forward and a craniotomy is performed to expose the dura. The dura is incised and a Torkildsen shunt is placed in the lateral ventricle. The terminal end of the catheter is then placed in the cisterna magna to bypass the cerebral aqueduct obstruction. This procedure has largely been replaced with other shunt procedures including neuroendoscopic third ventricle ventriculocisternography.

● New Code   ▲ Revised Code

Nervous System

62190-62192

62190   Creation of shunt; subarachnoid/subdural-atrial, -jugular, -auricular

62192   Creation of shunt; subarachnoid/subdural-peritoneal, -pleural, other terminus

A shunt is placed in the subarachnoid or subdural space in the brain to drain excess cerebrospinal fluid. In 62190, the shunt terminates in the right atrium of the heart, the atrial appendage (auricle), or the jugular vein. A curved skin incision is made in scalp to create a skin flap. The scalp is flapped forward and a single burr hole created with a perforator. A second incision is then made in the skin of neck for access to the jugular vein or common facial vein. A needle is inserted into the selected vein and a guidewire and vessel dilator is inserted through the needle into the jugular or facial vein. The dura is opened using pinhole cautery and the shunt (catheter) is then placed into the subarachnoid or subdural space. The proximal catheter and distal catheter are then connected to the shunt valve and the shunt valve is tested to ensure that cerebrospinal fluid (CSF) is flowing through the valve. If the shunt system is functioning properly, the distal catheter is then tunneled from the head into the neck. A cannula is placed under the scalp at the site of the coronal flap and advanced through the subgaleal space of the head and then between the subcuticular layer of the skin and the fascia of the superficial muscles of the neck. The distal catheter is advanced over the previously placed guidewire into the jugular vein. The catheter may terminate in the jugular vein or be advanced through the wall of the jugular and terminate in the right atrium or atrial appendage (auricle). In 62192, the shunt terminates in the peritoneum, pleural cavity, or other site in the body. The procedure is performed as described above except that the second incision is made in the skin of the chest or abdomen and the pleural space or peritoneum is exposed. The cannula is advanced between the subcuticular layer of the skin and the fascia of the superficial muscles of the neck and chest for a subarachnoid/subdural-pleural shunt. If the shunt terminates in the peritoneum, the cannula is advanced to abdomen. The terminal (distal) end of the catheter is then passed through the tunnel and positioned in the pleural space, peritoneum, or other prepared site.

62194

62194   Replacement or irrigation, subarachnoid/subdural catheter

An obstructed or malfunctioning subarachnoid or subdural catheter is irrigated or replaced. To irrigate the catheter, a needle is inserted into the catheter tubing. Aspiration may first be attempted to dislodge small obstructing particles. If this fails a second needle is inserted and the catheter is irrigated and aspirated simultaneously. If the obstruction cannot be eliminated by irrigation and aspiration, the catheter is removed and replaced. A skin incision is made over the malfunctioning catheter. The proximal catheter is disconnected from the shunt valve. A guidewire is inserted into the proximal catheter and advanced to subarachnoid or subdural space. The catheter is removed over the guidewire and a new catheter advanced into the subarachnoid or subdural space. The guidewire is removed and the new catheter secured and connected to the valve component.

62200

62200   Ventriculocisternostomy, third ventricle

An open ventriculocisternostomy is performed to create a communication (opening) between the third ventricle and the subarachnoid space (cistern). A circular incision is made in the scalp in the right frontal area and a skin flap is moved forward. A craniotomy is then created, the dura is opened, and the frontal horn of the lateral ventricle is identified. The lateral ventricle is catheterized and intracranial pressures are taken. The catheter is then advanced into the third ventricle and the floor is punctured to create an opening between the third ventricle and the subarachnoid cistern. The opening is enlarged until good flow of cerebrospinal fluid (CSF) is evidenced. If good CSF flow is not seen, the prepontine cistern is explored and any arachnoid bands obstructing flow are lysed. If an imperforate membrane of Liliequist is identified, it is disrupted. A second communication may be created if good flow of CSF is not seen following disruption of the obstruction. After good communication is verified, closing intracranial pressures are obtained. If pressures are elevated, an external ventricular drain is placed.

62201

62201   Ventriculocisternostomy, third ventricle; stereotactic, neuroendoscopic method

A stereotactic neuroendoscopic third ventricle ventriculocisternostomy, also referred to as endoscopic third ventriculostomy (ETV), is performed. The scalp is incised; a skin flap is created and retracted; and a single burr hole is created in the skull with a perforator. The dura is then perforated using pinhole cautery. A neuroendoscope and ventricular catheter system are introduced into the frontal horn of the lateral ventricle. The neuroendoscope is removed leaving the ventricular catheter in place and intracranial pressures are measured. The neuroendoscope is reinserted, the foramen of Monro is visualized, and the ventricular catheter is then advanced into the third ventricle. The basilar artery is identified. Care is taken to avoid puncturing the basilar artery as the floor of the third ventricle is opened (fenestrated) using the neuroendoscope, which is then passed into the subarachnoid space (cistern). The opening in the floor of the third ventricle is enlarged using the ventricular

catheter. The catheter and neuroendoscope are then withdrawn to the third ventricle and flow of CSF is verified as evidenced by CSF pulsation. If good CSF flow is not evidenced, a second opening may be created or the prepontine cistern may be explored and any obstructing arachnoid bands or an imperforate Liliequist's membrane disrupted using the ventricular catheter to perform gentle dissection. After good communication is verified, closing intracranial pressures are obtained. If the pressures are elevated, an external ventricular drain is placed.

62220-62223

62220   Creation of shunt; ventriculo-atrial, -jugular, -auricular

62223   Creation of shunt; ventriculo-peritoneal, -pleural, other terminus

A shunt is placed in a ventricle in the brain, usually the lateral ventricle, to drain excess cerebrospinal fluid from the brain into the right atrium of the heart, the atrial appendage (auricle), or the jugular vein. A curved skin incision is made in scalp to create a skin flap. The scalp is flapped forward and a single burr hole created with a perforator. The dura is perforated using pinhole cautery. A second incision is then made in the skin of neck for access to the jugular vein or common facial vein. A needle is inserted into the selected vein and a guidewire and vessel dilator is inserted through the needle into the jugular or facial vein. Using a stylet, the ventricular shunt (catheter) is then placed through the previously created opening in the dura, advanced through the pia, into the gray and white matter, through the ependymal lining, and positioned in the lateral ventricle. The stylet is then removed. The ventricular (proximal) catheter and distal catheter are then connected to the shunt valve and the shunt valve is tested to ensure that cerebrospinal fluid (CSF) is flowing through the valve. If the shunt system is functioning properly, the distal catheter is then tunneled from the head into the neck. A cannula is placed under the scalp at the site of the coronal flap and advanced through the subgaleal space of the head and then between the subcuticular layer of the skin and the fascia of the superficial muscles of the neck. The distal catheter is then advanced over the previously placed guidewire into the jugular vein. The catheter may terminate in the jugular vein or be advanced through the wall of the jugular and terminate in the right atrium or atrial appendage (auricle). Use code 62223 when a shunt is placed in a ventricle in the brain to drain excess cerebrospinal fluid from the brain into the peritoneum, pleural cavity, or other site in the body. The procedure is performed as described above except that the second incision is made in the skin of the chest or abdomen and the pleural space or peritoneum is exposed. The cannula is advanced between the subcuticular layer of the skin and the fascia of the superficial muscles of the neck and chest for a ventriculo-pleural shunt. If the shunt terminates in the peritoneum, the cannula is advanced to abdomen. The terminal (distal) end of the catheter is then passed through the tunnel and positioned in the pleural space, peritoneum, or other prepared site.

62225

62225   Replacement or irrigation, ventricular catheter

An obstructed or malfunctioning ventricular catheter is irrigated or replaced. To irrigate the catheter, a needle is inserted into the catheter tubing. Aspiration may first be attempted to dislodge small obstructing particles. If this fails a second needle is inserted and the catheter is irrigated and aspirated simultaneously. If the obstruction cannot be eliminated by irrigation and aspiration, the catheter is removed and replaced. A skin incision is made over the malfunctioning catheter. The proximal catheter is disconnected from the shunt valve. A guidewire is inserted into the proximal catheter and advanced into the ventricle. The catheter is removed over the guidewire and a new catheter advanced into the ventricle. The guidewire is removed and the new catheter secured and connected to the valve component.

62230

62230   Replacement or revision of cerebrospinal fluid shunt, obstructed valve, or distal catheter in shunt system

A malfunctioning or obstructed cerebrospinal fluid (CSF) shunt, valve, or distal catheter is replaced or revised. The shunt, valve, or distal catheter can become obstructed with protein deposits when there is excess protein in the CSF. Another cause of malfunction of the distal catheter is if it becomes dislodged. This is particularly common when the shunt terminates in the peritoneum. The shunt system is evaluated to determine which component is obstructed or malfunctioning. If the ventricular shunt is malfunctioning it may be repositioned or replaced. A skin incision is made over the malfunctioning shunt. A guidewire is advanced through the catheter to the proximal end. The catheter may be advanced or retracted. Flow of CSF is evaluated. If repositioning the catheter does not correct the malfunction, the proximal catheter is disconnected from the shunt valve. A guidewire is inserted into the proximal catheter and advanced into the ventricle. The catheter is removed over the guidewire and a new catheter advanced into the ventricle. The guidewire is removed and the new catheter secured and connected to the valve component. If the valve is malfunctioning or obstructed, the shunt may be flushed to help dislodge any protein deposits that are obstructing the valve. If this is not effective, the valve is disconnected from the proximal and distal catheters, and they are connected to a replacement valve. If the distal catheter is malfunctioning, it may be irrigated to relieve the obstruction. Alternatively, a guidewire may be inserted and the end of the distal catheter

Nervous System

repositioned in an attempt to relieve the obstruction. If this does not work, the distal catheter is removed over the guidewire and a new catheter advanced over the guidewire. Contrast is injected as needed and the position of the catheter checked. The revised or replaced components are then secured to surrounding skin and subcutaneous tissues.

62252

62252   Reprogramming of programmable cerebrospinal shunt

A programmable cerebrospinal fluid (CSF) shunt is reprogrammed. This non-invasive procedure is used to adjust pressure settings in a previously placed intracranial CSF shunt and can correct over- or under-drainage of CSF in a patient with hydrocephalus. These types of shunts are also used in patients with fluid-filled cysts or other fluid accumulations in the brain and reprogramming may be used to treat under-drainage in these patients. Reprogramming is also required following MRI. The previously implanted valve on the CSF shunt is palpated through the skin. The valve is typically located behind the ear. The transmitter head of the programmer is placed over the valve. The programming console is set to the desired pressure and an electromagnetic transmitter device is used to send a coded magnetic signal through the skin to the valve to reset the pressure setting. Following reprogramming, a separately reportable radiograph is obtained to verify that the pressure setting has been reset. The physician may repeat the procedure if the radiograph reveals that the desired setting has not been achieved.

62256-62258

62256   Removal of complete cerebrospinal fluid shunt system; without replacement
62258   Removal of complete cerebrospinal fluid shunt system; with replacement by similar or other shunt at same operation

A cerebrospinal fluid shunt system may be removed if it was placed temporarily or for a complication such as obstruction or infection. In 62256, the shunt system is removed without replacement. The shunt valve is exposed. The proximal and distal catheters are detached from the shunt valve and the shunt valve is removed. The proximal and distal catheters are then removed. To remove the proximal catheter a skin incision is made over the shunt. Overlying soft tissues are dissected and any anchoring sutures are cut. A guidewire is advanced through the catheter to the proximal end. The catheter is removed over the guidewire. A temporary drain may be placed over the guidewire or the guidewire may be removed and the dura closed. To remove the distal catheter, a guidewire is placed. The subcutaneous tunnel is opened and the shunt is dissected free of the tunnel and the terminal end removed. In 62258, the shunt system is removed as described above and replaced with a new shunt system during the same surgical session. After removing the shunt valve and the existing proximal catheter over the guidewire, a new catheter is inserted into the ventricle, subarachnoid or subdural space. The new proximal catheter and new distal catheter are then connected to the new shunt valve and the shunt valve is tested to ensure that cerebrospinal fluid (CSF) is flowing through the valve. If the shunt system is functioning properly, the distal catheter is then advanced into the termination site over the guidewire that was placed when the existing distal catheter was removed. Alternatively, if the distal catheter is rerouted to a new termination site, a cannula is placed under the scalp. If the new termination site is the jugular, right atrium, or atrial appendage, the cannula is advanced through the subgaleal space of the head and then between the subcuticular layer of the skin and the fascia of the superficial muscles of the neck. The distal catheter is then advanced over a previously placed guidewire into the jugular vein. The catheter may remain in the jugular vein or be advanced through the wall of the jugular and terminate in the right atrium or atrial appendage (auricle). If the shunt terminates in the peritoneum, pleural cavity, or other site in the body, the procedure is performed as described above except that the second incision is made in the skin of the chest or abdomen and the pleural space or peritoneum is exposed. The cannula is advanced between the subcuticular layer of the skin and the fascia of the superficial muscles of the neck and chest for a subarachnoid/subdural-pleural shunt. If the shunt terminates in the peritoneum, the cannula is advanced to abdomen. The terminal (distal) end of the catheter is then passed through the tunnel and positioned in the pleural space, peritoneum, or other prepared site.

62263-62264

62263   Percutaneous lysis of epidural adhesions using solution injection (eg, hypertonic saline, enzyme) or mechanical means (eg, catheter) including radiologic localization (includes contrast when administered), multiple adhesiolysis sessions; 2 or more days
62264   Percutaneous lysis of epidural adhesions using solution injection (eg, hypertonic saline, enzyme) or mechanical means (eg, catheter) including radiologic localization (includes contrast when administered), multiple adhesiolysis sessions; 1 day

One or more substances used to lyse adhesions are injected via an indwelling epidural catheter. The skin is cleansed over the planned injection site and a local anesthetic is administered. Using fluoroscopic or other radiological guidance as needed, a spinal needle is advanced into the epidural space or caudal vertebral space at the desired vertebral level. A catheter is advanced over the needle into the epidural space and the needle is withdrawn. The catheter is manipulated through the bands of scar tissue to the target

spinal nerve or nerve root. Contrast is injected to confirm proper placement of the catheter and to evaluate nerve roots and spinal nerves in the area. Free flow of contrast within the epidural space is confirmed. The number of injections and the substances that will be used to lyse the adhesions is determined. Typically, hyalurinase, a local anesthetic and a steroid are injected followed by an injection of hypertonic saline 30-minutes later. The catheter is secured. The first injection or series of injections is administered. Before each injection or series of injections, contrast is again injected and the catheter position checked. The epidural space at the injection site is evaluated and the destruction of scar tissue and amount of opening of the epidural space around the target nerves or nerve roots is also noted prior to each injection. Use 62263 when a series of injections are administered over two or more days. Use 62264 when injections are administered over a single day.

62267

62267   Percutaneous aspiration within the nucleus pulposus, intervertebral disc, or paravertebral tissue for diagnostic purposes

The physician performs a diagnostic percutaneous aspiration within the nucleus pulposus, intervertebral disc, or paravertebral tissue. Fluid is aspirated or cells are harvested to evaluate infectious discitis, spinal or paravetral fluid accumulations, or other conditions. The skin is cleansed and a local anesthetic is administered at the planned puncture site. The needle is then inserted into the disc or paraspinal tissue using separately reportable image guidance. Fluid and/or tissue is aspirated. The needle is moved as needed and additional fluid or tissue samples are aspirated. The needle is removed and the fluid or tissue is sent for laboratory analysis.

62268

62268   Percutaneous aspiration, spinal cord cyst or syrinx

A cyst or syrinx, also called a syringomyelia, is a fluid filled cavity in the spinal cord. It results when cerebrospinal fluid (CSF) that normally flows around the spinal cord becomes trapped in a small cavity in the spinal canal. The cyst or syrinx can enlarge over time damaging the spinal cord and causing pain, weakness, and stiffness in the back and/or extremities. The skin is cleansed and a local anesthetic is administered at the planned puncture site. The needle is then inserted into the fluid filled sac using separately reportable image guidance. Fluid is aspirated. The needle may be repositioned and additional fluid aspirated. When the fluid has been evacuated from the space, the needle is removed.

62269

62269   Biopsy of spinal cord, percutaneous needle

The skin is cleansed and a local anesthetic is administered at the planned puncture site. The biopsy needle is then inserted into the spinal canal using separately reportable ultrasound, fluoroscopic or CT guidance. On or more tissue samples from the spinal cord are obtained and sent to the laboratory for separately reportable pathological examination.

62270-62272

62270   Spinal puncture, lumbar, diagnostic
62272   Spinal puncture, therapeutic, for drainage of cerebrospinal fluid (by needle or catheter)

A lumbar spinal puncture is performed for diagnostic or therapeutic purposes. In 62270, a diagnostic lumbar puncture is performed for symptoms that may be indicative of an infection, such as meningitis; a malignant neoplasm; bleeding, such as subarachoid hemorrhage; multiple sclerosis; Guillain-Barre syndrome. It may also be performed to measure cerebrospinal fluid (CSF) pressure. The skin over the lumbar spine is disinfected and a local anesthetic administered. A lumbar puncture needle is then inserted into the spinal canal and CSF specimens collected. The CSF specimens are sent to the laboratory for separately reportable evaluation. In 62272, a therapeutic spinal puncture is performed for elevated CSF pressure and CSF is drained using a needle or catheter placed as described above. CSF pressure is monitored during the drainage procedure and when the desired pressure is reached, the needle or catheter is removed.

62273

62273   Injection, epidural, of blood or clot patch

The physician injects a blood or clot patch into the epidural space. Epidural blood patches are used to treat the complication of severe headache caused by a leak of spinal fluid into the epidural space following epidural anesthesia or diagnostic or therapeutic spinal punctures. The skin over the lower back is disinfected and local anesthetic injected. A separate site is prepped for a venipuncture and an intravenous catheter is placed in the vein. The epidural needle is placed in the epidural space near the site of the previous puncture site. Blood is withdrawn from the venous catheter and the blood is then injected into the epidural space. The patient rests for approximately 30 minutes while the blood forms a patch over the CSF leak.

Nervous System

62280-62282

62280 Injection/infusion of neurolytic substance (eg, alcohol, phenol, iced saline solutions), with or without other therapeutic substance; subarachnoid

62281 Injection/infusion of neurolytic substance (eg, alcohol, phenol, iced saline solutions), with or without other therapeutic substance; epidural, cervical or thoracic

62282 Injection/infusion of neurolytic substance (eg, alcohol, phenol, iced saline solutions), with or without other therapeutic substance; epidural, lumbar, sacral (caudal)

This procedure may also be referred to as a neurolytic block. Neurolytic substances such as alcohol, phenol, or iced saline destroy neural structures involved in pain perception and provide long-lasting pain relief. Types of conditions treated include chronic, intractable, non-terminal pain that is not responsive to other pain management modalities or cancer pain. Neurolytic blocks can be performed by injection or infusion of a neurolytic substance into the subarachnoid space which lies between the arachnoid mater and pia mater, or into the epidural space which lies between the bone and the outermost membrane covering the spinal cord or dura mater. The patient is positioned on an x-ray table with the back exposed. The site where the injection is to be performed is cleansed and a local anesthetic administered. Using separately reportable fluoroscopic guidance, a spinal needle or cannula is inserted into the subarachnoid or epidural space. A small amount of contrast is injected to ensure that the needle or cannula is properly positioned. The neurolytic substance is then injected or infused. Use 62280 for a subarachnoid injection or infusion at any level of the spine; use 62281 for an epidural injection or infusion in the cervical or thoracic region; and use 62282 for an epidural injection or infusion in the lumbar or sacral (caudal) region.

62284

62284 Injection procedure for myelography and/or computed tomography, lumbar (other than C1-C2 and posterior fossa)

The spinal canal (subarachnoid space) is injected with contrast material to visualize structures including the spinal cord and spinal nerve roots for separately reportable myelography and/or computed tomography (CT). This code is used to report injection procedures of the lumbar region of the spine. The patient is placed face-down on the examination table. The spine is visualized using separately reportable fluoroscopy. The skin over the planned injection site, usually the lower lumbar spine, is cleansed and a local anesthetic is injected. The patient may be repositioned if needed on the side or in a sitting position. A needle is then inserted into the subarachnoid space and contrast material is then injected. The X-ray table is tilted so that contrast material will move through the subarachnoid space enhancing visualization of the spinal cord and spinal nerve roots.

62287

▲ **62287** Decompression procedure, percutaneous, of nucleus pulposus of intervertebral disc, any method utilizing needle based technique to remove disc material under fluoroscopic imaging or other form of indirect visualization, with discography and/or epidural injection(s) at the treated level(s), when performed, single or multiple levels, lumbar

Percutaneous decompression of the nucleus pulposus of a herniated lumbar intervertebral disc is done by needle based technique to remove disc material using fluoroscopic imaging or other form of indirect visualization. Percutaneous disc decompression is done for patients with a contained herniated disc that is bulging without rupture. Different percutaneous procedures include manual, automated, and radiofrequency or laser methods. All types of procedures involve inserting small instruments through a needle placed between the vertebrae into the middle of the disc. Radiographic monitoring, such as fluoroscopy, is used to guide the instruments as herniated tissue is removed. Laser instruments burn or evaporate the disc. One method called coblation nucleoplasty uses low frequency radiowaves to carve tunnels in the disc by causing tissue to disintegrate into gases at the molecular level. Using fluoroscopic guidance, the needle is advanced through the skin and into the disc using a trajectory that avoids the spinal canal. Small amounts of contrast may be injected to ensure that the needle is properly positioned in the disc. A nucleoplasty cannula is then advanced through the needle and into the disc. The nucleoplasty catheter is activated and the nucleus pulposus is vaporized. As the catheter is withdrawn, coagulation is used to shrink the channel created by the coblation process which further decompresses the disc. Usually 6-12 channels are created using this technique. Another method, called DISC nucleoplasty, uses special plasma technology, instead of heat energy, to remove the tissue from the center of the disc. A SpineWand is inserted through a needle into the center of the disc. A series of channels are made to remove tissue precisely and without trauma. As tissue is removed from the nucleus, the disc is decompressed and the pressure exerted on the nearby nerve root is relieved. Use this code for percutaneous decompression of single or multiple lumbar levels.

62290-62291

62290 Injection procedure for discography, each level; lumbar

62291 Injection procedure for discography, each level; cervical or thoracic

Discography is performed to determine if an intervertebral disc abnormality is the cause of back pain. The patient is positioned on the side and the site of the injection is cleansed with an antiseptic solution. A local anesthetic is injected. Using separately reportable fluoroscopic supervision, a large bore needle is advanced through the skin to the disc. A discography needle is advanced through the first needle and into the center of the disc. Contrast is injected and separately reportable radiographs obtained. The procedure may be repeated on multiple discs and is reported for each level injected. Use 62290 for each lumbar disc injected; use 62291 for each cervical or thoracic disc injected.

62292

62292 Injection procedure for chemonucleolysis, including discography, intervertebral disc, single or multiple levels, lumbar

Chemonucleolysis involves the injection of the enzyme chymopapain into the gelatinous center of the intervertebral disc to treat herniated nucleus pulposus. This enzyme dissolves the gelantinous nucleus pulposus. The patient is positioned on the side and the site of the injection is cleansed with an antiseptic solution. A local anesthetic is injected. Using separately reportable fluoroscopic supervision, a large bore needle is advanced through the skin to the disc. A discography needle is advanced through the first needle and into the center of the disc. Saline or water may be injected to ensure that the correct disc has been penetrated. The saline or water injection will reproduce the patient's pain. Alternatively, contrast may be injected and separately reportable radiographs obtained. Once placement in the correct disc has been verified, a small test dose of chymopapain is injected to determine whether the patient is hypersensitive to the enzyme. The patient is observed for 10-15 minutes and if no adverse effects are noted, a full dose of chymopapain is injected. The procedure may be repeated on multiple lumbar discs.

62294

62294 Injection procedure, arterial, for occlusion of arteriovenous malformation, spinal

Endovascular occlusion is performed to treat a spinal anteriorvenous malformation (AVM). An AVM is a congenital malformation of blood vessels characterized by a tangled web of arteries and veins connected by abnormal connections called fistulas. Less common are acquired AVMs that form between an artery and vein following an injury or infection. The skin over the access artery, usually the femoral artery, is prepped. The artery is punctured with a needle. A sheath is placed over the needle and the needle removed. A guidewire is inserted through the sheath and advanced through the access artery to the aorta and then into the spinal artery that feeds the AVM. A catheter is threaded over the guidewire and the guidewire is withdrawn. The spinal artery is then occluded by injecting the artery with a liquid tissue adhesive, micro-coils, micro-particles, or other material. Following the occlusion procedure, contast is injected to ensure that the AVM is completely occluded. The catheter and sheath are removed and a pressure dressing applied over the access artery.

62302-62305

62302 Myelography via lumbar injection, including radiological supervision and interpretation; cervical

62303 Myelography via lumbar injection, including radiological supervision and interpretation; thoracic

62304 Myelography via lumbar injection, including radiological supervision and interpretation; lumbosacral

62305 Myelography via lumbar injection, including radiological supervision and interpretation; 2 or more regions (eg, lumbar/thoracic, cervical/thoracic, lumbar/cervical, lumbar/thoracic/cervical)

Myelography is an imaging technique that provides a detailed picture of the spinal canal, spinal cord, and spinal nerve roots using real time fluoroscopy and x-rays. The procedure is done under the direct supervision of a radiologist and may be used to diagnose intervertebral disc herniation, spinal stenosis, tumors, infection, inflammation, and other lesions caused by disease or trauma. The patient is positioned lying on the abdomen or side. Under fluoroscopy, a spinal needle is advanced into the spinal canal at the lumbar region until a free flow of cerebrospinal fluid (CSF) is observed. A contrast material (non-ionic dye) is injected through the needle into the subarachnoid space and the needle is withdrawn. The procedure table is slowly tilted up or down to allow the contrast dye to flow within the subarachnoid space. The flow of dye is monitored using fluoroscopy and x-rays may then be obtained to document abnormalities. When the procedure is complete, the table is returned to a horizontal position and the patient is allowed to assume a comfortable position. Code 62302 is used for examination of the cervical region of the spine; code 62303 for the thoracic region; code 62304 for the lumbosacral area; and code 62305 is reported when 2 or more areas of the spine are examined.

Nervous System

62350-62351

62350 Implantation, revision or repositioning of tunneled intrathecal or epidural catheter, for long-term medication administration via an external pump or implantable reservoir/infusion pump; without laminectomy

62351 Implantation, revision or repositioning of tunneled intrathecal or epidural catheter, for long-term medication administration via an external pump or implantable reservoir/infusion pump; with laminectomy

Implantation, revision, or repositioning of an intrathecal or epidural catheter may be performed with or without a laminectomy. In 62350, the procedure is performed without a laminectomy. For initial implantation, the overlying skin is cleansed with an antiseptic solution and a local anesthetic injected. A spinal needle is inserted into the skin and advanced into the intrathecal or epidural space. A catheter is then threaded through the needle and the catheter tip advanced cephalad to the selected level for pain control or other medication administration. The catheter is then tunneled subcutaneously approximately 5-10 cm away from the insertion site. The catheter is secured with sutures. The catheter is then connected to an external pump or an implantable reservoir or infusion pump. If revision of the catheter is performed the catheter is exposed and the connection site at the reservoir or pump is inspected. The catheter may be disconnected and trimmed and reconnected or other revisions made. If repositioning is performed, the catheter is disconnected from the internal or external pump or reservoir. The catheter is manipulated into a different site within the intrathecal or epidural space. The revised or repositioned catheter is secured with sutures and reconnected to the pump or reservoir. In 62351, the procedure is performed with a laminectomy. The skin is incised over the catheter placement site and extended down to the spinous processes. Muscle is retracted off the lamina and facet joint. A bone drill is used to remove part or all of the lamina. The intrathecal or epidural catheter is implanted, revised, or repositioned as described above. The catheter is tunneled through the subcutaneous tissue and connected to the pump or reservoir. The surgical wound is closed.

62355

62355 Removal of previously implanted intrathecal or epidural catheter

The previously placed intrathecal or epidural catheter is exposed at the distal aspect of the tunnel and disconnected from the pump or reservoir. Distal sutures are removed. The tunneled portion of the catheter is then palpated from the pump or reservoir site to the site where it enters the spinal canal. A small incision is made over the site where the catheter enters the spinal canal. The subcutaneous tunneled portion of the catheter is removed. Proximal sutures are removed. The catheter is then removed from the intrathecal or epidural space. The skin is closed with a suture or steristrips.

62360-62362

62360 Implantation or replacement of device for intrathecal or epidural drug infusion; subcutaneous reservoir

62361 Implantation or replacement of device for intrathecal or epidural drug infusion; nonprogrammable pump

62362 Implantation or replacement of device for intrathecal or epidural drug infusion; programmable pump, including preparation of pump, with or without programming

For initial implantation of a subcutaneous reservoir or pump, the skin is incised, typically in the lateral aspect of the lower abdomen. A subcutaneous pocket is fashioned. The subcutaneous reservoir or pump is connected to the catheter and placed in the pocket. The skin is closed over the device. For replacement of a subcutaneous reservoir or pump, the old device is first removed in a separately reportable procedure. The new device is then inserted. Use 62360 for placement of a subcutaneous reservoir. Use 62361 for placement of a nonprogrammable pump. Use 62362 for placement of a programmable pump. Placement of a programmable pump requires preparation of the pump. The reservoir and alarm status is checked to ensure that the pump will function properly once implanted. Dosing, continuous infusion rate and/or time intervals for bolus infusion may be programmed at this time.

62365

62365 Removal of subcutaneous reservoir or pump, previously implanted for intrathecal or epidural infusion

An incision is made in the skin over the implanted reservoir or pump. The device is exposed and dissected free of subcutaneous tissue. The device is disconnected from the intrathecal or epidural catheter and removed. Separately reportable procedures are then performed either to remove the catheter or to replace the reservoir or pump.

62367-62368

62367 Electronic analysis of programmable, implanted pump for intrathecal or epidural drug infusion (includes evaluation of reservoir status, alarm status, drug prescription status); without reprogramming or refill

62368 Electronic analysis of programmable, implanted pump for intrathecal or epidural drug infusion (includes evaluation of reservoir status, alarm status, drug prescription status); with reprogramming

A previously placed programmable implanted intrathecal or epidural drug infusion pump is evaluated using electronic analysis. A connection is established between the programmable pump and the interrogation device. The interrogation device provides information on reservoir status, alarm status and drug flow rates, which are evaluated to ensure that these are within normal parameters. The physician reviews the data obtained by the interrogation device and provides a written report of findings. In 62367, the pump is not reprogrammed or refilled. In 62368, the physician reprograms the pump using a telemetry device. Reprogramming may include adjusting alarm parameters and drug flow rates. The new settings are verified with the interrogation device. The pump is not refilled

62369-62370

62369 Electronic analysis of programmable, implanted pump for intrathecal or epidural drug infusion (includes evaluation of reservoir status, alarm status, drug prescription status); with reprogramming and refill

62370 Electronic analysis of programmable, implanted pump for intrathecal or epidural drug infusion (includes evaluation of reservoir status, alarm status, drug prescription status); with reprogramming and refill (requiring skill of a physician or other qualified health care professional)

A previously placed programmable, implanted intrathecal or epidural drug infusion pump is evaluated using electronic analysis. A connection is established between the programmable pump and the interrogation device. The interrogation device provides information on reservoir status, alarm status, and drug flow rates, which are evaluated to ensure that these are within normal parameters. The technician or physician reviews the data obtained by the interrogation device and determines that reprogramming is needed. Reprogramming is performed using a telemetry device and may include adjusting alarm parameters and drug flow rates. The new settings are verified with the interrogation device. The pump is also refilled. A written report of findings is provided. Use 62369 when the evaluation, reprogramming, and refilling of the pump is performed by a technician. Use 62370 when the skill of a physician or other qualified health care professional is required.

63001-63011

63001 Laminectomy with exploration and/or decompression of spinal cord and/or cauda equina, without facetectomy, foraminotomy or discectomy (eg, spinal stenosis), 1 or 2 vertebral segments; cervical

63003 Laminectomy with exploration and/or decompression of spinal cord and/or cauda equina, without facetectomy, foraminotomy or discectomy (eg, spinal stenosis), 1 or 2 vertebral segments; thoracic

63005 Laminectomy with exploration and/or decompression of spinal cord and/or cauda equina, without facetectomy, foraminotomy or discectomy (eg, spinal stenosis), 1 or 2 vertebral segments; lumbar, except for spondylolisthesis

63011 Laminectomy with exploration and/or decompression of spinal cord and/or cauda equina, without facetectomy, foraminotomy or discectomy (eg, spinal stenosis), 1 or 2 vertebral segments; sacral

Laminectomy (lamina excision) is performed to determine the cause of back pain and to relieve pressure on the spinal cord, spinal nerve roots, and/or cauda equina. The lamina is the portion of the vertebra that forms posterior aspect of the vertebral arch. A posterior skin incision is made over the affected portion of the spine. Overlying fat and muscle are retracted off the lamina. The lamina is excised. The underlying paired ligaments (ligamentum flavum) that bind the lamina of contiguous vertebrae together are also excised. The spinal canal is exposed and explored. The spinal canal is exposed and explored. Adhesions between the dura and ligamentum flavum are lysed. The spinal nerve roots and/or cauda equina are carefully dissected and freed within the intervertebral foramen. The procedure may be performed on a single vertebra or two contiguous vertebrae. Separately reportable arthrodesis is performed as needed to stabilize the spine. Laminectomy of 1 or 2 vertebral segments of the cervical spine is reported with 63001, thoracic spine with 63003, lumbar spine with 63005, and sacral spine with 63011.

63012

63012 Laminectomy with removal of abnormal facets and/or pars inter-articularis with decompression of cauda equina and nerve roots for spondylolisthesis, lumbar (Gill type procedure)

Spondylolisthesis is a condition in which one of the lower lumbar vertebral bodies, usually the fifth vertebral body, slips forward on the vertebral body below it. The condition begins with spondylolysis, which refers to degeneration or deficient development of the pars interarticularis of the slipped vertebra. The pars interarticularis is the segment of bone between the superior and inferior articular facets. A posterior skin incision is made over the affected vertebrae of the lumbar spine. Overlying fat and muscle are retracted off the

Nervous System

● New Code   ▲ Revised Code

lamina. The lamina is excised. The underlying paired ligaments (ligamentum flavum) that bind the lamina of contiguous vertebrae together are also excised. The superior and inferior articular facets and the pars interarticularis are inspected and smoothed or excised as needed. The spinal canal is exposed and explored. Adhesions between the dura and ligamentum flavum are lysed. The spinal nerve roots and/or cauda equina are carefully dissected and freed within the intervertebral foramen. The surgical wound is closed in layers.

63015-63017

63015   **Laminectomy with exploration and/or decompression of spinal cord and/or cauda equina, without facetectomy, foraminotomy or discectomy (eg, spinal stenosis), more than 2 vertebral segments; cervical**

63016   **Laminectomy with exploration and/or decompression of spinal cord and/or cauda equina, without facetectomy, foraminotomy or discectomy (eg, spinal stenosis), more than 2 vertebral segments; thoracic**

63017   **Laminectomy with exploration and/or decompression of spinal cord and/or cauda equina, without facetectomy, foraminotomy or discectomy (eg, spinal stenosis), more than 2 vertebral segments; lumbar**

Laminectomy (lamina excision) is performed to determine the cause of back pain and to relieve pressure on the spinal cord, spinal nerve roots, and/or cauda equina. The lamina is the portion of the vertebra that forms posterior aspect of the vertebral arch. A posterior skin incision is made over the affected portion of the spine. Overlying fat and muscle are retracted off the lamina. The lamina is excised. The underlying paired ligaments (ligamentum flavum) that bind the lamina of contiguous vertebrae together are also excised. The spinal canal is exposed and explored. The spinal canal is exposed and explored. Adhesions between the dura and ligamentum flavum are lysed. The spinal nerve roots and/or cauda equina are carefully dissected and freed within the intervertebral foramen. The procedure is performed on more than two contiguous vertebrae. Separately reportable arthrodesis is performed as needed to stabilize the spine. Laminectomy of more than 2 vertebral segments of the cervical spine is reported with 63015, thoracic spine with 63016, and lumbar spine with 63017.

63020-63035

63020   **Laminotomy (hemilaminectomy), with decompression of nerve root(s), including partial facetectomy, foraminotomy and/or excision of herniated intervertebral disc; 1 interspace, cervical**

63030   **Laminotomy (hemilaminectomy), with decompression of nerve root(s), including partial facetectomy, foraminotomy and/or excision of herniated intervertebral disc; 1 interspace, lumbar**

63035   **Laminotomy (hemilaminectomy), with decompression of nerve root(s), including partial facetectomy, foraminotomy and/or excision of herniated intervertebral disc; each additional interspace, cervical or lumbar (List separately in addition to code for primary procedure)**

A posterior approach laminotomy or hemilaminectomy with nerve root decompression is carried out on one interspace, including partial facetectomy, foraminotomy, and/or excision of a herniated intervertebral disc. A laminotomy is an incision into the lamina of the vertebral arch to open the space and decompress the spinal cord or nerve roots. It is sometimes performed as a hemilaminectomy, removing a portion of the lamina from the left or right side, usually with a portion of the facet joint also. The skin incision is marked out and carried down to the spinous processes. Muscle is retracted off the lamina and facet joint. The level is verified radiographically, and an operating microscope is brought in. A bone drill is used to remove part of the lamina and the facet joint (partial facetectomy) to allow more room for the compressed nerve(s). The ligamentum flavum attaching the vertebral lamina may be removed to expose the dura and compressed nerves. The openings under the facet joints where the nerve runs through are checked, and a portion of the bone around the opening may be removed for additional pressure relief, if necessary (foraminotomy). Ruptured disc fragments or bulging nucleus pulposus is also removed to decompress the nerve(s). The surgical wound is closed in layers. Code 63020 reports one cervical interspace; code 63030 reports one lumbar interspace; and code 63035 is used for each additional interspace, either cervical or lumbar.

63040-63044

63040   **Laminotomy (hemilaminectomy), with decompression of nerve root(s), including partial facetectomy, foraminotomy and/or excision of herniated intervertebral disc, reexploration, single interspace; cervical**

63042   **Laminotomy (hemilaminectomy), with decompression of nerve root(s), including partial facetectomy, foraminotomy and/or excision of herniated intervertebral disc, reexploration, single interspace; lumbar**

63043   **Laminotomy (hemilaminectomy), with decompression of nerve root(s), including partial facetectomy, foraminotomy and/or excision of herniated intervertebral disc, reexploration, single interspace; each additional cervical interspace (List separately in addition to code for primary procedure)**

63044   **Laminotomy (hemilaminectomy), with decompression of nerve root(s), including partial facetectomy, foraminotomy and/or excision of herniated intervertebral disc, reexploration, single interspace; each additional lumbar interspace (List separately in addition to code for primary procedure)**

Laminotomy (hemilaminectomy) for re-exploration of a previously explored cervical (63040, 63043) or lumbar (63042, 63044) disc space is performed with decompression of nerve roots. This procedure may include partial facetectomy, foraminotomy, and/or excision of herniated intervertebral disc. The previous skin incision is reopened and the disc space is exposed. Scar tissue over the laminae is removed and the laminotomy is enlarged. Scar tissue within the disc space is dissected. The nerve root is identified and explored. Scar tissue and bony spurs are removed. A portion of the flat articular surface (facet) of the vertebra may be excised (facetectomy). The foramen is enlarged as needed (foraminotomy). If a herniated disc is found, disc material is curetted from the disc space to decompress the nerve root. Upon completion of the procedure, bleeding is controlled by coagulation; the wound is irrigated; and incisions are closed. Use 63040 for laminotomy and re-exploration of a single cervical interspace and 63043 for each additional cervical interspace. Use 63042 for laminotomy and re-exploration of a single lumbar interspace and 63044 for each additional lumbar interspace.

63045-63048

63045   **Laminectomy, facetectomy and foraminotomy (unilateral or bilateral with decompression of spinal cord, cauda equina and/or nerve root[s], [eg, spinal or lateral recess stenosis]), single vertebral segment; cervical**

63046   **Laminectomy, facetectomy and foraminotomy (unilateral or bilateral with decompression of spinal cord, cauda equina and/or nerve root[s], [eg, spinal or lateral recess stenosis]), single vertebral segment; thoracic**

63047   **Laminectomy, facetectomy and foraminotomy (unilateral or bilateral with decompression of spinal cord, cauda equina and/or nerve root[s], [eg, spinal or lateral recess stenosis]), single vertebral segment; lumbar**

63048   **Laminectomy, facetectomy and foraminotomy (unilateral or bilateral with decompression of spinal cord, cauda equina and/or nerve root[s], [eg, spinal or lateral recess stenosis]), single vertebral segment; each additional segment, cervical, thoracic, or lumbar (List separately in addition to code for primary procedure)**

Laminectomy (lamina excision) is performed to determine the cause of back pain and to relieve pressure on the spinal cord, spinal nerve roots, and/or cauda equina. The lamina is the portion of the vertebra that forms posterior aspect of the vertebral arch. A posterior skin incision is made over the affected portion of the spine down to the spinous process. Overlying fat and muscle are retracted off the lamina. The lamina is excised. The underlying paired ligaments (ligamentum flavum) that bind the lamina of contiguous vertebrae together are also excised. The superior and inferior articular facets and the pars interarticularis are inspected. The openings under the facet joints where the spinal nerves emerge are explored and bone is removed as needed to decompress the nerve roots. The spinal canal is exposed and explored. The intervertebral foramen is enlarged to decompress the spinal cord. Adhesions between the dura and ligamentum flavum are lysed. The spinal nerve roots and/or cauda equina are carefully dissected and freed within the intervertebral foramen. The surgical wound is closed in layers. Separately reportable arthrodesis is performed as needed to stabilize the spine. Laminectomy, facetectomy, and foraminotomy of a single vertebral segment of the cervical spine are reported with 63045, thoracic spine with 63046, and lumbar spine with 63047, and each additional cervical, thoracic or lumbar segment is reported with 63048.

63050-63051

63050   **Laminoplasty, cervical, with decompression of the spinal cord, 2 or more vertebral segments**

63051   **Laminoplasty, cervical, with decompression of the spinal cord, 2 or more vertebral segments; with reconstruction of the posterior bony elements (including the application of bridging bone graft and non-segmental fixation devices [eg, wire, suture, mini-plates], when performed)**

Cervical laminoplasty is performed to treat spinal stenosis. The aim of the procedure is to put pressure on the spinal cord while maintaining posterior stability of the spine. This is accomplished by partially cutting the bony posterior elements on one side to create

● New Code   ▲ Revised Code   © 2017 DecisionHealth

Nervous System

a hinge and completely cutting posterior bone on the opposite side to form a partially opened door. A posterior incision is made over the cervical spine. Paraspinous muscles are retracted and the laminae, spinous processes, and facet joints over the affected vertebral bodies are exposed. Complete osteotomy of 2 or more vertebral segments is performed on the side that will form the open door component. The ligamentum flavum is divided. On the opposite side a hinge is created by scoring each vertebra with a drill at the junction of the facet and lamina. An elevator is used to open the side on which the complete ostetomy has been performed, relieving pressure on the spinal cord. In 63050, reconstruction of the bony elements is not performed. In 63051, reconstruction using bone grafts and/or a nonsegmental fixation device is performed following the laminoplasty. If bone grafts are used, the separately reportable bone allografts or autografts are configured to fit the bony defects. The bone grafts are then placed into the defects in each vertebra on the side of the complete osteotomy to maintain the opening. Fixation devices, such as wire, suture, or mini-plastes are then applied as needed across the osteotomy to secure the bone grafts. The surgical wound is closed in layers.

63055-63057

63055 Transpedicular approach with decompression of spinal cord, equina and/or nerve root(s) (eg, herniated intervertebral disc), single segment; thoracic

63056 Transpedicular approach with decompression of spinal cord, equina and/or nerve root(s) (eg, herniated intervertebral disc), single segment; lumbar (including transfacet, or lateral extraforaminal approach) (eg, far lateral herniated intervertebral disc)

63057 Transpedicular approach with decompression of spinal cord, equina and/or nerve root(s) (eg, herniated intervertebral disc), single segment; each additional segment, thoracic or lumbar (List separately in addition to code for primary procedure)

A transpedicular approach requires removal of part of one of the two pedicles. The pedicles are short, thick bone processes that project posteriorly from the body of the vertebra and unite with the lamina to form the vertebral arch, which contain the spinal cord. A skin incision is made at the lateral margin of the spinous process of the affected cervical disc. The paraspinal muscles are elevated off the spinous process, lamina and tranverse process. The lamina and facet joint are exposed. The medial portion of the facet and the lateral portion of the lamina are removed using a high-speed drill. The pedicle is partially removed and the lateral margin of the spinal cord exposed. The spinal nerve root and herniated portion of the intervertebral disc are identified. Any bone spurs at the site of the herniation are excised and a cavity is created. The cavity is enlarged and ruptured disc fragments or bulging nucleus pulposus impinging on the spinal cord, nerve root, and/or cauda equina are removed. Additional bone is removed as needed to relieve pressure on the nerve. Bleeding is controlled and the surgical wound is closed in layers. Use code 63055 for transpedicular decompression of a single segment of the thoracic spine; use 63056 for a single segment of the lumbar spine, and 63057 for each additional thoracic or lumbar segment.

63064-63066

63064 Costovertebral approach with decompression of spinal cord or nerve root(s) (eg, herniated intervertebral disc), thoracic; single segment

63066 Costovertebral approach with decompression of spinal cord or nerve root(s) (eg, herniated intervertebral disc), thoracic; each additional segment (List separately in addition to code for primary procedure)

A costovertebral approach involves partial rib excision and removal of the transverse process on the affected side of the vertebra so that a ventral window can be created for visualization of the spinal cord and nerve roots. The transverse processes extend laterally from the neural arch at the point where the pedicles and lamina join on each side of the vertebra. The transverse processes of the thoracic spine are longer and heavier than those in other regions and have facets that articulate with the tubercles (heads) of the ribs. A semilunar skin incision is made at the appropriate level over the thoracic spine and extended over the posterior aspect of the rib. Overlying soft tissue and muscle are dissected and the posterior aspect of the rib exposed. The paraspinal muscles are elevated off the spinous process, lamina and tranverse process. The lamina and facet joint are exposed. A portion of the rib and transverse process are removed using a high-speed drill to create a window. The spinal cord and nerve roots are exposed. The intervertebral disc is exposed and any herniation noted. Bone spurs are excised and a cavity is created. The cavity is enlarged and any ruptured disc fragments or bulging nucleus pulposus impinging on the spinal cord and/or nerve root are removed. Additional bone is removed as needed to relieve pressure on the nerve. Bleeding is controlled and the surgical wound is closed in layers. Use 63064 for a single thoracic vertebral segment and 63066 for each additional thoracic vertebral segment.

63075-63076

63075 Discectomy, anterior, with decompression of spinal cord and/or nerve root(s), including osteophytectomy; cervical, single interspace

63076 Discectomy, anterior, with decompression of spinal cord and/or nerve root(s), including osteophytectomy; cervical, each additional interspace (List separately in addition to code for primary procedure)

Anterior discectomy of the cervical spine is performed through a skin incision in the anterior aspect of the neck. The soft tissues and muscles overlying the cervical spine are dissected. The trachea and esophagus are retracted away from the surgical site. The affected portion of the cervical spine exposed. The intervertebral disc is exposed and carefully removed with the aid of the surgical microscope. Bone spurs and any bone impinging on the nerve roots are also removed, along with the ligament that covers the spinal cord. If a separately reportable bone graft is needed, the bone is contoured for placement of the graft. Separately reportable internal fixation may also be used to stabilize the spine. Upon completion of the procedure bleeding is controlled and soft tissues and skin are closed in layers. Use 63075 for a single cervical interspace and 63076 for each additional interspace.

63077-63078

63077 Discectomy, anterior, with decompression of spinal cord and/or nerve root(s), including osteophytectomy; thoracic, single interspace

63078 Discectomy, anterior, with decompression of spinal cord and/or nerve root(s), including osteophytectomy; thoracic, each additional interspace (List separately in addition to code for primary procedure)

Anterior discectomy of the thoracic spine is performed using a thoracic approach, which requires a thoracotomy. Typically a team approach is used with the exposure being performed by a thoracic surgeon and the discectomy performed by a spine surgeon. The skin over the thorax is incised to allow access to the appropriate level of the thoracic spine. Overlying muscles are dissected and a rib is resected. Rib spreaders are used to allow adequate exposure of the spine. The affected portion of the thoracic spine is exposed. The intervertebral disc is exposed and carefully removed with the aid of the surgical microscope. Bone spurs and any bone impinging on the nerve roots are also removed along with the ligament that covers the spinal cord. If a separately reportable bone graft is needed, the bone is contoured for placement of the graft. Separately reportable internal fixation may also be used to stabilize the spine. Upon completion of the procedure bleeding is controlled, a chest tube is placed, and the thorax is closed in layers. Use 63077 for a single thoracic interspace and 63078 for each additional interspace.

63081-63082

63081 Vertebral corpectomy (vertebral body resection), partial or complete, anterior approach with decompression of spinal cord and/or nerve root(s); cervical, single segment

63082 Vertebral corpectomy (vertebral body resection), partial or complete, anterior approach with decompression of spinal cord and/or nerve root(s); cervical, each additional segment (List separately in addition to code for primary procedure)

Vertebral corpectomy involves removal of the vertebral body as well as the vertebral discs above and below the vertebra. The procedure is typically performed to treat severe spinal stenosis with bone spurs arising from the vertebral body as well as the vertebral arch. The procedure may also be performed to treat fracture, tumor or infection of the spine. Often multiple vertebral segments are involved. The cervical spine is exposed via an anterior approach, beginning with a skin incision in the anterior aspect of the neck. The soft tissues and muscles overlying the cervical spine are dissected. The trachea and esophagus are retracted. The affected segment of the cervical spine is exposed. The intervertebral discs above and below the vertebral body are removed first with the aid of the surgical microscope. The discs are carefully dissected from surrounding tissue and removed. Bone spurs and any bone impinging on the nerve roots are also removed along with the ligament that covers the spinal cord. The vertebral body is then excised. Separately reportable bone grafting and fusion procedures are performed. The bone graft is placed in the surgical defect to support the anterior aspect of the spine where the discs and vertebral body have been removed. Surrounding bone is contoured for placement of the graft and to ensure fusion of the graft and adjacent bone. Separately reportable internal fixation may also be used to stabilize the spine. Upon completion of the procedure, bleeding is controlled and soft tissues and skin are closed in layers. Use 63081 for a single cervical segment and 63082 for each additional cervical segment.

Nervous System

63085-63086

63085 Vertebral corpectomy (vertebral body resection), partial or complete, transthoracic approach with decompression of spinal cord and/or nerve root(s); thoracic, single segment

63086 Vertebral corpectomy (vertebral body resection), partial or complete, transthoracic approach with decompression of spinal cord and/or nerve root(s); thoracic, each additional segment (List separately in addition to code for primary procedure)

Vertebral corpectomy involves removal of the vertebral body as well as the vertebral discs above and below the vertebra. The procedure is typically performed to treat severe spinal stenosis with bone spurs, arising from the vertebral body as well as the vertebral arch. The procedure may also be performed to treat fracture, tumor or infection of the spine. Often multiple vertebral segments are involved. Vertebral corpectomy of the thoracic spine is performed using a transthoracic approach, which requires a thoracotomy. Typically a co-surgeon or team approach is used, with the exposure being performed by a thoracic surgeon and the corpectomy performed by a spine surgeon. The skin over the thorax is incised to allow access to the appropriate levels of the thoracic spine. Overlying muscles are dissected and one or more ribs are resected. Rib spreaders are used to allow adequate exposure of the spine. The affected portion of the thoracic spine is exposed. The intervertebral discs above and below the vertebral body are removed first with the aid of the surgical microscope. The discs are carefully dissected from surrounding tissue and removed. Bone spurs and any bone impinging on the nerve roots are also removed along with the ligament that covers the spinal cord. The vertebral body is then excised. Separately reportable bone grafting and fusion procedures are performed. The bone graft is placed in the surgical defect to support the anterior aspect of the spine where the discs and vertebral body have been removed. Surrounding bone is contoured for placement of the graft and to ensure fusion of the graft and adjacent bone. Separately reportable internal fixation may also be used to stabilize the spine. Upon completion of the procedure bleeding is controlled, a chest tube is placed, and the thorax is closed in layers. Use 63085 for a single thoracic segment and 63086 for each additional thoracic segment.

63087-63088

63087 Vertebral corpectomy (vertebral body resection), partial or complete, combined thoracolumbar approach with decompression of spinal cord, cauda equina or nerve root(s), lower thoracic or lumbar; single segment

63088 Vertebral corpectomy (vertebral body resection), partial or complete, combined thoracolumbar approach with decompression of spinal cord, cauda equina or nerve root(s), lower thoracic or lumbar; each additional segment (List separately in addition to code for primary procedure)

Vertebral corpectomy involves removal of the vertebral body as well as the vertebral discs above and below the vertebra. The procedure is typically performed to treat severe spinal stenosis with bone spurs arising from the vertebral body as well as the vertebral arch. The procedure may also be performed to treat fracture, tumor or infection of the spine. Often multiple vertebral segments are involved. Vertebral corpectomy of the lower thoracic or lumbar spine is performed using a combined thoracolumbar approach. Typically a co-surgeon team approach is used, with the exposure being performed by a thoracic surgeon and the corpectomy performed by a spine surgeon. The skin over the thorax is incised to allow access to the appropriate levels of the thoracic spine. Overlying muscles are dissected and one or more ribs are resected. Rib spreaders are used to allow adequate exposure of the thoracic spine. The thoracic incision is extended over the abdomen to allow adequate exposure of all diseased or damaged lower thoracic and lumbar segments. Once the spine is adequately exposed, intervertebral discs above and below the vertebral body are removed with the aid of the surgical microscope. The discs are carefully dissected from surrounding tissue and removed. Bone spurs and any bone impinging on the nerve roots are also removed, along with the ligament that covers the spinal cord. The vertebral body is then excised. Separately reportable bone grafting and fusion procedures are performed. The bone graft is placed in the surgical defect to support the anterior aspect of the spine where the discs and vertebral body have been removed. Surrounding bone is contoured for placement of the graft and to ensure fusion of the graft and adjacent bone. Separately reportable internal fixation may also be used to stabilize the spine. Upon completion of the procedure bleeding is controlled, a chest tube is placed, and the thorax and abdomen are closed in layers. Use 63087 for a single lower thoracic or lumbar segment and 63088 for each additional segment.

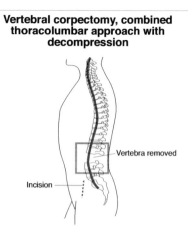

Vertebral corpectomy, combined thoracolumbar approach with decompression

Vertebra removed

Incision

Lower thoracic or lumbar, single segment (63087);
lower thoracic or lumbar, each additional segment (63088)

63090-63091

63090 Vertebral corpectomy (vertebral body resection), partial or complete, transperitoneal or retroperitoneal approach with decompression of spinal cord, cauda equina or nerve root(s), lower thoracic, lumbar, or sacral; single segment

63091 Vertebral corpectomy (vertebral body resection), partial or complete, transperitoneal or retroperitoneal approach with decompression of spinal cord, cauda equina or nerve root(s), lower thoracic, lumbar, or sacral; each additional segment (List separately in addition to code for primary procedure)

Vertebral corpectomy involves removal of the vertebral body as well as the vertebral discs above and below the vertebra. The procedure is typically performed to treat severe spinal stenosis with bone spurs arising from the vertebral body as well as the vertebral arch. The procedure may also be performed to treat fracture, tumor or infection of the spine. Often multiple vertebral segments are involved. Vertebral corpectomy of the lower thoracic, lumbar, or sacral spine is performed using an anterior or anterolateral approach. A co-surgeon or team approach may be used, with the exposure being performed by a general surgeon and the corpectomy performed by a spine surgeon. If a transperitoneal (anterior) approach is used, the abdomen is incised and the peritoneum entered. The bowel is moved out of the way. If a retroperitoneal (anterolateral) approach is used, a flank incision is made. Surrounding tissues are dissected taking care to protect vital structures. All diseased or damaged lower thoracic, lumbar and/or sacral segments are exposed. Intervertebral discs above and below the vertebral body are removed with the aid of the surgical microscope. The discs are carefully dissected from surrounding tissue and removed. Bone spurs and any bone impinging on the nerve roots and/or cauda equina is also removed, along with the ligament that covers the spinal cord. The vertebral body is then excised. Separately reportable bone grafting and fusion procedures are performed. The bone graft is placed in the surgical defect to support the anterior aspect of the spine where the discs and vertebral body have been removed. Surrounding bone is contoured for placement of the graft and to ensure fusion of the graft and adjacent bone. Separately reportable internal fixation may also be used to stabilize the spine. Upon completion of the procedure bleeding is controlled, drains placed as needed, and the surgical wound is closed in layers. Use 63090 for a single lower thoracic, lumbar, or sacral segment and 63091 for each additional segment.

63101-63103

63101 Vertebral corpectomy (vertebral body resection), partial or complete, lateral extracavitary approach with decompression of spinal cord and/or nerve root(s) (eg, for tumor or retropulsed bone fragments); thoracic, single segment

63102 Vertebral corpectomy (vertebral body resection), partial or complete, lateral extracavitary approach with decompression of spinal cord and/or nerve root(s) (eg, for tumor or retropulsed bone fragments); lumbar, single segment

63103 Vertebral corpectomy (vertebral body resection), partial or complete, lateral extracavitary approach with decompression of spinal cord and/or nerve root(s) (eg, for tumor or retropulsed bone fragments); thoracic or lumbar, each additional segment (List separately in addition to code for primary procedure)

Vertebral corpectomy involves removal of the vertebral body as well as the vertebral discs above and below the vertebra. In this procedure a lateral extracavity approach is used. This approach is more commonly used to treat tumor or fractures with retropulsed bone fragments, although it may also be used for severe spinal stenosis and infection. A co-surgeon or team approach may be used with the exposure being performed by a general or thoracic surgeon and the corpectomy performed by a spine surgeon. The skin of the back is incised in the midline over the involved vertebral segments and then carried laterally to allow exposure of the paraspinal muscles. Overlying muscles are elevated and the spinous processes and laminae exposed. The paraspinal muscle bundle is divided lateral to the spine and elevated off the ribs. The tumor, fracture, or other condition is identified using intraoperative imaging as needed. The ribs may be resected. The intercostal nerves are identified and protected. The spinous processes, facets, and pedicles are removed using a high-speed drill. The dural sac is exposed, along with the lateral aspect of the vertebral body. For a thoracic corpectomy, the parietal pleura are retracted as needed to allow more complete exposure of the vertebral body. The nerve root may be divided or retracted superiorly to allow better visualization of the vertebra. The vertebral body is partially or completely excised. The discs inferior and superior to the vertebral body are also removed. Any remaining tumor tissue, bone fragments, bone spurs or other lesions are removed. The site is then prepared for separately reportable bone grafts, fusion, and internal fixation devices. Use 63101 for vertebral corpectomy of a single thoracic segment, 63102 for a single lumbar segment, and 63103 for each additional thoracic or lumbar segment.

63170

63170   Laminectomy with myelotomy (eg, Bischof or DREZ type), cervical, thoracic, or thoracolumbar

Laminectomy with incision of the spinal cord is performed to treat intractable pain due to malignant neoplasm or neuropathic pain due to spinal nerve root avulsion, or pain, more specifically "end zone" or "boundary pain", following spinal cord injury. The skin is incised over the cervical, thoracic or thoracolumbar region where the myelotomy will be performed and extended down to the spinous processes. Muscle is retracted off the lamina and facet joint. A bone drill is used to remove part or all of the lamina and the spinal cord is exposed. The appropriate region of the spinal cord is then incised. A DREZ myelotomy, also referred to as DREZ lesioning, uses an incision that disrupts input and outflow in the superficial layers of the spinal cord dorsal horn. The incision is made where nerve fibers that send pain impulses from the affected body area to the spinal cord terminate and where some nerve fibers that send motor impulses to the trunk or extremity originate. This prevents pain stimuli from reaching the brain and some motor stimuli from reaching body part if pain is complicated by spasticity. A Bishop myelotomy is used to treat spasticity of the lower extremities. Bishop myelotomy involves making a longitudinal incision in the spinal cord through the lateral column.

63172-63173

63172   Laminectomy with drainage of intramedullary cyst/syrinx; to subarachnoid space
63173   Laminectomy with drainage of intramedullary cyst/syrinx; to peritoneal or pleural space

An intramedullary cyst or syrinx is a rare lesion consisting of a fluid-filled cavity within the spinal cord. The skin is incised over the cervical, thoracic or thoracolumbar region where the intramedullary cyst or syrinx is located and extended down to the spinous processes. Muscle is retracted off the lamina and facet joint. A bone drill is used to remove part or all of the lamina, the spinal cord is exposed and the cyst or syrinx evaluated. The lesion is incised and drained. A drain is placed in the lesion. The drain is tunneled is secured. In 63172, a short drain is placed that terminates in the subarachnoid space which is the space between the arachnoid, the middle membrane covering the spinal cord, and the pia mater, the innermost membrane that is adherent to the spinal cord. In 63173, the drain is tunneled to the planned exit site in the peritoneal or pleural cavity. The peritoneum or pleura is incised and the drain is placed into the peritoneal or pleural cavity. The drain is secured and the surgical incisions are closed.

63180-63182

63180   Laminectomy and section of dentate ligaments, with or without dural graft, cervical; 1 or 2 segments
63182   Laminectomy and section of dentate ligaments, with or without dural graft, cervical; more than 2 segments

The dentate ligaments are lateral extensions of the pia mater, which is the innermost membrane of the three membranes covering the spinal cord. The dentate ligaments extend through the arachnoid, the middle membrane and attach to the dura mater, the outermost membrane. There are 21 dentate ligaments on each side of the spinal cord located in the region from C1 to T12. The dentate ligaments create a longitudinal plane that separates the spinal cord into anterior and posterior regions. The ligaments spread out between the nerve roots, and the plane created by the ligaments divides the dorsal and ventral nerve roots. If the dentate ligaments become thickened or fibrosis occurs, they can impinge on the corresponding nerve roots causing pain. Sectioning of the dentate ligaments is performed only on ligaments in the cervical spine. The skin is incised over the cervical region where the dentate ligament is impinging on the nerve roots. The incision is extended down to the spinous processes. Muscle is retracted off the lamina and facet joint. A bone drill is used to remove part or all of the lamina, the spinal cord is exposed and the affected nerve roots identified. The dura is incised over the thickened dentate ligament. The dentate ligaments are sectioned (cut) to relieve pressure on the dorsal and ventral nerve roots. Once the

nerve roots are freed from the impinging ligament, the dural incision is closed with sutures or a graft is used to patch the dural membrane. Use 63180 when dentate ligaments at one or two levels of the spine are sectioned. Use 63182 when the procedure is performed on more than two levels.

63185-63190

63185   Laminectomy with rhizotomy; 1 or 2 segments
63190   Laminectomy with rhizotomy; more than 2 segments

Rhizotomy is performed to treat spasticity that has not responded to oral medications or less invasive treatment modalities, such as facet joint or nerve root injections of botulinum toxin, phenol, or alcohol. The procedure is most commonly used to treat severe lower extremity spasticity caused by cerebral palsy. The skin is incised over the spine in the region where the rhizotomy will be performed. The incision is extended down to the spinous processes. Muscle is retracted off the lamina and facet joint. A bone drill is used to remove part or all of the lamina, and the spinal cord and nerve roots are exposed. Electrical stimulation is applied selectively to individual nerve rootlets to identify the motor nerve rootlets that are causing the spasticity and the nerve rootlets are cut. Use 63185 when the procedure is performed on one or two vertebral segments. Use 63190 when rhizotomy is performed on more than two vertebral segments.

63191

63191   Laminectomy with section of spinal accessory nerve

The spinal accessory nerve, also referred to as cranial nerve XI (CN XI), is primarily a motor nerve that originates from nerve cell bodies located in the cervical spinal cord and caudal medulla. The nerve fibers innervate the sternocleidomastoid and trapezius muscles in the neck and back. Sectioning of the spinal accessory nerve fibers is performed to treat severe spasmodic torticollis also referred to as cervical dystonia. Spasmodic torticollis is believed to be caused by increased motor nerve signals that cause muscle spasm and malposition of the head along with pain and numbness that may extend into the shoulder, arm and hand. The skin is incised over one or more cervical vertebrae. The incision is extended down to the spinous processes. Muscle is retracted off the lamina and facet joint. A bone drill is used to remove part or all of the lamina, the spinal cord is exposed and the spinal accessory nerve identified. Electrical stimulation is applied selectively to individual spinal accessory nerve fibers to identify the motor fibers that are causing the spasticity and pain. The nerve fibers are then cut.

63194-63195

63194   Laminectomy with cordotomy, with section of 1 spinothalamic tract, 1 stage; cervical
63195   Laminectomy with cordotomy, with section of 1 spinothalamic tract, 1 stage; thoracic

Cordotomy is performed to selectively destroy the anterior spinothalamic tract, which is the primary pain-transmitting pathway of the spinal cord. The procedure may be performed in a single operation or a two-stage procedure, unilaterally or bilaterally. The spinothalamic tract is located on both sides of the spine in the anterolateral aspect of the spinal cord. The spinothalamic tract on one side of the spinal cord carries sensory stimuli from the opposite side of the body to the brain. With the advent of new pain treatment modalities, cordotomy is rarely performed today except for severe unilateral pain due to malignancy in terminally ill patients. The skin is incised over vertebra in the cervical or thoracic spine where the spinothalamic tract is to be destroyed. The incision is extended down to the spinous processes. Muscle is retracted off the lamina and facet joint. A bone drill is used to remove part or all of the lamina, and the spinal cord is exposed. The spinothalamic tract is identified and cut. Use 63194 for a unilateral single-stage cordotomy of the cervical spine or 63195 if a unilateral procedure is performed on the thoracic spine.

63196-63197

63196   Laminectomy with cordotomy, with section of both spinothalamic tracts, 1 stage; cervical
63197   Laminectomy with cordotomy, with section of both spinothalamic tracts, 1 stage; thoracic

Cordotomy is performed to selectively destroy the anterior spinothalamic tract which is the primary pain-transmitting pathway of the spinal cord. The procedure may be performed in a single operation or a two stage procedure, and it may be performed unilaterally or bilaterally. The spinothalamic tract is located on both sides of the spine in the anterolateral aspect of the spinal cord. The spinothalamic tract on one side of the spinal cord carries sensory stimuli from the opposite side of the body to the brain. With the advent of new pain treatment modalities, cordotomy is rarely performed today except for severe unilateral pain due to malignancy in terminally ill patients. The skin is incised over vertebra in the cervical or thoracic spine where the spinothalamic tract is to be destroyed. The incision is extended down to the spinous processes. Muscle is retracted off the lamina and facet joint. A bone drill is used to remove part or all of the lamina, and the spinal cord is exposed. The spinothalamic tract is identified and cut. Use 63196 for a bilateral single-stage cordotomy in the cervical spine or 63197 if a bilateral procedure is performed on the thoracic spine.

Nervous System

63198-63199

63198 Laminectomy with cordotomy with section of both spinothalamic tracts, 2 stages within 14 days; cervical

63199 Laminectomy with cordotomy with section of both spinothalamic tracts, 2 stages within 14 days; thoracic

Cordotomy is performed to selectively destroy the anterior spinothalamic tract, which is the primary pain-transmitting pathway of the spinal cord. The procedure may be performed in a single operation or a two-stage procedure, unilaterally or bilaterally. The spinothalamic tract is located on both sides of the spine in the anterolateral aspect of the spinal cord. The spinothalamic tract on one side of the spinal cord carries sensory stimuli from the opposite side of the body to the brain. With the advent of new pain treatment modalities, a cordotomy is rarely performed today except for severe unilateral pain due to malignancy in terminally ill patients. The skin is incised over vertebra in the cervical or thoracic spine where the spinothalamic tract is to be destroyed. The incision is extended down to the spinous processes. Muscle is retracted off the lamina and facet joint. A bone drill is used to remove part or all of the lamina, and the spinal cord is exposed. The spinothalamic tract is identified and cut. Use 63198 for a bilateral two-stage cordotomy of the cervical spine with the second stage being performed within 14 days of the first stage or 63199 if a two-stage procedure is performed on the thoracic spine.

63200

63200 Laminectomy, with release of tethered spinal cord, lumbar

Normally the distal aspect of the spinal cord, called the conus medullaris, floats freely in the spinal fluid that surrounds it. A tethered spinal cord is a condition where the end of the spinal cord is immobile due to attachment to the tissues that form the spinal canal. The condition is typically a congenital anomaly that is often associated with spina bifida and myelomeningocele; however, it can occur alone or it can result from trauma to the spinal cord. Tethering causes the spinal cord to stretch during movement and as a child grows. This stretching causes neurologic symptoms such as muscle weakness, sensory disturbances, loss of bladder and bowel control, and orthopedic deformities. The skin is incised over vertebra in the lumbar spine where the spinal cord is tethered. The incision is extended down to the spinous processes. Muscle is retracted off the lamina and facet joint. A bone drill is used to remove part or all of the lamina and the tethered end of the spinal cord is exposed. The dura mater is incised. The spinal cord is gently teased away from surrounding tissue, scar tissue, and/or fat with the aid of an operating microscope. When the spinal cord has been completely mobilized, the overlying meninges are closed with sutures or a dural patch graft.

63250-63252

63250 Laminectomy for excision or occlusion of arteriovenous malformation of spinal cord; cervical

63251 Laminectomy for excision or occlusion of arteriovenous malformation of spinal cord; thoracic

63252 Laminectomy for excision or occlusion of arteriovenous malformation of spinal cord; thoracolumbar

Spinal cord arteriovenous malformation (AVM) is an extremely rare congenital anomaly that is characterized by abnormally tangled arteries and veins on, in or near the spinal cord. An AVM may prevent oxygenated blood from reaching all the cells and tissues in and around the spinal cord causing the tissue to die. Other complications of AVM include rupture of weakened blood vessels or compression of the spinal cord. The skin is incised over the cervical, thoracic or thoracolumbar region where the AVM is located and extended down to the spinous processes. Muscle is retracted off the lamina and facet joint. A bone drill is used to remove part or all of the lamina, and the spinal cord is exposed. The AVM is located. Blood vessels supplying the AVM are located and suture ligated The AVM may be excised or permanently occluded using sutures or clamps. Use 63250 for an AVM in the cervical region, 63251 for an AVM in the thoracic region, or 63252 for one in the thoracolumbar region.

63265-63268

63265 Laminectomy for excision or evacuation of intraspinal lesion other than neoplasm, extradural; cervical

63266 Laminectomy for excision or evacuation of intraspinal lesion other than neoplasm, extradural; thoracic

63267 Laminectomy for excision or evacuation of intraspinal lesion other than neoplasm, extradural; lumbar

63268 Laminectomy for excision or evacuation of intraspinal lesion other than neoplasm, extradural; sacral

Non-neoplastic intraspinal lesions include infectious lesions such as those caused by tuberculosis, syphilis, cytomegalovirus, herpes simplex virus, bacteria, or parasites; non-infectious lesions include those caused by sarcoid, multiple sclerosis, or systemic lupus erythematosis; and inflammatory lesions, which may be caused by idiopathic necrotizing or radiation myelopathy. In this procedure, a non-neoplastic intraspinal lesion located outside the dura mater (extradural) is excised or evacuated. The skin is incised over the cervical,

thoracic, lumbar, or sacral region where the intraspinal lesion is located and extended down to the spinous processes. Muscle is retracted off the lamina and facet joint. A bone drill is used to remove part or all of the lamina, and the spinal cord is exposed. The lesion is identified. The extent of the lesion is explored and determined to be limited to tissue outside the dura mater. A tissue sample may be obtained and sent for a separate pathology examination. Once the nature of the lesion has been determined, it is carefully dissected away from surrounding tissue. Dissection may be performed with the help of an operating microscope which is reported separately. When it is completely free of all surrounding tissue, it is removed. Alternatively, the lesion may be evacuated using a suction device. Use 63265 for a non-neoplastic intraspinal lesion in the cervical region, 63266 for one in the thoracic region, 63267 for one in the lumbar region, or 63268 for one in the sacral region.

63270-63273

63270 Laminectomy for excision of intraspinal lesion other than neoplasm, intradural; cervical

63271 Laminectomy for excision of intraspinal lesion other than neoplasm, intradural; thoracic

63272 Laminectomy for excision of intraspinal lesion other than neoplasm, intradural; lumbar

63273 Laminectomy for excision of intraspinal lesion other than neoplasm, intradural; sacral

Non-neoplastic intraspinal lesions include infectious lesions such as those caused by tuberculosis, syphilis, cytomegalovirus, herpes simplex virus, bacteria, or parasites; non-infectious lesions include those caused by sarcoid, multiple sclerosis, or systemic lupus erythematosis; and inflammatory lesions, which may be caused by idiopathic necrotizing or radiation myelopathy. In this procedure, a non-neoplastic intraspinal lesion located within the dura mater (intradural) is excised. The skin is incised over the cervical, thoracic, lumbar, or sacral region where the intraspinal lesion is located and extended down to the spinous processes. Muscle is retracted off the lamina and facet joint. A bone drill is used to remove part or all of the lamina, and the spinal cord is exposed. The lesion is identified within the dura mater. The dura is incised over the site of the lesion. The extent of the lesion is explored. A tissue sample may be obtained and sent for separately pathology examination. Once the nature of the lesion has been determined, it is carefully dissected away from surrounding tissue with the help of an operating microscope. When it is completely free of all surrounding tissue it is removed. Use 63270 for a non-neoplastic intraspinal intradural lesion in the cervical region; 63271 for one in the thoracic region; 63272 for one in the lumbar region; or 63273 for one in the sacral region.

63275-63278

63275 Laminectomy for biopsy/excision of intraspinal neoplasm; extradural, cervical

63276 Laminectomy for biopsy/excision of intraspinal neoplasm; extradural, thoracic

63277 Laminectomy for biopsy/excision of intraspinal neoplasm; extradural, lumbar

63278 Laminectomy for biopsy/excision of intraspinal neoplasm; extradural, sacral

An intraspinal neoplasm may be benign, malignant or of uncertain behavior. In this procedure, a neoplastic intraspinal tumor located outside the dura mater (extradural) is biopsied or excised. The skin is incised over the cervical, thoracic, lumbar, or sacral region where the tumor is located. The incision is extended down to the spinous processes. Muscle is retracted off the lamina and facet joint. A bone drill is used to remove part or all of the lamina, and the spinal cord is exposed. The tumor is identified. The extent of the tumor is explored and determined to be limited to tissue outside the dura mater. A tissue sample may be obtained and sent for separately pathology examination. Following the tissue biopsy, the physician may close the surgical site or excise the tumor. If the tumor can be excised, it is carefully dissected away from surrounding tissue with the help of an operating microscope. When it is completely free of all surrounding tissue, it is removed. Use 63275 for a neoplastic intraspinal tumor in the cervical region; 63276 for one in the thoracic region; 63277 for one in the lumbar region; or 63278 for one in the sacral region.

63280-63283

63280 Laminectomy for biopsy/excision of intraspinal neoplasm; intradural, extramedullary, cervical

63281 Laminectomy for biopsy/excision of intraspinal neoplasm; intradural, extramedullary, thoracic

63282 Laminectomy for biopsy/excision of intraspinal neoplasm; intradural, extramedullary, lumbar

63283 Laminectomy for biopsy/excision of intraspinal neoplasm; intradural, sacral

An intraspinal neoplasm may be benign, malignant or uncertain behavior. In this procedure, a neoplastic intraspinal tumor located within the dura mater (intradural) but outside of the spinal cord (extramedullary) is biopsied or excised. The tumor does not extend outside the dura into the extradural tissues. The skin is incised over the cervical, thoracic, lumbar, or sacral region where the tumor is located. The incision is extended down to the spinous processes. Muscle is retracted off the lamina and facet joint. A bone drill is used to remove part or all of the lamina, and the spinal cord is exposed. The tumor is identified within the dura mater. The dura is incised over the site of the tumor. The tumor is determined to lie outside of the spinal cord. A tissue sample may be obtained and sent for separately pathology examination. Following the tissue biopsy, the physician may close the surgical site or excise the tumor. If the tumor can be excised, it is carefully dissected away from surrounding tissue with the help of an operating microscope. When it is completely free of all surrounding tissue it is removed. The dura is then closed with sutures or a dural patch graft. Use 63280 for a neoplastic intraspinal tumor in the cervical region; 63281 for one in the thoracic region; 63282 for one in the lumbar region; or 63283 for one in the sacral region.

63285-63287

63285   Laminectomy for biopsy/excision of intraspinal neoplasm; intradural, intramedullary, cervical

63286   Laminectomy for biopsy/excision of intraspinal neoplasm; intradural, intramedullary, thoracic

63287   Laminectomy for biopsy/excision of intraspinal neoplasm; intradural, intramedullary, thoracolumbar

An intraspinal neoplasm may be benign, malignant or uncertain behavior. In this procedure, a neoplastic intraspinal tumor located within the dura mater (intradural) and extending into the tissues of the spinal cord (intramedullary) is biopsied or excised. The tumor does not extend outside the dura into the extradural tissues. The skin is incised over the cervical, thoracic, or lumbar region where the tumor is located. The incision is extended down to the spinous processes. Muscle is retracted off the lamina and facet joint. A bone drill is used to remove part or all of the lamina, and the spinal cord is exposed. The tumor is identified within the dura mater. The dura is incised over the site of the tumor. The tumor is determined to extend into tissues of the spinal cord. A tissue sample may be obtained and sent for separately pathology examination. Following the tissue biopsy, the physician may close the surgical site or excise the tumor. If the tumor can be excised, it is carefully dissected away from surrounding tissue with the help of an operating microscope. When it is completely free of all surrounding tissue, it is removed. The dura is then closed with sutures or a dural patch graft. Use 63285 for a neoplastic intraspinal tumor in the cervical region; 63286 for one in the thoracic region; or 63287 for one in the thoracolumbar region.

63290

63290   Laminectomy for biopsy/excision of intraspinal neoplasm; combined extradural-intradural lesion, any level

An intraspinal neoplasm may be benign, malignant or uncertain behavior. In this procedure, the tumor is located outside the dura mater with extension of the tumor into the dura. The tumor is biopsied or excised. The skin is incised over the cervical, thoracic, lumbar, or sacral region where the tumor is located. The incision is extended down to the spinous processes. Muscle is retracted off the lamina and facet joint. A bone drill is used to remove part or all of the lamina, and the spinal cord is exposed. The tumor outside the dura mater is located, evaluated, and determined to extend beyond the dura mater. The dura is incised over the site of the lesion. A tissue sample may be obtained and sent for separately pathology examination. Following the tissue biopsy, the physician may close the surgical site or excise the tumor. If the tumor can be excised, it is carefully dissected away from surrounding tissue with the help of an operating microscope. When it is completely free of all surrounding tissue it is removed. The dura is then closed with sutures or a dural patch graft. Use 63290 for an extradural-intradural intraspinal neoplasm at any level of the spine.

63295

63295   Osteoplastic reconstruction of dorsal spinal elements, following primary intraspinal procedure (List separately in addition to code for primary procedure)

Osteoplastic reconstruction of dorsal spine elements is an additional procedure that may be performed following an intraspinal procedure. Reconstruction is more often needed in pediatric patients due to the high incidence of kyphotic spinal deformity following intraspinal procedures. Following completion of the intraspinal procedure, the dorsal elements of the spine that have removed during the laminectomy or other surgical approach are reconstructed. The laminae, spinous processes, and supporting ligaments are returned to their normal anatomic position. A drill is used to prepare the laminae and spinous processes for the internal fixation devices. Heavy sutures, wires, mini-plates, or other internal fixation is the used to secure the bone and ligaments into normal anatomic position.

63300

63300   Vertebral corpectomy (vertebral body resection), partial or complete, for excision of intraspinal lesion, single segment; extradural, cervical

Vertebral corpectomy involves removal of the vertebral body as well as the vertebral discs above and below the vertebra. In this procedure, vertebral corpectomy is performed to excise a lesion or tumor that is located within the spinal canal (intraspinal) but outside the dura mater (extradural). Resection is performed on only one vertebral segment in

the cervical spine. The cervical spine is exposed via an anterior approach beginning with a skin incision in the anterior aspect of the neck. The soft tissues and muscles overlying the cervical spine are dissected. The trachea and esophagus are retracted. The affected segment of the cervical spine is exposed. The intervertebral discs above and below the vertebral body are removed first with the aid of the surgical microscope. The discs are carefully dissected from surrounding tissue and removed. The vertebral body is excised and the lesion or tumor in the spinal canal identified and explored. It is determined that the lesion or tumor lies outside the dura. The lesion or tumor is carefully dissected free of surrounding tissues with the aid of an operating microscope. Once the lesion or tumor has been completely excised, separately reportable bone grafting and fusion procedures are performed. The bone graft is placed in the surgical defect to support the anterior aspect of the spine where the discs and vertebral body have been removed. Surrounding bone is contoured for placement of the graft and to ensure fusion of the graft and adjacent bone. Separately reportable spine instrumentation may also be used to stabilize the spine. Upon completion of the procedure, bleeding is controlled and soft tissues and skin are closed in layers.

63301-63302

63301   Vertebral corpectomy (vertebral body resection), partial or complete, for excision of intraspinal lesion, single segment; extradural, thoracic by transthoracic approach

63302   Vertebral corpectomy (vertebral body resection), partial or complete, for excision of intraspinal lesion, single segment; extradural, thoracic by thoracolumbar approach

Vertebral corpectomy involves removal of the vertebral body as well as the vertebral discs above and below the vertebra. In this procedure, vertebral corpectomy is performed to excise a lesion or tumor that is located within the spinal canal (intraspinal) but outside the dura mater (extradural). Resection is performed on only one vertebral segment in the thoracic spine. The thoracic spine is exposed using either a transthoracic approach (63301) or a thoracolumbar approach (63302), both of which require a thoracotomy. Typically a co-surgeon or team approach is used with the exposure being performed by a thoracic surgeon and the corpectomy performed by a spine surgeon. The skin over the thorax is incised to allow access to the appropriate levels of the thoracic spine. Overlying muscles are dissected. In 63301, one or more of the upper ribs are resected. Rib spreaders are used to allow adequate exposure of the spine. The pleura are incised and the affected portion of the thoracic spine is exposed. In 63302, the incision is made at the 10th rib and extended across the abdomen. The rib is cut at the costochondral junction and resected. The pleural cavity is opened along the bed of the 10th rib and the appropriate level of the thoracic spine exposed. The intervertebral discs above and below the vertebral body are removed first with the aid of the surgical microscope. The discs are carefully dissected from surrounding tissue and removed. The vertebral body is excised and the lesion or tumor in the spinal canal identified and explored. It is determined that the lesion or tumor lies outside the dura. The lesion or tumor is carefully dissected free of surrounding tissues with the aid of an operating microscope. Once the lesion or tumor has been completely excised, separately reportable bone grafting and fusion procedures are performed. The bone graft is placed in the surgical defect to support the anterior aspect of the spine where the discs and vertebral body have been removed. Surrounding bone is contoured for placement of the graft and to ensure fusion of the graft and adjacent bone. Separately reportable spine instrumentation may also be used to stabilize the spine. Upon completion of the procedure, bleeding is controlled and soft tissues and skin are closed in layers.

63303

63303   Vertebral corpectomy (vertebral body resection), partial or complete, for excision of intraspinal lesion, single segment; extradural, lumbar or sacral by transperitoneal or retroperitoneal approach

Vertebral corpectomy involves removal of the vertebral body as well as the vertebral discs above and below the vertebra. In this procedure, vertebral corpectomy is performed to excise a lesion or tumor that is located within the spinal canal (intraspinal) but outside the dura mater (extradural). Resection is performed on only one vertebral segment in the lumbar or sacral spine. If a transperitoneal (anterior) approach is used, the abdomen is incised and the peritoneum entered. The bowel is moved out of the way. If a retroperitoneal (anterolateral) approach is used, a flank incision is made. Surrounding tissues are dissected taking care to protect vital structures. The affected lumbar or sacral segment is exposed. The intervertebral discs above and below the vertebral body are removed first with the aid of the surgical microscope. The discs are carefully dissected from surrounding tissue and removed. The vertebral body is excised and the lesion or tumor in the spinal canal identified and explored. It is determined that the lesion or tumor lies outside the dura. The lesion or tumor is carefully dissected free of surrounding tissues with the aid of an operating microscope. Once the lesion or tumor has been completely excised, separately reportable bone grafting and fusion procedures are performed. The bone graft is placed in the surgical defect to support the anterior aspect of the spine where the discs and vertebral body have been removed. Surrounding bone is contoured for placement of the graft and to ensure fusion of the graft and adjacent bone. Separately reportable spinal

Nervous System

instrumentation may also be used to stabilize the spine. Upon completion of the procedure, bleeding is controlled and soft tissues and skin are closed in layers.

63304

63304   Vertebral corpectomy (vertebral body resection), partial or complete, for excision of intraspinal lesion, single segment; intradural, cervical

Vertebral corpectomy involves removal of the vertebral body as well as the vertebral discs above and below the vertebra. In this procedure, vertebral corpectomy is performed to excise a lesion or tumor that is located within the spinal canal (intraspinal) and extends into or lies within the dura mater (intradural). Resection is performed on only one vertebral segment in the cervical spine. The cervical spine is exposed via an anterior approach beginning with a skin incision in the anterior aspect of the neck. The soft tissues and muscles overlying the cervical spine are dissected. The trachea and esophagus are retracted. The affected segment of the cervical spine is exposed. The intervertebral discs above and below the vertebral body are removed first with the aid of the surgical microscope. The discs are carefully dissected from surrounding tissue and removed. The vertebral body is excised and the lesion or tumor in the spinal canal identified and explored. If it is determined that the lesion or tumor lies within or extends into the dura, the dura is incised. The lesion or tumor is carefully dissected free of surrounding tissues with the aid of an operating microscope and removed. The dura is then repaired with sutures or a dural graft. Separately reportable bone grafting and fusion procedures are performed. The bone graft is placed in the surgical defect to support the anterior aspect of the spine where the discs and vertebral body have been removed. Surrounding bone is contoured for placement of the graft and to ensure fusion of the graft and adjacent bone. Separately reportable spine instrumentation may also be used to stabilize the spine. Upon completion of the procedure, bleeding is controlled and soft tissues and skin are closed in layers.

63305-63306

63305   Vertebral corpectomy (vertebral body resection), partial or complete, for excision of intraspinal lesion, single segment; intradural, thoracic by transthoracic approach

63306   Vertebral corpectomy (vertebral body resection), partial or complete, for excision of intraspinal lesion, single segment; intradural, thoracic by thoracolumbar approach

Vertebral corpectomy involves removal of the vertebral body as well as the vertebral discs above and below the vertebra. In this procedure, vertebral corpectomy is performed to excise a lesion or tumor that is located within the spinal canal (intraspinal) and within or extending into the dura mater (intradural). Resection is performed on only one vertebral segment in the thoracic spine. The thoracic spine is exposed using either a transthoracic approach (63305) or a thoracolumbar approach (63306) both of which require a thoracotomy. Typically a co-surgeon or team approach is used with the exposure being performed by a thoracic surgeon and the corpectomy performed by a spine surgeon. The skin over the thorax is incised to allow access to the appropriate levels of the thoracic spine. Overlying muscles are dissected. In 63305, one or more of the upper ribs are resected. Rib spreaders are used to allow adequate exposure of the spine. The pleura are incised and the affected portion of the thoracic spine is exposed. In 63306, the incision is made at the 10th rib and extended across the abdomen. The rib is cut at the costochondral junction and resected. The pleural cavity is opened along the bed of the 10th rib and the appropriate level of the thoracic spine exposed. The intervertebral discs above and below the vertebral body are removed first with the aid of the surgical microscope. The discs are carefully dissected from surrounding tissue and removed. The vertebral body is excised and the lesion or tumor in the spinal canal identified and explored. If it is determined that the lesion or tumor lies within or extends into the dura, the dura is incised. The lesion or tumor is carefully dissected free of surrounding tissues with the aid of an operating microscope and removed. The dura is then repaired with sutures or a dural graft. Separately reportable bone grafting and fusion procedures are performed. The bone graft is placed in the surgical defect to support the anterior aspect of the spine where the discs and vertebral body have been removed. Surrounding bone is contoured for placement of the graft and to ensure fusion of the graft and adjacent bone. Separately reportable spine instrumentation may also be used to stabilize the spine.

63307

63307   Vertebral corpectomy (vertebral body resection), partial or complete, for excision of intraspinal lesion, single segment; intradural, lumbar or sacral by transperitoneal or retroperitoneal approach

Vertebral corpectomy involves removal of the vertebral body as well as the vertebral discs above and below the vertebra. In this procedure, vertebral corpectomy is performed to excise a lesion or tumor that is located within the spinal canal (intraspinal) and within or extending into the dura mater (intradural). Resection is performed on only one vertebral segment in the lumbar or sacral spine. If a transperitoneal (anterior) approach is used, the abdomen is incised and the peritoneum entered. The bowel is moved out of the way. If a retroperitoneal (anterolateral) approach is used, a flank incision is made. Surrounding tissues are dissected taking care to protect vital structures. The affected lumbar or

sacral segment is exposed. The intervertebral discs above and below the vertebral body are removed first with the aid of the surgical microscope. The discs are dissected from surrounding tissue and removed. The vertebral body is excised and the lesion or tumor in the spinal canal identified and explored. If it is determined that the lesion or tumor lies within or extends into the dura, the dura is incised. The lesion or tumor is carefully dissected free of surrounding tissues with the aid of an operating microscope and removed. The dura is then repaired with sutures or a dural graft. Separately reportable bone grafting and fusion procedures are performed. The bone graft is placed in the surgical defect to support the anterior aspect of the spine where the discs and vertebral body have been removed. Surrounding bone is contoured for placement of the graft and to ensure fusion of the graft and adjacent bone. Separately reportable spine instrumentation may also be used to stabilize the spine.

63308

63308   Vertebral corpectomy (vertebral body resection), partial or complete, for excision of intraspinal lesion, single segment; each additional segment (List separately in addition to codes for single segment)

Following exposure of the spine as described in the primary procedure, it is determined that vertebral body resection on more than one vertebral segment is required. The first vertebral segment and superior and inferior intervertebral discs are excised as described in the primary procedure. One or more additional contiguous vertebral segments are resected in the same manner. The intervertebral discs above and below the vertebral body are removed first followed by removal of vertebral body. Use 63308 for each additional vertebral body resection.

63600-63615

63600   Creation of lesion of spinal cord by stereotactic method, percutaneous, any modality (including stimulation and/or recording)

63610   Stereotactic stimulation of spinal cord, percutaneous, separate procedure not followed by other surgery

63615   Stereotactic biopsy, aspiration, or excision of lesion, spinal cord

CT and MRI scans are obtained prior to surgery using advanced computer systems that can locate the spinal cord abnormality. A three-dimensional image of the spine is created and the surgeon determines the safest, most direct approach to the area of interest. A small incision is made over the spine. Using a surgical navigation system, specialized instruments, and the three-dimensional image of the spine, the surgeon optically tracks the surgical instruments as the instruments are manipulated toward the abnormality. In 63600, a lesion of the spinal cord is created to block the transmission of pain impulses to the brain. Electrodes are strategically placed along the spinal cord and attached to a generator. Electrical impulses are generated to stimulate the spinal cord and recordings obtained as needed. The site where the lesion will be created is identified. A thermal, electrical or radiofrequency device is then advanced to the selected location and fired destroying the targeted region of the spinal cord. In 63610, electrodes are placed at the selected site in the spine and impulses generated to stimulate the spinal cord. No other surgical procedures are performed. In 63615, a biopsy, aspiration, or excision of a spinal cord lesion is performed. Using stereotactic guidance, the spinal cord lesion is identified. A biopsy forceps, aspiration device or surgical blade is advanced to the lesion. If a biopsy is performed, a tissue sample is obtained using the biopsy forceps. If fluid or cells are needed, an aspiration device is used to obtain the fluid or cell samples. If the lesion is to be removed, the surgical blade is used to carefully remove the entire lesion. Following completion of the procedure, all instruments are removed and the small incision is closed.

63620-63621

63620   Stereotactic radiosurgery (particle beam, gamma ray, or linear accelerator); 1 spinal lesion

63621   Stereotactic radiosurgery (particle beam, gamma ray, or linear accelerator); each additional spinal lesion (List separately in addition to code for primary procedure)

Stereotactic radiosurgery using a particle beam, gamma ray, or linear accelerator is performed on a single spinal lesion. Stereotactic radiosurgery delivers a very high radiation dose to a precise location using multiple intersecting beams of radiation. Particle beam or cyclotron technology has limited use in the United States. Gamma ray technology uses a gamma knife composed of 201 beams of highly focused gamma rays to treat small to medium-sized lesions. Linear accelerator (LINAC) technology uses high energy X-ray photons or electrons in curving paths and can be used to treat larger lesions. During a separately reportable planning procedure, the lesion is visualized using three-dimensional MRI or CT scans. Spinal lesions are treated using a frameless technique. If the lesion is in the cervical spine, a molded face mask may be used to stabilize the head and neck. If the lesion is in the thoracic or lumbar spine, gold fiducial markers are placed into the pedicles adjacent to the lesion. The implanted fiducials are used to direct the radiation beams. An immobilization device such as an alpha cradle may also be used. The required treatment is defined and includes determination of lesion location and volume, identification of surrounding structures and assessment of risk of damage to these structures, and dose computation. If a gamma knife is used, the patient is placed on the gamma bed. The

Nervous System

gamma bed moves backward into the treatment area and is locked into the radiation source. The radiation dose is delivered. If a linear accelerator is used, a computer is used in conjunction with a micro-multileaf collimator attached to the linear accelerator, which arranges and shapes high-energy radiation beams in the exact configuration of the lesion. The gantry rotates around the patient and delivers the planned radiation dose to the lesion. Use code 63620 for a single spinal lesion and code 63621 for each additional spinal lesion.

63650-63655

63650 Percutaneous implantation of neurostimulator electrode array, epidural
63655 Laminectomy for implantation of neurostimulator electrodes, plate/paddle, epidural

Placement of an implantable spinal cord stimulation system is performed to treat chronic back and/or leg pain. Electrical stimulation of the spinal cord alleviates pain by activating pain-inhibiting neurons and inducing a tingling sensation that masks pain sensations. In 63650, percutaneous placement of an electrode array in the epidural space is performed. Using separately reportable fluoroscopic guidance, a small incision is made in the skin over the planned insertion site. The vertebra is exposed and a small portion of the lamina removed (laminotomy). The electrode array, also referred to as leads, are advanced into the epidural space and secured with sutures. The patient is then awakened and the array tested to ensure that the neurostimulator is properly placed and that there is no pain from the electrode array implant itself. The neurostimulator will be tested at various settings and once the optimal settings are determined they will be used to program the pulse generator or receiver that will be implanted in a separately reportable procedure. The lead wires are then tunneled to the pulse generator/receiver pocket where they are attached to the generator/receiver. In 63655, an electrode plate or paddle is placed in the epidural space using an open technique requiring a laminectomy. An incision between 2-5 inches in length is made over the spine. Overlying soft tissue is dissected and the lamina exposed. Part or all of the lamina is excised to allow access to the epidural space. The plate or paddle is positioned in the epidural space and secured to the spine. Once the plate or paddle is in place, the patient is awakened and the device is tested. Tunneling of the leads to the pulse generator/receiver pocket and connection of the leads is performed as described above.

63661-63662

63661 Removal of spinal neurostimulator electrode percutaneous array(s), including fluoroscopy, when performed
63662 Removal of spinal neurostimulator electrode plate/paddle(s) placed via laminotomy or laminectomy, including fluoroscopy, when performed

An implantable spinal cord stimulation system used to treat chronic back and/or leg pain. Electrical stimulation of the spinal cord alleviates pain by activating pain-inhibiting neurons and inducing a tingling sensation that masks pain sensations. Typically a temporary electrode array, plate, or paddle is placed to determine the effectiveness of the device in alleviating pain. The temporary device is eventually removed and if effective replaced with a permanent device or if ineffective it is removed without replacement. In 63661, percutaneous removal of an electrode array in the epidural space is performed. The subcutaneous pocket containing the generator/receiver is opened and the leads are disconnected. Using fluoroscopic guidance as needed, a small incision is made in the skin over the insertion site. The vertebra is exposed and the electrode array, also referred to as leads, are located and removed from the epidural space. The leads are dissected free of the subcutaneous tunnel, and removed. If a permanent electrode array is to be placed this is performed in a separately reportable procedure. If the electrode array is not being replaced, the incisions are closed. In 63662, an electrode plate or paddle that has been placed via a laminotomy or laminectomy is removed from the epidural space. The subcutaneous pocket containing the generator/receiver is opened and the leads are disconnected. Using fluoroscopic guidance as needed, an incision is made over the spine. Overlying soft tissue is dissected and the lamina exposed. The plate or paddle is located in the epidural space and removed. The leads are dissected free of the subcutaneous tunnel, and removed. If a permanent electrode plate or paddle is to be placed this is performed in a separately reportable procedure. If the electrode plate or paddle is not being replaced, the incisions are closed.

63663-63664

63663 Revision including replacement, when performed, of spinal neurostimulator electrode percutaneous array(s), including fluoroscopy, when performed
63664 Revision including replacement, when performed, of spinal neurostimulator electrode plate/paddle(s) placed via laminotomy or laminectomy, including fluoroscopy, when performed

An implantable spinal cord stimulation system is used to treat chronic back and/or leg pain. Electrical stimulation of the spinal cord alleviates pain by activating pain-inhibiting neurons and inducing a tingling sensation that masks pain sensations. In 63663, revision including replacement of an electrode array in the epidural space is performed. Using separately reportable fluoroscopic guidance, a small incision is made in the skin over the insertion site. The electrode array is located and explored to determine whether it needs to be repositioned or removed and replaced. If it needs to be repositioned, any sutures are

removed and the array is then moved as needed to obtain optimal pain control. If the array needs to be replaced it is removed in a separately reportable procedure. The new array is then advanced into the epidural space and secured with sutures. The patient is awakened and the revised or new array tested to ensure that the neurostimulator is properly placed and that there is no pain from the electrode array implant itself. The neurostimulator will be tested at various settings and once the optimal settings are determined they will be used to program the pulse generator or receiver that will be implanted in a separately reportable procedure. The lead wires are then tunneled to the pulse generator/receiver pocket where they are attached to the generator/receiver. In 63664, an electrode plate or paddle that has been placed via a laminotomy or laminectomy in the epidural space is revised and replaced as needed. An incision between 2-5 inches in length is made over the spine. Overlying soft tissue is dissected and the plate or paddle exposed and freed from the spine. If revision is performed, the plate or paddle is repositioned in the epidural space and secured to the spine. If the plate or paddle must be replaced it is removed in a separately reportable procedure. A new plate or paddle is then placed in the epidural space and secured to the spine. Once the plate or paddle is in place, the patient is awakened and testing of the device, tunneling of the leads to the pulse generator/receiver pocket, and connection of the leads is performed as described above.

63685-63688

63685 Insertion or replacement of spinal neurostimulator pulse generator or receiver, direct or inductive coupling
63688 Revision or removal of implanted spinal neurostimulator pulse generator or receiver

An implantable generator for spinal cord stimulation (SCS) generates electrical impulses to implanted electrodes in the spine. An implantable receiver receives electrical impulses from an external generator and then transmits those signals to the electrodes. In 63685, a pulse generator or receiver is inserted or replaced. For initial insertion, an incision is made in the skin overlying the planned insertion site for the neurostimulator pulse generator or receiver. A subcutaneous pocket is fashioned. The electrodes, which have been implanted and tunneled to the pocket in the separately reportable procedure, are connected to the generator or receiver and tested. Stimulation parameters are set and the device is placed in the skin pocket, which is closed with sutures. Replacement is performed in the same manner except that the existing generator or receiver is removed first by incising the skin over the existing generator or receiver. The skin pocket is opened and the existing device exposed. The electrodes are disconnected. The generator or receiver is dissected free of surrounding tissue and removed. The new generator or receiver is connected to the electrodes and tested. In 63688, an existing generator or receiver is revised or removed. Revision involves opening the skin pocket and removing the generator or receiver. The device is then evaluated and adjustments made as needed to ensure proper functioning. Removal is accomplished by exposing the device, disconnecting the electrodes (which are removed in a separate procedure) and closing the skin pocket.

63700-63702

63700 Repair of meningocele; less than 5 cm diameter
63702 Repair of meningocele; larger than 5 cm diameter

A meningocele is a form of spina bifida, which is a congenital anomaly of the neural tube. In spina bifida, the neural tube does not close properly during the first month of fetal development. Meningocele is characterized by normal development of the spinal cord but with protrusion of meninges through a defect in the spine. A thin membrane may cover the defect. An incision is made in membrane (sac) covering the meninges and any excess fluid is drained. The skin is closed in layers over the protruding meninges. If direct closure is not possible, a skin flap may be created from the skin of the back or buttocks. The flap is then rotated to cover the defect and sutured to surrounding tissue. Use 63700 if the defect is less than 5 cm in diameter; use 63702 if it is 5 cm or larger.

63704-63706

63704 Repair of myelomeningocele; less than 5 cm diameter
63706 Repair of myelomeningocele; larger than 5 cm diameter

A myelomeningocele is a form of spina bifida, which is a congenital anomaly of the neural tube. In spina bifida, the neural tube does not close properly during the first month of fetal development. Myelomeningocele is the most severe form and is characterized by protrusion of the spinal cord and meninges from a defect in the spine. A thin membrane may cover the defect. An incision is made in membrane (sac) covering the spinal cord and meninges and any excess fluid is drained. The dura mater is then closed over the spinal cord with sutures. The skin is closed in layers over the protruding meninges, spinal cord and nerves. If direct closure is not possible, a skin flap may be created from the skin of the back or buttocks. The flap is rotated to cover the defect and sutured to surrounding tissue. Use 63704 if the defect is less than 5 cm in diameter; use 63706 if it is 5 cm or larger.

Nervous System

63707-63709

63707   **Repair of dural/cerebrospinal fluid leak, not requiring laminectomy**
63709   **Repair of dural/cerebrospinal fluid leak or pseudomeningocele, with laminectomy**

A cerebrospinal fluid (CSF) leak in the spinal region may be due to trauma or a complication of a surgical procedure on the spine. The leak typically results from a tear or laceration of the spinal meninges that does not heal, resulting in cutaneous fistula formation. In some cases, fluid leaks into soft tissues without cutaneous fistula formation. A fibrous capsule forms in the soft tissue. If the dura has been lacerated but the arachnoid remains intact it can hemiate through the dural laceration forming a pseudomeningocele. In 63707, the leak is repaired without a laminectomy. Following a separately reportable imaging procedure to determine the exact location of the leak, the skin is incised over the affected spine segment. The area of the leak is located. A nonabsorbable suture is used for primary closure. Fibrin sealant may be used to reinforce the sutures and obtain a watertight seal. In 63709, a leak or pseudomeningocele is repaired with a laminectomy. The skin is incised over the cervical, thoracic, lumbar, or sacral region where the CSF leak is located and extended down to the spinous processes. Muscle is retracted off the lamina and facet joint. A bone drill is used to remove part or all of the lamina, and the spinal cord is exposed. If the leak is due to a rent, hole or other defect in the meninges, it is repaired with suture. Alternatively, a muscle pledget may be used along with gelfoam and fibrin sealant. If a pseudomeningocele is present, the pseudomeningocele is incised. Any nerve roots present in the defect are freed and reduced into the dura. The dura is then sutured as described above.

63710

63710   **Dural graft, spinal**

A dural graft is used to repair a defect in the dura mater of the spine. The defect is exposed and prepared for graft placement. Depending on the size of the defect, the physician may use an autologous tissue graft, bovine pericardium, dura from a cadaver or synthetic material. The graft is configured to cover the defect and sutured into place. There are several choices for what to use as a dural graft: tissue taken from the patient's own body (autologous pericranium), bovine pericardium, dura taken from a cadaver, or a synthetic material.

63740-63741

63740   **Creation of shunt, lumbar, subarachnoid-peritoneal, -pleural, or other; including laminectomy**
63741   **Creation of shunt, lumbar, subarachnoid-peritoneal, -pleural, or other; percutaneous, not requiring laminectomy**

A lumbar subarachnoid shunt is used to treat communicating hydrocephalus. Cerebrospinal fluid (CSF) may be shunted to the peritoneal cavity, pleural cavity or other location. In 63740, the spinal cord is exposed using a laminectomy and a lumbar subarachnoid shunt is created. The skin is incised over the lumbar spine where the shunt will be created and extended down to the spinous processes. Muscle is retracted off the lamina and facet joint. A bone drill is used to remove part or all of the lamina, and the spinal cord is exposed. The meninges are opened and the catheter placed in the subarachnoid space. A tunnel is created from the laminectomy site to the peritoneum, pleura or other site. The catheter is passed through the tunnel and into the selected terminal location. In 63741, the subarachnoid shunt is placed percutaneously. The skin over the planned puncture site is cleansed. A spinal needle with a Huber tip is inserted into through the selected intervertebral space and into the spinal canal using separately reportable imaging guidance. The meninges are punctured and a catheter is passed through the spinal needle into the subarachnoid space. A catheter passer and trocar are used to pass the terminal end of the catheter into the pleural or peritoneal space other termination site.

63744-63746

63744   **Replacement, irrigation or revision of lumbosubarachnoid shunt**
63746   **Removal of entire lumbosubarachnoid shunt system without replacement**

If a lumbar subarachnoid shunt becomes obstructed, infected, or other complications occur, the shunt may be replaced, irrigated, revised or the entire shunt system may be removed. In 63744, the shunt is replaced, irrigated, or revised. To replace the shunt, the skin is incised in the skin over the lumbar spine. The catheter is opened and a guidewire advanced through the catheter into the subarachnoid space. The existing catheter is removed over the guidewire. A new catheter is advanced over the guidewire and into the subarachnoid space and the guidewire is removed. The guidewire is then passed through the distal portion of the catheter into the terminal end. The distal portion of the catheter is removed over the guidewire and the new catheter passed over the guidewire into the terminal site, in the peritoneal or pleural cavity or other location. A connector is used to secure the proximal and distal catheter segments. To irrigate an obstructed shunt, the shunt is exposed and punctured with a needle. Sterile saline is then used to flush out the shunt. Once patency has been restored, the needle is removed and the skin closed over the shunt. To revise a shunt, a portion of the catheter is removed as described above. The removed segment is replaced and spliced together with the remaining segment of catheter

using a connector. In 63746, the entire shunt system is completely removed. An incision is made in the skin over the lumbar spine at the level of the shunt. Overlying soft tissues are dissected and the shunt catheter is exposed. Any anchoring sutures are cut and the shunt is removed from the spinal canal. The subcutaneous tunnel is opened and the shunt is dissected free of the tunnel and the terminal end removed.

64400-64405

64400   **Injection, anesthetic agent; trigeminal nerve, any division or branch**
64402   **Injection, anesthetic agent; facial nerve**
64405   **Injection, anesthetic agent; greater occipital nerve**

Injection of an anesthetic agent, also referred to as a nerve block, may be performed as either a diagnostic or therapeutic measure. In 64400, any division or branch of the trigeminal nerve is injected. The most common indication for injection of the trigeminal nerve is trigeminal neuralgia, which is characterized by shock-like stabbing pain, also referred to as lancinating pain. The trigeminal nerve divisions or branches may be injected using an intraoral or transcutaneous approach depending on the division or branch being injected. A needle is introduced into the trigeminal nerve at the base of the skull or along any of the divisions or branches. An anesthetic agent such as glycol is injected. The patient is asked to assess the degree of pain relief. In 64402, the facial nerve is injected. The facial nerve, also referred to as cranial nerve VII (CN VII), is a mixed nerve with both motor and sensory components and assists with facial expression. The nerve may be injected to treat muscle spasms or to interrupt transmission of sensory stimuli. The skin is cleansed over the facial nerve and an anesthetic is injected. In 64405, the greater occipital nerve is injected. The greater occipital nerves originate between the second and third vertebrae of the spine and supply the top of the scalp and the region above the ears and over the salivary glands. Injecting the nerve near the base of the skull treats occipital neuralgia.

64408

64408   **Injection, anesthetic agent; vagus nerve**

Injection of an anesthetic agent, also referred to as a nerve block, may be performed as either a diagnostic or therapeutic measure. The vagus nerve, also referred to as cranial nerve X (CN X), is a mixed nerve that originates in the medulla and exits the skull at the jugular foramen. The motor portion innervates muscles of the pharynx, larynx, respiratory tract, heart, stomach, small intestine, most of large intestine and gallbladder. The sensory portion transmits sensation from the same structures that the motor portion innervates. The skin over the styloid process of the temporal bone is cleansed. A needle is advanced perpendicular to the skin until the styloid process is encountered. The needle is then retracted slightly and repositioned in a slightly inferior trajectory. The needle is advanced in this position until it is approximately 0.5 cm deeper than the point at which the styloid process was encountered. Positioning is checked by aspiration. If no blood or cerebral spinal fluid is aspirated, the anesthetic agent is injected.

64410

64410   **Injection, anesthetic agent; phrenic nerve**

Injection of an anesthetic agent, also referred to as a nerve block, may be performed as either a diagnostic or therapeutic measure. The phrenic nerve is a mixed spinal nerve originating from C4. It innervates muscles of the diaphragm and carries sensory information from the pleura, lungs, and pericardium. The skin over the C4 region of the spine is cleansed. A needle is inserted into the phrenic nerve, aspirated to ensure that it is not in a blood vessel, and an anesthetic agent is then injected.

64413

64413   **Injection, anesthetic agent; cervical plexus**

The cervical plexus is formed by then anterior rami of the C1-C4 nerve roots. It is located anterior to the cervical spine and posterior to the sternocleidomastoid muscle. The posterior border sternocleidomastoid is identified in the neck and marked. The planned injection site(s) is also marked. For a superficial cervical plexus block, a single injection is typically given at the midpoint of the sternocleidomastoid muscle. For a deep cervical plexus block, multiple injections between C2 and C6 may be given. The needle is inserted and aspirated to ensure that the needle is not in a blood vessel or for a deep block to ensure that it has not penetrated the subarachnoid space. The anesthetic is then injected. If multiple injections are performed, this is repeated until the desired level of anesthesia or analgesia has been attained.

64415-64416

64415   **Injection, anesthetic agent; brachial plexus, single**
64416   **Injection, anesthetic agent; brachial plexus, continuous infusion by catheter (including catheter placement)**

The physician makes a single injection of a drug to numb the nerves in the arm. For code 64416, an anesthetic is injected into the brachial plexus by continuous infusion. The arm is abducted with the elbow flexed and the hand above the shoulder. The skin is cleansed and anesthetized before a needle is placed in the infraclavicular or supraclavicular region and advanced into position in the brachial plexus sheath. Proper placement of the needle

   ● New Code   ▲ Revised Code

is verified with electrical nerve stimulation and/or with the onset of numbness, tingling, or prickling sensations, or through separately reportable ultrasound imaging. The cannula for the nerve block is then threaded over the needle through the brachial plexus sheath. The needle is removed when the cannula is in position. Next, the epidural-type catheter for administering the anesthetic is threaded through the cannula into position in the brachial plexus sheath. The nerve block into the brachial plexus is then injected using a local anesthetic medication like lidocaine or bupivacaine. The function of the nerve block is determined, and the continuous infusion is started.

64417-64418

64417   Injection, anesthetic agent; axillary nerve
64418   Injection, anesthetic agent; suprascapular nerve

Injection of an anesthetic agent, also referred to as a nerve block, may be performed as either a diagnostic or therapeutic measure. In 64417, an axillary nerve block is performed. The axillary nerve originates from the brachial plexus at the level of the axilla. It divides into anterior and posterior trunks. The anterior trunk branches and supplies the middle and anterior surface of the deltoid. The posterior trunk branches supply the teres minor and posterior deltoid muscle. In 64418, a subscapular nerve block is performed. The subscapular nerve arises from the brachial plexus and divides into upper and lower branches. The upper branch supplies the upper part of the subscapularis muscle and the lower part branches and one branch supplies the lower part of the subscapularis and another the teres major. The skin over the planned injection site is cleansed. A needle is inserted into the axillary or subscapular nerve, aspirated to ensure that it is not in a blood vessel, and an anesthetic is injected.

64420-64421

64420   Injection, anesthetic agent; intercostal nerve, single
64421   Injection, anesthetic agent; intercostal nerves, multiple, regional block

The intercostal nerves are mixed nerves that supply the skin and muscles of the upper extremities, thorax, and abdominal wall. The intercostal nerves exit the posterior aspect of the intercostal membrane just distal to the intervertebral foramen and then enter the intercostal groove running parallel to the rib. Branches of the intercostal nerves may be found between the ribs. Intercostal nerves are most often blocked along the posterior axillary line or just lateral to the paraspinal muscles at the angle of the rib. The planned injection site(s) is identified and marked along the inferior border of the rib(s). The needle is introduced underneath the inferior border of the rib and advanced until it reaches the subcostal groove. The anesthetic agent is then injected. Use 64420 for injection of a single intercostal nerve. Use 64421 if multiple intercostal nerves are injected.

64425

64425   Injection, anesthetic agent; ilioinguinal, iliohypogastric nerves

The ilioinguinal and iliohypogastric nerves arise from L1. Both nerves emerge from the upper part of the lateral border of the psoas major muscle and then penetrate the transversus abdominus muscle just above and medial to the anterior superior iliac spine. The nerves run between the transversus abdominus and the internal oblique muscles for a short distance then penetrate the internal oblique. They run between the internal and external oblique muscles before branching and penetrating the external oblique muscle where branches provide skin sensation. The anterior superior iliac spine is located and the planned injection site medial and superior to it is marked. A needle is positioned perpendicular to the skin and the skin is punctured. The needle is advanced through the external oblique muscle and into the space between the internal and external oblique. The needle is aspirated to ensure that the needle is not in a blood vessel and the anesthetic agent is injected between the oblique muscles. The needle is then advanced through the internal oblique muscle into the space between the internal oblique and transversus abdominus. The space is aspirated and injected as described above. The needle is withdrawn and inserted at a 45-degree angle laterally and the procedure repeated.

64430

64430   Injection, anesthetic agent; pudendal nerve

The physician performs a pudendal nerve block by injecting an anesthetic agent into the nerve. Pudendal nerve block is used during the second stage of labor to provide pain relief, for pelvic floor relaxation when forceps delivery is needed, and to provide anesthesia of the perineum for creation or repair of an episiotomy. The block may be administered via a transvaginal or transcutaneous perineal approach. Using a transvaginal approach, the ischial spine on the first side to be injected is palpated. A Huber needle is used to limit the depth of submucosal penetration. The needle is passed through the sacrospinous ligament and advanced about 1 cm. The physician ensures that the needle is in the proper location and that it has not penetrated the pudendal vessels by pulling back on the syringe. If blood is aspirated the needle is repositioned. Aspiration is again performed and if no blood is present, the anesthetic is injected. The procedure is repeated on the opposite side. Using a transcutaneous perineal approach, the ischial tuberosity is palpated and the needle introduced slightly medial to the tuberosity. The needle is advanced approximately 2.5 cm. Aspiration is performed to ensure that the needle is not in a blood vessel and then the

anesthetic is injected. The needle is withdrawn and directed into the deep superficial tissue of the vulva and anesthetic is again injected to block the ilioinguinal and genitofemoral components of the pudendal nerve. This is repeated on the opposite side.

64435

64435   Injection, anesthetic agent; paracervical (uterine) nerve

Paracervical nerve block is used to reduce pain during the first stage of labor. An 18.5 cm needle with a security tip is used to administer the injection. The needle is advanced transvaginally just deep to the lateral fornices of the vagina and into the broad ligament. The needle is aspirated to ensure that it is not in a blood vessel. The anesthetic agent is injected at various sites along the broad ligament. The procedure is repeated on the opposite side.

64445

64445   Injection, anesthetic agent; sciatic nerve, single

The thigh is flexed at the hip. A line is marked from the back of the knee to a point between the greater trochanter and the ischial tuberosity. The skin is cleansed. A needle is introduced just above the marked line to test the sciatic nerve using electrical nerve stimulation. After a motor response in the ankle, foot, or toes has been elicited, a sciatic nerve block is performed using a single injection of an anesthetic agent.

64446

64446   Injection, anesthetic agent; sciatic nerve, continuous infusion by catheter (including catheter placement)

The thigh is flexed at the hip. A line is marked from the back of the knee to a point between the greater trochanter and the ischial tuberosity. The skin is cleansed and anesthetized before a needle is introduced just above the marked line to test the sciatic nerve and elicit a motor response in the ankle, foot, or toes. Next, an insulated, epidural-type needle is inserted to intersect with the tip of the first. A catheter is then threaded through the epidural needle and out the tip. Electrical nerve stimulation is tested again through the catheter. The epidural needle is removed when the cannula is secured in position. The nerve block is then injected into the sciatic nerve using a local anesthetic medication like lidocaine or bupivacaine. The function of the nerve block is determined, and continuous infusion is started.

64447

64447   Injection, anesthetic agent; femoral nerve, single

The groin is cleansed and prepped with a small amount of local anesthetic on the affected side. The planned injection site is marked. A needle is introduced and electrical nerve stimulation performed to ensure that the needle is properly positioned. A femoral nerve block is performed using a single injection of an anesthetic agent.

64448

64448   Injection, anesthetic agent; femoral nerve, continuous infusion by catheter (including catheter placement)

An anesthetic is injected into the femoral nerve by continuous infusion. The patient's groin is cleansed and prepped with a small amount of local anesthetic on the affected side. An insulated needle is inserted within a long cannula, and the needle is placed through the anesthetized area of skin near the femoral artery and the inguinal ligament into the femoral nerve sheath. Proper placement of the needle is verified with electrical nerve stimulation and/or with the onset of numbness, tingling, or prickling sensations, or through separately reportable ultrasound imaging. The cannula is then advanced over the needle into the femoral nerve sheath. A long-acting local anesthetic like bupivicaine with epinephrine is carefully injected through the cannula and monitored for nerve block function. Periodic aspiration is performed to ensure that there is no possibility of intravascular injection. An epidural catheter is then threaded through the cannula and secured in position. The cannula is removed. Continuous infusion is started.

64449

64449   Injection, anesthetic agent; lumbar plexus, posterior approach, continuous infusion by catheter (including catheter placement)

The needle insertion site is marked near the area between the iliac crests. The skin of the lower back is cleansed and prepped with a small amount of local anesthetic placed into deeper tissues. A special needle connected to a peripheral nerve stimulator is advanced into the psoas compartment. Proper positioning of the needle is verified by stimulating the lumbar plexus, which results in elevation of the patella and contraction of the quadriceps and sartorius. Aspiration is done to test for blood and cerebrospinal fluid, and a test dose of anesthesia is given to rule out intravenous or intrathecal injection. An infusion catheter is inserted through the needle after a small amount of local anesthetic is injected for the block. The function of the block is checked for analgesia of the left leg and hip. The correct catheter position is also verified for intravenous or intrathecal placement and secured in place. Continuous infusion of a dilute local anesthetic is started.

● New Code   ▲ Revised Code

Nervous System

64450

64450   Injection, anesthetic agent; other peripheral nerve or branch

An anesthetic agent is injected into a peripheral nerve or branch not specifically described by another code. This procedure may also be referred to as a peripheral nerve block. Generally this is performed on peripheral nerves or branches in the arm or leg. The specific nerve or branch is identified. The skin over the planned puncture site is disinfected. The needle is inserted, aspirated to ensure it is not in a blood vessel, and the anesthetic is injected.

64455

64455   Injection(s), anesthetic agent and/or steroid, plantar common digital nerve(s) (eg, Morton's neuroma)

With the patient in a supine position, the knee is flexed and supported with a pillow and the foot is maintained in a relaxed neutral position. The interdigital spaces are palpated and any tenderness or fullness is noted. The needle is inserted on the dorsal foot surface in a distal to proximal direction at a point 1-2 cm proximal to the web space and in line with the metatarsophalangeal joints. The needle is held at an angle of approximately 45 degrees and advanced through the mid-web space into the area of fullness at the plantar aspect of the foot. The needle is advanced until it tents the skin and then withdrawn to the tip of the neuroma. Taking care to avoid the plantar fat pad, an anesthetic agent is injected first to confirm the diagnosis, followed by steroid injection. A steroid/anesthetic mix may be used. One or more common digital nerves may be injected.

64461-64463

- **64461   Paravertebral block (PVB) (paraspinous block), thoracic; single injection site (includes imaging guidance, when performed)**
- **64462   Paravertebral block (PVB) (paraspinous block), thoracic; second and any additional injection site(s) (includes imaging guidance, when performed) (List separately in addition to code for primary procedure)**
- **64463   Paravertebral block (PVB) (paraspinous block), thoracic; continuous infusion by catheter (includes imaging guidance, when performed)**

A procedure is performed to administer endovascular intracranial pharmacologic agent(s) other than for thrombolysis. These agents may include papaverine, nicardipine, and verapamil used to treat arterial vasospasm following stroke. Access to intracranial blood vessels is established through a peripheral artery. A needle is introduced into the artery under fluoroscopic guidance; a thin wire is threaded through the needle and advanced to the targeted vascular area. If diagnostic angiography is performed, a catheter is introduced over the guidewire and the guidewire is removed. Dye is injected to obtain detailed images of the intracranial blood vessels. The guidewire is then reinserted and the angiography catheter is removed. An infusion catheter is introduced over the guidewire to the targeted vascular territory and the pharmacologic agent is delivered as prolonged continuous infusion. The catheter may be moved to access additional vascular territories (61651) with subsequent delivery of pharmacologic agents before being removed at the end of the treatment period. These codes include diagnostic angiography and imaging guidance.

64479-64480

64479   Injection(s), anesthetic agent and/or steroid, transforaminal epidural, with imaging guidance (fluoroscopy or CT); cervical or thoracic, single level

64480   Injection(s), anesthetic agent and/or steroid, transforaminal epidural, with imaging guidance (fluoroscopy or CT); cervical or thoracic, each additional level (List separately in addition to code for primary procedure)

A transforaminal epidural injection allows for a very selective injection around a specific nerve root. Nerve roots exit the spinal canal through the foraminae, which are small openings between the vertebrae. The skin is cleansed and prepped over the affected cervical or thoracic vertebra. Using CT or fluoroscopic imaging, a needle is advanced through the skin and into the foramen. A small amount of radiopaque contrast material may be injected to enhance fluoroscopic images and to confirm proper placement of the spinal needle. The anesthetic and/or steroid is then injected around the nerve root. Use 64479 for transforaminal epidural injection at a single cervical or thoracic level. Use 64480 for each additional level injected.

64483-64484

64483   Injection(s), anesthetic agent and/or steroid, transforaminal epidural, with imaging guidance (fluoroscopy or CT); lumbar or sacral, single level

64484   Injection(s), anesthetic agent and/or steroid, transforaminal epidural, with imaging guidance (fluoroscopy or CT); lumbar or sacral, each additional level (List separately in addition to code for primary procedure)

A transforaminal epidural injection allows very selective injection around a specific nerve root. Nerve roots exit the spinal canal through the foraminae, which are small openings between the vertebrae. The skin is cleansed and prepped over the affected lumbar or sacral vertebra. Using CT or fluoroscopic imaging, a needle is advanced through the skin and into the foramen. A small amount of radiopaque contrast material may be injected to enhance fluoroscopic images and to confirm proper placement of the spinal needle.

The anesthetic and/or steroid is then injected around the nerve root. Use 64483 for transforaminal epidural injection at a single lumbar or sacral level. Use 64484 for each additional level injected.

64486

64486   Transversus abdominis plane (TAP) block (abdominal plane block, rectus sheath block) unilateral; by injection(s) (includes imaging guidance, when performed)

A unilateral transversus abdominis plane (TAP) block provides peripheral anesthesia to nerves in the anterior abdominal wall at the level of T6-L1 and may be used as an adjunct therapy for postoperative pain control. The TAP block can be performed preoperatively, intraoperatively, or postoperatively and is most effective when the surgical incision is located to the right or left of midline. A single injection of a long acting local anesthetic such as bupivacane can provide pain relief up to 36 hours. When using a blind approach, the triangle of Petit is identified and a needle is inserted perpendicular to the skin, cephalad to the iliac crest, and near the midaxillary line. The needle is advanced through the external and internal abdominal oblique muscles and into the fascia above the transversus abdominis muscle. Local anesthetic is injected at measured intervals following aspiration to ensure that the needle is not within a blood vessel. The needle is then removed. The procedure can also be performed using ultrasound guidance which allows the physician to visualize the layers of muscle and fascia and the hypoechoic spread of fluid when the anesthetic is injected.

64487

64487   Transversus abdominis plane (TAP) block (abdominal plane block, rectus sheath block) unilateral; by continuous infusion(s) (includes imaging guidance, when performed)

A unilateral transversus abdominis plane (TAP) block provides peripheral anesthesia to nerves in the anterior abdominal wall at the level of T6-L1 and may be used as an adjunct therapy for postoperative pain control. The TAP block can be performed preoperatively, intraoperatively, or postoperatively and is most effective when the surgical incision is located to the right or left of midline. A continuous infusion of local anesthetic such as bupivacane can provide extended pain relief for 36-72 hours. The procedure is performed using ultrasound guidance which allows the physician to visualize the layers of muscle and fascia and the hypoechoic spread of fluid following injection. A Touhy needle is inserted into the skin and advanced through the external and internal abdominal oblique muscles into the fascia directly above the transversus abdominis muscle. This layer of fascia, called the transversus abdominis plane (TAP) is hydrodissected with 10 ml of isotonic saline. An epidural catheter is introduced through the Touhy needle and advanced 10-20 cm into the TAP. The Touhy needle is removed and the epidural catheter is connected to tubing. A bolus injection of local anesthetic is given and monitored by ultrasound. Once placement has been confirmed, the epidural catheter is secured to the skin and continuous infusion or intermittent bolus injections of anesthetic are administered to the patient.

64488

64488   Transversus abdominis plane (TAP) block (abdominal plane block, rectus sheath block) bilateral; by injections (includes imaging guidance, when performed)

The transversus abdominis plane (TAP) block provides peripheral anesthesia to nerves in the anterior abdominal wall at the level of T6-L1 and may be used as an adjunct therapy for postoperative pain control. A bilateral TAP block can be performed preoperatively, intraoperatively, or postoperatively and may be used when the surgical incision is in the midline of the abdomen. A single injection of a long acting local anesthetic such as bupivacane can provide pain relief for up to 36 hours. When using a blind approach, the triangle of Petit is identified on either the right or left side and a needle is inserted perpendicular to the skin, cephalad to the iliac crest, and near the midaxillary line. The needle is advanced through the external and internal abdominal oblique muscles and into the fascia above the transversus abdominis muscle. Local anesthetic is injected at measured intervals following aspiration to ensure that the needle is not within a blood vessel. The needle is then removed and the procedure is repeated on the opposite side. The procedure can also be performed using ultrasound guidance which allows the physician to visualize the layers of muscle and fascia and the hypoechoic spread of fluid when the anesthetic is injected.

64489

64489   Transversus abdominis plane (TAP) block (abdominal plane block, rectus sheath block) bilateral; by continuous infusions (includes imaging guidance, when performed)

The transversus abdominis plane (TAP) block provides peripheral anesthesia to nerves in the anterior abdominal wall at the level of T6-L1 and may be used as an adjunct therapy for postoperative pain control. A bilateral TAP block can be performed preoperatively, intraoperatively, or postoperatively and may be used when the surgical incision is in the midline of the abdomen. A continuous infusion of local anesthetic such as bupivacane can provide extended pain relief for 36-72 hours. The procedure is performed using ultrasound

Nervous System

guidance which allows the physician to visualize the layers of muscle and fascia and the hypoechoic spread of fluid following injection. A Touhy needle is inserted into the skin on either the right or left side and advanced through the external and internal abdominal obliques to the fascia directly above the transversus abdominis muscle. This layer of fascia, called the transversus abdominis plane (TAP) is hydrodissected with 10 ml of isotonic saline. An epidural catheter is introduced through the Touhy needle and advanced 10-20 cm into the TAP. The Touhy needle is removed and the epidural catheter is connected to tubing. A bolus injection of local anesthetic is given and monitored by ultrasound. Once placement has been confirmed, the epidural catheter is secured to the skin and the procedure is repeated on the opposite side. Once both catheters are in place, continues infusion or intermittent bolus injections of the anesthetic are administered to the patient.

64490-64492

64490 Injection(s), diagnostic or therapeutic agent, paravertebral facet (zygapophyseal) joint (or nerves innervating that joint) with image guidance (fluoroscopy or CT), cervical or thoracic; single level

64491 Injection(s), diagnostic or therapeutic agent, paravertebral facet (zygapophyseal) joint (or nerves innervating that joint) with image guidance (fluoroscopy or CT), cervical or thoracic; second level (List separately in addition to code for primary procedure)

64492 Injection(s), diagnostic or therapeutic agent, paravertebral facet (zygapophyseal) joint (or nerves innervating that joint) with image guidance (fluoroscopy or CT), cervical or thoracic; third and any additional level(s) (List separately in addition to code for primary procedure)

Paravertebral facet joints, also called zygapophyseal joints, are located on the back (posterior) of the spine on each side of the vertebra at the point where one verebra overlaps the next. Facet joint pain may is associated with post laminectomy syndrome or other spine surgery due to destabilization of the spinal joints, scar tissue formation, or recurrent disc herniation. Other causes include spondylosis, spondylolisthesis, and arthritis. Using fluoroscopic or CT guidance, a diagnostic or therapeutic facet joint injection or injection of nerves innervating the joint is performed. The skin overlying the facet joint is prepped and a local anesthetic injected. A spinal needle is directed into the facet joint space until bone or cartilage is encountered. A small amount of contrast material is injected to verify that the needle is correctly positioned. This is followed by injection of a local anesthetic and/or steroid. Diagnostic facet joint injection uses a local anesthetic to identify the specific area generating the pain. If the patient experiences pain relief for a significant period of time following a diagnostic injection, the physician will perform a therapeutic injection on a subsequent date of service using a long acting local anesthetic in conjunction with a steroid. Use 64490 for a single cervical or thoracic facet joint injection; use 64491 for the second level; use 64492 for the third and any additional cervical or thoracic levels injected.

64493-64495

64493 Injection(s), diagnostic or therapeutic agent, paravertebral facet (zygapophyseal) joint (or nerves innervating that joint) with image guidance (fluoroscopy or CT), lumbar or sacral; single level

64494 Injection(s), diagnostic or therapeutic agent, paravertebral facet (zygapophyseal) joint (or nerves innervating that joint) with image guidance (fluoroscopy or CT), lumbar or sacral; second level (List separately in addition to code for primary procedure)

64495 Injection(s), diagnostic or therapeutic agent, paravertebral facet (zygapophyseal) joint (or nerves innervating that joint) with image guidance (fluoroscopy or CT), lumbar or sacral; third and any additional level(s) (List separately in addition to code for primary procedure)

Paravertebral facet joints, also called zygapophyseal joints, are located on the back (posterior) of the spine on each side of the vertebra at the point where one verebra overlaps the next. Facet joint pain may is associated with post laminectomy syndrome or other spine surgery due to destabilization of the spinal joints, scar tissue formation, or recurrent disc herniation. Other causes include spondylosis, spondylolisthesis, and arthritis. Using fluoroscopic or CT guidance, a diagnostic or therapeutic facet joint injection or injection of nerves innervating the joint is performed. The skin overlying the facet joint is prepped and a local anesthetic injected. A spinal needle is directed into the facet joint space until bone or cartilage is encountered. A small amount of contrast material is injected to verify that the needle is correctly positioned. This is followed by injection of a local anesthetic and/or steroid. Diagnostic facet joint injection uses a local anesthetic to identify the specific area generating the pain. If the patient experiences pain relief for a significant period of time following a diagnostic injection, the physician will perform a therapeutic injection on a subsequent date of service using a long acting local anesthetic in conjunction with a steroid. Use 64493 for a single lumbar or sacral facet joint injection; use 64494 for the second level; use 64495 for the third and any additional lumbar or sacral levels injected.

64505

64505 Injection, anesthetic agent; sphenopalatine ganglion

The sphenopalatine ganglion, also referred to as the pterygopalatine, nasal, or Meckel's ganglion, is located in the pterygopalatine fossa. This fossa lays at the back of the nose between the pterygoid process, the maxilla and palatine bones. A thin layer of connective tissue and mucous membrane covers the sphenopalatine ganglion. A sphenopalatine ganglion block is used to treat mixed type headaches, facial pain, and myofascial pain in the neck and upper back. Using a transnasal approach, the anterior aspect of the nasal turbinate is anesthetized using an aerosol spray. A cannula is inserted into the nose, passed along the upper border of the inferior turbinate, and directed backwards and advanced to the upper posterior wall of the nasopharynx. The anesthetic is infiltrated into the back of the nose. Alternatively, applicators saturated with lidocaine may be inserted into each nostril. The applicators are then advanced to the back of the nose. The lidocaine is absorbed through the mucous membrane anesthetizing the sphenopalatine ganglion.

64508

64508 Injection, anesthetic agent; carotid sinus (separate procedure)

The carotid sinus is a slightly enlarged area located in the common carotid artery where the artery divides into the internal and external carotids. This region contains baroreceptors that help the body respond to changes in blood pressure. When blood pressure increases, baroreceptors are stimulated causing reduction in blood pressure, dilation of blood vessels, and reduced heart rate. However, in some individuals, the response is excessive and may be triggered by mild pressure on the neck caused by turning the head or a shirt with a tight collar. The excessive sensitivity causes a rapid decline in blood pressure, dizziness, and fainting. Injection of anesthetic is performed to prevent a hypersensitivity reaction. The skin over the common carotid is prepped. A needle is inserted into the skin over the carotid sinus and advanced to a point just outside the blood vessel. The needle is aspirated to ensure that it is not in the blood vessel and the anesthetic agent is injected. The patient is monitored while the anesthetic takes effect.

64510

64510 Injection, anesthetic agent; stellate ganglion (cervical sympathetic)

A stellate ganglion block is performed to diagnose or treat sympathetic nerve mediated pain in the head, neck, chest or arm caused by conditions such as reflex sympathetic dystrophy, nerve injury, herpes zoster, or intractable angina. The front of the neck in the region of the voice box is palpated to identify the correct location for needle placement. The neck is prepped and the needle inserted into the skin and then advanced into the deeper tissues. When the needle is in the correct location, an anesthetic is injected. The patient is monitored for 10-20 minutes while the anesthetic takes effect.

64517

64517 Injection, anesthetic agent; superior hypogastric plexus

A superior hypogastric plexus block is performed to relieve intractable pain in the pelvic region. This type of pain is often due to malignant primary and metastatic neoplasms in the pelvic region. The back is prepped over the L5-S1 interspace. Using separately reportable radiologic guidance, a spinal needle is inserted into the skin, passed through the L5-S1 interspace, and positioned anterolateral to the interspace. The needle is aspirated to ensure that the tip is located outside the ureters, spinal canal and blood vessels. Radiographic contrast is injected to ensure that the needle is properly placed in the prevertebral space anterior to the psoas muscle fascia. The needle is aspirated again and then a local anesthetic is injected.

64520

64520 Injection, anesthetic agent; lumbar or thoracic (paravertebral sympathetic)

Thoracic or lumbar paravertebral nerve block is used to treat acute or chronic pain in the thoracic or abdominal regions. The paravertebral space is a wedge-shaped area immediately adjacent to the vertebral bodies on either side of the spine where the spinal nerves emerge from the intervertebral foramen. Injection of a local anesthetic in this region produces unilateral motor, sensory, and sympathetic nerve blocks. The level of the blocks is determined, and the superior aspect of the spinous process is identified and marked. A needle entry site is marked approximately 2.5 cm lateral to the superior aspect of the spinous process. A local anesthetic is injected at the planned needle insertion site. A spinal epidural needle with tubing attached to a syringe is then inserted through the skin and advanced until contact is made with the transverse process. The needle is then withdrawn to the subcutaneous tissue and angled so that is can be walked off the lower (caudad) edge of the transverse process. The needle is reinserted and advanced into the paravertebral space. The needle is aspirated to ensure that it is not in the spinal canal or a blood vessel. The anesthetic is injected.

Nervous System

64530

64530   Injection, anesthetic agent; celiac plexus, with or without radiologic monitoring

The celiac nerve plexus is a network of nerves located anterior to the aorta at the level of the T12 vertebra. The celiac plexus transmits nerve impulses from the pancreas, liver, gall bladder stomach and intestine to the brain. Celiac plexus block in performed to treat chronic pain due to disease or injury of these organs including malignant neoplasm, inflammation (pancreatitis), or other conditions. The skin of the back over the T12 vertebra is prepped. A local anesthetic is injected. Using radiological guidance, a needle is advanced into celiac plexus, which is the region immediately superior to the celiac artery. The needle is aspirated to ensure that the tip is not in a blood vessel. Contrast is injected to ensure that the needle is in the proper location. The needle is aspirated again and anesthetic is injected.

64550

64550   Application of surface (transcutaneous) neurostimulator

Transcutaneous electrical nerve stimulation (TENS) is used to block the input of pain messages to the brain. A TENS unit consists of a generator, battery, and electrodes. The generator is programmed to deliver stimuli that interrupt the transmission of pain impulses. Three parameters, amplitude, pulse width, and pulse rate are programmed and adjusted to provide the best pain control. Amplitude is the strength of the stimulus, pulse width the duration of the stimuli, and pulse rate the frequency of the stimulus. Electrodes are placed on the skin over the painful area, cutaneous nerves or trigger points depending on which site provides the best pain relief. The patient is provided with a treatment plan and instructed on the use of the TENS unit.

64553

64553   Percutaneous implantation of neurostimulator electrode array; cranial nerve

When implanting a neurostimulator electrode array, the exact procedure depends on which of the cranial nerves is being stimulated. One of the more common sites is the vagus nerve to help control epileptic seizures. For percutaneous vagus nerve neurostimulator electrode array placement, the planned insertion site in the neck is prepped. Anatomical landmarks are located and separately reportable ultrasound guidance is used as needed to facilitate correct placement of the electrodes. An electrically insulated needle is inserted into the side of the neck and advanced parallel to the vagus nerve until it is positioned near the carotid sheath. A power source is connected to the needle, stimulation is applied, and motor and sensory responses are evaluated as the position of the needle is changed until the desired response is achieved. The needle is disconnected from the power source. An electrode array is then passed through the lumen of the needle and positioned in the desired location next to the vagus nerve. The needle is removed, leaving the electrode array in place, which is then attached to an external generator/receiver.

64555

64555   Percutaneous implantation of neurostimulator electrode array; peripheral nerve (excludes sacral nerve)

When implanting a neurostimulator electrode array, the exact procedure depends on which of the peripheral nerves is being stimulated. The planned insertion site is prepped. Anatomical landmarks are located and separately reportable ultrasound guidance is used as needed to facilitate correct placement of the electrodes. An electrically insulated needle is inserted into the skin and advanced parallel to the peripheral nerve. A power source is connected to the needle, stimulation is applied, and motor and sensory responses are evaluated as the position of the needle is changed until the desired response is achieved. The needle is disconnected from the power source. An electrode array is then passed through the lumen of the needle and positioned in the desired location next to the peripheral nerve. The needle is removed leaving the electrode array in place, which is then attached to an external generator/receiver.

64561

64561   Percutaneous implantation of neurostimulator electrode array; sacral nerve (transforaminal placement) including image guidance, if performed

A neurostimulator electrode array is placed for direct transforaminal sacral nerve stimulation, which is used to treat voiding dysfunction, including urge incontinence, urgency, frequency, and nonobstructive retention. The sacral foramen are located using bony landmarks or with imaging guidance such as fluoroscopy. The skin is prepped and a local anesthetic is injected into the skin and the periosteum of the sacrum. Percutaneous placement is accomplished using an electrically insulated spinal needle advanced through the skin and deeper tissues into the selected sacral foramen. A power source is connected to the needle, stimulation is applied, and motor and sensory responses are evaluated as the position of the needle is changed until the desired response is achieved. The needle is disconnected from the power source. An electrode array is then passed through the lumen of the needle and positioned in the desired location next to the sacral nerve. The needle

is removed leaving the electrode array in place, which is then attached to an external generator/receiver.

64565

64565   Percutaneous implantation of neurostimulator electrode array; neuromuscular

When implanting a neurostimulator electrode array, the exact procedure depends on the location of the neuromuscular site to be stimulated. The planned insertion site is prepped. Anatomical landmarks are located and separately reportable ultrasound guidance is used as needed to facilitate correct placement of the electrode array. An electrically insulated needle is inserted into the skin and advanced to the neuromuscular site to be stimulated. A power source is connected to the needle, stimulation is applied, and responses are evaluated as the position of the needle is changed until the desired response is achieved. The needle is disconnected from the power source. An electrode array is then passed through the lumen of the needle and positioned in the desired neuromuscular location. The needle is removed leaving the electrode array in place. The electrode is tested and the correct position is verified. The electrode array is then attached to an external generator/receiver.

64566

64566   Posterior tibial neurostimulation, percutaneous needle electrode, single treatment, includes programming

Posterior tibial neurostimulation (PTNS) is used to treat voiding dysfunction in patients who have failed other treatment modalities. The posterior tibial nerve is located near the ankle. It is a nerve branch derived from the lumbar-sacral nerves (L4-S3). Neurostimulation of the posterior tibial nerve is believed to alter its function thereby improving voiding function and control. The skin just above the ankle over the tibial nerve is cleansed. The neurostimulator is programmed. A fine needle electrode is inserted adjacent to the nerve and low voltage electrical stimulation is delivered using the prescribed voltage for the prescribed amount of time. This code reports a single treatment session. Most patients receive once a week sessions over a 10-12 week period.

64568

64568   Incision for implantation of cranial nerve (eg, vagus nerve) neurostimulator electrode array and pulse generator

For placement of a neurostimulator electrode array and pulse generator, the exact implantation procedure depends on which cranial nerve is being stimulated. One of the more common sites for electrode placement is the vagus nerve to help control epileptic seizures. For open vagus nerve neurostimulator electrode array placement, the planned insertion site in the neck is prepped. The skin is incised and soft tissues are dissected to expose the vagus nerve and carotid artery sheath. The electrode array is then positioned in the desired location next to the vagus nerve. The electrode array is connected to a power source; stimulation is applied; and motor responses are evaluated. The electrode array is repositioned and retested until the desired responses are attained. The electrodes are then secured in place. An incision is made in the skin and a subcutaneous pocket is developed. The pulse generator is placed in the subcutaneous pocket. The electrode array wires are tunneled to the generator and connected. The generator and leads are tested and the pocket is closed. Tissues in the neck are closed in layers over the electrode array.

64569-64570

64569   Revision or replacement of cranial nerve (eg, vagus nerve) neurostimulator electrode array, including connection to existing pulse generator

64570   Removal of cranial nerve (eg, vagus nerve) neurostimulator electrode array and pulse generator

A neurostimulator electrode array is revised/replaced (64569) or removed along with the pulse generator (64570). The exact procedure depends on which cranial nerve is being stimulated. One of the more common sites for electrode placement is the vagus nerve to help control epileptic seizures. In 64569, the skin is incised and soft tissues are dissected to expose the electrode array and/or the pulse generator. Defective components are repaired or the array is replaced. The electrode array is then placed in the desired location next to the vagus nerve. The new or repaired electrode array is connected to the power source; stimulation is applied; and motor responses are evaluated. The electrode array is repositioned and retested until the desired responses are attained. The electrode array is then secured in place. If a new electrode array has been implanted, the electrode array wires are tunneled to the generator and connected. The generator and leads are tested and the pocket is then closed. Tissues in the neck are closed in layers over the electrode array. In 64570, the electrode array and pulse generator are exposed. The generator is detached from the array wires. The generator is removed and the subcutaneous pocket is closed. The electrode array is dissected free of surrounding tissues and the array and wires are removed. Incisions are closed.

● New Code   ▲ Revised Code

64575

64575   Incision for implantation of neurostimulator electrode array; peripheral nerve (excludes sacral nerve)

For placement of a neurostimulator electrode array, the exact procedure depends on which peripheral nerve is being stimulated. For open placement of a peripheral nerve neurostimulator electrode array, the planned insertion site is prepped and the skin is incised. Soft tissues are dissected to expose the targeted peripheral nerve. An electrode array is then positioned in the desired location next to the peripheral nerve and connected to a power source. Stimulation is applied and motor responses are evaluated. The electrode array is repositioned and retested until the desired responses are attained. The electrode array is then secured and tunneled to the generator/receiver which is implanted in a separately reportable procedure. Tissues are closed in layers over the electrode array.

64580

64580   Incision for implantation of neurostimulator electrode array; neuromuscular

The exact procedure for implanting a neurostimulator electrode array depends on which neuromuscular site is being stimulated. For open neuromuscular neurostimulator electrode array placement, the planned insertion site is prepped and the skin is incised. Soft tissues are dissected. An electrode array is positioned in the desired location for neuromuscular stimulation and connected to a power source. Electrical stimulation is then applied and the targeted neuromuscular responses are evaluated. The electrode array is repositioned and retested until the desired responses are attained. The electrode array is then secured and tunneled to the generator/receiver which is implanted in a separately reportable procedure. Tissues are closed in layers over the electrode array.

64581

64581   Incision for implantation of neurostimulator electrode array; sacral nerve (transforaminal placement)

Direct transforaminal sacral nerve stimulation is used to treat voiding dysfunction, including urge incontinence, urgency, frequency, and nonobstructive urinary retention. For open transforaminal implantation of a sacral nerve neurostimulator electrode array, the skin is prepped and a local anesthetic is injected into the skin and periosteum of the sacrum. The skin over the sacrum is incised in the midline. Overlying tissue is dissected and the sacrum is exposed. A foramen needle is inserted into the selected sacral foramen. A power source is connected to the needle; stimulation is applied; and the motor responses are evaluated as the position of the needle is changed until the desired response is achieved. The needle is disconnected from the power source and removed. An electrode array is then passed through the foramen and positioned in the desired location next to the sacral nerve. Correct placement is verified by testing motor response to stimulation. The electrode array is tunneled to the site of the generator/receiver which is implanted in a separately reportable procedure. The presacral fascia is closed over the electrode array, followed by closure of the subcutaneous tissue and skin.

64585

64585   Revision or removal of peripheral neurostimulator electrode array

The exact revision or removal procedure depends on the location of the existing peripheral neurostimulator electrode array. A skin incision is made over the existing array. Soft tissues are dissected and the electrode array is exposed. The device is inspected and detached from the generator/receiver. The array is tested and any malfunctioning components are replaced. The array is then positioned in the desired location next to the peripheral nerve. Correct placement is verified by testing motor response to stimulation. The electrode array is reconnected to the generator/receiver. Alternatively, the array may be removed and the surgical wound closed in layers.

64590

64590   Insertion or replacement of peripheral or gastric neurostimulator pulse generator or receiver, direct or inductive coupling

The physician incises or replaces a pulse generator or receiver under the skin. The device is connected to an electrode(s) using direct or inductive coupling, and is used to stimulate peripheral nervous tissue, or gastric tissue.

64595

64595   Revision or removal of peripheral or gastric neurostimulator pulse generator or receiver

The physician removes or revises a pulse generator or receiver which is located under the skin and connected to an electrode used to stimulate peripheral nervous tissue or gastric tissue.

64600-64610

64600   Destruction by neurolytic agent, trigeminal nerve; supraorbital, infraorbital, mental, or inferior alveolar branch
64605   Destruction by neurolytic agent, trigeminal nerve; second and third division branches at foramen ovale
64610   Destruction by neurolytic agent, trigeminal nerve; second and third division branches at foramen ovale under radiologic monitoring

Destruction of a nerve is performed to treat chronic pain and may be performed by injection of a chemical neurolytic agent or using thermal, electrical or radiofrequency techniques. The most common technique used today is radiofrequency destruction, although the other techniques may also be used for certain pain syndromes. Prior to the destruction procedure, an electrode needle is introduced through the skin and advanced toward the targeted neural tissue. The needle is connected to a generator for motor and sensory testing performed to ensure that the needle is correctly positioned at the nerve responsible for the pain. Once the correct nerve pathway has been identified, the nerve is destroyed. If a chemical agent is used, the chemical agent is injected along the nerve pathway. Neurolytic chemical agents include: phenol, ethyl alcohol, glycerol, ammonium salt compounds and hypertonic or hypotonic solutions. Thermal or electrical modalities involve the use of a probe or needle that is inserted through the skin and activated to produce heat and destroy nerve tissue. To perform radiofrequency nerve destruction, an electrode needle is introduced through the skin and advanced toward the targeted neural tissue. The electrode is adjusted as needed until correct positioning is achieved. The radiofrequency device is then activated and an electric current generated that produces heat at the tip of the electrode and destroys the targeted nerve tissue. Use 64600 for destruction of the supraorbital, infraorbital, mental, or inferior alveolar branch of the trigeminal nerve. For second or third division branches of the trigeminal nerve at the foramene ovale use 64605 when the procedure is performed without the use of radiologic monitoring; use 64610 when the procedure is performed with radiologic monitoring.

64611

64611   Chemodenervation of parotid and submandibular salivary glands, bilateral

Chemodenervation of the salivary glands is performed to treat excessive salivation and drooling, also referred to as sialorrhea. Sialorrhea can be a problem for individuals with some types of neurological conditions such as cerebral palsy, Parkinson's disease, and late effects of cerebrovascular accident (stroke). Imaging guidance is used as needed to locate the salivary glands. Type A botulinum toxin is injected directly into both the parotid and submandibular glands on each side. One or more injections may be required in each gland to accomplish the denervation.

64612

64612   Chemodenervation of muscle(s); muscle(s) innervated by facial nerve, unilateral (eg, for blepharospasm, hemifacial spasm)

Chemodenervation is performed on muscles innervated by the facial nerve unilaterally to treat involuntary muscle contractions or muscle spasms, such as blepharospasm or for treatment of hemifacial pain. Injection of botulinum toxin (type A or B) directly into a muscle produces temporary muscle paralysis by blocking the release of acetylcholine at the peripheral nerve endings which interrupts neuromuscular transmission of nerve impulses. The muscle and the specific muscle sites to be injected are determined either by use of electromyography or by examining and palpating the facial muscles and noting the location of the muscle spasm. The side of the face to be treated is prepped. The affected muscle or muscle group is then injected at carefully selected sites to accomplish the denervation.

64615

64615   Chemodenervation of muscle(s); muscle(s) innervated by facial, trigeminal, cervical spinal and accessory nerves, bilateral (eg, for chronic migraine)

Chemical denervation involves the injection of a toxin (type A botulinum) directly into a muscle to produce temporary muscle paralysis by blocking the release of acetylcholine. Botulinum toxin injections have been shown to be effective in the prevention of migraines by blocking the neurotransmitter responsible for muscle contractions and pain. To perform chemical denervation of the muscles innervated by the facial, trigeminal, cervical spinal and accessory nerves small doses of Botox are injected bilaterally into muscles of the forehead, the side and back of the head, and the neck and shoulders.

64616

64616   Chemodenervation of muscle(s); neck muscle(s), excluding muscles of the larynx, unilateral (eg, for cervical dystonia, spasmodic torticollis)

Chemodenervation is performed on neck muscles unilaterally to treat involuntary muscle contractions or muscle spasms in the neck. This condition may be referred to as cervical dystonia or spasmodic torticollis. Injection of botulinum toxin (type A or B) directly into a muscle produces temporary muscle paralysis by blocking the release of acetylcholine at the peripheral nerve endings which interrupts neuromuscular transmission of nerve impulses. The muscle and the specific muscle sites to be injected are determined either by use of electromyography or by examining the position of the head, palpating the neck

Nervous System

muscles, and noting the location of the muscle spasm. The side of the neck to be treated is prepped. The affected muscle or muscle group is then injected at carefully selected sites to accomplish the denervation.

64617

64617 **Chemodenervation of muscle(s); larynx, unilateral, percutaneous (eg, for spasmodic dysphonia), includes guidance by needle electromyography, when performed**

Chemodenervation is performed to treat involuntary muscle contractions or muscle spasms in the vocal cord muscles of the larynx. These muscle spasms result from a neurological condition that manifests as spasmodic dysphonia, also referred to as laryngeal dystonia, or spastic dysphonia, which affects speech quality. Injection of botulinum toxin (type A or B) directly into a muscle produces temporary muscle paralysis by blocking the release of acetylcholine at the peripheral nerve endings which interrupts neuromuscular transmission of nerve impulses. The muscle sites to be injected are determined by electromyography (EMG). A hollow EMG needle connected to the EMG recorder is used to perform the injection. The patient may be supine or seated with the head extended. The thyroid and cricoid cartilages are located by palpation and the midline of the cricothyroid membrane is identified. For abductor spasmodic dysphonia, the needle is placed percutaneously into the thyroarytenoid muscle and the desired amount of botulin toxin is injected. For adductor spasmodic dysphonia, the needle is placed percutaneously and botulinum toxin is injected into the posterior cricoarytenoid muscle. The injection is typically performed on one side at the first visit and then on the opposite side on a subsequent visit with the visits spaced approximately two weeks apart. Code 64617 reports a unilateral procedure.

64620

64620 **Destruction by neurolytic agent, intercostal nerve**

Destruction of an intercostal nerve is performed to treat chronic pain and may be performed by injection of a chemical neurolytic agent or using thermal, electrical or radiofrequency techniques. The most common technique used today is radiofrequency destruction, although the other techniques may also be used for certain pain syndromes. Prior to the destruction procedure, an electrode needle is introduced through the skin and advanced toward the targeted neural tissue. The needle is connected to a generator for motor and sensory testing performed to ensure that the needle is correctly positioned at the nerve responsible for the pain. Once the correct nerve pathway has been identified, the nerve is destroyed. If a chemical agent is used, the chemical agent is injected along the nerve pathway. Neurolytic chemical agents include: phenol, ethyl alcohol, glycerol, ammonium salt compounds and hypertonic or hypotonic solutions. Thermal or electrical modalities involve the use of a probe or needle that is inserted through the skin and activated to produce heat and destroy nerve tissue. To perform radiofrequency nerve destruction, an electrode needle is introduced through the skin and advanced toward the targeted neural tissue. The electrode is adjusted as needed until correct positioning is achieved. The radiofrequency device is then activated and an electric current generated that produces heat at the tip of the electrode and destroys the targeted nerve tissue.

64630

64630 **Destruction by neurolytic agent; pudendal nerve**

The pudendal nerve controls sensation in the area between the genitals and the anus, the rectum, and the external genitalia. Destruction of the pudendal nerve is performed to treat chronic pain and may be performed by injection of a chemical neurolytic agent or using thermal, electrical or radiofrequency techniques. The most common technique used today is radiofrequency destruction, although the other techniques may also be used for certain pain syndromes. Prior to the destruction procedure, an electrode needle is introduced through the skin and advanced toward the targeted neural tissue. The needle is connected to a generator for motor and sensory testing performed to ensure that the needle is correctly positioned at the nerve responsible for the pain. Once the correct nerve pathway has been identified, the nerve is destroyed. If a chemical agent is used, the chemical agent is injected along the nerve pathway. Neurolytic chemical agents include: phenol, ethyl alcohol, glycerol, ammonium salt compounds and hypertonic or hypotonic solutions. Thermal or electrical modalities involve the use of a probe or needle that is inserted through the skin and activated to produce heat and destroy nerve tissue. To perform radiofrequency nerve destruction, an electrode needle is introduced through the skin and advanced toward the targeted neural tissue. The electrode is adjusted as needed until correct positioning is achieved. The radiofrequency device is then activated and an electric current generated that produces heat at the tip of the electrode and destroys the targeted nerve tissue.

64632

64632 **Destruction by neurolytic agent; plantar common digital nerve**

This procedure is performed to treat pain in the interdigital space caused by conditions such as Morton's neuroma. With the patient in a supine position, the knee is flexed and supported with a pillow and the foot is maintained in a relaxed neutral position. The interdigital spaces are palpated and any tenderness or fullness is noted. The needle is

inserted on the dorsal foot surface in a distal to proximal direction at a point 1-2 cm proximal to the web space and in line with the metatarsophalangeal joints. The needle is held at an angle of approximately 45 degrees and advanced through the mid web space at the plantar aspect of the foot. The needle is advanced until it tents the skin and then withdrawn approximately 1 cm. Taking care to avoid the plantar fat pad, a neurolytic agent such as ethyl alcohol is injected in an alcohol/anesthetic mix. Alcohol causes chemical neurolysis of the plantar common digital nerve due to dehydration, necrosis, and precipitation of protoplasm.

64633-64636

64633 **Destruction by neurolytic agent, paravertebral facet joint nerve(s), with imaging guidance (fluoroscopy or CT); cervical or thoracic, single facet joint**

64634 **Destruction by neurolytic agent, paravertebral facet joint nerve(s), with imaging guidance (fluoroscopy or CT); cervical or thoracic, each additional facet joint (List separately in addition to code for primary procedure)**

64635 **Destruction by neurolytic agent, paravertebral facet joint nerve(s), with imaging guidance (fluoroscopy or CT); lumbar or sacral, single facet joint**

64636 **Destruction by neurolytic agent, paravertebral facet joint nerve(s), with imaging guidance (fluoroscopy or CT); lumbar or sacral, each additional facet joint (List separately in addition to code for primary procedure)**

Paravertebral facet joints, also called zygapophyseal joints, are located on the posterior aspect of the spine on each side of the vertebra at the point where one vertebra overlaps the next. Using fluoroscopic or CT guidance, the paravertebral facet joint nerve is destroyed using a neurolytic agent. The skin overlying the facet joint is prepped and a local anesthetic is injected. If a chemical neurolytic agent is used, a spinal needle is directed into the facet joint space until bone or cartilage is encountered. A small amount of contrast material is injected to verify that the needle is correctly positioned. This may be followed by injection of a local anesthetic and/or steroid. The selected chemical neurolytic agent is then injected along the nerve pathway. Neurolytic chemical agents include: phenol, ethyl alcohol, glycerol, ammonium salt compounds, and hypertonic or hypotonic solutions. Thermal or electrical modalities for neurolysis involve the use of a probe, needle, or electrode inserted through the skin and activated to produce heat and destroy nerve tissue. Using fluoroscopic or CT guidance, an electrode needle is introduced through the skin and advanced toward the targeted neural tissue. The needle is connected to a generator for performing motor and sensory testing to ensure that the needle is correctly positioned along the facet joint nerve. Once the correct nerve pathway has been identified, the nerve is destroyed. The probe, needle, or electrode is activated and an electric current is generated that produces heat at the tip of the device and destroys the targeted nerve tissue. Use 64633 for a single cervical or thoracic facet joint nerve; use 64634 for each additional cervical or thoracic level. Use 64635 for a single lumbar or sacral facet joint nerve; use 64636 for each additional lumbar or sacral level.

64640

64640 **Destruction by neurolytic agent; other peripheral nerve or branch**

Destruction of a nerve is performed to treat chronic pain and may be performed by injection of a chemical neurolytic agent or using thermal, electrical or radiofrequency techniques. The most common technique used today is radiofrequency destruction, although the other techniques may also be used for certain pain syndromes. Prior to the destruction procedure, an electrode needle is introduced through the skin and advanced toward the targeted neural tissue. The needle is connected to a generator for motor and sensory testing performed to ensure that the needle is correctly positioned at the nerve responsible for the pain. Once the correct nerve pathway has been identified, the nerve is destroyed. If a chemical agent is used, the chemical agent is injected along the nerve pathway. Neurolytic chemical agents include: phenol, ethyl alcohol, glycerol, ammonium salt compounds and hypertonic or hypotonic solutions. Thermal or electrical modalities involve the use of a probe or needle that is inserted through the skin and activated to produce heat and destroy nerve tissue. To perform radiofrequency nerve destruction, an electrode needle is introduced through the skin and advanced toward the targeted neural tissue. The electrode is adjusted as needed until correct positioning is achieved. The radiofrequency device is then activated and an electric current generated that produces heat at the tip of the electrode and destroys the targeted nerve tissue. Use 64640 for destruction of a peripheral nerve or branch that does not have a more specific code listed.

64642-64643

64642 **Chemodenervation of one extremity; 1-4 muscle(s)**
64643 **Chemodenervation of one extremity; each additional extremity, 1-4 muscle(s) (List separately in addition to code for primary procedure)**

Chemodenervation is performed on the muscles of one extremity to treat involuntary muscle contractions or muscle spasms such as those due to dystonia, cerebral palsy, or multiple sclerosis. Injection of botulinum toxin (type A or B) directly into a muscle produces temporary muscle paralysis by blocking the release of acetylcholine at the peripheral nerve endings which interrupts neuromuscular transmission of nerve impulses. The muscle and muscle sites to be injected are determined either by use of electromyography or by

Nervous System

● New Code   ▲ Revised Code

examining the affected extremity, palpating the muscles, and noting the location of the muscle spasm. The extremity to be treated is prepped. The affected muscle or muscle group is then injected at carefully selected sites to accomplish the denervation. Use 64642 for 1-4 muscles of one extremity and 64643 for 1-4 muscles in each additional extremity.

64644-64645

64644 **Chemodenervation of one extremity; 5 or more muscles**
64645 **Chemodenervation of one extremity; each additional extremity, 5 or more muscles (List separately in addition to code for primary procedure)**

Chemodenervation is performed on the muscles of one extremity to treat involuntary muscle contractions or muscle spasms such as those due to dystonia, cerebral palsy, or multiple sclerosis. Injection of botulinum toxin (type A or B) directly into a muscle produces temporary muscle paralysis by blocking the release of acetylcholine at the peripheral nerve endings which interrupts neuromuscular transmission of nerve impulses. The muscle and muscle sites to be injected are determined either by use of electromyography or by examining the affected extremity, palpating the muscles, and noting the location of the muscle spasm. The extremity to be treated is prepped. The affected muscles or muscle group(s) are then injected at carefully selected sites to accomplish the denervation. Use 64644 for 5 or more muscles of one extremity and 64645 for 5 or more muscles in each additional extremity.

64646-64647

64646 **Chemodenervation of trunk muscle(s); 1-5 muscle(s)**
64647 **Chemodenervation of trunk muscle(s); 6 or more muscles**

Chemodenervation is performed on the muscles of the trunk to treat involuntary muscle contractions or muscle spasms such as those due to dystonia, cerebral palsy, or multiple sclerosis. Injection of botulinum toxin (type A or B) directly into a muscle produces temporary muscle paralysis by blocking the release of acetylcholine at the peripheral nerve endings which interrupts neuromuscular transmission of nerve impulses. The muscle and muscle sites to be injected are determined either by use of electromyography or by examining the trunk, palpating the muscles, and noting the location of the muscle spasm. The trunk is prepped. The affected muscle(s) or muscle group is then injected at carefully selected sites to accomplish the denervation. Use 64646 for 1-5 muscles of the trunk and 64647 for 6 or more muscles in the trunk.

64650-64653

64650 **Chemodenervation of eccrine glands; both axillae**
64653 **Chemodenervation of eccrine glands; other area(s) (eg, scalp, face, neck), per day**

The eccrine glands are sweat glands and are located over most parts of the body. Chemodenervation of the eccrine glands is performed to treat severe focal hyperhidrosis. Focal hyperhidrosis is profuse, localized sweating. Common sites for chemodenervation include the axillary region, scalp, face, neck, and palms of the hands. The locations of excessive sweating are identified by painting the region with an iodine solution and then dusting the area with starch powder. After 10-15 minutes the presence of sweat causes the prepped areas to turn dark purple. The reactive area is then marked and the starch-iodine compound removed. The area is prepped with an antibacterial solution. The reconstituted botulinum toxin type A is then placed in syringes and injected into the dermis over the previously identified region at 1.5-2 cm intervals. Use 64650 for chemodenervation of eccrine glands in both axillae. Use 64653 for chemodenervation of eccrine glands in other areas. Code 64653 is reported once per day regardless of how many other areas are treated.

64680

64680 **Destruction by neurolytic agent, with or without radiologic monitoring; celiac plexus**

The celiac plexus is located in the retroperitoneum of the upper abdomen at the level of the T12-L1 vertebra lying anterior to the crura of the diaphragm. The celiac plexus surrounds the abdominal aorta, celiac and superior mesenteric arteries. Destruction of the celiac plexus is performed to treat pain due to metastatic cancer as well as nonmalignant pain, such as pain due to acute and chronic pancreatitis. Destruction may be performed by injection of a chemical neurolytic agent or using thermal, electrical or radiofrequency techniques. This procedure may be performed with or without radiologic monitoring. If radiologic monitoring is used, two needles are inserted on each side of the upper abdomen and directed toward the body of L1. Alternatively, the needles may be directed toward T12 if neurolysis is performed only on the splanchic nerves. Contrast is then injected to confirm proper needle placement. If a chemical agent is used, the chemical agent is injected. Neurolytic chemical agents include: phenol, ethyl alcohol, glycerol, ammonium salt compounds and hypertonic or hypotonic solutions. Thermal or electrical modalities involve the use of a probe or needle that is inserted through the skin and activated to produce heat and destroy nerve tissue. To perform radiofrequency nerve destruction, an electrode needle is introduced through the skin and advanced toward the targeted neural tissue. The electrode is adjusted as needed until correct positioning is achieved. The radiofrequency

device is then activated and an electric current generated that produces heat at the tip of the electrode and destroys the targeted nerve tissue.

64681

64681 **Destruction by neurolytic agent, with or without radiologic monitoring; superior hypogastric plexus**

The superior hypogastric plexus is a bilateral structure located in the retroperitoneum between the L5 and S1 vertebrae. Destruction of the superior hypogastric plexus is performed to treat pain due to a metastatic cancer in the pelvic region as well as nonmalignant chronic pain. Destruction may be performed by injection of a chemical neurolytic agent or using thermal, electrical or radiofrequency techniques. This procedure may be performed with or without radiologic monitoring. If radiologic monitoring is used, a needle is inserted into the ventral lateral surface of the spine at the L5-S1 interspace. Contrast is then injected to confirm proper needle placement in the prevertebral space just ventral to the psoas fascia. If a chemical agent is used, the chemical agent is injected. Neurolytic chemical agents include: phenol, ethyl alcohol, glycerol, ammonium salt compounds and hypertonic or hypotonic solutions. Thermal or electrical modalities involve the use of a probe or needle that is inserted through the skin and activated to produce heat and destroy nerve tissue. To perform radiofrequency nerve destruction, an electrode needle is introduced through the skin and advanced toward the targeted neural tissue. The electrode is adjusted as needed until correct positioning is achieved. The radiofrequency device is then activated and an electric current generated that produces heat at the tip of the electrode and destroys the targeted nerve tissue.

64702-64704

64702 **Neuroplasty; digital, 1 or both, same digit**
64704 **Neuroplasty; nerve of hand or foot**

Neuroplasty is performed to treat nerve entrapment, which may be caused by inflammation of surrounding tissues, a tumor or mass, or scar tissue and adhesion formation. The skin over the nerve is incised and soft tissues are dissected. The nerve is identified and any scar tissue or adhesions are dissected free of the nerve. Other structures such as fascia or ligaments may be divided to release pressure on the nerve. Once the nerve is completely freed of surrounding tissue and impinging structures, the soft tissues are closed in layers. In 64702, neuroplasty is performed on one or both digital nerves in the same digit of the hand or foot. In 64704, neuroplasty of a nerve of the hand or foot is performed.

64708-64712

64708 **Neuroplasty, major peripheral nerve, arm or leg, open; other than specified**
64712 **Neuroplasty, major peripheral nerve, arm or leg, open; sciatic nerve**

Neuroplasty is performed to treat nerve entrapment, which may be caused by inflammation of surrounding tissues, a tumor or mass, or scar tissue and adhesion formation. The skin over the nerve is incised and soft tissues are dissected. The nerve is identified and any scar tissue or adhesions are dissected free of the nerve. Other structures such as fascia or ligaments may be divided to release pressure on the nerve. Once the nerve is completely freed of surrounding tissue and impinging structures, the soft tissues are closed in layers. In 64708, neuroplasty is performed on a major peripheral nerve of the arm or leg other than one specified. In 64712, neuroplasty of the sciatic nerve is performed.

64713

64713 **Neuroplasty, major peripheral nerve, arm or leg, open; brachial plexus**

The brachial plexus is a network of nerves that sends signals from the spine to the shoulder, arm, and hand. Injury can occur as a result of blunt force, such as that occurring in contact sports, an auto accident, or a fall. The brachial plexus can also be damaged during the birth process or from inflammation, or a tumor. Damage to the brachial plexus can cause formation of scar tissue and adhesions that entrap and compress the nerves. A supraclavicular approach is used to expose the proximal aspect of the brachial plexus. The omohyoid muscle is divided. Electrophysiological tests are performed as needed to assess nerve function of exposed nerves and nerve roots as well as to determine which nerves are compressed. Compressed nerves in the brachial plexus are dissected free of scar tissue and other structures causing the compression. Once affected nerves are completely freed, the overlying soft tissues are closed in layers.

64714

64714 **Neuroplasty, major peripheral nerve, arm or leg, open; lumbar plexus**

The lumbar plexus is a network of nerves originating from the L1-L4 nerve roots that sends signals to the back, abdomen, groin, thighs, knees, and calves. Injury can occur as a result of blunt force, such as that occurring in contact sports, an auto accident, or a fall. The lumbar plexus can also be damaged by an inflammatory process or a tumor. Injury or other disease processes can cause formation of scar tissue and adhesions that entrap and compress nerves contained in the lumbar plexus. An incision is made in the lower back over the affected side. Soft tissues are divided. The lumbar plexus is exposed. Electrophysiological tests are performed as needed to assess nerve function of exposed nerves and nerve roots as well as to determine which nerves are compressed. Compressed

Nervous System

nerves in the lumbar plexus are dissected free of scar tissue and other structures causing the compression. Once affected nerves are completely freed, the overlying soft tissues are closed in layers.

64716

64716   Neuroplasty and/or transposition; cranial nerve (specify)

Neuroplasty and/or transposition of a cranial nerve is performed to treat nerve entrapment, which may be caused by inflammation of surrounding tissues, a tumor or mass, or scar tissue and adhesion formation. The skin over the nerve is incised and soft tissues are dissected. The nerve is identified and any scar tissue or adhesions are dissected free of the nerve. Other structures such as fascia or ligaments may be divided to release pressure on the nerve. If needed the nerve may be relocated to relieve the nerve compression. Once the nerve is completely freed of surrounding tissue and impinging structures, the soft tissues are closed in layers.

64718-64719

64718   Neuroplasty and/or transposition; ulnar nerve at elbow
64719   Neuroplasty and/or transposition; ulnar nerve at wrist

Neuroplasty and/or transposition of the ulnar nerve at the elbow or wrist is performed to treat nerve entrapment and compression of the nerve. The ulnar nerve passes under the collarbone, travels along the inner aspect of the arm, passes through the cubital tunnel in the inner aspect of the elbow, and then travels under the muscles of the inner arm and through Guyon's canal which is another tunnel in the wrist before entering the hand. In 64718, the ulnar nerve is decompressed at the elbow. An incision is made along the inner aspect of the elbow over the ulnar nerve and soft tissues are dissected. The ulnar nerve is identified and any scar tissue or adhesions are dissected free of the nerve. An anterior transposition may also be performed. This involves relocating the ulnar nerve from its usual position behind the elbow to a position in front of the elbow. The nerve can be moved to a subcutaneous position beneath the skin and fat but above the muscle or it can be moved to a position under the muscle. Once the nerve is completely freed of surrounding tissue and impinging structures, the soft tissues are closed in layers. In 64719, the ulnar nerve is decompressed at the wrist. A zigzag incision is made at the base of the palm on the little finger side and extended over the wrist. The roof of Guyon's canal is incised and scar tissue, adhesions or other impinging structures divided. Once the nerve is completely freed, overlying soft tissues are closed in layers.

64721

64721   Neuroplasty and/or transposition; median nerve at carpal tunnel

This procedure is performed to treat carpal tunnel syndrome (CTS) which results from median nerve compression within the carpal tunnel, a narrow passageway within the wrist between the carpal bones and carpal ligament. A regional or general anesthetic is administered. The skin is incised over the carpal tunnel in the palm of the hand and extended as needed over the wrist. The palmar fascia is exposed and incised. The carpal ligament is exposed. The median nerve and flexor tendons are identified and protected. The carpal ligament is then divided using scissors or a scalpel which releases the pressure on the median nerve. The nerve may also be relocated within the carpal tunnel to relieve the compression. The palmar fascia and skin are closed in layers.

64722

64722   Decompression; unspecified nerve(s) (specify)

TDecompression is performed to treat nerve entrapment, which may be caused by inflammation of surrounding tissues, a tumor or mass, or scar tissue and adhesion formation. The skin over the nerve is incised and soft tissues are dissected. The nerve is identified and any scar tissue or adhesions are dissected free of the nerve. Other structures such as fascia or ligaments may be divided to release pressure on the nerve. Once the nerve is completely freed of surrounding tissue and impinging structures, the soft tissues are closed in layers. Use 64722 for decompression of any nerve that does not have a more specific code.

64726

64726   Decompression; plantar digital nerve

The plantar aspect of the foot is innervated by the medial and lateral plantar nerves. The medial plantar nerve gives rise to the first through third common digital nerves, and the lateral plantar nerve to the fourth common digital nerve. Decompression is performed to treat nerve entrapment involving one of the plantar digital nerves. Entrapment may be caused by inflammation of surrounding tissues, a tumor or mass, or scar tissue and adhesion formation. The skin of the plantar aspect of the foot over the affected nerve is incised and soft tissues are dissected. The nerve is identified and scar tissue or adhesions are dissected free of the nerve. Other structures such as fascia or ligaments may also be divided to release pressure on the nerve. Once the nerve is completely freed of surrounding tissue and impinging structures, the soft tissues are closed in layers.

64727

64727   Internal neurolysis, requiring use of operating microscope (List separately in addition to code for neuroplasty) (Neuroplasty includes external neurolysis)

Internal neurolysis is performed to treat scarring and swelling occurring internally, that is within the outer nerve sheath. During a separately reportable neuroplasty procedure, the outer nerve sheath is incised using a microscope to improve visualization of the nerve. The nerve is inspected. If the nerve is swollen, opening the outer sheath alone will help relieve the nerve compression and promote blood flow to the nerve. If scar tissue is present within the outer sheath it is carefully dissected. The outer sheath is left open.

64732-64734

64732   Transection or avulsion of; supraorbital nerve
64734   Transection or avulsion of; infraorbital nerve

Transection or avulsion involves severing and/or removing a portion of the nerve and is performed to treat chronic pain. In 64732, transection or avulsion of the supraorbital nerve is performed. The supraorbital nerve is a branch of the frontal nerve. It exits the skull at the supraorbital foramen or groove, provides palpebral filaments to the upper eyelid, and then travels along the forehead dividing into medial and lateral branches that supply the scalp. An incision is made over the eyebrow. Soft tissues are dissected and the supraorbital nerve identified as it exits the supraorbital foramen. The nerve is isolated with a nerve hook. A fine rongeur may be used to remove the lip of bone over the supraorbital foramen to provide better exposure of the supraorbital nerve. Transection is performed by grasping the nerve and dividing it proximally. The nerve is then avulsed by twisting the nerve over a hemostat. This will usually sever the nerve within the foramen. Alternatively, the nerve may be stretched, ligated and divided first distally and then proximally. The proximal end of the nerve will then retract into the foramen. In 64734, transection of the infraorbital nerve is performed. The infraorbital nerve is a branch of the maxillary nerve. The maxillary nerve enters the face through the infraorbital canal where it becomes the infraorbital nerve and supplies sensory branches to the lower eyelid, side of the nose and upper lip. The infraorbital nerve may be approached intraorally or extraorally. Using an extraoral approach, an incision is made in a skin crease in the infraorbital rim. The infraorbital nerve is identified as it exits the infraorbital canal and transection or avulsion performed using the same techniques described above.

64736-64738

64736   Transection or avulsion of; mental nerve
64738   Transection or avulsion of; inferior alveolar nerve by osteotomy

Transection or avulsion involves severing and/or removing a portion of the nerve and is performed to treat chronic pain. In 64736, transection or avulsion of the mental nerve is performed. The mental nerve is a branch of the inferior alveolar nerve. It begins at the mental foramen where it exits the mandible and divides into three branches that innervate the skin of the chin and skin and mucous membrane of the lower lip. The mental nerve may be approached intraorally or extraorally. Using an extraoral approach an incision is made below and parallel to the angle of the mandible. The masseter muscle is exposed and split in line with its fibers to expose the lateral surface of the mandible. The mental nerve is identified and isolated. Transection is performed by grasping the nerve and dividing it proximally. The nerve may then be avulsed by twisting the nerve over a hemostat. This will usually sever the nerve within the foramen. Alternatively, the nerve may be stretched, ligated and divided first distally and then proximally. The proximal end of the nerve will then retract into the foramen. In 64738, transection or avulsion of the inferior alveolar nerve is performed by osteotomy. The inferior alveolar nerve may be approached intraorally or extraorally. If an extraoral approach is used the mental nerve and foramen are exposed as described above. The periosteum is incised over the mandibular ramus. The bone is incised or an opening created using a drill. Drilling continues through the cortical bone until the denser bone covering the neural canal is encountered. The neural canal is opened. The inferior alveolar nerve is exposed and transected or avulsed as described above.

64740

64740   Transection or avulsion of; lingual nerve

Transection or avulsion involves severing and/or removing a portion of the nerve and is performed to treat chronic pain. The lingual nerve is a branch of the mandibular nerve. It innervates the anterior two-thirds of the tongue and lingual surface of the mandibular gingiva. Using an intraoral approach, the lingual nerve is exposed and isolated. Transection is performed by grasping the nerve and dividing it proximally. The nerve may then be avulsed by twisting the nerve over a hemostat. Alternatively, the nerve may be stretched, ligated and divided first distally and then proximally.

64742

64742   Transection or avulsion of; facial nerve, differential or complete

Transection or avulsion involves severing and/or removing a portion of the nerve and is performed to treat chronic pain. The facial nerve, also known as cranial nerve VII (CN VII), is a mixed nerve containing both sensory and motor fibers. The motor fibers are responsible for facial expression. The facial nerve has intracranial, intratemporal and extratemporal components. The extratemporal portion begins where the nerve exits the stylomastoid foramen and this portion then branches into the temporal, zygomatic, buccal, marginal mandibular, and cervical branches. A differential or complete transection of the facial nerve may be performed. The branch of the facial nerve to be transected or avulsed is exposed and isolated. To perform a complete transection the nerve is grasped and divided. The nerve may then be avulsed by twisting the proximal segment of the nerve over a hemostat. Alternatively, the nerve may be stretched, ligated and divided first distally and then proximally. To perform a differential transection, the motor or sensory nerve fibers are isolated and only the selected fibers are transected or avulsed.

64744

64744   Transection or avulsion of; greater occipital nerve

Transection or avulsion involves severing and/or removing a portion of the nerve and is performed to treat chronic pain. The greater occipital nerve is a spinal nerve that arises between the first and second cervical vertebrae. After emerging from the suboccipital triangle it ascends and innervates the skin of the posterior aspect of the scalp to the top of the head. A skin incision is made over the posterolateral aspect of C2. Soft tissues are dissected and the greater occipital nerve is identified as it emerges from the transverse process of C2 and the inferior oblique muscle. The greater occipital nerve is isolated. Transection is performed by grasping the nerve and dividing it. The nerve may then be avulsed by twisting the nerve over a hemostat. Alternatively, the nerve may be stretched, ligated and divided first distally and then proximally. The proximal end of the nerve will retract into deeper tissues. Soft tissues are closed in layers.

Transection or avulsion of greater occipital nerve

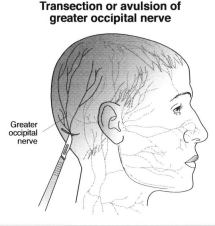

Greater occipital nerve

64746

64746   Transection or avulsion of; phrenic nerve

Transection or avulsion involves severing and/or removing a portion of the nerve and is performed to treat chronic pain. The phrenic nerve originates primarily from the 4th cervical nerve, but also contains fibers from the 3rd and 5th cervical nerves. The right and left phrenic nerves follow different paths. The right phrenic nerve lies deep to the scalene muscles in the neck and passes under the clavicle. It passes through the root of the right lung in the chest to the caval opening in the diaphragm at the level of the eighth thoracic vertebra. The left phrenic nerve follows the same route along the scalene muscle, passes into the thoracic cavity, travels downward over the left ventricle, and then enters the diaphragm. Transection is performed by grasping the nerve and dividing it. The nerve may then be avulsed by twisting the nerve over a hemostat. Alternatively, the nerve may be stretched, ligated and divided first distally and then proximally. The proximal end of the nerve will retract into deeper tissues.

64755-64760

64755   Transection or avulsion of; vagus nerves limited to proximal stomach (selective proximal vagotomy, proximal gastric vagotomy, parietal cell vagotomy, supra- or highly selective vagotomy)
64760   Transection or avulsion of; vagus nerve (vagotomy), abdominal

The vagus nerve is the tenth cranial nerve. It arises from the brainstem and travels through the neck, thorax, and abdomen, giving rise to multiple branches along its path. At the stomach, the vagus nerve divides into branches that innervate different parts of the stomach and upper digestive tract. Cutting of the vagus nerve is performed to decrease excessive acid production in the stomach to help prevent peptic ulcers. In 64755, the vagus nerves proximal to the stomach are transected. This procedure may be referred to as a selective proximal vagotomy, proximal gastric vagotomy, parietal cell vagotomy, supra or highly selective vagotomy (HSV). A midline upper abdominal incision is used to expose the stomach and vagus nerve. To perform a selective vagotomy, the main vagal trunks are

identified and dissected up to the branch leading to the biliary tree. This branch is followed to the hepatic branch and the nerve is transected as close to the hepatic branch as possible. To perform a highly selective vagotomy, the vagal nerve is identified and followed to the Latarjet's nerve branches, also referred to as the parietal cell branches. These branches are divided beginning at the esophagogastric junction and continuing along the lesser curvature of the stomach. In 64760, a truncal vagotomy is performed through an abdominal approach. A midline upper abdominal incision is used to expose the stomach and vagus nerve. The vagus nerve is identified and freed from surrounding structures. The main vagal trunks are located and divided.

64763-64766

64763   Transection or avulsion of obturator nerve, extrapelvic, with or without adductor tenotomy
64766   Transection or avulsion of obturator nerve, intrapelvic, with or without adductor tenotomy

The obturator nerve arises from the lumbar plexus, traverses the brim of the pelvis, enters the obturator canal, and extends into the thigh. In 64763, an extrapelvic transection or avulsion is performed. The skin is incised over the lateral aspect of the hip and subcutaneous tissues dissected. The adductor tendon is exposed and incised as needed. The anterior branch of the obturator nerve is exposed. The anterior branch is then transected (divided) or forcefully separated (avulsed) at its junction with the main obturator nerve. In 64766, an intrapelvic transection or avulsion is performed using an extraperitoneal approach. A skin incision is made in the right or left lower quadrant of the abdomen depending on which hip is affected. The external oblique muscle is divided above the inguinal ligament. The internal oblique and transverse abdominis muscles are split. The peritoneum and urinary bladder are retracted to permit exposure of the intrapelvic course of obturator nerve. An intrapelvic segment of the obturator nerve is then transected (divided) or forcefully separated (avulsed) from surrounding tissue.

64771-64772

64771   Transection or avulsion of other cranial nerve, extradural
64772   Transection or avulsion of other spinal nerve, extradural

Transection or avulsion involves severing and/or removing a portion of the nerve and is performed to treat chronic pain. Transection or avulsion of a cranial or spinal nerve not described by a more specific code is performed. This procedure is performed outside the dural membrane that covers the brain and spinal cord. A skin incision is made and soft tissues dissected to access the cranial or spinal nerve. The nerve is isolated. Transection is performed by grasping the nerve and dividing it. The nerve may then be avulsed by twisting the nerve over a hemostat. Alternatively, the nerve may be stretched, ligated and divided first distally and then proximally. The proximal end of the nerve will retract into deeper tissues. Soft tissues are closed in layers. Use 64771 for transection or avulsion of a cranial nerve and 64772 for a spinal nerve.

64774

64774   Excision of neuroma; cutaneous nerve, surgically identifiable

A cutaneous nerve is a nerve that innervates the skin. These nerves can develop painful benign lesions called neuromas. A skin incision is made over the site of the neuroma. The neuroma is exposed, dissected free of surrounding tissue and excised. The incision is closed.

64776-64778

64776   Excision of neuroma; digital nerve, 1 or both, same digit
64778   Excision of neuroma; digital nerve, each additional digit (List separately in addition to code for primary procedure)

The digital nerves innervate the fingers and toes. In the hand, the median nerve divides into lateral and medial branches. These branches divide again becoming the digital nerves. The lateral digital nerve divides into three branches, two of which innervate the thumb and one that innervates the radial side of the index finger. The medial digital nerve divides into two common palmar digital nerves that innervate the fingers. The common palmar digital nerves then divide into two branches at the end of the fingers. In the foot, the medial and lateral plantar nerves divide several times and eventually become the digital nerves of the toes with two branches in each of the toes. These nerves can develop painful benign lesions called neuromas. A skin incision is made over the site of the neuroma. The neuroma is exposed, dissected free of surrounding tissue and excised. The incision is closed. Use 64776 for excision of a neuroma of one or both digital nerves in the same finger or toe. Use 64778 for excision of a neuroma of one or both digital nerves in each additional finger or toe.

Nervous System

64782-64783

64782 Excision of neuroma; hand or foot, except digital nerve
64783 Excision of neuroma; hand or foot, each additional nerve, except same digit (List separately in addition to code for primary procedure)

The nerves of the hand or foot can develop painful benign lesions called neuromas. A skin incision is made over the site of the neuroma. The neuroma is exposed, dissected free of surrounding tissue and excised. The incision is closed. Use 64782 for excision of a neuroma affecting a single nerve other than the digital nerve in the hand or foot. Use 64783 for excision of a neuroma of each additional nerve in the hand or foot other than the digital nerves.

64784-64786

64784 Excision of neuroma; major peripheral nerve, except sciatic
64786 Excision of neuroma; sciatic nerve

The major peripheral nerves can develop painful benign lesions called neuromas. A skin incision is made over the site of the neuroma. Overlying soft tissues are dissected and the neuroma is exposed. The neuroma is dissected free of surrounding tissue and excised. The incision is closed. Use 64784 for excision of a neuroma of a major peripheral nerve other than the sciatic. Use 64786 for excision of a neuroma of the sciatic nerve.

64787

64787 Implantation of nerve end into bone or muscle (List separately in addition to neuroma excision)

Implantation of the nerve end in bone or muscle following excision of a neuroma inhibits scar tissue formation and protects the nerve end from recurrent trauma which is also a cause of neuroma formation. The neuroma is excised in a separately reportable procedure. The nerve is dissected proximally until enough nerve has been freed from surrounding tissue to allow relocation of the nerve in nearby muscle or bone. If the nerve end is implanted in muscle tissue, a small incision is made in line with the muscle fibers. The nerve is implanted and secured with sutures. If the nerve is implanted in bone, overlying soft tissue is dissected and the bone exposed. The periosteum is incised. A small drill is used to create a hole through the compact bone and into the medullary canal. The nerve end is then inserted through the drill hole into the medullary canal.

64788-64792

64788 Excision of neurofibroma or neurolemmoma; cutaneous nerve
64790 Excision of neurofibroma or neurolemmoma; major peripheral nerve
64792 Excision of neurofibroma or neurolemmoma; extensive (including malignant type)

Neurofibromas are tumors that involve nerve fibers. They arise from proliferation of Schwann cells and are one of the most common types of peripheral nerve tumors. While they sometimes occur as solitary tumors, the tumors more frequently occur in multiples as part of neurofibromatosis. Neurofibromatosis is a genetic disorder that varies greatly from very mild with limited tumors to severe with widespread debilitating tumor formation. Neurofibromas are typically benign but plexiform neurofibromas do have the potential to transform into malignant neoplasms. Plexiform neurofibromas are large neurofibromas that involve a long segment of a nerve or nerves. Neurolemmas are neoplasms of the outermost sheath or neurolemma of Schwann cells. In 64788 a cutaneous nerve neurofibroma or neurolemma is excised. A skin incision is made over the site of the tumor. The tumor is exposed, dissected free of surrounding tissue and excised. The incision is closed. In 64790, a neurofibroma or neurolemma is excised from a major peripheral nerve. The peripheral nerve is exposed. The segment of the nerve containing the tumor is dissected free of surrounding tissue. If the tumor is a neurofibroma, the nerve sheath is incised and the tumor is meticulously dissected from the nerve fibers. Following removal of the tumor the nerve sheath is closed. If the tumor is a neurolemma, the involved segment of the nerve sheath is excised. In 64792, extensive or malignant tumors are excised. The technique is similar to that described for 64790 except that the procedure may involve multiple tumors in the same region or may require more extensive dissection for excision of a malignant lesion.

64795

64795 Biopsy of nerve

A nerve biopsy may be performed to evaluate a nerve lesion or to help diagnosis the cause of pain, weakness, or numbness when a definitive diagnosis cannot be made using other diagnostic modalities such as history and clinical examination, laboratory tests and radiology studies. A skin incision is made over the nerve to be biopsied. Overlying soft tissues are dissected. A tissue sample is taken from the nerve lesion or a small segment of the nerve is excised and sent to the laboratory for separately reportable pathology examination. The overlying soft tissue and skin is closed in layers.

64802-64804

64802 Sympathectomy, cervical
64804 Sympathectomy, cervicothoracic

The sympathetic nervous system controls involuntary functions such as sweating, blushing, and salivation. Sympathectomy involves destruction or excision of sympathetic nerve fibers. In 64802, a cervical sympathectomy is performed which is usually done to increase blood supply in the internal carotid arteries. In 64804 a cervicothoracic sympathectomy is performed. An incision is made in the neck or chest at the level where the cervical or cervicothoracic sympathetic chain will be divided. Tissues are dissected and for cervicothoracic sympathectomy the lung may be deflated to allow better visualization of thoracic structures. The sympathetic chain is located and divided using electrocautery to cut and coagulate the chain. Alternatively, a segment of chain may be removed. The ganglia are completely obliterated which completely severs the sympathetic chain. For cervicothoracic sympathectomy, the pleura may be divided lateral to the chain and any aberrant nerve bundles located and severed. The sympathetic nerve bundles are separated and the ends are cauterized to prevent regrowth. The level of the transection is dependent on the condition being treated with division for hyperhidrosis at levels T2-T5, for thoracic outlet syndrome and reflex sympathetic dystrophy at levels T1-T3, and for chronic pancreatic pain at levels T4-T10. When the transection is complete, the lungs are expanded, a chest tube is placed and the chest incision is closed.

64809-64818

64809 Sympathectomy, thoracolumbar
64818 Sympathectomy, lumbar

The sympathetic nervous system controls involuntary functions such as sweating, blushing, and salivation. Sympathectomy involves destruction or excision of sympathetic nerve fibers. In 64809, a thoracolumbar sympathectomy is performed usually to treat malignant hypertension. In 64818, a lumbar sympathectomy is performed usually to treat hyperhidrosis of the feet. An incision is made in the lateral aspect of the chest and carried down to the iliac crest for a thoracolumbar sympathectomy or in the lower abdomen for a lumbar sympathectomy. Tissues are dissected. The sympathetic chain is located and divided using electrocautery to cut and coagulate the chain. Alternatively, a segment of chain may be removed. The ganglia are completely obliterated which completely severs the sympathetic chain. Additional dissection may be performed lateral to the chain and any aberrant nerve bundles located and severed. The sympathetic nerve bundles are separated and the ends are cauterized to prevent regrowth. When the transection is complete, the incision is closed in layers.

64820-64823

64820 Sympathectomy; digital arteries, each digit
64821 Sympathectomy; radial artery
64822 Sympathectomy; ulnar artery
64823 Sympathectomy; superficial palmar arch

Sympathectomy of the digital, superficial palmar arch, radial, and/or ulnar arteries may be performed to improve blood flow to the digits and may be used to treat severe ischemia due to Raynaud's syndrome, scleroderma, or other diseases. In 64820, digital artery sympathectomy of the hand is performed. A zigzag incision is made over the base of the finger and carried down into the palm. Using an operating microscope as needed, the common digital artery is separated from the adjacent digital nerve and stripped of adventitia beginning at the superficial arch and carrying the dissection distally. Separating the common digital artery from the adjacent digital nerve severs the sympathetic connections. Once the common digital artery and the adjacent digital nerve have been completely separated, the incisions are closed in layers. Report 64820 for each digit on which the procedure is performed. In 64821 and 64822, radial and/or ulnar artery sympathectomy is performed. The radial and/or ulnar artery is exposed at the wrist using an operating microscope as needed. The nerve connections are divided and the adventitia stripped from a 1-4 cm segment of the adjacent artery. Use 64821 for radial artery sympathectomy and 64822 for ulnar artery sympathectomy. In 64823, sympathectomy of the superficial palmar arch is performed. A transverse incision is made in the distal palmar flexion crease. Using microscopic technique as needed, the nerve connections are divided and the adventitia stripped from the superficial palmar arch.

64831-64832

64831 Suture of digital nerve, hand or foot; 1 nerve
64832 Suture of digital nerve, hand or foot; each additional digital nerve (List separately in addition to code for primary procedure)

A severed digital nerve is repaired with sutures. Suture repair of the nerve, also referred to as end-to-end closure, can be accomplished using several different techniques. Digital nerve repair is usually accomplished by epineural closure. The two ends of the transected nerve are exposed. Several sutures are placed in the epineurium of each of the two ends. Sutures are then placed so that nerve ends are approximated but not under tension. Use 64831 for suture repair of a single digital nerve in the hand or foot. Use 64832 for suture of each additional digital nerve in the hand or foot.

● New Code   ▲ Revised Code   CPT © 2016 American Medical Association. All Rights Reserved.   © 2017 DecisionHealth

Nervous System

64834-64837

64834   Suture of 1 nerve; hand or foot, common sensory nerve
64835   Suture of 1 nerve; median motor thenar
64836   Suture of 1 nerve; ulnar motor
64837   Suture of each additional nerve, hand or foot (List separately in addition to code for primary procedure)

A single common sensory nerve in the hand or foot is sutured in 64834. Suture repair of the nerve, also referred to as end-to-end closure, can be accomplished using several different techniques. For more distal injuries, an epineural closure may be performed. The two ends of the transected nerve are exposed. Several sutures are placed in the epineurium of each of the two ends. Sutures are then placed so that nerve ends are approximated but not under tension. For more proximal injuries, a perineural closure may be performed. The two ends of the transected nerve are exposed. The epineurium of each of the two ends is pulled back to expose the individual fascicles of axons. Fascicles that perform the same function (sensory, motor) are identified and approximated by end-to-end closure. Fascicles are then sutured together with a single suture placed through the perineurium. A second suture may be required if rotation occurs and fascicles are no longer aligned. The closure is performed by suturing the deeper fascicles first and then moving toward the nerve surface until all structures are repaired. A variation of the perineural technique is to repair a number of tightly grouped fascicles using several sutures to approximate and close the entire group. Use 64835 for suture repair of the median thenar nerve and 64836 for suture repair of the ulnar nerve. Use 64837 for suture of each additional nerve in the hand or foot.

64840

64840   Suture of posterior tibial nerve

Suture repair of the posterior tibial nerve, also referred to as end-to-end closure, can be accomplished using several different techniques. For more distal injuries, an epineural closure may be performed. The two ends of the transected nerve are exposed. Several sutures are placed in the epineurium of each of the two ends. Sutures are then placed so that nerve ends are approximated but not under tension. For more proximal injuries, a perineural closure may be performed. The two ends of the transected nerve are exposed. The epineurium of each of the two ends is pulled back to expose the individual fascicles of axons. Fascicles that perform the same function (sensory, motor) are identified and approximated by end-to-end closure. Fascicles are then sutured together with a single suture placed through the perineurium. A second suture may be required if rotation occurs and fascicles are no longer aligned. The closure is performed by suturing the deeper fascicles first and then moving toward the nerve surface until all structures are repaired. A variation of the perineural technique is to repair a number of tightly grouped fascicles using several sutures to approximate and close the entire group.

64856-64857

64856   Suture of major peripheral nerve, arm or leg, except sciatic; including transposition
64857   Suture of major peripheral nerve, arm or leg, except sciatic; without transposition

Suture repair of a major peripheral nerve in the arm or leg other than the sciatic nerve, also referred to as end-to-end closure, can be accomplished using several different techniques. For more distal injuries, an epineural closure may be performed. The two ends of the transected nerve are exposed. Prior to repair, the injured nerve may be transposed to a new position. The injured nerve is dissected from surrounding tissues proximal and distal to the site of the injury. The nerve is then rerouted as needed to allow a tension free repair. The repair is then performed. Several sutures are placed in the epineurium of each of the two ends. Sutures are placed so that nerve ends are approximated but not under tension. For more proximal injuries, a perineural closure may be performed. The two ends of the transected nerve are exposed. The epineurium of each of the two ends is pulled back to expose the individual fascicles of axons. Fascicles that perform the same function (sensory, motor) are identified and approximated by end-to-end closure. Fascicles are then sutured together with a single suture placed through the perineurium. A second suture may be required if rotation occurs and fascicles are no longer aligned. The closure is performed by suturing the deeper fascicles first and then moving toward the nerve surface until all structures are repaired. A variation of the perineural technique is to repair a number of tightly grouped fascicles using several sutures to approximate and close the entire group. Use 64856 for suture repair with nerve transposition. Use 64857 for nerve repair without nerve transposition.

64858

64858   Suture of sciatic nerve

Suture repair of the sciatic nerve, also referred to as end-to-end closure, can be accomplished using several different techniques. For more distal injuries, an epineural closure may be performed. The two ends of the transected nerve are exposed. Prior to repair, the injured nerve may be transposed to a new position. The injured nerve is dissected from surrounding tissues proximal and distal to the site of the injury. The nerve is then rerouted as needed to allow a tension free repair. The repair is then performed.

Several sutures are placed in the epineurium of each of the two ends. Sutures are placed so that nerve ends are approximated but not under tension. For more proximal injuries, a perineural closure may be performed. The two ends of the transected nerve are exposed. The epineurium of each of the two ends is pulled back to expose the individual fascicles of axons. Fascicles that perform the same function (sensory, motor) are identified and approximated by end-to-end closure. Fascicles are then sutured together with a single suture placed through the perineurium. A second suture may be required if rotation occurs and fascicles are no longer aligned. The closure is performed by suturing the deeper fascicles first and then moving toward the nerve surface until all structures are repaired. A variation of the perineural technique is to repair a number of tightly grouped fascicles using several sutures to approximate and close the entire group. Following repair of the nerve, overlying soft tissues and skin are closed in layers.

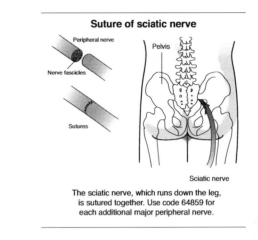

Suture of sciatic nerve

Peripheral nerve

Nerve fascicles

Sutures

Pelvis

Sciatic nerve

The sciatic nerve, which runs down the leg, is sutured together. Use code 64859 for each additional major peripheral nerve.

64859

64859   Suture of each additional major peripheral nerve (List separately in addition to code for primary procedure)

Following the first separately reported major peripheral nerve repair in the arm or leg, one or more additional nerves are repaired. Suture repair of the nerve, also referred to as end-to-end closure, can be accomplished using several different techniques. For more distal injuries, an epineural closure may be performed. The two ends of the transected nerve are exposed. Prior to repair, the injured nerve may be transposed to a new position. The injured nerve is dissected from surrounding tissues proximal and distal to the site of the injury. The nerve is then rerouted as needed to allow a tension free repair. The repair is then performed. Several sutures are placed in the epineurium of each of the two ends. Sutures are placed so that nerve ends are approximated but not under tension. For more proximal injuries, a perineural closure may be performed. The two ends of the transected nerve are exposed. The epineurium of each of the two ends is pulled back to expose the individual fascicles of axons. Fascicles that perform the same function (sensory, motor) are identified and approximated by end-to-end closure. Fascicles are then sutured together with a single suture placed through the perineurium. A second suture may be required if rotation occurs and fascicles are no longer aligned. The closure is performed by suturing the deeper fascicles first and then moving toward the nerve surface until all structures are repaired. A variation of the perineural technique is to repair a number of tightly grouped fascicles using several sutures to approximate and close the entire group. Report 64859 each additional major peripheral nerve repair after the first.

64861-64862

64861   Suture of; brachial plexus
64862   Suture of; lumbar plexus

The brachial and lumbar plexus are networks of nerves that start in the spinal cord. The brachial plexus controls movement and sensation in the upper extremity, while the lumbar plexus, also referred to as the lumbosacral plexus, controls movement and sensation in the lower extremity. Suture repair is typically performed for piercing type injuries involving a sharp object. The site of the injury of the brachial or lumbar plexus is exposed and explored to determine the extent of injury. Damaged tissue is debrided. Separately reportable intraoperative nerve function testing and monitoring is performed as needed. Using separately reportable microscopic technique as needed, severed nerves in the brachial or lumbar plexus are repaired. Suture repair of the nerve, also referred to as end-to-end closure, can be accomplished using several different techniques. The injured nerves are dissected from surrounding tissues proximal and distal to the site of the injury. To perform an epineural repair, several sutures are placed in the epineurium of each of the two ends. Sutures are placed so that nerve ends are approximated but not under tension. Alternatively, a perineural closure may be performed. The two ends of the transected nerve are exposed. The epineurium of each of the two ends is pulled back to expose the individual fascicles of axons. Fascicles that perform the same function (sensory, motor) are

Nervous System

identified and approximated by end-to-end closure. Fascicles are then sutured together with a single suture placed through the perineurium. A second suture may be required if rotation occurs and fascicles are no longer aligned. The closure is performed by suturing the deeper fascicles first and then moving toward the nerve surface until all structures are repaired. A variation of the perineural technique is to repair a number of tightly grouped fascicles using several sutures to approximate and close the entire group. Each severed nerve in the brachial or lumbar plexus is repaired separately. Use 64861 for suture repair of nerves in the brachial plexus and 64862 for nerves in the lumbar plexus.

64864-64865

64864   **Suture of facial nerve; extracranial**
64865   **Suture of facial nerve; infratemporal, with or without grafting**

The facial nerve which is cranial nerve VII (CN VII) is the nerve of facial expression. The facial nerve also has somatosensory and secretomotor fibers. In 64864, the extracranial portion of the facial nerve is repaired with sutures. The extracranial portion of the facial nerve begins where it exits the skull through the stylomastoid foramen. After exiting the skull, the facial nerve gives off several rami and then divides into its main branches. The extracranial facial nerve is exposed and explored to determine the extent of injury. Damaged tissue is debrided. Separately reportable intraoperative nerve function testing and monitoring is performed as needed. Using separately reportable microscopic technique as needed, the nerve ends are approximated and repaired. Suture repair of the nerve, also referred to as end-to-end closure, can be accomplished using several different techniques. The two ends of the transected nerve are exposed. The injured nerve is dissected from surrounding tissues proximal and distal to the site of the injury. For an epineural repair, several sutures are placed in the epineurium of each of the two ends. Sutures are placed so that nerve ends are approximated but not under tension. Alternatively, a perineural closure may be performed. The two ends of the transected nerve are exposed. The epineurium of each of the two ends is pulled back to expose the individual fascicles of axons. Fascicles that perform the same function (sensory, motor) are identified and approximated by end-to-end closure. Fascicles are then sutured together with a single suture placed through the perineurium. A second suture may be required if rotation occurs and fascicles are no longer aligned. The closure is performed by suturing the deeper fascicles first and then moving toward the nerve surface until all structures are repaired. A variation of the perineural technique is to repair a number of tightly grouped fascicles using several sutures to approximate and close the entire group. Overlying soft tissues and skin are repaired in layers. In 64865, the infratemporal portion of the facial nerve is repaired with or without grafting. End-to-end suture repair of the intratemporal portion of the facial nerve is performed as described above. If a nerve graft is required to facilitate a tension-free anastomosis, either the great auricular nerve or sural nerve is typically used. Less commonly the medial antebrachial cutaneous nerve is used. After determining the length of the nerve graft required, the donor nerve is exposed and dissected free of surrounding tissue. The graft is divided proximally and distally and harvested. The nerve graft is then sutured to the facial nerve ends using one of the suturing techniques described above.

64866-64868

64866   **Anastomosis; facial-spinal accessory**
64868   **Anastomosis; facial-hypoglossal**

Facial nerve reconstruction is performed by anastomosis of the facial-spinal accessory nerves or facial-hypoglossal nerves. An incision is made just in front of the auricle of the ear, carried down around the ear lobe, and extended along the mandible. A skin flap is elevated and the parotid gland is exposed. The inferior aspect of the parotid gland is dissected off the sternocleidomastoid muscle. Dissection continues to the digastric muscle. The tissue anterior to the tip and superior to the tragus is carefully dissected and the facial nerve is identified as it exits the stylomastoid foramen. Using separately reportable microsurgical technique as needed, the facial nerve is dissected to the point of the injury or damage and transected distal to this point. In 64866, the nerves of the face are reinnervated by a facial-spinal accessory nerve anastomosis. The spinal accessory nerve is located by following the posterior belly of the digastric muscle to its midpoint in the neck where the spinal accessory nerve crosses the jugular vein. The spinal accessory nerve is dissected distally until enough length has been attained to achieve a tension-free anastomosis with the facial nerve. The spinal nerve is transposed and sutured to the distal end of the facial nerve using a perineural or epineural technique. In 64868, the nerves of the face are reinnervated by a facial-hypoglossal anastomosis. The hypoglossal nerve is exposed by following the digastric muscle belly toward the hyoid bone until it is located. Distal dissection of the hypoglossal nerve continues until sufficient length has been freed. The hypoglossal nerve is then transected distally and transposed to meet the healthy distal segment of the facial nerve. The nerve ends are anastomosed using a perineural or epineural technique.

64872-64876

64872   **Suture of nerve; requiring secondary or delayed suture (List separately in addition to code for primary neurorrhaphy)**
64874   **Suture of nerve; requiring extensive mobilization, or transposition of nerve (List separately in addition to code for nerve suture)**
64876   **Suture of nerve; requiring shortening of bone of extremity (List separately in addition to code for nerve suture)**

In some instances, suture repair of a nerve requires additional separately reportable services. In 64872, a secondary or delayed suture repair is performed. The injured nerve is exposed. External neurolysis is performed. This involves freeing the nerve from any adhesions or scar tissue, which is usually performed under separately reportable microscopic visualization. Once the nerve has been freed, the suture repair is performed. In 64874, extensive mobilization or transposition of the nerve is required to allow a tension-free suture repair of the nerve. The injured nerve is freed from surrounding tissue distally and proximally until sufficient mobilization is achieved and a tension-free repair can be performed. If mobilization alone does not allow a tension-free repair, the nerve may be rerouted. This may involve creating a soft tissue tunnel for the nerve. In 64876, an osteoplasty is performed to shorten the bone of an extremity so that the nerve can be repaired. The extremity bone is exposed and the sites of the bone cuts are identified. The bone is cut and a segment of the bone is excised. The remaining distal and proximal portions of the bone are then brought into contact with each other and internal fixation is applied to stabilize the reconfigured bone. Alternatively, a separately reportable external fixation device may be applied.

64885-64886

64885   **Nerve graft (includes obtaining graft), head or neck; up to 4 cm in length**
64886   **Nerve graft (includes obtaining graft), head or neck; more than 4 cm length**

A nerve in the head or neck is repaired using a nerve graft in order to allow a tension-free repair of the injured nerve. The injured nerve is exposed and the extent of injury evaluated. Damaged tissue is debrided as needed. Separately reportable nerve testing and monitoring may be performed to help evaluate nerve function. The healthy proximal and distal nerve segments are dissected free of surrounding tissue and the length of the nerve graft is determined. The nerve graft is then harvested. The donor nerve is exposed and the desired length dissected free of surrounding tissue. The graft is divided proximally and distally and harvested. The nerve graft is then sutured to the severed nerve ends. End-to-end anastomosis of the graft can be accomplished using several different techniques. For an epineural repair, several sutures are placed in the epineurium of one end of the severed nerve and the graft. The nerve end and graft are then approximated and the sutures secured. The other end of the injured nerve and the graft are then sutured in the same manner. Alternatively, a perineural closure may be performed. The epineurium of the graft and severed nerve ends are pulled back to expose the individual fascicles of axons. Fascicles that perform the same function (sensory, motor) are identified and approximated by end-to-end closure. Fascicles are then sutured together with a single suture placed through the perineurium. A second suture may be required if rotation occurs and fascicles are no longer aligned. The closure is performed by suturing the deeper fascicles first and then moving toward the nerve surface until all structures are repaired. A variation of the perineural technique is to repair a number of tightly grouped fascicles using several sutures to approximate and close the entire group. Overlying soft tissues and skin are repaired in layers. Use 64885 if the nerve graft is 4 cm or less. Use 64886 if it is more than 4 cm.

Nerve graft, head or neck

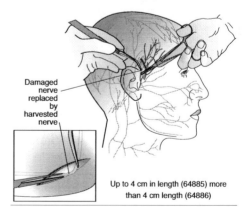

Damaged nerve replaced by harvested nerve

Up to 4 cm in length (64885) more than 4 cm length (64886)

   ● New Code   ▲ Revised Code

64890-64891

64890 Nerve graft (includes obtaining graft), single strand, hand or foot; up to 4 cm length

64891 Nerve graft (includes obtaining graft), single strand, hand or foot; more than 4 cm length

A nerve in the hand or foot is repaired using a single strand nerve graft in order to allow a tension-free repair of the injured nerve. The injured nerve is exposed and the extent of injury evaluated. Damaged tissue is debrided as needed. Separately reportable nerve testing and monitoring may be performed to help evaluate nerve function. Using separately reportable microscopic visualization, the healthy proximal and distal nerve segments are dissected free of surrounding tissue and the length of the nerve graft is determined. A single strand nerve graft is then harvested. The donor nerve is exposed and the desired length dissected free of surrounding tissue. The graft is divided proximally and distally and harvested. The single strand nerve graft is then sutured end-to-end to the severed nerve ends. Overlying soft tissues and skin are repaired in layers. Use 64890 if the single strand nerve graft is 4 cm or less. Use 64891 if it is more than 4 cm.

64892-64893

64892 Nerve graft (includes obtaining graft), single strand, arm or leg; up to 4 cm length

64893 Nerve graft (includes obtaining graft), single strand, arm or leg; more than 4 cm length

A nerve in the arm or leg is repaired using a single strand nerve graft in order to allow a tension-free repair of the injured nerve. The injured nerve is exposed and the extent of injury evaluated. Damaged tissue is debrided as needed. Separately reportable nerve testing and monitoring may be performed to help evaluate nerve function. Using separately reportable microscopic visualization, the healthy proximal and distal nerve segments are dissected free of surrounding tissue and the length of the nerve graft is determined. The nerve graft is then harvested. The donor nerve is exposed and the desired length dissected free of surrounding tissue. The graft is divided proximally and distally and harvested. The single strand nerve graft is then sutured end-to-end to the severed nerve ends. Overlying soft tissues and skin are repaired in layers. Use 64892 if the single strand nerve graft is 4 cm or less. Use 64893 if it is more than 4 cm.

64895-64896

64895 Nerve graft (includes obtaining graft), multiple strands (cable), hand or foot; up to 4 cm length

64896 Nerve graft (includes obtaining graft), multiple strands (cable), hand or foot; more than 4 cm length

A nerve in the hand or foot is repaired using a multiple strand nerve graft in order to allow a tension-free repair of the injured nerve. The injured nerve is exposed and the extent of injury evaluated. Damaged tissue is debrided as needed. Separately reportable nerve testing and monitoring may be performed to help evaluate nerve function. Using separately reportable microscopic visualization, the healthy proximal and distal nerve segments are dissected free of surrounding tissue and the length of the nerve graft is determined. The nerve graft is then harvested. The donor nerve is exposed and the desired length dissected free of surrounding tissue. The graft is divided proximally and distally and harvested. Multiple strands of the donor nerve are then sutured end-to-end to the severed nerve ends. Overlying soft tissues and skin are repaired in layers. Use 64895 if the multiple strand nerve graft is 4 cm or less. Use 64896 if it is more than 4 cm.

64897-64898

64897 Nerve graft (includes obtaining graft), multiple strands (cable), arm or leg; up to 4 cm length

64898 Nerve graft (includes obtaining graft), multiple strands (cable), arm or leg; more than 4 cm length

A nerve in the arm or leg is repaired using a multiple strand nerve graft in order to allow a tension-free repair of the injured nerve. The injured nerve is exposed and the extent of injury evaluated. Damaged tissue is debrided as needed. Separately reportable nerve testing and monitoring may be performed to help evaluate nerve function. Using separately reportable microscopic visualization, the healthy proximal and distal nerve segments are dissected free of surrounding tissue and the length of the nerve graft is determined. The nerve graft is then harvested. The donor nerve is exposed and the desired length dissected free of surrounding tissue. The graft is divided proximally and distally and harvested. Multiple strands of the donor nerve are then sutured end-to-end to the severed nerve ends. Overlying soft tissues and skin are repaired in layers. Use 64897 if the multiple strand nerve graft is 4 cm or less. Use 64898 if it is more than 4 cm.

64901-64902

64901 Nerve graft, each additional nerve; single strand (List separately in addition to code for primary procedure)

64902 Nerve graft, each additional nerve; multiple strands (cable) (List separately in addition to code for primary procedure)

Following repair of the first nerve using a nerve graft, additional nerves are repaired using single or multiple strand grafts. The injured nerve is exposed and the extent of injury evaluated. Damaged tissue is debrided as needed. Separately reportable nerve testing and monitoring may be performed to help evaluate nerve function. Using separately reportable microscopic visualization, the healthy proximal and distal nerve segments are dissected free of surrounding tissue and the length of the nerve graft is determined. The nerve graft is then harvested. The donor nerve is exposed and the desired length dissected free of surrounding tissue. The graft is divided proximally and distally and harvested. Single or multiple strands of the donor nerve are then sutured end-to-end to the severed nerve ends. Overlying soft tissues and skin are repaired in layers. Use 64901 for each additional nerve repaired with a single strand graft. Use 64902 for each additional nerve repaired with a multiple strand graft.

64905-64907

64905 Nerve pedicle transfer; first stage

64907 Nerve pedicle transfer; second stage

A nerve pedicle transfer involves transfer of a nerve and muscle pedicle with the motor endplate of the nerve in a staged procedure. In 64905, the pedicle is developed and transferred to the donor site. An incision is made over the injured nerve. Skin, fascial or muscle flaps are raised as needed. The injured nerve and involved branches are exposed. The incision is extended or a second incision is made over the site where the nerve pedicle is to be harvested. Using microscopic visualization, the donor nerve and the motor endplate are dissected from surrounding tissue along with muscle tissue. A tunnel is created from the donor site to the injured nerve and the nerve pedicle is pulled through the tunnel to the site of the injury. The nerve pedicle is then secured with sutures to the injury site. In 64907, after nerve axons have regenerated and nerve function has been restored, the nerve pedicle is severed at the site of origin.

64910-64911

64910 Nerve repair; with synthetic conduit or vein allograft (eg, nerve tube), each nerve

64911 Nerve repair; with autogenous vein graft (includes harvest of vein graft), each nerve

Nerve repair using either a synthetic conduit or vein allograft (eg, nerve tube) is done on one nerve (64910). When nerve function is lost through injury, the distal nerve portion dies and degenerates. The proximal portion can regenerate to establish nerve function, but if the gap is too great, a graft must be inserted between the proximal and distal nerve stumps to guide the regenerating axons. This code reports the creation of either a biological nerve tube allograft from human vein or the placement of an artificial guidance channel between the ends of a severed peripheral nerve for regeneration and repair. A synthetic, tubular nerve guidance conduit is made from polymers like poly-L-lactic acid and plated with populations of cultured Schwann cells that adhere to the acidic polymer. Schwann cells compose the natural insulating myelin sheath wrapped around nerve axons. The impregnated synthetic guidance tube provides a biocompatible environment for promoting robust nerve regeneration in a specific direction. Harvested vein grafts are pulled through and turned inside out before being sutured between the severed nerve stumps because the inside layer of the vein wall is rich in collagen, which has the best success for regenerating nerves. New capillaries form in the vein graft and neurites from the proximal stump grow in around them to repair the connection. Report code 64911 for nerve repair on one nerve that is done using an autogenous piece of vein harvested from the patient first before being surgically planted between two severed nerve ends.

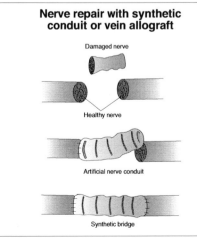

Nerve repair with synthetic conduit or vein allograft

Damaged nerve

Healthy nerve

Artificial nerve conduit

Synthetic bridge

Nervous System

Eye and Occular Adnexa

65091-65093

65091 Evisceration of ocular contents; without implant
65093 Evisceration of ocular contents; with implant

Evisceration of the eye is performed to treat eye infections that are unresponsive to antibiotics and for pain control or to improve the appearance in a blind eye. The cornea is excised and the ocular contents exposed. An ocular curette is then inserted into the space between the uveal tract and sclera. The ocular contents including the retina, uveal tract, vitreous and lens are then scraped away from the scleral shell. Bleeding from the vortex veins and central retinal artery is controlled with electrocautery and/or pressure. The scleral shell is carefully inspected and a swab used to remove any remaining uveal tissue. In 65091, evisceration is performed without placement of an implant. In 65093, an appropriately sized implant is inserted into the scleral shell. The sclera is then closed over the anterior surface of the implant in a layered fashion to prevent contraction of the sclera and extrusion of the implant.

65101-65105

65101 Enucleation of eye; without implant
65103 Enucleation of eye; with implant, muscles not attached to implant
65105 Enucleation of eye; with implant, muscles attached to implant

Enucleation of the eye is performed to treat tumors of the eye such as intraocular melanoma or retinoblastoma and for severe trauma to the eye. The globe is measured and the length of the optic nerve determined. The globe is illuminated and a dissecting microscope used to help visualize orbital structures and identify the extent of the lesion or trauma. A limbal incision is made around the conjunctiva and Tenon's capsule. The extraocular muscles are exposed and divided. The optic nerve is located and divided. The globe is removed. In 65101, an enucleation is performed without placement of an implant. In 65103, an appropriately sized implant is placed in the muscle cone without attachment to extraocular muscles. In 65105, an implant is placed in the muscle cone and the extraocular muscles are sutured to the implant.

65110-65114

65110 Exenteration of orbit (does not include skin graft), removal of orbital contents; only
65112 Exenteration of orbit (does not include skin graft), removal of orbital contents; with therapeutic removal of bone
65114 Exenteration of orbit (does not include skin graft), removal of orbital contents; with muscle or myocutaneous flap

Exenteration is performed primarily for orbital tumors or intraocular tumors that extend into the orbit or extraorbital structures, such as the eyelids or bone surrounding the eye. If the eyelid anatomy is free of disease, full thickness incisions are made through the entire eyelid just above the upper lashline and just below the loser lash line. If only the skin of the eyelid is preserved, the skin is incised just above the upper lash line and just below the lower lash line. The skin of the eyelid is dissected from underlying subcutaneous tissue and both superiorly and inferiorly to the level of the orbital rim. If the eyelids are completely removed full-thickness incisions are made through the skin and soft tissue along the orbital rim. The periosteum of the orbital rim is then dissected off of underlying bone in a circular fashion until the entire the globe and orbital contents have been completely freed. The entire globe and orbital contents are then removed. Underlying bony structures are inspected for evidence of tumor extension. If tumor is present in the bones of the orbits is, boney tissue is excised as well. If the entire eyelids or skin of the eyelids have been preserved, the eyelids are closed in layers. If the eyelids have been completely excised separately reportable skin grafts may be used to close the defect. Use 65110 when no bone is removed and the defect can be closed without the use of muscle or myocutaneous flaps. Use 65112 when bone is removed. Use 65114 when muscle or myocutaneous flap is used to close the surgical defect. A free muscle or myocutaneous flap is developed taking care to preserve blood supply to the flap. Commonly used free muscle flaps include the abdominus rectus or latissimus dorsi muscles. The free flap is trimmed to the desired size and shape. Blood vessels in the free flap are sutured to blood vessels surrounding the eye. The edges of the flap are secured with sutures.

65125

65125 Modification of ocular implant with placement or replacement of pegs (eg, drilling receptacle for prosthesis appendage) (separate procedure)

The ocular implant is removed in a separately reportable procedure. The ocular implant is then modified to improve the fit in the eye socket. Pegs are removed as needed and new

holes drilled for repositioning of the pegs. Additional pegs may be placed to better secure the implant within the eye socket.

65130

65130 Insertion of ocular implant secondary; after evisceration, in scleral shell

If the remaining scleral shell has been closed, it is opened. An appropriately sized implant is selected and placed in the sclera shell. The sclera is then closed over the anterior surface of the implant in a layered fashion to prevent contraction of the sclera and extrusion of the implant.

65135-65140

65135 Insertion of ocular implant secondary; after enucleation, muscles not attached to implant
65140 Insertion of ocular implant secondary; after enucleation, muscles attached to implant

If the eyelid has been closed with sutures it is opened and the muscle cone inspected. An appropriately sized ocular implant is selected and placed in the muscle cone. In 65135, the implant is not attached to the extraocular muscles. Ocular implants are composed of porous material, such as mesh or biosynthetic material. Surrounding tissue will eventually grown into the porous implant and secure it within the muscle cone. In 65140, the muscles are secured to the implant with sutures. The sutures can be easily placed through the porous implant material. The eye muscle tissue will eventually grow into the implant.

65150-65155

65150 Reinsertion of ocular implant; with or without conjunctival graft
65155 Reinsertion of ocular implant; with use of foreign material for reinforcement and/or attachment of muscles to implant

The scleral shell or muscle cone is exposed. The ocular implant is then reinserted in the scleral shell or muscle cone. In 65150, if the patient has had a previous evisceration procedure, the sclera is closed over the anterior surface of the implant in a layered fashion to prevent contraction of the sclera and extrusion of the implant. Alternatively, a conjunctival graft may be used to secure and/or cover the implant. If the patient has had an enucleation procedure, a conjunctival graft may be fashioned and used to secure and/ or completely cover the implant. In 65155, synthetic material such as pegs or mesh is used to secure the implant and attach extraocular muscles.

65175

65175 Removal of ocular implant

The ocular implant is exposed. If the patient has had a previous evisceration procedure, the scleral shell that has been secured over the anterior aspect of the implant is opened. The ocular implant is then dissected free of sclera and removed. If the patient has had a previous enucleation procedure, any overlying tissue or synthetic grafts are removed. The ocular implant is then dissected free of surrounding tissue and removed.

65205-65210

65205 Removal of foreign body, external eye; conjunctival superficial
65210 Removal of foreign body, external eye; conjunctival embedded (includes concretions), subconjunctival, or scleral nonperforating

A foreign body is removed from the conjunctiva, subconjunctiva, or sclera. The conjunctiva is the mucous membrane covering the anterior surface of the eyeball (bulbar conjunctiva) and the posterior surface of the eyelid (palpebral conjunctiva). The subconjunctiva is the tissue immediately below the conjunctiva. The sclera, also referred to as the white of the eye, is the fibrous layer that forms the outer envelope of the eye. The eye is examined and the foreign body identified. Anesthetic eye drops are applied as needed. In 65205, a superficial conjunctival foreign body is removed using saline irrigation or a cotton swab. In 65210, an embedded foreign body is removed from the conjunctiva, subconjunctiva, or sclera using a cotton tipped swab or forceps. The eye is copiously irrigated with saline solution following removal of the foreign body.

65220-65222

65220 Removal of foreign body, external eye; corneal, without slit lamp
65222 Removal of foreign body, external eye; corneal, with slit lamp

A foreign body is removed from the cornea. The cornea is the transparent tissue that covers the anterior aspect of the eye. The cornea refracts light helping the eye to focus. Anesthetic drops are instilled into the eye. The physician checks visual acuity and performs a funduscopy to locate the foreign body. A slit lamp, which is an instrument used to

CPT © 2016 American Medical Association. All Rights Reserved.   ● New Code   ▲ Revised Code   **457** illuminate and provide a magnified, three-dimensional view of the eye, may be also be used. A superficial corneal foreign body may be removed with a moistened cotton swab. An embedded foreign body is removed under magnification with an ophthalmic spud or needle. If a metallic foreign body has left a rust ring, the rust impregnated corneal tissue is removed using a corneal burr. The eye is flushed with saline solution to remove any foreign body fragments. The corneal defect caused by the foreign body is treated like a corneal abrasion using antibiotic ointment and an eye patch. Use 65220 if the foreign body is removed without a slit lamp and 65222 if a slit lamp is used.

65235

65235   Removal of foreign body, intraocular; from anterior chamber of eye or lens

The anterior chamber lies behind the cornea and in front of the iris and lens. The anterior chamber is filled with a clear watery fluid called aqueous humor. The injury to the eye is inspected and the location of the intraocular foreign body determined to be in the anterior chamber or lens without penetration into deeper structures of the eye. The site of entry is located and the wound enlarged as needed. Alternatively, a separate incision may be made to provide access to the foreign body. A metallic foreign body is removed using a magnet. A non-metallic foreign body is removed using forceps. The wound is closed with sutures as needed.

65260-65265

65260   Removal of foreign body, intraocular; from posterior segment, magnetic extraction, anterior or posterior route

65265   Removal of foreign body, intraocular; from posterior segment, nonmagnetic extraction

The posterior segment of the eye is a large cavity that lies between the lens and the retina. It is filled vitreous humor, a soft jellylike substance. The injury to the eye is inspected and the location of the intraocular foreign body determined to be in the posterior segment. The site of entry is located and the wound enlarged as needed. Alternatively, a separate incision may be made to provide access to the foreign body. Use 65260 for a metallic foreign body that is removed using a magnet and 65265 for a non-metallic foreign body that is removed using forceps or other technique. The wound is closed with sutures as needed.

65270

65270   Repair of laceration; conjunctiva, with or without nonperforating laceration sclera, direct closure

The conjunctiva is a transparent mucous membrane that covers the sclera (white of the eye) and the inner surface of the eyelids. Local anesthetic is administered. The eye is carefully examined and the injury determined to be limited to the conjunctiva. A partial thickness laceration of the sclera may also be present; however, there is no penetration of the globe. The edges of the laceration are debrided as needed. If the sclera is lacerated, it is closed first with absorbable suture material followed by direct repair of the conjunctival laceration.

65272-65273

65272   Repair of laceration; conjunctiva, by mobilization and rearrangement, without hospitalization

65273   Repair of laceration; conjunctiva, by mobilization and rearrangement, with hospitalization

The conjunctiva is a transparent mucous membrane that covers the sclera (white of the eye) and the inner surface of the eyelids. Local anesthetic is administered. The eye is carefully examined to ensure that there is no injury to the globe. The edges of the laceration are debrided as needed. The conjunctiva is mobilized and rearranged to relieve tension on the edges of the laceration. A flap may be developed to ensure adequate coverage of the defect. The defect is repaired using absorbable sutures. Use 65272 when the injury does not require hospitalization and 65273 when hospitalization is required.

65275

65275   Repair of laceration; cornea, nonperforating, with or without removal foreign body

The cornea is a clear dome of tissue located at the front of the eye. It covers and protects the uvea, a three layer (iris, ciliary body, choroid) pigmented area that encircles the black pupil. A non-perforating laceration does not violate the globe (fluid filled cavity behind the cornea and sclera). The eye is irrigated to remove foreign bodies and dirt and examined using a slit-lamp (ophthalmic microscope). A Seidel test using fluorescein dye may be performed. The laceration is sutured using tight, longer sutures at the periphery of the laceration to compress and flatten the area and steepen the center of the cornea followed by shorter, appositional sutures in the central cornea. Antibiotic and/or steroid ophthalmic drops may be instilled and the eye is patched.

65280

65280   Repair of laceration; cornea and/or sclera, perforating, not involving uveal tissue

The sclera is the opaque, white, outer layer of the eye made up of fibrous tissue and collagen. It extends from the cornea at the front of the eye to the optic nerve at the back of the eye. A thin transparent membrane called the conjunctiva covers the sclera at the front of the eye. The cornea is a clear dome of tissue also located at the front of the eye. It covers and protects the uvea, a three layer (iris, ciliary body, choroid) pigmented area that encircles the black pupil. The margin of the cornea and sclera is called the limbus. A perforating laceration, also called a full thickness laceration, of the cornea and/or sclera is repaired. The eye is irrigated to remove foreign bodies and dirt and examined using a slit-lamp (ophthalmic microscope). A Seidel test using fluorescein dye may be performed. Using fine nylon suture, the first stitch is placed at the limbus to anatomically approximate the wound. Next the corneal wound is sutured, followed by the sclera. The conjunctiva is closed with fine nylon suture. Antibiotic and/or steroid ophthalmic drops may be instilled and the eye is patched.

65285

65285   Repair of laceration; cornea and/or sclera, perforating, with reposition or resection of uveal tissue

Repair of a perforating corneal and/or scleral laceration with reposition or resection of uveal tissue is accomplished using conventional sutures. The goal of treatment is to ensure a watertight globe, reestablish original eye anatomy, and restore or preserve visual function. The corneal component is approached first. Vitreous or lens fragments are cut flush with the cornea. A limbal incision is made and working through that incision, uveal or retinal fragments are repositioned with a sweeping technique. The uveal surface and wound are checked for epithelial tissue, which is carefully peeled off if it is present. The corneal laceration is then closed. The anterior and posterior edges of the cornea are opposed using long tight sutures at the periphery and shorter, wider, central sutures preserving the natural curvature of the structure and avoiding entrapment of the iris. The scleral laceration is addressed next. Using gentle periotomy, the conjunctiva adjacent to the laceration is carefully dissected to explore the wound. Vitreous tissue that has prolapsed is excised, viable uveal/retinal tissue is repositioned and the sclera is closed with sutures. A deeply penetrating scleral wound can be left alone to heal. A paracentesis may be created and sterile water injected through it to fill the anterior chamber and check the globe for a watertight seal. At the end of the surgical procedure, antibiotics may be injected directly into the conjunctiva or other areas of the eye, and the eye is covered with a sterile dressing and eye shield.

65286

65286   Repair of laceration; application of tissue glue, wounds of cornea and/or sclera

Repair of a superficial corneal and/or scleral laceration may be accomplished using an application of liquid tissue adhesive (fibrin, chondroitin, isobutyl cyanoacrylate) and a bandage contact lens. The goal of treatment is to ensure a watertight globe, reestablish original eye anatomy, and restore or preserve visual function. The eye is irrigated and the wound is carefully examined under a slit-lamp or operating microscope. The edges of the laceration are manually approximated and liquid tissue adhesive is brushed over the wound. The liquid undergoes a chemical reaction when it comes in contact with moisture and polymerizes to bind the epithelium together and allow healing to take place in the underlying tissue. A bandage contact lens may be applied over the liquid tissue adhesive. The lens provides pressure patching over a large surface area to protect the eye from the mechanical trauma of lid closure and helps to relieve pain.

65290

65290   Repair of wound, extraocular muscle, tendon and/or Tenon's capsule

Repair of a wound, extraocular muscle, tendon and/or Tenon's capsule is accomplished using conventional sutures. The eye is carefully examined under slit-lamp or operating microscope to evaluate the wound and damage to eye structures. The eyeball is suspended in the orbit enveloped inside of Tenon's capsule, a fibrous tissue that covers the eyeball from the entrance of the optic nerve to the corneal limbus and attaches firmly to the conjunctiva. Three paired extraocular muscles—the horizontal rectus, vertical rectus, and oblique muscles are attached to the sclera/globe by broad thin tendons. A wound to the eye surface on the cornea or sclera may disrupt the integrity of muscle(s), tendon(s) and/ or Tenon's capsule. The ends of a transected muscle or tendon are located, reapproximated, and repaired using suture. Tenon's capsule is carefully dissected to expose foreign bodies and trapped tissue and is then closed with sutures. At the end of the surgical procedure, antibiotics may be injected directly into the conjunctiva or other areas of the eye and the eye is covered with a sterile dressing and eye shield.

65400

65400   Excision of lesion, cornea (keratectomy, lamellar, partial), except pterygium

Corneal lesions that require excision can include dystrophic, degenerative, and hypertrophic or scar tissue. Using a slit lamp or operating microscope, the lesion is visualized. Surface epithelial cells are gently debrided from the cornea using blunt forceps, spatula, or sponge to delineate the margins of the lesion and expose the deeper corneal epithelium and subepithelial fibrous and fibrovascular tissue. Blunt or sharp dissection of the deeper lesion is then carried out and the surface of the cornea may be polished using a diamond burr. A bandage contact lens is inserted at the conclusion of the procedure to facilitate healing and regeneration of corneal epithelial cells from limbic stem cells.

65410

65410   Biopsy of cornea

A surgical blade or aspiration cutter is used to obtain a tissue sample from the cornea or from a corneal lesion. A small incision is made over the area to be biopsied. If a surgical blade is used, a small amount of tissue is excised from the cornea or corneal lesion. If an aspiration cutter is used, a probe is introduced through the incision. Tissue samples are obtained and submitted for pathology examination.

65420-65426

65420   Excision or transposition of pterygium; without graft
65426   Excision or transposition of pterygium; with graft

The physician performs an excision or transposition of a pterygium without the use of a graft, also referred to as a simple excision or bare sclera technique. A pterygium is a raised, triangular growth of conjunctiva at the corner of the eye that extends into the sclera and may also invade the cornea. If the ptyergium extends into the central cornea, it is removed surgically. The pterygium is dissected free of underlying sclera and corneal tissue and a simple excision performed. The sclera is left open to heal. In 65426, the pterygium is removed and the scleral defect repaired using a graft. The pterygium is dissected down to the level of the Tenon's capsule and the fibrous tissue forming the pterygium is removed. An autograft, such as a free conjunctival graft, is then harvested from under the eyelid of the patient and used to repair the defect. Alternatively, an allograft, such as an amniotic membrane graft obtained from a tissue bank, may be used. The graft is sutured onto the conjunctiva or secured using fibrin tissue glue.

65430

65430   Scraping of cornea, diagnostic, for smear and/or culture

The eye is examined with the help of a slit lamp, magnifiers, loupe, or operating microscope. Eye drops are instilled to numb the eye. The cornea or corneal lesion is then scraped using a sterile kimura spatula or surgical blade. If the tissue sample is obtained from a corneal lesion, samples are obtained from the base and sides of the lesion. The tissue sample is applied to one or more prepared glass slides and separately reportable microscopic examination is done.

65435-65436

65435   Removal of corneal epithelium; with or without chemocauterization (abrasion, curettage)
65436   Removal of corneal epithelium; with application of chelating agent (eg, EDTA)

The physician removes the corneal epithelium with or without the use of chemocauterization using abrasion or curettage. The procedure is performed to remove a diseased, eroded, damaged, or dystrophied layer of epithelium from the cornea of the eye. The soft epithelial layer of the cornea is removed using a brushing or scraping instrument. The surface epithelium is separated and removed from the underlying and harder Bowman's layer. A chemical may then be applied to cauterize the newly exposed underlying tissue. In 65436, the corneal epithelium is removed and a chelating agent such as ethylenediaminetetraacetic acid (EDTA) applied. The epithelium is removed with a sponge or blade. The chelating agent is then applied using surgical sponges or a reservoir such as a corneal trephine or well. Additional scraping may be performed to remove calcifications or deposits from the Bowman's layer following application of the chelating agent.

65450

65450   Destruction of lesion of cornea by cryotherapy, photocoagulation or thermocauterization

Eye drops are instilled to numb the eye. Cryotherapy involves applying a freezing probe directly to the lesion. The extreme cold destroys the lesion. Photocoagulation is performed using a laser. The laser beam is fired at the cornea and destroys the lesion. Thermocauterization is performed by touching the lesion with a heat probe to destroy it by burning.

65600

65600   Multiple punctures of anterior cornea (eg, for corneal erosion, tattoo)

Multiple punctures of the anterior cornea are performed to treat recurrent corneal erosion or a disfiguring corneal scar. Eye drops are instilled to numb the eye. To treat corneal erosion, a 23-25 gauge bent needle is used to puncture the anterior corneal stroma. The small puncture wounds in the cornea promote healing of the erosion by causing intentional scarring of the cornea. Alternatively, puncturing of the anterior cornea may be performed to treat a disfiguring corneal scar following surgery or other trauma. Multiple punctures are performed as described above and an ink stain is applied until the desired cosmetic effect is attained.

65710

65710   Keratoplasty (corneal transplant); anterior lamellar

Anterior lamellar keratoplasty is performed to replace the diseased, or scarred, partial thickness portion of the anterior cornea selectively, leaving the rest of the healthy cornea undisturbed. The anterior corneal surface is trephined to a depth of 400 micrometers. A 25-gauge bent needle attached to a syringe is inserted with the bevel downward into the corneal stroma, through the trephine cut. Air is then injected to form a big bubble and to detach the deep stromal layers from Descemet's membrane and facilitate lamellar dissection. The anterior stromal disc is then removed with a rounded blade. The anterior chamber is entered and aqueous humor is partially released before a miotic agent is injected. A bubble test is performed to see if the big bubble is properly formed by injecting a small amount of air into the anterior chamber. If it stays within the periphery, pushed by the convex shape of the detached Descement's membrane, the big bubble has formed in the cornea. A small, oblique incision is made in the corneal stromal surface to collapse the big bubble. The small bubble in the anterior chamber migrates to the central area. Viscoelastic material is then used to fill the space between Descement's membrane and the detached stroma and to separate the tissue. Microscissors are used to excise the remaining deep corneal stroma and expose the smooth membrane surface. The donor cornea is trephined, stripped of its Descement's membrane and epithelium, placed into host cornea bed, and sutured into place.

65730

65730   Keratoplasty (corneal transplant); penetrating (except in aphakia or pseudophakia)

This is a full-thickness corneal transplant procedure that may be done for conditions such as viral keratitis, keratoconus, and Fuch's endothelial dystrophy, bullous keratopathy, or corneal scarring and dystrophy due to trauma or keratitis. The patient's eyes are miosed before the surgery to prevent damage to the lens and avoid causing cataract. The recipient cornea is trephined with a manual, motorized, or vacuum trephine. In order to avoid rapid decompression of the eye, only a partial-thickness trephination cut is made first, followed by a full-thickness cut to remove damaged cornea. The size of the graft is decided, and the donor corneoscleral graft button is cut with the epithelial side up in a concave setting until it is 0.5mm larger than the recipient bed. The donor button is fitted and stitched into place using radially interrupted sutures placed at 12, 3, 6, and 9 o'clock positions, or with a single continuous running suture. The volume in the anterior chamber is recreated with a balanced salt solution injection.

65750-65755

65750   Keratoplasty (corneal transplant); penetrating (in aphakia)
65755   Keratoplasty (corneal transplant); penetrating (in pseudophakia)

Keratoplasty is a procedure used to improve visual acuity by replacing diseased or damaged corneal tissue with clear, healthy tissue from a donor. Using an operating microscope to visualize the eye, a trephine is used to remove a circular section of the patient's cornea. The anterior chamber is filled with viscoelastic fluid and a similar circle cut from the donor tissue is placed epithelial side down on the recipient eye and sutured in place. Antibiotic eye drops may be instilled, and the eye is covered with a patch and/or shield. Code 65750 includes penetrating keratoplasty for corneal edema following cataract extraction. Code 65755 includes penetrating keratoplasty with the presence of a pseudophakia intraocular lens.

65756

65756   Keratoplasty (corneal transplant); endothelial

There are two techniques commonly used-deep lamellar endothelial keratoplasty (DLEK) and Descemet's stripping endothelial keratoplasty (DSEK). Endothelial keratoplasty is used to treat endothelial dysfunction, which includes conditions such as Fuchs dystrophy, pseudophakic bullous keratopathy (PBK), aphakic bullous keratopathy (ABK), and posterior polymorphous dystrophy (PPMD). The conjunctival tissue is incised around the whole circumference of the cornea (peritomy) using scissors and forceps. A 5 mm scleral tunnel is created beginning 1.5 mm from the limbus. Paracentesis is performed on each side of the scleral tunnel. The anterior chamber is filled with viscoelastic (Healon). If DLEK technique is used, the posterior corneal stroma is dissected away. A keratome is used to enter the anterior chamber and the posterior cornea is removed by scissor dissection. The Healon

CPT © 2016 American Medical Association. All Rights Reserved.
● New Code   ▲ Revised Code

Eye and Ocular Adnexa

is removed from the anterior chamber by irrigation and aspiration. A temporary suture is placed in the sclera tunnel. The prepared donor lenticle is folded and grasped with forceps. The temporary suture in the sclera tunnel is removed and the donor lenticle is placed into the anterior chamber. The sclera tunnel is closed and the lenticle is unfolded by infiltrating air into the anterior chamber. The lenticle is tucked into place using hooks; the anterior chamber is filled with balanced saline solution; and the conjunctiva is closed. If DSEK technique is used, the Descemet's membrane is first scored with a Sinskey hook and then stripped using a hook, strippers, or an irrigation/aspiration device. The edge is roughened and the prepared lenticle is folded and placed in the anterior chamber. The sclera tunnel is closed and the lenticle is unfolded and positioned by infiltrating air into the anterior chamber. Fluid is massaged out of the interface. The pupil is dilated and the conjunctiva is closed.

65757

65757   Backbench preparation of corneal endothelial allograft prior to transplantation (List separately in addition to code for primary procedure)

The physician prepares a corneal endothelial allograft in a backbench (back table) procedure prior to transplantation. The donor tissue may be prepared using a microkeratome in an automated technique or it may be prepared manually without the use of a microkeratome. Using an automated microkeratome system, the artificial anterior chamber is filled with preservation solution. The donor tissue endothelium is coated with a thin layer of Healon and placed in the artificial anterior chamber. The artificial chamber is pressurized and the epithelial cells are wiped from the surface of the cornea. The horizontal meridian of the donor tissue is marked so that it can be properly oriented during transplantation. The microkeratome head is mounted on the guide ring, positioned for resection, and then passed over the donor cornea. A free cap of anterior tissue is resected and held above the blade on the microkeratome head. The residual stromal bed is dried using sponges and the diameter and smoothness of the cut is evaluated. The anterior tissue cap is placed back in position using the previously placed reference marks. The exact center of the anterior tissue cap is marked and maintained in position until it adheres to the stromal bed. Alternatively, the donor tissue may be prepared without the use of a microkeratome. The donor tissue is placed in the artificial anterior chamber as described above. A diamond knife is set to the proper depth and a curved incision is made in the peripheral donor limbal area next to the edge of the metal cap of the artificial anterior chamber. Deeper stromal tissue is cut using a crescent blade until the desired plane has been reached. Dissectors are then used to continue all the way to the limbus of the donor tissue. A second manual technique uses a suction trephine placed on the surface of the donor tissue with suction applied. Trephination is carried down to the desired depth. The trephine is removed and the cut inspected to ensure it is of the proper depth. The donor tissue is now dismounted from the artificial anterior chamber and removed from the post, taking care not to damage the endothelium. The donor sclera is irrigated above and below the endothelial surface to remove any residual Healon. The donor tissue is placed on a standard punch trephine block, taking care to properly position the tissue using the previously placed central ink mark. The donor tissue is folded along the horizontal meridian prior to transplantation. The physician now proceeds with the separately reportable endothelial corneal transplant procedure.

65760

65760   Keratomileusis

Keratomileusis is a type of keratoplasty in which the cornea is surgically reshaped to the desired curvature and sutured back in place to correct a refractive error and improve visual acuity. Using an operating microscope to visualize the eye, the anterior lamella is peeled back and a section of corneal tissue is removed and frozen. The posterior surface of the corneal tissue is reshaped using a lathe, laser, or knife blade, and the tissue is sutured back into place. At the conclusion of the procedure, the eye may be covered with a patch or shield.

65765

65765   Keratophakia

Keratophakia is a type of keratoplasty in which a piece of frozen donor cornea is shaped to the desired curvature and inserted between layers of the recipient cornea to correct a refractive error and improve visual acuity in patients with aphakia, myopia, presbyopia, and stigmatism. Using an operating microscope to visualize the eye, the anterior lamella is peeled back and an implant of donor corneal tissue that has been reshaped to the correct curvature for the patient, or an intraocular lens, is placed deep within the corneal stroma and sutured in place. At the conclusion of the procedure, the eye may be covered with a patch or shield.

65767

65767   Epikeratoplasty

The corneal epithelium in the damaged or thinned region of the cornea is removed. Donor corneal tissue that has been reshaped and freeze dried is obtained and is used to fill the corneal defect in the recipient. The corneal graft is secured with sutures. The eyelids may

be temporarily sutured closed to allow the patient's corneal tissue to grow into and over the surface of the graft. Usually within 4-5 days the corneal epithelium has healed and the eyelid sutures are removed. The patient continues to use eye drops or ointment until the graft is completely stabilized by the overgrowth of new corneal epithelium which usually takes 2-3 months.

65770

65770   Keratoprosthesis

A keratoprosthesis is a synthetic substitute used to replace the cornea, usually due to human donor corneal transplant failure or when a donor transplant is not likely to succeed. The synthetic corneal transplant consists of a clear plastic prosthetic graft that takes the place of the cornea. The prosthesis is sutured into human donor tissue that is then sutured to the patient's damaged cornea. Once the keratoprosthesis is properly positioned and secured with sutures a soft contact lens is placed over the eye and must be worn continuously (24 hours a day) every day.

65771

65771   Radial keratotomy

Radial keratotomy is performed to correct nearsightedness. This procedure is no longer commonly performed having been replaced with photorefractive keratectomy (PRK), laser in situ keratomileusis (LASIK), or epi-LASIK. The eye is first mapped using a slit lamp and markings placed. The number and location of incisions is determined based on the severity of the patient's nearsightedness. The patient is then positioned supine and the eye prepped and draped. A topical anesthetic is applied to the eye. The cornea is irrigated with saline and a viscolubricant eye solution may be instilled. The globe of the eye is secured using a suction device or forceps. Incisions are then made in the cornea from the center of the cornea to the outer edge using a diamond blade that has been precisely calibrated to achieve the necessary depth of incision. As incisions are made, the cornea relaxes and flattens bringing the central aspect of the cornea closer to the retina which in turn corrects nearsightedness. Upon completion of the procedure the eye may be covered with soft bandage or patch or a contact lens bandage may be applied.

65772

65772   Corneal relaxing incision for correction of surgically induced astigmatism

Astigmatism occurs when the naturally spherical (round) cornea takes on an oval configuration. This change in shape causes vision to become less sharp (blurry). Surgically induced astigmatism may occur following cataract removal or refractive procedures such as LASIK. A low degree if astigmatism can be corrected using peripheral corneal relaxing incisions (PCRI) or limbal relaxing incisions (LRI). The eye is first mapped using a slit lamp and markings placed. The patient is then positioned supine and the eye prepped and draped. The cornea is anesthetized using a topical anesthetic. The cornea is irrigated with saline and a viscolubricant eye solution may be instilled. The globe of the eye is secured using a suction device or forceps and a diamond knife is used to incise the previously marked areas around the axis of the cornea. These small incisions allow the cornea to return to a more natural, spherical shape and vision to be sharper or clearer. At the conclusion of the procedure a corneal contact lens bandage may be placed, antibiotic eye drops are instilled and the eye is then patched.

65775

65775   Corneal wedge resection for correction of surgically induced astigmatism

Astigmatism occurs when the naturally spherical (round) cornea takes on an oval configuration. This change in shape causes vision to become less sharp (blurry). Surgically induced astigmatism may occur following cataract removal or refractive procedures such as LASIK. A high degree if astigmatism is usually corrected using corneal wedge resection. The eye is first mapped using a slit lamp and markings placed. The patient is then positioned supine and the eye is prepped and draped. The cornea is anesthetized using a topical anesthetic. The cornea is irrigated with saline and a viscolubricant eye solution may be instilled. The globe of the eye is secured using a suction device or forceps and a diamond knife is used to incise the previously marked area of the cornea. A sliver of corneal tissue is excised and the wound closed with 10-0 nylon. The removal of small section of tissue allows the cornea to return to a more natural, spherical shape and vision to be sharper or clearer. At the conclusion of the procedure a corneal contact lens bandage may be applied, antibiotic eye drops are instilled and the eye is then patched.

65778-65779

65778   Placement of amniotic membrane on the ocular surface; without sutures
65779   Placement of amniotic membrane on the ocular surface; single layer, sutured

Amniotic membrane, previously harvested from placental tissue and dried, is placed on the ocular surface of the eye to promote wound healing. The eye is irrigated with normal saline and antibiotic drops are used as needed for 24-48 hours before applying the amniotic membrane. Anesthetic eye drops and/or facial nerve block is used to anesthetize the eye. An eye speculum is applied to the eye to keep it open. In 65778, a self-retaining amniotic membrane graft is applied. This method of graft placement may also be referred to as spreading or sutureless. A dried piece of amniotic membrane approximately the size of the conjunctival sac is obtained from the tissue bank. A circular opening is cut into the membrane so that uninvolved portions of the cornea are not covered. Covering the entire cornea can result in temporary hazy vision in the affected eye. The amniotic membrane is then spread over the wound as well as the healthy conjunctiva. The membrane is spread from the upper fornix with the patient looking down and then over the lower fornix with the patient looking up. The eye speculum is removed. Liquid paraffin is used to seal the eye closed and both eyes are bandaged closed for 24-48 hours to allow the amniotic membrane to be absorbed. In 65779, the amniotic membrane is sutured over the wound. A dried piece of amniotic membrane conforming to the size and shape of the wound is obtained from the tissue bank. A suture is passed through each corner of the membrane graft. The graft is placed over the wound and the previously placed membrane sutures are passed through the conjunctiva to secure the graft to the eye. The speculum is removed, liquid paraffin is used to seal the eye closed, and both eyes are bandaged closed for 24-48 hours. The sutures are removed three days after the membrane placement.

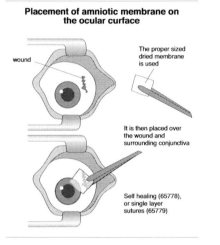

Placement of amniotic membrane on the ocular curface

wound

The proper sized dried membrane is used

It is then placed over the wound and surrounding conjunctiva

Self healing (65778), or single layer sutures (65779)

65780

65780   Ocular surface reconstruction; amniotic membrane transplantation, multiple layers

This procedure is performed to treat damage to the ocular surface caused by injury or a disease process. When the repair is performed by amniotic membrane reconstruction, the physician may use an inlay or overlay technique or for deeper defects the amniotic membrane may be used as a filler to repair the ocular surface. Amniotic membrane grafts act as a basement membrane over which epitheliazation takes place. The amniotic membrane graft is obtained from the tissue bank and prepared for transplant. The corneal epithelium is debrided as needed. The graft material is trimmed to the size of the corneal defect. Using an inlay technique, the graft is carefully placed in the defect taking care not to extend the graft edges beyond the defect. The graft is secured with interrupted sutures. Using an overlay technique, the entire corneal surface including the limbus is covered with the amniotic membrane graft. The overlay graft protects the underlying damaged epithelium while at the same time allowing oxygen and moisture to reach it, which promotes regeneration of the epithelium and healing of the cornea. Deeper defects may require amniotic membrane filler graft which is a multilayered amniotic membrane graft. Once the multilayered graft has been placed in the defect and secured with sutures, it may be covered with an inlay or overlay graft.

65781

65781   Ocular surface reconstruction; limbal stem cell allograft (eg, cadaveric or living donor)

This procedure is performed to treat damage to the cornea caused by injury or a disease process. Limbal stem cell allograft is performed only on patients with severe damage to the ocular surface causing inability of the eye to heal itself. Limbal stem cells arise from the white outer coating of eyeball, also referred to as the limbus. The limbal stem cells give rise to corneal epithelial cells which form the outermost layer of the cornea and act as a protective barrier to germs and other contaminants. If a live donor allograft is used, the limbal cells are harvested in a strip from the eye of the donor in a separately reportable procedure. Alternatively, previously harvested limbal stem cells from a cadaver may be used. In the patient receiving the transplant, the corneal epithelium is debrided to remove the damaged epithelial stem cells and the transplant bed is prepared for the allograft. The conjunctiva is resected and the sclera exposed to a point 4-5 mm beyond the limbus. The limbal stem cell allograft is then placed in the prepared transplant bed and secured with sutures. Antibiotic and corticosteroid ointments are applied to the surgical wound. The eye is patched and covered with an eye shield.

65782

65782   Ocular surface reconstruction; limbal conjunctival autograft (includes obtaining graft)

This procedure is performed to treat damage to the cornea caused by injury or a disease process. Limbal conjunctival autograft is performed only on patients with severe damage to the ocular surface causing inability of the eye to heal itself. The limbus is the white outer coating of the eyeball. The limbus contains stem cells that give rise to corneal epithelial cells which form the outermost layer of the cornea and act as a protective barrier to germs and other contaminants. If only one eye is damaged the physician obtains a graft from the patient's healthy eye. The limbal conjunctival autograft is harvested in a strip from the healthy eye. The corneal epithelium of the damaged eye is debrided to remove the damaged epithelial stem cells and the transplant bed is prepared for the allograft. The conjunctiva is resected and the sclera is exposed to a point 4-5 mm beyond the limbus. The limbal conjunctival autograft is then placed in the prepared transplant bed and secured with sutures. Antibiotic and corticosteroid ointments are applied to the surgical wound. The eye is patched and covered with an eye shield.

65785

65785   Implantation of intrastromal corneal ring segments

Intrastromal corneal ring segments are micro-thin, flexible, crescent-shaped plastic inserts made of polymethylmethacrylate in a range of thicknesses which can be implanted into the periphery of the cornea to improve visual acuity. A small incision is made in the cornea and channels are created with a laser or special dissecting device. One or two corneal ring implant segments are then placed within each channel, selecting the appropriate thicknesses for the degree of correction needed. The implants flatten the curvature of the anterior cornea and physically alter its shape, which affects the refraction in the eye and improves vision. Intrastromal corneal ring segments are used to correct myopia and astigmatism, most often in patients who have undergone refractive laser surgery and have associated corneal ectasia or keratoconus.

65800

65800   Paracentesis of anterior chamber of eye (separate procedure); with removal of aqueous

Removal of aqueous from the anterior chamber of the eye may be performed as a diagnostic or therapeutic procedure. Diagnostic removal of aqueous is performed for a condition such as uveitis to diagnose infectious organisms. Therapeutic removal of aqueous may be performed to lower intraocular pressure. Eye drops are instilled to numb the eye. The patient is positioned at the slit lamp. A needle attached to a syringe or an aqueous pipette is inserted at the paralimbal aspect of the cornea above and parallel to the iris. If a needle and syringe is used, the plunger is pulled and aqueous is aspirated into the syringe. If an aqueous pipette is used, the suction-infusion bulb that was compressed at the time of insertion in order to create a vacuum is released and aqueous is aspirated.

65810

65810   Paracentesis of anterior chamber of eye (separate procedure); with removal of vitreous and/or discission of anterior hyaloid membrane, with or without air injection

The physician repairs a condition in which the aqueous fluid in the front chamber of the eye pushes forward between the cornea and the lens. The physician may remove some of the fluid and/or remove part of the membrane that separates the fluid from the rest of the eye. The physician may also inject air into the eye to equalize the pressure in the eye.

65815

65815   Paracentesis of anterior chamber of eye (separate procedure); with removal of blood, with or without irrigation and/or air injection

This procedure is done to treat hyphema, which is a collection of blood in the anterior chamber of the eye, usually resulting from trauma. Eye drops are instilled to numb the eye. Two paracentesis sites are created using a knife blade. A needle or cannula is inserted into one of the sites and loose blood is irrigated from the eye with balanced saline solution. Intraocular pressure is monitored during the procedure. If a blood clot is present and the removal of loose blood does not reduce the intraocular pressure, the paracentesis site may be enlarged slightly and the blood clot removed using irrigation and aspiration. Following the irrigation aspiration procedure, air may be injected into the eye to stabilize eye pressure.

65820

65820   Goniotomy

The physician performs a goniotomy, used to treat congenital glaucoma in children. Congenital glaucoma can cause developmental arrest of the iris and ciliary body, which may then lead to obstruction of the trabecular network, preventing drainage of aqueous fluid from the eye and causing increased intraocular pressure. Mitotic eye drops are administered to constrict the pupil. The eye is then stabilized using forceps or sutures. The cornea is punctured and a viscoelastic tube is placed in the anterior chamber

CPT © 2016 American Medical Association. All Rights Reserved.   ● New Code   ▲ Revised Code through which fluid is introduced. A gonioscopy lens is placed on the eye and the anterior trabecular meshwork is incised using a needle or knife blade. The tubing is then removed; sterile saline is injected; and the corneal puncture site to the anterior chamber is closed.

65850

65850   Trabeculotomy ab externo

This procedure is performed to treat congenital and open angle glaucoma. An ab externo approach involves opening the trabecular meshwork in front of Schlemm's canal. Mitotic eye drops are administered to constrict the pupil. A slit lamp and gonioscopy lens are used to guide the trabeculotome as it is introduced into Schlemm's canal. The trabeculotome is rotated as it is advanced into the anterior chamber and an opening is created in the trabecular meshwork to release intraocular pressure. The trabeculotome is removed.

65855

65855   Trabeculoplasty by laser surgery

The procedure may also be referred to as argon laser trabeculoplasty (ALT) or selective laser trabeculoplasty (SLT). This procedure is performed for primary open angle glaucoma, pseudoexfoliation syndrome, and pigmentary dispersion syndrome. Eye drops are administered to constrict the pupil, decrease the amount of fluid in the eyes, and prevent elevation of eye pressure. A slit lamp and gonioscopy lens are used to guide the laser beam into the trabecular meshwork. The laser is activated and small burns are made in the trabecular meshwork. The treatment typically involves creating 40 to 80 burns over 180 degrees of trabecular meshwork.

65860

65860   Severing adhesions of anterior segment, laser technique (separate procedure)

Adhesions in the anterior segment are severed using laser technique. Eye drops are administered to numb the eye. A slit lamp and gonioscopy lens are used to guide the laser beam. The laser is activated and scar tissue in the anterior segment is severed.

65865-65880

65865   Severing adhesions of anterior segment of eye, incisional technique (with or without injection of air or liquid) (separate procedure); goniosynechiae

65870   Severing adhesions of anterior segment of eye, incisional technique (with or without injection of air or liquid) (separate procedure); anterior synechiae, except goniosynechiae

65875   Severing adhesions of anterior segment of eye, incisional technique (with or without injection of air or liquid) (separate procedure); posterior synechiae

65880   Severing adhesions of anterior segment of eye, incisional technique (with or without injection of air or liquid) (separate procedure); corneovitreal adhesions

Adhesions in the anterior segment are severed using an incisional technique with or without injection of air or liquid. In 65865, goniosynechiae are incised. Goniosynechiae are adhesions of the iris to the posterior surface of the cornea in the iridocorneal angle of the anterior chamber. Goniosynechiae are associated with angle closure glaucoma. An incision is made in the cornea and a needle or knife blade used to severe the adhesive tissue connecting the iris to the posterior surface of the cornea. Air or fluid may be injected to stabilize pressure in the eye if aqueous fluid is lost during the procedure. In 65870, adhesions between the iris and anterior segment structures other than the cornea are severed using a needle or knife blade. In 65875, posterior synechiae are severed using a needle or knife blade. Posterior synechiae are adhesions between the iris and lens capsule. In 65880, corneovitreal adhesions are severed using a needle or knife blade. Corneovitreal adhesions are adhesions between the cornea and vitreous matter filling the anterior segment.

65900

65900   Removal of epithelial downgrowth, anterior chamber of eye

Epithelial downgrowths (ingrowths) are a complication of surgical or nonsurgical trauma to the eye. The corneal or conjunctival epithelium gains access to the anterior (inner) chamber of the eye and grows on the back of the cornea, trabecular meshwork and/or anterior surface of the iris. The condition may also present as a fluid filled cystic lesion or as free-floating epithelial cells. Symptoms can include pain, increased intraocular pressure (glaucoma) and inflammation. The eye is anesthetized using a topical ophthalmic anesthetic. Using an operative microscope or slit lamp the flap edge from the previous incision or traumatic wound is located and opened using a Sinskey hook or similar instrument. If the area of downgrowth is extensive a cyclodialysis spatula may be used to further elevate the flap. The stromal bed is scraped with a blade or knife and the flap replaced. Alternatively, epithelial tissue can be removed surgically using direct electrocautery or photocoagulation. If the downgrowth presents as a cystic lesion, cyst aspiration with cauterization, diathermy or injection of sclerosing agents or alcohol may be performed. Following removal of the downgrowths, the eye is irrigated, a corneal contact

lens bandage may be placed followed by the instillation of antibiotic and/or steroid eye drops. The eye is then patched.

65930

65930   Removal of blood clot, anterior segment of eye

A blood clot or hyphema in the anterior segment of the eye may result from blunt or penetrating trauma to the exposed area of the eye, as a complication from intraocular surgery or spontaneously in the form of neovascularization in patients with diabetes mellitus, ischemic disease, acatrix formation, ocular neoplasm or uveitis. Red blood cells suspend in the aqueous humor forming the clot which then leads to inflammation, increased intraocular pressure and pain. Blood staining the cornea eventually leads to visual impairment if the clot is not removed. The patient is positioned supine and an operating microscopic put in place. An incision is made in the clear cornea using a diamond blade parallel to the plane of the iris. A 20 gauge Ocutome is attached to an infusion of balanced salt solution plus (BSS-Plus) and placed into the anterior chamber of the eye. The chamber is irrigated with this fluid to break up the clot and the fluid and blood are then aspirated using suction. An air bubble is placed into the chamber at the completion of the procedure and the incision in the cornea is closed with 10-0 suture. Antibiotic eye drops may be instilled and the eye is then patched.

66020-66030

66020   Injection, anterior chamber of eye (separate procedure); air or liquid

66030   Injection, anterior chamber of eye (separate procedure); medication

The anterior chamber of the eye is the area between the iris (outer layer of the cornea) and the endothelium (inner layer of the cornea). The anterior chamber is filled with clear gelatinous fluid called the aqueous humor. In 66020, air or liquid is injected into the anterior chamber. The patient is positioned supine with head and neck supported. A topical ophthalmic anesthetic applied and the eye is then cleansed with antiseptic. An eyelid speculum is placed and injection site marked. A fine needle with attached syringe is inserted through the cornea toward the mid-vitreous cavity. Air or liquid is then injected into the cavity. The needle is withdrawn, antibiotic eye drops instilled and the eye may be patched. In 66030, medication is injected into the anterior chamber using the same technique described above.

66130

66130   Excision of lesion, sclera

Lesions of the sclera are usually benign in nature. They can include pingueculae found most often in the open space between the eyelids and characterized by a yellowish color and slight elevation. Pigmented lesions that arise from melanocytes and non-melanocytes can be acquired or congenital. Scleral lesions may be removed for cosmetic reasons or when they become enlarged and cause discomfort. A topical ophthalmic anesthetic is applied and the eye is prepped with an antibacterial solution. An eyelid speculum is inserted and the lesion is excised. Separately reportable tissue grafting may be performed to repair the surgical defect resulting from the excision. At the conclusion of the procedure, the cytotoxic (anti-cancer) drug Mitomycin C may be applied briefly to reduce scarring and then flushed away.

66150

66150   Fistulization of sclera for glaucoma; trephination with iridectomy

Scleral fistulization to treat glaucoma is performed using trephination with iridectomy. The eye is visualized under an operating microscope and an incision is made in the conjunctiva near the limbus to expose the sclera. A flap is created in the sclera and a surgical instrument called a trephine is used to remove a small disc of tissue from the iris. The opening in the iris (iridectomy) allows fluid to flow between the anterior and posterior chambers of the eye, lowering the intraocular pressure. The scleral incision is closed with sutures followed by closure of the conjunctiva.

66155

66155   Fistulization of sclera for glaucoma; thermocauterization with iridectomy

Scleral fistulization to treat glaucoma is performed using thermocauterization with iridectomy. The eye is visualized under an operating microscope and an incision is made in the conjunctiva near the limbus to expose the sclera. An opening is created in the area of the pars plana of the ciliary body and a Fugo blade is used to dissolve tissue bands and create a small hole in the iris (iridectomy). The vascular ciliary body bleeds minimally when a Fugo blade is employed because it utilizes plasma energy around an ablation filament creating thermocauterization of the tissue as it cuts. The iridectomy allows fluid to drain from the posterior chamber into the subconjunctival lymphatics and lowers intraocular pressure. The scleral incision is closed with sutures followed by closure of the conjunctiva.

● New Code   ▲ Revised Code

66160

66160   **Fistulization of sclera for glaucoma; sclerectomy with punch or scissors, with iridectomy**

Scleral fistulization to treat glaucoma is performed using sclerectomy with iridectomy. The eye is visualized under an operating microscope and an incision is made in the conjunctiva. The sclera is incised close to the limbus, and using a punch or scissors, a scleral lip is excised. The iris is opened with forceps to create a smooth, inverted iris flap (iridectomy) under the sclera. The iridectomy allows fluid to drain from the posterior chamber and lowers intraocular pressure. The scleral incision is closed with sutures followed by closure of the conjunctiva.

66170-66172

66170   **Fistulization of sclera for glaucoma; trabeculectomy ab externo in absence of previous surgery**

66172   **Fistulization of sclera for glaucoma; trabeculectomy ab externo with scarring from previous ocular surgery or trauma (includes injection of antifibrotic agents)**

The physician creates a new drainage tube for eye fluids through the fibrous covering of the eye. This is done to treat a condition in which fluid drains from the front chamber of the eye slower than new fluid is produced. The physician removes some of the tissue connecting the iris to the fibrous membrane that surrounds the eye, leaving a passage for fluid to drain into the space between the fibrous membrane and the other structures of the eye. Code 66172 if this procedure is performed after a previous eye surgery to reduce scar tissue.

66174-66175

66174   **Transluminal dilation of aqueous outflow canal; without retention of device or stent**

66175   **Transluminal dilation of aqueous outflow canal; with retention of device or stent**

Transluminal dilation of the aqueous outflow canal (Schlemm's canal) without retention is performed to treat open angle glaucoma. This procedure is also referred to as glaucoma canaloplasty or enhanced viscocanalostomy. The procedure reduces intraocular pressure (IOP) in patients with glaucoma by forcibly opening Schlemm's canal to restore natural drainage of fluid from the eye. A scleral flap is created. The canal is exposed and deroofed. The scleral flap may be extended to expose Descemet's membrane and a window (Descemet's window) is created. The canal is then intubated with a flexible hollow microcatheter with a lighted tip. The lighted tip illuminates the canal as the microcatheter is advanced. A viscoelastic, such as high viscosity sodium hyaluronate, is instilled to dilate the canal and facilitate advancement of the microcatheter. After it has been passed through the entire length of the canal, the microcatheter is withdrawn. The scleral flap is closed. Use 66174 when the procedure is performed without retention of a device or stent. Use 66175 when transluminal dilation of the aqueous outflow canal is performed with retention of a device or stent. The procedure is performed as described above except that a device, such as a suture, or a stent is left in the canal. After the microcannula has been passed through the entire length of the canal, either a flexible stent or a suture is advanced along the path of the microcannula through the full length of the canal as well. The flexible stent or suture is left in the canal and the microcannula is withdrawn. If a suture is used to permanently open the canal, the suture is tied off and left in place. The suture cinches and stretches the trabecular meshwork inward and opens the canal.

66179-66180

66179   **Aqueous shunt to extraocular equatorial plate reservoir, external approach; without graft**

66180   **Aqueous shunt to extraocular equatorial plate reservoir, external approach; with graft**

Normal outflow of vitreous fluid begins at the aqueous humor and passes through the trabecular meshwork, enters Schlemm's canal (a space lined with endothelial cells) finally draining into the collector channel and the aqueous veins. An aqueous shunt to extraocular reservoir (Molteno, Schocket, Denver-Krupin) bypasses the trabecular meshwork and Schlemm's canal. The shunt is used to reduce intraocular pressure (IOP) when traditional medical (pharmacological) or surgical (trabeculectomy) therapy have failed. This procedure is most often implemented when increased intraocular pressure (IOP) is caused by iris swelling, abnormal vessel formation or iridocorneal endothelial (ICE) syndrome. With the patient supine and under general anesthesia, a small silicon tube is implanted into the anterior chamber of the eye allowing vitreous fluid to drain through the tube and collect in a tiny plate sutured on the anterior eye between the sclera and the conjunctiva (usually in the area of the upper eye lid). After collecting in the plate, the vitreous fluid is then absorbed by blood vessels on the surface of the anterior eye. In 66180, a scleral or corneal patch graft from donor tissue may be placed over the plate to keep it in position and reduce the incidence of conjunctival ulceration. At the conclusion of the procedure, the cytotoxic (anti-cancer) drug Mitomycin C may be applied briefly to reduce scarring and then flushed away. A contact lens bandage may be applied and antibiotic and/or steroid drops may be instilled. The eye is then patched.

66183

66183   **Insertion of anterior segment aqueous drainage device, without extraocular reservoir, external approach**

Insertion of an anterior segment aqueous drainage device is used to treat chronic or progressive open angle glaucoma. Using an external approach, which may also be described as non-penetrating deep sclerectomy, the conjunctiva is incised and a scleral flap is created with the base of the flap located at the corneoscleral junction (limbus). An incision is made into the anterior chamber and aqueous flow is established. A miniature drainage device (shunt), about the size of a grain of rice, is implanted between the anterior chamber and under the scleral flap in order to facilitate drainage of aqueous humor from the anterior chamber to the space under the conjunctiva. The scleral flap is secured with sutures and the conjunctival incision is closed.

66184-66185

66184   **Revision of aqueous shunt to extraocular equatorial plate reservoir; without graft**

66185   **Revision of aqueous shunt to extraocular equatorial plate reservoir; with graft**

A number of conditions may require revision of aqueous shunt to extraocular plate reservoir. With the sudden drop in intraocular pressure (IOP) from the newly created drainage system, the anterior chamber may decrease the amount of fluid it produces. This can be treated by priming the pump with a viscoelastic fluid to raise IOP in the anterior chamber and stimulate the production of vitreous humor. However, some conditions require revision of the shunt, including corneal damage, small cataracts, infection, and bleeding. The most common problem requiring revision of the aqueous shunt is the build up of scar tissue at the posterior plate. An incision is made in the conjunctival tissue over the plate. The scar tissue is then removed. Once the scar tissue is removed, the conjunctival incision is sutured closed. In 66185, a scleral or corneal patch graft from donor tissue may be placed over the plate to keep it in position after the revision and reduce the incidence of conjunctival ulceration. At the conclusion of the procedure, the cytotoxic (anti-cancer) drug Mitomycin C may be applied briefly to reduce recurrence of scarring and then flushed away. A contact lens bandage may be applied and antibiotic and/or steroid drops may be instilled. The eye is then patched.

66220-66225

66220   **Repair of scleral staphyloma; without graft**

66225   **Repair of scleral staphyloma; with graft**

A staphyloma is a protrusion of uveal tissue through a weak area of the sclera or cornea. Staphylomas usually arise in an area that has been injured or weakened by disease or inflammation. There are five areas in which staphylomas are found. Anterior segment staphylomas involve the cornea and adjacent scleral tissue. Intercalary or limbal staphylomas are found at the margin where the cornea and sclera meet and often present with secondary angle closure glaucoma or corneal astigmatism. Ciliary staphylomas are located in an area lined with ciliary bodies approximately 2-3 mm from the limbus. Equatorial staphylomas are found in a region perforated by vortex veins. Posterior or macular staphylomas are located at the back of the eye and are diagnosed by ophthalmoscopy often after the patient presents with myopia. In 66220, the protruding tissue is excised and the sclera is closed with sutures. In 66225, the protruding tissue is excised and then weak region of the sclera is reinforced with a tissue graft, such as an allogenic fascial graft fixed with fibrin tissue glue.

66250

66250   **Revision or repair of operative wound of anterior segment, any type, early or late, major or minor procedure**

The physician revises or repairs any type of wound to the front of the eye that resulted from surgery.

66500-66505

66500   **Iridotomy by stab incision (separate procedure); except transfixion**

66505   **Iridotomy by stab incision (separate procedure); with transfixion as for iris bombe**

Stab incision iridotomy with or without transfixion may be used to treat glaucoma, iris atrophy, papillary membrane adhesions, and aniridia. Using an operating microscope to visualize the eye, a stab incision is made through the conjunctiva and into the lamellar sclera. A superficial tunnel is then carefully dissected using a side-to-side technique up to the limbus. The dissection is extended into the lamellar cornea and the anterior chamber is entered horizontally. The blade is withdrawn in a single, smooth movement to open the tunnel. An ophthalmic viscoelastic fluid is injected through the tunnel and the globe is rotated downward allowing a membrane punch to slide along the tunnel and into the anterior chamber. The posterior lip of the corneal section is grasped and punched. To compromise the tunnel, additional punches may be taken in clear cornea and extended up to the limbus. The anterior chamber is then irrigated through the tunnel to remove excess viscoelastic fluid and monitor for leakage. The conjunctival incision is closed with

Eye and Ocular Adnexa

sutures. Code 66505 includes iridotomy by stab incision with transfixion as for iris bombe, a condition in which there is apposition of the iris to the anterior chamber blocking the flow of aqueous fluid from the posterior chamber. The increased pressure in the posterior chamber causes anterior bowing, or bulging of the iris and obstruction of the trabecular meshwork. Transfixion restores communication between the anterior and posterior chamber, returning the iris to its normal position, while reducing tension.

66600-66605

66600   Iridectomy, with corneoscleral or corneal section; for removal of lesion
66605   Iridectomy, with corneoscleral or corneal section; with cyclectomy

The physician performs an iridectomy for removal of a lesion with a corneoscleral or corneal section. Iridectomy involves excising or removing a small, full thickness section of the iris. A local anesthetic is applied to the eye. An incision is made in the cornea or at the limbus of the sclera. The lesion on the iris is excised along with a margin of healthy tissue. In 66605, the physician performs an iridectomy with a cyclectomy. In this procedure the physician removes a portion of the ciliary body, which lies immediately behind the iris, along with a small full-thickness section of the iris. The ciliary body produces aqueous humor, the clear fluid that fills the front of the eye, and also controls accommodation by contracting and relaxing to allow the ability of the eye to focus on a close or distant object. Cyclectomy may be performed to remove a lesion on the ciliary body. A local anesthetic is applied to the eye. An incision is made in the cornea or at the limbus of the sclera. A section of iris is excised along with a portion of the underlying ciliary body.

66625-66630

66625   Iridectomy, with corneoscleral or corneal section; peripheral for glaucoma (separate procedure)
66630   Iridectomy, with corneoscleral or corneal section; sector for glaucoma (separate procedure)

A portion of the iris is removed to treat glaucoma. Removing a portion of the iris allows fluid to drain from the anterior chamber to the posterior chamber, thereby reducing intraocular pressure (IOP). This procedure is typically performed for angle-closure glaucoma when laser iridotomy fails to achieve the necessary reduction in IOP. A topical anesthetic is applied to the eye. An incision is made in the cornea usually at the limbus where the cornea and sclera join. In 66625, a small full-thickness section of the iris is excised. In 66630, a larger full-thickness wedge-shaped section of the iris is excised. The corneal incision is typically not closed because it will close and heal on its own. Antibiotic drops may be applied along with a contact lens bandage and/or an eye patch.

66635

66635   Iridectomy, with corneoscleral or corneal section; optical (separate procedure)

The physician performs an optical iridectomy with corneoscleral or corneal section. Iridectomy involves excising or removing a small, full-thickness section of the iris. Optical iridectomy is performed to create an artificial pupil in the eye by removing a section of iris at the center of the eye. A local anesthetic is applied to the eye. An incision is made in the cornea or at the limbus of the sclera. Iris forceps or an iris hook is introduced through the corneal or limbal incision and the edge of the pupil is grasped. Iridectomy forceps are then introduced and the iris is grasped near the edge of the pupil and drawn out through the corneal or limbal incision. Iridectomy scissors are used to snip off a small fragment of iris. Excision of the iris continues in a radial fashion to form an artificial pupil at the center of the eye.

66680

66680   Repair of iris, ciliary body (as for iridodialysis)

An injury to the iris or ciliary body, such as one that results in iridodialysis, is repaired. Iridodialysis refers to separation of the iris root from the ciliary body or scleral spur. This results in an irregular D-shaped pupil. A miotic agent is used to constrict the pupil. A corneal incision is made and any synechiae are lysed to fully mobilization the iris leaflets. If the injury extends into the iris sphincter it is repaired first. The edges are carefully approximated to ensure a centrally located pupil. The remainder of the iris injury is repaired with sutures by passing the needle through a paracentesis tract in the anterior chamber and then through the iris. The needle passes through the proximal and distal leaflets of the iris and then out through the peripheral cornea. If iridodialysis has occurred the iris root is reattached to the ciliary body or scleral spur. The sutures are then tied and buried in the anterior chamber.

66682

66682   Suture of iris, ciliary body (separate procedure) with retrieval of suture through small incision (eg, McCannel suture)

A small incision is made in the conjunctiva at the limbus adjacent to the site of injury in the iris and/or ciliary body. Suture material is threaded through the first needle. The needle is then inserted at a point 180 degrees from the site of the injury in the iris. The needle is passed through the cornea, anterior chamber, iris base, iris root and sclera exiting at the

site of the injury. Several centimeters of suture are pulled through the wound. The suture material is left attached to the needle. The needle is then retracted back into the anterior chamber and a second pass is made through the iris root on the other side of the defect. The needle and suture material are again brought through the sclera a short distance from the first exit site. The two ends of the suture material are then tied over the sclera and the knot is buried. The conjunctival incision is closed. This type of suture repair may be referred to as a McCannel double arm suture

66700

66700   Ciliary body destruction; diathermy

The ciliary body is located just behind the iris. The two primary functions of the ciliary body include production of aqueous humor, which is the clear fluid that fills the anterior chamber, and accommodation, which changes the shape of the crystalline lens allowing the eye to focus on near or far objects. Destruction of the ciliary body is performed to treat glaucoma which has failed to respond to medication and other more conservative surgical procedures. Destruction of the ciliary body reduces inflow of aqueous to the anterior chamber thereby reducing intraocular pressure. A local periocular anesthetic is administered. A lid speculum is placed on the eye to hold the eyelids open. Diathermy, also referred to as electrodiathermy, uses an extra-ocular transcleral or transconjunctival approach. Alternatively, a scleral flap may be elevated to access the ciliary body. The ciliary body is destroyed using a heat probe.

66710-66711

66710   Ciliary body destruction; cyclophotocoagulation, transscleral
66711   Ciliary body destruction; cyclophotocoagulation, endoscopic

The ciliary body is located just behind the iris. The two primary functions of the ciliary body include production of aqueous humor, which is the clear fluid that fills the anterior chamber, and accommodation, which changes the shape of the crystalline lens allowing the eye to focus on near or far objects. Destruction of the ciliary body is performed to treat glaucoma which has failed to respond to medication and other more conservative surgical procedures. Partial destruction of the ciliary body reduces inflow of aqueous to the anterior chamber thereby reducing intraocular pressure. A local periocular anesthetic is administered. A lid speculum is placed on the eye to hold the eyelids open. In 66710, the ciliary body is destroyed using cyclophotocoagulation via an extra-ocular transcleral approach. The laser probe is positioned over the ciliary body. No incisions are made. The laser energy travels through the sclera to the ciliary body and partially destroys it. The physician must preserve enough of the ciliary body to allow some production of aqueous, but must destroy enough to reduce intraocular pressure. In 66711, the procedure is performed using an endoscope. An incision is made in the temporal aspect of the cornea. Viscoelastic material is injected into the anterior chamber over the pupil and lens and under the iris to allow better visualization of the ciliary body processes. The endoscope is inserted through the corneal incision. The ciliary processes are coagulated using laser energy. The endoscope is withdrawn. A second corneal incision is made to allow access to another section of the ciliary body and the ciliary processes are destroyed in the same manner. This continues until a sufficient amount of the ciliary body has been destroyed. The viscoelastic material is removed by irrigation and aspiration. A balanced saline solution is in injected to replace the viscoelastic material. The incisions are checked for fluid leakage and repaired with sutures as needed.

66720

66720   Ciliary body destruction; cryotherapy

The ciliary body is located just behind the iris. The two primary functions of the ciliary body include production of aqueous humor, which is the clear fluid that fills the anterior chamber, and accommodation, which changes the shape of the crystalline lens allowing the eye to focus on near or far objects. Destruction of the ciliary body is performed to treat glaucoma which has failed to respond to medication and other more conservative surgical procedures. Partial destruction of the ciliary body reduces inflow of aqueous to the anterior chamber thereby reducing intraocular pressure. A local periocular anesthetic is administered. A lid speculum is placed on the eye to hold the eyelids open. Cryotherapy nonselectively destroys ciliary body tissue. A cryoprobe is used to rapidly freeze part of the ciliary body. The tissue is then slowly thawed. The freeze-thaw cycle is repeated until the desired amount of ciliary body tissue has been destroyed.

66740

66740   Ciliary body destruction; cyclodialysis

The ciliary body is located just behind the iris. The two primary functions of the ciliary body include the production of aqueous humor, which is the clear fluid that fills the anterior chamber, and accommodation, which changes the shape of the crystalline lens allowing the eye to focus on near or far objects. Destruction of the ciliary body is performed to treat glaucoma which has failed to respond to medication and other more conservative surgical procedures. A local periocular anesthetic is administered. A lid speculum is placed on the eye to hold the eyelids open. Cyclodialysis involves separating the ciliary body from the scleral spur. This creates a communication between the anterior chamber and suprachoroidal space that allows aqueous to flow out of the anterior chamber thereby reducing intraocular pressure.

66761

66761   Iridotomy/iridectomy by laser surgery (eg, for glaucoma) (per session)

Iridotomy or iridectomy is performed to treat closed angle glaucoma. An intraocular pressure lowering eye drop is administered one hour prior to surgery and again immediately prior to surgery. Eye drops are administered to constrict the pupil. The patient is seated at the laser and an iridotomy contact lens is placed on the upper part of the front of the eye to magnify the lens and improve accuracy of laser beam projection. The laser is aimed at the 11:00 or 1:00 position and laser pulses are applied to the iris until a hole is formed. Once the laser has completely penetrated the iris, aqueous fluid begins to flow out of the anterior chamber. Following the laser procedure, the anterior chamber angle is examined using a gonioscope to ensure that the hole is wide enough to allow drainage of aqueous and lower the intraocular pressure. Multiple sessions may be required to ensure adequate drainage of aqueous and each session is reported separately.

66762

66762   Iridoplasty by photocoagulation (1 or more sessions) (eg, for improvement of vision, for widening of anterior chamber angle)

This procedure is performed to treat closed angle glaucoma and plateau iris. Eye drops are administered to constrict the pupil. The patient is seated at the laser and the physician carefully inspects the iris for areas of pigmentation at the periphery. Multiple laser burns are then placed around the periphery of the iris in the pigmented areas if possible. As the laser burns are placed the physician observes the iris which will contract as tissue shrinks in response to the laser treatment. Twenty or more laser burns may be required to open the anterior chamber angle allowing better drainage of aqueous. Following the laser procedure, the anterior chamber angle is examined using a gonioscope to ensure that it wide enough to allow drainage of aqueous and lower intraocular pressure.

66770

66770   Destruction of cyst or lesion iris or ciliary body (nonexcisional procedure)

Cysts or lesions of the iris or ciliary body can be primary (no known cause) or secondary (following trauma). Asymptomatic cysts and lesions are usually found during a routine eye examination and require no treatment. Cysts or lesions that block the visual axis (pupil) can cause secondary glaucoma (increased intraocular pressure) and/or loss of visual acuity. The most common site of cysts or lesions is the pigmented iris epithelium from the central pupillary margin to the peripheral iris. Less commonly a cyst or lesion will arise from the stroma which is lined with non-keratinized squamous epithelium. Infants and children are more likely to have cysts or lesions in the stromal area. Destruction of a cyst or lesion can be accomplished under local or general anesthesia. Cysts are usually treated by inserting a fine gauge needle into the base, aspirating the fluid and replacing the volume with ethyl alcohol (ETOH) x 1 minute. The ETOH solution is then aspirated back out allowing the cyst to collapse. Cysts and lesions may also be treated using endodiathermy (heat), cryotherapy (cold) and laser photocoagulation.

66820-66821

66820   Discission of secondary membranous cataract (opacified posterior lens capsule and/or anterior hyaloid); stab incision technique (Ziegler or Wheeler knife)
66821   Discission of secondary membranous cataract (opacified posterior lens capsule and/or anterior hyaloid); laser surgery (eg, YAG laser) (1 or more stages)

A secondary membranous cataract, also referred to as an after-cataract, is treated by discission using a stab incision technique (Ziegler or Wheeler knife). This procedure is performed when the remaining posterior portion of the lens capsule or the anterior hyaloid membrane that covers the anterior outer surface of the vitreous body in the posterior cavity of the eye becomes opacified or cloudy and impairs vision. This condition is sometimes referred to as posterior capsule opacification (PCO). A small surgical needle with a knife-like tip is inserted through the edge of the cornea and advanced into the posterior lens capsule and/or the anterior hyaloid membrane beneath the lens capsule. The posterior lens capsule and/or anterior hyaloid are incised using the small needle-knife and the secondary membranous cataract is opened providing an area of clear vision. In 66821, the secondary membranous cataract is opened by laser surgery in one or more stages. This procedure may also be referred to as a YAG laser capsulotomy. Eye drops may be used to dilate the pupil. A test shot is placed with the laser to mark the center of the pupil on the posterior capsule. Using a slit-lamp microscope, the laser is aimed at the posterior capsule and fired in a pattern that opens the center to provide an area of clear vision. More than one session may be required to create an adequate sized opening in the center of the posterior lens.

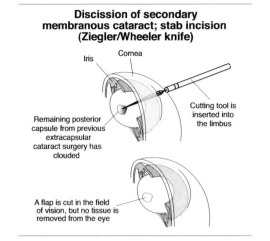

Discission of secondary membranous cataract; stab incision (Ziegler/Wheeler knife)

Iris

Cornea

Cutting tool is inserted into the limbus

Remaining posterior capsule from previous extracapsular cataract surgery has clouded

A flap is cut in the field of vision, but no tissue is removed from the eye

66825

66825   Repositioning of intraocular lens prosthesis, requiring an incision (separate procedure)

An intraocular lens (IOL) prosthesis may require repositioning when a toric lens is off axis, a multifocal lens or sulcus-fixated lens in decentered, or a single-piece haptic lens escapes from the capsular bag. Using an operating microscope, a scleral incision is made and the IOL is located and elevated using a vitreoretinal pick or hook. The IOL is then grasped with forceps and brought to the posterior chamber. Using a Sinskey hook inserted either through the sclerotomy or a limbic stab incision, the IOL is rotated into place. If there is inadequate capsular support, transcleral sutures or iris sutures may be placed. The scleral incision is closed with sutures and a patch or shield is placed over the eye.

66830

66830   Removal of secondary membranous cataract (opacified posterior lens capsule and/or anterior hyaloid) with corneo-scleral section, with or without iridectomy (iridocapsulotomy, iridocapsulectomy)

Secondary membranous cataracts are a complication of cataract surgery. After a cataract is removed from the anterior chamber and replaced with an intraocular lens, epithelial and fibroblastic cells from the cataract may remain and proliferate on the anterior surface of the posterior capsule, forming a hazy membrane. The posterior capsule is incised and the tissue is separated and retracted. A vitreous cutter or needle/hook is used to manually remove the tissue. Access to the posterior capsule may require an incision through the iris and capsular membrane surrounding the lens of the eye (iridectomy, iridocapsulotomy, iridocapsulectomy). The pressure is checked in the anterior chamber and fluid may be injected to inflate the chamber to a normal intraocular pressure. The instruments are removed and the wound(s) are checked for fluid leakage. Sutures may be placed if required to close the incision.

66840

66840   Removal of lens material; aspiration technique, 1 or more stages

To remove lens material by aspiration technique, the eye is visualized using an operating microscope and the anterior chamber is accessed with a needle or blade, creating one or more paracenteses. An irrigation and aspiration tool is inserted into the anterior chamber through the paracentesis and the lens material is gently pulled from the periphery to the pupillary center and aspirated. The pressure is checked in the anterior chamber and fluid may be injected to inflate the chamber to a normal intraocular pressure. The instruments are removed and the wound(s) is checked for fluid leakage. Sutures may be placed if required to close the incision(s).

66850

66850   Removal of lens material; phacofragmentation technique (mechanical or ultrasonic) (eg, phacoemulsification), with aspiration

To remove lens material by phacoemulsification aspiration technique, the eye is visualized using an operating microscope and the anterior chamber is accessed with a needle or blade, creating one or more paracenteses. A probe is inserted through the paracentesis into the anterior chamber and the lens material is broken up using ultrasound. The probe is removed and an irrigation and aspiration tool is inserted into the anterior chamber through the paracentesis. The fragmented pieces of lens material are gently pulled from the periphery to the pupillary center and aspirated. The pressure is checked in the anterior chamber and fluid may be injected to inflate the chamber to a normal intraocular pressure. The instruments are removed and the wound(s) are checked for fluid leakage. Sutures may be placed if required to close the incision(s).

Eye and Ocular Adnexa

66852

66852   Removal of lens material; pars plana approach, with or without vitrectomy

To remove lens material using a pars plana approach, with or without vitrectomy, the eye is visualized using an operating microscope. The posterior segment is accessed through a pars plana incision, opening the conjunctiva and Tenon's layer to expose the sclera. Hemostasis is achieved with cautery; the sclera is marked at the inferotemporal quadrant; and two sutures are placed on either side of the mark. Using a microvitreoretinal (MVR) blade, the sclera is incised at the mark between the two sutures. An infusion line is inserted and secured with the sutures, then visualized with a light pipe. It may be necessary to make a second sclerotomy in the inferotemporal quadrant to position the infusion line correctly. Superior sclerotomies are then made using the MVR blade, and a light pipe and vitreo cutter are passed through into the posterior segment. The lens material is removed using irrigation and aspiration. Vitreous fluid (vitrectomy) may be removed with the lens material. The intraocular pressure is monitored and maintained to ensure that the eye stays formed during the irrigation and aspiration. Fluid may be injected to inflate the chamber to a normal intraocular pressure at the conclusion of the procedure. Instruments are removed, and the sclerotomies are closed with suture and checked for fluid leakage. The infusion line is removed and closed with the previously placed sutures, followed by closure of the conjunctiva.

66920-66930

66920   Removal of lens material; intracapsular
66930   Removal of lens material; intracapsular, for dislocated lens

An incision is made at the corneoscleral junction. The lens capsule is exposed. Medication is injected to dissolve the zonal fibers that hold the lens in place. A cryoprobe is inserted and the lens is frozen. The probe is withdrawn and the natural lens and lens capsule are removed. The surgical wound is repaired with sutures. Temporary sutures are placed through the upper and lower eyelids to keep the eye closed until the eye has healed. A soft bandage or patch may also be applied to the eye. Use 66920 when intracapsular removal of lens material is performed for a condition other than a dislocated lense. Use 66930 when the procedure is performed to remove a dislocated natural lens and lens capsule.

66940

66940   Removal of lens material; extracapsular (other than 66840, 66850, 66852)

To remove lens material using extracapsular technique, the eye is visualized using an operating microscope and an incision is made in the cornea close to the scleral border. A circular tear is made in the front of the lens capsule and the capsule is opened. Lens material is removed using instruments and/or suction, and the incision is closed with sutures.

66982

66982   Extracapsular cataract removal with insertion of intraocular lens prosthesis (1-stage procedure), manual or mechanical technique (eg, irrigation and aspiration or phacoemulsification), complex, requiring devices or techniques not generally used in routine cataract surgery (eg, iris expansion device, suture support for intraocular lens, or primary posterior capsulorrhexis) or performed on patients in the amblyogenic developmental stage

Complex extracapsular cataract removal is performed with insertion of intraocular lens (IOL) prosthesis using manual or mechanical technique. A complex procedure uses devices or techniques not generally used in routine cataract surgery and may be required for children because primary posterior capsulotomy or capsulorrhexis is required which complicates insertion of the intraocular lens. Additionally, the anterior capsule in children is more difficult to open (tear) and the cortex is difficult to remove because of adhesion of the lens. Complexity of the cataract procedure may also be increased for patients with certain conditions, such as uveitis, glaucoma, pseudoexfoliation syndrome, or Marfan syndrome. Patients who have had prior intraocular surgery, who have experienced other trauma to the eye, and those with dense, hard, and/or white cataracts may also require a more complex procedure. Complex techniques include the use of an iris expansion device, suture support for the intraocular lens, or primary posterior capsulorrhexis. An incision is made in the corneoscleral junction (fornix) for insertion of the phacoemusification device. A side port incision is made. An attempt is made to dilate the pupil, but may be unsuccessful. In this case, a spatula is inserted and posterior synechiae are lysed. Four incisions are made and an expansion device consisting of four hooks is inserted. The iris is retracted using the hooks. A circular tear is made in the anterior lens capsule. The lens capsule is opened and the phacoemulsification probe is inserted. Ultrasound is used to break up and remove the cataract. Once the cataract has been removed, the softer cortex surrounding the cataract is removed by suction. Viscoelastic material is injected into the lens capsule to maintain its shape. If the patient is a child, the posterior capsule may be incised (capsulotomy or capsulorrhexis) to facilitate insertion of the IOL. The IOL is inserted and the viscoelastic material is removed. The expansion hooks are removed and the incisions are checked for water tightness. Subconjunctival injection of water or saline is performed to restore intraocular pressure and the eye is dressed.

66983

66983   Intracapsular cataract extraction with insertion of intraocular lens prosthesis (1 stage procedure)

The physician performs an intracapsular cataract extraction (ICCE) with insertion of an intraocular lens (IOL) prosthesis. ICCE is rarely used today due to the development of more advanced extracapsular techniques. A large incision is made at the corneoscleral junction (fornix). The eye is injected with a substance that disolves the zonular fibers that hold the lens in place. A cryoprobe is placed on the lens and liquid nitrogen is applied to freeze the lens. The probe is then withdrawn with the attached native lens. When the native lens is removed, the IOL is implanted in front of the iris. The eyelid is then sutured closed to allow the eye to heal.

66984

66984   Extracapsular cataract removal with insertion of intraocular lens prosthesis (1 stage procedure), manual or mechanical technique (eg, irrigation and aspiration or phacoemulsification)

The physician removes a cloudy membrane which has formed over the surface of the lens, and inserts a prosthetic lens into the eye, using a mechanical device to aid in the procedure. Cutting and suction is used, or an ultrasonic device is, removing the lens in pieces. A bubble of air is injected into the anterior chamber for protection of the cornea. The intraocular lens is placed into eye and the incision may be closed with sutures, and water or saline is injected to re-establish intraocular pressure.

66985

66985   Insertion of intraocular lens prosthesis (secondary implant), not associated with concurrent cataract removal

A secondary intraocular lens (IOL) prosthesis may be placed over an existing IOL implant ("piggybacked") to correct refractive errors following previous cataract surgery. The cornea is incised and viscoelastic material is injected into the anterior chamber to protect the corneal endothelium. The ciliary sulcus space is then distended with viscoelastic material, and the IOL mounted on an injector is placed into the eye. The lead haptic may be placed directly into the ciliary sulcus with the trailing haptic inserted into the eye and tucked behind the iris, or the entire lens can be delivered completely into the anterior chamber and both haptics secured under the iris. The viscoelastic material is removed from the eye and the corneal incision is closed with suture or stromal hydration.

66986

66986   Exchange of intraocular lens

The exchange of a previously placed intraocular lens (IOL) may be required to correct refractive errors following cataract surgery. The cornea is incised to create a paracentesis, and the anterior chamber is inflated with viscoelastic. A capsulorrhexis needle is advanced and dispersive viscoelastic is injected to separate the anterior capsule from the IOL. A blunt spatula is then used to dissect the anterior capsule from the IOL. Viscoelastic is then injected under the IOL to dissect it from the posterior capsule and the IOL is lifted, injecting more dispersive viscoelastic as necessary. A second paracentesis may be required to access 360 degrees around the IOL and complete the dissection. The IOL is dialed out of the capsule and into the anterior chamber where it can be folded and removed or cut with scissors and removed in pieces. Using a lens injector, the exchange IOL may be inserted behind the first IOL, before it is removed or it can be inserted after removal of the first IOL. The viscoelastic is removed from the eye and the corneal incision(s) are closed with suture or stromal hydration.

66990

66990   Use of ophthalmic endoscope (List separately in addition to code for primary procedure)

An ophthalmic endoscope provides better visualization of the anterior chamber, lens, and posterior segment than an operating microscope for certain types of procedures. Two stab incisions are made in the limbus. A cannula is inserted through one stab incision and viscoelastic material injected as needed to improve visualization. The endoscope is then inserted through the second stab incision and the surgical site carefully examined. Information obtained during the endoscopic exam is used to help plan the best surgical course for the patient. The physician then proceeds with the corrective procedure using endoscopic visualization as needed.

67005-67010

67005   Removal of vitreous, anterior approach (open sky technique or limbal incision); partial removal
67010   Removal of vitreous, anterior approach (open sky technique or limbal incision); subtotal removal with mechanical vitrectomy

Vitreous is a clear gel-like substance that fills the posterior chamber of the eye. An anterior approach requires either an open sky technique or a limbal incision. Using an open sky technique, an incision is made in the cornea. Alternatively a curvalinear incision is made in the limbus which is the edge of the cornea where the cornea joins the sclera. Vitreous removal has three components, cutting of vitreous strands, suction, and infusion of saline. In 67005, a needle or scissors is used for partial removal of the vitreous. In 67010, a mechanical device is used to remove the vitreous, such rotoextractors or a VISC device. This procedure may also involve severing of membranes and adhesions to achieve subtotal removal of the vitreous.

67015

67015   Aspiration or release of vitreous, subretinal or choroidal fluid, pars plana approach (posterior sclerotomy)

Ocular fluid normally moves between the vitreous and the choroid through a membrane called the retinal pigment epithelium (RPE). The RPE actively pumps ions and water from the vitreous into the choroid without pooling. When there is an increase in inflow or a decrease in outflow, fluid may accumulate in the subretinal space, causing an increase in ocular pressure and placing the patient at risk for retinal detachment. Vitreous, subretinal, and/or choroidal fluid may be aspirated to relieve the intraocular pressure. Anesthetic drops are instilled and an antibacterial solution is used to wash the surface of the eye. An area in the pars plana is identified and marked. A small gauge needle attached to an empty syringe is inserted through the marked area into the posterior eye and the accumulated ocular fluid is aspirated. The needle is withdrawn and a cotton tipped applicator is used to apply pressure at the puncture site. The puncture site is checked for fluid leakage and antibiotic eye drops may be instilled.

67025

67025   Injection of vitreous substitute, pars plana or limbal approach (fluid-gas exchange), with or without aspiration (separate procedure)

The vitreous humor is a clear substance of non-uniform density located in the posterior eye behind the lens. It is firmly attached to the anterior retina at the vitreous base. The consistency of vitreous humor is gel-like in early years and becomes more fluid like as a person ages. Vitreous humor may be lost due to eye injury or during vitrectomy, and replacement of the fluid with a vitreous substitute is necessary to relieve traction on the retina and allow a scar to form. Anesthetic drops are instilled and an antibacterial solution is used to wash the surface of the eye. An injection site is identified and marked in the area of the pars plana or limbus. A small gauge needle attached to a syringe containing the vitreous substitute is inserted through the marked area into the posterior eye and the vitreous substitute is injected. Substances may include gas (sulfur hexafluoride, n-perfluorpropane), air, and/or oil (polydimetylsiloxane). The needle is withdrawn and a cotton tipped applicator is used to apply pressure to the puncture site, which is then checked for fluid leakage. Antibiotic eye drops may be instilled.

67027

67027   Implantation of intravitreal drug delivery system (eg, ganciclovir implant), includes concomitant removal of vitreous

Implantable intravitreal drug delivery systems provide sustained release of a drug/medication to the posterior segment of the eye. This system may be used to treat conditions such as cytomegalovirus (CMV), macular degeneration, uveitis, diabetic retinopathy and retinal venous occlusions. Non-biodegradable implants include Vitrasert (contains the antiviral drug ganciclovir) and Retisert (contains the corticosteroid drug fluocinolone acetate). These devices can be implanted using local anesthesia in the ophthalmologist's office or same day surgery center. A 4-6 mm incision is made in the pars plana (area between the iris and sclera) near the cornea. A portion of the vitreous gel is removed and replaced with the implant. A suture is placed through a hub or tab on the implant and secured to the sclera. The pars plana incision is closed and saline is injected into the eye to return the intraocular pressure to normal. There are a number of implants that can be inserted into the posterior eye without an incision or removal of the vitreous gel. These include Iluvien, a non-biodegradable intravitreal implant containing the corticosteroid fluocinolone acetate which is inserted using a 25 gauge needle through the area of the pars plana and the biodegradable intravitreal implant, Ozurdex (Posturdex) containing the corticosteroid dexamethasone which is inserted using a customized 22 gauge applicator.

67028

67028   Intravitreal injection of a pharmacologic agent (separate procedure)

Intravitreal injection of a pharmacologic agent (drug, medication) can be performed without an incision or removal of a portion of the vitreous gel. Intravitral injected medications include Lucentis (Ranibizumab) a monoclonal antibody fragment which blocks vascular endothelial growth factor (VEGF) and is approved to treat neovascular (wet) age related macular degeneration (AMD) and macular edema following retinal vein occlusion. Macugen (Pegaptonib sodium) and Eylea (Aflibercept) are VEGF antagonists also approved for the treatment of neovascular AMD. Avastin (Bevacizumab) a VEGF antagonist, is sometimes used "off label" to treat AMD by intravitreal injection. Intravitreal injections are performed outpatient in the physician's office. A topical ophthalmic anesthetic is placed in the eye and then the eye is cleansed with an antiseptic. An eyelid speculum is placed and the injections site(s) marked. A short 30 gauge needle is inserted into the mid-vitreous

cavity, medication is injected and the needle is removed. Antibiotic eye drops may be instilled and the eye may be patched following the procedure.

67030

67030   Discission of vitreous strands (without removal), pars plana approach

Vitreous strands may become incarcerated (trapped) in a corneoscleral wound or incision following surgery or trauma to the eye. This may lead to cystoid macular edema, loss of vision or the appearance of "floaters", dark shadowy areas in the visual field. With the patient supine and the eye prepped, an anterior limbal (pars plana) incision is made into the anterior chamber. The area is swept using a cyclodialysis spatula and the vitreous strands are pulled back into the posterior segment of the eye. The incision is then closed with 10-0 suture.

67031

67031   Severing of vitreous strands, vitreous face adhesions, sheets, membranes or opacities, laser surgery (1 or more stages)

The normal vitreous degenerates with age and the clear vitreous gel can dehydrate and clump together. These clumps (vitreous densities) cast shadows on the sensory retina causing "floaters" or dark shadowy areas in the visual field. Vitreous densities may also be caused by more complicated pathological conditions such as retinal tears and hemorrhage, inflammation and infection, diabetes and autoimmune disorders. Vitreolysis of the strands (vitreous densities) can be accomplished using a neodymium YAG laser. The procedure is performed in the physician's office with the patient seated before a slit lamp. A special contact lens is inserted to keep the eye immobile during the procedure. The laser beam is directed to the vitreous strand or area of density and concentrated energy vaporizes the material. The molecules are converted to a gas micro bubble which is absorbed and disappears within a few hours of the procedure.

67036–67040

67036   Vitrectomy, mechanical, pars plana approach
67039   Vitrectomy, mechanical, pars plana approach; with focal endolaser photocoagulation
67040   Vitrectomy, mechanical, pars plana approach; with endolaser panretinal photocoagulation

A mechanical vitrectomy using a pars plana approach is performed. The vitreous is a clear, gel-like substance that fills the center of the eye. Removal of the vitreous may be performed to treat hemorrhage, clear debris from the vitreous, remove scar tissue, or alleviate tension on the retina. Three tiny incisions are made in the eye in the pars plana, located in front of the ciliary body and behind the retina. A light pipe, an infusion port, and a vitrectomy device are then inserted. The inside of the eye is illuminated with the light pipe. The vitrectomy device, a microscopic oscillating cutting device, is activated and the vitreous gel is removed from the eye in a slow, controlled fashion. As the vitreous gel is removed, it is replaced with fluid through the infusion port to maintain proper pressure in the eye. When the vitreous has been extracted, the surgical instruments are removed. Use 67039 when repair of the retina using focal endolaser photocoagulation is also done. A mechanical vitrectomy is performed as described above. An endoprobe is then inserted and small focal lesions of the retina are repaired using endolaser photocoagulation. Use 67040 when repair of the retina using panretinal endolaser photocoagulation is done following the mechanical vitrectomy. An endoprobe is inserted and the entire retina is treated by photocoagulation.

67041

67041   Vitrectomy, mechanical, pars plana approach; with removal of preretinal cellular membrane (eg, macular pucker)

A mechanical vitrectomy with removal of the preretinal cellular membrane (macular pucker) is performed via pars plana approach. The vitreous is a clear, gel-like substance that fills the center of the eye. It is removed prior to surgical treatment of macular pucker, also referred to as epiretinal membrane or preretinal membrane. A macular pucker occurs when the vitreous detaches from the retina, causing microscopic damage resulting in scar tissue at the site of the detachment. This can cause blurred or distorted vision. Three tiny incisions are made in the eye in the pars plana, located in front of the ciliary body and behind the retina. A light pipe, an infusion port, and a vitrectomy device are then inserted. The inside of the eye is illuminated with the light pipe. The vitrectomy device, a microscopic oscillating cutting device, is activated and vitreous gel is removed from the eye in a slow, controlled fashion. As the vitreous gel is removed, it is replaced with fluid through the infusion port to maintain proper pressure in the eye. The central vitreous is removed and the vitreous base is accessed. Using high magnification, the edge of the cellular membrane is elevated. Microforceps are introduced and the preretinal cellular membrane is elevated further and removed. The retina is examined for tearing before the surgical tools are removed.

Eye and Ocular Adnexa

67042

67042   Vitrectomy, mechanical, pars plana approach; with removal of internal limiting membrane of retina (eg, for repair of macular hole, diabetic macular edema), includes, if performed, intraocular tamponade (ie, air, gas or silicone oil)

A mechanical vitrectomy with peeling of the internal limiting membrane (ILM) for repair of a macular hole or diabetic macular edema is performed using a pars plana approach. The vitreous is a clear, gel-like substance that fills the center of the eye. It is removed prior to surgical treatment of a macular hole or diabetic macular edema. A macular hole occurs when the vitreous detaches from the retina, causing a tear that results in fluid leaking into the hole at the site of the detachment. Diabetic macular edema is caused by leaking vessels, resulting in retinal swelling (edema). In the case of macular holes, ILM peeling is done to release macular traction and prevent recurrences with optimal visual recovery. Three tiny incisions are made in the eye in the pars plana, located in front of the ciliary body and behind the retina. A light pipe, an infusion port, and a vitrectomy device are then inserted. The inside of the eye is illuminated with the light pipe. The vitrectomy device, a microscopic oscillating cutting device, is activated and vitreous gel is removed from the eye in a slow, controlled fashion. As the vitreous gel is removed, it is replaced with fluid through the infusion port to maintain proper pressure in the eye. The posterior cortical vitreous is separated from the optic nerve head and posterior retina. Indocyanine green may be used to selectively stain the ILM, which is peeled by making a small opening and flap tear with vitreous forceps. A continuous, curvilinear tear is made completely around the macular hole. Air-fluid exchange is done by injecting hexafluoride gas and the retina is examined for tearing. The patient must remain in the prone position for several days and anatomic closure occurs in about a month's time.

67043

67043   Vitrectomy, mechanical, pars plana approach; with removal of subretinal membrane (eg, choroidal neovascularization), includes, if performed, intraocular tamponade (ie, air, gas or silicone oil) and laser photocoagulation

A mechanical vitrectomy with removal of the subretinal membrane for treatment of choroidal neovascularization (CNV) is performed using a pars plana approach. The vitreous is a clear, gel-like substance that fills the center of the eye. It is removed prior to surgical treatment of CNV-the growth of new blood vessels in the choroid resulting from a break in the structural layer beneath the retina (Bruch's membrane), which separates the choroidal or vascular layer from the retina. When a break occurs, the vascular in-growth of new blood vessels leak fluid or blood, causing distorted vision and scarring of the macula. CNV has a number of causes but occurs most often in patients with proliferative diabetic vitreoretinopathy, causing traction that results in retinal detachment, or giant retinal tears. CNV is a major cause of visual loss. Three tiny incisions are made in the eye in the pars plana, located in front of the ciliary body and behind the retina. A light pipe, an infusion port, and a vitrectomy device are then inserted. The inside of the eye is illuminated with the light pipe. The vitrectomy device, a microscopic oscillating cutting device, is activated and vitreous gel is removed from the eye in a slow, controlled fashion. As the vitreous gel is removed, it is replaced with fluid through the infusion port to maintain proper pressure in the eye. The retina is next incised (retinotomy) and the subretinal space is expanded. Using high magnification, microforceps are introduced and the neovascular membrane is grasped and carefully removed from the subretinal space and then from the eye. The retina is examined for tearing. An intraocular tamponade may be performed using air, gas, or silicone oil if needed to prevent fluid from leaking into the retina.

67101-67105

▲ **67101   Repair of retinal detachment, including drainage of subretinal fluid when performed; cryotherapy**

▲ **67105   Repair of retinal detachment, including drainage of subretinal fluid when performed; photocoagulation**

Retinal detachment occurs when the retina separates from its normal position and the inner layers of the retina pull away from the choroid. Detachment results in blurred vision and if left untreated may cause blindness. A lid speculum is used to open the eyelids and expose the eye. In 67101, a freezing probe is used to treat the retinal detachment. Cryotherapy is performed to the outer surface of the eye through an intact sclera over the site of the retinal detachment. The cryotherapy probe is used to create a series of ice balls around the area of detachment. A lamellar scleral dissection is performed over the site of the detachment. As the frozen area over and around the detachment heals, scar tissue develops that helps secure the retina to the choroid. In 67105, a laser beam (photocoagulation) is directed through a contact lens or specially designed ophthalmoscope to the site of the retinal detachment. The laser beam is used to burn the tissue around the detachment resulting in scarring that secures the retina to the underlying choroid. Following the cryotherapy or photocoagulation, the physician may drain subretinal fluid. The sclera is incised over the area of retinal elevation and the choroid is punctured. Subretinal fluid is drained. When sufficient fluid has been expressed, the puncture site is dried and inspected to ensure that it has sealed. The scleral incision is closed with sutures.

67107

67107   Repair of retinal detachment; scleral buckling (such as lamellar scleral dissection, imbrication or encircling procedure), including, when performed, implant, cryotherapy, photocoagulation, and drainage of subretinal fluid

Retinal detachment occurs when the retina separates from its normal position and the inner layers of the retina pull away from the choroid. Detachment results in blurred vision and if left untreated may cause blindness. A lid speculum is used to open the eyelids and expose the eye. Local anesthesia is administered. Scleral buckling is the most frequently performed procedure to treat retinal detachment. Scleral buckles are typically fabricated with silicone. Buckles come in a variety of types and shapes that are selected based on the size and location of the retinal defect. The retina is repaired as needed using a freezing probe (cryotherapy, cryopexy) or laser photocoagulation. Cryotherapy is performed to the outer surface of the eye through an intact sclera over the site of the retinal detachment. The cryotherapy probe is used to create a series of ice balls around the area of detachment. Alternatively, a laser beam (photocoagulation) is directed through a contact lens or specially designed ophthalmoscope to the site of the retinal detachment and used to burn the tissue around the detachment. As the frozen or burned area over and around the detachment heals, scar tissue develops that helps secure the retina to the choroid. Following the cryotherapy or laser photocoagulation, one of the rectus muscles is detached to access the sclera. The scleral buckle is then secured to the sclera. The buckle pushes the sclera toward the middle of the eye and relieves traction on the retina which allows the retina to settle against the choroid and heal. The physician may also drain subretinal fluid. The sclera is incised over the area of retinal elevation and the choroid is punctured. Subretinal fluid is drained. When sufficient fluid has been expressed, the puncture site is dried and inspected to ensure that it has sealed. The scleral incision is closed with sutures.

67108

67108   Repair of retinal detachment; with vitrectomy, any method, including, when performed, air or gas tamponade, focal endolaser photocoagulation, cryotherapy, drainage of subretinal fluid, scleral buckling, and/or removal of lens by same technique

Retinal detachment occurs when the retina separates from its normal position and the inner layers of the retina pull away from the choroid. Detachment results in blurred vision and if left untreated may cause blindness. A lid speculum is used to open the eyelids and expose the eye. Local anesthesia is administered. Vitreous is a clear gel-like substance that fills the center of the eye. It is removed prior to the repair of the retinal detachment. To perform mechanical vitrectomy, three small incisions are made in the pars plana. A light pipe, an infusion port, and a vitrectomy device are inserted. The eye is illuminated with the light pipe. The vitrectomy device, a microscopic oscillating cutting device, is activated and vitreous is removed from the eye in a slow, controlled fashion. As the vitreous is removed, it is replaced with fluid to maintain proper eye pressure. Following removal of vitreous, the retina is repaired as needed using a freezing probe (cryotherapy, cryopexy) or laser photocoagulation. The lens may be removed to provide better access to the retina. Cryotherapy is performed to the outer surface of the eye through an intact sclera over the site of the retinal detachment. The cryotherapy probe is used to create a series of ice balls around the area of detachment. Alternatively, a laser beam (photocoagulation) is directed through a contact lens or specially designed ophthalmoscope to the site of the retinal detachment and used to burn the tissue around the detachment. As the frozen or burned area over and around the detachment heals, scar tissue develops that helps secure the retina to the choroid. If a scleral buckle is needed, one of the rectus muscles is detached to access the sclera. The buckle is then secured to the sclera. The buckle pushes the sclera toward the middle of the eye and relieves traction on the retina which allows the retina to settle against the choroid and heal. An intraocular tamponade may be performed using air or gas to prevent fluid from leaking into the retina. The physician may also drain subretinal fluid. The sclera is incised over the area of retinal elevation and the choroid is punctured. Subretinal fluid is drained. When sufficient fluid has been expressed, the puncture site is dried and inspected to ensure that it has sealed. The scleral incision is closed with sutures.

67110

67110   Repair of retinal detachment; by injection of air or other gas (eg, pneumatic retinopexy)

Retinal detachment occurs when the retina separates from its normal position and the inner layers of the retina pull away from the choroid. Detachment results in blurred vision and if left untreated may cause blindness. A lid speculum is used to open the eyelids and expose the eye. Local anesthetic is administered. Pneumatic retinopexy involves injecting air or another gas into the vitreal cavity at the site of the retinal detachment. The sclera is punctured and a needle advanced into the vitreous cavity. A gas bubble is injected. The head is positioned so that the gas bubble will move toward the area of detachment. The gas bubble then pushes the retina back against the choroid. Laser photocoagulation or cryotherapy may also be performed to seal the area of detachment. The patient may need to maintain the head in a certain position as much as possible for several weeks following the injection.

67113

67113   Repair of complex retinal detachment (eg, proliferative vitreoretinopathy, stage C-1 or greater, diabetic traction retinal detachment, retinopathy of prematurity, retinal tear of greater than 90 degrees), with vitrectomy and membrane peeling, including, when performed, air, gas, or silicone oil tamponade, cryotherapy, endolaser photocoagulation, drainage of subretinal fluid, scleral buckling, and/or removal of lens

A complex retinal detachment is repaired using multiple modalities including vitrectomy and membrane peeling. Complex retinal detachments are tears greater than 90 degrees or those resulting from conditions such as proliferative vitreoretinopathy with stage C-1 or greater, diabetic traction retinal detachment, or retinopathy of prematurity. Retinal detachment is the separation of the inner layers of the retina from the underlying choroid, also referred to as the retinal pigment epithelium (RPE), a vascular membrane that contains branched pigment cells lying between the retina and sclera. The conjunctiva is incised around the periphery of the cornea (peritomy). Tenon's capsule is peeled back and the rectus muscle is isolated. A vitrectomy device is inserted into the sclera. Two additional incisions are made in the sclera for a light pipe and infusion port. The inside of the eye is illuminated with the light pipe. The vitrectomy device, a microscopic oscillating cutting device, is activated and vitreous gel is removed from the center of the eye in a slow, controlled fashion. As the vitreous gel is removed, it is replaced with fluid through the infusion port to maintain proper pressure in the eye. The cellular membrane is then meticulously removed from the retinal surface and the retina is examined for tears. The posterior aspect of the retina may be opened (retinotomy), the subretinal fluid drained, and replaced with air, gas, or silicone oil to reattach the retina. Tears in the retina and the retinotomy are repaired using cryotherapy and/or endolaser photocoagulation. The lens may be removed to provide better access to the retina. Cryotherapy is performed to the outer surface of the eye through an intact sclera over the site of the retinal detachment. The cryotherapy probe is used to create a series of ice balls around the area of detachment. Alternatively, a laser beam (photocoagulation) is directed through a contact lens or specially designed ophthalmoscope to the site of the retinal detachment and used to burn the tissue around the detachment. As the frozen or burned area over heals, scar tissue develops that helps secure the retina to the choroid. A scleral buckle comprised of silicone, rubber, sponge, or soft plastic, may also be secured to the sclera to relieve traction on the retinal detachment, allowing the retina to settle against the choroid and heal. Incisions in the sclera and conjunctiva are closed.

67115

67115   Release of encircling material (posterior segment)

Release of encircling material (scleral buckle) is typically performed for infection or intrusion of the buckle into the scleral tissue. A lid speculum is used to open the eyelids and expose the eye. Local anesthesia is administered. One of the rectus muscles is detached to access the sclera. The encircling material is then cut and removed. If the implant has intruded into the scleral tissue it is removed using a device such as a fragmatome which breaks up and aspirates the pieces of the device that have become embedded in the sclera. The rectus muscle is reattached.

67120-67121

67120   Removal of implanted material, posterior segment; extraocular
67121   Removal of implanted material, posterior segment; intraocular

A procedure is performed to remove extraocular or intraocular implanted material from the posterior segment of the eye. The posterior segment contains the anterior hyaloid membrane and the optical structures behind it including the vitreous humor, retina, choroid, and optic nerve. The most common materials removed are silicone oil and displaced intraocular lenses without performing a vitrectomy.

67141-67145

67141   Prophylaxis of retinal detachment (eg, retinal break, lattice degeneration) without drainage, 1 or more sessions; cryotherapy, diathermy
67145   Prophylaxis of retinal detachment (eg, retinal break, lattice degeneration) without drainage, 1 or more sessions; photocoagulation (laser or xenon arc)

Prophylaxis is performed on a break, hole, or tear or lattice degeneration of the retina. Prophylactic treatment is required to prevent retinal detachment. A lid speculum is used to open the eyelids and expose the eye. Local anesthetic is administered. In 67141, a freezing probe (cryotherapy, cryopexy) or heat probe (diathermy) is used to treat the retinal defect. Cryotherapy is performed to the outer surface of the eye through an intact sclera over the site of the retinal defect. The cryotherapy probe is used to create a series of ice balls around the area of the defect. Diathermy uses a radiofrequency current to generate heat and burn the region around the defect. A lamellar scleral dissection is performed over the site of the defect. Diathermy burns are placed in the sclera bed using a blunt tipped electrode. As the frozen or burned area over and around the break or degeneration heals, scar tissue develops that closes the defect and secures the retina to the choroid. In 67145, a laser beam (photocoagulation) is directed through a contact lens or specially designed

ophthalmoscope to the site of the retinal defect. The laser beam is used to burn the tissue around the defect resulting in scarring that secures the retina to the underlying choroid.

67208-67210

67208   Destruction of localized lesion of retina (eg, macular edema, tumors), 1 or more sessions; cryotherapy, diathermy
67210   Destruction of localized lesion of retina (eg, macular edema, tumors), 1 or more sessions; photocoagulation

A lid speculum is used to open the eyelids and expose the eye. In 67208, a freezing probe (cryotherapy, cryopexy) or heat probe (diathermy) is used to destroy a localized lesion of the retina, such as a tumor or macular edema. Visual acuity is checked. The pupil is dilated and a local anesthetic administered to the surface of the retina. Cryotherapy is performed to the outer surface of the eye through an intact sclera over the site of the retinal lesion. The cryotherapy probe is positioned and the probe cooled to the desired temperature. Ice ball formation is monitored. Once the ice ball has encompassed the entire lesion, the tissue is warmed. This is repeated until the entire lesion has been destroyed. Diathermy uses a radiofrequency current to generate heat. A lamellar scleral dissection is performed over the site of the lesion. Diathermy burns are placed in the scleral bed at the site of the lesion using a blunt tipped electrode and the lesion is completely destroyed. In 67210, a laser beam (photocoagulation) is directed through a contact lens or specially designed ophthalmoscope to the site of the lesion. The laser beam is used to destroy the entire lesion.

67218

67218   Destruction of localized lesion of retina (eg, macular edema, tumors), 1 or more sessions; radiation by implantation of source (includes removal of source)

A procedure is performed to insert (or remove) a radioactive implant in the eye to treat macular edema and localized lesions of the choroid, retina, or iris such as tumors like melanoma. This treatment may be referred to as plaque radiotherapy, plaque brachytherapy, radiation implant, or radioactive source implantation. The device consists of a custom made, sealed metal plaque containing small radioactive seeds. The radioactive seeds deliver a precise dose of radiation to a prescribed area for a period of 4-7 days, after which the device is removed. An incision is made in the conjunctiva and the plaque is centered over the lesion and sutured to the sclera to keep it in place. The conjunctiva is then sutured closed and the eye is covered with a lead shield. At the conclusion of the treatment, the conjunctiva is incised, the plaque is removed, and the conjunctiva is closed again with sutures.

67220

67220   Destruction of localized lesion of choroid (eg, choroidal neovascularization); photocoagulation (eg, laser), 1 or more sessions

Destruction of a localized lesion of the choroid is performed in one or more sessions using photocoagulation. Laser photocoagulation uses a laser to physically ablate abnormal choroidal tissue, such as a choroidal neovascularization (CNV), a disorder in which new blood vessels originating in the choroid break through the Bruch membrane into the subretinal pigment epithelium or subretinal space. CNV is a major cause of vision loss. The lesion is delineated using fluoroscein angiography and then destroyed using multiple laser burns. After each firing of the laser, the surgeon evaluates the burn area, the tissue's reaction to the burn, and the remaining extent of the lesion to be destroyed, including both thickness and diameter. The procedure is performed in one or more sessions during a defined treatment period that may occur at different encounters on different days.

67221-67225

67221   Destruction of localized lesion of choroid (eg, choroidal neovascularization); photodynamic therapy (includes intravenous infusion)
67225   Destruction of localized lesion of choroid (eg, choroidal neovascularization); photodynamic therapy, second eye, at single session (List separately in addition to code for primary eye treatment)

Destruction of a localized lesion of the choroid is performed using photodynamic therapy to ablate abnormal choroidal tissue, such as choroidal neovascularization (CNV), a disorder in which new blood vessels originating in the choroid break through the Bruch membrane into the subretinal pigment epithelium or subretinal space. CNV is a major cause of vision loss. Photodynamic therapy (PDT) uses a low-energy targeted laser light to activate a photoactive drug that is administered intravenously prior to PDT. The photoactive drug, Verteporfin, is administered by intravenous infusion over an approximate 10 min period 15 min prior to the initiation of PDT. The lesion is then destroyed using a contact lens and slit lamp to direct the low-energy laser at the targeted lesion. The procedure may be performed on one or both eyes during a single session. Use 67221 for PDT on the first eye and 67225 for PDT on the second eye performed during the same session.

Eye and Ocular Adnexa

67227

67227   Destruction of extensive or progressive retinopathy (eg, diabetic retinopathy), cryotherapy, diathermy

Extensive or progressive retinopathy (diabetic retinopathy) is destroyed using extreme cold (cryotherapy) or extreme heat (diathermy) in 67227, or treated using photocoagulation in 67228. Extensive or progressive (diabetic) retinopathy is characterized by damage to the blood vessels, which swell and leak blood or cause new blood vessels to form on the surface of the retina. Visual acuity is checked. The pupil is dilated and a local anesthetic is administered. The cryoprobe or diathermy probe is briefly placed on the surface of the eye overlying the periphery of the retina and the damaged blood vessels are destroyed by freezing or heat. When laser photocoagulation is used for treatment, it is administered by a technique referred to as scatter laser treatment or pan retinal photocoagulation (PRP), in which as many as 2,000 burns are placed in the mid-periphery and periphery of the retina, taking care to avoid the area of central vision, the macula. The burns destroy oxygen-deprived retinal tissue, seal leaking blood vessels, and prevent the formation of new blood vessels. The procedure may be performed using a slit lamp delivery system, which requires placement of a fundus contact lens, or indirect delivery system.

67228

67228   Treatment of extensive or progressive retinopathy (eg, diabetic retinopathy), photocoagulation

Extensive or progressive retinopathy (diabetic retinopathy) is destroyed using extreme cold (cryotherapy) or extreme heat (diathermy) in 67227, or treated using photocoagulation in 67228. Extensive or progressive (diabetic) retinopathy is characterized by damage to the blood vessels, which swell and leak blood or cause new blood vessels to form on the surface of the retina. Visual acuity is checked. The pupil is dilated and a local anesthetic is administered. The cryoprobe or diathermy probe is briefly placed on the surface of the eye overlying the periphery of the retina and the damaged blood vessels are destroyed by freezing or heat. When laser photocoagulation is used for treatment, it is administered by a technique referred to as scatter laser treatment or pan retinal photocoagulation (PRP), in which as many as 2,000 burns are placed in the mid-periphery and periphery of the retina, taking care to avoid the area of central vision, the macula. The burns destroy oxygen-deprived retinal tissue, seal leaking blood vessels, and prevent the formation of new blood vessels. The procedure may be performed using a slit lamp delivery system, which requires placement of a fundus contact lens, or indirect delivery system.

67229

67229   Treatment of extensive or progressive retinopathy, 1 or more sessions; preterm infant (less than 37 weeks gestation at birth), performed from birth up to 1 year of age (eg, retinopathy of prematurity), photocoagulation or cryotherapy

Extensive progressive retinopathy of a preterm infant (retinopathy of prematurity) is treated by photocoagulation or cryotherapy in one or more sessions. A preterm infant is defined as being less than 37 weeks gestation at birth. The procedure may be performed from birth up to one year of age. Retinopathy of prematurity (ROP), also referred to as retrolental fibroplasia, primarily affects premature infants that are less than 31 weeks gestation and weigh less than 1250 grams (2.75 pounds) at birth. ROP is characterized by the failure of blood vessels in the retina to reach the periphery and an abnormal proliferation of blood vessels where they terminate. These fragile blood vessels may leak, causing scarring and traction on the retina that may cause it to detach, resulting in vision impairment or blindness. A topical anesthetic is administered. Mydriatic drops are applied to dilate the pupil as needed. Scleral depression is applied to position the eye. Regions of normal, abnormal, and absent vascularization are identified. If cryotherapy (freezing) is used to destroy the abnormal vasculature or avascular regions in the retina, a cryoprobe is briefly placed on the surface of the eye overlying the regions of abnormal or absent vasculature in the retina. If laser photocoagulation is used, as many as 1,500 burns may be applied to the abnormal vasculature or avascular regions in the retina using an indirect ophthalmoscopic laser delivery system. Care is taken to avoid damage to the iris and crystalline lens. Both laser treatment and cryotherapy destroy the peripheral areas of the retina that have no normal vasculature. Care is taken to preserve the area of central vision (macula).

67250-67255

67250   Scleral reinforcement (separate procedure); without graft
67255   Scleral reinforcement (separate procedure); with graft

Scleral reinforcement is performed in a separate procedure to treat high myopia and help prevent damage to the macula associated with this condition. A lid speculum is used to open the eyelids and expose the eye. Local anesthesia is administered. The conjunctiva and Tenon's capsule are incised about 6 mm from the corneal limbus. The lateral, superior and inferior recti muscles are separated using a strabismus hook. Connective tissue is dissected away from the posterior pole and inferior oblique muscle. In 67250, the sclera is reinforced without the use of a graft. This involves creating an indentation in the posterior aspect of the sclera. In this procedure, the thinned weakened region of the posterior sclera is oversewn with a thick piece of rubber or sponge material which causes the posterior

region to indent or buckle. A strip of synthetic material may be used to create a sling, which provides additional support of the posterior sclera. The sling is passed under the separated muscles along the posterior pole of the eye. The sling is sutured to the anteromedial and anterolateral sclera. In 67255, a graft is used to reinforce the sclera. Once the posterior aspect of the sclera has been exposed, an allograft, usually donor sclera, is used to reinforce the weak sclera at the back of the eye. The graft is sutured to the healthy, stronger anterior sclera. The muscles are repaired and the Tenon's capsule and conjunctive closed.

67311-67316

67311   Strabismus surgery, recession or resection procedure; 1 horizontal muscle
67312   Strabismus surgery, recession or resection procedure; 2 horizontal muscles
67314   Strabismus surgery, recession or resection procedure; 1 vertical muscle (excluding superior oblique)
67316   Strabismus surgery, recession or resection procedure; 2 or more vertical muscles (excluding superior oblique)

The eye has six extraocular muscles that control eye movement. If a muscle is too strong, it can cause the eye to turn in, turn out, or rotate too high or too low. If a muscle is too weak, the eyes may be misaligned. For an extraocular muscle that is too strong, a recession procedure of the affected eye is performed. For an extraocular muscle that is too weak, a recession procedure of the opposing eye is performed. In a recession procedure, the extraocular muscle is detached from the eye and reattached farther back on the eye to weaken the strength of the stronger muscle relative to the opposing weaker muscle. Alternatively a resection procedure may be used to strengthen an eye muscle and correct misalignment of the eye. Resection involves detaching the eye muscle from the eye and reattaching it in a new location. A small incision is made in the conjunctiva over the extraocular muscle. The muscle is detached from the globe. The eye muscle is then reattached with sutures farther back on the globe or in a new location to correct the misalignment of the eyes. The incision in the conjunctiva is closed. Use 67311 if recession or resection is performed on either the lateral or medial rectus muscle. Use 67312 if the procedure is performed on both the lateral and medial rectus muscle of the same eye. Use 67314 if the procedure is performed on either the superior or inferior rectus muscle. Use 67316 if the procedure is performed on both the superior and inferior rectus muscles of the same eye.

67318

67318   Strabismus surgery, any procedure, superior oblique muscle

The superior oblique muscle of the eye attaches to the superolateral aspect of the globe, passes through a tendon called the trochlea at the medial (nasal) aspect of the orbit and then attaches to the posterior aspect of the orbit. Because this code is for any procedure on the superior oblique muscle the exact procedure performed will depend on the condition being treated. One procedure, called the Harada-Ito procedure, is used to treat misalignment of the eye due to cranial nerve IV palsy. An incision is made in the conjunctiva over the superior oblique muscle. The superior oblique tendon is split and the anterior fibers are moved in an anterior and lateral direction and reattached to the globe. The conjunctival incision is closed with sutures.

67320

67320   Transposition procedure (eg, for paretic extraocular muscle), any extraocular muscle (specify) (List separately in addition to code for primary procedure)

Transposition of the extraocular muscles involves detaching and moving an extraocular muscle to a new location on the globe. This type of procedure is performed at the time of another separately reportable strabismus procedure. It may be performed to treat paralysis or paresis of an extraocular muscle caused by damage to one of the cranial nerves (CN III, CN IV, or CN VI). A conjunctival incision is made over the extraocular muscle or muscles that are to be detached. The muscle(s) is detached from the globe, moved to a new position, and secured to the globe with sutures. The conjunctival incision is closed.

67331-67332

67331   Strabismus surgery on patient with previous eye surgery or injury that did not involve the extraocular muscles (List separately in addition to code for primary procedure)
67332   Strabismus surgery on patient with scarring of extraocular muscles (eg, prior ocular injury, strabismus or retinal detachment surgery) or restrictive myopathy (eg, dysthyroid ophthalmopathy) (List separately in addition to code for primary procedure)

Strabismus surgery on a patient who has had a previous procedure on the eye is technically more difficult. An incision is made in the conjunctiva over the affected extraocular muscle and the muscle insertion site is exposed. Scar tissue and adhesions are released and old suture material removed as needed. The separately reportable recession, resection or other strabismus procedure on the eye is then performed. Use 67331 for strabismus surgery on a patient with previous eye surgery or an eye injury that did not involve the extraocular muscles Use 67332 for strabismus surgery on a patient with scarring of the extraocular

Eye and Ocular Adnexa

muscles due to previous ocular injury or strabismus or retinal detachment surgery on patients with restrictive myopathy.

67334-67335

67334 Strabismus surgery by posterior fixation suture technique, with or without muscle recession (List separately in addition to code for primary procedure)

67335 Placement of adjustable suture(s) during strabismus surgery, including postoperative adjustment(s) of suture(s) (List separately in addition to code for specific strabismus surgery)

Two suture techniques that are sometimes used for strabismus surgery and increase the technical difficulty of the procedure include posterior fixation suture technique and adjustable sutures. In 67334, posterior fixation suture is performed. This suture technique is used to limit the action of the extraocular muscle or make the muscle work harder in its field of action without changing the primary position of the muscle. Posterior fixation suturing is usually used in the fixing eye. The extra work required of the muscle in the fixing eye causes extra innervation and has a straightening effect on the fellow eye. The eye muscle is exposed in a separately reportable primary procedure. Once the necessary components of the primary procedure have been completed the physician places posterior fixation sutures through the borders of the extraocular muscle. If posterior fixation is required on the lateral rectus muscle, the inferior oblique insertion is dissected from the lateral rectus muscle and the sutures are then placed. If posterior fixation is performed on the superior rectus, the fixation suture is placed behind the superior oblique muscle. If posterior fixation is performed on the inferior rectus, the inferior oblique and Lockwood's ligament are retracted and the fixation sutures placed. The primary procedure is completed and the operative incisions are closed. In 67335, adjustable sutures are placed. The eye muscle is exposed and a separately reportable recession or resection procedure is performed. Instead of placing permanent knots in the sutures, the physician places temporary suture knots. The physician then evaluates the eyes several hours after the surgery. Anesthetic eye drops are applied. If the eye alignment is good, permanent knots are tied. If the eye needs some additional realignment, the adjustable suture is used to modify the muscle tension. Once the eyes are aligned, permanent knots are tied.

67340

67340 Strabismus surgery involving exploration and/or repair of detached extraocular muscle(s) (List separately in addition to code for primary procedure)

During a separately reportable primary strabismus surgery, the physician explores the eye to find a detached extraocular muscle and/or repair it. Extraocular muscles may become detached following a previous recession or resection procedure, due to facial or ocular trauma, or during a surgical misadventure. The conjunctiva is incised over the affected extraocular muscle. Often there is extensive scar tissue from previous surgeries or from the eye injury that must be dissected. The orbit is explored and an attempt made to locate the eye muscle. If the eye muscle cannot be retrieved a separately reportable transposition procedure may be required. If the eye muscle is located it is carefully inspected to determine if it can be reattached. If it cannot be reattached due to traumatic injury or damage from previous surgeries, a separately reportable transposition procedure is performed. If it can be reattached the muscle is debrided and sutured to any remaining muscle at the insertion site or sutured to the globe in a new location. The primary strabismus procedure is then completed.

67343

67343 Release of extensive scar tissue without detaching extraocular muscle (separate procedure)

Eye movement may be affected by extensive scar tissue from a previous injury or previous eye surgery. An incision is made over the affected extraocular muscle. The muscle is exposed and inspected. Leaving the eye muscle attached to the globe, the surgeon addresses the scar tissue that is causing the impaired eye movement. Adhesions between the eye muscle and surrounding structures are lysed. The conjunctiva is closed.

67345

67345 Chemodenervation of extraocular muscle

Chemodenervation of extraocular muscles involves the injection of botulinum toxin type A (BTA) into one or more eye muscles which temporarily paralyzes the muscles. Chemodenervation is used to treat paralytic strabismus. The botulinum toxin is injected into the unopposed antagonist of the paralyzed muscle which causes paralysis of that muscle as well and corrects the strabismus. Injection is performed under electromyographic (EMG) control. An electrode is placed on the forehead. Anesthetic eye drops are administered and an eye speculum placed to keep the eyelids open. Additional local anesthetic is applied with a cotton swab at the planned conjunctival injection site. A needle electrode is attached to a syringe and to the EMG device. The needle is inserted through the conjunctiva and into the eye muscle close to the insertion site. The patient is instructed to move the eye and movement is monitored by the EMG device. The needle is adjusted as needed. Once the needle is properly placed the botulinum toxin is injected. Alternatively, the procedure may be performed under direct vision. The conjunctiva is incised over the

extraocular muscle. The muscle is engaged on a muscle hook and the botulinum toxin injected. The conjunctival incision is closed.

67346

67346 Biopsy of extraocular muscle

An extraocular muscle is biopsied. An ocular speculum is placed to hold the patient's eye open and incisions are made through the conjunctiva and sclera to expose the muscle. The target biopsy muscle is isolated and a small sampling of the muscle tissue is carefully removed so that the excision will not harm the overall function of the eye muscle. The wound is closed.

67400-67405

67400 Orbitotomy without bone flap (frontal or transconjunctival approach); for exploration, with or without biopsy

67405 Orbitotomy without bone flap (frontal or transconjunctival approach); with drainage only

The orbit is explored and other procedures, such as biopsy or drainage, performed via a frontal or transconjunctival approach without creating a bone flap. The exact procedure depends on the site of the lesion or other abnormality. A transconjunctival approach may be performed via an incision in the upper or lower conjunctival fornix. Soft tissues are dissected and the area of interest exposed. In 67400, the upper or lower aspect of the orbit is explored and any abnormalities noted. Tissue samples are obtained as needed and sent for separately reportable pathology evaluation. In 67405, a fluid collection is located, tissues incised, and the fluid is drained. Fluid samples may be sent for separately reportable laboratory evaluation. Soft tissues and the conjunctiva are closed in layers.

67412-67413

67412 Orbitotomy without bone flap (frontal or transconjunctival approach); with removal of lesion

67413 Orbitotomy without bone flap (frontal or transconjunctival approach); with removal of foreign body

The orbit is explored and other procedures, such as removal of a lesion or foreign body, performed via a frontal or transconjunctival approach without creating a bone flap. The exact procedure depends on the site of the lesion or foreign body. A transconjunctival approach may be performed via an incision in the upper or lower conjunctival fornix. Soft tissues are dissected and the area of interest exposed. In 67412, the upper or lower aspect of the orbit is explored and the lesion is located. The cystic or solid tumor is carefully dissected free of surrounding tissue taking care to remove all abnormal tissue along with a margin of normal tissue. The cystic or solid tumor is sent for separately reportable pathology evaluation. In 67413, a foreign body is located, grasped with forceps and removed. Alternatively, the foreign body may be carefully dissected from surrounding tissue and removed. The wound is flushed with sterile saline or antibiotic solution as needed. Soft tissues and the conjunctiva are closed in layers.

67414

67414 Orbitotomy without bone flap (frontal or transconjunctival approach); with removal of bone for decompression

The orbit is explored and orbital decompression with removal of bone performed via a frontal or transconjunctival approach without creating a bone flap. The exact procedure depends on the compartment of the eye requiring decompression. A transconjunctival approach may be performed via an incision in the upper or lower conjunctival fornix. Soft tissues are dissected and the area of interest exposed. The upper or lower aspect of the orbit is explored and the region requiring decompression identified. The orbital bone is exposed and the periosteum incised. Holes are drilled in the orbital bone and the holes are connected using an oscillating saw or osteotome. The area of bone causing the compression of the orbit is excised. Soft tissues and the conjunctiva are closed in layers.

67415

67415 Fine needle aspiration of orbital contents

A mass or lesion is evaluated using fine needle aspiration of orbital contents. The eyelid overlying the area of interest is cleansed. Local anesthetic eyedrops or gel may be used for patient comfort. The eye is held in place using firm pressure and the needle is inserted through the eyelid and into the mass or lesion. Once the needle is located in the desired region, the syringe plunger is retracted. The needle is moved back and forth within the desired region while maintaining negative pressure in the syringe. Once sufficient aspirate is obtained, the needle is removed and slides are prepared and a separately reportable evaluation of the fine needle aspirate is performed.

Eye and Ocular Adnexa

67420-67430

67420 Orbitotomy with bone flap or window, lateral approach (eg, Kroenlein); with removal of lesion

67430 Orbitotomy with bone flap or window, lateral approach (eg, Kroenlein); with removal of foreign body

The orbit is explored and definitive procedures such as removal of a lesion or foreign body performed via a lateral approach with creation of a bone flap or window. A lazy-S incision is made in the upper eyelid crease. The lateral rectus muscle is exposed and retracted. Soft tissues are dissected and the underlying zygomatic bone is exposed. The periosteum is incised and the edges undermined to expose the hard cortical bone of the zygoma. Holes are drilled and the holes connected using an oscillating saw to create a bone window or flap. The periorbita is incised. Underlying fat and soft tissue attachments are dissected and the orbit is exposed. In 67420, a lesion is removed. The lesion may be cystic or solid and may involve soft tissue and/or bony structures. The lesion is carefully dissected free of surrounding tissue taking care to remove all abnormal tissue along with a margin of normal tissue. The lesion is sent for separately reportable pathology evaluation. In 67430, a foreign body is located, grasped with forceps and removed. Alternatively, the foreign body may be carefully dissected from surrounding tissue and removed. The wound is flushed with sterile saline or antibiotic solution as needed. Orbital tissues are reapproximated and the periorbita is closed. The bone window or flap is replaced and secured with miniplates and screws. The periosteum is closed. Soft tissues and the skin of the eyelid are closed in layers.

67440

67440 Orbitotomy with bone flap or window, lateral approach (eg, Kroenlein); with drainage

The orbit is explored and drainage of a fluid collection performed via a lateral approach with creation of a bone flap or window. A lazy-S incision is made in the upper eyelid crease. The lateral rectus muscle is exposed and retracted. Soft tissues are dissected and the underlying zygomatic bone is exposed. The periosteum is incised and the edges undermined to expose the hard cortical bone of the zygoma. Holes are drilled and the holes connected using an oscillating saw to create a bone window or flap. The periorbita is incised. Underlying fat and soft tissue attachments are dissected and the orbit is exposed. The fluid collection is located, tissues incised, and the fluid drained. The operative site is flushed with sterile saline or antibiotic solution as needed. Orbital tissues are reapproximated and the periorbita is closed. The bone window or flap is replaced and secured with miniplates and screws. The periosteum is closed. Soft tissues and the skin of the eyelid are closed in layers.

67445

67445 Orbitotomy with bone flap or window, lateral approach (eg, Kroenlein); with removal of bone for decompression

The orbit is explored and orbital decompression with removal of bone performed via a lateral approach with creation of a bone flap or window. A lazy-S incision is made in the upper eyelid crease. The lateral rectus muscle is exposed and retracted. Soft tissues are dissected and the underlying zygomatic bone is exposed. The periosteum is incised and the edges undermined to expose the hard cortical bone of the zygoma. Holes are drilled and the holes connected using an oscillating saw to create a bone window or flap. The periorbita is incised. Underlying fat and soft tissue attachments are dissected and the orbit is exposed. Soft tissues are dissected and the area of interest exposed. The orbit is explored and the region requiring decompression identified. The orbital bone is exposed and the periosteum incised. Holes are drilled in the orbital bone and the holes are connected using an oscillating saw or osteotome. The area of bone causing the compression of the orbit is excised. Orbital tissues are reapproximated and the periorbita is closed. The zygomatic bone window or flap is replaced and secured with miniplates and screws. The periosteum is closed. Soft tissues and the skin of the eyelid are closed in layers.

67450

67450 Orbitotomy with bone flap or window, lateral approach (eg, Kroenlein); for exploration, with or without biopsy

The orbit is explored and tissue samples obtained as needed via a lateral approach with creation of a bone flap or window. A lazy-S incision is made in the upper eyelid crease. The lateral rectus muscle is exposed and retracted. Soft tissues are dissected and the underlying zygomatic bone is exposed. The periosteum is incised and the edges undermined to expose the hard cortical bone of the zygoma. Holes are drilled and the holes connected using an oscillating saw to create a bone window or flap. The periorbita is incised. Underlying fat and soft tissue attachments are dissected and the orbit is exposed. Soft tissues are dissected and the area of interest exposed. The orbit is explored and any abnormalities noted. Tissue samples are obtained as needed and sent for separately reportable pathology evaluation. Orbital tissues are reapproximated and the periorbita is closed. The zygomatic bone window or flap is replaced and secured with miniplates

and screws. The periosteum is closed. Soft tissues and the skin of the eyelid are closed in layers.

67500-67505

67500 Retrobulbar injection; medication (separate procedure, does not include supply of medication)

67505 Retrobulbar injection; alcohol

An injection into the retrobulbar region of the eye is performed. The skin over the lateral aspect of the lower lid is cleansed and a local anesthetic administered as needed. The needle is inserted through the skin of the eyelid slightly lateral of the midline of the eye. The needle is inserted straight down through the septum and then the needle is redirected upward until the needle is in the free space of the retrobulbar region. The plunger is withdrawn to ensure the needle is not in a blood vessel or other vital structure of the eye. The medication or alcohol mixture is then injected into the retrobulbar space. The needle is withdrawn. Gentle pressure is applied over the injection site. Use 67500 for injection of medication. Use 67505 for injection of alcohol.

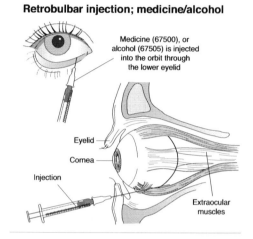

Retrobulbar injection; medicine/alcohol

Medicine (67500), or alcohol (67505) is injected into the orbit through the lower eyelid

Eyelid

Cornea

Injection

Extraocular muscles

67515

67515 Injection of medication or other substance into Tenon's capsule

The Tenon's capsule is a thin fascial sheath that envelopes the eyeball and separates it from the orbital fat. The inner surface is smooth and shiny and is separated from the outer surface of the sclera by a potential space called the episcleral or sub-Tenon's space. The fascial sheath and the sclera are actually attached to each other by fine bands of connective tissue. The anterior aspect of the fascial sheath is attached to the sclera about 1.5 cm posterior to the corneoscleral junction. In the posterior aspect the sheath fuses with the meninges around the optic nerve and with the sclera where the optic nerve exits the eyeball. The tendons of all six extrinsic eye muscles pierce the sheath and the fascial sheath forms a tubular sleeve around the tendons. To perform Tenon's capule injection, local anesthetic eye drops are administered. An eyelid speculum is placed to keep the lids open. As the patient looks upwards and outwards, the Tenon's capsule and sclera are grasped with a forceps. A small incision may be made. A blunt, curved sub-Tenon's capsule cannula is mounted on a syringe and inserted along the curvature of the sclera. The cannula is passed into the posterior sub-Tenon's space. The medication or other substance is injected. The cannula is removed and pressure applied over the globe so that the substance injected will spread throughout the capsule.

67550-67560

67550 Orbital implant (implant outside muscle cone); insertion

67560 Orbital implant (implant outside muscle cone); removal or revision

An orbital implant located outside the muscle cone is inserted, removed or revised. Implants placed outside the muscle cone are typically used for patients with extensive loss of tissue in the orbit due to trauma, surgery or radiation treatment. The physician works with an anaplastologist to determine the type and position of the implant. This procedure may be done in one or two stages. The first part of the procedure consists of placing one or more titanium implants into the bone to which the prosthesis will be attached. A skin incision is made at the planned implant site. Soft tissues are dissected and the orbital periosteum is exposed. One or more implant sites in the bone are prepared which involves incising the periosteum and then creating burr holes. The periosteum is incised in a cruciate fashion and the edges are raised. A drill is used to create a burr hole in the orbital bone. Soft tissues are then prepared. All hair follicles around the implant site are removed. The subcutaneous tissue is reduced to minimize skin mobility at the implant site. The periosteum is trimmed down to the innermost layer. The implant is then seated in the bone using a specially designed drill. This is repeated until all the implant components are in place. The soft tissue and skin around the implants is then closed. In a one-stage procedure healing abutments are placed until the implants have osseointegrated. The wound is dressed. In a two-stage procedure a cover screw is inserted into the implant and the soft tissue and skin is closed over the bone and the implants. Approximately 4-6 months later once the implants have osseointegrated. The skin is incised and the cover screws removed. The skin and soft tissues are repaired and abutments placed. Healing caps are attached to the abutments and a dressing applied. Once healing is complete the orbital implant, which has been fabricated in a separately reportable procedure, is attached to the abutments. Use 67550 for insertion of orbital implant. Use 67560 if complications arise and the orbital implant must be removed or revised. Removal is typically performed for infection. The abutments are removed. The bone implants are exposed and the removed. All infected tissue is debrided. A drain is placed as needed. Soft tissue and skin are closed around the drain. Revision may be required if there is excessive skin mobility at the implant site causing irritation. The abutments are removed and the implants are exposed and inspected. The subcutaneous tissue may be thinned to prevent mobility and irritation of the overlying skin or other revision measures performed. The skin is closed over the implants and the abutments replaced.

67570

67570   Optic nerve decompression (eg, incision or fenestration of optic nerve sheath)

Optic nerve decompression may be needed following a traumatic closed head injury causing traumatic optic neuropathy, papilledema accompanying psuedotumor cerebri, also referred to as idiopathic intracranial hypertension, or other condition causing compression of the optic nerve with associated loss of vision. The optic nerve may be approached via a transfrontal craniotomy, extranasal or intranasal transethmoidal approach, or lateral facial approach. If a transfrontal craniotomy is performed, the skin is incised over the affected eye and dissection carried down to the frontal bone. Burr holes are drilled and the holes connected using an oscillating saw or craniotome. A bone flap is elevated. The orbit is exposed and the optic nerve identified. The bone of the optic canal around the optic nerve is thinned as needed to widen the canal. The Zinn rings and the optic nerve sheath are incised to allow decompression of the nerve. Once the decompression is complete, the bone flap is replaced and secured with miniplates and screws. Soft tissue and skin are closed in layers. If an extranasal or intranasal ethmoidal approach is used, a total ethmoidectomy is performed and the orbital apex exposed. The optic nerve is located and exposed. The medial optic canal is enlarged with a burr followed by bone curettage. The nerve is then decompressed as described above.

67700

67700   Blepharotomy, drainage of abscess, eyelid

A blepharotomy is performed to drain an eyelid abscess. The skin overlying the abscess is cleansed and a local anesthetic injected. An incision is made over the area of greatest fluctuance and the abscess is drained.

67710

67710   Severing of tarsorrhaphy

The physician removes sutures that were previously placed in the eyelids to close them. Suturing of the eyelids, also referred to as tarsorrhaphy, is a rare procedure used to protect the eye following an eye injury, due to a corneal disease that has caused inflammation of the cornea, due to dendritic ulcers caused by a virus, or for other conditions that require closure of the eyelid. The sutures are cut and removed.

67715

67715   Canthotomy (separate procedure)

Canthotomy is typically performed on the lateral canthus to relieve pressure and swelling in the eye following trauma. The skin on the lateral aspect of the eye is crimped with a hemostat for 1-2 minutes to help achieve hemostasis and to mark the line of the incision. The hemostat is released and a forceps is used to elevate the skin around the lateral aspect of the eye. A scissors is used to make the incision beginning at the lateral canthus and extending laterally outward from the eye. If this does not relieve the pressure and swelling the lateral canthus tendon is exposed and divided. The incision is left open until the pressure and swelling subsides.

67800-67808

67800   Excision of chalazion; single
67801   Excision of chalazion; multiple, same lid
67805   Excision of chalazion; multiple, different lids
67808   Excision of chalazion; under general anesthesia and/or requiring hospitalization, single or multiple

The physician excises one or more chalazia. A chalazium is an inflammatory lesion of the eyelid caused by obstruction of a sebaceous gland that may be superficial or deep depending on which gland is blocked. Superficial chalazia may be removed under local anesthesia while deep chalazia may require a hospitalization and a general anesthetic. A vertical incision is made in the palpebral conjunctival surface. The chalazium is removed by

curettage or by dissecting the lesion from surrounding tissue. If a deep chalazium involving a meibomian gland is excised, the physician may cauterize or remove the meibomian gland. If the chalazium extends to the skin, it may be removed via an incision in the skin of the eyelid rather than the conjunctiva. For chalazia removed using a local anesthetic without hospitalization use 67800 for excision of a single chalazium, 67801 for multiple chalazia of the same eyelid, and 67805 for multiple chalazia involving both eyelids. When removal of one or more chalazia requires general anesthesia and/or hospitalization use 67808.

67810

67810   Incisional biopsy of eyelid skin including lid margin

An incisional biopsy of the eyelid is performed. The mass or lesion in the eyelid is identified. The skin is disinfected over the planned biopsy site and a local anesthetic is injected. An incision is made through the skin and a tissue sample obtained from the mass or lesion. The incision is closed with sutures. The tissue sample is sent to the laboratory for separately reportable histological evaluation.

67820-67835

67820   Correction of trichiasis; epilation, by forceps only
67825   Correction of trichiasis; epilation by other than forceps (eg, by electrosurgery, cryotherapy, laser surgery)
67830   Correction of trichiasis; incision of lid margin
67835   Correction of trichiasis; incision of lid margin, with free mucous membrane graft

Trichiasis is a common eyelid abnormality characterized by an inward orientation of the lashes toward the globe. This causes irritation of the eye. Treatment depends on whether only a segment of the eyelid is involved or whether the lashes on the entire eyelid are misdirected. Removal of the eyelashes, also called epilation, is typically performed when only a segment of the eyelid is involved, while incision with or without grafting is performed when a larger portion of the eyelid is affected. In 67820, the eyelashes are removed using forceps. The eyelid is everted. Each misdirected eyelash is grasped and removed under microscopic visualization. In 67825, the eyelashes are removed using another technique. Typically, the lashes along with the lash follicle are destroyed. If cryosurgery is performed the lash and follicle are destroyed by freezing with liquid nitrogen or a cryoprobe. If electrosurgery is used a thermal electrocautery device is used. Radiofrequency ablation uses a small gauge wire introduced alongside the lash down to the follicle. The radiofrequency device is activated and the tissue coagulated thereby destroying the lash and hair follicle. Alternatively an Argon laser may be used to destroy the lash and follicle. In 67830, the lid margin is strategically incised to release scar tissue that may have formed and to redirect the lashes away from the globe. The incision is left open to heal by secondary intention. In 67835, the lid margin is incised as described above and a free mucosal graft used to repair the defect. A split thickness mucous membrane graft is harvested from the lower lip or other site using a mucotome. The graft is configured to the desired size and shape to fit the defect in the lid margin. The graft is sutured to the lid margin at the site of the surgically created defect.

67840

67840   Excision of lesion of eyelid (except chalazion) without closure or with simple direct closure

A lesion of the eyelid other than a chalazion is excised without closure or with simple direct closure. The skin over the lesion is disinfected and a local anesthetic injected. An incision is made through the skin and the lesion excised along with a margin of healthy tissue. The excised tissue is sent to the laboratory for separately reportable histological evaluation. The incision may be left open to heal by secondary intention or sutured using simple, single layer, direct closure.

67850

67850   Destruction of lesion of lid margin (up to 1 cm)

The physician destroys a lesion of the lid margin of 1 cm or less. The lesion is examined and the most appropriate form of destruction determined. Local anesthesia is administered as needed. The lesion may be destroyed using a chemical compound, cryosurgery, electrosurgery or other technique. Cryosurgery is performed using liquid nitrogen to freeze the lesion. A series of freeze-thaw cycles may be required to completely destroy the lesion. Electrosurgery uses heat applied to the lesion(s) with a high frequency current that passes through a metal probe or needle.

67875

67875   Temporary closure of eyelids by suture (eg, Frost suture)

The upper and lower eyelids are temporarily sutured together usually following an injury. Suturing the eyelids together or passing sutures through the lower lid and then taping the suture ends to the forehead (Frost suture) protects the eye while the injury heals. To suture the upper and lower lids together sutures are placed through the upper and lower lid margins and the sutures are tied so that the eyelids will remain closed. Frost suture

Eye and Ocular Adnexa

involves passing sutures through the lower eyelid only. Tension is then applied to the suture ends to close the lower lid and the ends of the suture material are secured with tape to the forehead.

67880-67882

67880 **Construction of intermarginal adhesions, median tarsorrhaphy, or canthorrhaphy**

67882 **Construction of intermarginal adhesions, median tarsorrhaphy, or canthorrhaphy; with transposition of tarsal plate**

The eyelids consist of multiple tissue layers with the most superficial layer being the skin followed by the orbicularis muscle, tarsus, and conjunctiva. The tarsi, also referred to as the tarsal plates, are composed of dense fibrous tissue that gives the upper and lower eyelids their shape. The upper eyelid has a crescent shape and the lower eyelid has a rectangular shape. In 67880, a median tarsorrhaphy or canthorrhaphy is performed. Median tarsorrhaphy involves creating adhesions between the upper and lower lid margins at the midline. It is performed to protect the cornea. Canthorrhaphy is the creation of adhesions at the corners, also called the medial and lateral canthus, of the eye. To perform median tarsorrhaphy, a narrow strip of skin is excised from the upper and lower lids at the midline. The skin is incised just posterior to the eyelashes. The surgically created wounds in the upper and lower lid are then approximated and secured using interrupted sutures. Canthorrhaphy is performed in the same manner except a strip of skin is removed from the upper and lower lid at the medial or lateral canthus and the surgical wounds are then approximated and secured with sutures. In 67882, median tarsorrhaphy or canthorrhaphy is performed in conjunction with transposition of the tarsal plate. The tarsal plate is exposed and repositioned usually to allow better closure of the eyelid.

67900

67900 **Repair of brow ptosis (supraciliary, mid-forehead or coronal approach)**

The physician repairs a sagging eyelid by making an incision in the forehead and pulling the skin upwards. Brow ptosis repair may be performed to correct laxity of forehead muscles and the descent of periorbital soft tissue causing functional visual impairment in the peripheral and superior visual fields. The procedure can be approached through a supraciliary incision along the superior border of the eyebrow, through preexisting horizontal mid-forehead furrows, or through a coronal scalp incision along the hairline. For all approaches, the skin is carefully marked with the patient upright before local anesthetic is injected. The supraciliary approach is appropriate for unilateral or bilateral brow ptosis. The skin is incised along the marked line(s) above the eyebrow and extended to find the frontalis muscle. Excess skin and subcutaneous tissue are excised en bloc. For the mid-forehead approach, a skin incision is made along the marked line(s) and carried down through the subcutaneous tissue to expose the corrugator supercilii and procerus muscles. This muscle complex is removed by incising the subgalea at the level of the glabella. The skin is trimmed before approximating the superior and inferior edges of the incision and closing in layers. The coronal approach near the hairline starts at the midline and extends laterally on each side to the anterior or superior reflection of the ear, incising the skin and galea. The temporalis fascia is identified and spared along with the superficial temporalis vessels. The galea is retracted to expose the underlying pericranium and a coronal flap is developed while preserving the seventh nerve near the orbital rims. The flap is turned down to allow further dissection in the subgaleal avascular plane with preservation of the frontal branch of the facial nerve. A dissector is used to expose the supraorbital neovascular bundles and the flap is turned down completely to expose the supraorbital rim, periosteum over the zygomatic process of the frontal bone laterally, and the superior aspect of the nasal bone in the glabellar region medially. The procerus, corrugator supercilii, and orbital orbicularis muscles are then elevated with the forehead skin and frontalis muscle, and the muscle complex is completely excised. The skin is pulled superiorly and trimmed. Vertical incisions are made anteriorly in the coronal flaps and additional skin is trimmed. The apex of each incision is approximated to the posterior skin with sutures and excess skin and galea are trimmed as necessary. The galea is closed with sutures followed by closure of the skin with sutures or staples.

67901-67902

67901 **Repair of blepharoptosis; frontalis muscle technique with suture or other material (eg, banked fascia)**

67902 **Repair of blepharoptosis; frontalis muscle technique with autologous fascial sling (includes obtaining fascia)**

The physician repairs a blepharoptosis, which is a sagging of the upper eyelid caused by weakness of the levator palpebrae muscle, by frontalis muscle technique using suture or other material such as a silastic rod or banked fascia. A shield is placed over the cornea. A skin incision is made just above the central portion of the eyebrow. Three small subcutaneous incisions are made in the upper eyelid in the pretarsal region just below the lid crease, one located medially, one centrally and one in the lateral aspect. A needle is then passed through the incision above the eyebrow between the orbicularis and levator muscles and through the medial eyelid incision. A length of silastic rod or banked fascia may be threaded through the needle and retrieved through the incision above the eyebrow. The suture material, rod, or banked fascia is then threaded horizontally across the tarsus,

exiting at the previously made below crease incision in the central aspect of the eyelid. The suture material, rod, or banked fascia is then passed through the previously made below crease lateral eyelid incision. The suture, rod, or banked fascia is secured by taking an intratarsal bite along each of three below crease incisions. A needle is then passed through the incision above the eyebrow and the suture, rod, or banked fascia retrieved at the lateral aspect of the tarsus. If a silastic rod has been used, a silastic sleeve is placed over the incision above the eyebrow and the rod passed through the sleeve. The tension of the suture, rod, or banked fascia is adjusted to the proper tension and suture, banked fascia or rod and sleeve secured to the deep frontalis muscle. The skin incisions are closed. In 67902, the physician repairs a blepharoptosis using a frontalis muscle technique with an autologous fascial sling. A fascia lata graft is harvested from the lateral thigh using a fascia stripper. The repair is performed as described except that a silastic sleeve is not used. The lid level is adjusted and the fascia lata strip tied at each end. The fascial knot is reinforced at each end and anchored to the frontalis muscle on the upper edge of the incision above the eyebrow.

67903-67904

67903 **Repair of blepharoptosis; (tarso) levator resection or advancement, internal approach**

67904 **Repair of blepharoptosis; (tarso) levator resection or advancement, external approach**

The physician repairs a blepharoptosis, which is a sagging of the upper eyelid caused by weakness of the levator palpebrae muscle, by tarsolevator resection or advancement using an internal (67903) or external (67904) approach. A local anesthetic is injected into the upper eyelid. Measurements are taken to determine the amount of resection or advancement required. In 67903, the eyelid is everted and traction sutures placed in the upper eyelid. The planned incision lines are marked using previously obtained measurements and the conjunctiva incised for an internal approach. In 67904, a shield is placed over the cornea. An incision is made in the skin of the upper eyelid fold for an external approach. The anterior tarsal surface and levator aponeurosis are exposed by incising the orbicularis along the superior tarsal border and traversing the eyelid horizontally. Using the previously made measurements, the tarsal plate is incised and a spindle shaped section of tarsus and aponeurosis excised. A suture is placed anteriorly through the tarsus along the central portion of the superior edge and then passed through the superior edge of the levator aponeurosis. Two additional sutures are placed medially and laterally using the same technique. The sutures are temporarily tied and the lid contour assessed. The sutures are adjusted until an ideal lid shape is attained and the sutures are then permanently tied. The lid crease skin incision or conjunctival incision is closed.

67906

67906 **Repair of blepharoptosis; superior rectus technique with fascial sling (includes obtaining fascia)**

The physician repairs a blepharoptosis, which is a sagging of the upper eyelid caused by weakness of the levator palpebrae muscle, by a superior rectus technique with a fascial sling. A fascia lata graft is harvested from the lateral thigh using a fascia stripper. Alternatively, a length of banked fascia may be used. A skin incision is made over the superior rectus muscle of the eye. One or more small subcutaneous incisions are made in the upper eyelid in the pretarsal region just below the lid crease. A needle is then passed through the incision above the superior rectus. The fascial graft is threaded through the needle and retrieved through the incision over the superior rectus. The fascia is then threaded through the eyelid between the orbicularis and levator muscles and then horizontally across the tarsus, exiting in the upper eyelid. The fascia is then passed through the previously made incision(s) below the eyelid crease. The fascia is secured by taking an intratarsal bite along the crease incision(s). A needle is then passed through the incision over the superior rectus and the fascia is retrieved at the lateral aspect of the tarsus. The fascia is adjusted to the proper tension and secured in the superior rectus muscle. The skin incisions are closed. This code should be chosen carefully, as the superior rectus technique is considered outmoded and has been replaced by levator resection and advancement procedures.

67908

67908 **Repair of blepharoptosis; conjunctivo-tarso-Muller's muscle-levator resection (eg, Fasanella-Servat type)**

The physician repairs a blepharoptosis, which is a sagging of the upper eyelid caused by weakness of the levator palpebrae muscle, by conjunctivo-tarso-Muller's muscle levator resection, also referred to as a Muller muscle conjunctiva repair (MMCR) or Fasanella-Servat repair. The upper eyelid is everted and the tarsal plate is exposed. Three temporary traction sutures are placed close to the folded superior margin of the tarsal plate, one medially, one laterally, and one in the central aspect. These sutures lift and hold up the portion of the tarsal plate to be excised. The ends of the sutures are clamped with artery forceps. Three additional temporary traction sutures are placed close to the margin of the everted lid, emerging near the superior fornix aligned with the first three sutures. These three sutures lift and support the conjunctival and tarsal wedge for suturing. The planned incision lines are marked using previously obtained measurements. A blade breaker knife is used to make an incision in the form of a groove. Scissor tips are placed in the grove and the tarsal plate is excised. The wound is then repaired with a continuous buried suture temporarily tied at both ends. The lid shape is assessed and adjustments are made as needed until an ideal lid shape has been attained. The sutures are permanently tied with small knots that are buried at each end. The temporary traction sutures are removed and the lid crease skin incision is closed. If a modified or sutureless Fasanella-Servat repair is performed, a hemostat forceps is used to grasp the tarsoconjunctival Muller complex along the marked lines and the hemostat forceps is left in place for 60 seconds. When the hemostat is removed it leaves behind a broad ischemic groove of tissue that is then excised. Suture repair is not required as the compressed groove located at the site of the forceps acts as a mechanical suture.

67909

67909   Reduction of overcorrection of ptosis

Ptosis refers to sagging or drooping of the upper eyelid. Ptosis can be corrected surgically, but some patients experience an overcorrection of the ptosis. Overcorrection can make it impossible to completely close the eye which can cause dry eye and damage to the cornea. The old incision is reopened. The levator aponeurosis is exposed and released. The tension of the levator is adjusted until the eyelid is in a more normal position and the eyelid can be closed completely. The levator is then reattached more superiorly on the tarsus or to the Muller muscle or conjunctiva. The surgical wound is closed in layers.

67911

67911   Correction of lid retraction

The upper and lower eyelid can be affected by lid retraction. Lower eyelid retraction is caused by relaxation of the support system of the eye and also by shrinkage of the tissue layers that include skin, muscle, and retractor muscles. Lower lid retraction causes an inability to completely close the eye with exposure of the sclera below the cornea. Lower lid retraction may be due to aging, thyroid disease, or a complication of lower eyelid blepharoplasty. Upper lid retraction causes exposure of the sclera above the cornea and is most often caused by thyroid disease. The exact procedure performed for correction of lid retraction depends on whether the upper or lower eyelid is affected as well as the cause, extent, and any unique individual characteristics of the lid retraction. Correction of upper lid retraction is performed through a transconjunctival or transcutaneous approach. Mullers muscle is exposed and excised. The levator aponeurosis may also be resected. Adjustable sutures are then used to adjust the eyelid position. Alternatively an autogenous graft may be harvested usually from the hard palate or synthetic graft material may be used to support the eyelid and adjust the height. Lower lid retraction is corrected via a transconjunctival approach. Lower lid support structures may be reconstructed or reinforced. Repair may require skin grafting, placement of an another type of autogenous graft, or reinforcement with synthetic material. The lower lid height is adjusted as needed and the surgical wound is closed in layers.

67912

67912   Correction of lagophthalmos, with implantation of upper eyelid lid load (eg, gold weight)

Lagophthalmos affects the orbicularis muscle of the eyelid and is a form of facial paralysis that is characterized by the inability to completely close the upper eyelid. Surgical correction is performed when the paralysis is persistent or permanent and involves placement of a small pure gold weight in the upper eyelid. The upper eyelid is prepped and a local anesthetic injected. A small incision is made in the upper eyelid crease or just above the eyelashes. A small pocket is created inside the lid and an implant of the appropriate weight placed in the pocket. The weight is secured with sutures. The lid incision is closed. A protective eye pad is placed over the eyelid.

67914-67915

67914   Repair of ectropion; suture
67915   Repair of ectropion; thermocauterization

An ectropion is a condition where the lid margin is everted which means that it is turned outward and away from the globe. When the lid margin is everted the cornea is exposed, excessive tearing occurs, changes occur in the palpebral conjunctiva, and vision loss may occur. Ectropion is more common in the lower eyelid. A local anesthetic or nerve block is employed for pain control. In 67914, the ectropion is treated by suturing the eyelid at the site of the ectropion. Sutures are placed through the inferior border of the tarsus and exit at the skin surface near the orbital rim. The edges of the conjunctiva are approximated and secured with sutures. In 67915, thermocauterization is performed. A corneal protector is placed over the globe. The eyelid is everted and electrocautery applied at the junction of the conjunctiva and lower margin of the lower margin of the tarsus.

67916-67917

67916   Repair of ectropion; excision tarsal wedge
67917   Repair of ectropion; extensive (eg, tarsal strip operations)

An ectropion is a condition where the lid margin is everted which means that it is turned outward and away from the globe. When the lid margin is everted the cornea is exposed, excessive tearing occurs, changes occur in the palpebral conjunctiva, and vision loss may occur. Ectropion is more common in the lower eyelid. Local anesthesia is administered and supplemented with a nerve block as needed. A corneal shield is placed. In 67916, a tarsal wedge is excised. A V-shaped incision is made over the ectropion and a wedge of the tarsal plate is excised. The open wedge in the tarsal plate is then closed with sutures. The skin is closed. In 67917, an extensive repair is performed such as a tarsal strip procedure. The exact procedure performed depends on the site and severity of the ectropion. To perform a lateral tarsal strip procedure, the lateral canthus is incised and the lower lid mobilized. If excess skin is present it is excised. The lid margin is split and the meibomian orifices of the lateral strip are trimmed off. The lateral conjunctiva is inspected and scraped to prevent formation of epithelial inclusion cysts. The lateral strip of tarsus is sutured to periosteum of the lateral orbital rim near the Whitnall tubercle. The surgical wound is closed in layers.

67921-67922

67921   Repair of entropion; suture
67922   Repair of entropion; thermocauterization

Entropion is a condition in which the eyelid margin rotates inward toward the surface of the eye causing the eyelashes and eyelid to rub against the conjunctiva and cornea. The resulting irritation may progress to corneal abrasion and ulceration. Entropions are most commonly seen in the lower eyelid of elderly individuals. A local anesthetic is injected into the eyelid. In 67921, a suture repair of the entropion is performed. Paired full thickness sutures are placed from the conjunctival side of the eyelid just below the tarsal border, exiting out through the skin of the eyelid. The sutures are angled so that the exit site on the eyelid is closer to the lid margin, in order to cause eversion of the inverted eyelid. The externalized ends of the paired sutures are tied and remain in place for up to two weeks. Suture repair of an entropion is typically performed as a temporary measure until definitive, permanent repair of the entropion can be accomplished. In 67922, thermocauterization is performed. A corneal protector is placed over the globe. The eyelid is everted and electrocautery strategically applied so that when the burned tissue heals, scar tissue will form and the eyelid tissue will retract causing the inverted eyelid to assume a normal position against the globe.

67923-67924

67923   Repair of entropion; excision tarsal wedge
67924   Repair of entropion; extensive (eg, tarsal strip or capsulopalpebral fascia repairs operation)

Entropion is a condition in which the eyelid margin rotates inward toward the surface of the eye causing the eyelashes and eyelid to rub against the conjunctiva and cornea. The resulting irritation may progress to corneal abrasion and ulceration. Entropions are most commonly seen in the lower eyelid of elderly individuals. A local anesthetic is injected into the eyelid. Local anesthesia is administered and supplemented with a nerve block as needed. A corneal shield is placed. In 67923, a tarsal wedge is excised. A V-shaped incision is made over the entropion and a wedge of the tarsal plate is excised. The open wedge in the tarsal plate is then closed with sutures. The skin is closed. In 67924, an extensive repair is performed such as a tarsal strip procedure or capsulopalpebral fascia repair. The exact procedure performed depends on the site and severity of the entropion. To perform a lateral tarsal strip procedure, the lateral canthus is incised and the lower lid mobilized. If excess skin is present it is excised. The lid margin is split and the meibomian orifices of the lateral strip are trimmed off. The lateral conjunctiva is inspected and scraped to prevent formation of epithelial inclusion cysts. The lateral strip of tarsus is sutured to periosteum of the lateral orbital rim near the Whitnall tubercle. The surgical wound is closed in layers. If the entropion is due to horizontal and vertical laxity of the eyelid, medial and/or lateral canthal tightening may be performed using a tarsal strip procedure followed by vertical shortening and reattachment of the lower eyelid retractors to the inferior border of the tarsus.

67930-67935

67930   Suture of recent wound, eyelid, involving lid margin, tarsus, and/or palpebral conjunctiva direct closure; partial thickness
67935   Suture of recent wound, eyelid, involving lid margin, tarsus, and/or palpebral conjunctiva direct closure; full thickness

The eyelids consist of multiple tissue layers with the most superficial layer being the skin followed by the orbicularis muscle, tarsus, and conjunctiva. Repair of wounds involving more than the skin require layered closure. Anesthetic eye drops or other topical anesthetic is administered. The corneal protector is placed over the globe. The wound is cleansed and any debris removed. Damaged tissue is debrided. The lid margin is realigned by placing three marginal sutures. The first suture passes through the plane of the meibomian orifices. The other two sutures are placed anterior and posterior to the first. If the lid margin is

Eye and Ocular Adnexa

involved it is repaired with mattress sutures. Another technique is to use a single vertical mattress suture to realign the lid margin. If the tarsus is involved, sutures are placed through the tarsus with the knotted ends directed away from the cornea. If the palpebral conjunctiva is involved it is repaired with sutures. The skin is then closed. Use 67930 if the wound involves only a partial thickness injury extending only part of the way through the eyelid. Use 67935 if the wound extends through the entire eyelid.

67938

67938   Removal of embedded foreign body, eyelid

An embedded foreign body is removed from the eyelid. A topical anesthetic is administered. A corneal protector is placed over the globe. The wound is cleansed and any debris removed. The eyelid is inspected to try to identify the entry site of the foreign body. If the entry site cannot be identified a chalazion curette may be used to palpate the eyelid and help locate the foreign body. Once the foreign body is identified, the entry wound is enlarged or an incision is made in the eyelid and the foreign body is removed. The entry wound or incision is repaired with tissue glue or sutures.

67950

67950   Canthoplasty (reconstruction of canthus)

Canthoplasty is performed to reconstruct the medial or lateral canthus which is the point where the upper and lower eyelids meet. The medial canthus contains the medial canthal ligament that attaches to the orbit forming the bony attachment of the eyelids and the lacrimal drainage and collecting system. The lateral canthus consists of four structures, the lateral canthal tendon, Lockwood's ligament, cheek ligaments of the lateral rectus muscle, and the lateral horn of the levator aponeurosis. The exact procedure depends on which canthus is involved and the nature of the injury. If the medial canthus has been injured it may be reconstructed using a full thickness skin graft, upper eyelid transposition flap or a rotation or transposition flap from the glabella. If a skin graft is used it is harvested, prepared for grafting, and sutured over the defect. If a flap from the upper eyelid or glabella is used, the flap configuration is determined, the skin is incised and the incision is carried down to subcutaneous tissues. The flap is developed. Glabellar flaps require thinning to maintain the proper contour and skin thickness around the eye. If the medial canthal supports (ligaments and tendons) have been damaged they are reconstructed so that the eyelid will properly oppose the globe. The flap is then rotated or transferred and sutured to surrounding tissue. The flap must be configured in a way that allows reconstruction of the canthus and coverage of the defect. If the lateral canthus has been injured it is typically repaired with a cheek rotation flap. The location, shape and size of the flap depend on the characteristics of the defect and the available donor site. Extensive defects involving the ligaments may require development of a periosteal strip from the zygomatic arch to provide support to the lateral canthus. Once the supporting structures have been repaired, the flap is positioned and sutured over the defect and the donor site is repaired.

67961-67966

67961   Excision and repair of eyelid, involving lid margin, tarsus, conjunctiva, canthus, or full thickness, may include preparation for skin graft or pedicle flap with adjacent tissue transfer or rearrangement; up to one-fourth of lid margin

67966   Excision and repair of eyelid, involving lid margin, tarsus, conjunctiva, canthus, or full thickness, may include preparation for skin graft or pedicle flap with adjacent tissue transfer or rearrangement; over one-fourth of lid margin

A lesion of the eyelid involving the lid margin, tarsus, conjunctiva, canthus, or the full thickness of the eyelid is excised and the surgical defect repaired using a skin graft or pedicle flap or some type of tissue transfer or rearrangement. Most lesions requiring excision of deeper eyelid tissues are malignant in nature and include basal cell carcinoma, squamous cell carcinoma, sebaceous carcinoma, and melanoma. The lesion is excised along with a margin of healthy tissue. Separately reportable pathological examination is performed to ensure that the margins are clean. If the margins are not clean the excision is extended until clean margins are obtained. The eyelid is then reconstructed. The technique varies based on whether the upper or lower eyelid is reconstructed and the site of the defect on the lid itself (medial, central or lateral aspect). If a skin graft is used an appropriate donor site is selected and the skin graft is harvested. The skin graft is prepared, placed over the defect and sutured in place. If a pedicle flap is used, the configuration of the flap is determined. The skin and deeper tissues are incised and the flap is elevated and rotated over the defect. The flap is secured with sutures. The defect created by the creation of the flap is closed in layers. Use 67961 for excision of a lesion and repair of the surgical defect involving up to one-fourth of the lid margin. Use 67966 when the surgical procedure involves over one-fourth of the lid margin.

67971-67975

67971   Reconstruction of eyelid, full thickness by transfer of tarsoconjunctival flap from opposing eyelid; up to two-thirds of eyelid, 1 stage or first stage

67973   Reconstruction of eyelid, full thickness by transfer of tarsoconjunctival flap from opposing eyelid; total eyelid, lower, 1 stage or first stage

67974   Reconstruction of eyelid, full thickness by transfer of tarsoconjunctival flap from opposing eyelid; total eyelid, upper, 1 stage or first stage

67975   Reconstruction of eyelid, full thickness by transfer of tarsoconjunctival flap from opposing eyelid; second stage

A tarsoconjunctival flap from the opposing eyelid is used to reconstruct the eyelid defect following trauma or extensive surgical excision of a lesion. This is known as a lid-sharing reconstruction technique. The exact technique depends on whether the upper or lower eyelid is being reconstructed. A common technique for reconstruction of the lower eyelid is the tarsoconjunctival bridge flap, also called a modified Hughes procedure. A traction suture is placed in the upper eyelid margin. The upper eyelid is everted and the tarsus and conjunctiva of the upper eyelid are incised horizontally 4 mm proximal to the lid margin. The tarsus and conjunctiva are dissected away from the levator aponeurosis and the Muller muscle to create the flap. The flap is advanced to the defect in the lower eyelid. The edges of the flap are sutured to the medial and lateral remnants of the lower lid tarsus and the lower lid conjunctiva. The flap is then covered by a skin graft harvested from the upper eyelid or retroauricular region. Alternatively, the locally based skin flap may be advanced over the tarsoconjunctival flap. The flap is left in place for 4-6 weeks to develop lower lid blood supply to the flap. In the second stage of the procedure a grooved director is inserted under the flap and anterior to the globe. The flap is divided. Conjunctiva is sutured to the reconstructed lower lid margin. The Muller muscle and levator aponeurosis are dissected away from the overlying skin and allowed to retract. The remainder of the pedicled upper lid flap is reattached to the upper lid. A common technique for reconstructing the upper eyelid is the Cutler-Beard procedure. A skin-muscle-conjunctival flap is developed using the lower lid leaving the lower lid margin intact. The flap is advanced into the defect of the upper lid and sutured to the defect margins using a technique similar to that used for lower lid defects. The flap is left in place for 6-8 weeks. During the second stage of the procedure the flap is divided at the planned reconstructed upper lid margin and the remainder of the pedicled flap reattached to the lower eyelid. Use 67971 for reconstruction of up to two-thirds of the upper or lower eyelid, 1 stage or first stage. Use 67973 for total lower eyelid reconstruction, 1 stage or first stage. Use 67974 for total upper eyelid, 1 stage or first stage. Use 67975 for the second stage of a two stage procedure.

68020

68020   Incision of conjunctiva, drainage of cyst

A conjunctival cyst is a thin walled, fluid filled sac located on the surface of the clear vascular tissue that covers the eye. The cyst may be congenital or acquired and usually results from friction to the tissue. To drain the cyst, ocular anesthetic eye drops are first instilled and the sac is grasped with forceps. The sac is then incised using a needle, scissors, knife blade, or curette and the fluid is drained. Hemostasis is achieved using electrocautery and the incision is closed with fibrin glue.

68040

68040   Expression of conjunctival follicles (eg, for trachoma)

Expression of conjunctival follicles is performed to treat follicular conjunctivitis. Follicular conjunctivitis is usually caused by a viral or bacterial infection with the most common type requiring expression or drainage of the follicles being caused by Chlamydia trachomatis. Anesthetic drops are administered or another type of local anesthetic applied as needed. The eyelid is everted and the follicles inspected. Manual pressure is applied to express purulent matter from the follicles.

68100

68100   Biopsy of conjunctiva

The physician biopsies the conjunctiva. The conjunctiva is the mucous membrane covering the anterior surface of the eyeball (bulbar conjunctiva) and the posterior surface of the eyelid (palpebral conjunctiva). A biopsy may be performed when there is a lesion present or to help diagnose the cause of persistent conjunctivitis. A conjunctival biopsy may also be performed to aid in the diagnosis of some systemic diseases such as sarcoidosis, ocular pemphigoid, Stevens-Johnson syndrome, or amyloidosis. Anesthetic eyedrops are instilled to numb the eye. A forceps is used to grasp the conjunctiva and a small piece of tissue is removed with scissors. The tissue sample is sent to the laboratory for separately reportable histological evaluation. Antibiotic ointment is applied to the biopsy site. An eye patch is applied as needed.

● New Code   ▲ Revised Code

68110-68130

68110   **Excision of lesion, conjunctiva; up to 1 cm**
68115   **Excision of lesion, conjunctiva; over 1 cm**
68130   **Excision of lesion, conjunctiva; with adjacent sclera**

Some of the more common types of conjunctival lesions requiring excision include benign squamous cell and limbal papillomas, and malignant primary acquired melanosis, conjunctival melanoma, and squamous cell carcinoma. Anesthetic drops or another type of local anesthesia is administered. The conjunctiva is inspected and the extent of the excision determined. The lesion is then excised along with a margin of healthy tissue. The tissue is sent for separately reportable pathological evaluation and to ensure that the margins are clear. Additional tissue is excised as needed including scleral tissue until clear margins have been obtained. Use 68110 for a conjunctival lesion up to 1 cm; use 68115 for a conjunctival lesion over 1 cm; and use 68130 for a lesion that requires excision of adjacent scleral tissue.

68135

68135   **Destruction of lesion, conjunctiva**

A lesion of the conjunctiva is destroyed. Destruction may be performed using a laser, electrocautery, cryotherapy, chemical agent, or other method. Anesthetic drops or another type of local anesthesia is administered. The conjunctival lesion is inspected and the most effective method of destruction determined. Laser destruction uses a laser beam focused on the lesion. Electrocautery destroys the lesion using a heat probe. Cryotherapy uses liquid nitrogen to freeze the lesion. Chemical destruction involves the use of a chemical or pharmacologic agent.

68200

68200   **Subconjunctival injection**

A subconjunctival injection is administered usually to treat severe inflammation or infection. Local anesthetic drops are administered. The site of the injection, usually the upper or lower fornix is identified. The needle is advanced through the conjunctiva and into the space between the conjunctiva and the sclera. The substance is then injected slowly which will cause a ballooning effect between the conjunctiva and sclera. The needle is removed, the eye closed, and an eye pad applied until the fluid disperses and the ballooning subsides. The eye pad may be secured and left in place for several hours.

68320-68325

68320   **Conjunctivoplasty; with conjunctival graft or extensive rearrangement**
68325   **Conjunctivoplasty; with buccal mucous membrane graft (includes obtaining graft)**

Conjunctivoplasty is performed to treat a number of conditions including redundant conjunctiva, lesions of the conjunctiva, and hyperemia of conjunctival blood vessels. A subconjunctival injection may be used to elevate the conjunctiva off of the sclera. The redundant or abnormal conjunctival tissue is excised. In 68320, the remaining conjunctiva is then rearranged or a conjunctival graft is harvested from the contralateral eye and used to repair the defect. If the conjunctiva is rearranged, one or more conjunctival flaps are configured, raised and repositioned over the sclera. The flap is secured with sutures or tissue glue. If a conjunctival graft from the contralateral eye is used, the conjunctival harvest site is marked with a pen or keratotomy marker. The conjunctiva at the donor site is elevated using a subconjunctival injection of balanced salt solution and a local anesthetic. The lateral borders of the graft are incised in a radial fashion. The tissue between the incisions at the lateral borders is undermined using blunt dissection. Dissection is carried in an anterior direction to the conjunctival insertion at the limbus and then beyond the limbus into the peripheral cornea. The conjunctival graft including the superficial epithelial corneal tissue is then excised. The donor site may be left to heal by secondary intention or the conjunctiva may be advanced to cover a portion of the donor site to minimize pain and inflammation. The graft is then placed over the surgically created defect in the opposite eye. In 68325, a buccal mucous membrane graft is used to repair the defect and is usually taken from the lower lip. A split thickness mucous membrane graft is harvested using a mucotome. The graft is configured to the desired size and shape to fit the defect in the conjunctiva. The graft is sutured to the conjunctiva and/or sclera.

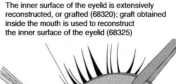

Conjunctivoplasty

The inner surface of the eyelid is extensively reconstructed, or grafted (68320); graft obtained inside the mouth is used to reconstruct the inner surface of the eyelid (68325)

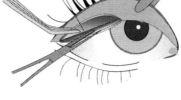

68326-68328

68326   **Conjunctivoplasty, reconstruction cul-de-sac; with conjunctival graft or extensive rearrangement**
68328   **Conjunctivoplasty, reconstruction cul-de-sac; with buccal mucous membrane graft (includes obtaining graft)**

Conjunctivoplasty with reconstruction of the cul-de-sac is performed to treat a number of conditions including redundant conjunctiva, lesions of the conjunctiva, and hyperemia of conjunctival blood vessels. The cul-de-sac, also referred to as the conjunctival fornix is the site where the conjunctiva of the globe meets the conjunctiva of the eyelid. A subconjunctival injection may be used to elevate the conjunctiva off of the sclera. The redundant or abnormal conjunctival tissue is excised. In 68326, the remaining conjunctiva is then rearranged or a conjunctival graft is harvested from the contralateral eye and used to repair the defect including the defect in the cul-de-sac. If the conjunctiva is rearranged, one or more conjunctival flaps are configured, raised and repositioned over the sclera and cul-de-sac. The flap is secured with sutures or tissue glue. If a conjunctival graft from the contralateral eye is used, the conjunctival harvest site is marked with a pen or keratotomy marker. The conjunctiva at the donor site is elevated using a subconjunctival injection of balanced salt solution and a local anesthetic. The lateral borders of the graft are incised in a radial fashion. The tissue between the incisions at the lateral borders is undermined using blunt dissection. Dissection is carried in an anterior direction to the conjunctival insertion at the limbus and then beyond the limbus into the peripheral cornea. The conjunctival graft including the superficial epithelial corneal tissue is then excised. The donor site may be left to heal by secondary intention or the conjunctiva may be advanced to cover a portion of the donor site to minimize pain and inflammation. The graft is then placed over the surgically created conjunctival defect in the opposite eye. In 68328, a buccal mucous membrane graft is used to repair a conjunctival defect that includes the cul-de-sac. The graft is usually taken from the lower lip. A split thickness mucous membrane graft is harvested using a mucotome. The graft is configured to the desired size and shape to fit the defect in the conjunctiva including the defect in the cul-de-sac. The graft is sutured to the conjunctiva and/or sclera including the defect in the cul-de-sac.

68330-68340

68330   **Repair of symblepharon; conjunctivoplasty, without graft**
68335   **Repair of symblepharon; with free graft conjunctiva or buccal mucous membrane (includes obtaining graft)**
68340   **Repair of symblepharon; division of symblepharon, with or without insertion of conformer or contact lens**

A symblepharon is the formation of adhesions or scar tissue between the palpebral conjunctiva of the eyelid and the bulbar conjunctiva of the globe and is typically secondary to trauma or infection. Symblepharon formation can affect eye movement, prevent the eyelids from closing or opening completely, and can cause double vision. In 68330, a symblepharon is repaired without a graft. The adhesions between the palpebral and bulbar conjunctiva are released and the fibrous tissue is carefully dissected from normal conjunctiva and excised. Adjacent healthy conjunctiva is advanced over the site where the adhesions were excised and secured with sutures. In 68335, the symblepharon is excised as described above and a free conjunctival graft or buccal mucous membrane graft is used to repair the defect. If a conjunctival graft from the contralateral eye is used, the conjunctival harvest site is marked with a pen or keratotomy marker. The conjunctiva at the donor site is elevated using a subconjunctival injection of balanced salt solution and a local anesthetic. The lateral borders of the graft are incised in a radial fashion. The tissue between the incisions at the lateral borders is undermined using blunt dissection. Dissection is carried in an anterior direction to the conjunctival insertion at the limbus and then beyond the limbus into the peripheral cornea. The conjunctival graft including the superficial epithelial corneal tissue is then excised. The donor site may be left to heal

Eye and Ocular Adnexa

by secondary intention or the conjunctiva may be advanced to cover a portion of the donor site to minimize pain and inflammation. The graft is then placed over the surgically created conjunctival defect in the opposite eye. If a buccal mucous membrane graft is used to repair a conjunctival defect, the graft is usually taken from the lower lip. A split thickness mucous membrane graft is harvested using a mucotome. The graft is configured to the desired size and shape to fit the defect in the conjunctiva. The graft is sutured to the conjunctiva and/or sclera including the defect in the cul-de-sac. In 68340, the symblepharon is divided. The adhesions between the palpebral and bulbar conjunctiva are released and the fibrous tissue is carefully dissected from normal conjunctiva and excised. The site may be left open to heal by secondary intention or a conformer or contact lens inserted. If a conformer or contact lens is inserted, the eye is measured and a properly sized conformer or lens is selected and inserted into the eye to maintain separation between the conjunctiva of the lid and the globe while the conjunctiva heals. The conformer or lens is permanently removed 4-12 weeks later.

68360-68362

68360   Conjunctival flap; bridge or partial (separate procedure)
68362   Conjunctival flap; total (such as Gunderson thin flap or purse string flap)

A conjunctival flap either partial or total may be used for treatment of corneal ulcers. Anesthetic eye drops are administered. An eye speculum is inserted and any diseased tissue is excised. The size and location of the defect is evaluated and the optimal site and configuration of the flap is determined. In 68360, a bridge or partial conjunctival flap is used. A subconjunctival injection containing lidocaine and epinephrine is injected to elevate the conjunctiva that will be used to configure the flap. Incisions are strategically placed and the flap is raised and mobilized. The flap is rotated over the defect taking care to maintain blood supply to the flap. The flap is secured with sutures. In 68362, a total conjunctival flap, also referred to as a Gunderson thin flap is prepared. A 360 degree peritomy is performed. Tissue from the upper bulbar conjunctiva is mobilized. Damaged corneal epithelium is excised. The flap is secured to the lower limbal conjunctiva. This type of flap covers the entire cornea.

68371

68371   Harvesting conjunctival allograft, living donor

The eye from which the conjunctival allograft is to be obtained is prepped and draped and the conjunctival harvest sites marked with a pen or keratotomy marker. The conjunctiva at the donor site is elevated using a subconjunctival injection of balanced salt solution and a local anesthetic. The lateral borders of the graft are incised in a radial fashion. The tissue between the incisions at the lateral borders is undermined using blunt dissection. Dissection is carried in an anterior direction to the conjunctival insertion at the limbus and then beyond the limbus into the peripheral cornea. The conjunctival graft including the superficial epithelial corneal tissue is then excised. The donor site may be left to heal by secondary intention or the conjunctiva may be advanced to cover a portion of the donor site to minimize pain and inflammation at the donor site. The graft is placed in preservation solution with the epithelial side up and transported to the recipient surgical suite.

68400-68420

68400   Incision, drainage of lacrimal gland
68420   Incision, drainage of lacrimal sac (dacryocystotomy or dacryocystostomy)

An abscess or other accumulation of fluid in the lacrimal gland or lacrimal sac is treated with incision and drainage. In 68400, the upper eyelid is cleansed and a local anesthetic is administered as needed. The area of fluctuance in the lacrimal gland is incised and drained. Any loculations are disrupted using blunt and sharp dissection. The area is flushed with antibiotic solution as needed. The incision may be left open or a drain may be placed and the skin closed around the drain. In 68420, the inner aspect of the lower eyelid is cleansed and a local anesthetic administered as needed. A stab incision is made over the area of fluctuance and fluid is drained.

68440

68440   Snip incision of lacrimal punctum

Stenosis of the lacrimal punctum is treated by using a snipping procedure to widen the opening. This procedure may also be referred to as a one-snip, two-snip or three-snip procedure, or a snip punctoplasty. Stenosis may result from an infection, a rare systemic condition such as porphyria cutanea tarda or acrodermatitis enteropathica, trauma, thermal or chemical burn, topical or systemic chemotherapy, or radiation therapy. The skin around the eye is cleansed and a local anesthetic injected subcutaneously below the lower punctum. The punctum is located and dilated. Toothed microforceps are inserted through the punctum and the posterior wall of the ampulla grasped. Vannas scissors are passed into the ampulla. A one-snip procedure involves a single vertical snip down the posterior aspect of the ampulla. A two-snip procedure uses a second snip down the canalicula. A three-snip procedure uses two downward snips along the posterior aspect of the ampulla and a third across the bottom joining the two downward snips.

68500-68505

68500   Excision of lacrimal gland (dacryoadenectomy), except for tumor; total
68505   Excision of lacrimal gland (dacryoadenectomy), except for tumor; partial

Part or all of the lacrimal (tear) gland is excised for a condition other than a tumor. The skin is cleansed over the eye. A local anesthetic is injected. An incision is made over the temporal aspect of the eye. The temporal muscle is exposed and retracted laterally to the expose the lacrimal gland. In 68500, the entire lacrimal gland is dissected free of surrounding tissue and excised. In 68505, part of the lacrimal gland, usually the palpebral lobe is dissected and excised. The operative wound is closed in layers.

68510

68510   Biopsy of lacrimal gland

The skin is cleansed over the eye. A local anesthetic is injected. An incision is made over the temporal aspect of the eye. The temporal muscle is exposed and retracted laterally to the expose the lacrimal gland. The lacrimal gland is inspected. One or more tissue samples are obtained from the lacrimal gland and sent to the laboratory for separately reportable pathology examination. The operative wound is closed in layers.

68520

68520   Excision of lacrimal sac (dacryocystectomy)

The skin around the eye is cleansed. A local anesthetic is injected subcutaneously around the lacrimal sac. An incision is made over the inner aspect of the lower eyelid, and the lacrimal sac, nasolacrimal duct, and canaliculi are exposed. The lacrimal sac is excised. The proximal end of the nasolacrimal duct is cauterized. The canaliculi are probed and if the superior or inferior canaliculus is patent they are cauterized. If a fistula is present it is also excised. The surgical wound is closed and a dressing applied.

68525

68525   Biopsy of lacrimal sac

The skin around the eye is cleansed. A local anesthetic is injected subcutaneously around the lacrimal sac. An incision is made over the inner aspect of the lower eyelid, and the lacrimal sac, nasolacrimal duct, and canaliculi exposed. The lacrimal sac and surrounding structures are inspected. One or two tissue samples are obtained from the lacrimal sac and sent to the laboratory for separately reportable pathology examination. The operative wound is closed in layers.

68530

68530   Removal of foreign body or dacryolith, lacrimal passages

A foreign body or dacryolith is removed from the lacrimal passages. A dacryolith is a concretion or stone that has formed in the lacrimal system. An incision is made over the affected lacrimal passage and the foreign body or dacryolith is located. An incision is made into the affected lacrimal structure and the foreign body or dacryolith is removed. The lacrimal structure is repaired with sutures.

68540-68550

68540   Excision of lacrimal gland tumor; frontal approach
68550   Excision of lacrimal gland tumor; involving osteotomy

The lacrimal gland is a bilobed gland located in the superotemporal aspect of the orbit. The two lobes consisting of the larger orbital lobe and smaller palpebral lobe are separated by the lateral horn of the levator aponeurosis. The palpebral lobe can be identified in the lateral fornix with the lid everted on an external eye exam. The orbital lobe lies behind the orbital bone and is not visible on external eye exam. Lesions of the lacrimal gland may be inflammatory or neoplastic. Inflammatory lesions include dacryoadenitis, sarcoidosis, and orbital inflammatory pseudotumor. Benign neoplastic lesions include pleomorphic adneoma, benign reactive lymphoid hyperplasia, and oncocytomas. Malignant neoplastic lesions include adenoid cystic carcinoma, squamous cell carcinoma, adenocarcinoma, mucoepidermoid carcinoma, and malignant lymphomas. In 68540, using an anterior or frontal approach, the eyelid is sutured closed and a skin incision is made over crease of the upper eyelid. Soft tissues are dissected and the lacrimal gland is exposed. The lacrimal gland is dissected free of surrounding tissues and excised. Separately reportable frozen sections are evaluated by a pathologist to determine if the margins are clean. If the margins are not clean surrounding tissue is excised until the margins are clean. The surgical wound is closed in layers. In 68550, the tumor excision is performed as described above except that any involved bone is also excised using a bone saw or osteotome.

68700

68700   Plastic repair of canaliculi

An injury to the canaliculus is repaired. The canaliculi are the mucosal ducts at the medial aspect of the eye that drain tears from the eye. The punctum is dilated and a probe passed through the punctum into the canaliculus. The severed ends of the canaliculus are identified. A surgical microscope or loupes may be used to provide better visualization. The ends are reapproximated and repaired with sutures.

68705

68705   Correction of everted punctum, cautery

The inferior punctum is normally oriented posteriorly and is in contact with the globe. An everted punctum turns outward and away from the globe. A probe is passed through the punctum and into the canaliculus. The lower lid is everted and strategically cauterized so that when the cautery site heals and scar tissue forms, the tissue will contract and pull the punctum back into a more normal posterior position that is in contact with the globe.

68720

68720   Dacryocystorhinostomy (fistulization of lacrimal sac to nasal cavity)

Dacryocystorhinostomy is performed to treat epiphora (excessive tearing) caused by blockage of the lacrimal passages. The nose is packed for 10 minutes with a solution containing epinephrine and xylocaine. A fiberoptic light probe is passed through the punctum, into the upper or lower canaliculus and then into the lacrimal sac. The light can be seen through the nose mucosa at the posterior end of the lacrimal sac. A 1 cm diameter circle of nasal mucosa is excised and the underlying bone exposed. The bone is removed with a drill. The lacrimal sac is opened. Metal stents attached to Silastic tubing are passed through the upper and lower canaliculi and the distal ends guided into the nasal passage. The metal stents are severed and the tubing is secured with sutures. The tubing keeps the lacrimal sac open so that tears drain into the nose.

68745-68750

68745   Conjunctivorhinostomy (fistulization of conjunctiva to nasal cavity); without tube

68750   Conjunctivorhinostomy (fistulization of conjunctiva to nasal cavity); with insertion of tube or stent

Conjunctivorhinostomy is performed to treat epiphora (excessive tearing) caused by blockage of the upper lacrimal structures including the punctum and canaliculi. An incision is made in the lower lid conjunctival sac and mucosal flaps are raised. In 68745, the frontal process of the maxillary bone is perforated and a passageway opened between the conjunctival sac and nasal fossa. In 68750, a tube is passed through the surgically created mucosal opening under the soft tissues of the face over the maxillary bone and into the nasal atrium. This creates a passageway from the lacrimal lake to the nasal atrium. The tube is secured with sutures.

68760-68761

68760   Closure of the lacrimal punctum; by thermocauterization, ligation, or laser surgery

68761   Closure of the lacrimal punctum; by plug, each

The lacrimal punctum is closed to treat dry eye syndrome. Anesthetic eye drops or other local anesthesia is applied to the conjunctiva near the punctum. In 68760, the punctum is closed by thermocauterization, ligation, or laser surgery. If thermocauterization is used, the electrocautery device is activated and the punctum burned to cause scarring and closure of the punctum. Ligation involves suturing the punctum closed. Laser surgery involves activating the laser and destroying the punctual opening. In 68761, a plug is placed in the punctum. The punctum is inspected and dilated as needed. The lid is pulled away from the globe. The implant is grasped with fine forceps and inserted into the punctum and the lid is manipulated until the plug is in the proper position.

68770

68770   Closure of lacrimal fistula (separate procedure)

Lacrimal fistulas may be congenital or acquired. Congenital fistulas may be open or closed. Open fistulous tracts appear as a small hole inferior to the medial canthus, and tears or other fluid drains from the fistula onto the skin. Closed fistulous tracts end in a blind sac and do not drain. Acquired fistulas may result from trauma or disease such as an infection. A local anesthetic is administered and the fistulous tract inspected. The fistula is then obliterated using electrocautery, laser surgery, or other technique.

68801

68801   Dilation of lacrimal punctum, with or without irrigation

Dilation of the lacrimal punctum is performed to treat stenosis or obstruction. A local anesthetic is administered. The punctum is inspected. A dilator is passed into the punctum and the narrowed region is dilated. The dilator is removed and the punctum is cannulated and flushed as needed with an irrigation solution.

68810-68816

68810   Probing of nasolacrimal duct, with or without irrigation

68811   Probing of nasolacrimal duct, with or without irrigation; requiring general anesthesia

68815   Probing of nasolacrimal duct, with or without irrigation; with insertion of tube or stent

68816   Probing of nasolacrimal duct, with or without irrigation; with transluminal balloon catheter dilation

The nasolacrimal duct is probed with or without irrigation in 68810. Probing of the nasolacrimal duct (NLD), also called the tear duct, is typically done to treat a congenital obstruction in children or, less commonly, to treat an acquired obstruction in adults. Congenital NLD obstruction is characterized by failure of the NLD to open into the nose. Most congenital obstructions resolve spontaneously by 12 months of age. If the NLD is still obstructed at 12 months, it may be treated by inserting a probe into the duct to identify and open the area of obstruction or stenosis. The puncta are dilated. A probe is inserted and passed through the duct until it can be visualized in the nose or can be touched by a second probe passed through the nasal punctum. The probe(s) is removed. The duct may be irrigated with saline solution containing fluoroscein dye to flush debris or an obstructing stone or concretion from the duct. Use 68811 if the procedure is performed under general anesthesia. Use 68815 if probing and irrigation is followed by insertion of a tube or stent, also referred to as silicone tube intubation, placed in the tear duct to stretch it. The tube is left in place for approximately six months and removed in a separately reportable procedure. Use 68816 if the probing and irrigation is followed by transluminal balloon dilation. A deflated balloon catheter is inserted into the nasolacrimal duct through the opening in the corner of the eye. The presence of the catheter is the duct is confirmed and the balloon is inflated to expand the tear duct for 90 seconds. The balloon is then deflated and reinflated for 60 seconds. The balloon is retracted to a point slightly higher in the duct and two inflation/deflation cycles are again performed before the deflated balloon catheter is removed.

68840

68840   Probing of lacrimal canaliculi, with or without irrigation

The canaliculi are the mucosal ducts at the medial aspect of the eye that drain tears from the eye. There are two canaliculi in each eye, one in the upper and lower lid referred to as the superior and inferior canaliculi respectively. A local anesthetic is administered. The punctum is dilated and a probe passed through the punctum into the superior and/or inferior canaliculus. The superior and/or inferior canaliculus are cannulated and flushed as needed with an irrigation solution.

68850

68850   Injection of contrast medium for dacryocystography

Dacryocystography is a radiologic examination performed on the nasolacrimal ducts, (tear ducts) after the injection of a contrast medium, to evaluate excessive tearing and assess patency or other pathology of the lacrimal drainage system. Dacryocystography is also used for pre- and post-operative evaluation. The patient may initially have separately reportable panoramic radiography of the face. Anesthetic drops are instilled into the eyes, the lacrimal canaliculi are cannulated, and water-soluble or oil-based contrast medium is injected. Radiographic images are obtained at different degrees or oblique angles to show the lacrimal pathways. This code reports the contrast medium injection and necessary cannulation portion of the procedure only.

       ● New Code   ▲ Revised Code

Eye and Ocular Adnexa

69000-69005

69000 Drainage external ear, abscess or hematoma; simple
69005 Drainage external ear, abscess or hematoma; complicated

An abscess or hematoma of the external ear is drained. The site is gently cleansed with a disinfectant. An incision is made in the center of the abscess or hematoma. The abscess or hematoma is drained and the site irrigated with a sterile solution. The skin may be closed or left open to drain. A tube may be inserted to facilitate drainage. Code 69000 is used for a simple procedure. Code 69005 is used for a complicated procedure. Treatment of a complicated abscess or hematoma may include sterile gauze packing of the site to help the wound heal.

69020

69020 Drainage external auditory canal, abscess

An abscess of the external auditory canal (EAC) is drained. An otoscopic examination of the external ear canal is performed and the abscess identified. An operating head is placed on the otoscope and surgical instruments passed through the speculum. The site is cleansed with disinfectant. The abscess is incised and drained. The abscess site is irrigated with sterile solution. Topical antibiotics may be applied. The skin may be closed or left open to drain. The ear canal may be packed with sterile gauze.

69090

69090 Ear piercing

An ear piercing procedure is performed. The skin of the ear at the site to be pierced is cleansed with disinfectant. A hollow medical needle is placed at the selected site. With the needle in place, the earring is pushed through the opening following the back of the needle. The needle is removed and the earring is secured.

69100-69105

69100 Biopsy external ear
69105 Biopsy external auditory canal

A biopsy of the external ear is performed, which may include skin, soft tissue, and cartilage. The external ear consists of the auricle (pinna). The skin over the biopsy site is cleansed with disinfectant. A tissue sample of the lesion along with normal tissue is removed and sent for pathological examination. The biopsy site may be closed or left to granulate without closure. In 69105, a biopsy of the external auditory canal (EAC), also called the external acoustic meatus, is performed. An otoscopic examination of the EAC is performed and the lesion identified. An operating head is placed on the otoscope and surgical instruments passed through the speculum. The site is cleansed with disinfectant. A tissue sample is obtained, which may include skin, soft tissue, cartilage, and bone. The biopsy site may be closed or left open to granulate. The ear canal may be packed with sterile gauze.

69110-69120

69110 Excision external ear; partial, simple repair
69120 Excision external ear; complete amputation

A partial excision of the external ear is performed with simple closure. The external ear consists of the auricle (pinna). An incision is made in the skin of the ear and carried down through the cartilage. The section of the external ear to be removed is excised. Bleeding is controlled. The surgical wound is closed by suture and a pressure dressing applied to prevent hematoma formation. In 69120, a complete amputation of the entire external ear is performed. An incision is made in the skin encircling the auricle and carried down through soft tissue and cartilage. The entire auricle is removed. Bleeding is controlled. The surgical wound may be closed or a separately reportable reconstruction of the ear performed.

69140-69145

69140 Excision exostosis(es), external auditory canal
69145 Excision soft tissue lesion, external auditory canal

The physician performs an excision of exostosis (es) of the external auditory canal (EAC). Exostoses are a bony abnormality of the EAC that cause gradual narrowing of the bony canal as a result of bone deposition on the canal wall. An otoscopic examination of the EAC is performed and the exotoses identified. An operating head is placed on the otoscope and surgical instruments passed through the speculum. The site is cleansed with disinfectant. A medially based canal skin flap is developed and reflected onto the tympanic membrane. The exostoses are drilled away using bone curettes and diamond burrs. The surgical site is covered by the previously created skin flap and closed. In 69145, the physician removes a

soft tissue lesion of the EAC. An otoscopic examination is performed as described above. The lesion is removed along with a margin of healthy tissue. Electrocautery may be used to control bleeding. The surgical wound may be closed or left open to granulate. The ear canal may be packed with sterile gauze.

69150-69155

69150 Radical excision external auditory canal lesion; without neck dissection
69155 Radical excision external auditory canal lesion; with neck dissection

The physician performs a radical excision of an external auditory canal lesion. Taking care to protect the facial nerve, an incision is made in the external auditory canal extending into the front of the ear to the parotid gland. The anterior portion of the external auditory canal lesion is excised along with portions of the parotid gland. Intraoperative frozen sections of surgical margins are sent for pathological examination. If margins are positive for tumor invasion, piecemeal resection of gross tumor extension is performed until all margins are free of all visible and microscopic evidence of tumor. The physician may remove skin, soft tissue, cartilage and bone. Separately reportable reconstruction of the external auditory canal with skin grafts is performed as needed. Code 69150 is used when radical excision is performed without radical neck dissection (RND). Code 69155 is used when a RND is also performed. Lymph node groups levels I-V are dissected free of surrounding tissue and excised. The sternocleidomastoid muscle and the internal jugular vein are removed. The submandibular gland on the affected side is removed. The anterior belly of the digastric muscle as well as the sternohyoid and sternothyroid muscles may also be removed.

69200-69205

69200 Removal foreign body from external auditory canal; without general anesthesia
69205 Removal foreign body from external auditory canal; with general anesthesia

A foreign body is removed from the external auditory canal. Techniques for removal depend on the type of foreign body and include mechanical extraction, irrigation, and suction. The ear is examined and the location and depth of the foreign body determined. Mechanical extraction is performed using an otoscope. Forceps are introduced through the otoscope lens and carefully advanced to the foreign body which is grasped and removed. Irrigation is performed by attaching an angiocatheter to a syringe. Irrigation fluid is warmed. A basin is placed under the ear to collect irrigation runoff. The angiocatheter is placed in the auditory canal and fluid is slowly injected to dislodge and wash out the foreign body. Suction is performed with a soft-tipped suction catheter using low suction. An otoscope is used to view the foreign body. The suction catheter is introduced through the otoscope and advanced to the foreign body. Suction is applied. The catheter is removed with the attached foreign body. Following removal of the foreign body the ear is inspected to ensure that there are no foreign body fragments remaining and that the tympanic membrane is intact. Use 69200 when the procedure is performed without anesthesia and 69205 when general anesthesia is used.

69209-69210

69209 Removal impacted cerumen using irrigation/lavage, unilateral
69210 Removal impacted cerumen requiring instrumentation, unilateral

Impacted cerumen is removed from the ear using irrigation/lavage to wash it out (69209), or instrumentation to clean it out (69210) through microsuction or mechanical removal. Cerumen is composed of lipids produced by the sebaceous glands of the external auditory canal to protect the lining of the canal. Impacted cerumen is an accumulation of hardened cerumen that obstructs the auditory canal causing discomfort in the ear, hearing impairment, tinnitus, and dizziness. The ears are examined using an otoscope or operating microscope. For irrigation, a syringe type tool is inserted into the ear canal to instill warm water or saline solution, soften the ear wax, and flush it out. For mechanical removal, the practitioner uses crocodile forceps, an aural speculum, wax hooks, probes of various sizes, and/or a suction device to remove the impacted cerumen under visualization with the patient semi-reclined or in supine position. Many times instrumentation must be used as the earwax may not be removed completely with irrigation alone.

69220-69222

69220 Debridement, mastoidectomy cavity, simple (eg, routine cleaning)
69222 Debridement, mastoidectomy cavity, complex (eg, with anesthesia or more than routine cleaning)

Periodic debridement may be required after mastoidectomy to keep the mastoid cavity free of debris or for persistent infection or drainage from the mastoid cavity. A mirror or rigid endoscope is used to visualize the mastoid cavity. The cavity may be flushed with a diluted hydrogen peroxide solution to loosen the debris. Debris is removed using a forceps or curette in one hand and a suction device in the other. The physician debrides the entire mastoid cavity while simultaneous suctioning the debris from the cavity. The middle ear is also cleaned as this is often a source of infection. Once the entire mastoid cavity has been debrided, it is inspected using a mirror or the endoscope. Any remaining hydrogen peroxide is suctioned out. The surface of the mastoid cavity is then dusted with boric acid and/or anti-fungal or anti-bacterial agents. Use 69220 for a simple or routine cleaning and 69222 for a complex cleaning such as one requiring the use of anesthesia or any cleaning that is other than routine such as cleaning due to infection.

69300

69300   Otoplasty, protruding ear, with or without size reduction

Otoplasty is performed for protruding ear with or without size reduction. An incision is made behind the ear in the skin fold between the ear and skull. The cartilage of the auricle, also referred to as the pinna, is exposed. The cartilage is trimmed and shaped to give the auricle a more desirable size, shape and form. The cartilage is then pinned back and secured with permanent sutures to maintain the auricle in a position closer to the skull. Excess skin is trimmed and the incision repaired with sutures.

69310

69310   Reconstruction of external auditory canal (meatoplasty) (eg, for stenosis due to injury, infection) (separate procedure)

The physician performs a reconstruction of the external auditory canal, also called a meatoplasty, for a condition such as stenosis following an injury or infection. The external auditory canal is inspected. Skin in the external auditory canal is excised. A drill is used to remove bone and increase the diameter of the canal. The eardrum is inspected to ensure that it is intact. Skin grafts are harvested and placed over the exposed bone in the external auditory canal.

69320

69320   Reconstruction external auditory canal for congenital atresia, single stage

The physician reconstructs the external auditory canal for congenital atresia which is the absence of an external ear canal and is also referred to as aural atresia. Aural atresia may be unilateral or bilateral. An incision is made in the skin where the external auditory canal will be constructed. Overlying bone is drilled out down to the level of the ossicles to create the canal. A small fascial graft is harvested and placed over the ossicles to create the eardrum. Skin grafts are also harvested and placed over the exposed bone in the canal.

69420-69421

69420   Myringotomy including aspiration and/or eustachian tube inflation
69421   Myringotomy including aspiration and/or eustachian tube inflation requiring general anesthesia

The physician performs a myringotomy including aspiration and Eustachian tube inflation. The Eustachian tube is a narrow tube that connects the middle ear to the back of the nose. It opens and closes in response to swallowing to equalize the pressure in the middle ear. It also drains mucus produced by the lining of the middle ear. If the Eustachian tube becomes blocked air is trapped in the middle ear. The lining of the middle ear absorbs the trapped air and creates negative pressure that retracts the tympanic membrane (eardrum). Chronic blockage also referred to as Eustachian tube dysfunction can result in an accumulation of fluid in the middle ear space that can cause hearing impairment. A small incision is made in the tympanic membrane (eardrum). Fluid within the middle ear is removed by suction aspiration. The Eustachian tube is opened by inflating it with air. Use 69420 when the procedure is performed without general anesthesia and 69421 when general anesthesia is required.

69424

69424   Ventilating tube removal requiring general anesthesia

The physician removes a previously placed ventilating (tympanostomy) tube under general anesthesia. Using an operating microscope, a small incision is made in the tympanic membrane at the junction with the ventilating tube to release tension on the tube. The tube is then dissected free of surrounding tissue and removed. Granulation (scar) tissue at the site of the tube is also removed to promote healing of the perforation site.

69433-69436

69433   Tympanostomy (requiring insertion of ventilating tube), local or topical anesthesia
69436   Tympanostomy (requiring insertion of ventilating tube), general anesthesia

The physician performs a tympanostomy with insertion of ventilating tube for chronic otitis media and/or Eustachian tube dysfunction. The Eustachian tube is a narrow tube that connects the middle ear to the back of the nose. It opens and closes in response to swallowing to equalize the pressure in the middle ear. It also drains mucus produced by the lining of the middle ear. If the Eustachian tube becomes blocked air is trapped in the middle ear. The lining of the middle ear absorbs the trapped air and creates negative

pressure that retracts the tympanic membrane (eardrum). Chronic blockage also referred to as Eustachian tube dysfunction can result in an accumulation of fluid in the middle ear space that can cause hearing impairment and chronic otitis media. A small incision is made in the tympanic membrane (eardrum). Fluid within the middle ear is removed by suction aspiration. The Eustachian tube is opened by inflating it with air. A tube is then placed into the opening in the tympanic membrane to maintain the opening. Use 69433 when the procedure is performed with local or topical anesthesia and 69436 when general anesthesia is required.

69440

69440   Middle ear exploration through postauricular or ear canal incision

If a postauricular approach is used, an incision is made in the skin fold behind the ear and the middle ear entered. If an ear canal approach is used, the meatus (ear canal) is incised and a tympanomeatal flap is developed and elevated and the middle ear entered. Bones of the middle ear are inspected which include the malleus, incus, and stapes. The articulations of these bones are evaluated. The oval and round windows are inspected. The Eustachian tube is also explored. No definitive procedures are performed. Any abnormal findings are noted. The postauricular incision is closed or the typanomeatal flap is replaced and the meatal incision closed with sutures.

69450

69450   Tympanolysis, transcanal

The meatus (ear canal) is incised and a tympanomeatal flap is developed and elevated and the middle ear entered. Adhesions and scar tissue between the tympanic membrane and bones of the middle ear or other structures are carefully dissected. The typanomeatal flap is replaced and the meatal incision closed with sutures.

69501

69501   Transmastoid antrotomy (simple mastoidectomy)

The mastoid antrum is a cavity in the petrous portion of the temporal bone. The posterior aspect of the mastoid antrum communicates with the mastoid air cells and the anterior aspect communicates with structures in the middle ear. Simple mastoidectomy is typically performed for an acute infection. The mastoid antrum is approached through the mastoid air cells. The antrum is exposed and purulent matter and debris removed along with infected tissue. A drain may be placed in the antrum for continued drainage.

69502-69511

69502   Mastoidectomy; complete
69505   Mastoidectomy; modified radical
69511   Mastoidectomy; radical

A mastoidectomy is performed to remove infected mastoid air cells. The mastoid process (bone) is located behind the ear and projects from the temporal bone of the skull. The mastoid air cells are located throughout the bone. An incision is made behind the ear and the mastoid bone is exposed. In 69502, a complete mastoidectomy is performed. This procedure is typically performed for acute infection. The mastoid bone is opened and the air cell system is completed removed along with purulent matter, debris, and infected tissue. A drain may be placed for continued drainage. In 69505, a modified radical mastoidectomy is performed. This procedure is typically performed for management of cholesteatoma. The mastoid is opened and the remaining air cells are completely removed. The posterior and superior walls of the external auditory canal are also removed to allow exposure of the mastoid and attic of the middle ear to the outside. The tympanic membrane and middle ear structures are preserved. In 69511, a radical mastoidectomy is performed. This procedure is performed for an extensive cholesteatoma. The procedure is the same as for a modified radical mastoidectomy except that structures of the epitympanum (upper portion of the tympanic cavity) which include the head of the malleus and body of the incus are removed. The stapes may also be removed but is preserved if possible. Removal of these structures allows exteriorization of the mastoid cavity and middle ear.

69530

69530   Petrous apicectomy including radical mastoidectomy

This procedure is performed for infections of the mastoid air cells that have spread to the petrous apex. An incision is made behind the ear and the mastoid bone is exposed. The mastoid bone is opened and the air cell system is completed removed along with purulent matter, debris, and infected tissue. Structures of the epitympanum (upper portion of the tympanic cavity) which include the head of the malleus and body of the incus are removed. The stapes may also be removed but is preserved if possible. Removal of these structures allows exteriorization of the mastoid cavity and middle ear. The petrous apex is exposed by removal of the anterior ear canal wall. The condyle of the mandible may be excised. The tensor muscle of the tympanic membrane is avulsed. The tensor semicanal is opened. The triangle between the carotid artery, the cochlea, and the middle fossa dura is dissected. The petrous apex is visualized and removed. A drain may be placed for continued drainage.

69535

69535   Resection temporal bone, external approach

A C-shaped incision is made beginning above the ear over the temporal bone, extending in a wide arc around the ear and down the neck. A flap is elevated to expose the temporal muscle, mastoid and neck structures. The temporal bone is exposed and the diseased portion excised. Once all diseased bone has been removed, the operative wound is repaired in layers.

69540

69540   Excision aural polyp

The physician excises an aural polyp which is a benign fleshy growth attached to the external ear canal or the eardrum. An incision is made around the polyp which is excised along with a margin of healthy tissue. The ear canal is packed with antibiotic and steroid soaked gauze or gelfoam and the excision site allowed to heal by secondary intention.

69550-69554

69550   Excision aural glomus tumor; transcanal

69552   Excision aural glomus tumor; transmastoid

69554   Excision aural glomus tumor; extended (extratemporal)

The physician excises an aural glomus tumor which is a benign tumor arising from the paraganglionic cells in glomus tissue near the temporal bone. Aural glomus tumors are subdivided into those that arise from the adventitia of the dome of the jugular bulb called glomus jugulare tumors and those that arise from glomus bodies along the tympanic branch of the glossopharyngeal nerve called glomus tympanicum tumors. There are three common approaches with the size and location of the tumor dictating the approach. In 69550, a transcanal approach is used to excise a tumor limited to the middle ear. The external auditory canal is entered and enlarged as needed. The meatus is incised and a tympanomeatal flap created. The middle ear is entered and the tumor is exposed. The tumor may be dissected from the surrounding middle ear structures or an Argon laser used to coagulate and destroy the tumor. In 69552, a transmastoid approach is used to excise a tumor that has extended from the middle ear into the mastoid bone. An incision is made behind the ear and the mastoid bone is exposed. The mastoid bone is entered and the mastoid cells are cleared of tumor tissue. The tumor can be dissected or an Argon laser used to destroy the tissue. In 69554, a tumor that has invaded the temporal bone is excised using an extended extratemporal approach. A C-shaped incision is made beginning above the ear over the temporal bone and extending in a wide arc around the ear and down the neck. A flap is elevated to expose the temporal muscle, mastoid bone and neck structures. A complete mastoidectomy along with removal of the mastoid tip is performed. The inferior tympanic bone is excised and the external auditory canal skeletonized. The internal carotid artery is exposed and protected. The internal jugular vein is exposed and ligated. The facial nerve is identified and protected. The tumor is dissected from surrounding structures and removed. Hearing is preserved if possible but depending on the exact location of the tumor, it is sometimes necessary to sacrifice the external auditory canal and structures of the middle ear.

69601-69603

69601   Revision mastoidectomy; resulting in complete mastoidectomy

69602   Revision mastoidectomy; resulting in modified radical mastoidectomy

69603   Revision mastoidectomy; resulting in radical mastoidectomy

A revision mastoidectomy is performed to remove infected mastoid air cells. The mastoid process (bone) is located behind the ear and projects from the temporal bone of the skull. The mastoid air cells are located throughout the bone. An incision is made behind the ear and the mastoid bone is exposed. The remaining mastoid air cells are inspected and the extent of the revision procedure determined. In 69601, the revision results in a complete mastoidectomy. This procedure is typically performed for acute infection. The air cell system is completely removed along with purulent matter, debris, and infected tissue. A drain may be placed for continued drainage. In 69602, the revision results in a modified radical mastoidectomy. This procedure is typically performed for management of recurrent cholesteatoma. The mastoid is opened and the remaining air cells are completely removed. The posterior and superior walls of the external auditory canal are also removed to allow exposure of the mastoid and attic of the middle ear to the outside. The tympanic membrane and middle ear structures are preserved. In 69603, the revision results in a radical mastoidectomy. This procedure is performed for a recurrent extensive cholesteatoma. The procedure is the same as for a modified radical mastoidectomy except the structures of the epitympanum (upper portion of the tympanic cavity) which include the head of the malleus and body of the incus are removed. The stapes may also be removed but is preserved if possible. Removal of these structures allows exteriorization of the mastoid cavity and middle ear.

69604

69604   Revision mastoidectomy; resulting in tympanoplasty

An incision is made behind the ear and the mastoid bone is exposed. The remaining mastoid air cells are inspected and the extent of the revision procedure determined. The

air cell system is completely removed along with purulent matter, debris, and infected tissue. The posterior and superior walls of the external auditory canal may also be removed to allow exposure of the mastoid and attic of the middle ear to the outside. If a more extensive (radical) mastoidectomy is required, the structures of the epitympanum (upper portion of the tympanic cavity) which include the head of the malleus and body of the incus are removed. The stapes may also be removed but is preserved if possible. Removal of these structures allows exteriorization of the mastoid cavity and middle ear. A drain may be placed behind the ear for continued drainage. The physician repairs the tympanic membrane. Tissue around the hole is rimmed until bleeding occurs. Depending on the exact location and size of the hole, simply rimming the hole may allow the edges to heal together. A larger hole may require a patch. A small amount of skin, fat, tendon, or fascia is harvested. The graft is prepared. Absorbable sponge material may be placed in the middle ear behind the hole to support the graft. The graft is placed over the hole, and absorbable sponge placed in the ear canal over the graft to hold the graft in place. The ear is packed with gauze.

69605

69605   Revision mastoidectomy; with apicectomy

This procedure is performed for recurrent infections of the mastoid air cells that have spread to the petrous apex. An incision is made behind the ear and the mastoid bone is exposed. The remaining mastoid air cells are inspected and the extent of the revision procedure determined. The air cell system is completely removed along with purulent matter, debris, and infected tissue. Structures of the epitympanum (upper portion of the tympanic cavity) which include the head of the malleus and body of the incus are removed. The stapes may also be removed but is preserved if possible. Removal of these structures allows exteriorization of the mastoid cavity and middle ear. The petrous apex is exposed by removal of the anterior ear canal wall. The condyle of the mandible may be excised. The tensor muscle of the tympanic membrane is avulsed. The tensor semicanal is opened. The triangle between the carotid artery, the cochlea, and the middle fossa dura is dissected. The petrous apex is visualized and removed. Once all infected tissue has been removed, incisions are closed. A drain may be placed to allow continued drainage.

69610

69610   Tympanic membrane repair, with or without site preparation of perforation for closure, with or without patch

The procedure may be performed through the ear canal or through a post-auricular incision. The hole is exposed and inspected. The middle ear structures are also inspected and any scar tissue in the middle ear removed. Tissue around the hole is rimmed until bleeding occurs. Depending on the exact location and size of the hole, simply rimming the hole may allow the edges to heal together. A larger hole may require a patch. A small amount of skin, fat, tendon, or fascia is harvested. The graft is prepared. Absorbable sponge material may be placed in the middle ear behind the hole to support the graft. The graft is placed over the hole and absorbable sponge placed in the ear canal over the graft to hold the graft in place. The ear is packed with gauze.

69620

69620   Myringoplasty (surgery confined to drumhead and donor area)

A myringoplasty is performed to repair a small hole (perforation) in the eardrum. This procedure is confined to the drumhead and donor area. The procedure may be performed through the ear canal or through a post-auricular incision. The hole is exposed and inspected. Tissue around the hole is rimmed until bleeding occurs. Depending on the exact location and size of the hole, simply rimming the hole may allow the edges to heal together. If a patch is required, a fat graft is typically harvested. The graft is prepared. Absorbable sponge material may be placed in the middle ear behind the hole to support the graft. The graft is then placed over the hole and absorbable sponge placed in the ear canal over the graft to hold the graft in place. The ear is packed with gauze.

69631-69633

69631   Tympanoplasty without mastoidectomy (including canalplasty, atticotomy and/or middle ear surgery), initial or revision; without ossicular chain reconstruction

69632   Tympanoplasty without mastoidectomy (including canalplasty, atticotomy and/or middle ear surgery), initial or revision; with ossicular chain reconstruction (eg, postfenestration)

69633   Tympanoplasty without mastoidectomy (including canalplasty, atticotomy and/or middle ear surgery), initial or revision; with ossicular chain reconstruction and synthetic prosthesis (eg, partial ossicular replacement prosthesis [PORP], total ossicular replacement prosthesis [TORP])

A tympanoplasty without mastoidectomy is performed. This procedure may be an initial procedure or a revision of a previous tympanoplasty and may include a canalplasty, atticotomy, and/or middle ear surgery. Tympanoplasties are classified by type depending on whether only the tympanic membrane requires repair or whether some or all of the bones (ossicles) also require repair. In 69631, the procedure is performed without ossicular chain reconstruction. The procedure may be performed through the ear canal or through a

Auditory System

post-auricular incision. If the external auditory canal is stenosed from repeated infection, a canalplasty is performed. A drill is used to remove bone and increase the diameter of the canal. The hole in the tympanic membrane is exposed and inspected. The middle ear structures are also inspected and any scar tissue in the middle ear removed. The tympanic attic may be opened (atticotomy) by removing the scutum (a thin plate of bone overlying the attic) or if a larger atticotomy is required by drilling the posterosuperior bony ear canal. Tissue around the hole in the tympanic membrane is rimmed until bleeding occurs. Depending on the exact location and size of the hole, simply rimming the hole may allow the edges to heal together. A larger hole may require a patch. A small amount of skin, fat, tendon, or fascia is harvested. The graft is prepared. Absorbable sponge material may be placed in the middle ear behind the hole to support the graft. The graft is then placed over the hole. If a canalplasty has been performed, skin grafts are harvested and placed over the exposed bone in the external auditory canal. An absorbable sponge is placed in the ear canal over the tympanic membrane graft to hold the graft in place. The ear is packed with gauze. In 69632, an ossicular chain reconstruction is performed in addition to the procedures above. The physician inspects the ossicles and determines that one or more these bones require reconstruction. Tissue grafts are harvested and the incus, malleus, and/or stapes are reconstructed. In 69633, the ossicular chain reconstruction is performed using a synthetic prosthesis. A partial ossicular replacement prosthesis (PORP) or total ossicular replacement prosthesis (TORP) may be used.

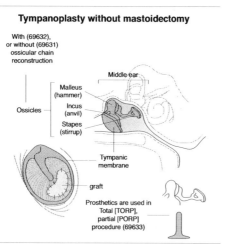

Tympanoplasty without mastoidectomy

69635-69637

69635 Tympanoplasty with antrotomy or mastoidotomy (including canalplasty, atticotomy, middle ear surgery, and/or tympanic membrane repair); without ossicular chain reconstruction

69636 Tympanoplasty with antrotomy or mastoidotomy (including canalplasty, atticotomy, middle ear surgery, and/or tympanic membrane repair); with ossicular chain reconstruction

69637 Tympanoplasty with antrotomy or mastoidotomy (including canalplasty, atticotomy, middle ear surgery, and/or tympanic membrane repair); with ossicular chain reconstruction and synthetic prosthesis (eg, partial ossicular replacement prosthesis [PORP], total ossicular replacement prosthesis [TORP])

A tympanoplasty with antrotomy or mastoidotomy is performed. This procedure may include a canalplasty, atticotomy, middle ear surgery, and/or tympanic membrane repair. Tympanoplasties are classified by type depending on whether only the tympanic membrane requires repair or whether some or all of the bones (ossicles) also require repair. This procedure also involves drilling an osseous channel into the temporal bone to the antrum (antrotomy) or into the mastoid bone (mastoidotomy) for drainage. In 69635, the procedure is performed without ossicular chain reconstruction. The procedure may be performed through the ear canal or through a post-auricular incision. If the external auditory canal is stenosed from repeated infection, a canalplasty is performed. A drill is used to remove bone and increase the diameter of the canal. The hole in the tympanic membrane is exposed and inspected. The middle ear structures are also inspected and any scar tissue in the middle ear removed. The tympanic attic may be opened (atticotomy) by removing the scutum (a thin plate of bone overlying the attic) or if a larger atticotomy is required by drilling the posterosuperior bony ear canal. An osseous channel is drilled into the antrum or mastoid cavity for drainage. The tympanic membrane is repaired. Tissue around the hole in the tympanic membrane is rimmed until bleeding occurs. Depending on the exact location and size of the hole, simply rimming the hole may allow the edges to heal together. A larger hole may require a patch. A small amount of skin, fat, tendon, or fascia is harvested. The graft is prepared. Absorbable sponge material may be placed in the middle ear behind the hole to support the graft. The graft is then placed over the hole. If a canalplasty has been performed, skin grafts are harvested and placed over the exposed bone in the external auditory canal. An absorbable sponge is placed in the ear canal over

the tympanic membrane graft to hold the graft in place. The ear is packed with gauze. In 69636, an ossicular chain reconstruction is performed in addition to the procedures above. The physician inspects the ossicles and determines that one or more of these bones require reconstruction. Tissue grafts are harvested and the incus, malleus, and/or stapes are reconstructed. In 69637, the ossicular chain reconstruction is performed using a synthetic prosthesis. A partial ossicular replacement prosthesis (PORP) or total ossicular replacement prosthesis (TORP) may be used.

69641-69642

69641 Tympanoplasty with mastoidectomy (including canalplasty, middle ear surgery, tympanic membrane repair); without ossicular chain reconstruction

69642 Tympanoplasty with mastoidectomy (including canalplasty, middle ear surgery, tympanic membrane repair); with ossicular chain reconstruction

A tympanoplasty with mastoidectomy is performed. This procedure may include a canalplasty, middle ear surgery, and/or tympanic membrane repair. Tympanoplasties are classified by type depending on whether only the tympanic membrane requires repair or whether some or all of the bones (ossicles) also require repair. This procedure includes a mastoidectomy which is performed as follows. An incision is made behind the ear and the mastoid bone is exposed. The mastoid air cells are inspected and the extent of the procedure determined. In this case a simple mastoidectomy is performed. The antrum is exposed and purulent matter and debris removed along with infected tissue. A drain may be placed behind the ear. In 69641, the procedure is performed without ossicular chain reconstruction. The procedure may be performed through the ear canal or through a post-auricular incision. If the external auditory canal is stenosed from repeated infection, a canalplasty is performed. A drill is used to remove bone and increase the diameter of the canal. The hole in the tympanic membrane is exposed and inspected. The middle ear structures are also inspected and any scar tissue in the middle ear removed. The tympanic membrane is repaired. Tissue around the hole in the tympanic membrane is rimmed until bleeding occurs. Depending on the exact location and size of the hole, simply rimming the hole may allow the edges to heal together. A larger hole may require a patch. A small amount of skin, fat, tendon, or fascia is harvested. The graft is prepared. Absorbable sponge material may be placed in the middle ear behind the hole to support the graft. The graft is then placed over the hole. If a canalplasty has been performed, skin grafts are harvested and placed over the exposed bone in the external auditory canal. An absorbable sponge is placed in the ear canal over the tympanic membrane graft to hold the graft in place. The ear is packed with gauze. In 69642, an ossicular chain reconstruction is performed in addition to the procedures above. The physician inspects the ossicles and determines that one or more of these bones require reconstruction. Tissue grafts are harvested and the incus, malleus, and/or stapes are reconstructed.

69643-69644

69643 Tympanoplasty with mastoidectomy (including canalplasty, middle ear surgery, tympanic membrane repair); with intact or reconstructed wall, without ossicular chain reconstruction

69644 Tympanoplasty with mastoidectomy (including canalplasty, middle ear surgery, tympanic membrane repair); with intact or reconstructed canal wall, with ossicular chain reconstruction

A tympanoplasty with mastoidectomy is performed with an intact or reconstructed wall. This procedure may include a canalplasty, middle ear surgery, and/or tympanic membrane repair. Tympanoplasties are classified by type depending on whether only the tympanic membrane requires repair or whether some or all of the bones (ossicles) also require repair. This procedure includes a mastoidectomy using a wall up (intact wall) technique or with reconstruction of the wall following the mastoidectomy. An incision is made behind the ear and the mastoid bone is exposed. The mastoid air cells are inspected and the extent of the procedure determined. The air cell system is completely removed along with purulent matter, debris, and infected tissue. If the posterior and superior walls of the external auditory canal are removed to allow exposure of the mastoid and attic of the middle ear to the outside they are reconstructed following the mastoidectomy. A drain may be placed behind the ear. In 69643, the procedure is performed without ossicular chain reconstruction. The procedure may be performed through the ear canal or through a post-auricular incision. If the external auditory canal is stenosed from repeated infection, a canalplasty is performed. A drill is used to remove bone and increase the diameter of the canal. The hole in the tympanic membrane is exposed and inspected. The middle ear structures are also inspected and any scar tissue in the middle ear removed. The tympanic membrane is repaired. Tissue around the hole in the tympanic membrane is rimmed until bleeding occurs. Depending on the exact location and size of the hole, simply rimming the hole may allow the edges to heal together. A larger hole may require a patch. A small amount of skin, fat, tendon, or fascia is harvested. The graft is prepared. Absorbable sponge material may be placed in the middle ear behind the hole to support the graft. The graft is then placed over the hole. If a canalplasty has been performed, skin grafts are harvested and placed over the exposed bone in the external auditory canal. An absorbable sponge is placed in the ear canal over the tympanic membrane graft to hold the graft in place. The ear is packed with gauze. In 69644, an ossicular chain reconstruction is performed in

Auditory System

addition to the procedures above. The physician inspects the ossicles and determines that one or more of these bones require reconstruction. Tissue grafts are harvested and the incus, malleus, and/or stapes are reconstructed.

69645-69646

69645 Tympanoplasty with mastoidectomy (including canalplasty, middle ear surgery, tympanic membrane repair); radical or complete, without ossicular chain reconstruction

69646 Tympanoplasty with mastoidectomy (including canalplasty, middle ear surgery, tympanic membrane repair); radical or complete, with ossicular chain reconstruction

A tympanoplasty with mastoidectomy is performed. This procedure may include a canalplasty, middle ear surgery, and/or tympanic membrane repair. Tympanoplasties are classified by type depending on whether only the tympanic membrane requires repair or whether some or all of the bones (ossicles) also require repair. This procedure includes a complete or radical mastoidectomy using a wall down technique. This involves removing bone from the back of the ear canal to create a single cavity that includes the mastoid and ear canal. An incision is made behind the ear and the mastoid bone is exposed. The mastoid air cells are inspected and the extent of the procedure determined. The air cell system is completely removed along with purulent matter, debris, and infected tissue. The posterior and superior walls of the external auditory canal are also removed to allow exposure of the mastoid and attic of the middle ear to the outside. If a more extensive (radical) mastoidectomy is required, the structures of the epitympanum (upper portion of the tympanic cavity) which include the head of the malleus and body of the incus are removed. The stapes may also be removed but is preserved if possible. Removal of these structures allows exteriorization of the mastoid cavity and middle ear. A drain may be placed behind the ear. In 69645, the procedure is performed without ossicular chain reconstruction. The procedure may be performed through the ear canal or through a post-auricular incision. If the external auditory canal is stenosed from repeated infection, a canalplasty is performed. A drill is used to remove bone and increase the diameter of the canal. The hole in the tympanic membrane is exposed and inspected. The middle ear structures are also inspected and any scar tissue in the middle ear removed. The tympanic membrane is repaired. Tissue around the hole in the tympanic membrane is rimmed until bleeding occurs. Depending on the exact location and size of the hole, simply rimming the hole may allow the edges to heal together. A larger hole may require a patch. A small amount of skin, fat, tendon, or fascia is harvested. The graft is prepared. Absorbable sponge material may be placed in the middle ear behind the hole to support the graft. The graft is then placed over the hole. If a canalplasty has been performed, skin grafts are harvested and placed over the exposed bone in the external auditory canal. An absorbable sponge is placed in the ear canal over the tympanic membrane graft to hold the graft in place. The ear is packed with gauze. In 69646, an ossicular chain reconstruction is performed in addition to the procedures above. The physician inspects the ossicles and determines that one or more of these bones require reconstruction. Tissue grafts are harvested and the incus, malleus, and/or stapes are reconstructed.

69650

69650 Stapes mobilization

A stapes mobilization is performed to restore movement to the stapes bone which has become fixed. Normally the stapes vibrates freely and transmits sound into the inner ear. However, when the stapes becomes fixed due to abnormal bone growth on the walls of the inner ear, a condition called otosclerosis, conductive hearing loss occurs. An incision is made in the posterior aspect of the external ear canal wall and tympanomeatal flap created. The flap is elevated and the ossicles of the middle ear exposed and inspected. Simple stapes mobilization involves use of a hook placed against the long process of the incus. The hook is moved in the direction of the stapes tendon to release any attachments that are causing fixation of the stapes. Upon completion of the procedure, the tympanomeatal flap is replaced and the meatal incision closed with sutures.

69660-69661

69660 Stapedectomy or stapedotomy with reestablishment of ossicular continuity, with or without use of foreign material

69661 Stapedectomy or stapedotomy with reestablishment of ossicular continuity, with or without use of foreign material; with footplate drill out

A stapedectomy or stapedotomy is performed with reestablishement of ossicular continuity with or without the use of foreign material (69660) or with footplate drillout (69661) is performed. Normally the stapes vibrates freely and transmits sound into the inner ear. However, when the stapes becomes fixed due to abnormal bone growth on the walls of the inner ear, a condition called otosclerosis, conductive hearing loss occurs. Stapedectomy or stapedotomy is performed to treat stapes fixation due to otosclerosis. An incision is made in the posterior ear canal wall and tympanomeatal flap created. The flap is elevated and the ossicles of the middle ear exposed and inspected. In 69660, part or all of the stapes is excised (stapedectomy) or the stapes is drilled (stapedotomy). The exact procedure depends on the location and extent of the otosclerosis. If part or all of the stapes is removed, it is replaced with a synthetic prosthesis. In 69661, the stapedectomy

or stapedotomy procedure is performed as described above along with a footplate drillout. The upper portion of the stapes is removed by downfracturing the stapes. This leaves the fixed footplate frozen in the oval window. A laser or drill is used to make a small hole in the footplate. A prosthetic rod is placed over the incus and into the hole in the footplate. The physician then confirms that movement is transmitted from the incus and prosthesis into the inner ear. Any surgically created oval window defects are repaired which might require the use of a mesodermal graft or placement of gelfilm or gelfoam. Upon completion of the procedure, the tympanomeatal flap is replaced and the meatal incision closed with sutures.

69662

69662 Revision of stapedectomy or stapedotomy

Normally the stapes vibrates freely and transmits sound into the inner ear. However, when the stapes becomes fixed due to abnormal bone growth on the walls of the inner ear, a condition called otosclerosis, conductive hearing loss occurs. Stapedectomy or stapedotomy is performed to treat stapes fixation due to otosclerosis. An incision is made in the posterior ear canal wall and tympanomeatal flap created. The flap is elevated and the ossicles of the middle ear exposed. The stapes is inspected and the physician determines what type of revision procedure is required. A previously placed prosthesis that has become broken or dislodged is removed and replaced. Alternatively, if a partial prosthesis has been used, the remainder of the stapes may be removed and complete prosthesis placed. The physician then confirms that movement is transmitted from the incus and prosthesis into the inner ear. Any surgically created oval window defects are repaired which might require the use of a mesodermal graft or placement of gelfilm or gelfoam. Upon completion of the procedure, the tympanomeatal flap is replaced and the meatal incision closed with sutures.

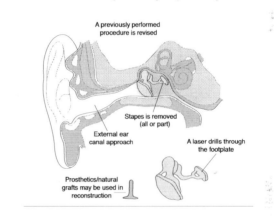

Revision of stapedectomy/stapedotomy

A previously performed procedure is revised

Stapes is removed (all or part)

External ear canal approach

A laser drills through the footplate

Prosthetics/natural grafts may be used in reconstruction

69666-69667

69666 Repair oval window fistula

69667 Repair round window fistula

The physician repairs a fistula in the oval window (69666) or round window (69667). These fistulas are abnormal communications or passages between the middle and inner ear. An incision is made in the posterior ear canal wall and tympanomeatal flap created. The flap is elevated and the affected window exposed. The fistula is repaired repaired using a mesodermal or other soft tissue graft. Upon completion of the procedure, the tympanomeatal flap is replaced and the meatal incision closed with sutures.

69670

69670 Mastoid obliteration (separate procedure)

This procedure is performed to reduce the size the mastoid cavity that was created during a previous mastoidectomy procedure. The mastoid cavity is exposed using a postauricular approach. The physician then creates a local flap or harvests a free flap or graft of bone, cartilage, and/or fat and places it in the mastoid cavity. One method is to use autogenous cranial bone. The bone graft is processed and mixed with antibiotic solution to form a paste. The cavity is filled with the bone graft material. The processed cranial bone graft induces formation of new bone that fills the mastoid cavity and epitympanic spaces resulting in complete obliteration of the cavity. Following placement of the graft, the postauricular incision is closed.

69676

69676 Tympanic neurectomy

This procedure is performed to treat excessive saliva secretion from the parotid gland and resulting parotid fistulas. The tympanic nerve is a branch of the glossopharyngeal nerve. The

● New Code   ▲ Revised Code

Auditory System

tympanic nerve branch begins inside the skull (cranium) and exits at the jugular foramen. It passes by the glossopharyngeal ganglion and re-enters the skull through the tympanic canaliculus. It then enters the tympanic cavity where it forms a plexus in the middle ear. From the plexus, it travels through a canal and into the middle cranial fossa where it exits beside the greater petrosal nerve. At the point where it exits the cranial fossa, it becomes the lesser petrosal nerve. The nerve is approached through the ear canal. The canal is incised and a tympanomeatal flap created. The tympanic nerve is exposed where it enters the tympanic cavity. The nerve is excised. The tympanomeatal flap is replaced and the ear canal incision closed.

69700

69700   Closure postauricular fistula, mastoid (separate procedure)

A postauricular mastoid cutaneous fistula is closed. This type of fistula may result from chronic infection of the middle ear or mastoid air cells or may be complication of previous ear or mastoid surgery. The entire fistula may be excised or the edges of the opening may be freshened to create a raw surface. A skin flap is created below the fistula with a pedicle located at the upper aspect of the flap. The flap is rotated upward and placed in the fistula with the skin surface facing inward and secured with sutures. The raw freshened edges of the fistulous opening are then closed over the raw surface of the skin flap. This creates an epithelial covering on both the inside and outside of the fistulous tract. Another method of closure involves creation of periosteal flaps that are used to cover the fistula and then covering the periosteal flaps with skin flaps.

69710

69710   Implantation or replacement of electromagnetic bone conduction hearing device in temporal bone

The physician implants or replaces an electromagnetic bone conduction hearing device in the temporal bone. These devices are also called bone-anchored hearing aids (BAHA). This type of hearing aid collects sound waves and transmits the sound waves to an oscillator that vibrates against the skull. The inner ear is able to pick up the vibration and interpret the sound. These devices were designed for people who cannot use traditional hearing aids such as individuals with congenital atresia of the auditory canal. The device is implanted by making an incision behind the ear over the temporal bone. The bone is exposed and the device which consists of a tiny box is anchored to the temporal bone using a titanium rod that is screwed into the bone. If the device is being replaced, the existing device is exposed and removed. The new device is placed as described above.

69711

69711   Removal or repair of electromagnetic bone conduction hearing device in temporal bone

The physician removes or repairs an electromagnetic bone conduction hearing device in the temporal bone. These devices are also called bone anchored hearing aids (BAHA). This type of hearing aid collects sound waves and transmits the sound waves to an oscillator that vibrates against the skull. The inner ear is able to pick up the vibration and interpret the sound. These devices were designed for people who cannot use traditional hearing aids such as individuals with congenital atresia of the auditory canal. To remove the device, a small incision is made over the device and the device is exposed. The titanium rod that attaches the device to the temporal bone is removed from the bone and the device is removed. The physician then inspects the malfunctioning device. If the device can be repaired, the necessary repairs are made and the repaired device is again secured to the temporal bone using the titanium rod.

69714–69715

69714   Implantation, osseointegrated implant, temporal bone, with percutaneous attachment to external speech processor/cochlear stimulator; without mastoidectomy

69715   Implantation, osseointegrated implant, temporal bone, with percutaneous attachment to external speech processor/cochlear stimulator; with mastoidectomy

An osseointegrated implant is placed in the temporal bone and attached percutaneously to an external speech processor or cochlear stimulator. This type of implant is used to re-establish hearing in patients with hearing loss due to disease of the middle ear and cochlea. The skin overlying the planned implantation site is measured and marked to allow optimal placement of the implant. The skin is incised and the mastoid complex is exposed. Skin and periosteal flaps are created. A pilot hole is drilled in the bone and enlarged until the opening can accommodate the implant, which is placed in the prepared implantation site and secured. The skin flap is perforated to allow attachment to the external speech processor or cochlear stimulator. The surrounding soft tissues are then reduced in thickness prior to closure of the wound over the implant. In 69714, the procedure is performed without mastoidectomy. In 69715, following exposure of the mastoid complex, a mastoidectomy is performed to remove infected and diseased air cells and to expose non-aerated segments of the mastoid prior to implanting the device.

69717-69718

69717   Replacement (including removal of existing device), osseointegrated implant, temporal bone, with percutaneous attachment to external speech processor/cochlear stimulator; without mastoidectomy

69718   Replacement (including removal of existing device), osseointegrated implant, temporal bone, with percutaneous attachment to external speech processor/cochlear stimulator; with mastoidectomy

An osseointegrated implant is replaced in the temporal bone and attached percutaneously to an external speech processor or cochlear stimulator. This procedure includes removal of the existing device. This type of implant is used to re-establish hearing in patients with hearing loss due to disease of the middle ear and cochlea. The skin overlying the implant is measured, marked, and incised. The mastoid complex is exposed. Skin and periosteal flaps are created. The subcutaneous tissue surrounding the implant is incised; the bone is drilled out; and the existing implant is removed. The hole is shaped to accommodate the new implant, which is placed in the prepared implantation site and secured. The skin flap is perforated to allow attachment to the external speech processor or cochlear stimulator. The surrounding soft tissues are then reduced in thickness to allow closure of the wound over the implant. In 69717, the procedure is performed without mastoidectomy. In 69718, following exposure of the mastoid complex, a mastoidectomy is performed to remove infected and diseased air cells and to expose non-aerated segments of the mastoid prior to implanting the device.

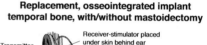

Replacement, osseointegrated implant temporal bone, with/without mastoidectomy

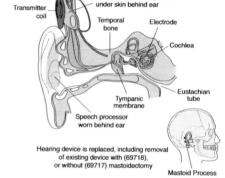

Hearing device is replaced, including removal of existing device with (69718), or without (69717) mastoidectomy

69720-69725

69720   Decompression facial nerve, intratemporal; lateral to geniculate ganglion

69725   Decompression facial nerve, intratemporal; including medial to geniculate ganglion

Decompression is performed in patients with facial nerve paralysis whose nerve function is deteriorating. The facial nerve is divided into intracranial, intratemporal, and extratemporal regions. The intratemporal region begins where the nerve enters the internal acoustic meatus and ends where it exits the stylomastoid foramen. The intratemporal region of the facial nerve contains the meatal, labyrinthine, tympanic, and vertical segments. In 69720, decompression is performed lateral to the geniculate ganglion which is contained in the tympanic segment. An incision is made behind the ear and a mastoidectomy performed to allow access to the nerve. The nerve is exposed along its vertical segment to the stylomastoid foramen. Bone overlying the nerve is removed with a burr. The tympanic cavity is approached through the facial recess and bone overlying the tympanic segment is also removed. The nerve sheath is exposed and incised to decompress the nerve lateral to the geniculate ganglion. In 69725, decompression continues to a point medial to the geniculate ganglion. Once the facial nerve has been exposed in the tympanic cavity, the geniculate ganglion is exposed and decompression continues medially within the cavity.

69740-69745

69740   Suture facial nerve, intratemporal, with or without graft or decompression; lateral to geniculate ganglion

69745   Suture facial nerve, intratemporal, with or without graft or decompression; including medial to geniculate ganglion

The physician sutures the facial nerve in the intratemporal region with or without nerve grafting and with or without decompression. The facial nerve is divided into intracranial, intratemporal, and extratemporal regions. The intratemporal region begins where the nerve enters the internal acoustic meatus and ends where it exits the stylomastoid foramen. The intratemporal region of the facial nerve contains the meatal, labyrinthine, tympanic, and vertical segments. In 69740, the facial nerve is sutured at a point lateral to the geniculate ganglion which is contained in the tympanic segment. An incision is made behind the ear and a mastoidectomy performed to access the nerve. The nerve is exposed along its

Auditory System

vertical segment to the stylomastoid foramen. Bone overlying the nerve is removed with a burr. The tympanic cavity is approached through the facial recess and bone overlying the tympanic segment is also removed. The nerve is exposed and inspected and the damaged or severed portion identified. The sheath may be exposed beyond the point of the injury so that the nerve can be decompressed by incising the nerve sheath lateral to the geniculate ganglion. The nerve is then repaired with fine microfilament sutures using microinstruments and an operating microscope. If a nerve graft is required it is harvested and secured to the remaining facial nerve segments using 2-3 sutures placed through the epineurium. In 69745, repair and decompression is performed at a point medial to the geniculate ganglion. Once the facial nerve has been exposed in the tympanic cavity, the geniculate ganglion is exposed and the nerve is followed medially to the point where the injury occurred. The nerve is repaired as described above.

69801

69801   Labyrinthotomy, with perfusion of vestibuloactive drug(s); transcanal

This procedure is performed to treat Meniere's disease. The inner ear, also called the labyrinth, is a series of canals or cavities contained in the petrous portion of the temporal bone. The labyrinth consists of an outer layer called the bony labyrinth and an inner layer called the membranous labyrinth. Areas within the labyrinth are divided into the vestibule, cochlea, and semicircular canals. The inner ear is accessed using a transcanal approach. An incision is made in the posterior aspect of the ear canal and a tympanomeatal flap is elevated. An incision is made behind the ear and the mastoid bone is exposed. Using an operating microscope and microscopic surgical tools, the physician traverses the middle ear and opens the bony and membranous labyrinth. A needle or catheter is then placed in the inner ear and drugs are instilled to help alleviate symptoms of Meniere's disease.

69805-69806

69805   Endolymphatic sac operation; without shunt
69806   Endolymphatic sac operation; with shunt

An endolymphatic sac operation is performed with or without a shunt. The procedure is performed to treat Meniere's disease which is a disorder of the inner ear causing episodes of vertigo, fluctuating hearing loss, tinnitus, and fullness in the ear. The mastoid bone is opened. In 69805, the sigmoid sinus, a small S-shaped cavity behind the mastoid bone, is denuded of bone except for a small rectangle called Bill's island. Removing the bone allows the endolymphatic sac to expand relieving pressure thought to cause Meniere's disease symptoms. In 69806, a shunt is placed. Following removal of the bone, the endolymphatic sac is exposed behind the semicircular canal. The sac is incised and a shunt tube inserted. The shunt which drains to the mastoid cavity or subarachnoid space has a one-way valve that allows fluid to seep out of the sac without allowing fluid back in.

69820-69840

69820   Fenestration semicircular canal
69840   Revision fenestration operation

The physician performs a fenestration of the semicircular canal (69820) or a revision of a fenestration procedure (69840). This procedure was used in the past to treat conductive hearing loss but is not commonly performed today. In 69820, the semicircular canal is exposed using a transmastoid approach. A mastoidectomy is performed using a wall down technique. This involves removing bone from the back of the ear canal to create a single cavity that includes the mastoid and ear canal. The lateral semicircular canal is identified. A fenestration, which is a small hole or opening, is then made in the semicircular canal. A fascial graft is placed over the fenestration. The fenestration allows sound to enter the ear, bypass the fixed stapes footplate and transmit sound through the lateral semicircular canal and through the cochlea. In 69840, a previously performed fenestration is revised. This might involve reopening the existing fenestration, replacing the fascial graft, or creating a new fenestration.

69905-69910

69905   Labyrinthectomy; transcanal
69910   Labyrinthectomy; with mastoidectomy

A labyrinthectomy is performed. The inner ear also called the labyrinth is a series of canals or cavities contained in the petrous portion of the temporal bone. The labyrinth consists of an outer layer called the bony labyrinth and an inner layer called membranous labyrinth. Areas within the labyrinth are divided into the vestibule, cochlea, and semicircular canals. Labyrinthectomy is performed to treat Meniere's disease and is effective because it removes the structures that affect balance. It is only used on patients with no significant hearing left in the ear as removal of the inner ear structures results in complete deafness in the affected ear. In 69905, the inner ear is accessed using a transcanal approach. An incision is made in the posterior aspect of the canal and a tympanomeatal flap elevated. An incision is made behind the ear and the mastoid bone exposed. Using an operating microscope and microscopic surgical tools the physician traverses the middle ear and opens the bony and membranous labyrinth. In 69910, the inner ear is accessed using a transmastoid approach with a mastoidectomy. An incision is made behind the ear and the mastoid bone opened. The air cell system within the mastoid bone is completely removed

to allow access to the inner ear. The labyrinth is opened. The bony and membranous labyrinth is then completely excised.

69915

69915   Vestibular nerve section, translabyrinthine approach

Vestibular nerve section is performed to treat severe recurrent attacks of vertigo. A C-shaped incision is made beginning above the ear and is carried around behind the ear. The mastoid bone is entered and a complete mastoidectomy performed using a high speed drill and a variety of burs. The antrum and incus are identified. Bone overlying the sigmoid sinus is removed and the sinus is skeletonized. Bone is removed posteriorly over the suboccipital dura. A labyrinthectomy is performed. The facial nerve is exposed and protected. Dissection continues to the ampullated end of the internal auditory canal where the superior vestibular nerve exits in the lateral aspect of the canal. The superior vestibular nerve is cut (sectioned). Dissection continues and the saccule, utricle, and posterior semicircular canal are identified. The inferior vestibular nerve is identified as it exits the lateral end of the internal auditory canal. The inferior vestibular nerve is sectioned. The surgical wound is irrigated and the incision closed in layers.

69930

69930   Cochlear device implantation, with or without mastoidectomy

A cochlear implant is an electronic device that can restore useful hearing in patients with severe bilateral sensorineural hearing loss. Cochlear implants work by transforming speech and other sounds into electrical energy that then stimulate auditory nerve fibers in the inner ear. The cochlear device has both an internal and external component. Surgery is performed to implant the internal processor. A C-shaped incision is made beginning above the ear and is carried around behind the ear. If a mastoidectomy is performed, the mastoid bone is entered and the mastoid air cells removed using a high speed drill and a variety of burs. If a mastoidectomy is not performed, the surgeon drills through the mastoid bone to the inner ear. The electrode array is then inserted into the cochlea. A small depression is created in the mastoid bone and the receiver/stimulator is placed in the depression and secured to the skull. The incision is closed in layers. This internal processor is then used with external components including a microphone, a speech processor that digitizes the sound into electrical signals, transmitting cables, and a transmitting coil that sends the electrical signals across the skin to the implanted receiver/stimulator.

69950

69950   Vestibular nerve section, transcranial approach

The physician performs a vestibular nerve section using a transcranial approach, also referred to as a middle cranial fossa approach. Vestibular nerve section is performed to treat severe recurrent attacks of vertigo. A long curvilinear incision is made over the temporal bone on the affected side. A lateral craniectomy is performed and the temporal lobe is exposed and retracted medially to allow access to the superior surface of the temporal bone. The internal auditory canal is identified and opened. The superior and inferior vestibular nerves are located and cut (sectioned). The surgical wound is irrigated. The bone flap is replaced and secured. The soft tissues are closed.

69955

69955   Total facial nerve decompression and/or repair (may include graft)

The facial nerve is divided into intracranial, intratemporal, and extratemporal regions. Exposure begins with an incision behind the ear and a mastoidectomy to access the nerve. The nerve is exposed along its vertical segment to the stylomastoid foramen. Bone overlying the nerve is removed with a burr. The tympanic cavity is approached through the facial recess and bone overlying the tympanic segment is also removed. The labyrinthine portion is exposed next. The postauricular incision may be extended in a posterosuperior direction or a separate incision may be made behind and above the ear. The skin is elevated and the temporal muscle fascia exposed. The muscle and underlying periosteum are incised and elevated. A temporal bone flap is created and elevated. Elevation continues to the petrous ridge where the arcuate eminence and greater petrosal nerve are exposed. Bone is then dissected until the previously dissected tympanic cavity is reached. The nerve is then inspected and tested. Neurolysis may be performed to free the nerve from surrounding tissue or the nerve sheath may be incised and the nerve decompressed. Any injured sections are repaired with fine microfilament sutures using microinstruments and an operating microscope. If nerve grafting is required nerve grafts are harvested and used to replace the injured segments. Once the repair is complete, bone flaps are used to repair surgical defects in the tympanic cavity and internal auditory canal to prevent herniation of the temporal lobe into the middle ear. Dural defects are repaired with temporalis fascia grafting. The temporal bone flap is then replaced and secured with sutures. Overlying tissues are closed in layers.

69960

69960   Decompression internal auditory canal

Decompression of the internal auditory canal is performed. This typically requires a middle fossa approach. A long curvilinear incision is made over the temporal bone on the affected

Auditory System

side. A lateral craniectomy is performed and the temporal lobe is exposed and retracted medially to allow access to the superior surface of the temporal bone. The internal auditory canal is identified and opened. Structures around and within the internal auditory canal that are being compressed are released from surrounding tissue to relieve pressure that may be causing pain or other symptoms. Following the decompression procedure, the bone flap is replaced and secured. The soft tissues are closed.

69970

69970   Removal of tumor, temporal bone

The physician removes a tumor of the temporal bone. Tumors of the temporal bone, whether benign or malignant, are rare. The temporal bone is divided into 3 parts, the squamous, tympanic, and petrous portions. The squamous portion includes a small portion of the bony external ear canal, the zygomatic process and mandibular fossa, and a portion of the the mastoid process. The superior aspect of the squamous portion also protects the temporal lobe and abuts the parietal and occipital bones. The tympanic portion forms most of the bony ear canal and the posterior wall of the mandibular fossa. The petrous portion contains the otic capsule and the internal auditory canal. The middle ear lies between the squamous, tympanic and petrous portions. The exact procedure depends on the site and extent of the lesion. There are three common approaches which include lateral temporal bone resection (LTBR), subtotal temporal bone resection (STBR) and total temporal bone resection. The physician exposes the involved portions of the temporal bone. The bone is then resected along with involved structures of the external, middle and internal ear.

69990

69990   Microsurgical techniques, requiring use of operating microscope (List separately in addition to code for primary procedure)

The physician performs microsurgical techniques using an operating microscope during a separately reportable procedure. Microsurgery is typically used for anastomosis of small blood vessels and nerves as well as for tissue reconstruction. The surgeon visualizes the blood vessels, nerves or individual nerve fibers, or other tissue through the operating microscope. Using a foot pedal, the microscope is focused and manipulated during the course of the microscopic portion of the surgery. Using the operating microscope and microsurgical tools, physician dissects and mobilizes blood vessels, nerves, or other tissues, meticulously controlling any bleeding. The physician then repairs the blood vessels, nerves or other tissues using the operating microscope which allows exact approximation of blood vessels, nerves, and tissue planes.

Microsurgical techniques, requiring use of operating microscope

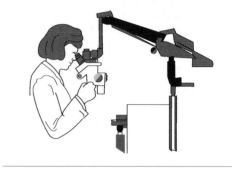

● New Code   ▲ Revised Code

Radiology

70010

70010   Myelography, posterior fossa, radiological supervision and interpretation

Posterior fossa myelography is used mainly for evaluating the cerebellopontine angles when an acoustic neuroma is suspected. Myelography is a type of diagnostic imaging that uses contrast material injected into the subarachnoid space around the spinal cord and nerve roots with real-time fluoroscopic x-ray imaging. For imaging the posterior fossa, the patient lies on the side to be imaged with legs Velcro strapped onto a footboard. After contrast is injected through a lumbar puncture, the table is tilted and the head is flexed and extended so the bolus of opaque dye flows to the upper cervical canal. The contrast material flows through the foramen magnum and pools in the dependent cerebellopontine cistern and internal auditory canal. When the contrast has reached the target area, the table is returned to a horizontal position, the patient's head is gently maneuvered to bring the petrous ridge parallel to the top of the film, and images are taken.

70015

70015   Cisternography, positive contrast, radiological supervision and interpretation

Cisternography is a radiographic examination of the basal cisterns of the brain following the injection of contrast medium in the subarachnoid space. Positive contrast medium used in this procedure is iodinated. It has an increased absorption of x-rays and shows up as white-grey. This procedure is used to evaluate suspected cases of normal pressure hydrocephalus (NPH) or cerebral atrophy. The physician injects the contrast medium intrathecally through lumbar puncture. Radiographic images are then taken over a period of hours or even days, following the flow of the contrast agent. In a normal patient, the contrast medium will rise to the basal cisterns of the brain in 1-3 hours and then flow over and collect in the sagittal area in 12-24 hours. The cisterns are usually clear in 24 hours and the ventricles are not visualized during the series. In a patient with NPH, reabsorption of cerebral spinal fluid is impaired, the flow is reversed, and the ventricles are visualized early in the series, persisting for up to 48 hours, with almost no flow of the tracer into the sagittal area. Ventricular reflux also occurs in isolated cerebral atrophy.

70030

70030   Radiologic examination, eye, for detection of foreign body

A radiologic examination to locate a foreign body that has become lodged in the eye tissue is performed. Plain films that produce a 2D image of the eye are typically obtained only when a metallic foreign body is suspected as other types of foreign bodies do not show up on plain films. One or more views may be obtained of the eye. The physician reviews the images and provides a written report of findings.

70100-70110

70100   Radiologic examination, mandible; partial, less than 4 views
70110   Radiologic examination, mandible; complete, minimum of 4 views

Plain films are obtained of the mandible (lower jaw). Plain films produce a 2D image of the structures. The exact views obtained depend on the condition being evaluated. Because disease and injuries of the jaw can affect the teeth and their roots, views are obtained that allow evaluation of these structures. A dental periapical view provides fine detail of the teeth and their roots. A dental occlusal view is obtained to evaluate fractures and determine whether the mandible is vertically displaced. A Caldwell or coronal view shows any displacement of the mandible in the horizontal plane. Oblique views allow evaluation of the ramus angle and the posterior body of the mandible. The Towne view allows evaluation of the condylar and subcondylar regions. Use 70100 for a partial radiologic examination on the mandible defined as less than four views. Use 70110 for a complete radiologic exam defined as a minimum of four views. The physician reviews the radiographs for abnormalities, including traumatic injuries, bony projections or growths, and other evidence of disease, and provides a written report of the findings.

70120-70130

70120   Radiologic examination, mastoids; less than 3 views per side
70130   Radiologic examination, mastoids; complete, minimum of 3 views per side

The physician performs a radiologic examination on the mastoids, the bony prominences located directly behind the ears that house the middle and inner ear structures. The mastoids are made of spongy bone and contain many air cells. X-ray imaging uses indirect ionizing radiation to take pictures inside the body. X-rays work on non-uniform material, such as human tissue, because of the different density and composition of the object, which allows some of the x-rays to be absorbed and some to pass through and be captured behind the object on a detector. This produces a 2D image of the structures. Report

70120 when less than 3 different X-ray images are taken on each side. Report 70130 for a complete radiologic exam of the mastoids, which requires at least 3 different views taken of each side. The physician reviews the radiographs for evidence of disease causing changes to the honeycomb-like bony structure of the mastoids, such as a chronic infection.

70134

70134   Radiologic examination, internal auditory meati, complete

The physician performs a complete radiologic examination on the internal auditory meati, which are canals in the temporal bone through which cranial nerves VII and VIII are carried to the middle and inner ear. X-ray imaging uses indirect ionizing radiation to take pictures inside the body. X-rays work on non-uniform material, such as human tissue, because of the different density and composition of the object, which allows some of the x-rays to be absorbed and some to pass through and be captured behind the object on a detector. This produces a 2D image of the structures. The physician reviews the radiographs and looks for evidence of disease, such as infection, narrowing, or tumor growth.

70140-70150

70140   Radiologic examination, facial bones; less than 3 views
70150   Radiologic examination, facial bones; complete, minimum of 3 views

The physician performs a complete radiologic examination on the facial bones in 70150 by taking at least three different X-ray images, covering the entire face. The main facial bones include the maxilla, mandible, frontal bone, nasal bones, and zygoma. X-ray uses indirect ionizing radiation to take pictures inside the body. X-rays work on non-uniform material, such as human tissue, because of the different density and composition of the object, which allows some of the x-rays to be absorbed and some to pass through and be captured behind the object on a detector. This produces a 2D image of the structures. Report 70140 when less than 3 different views are taken of the facial bones. The physician reviews the radiographs for abnormalities, including traumatic injuries, bony projections or growths, infections, and other evidence of disease.

70160

70160   Radiologic examination, nasal bones, complete, minimum of 3 views

The paired nasal bones are two small oblong bones that are fused at the midline of the nose. These two bones form the upper aspect of the bridge of the nose. Other structures that are imaged during radiographic studies of the nose include the vomer, which is a triangular bone that forms the lower part of the nasal septum; the nasal septum, which is composed primarily of cartilage; the perpendicular plate of the ethmoid bone; and other facial bones surrounding the nose. Images may be obtained with the patient standing or in a semi-prone position. Right and left lateral images and a Waters view are obtained. Lateral projections demonstrate the bridge of the nose, the anterior nasal spine of the maxilla, and the frontonasal suture. The Waters view, also referred to as the parietoacanthial or occipitomental view, demonstrates the orbits, maxillae, zygomatic arches, dorsal pyramind, lateral nasal walls, and the septum. Additional views are obtained as needed. The physician reviews the radiographs for abnormalities, including traumatic injuries, boney projections or growths, or other evidence of disease. The physician provides a written report of findings.

70170

70170   Dacryocystography, nasolacrimal duct, radiological supervision and interpretation

Dacryocystography is a radiologic examination performed on the nasolacrimal ducts (tear ducts) after the injection of contrast medium, to evaluate excessive tearing and assess patency or other pathology of the lacrimal drainage system. Dacryocystography is also used for pre- and post-operative evaluation. The patient may initially have separately reportable panoramic radiography of the face. Anesthetic drops are instilled into the eyes, the lacrimal canaliculi are cannulated, and water-soluble or oil-based contrast medium is injected. Radiographic images are obtained at different degrees or oblique angles to show the lacrimal pathways. The physician reviews the images and looks for evidence of pathology, such as stenosis, blockages, growths, or fistulae. A written report of findings is provided. This code reports the radiologic supervision and interpretation components of the procedure only.

70190-70200

70190   Radiologic examination; optic foramina
70200   Radiologic examination; orbits, complete, minimum of 4 views

The physician performs a radiologic examination on the optic foramina in 70190, which are the paired canals, or openings, in the sphenoid bone through which the optic nerve and ophthalmic artery pass. X-ray imaging uses indirect ionizing radiation to take pictures inside the body. X-rays work on non-uniform material, such as human tissue, because of the different density and composition of the object, which allows some of the x-rays to be absorbed and some to pass through and be captured behind the object on a detector. This produces a 2D image of the structures. X-rays are taken of the orbits in different positions, including the parieto-orbital oblique view, lateral views, occipitomental projections, and an inclined PA or Caldwell view, allowing the orbital structures to be viewed unobstructed by the petrous ridges. This may be done with the eyes looking up and down. Report 70200 when the physician performs a complete radiologic examination on the orbits, the bony sockets or cavities of the skull where the eye and ocular appendages are located. The physician reviews the images and looks for evidence of disease.

70210-70220

70210   Radiologic examination, sinuses, paranasal, less than 3 views
70220   Radiologic examination, sinuses, paranasal, complete, minimum of 3 views

The physician performs a radiologic examination of the paranasal sinuses. X-rays are taken of the sinuses which are paired, hollow, air-filled spaces or cavities within the facial bones surrounding the nasal cavity that consist of the frontal sinuses in the lower forehead, maxillary sinuses in the cheekbones, ethmoid sinuses beside the upper nose, or the sphenoid sinuses behind the nose. X-ray imaging uses indirect ionizing radiation to take pictures inside the body. X-rays work on non-uniform material, such as human tissue, because of the different density and composition of the object, which allows some of the x-rays to be absorbed and some to pass through and be captured behind the object on a detector. This produces a 2D image of the structures. If less than 3 views are taken, report 70210. Use 70220 when at least 3 views are taken for a complete exam. The physician reviews the images for infections, tumor-like lesions, or fibro-osseous lesions. Conventional radiology does not permit a detailed study of the paranasal sinuses and has largely been replaced by CT or MRI imaging.

70240

70240   Radiologic examination, sella turcica

The physician performs a radiologic examination of the sella turcica, a saddle-shaped depression in the upper surface of the sphenoid bone in the middle of the skull base where the pituitary gland sits. X-ray imaging uses indirect ionizing radiation to take pictures inside the body. X-rays work on non-uniform material, such as human tissue, because of the different density and composition of the object, which allows some of the x-rays to be absorbed and some to pass through and be captured behind the object on a detector. This produces a 2D image of the structures. The physician reviews the image for any pathological anatomy in the sella turcica.

70250-70260

70250   Radiologic examination, skull; less than 4 views
70260   Radiologic examination, skull; complete, minimum of 4 views

The physician performs a radiologic examination of the skull bones by taking up to three different X-ray images in 70250 or four or more images in 70260. Sponges or other supports may be placed around the head to keep it still as the head is turned various ways to obtain different views. X-ray uses indirect ionizing radiation to take pictures inside the body. X-rays work on non-uniform material, such as human tissue, because of the different density and composition of the object, which allows some of the x-rays to be absorbed and some to pass through and be captured behind the object on a detector. This produces a 2D image of the structures. The physician reviews the radiographs for developmental abnormalities, traumatic fractures or dislocations, bony projections or growths, and to detect progressive changes in skull dimensions.

70300-70320

70300   Radiologic examination, teeth; single view
70310   Radiologic examination, teeth; partial examination, less than full mouth
70320   Radiologic examination, teeth; complete, full mouth

The physician performs a radiologic examination of the teeth by using various types of dental x-rays. A bitewing x-ray is commonly done for a single view and shows the upper and lower back teeth, how they come together, any decay between teeth, and any bone loss occurring in gum disease or infection. Periapical x-rays are often done for a full mouth series and show the entire tooth from the crown to the end of the root and the supporting bone structures. Periapical x-rays are used to see what is occurring below the gum line, such as crowded or impacted teeth, broken tooth roots, abscesses, or other disease changes. Occlusal x-rays show the roof and floor of the mouth and demonstrate teeth that haven't broken through the gums, extra teeth, cleft palates, jaw fractures, foreign objects, and cysts or abscesses. Report 70300 for a single view of the teeth; 70310 for a partial examination that covers less than the full mouth; and 70320 for a full mouth series of x-rays.

70328-70330

70328   Radiologic examination, temporomandibular joint, open and closed mouth; unilateral
70330   Radiologic examination, temporomandibular joint, open and closed mouth; bilateral

A diagnostic radiology exam is done of the temporomandibular joint. X-rays are taken of the joint with the jaw open and closed. X-ray uses indirect ionizing radiation to take pictures inside the body. X-rays work on non-uniform material, such as human tissue, because of the different density and composition of the object, which allows some of the x-rays to be absorbed and some to pass through and be captured behind the object on a detector. This produces a 2D image of the structures. The physician reviews the images for narrowing of the joint spaces, changes in the articular surfaces, such as erosion and abnormal condylar contours, or other internal derangements or dislocation. Degenerative joint disease is the most common disease of the temporomandibular joint. Report 70328 for a radiologic exam on one side only and 70330 for both sides.

70332

70332   Temporomandibular joint arthrography, radiological supervision and interpretation

Arthrography of the temporomandibular joint (TMJ) is a type of diagnostic imaging that uses radioactive iodine injected into the joint for visualizing the contours of soft tissues within the joint space. This is done to diagnose internal derangement in temporomandibular joint disease. TMJ arthrography technique is usually accomplished using a single 27-gauge needle to inject contrast material into the upper and lower compartments of each joint. The contrast appears greyish or whitish with imaging, such as videofluoroscopy, and helps provide accurate information regarding displacement or abnormal morphology of the meniscus, perforation of the disk or meniscal attachments, joint capsule adhesions, and abnormal shape or function of the disk.

70336

70336   Magnetic resonance (eg, proton) imaging, temporomandibular joint(s)

Magnetic resonance imaging is done on the temporomandibular joint (TMJ). Magnetic resonance is a noninvasive, non-radiating imaging technique that uses the magnetic properties of hydrogen atoms in the body. The patient is placed on a motorized table within a large MRI tunnel scanner that contains the magnet. The powerful magnetic field forces the hydrogen atoms to line up. Radiowaves are then transmitted within the strong magnetic field. Protons in the nuclei of different types of tissues emit a specific radiofrequency signal that bounces back to the computer, which processes the signals and converts the data into tomographic, 3D images with very high resolution. MRI provides reliable information for diagnosing internal derangement of the TMJ, and intrinsic degeneration or displacement of the meniscus. MRI is also used for imaging TMJ effusions, failed implants, vascular necrosis, tendinitis, muscle atrophy and other anomalous muscular development, and soft tissue lesions, contusions, and hematomas.

70350

70350   Cephalogram, orthodontic

A cephalogram assists in diagnosing and planning for orthodontic treatment. A cephalogram is a radiological film of the patient's head. Frontal cephalograms are a full view of the face and are used to examine facial asymmetry. A lateral cephalogram is a full skull x-ray of the patient's profile and is used to detail the occlusion and the relationship between occlusion and skeletal structures. It also shows soft tissue position in relation to facial appearance and inclining of teeth. More quantitative evaluations of dento-facial deformities and facial asymmetry are achieved using both frontal and lateral cephalograms and then calculating orthodontic landmarks by correcting for distortion and magnification. This allows the orthodontist to calculate measurements of the teeth, jaws, soft tissue, and facial relationships to determine an appropriate treatment plan for correcting problems and achieving facial harmony.

70355

70355   Orthopantogram (eg, panoramic x-ray)

An orthopantogram is used in orthodontic diagnostic examinations. This is a radiograph taken extraorally that shows a panoramic view of the upper and lower jaws, the upper sinus area, the entire dentition, the relationship of all the teeth to each other, and the alveolar bone on one single film. Orthopantograms are used to locate missing, extra, or impacted teeth, view the condition of the tooth roots, determine the amount of supporting bone, and evaluate the position and development of non-erupted permanent teeth.

70360

70360   Radiologic examination; neck, soft tissue

X-rays are taken to evaluate the soft tissue of the neck. X-ray uses indirect ionizing radiation to take pictures inside the body. X-rays work on non-uniform material, such as human tissue, because of the different density and composition of the object, which allows some of the x-rays to be absorbed and some to pass through and be captured behind the object on a detector. This produces a 2D image of the structures. Frontal and lateral views of the neck may be taken for better evaluation. The physician reviews the radiographs to determine any asymmetry or enlargement on one side or the other, the caliber and contour of the trachea, and any soft tissue swelling that may involve the adenoids, tonsils, epiglottis, or aryepiglottic folds.

70370

70370   Radiologic examination; pharynx or larynx, including fluoroscopy and/or magnification technique

A radiologic exam of the pharynx or larynx is done. X-rays are taken using indirect ionizing radiation to take pictures inside the body. X-rays work on non-uniform material, such as human tissue, because of the different density and composition of the object, which allows some of the x-rays to be absorbed and some to pass through and be captured behind the object on a detector. This produces a 2D image of the structures. Posteroanterior and lateral views are standard. Oblique images may also be taken to provide more information on suspected or known pharyngeal or laryngeal disease or abnormal anatomy when standard views appear normal. Even though 70370 includes fluoroscopy and magnification techniques, it does not include evaluation of any dynamic movements involved in speech. The code reports only diagnostic x-ray evaluation of the pharynx or larynx to visualize any pathology or aberrant anatomy.

70371

70371   Complex dynamic pharyngeal and speech evaluation by cine or video recording

Dynamic evaluation of pharyngeal and speech movement is done using cine or video recording. This is often done on pediatric patients with speech delay and is most often reported for speech evaluation. This involves complex dynamic study of the movements of the pharynx, mouth, tongue, and tissues of the throat as patients are asked to say words. Fluoroscopy is used to record how the tongue, palate, pharynx, and soft tissues of the mouth are functioning during speech as words are repeated. The speech pathologist and radiologist then evaluate the moving recording for problems related to speech disturbances.

70380

70380   Radiologic examination, salivary gland for calculus

Sialoliths are stones within the salivary glands or ducts that appear radiopaque on diagnostic radiologic imaging. Large sialoliths are most often reported in the body of salivary glands and rarely in the ducts. An x-ray examination is done on the salivary gland to visualize a suspected calculus. X-rays use indirect ionizing radiation to take pictures inside the body. X-rays work on non-uniform material, such as human tissue, because of the different density and composition of the object, which allows some of the x-rays to be absorbed and some to pass through and be captured behind the object on a detector. This produces a 2D image of the structures. Panoramic and occlusal views may be taken. A panoramic view shows the entire extraoral jaw and facial area. An occlusal view shows submandibular spaces of the mouth. The physician reviews the images to locate the suspected stone for subsequent removal.

70390

70390   Sialography, radiological supervision and interpretation

Sialography is a diagnostic radiographic examination of the salivary ducts and glands. A small amount of opaque dye is injected into the salivary gland duct via a small, flexible catheter inserted through the mouth and into the duct. An x-ray may be taken before the injection to insure that no stones would block the flow of contrast. After the injection, the patient is given something to stimulate the production of saliva, such as lemon juice, as x-rays are then taken from a number of different positions to visualize the drainage of saliva into the mouth. The physician reviews the pictures for signs of small stones, strictures, ectasia, or other signs of disease.

70450-70470

70450   Computed tomography, head or brain; without contrast material
70460   Computed tomography, head or brain; with contrast material(s)
70470   Computed tomography, head or brain; without contrast material, followed by contrast material(s) and further sections

Computerized tomography, also referred to as a CT scan, uses special x-ray equipment and computer technology to produce multiple cross-sectional images of the region being studied. In this study, CT scan of the head or brain is performed. The patient is positioned on the CT examination table. An initial pass is made through the CT scanner to determine the starting position of the scans after which the CT scan is performed. As the table moves slowly through the scanner, numerous x-ray beams and electronic x-ray detectors rotate around the body region being

examined. The amount of radiation being absorbed is measured. As the beams and detectors rotate around the body, the table is moved through the scanner. A computer program processes the data and renders the data in two-dimensional cross-sectional images of the body region being examined. This data is displayed on a monitor. The physician reviews the data as it is being obtained and may request additional sections to provide more detail of areas of interest. Use 70450 for CT of the head or brain without intravenous contrast material. Use 70460 when intravenous contrast material is administered before the CT scanning beings. Use 70470 when CT is first performed without intravenous contrast followed by the administration of intravenous contrast and acquisition of additional sections. The physician reviews the CT scan, notes any abnormalities, and provides a written interpretation of the

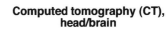

Computed tomography (CT), head/brain

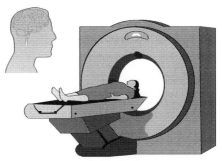

Without (70450), or with (70460) contrast material; further contrast procedures (70470)

findings.

70480-70482

70480   Computed tomography, orbit, sella, or posterior fossa or outer, middle, or inner ear; without contrast material
70481   Computed tomography, orbit, sella, or posterior fossa or outer, middle, or inner ear; with contrast material(s)
70482   Computed tomography, orbit, sella, or posterior fossa or outer, middle, or inner ear; without contrast material, followed by contrast material(s) and further sections

Computerized tomography, also referred to as a CT scan, uses special x-ray equipment and computer technology to produce multiple cross-sectional images of the region being studied. In this study, CT scan of the eye socket (orbit); region that houses the pituitary gland (sella); region at the base of the skull (posterior fossa); or any portion of the ear (outer, middle, or inner) is obtained. The patient is positioned on the CT examination table. An initial pass is made through the CT scanner to determine the starting position of the scans, after which the CT scan is performed. As the table moves slowly through the scanner, numerous x-ray beams and electronic x-ray detectors rotate around the body region being examined. The amount of radiation being absorbed is measured. As the beams and detectors rotate around the body, the table is moved through the scanner. A computer program processes the data and renders the data in two-dimensional cross-sectional images of the body region being examined. This data is displayed on a monitor. The physician reviews the data as it is being obtained and may request additional sections to provide more detail of areas of interest. Use 70480 for CT of the head or brain without intravenous contrast material. Use 70481 when intravenous contrast material is administered before the CT scanning beings. Use 70482 when CT is first performed without intravenous contrast followed by the administration of intravenous contrast and acquisition of additional sections. The physician reviews the CT scan, notes any abnormalities, and provides a written interpretation of the findings.

70486-70488

70486   Computed tomography, maxillofacial area; without contrast material
70487   Computed tomography, maxillofacial area; with contrast material(s)
70488   Computed tomography, maxillofacial area; without contrast material, followed by contrast material(s) and further sections

Computerized tomography, also referred to as a CT scan, uses special x-ray equipment and computer technology to produce multiple cross-sectional images of the region being studied. In this study, CT scan of the maxillofacial area is obtained. The maxillofacial area includes the forehead (frontal bone), sinuses, nose and nasal bones, jaw (maxilla and mandible). The only facial region not included in this study is the orbit. The patient is positioned on the CT examination table. An initial pass is made through the CT scanner to determine the starting position of the scans, after which the CT scan is performed. As the table moves slowly through the scanner, numerous x-ray beams and electronic x-ray detectors rotate around the body region being examined. The amount of radiation being absorbed is measured. As the beams and detectors rotate around the body, the table is moved through the scanner. A computer program processes the data and renders the data in two-dimensional cross-sectional images of the body region being examined. This data is displayed on a monitor. The physician reviews the data as it is being obtained and may request additional sections to provide more detail of areas of interest. Use 70486 for CT of the head or brain without intravenous contrast material. Use 70487 when intravenous contrast material is administered before the CT scanning beings. Use 70488 when CT is first performed without intravenous contrast followed by the administration of intravenous contrast and acquisition of additional sections. The physician reviews the CT scan, notes any abnormalities, and provides a written interpretation of the findings.

70490-70492

70490 Computed tomography, soft tissue neck; without contrast material

70491 Computed tomography, soft tissue neck; with contrast material(s)

70492 Computed tomography, soft tissue neck; without contrast material followed by contrast material(s) and further sections

Computerized tomography, also referred to as a CT scan, uses special x-ray equipment and computer technology to produce multiple cross-sectional images of the region being studied. In a CT scan of the soft tissues of the neck, the patient is positioned on the CT examination table. An initial pass is made through the CT scanner to determine the starting position of the scans, after which the CT scan is performed. As the table moves slowly through the scanner, numerous x-ray beams and electronic x-ray detectors rotate around the body region being examined. The amount of radiation being absorbed is measured. As the beams and detectors rotate around the body, the table is moved through the scanner. A computer program processes the data and renders the data in two-dimensional cross-sectional images of the body region being examined. This data is displayed on a monitor. The physician reviews the data as it is being obtained and may request additional sections to provide more detail of areas of interest. Use 70490 for CT of the head or brain without intravenous contrast material. Use 70491 when intravenous contrast material is administered before the CT scanning beings. Use 70492 when CT is first performed without intravenous contrast followed by the administration of intravenous contrast and acquisition of additional sections. The physician reviews the CT scan, notes any abnormalities, and provides a written interpretation of the findings.

70496

70496 Computed tomographic angiography, head, with contrast material(s), including noncontrast images, if performed, and image postprocessing

A computed tomographic angiography (CTA) of the head is performed with contrast material including image postprocessing. Noncontrast images may also be obtained and are included when performed. CTA provides images of the blood vessels using a combination of computed tomography (CT) and angiography with contrast material. When angiography is performed using CT, multiple images are obtained and processed on a computer to create detailed, two-dimensional, cross-sectional views of the blood vessels. These images are then displayed on a computer monitor. The patient is positioned on the CT table. An intravenous line is inserted into a blood vessel, usually in the arm or hand. Non-contrast images may be obtained. A small dose of contrast is injected and test images are obtained to verify correct positioning. The CTA is then performed. Contrast is injected at a controlled rate and the CT table moves through the CT machine as the scanning is performed. After completion of the CTA, the radiologist reviews and interprets the CTA images of the head.

Computed tomographic angiography

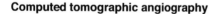

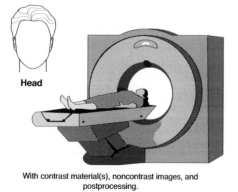

Head

With contrast material(s), noncontrast images, and postprocessing.

70498

70498 Computed tomographic angiography, neck, with contrast material(s), including noncontrast images, if performed, and image postprocessing

A computed tomographic angiography (CTA) of the neck is performed with contrast material including image postprocessing. Noncontrast images may also be obtained and are included when performed. CTA provides images of the blood vessels using a combination of computed tomography (CT) and angiography with contrast material. When angiography is performed using CT, multiple images are obtained and processed on a computer to create detailed, two-dimensional, cross-sectional views of the blood vessels. These images are then displayed on a computer monitor. The patient is positioned on the CT table. An intravenous line is inserted into a blood vessel, usually in the arm or hand. Non-contrast images may be obtained. A small dose of contrast is injected and test images are obtained to verify correct positioning. The CTA is then performed. Contrast is injected at a controlled rate and the CT table moves through the CT machine as the scanning is performed. After completion of the CTA, the radiologist reviews and interprets the CTA images of the neck.

70540-70543

70540 Magnetic resonance (eg, proton) imaging, orbit, face, and/or neck; without contrast material(s)

70542 Magnetic resonance (eg, proton) imaging, orbit, face, and/or neck; with contrast material(s)

70543 Magnetic resonance (eg, proton) imaging, orbit, face, and/or neck; without contrast material(s), followed by contrast material(s) and further sequences

Magnetic resonance imaging is done on the orbit, the face, and/or the neck. MRI is a noninvasive, non-radiating imaging technique that uses the magnetic properties of hydrogen atoms in the body. The patient is placed on a motorized table within a large MRI tunnel scanner that contains the magnet. The powerful magnetic field forces the hydrogen atoms to line up. Radiowaves are then transmitted within the strong magnetic field. Protons in the nuclei of different types of tissues emit a specific radiofrequency signal that bounces back to the computer, which processes the signals and converts the data into tomographic, 3D images with very high resolution. Orbital MRI provides reliable information for diagnosing tumors of the eye; infection or inflammation of the lacrimal glands and other soft tissues around the eye as well as osteomyelitis of nearby bone; damage or deterioration of the optic nerve; vascular edema or hemangioma of the eye area; and orbital muscular disorders. It is often performed in cases of trauma. MRI of the face and neck region is used to detect problems and abnormalities occurring outside the skull in the mouth, tongue, pharynx, nasal and sinus cavities, salivary glands, and vocal cords. MRI provides information on the presence and extent of tumors, masses, or lesions; infection, inflammation, and swelling of soft tissue; vascular edema or lesions; muscular abnormalities; and vocal cord paralysis. When MRI of the orbit, face, or neck is performed without intravenous contrast material, report 70540. When contrast dye, such as gadolinium is injected before the imaging is done, report 70542; and use 70543 when MRI is first performed without intravenous contrast followed by the administration of intravenous contrast and acquisition of additional images. The physician reviews the MRI, notes any abnormalities, and provides a written interpretation of the findings.

70544-70546

70544 Magnetic resonance angiography, head; without contrast material(s)

70545 Magnetic resonance angiography, head; with contrast material(s)

70546 Magnetic resonance angiography, head; without contrast material(s), followed by contrast material(s) and further sequences

Magnetic resonance angiography (MRA) is performed on the head without contrast materials (70544), with contrast materials (70545), and without contrast materials followed by contrast materials (70546). MRA is a noninvasive radiology procedure used to evaluate arterial and venous vessels for conditions such as atherosclerotic stenosis, arterial dissection, acute thrombosis, aneurysms or pseudo-aneurysms, vascular loops, vascular malformations/tumors, or arterial causes of pulsatile tinnitus. MRA may be performed following vascular surgery on the intracranial vessels to assess vascular status. MRA uses a magnetic field and pulses of radiowave energy to provide images of the blood vessels. Multiple images, 1-2 mm in thickness, are obtained and then processed using an array algorithm to produce maximum intensity projections (MIPs). MIPs are similar to subtraction angiograms. Areas of interest are identified by the radiologist and coned down to produce detailed views of the arteries. This post-processing of the images is performed by a technologist. The MIPs are reviewed by the radiologist along with the initial MRA images. The radiologist provides a written interpretation of findings. In 70544, MRA is performed without contrast materials. In 70545, an intravenous line is placed and contrast material is administered prior to the MRA. In 70546, MRA is first performed without contrast, followed by contrast administered intravenously, and additional MRA images.

70547-70549

70547 Magnetic resonance angiography, neck; without contrast material(s)

70548 Magnetic resonance angiography, neck; with contrast material(s)

70549 Magnetic resonance angiography, neck; without contrast material(s), followed by contrast material(s) and further sequences

Magnetic resonance angiography (MRA) is performed on the neck without contrast materials (70547), with contrast materials (70548), and without contrast materials followed by contrast materials (70549). MRA is a noninvasive radiology procedure used to evaluate arterial and venous vessels for conditions such as atherosclerotic stenosis, arterial dissection, acute thrombosis, aneurysms or pseudo-aneurysms, vascular loops, vascular malformations/tumors, or arterial causes of pulsatile tinnitus. MRA may be performed following vascular surgery on the neck vessels to assess vascular status. MRA uses a magnetic field and pulses of radiowave energy to provide images of the blood vessels. Multiple images of 1-2 mm in thickness are obtained and then processed using an array algorithm to produce maximum intensity projections (MIPs). MIPs are similar to subtraction angiograms. Areas of interest are identified by the radiologist and coned down to produce detailed views of the arteries. This post-processing of the images is performed by a technologist. The MIPs are reviewed by the radiologist along with the initial MRA images. The radiologist provides a written interpretation of findings. In 70547, MRA is performed without contrast materials. In 70548, an intravenous line is placed and contrast material is administered prior to the MRA. In 70549, MRA is first performed without contrast, followed by contrast administered intravenously, and additional MRA images.

70551-70553

70551 Magnetic resonance (eg, proton) imaging, brain (including brain stem); without contrast material

70552 Magnetic resonance (eg, proton) imaging, brain (including brain stem); with contrast material(s)

70553 Magnetic resonance (eg, proton) imaging, brain (including brain stem); without contrast material, followed by contrast material(s) and further sequences

Magnetic resonance imaging is done on the brain. MRI is a noninvasive, non-radiating imaging technique that uses the magnetic properties of hydrogen atoms in the body. The patient is placed on a motorized table within a large MRI tunnel scanner that contains the magnet. The powerful magnetic field forces the hydrogen atoms to line up. Radiowaves are then transmitted within the strong magnetic field. Protons in the nuclei of different types of tissues emit a specific radiofrequency signal that bounces back to the computer, which processes the signals and converts the data into tomographic, 3D images with very high resolution. MRI of the brain provides reliable information for diagnosing the presence, location, and extent of tumors, cysts, or other masses; swelling and infection; vascular disorders or malformations, such as aneurysms and intracranial hemorrhage; disease of the pituitary gland; stroke; developmental and structural anomalies of the brain; hydrocephalus; and chronic conditions and diseases affecting the central nervous system such as headaches and multiple sclerosis. When MRI of the brain is performed without intravenous contrast material, report 70551. When contrast dye, such as gadolinium is injected before the imaging is done, report 70552; and use 70553 when MRI is first performed without contrast followed by the administration of intravenous contrast and acquisition of additional images. The physician reviews the MRI, notes any abnormalities, and provides a written interpretation of the findings.

70554-70555

70554 Magnetic resonance imaging, brain, functional MRI; including test selection and administration of repetitive body part movement and/or visual stimulation, not requiring physician or psychologist administration

70555 Magnetic resonance imaging, brain, functional MRI; requiring physician or psychologist administration of entire neurofunctional testing

Functional magnetic resonance imaging (fMRI) uses a magnetic field, radio frequency pulses and a computer to produce detailed pictures of internal body structures. The magnetic field is produced by passing an electric current through wire coils. Other coils, located in the machine, send and receive radio waves, producing signals that are detected by the coils. The head is usually placed in a brace to hold it still. During an fMRI exam, a number of small tasks are performed by the patient, such as tapping a thumb against each of the fingers on the same hand, rubbing a block of sandpaper, or answering simple questions. The images are examined on a computer monitor, and printed or copied to CD. A computer processes the signals and generates a series of images each of which shows a thin slice of the brain. The images are then studied from different angles by the physician. The fMRI is performed to examine anatomy of the brain, to determine precisely which part of the brain is handling critical functions such as thought, speech, movement and sensation, help assess the effects of stroke, trauma or degenerative disease (e.g., Alzheimer's), monitor the growth and function of brain tumors, and/or guide the planning of surgery, radiation therapy, or other surgical treatments for the brain.

70557-70559

70557 Magnetic resonance (eg, proton) imaging, brain (including brain stem and skull base), during open intracranial procedure (eg, to assess for residual tumor or residual vascular malformation); without contrast material

70558 Magnetic resonance (eg, proton) imaging, brain (including brain stem and skull base), during open intracranial procedure (eg, to assess for residual tumor or residual vascular malformation); with contrast material(s)

70559 Magnetic resonance (eg, proton) imaging, brain (including brain stem and skull base), during open intracranial procedure (eg, to assess for residual tumor or residual vascular malformation); without contrast material(s), followed by contrast material(s) and further sequences

Magnetic resonance imaging is done on the brain during open intracranial surgery. MRI is a noninvasive, non-radiating imaging technique that uses the magnetic properties of hydrogen atoms in the body. The patient is placed on a motorized table within a large MRI tunnel scanner that contains the magnet. The powerful magnetic field forces the hydrogen atoms to line up. Radiowaves are then transmitted within the strong magnetic field. Protons in the nuclei of different types of tissues emit a specific radiofrequency signal that bounces back to the computer, which processes the signals and converts the data into tomographic, 3D images with very high resolution. Intraoperative MRI of the brain is done during open intracranial procedures performed in a specialized operative imaging suite that has an MRI scanner in the room. This allows the neurosurgeon to rotate the patient into the tunnel scanner at any point during the surgery to see the brain tumor clearly, assess whether the tumor has been completely removed, or to help place deep brain neurostimulator systems. The use of MRI during intracranial surgery greatly enhances surgical accuracy and reduces the risk of damage to other parts of the brain while reaching and resecting the tumor, or placing a neurostimulator to treat conditions such as Parkinson's, epilepsy, dystonia, and essential tremor . Intraoperative MRI also helps ensure surgical success by helping the surgeon confirm complete removal of the brain lesion, vascular malformation, or pituitary tumor. When MRI is performed without contrast material, report 70557. When imaging is performed after injection of a contrast dye, such as gadolinium, report 70558; and use 70559 when intraoperative MRI is first performed without contrast followed by the administration of contrast and acquisition of additional images.

71010-71015

71010 Radiologic examination, chest; single view, frontal

71015 Radiologic examination, chest; stereo, frontal

Chest radiographs (x-rays) provide images of the heart, lungs, bronchi, major blood vessels (aorta, vena cava, pulmonary vessels), and bones, (sternum, ribs, clavicle, scapula, spine). In 71010, a single frontal view of the chest is obtained. The patient is positioned facing the x-ray machine and a small burst of radiation is delivered to create the x-ray image. In 71015, a stereo frontal examination of the chest is performed. Stereoradiography involves taking two images of the internal body structure from slightly different angles. The two images are then viewed through a device that allows the two combined images to be viewed as one and provides a 3D image of the body structure. Images are recorded on hard copy film or stored electronically as digital images. The physician reviews the images, notes any abnormalities and provides a written interpretation of the findings.

71020-71023

71020 Radiologic examination, chest, 2 views, frontal and lateral

71021 Radiologic examination, chest, 2 views, frontal and lateral; with apical lordotic procedure

71022 Radiologic examination, chest, 2 views, frontal and lateral; with oblique projections

71023 Radiologic examination, chest, 2 views, frontal and lateral; with fluoroscopy

A radiologic examination of the chest is performed. Chest radiographs (X-rays) provide images of the heart, lungs, bronchi, major blood vessels (aorta, vena cava, pulmonary vessels), and bones, (sternum, ribs, clavicle, scapula, spine). In 71020, two views, frontal and lateral, are obtained. The patient is positioned facing the X-ray machine for the frontal view and then turned with the side of the chest positioned in front for the lateral view. A small burst of radiation is delivered for each X-ray and the images are recorded on hard copy film or stored electronically as digital images. In 71021, frontal and lateral images are obtained as described above along with an apical lordotic view that provides better visualization of the apical (top) regions of the lungs. The patient is positioned with the back arched so that the tops of the lungs can be X-rayed. In 71022, frontal and lateral images are obtained with oblique projections, which may be obtained to evaluate a pulmonary or mediastinal mass or opacity or to provide additional images of the heart and great vessels. There are four positions used for oblique views: right and left anterior oblique, and right and left posterior oblique. Anterior oblique views are obtained with the patient standing and the chest rotated 45 degrees. The arm closest to the X-ray cassette is flexed with the hand resting on the hip. The opposite arm is raised as high as possible. The part of the chest farthest away from the X-ray cassette is the area being studied. Posterior oblique views are typically obtained only when the patient is too ill to stand or lay prone for anterior oblique views. In 71023, frontal and lateral views are obtained with fluoroscopy. Fluoroscopy is performed to evaluate motion and function of chest structures including the

 ● New Code ▲ Revised Code

Radiology

lungs, diaphragm, and other structures of the respiratory tract. A continuous X-ray beam is passed through the chest, transmitted to a monitor, and the motion of chest structures is studied in detail.

71030-71034

71030   **Radiologic examination, chest, complete, minimum of 4 views**
71034   **Radiologic examination, chest, complete, minimum of 4 views; with fluoroscopy**

Chest radiographs (x-rays) provide images of the heart, lungs, bronchi, major blood vessels (aorta, vena cava, pulmonary vessels), and bones, (sternum, ribs, clavicle, scapula, spine). In 71030, a minimum of 4 views is obtained. The most common views are frontal (also referred to as anteroposterior or AP), posteroanterior (PA), and lateral. To obtain a frontal view, the patient is positioned facing the x-ray machine. A PA view is obtained with the patient's back toward the x-ray machine. For a lateral view, the patient is positioned with side of the chest toward the machine. Other views that may be obtained include apical lordotic and oblique. An apical lordotic image provides better visualization of the apical (top) regions of the lungs. The patient is positioned with the back arched so that the tops of the lungs can be x-rayed. Oblique views may be obtained to evaluate a pulmonary or mediastinal mass or opacity or to provide additional images of the heart and great vessels. There are four positions used for oblique views including right anterior oblique, left anterior oblique, right posterior oblique, and left posterior oblique. Anterior oblique views are obtained with the patient standing and the chest rotated 45 degrees. The arm closest to the x-ray cassette is flexed with the hand resting on the hip. The opposite arm is raised as high as possible. The part of the chest farthest away from the x-ray cassette is the area that is being studied. Posterior oblique views are typically obtained only when the patient is too ill to stand or lay prone for anterior oblique views. To obtain an expiratory view, the patient exhales and images are obtained. Images are recorded on hard copy film or stored electronically as digital images. The physician reviews the images, notes any abnormalities, and provides a written interpretation of the findings. In 71034, a minimum of 4 views is obtained with fluoroscopy. Fluoroscopy is performed to evaluate motion and function of chest structures including the lungs, diaphragm, and other structures of the respiratory tract. A continuous x-ray beam is passed through the chest, transmitted to a monitor, and motion of chest structures studied in detail.

71035

71035   **Radiologic examination, chest, special views (eg, lateral decubitus, Bucky studies)**

Special views of the chest, such as lateral decubitus or Bucky views, may be needed to help diagnose some conditions. A lateral decubitus view is obtained with the patient lying on the side; the patient's head resting on one arm, and the other arm is raised over the head with the elbow bent. Lateral decubitus views may be obtained with the patient lying on either side and should be specifically identified as right lateral decubitus or left lateral decubitus. Lateral decubitus x-rays are helpful in identifying fluid accumulation in the lungs and may be performed if the patient complains of painful respiration or for clinical indicators, such as a friction rub. Bucky studies are obtained using a special screen-film radiology device. Other special views not represented by a more specific code may also be reported with this code. The physician reviews the images, notes any abnormalities, and provides a written interpretation of the findings. Code 71035 represents a single special view and should be reported for each special image obtained.

71100-71111

71100   **Radiologic examination, ribs, unilateral; 2 views**
71101   **Radiologic examination, ribs, unilateral; including posteroanterior chest, minimum of 3 views**
71110   **Radiologic examination, ribs, bilateral; 3 views**
71111   **Radiologic examination, ribs, bilateral; including posteroanterior chest, minimum of 4 views**

Rib radiographs (x-rays) are typically obtained following trauma to the rib cage to determine if fractures or other internal injuries are present. The most common views of the ribs are anteroposterior (AP) (frontal) and oblique. There are four positions used for oblique views: right anterior oblique, left anterior oblique, right posterior oblique, and left posterior oblique. Anterior oblique views are obtained with the patient standing and the chest rotated 45 degrees. The arm closest to the x-ray cassette is flexed with the hand resting on the hip. The opposite arm is raised as high as possible. The part of the chest farthest away from the x-ray cassette is the area that is being studied. Posterior oblique views are typically obtained only when the patient is too ill to stand or lay prone for anterior oblique views. In 71100, 2 images of the ribs on one side of the chest are obtained. In 71101, 3 images of the ribs on one side of the chest are obtained, with one view being posteroanterior (PA). In a posteroanterior view, the patient is positioned with the back toward the x-ray machine. In 71110, images of the ribs are obtained on both sides of the chest with a total of 3 images being obtained. In 71111, images of the ribs on both sides of the chest are obtained. A minimum of 4 views is obtained with one view being posteroanterior. The physician reviews the images, notes any abnormalities, and provides a written interpretation of the findings.

71120

71120   **Radiologic examination; sternum, minimum of 2 views**

A diagnostic x-ray examination of the sternum, or breast bone, is done with a minimum of 2 views taken. X-ray uses indirect ionizing radiation to take pictures inside the body. X-rays work on non-uniform material, such as human tissue, because of the different density and composition of the object, which allows some of the x-rays to be absorbed and some to pass through and be captured behind the object on a detector. This produces a 2D image of the structures. Bones appear white while soft tissue and fluids appear shades of grey. Sternal x-rays are most often taken to look for fractures after a blow to the chest, particularly when an initial chest x-ray shows nothing, but the patient still feels pain in the chest area after a car accident, sports injury, assault, or even resuscitation measures. The physician reviews the images for signs of fracture or other injury.

71130

71130   **Radiologic examination; sternoclavicular joint or joints, minimum of 3 views**

Radiographs of the sternoclavicular (SC) joint are typically obtained to diagnose dislocation or other injury to the SC joint. The most common views include anteroposterior (AP) (frontal), Heinig view, Hobbs view, and serendipity view. In an AP view, the patient's chest the patient is positioned facing the x-ray machine. To obtain a Heinig view, the patient is in supine position. The x-ray is directed tangential to the injured sternoclavicular joint and parallel to the opposite clavicle. The cassette is placed on the opposite shoulder centered on the manubrium. To obtain a Hobbs view, the patient is seated at the x-ray table with an x-ray cassette on the table. The patient must lean forward over the table with the anterior rib cage positioned against the cassette. The x-ray beam is directed from above toward the nape of the neck. To obtain a serendipity view, the patient lies prone on the x-ray table with the cassette centered under the upper shoulder and neck. The x-ray beam is centered over the sternum and directed at a 40-degree angle from vertical. A minimum of three views of the sternoclavicular joints is obtained. The physician reviews the images, notes any abnormalities, and provides a written interpretation of the findings.

71250-71270

71250   **Computed tomography, thorax; without contrast material**
71260   **Computed tomography, thorax; with contrast material(s)**
71270   **Computed tomography, thorax; without contrast material, followed by contrast material(s) and further sections**

Diagnostic computed tomography (CT) is done on the thorax. CT uses multiple, narrow x-ray beams aimed around a single rotational axis, taking a series of 2D images of the target structure from multiple angles. Contrast material is used to enhance the images. Computer software processes the data and reconstructs a 3D image. Thin, cross-sectional 2D and 3D slices are then produced of the targeted organ or area. The patient is placed inside the CT scanner on the table and images are obtained of the thorax to look for problems or disease in the lungs, heart, esophagus, soft tissue, or major blood vessels of the chest, such as the aorta. In 71250, no contrast medium is used. In 71260, an iodine dye is used to see the target area better, and in 71270, images are first taken without contrast and again after the administration of the dye. The physician reviews the images to look for suspected disease such as infection, lung cancer, pulmonary embolism, aneurysms, and metastatic cancer to the chest from other areas.

71275

71275   **Computed tomographic angiography, chest (noncoronary), with contrast material(s), including noncontrast images, if performed, and image postprocessing**

A computed tomographic angiography (CTA) of the noncoronary vessels of the chest is performed with contrast material including image postprocessing. Noncontrast images may also be obtained and are included when performed. CTA provides images of the blood vessels using a combination of computed tomography (CT) and angiography with contrast material. When angiography is performed using CT, multiple images are obtained and processed on a computer to create detailed, two-dimensional, cross-sectional views of the blood vessels. These images are then displayed on a computer monitor. The patient is positioned on the CT table. An intravenous line is inserted into a blood vessel, usually in the arm or hand. Non-contrast images may be obtained. A small dose of contrast is injected and test images are obtained to verify correct positioning. The CTA is then performed. Contrast is injected at a controlled rate and the CT table moves through the CT machine as the scanning is performed. After completion of the CTA, the radiologist reviews and interprets the CTA images of the noncoronary vessels of the chest.

71550-71552

71550 Magnetic resonance (eg, proton) imaging, chest (eg, for evaluation of hilar and mediastinal lymphadenopathy); without contrast material(s)

71551 Magnetic resonance (eg, proton) imaging, chest (eg, for evaluation of hilar and mediastinal lymphadenopathy); with contrast material(s)

71552 Magnetic resonance (eg, proton) imaging, chest (eg, for evaluation of hilar and mediastinal lymphadenopathy); without contrast material(s), followed by contrast material(s) and further sequences

Magnetic resonance imaging (MRI) is done on the chest. MRI is a noninvasive, non-radiating imaging technique that uses the magnetic properties of nuclei within hydrogen atoms of the body. The powerful magnetic field forces the hydrogen atoms to line up. Radiowaves are then transmitted within the strong magnetic field. Protons in the nuclei of different types of tissues emit a specific radiofrequency signal that bounces back to the computer, which records the images. The computer processes the signals and coverts the data into tomographic, 3D, sectional images in slices with very high resolution. The patient is placed on a motorized table within a large MRI tunnel scanner that contains the magnet. The physician reviews the images to diagnose disease such as abnormal growths, view lymph nodes and vessels, evaluate lymphadenopathy or blood flow, or see if cancer has spread to the chest. In 71550, no contrast medium is used. In 71551, an iodine dye is used to see the chest area better, and in 71552, images are first taken without contrast and again after the administration of the dye.

71555

71555 Magnetic resonance angiography, chest (excluding myocardium), with or without contrast material(s)

Magnetic resonance angiography (MRA) is performed on the chest with or without contrast material. MRA is a noninvasive diagnostic radiology procedure that uses a high-powered magnetic field and pulses of radiowave energy to provide images of the blood vessels. MRA of the chest is done to identify aortic aneurysms, detect injury to blood vessels in trauma patients, evaluate arteries that may be feeding a tumor prior to chemoembolization or radiation therapy, identify dissection in the aorta or its major branches, demonstrate the extent of atherosclerosis prior to surgery, assess vascular status following surgery, screen for arterial disease in those with a family history, and detect pulmonary embolism. Multiple images of 1-2mm in thickness are obtained and processed to provide maximum intensity projections (MIPs), which are similar to subtraction angiograms. Areas of interest are identified by the radiologist and then coned down to produce detailed views of the vessels. This post-processing of the images is performed by a technologist. The radiologist reviews the MIPs along with the initial MRA images and provides a written report of findings. For some of the images, an intravenous line may be placed and contrast dye administered for enhancing visualization.

72020

72020 Radiologic examination, spine, single view, specify level

A diagnostic x-ray is taken of one area of the spine. X-ray uses indirect ionizing radiation to take pictures inside the body. X-rays work on non-uniform material, such as human tissue, because of the different density and composition of the object, which allows some of the x-rays to be absorbed and some to pass through and be captured behind the object on a detector. This produces a 2D image of the structures. This code reports a single view of the spine to look for abnormalities or problems related to injury or pain and must be specified for the level.

72040-72052

72040 Radiologic examination, spine, cervical; 2 or 3 views
72050 Radiologic examination, spine, cervical; 4 or 5 views
72052 Radiologic examination, spine, cervical; 6 or more views

A radiologic exam is done of the cervical spine. Anteroposterior and lateral views are the most common projections taken. X-ray uses indirect ionizing radiation to take pictures inside the body. X-rays work on non-uniform material, such as human tissue, because of the different density and composition of the object, which allows some of the x-rays to be absorbed and some to pass through and be captured behind the object on a detector. This produces a 2D image of the structures. When 2-3 views or less are taken of the cervical spine, report 72040. If 4 or 5 views are taken, report 72050. A cervical spine x-ray examination with 6 or more views is reported with 72052.

72070-72074

72070 Radiologic examination, spine; thoracic, 2 views
72072 Radiologic examination, spine; thoracic, 3 views
72074 Radiologic examination, spine; thoracic, minimum of 4 views

A radiologic exam is done of the thoracic spine. X-ray uses indirect ionizing radiation to take pictures inside the body. X-rays work on non-uniform material, such as human tissue, because of the different density and composition of the object, which allows some of the x-rays to be absorbed and some to pass through and be captured behind the object on a detector. This produces a 2D image of the structures. X-rays are taken of the thoracic spine to evaluate for back pain or suspected disease or injury. Films are taken from differing views that commonly include anteroposterior, lateral, posteroanterior, and a swimmer's view for the upper thoracic spine in which the patient reaches up with one arm and down with the other as if taking a swimming stroke. Report 72070 for 2 views of the thoracic spine; 72072 for 3 views; and 72074 for a minimum of 4 views of the thoracic spine.

72080

72080 Radiologic examination, spine; thoracolumbar junction, minimum of 2 views

A radiologic x-ray exam is done of the thoracolumbar junction of the spine. X-ray uses indirect ionizing radiation to take pictures inside the body. X-rays work on non-uniform material, such as human tissue, because of the different density and composition of the object, which allows some of the x-rays to be absorbed and some to pass through and be captured behind the object on a detector. This produces a 2D image of the structures. A minimum of two views are taken of the thoracolumbar junction of the spine to evaluate for back pain or suspected disease or injury. X-ray films are commonly taken from frontal and lateral views or posteroanterior and lateral views.

72081-72084

72081 Radiologic examination, spine, entire thoracic and lumbar, including skull, cervical and sacral spine if performed (eg, scoliosis evaluation); one view

72082 Radiologic examination, spine, entire thoracic and lumbar, including skull, cervical and sacral spine if performed (eg, scoliosis evaluation); 2 or 3 views

72083 Radiologic examination, spine, entire thoracic and lumbar, including skull, cervical and sacral spine if performed (eg, scoliosis evaluation); 4 or 5 views

72084 Radiologic examination, spine, entire thoracic and lumbar, including skull, cervical and sacral spine if performed (eg, scoliosis evaluation); minimum of 6 views

A diagnostic radiographic examination is done of the entire thoracic and lumbar spine for a scoliosis evaluation. This study is done to assess scoliosis, such as the type of scoliosis, and the location and degree of curvature. X-ray uses indirect ionizing radiation to take pictures inside the body. X-rays work on non-uniform material, such as human tissue, because of the different density and composition of the object, which allows some of the x-rays to be absorbed and some to pass through and be captured behind the object on a detector. This produces a 2D image of the structures. Code 72081 reports a single view x-ray of the entire thoracic and lumbar spine; code 72082 reports 2 or 3 views; code 72083 reports 4 or 5 views; and 72084 reports a spinal evaluation with a minimum of 6 views being taken. Posteroanterior, frontal, and lateral views are commonly taken of the spine while in an erect, standing, or upright position to help assess lateral curvature. The patient stands in front of a vertical grid with the knees together in full extension. The field of view includes the entire thoracic and lumbar spine and also the cervical and sacral spinal areas as well as the skull, whenever necessary. The vertebral bodies above and below the apex of the spinal curve that are the most tilted are measured by intersecting lines to give the degree of curvature. Lateral projections for viewing scoliosis may be taken with the patient's arms placed straight out in front for a better view of the curvature. Other views may also be taken of the spine while the patient is lying down face up.

72100-72114

72100 Radiologic examination, spine, lumbosacral; 2 or 3 views
72110 Radiologic examination, spine, lumbosacral; minimum of 4 views
72114 Radiologic examination, spine, lumbosacral; complete, including bending views, minimum of 6 views

A radiologic exam is done of the lumbosacral spine. Frontal, posteroanterior, and lateral views are the most common projections taken. X-ray uses indirect ionizing radiation to take pictures inside the body. X-rays work on non-uniform material, such as human tissue, because of the different density and composition of the object, which allows some of the x-rays to be absorbed and some to pass through and be captured behind the object on a detector. This produces a 2D image of the structures. When 2 or 3 views are taken of the lumbosacral spine, report 72100. If at least 4 views are taken, report 72110. A complete lumbosacral spine exam (72114) includes a minimum of 6 views, which may include views taken from oblique angles as well as in bending positions, flexion and extension. Lateral bending positions may also be taken with the patient sitting on a stool with the back against a contact to avoid moving the torso forward. The patient flexes the back over to each side as far as possible without losing contact with the stool. The complete exam is often done by taking anteroposterior and lateral views first, particularly to 'clear' the spine before the technologist moves the patient into position for oblique angles and bending views if evaluating for trauma.

72120

72120 Radiologic examination, spine, lumbosacral; bending views only, 2 or 3 views

A radiologic exam of the lumbosacral spine is done taking 2 or 3 views with the patient in bending positions only. X-ray uses indirect ionizing radiation to take pictures inside the body. X-rays work on non-uniform material, such as human tissue, because of the different density and composition of the object, which allows some of the x-rays to be absorbed and some to pass through and be captured behind the object on a detector. This produces a 2D image of the structures. Biomechanical dysfunction of the lumbar spine is revealed with lateral bending views. The patient is placed sitting on a stool with the back against a contact to avoid moving the torso forward. The patient flexes the back over to each side as far as possible without losing contact with the stool. Sitting instead of standing helps block out effects of gross musculature. These views are helpful when plain films seem normal and symptoms of dysfunction are not explained. Flexion or extension bending views may also be taken with the patient standing, such as bending over forward with the knees straight and the arms dangling.

72125-72127

72125 Computed tomography, cervical spine; without contrast material
72126 Computed tomography, cervical spine; with contrast material
72127 Computed tomography, cervical spine; without contrast material, followed by contrast material(s) and further sections

Diagnostic computed tomography (CT) is done on the cervical spine. CT uses multiple, narrow x-ray beams aimed around a single rotational axis, taking a series of 2D images of the target structure from multiple angles. Contrast material is used to enhance the images. Computer software processes the data and produces several images of thin, cross-sectional 2D slices of the targeted organ or area. Three-dimensional models of the spine can be created by stacking multiple, individual 2D slices together. The patient is placed inside the CT scanner on the table and images are obtained of the cervical spine. In 72125, no contrast medium is used. In 72126, an iodine contrast dye is injected either intrathecally into the C1-C2 or other cervical level, or administered intravenously to see the target area better before images are taken .If intrathecal injection is performed it is reported separately. In 72127, images are taken without contrast and again after the administration of the contrast. The physician reviews the images to look for suspected problems with the spine such as bone disease, fractures or other injuries, or birth defects of the spine in children.

72128-72130

72128 Computed tomography, thoracic spine; without contrast material
72129 Computed tomography, thoracic spine; with contrast material
72130 Computed tomography, thoracic spine; without contrast material, followed by contrast material(s) and further sections

Diagnostic computed tomography (CT) is done on the thoracic spine. CT uses multiple, narrow x-ray beams aimed around a single rotational axis, taking a series of 2D images of the target structure from multiple angles. Contrast material is used to enhance the images. Computer software processes the data and produces several images of thin, cross-sectional 2D slices of the targeted organ or area. Three-dimensional models of the spine can be created by stacking multiple, individual 2D slices together. The patient is placed inside the CT scanner on the table and images are obtained of the thoracic spine. In 72128, no contrast medium is used. In 72129, an iodine contrast dye is injected either intrathecally or administered intravenously to see the target area better before images are taken. If intrathecal injection is performed it is reported separately. In 72130, images are taken without contrast and again after the administration of the contrast. The physician reviews the images to look for suspected problems with the spine such as bone disease, and evaluate for fractures or other injuries as well as birth defects of the spine in children.

72131-72133

72131 Computed tomography, lumbar spine; without contrast material
72132 Computed tomography, lumbar spine; with contrast material
72133 Computed tomography, lumbar spine; without contrast material, followed by contrast material(s) and further sections

Diagnostic computed tomography (CT) is done on the lumbar spine. CT uses multiple, narrow x-ray beams aimed around a single rotational axis, taking a series of 2D images of the target structure from multiple angles. Contrast material is used to enhance the images. Computer software processes the data and produces several images of thin, cross-sectional 2D slices of the targeted organ or area. Three-dimensional models of the spine can be created by stacking multiple, individual 2D slices together. The patient is placed inside the CT scanner on the table and images are obtained of the lumbar spine. In 72131, no contrast medium is used. In 72132, an iodine contrast dye is injected either intrathecally or administered intravenously to see the target area better before images are taken. If intrathecal injection is performed it is reported separately. In 72133, images are taken without contrast and again after the administration of the contrast. The physician reviews the images to look for suspected problems with the spine such as bone disease, and evaluate for fractures or other injuries as well as birth defects of the spine in children.

72141-72142

72141 Magnetic resonance (eg, proton) imaging, spinal canal and contents, cervical; without contrast material
72142 Magnetic resonance (eg, proton) imaging, spinal canal and contents, cervical; with contrast material(s)

Magnetic resonance imaging (MRI) is done on the cervical spinal canal and contents. MRI is a noninvasive, non-radiating imaging technique that uses the magnetic properties of nuclei within hydrogen atoms of the body. The powerful magnetic field forces the hydrogen atoms to line up. Radiowaves are then transmitted within the strong magnetic field. Protons in the nuclei of different types of tissues emit a specific radiofrequency signal that bounces back to the computer, which records the images. The computer processes the signals and converts the data into tomographic, 3D, sectional images in slices with very high resolution. The patient is placed on a motorized table within a large MRI tunnel scanner that contains the magnet. MRI scans of the spine are often done when conservative treatment of back/neck pain is unsuccessful and more aggressive treatments are considered or following surgery. In 72141, no contrast medium is used. In 72142, a contrast dye is administered first to see the spinal area better before images are taken. The physician reviews the images to look for specific information that may correlate to the patient's symptoms, such as abnormal spinal alignment; disease or injury of vertebral bodies; intervertebral disc herniation, degeneration, or dehydration; the size of the spinal canal to accommodate the cord and nerve roots; pinched or inflamed nerves; or any changes since surgery.

72146-72147

72146 Magnetic resonance (eg, proton) imaging, spinal canal and contents, thoracic; without contrast material
72147 Magnetic resonance (eg, proton) imaging, spinal canal and contents, thoracic; with contrast material(s)

Magnetic resonance imaging (MRI) is done on the thoracic spinal canal and contents. MRI is a noninvasive, non-radiating imaging technique that uses the magnetic properties of nuclei within hydrogen atoms of the body. The powerful magnetic field forces the hydrogen atoms to line up. Radiowaves are then transmitted within the strong magnetic field. Protons in the nuclei of different types of tissues emit a specific radiofrequency signal that bounces back to the computer, which records the images. The computer processes the signals and converts the data into tomographic, 3D, sectional images in slices with very high resolution. The patient is placed on a motorized table within a large MRI tunnel scanner that contains the magnet. MRI scans of the spine are often done when conservative treatment of back/neck pain is unsuccessful and more aggressive treatments are considered or following surgery. In 72146, no contrast medium is used. In 72147, a contrast dye is administered first to see the spinal area better before images are taken. The physician reviews the images to look for specific information that may correlate to the patient's symptoms, such as abnormal spinal alignment; disease or injury of vertebral bodies; intervertebral disc herniation, degeneration, or dehydration; the size of the spinal canal to accommodate the cord and nerve roots; pinched or inflamed nerves; or any changes since surgery.

72148-72149

72148 Magnetic resonance (eg, proton) imaging, spinal canal and contents, lumbar; without contrast material
72149 Magnetic resonance (eg, proton) imaging, spinal canal and contents, lumbar; with contrast material(s)

Magnetic resonance imaging (MRI) is done on the lumbar spinal canal and contents. MRI is a noninvasive, non-radiating imaging technique that uses the magnetic properties of nuclei within hydrogen atoms of the body. The powerful magnetic field forces the hydrogen atoms to line up. Radiowaves are then transmitted within the strong magnetic field. Protons in the nuclei of different types of tissues emit a specific radiofrequency signal that bounces back to the computer, which records the images. The computer processes the signals and coverts the data into tomographic, 3D, sectional images in slices with very high resolution. The patient is placed on a motorized table within a large MRI tunnel scanner that contains the magnet. MRI scans of the spine are often done when conservative treatment of back pain is unsuccessful and more aggressive treatments are considered or following surgery. In 72148, no contrast medium is used. In 72149, a contrast dye is administered first to see the spinal area better before images are taken. The physician reviews the images to look for specific information that may correlate to the patient's symptoms, such as abnormal spinal alignment; disease or injury of vertebral bodies; intervertebral disc herniation, degeneration, or dehydration; the size of the spinal canal to accommodate the cord and nerve roots; pinched or inflamed nerves; or any changes since surgery.

72156-72158

72156 Magnetic resonance (eg, proton) imaging, spinal canal and contents, without contrast material, followed by contrast material(s) and further sequences; cervical

72157 Magnetic resonance (eg, proton) imaging, spinal canal and contents, without contrast material, followed by contrast material(s) and further sequences; thoracic

72158 Magnetic resonance (eg, proton) imaging, spinal canal and contents, without contrast material, followed by contrast material(s) and further sequences; lumbar

Magnetic resonance imaging (MRI) is done on the cervical, thoracic, or lumbar spinal canal and contents. MRI is a noninvasive, non-radiating imaging technique that uses the magnetic properties of nuclei within hydrogen atoms of the body. The powerful magnetic field forces the hydrogen atoms to line up. Radiowaves are then transmitted within the strong magnetic field. Protons in the nuclei of different types of tissues emit a specific radiofrequency signal that bounces back to the computer, which records the images. The computer processes the signals and coverts the data into tomographic, 3D, sectional images in slices with very high resolution. The patient is placed on a motorized table within a large MRI tunnel scanner that contains the magnet. MRI scans of the spine are often done when conservative treatment of back/neck pain is unsuccessful and more aggressive treatments are considered or following surgery. Images are taken first without contrast and again after the administration of contrast to see the spinal area better. The physician reviews the images to look for specific information that may correlate to the patient's symptoms, such as abnormal spinal alignment; disease or injury of vertebral bodies; intervertebral disc herniation, degeneration, or dehydration; the size of the spinal canal to accommodate the cord and nerve roots; pinched or inflamed nerves; or any changes since surgery. Use 72156 for MRI of the cervical spine, 72157 for the thoracic spine, and 72158 for the lumbar spine.

72159

72159 Magnetic resonance angiography, spinal canal and contents, with or without contrast material(s)

Magnetic resonance angiography (MRA) is performed on the spinal canal and contents with or without contrast material. MRA is a noninvasive diagnostic radiology procedure that uses a high-powered magnetic field and pulses of radiowave energy to provide images of the blood vessels. MRA of the spinal canal is done to assess vascular malformations or lesions of the spinal cord, such as dural arteriovenous fistulas, and intramedullary glomus type arteriovenous malformations. Multiple images of 1-2mm in thickness are obtained and processed to provide maximum intensity projections (MIPs), which are similar to subtraction angiograms. Areas of interest are identified by the radiologist and then coned down to produce detailed views of the vessels. This post-processing of the images is performed by a technologist. The radiologist reviews the MIPs along with the initial MRA images and provides a written report of findings. For some of the images, an intravenous line may be placed and contrast dye administered to enhance visualization.

72170-72190

72170 Radiologic examination, pelvis; 1 or 2 views
72190 Radiologic examination, pelvis; complete, minimum of 3 views

A diagnostic x-ray examination of the pelvis is done. X-ray uses indirect ionizing radiation to take pictures inside the body. X-rays work on non-uniform material, such as human tissue, because of the different density and composition of the object, which allows some of the x-rays to be absorbed and some to pass through and be captured behind the object on a detector. This produces a 2D image of the structures. Bones appear white while soft tissue and fluids appear shades of grey. Pelvic x-rays are taken when the patient complains of pain and/or injury in the area of the pelvis or hip joints to assess for fractures and detect arthritis or bone disease. The patient is placed on a table and different views of the pelvis are taken by having the patient position the legs and feet differently, such as turning the feet inward to point at each other, or bending the knees outward with the soles of the feet together in a 'frog-leg' position. Report 72170 for 1-2 views and 72190 for 3 or more views for a complete pelvic x-ray exam.

72191

72191 Computed tomographic angiography, pelvis, with contrast material(s), including noncontrast images, if performed, and image postprocessing

A computed tomographic angiography (CTA) of the pelvis is performed with contrast material including image postprocessing. Noncontrast images may also be obtained and are included when performed. CTA provides images of the blood vessels using a combination of computed tomography (CT) and angiography with contrast material. When angiography is performed using CT, multiple images are obtained and processed on a computer to create detailed, two-dimensional, cross-sectional views of the blood vessels. These images are then displayed on a computer monitor. The patient is positioned on the CT table. An intravenous line is inserted into a blood vessel, usually in the arm or hand. Non-contrast images may be obtained. A small dose of contrast is injected and test images

are obtained to verify correct positioning. The CTA is then performed. Contrast is injected at a controlled rate and the CT table moves through the CT machine as the scanning is performed. After completion of the CTA, the radiologist reviews and interprets the CTA images of the pelvis.

72192-72194

72192 Computed tomography, pelvis; without contrast material
72193 Computed tomography, pelvis; with contrast material(s)
72194 Computed tomography, pelvis; without contrast material, followed by contrast material(s) and further sections

Diagnostic computed tomography (CT) is done on the pelvis to provide detailed visualization of the organs and structures within or near the pelvis, such as kidneys, bladder, prostate, uterus, cervix, vagina, lymph nodes, and pelvic bones. CT uses multiple, narrow x-ray beams aimed around a single rotational axis, taking a series of 2D images of the target structure from multiple angles. Contrast material is used to enhance the images. Computer software processes the data and produces several images of thin, cross-sectional 2D slices of the targeted organ or area. Three-dimensional models of organs within the pelvis can be created by stacking multiple, individual 2D slices together. The patient is placed inside the CT scanner on the table and images are obtained of the pelvis area. In 72192, no contrast medium is used. In 72193, an iodine contrast dye is administered intravenously to see the target area better before images are taken. In 72194, images are taken without contrast and again after the administration of the contrast. The physician reviews the images to gather information for specified purposes such as diagnosing or monitoring cancer, evaluating the pelvic bones for fractures or other injury following trauma, locating abscesses or masses found during physical exam, finding the cause of pelvic pain, providing more detailed information before surgery, and evaluating the patient after surgery.

72195-72197

72195 Magnetic resonance (eg, proton) imaging, pelvis; without contrast material(s)
72196 Magnetic resonance (eg, proton) imaging, pelvis; with contrast material(s)
72197 Magnetic resonance (eg, proton) imaging, pelvis; without contrast material(s), followed by contrast material(s) and further sequences

Magnetic resonance imaging (MRI) is done on the pelvis and organs within the pelvic area. MRI is a noninvasive, non-radiating imaging technique that uses the magnetic properties of nuclei within hydrogen atoms of the body. The powerful magnetic field forces the hydrogen atoms to line up. Radiowaves are then transmitted within the strong magnetic field. Protons in the nuclei of different types of tissues emit a specific radiofrequency signal that bounces back to the computer, which records the images. The computer processes the signals and converts the data into tomographic, 3D, sectional images in slices with very high resolution. The patient is placed on a motorized table within a large MRI tunnel scanner that contains the magnet. Small coils that help transmit and receive the radiowaves may be placed around the hip area. MRI scans of the pelvis are often done for injury, trauma, birth defects, or unexplained hip or pelvic pain. In 72195, no contrast medium is used. In 72196, an iodine contrast dye is administered intravenously to see the target area better before images are taken. In 72197, images are taken without contrast and again after the administration of contrast. The physician reviews the images to look for information that may correlate to the patient's signs or symptoms. Pelvic MRI may be done on males to evaluate lumps or swelling of the testicles or scrotum and locate an undescended testicle that does not appear on ultrasound. For females, an MRI scan may be used to evaluate abnormal vaginal bleeding, endometriosis, a pelvic mass, or unexplained infertility.

72198

72198 Magnetic resonance angiography, pelvis, with or without contrast material(s)

Magnetic resonance angiography (MRA) is performed on the pelvis with or without contrast material. MRA is a noninvasive diagnostic radiology procedure that uses a high-powered magnetic field and pulses of radiowave energy to provide images of the blood vessels. MRA of the pelvis is done to assess vascular problems or disease such as narrowed or blocked arteries, venous blood clots, the extent of atherosclerosis, and ischemic areas. It is also done to evaluate blood flow from the hips in cases of claudication in the legs. Multiple images of 1-2mm in thickness are obtained and processed to provide maximum intensity projections (MIPs), which are similar to subtraction angiograms. Areas of interest are identified by the radiologist and then coned down to produce detailed views of the vessels. This post-processing of the images is performed by a technologist. The radiologist reviews the MIPs along with the initial MRA images and provides a written report of findings. For some of the images, an intravenous line may be placed and contrast dye administered for enhancing visualization.

72200-72202

72200 Radiologic examination, sacroiliac joints; less than 3 views
72202 Radiologic examination, sacroiliac joints; 3 or more views

A radiologic examination of the sacroiliac (SI) joints is performed. This is the area where the left and right winged pelvic bones join with the sacrum in the back to form the posterior portion of the pelvic ring. Because of its complex anatomy and irregular surfaces, the sacroiliac joint can be difficult to image. An anteroposterior (AP) view with the patient supine and knees or hips flexed, if possible, is typically done first for routine exam, along with left and right oblique views with the patient recumbent and rotated 25-30 degrees from the AP position. When imaging SI joints, the oblique views take the x-ray of the side that is up, although the patient is positioned for the opposite side down. Posteroanterior views may also be taken with the patient prone. X-rays are taken of the sacroiliac joints to help diagnose spondyloarthropathies in rheumatic disease, inflammatory lesions affecting the joint, sacroiliitis, ankylosing spondylitis, juvenile spondyloarthopathy, arthritis associated with inflammatory bowel disease, psoriatic arthritis, and reactive arthritis, as well as fractures or dislocations. X-ray imaging uses indirect ionizing radiation to take pictures inside the body. X-rays work on non-uniform material, such as human tissue, because of the different density and composition of the object, which allows some of the x-rays to be absorbed and some to pass through and be captured behind the object on a detector. This produces a 2D image of the structures. If less than 3 views are taken, report 72200. Use 72202 when 3 views or more are taken for a complete exam.

72220

72220 Radiologic examination, sacrum and coccyx, minimum of 2 views

A radiologic examination of the sacrum and coccyx is done with at least 2 views obtained. X-ray imaging uses indirect ionizing radiation to take pictures inside the body. X-rays work on non-uniform material, such as human tissue, because of the different density and composition of the object, which allows some of the x-rays to be absorbed and some to pass through and be captured behind the object on a detector. This produces a 2D image of the structures. Routine views include an anteroposterior (AP) or posteroanterior (PA) view of the sacrum, an AP or PA view of the coccyx, and lateral sacrum/coccyx views. For the sacral view, the patient's pelvis needs to be positioned correctly so the sacrum and sacroiliac joints are symmetrical. Because the coccyx has a forward curvature in relation to the sacrum, it is not automatically visualized when taking an AP view of the sacrum, and so another positioning is done for the coccyx. For lateral views, the patient stands sideways with feet shoulder width apart and arms crossed at the shoulders. Lateral imaging shows the entire 5th lumbar vertebra, the sacrum, and the coccyx. Good sacrum and coccyx imaging requires patient preparation with an empty bladder, clean colon, and removal of clothing in favor of wearing a gown. This is due to the difficulty these obstructions can cause in achieving a good radiographic image. Shielding is done for males, but is not possible for female patients.

72240-72270

72240 Myelography, cervical, radiological supervision and interpretation
72255 Myelography, thoracic, radiological supervision and interpretation
72265 Myelography, lumbosacral, radiological supervision and interpretation
72270 Myelography, 2 or more regions (eg, lumbar/thoracic, cervical/thoracic, lumbar/cervical, lumbar/thoracic/cervical), radiological supervision and interpretation

Myelography is a type of diagnostic imaging that uses contrast material injected into the subarachnoid space and real-time fluoroscopic x-ray imaging. After introducing a needle into the spinal canal and injecting contrast material into the subarachnoid space, the radiologist evaluates the spinal cord, spinal canal, nerve roots, meninges, and blood vessels in real time as contrast flows through the space around the spinal cord and nerve roots. Permanent x-ray images may also be taken. Spinal myelography is used to diagnose intervertebral disc herniation, meningeal inflammation, spinal stenosis, tumors, and other spinal lesions caused by infection or previous trauma. Report 72240 for myelography of the cervical spine, 72255 for thoracic myelography, 72265 for lumbosacral myelography, and 72270 when two or more regions of the spine are examined together.

72275

72275 Epidurography, radiological supervision and interpretation

Images of the epidural space surrounding the spinal cord are documented under radiological supervision while a therapeutic or diagnostic epidurography is performed. The radiologist also provides a formal radiologic report of the procedure after it is performed. The injection portion of the procedure to perform the epidurography is done by cleansing the skin over the targeted spinal region with an antiseptic solution and then injecting a local anesthetic. A spinal needle is inserted into the skin and advanced into the epidural space. Contrast may be injected to confirm proper needle placement or to perform the procedure itself. A diagnostic or therapeutic substance, such as an anesthetic, antispasmodic, opioid, steroid, or neurolytic substance is injected into the epidural space. Images are taken. Following injection, the patient is monitored for 15-20 minutes to ensure that there are no adverse effects. Report 72275 for radiological supervision during the

procedure that includes documented imaging and provision of a formal interpretation of the procedure by the radiologist.

72285

72285 Discography, cervical or thoracic, radiological supervision and interpretation

Images of a cervical or thoracic intervertebral disc are documented under radiological supervision while a discography is performed. A formal interpretation of the procedure is also provided. Discography is done to determine if an intervertebral disc abnormality is the cause of back pain. To perform the injection portion of the discography, the patient is positioned on the side and the site of the injection is cleansed with an antiseptic solution. A local anesthetic is injected. A large bore needle is advanced through the skin to the targeted cervical or thoracic disc. A discography needle is advanced through the first needle and into the center of the disc. Contrast is injected and radiographs are obtained under supervision. Report 72285 for radiological supervision during the discography procedure and provision of a written interpretation after completion.

72295

72295 Discography, lumbar, radiological supervision and interpretation

Images of a lumbar intervertebral disc are documented under radiological supervision while a discography is performed. A formal interpretation of the procedure is also provided. Discography is done to determine if an intervertebral disc abnormality is the cause of back pain. To perform the injection portion of the discography, the patient is positioned on the side and the site of the injection is cleansed with an antiseptic solution. A local anesthetic is injected. A large bore needle is advanced through the skin to the targeted lumbar disc. A discography needle is advanced through the first needle and into the center of the disc. Contrast is injected and radiographs are obtained under supervision. Report 72295 for radiological supervision during the discography procedure and provision of a written interpretation after completion.

73000

73000 Radiologic examination; clavicle, complete

A complete radiologic examination of the clavicle is performed to determine fractures or dislocations. The most common type of fracture involves the middle third of the clavicle, followed by the lateral third distal to the coracoclavicular ligament. The least common type of clavicular fracture involves the proximal third. X-ray imaging uses indirect ionizing radiation to take pictures inside the body. X-rays work on non-uniform material, such as human tissue, because of the different density and composition of the object, which allows some of the x-rays to be absorbed and some to pass through and be captured behind the object on a detector. This produces a 2D image of the structures. Radiographs are taken according to the suspected location of the injury. Standard evaluation includes an anteroposterior view focused on the midshaft wide enough to assess the acromioclavicular and sternoclavicular joints. Oblique views are also obtained with a cephalic tilt of 20-60 degrees.

73010

73010 Radiologic examination; scapula, complete

A complete radiologic examination of the scapula is performed. Fractures of the scapula are not very common and are sometimes found even when there is no clinical suspicion of injury. Parts of the scapula include the body, acromion, spine, coracoid, neck, and glenoid. The acromion and the coracoid form a 'Y' shape where they join with the body of the scapula. The lateral scapula view, also called the 'Y' view, is the standard view that may be taken by different techniques for a complete examination, including the anteroposterior (AP) or posteroanterior (PA) technique views, further dependent on arm position. With the patient in an oblique AP or PA position, lateral views may be taken with the hand on the hip, the arm by the side, and the hand of the target side placed on the opposite shoulder. X-ray imaging uses indirect ionizing radiation to take pictures inside the body. X-rays work on non-uniform material, such as human tissue, because of the different density and composition of the object, which allows some of the x-rays to be absorbed and some to pass through and be captured behind the object on a detector. This produces a 2D image of the structures.

73020-73030

73020 Radiologic examination, shoulder; 1 view
73030 Radiologic examination, shoulder; complete, minimum of 2 views

A radiologic examination of the shoulder is done. The shoulder is the junction of the humeral head and the glenoid of the scapula. Standard views include the anteroposterior (AP) view and the lateral 'Y' view, named because of the Y shape formed by the scapula when looking at it from the side. An axial view can also be obtained for further assessment when the patient is able to hold the arm in abduction. X-ray imaging uses indirect ionizing radiation to take pictures inside the body. X-rays work on non-uniform material, such as human tissue, because of the different density and composition of the object, which allows some of the x-rays to be absorbed and some to pass through and be captured behind the object on a detector. This produces a 2D image of the structures. Report 73020 for a single view and 73030 for a complete exam when a minimum of 2 views is taken.

73040

73040   Radiologic examination, shoulder, arthrography, radiological supervision and interpretation

Radiographic arthrography is performed on the shoulder. Intra-articular images of the shoulder are documented under radiological supervision while arthrography is performed. A formal interpretation of the procedure is also provided. For the injection portion of the procedure, the skin over the injection site is cleansed and a local anesthetic is injected. A needle may be inserted into the joint and fluid aspirated with a syringe. The radiopaque substance is then injected into the shoulder joint, usually under fluoroscopic guidance, which is included, and the joint is exercised to help distribute the radiopaque substance. Once the contrast has been distributed throughout the joint, the radiographic images are obtained. Report 73040 for the radiological supervision provided during the arthrography procedure and the provision of a written interpretation after completion.

73050

73050   Radiologic examination; acromioclavicular joints, bilateral, with or without weighted distraction

A radiologic examination of the acromioclavicular (AC) joints is done bilaterally. X-ray imaging uses indirect ionizing radiation to take pictures inside the body. X-rays work on non-uniform material, such as human tissue, because of the different density and composition of the object, which allows some of the x-rays to be absorbed and some to pass through and be captured behind the object on a detector. This produces a 2D image of the structures. AC joint injuries can be assessed using the standard anteroposterior (AP) view. Bilateral exams include a comparison view taken of the opposite shoulder. An AP view of the AC joint is taken with the patient's head inclined about 15 degrees along the spine of the scapula. Formerly, stress or weighted images were used to distinguish between partial and complete ligamentous tears, which are now both treated nonsurgically, so the value of weighted distraction images has fallen by the wayside, and they have basically been left out of current practice.

73060

73060   Radiologic examination; humerus, minimum of 2 views

A radiologic examination of the humerus is done with a minimum of 2 views taken. X-ray imaging uses indirect ionizing radiation to take pictures inside the body. X-rays work on non-uniform material, such as human tissue, because of the different density and composition of the object, which allows some of the x-rays to be absorbed and some to pass through and be captured behind the object on a detector. This produces a 2D image of the structures. The surgical neck of the humerus is the most common site of fracture. Shaft fractures are often associated with some kind of pathological lesion. X-rays of the humerus can be taken to detect deformities or lesions in the upper arm, such as cysts, tumors, late stage infection, or other diseases as well as a broken bone. The standard views of the humerus include the front to back anteroposterior view and the side, or lateral view.

73070-73080

73070   Radiologic examination, elbow; 2 views
73080   Radiologic examination, elbow; complete, minimum of 3 views

A radiologic examination of the elbow is done. X-ray imaging uses indirect ionizing radiation to take pictures inside the body. X-rays work on non-uniform material, such as human tissue, because of the different density and composition of the object, which allows some of the x-rays to be absorbed and some to pass through and be captured behind the object on a detector. This produces a 2D image of the structures. X-rays of the elbow are usually considered necessary to assess for fractures or dislocations when the normal range of motion for extension, flexion, supination, and pronation cannot be carried out. Most acute disruptions of the elbow joint can be diagnosed by conventional x-ray examination, with the minimum number of views including the front to back anteroposterior projection with the elbow in as full extension as possible, and the side, or lateral image taken in flexion. A complete series of images also includes an oblique view of the radial head-capitellar image to help diagnose suspected subtle fractures involving the radial head or in cases of acute pain and trauma. The patient needs to be able to hold the elbow in full extension for the front view and in 90 degree flexion for the oblique and lateral views as much as possible. Report 73070 for a radiologic exam of the elbow with 2 views, and 73080 for an exam with at least 3 different projections.

73085

73085   Radiologic examination, elbow, arthrography, radiological supervision and interpretation

Radiographic arthrography is performed on the elbow. Intra-articular images of the elbow joint are documented under radiological supervision while arthrography is performed. A formal interpretation of the procedure is also provided. For the injection portion of the procedure, the skin over the injection site is cleansed and a local anesthetic is injected.

A needle may be inserted into the joint and fluid aspirated with a syringe. The radiopaque substance is then injected into the elbow joint, usually under fluoroscopic guidance, which is included, and the joint is exercised to help distribute the radiopaque substance. Once the contrast has been distributed throughout the joint, the radiographic images are obtained. Report 73085 for the radiological supervision provided during the arthrography procedure and the provision of a written interpretation after completion.

73090

73090   Radiologic examination; forearm, 2 views

A radiologic examination of the forearm is done. X-ray imaging uses indirect ionizing radiation to take pictures inside the body. X-rays work on non-uniform material, such as human tissue, because of the different density and composition of the object, which allows some of the x-rays to be absorbed and some to pass through and be captured behind the object on a detector. This produces a 2D image of the structures. Frontal views, or back to front (PA) views and lateral views are necessary to show the radius and ulna and assess the extent and direction of injury. Since the radius and ulna are anatomically connected at both ends of the bones with ligaments, the two bones function in a manner that makes the forearm considered as a single unit when assessing injury. The two standard views taken for x-ray examination of the forearm include the anteroposterior (AP) view, and the lateral view.

73092

73092   Radiologic examination; upper extremity, infant, minimum of 2 views

An upper extremity x-ray exam of an infant is done with at least 2 views. In such a young child, an x-ray of the upper extremity looks at the wrist, forearm, elbow, upper arm, and shoulder, and may include the fingers and hand as well. The radiographs may be taken to look for fractures, dislocations, deformities, arthritis, and pathological lesions such as pockets of infection, bone tumors, and cysts which may be the cause of swelling and pain. The difficulty in infant exams is the need for the patient to be restrained and the arm to be held still without anything blocking the view. Tools used to help ensure a good diagnostic image include sponges, sandbags, Velcro, medical tape, objects of distraction, and wooden blocks used strategically with the young patient. X-ray imaging uses indirect ionizing radiation to take pictures inside the body. X-rays work on non-uniform material, such as human tissue, because of the different density and composition of the object, which allows some of the x-rays to be absorbed and some to pass through and be captured behind the object on a detector. This produces a 2D image of the structures. Any movement will blur the images. Two to four projections are taken, often depending on the size of the patient.

73100-73110

73100   Radiologic examination, wrist; 2 views
73110   Radiologic examination, wrist; complete, minimum of 3 views

A radiologic examination of the wrist is done. X-ray imaging uses indirect ionizing radiation to take pictures inside the body. X-rays work on non-uniform material, such as human tissue, because of the different density and composition of the object, which allows some of the x-rays to be absorbed and some to pass through and be captured behind the object on a detector. This produces a 2D image of the structures. The radiographs may be taken to look for conditions such as fractures, dislocations, deformities, arthritis, foreign body, infection, or tumor. Wrist standard views include the front to back anteroposterior (AP) or back to front posteroanterior (PA) projection; the lateral view with the elbow flexed and the hand and wrist placed thumb up; and oblique views. Oblique views are obtained with the hand and wrist either supinated or pronated with the hand slightly flexed so the carpal target area lies flat, and then rotating the wrist 45 degrees externally or internally. A more specialized image may be obtained for assessing carpal tunnel. For the carpal tunnel view, the forearm is pronated with the palm down, and the wrist is hyperextended as far as possible by grasping the fingers with the opposite hand and gently hyperextending the joint until the metacarpals and fingers are in a near vertical position. Report 73100 for an x-ray exam consisting of 2 views, and 73110 for a complete wrist exam with a minimum of 3 views.

73115

73115   Radiologic examination, wrist, arthrography, radiological supervision and interpretation

Radiographic arthrography is performed on the wrist. Intra-articular images of the wrist are documented under radiological supervision while arthrography is performed. A formal interpretation of the procedure is also provided. For the injection portion of the procedure, the skin over the injection site is cleansed and a local anesthetic is injected. A needle may be inserted into the joint and fluid aspirated with a syringe. The radiopaque substance is then injected into the wrist, usually under fluoroscopic guidance, which is included, and the joint is exercised to help distribute the radiopaque substance. Once the contrast has been distributed throughout the joint, the radiographic images are obtained. Report 73115 for the radiological supervision provided during the arthrography procedure and the provision of a written interpretation after completion.

73120-73130

73120 Radiologic examination, hand; 2 views
73130 Radiologic examination, hand; minimum of 3 views

A radiologic examination of the hand is done. X-ray imaging uses indirect ionizing radiation to take pictures inside the body. X-rays work on non-uniform material, such as human tissue, because of the different density and composition of the object, which allows some of the x-rays to be absorbed and some to pass through and be captured behind the object on a detector. This produces a 2D image of the structures. The radiographs may be taken to look for conditions such as fractures, dislocations, deformities, degenerative bone conditions, osteomyelitis, arthritis, foreign body, or tumors. Hand x-rays are also used to help determine the 'bone age' of children and assess whether any nutritional or metabolic disorders may be interfering with proper development. The posteroanterior projection is taken with the palm down flat and may show not only the metacarpals, phalanges, and interphalangeal joints, but the carpal bones, radius, and ulna as well. Lateral views may be taken with the hand placed upright, resting upon the ulnar side of the palm and little finger with the thumb on top, ideally with the fingers supported by a sponge and splayed to avoid overlap. Oblique views can be obtained with the hand placed palm down and rolled slightly to the outside with the fingertips still touching the film surface. The beam is angled perpendicular to the cassette for oblique projections and aimed at the middle finger metacarpophalangeal joint. Report 73120 for a radiologic exam with 2 views taken of the hand and 73130 for an x-ray exam in which a minimum of 3 different projections is obtained.

73140

73140 Radiologic examination, finger(s), minimum of 2 views

A radiologic examination of the finger(s) is done with at least 2 different projections taken. X-ray imaging uses indirect ionizing radiation to take pictures inside the body. X-rays work on non-uniform material, such as human tissue, because of the different density and composition of the object, which allows some of the x-rays to be absorbed and some to pass through and be captured behind the object on a detector. This produces a 2D image of the structures. The radiographs may be taken to look for conditions such as fractures, interphalangeal (IP) joint dislocations, deformities, degenerative bone conditions, osteomyelitis, arthritis, foreign body, or tumors. The posteroanterior projection is taken with the palm down flat, fingers extended, and slightly apart to show the metacarpals, phalanges, and IP joints of the target finger(s). Anteroposterior views are taken with the back of the hand placed on the film and the x-ray beam going from palmar to dorsal direction. Lateral views are taken with the ulnar side of the hand on the film cassette and the fingers spread apart to avoid overlap, sometimes supported from underneath. Oblique views can be obtained with the hand placed palm down and the radial side rotated 45 degrees up away from the surface, with the fingers extended and spread apart.

73200-73202

73200 Computed tomography, upper extremity; without contrast material
73201 Computed tomography, upper extremity; with contrast material(s)
73202 Computed tomography, upper extremity; without contrast material, followed by contrast material(s) and further sections

Diagnostic computed tomography (CT) is done on the upper extremity to provide detailed visualization of the tissues and bone structure of the arm. CT uses multiple, narrow x-ray beams aimed around a single rotational axis, taking a series of 2D images of the target structure from multiple angles. Contrast material is used to enhance the images. Computer software processes the data and produces several images of thin, cross-sectional 2D slices of the targeted organ or area. Three-dimensional models of the arm can be created by stacking multiple, individual 2D slices together. The patient is placed inside the CT scanner on the table and images are obtained of the upper extremity. In 73200, no contrast medium is used. In 73201, an iodine contrast dye is administered intravenously to see the target area better before images are taken. In 73202, CT is first performed without contrast followed by the administration of contrast and acquisition of additional sections. The physician reviews the CT scan, notes any abnormalities, and provides a written interpretation of the findings. The physician reviews the images to look for suspected problems with the arm such as locating tumors, abscesses, or masses; evaluating the bones for degenerative conditions, fractures, or other injury following trauma; and finding the cause of pain or swelling.

73206

73206 Computed tomographic angiography, upper extremity, with contrast material(s), including noncontrast images, if performed, and image postprocessing

A computed tomographic angiography (CTA) of the upper extremity is performed with contrast material including image postprocessing. Noncontrast images may also be obtained and are included when performed. CTA provides images of the blood vessels using a combination of computed tomography (CT) and angiography with contrast material. When angiography is performed using CT, multiple images are obtained and processed on a computer to create detailed, two-dimensional, cross-sectional views of the blood vessels. These images are displayed on a computer monitor. The patient is positioned on the CT table. An intravenous line is inserted into a blood vessel, usually in the arm or hand. Non-contrast images may be obtained. A small dose of contrast is injected and test images are obtained to verify correct positioning. The CTA is then performed. Contrast is injected at a controlled rate and the CT table moves through the CT machine as the scanning is performed. After completion of the CTA, the radiologist reviews and interprets the CTA images of the upper extremity.

73218-73220

73218 Magnetic resonance (eg, proton) imaging, upper extremity, other than joint; without contrast material(s)
73219 Magnetic resonance (eg, proton) imaging, upper extremity, other than joint; with contrast material(s)
73220 Magnetic resonance (eg, proton) imaging, upper extremity, other than joint; without contrast material(s), followed by contrast material(s) and further sequences

Magnetic resonance imaging is done on the upper or lower arm, other than a joint. Magnetic resonance is a noninvasive, non-radiating imaging technique that uses the magnetic properties of hydrogen atoms in the body. The patient is placed on a motorized table within a large MRI tunnel scanner that contains the magnet. The powerful magnetic field forces the hydrogen atoms to line up. Radiowaves are then transmitted within the strong magnetic field. Protons in the nuclei of different types of tissues emit a specific radiofrequency signal that bounces back to the computer, which processes the signals and converts the data into tomographic, 3D images with very high resolution. The patient is placed on a motorized table within a large MRI tunnel scanner that contains the magnet. Small coils that help transmit and receive the radiowaves may be placed around the arm. MRI scans of the arm are often done for injury, trauma, or unexplained pain and provide clear images of areas that may be difficult to see on CT. In 73218, no contrast medium is used. In 73219, an iodine contrast dye is administered intravenously to see the target area better before images are taken. In 73220, images are taken without contrast and again after the administration of contrast. The physician reviews the images to look for information that may correlate to the patient's signs or symptoms. MRI provides reliable information for diagnosing tendinitis; muscle atrophy and other anomalous muscular development; lesions of soft tissue and bone; osteomyelitis; contusions, hematomas, and other masses that can be palpated on exam; and broken bones or other abnormal findings on x-ray or bone scan.

73221-73223

73221 Magnetic resonance (eg, proton) imaging, any joint of upper extremity; without contrast material(s)
73222 Magnetic resonance (eg, proton) imaging, any joint of upper extremity; with contrast material(s)
73223 Magnetic resonance (eg, proton) imaging, any joint of upper extremity; without contrast material(s), followed by contrast material(s) and further sequences

Magnetic resonance imaging is done on a joint of the upper or lower arm. Magnetic resonance is a noninvasive, non-radiating imaging technique that uses the magnetic properties of hydrogen atoms in the body. The patient is placed on a motorized table within a large MRI tunnel scanner that contains the magnet. The powerful magnetic field forces the hydrogen atoms to line up. Radiowaves are then transmitted within the strong magnetic field. Protons in the nuclei of different types of tissues emit a specific radiofrequency signal that bounces back to the computer, which processes the signals and converts the data into tomographic, 3D images with very high resolution. The patient is placed on a motorized table within a large MRI tunnel scanner that contains the magnet. Small coils that help transmit and receive the radiowaves may be placed around the joint. MRI scans on joints of the upper extremity are often done for injury, trauma, unexplained pain, redness, or swelling, and freezing of a joint with loss of motion. MRI scans provide clear images of areas that may be difficult to see on CT. In 73221, no contrast medium is used. In 73222, an iodine contrast dye is administered into the joint to see the target area better before images are taken. In 73223, images are taken without contrast and again after the administration of contrast. The physician reviews the images to look for information that may correlate to the patient's signs or symptoms. MRI provides reliable information on the presence and extent of tumors, masses, or lesions in the joint; infection, inflammation, and swelling of soft tissue; muscle atrophy and other anomalous muscular development; and joint effusion and vascular necrosis.

73225

73225 Magnetic resonance angiography, upper extremity, with or without contrast material(s)

Magnetic resonance angiography (MRA) is performed on the upper or lower arm with or without the use of contrast material. MRA is a noninvasive radiology procedure used to evaluate arterial and venous vessels for conditions such as atherosclerotic stenosis, arterial dissection, acute thrombosis, aneurysms or pseudo-aneurysms, vascular loops, and vascular malformations or tumors. MRA uses a magnetic field and pulses of radiowave energy to provide images of the blood vessels. Multiple images, 1-2 mm in thickness, are obtained and then processed using an array algorithm to produce maximum intensity projections (MIPs). MIPs are similar to subtraction angiograms. Areas of interest are identified by the radiologist and coned down to produce detailed views of the arteries. This post-processing of the images is performed by a technologist. The MIPs are reviewed by the radiologist along with the initial MRA images. The radiologist provides a written interpretation of findings.

73501-73503

73501   **Radiologic examination, hip, unilateral, with pelvis when performed; 1 view**
73502   **Radiologic examination, hip, unilateral, with pelvis when performed; 2-3 views**
73503   **Radiologic examination, hip, unilateral, with pelvis when performed; minimum of 4 views**

A radiologic examination of the hip is done on either the left or the right side, which may also include the pelvis. X-ray imaging uses indirect ionizing radiation to take pictures inside the body. X-rays work on non-uniform material, such as human tissue, because of the different density and composition of the object, which allows some of the x-rays to be absorbed and some to pass through and be captured behind the object on a detector. This produces a 2D image of the structures. The radiographs may be taken to look for conditions such as fractures, dislocations, deformities, degenerative bone conditions, osteomyelitis, arthritis, foreign body, infection, or tumor. Hip standard views that are taken most frequently include the front to back anteroposterior view taken with the patient lying supine and the legs straight, rotated slightly inward; the lateral 'frog-leg' view, taken with the hips flexed and abducted and the knees flexed with the soles of the feet placed together; a cross table view with the unaffected hip and knee flexed at a 90 degree angle out of the way and the beam aimed perpendicular to the long axis of the femur on the affected side. Another type of lateral view is taken with the hip flexed 45 degrees and abducted 45 degrees and the beam aimed perpendicular to the table. Report 73501 for an x-ray exam of either the left or the right hip consisting of only 1 view; report 73502 for a hip exam on one side only with 2-3 views and code 73503 for a hip exam with a minimum of 4 views taken.

73521-73523

73521   **Radiologic examination, hips, bilateral, with pelvis when performed; 2 views**
73522   **Radiologic examination, hips, bilateral, with pelvis when performed; 3-4 views**
73523   **Radiologic examination, hips, bilateral, with pelvis when performed; minimum of 5 views**

A radiologic examination is done on both the left and the right hip, which may also include the pelvis. X-ray imaging uses indirect ionizing radiation to take pictures inside the body. X-rays work on non-uniform material, such as human tissue, because of the different density and composition of the object, which allows some of the x-rays to be absorbed and some to pass through and be captured behind the object on a detector. This produces a 2D image of the structures. The radiographs may be taken to look for conditions such as fractures, dislocations, deformities, degenerative bone conditions, osteomyelitis, arthritis, foreign body, infection, or tumor. Hip standard views that are taken most frequently include the front to back anteroposterior view taken with the patient lying supine and the legs straight, rotated slightly inward; the lateral 'frog-leg' view, taken with the hips flexed and abducted and the knees flexed with the soles of the feet placed together; a cross table view with the unaffected hip and knee flexed at a 90 degree angle out of the way and the beam aimed perpendicular to the long axis of the femur on the affected side. Another type of lateral view is taken with the hip flexed 45 degrees and abducted 45 degrees and the beam aimed perpendicular to the table. A front to back view of the hips in a pelvic view is often taken with the patient supine and both legs rotated slightly inward about 15 degrees. Report 73521 for an x-ray exam of both hips consisting of 2 projections; report 73522 for a bilateral hip x-ray exam with 3-4 views; and 73523 for a bilateral hip exam with a minimum of 5 views. The views taken may include a pelvic view.

73525

73525   **Radiologic examination, hip, arthrography, radiological supervision and interpretation**

Radiographic arthrography is performed on the hip to evaluate the joint's anatomy, particularly to view the acetabular labrum, articular ligaments, and cartilaginous structures. Intra-articular images of the hip joint are documented under radiological supervision while arthrography is performed. A formal interpretation of the procedure is also provided. For the injection portion of the procedure, the skin over the injection site is cleansed and a local anesthetic is injected. A needle may be inserted into the joint and fluid aspirated with a syringe. The radiopaque substance is then injected into the hip joint, usually under fluoroscopic guidance, which is included, and the joint is exercised to help distribute the radiopaque substance. Once the contrast has been distributed throughout the joint, the radiographic images are obtained. Report 73525 for the radiological supervision provided during the arthrography procedure and the provision of a written interpretation after completion.

73551-73552

73551   **Radiologic examination, femur; 1 view**
73552   **Radiologic examination, femur; minimum 2 views**

A radiologic examination of the femur is done between the hip and the knee. X-ray imaging uses indirect ionizing radiation to take pictures inside the body. X-rays work on non-uniform material, such as human tissue, because of the different density and composition of the object, which allows some of the x-rays to be absorbed and some to pass through and be captured behind the object on a detector. This produces a 2D image of the structures. The radiographs may be taken to look for the cause of pain, limping, or swelling, conditions such as fractures, dislocations, deformities, degenerative bone conditions, osteomyelitis, arthritis, foreign body, and cysts or tumors. X-rays may also be used to determine whether the femur is in satisfactory alignment following fracture treatment. Femur standard views that are taken most frequently include the front to back anteroposterior view and the lateral view from the side. Report 73551 for a single view of the femur, and code 73552 for an x-ray exam of the femur with a minimum of 2 views being taken.

73580

73580   **Radiologic examination, knee, arthrography, radiological supervision and interpretation**

Radiographic arthrography is performed on the knee. Intra-articular images of the knee joint are documented under radiological supervision while arthrography is performed. A formal interpretation of the procedure is also provided. For the injection portion of the procedure, the skin over the injection site is cleansed and a local anesthetic is injected. A needle may be inserted into the joint and fluid aspirated with a syringe. The radiopaque substance is then injected into the knee joint, usually under fluoroscopic guidance, which is included, and the joint is exercised to help distribute the radiopaque substance. Once the contrast has been distributed throughout the joint, the radiographic images are obtained. Report 73580 for the radiological supervision provided during the arthrography procedure and the provision of a written interpretation after completion.

73615

73615   **Radiologic examination, ankle, arthrography, radiological supervision and interpretation**

Radiographic arthrography is performed on the ankle. Intra-articular images of the ankle joint are documented under radiological supervision while arthrography is performed. A formal interpretation of the procedure is also provided. For the injection portion of the procedure, the skin over the injection site is cleansed and a local anesthetic is injected. A needle may be inserted into the joint and fluid aspirated with a syringe. The radiopaque substance is then injected into the ankle joint, usually under fluoroscopic guidance, which is included, and the joint is exercised to help distribute the radiopaque substance. Once the contrast has been distributed throughout the joint, the radiographic images are obtained. Report 73615 for the radiological supervision provided during the arthrography procedure and the provision of a written interpretation after completion.

73700-73702

73700   **Computed tomography, lower extremity; without contrast material**
73701   **Computed tomography, lower extremity; with contrast material(s)**
73702   **Computed tomography, lower extremity; without contrast material, followed by contrast material(s) and further sections**

Diagnostic computed tomography (CT) is done on the lower extremity to provide detailed visualization of the tissues and bone structure of the leg. CT uses multiple, narrow x-ray beams aimed around a single rotational axis, taking a series of 2D images of the target structure from multiple angles. Contrast material is used to enhance the images. Computer software processes the data and produces several images of thin, cross-sectional 2D slices of the targeted organ or area. Three-dimensional models of the leg can be created by stacking multiple, individual 2D slices together. The patient is placed inside the CT scanner on the table and images are obtained of the lower extremity. In 73700, no contrast medium is used. In 73701, an iodine contrast dye is administered intravenously to see the target area better before images are taken. In 73702, CT is first performed without contrast followed by the administration of contrast and acquisition of additional sections. The physician reviews the CT scan, notes any abnormalities, and provides a written interpretation of the findings. The physician reviews the images to look for suspected problems with the leg such as locating tumors, abscesses, or masses; evaluating the bones for degenerative conditions, fractures, or other injury following trauma; and finding the cause of pain or swelling.

73706

73706   **Computed tomographic angiography, lower extremity, with contrast material(s), including noncontrast images, if performed, and image postprocessing**

A computed tomographic angiography (CTA) of the lower extremity is performed with contrast material including image postprocessing. Noncontrast images may also be obtained and are included when performed. CTA provides images of the blood vessels using a combination of computed tomography (CT) and angiography with contrast material. When angiography is performed using CT, multiple images are obtained and processed on a computer to create detailed, two-dimensional, cross-sectional views of the blood vessels. These images are then displayed on a computer monitor. The patient is positioned on the CT table. An intravenous line is inserted into a blood vessel, usually in the arm or hand. Non-contrast images may be obtained. A small dose of contrast is injected and test images are obtained to verify correct positioning. The CTA is then performed. Contrast is injected at a controlled rate and the CT table moves through the CT machine as the scanning is performed. After completion of the CTA, the radiologist reviews and interprets the CTA images of the lower extremity.

73718-73720

73718 Magnetic resonance (eg, proton) imaging, lower extremity other than joint; without contrast material(s)

73719 Magnetic resonance (eg, proton) imaging, lower extremity other than joint; with contrast material(s)

73720 Magnetic resonance (eg, proton) imaging, lower extremity other than joint; without contrast material(s), followed by contrast material(s) and further sequences

Magnetic resonance imaging is done on the upper or lower leg, other than a joint. Magnetic resonance is a noninvasive, non-radiating imaging technique that uses the magnetic properties of hydrogen atoms in the body. The patient is placed on a motorized table within a large MRI tunnel scanner that contains the magnet. The powerful magnetic field forces the hydrogen atoms to line up. Radiowaves are then transmitted within the strong magnetic field. Protons in the nuclei of different types of tissues emit a specific radiofrequency signal that bounces back to the computer, which processes the signals and converts the data into tomographic, 3D images with very high resolution. The patient is placed on a motorized table within a large MRI tunnel scanner that contains the magnet. Small coils that help transmit and receive the radiowaves may be placed around the leg. MRI scans of the leg are often done for injury, trauma, or unexplained pain and provide clear images of areas that may be difficult to see on CT. In 73718, no contrast medium is used. In 73719, an iodine contrast dye is administered intravenously to see the target area better before images are taken. In 73720, images are taken without contrast and again after the administration of contrast. The physician reviews the images to look for information that may correlate to the patient's signs or symptoms. MRI provides reliable information for diagnosing tendinitis; muscle atrophy and other anomalous muscular development; lesions of soft tissue and bone; osteomyelitis; contusions, hematomas, and other masses that can be palpated on exam; and broken bones or other abnormal findings on x-ray or bone scan.

73721-73723

73721 Magnetic resonance (eg, proton) imaging, any joint of lower extremity; without contrast material

73722 Magnetic resonance (eg, proton) imaging, any joint of lower extremity; with contrast material(s)

73723 Magnetic resonance (eg, proton) imaging, any joint of lower extremity; without contrast material(s), followed by contrast material(s) and further sequences

Magnetic resonance imaging is done on a joint of the upper or lower leg. Magnetic resonance is a noninvasive, non-radiating imaging technique that uses the magnetic properties of hydrogen atoms in the body. The patient is placed on a motorized table within a large MRI tunnel scanner that contains the magnet. The powerful magnetic field forces the hydrogen atoms to line up. Radiowaves are then transmitted within the strong magnetic field. Protons in the nuclei of different types of tissues emit a specific radiofrequency signal that bounces back to the computer, which processes the signals and converts the data into tomographic, 3D images with very high resolution. The patient is placed on a motorized table within a large MRI tunnel scanner that contains the magnet. Small coils that help transmit and receive the radiowaves may be placed around the joint. MRI scans on joints of the lower extremity are often done for injury, trauma, unexplained pain, redness, or swelling, and freezing of a joint with loss of motion. MRI scans provide clear images of areas that may be difficult to see on CT. In 73721, no contrast medium is used. In 73722, an iodine contrast dye is administered into the joint to see the target area better before images are taken. In 73723, images are taken without contrast and again after the administration of contrast. The physician reviews the images to look for information that may correlate to the patient's signs or symptoms. MRI provides reliable information on the presence and extent of tumors, masses, or lesions within the joint; infection, inflammation, and swelling of soft tissue; muscle atrophy and other anomalous muscular development; and joint effusion and vascular necrosis.

73725

73725 Magnetic resonance angiography, lower extremity, with or without contrast material(s)

Magnetic resonance angiography (MRA) is performed on the upper or lower leg with or without the use of contrast material. MRA is a noninvasive radiology procedure used to evaluate arterial and venous vessels for conditions such as atherosclerotic stenosis,

arterial dissection, acute thrombosis, aneurysms or pseudo-aneurysms, vascular loops, and vascular malformations or tumors. MRA uses a magnetic field and pulses of radiowave energy to provide images of the blood vessels. Multiple images, 1-2 mm in thickness, are obtained and then processed using an array algorithm to produce maximum intensity projections (MIPs). MIPs are similar to subtraction angiograms. Areas of interest are identified by the radiologist and coned down to produce detailed views of the arteries. This post-processing of the images is performed by a technologist. The MIPs are reviewed by the radiologist along with the initial MRA images. The radiologist provides a written interpretation of findings.

74150-74170

74150 Computed tomography, abdomen; without contrast material

74160 Computed tomography, abdomen; with contrast material(s)

74170 Computed tomography, abdomen; without contrast material, followed by contrast material(s) and further sections

Diagnostic computed tomography (CT) is done on the abdomen to provide detailed visualization of the tissues and organs within the abdominal area. CT uses multiple, narrow x-ray beams aimed around a single rotational axis, taking a series of 2D images of the target structure from multiple angles. Contrast material is used to enhance the images. Computer software processes the data and produces several images of thin, cross-sectional 2D slices of the targeted organ or area. Three-dimensional models can be created by stacking multiple, individual 2D slices together. The patient is placed inside the CT scanner on the table and images are obtained of the abdomen. In 74150, no contrast medium is used. In 74160, an iodine contrast dye is administered intravenously to see the target area better before images are taken. In 74170, CT is first performed without contrast followed by the administration of contrast and acquisition of additional sections. The physician reviews the images for the cause of abdominal pain, swelling, and fever; for other suspected problems such as appendicitis and kidney stones; for locating tumors, abscesses, or masses; or for evaluating the abdominal area for hernias, infections, or internal injury. The physician reviews the CT scan, notes any abnormalities, and provides a written interpretation of the findings.

74174

74174 Computed tomographic angiography, abdomen and pelvis, with contrast material(s), including noncontrast images, if performed, and image postprocessing

Computed tomographic angiography (CTA) provides images of the blood vessels using a combination of computed tomography (CT) and angiography with contrast material. When angiography is performed using CT, multiple images are obtained and processed on a computer to create detailed, two-dimensional, cross-sectional views of the blood vessels. These images are then displayed on a computer monitor. The patient is positioned on the CT table. An intravenous line is inserted into a blood vessel, usually in the arm or hand. Non-contrast images of the abdomen and pelvis are obtained as needed. A small dose of contrast is injected and test images are obtained to verify correct positioning. The CTA of the abdomen and pelvis is then performed. Contrast is injected at a controlled rate and the CT table moves through the CT machine as the scanning is performed. After completion of the CTA, the radiologist reviews and interprets the CTA images of the blood vessels of the abdomen and pelvis.

74175

74175 Computed tomographic angiography, abdomen, with contrast material(s), including noncontrast images, if performed, and image postprocessing

A computed tomographic angiography (CTA) of the abdomen is performed with contrast material including image postprocessing. Noncontrast images may also be obtained and are included when performed. CTA provides images of the blood vessels using a combination of computed tomography (CT) and angiography with contrast material. When angiography is performed using CT, multiple images are obtained and processed on a computer to create detailed, two-dimensional, cross-sectional views of the blood vessels. These images are then displayed on a computer monitor. The patient is positioned on the CT table. An intravenous line is inserted into a blood vessel, usually in the arm or hand. Non-contrast images may be obtained. A small dose of contrast is injected and test images are obtained to verify correct positioning. The CTA is then performed. Contrast is injected at a controlled rate and the CT table moves through the CT machine as the scanning is performed. After completion of the CTA, the radiologist reviews and interprets the CTA images of the blood vessels of the abdomen.

74176-74178

74176 Computed tomography, abdomen and pelvis; without contrast material

74177 Computed tomography, abdomen and pelvis; with contrast material(s)

74178 Computed tomography, abdomen and pelvis; without contrast material in one or both body regions, followed by contrast material(s) and further sections in one or both body regions

Computerized tomography, also referred to as a CT scan, uses special x-ray equipment and computer technology to produce multiple cross-sectional images of the abdomen and pelvis. The patient is positioned on the CT examination table. An initial pass is made through the CT scanner to determine the starting position of the scans. The CT scan is then performed. As the table moves slowly through the scanner, numerous x-ray beams and electronic x-ray detectors rotate around the abdomen and pelvis. The amount of radiation being absorbed is measured. As the beams and detectors rotate around the body, the table is moved through the scanner. A computer program processes the data which is then displayed on the monitor as two-dimensional cross-sectional images of the abdomen or pelvis. The physician reviews the data and images as they are obtained and may request additional sections to provide more detail on areas of interest. Use 74176 for CT scan of the abdomen and pelvis without intravenous contrast material. Use 74177 for CT scan of the abdomen and pelvis in which intravenous contrast material is administered before CT scanning begins and contrast enhanced images are obtained. Use 74178 when CT is first performed without intravenous contrast followed by the administration of intravenous contrast and acquisition of additional sections. The physician reviews the CT scan, notes any abnormalities, and provides a written interpretation of the findings.

74181-74183

74181   Magnetic resonance (eg, proton) imaging, abdomen; without contrast material(s)

74182   Magnetic resonance (eg, proton) imaging, abdomen; with contrast material(s)

74183   Magnetic resonance (eg, proton) imaging, abdomen; without contrast material(s), followed by with contrast material(s) and further sequences

Magnetic resonance imaging is done on the abdomen. Magnetic resonance is a noninvasive, non-radiating imaging technique that uses the magnetic properties of hydrogen atoms in the body. The patient is placed on a motorized table within a large MRI tunnel scanner that contains the magnet. The powerful magnetic field forces the hydrogen atoms to line up. Radiowaves are then transmitted within the strong magnetic field. Protons in the nuclei of different types of tissues emit a specific radiofrequency signal that bounces back to the computer, which processes the signals and converts the data into tomographic, 3D images with very high resolution. The patient is placed on a motorized table within a large MRI tunnel scanner that contains the magnet. Small coils that help transmit and receive the radiowaves may be placed around the abdomen. MRI is often done for trauma and suspected internal injury, and unexplained abdominal pain, swelling, and fever. MRI scans provide clear images of areas that may be difficult to see on CT. In 74181, no contrast medium is used. In 74182, an iodine contrast dye is administered to see the target area better before images are taken. In 74183, images are taken without contrast and again after the administration of contrast. The physician reviews the images to look for information that may correlate to the patient's signs or symptoms, such as the location of tumors, abscesses, or masses; the presence of kidney stones, hernias, appendicitis or other infections, and internal injury.

74210-74220

74210   Radiologic examination; pharynx and/or cervical esophagus

74220   Radiologic examination; esophagus

Oral contrast material is swallowed and the passage of the contrast is observed fluoroscopically as it passes through the pharynx and/or esophagus. Once the lumen of the pharynx and/or esophagus is completely coated with contrast material, still radiographic images are obtained. The physician reviews the images, notes any abnormalities, and provides a written interpretation of the findings. Use 74210 for radiologic examination of the pharynx and/or cervical esophagus. Use 74220 for radiologic examination of the entire esophagus.

74246-74249

74246   Radiological examination, gastrointestinal tract, upper, air contrast, with specific high density barium, effervescent agent, with or without glucagon; with or without delayed images, without KUB

74247   Radiological examination, gastrointestinal tract, upper, air contrast, with specific high density barium, effervescent agent, with or without glucagon; with or without delayed images, with KUB

74249   Radiological examination, gastrointestinal tract, upper, air contrast, with specific high density barium, effervescent agent, with or without glucagon; with small intestine follow-through

A radiologic examination of the upper gastrointestinal (GI) tract images the esophagus, stomach, and duodenum, the first portion of the small intestine. X-ray imaging uses indirect ionizing radiation to take pictures of non-uniform material, such as human tissue, because of its different density and composition, which allows some of the x-rays to be absorbed and some to pass through and be captured behind the object on a detector. This produces a 2D image of the structures. A radiologic examination of the upper GI tract may be used to diagnose ulcers, tumors, inflammation, hiatal hernia, scarring, obstruction, and abnormal position or configuration of the organs. Patients may present with symptoms such as difficulty swallowing, chest or abdominal pain, vomiting, reflux, indigestion, or blood in the stool. A radiologic examination of the GI tract will often begin with a single, front to back anteroposterior (AP) scout film obtained in an erect or supine position that

includes imaging of the kidneys, ureter, and bladder—known as a KUB. For this air contrast study, the patient ingests a substance that will cause a buildup of air in the stomach as it is digested, along with a barium sulfate mixture that will coat the esophagus and the stomach. The patient may also be given glucagon to relax the muscles of the targeted area to be examined. X-ray images of the esophagus and stomach are taken as indicated and examined. Delayed images may be required if movement is very slow or to verify emptying of the contrast. All images from this procedure may not be available for immediate viewing. Use code 74246 if the procedure is performed without a KUB. Use code 74247 if a KUB of the abdominal region is also taken during the procedure. Use code 74249 when x-ray images of the small intestine are also obtained after the barium sulfate mixture has reached that area.

74261-74262

74261   Computed tomographic (CT) colonography, diagnostic, including image postprocessing; without contrast material

74262   Computed tomographic (CT) colonography, diagnostic, including image postprocessing; with contrast material(s) including non-contrast images, if performed

CT colonography, also referred to as virtual colonoscopy, is performed as a diagnostic procedure in a patient exhibiting signs or symptoms related to bowel disease. A bowel prep is performed the night before the procedure to clear the bowel of stool. The patient is positioned on the CT table. A small flexible tube is inserted through the anus and advanced approximately 2 inches into the rectum. Air or carbon dioxide gas is then pumped into the colon using a manual or electronic pump. Images are obtained to ensure that the colon is adequately distended. In 74261, non-contrast CT images of the abdomen and pelvis are then obtained. The patient is placed in a supine position and a first pass is made through the CT scanner and CT images are obtained. The patient is then placed prone and a second pass is made and images obtained. In 74262, CT colonography is performed with contrast materials. If indicated, the physician may first obtain non-contrast images as described above. Contrast material is then injected intravenously and contrast images are obtained in supine and prone positions in the same manner as the non-contrast images. The non-contrast and/or contrast CT images are reviewed. 3D reconstructions of the colon are created and adjustments made as needed to the 3D reconstructions to obtain the best visualization of the colon. These images are compared to any previously obtained radiological studies. The physician interprets the CT images and provides a written report of findings.

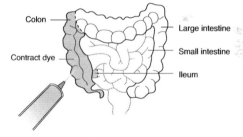

Computed tomographic (CT) colonography diagnostic including image postprocessing

Colon — Large intestine — Small intestine — Ileum — Contract dye

In 74261, non-contrast CT images of the abdomen and pelvis are obtained. In 74262, CT colonography is performed with contrast materials.

74263

74263   Computed tomographic (CT) colonography, screening, including image postprocessing

CT colonography, also referred to as virtual colonoscopy, is performed to screen for polyps or other masses or lesions in the colon. A bowel prep is performed the night before the procedure to clear the bowel of stool. The patient is positioned on the CT table. A small flexible tube is inserted through the anus and advanced approximately 2 inches into the rectum. Air or carbon dioxide gas is then pumped into the colon using a manual or electronic pump. Images are obtained to ensure that the colon is adequately distended. Non-contrast CT images of the abdomen and pelvis are then obtained. The patient is placed in a supine position and a first pass is made through the CT scanner and CT images are obtained. The patient is then placed prone and a second pass is made and images obtained. The CT images are reviewed. 3D reconstructions of the colon are created and adjustments made as needed to the 3D reconstructions to obtain the best visualization of the colon. These images are compared to any previously obtained radiological studies. The physician interprets the CT images and provides a written report of findings.

74270

74270 Radiologic examination, colon; contrast (eg, barium) enema, with or without KUB

A radiological examination of the colon is performed using any type of contrast agent enema, such as a barium or water-soluble contrast enema. The enema is given to instill the contrast agent, which coats the lining of the colon. Fluoroscopy and x-ray images are taken to study to colon and look for abnormalities, such as growths or inflammation, and help diagnose conditions such as cancer or colitis. After the patient voids the colon, more x-rays are taken, which may include the abdomen when a KUB is also done.

74290

74290 Cholecystography, oral contrast

Cholecystography with oral contrast is a radiologic procedure used to examine the gallbladder. The gallbladder is located in the upper right quadrant of the abdomen and stores bile, a fluid that aids in the digestion of fats. A contrast dye is ingested orally a few hours prior to the study. The dye is excreted by the liver and collects in the gallbladder, giving it an opaque appearance on x-ray film. Cholecystography is performed using fluoroscopy with the patient resting supine on the procedure table. Films are taken at intervals to record the findings. Gallstones will appear as darker images within the gallbladder and/or bile ducts. Tumors, polyps, inflammation, infection, and dysfunction may also be visible. The patient may be given a special liquid to drink during the study to stimulate the gallbladder to release bile.

74340

74340 Introduction of long gastrointestinal tube (eg, Miller-Abbott), including multiple fluoroscopies and images, radiological supervision and interpretation

A procedure is performed to insert a long gastrointestinal tube under fluoroscopic guidance. A single or double lumen tube is inserted through the patient's nose or mouth and into the stomach. Gastric secretions are aspirated for testing or to decompress the stomach. Irrigation fluids or contrast medium may be instilled to isolate areas of damage or produce clear radiologic images. If a double lumen tube is used, a balloon at the tip of one lumen can be inflated to assist with peristaltic advancement of the tube through the pylorus and into the duodenum. A guidewire or stylet can also be inserted through the lumen and used to manipulate the tube inside the stomach through the pylorus and into the duodenum. Multiple fluoroscopic images are obtained to verify placement of the tube in the stomach, advancement into the small intestine, and documentation of any obstruction or abnormal pathology. This includes all radiological supervision and interpretation of images for the procedure.

74420

74420 Urography, retrograde, with or without KUB

The physician introduces a special dye into the kidneys and the tubes that carry urine from the kidneys to the bladder (ureters). The dye is inserted so it enters the kidneys and ureters against the normal flow of liquid through these structures. The physician then takes and examines an X-ray image of these structures. The physician may also take a general X-ray image of the abdomen during the procedure.

74445

74445 Corpora cavernosography, radiological supervision and interpretation

Cavernosography involves the injection of contrast medium into the corpora cavernosa to examine radiographically the structure of the corpora cavernosa and the veins that drain blood from it. During a separately reportable injection procedure, a 19-22 gauge needle is inserted into the tissue of the corpora cavernosa on the dorsal lateral aspect proximal to the glans penis and contrast medium injected. Radiographic images are taken immediately from two angles, anterior/posterior and lateral/oblique. The radiologist supervises the injection procedure and provides a written interpretation of the procedure.

74710

74710 Pelvimetry, with or without placental localization

Pelvimetry is performed with or without placental location. This test used to be performed routinely in pregnant women to identify cephalopelvic disproportion (CPD), or the ability to deliver a baby in breech position; however, it is rarely performed today. CPD refers to a condition in which the woman's pelvis is too small compared to the size of the fetal head to allow vaginal delivery. With the patient standing, a lateral view of the pelvis and pregnant uterus is obtained. Sagittal views may also be obtained. The physician then measures the pelvic inlet and outet and compares those measurements to measurements of the fetal head. If the fetus is in breech position, the physician evaluates the size of the pelvic inlet and outlet to determine whether the patient can safely attempt a breech delivery. The location of the placenta may also be determined.

74712-74713

74712 Magnetic resonance (eg, proton) imaging, fetal, including placental and maternal pelvic imaging when performed; single or first gestation
74713 Magnetic resonance (eg, proton) imaging, fetal, including placental and maternal pelvic imaging when performed; each additional gestation (List separately in addition to code for primary procedure)

Fetal magnetic resonance imaging (MRI) is done to evaluate disorders or anomalies suspected on ultrasound. Fetal MRI is performed only in the 2nd and 3rd trimesters, due to the exceptionally small fetus size in the first trimester. MRI provides much more detailed images than ultrasound, enabling a more thorough assessment and diagnosis of fetal abnormalities, particularly providing information about the developing brain, chest, and abdomen. MRI is also safer than imaging modalities that use radiation. Magnetic resonance is a noninvasive, non-radiating imaging technique that uses the magnetic properties of hydrogen atoms in the body. The pregnant patient is placed lying comfortably on a motorized exam table that enters a large MRI tunnel scanner containing the magnet. Radiowaves are then transmitted from a scanner within the strong magnetic field, which forces the hydrogen atoms in the body to line up out of normal position. As the nuclei realign themselves into proper position, the protons in the nuclei of different types of tissues emit a specific radiofrequency signal that bounces back to the computer, which processes the signals and converts the data into tomographic, 3D images of the baby with very high resolution. A microphone in the scanner allows the mother to talk to the technologist during the procedure, which normally takes 30-40 minutes. Normal use of the magnetic field and radiowaves has shown no adverse effects.

74740

74740 Hysterosalpingography, radiological supervision and interpretation

The physician performs radiological supervision and interpretation of hysterosalpingography. In a separately reportable procedure, a catheter is inserted through the cervix and into the uterus. The patient is then situated under a fluoroscopy device. As contrast is instilled in the uterus, fluoroscopic images are obtained. The physician reviews these images for evidence of cysts, tumors, or other malformations of the uterus or fallopian tubes. Following completion of the procedure, the catheter is removed and the physician provides a written interpretation of the findings.

74742

74742 Transcervical catheterization of fallopian tube, radiological supervision and interpretation

Radiological supervision and interpretation of transcervical catheterization of the Fallopian tubes is performed. The patient is situated under a fluoroscopy device. In a separately reportable procedure, a catheter is inserted through the cervix into the uterus and advanced into the tubal ostium under fluoroscopic monitoring. The physician reviews the imaging as contrast is instilled into the fallopian tubes and notes any obstructions or abnormalities. If an obstruction is present, the physician supervises a separately reportable recanalization procedure. The catheterization is repeated on the opposite side as needed. Following completion of the procedure, the catheter is removed and the physician provides a written interpretation of the findings.

74775

74775 Perineogram (eg, vaginogram, for sex determination or extent of anomalies)

A perineogram or vaginogram is performed to identify and determine the extent of anomalies, such as anorectal angle anomalies causing fecal incontinence, and anomalies of the pelvic floor and vagina. The test can also detect rectocele, enterocele, and rectal prolapse. Nonionic contrast material is injected into the peritoneum using separately reportable fluoroscopic guidance. Anteroposterior (AP) and lateral radiographs are obtained. A barium paste enema is administered followed by injection of liquid barium into the vagina. The patient is placed on a commode and lateral radiographs are again obtained with the patient at rest and with maximum anal squeeze. The patient then evacuates the barium from the rectum as the physician observes on a videomonitor. A final lateral radiograph is also taken as the patient evacuates the barium.

75557-75559

75557 Cardiac magnetic resonance imaging for morphology and function without contrast material
75559 Cardiac magnetic resonance imaging for morphology and function without contrast material; with stress imaging

Cardiac magnetic resonance (CMR) imaging for morphology and function is performed without contrast. CMR uses a large magnet, radiofrequencies, and a computer to produce detailed still and moving images of the heart. CMR is performed to evaluate the structures (morphology) and function of the heart, valves, and major vessels, and to diagnose and manage coronary artery disease and other disorders of the cardiovascular system. CMR is also used to determine the extent of damage caused by a heart attack or other progressive heart disease, and to develop or revise a plan of care for treatment of cardiovascular problems and to monitor progress. Based on patient history and presenting symptoms, the setup is supervised for the necessary anatomic imaging planes. In 75557, the initial

Radiology

study images are reviewed and any additional planes or sequences requested and obtained. An independent workstation is used to create reconstructions of the anatomy, including structures of the heart and major vessels. Adjustments and enhancements are made to the reconstructions to optimize visualization of anatomy and identify areas of disease. The source and reformatted images are reviewed and interpreted including motion (cinematography) review for structural findings in multiple planes, evaluation of biventricular function with ejection fraction and a description of any wall motion abnormalities, as well as comparison with any available prior studies. A dictated report of findings is provided. In 75559, CMR is performed as described above and stress imaging is also performed. Pharmacologic stress imaging sequences are obtained to evaluate wall motion, which typically includes multiple cardiac segments at incremental levels of stress. These sequences are reviewed, adjusted, and enhanced for optimal visualization of any abnormal wall function. The sequences are interpreted and a report of the findings is provided.

75561-75563

75561   Cardiac magnetic resonance imaging for morphology and function without contrast material(s), followed by contrast material(s) and further sequences

75563   Cardiac magnetic resonance imaging for morphology and function without contrast material(s), followed by contrast material(s) and further sequences; with stress imaging

Cardiac magnetic resonance (CMR) imaging for morphology and function is performed without contrast followed by contrast and further sequences. CMR uses a large magnet, radiofrequencies, and a computer to produce detailed still and moving images of the heart. CMR is performed to evaluate the structures (morphology) and function of the heart, valves, and major vessels, and to diagnose and manage coronary artery disease and other disorders of the cardiovascular system. CMR is also used to determine the extent of damage caused by a heart attack or other progressive heart disease, and to develop or revise a plan of care for treatment of cardiovascular problems and to monitor progress. Based on patient history and presenting symptoms, the setup is supervised for the necessary anatomic imaging planes. The initial study images are reviewed and any additional planes or sequences requested and obtained. An independent workstation is used to supervise and create reconstructions of the anatomy, including structures of the heart and major vessels. Adjustments and enhancements are made to the reconstructions to optimize visualization of anatomy and identify areas of disease. The source and reformatted images are reviewed and interpreted including motion (cinematography) review for structural findings in multiple planes, evaluation of biventricular function with ejection fraction and a description of any wall motion abnormalities, as well as comparison with any available prior studies. Intravenous contrast media is administered and additional images obtained, reviewed, adjusted and enhanced. The post-contrast images are reviewed and interpreted. A dictated report of findings is provided. Use 75561 when the procedure is performed without stress images. Use 75563 when stress imaging is performed. Pharmacologic stress imaging sequences are obtained to evaluate wall motion, which typically includes multiple cardiac segments at incremental levels of stress. These sequences are reviewed, adjusted, and enhanced for optimal visualization of any abnormal wall function, ischemia, and myocardial viability. The sequences are interpreted and a report of the findings is provided.

75565

75565   Cardiac magnetic resonance imaging for velocity flow mapping (List separately in addition to code for primary procedure)

Velocity flow mapping is performed at the time of separately reportable cardiac magnetic resonance (CMR) study to evaluate blood flow and velocity through the heart and great vessels. A clinician obtains flow and velocity sequences using appropriate protocols for conditions such as valve disease, congenital heart disease, or other vascular anomalies. These sequences are reconstructed to create 3D images of the blood flow pattern and velocity. A computer software program maps and analyzes the sequences. These sequences are reviewed, adjusted, and enhanced for optimal visualization and quantification of function. The sequences are interpreted and a report of the findings is provided.

75571

75571   Computed tomography, heart, without contrast material, with quantitative evaluation of coronary calcium

Computed tomography of the heart aims multiple, narrow X-ray beams around a single rotational axis, taking a series of 2D images of the target structure from multiple angles. No contrast is used in this heart study. A computer software program then processes the data and reconstructs a 3D image and the heart and great vessels. Thin, cross-sectional 2D and 3D images (slices) are also produced by the software program. Quantitative evaluation of coronary calcium involves measuring and scoring the amount of calcified plaque in the coronary arteries. This is done to detect the extent of heart disease, predict future cardiac events, such as myocardial infarction, and to determine the need for cardiac inventions, such as cardiac bypass surgery or percutaneous coronary artery angioplasty. Minimal plaque burden with possible mild stenosis has a calcium score of 11-100; moderate

plaque burden with moderate stenosis has a score of 101-400; extensive plaque burden with at least one major stenosis has a score over 400. The physician reviews and interprets the CT images, image reconstructions, and coronary calcium data and provides a written report of findings.

75572

75572   Computed tomography, heart, with contrast material, for evaluation of cardiac structure and morphology (including 3D image postprocessing, assessment of cardiac function, and evaluation of venous structures, if performed)

Computed tomography of the heart aims multiple, narrow X-ray beams around a single rotational axis, taking a series of 2D images of the target structure from multiple angles. CT of the heart is performed to evaluate the structures (morphology) and function of the heart, valves, and major vessels, and to diagnose and manage coronary artery disease and other disorders of the cardiovascular system. It is also used to determine the extent of damage caused by a heart attack or other progressive heart disease, and to develop or revise a plan of care for treatment of cardiovascular problems and to monitor progress. Based on patient history and presenting symptoms, the setup is supervised for the necessary anatomic imaging planes. An intravenous line is placed and contrast is injected prior to obtaining CT images. The contrast material enhances images of heart and great vessels. CT images are then obtained. The initial study images are reviewed and additional images obtained as needed. A computer software program then processes the data and reconstructs a 3D image and the heart and great vessels. Thin, cross-sectional 2D and 3D images (slices) are also produced by the software program. The physician reviews and evaluates cardiac structure and function using the source and reconstructed CT images. Venous structures may also be evaluated. A dictated report of findings is provided.

75573

75573   Computed tomography, heart, with contrast material, for evaluation of cardiac structure and morphology in the setting of congenital heart disease (including 3D image postprocessing, assessment of LV cardiac function, RV structure and function and evaluation of venous structures, if performed)

Computed tomography of the heart aims multiple, narrow X-ray beams around a single rotational axis, taking a series of 2D images of the target structure from multiple angles. CT of the heart for congenital heart disease is performed to evaluate the structures (morphology) and function of the heart, valves, and major vessels. Noncontrast images are obtained first, if indicated. Contrast material is then injected via a previously placed intravenous line and images obtained with contrast. The contrast material enhances images of heart and great vessels. The initial study images are reviewed and additional images obtained as needed. A computer software program is then used to process all the data and reconstruct 3D images of the heart and great vessels. Thin, cross-sectional 2D and 3D images (slices) are also produced by the software program. The physician reviews and evaluates cardiac structure and morphology and asses cardiac function. Venous structures may also be evaluated. A dictated report of findings is provided.

75574

75574   Computed tomographic angiography, heart, coronary arteries and bypass grafts (when present), with contrast material, including 3D image postprocessing (including evaluation of cardiac structure and morphology, assessment of cardiac function, and evaluation of venous structures, if performed)

A computed tomography angiography (CTA) is used to evaluate the heart, coronary arteries and bypass grafts. An intravenous line is placed and an injection of contrast is administered. The patient is also given a nitroglycerin tablet to place under the tongue. Nitroglycerin dilates the blood vessels for better visualization during the angiography procedure. A CT scanner is then used to obtain images of the heart, coronary arteries and bypass grafts. CTA is used specifically to evaluate blood flow and to identify any plaque deposits, or narrowing or obstruction of coronary arteries or bypass grafts. The CT scanner aims multiple, narrow X-ray beams around a single rotational axis, taking a series of 2D images of the heart from multiple angles. The initial study images are reviewed and additional images obtained as needed. A computer software program is then used to process all the data and reconstruct 3D images of the heart, coronary arteries, bypass grafts and other venous structures. Thin, cross-sectional 2D and 3D images (slices) are also produced by the software program. The physician reviews and evaluates cardiac structure and morphology and asses cardiac function. A dictated report of findings is provided.

75635

75635   Computed tomographic angiography, abdominal aorta and bilateral iliofemoral lower extremity runoff, with contrast material(s), including noncontrast images, if performed, and image postprocessing

A computed tomographic angiography (CTA) of the abdominal aorta with bilateral iliofemoral lower extremity run-off is performed with contrast material including image postprocessing. Noncontrast images may also be obtained and are included when performed. CTA provides images of the blood vessels using a combination of computed

Radiology

tomography (CT) and angiography with contrast material. When angiography is performed using CT, multiple images are obtained and processed on a computer to create detailed, two-dimensional, cross-sectional views of the blood vessels. These images are then displayed on a computer monitor. The patient is positioned on the CT table. An intravenous line is inserted into a blood vessel, usually in the arm or hand. Non-contrast images may be obtained. A small dose of contrast is injected and test images are obtained to verify correct positioning. The CTA is then performed. Contrast is injected at a controlled rate and the CT table moves through the CT machine as the scanning is performed. After completion of the CTA, the radiologist reviews and interprets the CTA images of the abdominal aorta with bilateral iliofemoral lower extremity runoff.

75801-75803

75801   Lymphangiography, extremity only, unilateral, radiological supervision and interpretation

75803   Lymphangiography, extremity only, bilateral, radiological supervision and interpretation

The physician performs radiological supervision and interpretation of a lymphangiography of the extremities. A separately reportable injection procedure for lymphangiography is performed. The skin of the foot is cleansed and blue indicator dye is injected between several toes. The provider waits and observes the dye as it spreads into the small lymph vessels of the foot, which takes 15-30 minutes. When there is good delineation of the lymph vessels in the foot, a local anesthetic is injected over one of the larger lymph vessels. The skin is incised and the lymph vessel exposed. A needle or catheter is inserted into the exposed lymph vessel and contrast media injected. Radiographs are obtained of the lymph vessels in the extremity over a period of 1-2 hours as the contrast travels through the lymph vessels of the leg. The physician reviews the radiographs and provides a written interpretation of the results. Use 75801 for a unilateral lymphangiogram of the extremities and 75803 if a bilateral imaging procedure is performed.

75805-75807

75805   Lymphangiography, pelvic/abdominal, unilateral, radiological supervision and interpretation

75807   Lymphangiography, pelvic/abdominal, bilateral, radiological supervision and interpretation

The physician performs radiological supervision and interpretation of a lymphangiography of the abdomen and/or pelvis. A separately reportable injection procedure for lymphangiography is performed. The skin of the foot is cleansed and blue indicator dye is injected between several toes. The provider waits and observes the dye as it spreads into the small lymph vessels of the foot which takes 15-30 minutes. When there is good delineation of the lymph vessels in the foot, a local anesthetic is injected over one of the larger lymph vessels. The skin is incised and the lymph vessel exposed. A needle or catheter is inserted into the exposed lymph vessel and contrast media injected. Radiographs are obtained of the lymph vessels on one or both sides of the abdomen and/or pelvis over a period of 1-2 hours. The physician reviews the radiographs and provides a written interpretation of the results. Use 75805 for a unilateral lymphangiogram of the abdomen/pelvis and 75807 if a bilateral imaging procedure is performed.

75810

75810   Splenoportography, radiological supervision and interpretation

The physician performs radiological supervision and interpretation during a separately reportable injection procedure for splenoportography. A sheathed needle is placed into the spleen under fluoroscopic guidance. The needle is removed and correct sheath positioning is verified by the presence of free blood return and a small test amount of contrast. Following the test injection, contrast media is injected into the spleen and recorded by cineangiography. The splenic veins are visualized and the contrast is observed as it drains from the splenic vasculature into the portal vein. Gelfoam plugs are inserted through the sheath to tamponade the entire needle tract. The sheath is removed and a dressing is applied. The physician reviews the radiographs and provides a written interpretation of the results.

75820-75822

75820   Venography, extremity, unilateral, radiological supervision and interpretation

75822   Venography, extremity, bilateral, radiological supervision and interpretation

The physician performs radiological supervision and interpretation during a separately reportable injection procedure for venography of an extremity. Following the injection of contrast media into the hand or foot, a series of radiographs are obtained at timed intervals. The physician observes the flow of blood through the veins in the extremity and supervises the radiological component of the procedure. The physician reviews the radiographs and provides a written interpretation of the results. Use 75820 for radiological supervision and interpretation of a unilateral extremity venography and 75822 for a bilateral procedure.

75825-75827

75825   Venography, caval, inferior, with serialography, radiological supervision and interpretation

75827   Venography, caval, superior, with serialography, radiological supervision and interpretation

The physician performs radiological supervision and interpretation during a separately reportable injection procedure for venography of the inferior or superior vena cava. The procedure may be performed with or without serialography. Following injection of contrast media into the superior or inferior vena cava or another blood vessel, such as the femoral vein, radiographs are obtained. If seriology is performed, a series of radiographs are obtained at timed intervals using a high speed camera. The physician observes the flow of blood through the superior or inferior vena cava and supervises the radiological component of the procedure. The physician reviews the radiographs and provides a written interpretation of the results. Use 75825 for venography of the inferior vena cava and 75827 for venography of the superior vena cava.

75885-75887

75885   Percutaneous transhepatic portography with hemodynamic evaluation, radiological supervision and interpretation

75887   Percutaneous transhepatic portography without hemodynamic evaluation, radiological supervision and interpretation

The physician performs radiological supervision and interpretation of transhepatic portography during a separately reportable portal vein catheterization and injection procedure. Following placement of the portal vein catheter and injection of radiopaque contrast material, radiographs are obtained of the portal vein and collateral veins. The physician observes the flow of blood through the portal vein and collateral veins and supervises the radiological component of the procedure. Any varices in the esophagus or stomach are also visualized and evaluated. The physician reviews the radiographs and provides a written interpretation of the results. In 75885, portography is performed with hemodynamic evaluation which includes measurement of portal vein blood pressure, flow gradients and flow velocity. In 75887, portography is performed without hemodynamic evaluation.

75889-75891

75889   Hepatic venography, wedged or free, with hemodynamic evaluation, radiological supervision and interpretation

75891   Hepatic venography, wedged or free, without hemodynamic evaluation, radiological supervision and interpretation

The physician performs radiological supervision and interpretation of hepatic venography with wedged or free hepatic venous pressures during a separately reportable hepatic vein catheterization and injection procedure. Following placement of the hepatic vein catheter and injection of radiopaque contrast material, radiographs are obtained of the hepatic vein and its branches. The physician observes the flow of blood through the hepatic vein and branches and supervises the radiological component of the procedure. Wedged or free hepatic venous pressures are obtained. A balloon-tipped catheter is introduced into a distal hepatic vein branch. Free hepatic pressure is obtained without distending the balloon. Wedged hepatic venous pressure is obtained by inflating the balloon and wedging it in a distal hepatic vein branch and then obtaining pressures. Alternatively, an end-hole catheter can be used and free hepatic pressure obtained. The physician then wedges the tip of the end-hole catheter in the distal hepatic vein. The physician ensures proper wedging of the end-hole catheter using fluoroscopic imaging and an injection of contrast the produces parenchymal blushing with no reflux of contrast along the catheter. The physician reviews the radiographs and provides a written interpretation of the results. In 75889, hepatic venography is performed with hemodynamic evaluation which includes measurement flow gradients and flow velocity. The physician may calculate the hepatic venous pressure gradient to estimate portal venous pressure. In 75891, hepatic venography is performed without hemodynamic evaluation.

75893

75893   Venous sampling through catheter, with or without angiography (eg, for parathyroid hormone, renin), radiological supervision and interpretation

The physician performs radiological supervision and interpretation during a separately reportable venous catheterization for selective organ blood sampling with or without angiography. The physician supervises the radiographic component of catheter placement in the selected vein. Separately reportable organ blood samples are obtained. Separately reportable injection of radiopaque contrast may also be performed. The physician observes the regional flow of blood through the veins and supervises the radiological component of the angiography procedure. The physician reviews the radiographs and provides a written interpretation of the results.

75898

75898   Angiography through existing catheter for follow-up study for transcatheter therapy, embolization or infusion, other than for thrombolysis

During a separately reportable transcatheter embolization or infusion procedure, follow-up angiograms are obtained to evaluate the outcome of the procedure. Using the existing catheter contrast is injected and images obtained of the treatment site. If an embolization procedure has been performed, the images should show partial or complete occlusion of the desired blood vessel(s). If an infusion procedure has been performed, the images should identify whether the desired results have been obtained. A written interpretation of the follow-up angiography is provided.

75952

75952   Endovascular repair of infrarenal abdominal aortic aneurysm or dissection, radiological supervision and interpretation

Radiological supervision and interpretation is performed during endovascular repair of an infrarenal abdominal aortic aneurysm or dissection. The radiological supervision and interpretation service includes angiography of the aorta and its branches prior to deployment of the endovascular prosthesis, fluoroscopic guidance during the delivery of endovascular components, and intraprocedural angiography to confirm position of the prosthesis, detect endoleaks, and evaluate runoff. A road-mapping angiography of the aortic anatomy is obtained prior to the endovascular aneurysm repair. Fluoroscopic guidance is performed throughout the procedure to assist in the placement of guidewires, catheters, endovascular prosthesis, and docking limbs when used. Fluoroscopic guidance is also performed as needed during balloon dilation to seat the prosthesis. A post-deployment aortogram is performed to evaluate prosthesis position, check for endoleaks, and verify patency of renal, hypogastric, lumbar, and inferior mesenteric arteries. The physician provides a written interpretation of all angiographic and fluoroscopic imaging.

75953

75953   Placement of proximal or distal extension prosthesis for endovascular repair of infrarenal aortic or iliac artery aneurysm, pseudoaneurysm, or dissection, radiological supervision and interpretation

Radiological supervision and interpretation is performed during placement of a proximal or distal extension prosthesis for endovascular repair of an infrarenal aortic or iliac artery aneurysm, pseudoaneurysm, or dissection. The radiological supervision and interpretation service includes angiography of the aorta and its branches prior to deployment of the endovascular extension prosthesis, fluoroscopic guidance during delivery of the extension prosthesis, and intraprocedural angiography to confirm the position of the prosthesis, detect endoleaks, and evaluate runoff. A road-mapping angiography of the aortic or iliac artery anatomy is obtained prior to delivery of the extension prosthesis. Fluoroscopic guidance is performed throughout the procedure to assist in placing guidewires, catheters, and the prosthesis. Fluoroscopic guidance is also performed as needed during balloon dilation to seat the extension prosthesis. A post-deployment aortogram or iliac artery angiogram is performed to evaluate prosthesis position, check for endoleaks, and verify patency of renal, hypogastric, lumbar, and inferior mesenteric arteries. The physician provides a written interpretation of all angiographic and fluoroscopic imaging.

75954

75954   Endovascular repair of iliac artery aneurysm, pseudoaneurysm, arteriovenous malformation, or trauma, using ilio-iliac tube endoprosthesis, radiological supervision and interpretation

Radiological supervision and interpretation is performed during endovascular repair of an iliac artery aneurysm, psuedoaneurysm, arteriovenous malformation, or traumatic injury. The radiological supervision and interpretation service includes angiography of the iliac artery and its branches prior to deployment of the endovascular prosthesis, fluoroscopic guidance during delivery of the prosthesis, and intraprocedural angiography to confirm the position of the prosthesis, detect endoleaks, and evaluate runoff. A road-mapping angiography of the iliac artery anatomy is obtained prior to the endovascular repair. Fluoroscopic guidance is performed throughout the procedure to assist in placing the guidewires, catheters, and prosthesis. Fluoroscopic guidance is also performed as needed during balloon dilation to seat the prosthesis. A post-deployment angiogram is performed to evaluate prosthesis position, check for endoleaks, and verify patency. The physician provides a written interpretation of all angiographic and fluoroscopic imaging.

75956-75957

75956   Endovascular repair of descending thoracic aorta (eg, aneurysm, pseudoaneurysm, dissection, penetrating ulcer, intramural hematoma, or traumatic disruption); involving coverage of left subclavian artery origin, initial endoprosthesis plus descending thoracic aortic extension(s), if required, to level of celiac artery origin, radiological supervision and interpretation

75957   Endovascular repair of descending thoracic aorta (eg, aneurysm, pseudoaneurysm, dissection, penetrating ulcer, intramural hematoma, or traumatic disruption); not involving coverage of left subclavian artery origin, initial endoprosthesis plus descending thoracic aortic extension(s), if required, to level of celiac artery origin, radiological supervision and interpretation

Radiological supervision and interpretation is performed during endovascular repair of descending thoracic aorta involving coverage (75956) or not involving coverage (75957) of left subclavian artery origin. This procedure includes placement of the initial endoprosthesis and any descending thoracic aortic extensions to the level of the celiac artery origin. Endovascular repair of the descending thoracic aorta may be performed for aneurysm, psuedoaneurysm, dissection, penetrating ulcer, intramural hematoma, or traumatic disruption. The radiological supervision and interpretation service includes angiography of the aorta and its branches prior to deployment of the endovascular prosthesis, fluoroscopic guidance during the delivery of endovascular prosthesis, and intraprocedural angiography to confirm position of the prosthesis, detect endoleaks, and evaluate runoff. A road-mapping angiography of the aortic anatomy is obtained prior to the endovascular repair. Fluoroscopic guidance is performed throughout the procedure to assist in the placement of guidewires, catheters, and endovascular prosthesis. Fluoroscopic guidance is also performed as needed during balloon dilation to seat the prosthesis and for placement of distal extension prosthesis. A post-deployment angiogram is performed to evaluate prosthesis position, to check for endoleaks, and to verify patency. The physician provides a written interpretation of all angiographic and fluoroscopic imaging.

75958-75959

75958   Placement of proximal extension prosthesis for endovascular repair of descending thoracic aorta (eg, aneurysm, pseudoaneurysm, dissection, penetrating ulcer, intramural hematoma, or traumatic disruption), radiological supervision and interpretation

75959   Placement of distal extension prosthesis(s) (delayed) after endovascular repair of descending thoracic aorta, as needed, to level of celiac origin, radiological supervision and interpretation

Radiological supervision and interpretation is performed during placement of a proximal or distal extension prosthesis for endovascular repair of the descending thoracic aorta. The radiological supervision and interpretation service includes angiography of the aorta and its branches prior to deployment of the endovascular extension prosthesis, fluoroscopic guidance during delivery of the prosthesis, and intraprocedural angiography to confirm the position of the prosthesis, detect endoleaks, and evaluate runoff. A road-mapping angiography of the aortic anatomy is obtained prior to delivery of the extension prosthesis. Fluoroscopic guidance is performed throughout the procedure to assist in placing guidewires, catheters, and prosthesis. Fluoroscopic guidance is also performed as needed during balloon dilation to seat the extension prosthesis. A post-deployment aortogram is performed to evaluate extension prosthesis position, check for endoleaks, and verify patency. The physician provides a written interpretation of all angiographic and fluoroscopic imaging. Use 75958 for radiological supervision and interpretation for placement of a proximal extension prosthesis and 75959 for a distal extension prosthesis.

75984

75984   Change of percutaneous tube or drainage catheter with contrast monitoring (eg, genitourinary system, abscess), radiological supervision and interpretation

Radiological supervision and interpretation is performed during a separately reportable change of a percutaneous tube or drainage catheter with the use of contrast monitoring. A tube of the genitourinary system, an abscess, or other type drainage catheter is visualized and changed using ultrasound, fluoroscopy, or computed tomography (CT). Contrast media is injected into the existing tube or drainage catheter to identify the current location and any malfunction. The existing tube or drainage catheter is visualized as it is removed. A replacement tube or drainage catheter is then placed under radiographic guidance through the existing tract. Contrast media is injected to verify correct placement of the replacement tube or drainage catheter.

Radiology

Radiology

76000-76001

76000 Fluoroscopy (separate procedure), up to 1 hour physician or other qualified health care professional time, other than 71023 or 71034 (eg, cardiac fluoroscopy)

76001 Fluoroscopy, physician or other qualified health care professional time more than 1 hour, assisting a nonradiologic physician or other qualified health care professional (eg, nephrostolithotomy, ERCP, bronchoscopy, transbronchial biopsy)

Fluoroscopic monitoring of a separately reportable procedure is performed. Fluoroscopy is an imaging technique used to obtained real-time moving images of internal structures using a device that consists of an x-ray source and a fluorescent screen. These devices include image intensifiers and video cameras that allow images to be recorded and displayed on a monitor. In 76000, the physician or other qualified health care professional provides fluoroscopic monitoring for up to one hour for a service or procedure that does not include the fluoroscopy service as part of the procedure. In 76001, fluoroscopy is provided by a physician or other qualified health care professional to assist a nonradiologic physician or other qualified health care professional in the performance of a procedure such as nephrostolithotomy, ERCP, bronchoscopy, or transbronchial biopsy. Report 76001 only if the fluoroscopy time is for more than 1 hour.

76010

76010 Radiologic examination from nose to rectum for foreign body, single view, child

A radiologic examination from nose to rectum is performed on a child for suspected ingestion or inhalation of a radiopaque foreign body. Ingestion or inhalation of foreign bodies is most common in children aged 6 mo -5 yrs, but can occur in younger or older children. Radiopaque items commonly ingested or inhaled include coins, small toys, batteries, safety pins, needles, and hairpins. Children who have swallowed or even inhaled foreign bodies are often asymptomatic initially. A single frontal plain film is taken to include the entire respiratory and digestive tract from the nose to the anus. The X-ray is reviewed for evidence of the foreign body. Close attention is paid to the esophagus and trachea where the foreign body can become lodged, causing obstruction. The stomach and intestines are also inspected; however, once a foreign body has passed into the stomach it is less likely to cause obstruction and will usually be passed from the bowel with feces. If the object is sharp, careful inspection is made to determine if the foreign body has perforated the respiratory or digestive tract. Also of concern are button batteries, which if located, are typically removed in a separately reportable procedure rather than being allowed to pass with feces.

76080

76080 Radiologic examination, abscess, fistula or sinus tract study, radiological supervision and interpretation

A radiologic examination of an abscess, fistula, or sinus tract is performed. Radiologic examination is performed on a draining abscess or a fistula or sinus tract to determine the size and location of abscess pocket or the site of origin of the fistula or sinus tract. A sterile catheter is inserted into the abscess pocket or advanced into the fistula or sinus tract under radiologic supervision. A separately reportable injection procedure is then performed and the distribution of the contrast material observed radiographically. The radiologist provides a written interpretation of the imaging component of the procedure.

76376-76377

76376 3D rendering with interpretation and reporting of computed tomography, magnetic resonance imaging, ultrasound, or other tomographic modality with image postprocessing under concurrent supervision; not requiring image postprocessing on an independent workstation

76377 3D rendering with interpretation and reporting of computed tomography, magnetic resonance imaging, ultrasound, or other tomographic modality with image postprocessing under concurrent supervision; requiring image postprocessing on an independent workstation

Separately reportable ultrasound, MRI, CT scan or other tomographic images are obtained. Using these images, complex 3D rendering is performed by a physician or a specially trained technologist. This may include shaded surface rendering, volumetric rendering, maximum intensity projections (MIPs), fusion imaging, and quantitative analysis of the images for treatment planning. If the 3D rendering and image postprocessing is performed by a technologist, concurrent physician supervision is required. An interpretation of the image postprocessing is provided in a written report. In 76376, complex 3D rendering is performed by the physician or a specially trained technologist under physician supervision without the use of an independent workstation. In 76377, complex 3D image rendering is performed by the physician or a specially trained technologist under physician supervision on an independent workstation.

76536

76536 Ultrasound, soft tissues of head and neck (eg, thyroid, parathyroid, parotid), real time with image documentation

An ultrasound examination of soft tissues of the head and neck is performed with image documentation. The thyroid, parathyroid, or parotid glands and surrounding soft tissue may be examined. Ultrasound visualizes the body internally using sound waves far above human perception bounce off interior anatomical structures. As the sound waves pass through different densities of tissue, they are reflected back to the receiving unit at varying speeds and converted into pictures displayed on screen. A linear scanner or mechanical sector scanner is used to evaluate the shape, size, border, internal architecture, distal enhancement, colorflow, and echogenicity of the soft tissue structures of the head and neck as well as any lesions or masses. The echogenicity is compared to that of the surrounding muscle tissue. The physician reviews the images and provides a written interpretation.

76604

76604 Ultrasound, chest (includes mediastinum), real time with image documentation

A real time ultrasound examination of chest including the mediastinum is performed with image documentation. Ultrasound may be used to evaluate mediastinum and surrounding soft tissue for lesions or masses. In children, ultrasound of the chest and mediastinum may also be used to definitively diagnose pneumonia, pleural effusion, diaphragmatic palsy, and bronchopulmonary sequestration following inconclusive findings on plain films. The patient is placed in a supine position with a pillow under the shoulders. The neck is extended slightly and the chin flexed. Acoustic coupling gel is applied to suprasternal and supraclavicular sites just lateral to the sternocleidomastoid bilaterally. The ultrasound probe is then used to obtain semicoronal, sagittal, parasagittal and oblique views of the soft tissues of the chest and mediastinum through suprasternal, paratracheal, and supraclavicular windows. Any abnormalities are evaluated to identify structure of origin, nature, internal architecture, and other characteristics that might provide a definitive diagnosis. The ultrasonic wave pulses directed at the soft tissues of the chest and mediastinum are imaged by recording the ultrasound echoes. The physician reviews the ultrasound images of the soft tissues of the chest and mediastinum and provides a written interpretation.

76641-76642

76641 Ultrasound, breast, unilateral, real time with image documentation, including axilla when performed; complete

76642 Ultrasound, breast, unilateral, real time with image documentation, including axilla when performed; limited

A real time ultrasound of the right or left breast is performed with image documentation, including the axillary area, when performed. Breast ultrasound is used to help diagnose breast abnormalities detected during a physical exam or on mammography. Ultrasound imaging can identify masses as solid or fluid-filled and can show additional structural features of the abnormal area and surrounding tissues. The patient is placed supine with the arm raised above the head on the side being examined. Acoustic coupling gel is applied to the breast and the transducer is pressed firmly against the skin of the breast. The transducer is then swept back and forth over the area of the abnormality and images are obtained. The ultrasonic wave pulses directed at the breast are imaged by recording the ultrasound echoes. Any abnormalities are evaluated to identify characteristics that might provide a definitive diagnosis. In 76641, a complete unilateral ultrasound examination of the breast is performed. All four quadrants as well as the area directly behind the areola are viewed and evaluated. In 76642, a focused ultrasound examination is done to assess only a specific area(s) or quadrant(s) of interest in the breast. The physician reviews the ultrasound images of the breast and provides a written interpretation.

76700-76705

76700 Ultrasound, abdominal, real time with image documentation; complete

76705 Ultrasound, abdominal, real time with image documentation; limited (eg, single organ, quadrant, follow-up)

A real time abdominal ultrasound is performed with image documentation. The patient is placed supine. Acoustic coupling gel is applied to the skin of the abdomen. The transducer is pressed firmly against the skin and swept back and forth over the abdomen and images obtained. The ultrasonic wave pulses directed at the abdomen are imaged by recording the ultrasound echoes. Any abnormalities are evaluated to identify characteristics that might provide a definitive diagnosis. The physician reviews the ultrasound images of the abdomen and provides a written interpretation. Code 76700 is used for a complete abdominal ultrasound, which includes real time scanning of the liver, gall bladder, common bile duct, pancreas, spleen, kidneys, upper abdominal aorta, and inferior vena cava. Code 76705 is used when a limited ultrasound examination is performed such as a single organ, single quadrant, or a follow-up scan.

Radiology

76770-76775

76770 Ultrasound, retroperitoneal (eg, renal, aorta, nodes), real time with image documentation; complete

76775 Ultrasound, retroperitoneal (eg, renal, aorta, nodes), real time with image documentation; limited

A real time retroperitoneal ultrasound is performed with image documentation. The patient is placed supine. Acoustic coupling gel is applied to the skin of the abdomen. The transducer is pressed firmly against the skin and swept back and forth over the abdomen and images obtained of the retroperitoneal area. The ultrasonic wave pulses directed at the retroperitoneum are imaged by recording the ultrasound echoes. Any abnormalities are evaluated to identify characteristics that might provide a definitive diagnosis. The physician reviews the ultrasound images of the retroperitoneum and provides a written interpretation. Code 76770 is used for a complete retroperitoneal ultrasound, which includes real time scanning of the kidneys, abdominal aorta, common iliac artery origins, and inferior vena cava. Alternatively, if ultrasonography is being performed to evaluate the urinary tract, examination of the kidneys and urinary bladder constitutes a complete exam. Code 76775 is used when a limited retroperitoneal ultrasound examination is performed.

76800

76800 Ultrasound, spinal canal and contents

An ultrasound examination of the spinal canal and contents is performed. Ultrasound visualizes the body internally using sound waves far above human perception bounced off interior anatomical structures. As the sound waves pass through different densities of tissue, they are reflected back to the receiving unit at varying speeds and converted into pictures displayed on screen. Transdermal spinal ultrasound is used primarily in evaluation of newborns and infants because of the minimal ossification of the spine and the short distance between the skin and the spinal subarachnoid space. Spinal ultrasound may be used intraoperatively in adults and older children but is generally not considered an effective diagnostic tool in these patients. With the newborn or infant placed in a prone position, the neck is flexed. Acoustic coupling gel is applied to the skin along the spine. The spinal canal and contents are examined using a linear probe in both the sagittal and axial plane along the entire length of the spine. The physician reviews the images and provides a written interpretation.

76801-76802

76801 Ultrasound, pregnant uterus, real time with image documentation, fetal and maternal evaluation, first trimester (< 14 weeks 0 days), transabdominal approach; single or first gestation

76802 Ultrasound, pregnant uterus, real time with image documentation, fetal and maternal evaluation, first trimester (< 14 weeks 0 days), transabdominal approach; each additional gestation (List separately in addition to code for primary procedure)

A real time transabdominal obstetrical ultrasound is performed with image documentation to evaluate the fetus and the pregnant uterus and surrounding pelvic structures of the mother during the first trimester. The first trimester is defined as a gestation period of less than 14 weeks 0 days. Obstetric ultrasound is performed to establish viability of the embryo or fetus, to determine whether a multiple gestation exists, to determine fetal age using measurements of the gestational sac and fetus, to evaluate the position of the fetus and placenta, to evaluate visible fetal and placental anatomic structure, to evaluate amniotic fluid volume, to evaluate the maternal uterus and adnexa. The mother presents with a full bladder. Acoustic coupling gel is applied to the skin of the lower abdomen. The transducer is pressed firmly against the skin and swept back and forth over the lower abdomen and images obtained of the pregnant uterus, surrounding pelvic structures, and fetus. The ultrasonic wave pulses directed at the fetus, pregnant uterus, and surrounding pelvic structures of the mother are imaged by recording the ultrasound echoes. Any abnormalities are evaluated. The physician reviews the ultrasound images of the fetus, pregnant uterus, and maternal pelvic structures, and provides a written interpretation. Code 76801 is used for a single gestation or the first gestation in a multiple pregnancy during the first trimester and code 76802 is used for each additional gestation.

76805-76810

76805 Ultrasound, pregnant uterus, real time with image documentation, fetal and maternal evaluation, after first trimester (> or = 14 weeks 0 days), transabdominal approach; single or first gestation

76810 Ultrasound, pregnant uterus, real time with image documentation, fetal and maternal evaluation, after first trimester (> or = 14 weeks 0 days), transabdominal approach; each additional gestation (List separately in addition to code for primary procedure)

A real time transabdominal obstetrical ultrasound is performed with image documentation to evaluate the fetus and the pregnant uterus and surrounding pelvic structures of the mother after the first trimester, which is defined as a gestation period equal to or greater than 14 weeks 0 days. Obstetric ultrasound is performed to establish viability of the fetus; to determine whether a multiple gestation exists; to determine fetal age using fetal measurements; to evaluate the position of the fetus and placenta; to survey fetal anatomy

including intracranial, spinal, abdominal, and heart with four chamber evaluation; to identify umbilical cord insertion site; to evaluate amniotic fluid volume; and to evaluate the maternal uterus and adnexa if visible. The mother presents with a full bladder. Acoustic coupling gel is applied to the skin of the lower abdomen. The transducer is pressed firmly against the skin and swept back and forth over the lower abdomen and images obtained of the pregnant uterus, surrounding pelvic structures, and fetus. The ultrasonic wave pulses directed at the fetus, pregnant uterus, and surrounding pelvic structures of the mother are imaged by recording the ultrasound echoes. Any abnormalities are evaluated. The physician reviews the ultrasound images of the fetus, pregnant uterus, and maternal pelvic structures, and provides a written interpretation. Code 76805 is used for a single gestation or the first gestation in a multiple pregnancy after the first trimester and code 76810 is used for each additional gestation.

76811-76812

76811 Ultrasound, pregnant uterus, real time with image documentation, fetal and maternal evaluation plus detailed fetal anatomic examination, transabdominal approach; single or first gestation

76812 Ultrasound, pregnant uterus, real time with image documentation, fetal and maternal evaluation plus detailed fetal anatomic examination, transabdominal approach; each additional gestation (List separately in addition to code for primary procedure)

A real time transabdominal obstetrical ultrasound is performed with image documentation to evaluate the fetus and the pregnant uterus and surrounding pelvic structures of the mother with a detailed fetal anatomic evaluation. Obstetric ultrasound is performed to establish viability of the fetus; to determine whether a multiple gestation exists; to determine fetal age using fetal measurements; to evaluate the position of the fetus and placenta; to survey fetal anatomy including intracranial, spinal, abdominal, and heart with four chamber evaluation; to identify umbilical cord insertion site; to evaluate amniotic fluid volume; and to evaluate the maternal uterus and adnexa if visible. In addition, a detailed fetal anatomic evaluation is performed which includes evaluation of the fetal brain and ventricles, face, heart and outflow tracts, chest anatomy, and abdominal organs; evaluation of limbs with an assessment of number, length, and architecture; evaluation of umbilical cord and placental details; and evaluation of other fetal anatomy as indicated. The mother presents with a full bladder. Acoustic coupling gel is applied to the skin of the lower abdomen. The transducer is pressed firmly against the skin and swept back and forth over the lower abdomen and images obtained of the pregnant uterus, surrounding pelvic structures, and fetus. The ultrasonic wave pulses directed at the fetus, pregnant uterus, and surrounding pelvic structures of the mother are imaged by recording the ultrasound echoes. Any abnormalities are evaluated. The physician reviews the ultrasound images of the fetus, pregnant uterus, and maternal pelvic structures, and provides a written interpretation. Code 76811 is used for an obstetric ultrasound with detailed fetal anatomic evaluation of a single gestation or the first gestation in a multiple pregnancy and code 76812 is used for each additional gestation.

76813-76814

76813 Ultrasound, pregnant uterus, real time with image documentation, first trimester fetal nuchal translucency measurement, transabdominal or transvaginal approach; single or first gestation

76814 Ultrasound, pregnant uterus, real time with image documentation, first trimester fetal nuchal translucency measurement, transabdominal or transvaginal approach; each additional gestation (List separately in addition to code for primary procedure)

Real time ultrasound imaging with documentation is performed in the first trimester to measure fetal nuchal translucency. The ultrasound is done either transabdominally or transvaginally. Real time ultrasound scanning displays both the two dimensional picture of the structure being viewed and movement as it occurs with time. Nuchal translucency refers to the ultrasonic detection of subcutaneous edema in the fetal neck. Measurement is taken of the maximum thickness of the sonographically lucent zone between the inside of the fetal skin and the outer side of the soft tissue that overlies the cervical spine or occipital bone. Increased nuchal translucency in the first trimester is associated with chromosomal defects and genetic abnormalities, such as Down Syndrome; trisomy 13 or 18; heart and great vessel anomalies; and skeletal dysplasias. Use 76813 for the single or first gestation and code 76814 for each additional gestation.

76815-76816

76815   **Ultrasound, pregnant uterus, real time with image documentation, limited (eg, fetal heart beat, placental location, fetal position and/or qualitative amniotic fluid volume), 1 or more fetuses**

76816   **Ultrasound, pregnant uterus, real time with image documentation, follow-up (eg, re-evaluation of fetal size by measuring standard growth parameters and amniotic fluid volume, re-evaluation of organ system(s) suspected or confirmed to be abnormal on a previous scan), transabdominal approach, per fetus**

A real time limited (76815) or follow-up (76816) transabdominal obstetrical ultrasound is performed with image documentation to evaluate the fetus and the pregnant uterus and surrounding pelvic structures of the mother. The mother presents with a full bladder. Acoustic coupling gel is applied to the skin of the lower abdomen. The transducer is pressed firmly against the skin and swept back and forth over the lower abdomen and images obtained of the pregnant uterus, surrounding pelvic structures, and fetus. The ultrasonic wave pulses directed at the fetus, pregnant uterus, and surrounding pelvic structures of the mother are imaged by recording the ultrasound echoes. Any abnormalities are evaluated. The physician reviews the ultrasound images of the fetus, pregnant uterus, and maternal pelvic structures, and provides a written interpretation. Code 76815 is used for a limited or "quick-look" examination to assess one or more of the following elements: fetal heart beat, placental location, fetal position, amniotic fluid. Code 76816 is used for a follow-up examination to reassess fetal size and interval growth or to re-evaluate one or more anatomic fetal abnormalities identified on a previous ultrasound.

76817

76817   **Ultrasound, pregnant uterus, real time with image documentation, transvaginal**

A real time transvaginal obstetrical ultrasound is performed with image documentation to evaluate the fetus, pregnant uterus, and surrounding maternal pelvic structures. Ultrasound visualizes the body internally using sound waves far above human perception bounced off interior anatomical structures. As the sound waves pass through different densities of tissue, they are reflected back to the receiving unit at varying speeds and converted into pictures displayed on screen. The patient is first asked to empty the bladder. A protective cover is placed over the transducer and acoustic coupling gel is applied to the cover. The transducer is inserted into the vagina and images of the fetus, pregnant uterus, and maternal structures are obtained from different orientations. Any abnormalities are evaluated. The physician reviews the images and provides a written interpretation.

76818-76819

76818   **Fetal biophysical profile; with non-stress testing**
76819   **Fetal biophysical profile; without non-stress testing**

A fetal biophysical profile (BPP) is performed. BPP uses ultrasound imaging to evaluate amniotic fluid volume, to observe chest movement (fetal breathing) and gross body movement, and to assess fetal body tone. Fetal heart rate monitoring may also be evaluated using a non-stress test (NST). BPP is used to predict the presence or absence of fetal asphyxia and to assess the risk of fetal death during the antenatal period. Real time ultrasound is used to measure amniotic fluid volume and to observe fetal movement, breathing and tone. The mother presents with a full bladder. Acoustic coupling gel is applied to the skin of the lower abdomen. The transducer is pressed against the skin and swept back and forth over the lower abdomen and general exam performed to identify the location of the fetus and the presence of cardiac activity. Placental position may also be noted. Following the general exam, amniotic fluid volume is assessed, gross fetal motion and tone are evaluated, and breathing movements are evaluated. A non-stress test (NST) may also be performed using a fetal monitor. NST typically requires a minimum of 30 minutes of fetal monitoring. A biophysical score (BPS) is calculated and the risk of fetal asphyxia and fetal death determined. The physician reviews the ultrasound images, reads the NST, determines the BPS, and provides a written interpretation. Code 76818 is used when BPP is performed with NST and code 76819 is used when BPP is performed without NST.

76820-76821

76820   **Doppler velocimetry, fetal; umbilical artery**
76821   **Doppler velocimetry, fetal; middle cerebral artery**

The physician performs fetal Doppler velocimetry to evaluate blood flow velocity within the umbilical artery. This procedure is used to determine the best timing for inducing labor or to diagnose and evaluate fetal anemia. The mother is positioned in a semi-recumbant position with a slight lateral tilt to minimize the risk of supine hypotension syndrome. Acoustic coupling gel is applied to the skin of the lower abdomen and the transducer pressed against the lower abdomen. The transducer is manipulated to obtain Doppler frequency shift waveforms from the umbilical artery. Continuous wave or pulsed wave Doppler interrogation is then used to assess umbilical artery blood flow by evaluating downstream impedance. The Doppler waveforms are displayed on a video monitor. The screen is frozen when appropriate signals are displayed, and measurements are performed.

These measurements are then used to calculate indices that characterize downstream impedance. The indices used include umbilical artery systolic-diastolic (S/D) ratio, resistance index (RI), or pulsatility index (PI). The physician reviews the ultrasound imaging, calculates indices, evaluates umbilical artery blood flow velocity, and provides a written report. Code 76821 is used for fetal Doppler velocimetry of the middle cerebral artery. The procedure is performed as described above except that middle cerebral artery Doppler waveforms are obtained and displayed on the video monitor. The screen is frozen and measurements performed to evaluate middle cerebral blood flow velocity. Measurements are used to calculate indices with the pulsatility index (PI) being the one most commonly used for the middle cerebral artery. The physician reviews the ultrasound imaging, calculates indices, evaluates middle cerebral artery blood flow velocity, and provides a written report.

76825-76826

76825   **Echocardiography, fetal, cardiovascular system, real time with image documentation (2D), with or without M-mode recording**

76826   **Echocardiography, fetal, cardiovascular system, real time with image documentation (2D), with or without M-mode recording; follow-up or repeat study**

The physician performs fetal echocardiography with real time image documentation (2D) with or without M-mode recording to assess the structure and function of the fetal heart. This test is performed during pregnancy to evaluate the unborn baby for suspected cardiovascular anomalies, particularly when there is a family history of congenital heart disease, the obstetrician has detected an abnormal fetal heart rhythm, anomalies of the heart or other major organ systems have been seen on a routine ultrasound, the mother has Type I diabetes or has taken drugs during pregnancy that are known to affect fetal heart development, or an amniocentesis is abnormal. Fetal echocardiography may be performed using abdominal or transvaginal ultrasound. If an abdominal ultrasound is performed, gel is applied to the abdomen and the transducer probe is moved over the abdomen to obtain images from different locations. If a transvaginal ultrasound is used, a transducer is inserted into the vagina to obtain images of the heart. Two-dimensional (2-D) echocardiography provides images of heart structure and motion. The 2-D echo appears as a cone-shaped image on a videomonitor and the heart structures and motion are observed in real-time, meaning that heart motion is observed as it is happening. This allows the physician to evaluate the heart structures as the heart is beating. Selective time-motion (M-mode) recordings are made as needed to allow dimensional measurement. M-mode displays more specific time-motion information from a stationary beam that is superimposed over the 2-D image. Depth is oriented along the vertical axis and time on the horizontal axis. M-mode is used to evaluate heart wall and septa thickness and timing of the opening and closing of aortic, mitral, and tricuspid valves. M-mode may also be used to evaluate the pericardium and aorta. Use 76825 for the initial study or 76826 for a follow-up or repeat study.

76827-76828

76827   **Doppler echocardiography, fetal, pulsed wave and/or continuous wave with spectral display; complete**

76828   **Doppler echocardiography, fetal, pulsed wave and/or continuous wave with spectral display; follow-up or repeat study**

The physician performs a fetal Doppler echocardiography including pulsed wave and/or continuous wave with spectral display. This test is performed during pregnancy to evaluate the unborn baby for suspected cardiovascular anomalies, particularly when there is a family history of congenital heart disease, the obstetrician has detected an abnormal fetal heart rhythm, anomalies of the heart or other major organ systems have been seen on a routine ultrasound, the mother has Type I diabetes or has taken drugs during pregnancy that are known to affect fetal heart development, or an amniocentesis is abnormal. Fetal Doppler echocardiography may be performed using abdominal or transvaginal ultrasound. If an abdominal ultrasound is performed, gel is applied to the abdomen and the transducer probe is moved over the abdomen to obtain images from different locations. If a transvaginal ultrasound is used, a transducer is inserted into the vagina to obtain images of the heart. Doppler technique is used to evaluate and measure the flow of blood through the heart chambers and valves. Doppler studies can determine how much blood is pumped out of each chamber as the heart beats and can also detect abnormal blood flow within the heart chambers. It can be used to identify anomalies of the atrial or ventricular septum as well as anomalies of the heart valves. Use 76827 for an initial complete study or 76828 for a follow-up or repeat study.

76830

76830   **Ultrasound, transvaginal**

A transvaginal ultrasound is performed to evaluate the non-pregnant uterus and other pelvic structures. Conditions that may be evaluated by transvaginal ultrasound include infertility, abnormal bleeding, unexplained pain, congenital anomalies of the ovaries and uterus, ovarian cysts and tumors, pelvic inflammatory disease, bladder abnormalities, and intrauterine device (IUD) location. The patient is asked to empty the bladder and then lies back with the feet in stirrups. A protective cover is placed over the transducer and acoustic coupling gel is applied. The transducer is inserted into the vagina. Images of the uterus, ovaries, and surrounding pelvic structures are obtained from different orientations of the transducer. The ultrasonic wave pulses directed at the pelvic structures are imaged by recording the ultrasound echoes. The uterus is examined and endometrial thickness is determined. The ovaries are examined and any ovarian masses are carefully evaluated. The bladder and other pelvic structures are examined and any abnormalities are noted. The physician reviews the transvaginal ultrasound images and provides a written interpretation.

76831

76831 **Saline infusion sonohysterography (SIS), including color flow Doppler, when performed**

The physician performs saline infused sonohysterography (SIS), including any required color flow Doppler. A vaginal probe is inserted into the vagina and a baseline transvaginal ultrasound is performed. The probe is removed and the physician inserts a catheter through the cervix and into the uterus in a separately reportable procedure. The vaginal probe is reinserted as the physician instills sterile saline into the uterus. The ultrasound probe is maneuvered and the entire uterine cavity surface is studied as the saline is infused. Any abnormalities are noted. Following completion of the procedure, the catheter is removed and the physician provides a written report of findings.

76856-76857

76856 **Ultrasound, pelvic (nonobstetric), real time with image documentation; complete**
76857 **Ultrasound, pelvic (nonobstetric), real time with image documentation; limited or follow-up (eg, for follicles)**

A real time pelvic (non-obstetric) ultrasound is performed with image documentation to evaluate the uterus and cervix, ovaries, fallopian tubes, and bladder. Conditions evaluated include pelvic pain, abnormal bleeding, and palpable masses, such as ovarian cysts, uterine fibroids, or other pelvic masses. The patient presents with a full bladder. Acoustic coupling gel is applied to the skin of the lower abdomen. The transducer is pressed firmly against the skin and swept back and forth over the lower abdomen and images obtained of the uterus, ovaries, and surrounding pelvic structures. The ultrasonic wave pulses directed at the pelvic structures are imaged by recording the ultrasound echoes. Any abnormalities are evaluated. The physician reviews the ultrasound images and provides a written interpretation. Use 76856 for an initial or complete pelvic ultrasound and 76857 for a limited or follow-up study.

76872-76873

76872 **Ultrasound, transrectal**
76873 **Ultrasound, transrectal; prostate volume study for brachytherapy treatment planning (separate procedure)**

The physician inserts an ultrasound probe through the rectum to view an ultrasound image of tissue inside the digestive tract. This imaging technique bounces waves through tissue in the body and a response is given to a receiving unit. The unit converts what is received into electrical pulses that are displayed on a screen. Code 76873 if the physician measures the size of the prostate, allowing the physician to determine the best course of brachytherapy, the implantation of radioactive beads for prostate cancer.

76881-76882

76881 **Ultrasound, extremity, nonvascular, real-time with image documentation; complete**
76882 **Ultrasound, extremity, nonvascular, real-time with image documentation; limited, anatomic specific**

Ultrasound, also referred to as sonography and echography, is a non-invasive imaging technique that uses high-frequency sound waves to evaluate tissues and structures. Nonvascular structures of the extremities that may be evaluated by ultrasound include subcutaneous tissue, fascia, muscle, tendons, ligaments, and joints. Common conditions that can be detected or evaluated by ultrasound include cystic lesions, solid tumors, abscesses, joint effusion, tendon tears, tendonitis, tenosynovitis, nerve compression, and stress fractures. Acoustic coupling gel is applied to the extremity to be examined. An ultrasound probe is placed against the skin and moved over the area to be examined as sound waves pass through and bounce off extremity tissues and structures. The sound waves are reflected back to the receiving unit at varying speeds and converted into images. Longitudinal, transverse, and oblique images are obtained. The physician reviews the images and provides a written interpretation. Use 76881 for a complete upper or lower extremity examination. A complete examination of the upper extremity includes ultrasound examination from the shoulder joint through the fingers. A complete examination of the lower extremity includes ultrasound examination from the hip joint through the toes. Use 76882 for a limited examination of one specific anatomic area of the extremity.

76885-76886

76885 **Ultrasound, infant hips, real time with imaging documentation; dynamic (requiring physician or other qualified health care professional manipulation)**
76886 **Ultrasound, infant hips, real time with imaging documentation; limited, static (not requiring physician or other qualified health care professional manipulation)**

Real time ultrasound images of the hips are obtained in an infant with suspected developmental dysplasia of the hip joints. The infant is placed on the exam table and coupling gel applied to the hip area. An ultrasound technician (sonographer) then uses a hand-held transducer to obtain real time images that are displayed on a computer screen. The transducer is moved over the hip region and images obtained of all hip joint structures. This is repeated on the opposite side. The ultrasound images are reviewed and a written interpretation of findings provided. In 76885, dynamic images are obtained. Dynamic images require manipulation of the hip joint by the physician or other qualified health care professional during the ultrasound. In 76886, static images are obtained. Static images do not require movement of the hip joint.

76930

76930 **Ultrasonic guidance for pericardiocentesis, imaging supervision and interpretation**

Ultrasound guidance (echocardiography guidance) with imaging supervision and interpretation is performed for a separately reportable pericardiocentesis procedure. Both 2D and Doppler studies are performed prior to the pericardiocentesis to evaluate the size, distribution, and hemodynamic effect of the pericardial effusion. The ideal entry site for the needle is identified. Generally this is the site of greatest fluid accumulation where the effusion is closest to the transducer. The intended point of entry is marked on the skin and the direction of the ultrasound beam is noted. Following skin preparation, a sheathed needle is introduced into the pericardial sac. The needle is withdrawn, leaving the sheath in place. Correct positioning of the needle in the pericardial sac may be confirmed using saline echo contrast monitored by ultrasound. A catheter is then placed into the pericardial sac, the position of the catheter is confirmed by ultrasound, and the effusion is drained. Following drainage of the pericardial fluid, ultrasound assessment of residual fluid is performed.

76932

76932 **Ultrasonic guidance for endomyocardial biopsy, imaging supervision and interpretation**

Ultrasound guidance (echocardiography guidance) with imaging supervision and interpretation is performed during a separately reportable endomyocardial biopsy procedure. The bioptome is introduced through a previously placed heart catheter and advanced into the right or left side of the heart under ultrasound guidance. Using continuous ultrasound guidance, the bioptome forceps are directed into the desired biopsy site and a tissue sample is obtained.

76941

76941 **Ultrasonic guidance for intrauterine fetal transfusion or cordocentesis, imaging supervision and interpretation**

Ultrasound guidance including imaging supervision and interpretation is provided for intrauterine fetal transfusion or cordocentesis. Fetal transfusion is performed when fetal red blood cells of an Rh-positive fetus are destroyed by the Rh-sensitized immune system of the mother. Another indication for transfusion is neonatal alloimmune thrombocytopenia caused by maternal antibodies directed against platelet-specific antigens. Cordocentesis, also referred to as percutaneous umbilical cord sampling, is performed to obtain a fetal blood sample to detect fetal anomalies, infection, thrombocytopenia, anemia, or isoimmunization. Prior to the transfusion or cordocentesis procedure, an abdominal ultrasound of the pregnant uterus is performed to determine the position of the fetus and locate the placenta and umbilical vein. Amniotic fluid level is also evaluated. Ultrasound imaging is then used continuously to monitor proper placement of the needle in the umbilical vein at the placental insertion for cordocentesis. Alternatively, transfusion may be performed with the needle inserted into the fetal abdomen. The subsequent transfusion or cordocentesis procedure is also monitored. The physician provides a written report of the imaging component of the procedure.

76942

76942 **Ultrasonic guidance for needle placement (eg, biopsy, aspiration, injection, localization device), imaging supervision and interpretation**

Ultrasound guidance including imaging supervision and interpretation is performed for needle placement during a separately reportable biopsy, aspiration, injection, or placement of a localization device. A local anesthetic is injected at the site of the planned needle or localization device placement. A transducer is then used to locate the lesion, site of the planned injection, or site of the planned placement of the localization device. The radiologist constantly monitors needle placement with the ultrasound probe to ensure the needle is properly placed. The radiologist also uses ultrasound imaging to monitor separately reportable biopsy, aspiration, injection, or device localization procedures. Upon completion of the procedure, the needle is withdrawn and pressure applied to control bleeding. A dressing is applied as needed. The radiologist then provides a written report of the ultrasound imaging component of the procedure.

76945

76945   Ultrasonic guidance for chorionic villus sampling, imaging supervision and interpretation

Ultrasound guidance including imaging supervision and interpretation is provided for chorionic villus sampling (CVS). Chorionic villi are tiny finger-shaped growths located in the placenta that contain the same genetic material as the fetus. CVS is performed to identify the presence of fetal genetic disorders such as Tay-Sachs disease, hemophilia, or Down syndrome. Prior to the CVS procedure, an ultrasound of the pregnant uterus is performed to determine the position of the fetus and locate the placenta. CVS may be performed transvaginally using a catheter that is passed through the cervix and into the placenta. Alternatively, the procedure can be performed by placing a needle through the mother's abdomen. Ultrasound imaging is then used continuously to monitor proper placement of the catheter or needle into the placenta and subsequent aspiration of a chorionic villus sample. The physician provides a written report of the imaging component of the procedure.

76946

76946   Ultrasonic guidance for amniocentesis, imaging supervision and interpretation

Ultrasound guidance including imaging supervision and interpretation is provided for amniocentesis. Amniocentesis is performed early in pregnancy to identify the presence of fetal chromosome disorders such as Down syndrome, structural defects such as spina bifida or anencephaly, and many other inherited disorders. Later in pregnancy it may be used to identify Rh incompatibility or infection, or to evaluate lung maturity. Prior to the amniocentesis procedure, an abdominal ultrasound of the pregnant uterus is performed to determine the position of the fetus and locate the placenta. Amniotic fluid level is evaluated and a pocket of amniotic fluid is identified. Ultrasound imaging is then used continuously to monitor the placement of the needle in the amniotic fluid pocket and subsequent aspiration of the amniotic fluid sample. The physician provides a written report of the imaging component of the procedure.

76948

76948   Ultrasonic guidance for aspiration of ova, imaging supervision and interpretation

Ultrasound guidance including imaging supervision and interpretation is provided for aspiration of ova. Mature ova are retrieved for use in an in vitro fertilization procedure. Approximately 35 hours after human chorionic gonadotropin (HCG) injection, mature ova are retrieved using ultrasound guidance via a transvaginal, transvesical, or percutaneous transabdominal approach. Using a transvaginal approach, the ultrasound probe and aspiration needle guide are advanced through the cervix, uterus, and fallopian tube into the ovary. Ultrasound guidance is used to direct the needle toward the follicle. The follicle is then punctured and fluid is aspirated along with the ovum. The ovum is then placed in sterile solution. This is repeated until all mature ova have been harvested. If ova cannot be retrieved via a transvaginal approach, a transvesical approach may be employed. The ultrasound probe and aspiration needle are passed through the urethra to the posterior bladder wall. The bladder wall is punctured and the needle is advanced into the ovary. The ova are retrieved under ultrasound guidance as described above. Alternatively, a percutaneous abdominal approach may be used. The aspiration needle is advanced through the abdomen to the ovary under ultrasound guidance and mature ova are aspirated. The physician provides a written report of the imaging component of the procedure.

76977

76977   Ultrasound bone density measurement and interpretation, peripheral site(s), any method

Ultrasound bone density measurement can only be performed on peripheral sites with bone density of the heel typically used. The heel is placed in the ultrasound device. The device uses a transmitting transducer that directs the ultrasonic wave through the heel and a receiving transducer that receives the ultrasonic wave. Several parameters that reflect bone density are then calculated by the device. The physician reviews the data and provides a written report.

76998

76998   Ultrasonic guidance, intraoperative

Intraoperative sonographic guidance is used to aid visualization during surgical procedures and may be used in a number of different kinds of operations on different body locations. Ultrasound is a noninvasive way of visualizing the body internally using sound waves far above human perception bounced off interior anatomical structures. As the sound waves

pass through different densities of tissue, they are reflected back to the receiving unit at varying speeds. The waves are then converted into electrical pulses which are instantly displayed as a picture on screen. This imaging helps the surgeon see target structures, determine location and depth of incisions, monitor surgical progression, etc. This code is not used for ultrasonic guidance specifically for tissue ablation as that is reported elsewhere.

77001

77001   Fluoroscopic guidance for central venous access device placement, replacement (catheter only or complete), or removal (includes fluoroscopic guidance for vascular access and catheter manipulation, any necessary contrast injections through access site or catheter with related venography radiologic supervision and interpretation, and radiographic documentation of final catheter position) (List separately in addition to code for primary procedure)

This code reports the radiological portion of fluoroscopic guidance used throughout the procedure of placing, replacing, or removing a central venous access device, or CVAD. This includes contrast injections through the access site or catheter, related venography supervision and interpretation, and radiographic verification of the final catheter position. A CVAD is a catheter inserted with its tip in the superior or inferior vena cava or the right atrium for purposes of administering large amounts of blood, fluid, or repeated transfusions, such as antibiotics or cytotoxic therapy. Central veins are those in the thorax with direct continuity to the right atrium. The most commonly used access veins are the internal and external jugular and subclavian veins. A CVAD may be a peripherally inserted central catheter, or PICC line, which is placed through the antecubital veins in the arm and advanced to the central vein with the tip in the superior vena cava. CVADs may also be nontunneled, which are placed more directly into the central vein by access through the chest wall in the clavicular area. These have multiple lumen access within the catheter and are used mainly in intensive care settings for therapies under three weeks. A tunneled CVAD is placed through a subcutaneous tunnel created from the venous access site on the chest wall to a more distant exit site in the skin of the abdomen. CVADs may also be a totally implantable port with a silicone catheter and septum placed in a subcutaneous pocket and accessed across the skin by a needle into the port. This code is reported in addition to the primary procedure.

77002

▲ 77002   Fluoroscopic guidance for needle placement (eg, biopsy, aspiration, injection, localization device) (List separately in addition to code for primary procedure)

This code reports the radiological portion of fluoroscopic guidance used in needle placement for biopsy, aspiration, injection, or localization type procedures. Fluoroscopy is a continuous, x-ray beam passed through the body part being examined and projected onto a TV-like monitor to create a kind of x-ray movie. This uses more radiation than standard x-rays and can image many different body systems to study a specific structure or organ, localize a tumor or foreign body, and also study movement within the body. The target area is identified with fluoroscopy and anesthetized. The appropriate type of needle is inserted under fluoroscopic guidance to perform the specified procedure such as removing aspirate or tissue samples for biopsy, injecting a therapeutic or diagnostic substance, or localizing a tumor or mass for further study. The primary procedural code reports the type of procedure and anatomic location.

77003

▲ 77003   Fluoroscopic guidance and localization of needle or catheter tip for spine or paraspinous diagnostic or therapeutic injection procedures (epidural or subarachnoid) (List separately in addition to code for primary procedure)

Fluoroscopic guidance is used to locate the target site for inserting a needle or catheter tip for spinal or paraspinous diagnostic or therapeutic injection procedures. Fluoroscopy is a continuous, x-ray beam passed through the body part being examined and projected onto a TV-like monitor to create a kind of x-ray movie. This uses more radiation than standard x-rays and can image many different body systems to locate a specific structure or organ, as well as study movement within the body. The needle or catheter tip is inserted and a small amount of contrast material is injected and observed fluoroscopically to ensure correct positioning for an epidural or subarachnoid injection. The separately reportable primary injection procedure may be performed for diagnostic or therapeutic purposes, including injection of an anesthetic, a steroid, or destruction by neurolytic agent. Under fluoroscopic guidance, the physician monitors the injection procedure as it is carried out and provides a written report of the radiological component of the procedure.

77011

77011   Computed tomography guidance for stereotactic localization

This code reports computed tomography guidance for stereotactic localization. Stereotactic localization is a method of determining a lesion's unique location within a certain volume by describing it in terms of specific x, y, and z coordinates in relation to an original point of reference. The position of the lesion remains fixed while an initial image is made at 0 degrees angulation. Another pair of images is obtained relative to the 0 degree position by moving the imaging detector or beams in a controlled fashion around the center of rotation plus and minus specified degrees. Basic geometry is used to determine the lesion location in a 3D coordinate system by these paired images in relation to the fixed origin. CT imaging is the method used to locate the lesion and determine its coordinates.

77012

77012   Computed tomography guidance for needle placement (eg, biopsy, aspiration, injection, localization device), radiological supervision and interpretation

This code reports the radiological supervision and interpretation portion of computed tomography guidance used in needle placement for biopsy, aspiration, injection, or localization procedures. The target area is localized using computed tomography and then anesthetized. The appropriate type of needle is inserted under CT guidance to perform the specified procedure such as removing aspirate or tissue samples for biopsy, injecting a therapeutic or diagnostic substance, or localizing a tumor or mass for further study. The surgical code reports the procedure and anatomic location. CT aims multiple, narrow x-ray beams around a single rotational axis, taking a large series of two-dimensional images of the target structure from multiple angles. The computer can digitally reconstruct the data into a three-dimensional image and produce thin, cross-sectional 2D or 3D images (slices) of the test object.

77013

77013   Computed tomography guidance for, and monitoring of, parenchymal tissue ablation

This code reports the radiological supervision and interpretation portion of computed tomography guidance used in tissue ablation procedures. The target area is localized using computed tomography and then anesthetized. The appropriate type of needle is inserted under CT guidance to perform the specified procedure such as removing aspirate or tissue samples for biopsy, injecting a therapeutic or diagnostic substance, or localizing a tumor or mass for further study. The surgical code reports the procedure and anatomic location. CT aims multiple, narrow x-ray beams around a single rotational axis, taking a large series of two-dimensional images of the target structure from multiple angles. The computer can digitally reconstruct the data into a three dimensional image and produce thin, cross-sectional 2D or 3D images (slices) of the test object.

77014

77014   Computed tomography guidance for placement of radiation therapy fields

This code reports computed tomographic guidance for placement of radiation therapy fields. This is an important part of treatment planning which maps out the volume of the area to receive radiation treatment. The patient remains very still while CT scanning is applied. CT aims multiple, narrow beams of x-ray around a single rotational axis, taking a large series of two-dimensional images of the target structure from multiple angles. The computer can digitally reconstruct the data into a three dimensional image and produce thin, cross-sectional 2D or 3D images (slices) of the test object. Cross-sectional images are acquired for the entire treatment area. Both normal and abnormal tissue within the therapy field is defined and the treatment parameters are set for the best application of the radiation beam.

77021

77021   Magnetic resonance guidance for needle placement (eg, for biopsy, needle aspiration, injection, or placement of localization device) radiological supervision and interpretation

This code reports the radiological supervision and interpretation portion of magnetic resonance imaging (MRI) used in needle placement for biopsy, aspiration, injection, or localization procedures. The target area is localized using magnetic resonance and then anesthetized. The appropriate type of needle is inserted under MRI guidance to perform the specified procedure such as removing aspirate or tissue samples for biopsy, injecting a therapeutic or diagnostic substance, or localizing a tumor or mass for further study. The surgical code reports the procedure and anatomic location. Magnetic resonance is a noninvasive, non-radiating imaging technique that uses the magnetic properties of hydrogen atoms in the body. The nuclei of hydrogen atoms emit radiofrequency signals when the body is exposed to radiowaves transmitted within a strong magnetic field. The computer processes the signals and converts the data into tomographic, 3D images with very high resolution. The needle being used with MRI guidance may have special metallic ringlets around it; be coated with contrast material; or have a signal receiving coil in its tip.

77022

77022   Magnetic resonance guidance for, and monitoring of, parenchymal tissue ablation

This code reports the radiological supervision and interpretation portion of magnetic resonance imaging (MRI) used in tissue ablation procedures. The target area is localized using magnetic resonance and then anesthetized. The appropriate type of needle is inserted under MRI guidance to perform the specified procedure such as removing

aspirate or tissue samples for biopsy, injecting a therapeutic or diagnostic substance, or localizing a tumor or mass for further study. The surgical code reports the procedure and anatomic location. Magnetic resonance is a noninvasive, non-radiating imaging technique that uses the magnetic properties of hydrogen atoms in the body. The nuclei of hydrogen atoms emit radiofrequency signals when the body is exposed to radiowaves transmitted within a strong magnetic field. The computer processes the signals and converts the data into tomographic, 3D images with very high resolution. The needle being used with MRI guidance may have special metallic ringlets around it; be coated with contrast material; or have a signal receiving coil in its tip.

77051-77052

77051   Computer-aided detection (computer algorithm analysis of digital image data for lesion detection) with further review for interpretation, with or without digitization of film radiographic images; diagnostic mammography (List separately in addition to code for primary procedure)

77052   Computer-aided detection (computer algorithm analysis of digital image data for lesion detection) with further review for interpretation, with or without digitization of film radiographic images; screening mammography (List separately in addition to code for primary procedure)

These codes report computer-aided lesion detection by algorithm analysis of image data obtained from mammographic films, with or without digitization of the radiographic images, including additional interpretive review. These are add-on codes to be used in conjunction with the primary procedure of diagnostic mammography for 77051 and screening mammography for 77052. In computer aided detection, the mammographic picture of the breast is used by scanning the x-ray film with a laser beam, usually converting the scanned image of the analog film into digital data for the computer first, then employing a methodical, step-by-step pattern of analyzing the data on video display for unusual or suspicious areas.

77053-77054

77053   Mammary ductogram or galactogram, single duct, radiological supervision and interpretation

77054   Mammary ductogram or galactogram, multiple ducts, radiological supervision and interpretation

These codes report the radiological supervision and interpretation portion of a mammary ductogram or galactogram for a single duct in 77053 or multiple ducts in 77054. A galactogram is radiographic imaging of the mammary duct(s) done after the injection of a radiopaque substance into the duct(s). A needle and cannula are first inserted into the duct for injection of the contrast agent. This is reported with a surgical procedure code. The needle and cannula are removed when the imaging is completed.

77058-77059

77058   Magnetic resonance imaging, breast, without and/or with contrast material(s); unilateral

77059   Magnetic resonance imaging, breast, without and/or with contrast material(s); bilateral

These codes report magnetic resonance imaging done on one breast in 77058 and both breasts in 77059, without and/or with contrast material(s). Magnetic resonance is a noninvasive, non-radiating imaging technique that uses the magnetic properties of hydrogen atoms in the body. The nuclei of hydrogen atoms emit radiofrequency signals when the body is exposed to radiowaves transmitted within a strong magnetic field. The computer processes the signals and converts the data into high resolution, tomographic, 3D sectional images of the inside of the body structure (i.e. the breast). The patient may be given a sedative to help her remain still while lying on a motorized table within a large MRI tunnel. Contrast material is sometimes injected for image enhancement.

77061-77063

77061   Digital breast tomosynthesis; unilateral

77062   Digital breast tomosynthesis; bilateral

77063   Screening digital breast tomosynthesis, bilateral (List separately in addition to code for primary procedure)

Digital breast tomosynthesis (DBT) provides a 3-dimensional picture of breast tissue using standard mammography equipment and sends the image to a computer for the radiologist to interpret. The patient is positioned as for standard mammography with breast tissue stabilized but not over compressed between two glass plates while top to bottom and then side to side views are obtained. The x-ray scanner moves around the breast in an arc and takes 11 images in 7 seconds. The images are sent to a computer and assembled for the radiologist to view in 3-dimension. DBT can provide earlier detection of breast cancer with greater accuracy. Its use may result in fewer unnecessary breast biopsies, aide in the detection of multiple tumors, and provide better imaging of very dense breast tissue. Code 77061 is used for unilateral DBT; code 77062 is used for bilateral DBT; and code 77063 is used when DBT is performed as a bilateral screening procedure in conjunction with another primary procedure.

Radiology

77065-77066

● **77065** Diagnostic mammography, including computer-aided detection (CAD) when performed; unilateral
● **77066** Diagnostic mammography, including computer-aided detection (CAD) when performed; bilateral

These codes report diagnostic mammography of one breast (77065) or both breasts (77066) with computer-aided lesion detection (CAD), when performed. Mammography is the radiographic imaging of the breast using low-dose ionizing radiation. The x-rays used in mammography have a longer wavelength that those typically used for bone imaging. The test is done to detect tumors or cysts in women who have symptoms of breast disease or a palpable mass. The breast is compressed between planes on a machine dedicated strictly to mammography. This evens out the dense tissue and holds the breast still for a better quality image. Computer-aided detection uses algorithm analysis of the image data obtained from the mammographic films, with or without digitization of the radiographic images. The mammographic picture of the breast is used by scanning the x-ray film with a laser beam, usually converting the scanned image of the analog film into digital data for the computer first, then employing a methodical, step-by-step pattern of analyzing the data on video display for unusual or suspicious areas.

77067

● **77067** Screening mammography, bilateral (2-view study of each breast), including computer-aided detection (CAD) when performed

Bilateral screening mammography is done with computer-aided lesion detection (CAD), when performed. Mammography is the radiographic imaging of the breast using low-dose ionizing radiation. The x-rays used in mammography have a longer wavelength than those typically used for bone imaging. A screening mammogram is done on asymptomatic women for early breast cancer detection when there are no known palpable masses. This is done on both breasts with two views taken on each side. The breast is compressed between planes on a machine dedicated strictly to mammography. This evens out the dense tissue and holds the breast still for a better quality image. Computer-aided detection uses algorithm analysis of the image data obtained from the mammographic films, with or without digitization of the radiographic images. The mammographic picture of the breast is used by scanning the x-ray film with a laser beam, usually converting the scanned image of the analog film into digital data for the computer first, then employing a methodical, step-by-step pattern of analyzing the data on video display for unusual or suspicious areas.

77071

77071 Manual application of stress performed by physician or other qualified health care professional for joint radiography, including contralateral joint if indicated

While wearing protective gloves, the physician or other qualified health care professional applies manual stress to the joint being x-rayed. The joint is held in the desired position while the x-rays are taken. The forced amount of stress applied to the joint allows visualization of the joint under conditions that would not appear on films taken in normal, routine positioning. Manual application of stress during joint x-ray is performed on the opposite (contralateral) joint as needed.

77072

77072 Bone age studies

Bone age studies are a method of estimating the skeletal development of children by using radiographic films. X-rays of the child's hand and wrist are taken and compared against "normal" reference x-rays of different ages. One method requires the systematic assessment of bone maturity of all the bones in the hand and wrist. Another method is a modified, rapid version of assessing bone maturity in which the overall appearance of one given radiograph is compared with the reference radiographs and the nearest match is selected to determine bone age. Growth retardation must be treated before the bones fuse, at which point, there is no more bone growth possible.

77073

77073 Bone length studies (orthoroentgenogram, scanogram)

Bone length studies are a method of measuring the length of long bones in skeletal limbs by radiographic films. This is often done to assess limb length discrepancy more accurately than external observational measurements. Various types of radiographic pictures of the long bones in question may be taken to determine limb length inequality. The classic orthoroentgenogram is made by incorporating three separate exposures of the hip, knee, and ankle joint. A scanogram is similar, but with a reduced exposure size to put all three exposures on one film cassette. A teleoroentgenogram is a single exposure anteroposterior radiograph film with a ruler integrated into the picture.

77074-77076

77074 Radiologic examination, osseous survey; limited (eg, for metastases)
77075 Radiologic examination, osseous survey; complete (axial and appendicular skeleton)
77076 Radiologic examination, osseous survey, infant

These codes report a radiological examination for surveying bones. Code 77074 reports a limited osseous study when a specific symptomatic or suspected disease site is examined by x-ray. This is not usually done for verifying the spread of cancer since nuclear bone dexa scanning studies have replaced regular x-ray for bone metastasis staging. Code 77075 reports a complete osseous survey that includes x-rays taken of both the axial (head and main trunk portion) and the appendicular skeleton (bones of the limbs). Use code 77076 for a radiological survey of bones performed on an infant. This may be done to look for evidence of child abuse, suspected disease, or bone lesions that may occur in a known illness.

77078

77078 Computed tomography, bone mineral density study, 1 or more sites; axial skeleton (eg, hips, pelvis, spine)

Computed tomography (CT) for bone mineral density study, also called quantitative computed tomography densitometry or QCT densitometry, is performed on one or more sites of the axial skeleton (pelvis, hips, and/or spine). Measuring bone mass or bone mineral density (BMD) is done to diagnose for bone disease, evaluate bone disease progression, or monitor the results of treatment, particularly for osteoporosis, which puts a bone at higher risk of fracture. CT aims multiple, narrow x-ray beams around a single rotational axis, taking a series of two-dimensional images of the target structure from multiple angles. The computer can digitally reconstruct the data into a three dimensional image and produce thin, cross-sectional 2D or 3D images (slices) of the test object. QCT is measured to be 2-3 times more accurate than bone DXA scanning due to the fact that it is three dimensional and can calculate a more exact measurement of bone density, which is mass divided by volume. Since DXA calculates BMD by the bone's attenuation of x-ray divided by the area of the site being scanned, there is no depth value in the calculation and that is where 3D QCT densitometry is capable of making a more accurate calculation.

77080-77081

77080 Dual-energy X-ray absorptiometry (DXA), bone density study, 1 or more sites; axial skeleton (eg, hips, pelvis, spine)
77081 Dual-energy X-ray absorptiometry (DXA), bone density study, 1 or more sites; appendicular skeleton (peripheral) (eg, radius, wrist, heel)

These codes report dual-energy x-ray absorptiometry (DXA) for bone density study. Measuring bone mass or bone mineral density (BMD) is done to diagnose for bone disease, evaluate bone disease progression, or monitor the results of treatment, particularly for osteoporosis, which puts a bone at higher risk of fracture. The radiation dose of DXA is around 1/30th of that in a standard chest x-ray. DXA involves aiming two x-ray beams of different energy levels at the bones in alternate pulses. Soft tissue absorption is subtracted out, and the BMD is determined by the bone's absorption of each beam in the projected area. The DXA scan measurement is then compared to a same sex standard of bone density at age 30, since the maximum BMD occurs at age 30 in both males and females. The difference between the measured BMD and the sex-matched, average 30-year-old standard is known as the T score. A T score between -1.0 and -2.4 diagnoses osteopenia, while a T score of -2.5 or less indicates osteoporosis. Use 77080 to report a DXA bone density study looking at one or more sites of the axial skeleton, such as the pelvis, hips, or spine. Use 77081 for assessment of one or more sites of the appendicular or peripheral skeleton, such as the radius, ulna, wrist, or heel.

77084

77084 Magnetic resonance (eg, proton) imaging, bone marrow blood supply

Magnetic resonance (proton) imaging is performed to examine bone marrow blood supply. Magnetic resonance is a noninvasive, non-radiating imaging technique that uses the magnetic properties of the nuclei within atoms in the body. The protons in the nuclei of different atoms, such as hydrogen, emit a certain radiofrequency signal when the body is exposed to radiowaves transmitted within a strong magnetic field. The computer processes the signals and converts the data into tomographic, 3D, sectional images with very high resolution. The patient is placed on a motorized table within a large MRI tunnel scanner for the images to be taken. Bone marrow contains both fat cells with a high water content along with non-fat cells. MRI gives information about changes occurring in the bone marrow based on the atomic action of different tissue composition and blood cell distribution within the medullary cavity of the bone. Avascular necrosis and metastatic tumors can be directly visualized because of the radiofrequency signal differences between the normal cell composition and distribution in bone marrow and abnormal, necrotic or neoplastic tissue.

77085

77085 Dual-energy X-ray absorptiometry (DXA), bone density study, 1 or more sites; axial skeleton (eg, hips, pelvis, spine), including vertebral fracture assessment

These codes report dual-energy x-ray absorptiometry (DXA) for bone density study. Measuring bone mass or bone mineral density (BMD) is done to diagnose for bone disease, evaluate bone disease progression, or monitor the results of treatment, particularly for osteoporosis, which puts a bone at higher risk of fracture. The radiation dose of DXA is around 1/30th of that in a standard chest x-ray. DXA involves aiming two x-ray beams of different energy levels at the bones in alternate pulses. Soft tissue absorption is subtracted out, and the BMD is determined by the bone's absorption of each beam in the projected area. The DXA scan measurement is then compared to a same sex standard of bone density at age 30, since the maximum BMD occurs at age 30 in both males and females. The difference between the measured BMD and the sex-matched, average 30-year-old standard is known as the T score. A T score between -1.0 and -2.4 diagnoses osteopenia, while a T score of -2.5 or less indicates osteoporosis. Use 77085 when looking at one or more sites of the axial skeleton, such as the pelvis, hips, or spine in combination with a specific assessment of the spinal vertebrae for vertebral fracture.

77086

77086 Vertebral fracture assessment via dual-energy X-ray absorptiometry (DXA)

Vertebral fractures are highly prevalent in the elderly but go unrecognized clinically in many individuals. Vertebral fracture assessment can be performed using dual-energy X-ray absorptiometry (DXA), a technique that aims two x-ray beams of different energy levels at the bones in alternate pulses with the addition of densitometers and special software. With the patient positioned supine or in left decubitus, the lateral spine is scanned using a rotating arm. The low level radiation exposure of DXA will show bone fractures but not other bone or soft tissue abnormalities. Vertebral fractures are graded I-III with a Grade I fracture characterized by a 20-24% decrease in vertebral height and a Grade III fracture with a 40% or greater decrease. The vertebral deformity location may also be noted and can include an endplate deformity (vertebral midheight), wedge deformity (anterior and midheight) and crush deformity (entire vertebrae).

77293

77293 Respiratory motion management simulation (List separately in addition to code for primary procedure)

Respiratory motion management simulation is used during the treatment planning phase of radiation therapy for malignant neoplasm. Organs in the chest, upper abdominal region, and retroperitoneum move during breathing. However, respiratory motion varies significantly between individuals. In addition, a patient's breathing pattern can vary in magnitude, length, and regularity during imaging and treatment sessions. Simulation of respiratory motion is used to create a radiation treatment plan that is modified for the patient's respiratory motion and pattern. Respiratory motion studies track the movement of the tumor, the host organ (organ where the tumor is located), and surrounding organs or structures. Organ motion can be detected using ultrasound, CT, magnetic resonance, or fluoroscopic imaging. A 2-D motion management simulation showing the tumor, host organ, and surrounding structures can be created using fluoroscopy. A 3-D reconstruction requires two simultaneous projections, visualization of the tumor and host organ, and visualization of surrogate markers, such as previously implanted fiducial markers, radiographic tracers (e.g. radiopharmaceuticals), and/or an anatomic marker, such as the diaphragm. Information from the respiratory motion management simulation is then used along with other clinical treatment planning modalities to modify and individualize the radiation treatment.

77295

77295 3-dimensional radiotherapy plan, including dose-volume histograms

A 3-dimensional (3-D) radiotherapy plan is used during the treatment planning phase for radiation treatment of malignant neoplasms. It involves creating a computer generated 3-D reconstruction of the tumor and critical structures near the tumor. The 3-D reconstruction uses direct CT scans and/or MRI data to generate the 3-D images. The computer generated 3-D reconstruction is used with dose-volume histograms (DVH) that provide a frequency distribution of average dose values over the 3-D reconstruction to determine the target dose that will be most effective in eradicating the tumor while at the same time sparing critical structures and surrounding healthy tissue. The 3-D reconstruction and dose-volume histograms allow adjustments to the radiation treatment plan based on the patient's specific or unique anatomy.

77306-77307

77306 Teletherapy isodose plan; simple (1 or 2 unmodified ports directed to a single area of interest), includes basic dosimetry calculation(s)
77307 Teletherapy isodose plan; complex (multiple treatment areas, tangential ports, the use of wedges, blocking, rotational beam, or special beam considerations), includes basic dosimetry calculation(s)

The teletherapy isodose plan is a patient specific procedure performed by a medical dosimetrist and/or qualified medical physicist under the direction of a radiation oncologist and is used to determine the amount, rate, and distribution of radiation from an external beam such as a linear accelerator or cobalt unit, that will be applied to treat tumors or other medical conditions. The plan includes a graphic display of the patient's anatomy and uses a dataset from digitally reconstructed radiographs to design the port locations where the body will receive the radiation. The basic dosimetry calculations may be done manually or by computer. Code 77306 is used for a simple teletherapy isodose plan with 1 or 2 unmodified ports with a single treatment area. Code 77307 is used when the teletherapy isodose plan is more complex and might include more than one treatment area, tangential ports, the use of wedges, custom blocking, rotational beams, or other special considerations.

77316-77318

77316 Brachytherapy isodose plan; simple (calculation[s] made from 1 to 4 sources, or remote afterloading brachytherapy, 1 channel), includes basic dosimetry calculation(s)
77317 Brachytherapy isodose plan; intermediate (calculation[s] made from 5 to 10 sources, or remote afterloading brachytherapy, 2-12 channels), includes basic dosimetry calculation(s)
77318 Brachytherapy isodose plan; complex (calculation[s] made from over 10 sources, or remote afterloading brachytherapy, over 12 channels), includes basic dosimetry calculation(s)

The brachytherapy isodose plan is a patient specific procedure performed by a medical dosimetrist and/or qualified medical physicist under the direction of a radiation oncologist. Brachytherapy provides localized, precise radiation by implanting (afterloading) seeds or pellets temporarily or permanently into body cavities and/or interstitial tissue. The isodose plan is used to determine the technique, the precise dose, and the type of radiation (iodine, palladium, cesium, iridium) applied to treat tumors or other medical conditions, and also to measure the amount of radiation that the surrounding tissue can tolerate. Temporary brachytherapy places a radioactive seed or pellet inside a catheter or tube (source) for a specific amount of time after which the seed or pellet is removed. The temporary technique may use a low-dose rate (LDR) with continuous treatment over 1-2 days (20-50 hours), a pulse-dose rate (PDR) which gives episodic doses of radiation, typically once each hour for several hours or days, or a high-dose rate (HDR) where the session length is usually 10-20 minutes and is repeated several times. In permanent brachytherapy, the implanted seeds/pellets shed their radioactive material over several months until it is completely gone. Following confirmation of the proper location of the radiation delivery device (source), the seeds or pellets are inserted (afterloaded) manually or by using a computer controlled machine. Code 77316 is used for a simple brachytherapy isodose plan using calculations from 1-4 sources, or remote afterloading of 1 channel. Code 77317 is used for an intermediate brachytherapy isodose plan with calculations made from 5-10 sources, or remote afterloading of 2-12 channels. Code 77318 is used for a complex brachytherapy isodose plan with calculations made from more than 10 sources, or remote afterloading of more than 12 channels.

77334

77334 Treatment devices, design and construction; complex (irregular blocks, special shields, compensators, wedges, molds or casts)

The physician builds and shapes special devices used in radiation therapy to protect healthy tissue from the radiation beams. The devices are designed for a radiation procedure involving highly complex blocking, custom shielding blocks, tangential ports, special wedges or compensators, three or more separate treatment areas, rotational or special beam considerations, combination of therapeutic modalities.

77338

77338 Multi-leaf collimator (MLC) device(s) for intensity modulated radiation therapy (IMRT), design and construction per IMRT plan

The multi-leaf collimator (MLC) device was originally used during radiation therapy as a replacement for conventional alloy block shaping to direct the radiation beam to the tumor and protect surrounding structures. It is now also used for intensity modulated radiation therapy (IMRT) to improve the efficiency of treatment delivery. Previously obtained plain radiographs and CT images are used to help design and construct an IMRT plan. The MLC device has between 20-80 movable leaves or shields that can block a fraction of the radiation beam. Using previously obtained images, a computer program is used to determine optimal positioning of the leaves so that the radiation beam can be delivered more precisely to the tumor. The computer programming takes into consideration the need to change the positions of the leaves during radiation delivery in response to the arc rotation of the beam thereby allowing IMRT. This data is stored in the computer and used at the time of radiation delivery to program the MLC device which then moves the leaves into the required configuration as radiation treatment is delivered. As the tumor shrinks, the IMRT plan may need to be revised and the computer reprogrammed. This code reports the design and construction of the IMRT plan and is reported for each IMRT plan.

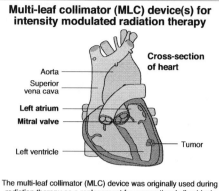

Multi-leaf collimator (MLC) device(s) for intensity modulated radiation therapy

The multi-leaf collimator (MLC) device was originally used during radiation therapy as a replacement for conventional alloy block shaping to direct the radiation beam to the tumor and protect surrounding structures.

77371

77371   Radiation treatment delivery, stereotactic radiosurgery (SRS), complete course of treatment of cranial lesion(s) consisting of 1 session; multi-source Cobalt 60 based

A complete course of radiation treatment is delivered to a cranial lesion(s) in one session with multi-source Cobalt 60 based stereotactic radiosurgery (SRS). Stereotactic radiosurgery does not actually remove the tumor, but utilizes an external beam of radiation like conventional radiotherapy to disrupt DNA of the tumor cells, damaging their ability to reproduce. Focused radiation beams are delivered very precisely to a specific area of the brain (or neck) in a single, high dose of radiation within one day, or a one-session treatment. The one-session treatment is called radiosurgery because its effect on the target is so dramatic that the changes are considered "surgical" in nature. Computer-aided planning pinpoints the exact three dimensional location. The patient is immobilized with skeletal fixation devices that completely restrict head movement, giving radiosurgery the most precise and accurate treatment capabilities while minimizing the amount of radiation passing through healthy tissue. This type of required immobilization limits radiosurgery to the head and neck. Cobalt 60 based, or photon beam, radiosurgery, also known as Gamma Knife surgery, is one of three different technologies available for SRS. Cobalt 60 based machines utilize multiple sources of radiation in a multitude of collimated beams with scalpel-like precision which lessens damage to healthy tissue and provides better targeting. This works well on smaller tumors and functional disorders of the brain. Cobalt 60 machines are dedicated to brain dysfunction or tumor treatment in one session and provide the preferred treatment for tumors, arteriovenous malformations, and dysfunctions such as trigeminal neuralgia.

77372

77372   Radiation treatment delivery, stereotactic radiosurgery (SRS), complete course of treatment of cranial lesion(s) consisting of 1 session; linear accelerator based

A complete course of radiation treatment is delivered to a cranial lesion(s) in one session with linear accelerator based stereotactic radiosurgery (SRS). Stereotactic radiosurgery does not actually remove the tumor, but utilizes an external beam of radiation like conventional radiotherapy to disrupt DNA of the tumor cells, damaging their ability to reproduce. Focused radiation beams are delivered very precisely to a specific area of the brain (or neck) in a single, high dose of radiation within one day, or a one-session treatment. The one-session treatment is called radiosurgery because its effect on the target is so dramatic that the changes are considered "surgical" in nature. Computer-aided planning pinpoints the exact three dimensional location. The patient is immobilized with skeletal fixation devices that completely restrict head movement, giving radiosurgery the most precise and accurate treatment capabilities while minimizing the amount of radiation passing through healthy tissue. This type of required immobilization limits radiosurgery to the head and neck. Linear accelerator based, or linac, radiosurgery is one of three different technologies available for SRS. Linac utilizes one large intense beam and moves during treatment, redirecting the beam in many arcs to lessen adverse effect on healthy tissue. This works well on larger tumors and can also be applied to other body areas. Linear accelerator machines are capable of delivering fractionated therapy over several days to other body areas as well as radiosurgical one-session treatment to the brain, which is reported with this code.

77373

77373   Stereotactic body radiation therapy, treatment delivery, per fraction to 1 or more lesions, including image guidance, entire course not to exceed 5 fractions

Stereotactic radiation therapy treatment is delivered to one or more lesions of the body, including image guidance. This code is reported per fraction, or treatment session, with the entire course not to exceed 5 fractions. Stereotactic radiotherapy (SRT) or fractionated stereotactic radiotherapy (FSR) consists of treatments that give a small fraction of the total radiation dose over a period of time as opposed to radiosurgery done in a single, one-session treatment. Computer-aided mapping pinpoints the exact three dimensional location of the target. A focused, external beam of radiation is delivered very precisely to a specific area to disrupt DNA of the tumor cells, damaging their ability to reproduce. The body part receiving treatment is immobilized with the use of removable frames, masks, or fitted casts or molds to limit movement and damage to healthy tissue. Stereotactic radiotherapy is performed with linear accelerator technology. Linear accelerator machines produce radiation in the form of high energy x-ray. They utilize one large intense beam and move during treatment, redirecting the beam in many arcs to lessen adverse effect on healthy tissue. This works well on larger tumors and can be applied to many body areas. Both MRI and CT imaging modalities are used with linear accelerator stereotactic radiotherapy. MRI is considered the gold standard of imaging guidance because of the unparalleled high resolution, 3D imaging within the body that it can provide, differentiating between normal and tumor tissue. Some linear accelerator technology can only be used with CT scanning, however.

77385-77386

77385   Intensity modulated radiation treatment delivery (IMRT), includes guidance and tracking, when performed; simple

77386   Intensity modulated radiation treatment delivery (IMRT), includes guidance and tracking, when performed; complex

Intensity modulated radiation treatment (IMRT) is planned by mapping the target area with CT or MRI imaging and then using a computerized calculation to produce a custom tailored radiation dose. IMRT is a radiotherapy technique that uses a computer controlled radiotherapy treatment machine to deliver precise doses of radiation from multiple, small, non-uniform beams that are manipulated to radiate a whole tumor, or a very specific area of the tumor, very precisely by conforming to its shape. By allowing the radiation to conform to a 3-dimensional shape, higher and more effective doses of radiation can be delivered to a focused area, thus minimizing destruction of healthy surrounding tissue and reducing side effects. A number of different technologies may be employed to generate IMRT and complexity varies with the target area or the technique used. Code 77385 is applied for simple IMRT that uses a minimal number of segments while still maintaining an acceptable dose of radiation. Prostate, breast, and other sites treated using a physical compensator are reported with 77385. Code 77386 is reported for complex IMRT that uses the maximum number of segments, multiple subfields, and/or higher intensity radiation doses. Any site not using physical compensator IMRT is reported with 77386. The technical component of image guidance or tracking is included.

77387

77387   Guidance for localization of target volume for delivery of radiation treatment delivery, includes intrafraction tracking, when performed

To improve treatment accuracy and decrease complications, real-time image guided radiotherapy may be used to localize the target volume for radiation delivery. Intra-fraction tracking allows for the adjustment of treatment beams while radiation is being delivered to compensate for movement of organs inside the body caused by breathing, cardiac or bowel movement, swallowing, or sneezing. The procedure usually requires the implantation of electromagnetic transponders around the tumor/target area and a 4-dimensional electromagnetic array machine (Calypso, RayPilot, AlignRT) positioned above the patient during treatment which activates and communicates with the transponders.

77401

77401   Radiation treatment delivery, superficial and/or ortho voltage, per day

Superficial and/or ortho voltage radiation therapy uses low dose energy ionizing radiation to treat non-melanoma skin cancers such as basal cell and squamous cell carcinomas and recurrent keloids on or near the skin surface. It may also be used as a palliative treatment for bony metastasis in shallow areas such as the ribs and sternum. Superficial radiation therapy uses 50-200 kV and penetrates to about 5 mm. Ortho voltage radiation therapy uses 200-500 kV and penetrates to a depth of 4-6 cm. Both can be performed in a physician's office without anesthesia. These procedures are simple, safe, and accurate with minimal side effects and may be used as an alternative to excision in patients who are poor surgical candidates due to complicating medical conditions. Superficial and/or ortho voltage may also be used when the skin lesion is in a hard to heal location such as on the legs or scalp, or in a highly visible area like the nose. A treatment plan is developed based on the size and depth of the lesion(s). The total radiation dose is divided into the total number of treatment sessions to arrive at the radiation dose per treatment. Treatments may be given 2-5 times per week until the total radiation dose has been delivered. Code 77401 is used to report superficial and/or ortho voltage radiation therapy to one or more skin sites/lesions per treatment day.

77402-77407

77407   Radiation treatment delivery, >1 MeV; intermediate

Conventional external beam radiation therapy is commonly used to destroy abnormal tissue, such as malignant tumors, and may be employed alone or in combination with surgery and/or chemotherapy for curative purposes or as a palliative measure to relieve symptoms. Treatment consists of a focused beam of radiation directed from outside the body to the targeted internal organ/tissue. A radiation oncologist determines the total radiation dose and divides that into smaller fractions which are delivered over a planned course of treatment. The intensity and duration of radiation therapy depends on the location, size, and type of tumor. Code 77402 is used for simple radiation treatment delivery of >1 MeV involving a single area, the use of one or two ports, and up to two simple blocks. Code 77407 is reported for intermediate radiation treatment delivery of >1 MeV involving any of the following criteria: two separate areas of treatment, the use of 3 or more ports on any one treatment site, or 3 or more simple blocks. Code 77412 is reported for complex radiation treatment delivery of >1 MeV involving any of the following criteria: 3 or more separate treatment sites, the use of custom blocking, wedges, tangential ports, electron beam, rotational beams, physical or virtual tissue compensators not congruent with IMRT, or field-in-field treatment for dose homogeneity. The amount of megavoltage is not a consideration for complexity level.

77402-77412

77402   Radiation treatment delivery, >1 MeV; simple
77412   Radiation treatment delivery, >1 MeV; complex

Conventional external beam radiation therapy is commonly used to destroy abnormal tissue, such as malignant tumors, and may be employed alone or in combination with surgery and/or chemotherapy for curative purposes or as a palliative measure to relieve symptoms. Treatment consists of a focused beam of radiation directed from outside the body to the targeted internal organ/tissue. A radiation oncologist determines the total radiation dose and divides that into smaller fractions which are delivered over a planned course of treatment. The intensity and duration of radiation therapy depends on the location, size, and type of tumor. Code 77402 is used for simple radiation treatment delivery of >1 MeV involving a single area, the use of one or two ports, and up to two simple blocks. Code 77407 is reported for intermediate radiation treatment delivery of >1 MeV involving any of the following criteria: two separate areas of treatment, the use of 3 or more ports on any one treatment site, or 3 or more simple blocks. Code 77412 is reported for complex radiation treatment delivery of >1 MeV involving any of the following criteria: 3 or more separate treatment sites, the use of custom blocking, wedges, tangential ports, electron beam, rotational beams, physical or virtual tissue compensators not congruent with IMRT, or field-in-field treatment for dose homogeneity. The amount of megavoltage is not a consideration for complexity level.

77424-77425

77424   Intraoperative radiation treatment delivery, x-ray, single treatment session
77425   Intraoperative radiation treatment delivery, electrons, single treatment session

Intraoperative radiation therapy (IORT) allows for intensive radiation to tumors as they are located during the surgical procedure. Because the tumor is exposed, other tissues and organs can be protected which limits or prevents radiation damage to normal healthy tissues and organs. Malignant tumors treated with IORT include gastric, pancreatic, colonic, rectal, and anal tumors. Cervical, uterine, ovarian, and prostatic tumors are also treated using IORT, as are tumors of the bladder and kidney, and soft tissue sarcomas. During a separately reportable surgical procedure, the surgeon removes as much of the tumor as possible. The surgeon moves healthy organs away from the radiation field. Special tubes are used to focus the radiation directly on the tumor. The radiation treatment is then delivered. Use 77424 for IORT using low energy x-ray radiation. This type of IORT is typically performed with a portable miniature x-ray source. Use 77425 for intraoperative electron radiation therapy (IOERT), which uses electron beams that allow for more precise delivery of radiation to the target site. Because the dose drops off rapidly underneath the target site when electron beams are used, less underlying healthy tissue is damaged. IOERT may be performed in a dedicated operating room with a radiation therapy machine and the required shield walls or in a standard operating room using a self-shielded, mobile, linear accelerator for IOERT.

77435

77435   Stereotactic body radiation therapy, treatment management, per treatment course, to 1 or more lesions, including image guidance, entire course not to exceed 5 fractions

Stereotactic radiation therapy treatment management is reported for the entire treatment course to one or more lesions, including image guidance for a course that does not exceed

5 fractions, or sessions. Stereotactic radiotherapy treatments give a small fraction of the total radiation dose over a period of time. Computer-aided planning pinpoints the exact three dimensional location of the target. A focused, external beam of radiation is delivered very precisely to a specific area while the patient is immobilized in removable frames, masks, or fitted casts or molds to limit movement and damage to healthy tissue. MRI or CT scanning is employed for imaging. Management of such treatment involves calculation and review of dosimetery, individual dose delivery, and the parameters or treatment; pre-treatment set-up, which includes positioning the patient, and assessing the placement of immobilization devices, and radiation blocks or wedges; coordinating the patient's care and evaluating the body's response to treatment; reviewing lab tests and imaging films.

77469

77469   Intraoperative radiation treatment management

Intraoperative radiation therapy (IORT) allows for intensive radiation to tumors as they are located during the surgical procedure. Because the tumor is exposed, other tissues and organs can be protected which limits or prevents radiation damage to normal healthy tissues and organs. Malignant tumors treated with IORT include gastric, pancreatic, colonic, rectal, and anal tumors. Cervical, uterine, ovarian, and prostatic tumors are also treated using IORT, as are tumors of the bladder and kidney, and soft tissue sarcomas. Management of IORT treatment involves calculation and review of dosimetry, individual dose delivery, and the parameters for treatment. Pre-treatment set-up, which includes positioning the patient and assessing the placement of immobilization devices, radiation blocks, or wedges is also included in the management for IORT as well as coordinating the patient's care and evaluating the patient's response to treatment afterwards, and reviewing lab tests and imaging films.

77470

77470   Special treatment procedure (eg, total body irradiation, hemibody radiation, per oral or endocavitary irradiation)

Radiation treatment management is performed for a special procedure, such as total body irradiation, hemibody radiation, per oral or endocavitary irradiation. These procedures require extensive planning to ensure proper dose delivery and to minimize damage to major organs and other structures. Total body irradiation gives a dose of radiation to the entire body and is often performed prior to a bone marrow transplant. Total body irradiation destroys both cancer cells and healthy tissue, and depending on the dose it may also completely destroy the body's immune system. Hemibody radiation, also referred to as systemic radiation, is radiation therapy to one side (right, left) or one half (upper, lower) of the body. Hemibody radiation is used to treat malignancies such as small cell lung cancer, advanced prostate cancer, and disseminated cancers. Hemibody radiation may be given on alternate sides or alternate halves of the body during a course of treatment for disseminated cancer or widespread metastases. Irradiating only one side or one half of the body at a time allows larger doses of radiation to be given than could be given with whole body radiation. Per oral irradiation uses a special per oral cone to delivery radiation to the oral cavity. Endocavitary irradiation delivers high-dose irradiation to a body cavity with limited penetration to surrounding structures. It is used to treat rectal cancer as well as other select cancers of internal organs and structures.

77520-77522

77520   Proton treatment delivery; simple, without compensation
77522   Proton treatment delivery; simple, with compensation

The physician administers radiation therapy to a patient by aiming a proton beam at a tumor. Proton beams are often used to treat tumors located beneath a good deal of healthy tissue, as the proton beam can be targeted accurately at the tumor without causing unnecessary damage to healthy tissue. The procedure is delivered to a single treatment area utilizing a single non-tangential/oblique port and a custom block. Code 77522 if the physician attaches a custom-made device to the machine delivering the radiation to properly control the dose of radiation that is administered.

77523

77523   Proton treatment delivery; intermediate

The physician administers radiation therapy to a patient by aiming a proton beam at a tumor. Proton beams are often used to treat tumors located beneath a good deal of healthy tissue, as the proton beam can be targeted accurately at the tumor without causing unnecessary damage to healthy tissue. The procedure is delivered to two or more treatment areas utilizing two or more ports or one or more tangential/oblique ports, with custom blocks and compensators.

77525

77525   Proton treatment delivery; complex

The physician administers radiation therapy to a patient by aiming a proton beam at a tumor. Proton beams are often used to treat tumors located beneath a good deal of healthy tissue, as the proton beam can be targeted accurately at the tumor without causing unnecessary damage to healthy tissue. The procedure is delivered to one or more treatment areas utilizing two or more ports per treatment area with matching or patching fields and/or multiple isocenters, with custom blocks and compensators.

77767-77768

77767 Remote afterloading high dose rate radionuclide skin surface brachytherapy, includes basic dosimetry, when performed; lesion diameter up to 2.0 cm or 1 channel

77768 Remote afterloading high dose rate radionuclide skin surface brachytherapy, includes basic dosimetry, when performed; lesion diameter over 2.0 cm and 2 or more channels, or multiple lesions

Remote afterloading is performed for high dose rate (HDR) radionuclide skin surface brachytherapy. HDR brachytherapy using skin applicators is employed to treat non-melanoma skin cancers, avoiding surgery and shortening the radiation treated needed. An appropriate size surface applicator that will allow for an acceptable margin is first selected after determining the lesion depth and basic isodose treatment planning. Surface applicators are then implanted in and around the cutaneous tumor in a separately reportable procedure. Applicators are then inspected for size, placement, and stability, and adjustments are made as needed. A transfer tube is selected and connected to the channel applicator in the remote afterloading machine. Only the patient remains in the room and is monitored visually and verbally throughout the procedure. The remote afterloading machine loads the selected radioactive source into the previously placed applicators. Timers in the machine control the duration of exposure to the radioactive source. When the procedure is complete, the radioactive source is retracted and contained safely in the afterloading machine, verified by use of a room radiation detector followed by a patient radiation survey. The empty applicators are then removed from the patient. HDR radionuclide surface brachytherapy is reported based on the number of catheters or channels used to deliver the radioactive source and the size of the cutaneous lesion. Report 77767 for 1 channel treatment or a lesion up to 2.0 cm. Report 77768 for a malignant skin lesion over 2.0 cm in diameter, multiple lesions, or treatment with 2 or more channels.

77770-77772

77770 Remote afterloading high dose rate radionuclide interstitial or intracavitary brachytherapy, includes basic dosimetry, when performed; 1 channel

77771 Remote afterloading high dose rate radionuclide interstitial or intracavitary brachytherapy, includes basic dosimetry, when performed; 2-12 channels

77772 Remote afterloading high dose rate radionuclide interstitial or intracavitary brachytherapy, includes basic dosimetry, when performed; over 12 channels

Remote afterloading is performed for high dose rate (HDR) radionuclide interstitial or intracavitary brachytherapy. Basic isodose planning performed to determine optimal placement and dose of the radioactive source is included. Empty cylinders or other applicators are implanted in and around the tumor in a separately reportable procedure. Applicators are then inspected for size, placement, and stability, and adjustments are made as needed. A transfer tube is selected and connected to the channel applicator in the remote afterloading machine. Only the patient remains in the room and is monitored visually and verbally throughout the procedure. The remote afterloading machine loads the selected radioactive source into the previously placed applicators. Timers in the machine control the duration of exposure to the radioactive source. When the procedure is complete, the radioactive source is retracted and contained safely in the afterloading machine, verified by use of a room radiation detector followed by a patient radiation survey. The empty applicators are then removed from the patient. HDR radionuclide brachytherapy work is measured based on the number of catheters or channels used to deliver the radioactive source. Use code 77770 for one channel, code 77771 for two to 12 channels, or 77772 for more than 12 channels.

78012

78012 Thyroid uptake, single or multiple quantitative measurement(s) (including stimulation, suppression, or discharge, when performed)

Thyroid uptake is performed to evaluate thyroid gland function. Single or multiple uptake measurements may be obtained to determine how much iodine is absorbed by the thyroid gland and how quickly. Radioactive iodine isotopes (I-123 or I-131) are administered orally in liquid or capsule form approximately 4 hours before the thyroid uptake imaging is performed. A stationary probe is positioned over the thyroid gland in the neck and images are obtained. A second thyroid uptake determination is typically performed 24 hours after the administration of the iodine. Additional images may be obtained following the administration of substances that stimulate and/or suppress thyroid function. The images are then reviewed by the physician and written interpretation of findings provided.

78013-78014

78013 Thyroid imaging (including vascular flow, when performed)
78014 Thyroid imaging (including vascular flow, when performed); with single or multiple uptake(s) quantitative measurement(s) (including stimulation, suppression, or discharge, when performed)

Thyroid imaging, also referred to as a thyroid scan, is a type of nuclear medicine study that is used to determine the size, shape and position of the thyroid. Radioactive iodine

isotopes are administered orally in the form of a liquid or capsule or intravenously. If the radioactive tracer is administered orally the imaging procedure is performed several hours or up to 24 hours later. If the radioactive tracer is administered intravenously, the imaging procedure is performed approximately 30 minutes later. The patient positioned supine on an exam table with the head tipped back and a series of images of the thyroid gland are obtained using a gamma camera. Images of the thyroid vasculature may also be obtained. The images are reviewed by the physician and a written report of findings provided. Thyroid imaging may be performed in conjunction with thyroid uptake. Thyroid uptake is performed to evaluate thyroid gland function. Single or multiple uptake measurements may be obtained to determine how much iodine is absorbed by the thyroid gland and how quickly. Radioactive iodine isotopes (I-123 or I-131) are administered orally in liquid or capsule form approximately 4 hours before the thyroid uptake imaging is performed. A stationary probe is positioned over the thyroid gland in the neck and images are obtained. A second thyroid uptake determination is typically performed 24 hours after the administration of the iodine. Additional images may be obtained following the administration of substances that stimulate and/or suppress thyroid function. The images are then reviewed by the physician and written interpretation of findings provided. Report code 78013 when thyroid imaging is performed alone. Report code 78014 both thyroid imaging and thyroid uptake studies are performed together.

78015-78018

78015 Thyroid carcinoma metastases imaging; limited area (eg, neck and chest only)
78016 Thyroid carcinoma metastases imaging; with additional studies (eg, urinary recovery)
78018 Thyroid carcinoma metastases imaging; whole body

A nuclear medicine study is performed to determine the site(s) and extent of thyroid cancer metastatic disease. Radioactive iodine isotopes, which are also referred to as radioactive tracers, are administered orally in the form of a liquid or capsule or intravenously. If the radioactive tracer is administered orally the imaging procedure is performed several hours or up to 24 hours later. If the radioactive tracer is administered intravenously, the imaging procedure is performed approximately 30 minutes later. The radioactive isotope releases gamma rays that are detected by a gamma camera, processed by a computer with images displayed on a computer screen. In 78015, a limited region, typically the neck and chest, is evaluated for metastatic disease. A series of images of the neck and chest or another limited region are obtained using the gamma camera. The gamma camera scans the region of interest and tracks the radioisotope. If metastatic disease is present, the scanner tracks how the metastatic sites process the radioactive isotope. The gamma images are then processed and displayed on a computer screen. The images are reviewed by the physician and a written report of findings provided. In 78016, additional studies, such as urinary recovery, are performed. In 78018, a whole body metastatic survey is performed. The patient lies supine on the exam table while the front of the body is scanned and then lies prone on the exam table so that the back of the body can be scanned.

78020

78020 Thyroid carcinoma metastases uptake (List separately in addition to code for primary procedure)

Thyroid uptake is performed to evaluate function of the metastatic disease. Single or multiple uptake measurements may be obtained to determine how much iodine is absorbed by the metastases and how quickly. Radioactive iodine isotopes (I-123 or I-131) are administered orally in liquid or capsule form approximately 4 hours before the thyroid uptake imaging is performed. A stationary probe is positioned over the site of the metastatic disease and images are obtained. The images are then reviewed by the physician and written interpretation of findings provided.

78070-78072

78070 Parathyroid planar imaging (including subtraction, when performed)
78071 Parathyroid planar imaging (including subtraction, when performed); with tomographic (SPECT)
78072 Parathyroid planar imaging (including subtraction, when performed); with tomographic (SPECT), and concurrently acquired computed tomography (CT) for anatomical localization

Parathyroid planar imaging is obtained following intravenous administration of the radiopharmaceutical TC-99 sestamibi. Initial planar images are obtained shortly after administration of the radiopharmaceutical to evaluate any increased radiotracer uptake in the parathyroid tissue as compared to the thyroid tissue. Additional images are obtained approximately 2 hours later to evaluate for any retained radiotracer in the parathyroids. If subtraction studies are performed, a second radiopharmaceutical taken up only by the thyroid gland (I-123 or TC-99 pertechnetate) is administered. Subtraction images of the parathyroid glands are then obtained. Multiple imaging modalities are often used to diagnose parathyroid disease. Recent advances in parathyroid planar imaging has combined 99mTc-sestamibi with SPECT and concurrently acquired CT to improve sensitivity by combining anatomic and functional information. Use code 78070 for parathyroid planar imaging alone. Use code 78071 when planar imaging is combined with tomographic (SPECT) studies. Use 78072 when planar imaging, tomographic (SPECT) studies and concurrent CT images for anatomical localization are performed.

78205-78206

78205   Liver imaging (SPECT)
78206   Liver imaging (SPECT); with vascular flow

The physician uses single photon emission computed tomography to obtain an in-depth, layered view of the liver. The physician injects radioactive sulfur into the patient, and uses SPECT imaging to examine the radioactive sulfur as it travels through the liver. The camera is moved in a circular motion around the patient's abdomen so that three-dimensional images of liver can be produced. Code 78206 if the physician monitors the blood flow through the liver during the procedure.

78215-78216

78215   Liver and spleen imaging; static only
78216   Liver and spleen imaging; with vascular flow

The physician injects the patient with radioactive sulfur, and watches through a special camera as the sulfur is absorbed into the liver and the spleen. The physician checks to see if any part of the liver or spleen is absorbing more or less sulfur than normal; this may be a sign of cancerous cells. Code 78216 if the physician monitors blood flow into the liver and the spleen during the procedure.

78226-78227

78226   Hepatobiliary system imaging, including gallbladder when present
78227   Hepatobiliary system imaging, including gallbladder when present; with pharmacologic intervention, including quantitative measurement(s) when performed

Hepatobiliary system nuclear imaging tracks the production and flow of bile from the liver to the small intestine using a radioactive tracer that highlights the liver, bile ducts, and gallbladder if the gallbladder has not been surgically removed. This procedure may also be referred to as a HIDA scan which stands for hepatobiliary iminodiacetic acid scan. The procedure is performed to evaluate liver function, specifically bile production and excretion, and to evaluate the drainage system (bile ducts) and gallbladder for obstruction, inflammation, or other abnormalities. An intravenous catheter is placed. The radioactive tracer is injected. A gamma camera travels back and forth over the abdomen and multiple images are obtained as the radioactive tracer flows through the bloodstream and is taken up by the bile-producing cells in the liver. Images are obtained continuously as the radioactive tracer, which is now contained in the bile, travels from the liver through the biliary ducts into the gallbladder, and then from the gallbladder through the common bile duct into the duodenum. The patient is monitored throughout the procedure. Upon completion, the physician reviews the images and provides a written report of findings. In 78227, the procedure is performed as described above except that during the procedure additional medications are administered. These medications may be given to enhance the gallbladder images or to trigger the gallbladder to empty. The physician may also perform a test called gallbladder ejection fraction which is a measurement of the rate at which bile is released from the gallbladder.

78265-78266

78265   Gastric emptying imaging study (eg, solid, liquid, or both); with small bowel transit
78266   Gastric emptying imaging study (eg, solid, liquid, or both); with small bowel and colon transit, multiple days

A gastric emptying imaging study with small bowel transit (78265), or small bowel and colon transit over multiple days (78266) is performed using scintigraphy and a radiolabeled isotope tracer(s). This noninvasive study measures gastric motility in the upper and lower gastrointestinal (GI) tract and may be used for known or suspected gastroparesis, dyspepsia, abdominal pain and bloating, chronic diarrhea or constipation, idiopathic intestinal pseudo-obstruction, scleroderma, celiac disease, or malabsorption syndrome. The study is performed by suspending a single or dual isotope tracer in a meal of solids and/or liquids, which the patient ingests orally. For infants or individuals who cannot or will not eat, the isotope tracer(s) is suspended in liquid and given via nasal feeding tube or gastrostomy tube. After a prescribed period of time, the patient is positioned on the imaging table with the gamma camera over the abdomen. Scanning is performed at specific intervals and the radioactive energy emitted is converted into an image to capture movement of the material through the GI tract. The physician interprets the study and provides a written report of the findings.

78267-78268

78267   Urea breath test, C-14 (isotopic); acquisition for analysis
78268   Urea breath test, C-14 (isotopic); analysis

The patient drinks a chemical called urea, which has been fortified with a radioactive carbon isotope in an attempt to diagnose a stomach infection. Bacteria from the infection (if any) will break down the urea, and the carbon isotope will be expelled by the patient.

The physician captures the patient's exhalations for later study. Code 78268 for the analysis of the exhalations to detect the carbon isotope.

78270-78272

78270   Vitamin B-12 absorption study (eg, Schilling test); without intrinsic factor
78271   Vitamin B-12 absorption study (eg, Schilling test); with intrinsic factor
78272   Vitamin B-12 absorption studies combined, with and without intrinsic factor

The patient swallows a capsule containing radioactive vitamin B-12. A urine sample is taken after a period of time to check for its presence. If it is not present, it has not been absorbed by the body. The physician injects the patient with more radioactive B-12, as well as intrinsic agent, and takes another urine sample. If the radioactive B-12 is present, it can determined why it is not being absorbed by the body. Code 78271 if the test is performed with the intrinsic agent. Code 78272 if the test is performed both with and without the intrinsic factor.

78291

78291   Peritoneal-venous shunt patency test (eg, for LeVeen, Denver shunt)

The imaging device is placed over the abdomen and thorax to allow visualization of the pump and shunt tubing. A separately reportable injection of a radiotracer, such as TC99m-SC or TC99m-MAA, is performed. If the patient has a LeVeen shunt, the abdomen is massaged to distribute the radiotracer. If the patient has a Denver shunt, the patient is instructed to pump the system. An anterior abdominal image is obtained immediately following radiotracer injection followed by a series of images of the anterior abdomen and thorax until an hour has elapsed. If the shunt is patent, visualization of the radionuclide in lungs and/or liver will typically occur within one hour of the injection procedure. If no lung or liver visualization has occurred after 60 minutes, delayed films are obtained 2-4 hours following injection. If no visualization occurs after 4 hours, the shunt is obstructed. The physician supervises the acquisition of images and provides a written interpretation of the test.

78300-78320

78300   Bone and/or joint imaging; limited area
78305   Bone and/or joint imaging; multiple areas
78306   Bone and/or joint imaging; whole body
78315   Bone and/or joint imaging; 3 phase study
78320   Bone and/or joint imaging; tomographic (SPECT)

The physician injects a solution consisting of radioactive calcium and white blood cells into a patient. This solution will concentrate on bone fractures and sites of bone disease, allowing the physician to diagnose when the radioactive solution is viewed through a special camera. Code 78305 if multiple areas are viewed. Code 78306 if the entire body is viewed. Code 78315 if the targeted areas are viewed in a three-phase scan. Code 78320 if the physician uses a single photon emission computed tomography (SPECT) machine to take a more detailed image of the targeted area.

78350-78351

78350   Bone density (bone mineral content) study, 1 or more sites; single photon absorptiometry
78351   Bone density (bone mineral content) study, 1 or more sites; dual photon absorptiometry, 1 or more sites

The physician places a device over the patient's bone that will emit a low-level radiation field over the bone. One or two photon beams are aimed at the targeted site to measure how quickly the radiation is absorbed by the bone, which allows the physician to measure bone density. This procedure may be performed on one or more sites on the patient's body. Code 78350 if one photon beam is used, and 78351 if two photon beams are used.

78451-78452

78451   Myocardial perfusion imaging, tomographic (SPECT) (including attenuation correction, qualitative or quantitative wall motion, ejection fraction by first pass or gated technique, additional quantification, when performed); single study, at rest or stress (exercise or pharmacologic)
78452   Myocardial perfusion imaging, tomographic (SPECT) (including attenuation correction, qualitative or quantitative wall motion, ejection fraction by first pass or gated technique, additional quantification, when performed); multiple studies, at rest and/or stress (exercise or pharmacologic) and/or redistribution and/or rest reinjection

Myocardial perfusion imaging is a nuclear medicine procedure used to evaluate the heart muscle and blood flow to the heart. An intravenous line is inserted into a vein in the hand or arm. ECG leads are placed and a blood pressure cuff is placed on the arm. The patient lies flat on a table in the procedure room for myocardial perfusion imaging performed at rest. For a stress study, the patient is either on a treadmill or bike or an injection of a pharmacologic agent is administered to stress the heart. A radionuclide, also called a tracer, is injected into the intravenous line and allowed to circulate. The radionuclide localizes in healthy heart tissue. Ischemic heart tissue does not absorb the radionuclide. Images of the heart and great vessels are obtained using single photon emission computed tomography (SPECT). When SPECT images are obtained, the scanner rotates around the body to obtain images in multiple planes. The physician evaluates heart wall motion to determine how effective the heart muscle is in pumping blood through the heart and to the peripheral vascular system. Ejection fraction, which is the percentage of blood pumped out of the heart to the peripheral vascular system, is measured using either a first pass or gated technique. In a first pass technique, images are obtained as the blood circulates through the heart during the first pass of the radionuclide. In a gated technique, a series of images are obtained between heart beats. Using electrical signals from the heart, the camera captures a series of images as the heart rests, creating very sharp, high resolution images. Additional images are obtained as needed. The physician reviews the images, calculates the ejection fraction and quantifies other parameters of heart function based on the distribution of the radionuclide. The physician then provides a written report of findings. In 78451, a single study is performed at rest or stress. In 78452, multiple studies are performed at rest and/or stress. Additional injections of radionuclide may be administered and the physician may perform redistribution and/or rest reinjection studies.

78453-78454

78453   Myocardial perfusion imaging, planar (including qualitative or quantitative wall motion, ejection fraction by first pass or gated technique, additional quantification, when performed); single study, at rest or stress (exercise or pharmacologic)

78454   Myocardial perfusion imaging, planar (including qualitative or quantitative wall motion, ejection fraction by first pass or gated technique, additional quantification, when performed); multiple studies, at rest and/or stress (exercise or pharmacologic) and/or redistribution and/or rest reinjection

Myocardial perfusion imaging is a nuclear medicine procedure used to evaluate the heart muscle and blood flow to the heart. An intravenous line is inserted into a vein in the hand or arm. ECG leads are placed on the chest and a blood pressure cuff is placed on the arm. The patient lies flat on a table in the procedure room for myocardial perfusion imaging performed at rest. For a stress study, the patient is either on a treadmill or bike or an injection of a pharmacologic agent is administered to stress the heart. A radionuclide, also called a tracer, is injected into the intravenous line and allowed to circulate. The radionuclide localizes in healthy heart tissue. Ischemic heart tissue does not absorb the radionuclide. Planar films of the heart and great vessels are then obtained. The physician evaluates heart wall motion to determine how effective the heart muscle is in pumping blood through the heart and to the peripheral vascular system. Ejection fraction, which is the percentage of blood pumped out of the heart to the peripheral vascular system, is measured using either a first pass or gated technique. In a first pass technique, images are obtained as the blood circulates through the heart during the first pass of the radionuclide. In a gated technique, a series of images are obtained between heart beats. Using electrical signals from the heart, the camera captures a series of images as the heart rests, creating very sharp, high resolution images. Additional images are obtained as needed. The physician reviews the images, calculates the ejection fraction and quantifies other parameters of heart function based on the distribution of the radionuclide. The physician then provides a written report of findings. In 78453, a single study is performed at rest or stress. In 78454, multiple studies are performed at rest and/or stress. Additional injections of radionuclide may be administered and the physician may perform redistribution and/or rest reinjection studies.

Myocardial perfusion imaging planar

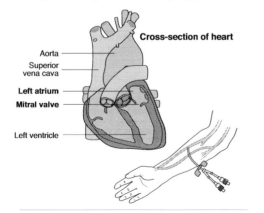

Cross-section of heart

Aorta
Superior vena cava
Left atrium
Mitral valve
Left ventricle

78466-78469

78466   Myocardial imaging, infarct avid, planar; qualitative or quantitative

78468   Myocardial imaging, infarct avid, planar; with ejection fraction by first pass technique

78469   Myocardial imaging, infarct avid, planar; tomographic SPECT with or without quantification

The physician injects the patient with a radioactive substance that will collect on heart tissue that has stopped functioning in the last 72 hours. The physician uses a special camera to observe any collections of the substance. Code 78468 if the physician uses the camera to watch the substance as it travels through the heart to diagnose any problems in overall heart function. Code 78469 if the physician views any collections of the substance on the heart with a SPECT camera, which produces highly detailed images of the heart. The camera is rotated around the patient to produce a three-dimensional view of the heart.

78481-78483

78481   Cardiac blood pool imaging (planar), first pass technique; single study, at rest or with stress (exercise and/or pharmacologic), wall motion study plus ejection fraction, with or without quantification

78483   Cardiac blood pool imaging (planar), first pass technique; multiple studies, at rest and with stress (exercise and/or pharmacologic), wall motion study plus ejection fraction, with or without quantification

Cardiac blood pool imaging is used to evaluate how effective the heart muscle is at pumping blood through the heart and to the peripheral vascular system. An intravenous line is inserted into a vein in the hand or arm. ECG leads are placed on the chest and a blood pressure cuff is placed on the arm. The patient lies flat on a table in the procedure room for myocardial perfusion imaging performed at rest. For a stress study, the patient is either on a treadmill or bike or an injection of a pharmacologic agent is administered to stress the heart. A radionuclide, also called a tracer, is injected into the intravenous line and allowed to circulate. Planar films of the heart and great vessels are then obtained. The physician evaluates heart wall motion to determine how effective the heart muscle is in pumping blood through the heart and to the peripheral vascular system. Ejection fraction, which is the percentage of blood pumped out of the heart to the peripheral vascular system, is measured using either a first pass technique. In a first pass technique, images are obtained as the blood circulates through the heart during the first pass of the radionuclide. The physician reviews the images, calculates the ejection fraction and may quantify other parameters of heart function based on the distribution of the radionuclide. The physician then provides a written report of findings. In 78481, a single study is performed at rest or with stress. In 78483, multiple studies at rest and with stress are performed.

78579-78582

78579   Pulmonary ventilation imaging (eg, aerosol or gas)
78580   Pulmonary perfusion imaging (eg, particulate)
78582   Pulmonary ventilation (eg, aerosol or gas) and perfusion imaging

Pulmonary nuclear imaging studies are performed to evaluate lung function. There are two components of lung function, ventilation and perfusion. Ventilation refers to the ability of air to reach all areas of the lung. Perfusion refers to the circulation of blood throughout lung tissue. Nuclear studies use radioactive tracers to highlight lung structures and blood flow. In 78579, pulmonary ventilation images are obtained. A gaseous radionuclide, such as xenon or technetium DTPA, contained in an aerosol is inhaled through a mouthpiece or mask. The patient inhales the aerosol taking as deep a breath as possible and then holds the breath as long as possible. Scintographic images are obtained and ventilation of the lungs is evaluated. The patient is monitored throughout the procedure and the physician reviews the images and provides a written report of findings upon completion. In 78580, pulmonary perfusion images are obtained. An intravenous catheter is placed and a radioactive tracer, such as technetium macro aggregated albumin (Tc99m-MAA), is injected. Multiple images of the lungs are obtained using a gamma camera, and the radioactive tracer is observed as blood circulates throughout the lungs. The patient is monitored through the procedure and the physician reviews the images and provides a written report of findings upon completion. In 78582, a two-phase ventilation and perfusion study is performed using the techniques described above.

78597-78598

78597   Quantitative differential pulmonary perfusion, including imaging when performed

78598   Quantitative differential pulmonary perfusion and ventilation (eg, aerosol or gas), including imaging when performed

Pulmonary nuclear imaging studies are performed to evaluate lung function. There are two components of lung function, ventilation and perfusion. Ventilation refers to the ability of air to reach all areas of the lung. Perfusion refers to the circulation of blood throughout lung tissue. Nuclear studies use radioactive tracers to highlight lung structures and blood flow. Quantitative differential pulmonary perfusion and ventilation studies compare and measure the accumulation of the radioactive tracer in different regions of the lung and/or compare and measure the accumulation of radioactive tracer in the lung and other regions of the body. In 78597, a quantitative differential perfusion study is performed. An intravenous catheter is placed and a radioactive tracer, such as technetium macro aggregated albumin (Tc99m-MAA), is injected. Multiple images of the lungs are obtained using a gamma camera. Images of other body regions may also be obtained for comparison as the radioactive tracer circulates through the lungs and other body regions. The amount of tracer that has accumulated in various regions of the lungs and other body areas is measured and compared. The patient is monitored through the procedure. The physician reviews the images and provides a written report of findings that includes measurements and comparisons of radionuclide accumulations. In 78598, a quantitative differential pulmonary perfusion and ventilation study is performed. To perform the ventilation component, a gaseous radionuclide, such as xenon or technetium DTPA, contained in an aerosol is inhaled through a mouthpiece or mask. The patient inhales the aerosol taking as deep a breath as possible and then holds the breath as long as possible. Scintigraphic images are obtained and ventilation of different lung regions is measured and then compared. The patient is monitored throughout the procedure. The physician reviews the images and provides a written report of findings including measurements and comparisons of radionuclide accumulations. The perfusion component of the scan is then performed as described above.

78600-78601

78600   Brain imaging, less than 4 static views
78601   Brain imaging, less than 4 static views; with vascular flow

Static nuclear imaging of the brain is performed with less than four views obtained, typically performed for brain death imaging. Static images are recorded at a single point in time. An intravenous injection of a radioactive tracer (radiopharmaceutical) is administered. Following injection, a radiation detector (usually a scintillation detector) is used to record the spatial distribution of the radiopharmaceutical in the brain. The images are interpreted and a written report is provided. Use 78601 when less than four static views are obtained with vascular flow imaging.

78605-78606

78605   Brain imaging, minimum 4 static views
78606   Brain imaging, minimum 4 static views; with vascular flow

Static nuclear imaging of the brain is performed with a minimum of four views obtained, typically performed for evaluation of the brain. Static images are recorded at a single point in time. An intravenous injection of a radioactive tracer (radiopharmaceutical) is administered. Following injection, a radiation detector (usually a scintillation detector) is used to record the spatial distribution of the radiopharmaceutical in the brain. The images are interpreted and a written report is provided. Use 78606 when a minimum of four static views are obtained with vascular flow imaging.

78607

78607   Brain imaging, tomographic (SPECT)

Tomographic (SPECT) imaging of the brain is performed. Single photon emission computed tomography (SPECT) studies are based on the decay of a single-photon emitting nuclide, such as technetium-99. Because blood flows at different rates in the brain depending on location and neural activity, SPECT imaging can identify areas of activity when specific tasks are performed. An intravenous injection of a radioactive tracer (radiopharmaceutical) is administered. Computed tomographic (CT) images of the brain are obtained and areas of activity and inactivity in the brain are studied. The physician provides an interpretation of the imaging and a written report of findings.

78609

78609   Brain imaging, positron emission tomography (PET); perfusion evaluation

The physician introduces a chemical substance into the patient that will decay and release positrons, which are then viewed with a PET scanner. The brain is targeted and images are taken when the substance has reached the brain. This allows the physician to determine the rate of blood flow to different parts of the brain as the radioactive substance is carried through the bloodstream.

78660

78660   Radiopharmaceutical dacryocystography

Radiopharmaceutical dacryocystography is a radiologic examination performed on the nasolacrimal ducts (tear ducts) after the injection of a radioisotope labeled medium to evaluate excessive tearing and assess patency or other pathology of the lacrimal drainage system. Types of radioisotopes used for dacryocystography include Indium and Technicium 99m. Anesthetic drops are instilled into the eyes, the lacrimal canaliculi are cannulated, and radioisotope labeled medium is injected. Radiographic images are obtained at different degrees or oblique angles to show the lacrimal pathways. The physician reviews the images and looks for evidence of pathology, such as stenosis, blockages, growths, or fistulae. A written report of findings is provided. This code reports the radiologic component of the procedure only.

78800-78804

78800   Radiopharmaceutical localization of tumor or distribution of radiopharmaceutical agent(s); limited area
78801   Radiopharmaceutical localization of tumor or distribution of radiopharmaceutical agent(s); multiple areas
78802   Radiopharmaceutical localization of tumor or distribution of radiopharmaceutical agent(s); whole body, single day imaging
78803   Radiopharmaceutical localization of tumor or distribution of radiopharmaceutical agent(s); tomographic (SPECT)
78804   Radiopharmaceutical localization of tumor or distribution of radiopharmaceutical agent(s); whole body, requiring 2 or more days imaging

The physician introduces a radioactive agent that will collect around a specific type of tumor. A limited area of the body is examined for accumulations of the substance, which indicates the presence of a tumor. Code 78801 if the physician examines multiple areas for signs of tumors, and 78802 if the entire body is examined. Code 78803 if the physician uses a SPECT camera to take very detailed images of the targeted area. The camera is rotated around the body to produce three-dimensional images of the targeted area. Code 78804 if the scanning process takes place over two or more days.

78805-78807

78805   Radiopharmaceutical localization of inflammatory process; limited area
78806   Radiopharmaceutical localization of inflammatory process; whole body
78807   Radiopharmaceutical localization of inflammatory process; tomographic (SPECT)

The physician introduces a radioactive agent into the patient that will collect around inflamed tissue. A limited area is examined for accumulations of the agent, which indicates the presence of inflamed tissue. Use 78806 is the entire body is examined; use 78807 if a tomographic (SPECT) procedure is performed.

78808

78808   Injection procedure for radiopharmaceutical localization by non-imaging probe study, intravenous (eg, parathyroid adenoma)

An intravenous injection procedure for radiopharmaceutical localization by a non-imaging probe study is performed. The injection of the radiopharmaceutical is performed prior to gamma probe localization during the surgical resection procedure in order to identify the sentinel node in breast cancer, melanoma, or other malignant tumors. It is also used during neck surgery for parathyroid tumors. The radiopharmaceutical is prepared and injected following regulatory and safety requirements and standards. The physician provides a written report of the injection procedure as well as an interpretation and report of the findings.

78811

78811   Positron emission tomography (PET) imaging; limited area (eg, chest, head/neck)

Positron emission tomography (PET) imaging, also referred to as PET scan, is performed on a limited body area such as the chest, head, or neck. PET imaging is a diagnostic imaging procedure that uses a radioactive substance (radioisotope) administered to the patient followed by acquisition of physiologic images that detect the emission of positrons from the radioactive substance in the body region being studied. PET imaging is used primarily for the detection of malignant lesions and to determine the effectiveness of treatment for malignancies. However, PET imaging is used for diagnosis and evaluation of other conditions as well. The radioisotopes used in PET imaging are short-lived and require the use of a cyclotron. The cyclotron produces the radioisotope immediately prior to the procedure and then the radioisotope is attached or tagged to a natural compound such as glucose. The radioisotope is administered intravenously or, less commonly, by inhalation. The radioisotope is then taken up by body tissues/organs. Normal and diseased tissues/organs accumulate the radioisotope at different rates and levels and so are displayed in the PET imaging as different colors or different levels of brightness. The patient is prepared for the PET imaging procedure. An intravenous line is placed. The radioisotope is administered. The patient is told to rest quietly until the radiosotope has been perfused to the body region(s) to be imaged. This may take 30 to 90 minutes. PET images are then obtained. The radiologist reviews the images, noting variations in radioisotope accumulation in the body region(s) studied. The current PET images are compared to any previously obtained radiological studies, interpreted, and a written report is provided.

78812

78812   Positron emission tomography (PET) imaging; skull base to mid-thigh

Positron emission tomography (PET) imaging, also referred to as PET scan, is performed from the skull base to mid-thigh. PET imaging is a diagnostic imaging procedure that uses a radioactive substance (radioisotope) administered to the patient followed by acquisition of physiologic images that detect the emission of positrons from the radioactive substance in the body region being studied. PET imaging is used primarily for the detection of malignant lesions and to determine the effectiveness of treatment for malignancies. However, PET imaging is used for diagnosis and evaluation of other conditions as well. The radioisotopes used in PET imaging are short-lived and require the use of a cyclotron. The cyclotron produces the radioisotope immediately prior to the procedure and then the radioisotope is attached or tagged to a natural compound such as glucose. The radioisotope is administered intravenously or, less commonly, by inhalation. The radioisotope is then taken up by body tissues/organs. Normal and diseased tissues/organs accumulate the radioisotope at different rates and levels and so are displayed in the PET imaging as different colors or different levels of brightness. The patient is prepared for the PET imaging procedure. An intravenous line is placed. The radioisotope is administered. The patient is told to rest quietly until the radiosotope has been perfused to the body region(s) to be imaged. This may take 30 to 90 minutes. PET images are then obtained. The radiologist reviews the images, noting variations in radioisotope accumulation in the body region(s) studied. The current PET images are compared to any previously obtained radiological studies, interpreted, and a written report is provided.

78813

78813   Positron emission tomography (PET) imaging; whole body

Positron emission tomography (PET) imaging, also referred to as PET scan, is performed on the whole body. PET imaging is a diagnostic imaging procedure that uses a radioactive substance (radioisotope) administered to the patient followed by acquisition of physiologic images that detect the emission of positrons from the radioactive substance in the body region being studied. PET imaging is used primarily for the detection of malignant lesions and to determine the effectiveness of treatment for malignancies. However, PET imaging is used for diagnosis and evaluation of other conditions as well. The radioisotopes used in PET imaging are short-lived and require the use of a cyclotron. The cyclotron produces the radioisotope immediately prior to the procedure and then the radioisotope is attached or tagged to a natural compound such as glucose. The radioisotope is administered intravenously or, less commonly, by inhalation. The radioisotope is then taken up by body tissues/organs. Normal and diseased tissues/organs accumulate the radioisotope at different rates and levels and so are displayed in the PET imaging as different colors or different levels of brightness. The patient is prepared for the PET imaging procedure. An intravenous line is placed. The radioisotope is administered. The patient is told to rest quietly until the radiosotope has been perfused to the body region(s) to be imaged. This may take 30 to 90 minutes. PET images are then obtained. The radiologist reviews the images, noting variations in radioisotope accumulation in the body region(s) studied. The current PET images are compared to any previously obtained radiological studies, interpreted, and a written report is provided.

78814

78814   Positron emission tomography (PET) with concurrently acquired computed tomography (CT) for attenuation correction and anatomical localization imaging; limited area (eg, chest, head/neck)

Tumor imaging using positron emission tomography (PET) concurrent with a computed tomography (CT) in order to get an accurate image of both the tumor's metabolism and its location, size, and shape.

78815

78815   Positron emission tomography (PET) with concurrently acquired computed tomography (CT) for attenuation correction and anatomical localization imaging; skull base to mid-thigh

Positron emission tomography (PET) imaging, also referred to as PET scan, is performed from the skull base to mid-thigh with a concurrently acquired computed tomography (CT) scan for correction and anatomical localization. PET imaging is a diagnostic imaging procedure that uses a radioactive substance (radioisotope) administered to the patient followed by acquisition of physiologic images that detect the emission of positrons from the radioactive substance in the body region being studied. PET imaging is used primarily for the detection of malignant lesions and to determine the effectiveness of treatment for malignancies. However, PET imaging is used for diagnosis and evaluation of other conditions as well. The radioisotopes used in PET imaging are short-lived and require the use of a cyclotron. The cyclotron produces the radioisotope immediately prior to the procedure and then the radioisotope is attached or tagged to a natural compound such as glucose. The radioisotope is administered intravenously or, less commonly, by inhalation. The radioisotope is then taken up by body tissues/organs. Normal and diseased tissues/organs accumulate the radioisotope at different rates and levels and so are displayed in the PET imaging as different colors or different levels of brightness. The patient is prepared for the PET imaging procedure. An intravenous line is placed. The radioisotope is administered. The patient is told to rest quietly until the radiosotope has been perfused to the body region(s) to be imaged. This may take 30 to 90 minutes. PET images are then obtained. CT images are obtained concurrently with the PET imaging to correct attenuation and localize anatomical structures. Attenuation of images occurs when the energy in a radiant source passes through body structures making the images less defined. Attenuation can diminish the intensity of the PET images. CT uses multiple x-ray beams combined with electronic detectors to produce a series of images (slices) that are processed on a

computer and displayed as two-dimensional images on a computer monitor. CT is used to enhance the PET images and localize specific anatomic structures. The radiologist reviews the PET and CT images, noting variations in radioisotope accumulation in the body region(s) studied. The current PET/CT images are compared to any previously obtained radiological studies, interpreted, and a written report is provided.

78816

78816   Positron emission tomography (PET) with concurrently acquired computed tomography (CT) for attenuation correction and anatomical localization imaging; whole body

Positron emission tomography (PET) imaging, also referred to as PET scan, is performed on the whole body with a concurrently acquired computed tomography (CT) scan for correction and anatomical localization. PET imaging is a diagnostic imaging procedure that uses a radioactive substance (radioisotope) administered to the patient followed by acquisition of physiologic images that detect the emission of positrons from the radioactive substance in the body region being studied. PET imaging is used primarily for the detection of malignant lesions and to determine the effectiveness of treatment for malignancies. However, PET imaging is used for diagnosis and evaluation of other conditions as well. The radioisotopes used in PET imaging are short-lived and require the use of a cyclotron. The cyclotron produces the radioisotope immediately prior to the procedure and then the radioisotope is attached or tagged to a natural compound such as glucose. The radioisotope is administered intravenously or, less commonly, by inhalation. The radioisotope is then taken up by body tissues/organs. Normal and diseased tissues/organs accumulate the radioisotope at different rates and levels and so are displayed in the PET imaging as different colors or different levels of brightness. The patient is prepared for the PET imaging procedure. An intravenous line is placed. The radioisotope is administered. The patient is told to rest quietly until the radiosotope has been perfused to the body region(s) to be imaged. This may take 30 to 90 minutes. PET images are then obtained. CT images are obtained concurrently with the PET imaging to correct attenuation and localize anatomical structures. Attenuation of images occurs when the energy in a radiant source passes through body structures, making the images less defined. Attenuation can diminish the intensity of the PET images. CT uses multiple x-ray beams combined with electronic detectors to produce a series of images (slices) that are processed on a computer and displayed as two-dimensional images on a computer monitor. CT is used to enhance the PET images and localize specific anatomic structures. The radiologist reviews the PET and CT images, noting variations in radioisotope accumulation in the body region(s) studied. The current PET/CT images are compared to any previously obtained radiological studies, interpreted, and a written report is provided.

80047-80048

80048 **Basic metabolic panel (Calcium, total)**
This panel must include the following:
Calcium, total (82310)
Carbon dioxide (bicarbonate) (82374)
Chloride (82435)
Creatinine (82565)
Glucose (82947)
Potassium (84132)
Sodium (84295)
Urea nitrogen (BUN) (84520)

80047 **Basic metabolic panel (Calcium, ionized)**
This panel must include the following:
Calcium, ionized (82330)
Carbon dioxide (bicarbonate) (82374)
Chloride (82435)
Creatinine (82565)
Glucose (82947)
Potassium (84132)
Sodium (84295)
Urea Nitrogen (BUN) (84520)

A basic metabolic blood panel is obtained that includes ionized calcium levels along with carbon dioxide (bicarbonate) (CO2), chloride, creatinine, glucose, potassium, sodium, and urea nitrogen (BUN). A basic metabolic panel with measurement of ionized calcium may be used to screen for or monitor overall metabolic function or identify imbalances. Ionized or free calcium flows freely in the blood, is not attached to any proteins, and represents the amount of calcium available to support metabolic processes such as heart function, muscle contraction, nerve function, and blood clotting. Total carbon dioxide (bicarbonate) (CO2) level is composed of CO2, bicarbonate (HCO3-), and carbonic acid (H2CO3) with the primary constituent being bicarbonate, a negatively charged electrolyte that works in conjunction with other electrolytes, such as potassium, sodium, and chloride, to maintain proper acid-base balance and electrical neutrality at the cellular level. Chloride is also a negatively charged electrolyte that helps regulate body fluid and maintain proper acid-base balance. Creatinine is a waste product excreted by the kidneys that is produced in the muscles while breaking down creatine, a compound used by the muscles to create energy. Blood levels of creatinine provide a good measurement of renal function. Glucose is a simple sugar and the main source of energy for the body, regulated by insulin. When more glucose is available than is required, it is stored in the liver as glycogen or stored in adipose tissue as fat. Glucose measurement determines whether the glucose/insulin metabolic process is functioning properly. Both potassium and sodium are positively charged electrolytes that work in conjunction with other electrolytes to regulate body fluid, stimulate muscle contraction, and maintain proper acid-base balance and both are essential for maintaining normal metabolic processes. Urea is a waste product produced in the liver by the breakdown of protein from a sequence of chemical reactions referred to as the urea or Krebs-Henseleit cycle. Urea is taken up by the kidneys and excreted in the urine. Blood urea nitrogen, BUN, is a measure of renal function, and helps monitor renal disease and the effectiveness of dialysis. Report 80048 for the same basic metabolic panel, but with total calcium measured instead of ionized calcium. Total calcium is a measurement of the total amount of both ionized (free) calcium and calcium attached (bound) to proteins circulating in the blood. The measurement can screen for or monitor a number of conditions, including those affecting the bones, heart, nerves, kidneys, and teeth.

80050

80050 **General health panel**
This panel must include the following:
Comprehensive metabolic panel (80053)
Blood count, complete (CBC), automated and automated differential WBC count (85025 or 85027 and 85004) OR Blood count, complete (CBC), automated (85027) and appropriate manual differential WBC count (85007 or 85009)
Thyroid stimulating hormone (TSH) (84443)

A general health panel is obtained that includes a comprehensive metabolic panel with albumin, bilirubin, total calcium, carbon dioxide, chloride, creatinine, glucose, alkaline phosphatase, potassium, total protein, sodium, alanine amino transferase (ALT) (SGPT), aspartate amino transferase (AST) (SGOT), urea nitrogen (BUN); a complete blood count with differential white count; and thyroid stimulating hormone (TSH). This test is used to evaluate electrolytes and fluid balance, liver and kidney function, and is used to help rule out conditions such as diabetes, thyroid disease, and anemia. Tests related to electrolytes and fluid balance include: carbon dioxide, chloride, potassium, and sodium. Tests specific to liver function include: albumin, bilirubin, alkaline phosphatase, ALT, AST, and total protein. Tests specific to kidney function: include BUN and creatinine. Calcium is needed to support metabolic processes such as heart function, muscle contraction, nerve function, and blood clotting. Glucose is the main source of energy for the body and is regulated by insulin. Glucose measurement determines whether the glucose/insulin metabolic process is functioning properly. A CBC is performed to test for anemia, infection, blood clotting disorders, as well as many other diseases. TSH is produced in the pituitary and helps to regulate two other thyroid hormones, T3 and T4, which in turn help regulate the body's metabolic processes.

80051

80051 **Electrolyte panel**
This panel must include the following:
Carbon dioxide (bicarbonate) (82374)
Chloride (82435)
Potassium (84132)
Sodium (84295)

An electrolyte panel is obtained to detect problems with fluid and electrolyte balance and monitor the health status of persons with acute or chronic medical conditions including high blood pressure, heart failure, and kidney or liver disease. The test measures electrically charged minerals such as sodium, potassium, and chloride found in body tissues and blood. Sodium is primarily found outside cells and maintains water balance in the tissues, as well as nerve and muscle function. Potassium is primarily found inside cells and affects heart rhythm, cell metabolism, and muscle function. Chloride moves freely in and out of cells to regulate fluid levels and help maintain electrical neutrality. Carbon dioxide, or bicarbonate, maintains body pH and the acid/base balance of the blood. A test called "anion gap" may be included in the electrolyte panel. Anion gap is a calculated value of the test components that measures the difference between the negatively charged ions (anions) and the positivity charged ions (cations). Anion gap values can be affected by many conditions such as metabolic disorders, starvation, and diabetes, or exposure to toxins. A blood sample is obtained by separately reportable venipuncture, heel or finger stick. Serum/plasma is tested using quantitative ion-selective electrode/enzymatic method.

80053

80053 **Comprehensive metabolic panel**
This panel must include the following:
Albumin (82040)
Bilirubin, total (82247)
Calcium, total (82310)
Carbon dioxide (bicarbonate) (82374)
Chloride (82435)
Creatinine (82565)
Glucose (82947)
Phosphatase, alkaline (84075)
Potassium (84132)
Protein, total (84155)
Sodium (84295)
Transferase, alanine amino (ALT) (SGPT) (84460) T
ransferase, aspartate amino (AST) (SGOT) (84450)
Urea nitrogen (BUN) (84520)

A comprehensive metabolic panel is obtained that includes albumin, bilirubin, total calcium, carbon dioxide, chloride, creatinine, glucose, alkaline phosphatase, potassium, total protein, sodium, alanine amino transferase (ALT) (SGPT), aspartate amino transferase (AST) (SGOT), and urea nitrogen (BUN). This test is used to evaluate electrolytes and fluid balance as well as liver and kidney function. It is also used to help rule out conditions such as diabetes. Tests related to electrolytes and fluid balance include: carbon dioxide, chloride, potassium, and sodium. Tests specific to liver function include: albumin, bilirubin, alkaline phosphatase, ALT, AST, and total protein. Tests specific to kidney function include: BUN and creatinine. Calcium is needed to support metabolic processes such as heart function, muscle contraction, nerve function, and blood clotting. Glucose is the main source of energy for the body and is regulated by insulin. Glucose measurement determines whether the glucose/insulin metabolic process is functioning properly.

80055

80055   Obstetric panel
    This panel must include the following:
    Blood count, complete (CBC), automated and automated differential WBC count (85025 or 85027 and 85004) OR Blood count, complete (CBC), automated (85027) and appropriate manual differential WBC count (85007 or 85009)
    Hepatitis B surface antigen (HBsAg) (87340)
    Antibody, rubella (86762)
    Syphilis test, non-treponemal antibody; qualitative (eg, VDRL, RPR, ART) (86592)
    Antibody screen, RBC, each serum technique (86850)
    Blood typing, ABO (86900) AND Blood typing, Rh (D) (86901)

An obstetric panel is obtained that includes a complete blood count (CBC) with differential white count; hepatitis B surface antigen (HBsAg), rubella antibody, qualitative syphilis test (VDRL, RPR, ART), red blood cell (RBC) antibody screen, and blood typing for ABO and Rh. This test is used to screen for conditions that could affect the mother and/or fetus, including anemia, blood clotting disorders, venereal disease, current hepatitis B infection, current infection or immunity to rubella, and blood incompatibilities between mother and fetus. A CBC is performed to test for anemia, infection, blood clotting disorders, as well as many other conditions. HBsAG is a protein produced by hepatitis B virus (HBV) and the earliest indicator of an acute HBV infection. This antigen is also present in individuals with chronic HBV infection. Rubella antibody test is performed to determine whether the patient has immunity to German measles, a virus that can cause fetal anomalies. Syphilis test is performed to diagnose a current infection, which can also cause fetal anomalies. ABO and Rh blood typing is performed to identify the mother's blood type, to determine the possibility of incompatibility between mother and fetus, and in anticipation of the need for transfusion. RBC antibody screen is performed in anticipation of the need for a blood transfusion to identify RBC antibodies other than those to A or B antigens.

80061

80061   Lipid panel
    This panel must include the following:
    Cholesterol, serum, total (82465)
    Lipoprotein, direct measurement, high density cholesterol (HDL cholesterol) (83718)
    Triglycerides (84478)

A lipid panel is obtained to assess the risk for cardiovascular disease and to monitor appropriate treatment. Lipids are comprised of cholesterol, protein, and triglycerides. They are stored in cells and circulate in the blood. Lipids are important for cell health and as an energy source. A lipid panel should include a measurement of triglycerides and total serum cholesterol and then calculate to find the measurement of high density lipoprotein (HDL-C), low density lipoprotein (LDL-C) and very low density lipoprotein (VLDL-C). HDL contains the highest ratio of cholesterol and is often referred to as "good cholesterol" because it is capable of transporting excess cholesterol in the blood to the liver for removal. LDL contains the highest ratio of protein and is considered "bad cholesterol" because it transports and deposits cholesterol in the walls of blood vessels. VLDL contains the highest ratio of triglycerides and high levels are also considered "bad" because it converts to LDL after depositing triglyceride molecules in the walls of blood vessels. A blood sample is obtained by separately reportable venipuncture or finger stick. Serum/plasma is tested using quantitative enzymatic method.

80069

80069   Renal function panel
    This panel must include the following:
    Albumin (82040)
    Calcium, total (82310)
    Carbon dioxide (bicarbonate) (82374)
    Chloride (82435)
    Creatinine (82565)
    Glucose (82947)
    Phosphorus inorganic (phosphate) (84100)
    Potassium (84132)
    Sodium (84295)
    Urea nitrogen (BUN) (84520)

A renal panel is obtained for routine health screening and to monitor conditions such as diabetes, renal disease, liver disease, nutritional disorders, thyroid and parathyroid function, and interventional drug therapies. Tests in a renal panel include glucose or blood sugar; electrolytes and minerals as sodium, potassium, chloride, total calcium, and phosphorus; the waste products blood urea nitrogen (BUN) and creatinine; a protein called albumin; and bicarbonate (carbon dioxide, CO2) responsible for acid base balance. Glucose is the main source of energy for the body and is regulated by insulin. High levels may indicate diabetes or impaired kidney function. Sodium is found primarily outside

cells and maintains water balance in the tissues, as well as nerve and muscle function. Potassium is primarily found inside cells and affects heart rhythm, cell metabolism, and muscle function. Chloride moves freely in and out of cells to regulate fluid levels and help maintain electrical neutrality. Calcium is needed to support metabolic processes, heart and nerve function, muscle contraction, and blood clotting. Phosphorus is essential for energy production, nerve and muscle function, and bone growth. Blood urea nitrogen (BUN) and creatinine are waste products from tissue breakdown that circulate in the blood and are filtered out by the kidneys. Albumin, a protein made by the liver, helps to nourish tissue and transport hormones, vitamins, drugs, and calcium throughout the body. Bicarbonate (HCO3) may also be referred to as carbon dioxide (CO2) maintains body pH or the acid/base balance. A specimen is obtained by separately reportable venipuncture. Serum/plasma is tested using quantitative chemiluminescent immunoassay or quantitative enzyme-linked immunosorbent assay.

80074

80074   Acute hepatitis panel
    This panel must include the following:
    Hepatitis A antibody (HAAb), IgM antibody (86709)
    Hepatitis B core antibody (HBcAb), IgM antibody (86705)
    Hepatitis B surface antigen (HBsAg) (87340)
    Hepatitis C antibody (86803)

An acute hepatitis panel is obtained to detect and diagnose acute or chronic viral liver infections. Hepatitis A virus (HAV) is highly contagious but usually causes only a mild illness. HAV is found in contaminated food and water but may also be spread person to person by close physical contact. It does not cause a chronic infection and a vaccine is available. Hepatitis B virus (HBV) is found in blood and body fluids and is the most common hepatitis virus contracted. It is a chronic infection and a vaccine is available against HBV. Hepatitis C virus is also found in blood and body fluids, and is chronic, however no vaccine is yet available to protect against this virus. Tests in an acute hepatitis panel should include Hepatitis A antibody, IgM antibody (HAAb IgM Ab), Hepatitis B core antibody, IgM antibody (HBcAb IgM Ab), Hepatitis B surface antigen (HBsAg), and Hepatitis C antibody (by CIA or Interp). Hepatitis A Virus antibody, IgM develops 2-3 weeks post exposure and remains elevated for 2-6 months. Hepatitis B Virus core antibody, IgM is produced in response to the presence of Hepatitis B core antigen. It will be elevated with acute initial infection and during flare up of disease activity in chronic infection. Hepatitis B Virus surface antigen is a protein located on the surface of HBV. Elevated levels of HBsAg may be an early sign of exposure to the virus or indicate an acute or chronic infection. When testing for Hepatitis C antibody, it is not possible to distinguish whether elevated levels are due to active acute infection or a chronic disease state unless differentiated by further testing. A specimen is obtained by separately reportable venipuncture. Serum/plasma is tested using quantitative chemiluminescent immunoassay.

80076

80076   Hepatic function panel
    This panel must include the following:
    Albumin (82040)
    Bilirubin, total (82247)
    Bilirubin, direct (82248)
    Phosphatase, alkaline (84075)
    Protein, total (84155)
    Transferase, alanine amino (ALT) (SGPT) (84460)
    Transferase, aspartate amino (AST) (SGOT) (84450)

A hepatic function panel is obtained to diagnose acute and chronic liver disease, inflammation, or scarring and to monitor hepatic function while taking certain medications. Tests in a hepatic function panel should include albumin (ALB), total and direct bilirubin, alkaline phosphatase (ALP), total protein (TP), alanine aminotransferase (ALT, SGPT), and aspartate aminotransferase (AST, SGOT). Albumin (ALB) is a protein made by the liver that helps to nourish tissue and transport hormones, vitamins, drugs, and calcium throughout the body. Bilirubin, a waste product from the breakdown of red blood cells, is removed by the liver in a conjugated state. Bilirubin is measured as total (all the bilirubin circulating in the blood) and direct (the conjugated amount only) to determine how well the liver is performing. Alkaline phosphatase (ALP) is an enzyme produced by the liver and other organs of the body. In the liver, cells along the bile duct produce ALP. Blockage of these ducts can cause elevated levels of ALP, whereas cirrhosis, cancer, and toxic drugs will decrease ALP levels. Circulating blood proteins include albumin (60% of total) and globulins (40% of total). By measuring total protein (TP) and albumin (ALB), the albumin/globulin (A/G) ratio can be determined and monitored. TP may decrease with malnutrition, congestive heart failure, hepatic disease, and renal disease and increase with inflammation and dehydration. Alanine aminotransferase (ALT, SGPT) is an enzyme produced primarily in the liver and kidneys. In healthy individuals ALT is normally low. ALT is released when the liver is damaged, especially with exposure to toxic substances such as drugs and alcohol. Aspartate aminotransferase (AST, SGOT) is an enzyme produced by the liver, heart, kidneys, and muscles. In healthy individuals AST is normally low. An AST/ALT ratio is often performed to determine if elevated levels are due to liver injury or damage to the heart or skeletal muscles. A specimen is obtained by separately reportable venipuncture. Serum/plasma is tested using quantitative enzymatic method or quantitative spectrophotometry.

80081

80081   Obstetric panel (includes HIV testing)
This panel must include the following:
Blood count, complete (CBC), and automated differential WBC count (85025 or 85027 and 85004) OR Blood count, complete (CBC), automated (85027) and appropriate manual differential WBC count (85007 or 85009)
Hepatitis B surface antigen (HBsAg) (87340)
HIV-1 antigen(s), with HIV-1 and HIV-2 antibodies, single result (87389)
Antibody, rubella (86762)
Syphilis test, non-treponemal antibody; qualitative (eg, VDRL, RPR, ART) (86592)
Antibody screen, RBC, each serum technique (86850)
Blood typing, ABO (86900) AND Blood typing, Rh (D) (86901)

A panel of laboratory tests is performed on maternal blood prior to or during pregnancy to identify and monitor certain medical conditions including infection, anemia, coagulopathy, or immune disorders that may affect the health of mother and baby. Code 80081 includes an automated complete blood count (CBC) with an automated differential WBC or manual differential white blood cell (WBC) count. A CBC includes measurement of hemoglobin (Hgb) and hematocrit (Hct), red blood cell (RBC) count, white blood cell (WBC) count, and platelet count. Hct refers to the volume of red blood cells (erythrocytes) in a given volume of blood and is usually expressed as a percentage of total blood volume. RBC count is the number of erythrocytes in a specific volume of blood. WBC count is the number of white blood cells (leukocytes) in a specific volume of blood. There are five types of WBCs: neutrophils, eosinophils, basophils, monocytes, and lymphocytes. In a differential, each of the five types is counted separately. Platelet count is the number of thrombocytes in the blood, responsible for blood clotting. The obstetric panel must also include Hepatitis B surface antigen (HBsAg), human immunodeficiency virus-1 (HIV-1) antigen with HIV-1 and HIV-2 antibodies, rubella antibody, syphilis non-treponemal antibody (VDRL, RPR, ART), RBC antibody screen, ABO and Rh D blood typing.

80150

80150   Amikacin
A blood test is performed to measure Amikacin levels at random, peak or trough times. Amikacin is an injectable aminoglycoside prescribed to treat severe or serious gram negative systemic bacterial infections. Blood level monitoring is necessary because the drug has the potential to cause auditory, vestibular, and renal toxicity and neuromuscular blockade (paralysis of muscles including those used for breathing). A random sample may be drawn any time. Peak and trough levels are time-dependant and are usually drawn 24 hours after initiating therapy and every 2-3 days thereafter. A trough level is drawn 30 minutes prior to intravenous infusion or intramuscular injection. A peak level is drawn 15-30 minutes after intravenous infusion is complete or 90 minutes after an intramuscular injection. A blood sample is obtained by separately reportable venipuncture. Blood serum is then tested using fluorescence polarization immunoassay.

80155

80155   Caffeine
A blood test is performed to measure caffeine levels. Caffeine (a methylxanthine) stimulates breathing and may be used to treat apnea in premature infants. Random blood samples are drawn to establish and maintain therapeutic levels of the drug. A blood sample is obtained by separately reportable venipuncture or heel stick. Serum/plasma is tested using quantitative enzyme multiplied immunoassay technique.

80156-80157

80156   Carbamazepine; total
80157   Carbamazepine; free
A laboratory test is performed to determine total (80156) or free (80157) carbamazepine levels. Carbamazepine, also referred to as Tegretol, is an anticonvulsant used to treat epilepsy and may also be used as an analgesic to treat trigeminal neuralgia. Carbamazepine, carbamazepine metabolite (10,11-epoxide), and free carbamazepine are routinely measured to determine optimal doses in patients with epilepsy as well as to monitor for carbamazepine toxicity. A blood sample is obtained by separately reportable venipuncture. Blood serum is then tested using one of several techniques including high performance liquid chromatography or fluorescent polarization immunoassay. Total carbamazepine tests the total amount present in the blood. Under normal circumstances, circulating carbamazepine is 75% protein bound. In some patients carbamazepine may be displaced from protein resulting in higher levels of free carbamazepine circulating in the blood. In these patients, lower levels of the drug may result in toxicity, so the unbound (free) levels must be monitored.

80158

80158   Cyclosporine
A blood test performed to measure cyclosporine levels. Cyclosporine, also known as Sandimmune, Gengraf, or Neoral can be administered in oral and injectable form and Restasis in ophthalmic solution, is an immunosuppressant drug that affects the ability of certain white blood cells in the body to recognize and respond to transplanted bone marrow and body organs such as kidney, liver, heart and lung. The drug may also be used to treat rheumatoid arthritis, psoriasis, aplastic anemia, Crohn's disease and increase tear production in keratoconjunctivitis sicca (severe dry eyes). For transplant patients the therapeutic levels may be assessed daily at the start of therapy, taper to 1-2 times per week and finally to once every 1-2 months. For routine monitoring the specimen is collected 12 hours after a dose. In new transplant patients peak levels may be drawn 2 hours after a dose and trough levels immediately prior to a dose. A blood sample is obtained by a separately reportable venipuncture. Whole blood is then tested using liquid chromatography-tandem mass spectrometry. Sandimmune may be tested with chromatographic or immunoassay technique and the results will be somewhat different. Make note of the technique used when comparing results with previous levels.

80159

80159   Clozapine
A blood test is performed to measure clozapine levels. Clozapine (Clozaril, FazaCol, Froidir, Leponex) is an atypical antipsychotic that changes the activity of certain chemicals in the brain. It is used to treat schizophrenia in patients who are unresponsive or intolerant to other drugs. Clozapine levels should be monitored by pre-dose (trough) blood draws. A blood sample is obtained by separately reportable venipuncture. Serum/plasma is tested using quantitative liquid chromatography-tandem mass spectrometry.

80162-80163

80162   Digoxin; total
80163   Digoxin; free
A laboratory test is performed to measure digoxin levels. Digoxin, also known as Lanoxin, is a cardiac glycoside that controls sodium and potassium levels in the cells. Digoxin is primarily prescribed to treat atrial fibrillation, atrial flutter, and congestive heart failure. The drug increases the strength of cardiac muscle contractions which increases cardiac output and lowers the heart rate and venous pressure. Digoxin has a narrow therapeutic window but antidotal treatment is available (Digibind, Digoxin Immune FAB). The test for total digoxin (80162) measures Fab fragment-bound (inactive) digoxin and free (active) digoxin. This test is primarily used to monitor digoxin therapy and should be drawn 8-12 hours following an oral dose. The test for free digoxin (80163) may be used to evaluate breakthrough digoxin toxicity in patients with renal failure, access the need for additional antidigoxin Fab, determine when to reintroduce digoxin therapy, and monitor patients with possible digoxin-like immune reactive factors. To measure free digoxin, a blood sample is obtained by separately reportable venipuncture 6-8 hours after the last dose. Serum is tested for total digoxin using immunoassay and for free digoxin using ultrafiltration followed by electrochemiluminescent immunoassay.

80164-80165

80164   Valproic acid (dipropylacetic acid); total
80165   Valproic acid (dipropylacetic acid); free
A laboratory test is performed to measure valproic acid (dipropylacetic acid, depakote). Valproic acid is an anticonvulsant that may be used to treat seizure disorders, manic phase of bipolar disorders, and migraine headaches. The drug works by changing certain chemicals neurotransmitters in the brain. The test for total valproic acid (80164) can be used to monitor drug therapy, assess patient compliance, and evaluate for potential toxicity. The test for free valproic acid (80165) may be used to evaluate the cause of toxicity when the total valproic acid concentration is within the normal range. Free valproic acid may be elevated in patients with an altered or unpredictable protein binding capacity. A blood sample is obtained by separately reportable venipuncture just prior to medication administration to obtain the trough level. Serum/plasma is tested for total valproic acid using fluorescence polarization immunoassay and for free valproic acid using quantitative enzyme multiplied immunoassay.

80168

80168   Ethosuximide
A blood test is performed to measure ethosuximide levels. Ethosuximide also known as Zarontin, is an anticonvulsant drug and is prescribed to treat seizures. The drug is administered orally and blood concentration levels are monitored at the start of treatment, at regular intervals to maintain therapeutic levels and when symptoms/breakthrough seizure activity occurs, indicating possible low therapeutic blood levels. A blood sample is obtained by a separately reportable venipuncture. Blood serum is then tested using enzyme immunoassay.

Pathology and Laboratory

80169

80169   Everolimus

A blood test is performed to measure everolimus levels. Everolimus (Zortress, Certican, Afinitor) is an immunosuppressive agent that is used to prevent organ rejection (Zortress, Certican) in patients with kidney or liver transplants and to treat certain cancers (Afinitor) including advanced renal cell carcinoma (aRCC), subependymal giant cell astrocytoma (SEGA) associated with tuberous sclerosis complex (TSC) when the patient cannot undergo curative surgical resection, progressive or metastatic pancreatic neuroendocrine tumors (PNET) not surgically removable, and advanced hormone-receptor positive HER2-negative breast cancer in post-menopausal women. Everolimus levels should be monitored by pre-dose (trough) blood draws. A blood sample is obtained by separately reportable venipuncture. Whole blood is tested using quantitative liquid chromatography-tandem mass spectrometry.

80170

80170   Gentamicin

A blood test is performed to measure gentamicin levels at random, peak and trough times. Gentamicin, also know as Garamycin, Cidomycin or Septopal is an injectable aminoglycoside prescribed to treat severe or serious bacterial infections. Blood level monitoring is necessary because the drug has the potential to cause auditory, vestibular and renal toxicity. A random sample may be drawn any time, peak and trough levels are time dependant and are usually drawn 24 hours after initiating therapy and every 2-3 days thereafter. A trough level is drawn 30 minutes prior to intravenous infusion or intramuscular injection. A peak level is drawn 15-30 minutes after intravenous infusion is complete or 90 minutes after an intramuscular injection. A blood sample is obtained by separately reportable venipuncture. Blood serum is then tested using fluorescence polarization immunoassay.

80171

80171   Gabapentin, whole blood, serum, or plasma

A blood test is performed to measure gabapentin levels. Gabapentin (Gabarone, Neurontin) is an analog of gamma-aminobutyric acid (GABA), a neurotransmitter produced by the brain, and is used to treat seizure disorders and chronic neuropathic pain. The drug may also be prescribed "off label" for migraine headaches and bipolar disorder. A blood sample is obtained by separately reportable venipuncture. Whole blood, serum, or plasma is tested using quantitative liquid chromatography-tandem mass spectrometry.

80173

80173   Haloperidol

A blood test is performed to monitor haloperidol level. Haloperidol, also referred to as Haldol, is used to treat schizophrenia and may also be used to treat tics and vocal utterances in Tourette's syndrome. A blood specimen is obtained by separately reportable venipuncture. Blood serum or plasma is tested using high performance liquid chromatography or gas chromatography. This test is performed to monitor haloperidol for optimal dosing and to prevent toxicity.

80175

80175   Lamotrigine

A blood test is performed to measure lamotrigine levels. Lamotrigine (Lamictal) is an anticonvulsant from the phenyltrizine class of medications and is used to treat seizure disorders and bipolar disorders. The drug may also be prescribed "off label" for peripheral neuropathy, migraine headaches and depression (without mania). A blood sample is obtained by separately reportable venipuncture. Serum/plasma is tested using quantitative enzyme immunoassay.

80176

80176   Lidocaine

A blood test is performed to measure lidocaine levels. Lidocaine, also know as Xylocaine is an anesthetic agent which acts as a central neural blockade (increasing cardiac output, peripheral resistance and mean arterial pressure) when administered intravenously for cardiac arrhythmia prophylaxis. Blood levels are assessed 12 hours after initiating therapy and then every 24 hours until medication is discontinued. A blood sample is obtained by a separately reportable venipuncture. Blood serum is then tested using fluorescence polarization immunoassay.

80177

80177   Levetiracetam

A blood test is performed to measure levetiracetam levels. Levetiracetam (Keppra) is an anticonvulsant medication used to treat seizure disorders. The drug may also be prescribed "off label" for neuropathic pain, Tourette syndrome, autism, bipolar disorder, anxiety disorder and Alzheimer's disease. A blood sample is obtained by separately reportable venipuncture. Serum/plasma is tested using quantitative enzyme immunoassay.

80178

80178   Lithium

A blood test is performed to measure lithium levels. Lithium (carbonate), also known as Eskalith or Lithobid, is a neurotransmitter that affects the flow of sodium through nerve and muscle cells. It is used to stabilize the manic phase in patients with bipolar disorder and may also be prescribed to treat cluster headaches and bipolar depression. Lithium has a very narrow therapeutic range and blood levels are monitored frequently at the beginning of therapy, when dose is being adjusted, for suspected high or low levels and then at regular intervals when on maintenance doses. Blood should be drawn 12 hours after the last dose. A blood sample is obtained by a separately reportable venipuncture. Blood serum is then tested using reflectance spectrophotometry.

80180

80180   Mycophenolate (mycophenolic acid)

A blood test is performed to measure mycophenolate levels. Mycophenolate (mycophenolic acid, CellCept, Myfortic) is an immunosuppressant agent used to prevent organ rejection in patients with kidney, liver, heart or lung transplants. Mycopenolate levels should be monitored by pre-dose (trough) blood draws. A blood sample is obtained by separately reportable venipuncture. Serum/plasma is tested for mycophenolic acid using high performance liquid chromatography or for mycophenolic acid and metabolites using quantitative tandem mass spectrometry.

80183

80183   Oxcarbazepine

A blood test is performed to measure Oxcarbazepine levels. Oxcarbazepine (Trileptal) is an anticonvulsant and mood stabilizing medication used to treat seizure disorders. The drug may also be prescribed "off label" for anxiety, mood disorders, and benign motor tics. A blood sample is obtained by separately reportable venipuncture. Serum/plasma is tested for oxcarbazepine metabolite using quantitative liquid chromatography-tandem mass spectrometry.

80184

80184   Phenobarbital

A blood test is performed to measure phenobarbital levels. Phenobarbital, also known as Luminal, is an anticonvulsant/hypnotic prescribed to treat seizures and insomnia by decreasing electrical activity in the brain. The drug may be administered orally or by injection. Blood concentration levels are monitored at regular intervals and also when breakthrough seizure activity or over sedation occurs, indicating possible high/low therapeutic blood levels. A blood sample is obtained by a separately reportable venipuncture. Blood serum is then tested using high performance liquid chromatography.

80185-80186

80185   Phenytoin; total
80186   Phenytoin; free

A blood test is performed to measure phenytoin total (80185) and phenytoin free (80186) levels. Phenytoin also known as Dilantin, Phenytek or Prompt, is an anticonvulsant prescribed to treat seizures and works by deceasing electrical activity in the brain. The drug may be administered orally or by injection. Phenytoin has a narrow therapeutic range and the patient should be monitored for both total and free phenytoin levels. Total phenytoin reflects the total serum concentration of the drug while free phenytoin levels reflect the unbound levels. Only the unbound levels are biologically active. Ninety (90) percent of the drug is typically highly bound and biologically inactive, but bound phenytoin is sensitive to displacement by other protein binding drugs which can elevate levels of free phenytoin in the blood. Blood concentration levels are monitored at regular intervals and also when breakthrough seizures occur, indicating possible low therapeutic levels. A blood sample is obtained by a separately reportable venipuncture. Blood serum is then tested using immunoassay.

80188

80188   Primidone

A blood test is performed to measure primidone levels. Primidone, also known as Mysoline, is an anticonvulsant prescribed to treat seizures and essential tremor and works by deceasing electrical activity in the brain. The drug is administered orally. Blood concentration levels are monitored at regular intervals and also when breakthrough seizures occur, indicating possible low therapeutic levels. A blood sample is obtained by a separately reportable venipuncture. Blood serum is then tested using fluorescence polarization immunoassay.

80190-80192

80190   Procainamide
80192   Procainamide; with metabolites (eg, n-acetyl procainamide)

A blood test is performed to measure procainamide (80190) and/or procainamide with metabolites, specifically n-acetyl procainamide (80192) levels. Procainamide, also known as Procan, Procanbid or Pronestyl is a cardiac antidysrhythmic drug that blocks abnormal electrical impulses in the heart. It is used to treat ventricular tachycardia and may be administered orally or by injection. Blood concentration levels are monitored at regular intervals to assess therapeutic drug levels. Procainamide may cause a condition known as antinuclear antibody formation with symptoms/syndrome similar to systemic lupus erythematosis. A blood sample is obtained by a separately reportable venipuncture. Blood serum is then tested using fluorescence polarization immunoassay.

80194

80194   Quinidine

A blood test is performed to measure quinidine levels. Quinidine, also known as Cardioquin, Quinora or Quinidex, has 2 pharmacological uses. The first is for ventricular and atrial cardiac dysrhythmia to block abnormal electrical impulses in the heart. The second is for treatment of malaria. The drug may be administered orally or by injection. Blood concentration levels are monitored at regular intervals to assess therapeutic drug levels. A blood sample is obtained by a separately reportable venipuncture. Blood serum is then tested using fluorescence polarization immunoassay.

80195

80195   Sirolimus

A blood test is performed to measure sirolimus levels. Sirolimus, also known as Rapamune is an immunosuppressant drug that affects the ability of certain white blood cells in the body to recognize and respond to transplanted body organs such as kidney, liver and heart. The drug is administered orally, either alone or in combination with other immunosuppressant drugs. Sirolimus has a narrow therapeutic range and blood levels may be assessed daily at the start of therapy, taper to 1-2 times week and finally to once every 1-2 months. For routine monitoring the specimen is collected as a trough level, immediately prior to a scheduled dose and at least 12 hours after the previous dose. A blood sample is obtained by a separately reportable venipuncture. Whole blood is then tested using liquid chromatography-tandem mass spectrometry. Sirolimus may be tested with chromatographic or immunoassay technique and the results will be somewhat different.

80197

80197   Tacrolimus

A blood test is performed to measure tacrolimus levels. Tacrolimus, also known as Prograf is an immunosuppressant drug that affects the ability of certain white blood cells in the body to recognize and respond to transplanted body organs such as kidney, liver, heart and lung. The drug is administered intravenously, either alone or in combination with other immunosuppressant drugs. Tacrolimus has a narrow therapeutic range and blood levels may be assessed daily at the start of therapy, taper to 1-2 times per week and finally to once every 1-2 months. For routine monitoring the specimen is collected as a trough level, immediately prior to a scheduled dose and at least 12 hours after the previous dose. A blood sample is obtained by a separately reportable venipuncture. Whole blood is then tested using liquid chromatography-tandem mass spectrometry. Prograf may be tested with chromatographic or immunoassay technique and the results will be somewhat different. Make note of the technique used when comparing results with previous levels.

80198

80198   Theophylline

A blood test is performed to measure theophylline levels. Theophylline, also known as Aminophylline, Uniphyl or Elixophylline can be administered orally or intravenously to relax the muscles of the lungs and chest, making them less reactive to allergens and bronchospasm. It is used to treat acute bronchitis and chronic respiratory conditions such as asthma and emphysema and may also be administered to neonates to treat apnea. A blood sample is obtained by separately reportable venipuncture. Serum is then tested using reflectance spectrophotometry.

80199

80199   Tiagabine

A blood test is performed to measure tiagabine levels. Tiagabine (Gabitril) is an anticonvulsant medication used as an adjunct treatment for partial seizure disorders in patients over the age of 12. The drug may also be prescribed "off label" for anxiety disorders and neuropathic pain. Tiagabine levels should be monitored by pre-dose (trough) blood draws. A blood sample is obtained by separately reportable venipuncture. Serum/plasma is tested using high performance liquid chromatography/tandem mass spectrometry.

80200

80200   Tobramycin

A blood test is performed to measure tobramycin levels. The levels may be measured at random, peak and trough times. Tobramycin is an injectable aminoglycoside prescribed to treat severe or serious bacterial infections. Blood level monitoring is necessary because the drug has the potential to cause auditory, vestibular and renal toxicity. A random sample may be drawn any time. Peak and trough levels are time dependant and are usually drawn 24 hours after initiating therapy and every 2-3 days thereafter. A trough level is drawn 5-90 minutes prior to intravenous infusion or intramuscular injection. A peak level is drawn 30 minutes after intravenous infusion is complete and 30-90 minutes after an intramuscular injection. A blood sample is obtained by separately reportable venipuncture. Blood serum is then tested using fluorescence polarization immunoassay.

80201

80201   Topiramate

A blood test is performed to measure topiramate levels. Topiramate, also known as Topamax is an anticonvulsant prescribed to treat seizures, migraine headaches and essential tremor and works by decasing electrical activity in the brain. The drug is administered orally. Blood concentration levels are monitored at regular intervals and also when breakthrough seizures occur, indicating possible low therapeutic levels. A blood sample is obtained by a separately reportable venipuncture. Blood serum is then tested using fluorescence polarization immunoassay.

80202

80202   Vancomycin

A blood test is performed to measure vancomycin levels at random, peak and trough times. Vancomycin, also known as Vancocin is a glycopeptide antibiotic prescribed to treat severe or serious bacterial infections. For systemic infections it is administered by intravenous infusion. For intestinal infections such as colitis or clostridium difficile it is taken orally. Blood level monitoring is necessary because the drug has the potential to cause auditory toxicity. A random sample may be drawn any time, peak and trough levels are time dependant and are usually drawn 24 hours after initiating therapy and every 2-3 days thereafter. A trough level is drawn 10 minutes prior to intravenous infusion. A peak level is drawn 1-2 hours after intravenous infusion is complete. A blood sample is obtained by separately reportable venipuncture. Blood serum is then tested using fluorescence polarization immunoassay.

80203

80203   Zonisamide

A blood test is performed to measure zonisamide levels. Zonisamide (Excegran, Zonegran) is a sulfonamide anticonvulsant medication used as an adjunct treatment for partial-onset seizures in adults. The drug may also be prescribed "off label" for migraine headaches, neuropathic pain and bipolar disorder. Zonisamide is currently in clinical trials for Parkinson's Disease under the trade name Tremode and for obesity under the trade name Empatic. Zonisamide levels should be monitored by pre-dose (trough) blood draws. A blood sample is obtained by separately reportable venipuncture. Serum/plasma is tested using quantitative enzyme multiplied immunoassay technique.

80299

80299   Quantitation of therapeutic drug, not elsewhere specified

A drug test is performed to detect the presence and quantity of any therapeutic drug not listed with a specific code for reporting purposes.

80320

80320   Alcohols

A laboratory test is performed to measure alcohol (ethanol, methanol, isopropanol) in blood or body fluids. In the clinical setting, the level of alcohol in serum, plasma, and whole blood may be used to diagnose, evaluate, and treat certain medical conditions, or used as part of drug abuse screening. Breath and saliva testing for alcohol is more often used in a point of care setting for medical or legal purposes. Alcohol distributes in body fluid in proportion to the water content of that fluid. Plasma and serum levels will be 12-18% higher than whole blood; saliva will be 7% higher than whole blood; and urine will be 30% higher than whole blood. Serum, plasma, whole blood, saliva, and/or urine may be tested using gas chromatography and/or enzymatic oxidation assay. Gas chromatography takes longer to perform but can quantitatively evaluate ethanol and also identify methanol and isopropanol. Enzymatic oxidation assay (EOA) is a rapid test using alcohol dehydrogenase to produce a visible color change when alcohol is present in a specimen. EOA may also be adapted for clinical chemistry instrumentation; however, it is not specific for ethanol and may miss methanol and isopropanol entirely.

Pathology and Laboratory

80321-80322

80321   Alcohol biomarkers; 1 or 2
80322   Alcohol biomarkers; 3 or more

A laboratory test is performed to measure alcohol biomarkers in serum, plasma, urine, saliva, or hair. Biomarkers include carbohydrate-deficient transferrin (CDT), fatty acid ethyl esters, ethyl sulfate, ethyl glucuronide, and phosphatidylethanol. The presence of alcohol biomarkers are an indication of alcohol exposure or ingestion and may be used to detect current drinking or recent relapse/binge drinking. CDT can be used as a marker for chronic alcoholism because it causes transient changes in the glycosylation pattern of transferrin. The level of CDT will normalize within a few weeks of alcohol abstinence. Serum is tested for CDT using standardized affinity chromatography or by rapid test using immunoaffinity liquid chromatography and electrospray mass spectrometry. Fatty acid ethyl esters (FAEE) are formed when fatty acids are exposed to alcohol. Measuring serum levels and/or hair samples for FAEE can help differentiate chronic alcohol abusers from binge drinkers. Samples are tested using gas chromatography/mass spectrometry. Ethyl sulfate (EtS) is usually tested in conjunction with ethyl glucuronide (EtG) to detect recent alcohol consumption. These biomarkers are broken down by different pathways in the body and when measured together will increase the sensitivity of the test. Urine and hair are tested for EtS and EtG using liquid chromatography-tandem mass spectrometry. The metabolite EtG may be present in urine for up to 80 hours post ingestion and in hair for 7-90 days. Phosphatidylethanol (PEth) measures an abnormal phospholipid formed on red blood cells following exposure to alcohol. PEth testing is helpful when identifying binge or prolonged drinking, and because it is less sensitive to small amounts of alcohol than EtS or EtG, it may be used to determine incidental exposure such as mouthwash and antibacterial hand cleaners. Serum is tested for PEth using high performance liquid chromatography-tandem mass spectrometry. Use code 80321 for identifying 1 or 2 alcohol biomarkers and 80322 when identifying 3 or more.

80323

80323   Alkaloids, not otherwise specified

A laboratory test is performed to measure alkaloids. Alkaloids are naturally occurring chemical compounds comprised of basic nitrogen atoms. The two most common forms are true alkaloids, which contain nitrogen in the heterocycle that originates from amino acids, and protoalkaloids that have nitrogen originating directly from the amino acids. Bacteria, fungi, plants, and animals can all produce alkaloid compounds that may be toxic to people, animals, and the environment. The pharmacological effects of alkaloids have been used for centuries in medications, for recreation drug use, and for entheogenic rituals. Alkaloid examples include local anesthetics, cocaine, caffeine, and nicotine (stimulants), morphine (analgesic), atropine (anti-cholinergic), quinidine (anti-arrhythmic), quinine (anti-malarial), berberine (antibacterial), vincristine (anti-neoplastic), reserpine (antihypertensive), ephedrine (bronchodilator), and the hallucinogens psilocin and mescaline. Serum and urine may be tested using high performance liquid chromatography/tandem mass spectrometry.

80324-80326

80324   Amphetamines; 1 or 2
80325   Amphetamines; 3 or 4
80326   Amphetamines; 5 or more

A laboratory test is performed to measure amphetamines in serum, urine, saliva, hair, and/or stool. Amphetamine is a broad representation of central nervous system stimulants used primarily to treat attention deficient hyperactivity disorder (ADHD) and narcolepsy. The designer drugs methylenedioxyamphetamine (MDA), methylenedioxymethamphetamine (MDMA, Ecstasy), and methylenedioxyethylamphetamine (MDEA, Eve) have a hallucinogenic as well as a stimulant effect on the central nervous system. Amphetamines can be very addictive and are often highly abused. The drug or its metabolites can be measured in blood or serum for up to 12 hours following ingestion, in urine for 2-5 days, in saliva for 1-5 days, and in hair for up to 90 days. Serum, urine, and stool are tested using high performance liquid chromatography/tandem mass spectrometry. Hair samples are tested using gas chromatography/mass spectrometry. Saliva is tested using rapid immunochromatographic assay. Code 80324 is used to test for 1 or 2 amphetamines. Code 80325 is used when testing for 3 or 4 amphetamines, and code 80326 is used when testing for 5 or more amphetamines.

80327-80328

80327   Anabolic steroids; 1 or 2
80328   Anabolic steroids; 3 or more

A laboratory test is performed to measure anabolic steroids in urine. Anabolic steroids (anabolic-androgenic steroids, AAS) are synthetic variants of the male sex hormone testosterone. These drugs may be prescribed to treat male hormone deficiency syndromes, delayed puberty, and muscle wasting diseases such as cancer and AIDS. Anabolic steroids are often abused by individuals to enhance performance or improve physical appearance. When anabolic steroids are abused, they may be combined with nonsteroidal compounds, called stacking, or used sporadically, known as cycling. In addition to increasing muscle

mass, steroids can cause mood swings and impaired judgment. Anabolic steroid compounds that can be identified in urine include bolasterone, boldenone, clenbuterol (and metabolite), clostebol, creatinine, drostanolone metabolite, epitestosterone, fluoxymesterone, methandienone (and metabolite), methenolone, methyltestosterone, nandrolone (and metabolite), norandrostenedione, norethandrolone (and metabolite), norethindrone, oxandrolone, oxymetholone metabolite, probenecid, stanozolol (and metabolite), testosterone, tetrahydrogestrinone, trenbolone metabolite and turinabol. A urine sample is obtained by separately reportable random void or catheterization. Urine is tested using qualitative colorimetry/high performance liquid chromatography/tandem mass spectrometry. Code 80327 is used when testing for 1 or 2 anabolic steroids. Code 80328 is used when identifying 3 or more anabolic steroid compounds.

80329-80331

80329   Analgesics, non-opioid; 1 or 2
80330   Analgesics, non-opioid; 3-5
80331   Analgesics, non-opioid; 6 or more

A laboratory test is performed to measure non-opioid analgesics in urine, serum, or plasma. Non-opioid analgesics include salicylates (aspirin), acetaminophen, the non-steroidal anti-inflammatory drugs (NSAIDS) ibuprofen and naproxen sodium, and selective cyclooxygenase-2 (COX-2) inhibitors (Celebrex). These drugs can be used to treat acute or chronic, mild to moderate pain and may be combined with opioids or other compounds to treat moderate to severe pain. In addition to relieving pain, many analgesics have anti-inflammatory and/or anti-pyretic properties. Salicylates in serum or plasma and acetaminophen in plasma are tested for using spectrophotometry. Ibuprofen in serum or plasma and naproxen sodium is tested for using high performance liquid chromatography. Code 80329 is used when testing for 1 or 2 non-opioid analgesic compounds. Code 80330 is used for 3-5 non-opioid analgesics, and code 80331 is used when identifying 6 or more.

80332-80334

80332   Antidepressants, serotonergic class; 1 or 2
80333   Antidepressants, serotonergic class; 3-5
80334   Antidepressants, serotonergic class; 6 or more

A laboratory test is performed to measure serotonergic antidepressants. Selective serotonin reuptake inhibitors (SSRIs) increase circulating levels of serotonin by inhibiting the reuptake of the neurotransmitter by the brain. They may be used to treat depression, anxiety disorders, chronic pain, and posttraumatic stress disorder (PTSD). Drugs in this class include citalopram (Celexa), escitalopram (Lexapro), fluvoxamine (Luvox), paroxetine (Paxil), fluoxetine (Prozac), and sertraline (Zoloft). A blood sample is obtained by separately reportable venipuncture. Serum or plasma is tested for citalopram, escitalopram, paroxetine, or sertraline using quantitative liquid chromatography-tandem mass spectrometry, for fluvoxamine using gas chromatography, and for fluoxetine using quantitative high performance liquid chromatography. Code 80332 is used when testing for 1 or 2 compounds; code 80333 is used for 3-5 compounds; and code 80334 is used when evaluating 6 or more serotonergic antidepressants.

80335-80337

80335   Antidepressants, tricyclic and other cyclicals; 1 or 2
80336   Antidepressants, tricyclic and other cyclicals; 3-5
80337   Antidepressants, tricyclic and other cyclicals; 6 or more

A laboratory test is performed to measure tricyclic and other cyclical antidepressants in urine, serum, or plasma. Tricyclic antidepressants (TCAs) and tetracyclic antidepressants (TeCAs) increase levels of the brain neurotransmitters, norepinephrine and serotonin while blocking acetylcholine. These drugs may be prescribed to treat depression, anxiety, fibromyalgia, chronic pain, and bedwetting. Tricyclic antidepressants include clomipramine (Anafranil), amitriptyline (Elavil), desipramine (Norpramin), nortriptyline (Pamelor), doxepin (Sinequan), and trimipramine (Surmontil). Tetracyclic antidepressants include amoxapin (Asendin), loxapin (Loxapac, Loxitan), mirtazapin (Remeron, Avanza), and maprotiline (Ludiomil). A blood sample is obtained by separately reportable venipuncture; urine sample by random void or catheterization. Urine, serum, or plasma is tested for all TCAs using quantitative liquid chromatography-tandem mass spectrometry. Serum or plasma is tested for the TeCA loxapin using high performance liquid chromatography. Urine, serum, or plasma is tested for amoxapin using quantitative high performance liquid chromatography. Serum or plasma is tested for maprotiline using quantitative gas chromatography and urine, serum, or plasma is tested for mirtazapin using quantitative gas chromatography/gas chromatography-mass spectrometry. Code 80335 is used when testing for 1 or 2 cyclical antidepressants; code 80336 is used for 3-5 compounds; and code 80337 is used when evaluating for 6 or more.

80338

80338   Antidepressants, not otherwise specified

A laboratory test is performed to measure antidepressants, not otherwise specified. The serotonin and norepinephrine reuptake inhibitor (SNRI) drugs venlafaxine (Effexor) and desvenlafaxine (Pristiq) may be prescribed to treat depression and can be tested for in serum or plasma using quantitative liquid chromatography-tandem mass spectrometry. The SNRI duloxetine (Cymbalta) is used to treat depression and chronic pain and can be tested for in serum or plasma using quantitative high performance liquid chromatography-tandem mass spectrometry. Atypical antidepressants include bupropion (Wellbutrin), used to treat depression and for smoking cessation, and trazodone, a powerful sleep aid. Both can be tested for in serum or plasma using quantitative liquid chromatography-tandem mass spectrometry.

80339-80341

80339 **Antiepileptics, not otherwise specified; 1-3**
80340 **Antiepileptics, not otherwise specified; 4-6**
80341 **Antiepileptics, not otherwise specified; 7 or more**

A laboratory test is performed to measure antiepileptics, not otherwise specified. Antiepileptics are used to treat seizure disorders and may also be prescribed to patients with chronic pain conditions like migraine or fibromyalgia. The mechanism of action can vary substantially between drugs in this category but they all function to change brain chemicals such as sodium channels, GABA receptors, NMDA receptors, calcium channels, AMPA receptors, and potassium channels, and to decrease the incidence of unusual electrical discharges that may trigger seizure activity or pain sensation. Primary analytical methods for testing urine, serum, or plasma for antiepileptics include high performance liquid chromatography, gas chromatography, liquid chromatography-tandem mass spectrometry, and immunoassays. Code 80339 is used when testing for 1-3 antiepileptics; code 80340 is used when testing for 4-6 compounds; and code 80341 is used when evaluating a sample for 7 or more antiepileptic drugs.

80342-80344

80342 **Antipsychotics, not otherwise specified; 1-3**
80343 **Antipsychotics, not otherwise specified; 4-6**
80344 **Antipsychotics, not otherwise specified; 7 or more**

A laboratory test is performed to measure antipsychotics, not otherwise specified. Antipsychotics are neuroleptic drugs that affect some neurotransmitters (dopamine, serotonin) and communication between nerve cells in the brain. Psychosis is often associated with schizophrenia and bipolar disorder and may cause delusions, auditory or visual hallucinations, and disordered thought processes. The use of neuroleptic antipsychotics will not cure these disorders but may substantially control the symptoms associated with them. Primary analytical methods for testing urine, serum, or plasma for antipsychotics include gas chromatography, gas chromatography-mass spectrometry, high performance liquid chromatography, and liquid chromatography-tandem mass spectrometry. Code 80342 is used when testing for 1-3 antipsychotics; code 80343 is used when testing a sample for 4-6 compounds; and code 80344 is used when evaluating a sample for 7 or more antipsychotics drugs.

80345

80345 **Barbiturates**

A laboratory test is performed to measure barbiturates in stool, serum, plasma, or urine. Barbiturates are a class of drugs that cause central nervous system depression and may be prescribed to treat anxiety, insomnia, or seizures, and are used to produce mild sedation and general anesthesia. Barbiturates decrease tension and calm the brain. They can be highly addictive and produce withdrawal symptoms including rebound effects on REM sleep. The effects of barbiturates may vary and drugs are usually assigned to a class (very short, short, medium, or long acting) in relationship to their half-life. Very short acting barbiturates include methohexital (Brevital), thiamylal (Surital), and thiopental (pentobarbital) and are used primarily for anesthesia. Short acting barbiturates include phentobarbital (Nembutal), amobarbital (Amytal), butabarbital (Butisol, Soneryl), secobarbital (Seconal), aprobarbital (Alurate). Medium acting drugs are talbutal (Lotusate), cyclobarbital (Phanodorn), and butalbital (Fiorinal, Fioricet); the long acting drugs are mephobarbital (Mebaral), methylphenobarbital (Prominal), and phenobarbital (Luminal). A blood sample is obtained by separately reportable venipuncture, urine specimen by random void or catheterization, and meconium stool is collected from a diaper. Serum or plasma and urine are tested using quantitative gas chromatography-mass spectrometry. Stool may be tested using multiple chromatography and mass spectrometry procedures.

80346-80347

80346 **Benzodiazepines; 1-12**
80347 **Benzodiazepines; 13 or more**

A laboratory test is performed to measure benzodiazepines in stool, urine, serum, or plasma. Benzodiazepines are a class of drugs with sedative, hypnotic, anxiolytic, anti-convulsive, and muscle relaxant capabilities. Some short acting benzodiazepines have amnesic-dissociative actions. They may be prescribed to treat anxiety, panic disorders, insomnia, alcohol withdrawal, or seizures, and may be used as preoperative or intra-operative anesthesia. Common benzodiazepines and their uses include chlordiazepoxide (Librium) for alcohol withdrawal; diazepam (Valium) for anxiety, panic disorders, seizures, and insomnia; flurazepam (Dalmane) for insomnia and preoperative anesthesia;

lorazepam (Ativan) for anxiety, insomnia, and seizures; temazepam (Restoril) for insomnia; clonazepam (Klonopin) for seizures and panic disorders; flunitrazepam (Rohipnol) for insomnia -often implicated as a "date rape" drug; alprazolam (Xanax) for anxiety and panic disorders; triazolam (Halcion) for insomnia, and midazolam (Versed) for preoperative and intra-operative anesthesia. A blood sample is obtained by separately reportable venipuncture, urine specimen by random void or catheterization; and meconium stool is collected from a diaper. Serum, plasma, and meconium are tested using quantitative liquid chromatography-tandem mass spectrometry. Urine is tested using quantitative high performance liquid chromatography-tandem mass spectrometry. Code 80346 is used when testing for 1-12 benzodiazepines and code 80347 is reported when identifying 13 or more.

80348

80348 **Buprenorphine**

A laboratory test is performed to measure buprenorphine and its metabolites in urine, serum, or plasma. Buprenorphine is a semi-synthetic opioid partial agonist used to treat opioid addiction and control acute or chronic pain in non-opioid tolerant persons. The drug is available in an oral form (Subutex, Suboxone, Zublolv) to treat opioid addiction, or as a sublingual preparation (Temgesic) for moderate to severe pain. It may also be injected (Buprenex) for acute pain or administered via transdermal patch (Norspan, Butrans) to treat chronic pain. A blood sample is obtained by separately reportable venipuncture, urine by random void or catheterization. Serum or plasma is tested using quantitative high performance liquid chromatography-tandem mass spectrometry. Urine is tested using quantitative liquid chromatography-tandem mass spectrometry.

80349

80349 **Cannabinoids, natural**

A laboratory test is performed to measure natural cannabinoids in meconium stool, urine, serum, or plasma. Cannabinoids occur naturally in the marijuana plant (Cannabis sativa). Tetrahydrocannabinoid, or THC, is the principal mind altering constituent of cannabis. When smoked or ingested, THC primarily affects the limbic system responsible for memory, cognition, and psychomotor performance, and the mesolimbic pathways responsible for the feeling of reward and pain perception. The chemical is fat soluble with a long elimination half-life. Cannabinoids may be detected in urine for several weeks and in serum or plasma for up to 12 hours. A blood sample is obtained by separately reportable venipuncture, urine sample by random void or catheterization, and meconium stool is collected from a diaper. Samples are tested for THC and its metabolite 9-carboxy-THC using quantitative liquid chromatography-tandem mass spectrometry.

80350-80352

80350 **Cannabinoids, synthetic; 1-3**
80351 **Cannabinoids, synthetic; 4-6**
80352 **Cannabinoids, synthetic; 7 or more**

A laboratory test is performed to measure synthetic cannabinoids in urine, saliva, or blood. Synthetic cannabinoids include the designer drugs "spice" and "K2". They may be referred to as "herbal incense", "potpourri", or "legal" marijuana. These chemicals affect the same receptors in the central nervous system as THC to produce similar psychoactive effects but are more likely to cause anxiety, agitation, and hallucinations in addition. Synthetic cannabinoids are usually assigned to three classes that include classical cannabinoids (HU-210), cyclohexylphenols, and aminoalkylindoles. These designer drugs are manufactured with continually changing chemical structures to avoid detection in commercially available tests. Synthetic cannabinoids will not be detected in immunoassay tests for THC. A blood sample is obtained by separately reportable venipuncture, a urine sample by random void or catheterization, and saliva is collected by swab or in a sample cup. Blood and saliva are tested using liquid chromatography-tandem mass spectrometry. Urine is screened using enzyme-linked immunosorbent assay and confirmed using high performance liquid chromatography-tandem mass spectrometry. Code 80350 is used when testing for 1-3 synthetic cannabinoids; code 80351 is used for 4-6 compounds; and code 80352 is used for 7 or more synthetic cannabinoids.

80353

80353 **Cocaine**

A laboratory test is performed to measure cocaine in meconium stool, urine, serum, or plasma. Cocaine is a highly addictive, central nervous system stimulant and anesthetic derived from the leaves of the coca plant. It is a "triple reuptake inhibitor" (TRI) that affects serotonin, norepinephrine, and dopamine receptors in the brain. The drug can be inhaled, injected, or absorbed topically. A blood sample is obtained by separately reportable venipuncture. Urine is collected by random void or catheterization, and meconium stool is collected from a diaper. Serum, plasma, meconium stool, and a positive urine screen are tested using quantitative gas chromatography-mass spectrometry/quantitative liquid chromatography-tandem mass spectrometry.

Pathology and Laboratory

80354

80354   Fentanyl

A laboratory test is performed to measure fentanyl in urine, serum, or plasma. Fentanyl is a potent synthetic opioid analgesic which has a rapid onset but short duration of action. It is often administered with benzodiazepines for conscious sedation. It may be used to treat acute postoperative pain, breakthrough pain associated with cancer or bone fractures, and chronic pain conditions. Fentanyl may be administered intravenously (Sublimaze), intrathecally with spinal or epidural anesthesia, via a transdermal patch (Duragesic), and orally in the form of a lollipop/lozenge (Actiq), buccal tablet (Fentora), or a sublingual spray. A blood sample is obtained by separately reportable venipuncture; urine specimen by random void or catheterization. Urine, serum, and plasma are tested using quantitative liquid chromatography-tandem mass spectrometry.

80355

80355   Gabapentin, non-blood

A laboratory test is performed to measure gabapentin in urine. Gabapentin (Neurontin) is an anticonvulsant, analgesic used to treat seizure disorders, neuropathic pain like diabetic neuropathy and post herpetic neuralgia, and restless leg syndrome. A urine sample is obtained by separately reportable random void or catheterization and tested using quantitative high performance liquid chromatography/tandem mass spectrometry.

80356

80356   Heroin metabolite

A laboratory test is performed to measure the heroin metabolite, 6-monoacetylmorphine (6-MAM) in urine, serum, or plasma. Heroin (diacetylmorphine) is a synthetic opioid made from morphine. Heroin is not an active chemical. The body rapidly converts heroin to 6-MAM in under 6 minutes, which is then quickly filtered by the kidneys and excreted in urine. The detection window to identify 6-MAM in urine is less than 24 hours. The small amount of remaining 6-MAM converts to morphine in under 40 minutes. A blood sample is obtained by separately reportable venipuncture; urine specimen by random void or catheterization. Serum and plasma are tested using quantitative liquid chromatography-tandem mass spectrometry. Urine is screened using qualitative enzyme immunoassay and a positive result is confirmed using quantitative high performance chromatography-tandem mass spectrometry.

80357

80357   Ketamine and norketamine

A laboratory test is performed to measure ketamine and its metabolite, norketamine in serum or plasma. Ketamine is an N-methyl-D-aspartate receptor (NMDAR) antagonist that can be injected, ingested, or inhaled. It is a potent analgesic, sedative, amnesic that is used clinically for anesthesia, pain management, and to treat bronchospasm. Ketamine can provide stable cardiovascular function with protection of airway reflexes making it a safe anesthesic choice for many patients. However, the dissociative effects of the drug have made it attractive to individuals for recreational use and abuse. A blood sample is obtained by separately reportable venipuncture. Serum or plasma is tested using quantitative gas chromatography-mass spectrometry.

80358

80358   Methadone

A laboratory test is performed to measure methadone in meconium stool, urine, serum, or plasma. Methadone is a synthetic opioid with a long duration of action and strong analgesic effect. It is most commonly prescribed as part of a medically supervised drug addiction detoxification and maintenance program but may also be used to treat severe chronic pain. Methadone can decrease the symptoms of withdrawal in persons who are opioid addicted without producing the pleasurable symptoms associated with opioid abuse. A blood sample is obtained by separately reportable venipuncture. A urine sample is obtained by random void or catheterization, and meconium stool is collected from a diaper. Urine, serum, plasma, and stool may all be tested using quantitative liquid chromatography-tandem mass spectrometry.

80359

80359   Methylenedioxyamphetamines (MDA, MDEA, MDMA)

A laboratory test is performed to measure 3, 4-methylenedioxyamphetamines (MDA), 3, 4-methylenedioxy-N-ethylamphetamine (MDEA, Ecstasy), or 3, 4-methylenedioxymethamphetamine (MDMA, Eve) in meconium stool, urine, serum, plasma, or saliva. MDA, MDEA, and MDMA are central nervous system stimulants with hallucinogenic, psychedelic, and empathogenic properties. There is no legitimate medical use for these drugs but they are often used or abused recreationally. A blood sample is obtained by separately reportable venipuncture. A urine sample is obtained by random void or catheterization. Saliva is obtained by oral swab or sample cup, and meconium stool is collected from a diaper. Serum, plasma, and stool are tested using quantitative high performance liquid chromatography-tandem mass spectrometry. Urine is screened using

enzyme immunoassay and confirmed using mass spectrometry. Saliva is screened using immunochromatography or reflectometry and confirmed using gas chromatography-mass spectrometry.

80360

80360   Methylphenidate

A laboratory test is performed to measure methylphenidate and its metabolite ritalinic acid. Methylphenidate (Ritalin, Methylin, Concerta) is a central nervous system psycho-stimulant used to treat attention deficit hyperactivity disorder (ADHD), narcolepsy, and postural orthostatic tachycardia syndrome. Methylphenidate works primarily by increasing the levels of the neurotransmitters dopamine and norepinephrine in the brain, allowing an individual to be better focused and in control of their actions. A blood sample is obtained by separately reportable venipuncture, and urine by random void or catheterization. Urine, serum, and plasma are tested using quantitative liquid chromatography-tandem mass spectrometry.

80361

80361   Opiates, 1 or more

A laboratory test is performed to measure opiates in meconium stool, urine, serum, or plasma. Opiates are the naturally occurring opioid alkaloids found in the resin of the opium poppy plant (Papaver somniferum) and include morphine, codeine, and thebaine. Naturally occurring hydromorphone and hydrocodone may rarely be detected in opium. Dihydrocodeine, oxymorphol, oxycodone, oxymorphone, and metopon are also occasionally found in trace amounts. The semi-synthetic versions of these compounds are more appropriately defined as opioids or opiate analogs. Opiates fall into the class of narcotic analgesics and are prescribed clinically to treat moderate to severe pain. Opiates are central nervous system depressants but also affect areas of the brain that mediate pleasure to produce a euphoric state along with pain relief. These drugs may be consumed by individuals for recreational abuse. A blood sample is obtained by separately reportable venipuncture. A urine sample is obtained by random void or catheterization, and meconium stool is collected from a diaper. All samples are confirmed using quantitative liquid chromatography-tandem mass spectrometry.

80362-80364

80362   Opioids and opiate analogs; 1 or 2
80363   Opioids and Opiate analogs; 3 or 4
80364   Opioids and Opiate analogs; 5 or more

A laboratory test is performed to measure opioids and opiate analogs in meconium stool, urine, serum, or plasma. Opioids and opiate analogs are a class of drugs comprised of any naturally occurring opiate (codeine, morphine, thebaine) or semi-synthetic opioid (hydromorphone, hydrocodone, oxycodone, oxymorphone, buprenorphine, meperidine, methadone, propoxphene, tapentadol, tramadol) that share a similar chemical structure and pharmacological effects. Opioids and opiate analogs are narcotic analgesic, central nervous system depressants prescribed clinically to treat moderate to severe, acute or chronic pain. These drugs also have an effect on areas of the brain that mediate pleasure and may produce a euphoric state along with pain relief. Opioids and opiate analogs may be abused by recreational drug users. A blood sample is obtained by separately reportable venipuncture. A urine sample is obtained by random void or catheterization, and meconium stool is collected from a diaper. Serum, plasma, urine, and stool are tested using quantitative liquid chromatography-tandem mass spectrometry. Code 80362 is used when testing for 1 or 2 opioids/opiate analogs; code 80363 is used for 3 or more; and code 80364 is used when evaluating a sample for 5 or more opioids/opiate analogs.

80365

80365   Oxycodone

A laboratory test is performed to measure oxycodone (oxymorphone) in urine, serum, or plasma. Oxycodone is a semi-synthetic opioid, narcotic analgesic that is used to treat moderate to severe, acute or chronic pain. The drug can be used alone or in combination with aspirin or acetaminophen. Oxycodone may be injected or ingested orally. A blood sample is obtained by separately reportable venipuncture; urine by random void or catheterization. Urine is screened using qualitative enzyme immunoassay and urine, serum, and plasma are tested by quantitative liquid chromatography-tandem mass spectrometry.

80366

80366   Pregabalin

A laboratory test is performed to measure pregabalin in urine, serum, or plasma. Pregabalin is marketed in the United States as Lyrica. It is an anticonvulsant prescribed to treat neuropathic pain like post herpetic neuralgia and diabetic peripheral neuropathy, chronic pain conditions such as fibromyalgia, and as an adjunct therapy in patients diagnosed with partial seizure disorder with or without secondary generalization. A blood sample is obtained by separately reportable venipuncture and urine by random void or catheterization. Urine, serum, and plasma are tested using quantitative high performance liquid chromatography/tandem mass spectrometry.

80367

80367   Propoxyphene

A laboratory test is performed to measure propoxyphene (dextropropoxyphene) in meconium stool, urine, serum, or plasma. Propoxyphene, an analgesic, antitussive often combined with aspirin or acetaminophen and marketed under the brand names Darvon or Darvocet, is no longer available in the United States. It was taken off the market in November 2010 because of fatal overdoses and cardiac arrhythmias. A blood sample is obtained by separately reportable venipuncture. A urine sample is obtained by random void or catheterization, and meconium stool is collected from a diaper. Samples are tested using quantitative high performance liquid chromatography-tandem mass spectrometry.

80368

80368   Sedative hypnotics (non-benzodiazepines)

A laboratory test is performed to measure non-benzodiazepine sedative hypnotics in urine, serum, or plasma. This class of psychoactive drugs provides the same benefits, side effects, and risks as benzodiazepines but has a very different chemical structure. Non-benzodiazepine drugs include eszopiclone (Lunesta), zaleplon (Sonata), Zolpidem (Ambien), Zolpidem tartrate (Interrmezzo sublingual), ramelteon (Rozerem), chloral hydrate (Nortec), dexmedetomidine hydrochloride (Precedex). Most drugs in this class induce sleep by binding to a specific benzodiazepine brain receptor called omega-1 and are believed to be less disruptive to REM sleep cycles than benzodiazepines. Eszopiclone differs somewhat by increasing gamma-aminobutyric acid (GABA) at receptor sites in the brain and ramelteon is a melatonin receptor stimulator. Non-benzodiazepine sedative hypnotics are used as short term treatment for insomnia, dexmedetomidine is used primarily for anesthesia. A blood sample is obtained by separately reportable venipuncture, and urine by random void or catheterization. Samples are tested for eszopiclone, zolpidem, and ramelteon using high performance liquid chromatography-tandem mass spectrometry. Zaleplon is tested for using high performance liquid chromatography alone. Serum and plasma are tested for chloral hydrate using gas chromatography and for dexmedetomidine using gas chromatography-mass spectrometry.

80369-80370

80369   Skeletal muscle relaxants; 1 or 2
80370   Skeletal muscle relaxants; 3 or more

A laboratory test is performed to measure skeletal muscle relaxants in urine, serum, or plasma. Skeletal muscle relaxants belong to several drug classes including neuromuscular blockers that prevent transmission of signals at the neuromuscular end plates causing paralysis (succinylcholine, pancuronium, botulinum toxins) and central nervous system spasmolytics that increase the inhibition of motor neurons, or decrease the level of excitation in the neocortex, brain stem, and/or spinal cord. Skeletal muscle relaxants may be used to treat conditions such as cerebral palsy, multiple sclerosis, spinal cord injury, low back pain, neck pain, fibromyalgia, myofacial pain syndrome, and tension headaches. Common antispasmotics include dantrolene (Dantruim), carisoprodol (Soma), baclofen (Lioresel), tizanidine (Zonaflex), cyclobenzaprine (Flexeril), metaxalone (Skelelaxin), methocarbamol (Robaxin), and chlorzoxazone (Parafon Forte). A blood sample is obtained by separately reportable venipuncture, and a urine sample by random void or catheterization. Samples are tested for baclofen and cyclobenzaprine using quantitative high performance liquid chromatrography/tandem mass spectrometry. Serum and plasma are tested for dantrolene using spectrofluorometry and for carisoprodol using quantitative gas chromatography-mass spectrometry. Code 80369 is reported for 1-2 relaxants, and 80370 for 3 or more.

80371

80371   Stimulants, synthetic

A laboratory test is performed to measure synthetic stimulates in urine. Synthetic stimulants include methylenedioxypyrovalerone (MDPV), mephedrone (Meph, MCat), Butylone (bk-MBDB), cathinone (Khat), ethylone (MDEC, bk-MDEA), benzylpiperazine (BZP), meta-chlorophenylpiperazine (mCPP) and 3-Trifluoromethylphenylpiperazine (TFMPP). There is no medical indication for synthetic stimulant use and these drugs are most commonly abused recreationally. Synthetic stimulants inhibit the removal of neurotransmitters (dopamine, norepinephrine, serotonin) at the brain synapses causing euphoria, excessive physical activity, wakefulness, hallucinations, and delusions that can often lead to violence toward self and others. A urine sample is obtained by random void or catheterization and screened using gas chromatography/mass spectrometry, or quantitative high performance liquid chromatography/tandem mass spectrometry when testing for MDPV.

80372

80372   Tapentadol

A laboratory test is performed to measure tapentadol in urine, serum, or plasma. Tapentadol is marketed under the brand name Nucynta. It is a central acting opioid analgesic that works as an agonist of the ¬μ-opioid receptor to inhibit the reuptake of norepinephrine. Tapentadol is used to treat moderate to severe acute pain as an alternative to opiates. It may also be prescribed in an extend release formula to treat

diabetic peripheral neuropathy. A blood sample is obtained by separately reportable venipuncture, and urine by random void or catheterization. Urine, serum, and plasma are tested using quantitative liquid chromatography-tandem mass spectrometry.

80373

80373   Tramadol

A laboratory test is performed to measure tramadol in urine, serum, or plasma. Tramadol may be marketed under the brand name Ultram. It is a central acting opioid analgesic that works as an agonist of the ¬μ-opioid receptor to inhibit the reuptake of norepinephrine and serotonin. Tramadol is used to treat moderate to moderate-severe acute or chronic pain as an alternative to opiates. It may also be prescribed in an extend release formula to treat fibromyalgia. A blood sample is obtained by separately reportable venipuncture, and urine by random void or catheterization. Urine, serum, and plasma are tested using quantitative liquid chromatography-tandem mass spectrometry.

80374

80374   Stereoisomer (enantiomer) analysis, single drug class

A laboratory test may be performed to analyze stereoisomers (enantiomers) in a single drug class. Stereoisomers are molecules that have the same sequence of bonded atoms that differ only by the three dimensional orientation of those atoms in space. An enantiomer is the reflected (mirror) image of two stereoisomers that cannot be superimposed, giving them asymmetric (chiral) centers. Enantiomers share some of the same biological properties but often have very different pharmacokinetic properties, affecting absorption, distribution, biotransformation, excretion, and quantitative/qualitative differences in pharmacologic or toxicologic effects. Drugs may be marketed as a chiral (racemic) mixture of enantiomers or as a pure substance. For example: the racemic R/S citalopram is marketed as Celexa and the S (only) citalopram is marketed as Lexapro. S-citalopram is the primary inhibitor of serotonin reuptake with R-citalopram having a much less potent affect. In some individuals, the S-citalopram (Lexapro) has been shown to have greater efficacy with less side effects when compared to R/S citalopram (Celexa). Testing blood, body tissue, or body fluids for enantiomers of a prescribed drug may help with dose determination, narrowing indicated uses, and assist in monitoring patients for drug side effects and efficacy.

80375-80377

80375   Drug(s) or substance(s), definitive, qualitative or quantitative, not otherwise specified; 1-3
80376   Drug(s) or substance(s), definitive, qualitative or quantitative, not otherwise specified; 4-6
80377   Drug(s) or substance(s), definitive, qualitative or quantitative, not otherwise specified; 7 or more

A laboratory test is performed to definitively, qualitatively, or quantitatively measure drug(s) or substance(s), not otherwise specified. The most common methodologies for testing drugs or substances are gas chromatography, liquid chromatography, tandem mass spectrometry or a combination of one or more of these. Code 80375 is used when testing for 1-3 drugs or substances; code 80376 is used when 4-6 drugs or compounds are tested; and code 80377 is used when identifying 7 or more drugs or compounds in a patient sample.

80400

80400   ACTH stimulation panel; for adrenal insufficiency
      This panel must include the following:
         Cortisol (82533 x 2)

An ACTH stimulation panel is performed to assess adrenal gland function for primary or secondary insufficiency. The adrenal glands are part of the endocrine system and are located just above each kidney. The outer layer of the gland, the adrenal cortex, produces cortisol, aldosterone, and androgen hormones. The inner layer of the gland, the medulla, produces adrenaline and noradrenaline (norepinephrine). Adrenal insufficiency may have a primary cause such as autoimmune adrenalitis, Addison's disease, congenital abnormalities, or tumors, or it may be secondary to pituitary or hypothalamus dysfunction. The adrenocorticotropic hormone (ACTH) stimulation test is ideally performed between 8 – 9 AM, following a fat free meal. A blood sample is obtained by separately reportable venipuncture and the sample is used to measure the baseline cortisol level. Cosyntropin (Cortosyn) 0.25 mg is injected intravenously (IV) and the patient is allowed to rest, undisturbed for 30-60 minutes. A second blood sample is obtained by separately reportable venipuncture and used to measure the 30-60 minute cortisol level. Serum/plasma is tested using quantitative chemiluminescent immunoassay.

Pathology and Laboratory

80402

80402   ACTH stimulation panel; for 21 hydroxylase deficiency
This panel must include the following:
Cortisol (82533 x 2)
17 hydroxyprogesterone (83498 x 2)

An ACTH stimulation panel is performed to assess adrenal gland function for enzyme deficiency and adrenal steroid biosynthesis disorders like congenital adrenal hyperplasia (CAH). The outer layer of the gland, the adrenal cortex, produces cortisol, aldosterone, and androgen hormones. The inner layer of the gland, the medulla, produces adrenaline and noradrenaline (norepinephrine). CAH is an inherited disorder that affects adrenal gland function due to a deficiency of enzymes necessary for the production of cortisol, aldosterone, and/or androgen hormones. CAH can be caused by a deficiency in the enzyme 21-hydroxylase, and can be tested for using the ACTH stimulation test and measuring cortisol and 17-hydroxyprogesterone. The test is ideally performed between 8 – 9 AM, following a fat free meal. A blood sample is obtained by separately reportable venipuncture and used to measure the baseline cortisol and 17-hydroxyprogesterone levels. Cosyntropin (Cortosyn) 0.25 mg is injected intravenously, and the patient is allowed to rest undisturbed for 30-60 minutes. A second blood sample is obtained and used to measure the 30-60 minute cortisol and 17-hydroxyprogesterone levels. Serum/plasma is tested for cortisol using quantitative chemiluminescent immunoassay and for 17-hydroxyprogesterone using quantitative high performance liquid chromatography-tandem mass spectrometry.

80406

80406   ACTH stimulation panel; for 3 beta-hydroxydehydrogenase deficiency
This panel must include the following:
Cortisol (82533 x 2) 17 hydroxypregnenolone (84143 x 2)

An ACTH stimulation panel is performed to assess adrenal gland function for enzyme deficiency and adrenal steroid biosynthesis disorders like congenital adrenal hyperplasia (CAH). The outer layer of the gland, the adrenal cortex, produces cortisol, aldosterone, and androgen hormones. The inner layer of the gland, the medulla, produces adrenaline and noradrenaline (norepinephrine). CAH is an inherited disorder that affects adrenal gland function due to a deficiency of enzymes necessary for the production of cortisol, aldosterone, and/or androgen hormones. CAH can be caused by a deficiency in the enzyme 3 beta-hydroxydehydrogenase, and can be tested for using the ACTH stimulation test and measuring cortisol and 17-hydroxypregnenolone. The test is ideally performed between 8 – 9 AM, following a fat free meal. A blood sample is obtained by separately reportable venipuncture and used to measure the baseline cortisol and 17-hydroxypregnenolone levels. Cosyntropin (Cortosyn) 0.25 mg is injected intravenously, and the patient is allowed to rest undisturbed for 30-60 minutes. A second blood sample is obtained and used to measure the 30-60 minute cortisol and 17-hydroxypregnenolone levels. Serum/plasma is tested for cortisol using quantitative chemiluminescent immunoassay and for 17-hydroxypregnenolone using quantitative high performance liquid chromatography-tandem mass spectrometry.

80408

80408   Aldosterone suppression evaluation panel (eg, saline infusion)
This panel must include the following:
Aldosterone (82088 x 2) Renin (84244 x 2)

A laboratory test is performed to assess aldosterone and renin levels in patients with suspected primary and/or secondary hyperaldosteronism. Primary hyperaldosteronism causes elevated aldosterone levels, sodium retention, potassium depletion, and elevated blood pressure. It can result from benign adrenal tumors, bilateral adrenal hyperplasia, or an unknown etiology. Secondary hyperaldosteronism is more common and renin levels will be elevated along with aldosterone. Causes of secondary hyperaldosteronism include renal artery stenosis, congestive heart failure, cirrhosis, kidney disease, and preeclampsia. Symptoms include urinary frequency, increased thirst, fatigue, muscle weakness or cramping, palpitations, and headache. The aldosterone suppression evaluation test measures aldosterone and renin at baseline and the changes that occur following an intravenous infusion of isotonic (0.9%) sodium chloride (NaCl) solution. Patient preparation includes a normal sodium diet (100-200 mEq/day) x 3 days and no medication known to affect the renin/aldosterone system. If the physician has specified a supine test, the baseline blood draw should be done between 8 – 10 am with the patient supine for a minimum of 2 hours before the blood draw and remaining supine until the test is over. If the test is ordered in the upright position, the baseline blood draw must be done before noon with the patient sitting or standing upright for at least 2 hours prior to the blood draw and remaining sitting or standing for the duration of the test. An IV line is established in a separately reportable procedure. A blood sample may be obtained from this IV line or by separately reportable venipuncture and used to measure the baseline aldosterone and renin levels. The IV infusion of sodium chloride is started at a rate of 500 ml/h x 4 hours for a total of 2L. At the end of the infusion, a second blood sample is obtained and used to measure the post infusion levels of aldosterone and renin. Serum/plasma is tested using quantitative radioimmunoassay or quantitative immunoradiometry.

80410

80410   Calcitonin stimulation panel (eg, calcium, pentagastrin)
This panel must include the following:
Calcitonin (82308 x 3)

A laboratory test is performed to diagnose and monitor medullary thyroid cancer (MTC), benign C-cell hyperplasia, and multiple endocrine neoplasia type 2 (MEN2). The calcitonin stimulation test measures the baseline calcitonin level and changes that occur following intravenous injection of calcium and/or pentagastrin. Calcitonin is a hormone produced by C-cells in the thyroid gland and regulates calcium levels in the blood. The thyroid is a butterfly shaped gland located at the base of the throat. In addition to calcitonin, the thyroid gland produces thyroxin (T4) and triiodothyronine (T3). An intravenous line is established by separately reportable procedure. A blood sample may be obtained from this IV line or by separately reportable venipuncture and used to measure the baseline calcitonin level. For calcium and pentagastrin stimulation, calcium 2mg/kg is injected intravenously over 1 minute followed by pentagastrin 0.5 mcg/kg via IV push. Additional blood samples for calcitonin levels are then collected at 1 and/or 2 minutes, and at 5 minutes post injection. For calcium stimulation only, calcium 2 mg/kg is injected intravenously over 1 minute or calcium 2.4 mg/kg is injected via IV push. Additional blood samples for calcitonin levels are then collected at 1 and/or 2 minutes, and at 5 minutes post injection. For pentagastrin stimulation only, pentagastrin 0.5 mg/kg is injected via IV push. Additional blood samples for calcitonin levels are then collected at 1 and/or 2 minutes, and at 5 minutes post injection. Serum/plasma is tested using quantitative chemiluminescent immunoassay.

80412

80412   Corticotropic releasing hormone (CRH) stimulation panel This panel must include the following: Cortisol (82533 x 6) Adrenocorticotropic hormone (ACTH) (82024 x 6)

A laboratory test is performed to diagnose and monitor primary (adrenal), secondary (pituitary), and tertiary (hypothalamic) adrenal insufficiency conditions and to differentiate pituitary Cushing syndrome from conditions such as primary adrenal hypercortisolism or ectopic corticotropin syndrome. The corticotropic releasing hormone (CRH) stimulation test measures the baseline cortisol and adrenocorticotropic hormone (ACTH) levels and the changes that occur following an intravenous injection of synthetic ovine CRH. The test can be done at any time of the day. The patient should fast for 4 hours prior to the test. An intravenous line is established by separately reportable procedure. A blood sample may be obtained from this IV line or by separately reportable venipuncture and used to measure the baseline cortisol and ACTH levels. Ovine CRH 1 mcg/kg is administered via IV push over 30 seconds for a total dose of 100 mcg. Additional blood samples for cortisol and ACTH levels are then collected 30, 45, 60, 90, and 120 minutes post injection by separately reportable venipuncture. Serum/plasma is tested using quantitative chemiluminescent immunoassay.

80414

80414   Chorionic gonadotropin stimulation panel; testosterone response
This panel must include the following:
Testosterone (84403 x 2 on 3 pooled blood samples)

A laboratory test is performed to evaluate infants with ambiguous genitalia and palpable gonads, males with delayed puberty or undescended testes and/or to confirm the presence of active testicular tissue. The chorionic gonadotropin stimulation test measures the baseline level of testosterone and testosterone levels following the injection of an evocative agent. The baseline sample is obtained by separately reportable venipuncture and consists of 3 blood samples, drawn 15-20 minutes apart which are pooled together to measure the testosterone level. An intramuscular or subcutaneous injection of human chorionic gonadotropin (hCG) 5,000 units is then administered as the evocative agent. Three days later, a post response sample is obtained by separately reportable venipuncture and consists of 3 blood samples, drawn 15-20 minutes apart which are pooled together to measure the testosterone level. Serum/plasma is tested using quantitative electrochemiluminescent immunoassay.

80415

80415   Chorionic gonadotropin stimulation panel; estradiol response
This panel must include the following:
Estradiol (82670 x 2 on 3 pooled blood samples)

A chorionic gonadotropin stimulation panel is performed to evaluate estradiol response. This test is performed to aid in diagnosis of female fertility disorders. A baseline estradiol level is obtained. Human chorionic gonadotropin (hCG) is then administered. Following hCG administration, estradiol levels are again obtained and compared to baseline levels to determine response to simulation with hCG. This test includes testing of estradiol levels twice on three pooled blood samples.

● New Code   ▲ Revised Code

80416

80416   Renal vein renin stimulation panel (eg, captopril)
This panel must include the following:
Renin (84244 x 6)

A laboratory test is performed to diagnose renovascular hypertension, which may be caused by renal artery stenosis (RAS), a narrowing of the renovascular bed often due to atherosclerotic plaque formation, or fibromuscular hyperplasia. When hypertension is caused by RAS it can be treated using angiotensin converting enzyme (ACE) inhibitors. Plasma renin activity will be increased in patients with renovascular hypertension. The renal vein renin stimulation test is performed to determine the baseline renin level in the kidneys and the changes that occur following administration of an ACE inhibiting medication, captopril. The patient discontinues diuretics and ACE inhibiting medications at least 14 days prior to the test and eats a normal sodium diet (100-200 mEq/day) x 3 days. Angiography is performed as a separately reportable procedure. The patient is positioned supine on the table, prepped and draped in the usual sterile manner. The renal veins are catheterized from a transfemoral or jugular approach using a 4 or 5 F cobra or shepard catheter with sidehole. Small injections of contrast are given to confirm catheter location. A baseline blood sample is obtained from the right and left renal veins to determine renin levels. Captopril 25-50 mg is administered and additional blood samples are then taken at timed intervals from the right and left veins to determine renin levels. Serum/plasma is tested using quantitative immunoradiometry.

80417

80417   Peripheral vein renin stimulation panel (eg, captopril)
This panel must include the following:
Renin (84244 x 2)

A laboratory test is performed to diagnose renovascular hypertension, which may be caused by renal artery stenosis (RAS), a narrowing of the renovascular bed often due to atherosclerotic plaque formation, or fibromuscular hyperplasia. When hypertension is caused by RAS it can be treated using angiotensin converting enzyme (ACE) inhibitors. Plasma renin activity will be increased in patients with renovascular hypertension. The peripheral vein renin stimulation test is performed to determine the baseline renin level in the peripheral circulating blood and the changes that occur following ingestion of an ACE inhibiting medication, captopril. The patient discontinues diuretics and ACE inhibiting medications at least 14 days prior to the test and eats a normal sodium diet (100-200 mEq/day) x 3 days. If the physician has specified a supine test, the baseline blood draw should be done between 8 - 10 am with the patient supine for a minimum of 2 hours before the blood draw and remaining supine until the test is over. If the test is ordered in the upright position, the baseline blood draw must be done before noon with the patient sitting or standing upright for at least 2 hours prior to the blood draw and remaining sitting or standing for the duration of the test. The baseline blood sample is obtained by separately reportable venipuncture. Captopril 25-50 mg is administered orally and the second blood sample is obtained 30 minutes later. Serum/plasma is tested using quantitative immunoradiometry.

80418

80418   Combined rapid anterior pituitary evaluation panel
This panel must include the following:
Adrenocorticotropic hormone (ACTH) (82024 x 4)
Luteinizing hormone (LH) (83002 x 4)
Follicle stimulating hormone (FSH) (83001 x 4)
Prolactin (84146 x 4)
Human growth hormone (HGH) (83003 x 4)
Cortisol (82533 x 4)
Thyroid stimulating hormone (TSH) (84443 x 4)

A laboratory test is performed to evaluate anterior pituitary function. The pituitary is a pea size endocrine gland located in the brain, behind the sinus cavity. It is divided into two regions, anterior and posterior. The posterior region is not glandular but contains axonal projections from the hypothalamus and stores oxytocin and vasopressin for later release. The anterior region of the pituitary gland produces and regulates hormones that influence bone growth and muscle mass, the body's response to stress, blood glucose levels, metabolism, secondary sex characteristics, fertility, and breast milk production. The combined rapid anterior pituitary evaluation test measures the level of adrenocorticotropic hormone (ACTH), luteinizing hormone (LH), follicle stimulating hormone (FSH), prolactin, human growth hormone (HGH), cortisol, and thyroid stimulating hormone (TSH) by comparing a baseline blood sample to levels following the intravenous administration of insulin, thyrotropin-releasing hormone (TRH), and gonadotropin-releasing hormone (GnRH). The patient should be fasting for 8 hours prior to the start of the test. An IV line is established by separately reportable procedure. A blood sample may be obtained from this IV line or by separately reportable venipuncture and used to measure the baseline blood levels of ACTH, LH, FSH, prolactin, HGH, cortisol, and TSH. Insulin, TRH, and GnRH are then administered by intravenous push. Blood sugar levels may be obtained and reported separately to verify adequate hypoglycemia is achieved before post injection

levels of the hormones are drawn. Some levels, such as cortisol and HGH, may be drawn at 15-30 minute intervals starting 15 minutes after insulin injection and ending 120 minutes later. Others levels may be drawn 2 hours, 4 hours, 6 hours, and 24 hours after GnRH administration. Serum/plasma is tested using quantitative chemiluminescent immunoassay.

80420

80420   Dexamethasone suppression panel, 48 hour
This panel must include the following:
Free cortisol, urine (82530 x 2) Cortisol (82533 x 2)
Volume measurement for timed collection (81050 x 2)

A laboratory test is performed to measure adrenal gland function in response to adrenocorticotropin hormone (ACTH) suppression. The dexamethasone suppression test is used to diagnose Cushing syndrome and further identify the cause. A 24-hour urine collection is obtained starting after the first morning void. The urine must be refrigerated during the collection period. At the end of the 24-hour collection period which includes the first morning void, the urine is labeled with the collection time and date and sent to the lab for volume measurement and testing for free cortisol levels. A baseline blood sample is obtained by separately reportable venipuncture for cortisol levels. Oral dexamethasone 2 mg is administered every 6 hours x 48 hours. Urine collection continues during this time. The urine must be refrigerated. Six hours after the last dose of dexamethasone, a blood sample is obtained by separately reportable venipuncture to measure cortisol levels, and the last voided urine is added to the 48-hour urine collection. The urine container is labeled with collection time and date and sent to the lab for volume measurement and testing for free cortisol levels. Urine is tested for cortisol using quantitative liquid chromatography-tandem mass spectrometry. Serum/plasma is tested for cortisol using quantitative chemiluminescent immunoassay.

80422

80422   Glucagon tolerance panel; for insulinoma
This panel must include the following:
Glucose (82947 x 3)
Insulin (83525 x 3)

A laboratory test is performed to diagnose and monitor insulinoma, a neuroendocrine tumor found in the pancreas in the islets of Langerhans where beta cells produce the hormone insulin. Insulin is necessary for the transport and storage of glucose and also plays a role in lipid metabolism. Insulinomas are the most common cause of hyperinsulinemia from an endogenous source. High levels of insulin will cause low levels of circulating glucose, or hypoglycemia. Symptoms of hypoglycemia can include sweating, palpitations, visual changes, dizziness, fainting, and seizures. The glucagon tolerance test measures circulating glucose and insulin levels at baseline and following an intravenous injection of glucagon, a polypeptide hormone normally secreted by pancreatic alpha cells that raises blood glucose levels by stimulating the liver to release glycogen stores. The patient should be fasting for at least 8 hours prior to the start of the test. An intravenous line is inserted by separately reportable procedure. A baseline blood sample may be obtained from this IV line or by separately reportable venipuncture for glucose and insulin levels. Glucagon 1 mg is administered via IV push and subsequent blood samples are obtained to test glucose and insulin levels post response. Serum/plasma is tested for glucose using quantitative enzymatic method, and insulin using chemiluminescent immunoassay.

80424

80424   Glucagon tolerance panel; for pheochromocytoma
This panel must include the following:
Catecholamines, fractionated (82384 x 2)

A laboratory test is performed to diagnose and monitor pheochromocytoma, a type of neuroendocrine tumor found in the adrenal medulla, specifically in the chromaffin cells that produce adrenaline and noradrenaline (norepinephrine). Adrenaline and noradrenaline are a type of hormone called catacholamines that help to regulate heart rate, blood pressure, and metabolism. Symptoms of high catecholamine levels can include elevated blood pressure, rapid and forceful heartbeat, sweating, headache, tremors, paleness, shortness of breath, and anxiety. It is not uncommon for symptoms to be very brief, lasting 15-20 minutes, occurring several times a day. The glucagon tolerance test measures circulating catecholamine levels at baseline and following an intravenous injection of glucagon, a polypeptide hormone normally secreted by the pancreatic alpha cells. An intravenous line is inserted by separately reportable procedure and the patient is allowed to rest supine for a minimum of 30 minutes. A baseline blood sample is obtained from the IV line for fractionated catacholamines, and then glucagon 1 mg is injected IV push. A second blood sample is obtained from the IV line two minutes post injection to test for fractionated catecholamine levels in response. Serum/plasma is tested using quantitative high performance liquid chromatography.

Pathology and Laboratory

80426

80426   Gonadotropin releasing hormone stimulation panel

This panel must include the following:
Follicle stimulating hormone (FSH) (83001 x 4)
Luteinizing hormone (LH) (83002 x 4)

A gonadotropin releasing hormone stimulation panel is performed to evaluate follicle stimulating hormone (FSH) and luteinizing hormone (LH) response. This test is performed to identify pituitary disorders in children with premature or delayed puberty. Baseline levels of FSH and LH are obtained. Gonatropin releasing hormone (GnRH) is administered. Following administration of GnRH, FSH and LH levels are again obtained to determine the response to stimulation with GnRH. This test includes testing of FSH and LH levels four times, which includes the baseline level and testing three times following administration of GnRH.

80428

80428   Growth hormone stimulation panel (eg, arginine infusion, l-dopa administration)

This panel must include the following:
Human growth hormone (HGH) (83003 x 4)

A laboratory test is performed to evaluate an individual with symptoms of low human growth hormone (HGH) levels. HGH is produced by the pituitary gland, a pea size endocrine gland located in the brain, behind the sinus cavity. HGH promotes proper linear bone growth in children from birth to puberty and regulates bone density, muscle mass, and lipid metabolism in children and adults. The growth hormone stimulation test measures the ability of the pituitary to release HGH when an evocative agent is introduced. The test may be ordered when a child is consistently small for age or when normal growth suddenly slows down or stops completely. The test may be ordered for an adult with evidence of decreased bone density, fatigue, poor exercise tolerance, and/or adverse changes in lipid levels. The patient should be fasting and refrain from exercise for at least 10 hours prior to the start of the test. An intravenous line is inserted by separately reportable procedure and the patient is allowed to rest supine for a minimum of 30 minutes. A baseline blood sample is obtained from the IV line or by separately reportable venipuncture for HGH levels. Arginine 0.5 g/kg is infused intravenously over 30 minutes OR a single dose of L-dopa 250-500 mg is taken orally. Additional blood samples are then obtained from the IV line or by venipuncture at 30 minute intervals up to 120 minutes post infusion/ingestion to monitor changes in HGH levels. Serum/plasma is tested using quantitative chemiluminescent immunoassay.

80430

80430   Growth hormone suppression panel (glucose administration)

This panel must include the following:
Glucose (82947 x 3)
Human growth hormone (HGH) (83003 x 4)

A laboratory test is performed to evaluate an individual with symptoms of elevated growth hormone levels. Human growth hormone (HGH) is produced by the pituitary gland, a pea size endocrine gland located in the brain, behind the sinus cavity. HGH promotes proper linear bone growth in children from birth to puberty and regulates bone density, muscle mass, and lipid metabolism in children and adults. Symptoms of excess HGH can include exaggerated length of long bones in children (gigantism), facial thickening, and enlarged hands and feet in adults (acromegaly). Elevated HGH is most commonly caused by benign pituitary tumors. The growth hormone suppression test measures the ability of the pituitary to slow down HGH release when an evocative agent is introduced. The patient should be fasting and refrain from exercise for at least 10 hours prior to the start of the test. An intravenous line is inserted by separately reportable procedure and the patient is allowed to rest supine for a minimum of 30 minutes. A baseline blood sample is obtained from the IV line or by separately reportable venipuncture for Human Growth Hormone levels. Glucose 75-100 grams is then administered orally. Additional blood samples are then obtained from the IV line or venipuncture to monitor changes in HGH and glucose levels. Serum/plasma is tested using quantitative chemiluminescent immunoassay.

80432

80432   Insulin-induced C-peptide suppression panel

This panel must include the following:
Insulin (83525)
C-peptide (84681 x 5) Glucose (82947 x 5)

A laboratory test is performed to evaluate the insulin production of beta cells. Insulin is a hormone produced by the pancreas in the islets of Langerhans and is necessary for the transport and storage of glucose and also plays a role in lipid metabolism. C-peptides are short chain amino acids released as a byproduct from biologically inactive proinsulin, when it splits from 2 molecules into a single insulin molecule and a single C-peptide molecule. The insulin-induced C-peptide suppression test can be used to diagnose insulinoma, (a tumor found in the beta cells of the pancreas), metabolic syndrome, and hypoglycemia caused by exogenous insulin administration. The patient should be fasting for at least 10 hours prior to the test. An intravenous line is inserted by separately reportable procedure. A baseline blood sample may be taken from the IV line or by separately reportable

venipuncture for insulin, C-peptide, and glucose levels. Insulin 0.05-0.075 U/kg diluted in normal saline is infused over two hours. Additional blood samples are drawn at 15-20 minute intervals to measure changes in C-peptide and glucose levels. Serum/plasma is tested for insulin and C-peptide using quantitative chemiluminescent immunoassay and for glucose using quantitative enzymatic method.

80434

80434   Insulin tolerance panel; for ACTH insufficiency

This panel must include the following:
Cortisol (82533 x 5)
Glucose (82947 x 5)

A laboratory test is performed to assess adrenocorticotropic hormone (ACTH) insufficiency. Low levels of ACTH can cause Cushing syndrome, Addison disease, secondary adrenal insufficiency, hypopituitarism and other conditions leading to an imbalance of cortisol. Cortisol is a steroid hormone produced by the adrenal glands that is important for glucose, protein, and lipid metabolism; for suppression of the immune system response; and to maintain normal blood pressure. A dynamic feedback system in the body called the hypothalamic-pituitary-adrenal axis regulates cortisol levels. In response to decreased cortisol in the circulating blood, the hypothalamus produces corticotropin-releasing hormone (CRH) stimulating the pituitary to produce ACTH and the adrenal glands to make more cortisol. The insulin tolerance test (ITT) is used to induce severe hypoglycemia. The normal response to hypoglycemia is pituitary release of ACTH, followed by a release of cortisol from the adrenal glands. Failure to see a rise in cortisol with adequate hypoglycemia is an indication of insufficient ACTH production by the pituitary gland. The patient should be fasting for at least 10 hours prior to the test. An intravenous line is inserted by separately reportable procedure and the patient is allowed to rest for a minimum of 30 minutes. A baseline blood sample may be obtained from the IV line or by separately reportable venipuncture for cortisol and glucose levels. Fast acting (regular) insulin is given via IV push. Additional blood samples are drawn from the IV line or venipuncture at 30, 60, 90, and 120 minutes to measure changes in cortisol and glucose levels. Serum/plasma is tested for cortisol using quantitative chemiluminescent immunoassay and for glucose using quantitative enzymatic method.

80435

80435   Insulin tolerance panel; for growth hormone deficiency

This panel must include the following:
Glucose (82947 x 5)
Human growth hormone (HGH) (83003 x 5)

A laboratory test is performed to assess human growth hormone (HGH) deficiency. Low levels of HGH can manifest in childhood or adulthood. The cause may be congenital or acquired. The most common cause of decreased HGH is pituitary or parasellar tumors. HGH deficiency can be partial or complete, transient or permanent. Characteristics of HGH deficiency include hypoglycemia and growth failure in children, and decreased lean body mass and bone density in both children and adults. The insulin tolerance test (ITT) is a provocative test used to induce severe hypoglycemia which should stimulate the pituitary gland to increase production of HGH. Failure to see a rise in HGH with adequate hypoglycemia is an indication of HGH deficiency. The patient should be fasting for at least 10 hours prior to the start of the test. An intravenous line is inserted by separately reportable procedure. A baseline blood sample may be taken from the IV line or by separately reportable venipuncture for HGH and glucose levels. Fast acting (regular) insulin is given via IV push. Additional blood samples are drawn from the IV line or venipuncture at 15, 30, 45, and 60 minutes to measure changes in HGH and glucose levels. Serum/plasma is tested for HGH using quantitative chemiluminescent immunoassay and for glucose using quantitative enzymatic method.

80436

80436   Metyrapone panel

This panel must include the following:
Cortisol (82533 x 2)
11 deoxycortisol (82634 x 2)

A laboratory test is performed to diagnose adrenal insufficiency. The metyrapone (Metopirone) test may be used when insulin or glucagon stress testing is contraindicated. Low levels of ACTH can cause Cushing syndrome, Addison disease, secondary adrenal insufficiency, hypopituitarism, and other conditions leading to an imbalance of cortisol. Cortisol is a steroid hormone produced by the adrenal glands that is important for glucose, protein, and lipid metabolism; for suppression of the immune system response; and to maintain normal blood pressure. A dynamic feedback system in the body called the hypothalamic-pituitary-adrenal axis regulates cortisol levels. In response to decreased cortisol in the circulating blood, the hypothalamus produces corticotropin-releasing hormone (CRH) stimulating the pituitary to produce ACTH and the adrenal glands to make more cortisol. Metyrapone inhibits an enzyme, causing cortisol synthesis to be blocked. This in turn stimulates ACTH secretion in the pituitary gland and increases plasma levels of 11-deoxycortisol. A baseline blood sample is obtained by separately reportable venipuncture for cortisol and 11-deoxycortisol levels. Metyrapone 30 mg/kg is administered orally at midnight with a snack. A blood sample is obtained between 8 - 9 am the next morning for cortisol and 11-deoxycortisol levels. Serum/plasma is tested for cortisol using quantitative chemiluminescent immunoassay and for 11-deoxycortisol using quantitative high performance liquid chromatography-tandem mass spectrometry.

80438-80439

80438   Thyrotropin releasing hormone (TRH) stimulation panel; 1 hour
This panel must include the following:
Thyroid stimulating hormone (TSH) (84443 x 3)

80439   Thyrotropin releasing hormone (TRH) stimulation panel; 2 hour
This panel must include the following:
Thyroid stimulating hormone (TSH) (84443 x 4)

(pituitary) and tertiary (hypothalamic) hypothyroidism. The hypothalamus releases thyrotropin releasing hormone (TRH) in response to low circulating levels of T4 and T3. TRH stimulates the pituitary to release thyroid stimulating hormone (TSH), which in turn causes the thyroid gland to manufacture and release T4 and T3. Thyrotropin releasing hormone (TRH) stimulation testing has largely been replaced by the thyroid stimulating hormone 3rd generation test due to the poor availability of the necessary drug (Protirelin). An intravenous line is inserted by separately reportable procedure. A baseline blood sample is obtained from the IV line or by separately reportable venipuncture for TSH levels. Protirelin (TRH) 200¬µg is administered via IV push. To test for TSH using TRH 1 hour stimulation panel (80438), additional blood samples are obtained at 20 and 60 minutes for TSH levels. To test for TSH using TRH 2 hour stimulation panel (80439), additional blood samples are obtained at 20, 60, and 120 minutes for TSH levels. Serum/plasma is tested using quantitative chemiluminescent immunoassay.

80500

80500   Clinical pathology consultation; limited, without review of patient's history and medical records

A limited clinical pathology consultation is a service rendered by a pathologist to provide additional interpretive judgment to one or more test results. The pathologist is provided with the patient's diagnosis but does not review the patient's medical history or medical records. The request for consultation must be made in writing by the attending physician and relate to test results that fall outside of an expected range. The consulting pathologist provides a written report of the findings to the requesting physician at the conclusion of the review.

80502

80502   Clinical pathology consultation; comprehensive, for a complex diagnostic problem, with review of patient's history and medical records

A comprehensive clinical pathology consultation is a service rendered by a pathologist to provide additional interpretive judgment to one or more test results when a complex diagnostic problem has been identified. The clinical pathologist is provided with the patient's diagnosis and does a complete review of the patient's medical history and all available medical records. The request for consultation must be made in writing by the attending physician and relate to test results that fall outside of an expected range. The consulting pathologist provides a written report of the findings to the requesting physician at the conclusion of the review.

81000-81003

81000   Urinalysis, by dip stick or tablet reagent for bilirubin, glucose, hemoglobin, ketones, leukocytes, nitrite, pH, protein, specific gravity, urobilinogen, any number of these constituents; non-automated, with microscopy

81001   Urinalysis, by dip stick or tablet reagent for bilirubin, glucose, hemoglobin, ketones, leukocytes, nitrite, pH, protein, specific gravity, urobilinogen, any number of these constituents; automated, with microscopy

81002   Urinalysis, by dip stick or tablet reagent for bilirubin, glucose, hemoglobin, ketones, leukocytes, nitrite, pH, protein, specific gravity, urobilinogen, any number of these constituents; non-automated, without microscopy

81003   Urinalysis, by dip stick or tablet reagent for bilirubin, glucose, hemoglobin, ketones, leukocytes, nitrite, pH, protein, specific gravity, urobilinogen, any number of these constituents; automated, without microscopy

A urinalysis is performed by dip stick or tablet reagent for bilirubin, glucose, hemoglobin, ketones, leukocytes, nitrite, pH, protein, specific gravity, and/or urobilinogen. Urinalysis can quickly screen for conditions that do not immediately produce symptoms such as diabetes mellitus, kidney disease, or urinary tract infection. A dip stick allows qualitative and semi-quantitative analysis using a paper or plastic stick with color strips for each agent being tested. The stick is dipped in the urine specimen and the color strips are then compared to a color chart to determine the presence or absence and/or a rough estimate of the concentration of each agent tested. Reagent tablets use an absorbent mat with a few drops of urine placed on the mat followed by a reagent tablet. A drop of distilled, deionized water is then placed on the tablet and the color change is observed. Bilirubin is a byproduct of the breakdown of red blood cells by the liver. Normally bilirubin

is excreted through the bowel, but in patients with liver disease, bilirubin is filtered by the kidneys and excreted in the urine. Glucose is a sugar that is normally filtered by the glomerulus and excreted only in small quantities in the urine. Excess sugar in the urine (glycosuria) is indicative of diabetes mellitus. The peroxidase activity of erythrocytes is used to detect hemoglobin in the urine which may be indicative of hematuria, myoglobinuria, or hemoglobinuria. Ketones in the urine are the result of diabetic ketoacidosis or calorie deprivation (starvation). A leukocyte esterase test identifies the presence of white blood cells in the urine. The presence of nitrites in the urine is indicative of bacteria. The pH identifies the acid-base levels in the urine. The presence of excessive amounts of protein (proteinuria) may be indicative of nephrotic syndrome. Specific gravity measures urine density and is indicative of the kidneys' ability to concentrate and dilute urine. Following dip stick or reagent testing, the urine sample may be examined under a microscope. The urine sample is placed in a test tube and centrifuged. The sediment is resuspended. A drop of the resuspended sediment is then placed on a glass slide, coverslipped, and examined under a microscope for crystals, casts, squamous cells, blood (white, red) cells, and bacteria. Use 81000 for a non-automated test with microscopy and 81001 for an automated test with microscopy. Use 81002 for a non-automated test without microscopy and 81003 for an automated test without microscopy.

81005

81005   Urinalysis; qualitative or semiquantitative, except immunoassays

A random urine sample is obtained. The specimen is then tested for the presence of any number of constituents using a technique such as colorimetry. If semi-quantitative analysis is performed, the amounts of the various constituents are estimated. Examples of commonly identified constituents in the urine include bilirubin, glucose, hemoglobin, ketones, leukocytes, nitrite, pH, protein, specific gravity, and urobilinogen.

81007

81007   Urinalysis; bacteriuria screen, except by culture or dipstick

This test is performed to detect the presence of potentially significant bacteria in the urine and to diagnose urinary tract infection, cystitis, or pyelonephritis. A first morning urine specimen is preferred, but a random sample may also be used. Clean catch mid-stream technique is used to obtain the specimen. The specimen is then tested for the presence of bacteria using any method except culture or dipstick.

81015

81015   Urinalysis; microscopic only

Microscopic analysis is performed to determine if sediment in the urine specimen is normal or indicative of an abnormality such as infection. Microscopy can be performed using a standard glass counting chamber and coverslips or a disposable system. Most laboratories use disposable systems. Urine from the sample is centrifuged to concentrate the sediment in a button at the bottom of the tube. The specimen is decanted leaving only 0.2-0.5 ml liquid. The sediment is resuspended. The sediment is placed in a test well and examined under a microscope at low power to identify crystals, casts, squamous cells, and other debris. The test well is 0.1 mm deep and contains a grid that measures 3x3 mm with 90 small squares in the grid. Each of the 90 small squares are grouped together in 1x1 mm squares which are the medium squares and each contains 9 small squares. Casts are usually counted at low power. The urine is then examined under high power for the presence of red blood cells (RBCs), white blood cells (WBCs), epithelial cells, bacteria, yeast, and crystals and each of the constituents is characterized and counted. Counts may be performed on a single small cell or all 90 cells may be counted depending on the concentration of each of the constituents in the specimen. For example, WBCs may be counted in only a single small square when high numbers of cells are present, 9 medium squares when moderate levels of cells are present, or the entire 90 cells when low cell counts are present. If a single small square is counted the results are multiplied by 90 to obtain the WBC count. If a medium square is counted (9 small cells) the results are multiplied by 10. If all 90 cells are counted, the total count is reported.

81020

81020   Urinalysis; 2 or 3 glass test

This test is performed to help diagnose the site and cause of inflammation of the urethra, particularly in males. First morning urine is collected in two or three glasses. Each glass is then tested for the presence of white blood cells (WBCs) as indicated by turbidity (cloudiness) of the specimen and red blood cells (RBCs). If the first glass is turbid and the second glass and third glass clear, urethritis is present in the anterior segment only. If all two or three glasses are turbid, both anterior and posterior urethritis is present. If only the anterior urethra is inflamed, the first glass will contain blood while the other two will not. If both anterior and posterior urethritis is present, all two or three glasses will contain blood.

81025

81025   Urine pregnancy test, by visual color comparison methods

Pregnancy tests detect the presence of human chorionic gonadotropin (hCG) in the urine. HCG is produced by the placenta and can be detected in urine shortly after the embryo attaches to the uterine lining. The test may be performed by collecting a urine specimen and dipping a stick treated to detect the presence of hCG in the urine. The presence of hCG is indicated by a color change in the treated section of the dipstick indicating a positive pregnancy test. If no color change occurs, the test is negative.

81161

81161 DMD (dystrophin) (eg, Duchenne/Becker muscular dystrophy) deletion analysis, and duplication analysis, if performed

Molecular genetic testing is performed for Duchenne/Becker muscular dystrophy to screen for a deletion defect in the dystrophin gene located at Xp21. Duchenne/Becker muscular dystrophies are the most common neuromuscular diseases diagnosed in childhood. These two types of muscular dystrophy are X-linked genetic diseases, so the disease primarily affects males although females with X chromosome abnormalities may also be affected. Duchenne muscular dystrophy is the more severe form of the disease usually manifesting by age 3, with loss of mobility by age 9 or 10, and death by age 20. Becker muscular dystrophy progresses more slowly but death usually occurs in the 30s or 40s. The test for Duchenne/Becker muscular dystrophy gene deletions may be performed using Southern blot technique with complementary DNA (cDNA) probes or by polymerase chain reaction (PCR) or another molecular genetic testing technique. Any testing for gene duplication related to Duchenne/Becker muscular dystrophy is included in code 81161.

81162

81162 BRCA1, BRCA2 (breast cancer 1 and 2) (eg, hereditary breast and ovarian cancer) gene analysis; full sequence analysis and full duplication/deletion analysis

Molecular genetic testing is performed to identify mutations on the BRCA1 gene located on chromosome 17 and the BRCA2 gene found on chromosome 13. Both genes are tumor suppressors which help to stabilize genetic material and prevent uncontrolled cell growth. Mutations are linked to an inherited increased risk for developing breast and certain other cancers in both men and women. BCRA1 mutations in women increase the risk of early onset breast cancer and also cervical, ovarian, uterine, pancreatic, and colon cancer. BCRA1 mutations in males increase the risk of breast cancer, pancreatic and testicular cancer. A mutation of BRCA2 in women increases the risk of pancreatic, stomach, gall bladder, and bile duct cancers, and melanoma. Males with a BCRA2 mutation have a higher rate of breast, pancreatic, and prostate cancer. A full sequence analysis of both BRCA1 and BRCA2 is performed along with a full duplication/deletion analysis for variants. Full sequence analysis compares gene segments to determine their similarities or differences and identify relationships. Intrinsic features are studied to find active and post-translational modification sites, gene structures, distribution of introns and extrons, and regulatory elements. Genetic markers can be found by identifying point mutations or single nucleotide polymorphisms (SNP). Variants not identified by the sequence analysis may be found using a duplication/deletion analysis. Since a normal gene should have 2 copies per cell (with the exception of sex chromosomes), zero or one copy indicates a deletion variant, and three or more copies is evidence of a duplication variant. This testing can be used to identify those with hereditary cancer or an increased risk of developing cancer, and guide treatment decisions based on inherited germ line mutations.

81200

81200 ASPA (aspartoacylase) (eg, Canavan disease) gene analysis, common variants (eg, E285A, Y231X)

Molecular genetic testing is performed to identify the specific mutation of the ASPA (aspartocylase) gene which causes Canavan disease. Canavan disease is an autosomal recessive inherited condition caused by mutations in the ASPA gene. Individuals with mutations of the ASPA gene from both parents develop Canavan disease. Individuals that receive the ASPA mutation from only one parent are carriers of the disease. People of Ashkenazi Jewish descent (Central and Eastern European) are most commonly affected. The ASPA gene is responsible for providing instructions in the creation of the enzyme aspartoacylase. In the brain, this enzyme is responsible for breaking down N-acetyl-L-aspartic acid (NAA) into two substances, aspartic acid and acetic acid. Although the exact function of NAA is not known, the production and breakdown of NAA appears to be critical for maintaining white matter (nerve fibers covered with myelin) in the brain. It is believed that NAA is essential for making certain lipids that are used to produce myelin. Mutations of the ASPA gene reduce or eliminate the enzymatic activity of aspartocylase which causes deterioration of white matter in the brain. There are more than 55 mutations of the ASPA gene that are known to cause Canavan disease. The two most common variants are E285A and Y231X. The E285A mutation, also referred to as Glu285Ala, replaces glutamic acid with alanine at the 285 position of the enzyme. The Y231X mutation, also referred to as Tyr231Ter, prematurely stops protein production leading to a nonfunctional version of the enzyme. DNA testing is performed to identify carriers of the disease and the specific ASPA gene mutation. DNA testing may also be performed to identify the specific ASPA gene mutation in individuals diagnosed with Canavan disease. Canavan disease affects all aspects of infant development including muscle control and tone, feeding, swallowing, and vision, and also causes mental retardation. Most individuals with Canavan disease die

before 18 months of age, although in milder forms of the disease the individual may survive into adolescence or young adulthood.

81201-81203

81201 APC (adenomatous polyposis coli) (eg, familial adenomatosis polyposis [FAP], attenuated FAP) gene analysis; full gene sequence

81202 APC (adenomatous polyposis coli) (eg, familial adenomatosis polyposis [FAP], attenuated FAP) gene analysis; known familial variants

81203 APC (adenomatous polyposis coli) (eg, familial adenomatosis polyposis [FAP], attenuated FAP) gene analysis; duplication/deletion variants

Molecular genetic testing is performed to identify the specific mutation of the adenomatous polyposis coli (APC) gene that causes familial adenomatosis polyposis (classic, attenuated FAP). FAP is an autosomal dominant inherited condition. Individuals who inherit a mutated APC gene from one parent will have the disease. The classic form of FAP is more severe than the attenuated form. APC gene mutation affects a tumor suppressor protein which allows overgrowth of cells and formation of polyps in the large intestine. This is a pre-malignant condition which usually progresses to colorectal cancer. The APC gene is located on chromosome 5. More than 700 mutations have been identified and cause an abnormally short, nonfunctional APC protein. Testing may involve full gene sequencing which is reported with code 81201. Testing for known familial variants is reported with 81202. One known familial variant of the APC gene causes Turcot syndrome, colorectal cancer with a medulloblastoma, a malignant brain tumor. Another variant which is found in the Ashkenazi Jewish population is replacement of the amino acid isoleucine with the amino acid lysine at position 1307 on the APC gene (Ile1307Lys or I1307K). This mutation is associated with an increased incidence of colon cancer. Testing for duplication/deletion variants is reported with 81203. The most common mutation is a deletion of five DNA nucleotides that change the sequence of amino acids on the APC gene.

81205

81205 BCKDHB (branched-chain keto acid dehydrogenase E1, beta polypeptide) (eg, maple syrup urine disease) gene analysis, common variants (eg, R183P, G278S, E422X)

Molecular genetic testing is performed to identify the specific mutation of the BCKDHB (branched-chain keto acid dehydrogenase E1, beta polypeptide) gene which causes Maple syrup urine disease. Maple syrup urine disease is an autosomal recessive inherited condition caused by mutations on the BCKDHB gene. Individuals with mutations of the BCKDHB gene from both parents develop maple syrup urine disease. Individuals that receive the BCKDHB mutation from only one parent are carriers of the disease. More than 40 mutations of the gene have been identified on chromosome 6 at the 14, 1 position. The incidence in newborns is estimated to be 1 in 185,000 worldwide. People of Ashkenazi Jewish descent (Central and Eastern European) are most commonly affected by two of the identified mutations (R183P, G278S) and a disproportionate number of cases have also been identified in Old Order Mennonite populations, with newborns affected at a rate of 1 in 380. The BCKDHB gene is responsible for providing instructions to create the beta subunit of an enzyme complex known as branched-chain alpha-keto acid dehydrogenase (BCKD). Two beta subunits connect with two alpha subunits produced from the BCKDHA gene forming a critical part of the enzyme complex known as the E1 component. This complex is most active in the inner membrane of the mitochondria (energy areas of a cell) and is responsible for a step in the catabolism of the amino acids leucine, isoleucine, and valine ingested from dietary protein (such as milk, meat and eggs). The disruption of the BCKD enzyme complex causes a build up of amino acids and their byproducts which are toxic to cells and tissue especially in the brain. The toxic byproducts are excreted in urine, giving it a sweet aroma characteristic of maple syrup. DNA testing is performed to identify carriers of the disease and the specific BCKDHB gene mutation. DNA testing may also be performed to identify the specific BCKDHB gene mutation in individuals diagnosed with Maple syrup urine disease. Symptoms associated with Maple syrup urine disease include feeding problems and developmental delays in infants, decreased appetite at all ages, lethargy, seizures, and coma. Symptoms may be exacerbated during times of physical stress such as infection/illness, fever or under nourishment. Treatment consists of a protein free diet and dialysis to reduce the level of toxic byproducts in the blood followed by a diet low in the branched-chain amino acids leucine, isoleucine and valine.

81206-81208

81206 BCR/ABL1 (t(9;22)) (eg, chronic myelogenous leukemia) translocation analysis; major breakpoint, qualitative or quantitative

81207 BCR/ABL1 (t(9;22)) (eg, chronic myelogenous leukemia) translocation analysis; minor breakpoint, qualitative or quantitative

81208 BCR/ABL1 (t(9;22)) (eg, chronic myelogenous leukemia) translocation analysis; other breakpoint, qualitative or quantitative

Molecular genetic testing is performed to identify a specific mutation of the BCR/ABL1 gene often found in patients diagnosed with chronic myelogenous leukemia (CML). The mutation is expressed as a reciprocal translocation, t(9;22), involving the BCR (breakpoint cluster region) gene on chromosome 22 (Philadelphia chromosome) and ABL1 (V-abl Abelson murine leukemia viral oncogene) located on chromosome 9. This fusion gene

Pathology and Laboratory

encodes an unregulated, cytoplasm targeted, tyrosine kinase that allows cell proliferation in the absence of cytokine regulation, predisposing an individual to certain cancers. Karyotyping and molecular testing (using rtPCR or FISH) is indicated at initial diagnosis to define tumor markers by which residual disease can later be measured (during and after treatment). The BCR gene has three separate breakpoint cluster regions. Use 81206 for identification of major breakpoint, occurring at p210 in a 5.8 kb major breakpoint cluster region (M-bcr) around exon b3. This results in a BCR-ABL1 p210 chimeric transcription of BCR at exon b2 or b3 fused with ABL1 exons 2 through 11. Use 81207 for identification of a minor breakpoint, occurring at p190 in the minor breakpoint cluster region (m-bcr) on intron 1 which results in the fusion of BCR exon 1 to the same ABL1 exons. Use 81208 for identification of other breakpoint cluster regions not specified as major or minor.

81209

81209   BLM (Bloom syndrome, RecQ helicase-like) (eg, Bloom syndrome) gene analysis, 2281del6ins7 variant

Molecular genetic testing is performed to identify the specific mutation of the BLM (Bloom syndrome, RecQ helicase-like) gene which causes Bloom syndrome. Bloom syndrome is an autosomal recessive inherited condition caused by mutations on the BLM gene. Individuals with mutations of the BLM gene from both parents develop Bloom syndrome. Individuals that receive the BLM mutation from only one parent are carriers of the disease. People of Ashkenazi Jewish descent (Central and Eastern European) are most commonly affected by the 2281del6ins7 or blmAsh variant. Over 70 mutations of the gene have been identified. BLM provides instructions to make the protein RecQ helicase, an enzyme which binds to DNA to temporarily unwind the double helix molecule so it can be copied into sister chromatids. Sister chromatids are two identical DNA structures attached to each other which exchange small sections of DNA. Mutations on the BLM gene affect genome stability and an increase in sister chromatid exchange takes place. Gaps or breaks in the DNA sequencing occur, impairing normal cellular activity and increasing cell death and slowing growth. The BLM enzyme suppresses sister chromatid exchange during copying which helps to maintain the stability of the DNA molecule and may also restart DNA copying when the process stalls. DNA testing is performed to identify carriers of the disease and the specific BLM gene mutation. DNA testing may also be performed to identify the specific BLM gene mutation in individuals diagnosed with Bloom syndrome. Characteristics of individuals with BLM mutation include short stature, facial rash (butterfly pattern on cheeks) or rash on back of hands induced by sun exposure, high pitched vocal quality, long narrow face with small mandible and prominent ears and nose, skin pigment changes (caf√©-au-lait spots), and telangiectasias (broken blood vessels) in skin and eyes. The BLM mutation may also cause disorders of the immune system especially an increased incidence of pneumonia, ear infections, and a predisposition to all types of cancers at an early age. Males often have hypo-gonadism with reduced or absent sperm and females have early onset menopause. Learning disabilities and mental retardation have also been identified.

81210

81210   BRAF (B-Raf proto-oncogene, serine/threonine kinase) (eg, colon cancer, melanoma), gene analysis, V600 variant(s)

Molecular genetic testing is performed to identify the specific mutation of the BRAF (B-Raf proto-oncogene, serine/threonine kinase) gene, V600 variant(s) associated with colorectal cancer and melanoma. The gene encodes a protein associated with the raf/mil family of serine/threonine protein kinases that regulate MAP kinase/ERK pathways affecting cell division, differentiation, and secretion. Proteins encoded by the BRAF gene are responsible for signaling cell growth. A mutation on the BRAF gene causes an alteration in the normal function of B-Raf protein, activating it and disrupting the pathways that signal cell division, differentiation, and secretion. The most common alteration involves replacement of the amino acid valine with the amino acid glutamic acid at position 600 on the BRAF gene. Chemical signals from outside the cell are transmitted continuously into the cell nucleus causing them to grow and divide uncontrollably. More than 30 mutations of the BRAF gene have been identified. Genetic testing may be performed to identify the specific BRAF gene mutation in individuals diagnosed with cancer as an aide to directed treatment, including the use of chemotherapeutic agents dabrafenib, trametinib, and vemurafenib.

81211-81213

81211   BRCA1, BRCA2 (breast cancer 1 and 2) (eg, hereditary breast and ovarian cancer) gene analysis; full sequence analysis and common duplication/deletion variants in BRCA1 (ie, exon 13 del 3.835kb, exon 13 dup 6kb, exon 14-20 del 26kb, exon 22 del 510bp, exon 8-9 del 7.1kb)

81212   BRCA1, BRCA2 (breast cancer 1 and 2) (eg, hereditary breast and ovarian cancer) gene analysis; 185delAG, 5385insC, 6174delT variants

81213   BRCA1, BRCA2 (breast cancer 1 and 2) (eg, hereditary breast and ovarian cancer) gene analysis; uncommon duplication/deletion variants

Molecular genetic testing is performed to identify specific mutations on the BRCA1 gene located on chromosome 17 and the BRCA2 gene found on chromosome 13. Both of these genes are tumor suppressors which help to stabilize genetic material and prevent uncontrolled growth of cells. Mutations are linked to an inherited increased risk for developing breast and certain other cancers in both men and women. BCRA1 mutations

in women increase the risk of early onset breast cancer and also cervical, ovarian, uterine, pancreatic, and colon cancer. This gene mutation in males increases the risk of breast cancer and to some extent pancreatic and testicular cancer. A mutation of BRCA2 in women increases the risk for pancreatic, stomach, gall bladder and bile duct cancers, and melanoma. In males with a BCRA2 mutation there is a higher rate of breast, pancreatic, and prostate cancer. In 81211, a full sequence analysis of both BRCA1 and BRCA2 is performed along with an analysis for common duplication and deletion variants found in the BRCA1 gene. Full sequence analysis compares gene segments to determine their similarities or differences and identify relationships. Intrinsic features are studied to find active and post translational modification sites, gene structures, distribution of introns and extrons, and regulatory elements. Genetic markers can be found by identifying point mutations or single nucleotide polymorphisms (SNP). A normal gene should have 2 copies per cell (with the exception of sex chromosomes). Zero or one copies would indicate a deletion variant and three or more copies would be evidence of a duplication variant. The most common variants in BRCA1 are: exon 13 del 3.835kb, exon 13 dup 6kb, exon 14-20 del 26kb, exon 22 del 510bp, exon 8-9 del 7.1kb. In 81212, an analysis is performed for three very specific variants that have been identified in Central and Eastern European populations of Ashkenazi Jews. Two are found on the BRCA1 gene, c. 68_69delAG (185delAG) and c. 5266dupC (5385insC) and one is located on the BRCA2 gene, c. 5946delT (6174delT). These variants are not limited to this population but they are found with increased frequency among individuals of Ashkenazi Jewish descent. In 82313, an analysis is performed for uncommon duplication or deletion variants, which may also be referred to as variants of uncertain significance (VUS). In VUS there may be missense or potential splice site changes on the gene which are often seen with greater frequency in minority or ethnic populations. It is estimated that half of all uncommon mutations that have been identified on BRCA 1 or BRCA2 have an unknown clinical significance.

81214-81215

81214   BRCA1 (breast cancer 1) (eg, hereditary breast and ovarian cancer) gene analysis; full sequence analysis and common duplication/deletion variants (ie, exon 13 del 3.835kb, exon 13 dup 6kb, exon 14-20 del 26kb, exon 22 del 510bp, exon 8-9 del 7.1kb)

81215   BRCA1 (breast cancer 1) (eg, hereditary breast and ovarian cancer) gene analysis; known familial variant

Molecular genetic testing is performed to identify a specific mutation of the BRCA1 "caretaker" gene located on chromosome 17 that encodes the breast cancer type 1 susceptibility protein responsible for repairing DNA found in breast and other tissue. When the gene is damaged or mutated, the protein is not able to repair (or destroy) the damaged DNA and this may predispose an individual to early onset breast cancer or ovarian and fallopian tube cancers at any age. In 81214, a full sequence analysis as well as an analysis for common duplication/deletion variants is performed. Full sequence analysis compares gene segments to determine their similarities or differences and identify relationships. Intrinsic features are studied to find active and post translational modification sites, gene structures, distribution of introns, extrons and regulatory elements. Genetic markers can be found by identifying point mutations or single nucleotide polymorphisms (SNP). A normal gene should have 2 copies per cell (with the exception of sex chromosomes). Zero or one copies would indicate a deletion variant and three (or more) copies would be evidence of a duplication variant. In 81215, a gene analysis for BRCA1 is performed for a known familial variant. When there is a family history of certain types of cancer (breast, ovarian, fallopian tube) it is advantageous to perform molecular genetic testing on all members of the family to determine the exact mutation(s) of the gene. This genetic mapping can determine common or familial variants among blood relatives and help to determine the risk factors for individuals identified as having a gene mutation.

81216-81217

81216   BRCA2 (breast cancer 2) (eg, hereditary breast and ovarian cancer) gene analysis; full sequence analysis

81217   BRCA2 (breast cancer 2) (eg, hereditary breast and ovarian cancer) gene analysis; known familial variant

Molecular genetic testing is performed to identify a specific mutation of the BRCA2 gene located on chromosome 13 that encodes the breast cancer type 2 susceptibility protein. BRCA2 is part of the tumor suppressor gene family which is responsible for error-free repair of chromosomal damage and DNA double strand breaks. When the gene is damaged or mutated, the protein cannot repair damaged DNA causing the damaged cells to proliferate uncontrollably forming malignant tumors. These cancers are found in male breast tissue and prostate, female breast and ovaries, both male and female skin (melanoma), and the pancreas. In 81216, full sequence analysis for BRCA2 is performed. Full sequence analysis compares gene segments to determine their similarities or differences and identify relationships. Intrinsic features are studied to find active and post translational modification sites, gene structures, and distribution of introns, extrons, and regulatory elements. Genetic markers can be found by identifying point mutations or single nucleotide polymorphisms (SNP). In 81217, a gene analysis for BRCA2 is performed for a known familial variant. When there is a family history of certain types of cancers (breast, ovarian, prostate, skin, pancreas) it is advantageous to perform molecular genetic testing on all members of the family to determine the exact mutation(s) of the gene. This genetic mapping can determine common or familial variants among blood relatives and help to determine the risk factors for individuals identified as having a gene mutation.

81220-81223

81220   CFTR (cystic fibrosis transmembrane conductance regulator) (eg, cystic fibrosis) gene analysis; common variants (eg, ACMG/ACOG guidelines)

81221   CFTR (cystic fibrosis transmembrane conductance regulator) (eg, cystic fibrosis) gene analysis; known familial variants

81222   CFTR (cystic fibrosis transmembrane conductance regulator) (eg, cystic fibrosis) gene analysis; duplication/deletion variants

81223   CFTR (cystic fibrosis transmembrane conductance regulator) (eg, cystic fibrosis) gene analysis; full gene sequence

Molecular genetic testing is performed to identify a specific mutation of the CFTR gene found on chromosome 7 and responsible for encoding the protein, cystic fibrosis transmembrane conductance regulator which causes cystic fibrosis. This chloride channel protein is found in epithelial cells which line the lung, liver, pancreas, digestive tract, reproductive organs, and sweat glands. Mutation causes a disruption of salt and water movement into and out of the cells producing a thick, sticky mucous which obstructs the airways and glands. Cystic fibrosis is one of the most common autosomal recessive diseases among Caucasians and is also found in high numbers among populations of Ashkenazi Jews. An individual who inherits a mutated CFTR gene from each parent will show mild to severe symptoms of the disease. An individual who inherits a mutated CFTR gene from only one parent will be a carrier of the disease. The severity of the disease is often determined by heterozygous or homozygous pairing of gene mutations. The homozygous pairing del508F/del508F is associated with severe manifestations of the disease. Pulmonary disease is a critical factor in the prognosis, with respiratory infections often leading to respiratory failure. Pancreatic insufficiency is present in about 85% of cases. Other problems can include sinusitis, nasal polyps, liver disease, and pancreatitis. The life expectancy for an individual with even mild forms of the disease is 30 years. In 81220, gene analysis for common CFTR variants is performed. The most common variant (70%) of CFTR gene mutations among all populations is identified as del508F and involves a deletion of 3 nucleotides resulting in a loss of the amino acid phenylalanine (F) at position 508 on the protein molecule. Other mutations common in Non-Hispanic Caucasian populations include: W1282X, G542X, G551D, 621+1G>T, N1303k. In Ashkenazi Jewish populations common mutations include: W1282X, G542X, 3842+10kbC>T, N1303k. In African-American populations common mutations include: G5510, G542X, 621+1G>T, R553x, del1507. In Hispanic populations common mutations include: R334W, G542X, 3849+10kbC>T, R553X, N1303k. The disease is found rarely in Asian populations and no common variants have been clearly identified. In 81221, as gene analysis for a known familial variant is performed. When there is a family history of CFTR gene mutation it is advantageous to perform molecular genetic testing on all members of the family to determine the exact mutation(s) of carriers and individuals with active disease. This genetic mapping can determine common or familial variants among blood relatives and help to determine the severity of the disease based on homozygous or heterozygous gene pairings. In 81222, a gene analysis is performed for duplication and deletion variants. A normal gene should have 2 copies per cell (with the exception of sex chromosomes). Zero or one copies would indicate a deletion variant and three (or more) copies would be evidence of a duplication variant. Variants such as CFTR exonic and whole gene deletions not identified by sequence analysis may be found using multiplex ligation-dependent probe amplification (MMLPA). In 81223, a full sequence analysis is performed. Full gene sequencing may identify more than 98% of CFTR mutations. This involves sequencing all exons, intron/extron borders, promoter regions, and specific intronic regions of the CFTR gene.

81224

81224   CFTR (cystic fibrosis transmembrane conductance regulator) (eg, cystic fibrosis) gene analysis; intron 8 poly-T analysis (eg, male infertility)

Molecular genetic testing is performed to identify a specific mutation of the CFTR gene found on chromosome 7 and responsible for encoding the protein, cystic fibrosis transmembrane conductance regulator which causes cystic fibrosis (CF) and congenital bilateral absence of the vas deferens (CBAVD). Males who present with azospermia, low semen ejaculatory volume, and absence of vas deferens on clinical exam or ultrasound are candidates for molecular genetic testing to determine if they are carriers of a CFTR gene mutation. An intron 8 poly-T analysis is a reflex test performed when a R117H mutation (or other disease causing mutation) is identified. The poly-T tract is a string of thymidine bases located on intron 8, with 3 common variants, 5T, a penetrant mutation variable and 7T and 9T, both polymorphic variants.

81225

81225   CYP2C19 (cytochrome P450, family 2, subfamily C, polypeptide 19) (eg, drug metabolism), gene analysis, common variants (eg, *2, *3, *4, *8, *17)

Molecular genetic testing is performed to identify a specific mutation of the CYP2C19 gene located on chromosome 10, responsible for encoding the cytochrome P450, family 2, subfamily C, polypeptide 19. This complex polypeptide is part of a mixed function oxidase

system that metabolizes xenobiotics (compounds foreign to the body such as drugs and toxins) and also bioactivates and synthesizes substances such as cholesterol, steroids, and other lipids. A large phenotypical variability factor is present due to genetic polymorphism. The common variants are categorized as normal-fully functional (*1), decreased or non-functioning (*2, *3), decreased or partial-functioning (*4, *5, *6, *7, *8), or increased-partial functioning (*17). Genetic testing may be ordered for individuals undergoing certain drug therapy (antiepileptics, proton pump inhibitors, antidepressants) to identify gene mutations which alter the metabolism of the compound leading to an adverse drug response or effect.

81226

81226   CYP2D6 (cytochrome P450, family 2, subfamily D, polypeptide 6) (eg, drug metabolism), gene analysis, common variants (eg, *2, *3, *4, *5, *6, *9, *10, *17, *19, *29, *35, *41, *1XN, *2XN, *4XN)

Molecular genetic testing is performed to identify a specific mutation of the CYP2D6 gene located on chromosome 22, responsible for encoding the cytochrome P450, family 2, subfamily D, polypeptide 6. This complex polypeptide is part of a mixed function oxidase system that metabolizes xenobiotics (compounds foreign to the body such as drugs and toxins) and also bioactivates and synthesizes substances such as cholesterol, steroids, and other lipids. A large phenotypical variability factor is present due to genetic polymorphism. The common variants are categorized as: Normal-fully functional (*1, *2 [except for *1xN and *2xN]), Partial functioning-Decreased (*9, *10, *17, *29, *41), Partial functioning-Increased (*1xN, *2xN), Non-functioning (*3, *4, *5, *6, *19, *4xN). Genetic testing may be ordered for individuals undergoing certain types of drug therapy (such as Tamoxifen for breast cancer) to identify gene mutations which alter the metabolism of the compound leading to an adverse drug response or effect.

81227

81227   CYP2C9 (cytochrome P450, family 2, subfamily C, polypeptide 9) (eg, drug metabolism), gene analysis, common variants (eg, *2, *3, *5, *6)

Molecular genetic testing is performed to identify a specific mutation of the CYP2C9 gene located on chromosome 10, responsible for encoding the cytochrome P450, family 2, subfamily C, polypeptide 9. This complex protein of monooxygenases catalyze the metabolism of xenobiotics (compounds foreign to the body such as drugs and toxins) and also bioactivates and synthesizes substances such as cholesterol, steroids, and other lipids. At least 50 single nucleotide polymorphisms (SNP) have been identified in coding regions associated with decreased enzyme activity. Adverse drug reactions are often a result of unexpected enzymatic alteration due to polymorphism. The common variants *2, *3, are associated with reduced warfarin metabolism. Individuals with this mutation require a lower dose of warfarin during anti-coagulation therapy and are at increased risk for bleeding. Low frequency variants *5, *6 have been identified in African-American populations and are associated with decreased activity for *5 and no activity for *6. Genetic testing may be ordered for individuals undergoing certain types of drug therapy (such as warfarin and phenytoin) to identify gene mutations which alter the metabolism of the compound, leading to toxicity at normal therapeutic dosages.

81228

81228   Cytogenomic constitutional (genome-wide) microarray analysis; interrogation of genomic regions for copy number variants (eg, bacterial artificial chromosome [BAC] or oligo-based comparative genomic hybridization [CGH] microarray analysis)

Molecular genetic testing is performed to identify specific gene mutations. Two techniques, cytogenomic constitutional (genome-wide) microarray analysis by bacterial artificial chromosome (BAC) and by oligo-based comparative genomic hybridization are now considered to be 1st tier diagnostic tools for postnatal evaluation of individuals with idiopathic mental retardation or developmental delay, autism spectrum disorders, and multiple congenital anomalies. In cytogenomic constitutional microarray, a short piece of human DNA is amplified and inserted into a bacterial artificial chromosome (BAC). The BAC is then able to sequence the genome and model the genetic disease(s) that are present in the individual. The DNA for this test can be harvested from products of conception (umbilical cord, cord blood), skin or peripheral blood samples. In microarray oligo-based comparative genomic hybridization, a test sample of human DNA and a reference sample of DNA are labeled with different fluorophores, hybridized to probes derived from known genes and non-coding regions of the genome, and printed on a glass slide. It is then possible to calculate the ratio of fluorescence intensity of the test DNA to the reference DNA and measure the copy number changes for a particular location in the genome. The DNA for this test may be obtained from primary cultured fibroblasts, saliva, and buccal swabs. Prenatal testing of cells obtained by amniocentesis and chorionic villus sampling (CVS) may also be examined using these techniques when it is determined by ultrasound or magnetic resonance imaging (MRI) that a fetus has congenital anomalies with significant risk for an unbalanced chromosome abnormality or when an apparently balanced rearrangement has been identified by G-band analysis.

Pathology and Laboratory

81229

81229 **Cytogenomic constitutional (genome-wide) microarray analysis; interrogation of genomic regions for copy number and single nucleotide polymorphism (SNP) variants for chromosomal abnormalities**

Molecular genetic testing is performed to identify specific gene mutations. Cytogenomic constitutional (genome-wide) microarray analysis using interrogation of genomic regions for copy number alterations (CNA) and single nucleotide polymorphism (SNP) are the preferred platform for testing cancer genomes. Cancer cells contain many CNAs. When SNP array is used, there is better detection due to higher resolution at the individual gene level. These techniques may also be used to test matched cohorts with or without disease in genome-wide association studies.

81235

81235 **EGFR (epidermal growth factor receptor) (eg, non-small cell lung cancer) gene analysis, common variants (eg, exon 19 LREA deletion, L858R, T790M, G719A, G719S, L861Q)**

Molecular genetic testing is performed to identify the specific mutation of the epidermal growth factor receptor (EGFR) gene that causes non-small-cell lung cancer (NSCLC). NSCLC is considered to be biologically aggressive and accounts for 85-90% of all lung cancers. A transmembrane glycoprotein found on cell surfaces binds epidermal growth factor receptors (EGFR). That binding activates ligands which transform EGFR from an inactive monomeric form to an active homodimer form. Mutations on the EGFR gene cause an overexpression and proliferation of cells in the tyrosine-kinase domain. Most mutations occur within four exons (18-21) on the EGFR gene. The most common mutations are an exon 19 LREA deletion (47%) and L858R, an exon 19 deletion and point mutation at exon 21 that replaces leucine with arginine (34%). A less common mutation but one that has been identified with poor response to chemotherapy is T790M, where threonine has been exchanged for methionine on exon 20. Mutations that account for approximately 3% of NSCLC include G719A which exchanges glycine for alanine in the kinase domain on exon 18, position 719 (also G719S, G719C). L861Q is identified in approximately 2% of mutations where leucine is changed to glutamine at position 861 on exon 21.

81240

81240 **F2 (prothrombin, coagulation factor II) (eg, hereditary hypercoagulability) gene analysis, 20210G>A variant**

Molecular genetic testing is performed to identify a specific mutation of the F2 (prothrombin, coagulation factor II) gene responsible for hereditary hypercoagulability. The 20210G>A variant, is a single point (guanine to adenine at the nucleotide 20210) autosomal dominant mutation which causes an elevation of plasma prothrombin. It is present in approximately 2% of the United States Caucasian population, predominantly in those of southern European ancestry. It is found equally in men and women and in all blood types. In an autosomal dominant mutation, the inheritance of one mutated gene (heterozygous) can predispose an individual to venous thrombosis (upper and lower extremities, cerebral, and intra-abdominal) and/or arterial thrombosis (myocardial infarction, stroke, limb ischemia, and splanchic). It is uncommon to inherit two mutated genes (homozygous), but it is possible. Women with the gene mutation (heterozygous or homozygous) may be at increased risk of developing deep vein thrombosis when using oral contraceptives and they may also experience an increased incidence of miscarriage, stillbirths, 2nd trimester fetal loss, placental abruption, and pre-eclampsia. Molecular genetic testing is indicated in women who have a history of infertility or fetal loss and in both men and women who develop deep vein thrombosis, pulmonary emboli, cerebral vein thrombosis, premature stroke, or myocardial infarction.

81241

81241 **F5 (coagulation factor V) (eg, hereditary hypercoagulability) gene analysis, Leiden variant**

Molecular genetic testing is performed to identify a specific mutation on the F5 (coagulation Factor V) gene responsible for hereditary hypercoagulability. The Leiden variant, also identified as c.1601G>A or pArg534Gln, involves the inactivation of Factor V by activated Protein C (APC). Factor V is a cofactor in the clotting cascade, allowing Factor X to active the enzyme thrombin which in turn cleaves fibrinogen to fibrin forming a clot. With the mutation of the F5 gene, Factor V is left active, leading to the over production of thrombin and excess fibrin resulting in hypercoagulation or clot formation. The Leiden variant is autosomal dominant and the mutation is a single nucleotide polymorphism (SNP) located on exon 10 in the form of a missense substitution of the amino acid arginine to glutamine. It is the most common hereditary hypercoagulability disorder among the Eurasian population with an estimated 5% of Caucasians in North America carrying a heterozygous gene mutation and 1 in 5000 with a homozygous gene mutation. In an autosomal dominant mutation, the inheritance of one mutated gene (heterozygous) can predispose an individual to venous thrombosis (most often lower extremity). The inheritance of two mutated genes (homozygous) may place women at increased risk of venous thrombosis when using oral contraceptives and they may also experience an increased incidence of miscarriage, still births, fetal growth retardation and placental

abruption. Molecular genetic testing is indicated in women who have a history of infertility or fetal loss and in both men and women who develop deep vein thrombosis or pulmonary emboli.

81242

81242 **FANCC (Fanconi anemia, complementation group C) (eg, Fanconi anemia, type C) gene analysis, common variant (eg, IVS4+4A>T)**

Molecular genetic testing is performed to identify a specific mutation on the FANCC (Fanconi anemia, complementation group C) gene responsible for Fanconi anemia, type C. Fanconi anemia is an autosomal recessive inherited condition caused by mutation of the FANCC gene on chromosome 9 at position 22,3. Individuals with mutation of the FANCC gene from both parents develop Fanconi anemia. Individuals who receive the FANCC mutation from only one parent are carriers of the disease. People of Ashkenazi Jewish descent (Central and Eastern European) are most commonly affected by the IVS4+4A>T variant and the disease manifestations may be more severe in this ethnic group. Proteins on the FANCC gene are responsible for delaying the onset of apoptosis (cell death/destruction) and promoting recombination and repair of DNA. Mutation of the FANCC gene causes cytogeneticity of cells, hypersensitivity to DNA damaging agents, chromosome instability, or breakage and defective DNA repair. Most individuals with Fanconi anemia have a lifespan of only 20-30 years due to pancytopenia and a predisposition to develop malignancies. Fanconi anemia is often referred to as aplastic anemia with congenital anomalies. Heart, kidney, skeletal anomalies, and/or patchy brown skin pigmentation may be present at birth or develop in childhood. The mutated gene prevents stem cells from making red blood cells, white blood cells, and platelets, leading to pancytopenia. Reproductive tumors often affect women. Leukemia and solid tumors of the oral cavity and esophagus are found in both women and men. Molecular genetic testing is indicated in individuals with symptoms associated with Fanconi anemia or when there is a family history of the disease.

81243-81244

81243 **FMR1 (fragile X mental retardation 1) (eg, fragile X mental retardation) gene analysis; evaluation to detect abnormal (eg, expanded) alleles**

81244 **FMR1 (Fragile X mental retardation 1) (eg, fragile X mental retardation) gene analysis; characterization of alleles (eg, expanded size and methylation status)**

Molecular genetic testing is performed to identify a specific mutation of the FMR1 gene located on the X chromosome responsible for coding the Fragile X mental retardation protein. The brain requires this protein to develop normal synapses (nerve cell connections), especially synaptic plasticity, which plays a role in learning and memory. A non-mutated protein is necessary for normal cognitive development and female reproductive function. Mutations may be responsible for Fragile X syndrome, mental retardation, autism spectrum disorders, premature ovarian failure, and Parkinson's disease. The protein is believed to bind RNA in association with polysomes and is possibly involved with mRNA trafficking from nucleus to cytoplasm. Fragile X is one of the most common inherited forms of mental retardation. The effects are more severe and more frequent in males than females. In 81243, a FMR1 gene analysis is performed to detect abnormal or expanded alleles. The normal protein sequencing for the FMR1 gene is a pattern of CGG (cytosine-guanine-guanine) with AGG (alanine-guanine-guanine) interrupting several times. This normal segment repeats between 4-44 times. When the segment repeats from 45-54 times, an individual is at borderline risk for expressing characteristics of the syndrome. Pre-mutation expression involves sequencing that repeats 55-200 times, and full mutation is demonstrated when there is >200 repetitions. Mutations that delete all or part of the FMR1 gene, or change a base pair of amino acids, disrupting its three dimensional shape or preventing protein synthesis is expressed in <1% of individuals with Fragile X syndrome. In 81244, a FMR1 gene analysis is performed to characterize the alleles including specific expansions and methylene status. Pre-mutation expression (55-200 sequencing repetitions) can be identified in both males and females placing them at an increased risk of developing conditions such as Fragile X associated tremor/autism syndrome (FXTAS). The syndrome develops later in life with progressive problems with movement (ataxia) and balance, tremors, memory loss, peripheral neuropathy, and mental and behavioral changes. Some individuals may display physical characteristics of Fragile X syndrome such as prominent ears and have an increased risk of developing anxiety and depression in their lifetime. Children may present with learning disabilities, mental retardation, and autism spectrum disorders (especially communication and social problems). Twenty percent of women with premutation expression will experience premature ovarian failure (POF) or occult primary ovarian insufficiency (egg depletion by the age of 40). The heterozygous pairing of normal/low FMR1 genes in a woman predisposes her to polycystic ovarian syndrome progressing to premature ovarian failure. Full mutation of the gene (200->1000 sequencing repetitions) causes gene instability and methylation or silencing of the fragile X mental retardation protein, and Fragile X syndrome. One third of males identified with Fragile X syndrome will have an autism spectrum disorder.

Pathology and Laboratory

81245

81245   FLT3 (fms-related tyrosine kinase 3) (eg, acute myeloid leukemia), gene analysis; internal tandem duplication (ITD) variants (ie, exons 14, 15)

Molecular genetic testing is performed to identify a specific mutation of the FLT3 (fms-related tyrosine kinase 3) gene associated with acute myeloid leukemia (AML). Genetic testing for this gene mutation is considered the standard of care for all patients diagnosed with AML. The absence or presence of the gene mutation can help predict the benefit of therapy and the risk of recurrence or disease progression. The mutation is present in at least 25% of all patients with AML and does not equate with having a poor cure rate. AML is the most common type of acute leukemia diagnosed, usually affecting men over the age of 65. It is rarely found in patients under the age of 40. Tyrosine kinase on the cell surface belonging to a larger group of growth factor receptors with an intracellular tyrosine kinase domain, encodes a class 3 tyrosine kinase receptor regulating hematopoiesis. The receptor is activated by binding of fms-related tyrosine kinase 3 ligand to the extracellular domain. This induces homodimer formation in the plasma membrane leading to autophosphorylation of the receptor with continuing receptor activation of the cytoplasmic effector molecules in the apoptosis, proliferation, and differentiation pathways of hematopoietic cells in the bone marrow. The mutations may then result in acute myeloid leukemia and also acute lymphoblastic leukemia.

81250

81250   G6PC (glucose-6-phosphatase, catalytic subunit) (eg, Glycogen storage disease, type 1a, von Gierke disease) gene analysis, common variants (eg, R83C, Q347X)

Molecular genetic testing is performed to identify a specific mutation of the G6PC (glucose-6-phosphatase, catalytic subunit) gene. Located on chromosome 17, as many as 85 mutations of the G6PC gene have been identified for the glycogen storage disease, type 1a, also known as von Gierke disease. Most change a single amino acid in the enzyme, glucose-6-phosphatase on the membrane of the endoplasmic reticulum. This membrane, located inside of cells, involves protein transport and processing along with the glucose-6-phosphate translocase protein (produced from the 5LC37A4 gene) to breakdown the glucose 6 phosphate sugar molecule forming a simple glucose sugar for energy use by the cell. This enzyme is the main regulator of glucose produced by the liver and is also active in the kidneys and intestine. Mutation impairs the glucose-6-phosphatase enzyme which then impairs the glucose 6 phosphate sugar molecule from breaking down into glucose, instead converting it into fat and glycogen. Fat and glycogen accumulation in the cell leads to tissue and organ damage, particularly in the kidneys and liver. The disease is autosomal recessive. Individuals with mutation of the G6PC gene from both parents develop von Gierke disease. Individuals who receive the G6PC mutation from only one parent are carriers of the disease. Symptoms of this inherited disorder include severe hypoglycemia, constant hunger, irritability, excess bleeding/bruising, fatigue, abdominal distention with thin extremities and puffy cheeks, inflammatory bowel disease, stunted growth, and delayed puberty. The disease is treated by restricting fructose (fruits) and galactose (dairy products), avoiding low blood glucose levels by eating starches such as uncooked cornstarch and taking allopurinol to decrease uric acid levels. Molecular genetic testing is indicated in individuals with symptoms associated with von Gierke disease or when there is a family history of the disorder.

81251

81251   GBA (glucosidase, beta, acid) (eg, Gaucher disease) gene analysis, common variants (eg, N370S, 84GG, L444P, IVS2+1G>A)

Molecular genetic testing is performed to identify a specific mutation of the GBA (glucosidase, beta, acid) gene responsible for causing Gaucher disease. Gaucher disease is classified as a lysosomal storage disease and results from a missing enzyme (glucocerebrosidase) necessary to break down the lipid substance, glucocerebroside, resulting in fat deposits in the liver, kidneys, spleen, bones, brain, and lungs. The disease is autosomal recessive. Individuals with mutation of the GBA gene from both parents develop Gaucher disease. Individuals who receive the GBA mutation from only one parent are carriers of the disease. There are at least 25 identified variants of the gene mutation with 4 seen most frequently, N370S, 84GG, L444P and IVS2+1G>A. The homozygous pairing of these variants can influence the disease manifestations. The pairing of N370S/N370S is most often seen in non-neuropathic, Type 1 and individuals can be asymptomatic or have very mild symptoms. When N370S is paired with any of the other 3 variants (or any of the 3 variants are paired together) the disease manifestations are more likely to be neuropathic Type 2 or 3. Type 2, also referred to as acute infantile neuropathic, begins in early infancy rapidly progressing with death occurring by age 2. Type 3, referred to as chronic neuropathic, has a better prognosis with affected individuals living to adulthood. People of Ashkenazi Jewish descent (Central and Eastern European) have an affected rate of 1 in 450, most commonly of the mutations 84GG and L444P. In the general population the affected rate is estimated to be 1 in 50,000-100,000. Symptoms of the disease include bone fracture, fatigue, heart valve problems, lung disease, brown discoloration of skin, yellow fat deposits in sclera, lymph node swelling, joint swelling, painful bone lesions, low platelet count, and severe edema in a newborn. The disease can be treated with enzyme replacement therapy using intravenous glucocerebrosidase (imiglucerase) or velaglucerase

alfa. Molecular genetic testing is indicated in individuals with symptoms associated with Gaucher disease or when there is a family history of the disorder.

81252-81253

81252   GJB2 (gap junction protein, beta 2, 26kDa, connexin 26) (eg, nonsyndromic hearing loss) gene analysis; full gene sequence

81253   GJB2 (gap junction protein, beta 2, 26kDa, connexin 26) (eg, nonsyndromic hearing loss) gene analysis; known familial variants

Molecular genetic testing is performed to identify the specific mutation of the gap junction protein, beta 2 (GJB2) gene that causes nonsyndromic hearing loss (NSHL). The GJB2 gene provides instructions for gap junction proteins (aka connexin proteins) that transport nutrients, ions and signaling molecules between cells. Connexin 26 is specific to cells in the inner ear (cochlea) and epidermis. The GJB2 gene is located on chromosome 13. There are at least 90 identified mutations of the GJB2 gene that cause NFNB1 deafness. NFNB1 is an autosomal recessive inherited condition. An individual who receives one mutated gene will be a carrier of the disease, an individual who receives two mutated genes will have the condition. The gene mutation most likely disturbs the conversion of sound waves to nerve impulses. Full gene sequence testing is reported with 81252. Testing for the known familial variants is reported with 81253. Known familial variants include 35delG or 30delG, with deletions of a base pair occurring between positions 30 and 35 and are found most often in Caucasian populations. In Asian populations the deletion of a base pair occurs most often at position 235 (235delC) and in Ashkenazi Jewish populations the deletion is usually located at position 167 (167delT). All of these deletions lead to an abnormally small protein that cannot bridge the functional gap between cells. Some mutations replace amino acids and lead to unstable or dysfunctional proteins that cannot form gap junctions. DFNA3 is an autosomal dominant inherited form of deafness that is caused by replacement of one amino acid for another. In an autosomal dominant condition, inheriting only one mutated gene will cause the disease.

81254

81254   GJB6 (gap junction protein, beta 6, 30kDa, connexin 30) (eg, nonsyndromic hearing loss) gene analysis, common variants (eg, 309kb [del(GJB6-D13S1830)] and 232kb [del(GJB6-D13S1854)])

Molecular genetic testing is performed to identify the specific mutation of the gap junction protein, beta 6 (GJB6) gene that causes nonsyndromic hearing loss. The GJB6 gene provides instructions for gap junction proteins (aka connexin proteins) that transport nutrients, ions and signaling molecules between cells. Connexin 30 is specific to cells in the brain, skin and inner ear (cochlea). The GJB6 gene is located on chromosome 13. Nonsyndromic deafness NFNB1 is an autosomal recessive inherited condition. An individual who receives one mutated gene will be a carrier of the disease, an individual who receives two mutated genes will have the condition. In some cases of NFNB1 there will be a deletion of a protein (amino acid building block) in both copies of the GJB6 gene (monogenic pattern). In other cases there is a deletion in only one copy of the GJB6 gene combined with a different mutation on the neighboring GJB2 gene (digenic pattern) which results in decreased functioning in the junctions, decreased potassium levels and hearing loss. These gene mutations most likely disturb the conversion of sound waves to nerve impulses. A less common nonsyndromic deafness DFNA3 is an inherited autosomal dominate disorder where only one copy of the GJB6 gene is altered by a change in the amino acid used to make connexin 30. The amino acid threonin is replaced with methionine at position 5 (Thr5Met). This change inhibits activity in the gap junction and the level of potassium in the cells.

81255

81255   HEXA (hexosaminidase A [alpha polypeptide]) (eg, Tay-Sachs disease) gene analysis, common variants (eg, 1278insTATC, 1421+1G>C, G269S)

Molecular genetic testing is performed to identify a specific mutation on the HEXA (hexosaminidase A [alpha polypeptide]) gene associated with Tay-Sachs disease (TSD). Tay-Sachs is a lysosomal storage disease involving glycosphingolipid, a GM2 ganglioside, which in the absence or near absence of the beta-hexosaminidase A enzyme, accumulates in the nerve cells of the brain causing premature cell death. The disease is autosomal recessive. Individuals with mutation of the HEXA gene from both parents develop Tay-Sachs disease. Individuals who receive the HEXA mutation from only one parent are carriers of the disease. The HEXA gene is found on chromosome 15 and more than 100 mutations have been identified. The most common variants are 1278insTATC, found almost exclusively in the Cajun population of Louisiana and people of Ashkenazi Jewish descent (Central and Eastern European) and 1421+1G>C. When these two mutations are paired homozygously, Acute Infantile TSD is expressed. Symptoms of Acute Infantile TSD begin between 3-6 months of age and are characterized by a deterioration of mental and physical abilities. The individual becomes blind and deaf. Muscles atrophy and finally paralysis sets in. Death usually occurs by age 4. A third mutation, G269S, when paired with one of 3 null alleles, 1421+1G>C, 1073+G>A or Tyr427IlefsX5, produces Subacute Juvenile or Adult/Late Onset TSD. Subacute Juvenile TSD is extremely rare with symptoms presenting between ages 2-10 in the form of cognitive, motor and speech difficulties, swallowing problems, spasticity, and gait disturbances. Death occurs between 5 and 15 years of age. Adult/Late Onset TSD is rare, appearing between the ages of 20-30 and is not usually fatal. Symptoms include speech and swallowing difficulties, muscle spasticity and unstable gait, cognitive decline and psychiatric illness such as bipolar or schizophrenic psychosis. Molecular genetic testing is indicated to distinguish pseudo deficiency alleles from mutations that cause disease in healthy individuals during population screening programs and to identify the specific mutation in individuals with symptoms associated with Tay-Sachs disease followed by genetic counseling for other family members.

81256

81256   HFE (hemochromatosis) (eg, hereditary hemochromatosis) gene analysis, common variants (eg, C282Y, H63D)

Molecular genetic testing is performed to identify a specific mutation on the HFE gene associated with hereditary hemochromatosis. Hemochromatosis is an iron overload disease caused by excessive absorption of dietary iron by the intestines. The HFE protein has no immunological function and when mutated, a disulfide bond fails and the HFE protein cannot form a complex with the stabilizing beta-2-microglobin. The HFE protein becomes degraded before incorporating into the cell membrane causing a strong transferrin signal which the intestine interprets as a deficit in iron and increases its absorption rate. The disease is autosomal recessive. Individuals with mutation of the HFE gene from both parents develop hereditary hemochromatosis. Individuals who receive the HFE mutation from only one parent are carriers of the disease. The HFE gene is found on chromosome 6 and has 2 common variants, C282Y and H63D (also expressed as 187 C+G). Found in 60-90% of individuals diagnosed with hemochromatosis, C282Y substitutes tyrosine for cysteine at the 282 amino acid position and most often expresses symptoms of the disease. The allele H63D may be almost asymptomatic when paired homozygously (H63D/H63D). Prolonged overload of iron causes damage to tissue and organs, especially the liver, pancreas and heart. Molecular genetic testing is indicated in individuals with symptoms associated with hemochromatosis or when there is a family history of the disease.

81257

81257   HBA1/HBA2 (alpha globin 1 and alpha globin 2) (eg, alpha thalassemia, Hb Bart hydrops fetalis syndrome, HbH disease), gene analysis, for common deletions or variant (eg, Southeast Asian, Thai, Filipino, Mediterranean, alpha3.7, alpha4.2, alpha20.5, and Constant Spring)

Molecular genetic testing is performed to identify a specific mutation of the HBA1 or HBA2 gene which encodes hemoglobin protein and is associated with a number of hemoglobin disorders. The genes are located on chromosome 16 in the alpha globin locus. There are many variants of the disorder, the most common world wide is alpha thalassemia, caused by absent or decreased alpha globin chain production due to deletion of alpha A genes as well as both HBA1 and HBA2. The variants SEA, THAI, FIL, MED and alpha20.5 have a deletion of HBA1 and HBA2 from the same chromosome. The variants alpha3.7 and alpha4.2 delete a single alpha gene and the variant Constant Spring (HbCS) has a common mutation in the termination codes of HBA2, elongating the protein structure by 31 amino acids. The disease is autosomal recessive. Individuals with mutation of the HBA1 or HBA2 gene from both parents develop hemoglobin disorders. Individuals who receive the HBA1 or HBA2 mutation from only one parent are carriers of the disease. There are two clinically significant forms of alpha thalassemia. The first is Hb Bart which causes hydrops fetalis syndrome due to a loss of all 4 alpha globin genes. It is associated with fetal and perinatal death, fetal edema, ascites, pleural/pericardial effusion and severe hypochromic anemia. The second is Hemoglobin H (HbH) disease due to a loss of 3 alpha genes. Symptoms include moderate microcytic hypochromic anemia, splenomegaly, and a propensity for acute hemolysis after oxidative stress, drug therapy, or infection. In the carrier states of alpha thalassemia, a loss of 2 genes may show mild microcytic anemia and is often misdiagnosed as iron deficiency anemia. The silent carrier has a loss of just a single alpha gene and is typically asymptomatic or has borderline anemia or very mild microcytosis present. Molecular genetic testing is indicated in individuals with symptoms associated with hemoglobin disorders, women who have fetal loss with evidence of hydrops fetalis syndrome or when there is a family history of the disease.

81260

81260   IKBKAP (inhibitor of kappa light polypeptide gene enhancer in B-cells, kinase complex-associated protein) (eg, familial dysautonomia) gene analysis, common variants (eg, 2507+6T>C, R696P)

Molecular genetic testing is performed to identify a specific mutation of the IKBKAP gene which provides instruction to make IKAP protein, part of a six protein elongation complex that interacts with enzymes necessary for transcription (the process of transferring information from one gene to the area of the cell responsible for making the protein). Two copies of the same IKBKAP gene code in each cell disrupts the information that the IKBKAP gene splices together when making a blueprint for production of the IKAP protein. This causes an inconsistent amount of IKAP protein to be manufactured by the cells. Brain cells are particularly vulnerable to underproduction of the protein. The disease is autosomal recessive. Individuals with mutation of the IKBKAP gene from both parents develop familial dysautonomia. Individuals who receive the IKBKAP mutation from only one parent are carriers of the disease. The disorder is found most commonly in people of Ashkenazi Jewish

descent (Central and Eastern European). Located on chromosome 9, the most common variants are IVS20(+6TC) which may also be expressed as 2507+6T>C accounting for nearly 99% of cases and R696P. The disease affects the autonomic nervous system which controls involuntary actions (breathing, digestion, tear production, regulation of heart rate, blood pressure, and body temperature) and the sensory nervous system (taste, pain, and temperature perception). Symptoms of the disorder begin during infancy or early childhood and include inability to maintain normal body temperature, poor feeding, vomiting, recurrent pneumonia, poor muscle tone, growth retardation, poor balance, frequent injury due to altered perception of pain, scoliosis, bone fractures, kidney and heart problems, dangerous drop in blood pressure when standing, or elevation in blood pressure when excited or stressed. Half the individuals identified with the disorder will die by the age of 40. Molecular genetic testing is indicated in individuals with symptoms associated with familial dysautonomia or when there is a family history of the disease.

81261-81262

81261   IGH@ (Immunoglobulin heavy chain locus) (eg, leukemias and lymphomas, B-cell), gene rearrangement analysis to detect abnormal clonal population(s); amplified methodology (eg, polymerase chain reaction)

81262   IGH@ (Immunoglobulin heavy chain locus) (eg, leukemias and lymphomas, B-cell), gene rearrangement analysis to detect abnormal clonal population(s); direct probe methodology (eg, Southern blot)

Molecular genetic testing is performed to identify specific gene mutations. The immunoglobulin heavy chain locus (IGH@) locus is found on chromosome 14. The function of immunoglobulin is to recognize foreign antigens and initiate the immune response. Each IGH molecule has 2 identical heavy chains and 2 identical light chains. Complete IGH gene rearrangement can occur during B-cell development by following a stage specific order. IGH@ gene mutations have been identified in blood and lymph cancers. The gene rearrangement analysis to detect abnormal clonal populations can be accomplished using amplified methodology, such as polymerase chain reaction (PCR,) or direct probe (Southern blot technique). In 81261, amplified methodology is used. This technique is fast, simple, and has the ability to be extensively modified to test a diverse array of genetic manipulations. It can be used to monitor an individual's response to treatment and predict the prognosis of a disease. In 81262, direct probe methodology, also referred to as Southern blot, is used. The Southern blot technique first separates DNA into fragments using electrophoresis. The DNA fragments are then transferred to a filler membrane where they are identified and tagged by probe hybridization.

81263

81263   IGH@ (Immunoglobulin heavy chain locus) (eg, leukemia and lymphoma, B-cell), variable region somatic mutation analysis

Molecular genetic testing is performed to identify specific gene mutations. The immunoglobulin heavy chain locus (IGH@) is found on chromosome 14. The function of immunoglobulin is to recognize foreign antigens and initiate the immune response. Each IGH molecule has 2 identical heavy chains and 2 identical light chains. Complete IGH gene rearrangement can occur during B-cell development by following a stage specific order. IGH@ gene mutations have been identified in blood and lymph cancers. The variable region somatic analysis uses DNA extracted from cell or tissue. Clonality is first confirmed by separately reportable polymerase chain reaction (PCR). The DNA is then reamplified using variable (V) heavy chain family specific primers. The amplifications can then be sequenced and compared with control germline IGH V gene segments to determine specific mutations.

81264

81264   IGK@ (Immunoglobulin kappa light chain locus) (eg, leukemia and lymphoma, B-cell), gene rearrangement analysis, evaluation to detect abnormal clonal population(s)

Molecular genetic testing is performed to identify specific gene mutations. The immunoglobulin kappa light chain locus (IGK@) is found on chromosome 2. The function of immunoglobulin is to recognize foreign antigens and initiate the immune response. Light chains are comprised of small polypeptide subunits that can be classified as either kappa (chromosome 2) or lambda (located on chromosome 22). IGK@ assays have been shown to detect clonal immunoglobulin gene rearrangements in blood and lymph tissue with greater accuracy than IGH@ assays using polymerase chain reaction (PCR). The IGKV configuration is less often targeted by somatic hypermutation than IGHV. IGK@ assay testing should be included with routine clonality analysis especially when diagnosing lymphatic neoplasms.

81265-81266

81265 Comparative analysis using Short Tandem Repeat (STR) markers; patient and comparative specimen (eg, pre-transplant recipient and donor germline testing, post-transplant non-hematopoietic recipient germline [eg, buccal swab or other germline tissue sample] and donor testing, twin zygosity testing, or maternal cell contamination of fetal cells)

81266 Comparative analysis using Short Tandem Repeat (STR) markers; each additional specimen (eg, additional cord blood donor, additional fetal samples from different cultures, or additional zygosity in multiple birth pregnancies) (List separately in addition to code for primary procedure)

Molecular genetic testing is performed to identify common gene sequencing between two individuals. Comparative analysis is performed using Short Tandem Repeat (STR) markers. STR is a pattern of 2 or more nucleotides that repeat themselves with the repeated sequences adjacent to each other. STR markers are typically found in the non-coding intron region of a gene. DNA markers are identified prior to transplant on both the donor and recipient and used to document engraftment and detect residual disease. DNA STR markers found in buccal mucosa may be compared when assessing homozygous or heterozygous genetic lines in twins. STR markers on 5 DNA segments are examined in fetal cells obtained during amniocentisis or chorionic villus sampling and compared with the same segments from a venous blood sample obtained from the mother to rule out maternal cell contamination of the fetal cells. Use 81265 to report testing of a patient and comparative specimen, such as pre-transplant recipient and donor germline testing, post-transplant non-hematopoietic recipient germline, donor testing, twin zyogosity testing, or maternal cell contamination of fetal cells. Use 81266 for each additional cord blood donor, each additional fetal sample from different cultures, or each additional zygosity in multiple birth pregnancies.

81267

81267 Chimerism (engraftment) analysis, post transplantation specimen (eg, hematopoietic stem cell), includes comparison to previously performed baseline analyses; without cell selection

Molecular genetic testing is performed to identify the extent of chimerism following hematopoietic stem cell transplantation. When testing for acquired chimerism (engraftment), genetic profiles of both the donor and the recipient are identified and the extent of donor cell proliferation in recipient blood, bone marrow, or other tissue is evaluated. While it is possible for complete conversion to donor cells to occur, it is also possible to have an immunologic tolerance to both cell lines. A mixture of donor and recipient cells does not indicate graft failure. Testing is performed by analyzing genomic polymorphisms called short tandem repeat (STR) loci. STR loci have core DNA sequences which are repeated on a particular gene locus. These DNA sequences store information within flanking regions which are used to create oligonucleotide primer pairs of the STR. The primer pairs are used in polymerase chain reaction (PCR) amplification test samples. Following amplification, the strands can be separated using electrophoresis gel or capillary electrophoresis (CE). This method (PCR based STR/CE) is advantageous because multiple strands can be tested at the same time using very small DNA samples. This method has also proved successful in analysis for graft failure, severe leukopenia, hematopoietic cell subset fractions, double cord blood donor units, and a second transplant from a different donor.

81268

81268 Chimerism (engraftment) analysis, post transplantation specimen (eg, hematopoietic stem cell), includes comparison to previously performed baseline analyses; with cell selection (eg, CD3, CD33), each cell type

Molecular genetic testing is performed to identify the extent of chimerism following hematopoietic stem cell transplantation. The population of CD3+ and CD33+ cells are prepared using monoclonal antibody coupled magnetic beads and then lysed. Testing for engraftment is then performed using gene amplification of variable number tandem repeat (VNTR) or short tandem repeat (STR) loci. The test is performed in three parts. First, a separately reportable pre-transplant analysis is done to determine which locus can be used for identification of the recipient and donor alleles. Second, a post-transplant sample is separated into CD3+ and CD33+ fractions. Third, post-transplant analysis is done to determine the amount of recipient and donor DNA present in blood, bone marrow, or other tissue. Report 81268 for each cell type analyzed.

81270

81270 JAK2 (Janus kinase 2) (eg, myeloproliferative disorder) gene analysis, p.Val617Phe (V617F) variant

Molecular genetic testing is performed to identify a specific mutation of the JAK2 gene which provides instructions to make a protein that promotes cell proliferation. This protein is part of the JAK/STAT pathway responsible for transmitting chemical signals from outside the cell to inside the cell nucleus and is especially important for controlling blood cell production in hematopoietic stem cells within bone marrow. Located on chromosome 9, this is a somatic gene mutation. It is an acquired mutation and not inherited from family members. The JAK2 mutation is found in 96% of individual with polycythemia vera, a

disease characterized by uncontrolled production of blood cells. The most common variant is V617F, in which the amino acid valine is replaced with the amino acid phenylalanine at position 617. The mutation keeps the JAK2 protein constantly activated, producing white and red blood cells and platelets in the bone marrow. The over production of these blood cells leads to abnormal blood clotting, slowed or sluggish circulatory rate, and decreased oxygen to the organs. The mutation is also found in individuals with essential thrombocytopenia (elevated platelet levels) and primary myelofibrosis (fibrotic bone marrow). Molecular genetic testing is indicated in individuals with symptoms associated with myeloproliferative disorder (MPD).

81272

81272 KIT (v-kit Hardy-Zuckerman 4 feline sarcoma viral oncogene homolog) (eg, gastrointestinal stromal tumor [GIST], acute myeloid leukemia, melanoma), gene analysis, targeted sequence analysis (eg, exons 8, 11, 13, 17, 18)

Molecular genetic testing is performed to identify the specific mutation of the KIT (v-kit Hardy-Zuckerman 4 feline sarcoma viral oncogene homolog) gene using targeted sequence analysis of exons 8,11,13,17, and 18 on chromosome 4. The KIT gene encodes a protein belonging to the tyrosine kinase family of receptors responsible for transmitting signals from cell surfaces into the cell through signal transduction. A stem cell factor binds to the tyrosine kinase receptor protein on certain cells which activates other proteins inside the cell through phosphorylation. This creates an activation cascade of proteins involved in cell proliferation, survival, and migration primarily in germ cells, hematopoietic stem cells, mast cells, gastrointestinal cells, and pigment-producing melanocytes. KIT mutations are associated with piebaldism, gastrointestinal stromal tumors (GIST), acute myeloid leukemia, sinonasal natural killer/T-cell lymphoma (NKTCL), and melanoma. Genetic testing is performed to identify the specific KIT gene mutation in individuals diagnosed with cancer to determine prognosis and response or resistance to specific cancer treatments or therapies.

81275

81275 KRAS (Kirsten rat sarcoma viral oncogene homolog) (eg, carcinoma) gene analysis; variants in exon 2 (eg, codons 12 and 13)

Molecular genetic testing is performed to identify a specific mutation of the KRAS gene which provides instruction to make the K-Ras protein primarily responsible for cell growth, division, maturation, and differentiation. This protein relays signals from outside the cell to the inside via signal transduction. The K-ras protein is a GTPase and works like a switch, turning on when bound to GTP and off when it converts GTP to GDP. In the mutation, a single protein building block causes prolonged activation and the cell grows and divides constantly. The KRAS gene is in the Ras family of oncogenes. It is found on chromosome 12, codon 12 or 13 (exon2). An autosomal dominant mutation on the KRAS gene can cause an atypical but severe form of Noonan syndrome. Symptoms of this mutation include low intellectual function, short statue, heart defects, and skeletal abnormalities. Another disorder that can be attributed to mutations of the KRAS gene is cardiofaciocutaneous (CFC) syndrome. Symptoms include low intellectual function, distinctive facial features, short stature, large head, and sparse hair. Somatic mutations of the KRAS gene have been identified in some cancers including tumors of the lung, pancreas, and colorectum. Molecular genetic testing is indicated in individuals with symptoms associated with Noonan or cardiofaciocutaneous (CFC) syndromes and in those diagnosed with specific cancers.

81287

81287 MGMT (O-6-methylguanine-DNA methyltransferase) (eg, glioblastoma multiforme), methylation analysis

Paraffin-embedded biopsy tissue samples are examined for MGMT (O-6-methylguanine-DNA methyltransferase) gene promoter methylation in patients diagnosed with glioblastoma, a common and aggressive malignant brain tumor. The presence of promoter methylation lends a more favorable outcome to treatment with alkylating chemotherapy agents, including Tremador (temozolomide). MGMT is a DNA repair enzyme that reverses alkylation of guanine. When MGMT expression is silenced (decreased) for promoter methylation, it allows alkylguanine DNA to accumulate which leads to incorrect base pairings with thymine and finally DNA damage and cell death. MGMT gene methylation can be assessed using methylation-specific polymerase-chain-reaction (PCR) or pyrosequencing methylation assay.

81290

81290 MCOLN1 (mucolipin 1) (eg, Mucolipidosis, type IV) gene analysis, common variants (eg, IVS3-2A>G, del6.4kb)

Molecular genetic testing is performed to identify a specific mutation of the MCOLN1 gene which provides instruction to make the mucolipin 1 protein responsible for the transport of fat and protein across the membrane of lysosomes and endosomes, structures that digest and recycle cellular material. A lysosomal storage disorder, mucolipidosis, type IV, results when the mutated gene fails to produce an adequate amount of functional mucolipin-1 causing a buildup of fat and protein inside the lysosomes/endosomes. The mucolipin-1 protein is necessary for the development and maintenance of brain/nerve cells, light sensitive retinal tissue in the eye, and cells that produce digestive acids. The disease is autosomal recessive. Individuals with mutation of the MCOLN1 gene from both parents develop Mucolipidosis, type IV. Individuals who receive the MCOLN1 mutation from only one parent are carriers of the disease. The disorder is found most commonly in people of Ashkenazi Jewish descent (Central and Eastern European). The gene is located on chromosome 19 and there are 2 common variants in the Ashkenazi Jewish population, c.406-2A>G which changes a nucleotide by splice mutation at intron 3 and prematurely stops production of mucolipin 1, and g.511_6943del which deletes a large piece of DNA on the MCOLN1 gene. Both of these mutations cause the mucolipin 1 protein to be abnormally short and non functional. Symptoms of typical mucolipidosis, type IV begin in the first year of life and include psychomotor delay, progressive vision loss, achlorhydia (decreased stomach acid), hypotonia leading to spasticity and muscle stiffness, elevated serum gastrin levels, and anemia. Individuals with the disorder have a shortened lifespan. Atypical mucolipidosis, type IV will display milder (Typical) symptoms beginning in the first decade of life. Molecular genetic testing is indicated in individuals with symptoms associated with lysosomal storage disorders or when there is a family history of the disease.

81291

81291   MTHFR (5,10-methylenetetrahydrofolate reductase) (eg, hereditary hypercoagulability) gene analysis, common variants (eg, 677T, 1298C)

Molecular genetic testing is performed to identify a specific mutation of the MTHFR gene which provides instruction to make the enzyme methylenetetrahydrofolate reductase. This enzyme is responsible for processing amino acids in a chemical reaction involving folate (folic acid) and other B vitamins to change 5,10-methylenetetrahydrofolate to 5-methyltetrahydrofolate as part of a multi-step process for converting the amino acid homocysteine to the amino acid methionine. The mutated enzyme is not able to assist in the conversion of homocysteine and this amino acid builds up in the blood leading to a disorder called hereditary hypercoagulability. The disease is autosomal recessive. Individuals with mutation of the MTHFR gene from both parents can develop hereditary hypercoagulability. Individuals who receive the MTHFR mutation from only one parent are carriers of the disease. The MTHFR gene is found on chromosome 1. Two mutation variants, 677T and 1298C are most often identified in individuals with elevated homocysteine levels and hypercoagulability disorders. Homocysteine is an irritant to blood vessels causing atherosclerosis which can then lead to increased venous blood clotting. Treatment for the disorder includes dietary supplementation of folate (folic acid) and vitamins B6 and B12. Molecular genetic testing is indicated in individuals with symptoms associated with hereditary hypercoagulability or when there is a family history of the disorder.

81292-81294

81292   MLH1 (mutL homolog 1, colon cancer, nonpolyposis type 2) (eg, hereditary non-polyposis colorectal cancer, Lynch syndrome) gene analysis; full sequence analysis

81293   MLH1 (mutL homolog 1, colon cancer, nonpolyposis type 2) (eg, hereditary non-polyposis colorectal cancer, Lynch syndrome) gene analysis; known familial variants

81294   MLH1 (mutL homolog 1, colon cancer, nonpolyposis type 2) (eg, hereditary non-polyposis colorectal cancer, Lynch syndrome) gene analysis; duplication/deletion variants

Molecular genetic testing is performed to identify a specific mutation on the MLH1 gene that places an individual at increased risk of developing colorectal and certain other cancers. The MLH1 gene is located on chromosome 3 and is one of a number of mismatch repair (MMR) genes responsible for providing instructions to proteins that repair DNA. The mutation prevents production of the MLH1 protein or alters it so that it cannot perform its function. This leads to an increase in the number of unrepaired DNA errors which accumulate over time, allowing cells to proliferate into tumors. Colorectal is the most common cancer caused by this mutation but tumors may also be found in the endometrium, ovaries, prostate, stomach, small intestine, liver, gallbladder duct, upper urinary tract, brain, and skin. These tumors are characterized by high micro satellite instability (MSI). The disease caused by MLH1 mutation is known as hereditary nonpolyposis colorectal cancer (HNPCC). Another name for HNPCC is Lynch syndrome and this mutation is identified in approximately 50% of individuals with this diagnosis. It is an autosomal dominant mutation. An individual needs to inherit only one mutated gene to have an increased risk of developing cancer. In 81292, a full sequence analysis is performed. Full sequence analysis compares gene segments to determine their similarities or differences and identify relationships. Intrinsic features are studied to find active and post translational modification sites, gene structures, and distribution of introns, extrons, and regulatory elements. Genetic markers can be found by identifying point mutations or single nucleotide polymorphisms (SNP). Most MLH1 mutations are considered to be point mutations where a single DNA protein base is altered. In 81293, MLH1 gene analysis is performed for known familial variants. When an individual has been identified with a MLH1 gene mutation, family members should undergo molecular genetic testing by age 18. This genetic mapping can determine common or familial variants among blood relatives and help to determine the risk factors for individuals identified as having the same or similar gene mutation. In 81294, MLH1 gene analysis is performed for deletion/duplication variants. A normal gene should have 2 copies per cell (with the exception of sex chromosomes). Zero or one copies would indicate a deletion variant and three (or more)

copies would be evidence of a duplication variant. The gene mutation commonly found in HNPCC is the loss of a protein or amine group.

81295-81297

81295   MSH2 (mutS homolog 2, colon cancer, nonpolyposis type 1) (eg, hereditary non-polyposis colorectal cancer, Lynch syndrome) gene analysis; full sequence analysis

81296   MSH2 (mutS homolog 2, colon cancer, nonpolyposis type 1) (eg, hereditary non-polyposis colorectal cancer, Lynch syndrome) gene analysis; known familial variants

81297   MSH2 (mutS homolog 2, colon cancer, nonpolyposis type 1) (eg, hereditary non-polyposis colorectal cancer, Lynch syndrome) gene analysis; duplication/deletion variants

Molecular genetic testing is performed to identify a specific mutation on the MSH2 gene that places an individual at increased risk of developing colorectal (and certain other) cancers. The MSH2 gene is located on chromosome 2 and is one of three mismatch repair (MMR) genes that form an active protein complex. This complex identifies DNA mistakes that take place during DNA replication and allows the MSH1/PMS2 protein complex to take over and make the repair. DNA errors which are not repaired accumulate over time, allowing cells to proliferate into tumors. Colorectal is the most common cancer caused by this mutation but tumors may also be found in the endometrium, ovaries, prostate, stomach, small intestine, liver, gallbladder duct, upper urinary tract, brain, and skin. These tumors are characterized by high micro satellite instability (MSI). The disease caused by MSH2 mutation is known as hereditary non-polyposis colorectal cancer (HNPCC). Another name for HNPCC is Lynch syndrome and this mutation is identified in approximately 40% of individuals with this diagnosis. It is an autosomal dominant mutation. An individual needs to inherit only one mutated gene to have an increased risk of developing cancer. In 81295, a full sequence analysis is performed. Full sequence analysis compares gene segments to determine their similarities or differences and identify relationships. Intrinsic features are studied to find active and post translational modification sites, gene structures, and distribution of introns, extrons, and regulatory elements. Genetic markers can be found by identifying point mutations or single nucleotide polymorphisms (SNP). Most MSH2 mutations are considered to be point mutations where a single DNA protein base is altered. In 81296, MSH2 gene analysis is performed for known familial variants. When an individual has been identified with a MSH2 gene mutation, molecular genetic testing should be performed on all family members. Those testing positive for the gene mutation should be counseled and offered clinical supervision. This genetic mapping can determine common or familial variants among blood relatives and help to determine the risk factors for individuals identified as having the same or similar gene mutation. In 81297, MSH2 gene analysis is performed for deletion/duplication variants. A normal gene should have 2 copies per cell (with the exception of sex chromosomes). Zero or one copies would indicate a deletion variant and three (or more) copies would be evidence of a duplication variant. The MSH2 gene mutation most often found in hereditary non-polyposis colorectal cancer (HNPCC) is the genomic deletion of protein alleles encompassing exons 1-6.

81298-81300

81298   MSH6 (mutS homolog 6 [E. coli]) (eg, hereditary non-polyposis colorectal cancer, Lynch syndrome) gene analysis; full sequence analysis

81299   MSH6 (mutS homolog 6 [E. coli]) (eg, hereditary non-polyposis colorectal cancer, Lynch syndrome) gene analysis; known familial variants

81300   MSH6 (mutS homolog 6 [E. coli]) (eg, hereditary non-polyposis colorectal cancer, Lynch syndrome) gene analysis; duplication/deletion variants

Molecular genetic testing is performed to identify a specific mutation on the MSH6 gene that places an individual at increased risk of developing colorectal and certain other cancers. The MSH6 gene is located on chromosome 2 and is one of three mismatch repair (MMR) genes that form an active protein complex. This complex identifies DNA mistakes that take place during DNA replication and allows the MSH1/PMS2 protein complex to take over and make the repair. DNA errors which are not repaired accumulate over time, allowing cells to proliferate into tumors. Colorectal is the most common cancer caused by this mutation but tumors may also be found in the endometrium, ovaries, prostate, stomach, small intestine, liver, gallbladder duct, upper urinary tract, brain, and skin. These tumors are characterized by low micro satellite instability (MSI). The disease caused by MSH6 mutation is known as hereditary non-polyposis colorectal cancer (HNPCC). Another name for HNPCC is Lynch syndrome and this mutation is identified in approximately 10% of individuals with this diagnosis. It is an autosomal dominant mutation. An individual needs to inherit only one mutated gene to have an increased risk of developing cancer. Characteristics of the MSH6 gene mutation includes older onset of both colorectal and endometrial cancers, an increased incidence of endometrial cancers when compared with MLH1 and MSH2 gene mutations, and colon tumors that are located in the left side of the abdomen. When an individual inherits two copies of the mutated gene (homozygous or compound heterozygous), they are at greater risk of developing childhood leukemia, lymphoma and brain tumors in addition to gastrointestinal cancer. Two mutations, c.3984_3987dup and c.1906G>C, have been identified with increased frequency in Ashkenazi Jewish populations with tumors appearing later in life. In 81298, a full sequence

Pathology and Laboratory

analysis is performed that compares gene segments to determine their similarities or differences and identify relationships. Intrinsic features are studied to find active and post translational modification sites, gene structures, and distribution of introns, extrons, and regulatory elements. Genetic markers can be found by identifying point mutations or single nucleotide polymorphisms (SNP). Most MSH6 mutations are considered to be point mutations where a single DNA protein base is altered. Immunohistochemistry may be used to determine the degree to which gene expression has been lost or compromised by mutation. In 81299, molecular genetic testing is performed for known familial variants. Family members of individuals who have been identified with a MSH6 gene mutation should be tested for known familial variants. Those testing positive for the gene mutation should be counseled and offered clinical supervision. This genetic mapping can determine common or familial variants among blood relatives and help to determine the risk factors for individuals identified as having the same or similar gene mutation. In 81300, molecular gene analysis for MSH6 duplication/deletion variants is performed. A normal gene should have 2 copies per cell (with the exception of sex chromosomes). Zero or one copies would indicate a deletion variant and three (or more) copies would be evidence of a duplication variant. The gene mutation commonly found in hereditary non-polyposis colorectal cancer (HNPCC) is the loss of a protein or amine group.

81301

81301   Microsatellite instability analysis (eg, hereditary non-polyposis colorectal cancer, Lynch syndrome) of markers for mismatch repair deficiency (eg, BAT25, BAT26), includes comparison of neoplastic and normal tissue, if performed

Microsatellite instability (MSI) is a condition manifested by damaged DNA when there is a defective DNA repair process. Microsatellites, also known as simple sequence repeats (SSRs), are DNA sequences that repeat at a set length unique to each individual. When mutation of a DNA repair gene is present, the sequences can develop errors causing an alteration in their length (making them longer or shorter than normal). MSI is the degree of difficulty that a cell has in repairing DNA errors. In 90% of hereditary non-polyposis colorectal cancer (HNPCC), also referred to as Lynch syndrome, MSI will be present in the tumor cells. This instability suggests the presence of a mismatch repair (MMR) gene mutation. Analysis of tumor cells in five different microsatellite regions (including BAT25 and BAT26) can determine if the tumor is unstable high (2 or more regions have DNA changes) or unstable low (only one region shows a change). A tumor is considered stable if there are no changes between tumor cell DNA and normal cell DNA. An MSI marker of unstable high suggests HNPCC is present and more complex molecular genetic testing is appropriate. Microsatellite stable (MSS) or unstable low, indicates an unlikely (although not impossible) presence of HNPCC. BAT25 and BAT26 are very sensitive markers, able to detect MSI when the sample of cells is low. MSI poses different clinicopathological features when compared to MSS including more insertion/deletion mutations in short nucleotide repeats. These differences can influence response to chemotherapeutic agents. Routine gene analysis to determine MSI/MSS of tumors is recommended for all individuals diagnosed with colon and certain other cancers.

81302-81304

81302   MECP2 (methyl CpG binding protein 2) (eg, Rett syndrome) gene analysis; full sequence analysis

81303   MECP2 (methyl CpG binding protein 2) (eg, Rett syndrome) gene analysis; known familial variant

81304   MECP2 (methyl CpG binding protein 2) (eg, Rett syndrome) gene analysis; duplication/deletion variants

Molecular genetic testing is performed to identify a specific mutation of the MECP2 gene which provides instructions to make a protein product essential to normal nerve cell functioning. This protein is found in all body cells and acts as a transcriptional repressor and activator in the brain. Neurons have especially high concentrations of MECP2 where it plays a role in forming synapses (connections) between nerve cells for communication. The MECP2 gene is located on the X chromosome and is predominantly a paternal linked autosomal dominant mutation. MECP2 mutations have been identified in most cases of Rett syndrome, a progressive, neurological/developmental disorder most often affecting females. In classic Rett syndrome, the individual has near normal growth and development for 6-18 months, and then severe problems with language, communication, learning, coordination, and brain function begin to emerge. Atypical forms may present at times, such as a mild form where speech is preserved and a severe form where there is no period of normal growth and development. Research has shown that in as many as 90% of classic Rett syndrome cases, there is no family history of the disorder and the syndrome arises from a new ("de novo") mutation of the gene. Because a few families have had more than one member identified with the disorder, the link to the X chromosome was established. Males with the mutation most often die in utero or during infancy. A small number of living males have been identified with classic Rett syndrome. These individuals most often have an extra X chromosome in some or all of their cells with a normal copy of MECP2 that produces enough of the protein MECP2 to support life. In 81302, full sequence MECP2 analysis is performed. Full sequence analysis compares gene segments to determine their similarities or differences and identify relationships. Intrinsic features are studied

to find active and post translational modification sites, gene structures, and distribution of introns, extrons, and regulatory elements. Genetic markers can be found by identifying point mutations or single nucleotide polymorphisms (SNP). Several types of mutations have been identified on the MECP2 gene in individuals diagnosed with Rett syndrome including point mutations where a single DNA protein (base pair) is altered and insertion/deletion mutations of DNA containing alleles. MECP2 mutations have also been found in some individuals with moderate to severe X linked mental retardation (XLMR), in some males with a severe brain dysfunction known as neonatal encephalopathy, in some individuals with manifestations of characteristics of both Rett syndrome and Angelman syndrome, and it has also been identified in a few cases of autism. In 81303, a molecular testing is performed for a known familial variant to MECP2. When an individual has been identified with an MECP2 gene mutation, molecular genetic testing should be performed on all family members. This genetic mapping can determine common or familial variants among blood relatives. In 81304, MECP2 gene analysis is performed for duplication/deletion variants. A normal gene should have 2 copies per cell (with the exception of sex chromosomes). Zero or one copies would indicate a deletion variant and three (or more) copies would be evidence of a duplication variant. The gene mutations commonly found in individuals with Rett syndrome include point mutations where a single DNA protein (base pair) is altered and insertion/deletion mutations of DNA containing alleles. A duplication mutation of MECP2 has been identified in a few individuals with a progressive life threatening brain disorder characterized by severe developmental delays, hypotonia (weak muscles), and seizures.

81310

81310   NPM1 (nucleophosmin) (eg, acute myeloid leukemia) gene analysis, exon 12 variants

Molecular genetic testing is performed to identify a specific mutation of the NPM1 gene on chromosome 5 which encodes nucleolar phosphoprotein B23 (numatrin). Located in the nucleolus but able to translocate to the nucleoplasm during periods of serum starvation or treatment with antineoplastic drugs, this protein is involved with the biosynthesis of ribosomes and may assist with the binding of single stranded nucleic acids and the transport of small proteins between the cell nucleus and the cytoplasm. Mutation of the gene is believed to promote tumor growth by affecting the activation mechanisms along the p53/ARF pathway. Genetic testing is useful as a prognostic indicator in newly diagnosed cases of acute myeloid leukemia.

81311

81311   NRAS (neuroblastoma RAS viral [v-ras] oncogene homolog) (eg, colorectal carcinoma), gene analysis, variants in exon 2 (eg, codons 12 and 13) and exon 3 (eg, codon 61)

Molecular genetic testing is performed to identify the specific mutation of the NRAS (neuroblastoma RAS viral [v-ras] ongogene homolog) gene for exon 2 (codons 12 and 13) and exon 3 (codon 61) variants located on chromosome 1 that are associated with colorectal cancers. The gene encodes a membrane-bound protein with GTPase activity. Mutations occurring on exon 2, codons 12 and 13 and exon 3, codon 61, disrupt the intrinsic pathway for RAS-GAP mediated GTP hydrolysis and the epidermal growth factor receptor (EGFR) cascade. Genetic testing is performed to identify the specific NRAS mutation in individuals diagnosed with colorectal carcinoma and evaluate the treatment option of monoclonal antibody therapy using cetuximab and panitumumab. These antibodies bind to EGRF and disrupt the downstream signaling pathway necessary for malignant cell proliferation, invasion, metastasis, and neovascularization.

81314

81314   PDGFRA (platelet-derived growth factor receptor, alpha polypeptide) (eg, gastrointestinal stromal tumor [GIST]), gene analysis, targeted sequence analysis (eg, exons 12, 18)

Molecular genetic testing is performed to identify the specific mutation of the PDGFRA (platelet-derived growth factor receptor, alpha polypeptide) gene using targeted sequence analysis of exons 12 and 18 on chromosome 4. The PDGFRA gene encodes a tyrosine kinase receptor protein which is responsible for transmitting signals from cell surfaces into the cell through signal transduction. Using phosphorylation, certain cells activate a cascade of proteins involved in cell growth, proliferation, adhesion, migration, differentiation, and apoptosis. PDGFRA mutations are most often associated with mesenchymal tumors of the stomach and small intestine known as gastrointestinal stromal tumors (GIST). Genetic testing is performed to identify the specific PDGFRA gene mutation in individuals diagnosed with cancer to evaluate for imatinib or sunitinib therapy resistance.

81315-81316

81315 PML/RARalpha, (t(15;17)), (promyelocytic leukemia/retinoic acid receptor alpha) (eg, promyelocytic leukemia) translocation analysis; common breakpoints (eg, intron 3 and intron 6), qualitative or quantitative

81316 PML/RARalpha, (t(15;17)), (promyelocytic leukemia/retinoic acid receptor alpha) (eg, promyelocytic leukemia) translocation analysis; single breakpoint (eg, intron 3, intron 6 or exon 6), qualitative or quantitative

Molecular genetic testing is performed to identify a specific mutation between PML (promyelocytic leukemia) and RARalpha (retinoic acid receptor alpha) resulting in a chimeric fusion of the two genes. In almost 99% of individuals diagnosed with acute myeloid leukemia (AML) the translocation between chromosome 15 (PML gene) and chromosome 17 (RARA) gene is present and forms a transcript isoform. The length of the isoform will either be short or long, depending on the PML breakpoint. In 81315, PML/RARalpha translocation analysis for common breakpoints is performed. A qualitative or quantitative test for common breakpoints can be accomplished by extracting RNA and examining by reverse transcription-polymerase chain reaction (RT-PCR) the PML/RARA fusion transcripts for long or short isoforms. A control sample of ABL gene is amplified and used to check for quality and referenced for relative quantification (reported as positive or negative). If the test is positive, the length of the isoform and the ratio of target (PML/RARA) to control (ABL) mRNA is reported. When retesting to assess effectiveness of therapy, monitor minimal residual disease (MRD), or predict early relapse, previously obtained samples can be compared to new samples and the quantitative change over time determined. Common breakpoints have been identified in breakpoint clusters regions (bcr) on intron 6 (bcr1) and intron 3 (bcr3) of PML. The RARA gene has a single breakpoint on intron 2. Bcr1 is the most common mutation occurring in 45-55% of individuals diagnosed with acute promyelocytic leukemia (APL) and is a long isoform. Bcr3 is a short isoform and is identified in 37-45% of APL cases. The location of a breakpoint cluster may be influenced by ethnicity. It has been documented that intron 6 breakpoints occur with greater frequency in Asian and Latin American populations, as compared to Caucasian populations. In 81316, PML/RARalpha translocation analysis for a single breakpoint is performed. The procedure is performed as described above except that qualitative or quantitative testing is performed on only a single breakpoint. Single breakpoints have been identified in breakpoint clusters regions (bcr) on intron 6 (bcr1), exon 6 (bcr2) and intron 3 (bcr3) of PML. The RARA gene has a single breakpoint on intron 2. Bcr2 is a rare variant isoform identified in only 8-10% of APL cases.

81317-81319

81317 PMS2 (postmeiotic segregation increased 2 [S. cerevisiae]) (eg, hereditary non-polyposis colorectal cancer, Lynch syndrome) gene analysis; full sequence analysis

81318 PMS2 (postmeiotic segregation increased 2 [S. cerevisiae]) (eg, hereditary non-polyposis colorectal cancer, Lynch syndrome) gene analysis; known familial variants

81319 PMS2 (postmeiotic segregation increased 2 [S. cerevisiae]) (eg, hereditary non-polyposis colorectal cancer, Lynch syndrome) gene analysis; duplication/deletion variants

Molecular genetic testing is performed to identify a specific mutation on the PMS2 gene that places an individual at increased risk of developing colorectal and certain other cancers. The PMS2 gene is located on chromosome 7 and is one of a number of mismatch repair (MMR) genes responsible for providing instructions to proteins that repair DNA. The mutation produces an abnormally short or inactivated PMS2 protein which is inefficient in repairing DNA. This leads to an increase in the number of unrepaired DNA errors which accumulate over time, allowing cells to proliferate into tumors. The disease caused by PMS2 mutation is known as hereditary non-polyposis colorectal cancer (HNPCC). Another name for HNPCC is Lynch syndrome. This particular mutation produces an uncommon variant of Lynch syndrome known as Turcot. Individuals with this mutation present with a brain tumor called glioblastoma, in addition to colorectal cancer. The PMS2 mutation is autosomal dominant. An individual needs to inherit only one mutated gene to have an increased risk of developing cancer. When an individual inherits two copies of the mutated gene (homozygous or compound heterozygous), they are at greater risk of developing childhood leukemia, lymphoma, and brain tumors in addition to gastrointestinal cancer. Some individuals will develop HNPCC "de novo" (new generation). In these individuals, the mutation was not inherited from a parent who carried it, but occurred in the germ cell (egg or sperm) of one parent or in the fertilized egg itself, making them the first generation for the mutation. In 81317, a full sequence PMS2 gene analysis is performed. Full sequence analysis compares gene segments to determine their similarities or differences and identify relationships. Intrinsic features are studied to find active and post translational modification sites, gene structures, and distribution of introns, extrons, and regulatory elements. Genetic markers can be found by identifying point mutations or single nucleotide polymorphisms (SNP). PMS2 mutations are uncommon and difficult to identify due to the presence of pseudogenes (dysfunctional PMS2 or similar relative which has lost its coding DNA or mRNA). Those that have been identified are deletion mutations. In 81318, genetic testing is performed for known familial variants. When an individual has been identified with a PMS2 gene mutation, it may be advantageous to test additional family members.

This genetic mapping can determine common or familial variants among blood relatives and help to determine the risk factors for individuals identified as having the same or similar gene mutation. In 81319, genetic testing is performed for PMS2 duplication/deletion variants. A normal gene should have 2 copies per cell (with the exception of sex chromosomes). Zero or one copies would indicate a deletion variant and three (or more) copies would be evidence of a duplication variant. The gene mutation identified on PMS2 which leads to hereditary non-polyposis colorectal cancer (HNPCC) is a deletion or loss of a protein or amine group. Immunohistochemistry (IHC) may be performed on tumor tissue to determine the presence or absence of certain proteins (amine groups).

81321-81323

81321 PTEN (phosphatase and tensin homolog) (eg, Cowden syndrome, PTEN hamartoma tumor syndrome) gene analysis; full sequence analysis

81322 PTEN (phosphatase and tensin homolog) (eg, Cowden syndrome, PTEN hamartoma tumor syndrome) gene analysis; known familial variant

81323 PTEN (phosphatase and tensin homolog) (eg, Cowden syndrome, PTEN hamartoma tumor syndrome) gene analysis; duplication/deletion variant

Molecular genetic testing is performed to identify the specific mutation of the phosphatase and tensin homolog (PTEN) gene that causes PTEN hamartoma tumor syndrome (Cowden syndrome). The PTEN gene is found on chromosome 10. Cowden syndrome is an autosomal dominant inherited condition. An individual who inherits a mutated PTEN gene from one parent will have the disease. PTEN is a (protein) enzyme found in tissue throughout the body. It acts as a tumor suppressor and regulates cell division. The enzyme modifies proteins and lipids by removing a phosphate group. It also controls migration and adhesion of cells to surrounding tissue and the formation of new blood vessels. There are at least 130 documented mutations of PTEN that cause Cowden hamartoma syndrome. The syndrome is characterized by multiple non-malignant tumors that are predisposed to becoming cancer especially when located in the breast, thyroid and uterus (endometrium). The mutation may change only a few DNA building blocks (nucleotides) or delete a large number. The changes to the enzyme may cause it to be defective and function poorly or it may be completely absent from the cells. Full sequence PTEN gene analysis is reported with 81321. Testing for known familial variants is reported with 81322. Three familial variants of PTEN have been identified in patients with breast cancer and include -903GA, -975GC and -1026CA. All of these variants are associated with aggressive tumors and poor treatment outcomes. Testing for duplication/deletion variants is reported with 81323.

81324-81326

81324 PMP22 (peripheral myelin protein 22) (eg, Charcot-Marie-Tooth, hereditary neuropathy with liability to pressure palsies) gene analysis; duplication/deletion analysis

81325 PMP22 (peripheral myelin protein 22) (eg, Charcot-Marie-Tooth, hereditary neuropathy with liability to pressure palsies) gene analysis; full sequence analysis

81326 PMP22 (peripheral myelin protein 22) (eg, Charcot-Marie-Tooth, hereditary neuropathy with liability to pressure palsies) gene analysis; known familial variant

Molecular genetic testing is performed to identify the specific mutation of the peripheral myelin protein 22 (PMP22) gene that causes Charcot-Marie-Tooth disease and hereditary neuropathy with liability to pressure palsies. The PMP22 gene is found on chromosome 17. Peripheral myelin protein is found in the sheath that covers nerve cells. This component helps to transmit impulses produced by Schwann cells also found in the sheath. PMP22 may also play a role in Schwann cell growth and differentiation. Mutations may be autosomal recessive, requiring a mutated gene from each parent to show signs of disease or autosomal dominant, where only one copy of the mutated gene will cause disease. 1A is the most common form of Charcot-Marie-Tooth disease and has an extra copy (duplication) of PMP22 gene. This causes an over production of PMP22 and prevents effective processing of the protein. A reduction in functional PMP22 leads to a decrease in myelin and the unprocessed PMP22 further disrupts Schwann cell function causing decreased muscle activation and relay of information along the nerve pathway. 1A may also result from addition, deletion or change in the amino acid sequencing on the PMP22 gene. The altered protein causes PMP to be processed more slowly or abnormally. This leads to impairment of the Schwann cells and demyelination of the nerves. Hereditary neuropathy with liability to pressure palsies usually involves reduced gene dosage (loss of one copy of the PMP22 gene). This reduction leads to low levels of circulating PMP22. The condition may also be caused by a mutation that results in an abnormally small, unstable protein which breaks down rapidly and leaves myelin unprotected. The unprotected myelin is then hypersensitive to pressure placed on the nerve. Duplication/deletion analysis is reported with code 81324. Full sequence gene analysis is reported with code 81325. Testing for known familial variants is reported with code 81326. A known familial variant of Charcot-Marie-Tooth is Type 1E. It is characterized by sensorineural hearing loss. The most common cause is replacement of the amino acid alanine with proline at position 67 (Ala67Pro).

81330

81330 **SMPD1(sphingomyelin phosphodiesterase 1, acid lysosomal) (eg, Niemann-Pick disease, Type A) gene analysis, common variants (eg, R496L, L302P, fsP330)**

Molecular genetic testing is performed to identify a specific mutation of the SMPD1 gene which provides instruction to make the enzyme acid sphingomyelinase. The enzyme is found in lysosomes, structures that digest and recycle cellular material, and is responsible for converting sphingomyelin to ceramide. This conversion of one lipid structure to another is required to maintain normal structure and function of cells and tissue. Found on chromosome 11, this gene mutation is parent specific and autosomal recessive, only the maternal copy of the gene is active. Niemann-Pick disease results from mutation of the SMPD1 gene. More than 100 mutations have been identified for types A and B, causing a reduction or absence of enzyme activity in the cells. This results in an abnormal accumulation of cholesterol, sphingomyelin and other lipids in the cells of the spleen, liver, and brain. A buildup of these substances causes a disruption of cell function and ultimately, cell destruction and death. Niemann-Pick, type A is identified disproportionately in people of Ashkenazi Jewish descent (Central and Eastern European). Three common variants are R496L in which arginine is changed to leucine at codon 496, fsP330 where a deletion of a single cytosine is found at codon 330, and L302P in which proline is substituted for leucine at codon 302. Symptoms begin during infancy and include feeding problems, abdominal swelling, a loss of motor skills that worsens over time, and a cherry red spot in the eye. Molecular genetic testing is indicated in individuals with symptoms associated with Niemann-Pick disease or when there is a family history of the disorder.

81331

81331 **SNRPN/UBE3A (small nuclear ribonucleoprotein polypeptide N and ubiquitin protein ligase E3A) (eg, Prader-Willi syndrome and/or Angelman syndrome), methylation analysis**

Methylation analysis is performed to identify uniparental disomy, a mutation of the SNRPN gene responsible for small nuclear ribonucleoprotein polypeptide N (Prader-Willi syndrome) and/or the UBE3A gene responsible for ubiquitin protein ligase E3A (Angelman syndrome). These mutations are most often splice variants or imprinting errors which are not inherited but rather random events that occur during the formation of reproductive cells (egg, sperm) or in early embryonic development. Prader-Willi syndrome results when a paternal segment is deleted from the SNRPN gene on chromosome 15 or 2 copies of the mother's chromosome are expressed (maternal uniparental disomy). Symptoms of the disorder appear in infancy and include small for gestational age (SGA) at birth, underdeveloped genitalia, feeding problems (weak suck/swallow), failure to thrive, weak cry, and floppy muscle tone. There may be skeletal abnormalities including small hands, skin irregularities such as bands, stripes, and lines and unusual facial features. In childhood, an intense, uncontrollable craving for food develops which leads to chronic overeating, obesity, respiratory failure, insulin resistance (Type 2 diabetes) and right sided heart failure. Angelman syndrome results when the maternal copy of the UBE3A gene fails to turn on in the brain because of a mutation or loss of the gene on chromosome 15 or when 2 copies of the father's chromosome are expressed (paternal uniparental disomy). Individuals with Angelman syndrome have a complex genetic disorder affecting the central nervous system that is characterized by developmental delays, speech impairments, ataxia (balance and movement problems), seizures, and microcephaly. Symptoms begin during the first year of life and progress through childhood and include hand flapping, hyperactivity, short attention span, and sleep disturbances. Genetic testing is indicated in individuals with symptoms of either Prader-Willi or Angelman syndromes.

81332

81332 **SERPINA1 (serpin peptidase inhibitor, clade A, alpha-1 antiproteinase, antitrypsin, member 1) (eg, alpha-1-antitrypsin deficiency), gene analysis, common variants (eg, *S and *Z)**

Molecular genetic testing is performed to identify a specific mutation of the SERPINA1 gene which provides instruction to make the protein alpha-1 antitrypsin, a serine protease inhibitor (serpine). Serpine is responsible for controlling chemical reactions by inhibiting certain enzymes. Alpha-1 antitrypsin (AAT) is produced in the liver and transported to the lungs via the bloodstream. When there is a deficiency of AAT, the enzyme neutrophil elastase, which is released from white blood cells in response to infection, attacks and destroys the alveoli (air sacs) in the lungs leading to a condition called emphysema. Found on chromosome 14, at least 120 mutations have been identified. Most alter the molecular structure by exchanging amino acids. The two most common variants are an "S" allele, which changes glutamic acid (glutamate) to valine at codon 264 and the "Z" allele (found in high numbers in individuals of North Western European descent), which changes glutamic acid (glutamate) to lysine at position 342. In addition to AAT deficiency, some mutations of the gene will cause unusual binding of AAT resulting in a large molecule unable to leave the liver, where it accumulates causing liver damage in addition to lung damage from inadequate protection against neutrophil elastase. Or the AAT molecule can be unusually small in size allowing the liver to break it down quickly making it unavailable to the lungs. This mutation spares the liver from damage but the lungs remain unprotected and emphysema can develop. Molecular genetic testing is indicated in individuals with symptoms associated with alpha-1 antitrypsin deficiency or when there is a family history of the disorder.

81340-81341

81340 **TRB@ (T cell antigen receptor, beta) (eg, leukemia and lymphoma), gene rearrangement analysis to detect abnormal clonal population(s); using amplification methodology (eg, polymerase chain reaction)**

81341 **TRB@ (T cell antigen receptor, beta) (eg, leukemia and lymphoma), gene rearrangement analysis to detect abnormal clonal population(s); using direct probe methodology (eg, Southern blot)**

Molecular genetic testing is performed to identify mutations of the T cell antigen receptor, beta (TRB@) gene located on chromosome 7 which are responsible for some forms of leukemia and lymphoma. T cell antigen receptors are constructed from independent gene segments, forming a structure similar to immunoglobulin genes. T cells recognize foreign antigens (small peptides) which are bound to major histocompatibility complex (MHC) molecules on the surface of antigen presenting cells (APC). The T cell antigen receptor is comprised of alpha/beta (95%) and gamma/delta (5%) chain receptor loci which DNA clones can also encode onto. These procedures test for the TRB@ which is the beta T cell antigen receptor. In 81340, TRB@ gene rarrangement analysis to detect abnormal clonal populations is performed using amplification methodology. The beta protein subunit chain of T cell antigen receptors is comprised of a limited number of variable (V) region segments. It is possible to identify the V region monoclonal antibodies and define the population of normal T cells by using an amplification methodology such as polymerase chain reaction (PCR), a form of molecular photocopying. PCR uses heat to separate (denature) the target DNA strand then primers are added to bracket the sequence under analysis. Taq polymerase is applied to priming site and extends the new (copied) DNA stand. This comprehensive gene expression analysis can be used to evaluate human T cell receptor beta variable (TCRBV) proteins and the body's immune response to a variety of problems, including blood cell and lymph system cancers. In 81341, testing is performed by direct probe methodology. The beta protein subunit chain of T cell antigen receptors is comprised of a limited number of variable (V) region segments. It is possible to identify the V region monoclonal antibodies and define the population of normal T cells by using a direct probe methodology such as Southern blot. Direct probe methodology uses radioactivity or an enzyme bound to a single strand DNA probe to distinguish base pairing and DNA sequencing of the gene. This comprehensive gene expression analysis can be used to evaluate human T cell receptor beta variable (TCRBV) proteins and the body's immune response to a variety of problems, including blood cell and lymph system cancers.

81342

81342 **TRG@ (T cell antigen receptor, gamma) (eg, leukemia and lymphoma), gene rearrangement analysis, evaluation to detect abnormal clonal population(s)**

Molecular genetic testing is performed to identify mutations of the T cell antigen receptor, gamma (TRG@) gene located on chromosome 7 which are responsible for some forms of leukemia and lymphoma. T cell antigen receptors are constructed from independent gene segments, forming a structure similar to immunoglobulin genes. T cells recognize foreign antigens (small peptides) which are bound to major histocompatibility complex (MHC) molecules on the surface of antigen presenting cells (APC). The T cell antigen receptor is comprised of alpha/beta (95%) and gamma/delta (5%) chain receptor loci which DNA clones can also encode onto. This test is for TRG@ which is the gamma T cell antigen receptor. The gamma protein subunit chain, a very small subset of T cell antigen receptors is found abundantly in intraepithelial lymphocytes located in the gut and to a lesser extent in skin. Gamma subunits of T cell antigen receptors also contain variable (V) regions of monoclonal and polyclonal antibodies that help define the cells. Non radioactive polymerase chain reaction-single strand conformational polymorphism (PCR-SSCP) along with histological and immunophenotypic analysis are the preferred methods to detect abnormal clonal populations. This comprehensive gene expression analysis can be used to evaluate human T cell receptor gamma variable proteins and the body's immune response to a variety of problems, including blood cell and lymph system cancers.

81350

81350 **UGT1A1 (UDP glucuronosyltransferase 1 family, polypeptide A1) (eg, irinotecan metabolism), gene analysis, common variants (eg, *28, *36, *37)**

Molecular genetic testing is performed to identify a specific mutation of the UGT1A1 gene responsible for encoding enzymes of the glucuronidation pathway. It is part of a complex locus that transforms small lipophilic molecules such as steroids, bilirubin, hormones, drugs and environmental toxins into water soluble metabolites that can be filtered by the kidney and excreted in urine. Individuals with this mutation may develop Gilbert's syndrome (aka, GS or Gilbert-Meulengracht syndrome) which manifests with elevated levels of bilirubin in the blood. The disease is autosomal recessive. Individuals with mutation of the UGT1A1 gene from both parents may develop Gilbert's syndrome and be at increased risk of irinotecan toxicity with chemotherapy. Individuals who receive the UGT1A1 mutation from only one parent are carriers of the disease. Carriers may produce less of the enzyme than non-carriers and may also be at risk for irinotecan toxicity with chemotherapy. The variant *28 is associated with a decrease of the UGT1A1 enzyme in the liver and Gilbert's syndrome. It is commonly found in Caucasians, Africans and to a lesser extent in Asian populations. Variants *36 and *37 are found predominately in individuals of African descent and are identified with ineffective metabolism and excretion of SN-38, broken down by glucuronidation in the liver by the enzyme UGT1A and excreted though the kidneys. Molecular genetic testing is performed on individuals undergoing chemotherapy with irinotecan to determine the need for reduced drug dosage. Irinotecan toxicity is associated with severe neutopenia (low white blood cell count) and diarrhea.

81355

81355 **VKORC1 (vitamin K epoxide reductase complex, subunit 1) (eg, warfarin metabolism), gene analysis, common variant(s) (eg, -1639G>A, c.173+1000C>T)**

Molecular genetic testing is performed to identify a specific mutation of the VKORC1 gene which encodes the enzyme, vitamin K epoxide reductase complex, subunit 1. Vitamin K is an essential component for blood clotting and this enzyme is responsible for reducing vitamin K 2,3-epoxide to its activated form. The variant -1639G>A is a single nucleotide polymorphism (SNP) in the promoter region of the VKORC1 gene which causes a decrease in functional copies of mature VKORC1 protein, limiting the enzyme available in the vitamin K cycle. This gene mutation is important to identify when an individual is undergoing long term treatment/prevention of thromboembolic events using the drug warfarin because it can affect warfarin metabolism by the body. When the ôGô allele is replaced by an ôAô allele (variant -1639) less warfarin is required for anti-coagulation due to a slowed metabolism of the drug and longer half-life in the circulatory system. Heterozygous inheritance of the mutated gene (copy of gene from one parent) may require a moderate dose adjustment of the drug warfarin. Homozygous inheritance of the mutated gene (copy of gene from each parent) may require a very low dose of the drug warfarin to achieve a therapeutic anti-coagulation state. The mutation is found commonly in Asian populations (as high as 90%) and in Caucasians (as high as 50%). Molecular genetic testing is performed on individuals undergoing warfarin therapy to determine the need for reduced drug dosing.

81370-81371

81370 **HLA Class I and II typing, low resolution (eg, antigen equivalents); HLA-A, -B, -C, -DRB1/3/4/5, and -DQB1**

81371 **HLA Class I and II typing, low resolution (eg, antigen equivalents); HLA-A, -B, and -DRB1 (eg, verification typing)**

The human leukocyte antigen (HLA) system forms part of the major histocompatibility complex (MHC). The MHC is responsible for self-recognition which means that it identifies the specific characteristics of an individual's cells and tissues and defends the body against foreign substances including microorganisms and nonself cells and tissues. HLAs are essential for the normal functioning of the immune system and are found on the short arm of chromosome 6. HLAs are comprised of two classes, Class I and Class II. Of these, Class I is the most important and loci A, B, and C are the most important loci within Class I. HLA Class II has 5 loci—DR, DQ, DP, DM, and DO with DR, DQ, and DP being the most important. Each HLA Class I and Class II locus has a number of variants called alleles. HLA alleles are designated first by the locus and then an asterisk (*) followed by two or more digits. The first two digits represent a specific group of alleles while subsequent digits provide more specific information (e.g., HLA-B*08:01) HLAs play a role in general immune response, disease defense, organ transplant rejections, and protection against or susceptibility to certain cancers and autoimmune diseases. All molecular methods for extracting DNA require the use of cell lysis and protein digestion prior to DNA extraction from a nucleated cell. Most molecular methods also use polymerase chain reaction (PCR) as part of the technique. Low resolution testing identifies antigen equivalents. One molecular technique for low resolution typing of HLA Class I and II is called PCR sequence specific priming (SSP). PCR SSP uses a panel of primer pairs to amplify groups of alleles. Low resolution may be performed using test kits or semi-automatic test systems. Use 81370 when low resolution testing for both Class I and Class II HLAs is performed. This test includes three Class I HLA loci, HLA-A, HLA-B, and HLA-C as well as five Class II loci, DRB1, DRB3, DRB4, DRB5, and DQB1. Use 81371 when low resolution verification typing is performed on two Class I HLA loci, HLA-A and HLA-B, as well as one Class II locus, DRB1.

81372-81374

81372 **HLA Class I typing, low resolution (eg, antigen equivalents); complete (ie, HLA-A, -B, and -C)**

81373 **HLA Class I typing, low resolution (eg, antigen equivalents); one locus (eg, HLA-A, -B, or -C), each**

81374 **HLA Class I typing, low resolution (eg, antigen equivalents); one antigen equivalent (eg, B*27), each**

The human leukocyte antigen (HLA) system forms part of the major histocompatibility complex (MHC). The MHC is responsible for self-recognition which means that it identifies the specific characteristics of an individual's cells and tissues and defends the body against foreign substances including microorganisms, and nonself cells and tissues. HLAs are essential for the normal functioning of the immune system and are found on the short arm of chromosome 6. HLAs are comprised of two classes, Class I and Class II. Of these,

Class I is the most important and loci, A, B, and C are the most important loci within Class I. Each HLA Class I locus has a number of variants called alleles. HLA alleles are designated first by the locus and then an asterisk (*) followed by two or more digits. The first two digits represent a specific group of alleles while subsequent digits provide more specific information (e.g., HLA-B*08:01) HLAs play a role in general immune response, disease defense, organ transplant rejections, and protection against or susceptibility to certain cancers and autoimmune diseases. All molecular methods for extracting DNA require the use of cell lysis and protein digestion prior to DNA extraction from a nucleated cell. Most molecular methods also use polymerase chain reaction (PCR) as part of the technique. Low resolution testing identifies antigen equivalents. One molecular technique for low resolution typing of HLA Class I is called PCR sequence specific priming (SSP). PCR SSP uses a panel of primer pairs to amplify groups of alleles. Low resolution may be performed using test kits or semi-automatic test systems. Use 81372 for complete low resolution HLA Class I typing which includes all three loci HLA-A, HLA-B, and HLA-C. Use 81373 when low resolution testing for a single HLA Class I locus is performed (HLA-A, HLA-B, or HLA-C). Use 81374 when low resolution testing is used to identify a specific Class I antigen equivalent, such as B*27.

81375-81377

81375 **HLA Class II typing, low resolution (eg, antigen equivalents); HLA-DRB1/3/4/5 and -DQB1**

81376 **HLA Class II typing, low resolution (eg, antigen equivalents); one locus (eg, HLA-DRB1, -DRB3/4/5, -DQB1, -DQA1, -DPB1, or -DPA1), each**

81377 **HLA Class II typing, low resolution (eg, antigen equivalents); one antigen equivalent, each**

The human leukocyte antigen (HLA) system forms part of the major histocompatibility complex (MHC). The MHC is responsible for self-recognition which means that it identifies the specific characteristics of an individual's cells and tissues and defends the body against foreign substances including microorganisms, and nonself cells and tissues. HLAs are essential for the normal functioning of the immune system and are found on the short arm of chromosome 6. HLAs are comprised of two classes, Class I and Class II. HLA Class II has 5 loci—DR, DQ, DP, DM, and DO with DR, DQ, and DP being the most important. Each HLA Class II locus has a number of variants called alleles. HLA alleles are designated first by the locus and then an asterisk (*) followed by two or more digits. The first two digits represent a specific group of alleles while subsequent digits provide more specific information (e.g., DRB1*15). Class II antigens are responsible for initiating general immune response. All molecular methods for extracting DNA require the use of cell lysis and protein digestion prior to DNA extraction from a nucleated cell. Most molecular methods also use polymerase chain reaction (PCR) as part of the technique. Low resolution testing identifies antigen equivalents. One molecular technique for low resolution typing of HLA Class II is called PCR sequence specific priming (SSP). PCR SSP uses a panel of primer pairs to amplify groups of alleles. Low resolution may be performed using test kits or semi-automatic test systems. Use 81375 when low resolution testing for all five HLA Class II loci is performed. This includes testing for DRB1, DRB3, DRB4, DRB5, and DQB1. Use 81376 for low resolution testing for a single HLA Class II locus (either DRB1, DRB3/4/5, DQB1, DQA1, DPB1, or DPA1). Use 81377 for low resolution testing for a single HLA Class II antigen equivalent, such as DRB1*15.

81378

81378 **HLA Class I and II typing, high resolution (ie, alleles or allele groups), HLA-A, -B, -C, and -DRB1**

The human leukocyte antigen (HLA) system forms part of the major histocompatibility complex (MHC). The MHC is responsible for self-recognition which means that it identifies the specific characteristics of an individual's cells and tissues and defends the body against foreign substances including microorganisms and nonself cells and tissues. HLAs are essential for the normal functioning of the immune system and are found on the short arm of chromosome 6. HLAs are comprised of two classes, Class I and Class II. Of these, Class I is the most important and loci, A, B, and C are the most important loci within Class I. HLA Class II has 5 loci—DR, DQ, DP, DM, and DO with DR, DQ, and DP being the most important. Each HLA Class I and Class II locus has a number of variants called alleles. HLA alleles are designated first by the locus and then an asterisk (*) followed by two or more digits. The first two digits represent a specific group of alleles while subsequent digits provide more specific information (e.g., HLA-B*08:01) HLAs play a role in general immune response, disease defense, organ transplant rejections, and protection against or susceptibility to certain cancers and autoimmune diseases. All molecular methods for extracting DNA require the use of cell lysis and protein digestion prior to DNA extraction from a nucleated cell. Most molecular methods also use polymerase chain reaction (PCR) as part of the technique. High resolution testing identifies specific alleles or allele groups. One molecular technique for high resolution typing of HLA Class I and II is called PCR sequence specific priming (SSP). PCR SSP uses a panel of primer pairs is to amplify groups of alleles. High resolution may be performed using test kits or semi-automatic test systems. Use 81378 when high resolution testing is performed for three Class I loci, HLA-A, HLA-B, and HLA-C as well as for Class II locus HLA-DRB1.

Pathology and Laboratory

81379-81381

81379 HLA Class I typing, high resolution (ie, alleles or allele groups); complete (ie, HLA-A, -B, and -C)

81380 HLA Class I typing, high resolution (ie, alleles or allele groups); one locus (eg, HLA-A, -B, or -C), each

81381 HLA Class I typing, high resolution (ie, alleles or allele groups); one allele or allele group (eg, B*57:01P), each

The human leukocyte antigen (HLA) system forms part of the major histocompatibility complex (MHC). The MHC is responsible for self-recognition which means that it identifies the specific characteristics of an individual's cells and tissues and defends the body against foreign substances including microorganisms and nonself cells and tissues. HLAs are essential for the normal functioning of the immune system and are found on the short arm of chromosome 6. HLAs are comprised of two classes, Class I and Class II. Of these, Class I is the most important and loci, A, B, and C are the most important loci within Class I. Each HLA Class I locus has a number of variants called alleles. HLA alleles are designated first by the locus and then an asterisk (*) followed by two or more digits. The first two digits represent a specific group of alleles while subsequent digits provide more specific information (e.g., HLA-B*08:01) HLAs play a role in general immune response, disease defense, organ transplant rejections, and protection against or susceptibility to certain cancers and autoimmune diseases. All molecular methods for extracting DNA require the use of cell lysis and protein digestion prior to DNA extraction from a nucleated cell. Most molecular methods also use polymerase chain reaction (PCR) as part of the technique. High resolution testing identifies specific alleles or allele groups. One molecular technique for high resolution typing of HLA Class I and II is called PCR sequence specific priming (SSP). PCR SSP uses a panel of primer pairs to amplify groups of alleles. High resolution may be performed using test kits or semi-automatic test systems. Use 81379 for complete high resolution HLA Class I typing which includes all three loci—HLA-A, HLA-B, and HLA-C. Use 81380 when high resolution testing for a single HLA Class I locus is performed (either HLA-A, HLA-B, or HLA-C). Use 81381 when high resolution testing is used to identify a specific Class I allele or allele group, such as HLA-B*57:01P .

81382-81383

81382 HLA Class II typing, high resolution (ie, alleles or allele groups); one locus (eg, HLA-DRB1, -DRB3/4/5, -DQB1, -DQA1, -DPB1, or -DPA1), each

81383 HLA Class II typing, high resolution (ie, alleles or allele groups); one allele or allele group (eg, HLA-DQB1*06:02P), each

The human leukocyte antigen (HLA) system forms part of the major histocompatibility complex (MHC). The MHC is responsible for self-recognition which means that it identifies the specific characteristics of an individual's cells and tissues and defends the body against foreign substances including microorganisms and nonself cells and tissues. HLAs are essential for the normal functioning of the immune system and are found on the short arm of chromosome 6. HLAs are comprised of two classes, Class I and Class II. HLA Class II has 5 loci—DR, DQ, DP, DM, and DO with DR, DQ, and DP being the most important. Each HLA Class II locus has a number of variants called alleles. HLA alleles are designated first by the locus and then an asterisk (*) followed by two or more digits. The first two digits represent a specific group of alleles while subsequent digits provide more specific information (e.g., DRB1*15). Class II antigens are responsible for initiating general immune response. All molecular methods for extracting DNA require the use of cell lysis and protein digestion prior to DNA extraction from a nucleated cell. Most molecular methods also use polymerase chain reaction (PCR) as part of the technique. High resolution testing identifies specific alleles or allele groups. One molecular technique for high resolution typing of HLA Class II is called PCR sequence specific priming (SSP). PCR SSP uses a panel of primer pairs to amplify groups of alleles. High resolution may be performed using test kits or semi-automatic test systems. Use 81382 when high resolution testing is used for a single HLA Class II locus and report for each locus typed, if more than one is done. Typically one or more of the following loci will be typed: HLA-DRB1, -DRB3/4/5, -DQB1, -DQA1, -DPB1, or -DPA1. Use 81383 for high resolution typing of each specific allele or allele group, such as HLA-DQB1*06:02P.

81400

81400 Molecular pathology procedure, Level 1 (eg, identification of single germline variant [eg, SNP] by techniques such as restriction enzyme digestion or melt curve analysis)

ACADM (acyl-CoA dehydrogenase, C-4 to C-12 straight chain, MCAD) (eg, medium chain acyl dehydrogenase deficiency), K304E variant ACE (angiotensin converting enzyme) (eg, hereditary blood pressure regulation), insertion/deletion variant

AGTR1 (angiotensin II receptor, type 1) (eg, essential hypertension), 1166A>C variant

BCKDHA (branched chain keto acid dehydrogenase E1, alpha polypeptide) (eg, maple syrup urine disease, type 1A), Y438N variant

CCR5 (chemokine C-C motif receptor 5) (eg, HIV resistance), 32-bp deletion mutation/794 825del32 deletion CLRN1 (clarin 1) (eg, Usher syndrome, type

3), N48K variant

DPYD (dihydropyrimidine dehydrogenase) (eg, 5-fluorouracil/5-FU and capecitabine drug metabolism), IVS14+1G>A variant

F2 (coagulation factor 2) (eg, hereditary hypercoagulability), 1199G>A variant

F5 (coagulation factor V) (eg, hereditary hypercoagulability), HR2 variant

F7 (coagulation factor VII [serum prothrombin conversion accelerator]) (eg, hereditary hypercoagulability), R353Q variant

F13B (coagulation factor XIII, B polypeptide) (eg, hereditary hypercoagulability), V34L variant

FGB (fibrinogen beta chain) (eg, hereditary ischemic heart disease), -455G>A variant

FGFR1 (fibroblast growth factor receptor 1) (eg, Pfeiffer syndrome type 1, craniosynostosis), P252R variant

FGFR3 (fibroblast growth factor receptor 3) (eg, Muenke syndrome), P250R variant

FKTN (fukutin) (eg, Fukuyama congenital muscular dystrophy), retrotransposon insertion variant

GNE (glucosamine [UDP-N-acetyl]-2-epimerase/N-acetylmannosamine kinase) (eg, inclusion body myopathy 2 [IBM2], Nonaka myopathy), M712T variant

Human Platelet Antigen 1 genotyping (HPA-1), ITGB3 (integrin, beta 3 [platelet glycoprotein IIIa], antigen CD61 [GPIIIa]) (eg, neonatal alloimmune thrombocytopenia [NAIT], post-transfusion purpura), HPA-1a/b (L33P)

Human Platelet Antigen 2 genotyping (HPA-2), GP1BA (glycoprotein Ib [platelet], alpha polypeptide [GPIba]) (eg, neonatal alloimmune thrombocytopenia [NAIT], post-transfusion purpura), HPA-2a/b (T145M)

Human Platelet Antigen 3 genotyping (HPA-3), ITGA2B (integrin, alpha 2b [platelet glycoprotein IIb of IIb/IIIa complex], antigen CD41 [GPIIb]) (eg, neonatal alloimmune thrombocytopenia [NAIT], post-transfusion purpura), HPA-3a/b (I843S)

Human Platelet Antigen 4 genotyping (HPA-4), ITGB3 (integrin, beta 3 [platelet glycoprotein IIIa], antigen CD61 [GPIIIa]) (eg, neonatal alloimmune thrombocytopenia [NAIT], post-transfusion purpura), HPA-4a/b (R143Q)

Human Platelet Antigen 5 genotyping (HPA-5), ITGA2 (integrin, alpha 2 [CD49B, alpha 2 subunit of VLA-2 receptor] [GPIa]) (eg, neonatal alloimmune thrombocytopenia [NAIT], post-transfusion purpura), HPA-5a/b (K505E)

Human Platelet Antigen 6 genotyping (HPA-6w), ITGB3 (integrin, beta 3 [platelet glycoprotein IIIa, antigen CD61] [GPIIIa]) (eg, neonatal alloimmune thrombocytopenia [NAIT], post-transfusion purpura), HPA-6a/b (R489Q)

Human Platelet Antigen 9 genotyping (HPA-9w), ITGA2B (integrin, alpha 2b [platelet glycoprotein IIb of IIb/IIIa complex, antigen CD41] [GPIIb]) (eg, neonatal alloimmune thrombocytopenia [NAIT], post-transfusion purpura), HPA-9a/b (V837M)

Human Platelet Antigen 15 genotyping (HPA-15), CD109 (CD109 molecule) (eg, neonatal alloimmune thrombocytopenia [NAIT], post-transfusion purpura), HPA-15a/b (S682Y)

IL28B (interleukin 28B [interferon, lambda 3]) (eg, drug response), rs12979860 variant

IVD (isovaleryl-CoA dehydrogenase) (eg, isovaleric acidemia), A282V variant

LCT (lactase-phlorizin hydrolase) (eg, lactose intolerance), 13910 C>T variant

NEB (nebulin) (eg, nemaline myopathy), exon 55 deletion variant

PCDH15 (protocadherin-related 15) (eg, Usher syndrome type 1F), R245X variant

SERPINE1 (serpine peptidase inhibitor clade E, member 1, plasminogen activator inhibitor -1, PAI-1) (eg, thrombophilia), 4G variant

SHOC2 (soc-2 suppressor of clear homolog) (eg, Noonan-like syndrome with loose anagen hair), S2G variant

SLCO1B1 (solute carrier organic anion transporter family, member 1B1) (eg, adverse drug reaction), V174A variant

SMN1 (survival of motor neuron 1, telomeric) (eg, spinal muscular atrophy), exon 7 deletion

SRY (sex determining region Y) (eg, 46,XX testicular disorder of sex development, gonadal dysgenesis), gene analysis

TOR1A (torsin family 1, member A [torsin A]) (eg, early-onset primary dystonia [DYT1]), 907_909delGAG (904_906delGAG) variant

Molecular pathology procedures are tests performed at the molecular level to diagnose, treat, and provide prognostic indicators for genetic disorders, cancer, infectious diseases, and in the case of transplant procedures, to identify tissue histocompatibility. Molecular pathology procedures vary in complexity. The levels take into account the amount of professional work and laboratory costs required to perform the procedure. Level I tests involve identification of single variants using a simple technique. One type of Level 1 test would be identification of a single germline variant, such as a single nucleotide variant (SNP) using restriction enzyme digestion or melt curve analysis. The molecular pathologist reviews the patient's medical history, clinical findings, and the results of other diagnostic tests and procedures. The Level 1 test is then performed. A number of Level 1 tests are specifically identified under this code. Molecular pathology procedures that are not specifically identified here but require similar levels of professional expertise, similar amounts of work and laboratory costs, and are performed by similar techniques but do not have a more specific code should also be reported with 81400. Following performance of the test, the molecular pathologist interprets the results and provides a detailed written report of findings.

81401

▲ 81401 **Molecular pathology procedure, Level 2 (eg, 2-10 SNPs, 1 methylated variant, or 1 somatic variant [typically using nonsequencing target variant analysis], or detection of a dynamic mutation disorder/triplet repeat)**

ABCC8 (ATP-binding cassette, sub-family C [CFTR/MRP], member 8) (eg, familial hyperinsulinism), common variants (eg, c.3898-9G>A [c.3992-9G>A], F1388del)

ABL1 (ABL proto-oncogene 1, non-receptor tyrosine kinase) (eg, acquired imatinib resistance), T315I variant

ACADM (acyl-CoA dehydrogenase, C-4 to C-12 straight chain, MCAD) (eg, medium chain acyl dehydrogenase deficiency), commons variants (eg, K304E, Y42H)

ADRB2 (adrenergic beta-2 receptor surface) (eg, drug metabolism), common variants (eg, G16R, Q27E)

AFF2 (AF4/FMR2 family, member 2 [FMR2]) (eg, fragile X mental retardation 2 [FRAXE]), evaluation to detect abnormal (eg, expanded) alleles

APOB (apolipoprotein B) (eg, familial hypercholesterolemia type B), common variants (eg, R3500Q, R3500W)

APOE (apolipoprotein E) (eg, hyperlipoproteinemia type III, cardiovascular disease, Alzheimer disease), common variants (eg, *2, *3, *4)

AR (androgen receptor) (eg, spinal and bulbar muscular atrophy, Kennedy disease, X chromosome inactivation), characterization of alleles (eg, expanded size or methylation status)

ATN1 (atrophin 1) (eg, dentatorubral-pallidoluysian atrophy), evaluation to detect abnormal (eg, expanded) alleles

ATXN1 (ataxin 1) (eg, spinocerebellar ataxia), evaluation to detect abnormal (eg, expanded) alleles

ATXN2 (ataxin 2) (eg, spinocerebellar ataxia), evaluation to detect abnormal (eg, expanded) alleles

ATXN3 (ataxin 3) (eg, spinocerebellar ataxia, Machado-Joseph disease), evaluation to detect abnormal (eg, expanded) alleles

ATXN7 (ataxin 7) (eg, spinocerebellar ataxia), evaluation to detect abnormal (eg, expanded) alleles

ATXN8OS (ATXN8 opposite strand [non-protein coding]) (eg, spinocerebellar ataxia), evaluation to detect abnormal (eg, expanded) alleles

ATXN10 (ataxin 10) (eg, spinocerebellar ataxia), evaluation to detect abnormal (eg, expanded) alleles

CACNA1A (calcium channel, voltage-dependent, P/Q type, alpha 1A subunit) (eg, spinocerebellar ataxia), evaluation to detect abnormal (eg, expanded) alleles

CBFB/MYH11 (inv(16)) (eg, acute myeloid leukemia), qualitative, and quantitative, if performed

CBS (cystathionine-beta-synthase) (eg, homocystinuria, cystathionine beta-synthase deficiency), common variants (eg, I278T, G307S)

CCND1/IGH (BCL1/IgH, t(11;14)) (eg, mantle cell lymphoma) translocation analysis, major breakpoint, qualitative, and quantitative, if performed

CFH/ARMS2 (complement factor H/age-related maculopathy susceptibility 2) (eg, macular degeneration), common variants (eg, Y402H [CFH], A69S [ARMS2])

CNBP (CCHC-type zinc finger, nucleic acid binding protein) (eg, myotonic dystrophy type 2), evaluation to detect abnormal (eg, expanded) alleles

CSTB (cystatin B [stefin B]) (eg, Unverricht-Lundborg disease), evaluation to detect abnormal (eg, expanded) alleles

CYP3A4 (cytochrome P450, family 3, subfamily A, polypeptide 4) (eg, drug metabolism), common variants (eg, *2, *3, *4, *5, *6)

CYP3A5 (cytochrome P450, family 3, subfamily A, polypeptide 5) (eg, drug metabolism), common variants (eg, *2, *3, *4, *5, *6)

DEK/NUP214 (t(6;9)) (eg, acute myeloid leukemia), translocation analysis, qualitative, and quantitative, if performed

DMPK (dystrophia myotonica-protein kinase) (eg, myotonic dystrophy, type 1), evaluation to detect abnormal (eg, expanded) alleles

E2A/PBX1 (t(1;19)) (eg, acute lymphocytic leukemia), translocation analysis, qualitative, and quantitative, if performed

EML4/ALK (inv(2)) (eg, non-small cell lung cancer), translocation or inversion analysis

ETV6/NTRK3 (t(12;15)) (eg, congenital/infantile fibrosarcoma), translocation analysis, qualitative, and quantitative, if performed

ETV6/RUNX1 (t(12;21)) (eg, acute lymphocytic leukemia), translocation analysis, qualitative, and quantitative, if performed

EWSR1/ATF1 (t(12;22)) (eg, clear cell sarcoma), translocation analysis,

qualitative, and quantitative, if performed

EWSR1/ERG (t(21;22)) (eg, Ewing sarcoma/peripheral neuroectodermal tumor), translocation analysis, qualitative, and quantitative, if performed

EWSR1/FLI1 (t(11;22)) (eg, Ewing sarcoma/peripheral neuroectodermal tumor), translocation analysis, qualitative, and quantitative, if performed

EWSR1/WT1 (t(11;22)) (eg, desmoplastic small round cell tumor), translocation analysis, qualitative, and quantitative, if performed

F11 (coagulation factor XI) (eg, coagulation disorder), common variants (eg, E117X [Type II], F283L [Type III], IVS14del14, and IVS14+1G>A [Type I]) FGFR3 (fibroblast growth factor receptor 3) (eg, achondroplasia, hypochondroplasia), common variants (eg, 1138G>A, 1138G>C, 1620C>A, 1620C>G)

FIP1L1/PDGFRA (del[4q12]) (eg, imatinib-sensitive chronic eosinophilic leukemia), qualitative, and quantitative, if performed FLG (filaggrin) (eg, ichthyosis vulgaris), common variants (eg, R501X, 2282del4, R2447X, S3247X, 3702delG)

FOXO1/PAX3 (t(2;13)) (eg, alveolar rhabdomyosarcoma), translocation analysis, qualitative, and quantitative, if performed

FOXO1/PAX7 (t(1;13)) (eg, alveolar rhabdomyosarcoma), translocation analysis, qualitative, and quantitative, if performed

FUS/DDIT3 (t(12;16)) (eg, myxoid liposarcoma), translocation analysis, qualitative, and quantitative, if performed

FXN (frataxin) (eg, Friedreich ataxia), evaluation to detect abnormal (expanded) alleles

GALC (galactosylceramidase) (eg, Krabbe disease), common variants (eg, c.857G>A, 30-kb deletion)

GALT (galactose-1-phosphate uridylyltransferase) (eg, galactosemia), common variants (eg, Q188R, S135L, K285N, T138M, L195P, Y209C, IVS2-2A>G, P171S, del5kb, N314D, L218L/N314D)

H19 (imprinted maternally expressed transcript [non-protein coding]) (eg, Beckwith-Wiedemann syndrome), methylation analysis

HBB (hemoglobin, beta) (eg, sickle cell anemia, hemoglobin C, hemoglobin E), common variants (eg, HbS, HbC, HbE)

HTT (huntingtin) (eg, Huntington disease), evaluation to detect abnormal (eg, expanded) alleles IGH@/BCL2 (t(14;18)) (eg, follicular lymphoma), translocation analysis; single breakpoint (eg, major breakpoint region [MBR] or minor cluster region [mcr]), qualitative or quantitative (When both MBR and mcr breakpoints are performed, use 81402)

KCNQ1OT1 (KCNQ1 overlapping transcript 1 [non-protein coding]) (eg, Beckwith-Wiedemann syndrome), methylation analysis

LRRK2 (leucine-rich repeat kinase 2) (eg, Parkinson disease), common variants (eg, R1441G, G2019S, I2020T) MED12 (mediator complex subunit 12) (eg, FG syndrome type 1, Lujan syndrome), common variants (eg, R961W, N1007S)

MEG3/DLK1 (maternally expressed 3 [non-protein coding]/delta-like 1 homolog [Drosophila]) (eg, intrauterine growth retardation), methylation analysis

MLL/AFF1 (t(4;11)) (eg, acute lymphoblastic leukemia), translocation analysis, qualitative, and quantitative, if performed

MLL/MLLT3 (t(9;11)) (eg, acute myeloid leukemia), translocation analysis, qualitative, and quantitative, if performed

MT-ATP6 (mitochondrially encoded ATP synthase 6) (eg, neuropathy with ataxia and retinitis pigmentosa [NARP], Leigh syndrome), common variants (eg, m.8993T>G, m.8993T>C)

MT-ND4, MT-ND6 (mitochondrially encoded NADH dehydrogenase 4, mitochondrially encoded NADH dehydrogenase 6) (eg, Leber hereditary optic neuropathy [LHON]), common variants (eg, m.11778G>A, m.3460G>A, m.14484T>C)

MT-ND5 (mitochondrially encoded tRNA leucine 1 [UUA/G], mitochondrially encoded NADH dehydrogenase 5) (eg, mitochondrial encephalopathy with lactic acidosis and stroke-like episodes [MELAS]), common variants (eg, m.3243A>G, m.3271T>C, m.3252A>G, m.13513G>A)

MT-RNR1 (mitochondrially encoded 12S RNA) (eg, nonsyndromic hearing loss), common variants (eg, m.1555A>G, m.1494C>T)

MT-TK (mitochondrially encoded tRNA lysine) (eg, myoclonic epilepsy with ragged-red fibers [MERRF]), common variants (eg, m.8344A>G, m.8356T>C)

MT-TL1 (mitochondrially encoded tRNA leucine 1 [UUA/G]) (eg, diabetes and hearing loss), common variants (eg, m.3243A>G, m.14709 T>C)

MT-TL1 MT-TS1, MT-RNR1 (mitochondrially encoded tRNA serine 1 [UCN], mitochondrially encoded 12S RNA) (eg, nonsyndromic sensorineural deafness [including aminoglycoside-induced nonsyndromic deafness]), common variants (eg, m.7445A>G, m.1555A>G)

MUTYH (mutY homolog [E. coli]) (eg, MYH-associated polyposis), common variants (eg, Y165C, G382D)

NOD2 (nucleotide-binding oligomerization domain containing 2) (eg, Crohn's disease, Blau syndrome), common variants (eg, SNP 8, SNP 12, SNP 13)

NPM1/ALK (t(2;5)) (eg, anaplastic large cell lymphoma), translocation

Pathology and Laboratory

analysis

PABPN1 (poly[A] binding protein, nuclear 1) (eg, oculopharyngeal muscular dystrophy), evaluation to detect abnormal (eg, expanded) alleles

PAX8/PPARG (t(2;3) (q13;p25)) (eg, follicular thyroid carcinoma), translocation analysis

PPP2R2B (protein phosphatase 2, regulatory subunit B, beta) (eg, spinocerebellar ataxia), evaluation to detect abnormal (eg, expanded) alleles

PRSS1 (protease, serine, 1 [trypsin 1]) (eg, hereditary pancreatitis), common variants (eg, N29I, A16V, R122H)

PYGM (phosphorylase, glycogen, muscle) (eg, glycogen storage disease type V, McArdle disease), common variants (eg, R50X, G205S)

RUNX1/RUNX1T1 (t(8;21)) (eg, acute myeloid leukemia) translocation analysis, qualitative, and quantitative, if performed

SMN1/SMN2 (survival of motor neuron 1, telomeric/survival of motor neuron 2, centromeric) (eg, spinal muscular atrophy), dosage analysis (eg, carrier testing) (For duplication/deletion analysis of SMN1/SMN2, use 81401) SS18/SSX1 (t(X;18)) (eg, synovial sarcoma), translocation analysis, qualitative, and quantitative, if performed

SS18/SSX2 (t(X;18)) (eg, synovial sarcoma), translocation analysis, qualitative, and quantitative, if performed

TBP (TATA box binding protein) (eg, spinocerebellar ataxia), evaluation to detect abnormal (eg, expanded) alleles

TPMT (thiopurine S-methyltransferase) (eg, drug metabolism), common variants (eg, *2, *3) TYMS (thymidylate synthetase) (eg, 5-fluorouracil/5-FU drug metabolism), tandem repeat variant

VWF (von Willebrand factor) (eg, von Willebrand disease type 2N), common variants (eg, T791M, R816W, R854Q)

Molecular pathology procedures are tests performed at the molecular level to diagnose, treat, and provide prognostic indicators for genetic disorders, cancer, infectious diseases, and in the case of transplant procedures, to identify tissue histocompatibility. Molecular pathology procedures vary in complexity. The levels take into account the amount of professional work and the laboratory costs required to perform the procedure. Level 2 tests involve identification of 2-10 single nucleotide variants (SNPs), 1 methylated variant, or 1 somatic variant (typically performed using non-sequencing target variant analysis), or detection of a dynamic mutation disorder/triplet repeat. The molecular pathologist reviews the patient's medical history, clinical findings, and results of other diagnostic tests and procedures. The Level 2 test is then performed. A number of Level 2 tests are specifically identified under this code. Molecular pathology procedures that are not specifically identified here but require similar levels of professional expertise, similar amounts of work and laboratory costs, and are performed by similar techniques but do not have a more specific code should also be reported with 81401. Following performance of the test, the molecular pathologist interprets the results and provides a detailed written report of the findings.

81402

81402   Molecular pathology procedure, Level 3 (eg, >10 SNPs, 2-10 methylated variants, or 2-10 somatic variants [typically using non-sequencing target variant analysis], immunoglobulin and T-cell receptor gene rearrangements, duplication/deletion variants of 1 exon, loss of heterozygosity [LOH], uniparental disomy [UPD])

Chromosome 18q- (eg, D18S55, D18S58, D18S61, D18S64, and D18S69) (eg, colon cancer), allelic imbalance assessment (ie, loss of heterozygosity)

COL1A1/PDGFB (t(17;22)) (eg, dermatofibrosarcoma protuberans), translocation analysis, multiple breakpoints, qualitative, and quantitative, if performed

CYP21A2 (cytochrome P450, family 21, subfamily A, polypeptide 2) (eg, congenital adrenal hyperplasia, 21-hydroxylase deficiency), common variants (eg, IVS2-13G, P30L, I172N, exon 6 mutation cluster [I235N, V236E, M238K], V281L, L307FfsX6, Q318X, R356W, P453S, G110VfsX21, 30-kb deletion variant)

ESR1/PGR (receptor 1/progesterone receptor) ratio (eg, breast cancer)

IGH@/BCL2 (t(14;18)) (eg, follicular lymphoma), translocation analysis; major breakpoint region (MBR) and minor cluster region (mcr) breakpoints, qualitative or quantitative

MEFV (Mediterranean fever) (eg, familial Mediterranean fever), common variants (eg, E148Q, P369S, F479L, M680I, I692del, M694V, M694I, K695R, V726A, A744S, R761H)

MPL (myeloproliferative leukemia virus oncogene, thrombopoietin receptor, TPOR) (eg, myeloproliferative disorder), common variants (eg, W515A, W515K, W515L, W515R)

TRD@ (T cell antigen receptor, delta) (eg, leukemia and lymphoma), gene rearrangement analysis, evaluation to detect abnormal clonal population

Uniparental disomy (UPD) (eg, Russell-Silver syndrome, Prader-Willi/Angelman

syndrome), short tandem repeat (STR) analysis

Molecular pathology procedures are tests performed at the molecular level to diagnose, treat, and provide prognostic indicators for genetic disorders, cancer, infectious diseases, and in the case of transplant procedures, to identify tissue histocompatibility. Molecular pathology procedures vary in complexity. The levels take into account the amount of professional work and the laboratory costs required to perform the procedure. Level 3 tests involve identification of more than 10 single nucleotide variants (SNPs), 2-10 methylated variants, or 2-10 somatic variants (typically performed using non-sequencing target variant analysis), immunoglobulin and T-cell receptor gene rearrangements, duplication/deletion variants of 1 exon, loss of heterozygosity [LOH], or uniparental disomy [UPD]). The molecular pathologist reviews the patient's medical history, clinical findings, and results of other diagnostic tests and procedures. The Level 3 test is then performed. A number of Level 3 tests are specifically identified under this code. Molecular pathology procedures that are not specifically identified here but require similar levels of professional expertise, similar amounts of work and laboratory costs, and are performed by similar techniques but do not have a more specific code should also be reported with 81402. Following performance of the test, the molecular pathologist interprets the results and provides a detailed written report of findings.

81403

▲ 81403   Molecular pathology procedure, Level 4 (eg, analysis of single exon by DNA sequence analysis, analysis of >10 amplicons using multiplex PCR in 2 or more independent reactions, mutation scanning or duplication/deletion variants of 2-5 exons

ANG (angiogenin, ribonuclease, RNase A family, 5) (eg, amyotrophic lateral sclerosis), full gene sequence

ARX (aristaless-related homeobox) (eg, X-linked lissencephaly with ambiguous genitalia, X-linked mental retardation), duplication/deletion analysis

CEL (carboxyl ester lipase [bile salt-stimulated lipase]) (eg, maturity-onset diabetes of the young [MODY]), targeted sequence analysis of exon 11 (eg, c.1785delC, c.1686delT)

CTNNB1 (catenin [cadherin-associated protein], beta 1, 88kDa) (eg, desmoid tumors), targeted sequence analysis (eg, exon 3) DAZ/SRY (deleted in azoospermia and sex determining region Y) (eg, male infertility), common deletions (eg, AZFa, AZFb, AZFc, AZFd) DNMT3A (DNA [cytosine-5-]-methyltransferase 3 alpha) (eg, acute myeloid leukemia), targeted sequence analysis (eg, exon 23)

EPCAM (epithelial cell adhesion molecule) (eg, Lynch syndrome), duplication/deletion analysis F8 (coagulation factor VIII) (eg, hemophilia A), inversion analysis, intron 1 and intron 22A F12 (coagulation factor XII [Hageman factor]) (eg, angioedema, hereditary, type III; factor XII deficiency), targeted sequence analysis of exon 9

FGFR3 (fibroblast growth factor receptor 3) (eg, isolated craniosynostosis), targeted sequence analysis (eg, exon 7) (For targeted sequence analysis of multiple FGFR3 exons, use 81404)

GJB1 (gap junction protein, beta 1) (eg, Charcot-Marie-Tooth X-linked), full gene sequence GNAQ (guanine nucleotide-binding protein G[q] subunit alpha) (eg, uveal melanoma), common variants (eg, R183, Q209)

HBB (hemoglobin, beta, beta-globin) (eg, beta thalassemia), duplication/deletion analysis

Human erythrocyte antigen gene analyses (eg, SLC14A1 [Kidd blood group], BCAM [Lutheran blood group], ICAM4 [Landsteiner-Wiener blood group], SLC4A1 [Diego blood group], AQP1 [Colton blood group], ERMAP [Scianna blood group], RHCE [Rh blood group, CcEe antigens], KEL [Kell blood group], DARC [Duffy blood group], GYPA, GYPB, GYPE [MNS blood group], ART4 [Dombrock blood group]) (eg, sickle-cell disease, thalassemia, hemolytic transfusion reactions, hemolytic disease of the fetus or newborn), common variants

HRAS (v-Ha-ras Harvey rat sarcoma viral oncogene homolog) (eg, Costello syndrome), exon 2 sequence

IDH1 (isocitrate dehydrogenase 1 [NADP+], soluble) (eg, glioma), common exon 4 variants (eg, R132H, R132C) IDH2 (isocitrate dehydrogenase 2 [NADP+], mitochondrial) (eg, glioma), common exon 4 variants (eg, R140W, R172M)

JAK2 (Janus kinase 2) (eg, myeloproliferative disorder), exon 12 sequence and exon 13 sequence, if performed

KCNC3 (potassium voltage-gated channel, Shaw-related subfamily, member 3) (eg, spinocerebellar ataxia), targeted sequence analysis (eg, exon 2)

KCNJ2 (potassium inwardly-rectifying channel, subfamily J, member 2) (eg, Andersen-Tawil syndrome), full gene sequence

KCNJ11 (potassium inwardly-rectifying channel, subfamily J, member 11) (eg, familial hyperinsulinism), full gene sequence

Killer cell immunoglobulin-like receptor (KIR) gene family (eg, hematopoietic stem cell transplantation), genotyping of KIR family genes

Known familial variant not otherwise specified, for gene listed in Tier 1 or Tier 2, or identified during a genomic sequencing procedure, DNA sequence

● New Code   ▲ Revised Code   CPT © 2016 American Medical Association. All Rights Reserved.   © 2017 DecisionHealth

analysis, each variant exon (For a known familial variant that is considered a common variant, use specific common variant Tier 1 or Tier 2 code)

MC4R (melanocortin 4 receptor) (eg, obesity), full gene sequence

MICA (MHC class I polypeptide-related sequence A) (eg, solid organ transplantation), common variants (eg, *001, *002)

MPL (myeloproliferative leukemia virus oncogene, thrombopoietin receptor, TPOR) (eg, myeloproliferative disorder), exon 10 sequence MT-RNR1 (mitochondrially encoded 12S RNA) (eg, nonsyndromic hearing loss), full gene sequence

MT-TS1 (mitochondrially encoded tRNA serine 1) (eg, nonsyndromic hearing loss), full gene sequence

NDP (Norrie disease [pseudoglioma]) (eg, Norrie disease), duplication/deletion analysis

NHLRC1 (NHL repeat containing 1) (eg, progressive myoclonus epilepsy), full gene sequence

PHOX2B (paired-like homeobox 2b) (eg, congenital central hypoventilation syndrome), duplication/deletion analysis

PLN (phospholamban) (eg, dilated cardiomyopathy, hypertrophic cardiomyopathy), full gene sequence

RHD (Rh blood group, D antigen) (eg, hemolytic disease of the fetus and newborn, Rh maternal/fetal compatibility), deletion analysis (eg, exons 4, 5, and 7, pseudogene) RHD (Rh blood group, D antigen) (eg, hemolytic disease of the fetus and newborn, Rh maternal/fetal compatibility), deletion analysis (eg, exons 4, 5, and 7, pseudogene), performed on cell-free fetal DNA in maternal blood (For human erythrocyte gene analysis of RHD, use a separate unit of 81403)

SH2D1A (SH2 domain containing 1A) (eg, X-linked lymphoproliferative syndrome), duplication/deletion analysis

SMN1 (survival of motor neuron 1, telomeric) (eg, spinal muscular atrophy), known familial sequence variant(s)

TWIST1 (twist homolog 1 [Drosophila]) (eg, Saethre-Chotzen syndrome), duplication/deletion analysis

UBA1 (ubiquitin-like modifier activating enzyme 1) (eg, spinal muscular atrophy, X-linked), targeted sequence analysis (eg, exon 15)

VHL (von Hippel-Lindau tumor suppressor) (eg, von Hippel-Lindau familial cancer syndrome), deletion/duplication analysis

VWF (von Willebrand factor) (eg, von Willebrand disease types 2A, 2B, 2M), targeted sequence analysis (eg, exon 28)

Molecular pathology procedures are tests performed at the molecular level to diagnose, treat, and provide prognostic indicators for genetic disorders, cancer, infectious diseases, and in the case of transplant procedures, to identify tissue histocompatibility. Molecular pathology procedures vary in complexity. The levels take into account the amount of professional work and the laboratory costs required to perform the procedure. Level 4 tests involve analysis of single exon by DNA sequence analysis, analysis of greater than 10 amplicons using multiplex polymerase chain reaction (PCR) in 2 or more independent reactions, mutation scanning or duplication/deletion variants of 2-5 exons. The molecular pathologist reviews the patient's medical history, clinical findings, and results of other diagnostic tests and procedures. The Level 4 test is then performed. A number of Level 4 tests are specifically identified under this code. Molecular pathology procedures that are not specifically identified here but require similar levels of professional expertise, similar amounts of work and laboratory costs, and are performed by similar techniques but do not have a more specific code should also be reported with 81403. Following performance of the test, the molecular pathologist interprets the results and provides a detailed written report of findings.

81404

81404 **Molecular pathology procedure, Level 5 (eg, analysis of 2-5 exons by DNA sequence analysis, mutation scanning or duplication/deletion variants of 6-10 exons, or characterization of a dynamic mutation disorder/triplet repeat by Southern blot analysis)**

ACADS (acyl-CoA dehydrogenase, C-2 to C-3 short chain) (eg, short chain acyl-CoA dehydrogenase deficiency), targeted sequence analysis (eg, exons 5 and 6)

AFF2 (AF4/FMR2 family, member 2 [FMR2]) (eg, fragile X mental retardation 2 [FRAXE]), characterization of alleles (eg, expanded size and methylation status)

AQP2 (aquaporin 2 [collecting duct]) (eg, nephrogenic diabetes insipidus), full gene sequence

ARX (aristaless related homeobox) (eg, X-linked lissencephaly with ambiguous genitalia, X-linked mental retardation), full gene sequence

AVPR2 (arginine vasopressin receptor 2) (eg, nephrogenic diabetes insipidus), full gene sequence

BBS10 (Bardet-Biedl syndrome 10) (eg, Bardet-Biedl syndrome), full gene

sequence

BTD (biotinidase) (eg, biotinidase deficiency), full gene sequence

C10orf2 (chromosome 10 open reading frame 2) (eg, mitochondrial DNA depletion syndrome), full gene sequence

CAV3 (caveolin 3) (eg, CAV3-related distal myopathy, limb-girdle muscular dystrophy type 1C), full gene sequence

CD40LG (CD40 ligand) (eg, X-linked hyper IgM syndrome), full gene sequence

CDKN2A (cyclin-dependent kinase inhibitor 2A) (eg, CDKN2A-related cutaneous malignant melanoma, familial atypical mole-malignant melanoma syndrome), full gene sequence

CLRN1 (clarin 1) (eg, Usher syndrome, type 3), full gene sequence

COX6B1 (cytochrome c oxidase subunit VIb polypeptide 1) (eg, mitochondrial respiratory chain complex IV deficiency), full gene sequence

CPT2 (carnitine palmitoyltransferase 2) (eg, carnitine palmitoyltransferase II deficiency), full gene sequence

CRX (cone-rod homeobox) (eg, cone-rod dystrophy 2, Leber congenital amaurosis), full gene sequence

CSTB (cystatin B [stefin B]) (eg, Unverricht-Lundborg disease), full gene sequence

CYP1B1 (cytochrome P450, family 1, subfamily B, polypeptide 1) (eg, primary congenital glaucoma), full gene sequence

DMPK (dystrophia myotonica-protein kinase) (eg, myotonic dystrophy type 1), characterization of abnormal (eg, expanded) alleles EGR2 (early growth response 2) (eg, Charcot-Marie-Tooth), full gene sequence

EMD (emerin) (eg, Emery-Dreifuss muscular dystrophy), duplication/deletion analysis

EPM2A (epilepsy, progressive myoclonus type 2A, Lafora disease [laforin]) (eg, progressive myoclonus epilepsy), full gene sequence

FGF23 (fibroblast growth factor 23) (eg, hypophosphatemic rickets), full gene sequence

FGFR2 (fibroblast growth factor receptor 2) (eg, craniosynostosis, Apert syndrome, Crouzon syndrome), targeted sequence analysis (eg, exons 8, 10)

FGFR3 (fibroblast growth factor receptor 3) (eg, achondroplasia, hypochondroplasia), targeted sequence analysis (eg, exons 8, 11, 12, 13)

FHL1 (four and a half LIM domains 1) (eg, Emery-Dreifuss muscular dystrophy), full gene sequence

FKRP (fukutin related protein) (eg, congenital muscular dystrophy type 1C [MDC1C], limb-girdle muscular dystrophy [LGMD] type 2I), full gene sequence

FOXG1 (forkhead box G1) (eg, Rett syndrome), full gene sequence

FSHMD1A (facioscapulohumeral muscular dystrophy 1A) (eg, facioscapulohumeral muscular dystrophy), evaluation to detect abnormal (eg, deleted) alleles

FSHMD1A (facioscapulohumeral muscular dystrophy 1A) (eg, facioscapulohumeral muscular dystrophy), characterization of haplotype(s) (ie, chromosome 4A and 4B haplotypes)

FXN (frataxin) (eg, Friedreich ataxia), full gene sequence

GH1 (growth hormone 1) (eg, growth hormone deficiency), full gene sequence

GP1BB (glycoprotein Ib [platelet], beta polypeptide) (eg, Bernard-Soulier syndrome type B), full gene sequence

HBA1/HBA2 (alpha globin 1 and alpha globin 2) (eg, alpha thalassemia), duplication/deletion analysis (For common deletion variants of alpha globin 1 and alpha globin 2 genes, use 81257)

HBB (hemoglobin, beta, Beta-Globin) (eg, thalassemia), full gene sequence

HNF1B (HNF1 homeobox B) (eg, maturity-onset diabetes of the young [MODY]), duplication/deletion analysis

HRAS (v-Ha-ras Harvey rat sarcoma viral oncogene homolog) (eg, Costello syndrome), full gene sequence

HSD3B2 (hydroxy-delta-5-steroid dehydrogenase, 3 beta- and steroid delta-isomerase 2) (eg, 3-beta-hydroxysteroid dehydrogenase type II deficiency), full gene sequence

HSD11B2 (hydroxysteroid [11-beta] dehydrogenase 2) (eg, mineralocorticoid excess syndrome), full gene sequence

HSPB1 (heat shock 27kDa protein 1) (eg, Charcot-Marie-Tooth disease), full gene sequence

INS (insulin) (eg, diabetes mellitus), full gene sequence

KCNJ1 (potassium inwardly-rectifying channel, subfamily J, member 1) (eg, Bartter syndrome), full gene sequence

KCNJ10 (potassium inwardly-rectifying channel, subfamily J, member 10) (eg, SeSAME syndrome, EAST syndrome, sensorineural hearing loss), full gene sequence

LITAF (lipopolysaccharide-induced TNF factor) (eg, Charcot-Marie-Tooth), full gene sequence

MEFV (Mediterranean fever) (eg, familial Mediterranean fever), full gene sequence

MEN1 (multiple endocrine neoplasia I) (eg, multiple endocrine neoplasia type

1, Wermer syndrome), duplication/deletion analysis

MMACHC (methylmalonic aciduria [cobalamin deficiency] cblC type, with homocystinuria) (eg, methylmalonic acidemia and homocystinuria), full gene sequence

MPV17 (MpV17 mitochondrial inner membrane protein) (eg, mitochondrial DNA depletion syndrome), duplication/deletion analysis

NDP (Norrie disease [pseudoglioma]) (eg, Norrie disease), full gene sequence

NDUFA1 (NADH dehydrogenase [ubiquinone] 1 alpha subcomplex, 1, 7.5kDa) (eg, Leigh syndrome, mitochondrial complex I deficiency), full gene sequence

NDUFAF2 (NADH dehydrogenase [ubiquinone] 1 alpha subcomplex, assembly factor 2) (eg, Leigh syndrome, mitochondrial complex I deficiency), full gene sequence

NDUFS4 (NADH dehydrogenase [ubiquinone] Fe-S protein 4, 18kDa [NADH-coenzyme Q reductase]) (eg, Leigh syndrome, mitochondrial complex I deficiency), full gene sequence

NIPA1 (non-imprinted in Prader-Willi/Angelman syndrome 1) (eg, spastic paraplegia), full gene sequence

NLGN4X (neuroligin 4, X-linked) (eg, autism spectrum disorders), duplication/deletion analysis

NPC2 (Niemann-Pick disease, type C2 [epididymal secretory protein E1]) (eg, Niemann-Pick disease type C2), full gene sequence

NROB1 (nuclear receptor subfamily O, group B, member 1) (eg, congenital adrenal hypoplasia), full gene sequence

PDX1 (pancreatic and duodenal homeobox 1) (eg, maturity-onset diabetes of the young [MODY]), full gene sequence

PHOX2B (paired-like homeobox 2b) (eg, congenital central hypoventilation syndrome), full gene sequence

PIK3CA (phosphatidylinositol-4,5-bisphosphate 3-kinase, catalytic subunit alpha) (eg, colorectal cancer), targeted sequence analysis (eg, exons 9 and 20)

PLP1 (proteolipid protein 1) (eg, Pelizaeus-Merzbacher disease, spastic paraplegia), duplication/deletion analysis

PQBP1 (polyglutamine binding protein 1) (eg, Renpenning syndrome), duplication/deletion analysis

PRNP (prion protein) (eg, genetic prion disease), full gene sequence

PROP1 (PROP paired-like homeobox 1) (eg, combined pituitary hormone deficiency), full gene sequence

PRPH2 (peripherin 2 [retinal degeneration, slow]) (eg, retinitis pigmentosa), full gene sequence

PRSS1 (protease, serine, 1 [trypsin 1]) (eg, hereditary pancreatitis), full gene sequence

RAF1 (v-raf-1 murine leukemia viral oncogene homolog 1) (eg, LEOPARD syndrome), targeted sequence analysis (eg, exons 7, 12, 14, 17)

RET (ret proto-oncogene) (eg, multiple endocrine neoplasia, type 2B and familial medullary thyroid carcinoma), common variants (eg, M918T, 2647_2648delinsTT, A883F)

RHO (rhodopsin) (eg, retinitis pigmentosa), full gene sequence

RP1 (retinitis pigmentosa 1) (eg, retinitis pigmentosa), full gene sequence

SCN1B (sodium channel, voltage-gated, type I, beta) (eg, Brugada syndrome), full gene sequence

SCO2 (SCO cytochrome oxidase deficient homolog 2 [SCO1L]) (eg, mitochondrial respiratory chain complex IV deficiency), full gene sequence

SDHC (succinate dehydrogenase complex, subunit C, integral membrane protein, 15kDa) (eg, hereditary paraganglioma-pheochromocytoma syndrome), duplication/deletion analysis

SDHD (succinate dehydrogenase complex, subunit D, integral membrane protein) (eg, hereditary paraganglioma), full gene sequence

SGCG (sarcoglycan, gamma [35kDa dystrophin-associated glycoprotein]) (eg, limb-girdle muscular dystrophy), duplication/deletion analysis

SH2D1A (SH2 domain containing 1A) (eg, X-linked lymphoproliferative syndrome), full gene sequence

SLC16A2 (solute carrier family 16, member 2 [thyroid hormone transporter]) (eg, specific thyroid hormone cell transporter deficiency, Allan-Herndon-Dudley syndrome), duplication/deletion analysis

SLC25A20 (solute carrier family 25 [carnitine/acylcarnitine translocase], member 20) (eg, carnitine-acylcarnitine translocase deficiency), duplication/deletion analysis

SLC25A4 (solute carrier family 25 [mitochondrial carrier; adenine nucleotide translocator], member 4) (eg, progressive external ophthalmoplegia), full gene sequence

SOD1 (superoxide dismutase 1, soluble) (eg, amyotrophic lateral sclerosis), full gene sequence

SPINK1 (serine peptidase inhibitor, Kazal type 1) (eg, hereditary pancreatitis), full gene sequence

STK11 (serine/threonine kinase 11) (eg, Peutz-Jeghers syndrome),

duplication/deletion analysis

TACO1 (translational activator of mitochondrial encoded cytochrome c oxidase I) (eg, mitochondrial respiratory chain complex IV deficiency), full gene sequence

THAP1 (THAP domain containing, apoptosis associated protein 1) (eg, torsion dystonia), full gene sequence

TOR1A (torsin family 1, member A [torsin A]) (eg, torsion dystonia), full gene sequence

TP53 (tumor protein 53) (eg, tumor samples), targeted sequence analysis of 2-5 exons

TTPA (tocopherol [alpha] transfer protein) (eg, ataxia), full gene sequence

TTR (transthyretin) (eg, familial transthyretin amyloidosis), full gene sequence

TWIST1 (twist homolog 1 [Drosophila]) (eg, Saethre-Chotzen syndrome), full gene sequence

TYR (tyrosinase [oculocutaneous albinism IA]) (eg, oculocutaneous albinism IA), full gene sequence

USH1G (Usher syndrome 1G [autosomal recessive]) (eg, Usher syndrome, type 1), full gene sequence

VHL (von Hippel-Lindau tumor suppressor) (eg, von Hippel-Lindau familial cancer syndrome), full gene sequence

VWF (von Willebrand factor) (eg, von Willebrand disease type 1C), targeted sequence analysis (eg, exons 26, 27, 37)

ZEB2 (zinc finger E-box binding homeobox 2) (eg, Mowat-Wilson syndrome), duplication/deletion analysis

ZNF41 (zinc finger protein 41) (eg, X-linked mental retardation 89), full gene sequence

Molecular pathology procedures are tests performed at the molecular level to diagnose, treat, and provide prognostic indicators for genetic disorders, cancer, infectious diseases, and in the case of transplant procedures, to identify tissue histocompatibility. Molecular pathology procedures vary in complexity. The levels take into account the amount of professional work and the laboratory costs required to perform the procedure. Level 5 tests involve analysis of 2-5 exons by DNA sequence analysis, mutation scanning or duplication/deletion variants of 6-10 exons, or characterization of a dynamic mutation disorder/triplet repeat by Southern blot analysis. The molecular pathologist reviews the patient's medical history, clinical findings, and results of other diagnostic tests and procedures. The Level 5 test is then performed. A number of Level 5 tests are specifically identified under this code. Molecular pathology procedures that are not specifically identified here but require similar levels of professional expertise, similar amounts of work and laboratory costs, and are performed by similar techniques but do not have a more specific code should also be reported with 81404. Following performance of the test, the molecular pathologist interprets the results and provides a detailed written report of findings.

81405

81405   Molecular pathology procedure, Level 6 (eg, analysis of 6-10 exons by DNA sequence analysis, mutation scanning or duplication/deletion variants of 11-25 exons, regionally targeted cytogenomic array analysis)

ABCD1 (ATP-binding cassette, sub-family D [ALD], member 1) (eg, adrenoleukodystrophy), full gene sequence

ACADS (acyl-CoA dehydrogenase, C-2 to C-3 short chain) (eg, short chain acyl-CoA dehydrogenase deficiency), full gene sequence

ACTA2 (actin, alpha 2, smooth muscle, aorta) (eg, thoracic aortic aneurysms and aortic dissections) (eg, familial hypertrophic cardiomyopathy), full gene sequence

ACTC1 (actin, alpha, cardiac muscle 1) (eg, familial hypertrophic cardiomyopathy), full gene sequence

ANKRD1 (ankyrin repeat domain 1) (eg, dilated cardiomyopathy), full gene sequence

APTX (aprataxin) (eg, ataxia with oculomotor apraxia 1), full gene sequence

AR (androgen receptor) (eg, androgen insensitivity syndrome), full gene sequence

ARSA (arylsulfatase A) (eg, arylsulfatase A deficiency), full gene sequence

BCKDHA (branched chain keto acid dehydrogenase E1, alpha polypeptide) (eg, maple syrup urine disease, type 1A), full gene sequence

BCS1L (BCS1-like [S. cerevisiae]) (eg, Leigh syndrome, mitochondrial complex III deficiency, GRACILE syndrome), full gene sequence

BMPR2 (bone morphogenetic protein receptor, type II [serine/threonine kinase]) (eg, heritable pulmonary arterial hypertension), duplication/deletion analysis CASQ2 (calsequestrin 2 [cardiac muscle]) (eg, catecholaminergic polymorphic ventricular tachycardia), full gene sequence

CASR (calcium-sensing receptor) (eg, hypocalcemia), full gene sequence

CDKL5 (cyclin-dependent kinase-like 5) (eg, early infantile epileptic encephalopathy), duplication/deletion analysis CHRNA4 (cholinergic receptor, nicotinic, alpha 4) (eg, nocturnal frontal lobe epilepsy), full gene sequence

CHRNB2 (cholinergic receptor, nicotinic, beta 2 [neuronal]) (eg, nocturnal frontal lobe epilepsy), full gene sequence

COX10 (COX10 homolog, cytochrome c oxidase assembly protein) (eg,

Pathology and Laboratory

mitochondrial respiratory chain complex IV deficiency), full gene sequence

COX15 (COX15 homolog, cytochrome c oxidase assembly protein) (eg, mitochondrial respiratory chain complex IV deficiency), full gene sequence

CYP11B1 (cytochrome P450, family 11, subfamily B, polypeptide 1) (eg, congenital adrenal hyperplasia), full gene sequence

CYP17A1 (cytochrome P450, family 17, subfamily A, polypeptide 1) (eg, congenital adrenal hyperplasia), full gene sequence

CYP21A2 (cytochrome P450, family 21, subfamily A, polypeptide2) (eg, steroid 21-hydroxylase isoform, congenital adrenal hyperplasia), full gene sequence

Cytogenomic constitutional targeted microarray analysis of chromosome 22q13 by interrogation of genomic regions for copy number and single nucleotide polymorphism (SNP) variants for chromosomal abnormalities (When performing genome-wide cytogenomic constitutional microarray analysis, see 81228, 81229) (Do not report analyte-specific molecular pathology procedures separately when the specific analytes are included as part of the microarray analysis of chromosome 22q13) (Do not report 88271 when performing cytogenomic microarray analysis)

DBT (dihydrolipoamide branched chain transacylase E2) (eg, maple syrup urine disease, type 2), duplication/deletion analysis

DCX (doublecortin) (eg, X-linked lissencephaly), full gene sequence

DES (desmin) (eg, myofibrillar myopathy), full gene sequence

DFNB59 (deafness, autosomal recessive 59) (eg, autosomal recessive nonsyndromic hearing impairment), full gene sequence

DGUOK (deoxyguanosine kinase) (eg, hepatocerebral mitochondrial DNA depletion syndrome), full gene sequence

DHCR7 (7-dehydrocholesterol reductase) (eg, Smith-Lemli-Opitz syndrome), full gene sequence

EIF2B2 (eukaryotic translation initiation factor 2B, subunit 2 beta, 39kDa) (eg, leukoencephalopathy with vanishing white matter), full gene sequence

EMD (emerin) (eg, Emery-Dreifuss muscular dystrophy), full gene sequence

ENG (endoglin) (eg, hereditary hemorrhagic telangiectasia, type 1), duplication/deletion analysis EYA1 (eyes absent homolog 1 [Drosophila]) (eg, branchio-oto-renal [BOR] spectrum disorders), duplication/deletion analysis

F9 (coagulation factor IX) (eg, hemophilia B), full gene sequence

FGFR1 (fibroblast growth factor receptor 1) (eg, Kallmann syndrome 2), full gene sequence

FH (fumarate hydratase) (eg, fumarate hydratase deficiency, hereditary leiomyomatosis with renal cell cancer), full gene sequence

FKTN (fukutin) (eg, limb-girdle muscular dystrophy [LGMD] type 2M or 2L), full gene sequence

FTSJ1 (FtsJ RNA methyltransferase homolog 1 [E. coli]) (eg, X-linked mental retardation 9), duplication/deletion analysis GABRG2 (gamma-aminobutyric acid [GABA] A receptor, gamma 2) (eg, generalized epilepsy with febrile seizures), full gene sequence

GCH1 (GTP cyclohydrolase 1) (eg, autosomal dominant dopa-responsive dystonia), full gene sequence

GDAP1 (ganglioside-induced differentiation-associated protein 1) (eg, Charcot-Marie-Tooth disease), full gene sequence

GFAP (glial fibrillary acidic protein) (eg, Alexander disease), full gene sequence

GHR (growth hormone receptor) (eg, Laron syndrome), full gene sequence

GHRHR (growth hormone releasing hormone receptor) (eg, growth hormone deficiency), full gene sequence

GLA (galactosidase, alpha) (eg, Fabry disease), full gene sequence

HBA1/HBA2 (alpha globin 1 and alpha globin 2) (eg, thalassemia), full gene sequence

HNF1A (HNF1 homeobox A) (eg, maturity-onset diabetes of the young [MODY]), full gene sequence

HNF1B (HNF1 homeobox B) (eg, maturity-onset diabetes of the young [MODY]), full gene sequence

HTRA1 (HtrA serine peptidase 1) (eg, macular degeneration), full gene sequence

IDS (iduronate 2-sulfatase) (eg, mucopolysacchridosis, type II), full gene sequence

IL2RG (interleukin 2 receptor, gamma) (eg, X-linked severe combined immunodeficiency), full gene sequence

ISPD (isoprenoid synthase domain containing) (eg, muscle-eye-brain disease, Walker-Warburg syndrome), full gene sequence

KRAS (Kirsten rat sarcoma viral oncogene homolog) (eg, Noonan syndrome), full gene sequence

LAMP2 (lysosomal-associated membrane protein 2) (eg, Danon disease), full gene sequence

LDLR (low density lipoprotein receptor) (eg, familial hypercholesterolemia), duplication/deletion analysis MEN1 (multiple endocrine neoplasia I) (eg, multiple endocrine neoplasia type 1, Wermer syndrome), full gene sequence

MMAA (methylmalonic aciduria [cobalamine deficiency] type A) (eg, MMAA-

related methylmalonic acidemia), full gene sequence

MMAB (methylmalonic aciduria [cobalamine deficiency] type B) (eg, MMAA-related methylmalonic acidemia), full gene sequence

MPI (mannose phosphate isomerase) (eg, congenital disorder of glycosylation 1b), full gene sequence

MPV17 (MpV17 mitochondrial inner membrane protein) (eg, mitochondrial DNA depletion syndrome), full gene sequence

MPZ (myelin protein zero) (eg, Charcot-Marie-Tooth), full gene sequence

MTM1 (myotubularin 1) (eg, X-linked centronuclear myopathy), duplication/deletion analysis MYL2 (myosin, light chain 2, regulatory, cardiac, slow) (eg, familial hypertrophic cardiomyopathy), full gene sequence

MYL3 (myosin, light chain 3, alkali, ventricular, skeletal, slow) (eg, familial hypertrophic cardiomyopathy), full gene sequence

MYOT (myotilin) (eg, limb-girdle muscular dystrophy), full gene sequence

NDUFS7 (NADH dehydrogenase [ubiquinone] Fe-S protein 7, 20kDa [NADH-coenzyme Q reductase]) (eg, Leigh syndrome, mitochondrial complex I deficiency), full gene sequence

NDUFS8 (NADH dehydrogenase [ubiquinone] Fe-S protein 8, 23kDa [NADH-coenzyme Q reductase]) (eg, Leigh syndrome, mitochondrial complex I deficiency), full gene sequence

NDUFV1 (NADH dehydrogenase [ubiquinone] flavoprotein 1, 51kDa) (eg, Leigh syndrome, mitochondrial complex I deficiency), full gene sequence

NEFL (neurofilament, light polypeptide) (eg, Charcot-Marie-Tooth), full gene sequence

NF2 (neurofibromin 2 [merlin]) (eg, neurofibromatosis, type 2), duplication/deletion analysis NLGN3 (neuroligin 3) (eg, autism spectrum disorders), full gene sequence

NLGN4X (neuroligin 4, X-linked) (eg, autism spectrum disorders), full gene sequence

NPHP1 (nephronophthisis 1 [juvenile]) (eg, Joubert syndrome), deletion analysis, and duplication analysis, if performed

NPHS2 (nephrosis 2, idiopathic, steroid-resistant [podocin]) (eg, steroid-resistant nephrotic syndrome), full gene sequence

NSD1 (nuclear receptor binding SET domain protein 1) (eg, Sotos syndrome), duplication/deletion analysis

OTC (ornithine carbamoyltransferase) (eg, ornithine transcarbamylase deficiency), full gene sequence

PAFAH1B1 (platelet-activating factor acetylhydrolase 1b, regulatory subunit 1 [45kDa]) (eg, lissencephaly, Miller-Dieker syndrome), duplication/deletion analysis

PARK2 (Parkinson protein 2, E3 ubiquitin protein ligase [parkin]) (eg, Parkinson disease), duplication/deletion analysis

PCCA (propionyl CoA carboxylase, alpha polypeptide) (eg, propionic acidemia, type 1), duplication/deletion analysis

PCDH19 (protocadherin 19) (eg, epileptic encephalopathy), full gene sequence

PDHA1 (pyruvate dehydrogenase [lipoamide] alpha 1) (eg, lactic acidosis), duplication/deletion analysis

PDHB (pyruvate dehydrogenase [lipoamide] beta) (eg, lactic acidosis), full gene sequence

PINK1 (PTEN induced putative kinase 1) (eg, Parkinson disease), full gene sequence

PLP1 (proteolipid protein 1) (eg, Pelizaeus-Merzbacher disease, spastic paraplegia), full gene sequence

POU1F1 (POU class 1 homeobox 1) (eg, combined pituitary hormone deficiency), full gene sequence

PRX (periaxin) (eg, Charcot-Marie-Tooth disease), full gene sequence

PQBP1 (polyglutamine binding protein 1) (eg, Renpenning syndrome), full gene sequence

PSEN1 (presenilin 1) (eg, Alzheimer disease), full gene sequence

RAB7A (RAB7A, member RAS oncogene family) (eg, Charcot-Marie-Tooth disease), full gene sequence

RAI1 (retinoic acid induced 1) (eg, Smith-Magenis syndrome), full gene sequence

REEP1 (receptor accessory protein 1) (eg, spastic paraplegia), full gene sequence

RET (ret proto-oncogene) (eg, multiple endocrine neoplasia, type 2A and familial medullary thyroid carcinoma), targeted sequence analysis (eg, exons 10, 11, 13-16) RPS19 (ribosomal protein S19) (eg, Diamond-Blackfan anemia), full gene sequence

RRM2B (ribonucleotide reductase M2 B [TP53 inducible]) (eg, mitochondrial DNA depletion), full gene sequence

SCO1 (SCO cytochrome oxidase deficient homolog 1) (eg, mitochondrial respiratory chain complex IV deficiency), full gene sequence

SDHB (succinate dehydrogenase complex, subunit B, iron sulfur) (eg, hereditary paraganglioma), full gene sequence

SDHC (succinate dehydrogenase complex, subunit C, integral membrane protein, 15kDa) (eg, hereditary paraganglioma-pheochromocytoma syndrome), full gene sequence

SGCA (sarcoglycan, alpha [50kDa dystrophin-associated glycoprotein]) (eg, limb-girdle muscular dystrophy), full gene sequence

SGCB (sarcoglycan, beta [43kDa dystrophin-associated glycoprotein]) (eg, limb-girdle muscular dystrophy), full gene sequence

SGCD (sarcoglycan, delta [35kDa dystrophin-associated glycoprotein]) (eg, limb-girdle muscular dystrophy), full gene sequence

SGCE (sarcoglycan, epsilon) (eg, myoclonic dystonia), duplication/deletion analysis

SGCG (sarcoglycan, gamma [35kDa dystrophin-associated glycoprotein]) (eg, limb-girdle muscular dystrophy), full gene sequence

SHOC2 (soc-2 suppressor of clear homolog) (eg, Noonan-like syndrome with loose anagen hair), full gene sequence

SHOX (short stature homeobox) (eg, Langer mesomelic dysplasia), full gene sequence

SIL1 (SIL1 homolog, endoplasmic reticulum chaperone [S. cerevisiae]) (eg, ataxia), full gene sequence

SLC2A1 (solute carrier family 2 [facilitated glucose transporter], member 1) (eg, glucose transporter type 1 [GLUT 1] deficiency syndrome), full gene sequence

SLC16A2 (solute carrier family 16, member 2 [thyroid hormone transporter]) (eg, specific thyroid hormone cell transporter deficiency, Allan-Herndon-Dudley syndrome), full gene sequence

SLC22A5 (solute carrier family 22 [organic cation/carnitine transporter], member 5) (eg, systemic primary carnitine deficiency), full gene sequence

SLC25A20 (solute carrier family 25 [carnitine/acylcarnitine translocase], member 20) (eg, carnitine-acylcarnitine translocase deficiency), full gene sequence

SMAD4 (SMAD family member 4) (eg, hemorrhagic telangiectasia syndrome, juvenile polyposis), duplication/deletion analysis

SMN1 (survival of motor neuron 1, telomeric) (eg, spinal muscular atrophy), full gene sequence

SPAST (spastin) (eg, spastic paraplegia), duplication/deletion analysis

SPG7 (spastic paraplegia 7 [pure and complicated autosomal recessive]) (eg, spastic paraplegia), duplication/deletion analysis

SPRED1 (sprouty-related, EVH1 domain containing 1) (eg, Legius syndrome), full gene sequence

STAT3 (signal transducer and activator of transcription 3 [acute-phase response factor]) (eg, autosomal dominant hyper-IgE syndrome), targeted sequence analysis (eg, exons 12, 13, 14, 16, 17, 20, 21)

STK11 (serine/threonine kinase 11) (eg, Peutz-Jeghers syndrome), full gene sequence

SURF1 (surfeit 1) (eg, mitochondrial respiratory chain complex IV deficiency), full gene sequence

TARDBP (TAR DNA binding protein) (eg, amyotrophic lateral sclerosis), full gene sequence

TBX5 (T-box 5) (eg, Holt-Oram syndrome), full gene sequence

TCF4 (transcription factor 4) (eg, Pitt-Hopkins syndrome), duplication/deletion analysis

TGFBR1 (transforming growth factor, beta receptor 1) (eg, Marfan syndrome), full gene sequence

TGFBR2 (transforming growth factor, beta receptor 2) (eg, Marfan syndrome), full gene sequence

THRB (thyroid hormone receptor, beta) (eg, thyroid hormone resistance, thyroid hormone beta receptor deficiency), full gene sequence or targeted sequence analysis of >5 exons

TK2 (thymidine kinase 2, mitochondrial) (eg, mitochondrial DNA depletion syndrome), full gene sequence

TNNC1 (troponin C type 1 [slow]) (eg, hypertrophic cardiomyopathy or dilated cardiomyopathy), full gene sequence

TNNI3 (troponin I, type 3 [cardiac]) (eg, familial hypertrophic cardiomyopathy), full gene sequence

TP53 (tumor protein 53) (eg, Li-Fraumeni syndrome, tumor samples), full gene sequence or targeted sequence analysis of >5 exons

TPM1 (tropomyosin 1 [alpha]) (eg, familial hypertrophic cardiomyopathy), full gene sequence

TSC1 (tuberous sclerosis 1) (eg, tuberous sclerosis), duplication/deletion analysis

TYMP (thymidine phosphorylase) (eg, mitochondrial DNA depletion syndrome), full gene sequence

VWF (von Willebrand factor) (eg, von Willebrand disease type 2N), targeted sequence analysis (eg, exons 18-20, 23-25)

WT1 (Wilms tumor 1) (eg, Denys-Drash syndrome, familial Wilms tumor), full gene sequence

ZEB2 (zinc finger E-box binding homeobox 2) (eg, Mowat-Wilson syndrome),

full gene sequence

Molecular pathology procedures are tests performed at the molecular level to diagnose, treat, and provide prognostic indicators for genetic disorders, cancer, infectious diseases, and in the case of transplant procedures, to identify tissue histocompatibility. Molecular pathology procedures vary in complexity. The levels take into account the amount of professional work and the laboratory costs required to perform the procedure. Level 6 tests involve regionally targeted cytogenomic array analysis, such as analysis of 6-10 exons by DNA sequence analysis, mutation scanning or duplication/deletion variants of 11-25 exons. The molecular pathologist reviews the patient's medical history, clinical findings, and results of other diagnostic tests and procedures. The Level 6 test is then performed. A number of Level 6 tests are specifically identified under this code. Molecular pathology procedures that are not specifically identified here but require similar levels of professional expertise, similar amounts of work and laboratory costs, and are performed by similar techniques but do not have a more specific code should also be reported with 81405. Following performance of the test, the molecular pathologist interprets the results and provides a detailed written report of findings.

81406

▲ 81406   **Molecular pathology procedure, Level 7 (eg, analysis of 11-25 exons by DNA sequence analysis, mutation scanning or duplication/deletion variants of 26-50 exons, cytogenomic array analysis for neoplasia)**

ACADVL (acyl-CoA dehydrogenase, very long chain) (eg, very long chain acyl-coenzyme A dehydrogenase deficiency), full gene sequence

ACTN4 (actinin, alpha 4) (eg, focal segmental glomerulosclerosis), full gene sequence

AFG3L2 (AFG3 ATPase family gene 3-like 2 [S. cerevisiae]) (eg, spinocerebellar ataxia), full gene sequence

AIRE (autoimmune regulator) (eg, autoimmune polyendocrinopathy syndrome type 1), full gene sequence

ALDH7A1 (aldehyde dehydrogenase 7 family, member A1) (eg, pyridoxine-dependent epilepsy), full gene sequence

ANO5 (anoctamin 5) (eg, limb-girdle muscular dystrophy), full gene sequence

APP (amyloid beta [A4] precursor protein) (eg, Alzheimer disease), full gene sequence

ASS1 (argininosuccinate synthase 1) (eg, citrullinemia type I), full gene sequence

ATL1 (atlastin GTPase 1) (eg, spastic paraplegia), full gene sequence

ATP1A2 (ATPase, Na+/K+ transporting, alpha 2 polypeptide) (eg, familial hemiplegic migraine), full gene sequence

ATP7B (ATPase, Cu++ transporting, beta polypeptide) (eg, Wilson disease), full gene sequence

BBS1 (Bardet-Biedl syndrome 1) (eg, Bardet-Biedl syndrome), full gene sequence

BBS2 (Bardet-Biedl syndrome 2) (eg, Bardet-Biedl syndrome), full gene sequence

BCKDHB (branched-chain keto acid dehydrogenase E1, beta polypeptide) (eg, maple syrup urine disease, type 1B), full gene sequence

BEST1 (bestrophin 1) (eg, vitelliform macular dystrophy), full gene sequence

BMPR2 (bone morphogenetic protein receptor, type II [serine/threonine kinase]) (eg, heritable pulmonary arterial hypertension), full gene sequence

BRAF (B-Raf proto-oncogene, serine/threonine kinase) (eg, Noonan syndrome), full gene sequence

BSCL2 (Berardinelli-Seip congenital lipodystrophy 2 [seipin]) (eg, Berardinelli-Seip congenital lipodystrophy), full gene sequence

BTK (Bruton agammaglobulinemia tyrosine kinase) (eg, X-linked agammaglobulinemia), full gene sequence

CACNB2 (calcium channel, voltage-dependent, beta 2 subunit) (eg, Brugada syndrome), full gene sequence

CAPN3 (calpain 3) (eg, limb-girdle muscular dystrophy [LGMD] type 2A, calpainopathy), full gene sequence

CBS (cystathionine-beta-synthase) (eg, homocystinuria, cystathionine beta-synthase deficiency), full gene sequence

CDH1 (cadherin 1, type 1, E-cadherin [epithelial]) (eg, hereditary diffuse gastric cancer), full gene sequence

CDKL5 (cyclin-dependent kinase-like 5) (eg, early infantile epileptic encephalopathy), full gene sequence

CLCN1 (chloride channel 1, skeletal muscle) (eg, myotonia congenita), full gene sequence CLCNKB (chloride channel, voltage-sensitive Kb) (eg, Bartter syndrome 3 and 4b), full gene sequence

CNTNAP2 (contactin-associated protein-like 2) (eg, Pitt-Hopkins-like syndrome 1), full gene sequence

COL6A2 (collagen, type VI, alpha 2) (eg, collagen type VI-related disorders), duplication/deletion analysis

CPT1A (carnitine palmitoyltransferase 1A [liver]) (eg, carnitine palmitoyltransferase 1A [CPT1A] deficiency), full gene sequence

CRB1 (crumbs homolog 1 [Drosophila]) (eg, Leber congenital amaurosis), full gene sequence

CREBBP (CREB binding protein) (eg, Rubinstein-Taybi syndrome), duplication/deletion analysis Cytogenomic microarray analysis, neoplasia (eg, interrogation of copy number, and loss-of-heterozygosity via single nucleotide polymorphism [SNP]-based comparative genomic hybridization [CGH] microarray analysis) (Do not report analyte-specific molecular pathology procedures separately when the specific analytes are included as part of the cytogenomic microarray analysis for neoplasia) (Do not report 88271 when performing cytogenomic microarray analysis)

DBT (dihydrolipoamide branched chain transacylase E2) (eg, maple syrup urine disease, type 2), full gene sequence

DLAT (dihydrolipoamide S-acetyltransferase) (eg, pyruvate dehydrogenase E2 deficiency), full gene sequence

DLD (dihydrolipoamide dehydrogenase) (eg, maple syrup urine disease, type III), full gene sequence

DSC2 (desmocollin) (eg, arrhythmogenic right ventricular dysplasia/cardiomyopathy 11), full gene sequence

DSG2 (desmoglein 2) (eg, arrhythmogenic right ventricular dysplasia/cardiomyopathy 10), full gene sequence

DSP (desmoplakin) (eg, arrhythmogenic right ventricular dysplasia/cardiomyopathy 8), full gene sequence

EFHC1 (EF-hand domain [C-terminal] containing 1) (eg, juvenile myoclonic epilepsy), full gene sequence

EIF2B3 (eukaryotic translation initiation factor 2B, subunit 3 gamma, 58kDa) (eg, leukoencephalopathy with vanishing white matter), full gene sequence

EIF2B4 (eukaryotic translation initiation factor 2B, subunit 4 delta, 67kDa) (eg, leukoencephalopathy with vanishing white matter), full gene sequence

EIF2B5 (eukaryotic translation initiation factor 2B, subunit 5 epsilon, 82kDa) (eg, childhood ataxia with central nervous system hypomyelination/vanishing white matter), full gene sequence

ENG (endoglin) (eg, hereditary hemorrhagic telangiectasia, type 1), full gene sequence

EYA1 (eyes absent homolog 1 [Drosophila]) (eg, branchio-oto-renal [BOR] spectrum disorders), full gene sequence

F8 (coagulation factor VIII) (eg, hemophilia A), duplication/deletion analysis

FAH (fumarylacetoacetate hydrolase [fumarylacetoacetase]) (eg, tyrosinemia, type 1), full gene sequence

FASTKD2 (FAST kinase domains 2) (eg, mitochondrial respiratory chain complex IV deficiency), full gene sequence

FIG4 (FIG4 homolog, SAC1 lipid phosphatase domain containing [S. cerevisiae]) (eg, Charcot-Marie-Tooth disease), full gene sequence

FTSJ1 (FtsJ RNA methyltransferase homolog 1 [E. coli]) (eg, X-linked mental retardation 9), full gene sequence

FUS (fused in sarcoma) (eg, amyotrophic lateral sclerosis), full gene sequence

GAA (glucosidase, alpha; acid) (eg, glycogen storage disease type II [Pompe disease]), full gene sequence

GALC (galactosylceramidase) (eg, Krabbe disease), full gene sequence

GALT (galactose-1-phosphate uridylyltransferase) (eg, galactosemia), full gene sequence

GARS (glycyl-tRNA synthetase) (eg, Charcot-Marie-Tooth disease), full gene sequence GCDH (glutaryl-CoA dehydrogenase) (eg, glutaricacidemia type 1), full gene sequence

GCK (glucokinase [hexokinase 4]) (eg, maturity-onset diabetes of the young [MODY]), full gene sequence

GLUD1 (glutamate dehydrogenase 1) (eg, familial hyperinsulinism), full gene sequence GNE (glucosamine [UDP-N-acetyl]-2-epimerase/N-acetylmannosamine kinase) (eg, inclusion body myopathy 2 [IBM2], Nonaka myopathy), full gene sequence

GRN (granulin) (eg, frontotemporal dementia), full gene sequence HADHA (hydroxyacyl-CoA dehydrogenase/3-ketoacyl-CoA thiolase/enoyl-CoA hydratase [trifunctional protein] alpha subunit) (eg, long chain acyl-coenzyme A dehydrogenase deficiency), full gene sequence

HADHB (hydroxyacyl-CoA dehydrogenase/3-ketoacyl-CoA thiolase/enoyl-CoA hydratase [trifunctional protein], beta subunit) (eg, trifunctional protein deficiency), full gene sequence

HEXA (hexosaminidase A, alpha polypeptide) (eg, Tay-Sachs disease), full gene sequence

HLCS (HLCS holocarboxylase synthetase) (eg, holocarboxylase synthetase deficiency), full gene sequence

HNF4A (hepatocyte nuclear factor 4, alpha) (eg, maturity-onset diabetes of the young [MODY]), full gene sequence IDUA (iduronidase, alpha-L-) (eg, mucopolysaccharidosis type I), full gene sequence

INF2 (inverted formin, FH2 and WH2 domain containing) (eg, focal segmental glomerulosclerosis), full gene sequence

IVD (isovaleryl-CoA dehydrogenase) (eg, isovaleric acidemia), full gene sequence

JAG1 (jagged 1) (eg, Alagille syndrome), duplication/deletion analysis

JUP (junction plakoglobin) (eg, arrhythmogenic right ventricular dysplasia/cardiomyopathy 11), full gene sequence

KAL1 (Kallmann syndrome 1 sequence) (eg, Kallmann syndrome), full gene sequence

KCNH2 (potassium voltage-gated channel, subfamily H [eag-related], member 2) (eg, short QT syndrome, long QT syndrome), full gene sequence

KCNQ1 (potassium voltage-gated channel, KQT-like subfamily, member 1) (eg, short QT syndrome, long QT syndrome), full gene sequence

KCNQ2 (potassium voltage-gated channel, KQT-like subfamily, member 2) (eg, epileptic encephalopathy), full gene sequence

LDB3 (LIM domain binding 3) (eg, familial dilated cardiomyopathy, myofibrillar myopathy), full gene sequence

LDLR (low density lipoprotein receptor) (eg, familial hypercholesterolemia), full gene sequence

LEPR (leptin receptor) (eg, obesity with hypogonadism), full gene sequence

LHCGR (luteinizing hormone/choriogonadotropin receptor) (eg, precocious male puberty), full gene sequence

LMNA (lamin A/C) (eg, Emery-Dreifuss muscular dystrophy [EDMD1, 2 and 3] limb-girdle muscular dystrophy [LGMD] type 1B, dilated cardiomyopathy [CMD1A], familial partial lipodystrophy [FPLD2]), full gene sequence LRP5 (low density lipoprotein receptor-related protein 5) (eg, osteopetrosis), full gene sequence

MAP2K1 (mitogen-activated protein kinase 1) (eg, cardiofaciocutaneous syndrome), full gene sequence

MAP2K2 (mitogen-activated protein kinase 2) (eg, cardiofaciocutaneous syndrome), full gene sequence

MAPT (microtubule-associated protein tau) (eg, frontotemporal dementia), full gene sequence

MCCC1 (methylcrotonoyl-CoA carboxylase 1 [alpha]) (eg, 3-methylcrotonyl-CoA carboxylase deficiency), full gene sequence

MCCC2 (methylcrotonoyl-CoA carboxylase 2 [beta]) (eg, 3-methylcrotonyl carboxylase deficiency), full gene sequence

MFN2 (mitofusin 2) (eg, Charcot-Marie-Tooth disease), full gene sequence

MTM1 (myotubularin 1) (eg, X-linked centronuclear myopathy), full gene sequence

MUT (methylmalonyl CoA mutase) (eg, methylmalonic acidemia), full gene sequence MUTYH (mutY homolog [E. coli]) (eg, MYH-associated polyposis), full gene sequence

NDUFS1 (NADH dehydrogenase [ubiquinone] Fe-S protein 1, 75kDa [NADH-coenzyme Q reductase]) (eg, Leigh syndrome, mitochondrial complex I deficiency), full gene sequence

NF2 (neurofibromin 2 [merlin]) (eg, neurofibromatosis, type 2), full gene sequence

NOTCH3 (notch 3) (eg, cerebral autosomal dominant arteriopathy with subcortical infarcts and leukoencephalopathy [CADASIL]), targeted sequence analysis (eg, exons 1-23)

NPC1 (Niemann-Pick disease, type C1) (eg, Niemann-Pick disease), full gene sequence

NPHP1 (nephronophthisis 1 [juvenile]) (eg, Joubert syndrome), full gene sequence

NSD1 (nuclear receptor binding SET domain protein 1) (eg, Sotos syndrome), full gene sequence

OPA1 (optic atrophy 1) (eg, optic atrophy), duplication/deletion analysis

OPTN (optineurin) (eg, amyotrophic lateral sclerosis), full gene sequence

PAFAH1B1 (platelet-activating factor acetylhydrolase 1b, regulatory subunit 1 [45kDa]) (eg, lissencephaly, Miller-Dieker syndrome), full gene sequence

PAH (phenylalanine hydroxylase) (eg, phenylketonuria), full gene sequence

PALB2 (partner and localizer of BRCA2) (eg, breast and pancreatic cancer), full gene sequence

PARK2 (Parkinson protein 2, E3 ubiquitin protein ligase [parkin]) (eg, Parkinson disease), full gene sequence

PAX2 (paired box 2) (eg, renal coloboma syndrome), full gene sequence

PC (pyruvate carboxylase) (eg, pyruvate carboxylase deficiency), full gene sequence

PCCA (propionyl CoA carboxylase, alpha polypeptide) (eg, propionic acidemia, type 1), full gene sequence

PCCB (propionyl CoA carboxylase, beta polypeptide) (eg, propionic acidemia), full gene sequence

PCDH15 (protocadherin-related 15) (eg, Usher syndrome type 1F), duplication/deletion analysis

PCSK9 (proprotein convertase subtilisin/kexin type 9) (eg, familial hypercholesterolemia), full gene sequence

PDHA1 (pyruvate dehydrogenase [lipoamide] alpha 1) (eg, lactic acidosis), full gene sequence

PDHX (pyruvate dehydrogenase complex, component X) (eg, lactic acidosis), full gene sequence

PHEX (phosphate-regulating endopeptidase homolog, X-linked) (eg, hypophosphatemic rickets), full gene sequence

PKD2 (polycystic kidney disease 2 [autosomal dominant]) (eg, polycystic kidney disease), full gene sequence

PKP2 (plakophilin 2) (eg, arrhythmogenic right ventricular dysplasia/cardiomyopathy 9), full gene sequence

PNKD (paroxysmal nonkinesigenic dyskinesia) (eg, paroxysmal nonkinesigenic dyskinesia), full gene sequence

POLG (polymerase [DNA directed], gamma) (eg, Alpers-Huttenlocher syndrome, autosomal dominant progressive external ophthalmoplegia), full gene sequence

POMGNT1 (protein O-linked mannose beta1,2-N acetylglucosaminyltransferase) (eg, muscle-eye-brain disease, Walker-Warburg syndrome), full gene sequence

POMT1 (protein-O-mannosyltransferase 1) (eg, limb-girdle muscular dystrophy [LGMD] type 2K, Walker-Warburg syndrome), full gene sequence

POMT2 (protein-O-mannosyltransferase 2) (eg, limb-girdle muscular dystrophy [LGMD] type 2N, Walker-Warburg syndrome), full gene sequence

PRKAG2 (protein kinase, AMP-activated, gamma 2 non-catalytic subunit) (eg, familial hypertrophic cardiomyopathy with Wolff-Parkinson-White syndrome, lethal congenital glycogen storage disease of heart), full gene sequence

PRKCG (protein kinase C, gamma) (eg, spinocerebellar ataxia), full gene sequence

PSEN2 (presenilin 2 [Alzheimer disease 4]) (eg, Alzheimer disease), full gene sequence

PTPN11 (protein tyrosine phosphatase, non-receptor type 11) (eg, Noonan syndrome, LEOPARD syndrome), full gene sequence

PYGM (phosphorylase, glycogen, muscle) (eg, glycogen storage disease type V, McArdle disease), full gene sequence

RAF1 (v-raf-1 murine leukemia viral oncogene homolog 1) (eg, LEOPARD syndrome), full gene sequence

RET (ret proto-oncogene) (eg, Hirschsprung disease), full gene sequence

RPE65 (retinal pigment epithelium-specific protein 65kDa) (eg, retinitis pigmentosa, Leber congenital amaurosis), full gene sequence

RYR1 (ryanodine receptor 1, skeletal) (eg, malignant hyperthermia), targeted sequence analysis of exons with functionally-confirmed mutations

SCN4A (sodium channel, voltage-gated, type IV, alpha subunit) (eg, hyperkalemic periodic paralysis), full gene sequence

SCNN1A (sodium channel, nonvoltage-gated 1 alpha) (eg, pseudohypoaldosteronism), full gene sequence

SCNN1B (sodium channel, nonvoltage-gated 1, beta) (eg, Liddle syndrome, pseudohypoaldosteronism), full gene sequence

SCNN1G (sodium channel, nonvoltage-gated 1, gamma) (eg, Liddle syndrome, pseudohypoaldosteronism), full gene sequence

SDHA (succinate dehydrogenase complex, subunit A, flavoprotein [Fp]) (eg, Leigh syndrome, mitochondrial complex II deficiency), full gene sequence

SETX (senataxin) (eg, ataxia), full gene sequence

SGCE (sarcoglycan, epsilon) (eg, myoclonic dystonia), full gene sequence

SH3TC2 (SH3 domain and tetratricopeptide repeats 2) (eg, Charcot-Marie-Tooth disease), full gene sequence

SLC9A6 (solute carrier family 9 [sodium/hydrogen exchanger], member 6) (eg, Christianson syndrome), full gene sequence

SLC26A4 (solute carrier family 26, member 4) (eg, Pendred syndrome), full gene sequence

SLC37A4 (solute carrier family 37 [glucose-6-phosphate transporter], member 4) (eg, glycogen storage disease type Ib), full gene sequence

SMAD4 (SMAD family member 4) (eg, hemorrhagic telangiectasia syndrome, juvenile polyposis), full gene sequence

SOS1 (son of sevenless homolog 1) (eg, Noonan syndrome, gingival fibromatosis), full gene sequence

SPAST (spastin) (eg, spastic paraplegia), full gene sequence

SPG7 (spastic paraplegia 7 [pure and complicated autosomal recessive]) (eg, spastic paraplegia), full gene sequence

STXBP1 (syntaxin-binding protein 1) (eg, epileptic encephalopathy), full gene sequence

TAZ (tafazzin) (eg, methylglutaconic aciduria type 2, Barth syndrome), full gene sequence

TCF4 (transcription factor 4) (eg, Pitt-Hopkins syndrome), full gene sequence

TH (tyrosine hydroxylase) (eg, Segawa syndrome), full gene sequence

TMEM43 (transmembrane protein 43) (eg, arrhythmogenic right ventricular

cardiomyopathy), full gene sequence

TNNT2 (troponin T, type 2 [cardiac]) (eg, familial hypertrophic cardiomyopathy), full gene sequence

TRPC6 (transient receptor potential cation channel, subfamily C, member 6) (eg, focal segmental glomerulosclerosis), full gene sequence

TSC1 (tuberous sclerosis 1) (eg, tuberous sclerosis), full gene sequence

TSC2 (tuberous sclerosis 2) (eg, tuberous sclerosis), duplication/deletion analysis

UBE3A (ubiquitin protein ligase E3A) (eg, Angelman syndrome), full gene sequence

UMOD (uromodulin) (eg, glomerulocystic kidney disease with hyperuricemia and isosthenuria), full gene sequence

VWF (von Willebrand factor) (von Willebrand disease type 2A), extended targeted sequence analysis (eg, exons 11-16, 24-26, 51, 52)

WAS (Wiskott-Aldrich syndrome [eczema-thrombocytopenia]) (eg, Wiskott-Aldrich syndrome), full gene sequence

Molecular pathology procedures are tests performed at the molecular level to diagnose, treat, and provide prognostic indicators for genetic disorders, cancer, infectious diseases, and in the case of transplant procedures, to identify tissue histocompatibility. Molecular pathology procedures vary in complexity. The levels take into account the amount of professional work and the laboratory costs required to perform the procedure. Level 7 tests involve analysis of 11-25 exons by DNA sequence analysis, mutation scanning or duplication/deletion variants of 26-50 exons, or cytogenomic array analysis for neoplasia. The molecular pathologist reviews the patient's medical history, clinical findings, and results of other diagnostic tests and procedures. The Level 7 test is then performed. A number of Level 7 tests are specifically identified under this code. Molecular pathology procedures that are not specifically identified here but require similar levels of professional expertise, similar amounts of work and laboratory costs, and are performed by similar techniques but do not have a more specific code should also be reported with 81406. Following performance of the test, the molecular pathologist interprets the results and provides a detailed written report of findings.

81407

81407   Molecular pathology procedure, Level 8 (eg, analysis of 26-50 exons by DNA sequence analysis, mutation scanning or duplication/deletion variants of >50 exons, sequence analysis of multiple genes on one platform)

ABCC8 (ATP-binding cassette, sub-family C [CFTR/MRP], member 8) (eg, familial hyperinsulinism), full gene sequence

AGL (amylo-alpha-1, 6-glucosidase, 4-alpha-glucanotransferase) (eg, glycogen storage disease type III), full gene sequence

AHI1 (Abelson helper integration site 1) (eg, Joubert syndrome), full gene sequence

ASPM (asp [abnormal spindle] homolog, microcephaly associated [Drosophila]) (eg, primary microcephaly), full gene sequence

CACNA1A (calcium channel, voltage-dependent, P/Q type, alpha 1A subunit) (eg, familial hemiplegic migraine), full gene sequence

CHD7 (chromodomain helicase DNA binding protein 7) (eg, CHARGE syndrome), full gene sequence

COL4A4 (collagen, type IV, alpha 4) (eg, Alport syndrome), full gene sequence

COL4A5 (collagen, type IV, alpha 5) (eg, Alport syndrome), duplication/deletion analysis COL6A1 (collagen, type VI, alpha 1) (eg, collagen type VI-related disorders), full gene sequence

COL6A2 (collagen, type VI, alpha 2) (eg, collagen type VI-related disorders), full gene sequence

COL6A3 (collagen, type VI, alpha 3) (eg, collagen type VI-related disorders), full gene sequence

CREBBP (CREB binding protein) (eg, Rubinstein-Taybi syndrome), full gene sequence

F8 (coagulation factor VIII) (eg, hemophilia A), full gene sequence

JAG1 (jagged 1) (eg, Alagille syndrome), full gene sequence

KDM5C (lysine [K]-specific demethylase 5C) (eg, X-linked mental retardation), full gene sequence

KIAA0196 (KIAA0196) (eg, spastic paraplegia), full gene sequence

L1CAM (L1 cell adhesion molecule) (eg, MASA syndrome, X-linked hydrocephaly), full gene sequence

LAMB2 (laminin, beta 2 [laminin S]) (eg, Pierson syndrome), full gene sequence

MYBPC3 (myosin binding protein C, cardiac) (eg, familial hypertrophic cardiomyopathy), full gene sequence

MYH6 (myosin, heavy chain 6, cardiac muscle, alpha) (eg, familial dilated cardiomyopathy), full gene sequence

MYH7 (myosin, heavy chain 7, cardiac muscle, beta) (eg, familial hypertrophic

● New Code ▲ Revised Code

cardiomyopathy, Liang distal myopathy), full gene sequence

MYO7A (myosin VIIA) (eg, Usher syndrome, type 1), full gene sequence

NOTCH1 (notch 1) (eg, aortic valve disease), full gene sequence

NPHS1 (nephrosis 1, congenital, Finnish type [nephrin]) (eg, congenital Finnish nephrosis), full gene sequence

OPA1 (optic atrophy 1) (eg, optic atrophy), full gene sequence

PCDH15 (protocadherin-related 15) (eg, Usher syndrome, type 1), full gene sequence

PKD1 (polycystic kidney disease 1 [autosomal dominant]) (eg, polycystic kidney disease), full gene sequence

PLCE1 (phospholipase C, epsilon 1) (eg, nephrotic syndrome type 3), full gene sequence

SCN1A (sodium channel, voltage-gated, type 1, alpha subunit) (eg, generalized epilepsy with febrile seizures), full gene sequence

SCN5A (sodium channel, voltage-gated, type V, alpha subunit) (eg, familial dilated cardiomyopathy), full gene sequence

SLC12A1 (solute carrier family 12 [sodium/potassium/chloride transporters], member 1) (eg, Bartter syndrome), full gene sequence

SLC12A3 (solute carrier family 12 [sodium/chloride transporters], member 3) (eg, Gitelman syndrome), full gene sequence

SPG11 (spastic paraplegia 11 [autosomal recessive]) (eg, spastic paraplegia), full gene sequence

SPTBN2 (spectrin, beta, non-erythrocytic 2) (eg, spinocerebellar ataxia), full gene sequence

TMEM67 (transmembrane protein 67) (eg, Joubert syndrome), full gene sequence

TSC2 (tuberous sclerosis 2) (eg, tuberous sclerosis), full gene sequence

USH1C (Usher syndrome 1C [autosomal recessive, severe]) (eg, Usher syndrome, type 1), full gene sequence

VPS13B (vacuolar protein sorting 13 homolog B [yeast]) (eg, Cohen syndrome), duplication/deletion analysis WDR62 (WD repeat domain 62) (eg, primary autosomal recessive microcephaly), full gene sequence

Molecular pathology procedures are tests performed at the molecular level to diagnose, treat, and provide prognostic indicators for genetic disorders, cancer, infectious diseases, and in the case of transplant procedures, to identify tissue histocompatibility. Molecular pathology procedures vary in complexity. The levels take into account the amount of professional work and the laboratory costs required to perform the procedure. Level 8 tests involve analysis of 26-50 exons by DNA sequence analysis, mutation scanning or duplication/deletion analysis of >50 exons, or sequence analysis of multiple genes on one platform. The molecular pathologist reviews the patient's medical history, clinical findings, and results of other diagnostic tests and procedures. The Level 8 test is then performed. A number of Level 8 tests are specifically identified under this code. Molecular pathology procedures that are not specifically identified here but require similar levels of professional expertise, similar amounts of work and laboratory costs, and are performed by similar techniques but do not have a more specific code should also be reported with 81407. Following performance of the test, the molecular pathologist interprets the results and provides a detailed written report of findings.

81408

81408   Molecular pathology procedure, Level 9 (eg, analysis of >50 exons in a single gene by DNA sequence analysis)

ABCA4 (ATP-binding cassette, sub-family A [ABC1], member 4) (eg, Stargardt disease, age-related macular degeneration), full gene sequence

ATM (ataxia telangiectasia mutated) (eg, ataxia telangiectasia), full gene sequence

CDH23 (cadherin-related 23) (eg, Usher syndrome, type 1), full gene sequence

CEP290 (centrosomal protein 290kDa) (eg, Joubert syndrome), full gene sequence

COL1A1 (collagen, type I, alpha 1) (eg, osteogenesis imperfecta, type I), full gene sequence

COL1A2 (collagen, type I, alpha 2) (eg, osteogenesis imperfecta, type I), full gene sequence

COL4A1 (collagen, type IV, alpha 1) (eg, brain small-vessel disease with hemorrhage), full gene sequence

COL4A3 (collagen, type IV, alpha 3 [Goodpasture antigen]) (eg, Alport syndrome), full gene sequence

COL4A5 (collagen, type IV, alpha 5) (eg, Alport syndrome), full gene sequence

DMD (dystrophin) (eg, Duchenne/Becker muscular dystrophy), full gene sequence

DYSF (dysferlin, limb girdle muscular dystrophy 2B [autosomal recessive]) (eg, limb-girdle muscular dystrophy), full gene sequence

FBN1 (fibrillin 1) (eg, Marfan syndrome), full gene sequence

ITPR1 (inositol 1,4,5-trisphosphate receptor, type 1) (eg, spinocerebellar ataxia), full gene sequence

LAMA2 (laminin, alpha 2) (eg, congenital muscular dystrophy), full gene

sequence

LRRK2 (leucine-rich repeat kinase 2) (eg, Parkinson disease), full gene sequence

MYH11 (myosin, heavy chain 11, smooth muscle) (eg, thoracic aortic aneurysms and aortic dissections), full gene sequence

NEB (nebulin) (eg, nemaline myopathy 2), full gene sequence

NF1 (neurofibromin 1) (eg, neurofibromatosis, type 1), full gene sequence

PKHD1 (polycystic kidney and hepatic disease 1) (eg, autosomal recessive polycystic kidney disease), full gene sequence

RYR1 (ryanodine receptor 1, skeletal) (eg, malignant hyperthermia), full gene sequence

RYR2 (ryanodine receptor 2 [cardiac]) (eg, catecholaminergic polymorphic ventricular tachycardia, arrhythmogenic right ventricular dysplasia), full gene sequence

or targeted sequence

analysis of > 50 exons USH2A (Usher syndrome 2A [autosomal recessive, mild]) (eg, Usher syndrome, type 2), full gene sequence

VPS13B (vacuolar protein sorting 13 homolog B [yeast]) (eg, Cohen syndrome), full gene sequence

VWF (von Willebrand factor) (eg, von Willebrand disease types 1 and 3), full gene sequence

Molecular pathology procedures are tests performed at the molecular level to diagnose, treat, and provide prognostic indicators for genetic disorders, cancer, infectious diseases, and in the case of transplant procedures, to identify tissue histocompatibility. Molecular pathology procedures vary in complexity. The levels take into account the amount of professional work and the laboratory costs required to perform the procedure. Level 9 tests involve analysis of more than 50 exons in a single gene by DNA sequence analysis. The molecular pathologist reviews the patient's medical history, clinical findings, and results of other diagnostic tests and procedures. The Level 9 test is then performed. A number of Level 9 tests are specifically identified under this code. Molecular pathology procedures that are not specifically identified here but require similar levels of professional expertise, similar amounts of work and laboratory costs, and are performed by similar techniques but do not have a more specific code should also be reported with 81408. Following performance of the test, the molecular pathologist interprets the results and provides a detailed written report of findings.

81432-81433

81432   Hereditary breast cancer-related disorders (eg, hereditary breast cancer, hereditary ovarian cancer, hereditary endometrial cancer); genomic sequence analysis panel, must include sequencing of at least 14 genes, including ATM, BRCA1, BRCA2, BRIP1, CDH1, MLH1, MSH2, MSH6, NBN, PALB2, PTEN, RAD51C, STK11, and TP53

81433   Hereditary breast cancer-related disorders (eg, hereditary breast cancer, hereditary ovarian cancer, hereditary endometrial cancer); duplication/ deletion analysis panel, must include analyses for BRCA1, BRCA2, MLH1, MSH2, and STK11

Molecular genetic testing is performed to identify hereditary breast cancer related disorders such as hereditary breast, ovarian, and endometrial cancers using a genomic sequence analysis panel (81432) or a duplication/deletion analysis panel (81433). Code 81432 includes at least 14 genes (ATM, BRCA1, BRCA2, BRIP1, CDH1, MLH1, MSH2, MSH6, NBN, PALB2, PTEN, RAD51C, STK11 and TP53) for genomic sequence analysis. Code 81433 must include analysis of BRCA1, BRCA2, MLH1, MSH2 and STK11 for duplication/deletion mutations. Genetic material (DNA) extracted from a specimen of whole blood is fragmented using sonication. The targeted gene segments are enriched using capture hybridization. Massively parallel sequencing and/or microarray analysis is applied to the target regions to detect gene mutations in a genomic sequencing analysis by comparing gene segments and determining similarities or differences. Genetic markers can be found by identifying point mutations or single nucleotide polymorphisms. In 81433, a genetic duplication/ deletion analysis is performed. A normal gene should have 2 copies per cell (with the exception of sex chromosomes). Zero or one copy indicates a deletion variant and three or more copies is evidence of a duplication variant. Variants not identified by sequence analysis may be found using a different type of probe amplification. Genetic testing is used to confirm a diagnosis of hereditary cancer and guide treatment decisions. It may also be used to identify family members who may be at increased risk for developing cancer due to inherited germ line mutations in their DNA.

81434

81434   Hereditary retinal disorders (eg, retinitis pigmentosa, Leber congenital amaurosis, cone-rod dystrophy), genomic sequence analysis panel, must include sequencing of at least 15 genes, including ABCA4, CNGA1, CRB1, EYS, PDE6A, PDE6B, PRPF31, PRPH2, RDH12, RHO, RP1, RP2, RPE65, RPGR, and USH2A

Molecular genetic testing is performed to identify hereditary retinal disorders including retinitis pigmentosa, Leber congenital amaurosis, and cone-rod dystrophy using a genomic

Pathology and Laboratory

sequence analysis panel. Hereditary retinal disorders may be present at birth or develop later in life and are characterized by vision loss, including night blindness and vision distortion. Targeted gene segments (exons) extracted from the DNA in a whole blood specimen are enriched using hybridization. The captured regions undergo next generation sequencing to detect gene mutations. Genetic testing may be used to confirm a clinical diagnosis for a syndromic or non-syndromic eye disorder or to identify adults who may carry familial germ line mutations in their DNA.

81435-81436

81435 Hereditary colon cancer disorders (eg, Lynch syndrome, PTEN hamartoma yndrome, Cowden syndrome, familial adenomatosis polyposis); genomic sequence analysis panel, must include sequencing of at least 10 genes, including APC, BMPR1A, CDH1, MLH1, MSH2, MSH6, MUTYH, PTEN, SMAD4, and STK11

81436 Hereditary colon cancer disorders (eg, Lynch syndrome, PTEN hamartoma syndrome, Cowden syndrome, familial adenomatosis polyposis); duplication/deletion analysis panel, must include analysis of at least 5 genes, including MLH1, MSH2, EPCAM, SMAD4, and STK11

A laboratory test is performed to identify genetic mutations associated with hereditary colon cancer disorders. Genetic testing may be indicated for individuals diagnosed with cancer and/or family members determined to be at risk for developing hereditary colon cancers including familial adenomatosis polyposis, Lynch syndrome (hereditary nonpolyposis colon cancer), PTEN hamartoma tumor syndrome, and Cowden syndrome. PTEN and Cowden syndrome are rare disorders characterized by the growth of multiple hamartomas, or benign tumor-like malformations, on various body areas and an increased risk of certain types of cancers. A blood, saliva, or stool sample is obtained by separately reportable procedure. The specimen is tested using genomic sequencing procedure to evaluate genetic material in totality or near totality. The panel examines at least 10 genes including adenomatous polyposis coli (APC) gene on chromosome 5 associated with familial adenomatosis polyposis, the mismatch repair genes MLH1, MSH2, and MSH6 associated with Lynch syndrome, the MUTYH gene (monallelic, biallelic) associated with polyposis, and the PTEN gene for variant mutations. Code 81435 uses full gene coding sequencing, usually to +/- 10 base pairs on the minimum 10 genes. Code 81436 includes the epithelial cell adhesion molecule (EPCAM) gene on chromosome 2 associated with Lynch syndrome, and takes the genomic sequencing procedure a step further for the analysis of the minimum 5 genes by using next generation sequencing or massively parallel sequencing to detect intragenic deletions or duplications at single exon resolution.

81442

81442 Noonan spectrum disorders (eg, Noonan syndrome, cardio-facio-cutaneous syndrome, Costello syndrome, LEOPARD syndrome, Noonan-like syndrome), genomic sequence analysis panel, must include sequencing of at least 12 genes, including BRAF, CBL, HRAS, KRAS, MAP2K1, MAP2K2, NRAS, PTPN11, RAF1, RIT1, SHOC2, and SOS1

Molecular genetic testing is performed to identify Noonan spectrum disorders (RASopathies) including Noonan syndrome, cardiofaciocutaneous syndrome, Costello syndrome, LEOPARD syndrome, and Noonan-like syndrome. RASopathies are a class of pediatric disorders linked to mutations in the mitogen-activated protein kinase (RAS/MAPK) pathways. These mutations interrupt the signal transductive cascade of certain types of tissue during embryonic and postnatal development. Characteristics of RASopathies often involve multiple body systems and the expression can be highly variable even among family members. There can be overlapping phenotypical features from RAS/MAPK pathway dysregulation including distinctive facial features, cardiac defects, cutaneous abnormalities, neurocognitive delay, and a predisposition to malignancies. The genomic sequence analysis panel must include at least 12 genes including BRAF, CBL, HRAS, KRAS, MAP2K1, MAP2K2, NRAS, PTPN11, RAF1, RIT1, SHOC2 and SOS1. The targeted gene segments (exons) extracted from the DNA in a whole blood specimen are enriched using hybridization. The captured regions undergo massively parallel sequencing to detect gene mutations. Genetic testing may be used to confirm a clinical diagnosis in a patient presenting with symptoms, to differentiate hereditary and acquired cardiomyopathy and arrhythmias, and to identify non-symptomatic family members who may carry familial germ line mutations in their DNA.

81445

81445 Targeted genomic sequence analysis panel, solid organ neoplasm, DNA analysis, and RNA analysis when performed, 5-50 genes (eg, ALK, BRAF, CDKN2A, EGFR, ERBB2, KIT, KRAS, NRAS, MET, PDGFRA, PDGFRB, PGR, PIK3CA, PTEN, RET), interrogation for sequence variants and copy number variants or rearrangements, if performed

Molecular genetic testing is performed on a solid organ neoplasm to identify sequence variants and copy number variants in the DNA and RNA of 5-50 genes including ALK, BRAF, CDKN2A, EGFR, ERBB2, KIT, KRAS, NRAS, MET, PDGFRA, PDGFRB, PGR, PIK3CA, PTEN, and RET. This targeted genomic sequence analysis panel can be used as an adjunct to tumor location, grade, stage, and underlying physical condition of the patient to make treatment

decisions following the diagnosis of cancer. The diversity of tumors at the molecular level can lead to clinical variability of treatment response. Genetic testing allows cancer treatment to be targeted based on the specific molecular genetic pathways of the tumor. A tumor sample is obtained by separately reportable surgical or needle biopsy. The panel analysis of cancer related genes allows for identification of mutations including base substitutions, duplications/deletions, copy number variations, and rearrangements in multiple genes at one time. Testing modalities may include next generation sequencing, immunohistochemistry, fluorescence in situ hybridization (FISH), pyrosequencing, quantitative PCR, and DNA/RNA fragment analysis.

81493

81493 Coronary artery disease, mRNA, gene expression profiling by real-time RT-PCR of 23 genes, utilizing whole peripheral blood, algorithm reported as a risk score

Gene expression profiling is performed on patients who present with stable symptoms suggestive of obstructive coronary artery disease (CAD) to obtain a risk score based on age, sex, and the level of messenger ribonucleic acid (mRNA) in 23 targeted genes. CAD and atherosclerotic disease (stroke, myocardial infarction) are linked to systemic inflammation involving monocytes, macrophages, CD4+ T-cells, and oxidized lipids with subsequent inflammatory response by endothelial, vascular, smooth muscle cells and circulating cells. Gene activity (production of mRNA) increases in response to environmental factors. Elevated levels of the signature genes contained in this test correlate with the presence of systemic inflammation and immune mediated disease, including CAD. A blood sample is obtained by separately reportable venipuncture. Whole blood is tested using real-time polymerase chain reaction (RT-PCR) to assess which genes are turned on (producing proteins or mRNA), or turned off (not producing proteins or mRNA). The results are analyzed using a computer software program to produce an algorithm risk score that correlates positively or negatively for the presence of inflammation and CAD.

81500-81503

81500 Oncology (ovarian), biochemical assays of two proteins (CA-125 and HE4), utilizing serum, with menopausal status, algorithm reported as a risk score

81503 Oncology (ovarian), biochemical assays of five proteins (CA-125, apolipoprotein A1, beta-2 microglobulin, transferrin, and pre-albumin), utilizing serum, algorithm reported as a risk score

Ovarian oncology biochemical assays are performed on women who present with pelvic or ovarian mass to evaluate their risk for ovarian cancer. In 81500, a blood test is performed to measure Cancer Antigen 125 (CA-125) and Human Epididymis Protein 4 (HE4) in women who present with a pelvic mass. This test is referred to as a Risk of Ovarian Malignancy Algorithm (ROMA) and uses a simple scoring system that includes age and menopausal status. The level of CA-125 and HE4 protein markers, offer excellent diagnostic prediction of ovarian cancer. A blood sample is obtained by separately reportable venipuncture. Serum is tested for CA-125 using quantitative electrochemiluminescentilmmunoassay and HE4 is tested using quantitative enzyme immunoassay. In 81503, a blood test is performed to measure Cancer Antigen 125 (CA-125), apolipoprotein A1 (APO A1), beta-2 microglobulin, transferrin and prealbumin in women age 18 or older who present with an ovarian adnexal mass. This test, called an OVA1 assay, is typically performed when surgery is planned and the patient has not yet been referred to an oncologist. A blood sample is obtained by separately reportable venipuncture. Serum is tested for CA-125 using quantitative electrochemiluminescent immunoassay, for APO A1 using quantitative nephelometry, and for beta-2 microglobulin, transferrin and prealbumin using quantitative immunoturbidimetry.

81504

81504 Oncology (tissue of origin), microarray gene expression profiling of > 2000 genes, utilizing formalin-fixed paraffin-embedded tissue, algorithm reported as tissue similarity scores

Microarray gene expression profiling uses molecular biology to query the expression of thousands of genes simultaneously, allowing for more accurate classification of tumors and better prediction of a patient's clinical outcome. In this test, predefined DNA oligonucleotide probes are covalently attached to a solid surface (such as a glass slide) forming a gene chip. Messenger RNA (mRNA) labeled with fluorophore targets is prepared with the tissue sample and hybridized to the complementary DNA (cDNA) sequences on the gene chip. The gene chip is then scanned to detect the presence and strength of the fluorescent labels at each of the probe-target hybrid spots. The level at any particular spot(s) provides quantitative information regarding the gene expression of that cDNA sequence. Computer programming software can then be used to measure the degree of similarity between the gene expression pattern of the patient's tissue sample and a database of tumor samples and assign a score using an algorithm.

81506

81506 **Endocrinology (type 2 diabetes), biochemical assays of seven analytes (glucose, HbA1c, insulin, hs-CRP, adiponectin, ferritin, interleukin 2-receptor alpha), utilizing serum or plasma, algorithm reporting a risk score**

A blood test is performed to measure glucose, hemoglobin A1c (HbA1c), insulin, high sensitivity C reactive protein (hs-CRP), adoponectin, ferritin and interleukin 2-receptor alpha (IL-2Ralpha). The levels of these seven analytes are assigned a risk score to correlate the probability of a patient developing Type II diabetes within a 5 year period. The risk score assigned may be used to implement an aggressive diabetes prevention regimen. A blood sample is obtained by separately reportable venipuncture. Serum is tested for glucose using quantitative enzymatic assay, for HbA1c using quantitative high performance liquid chromatography/boronate affinity, for insulin using quantitative ultrafiltration/quantitative chemiluminescent immunoassay, for hs-CRP using quantitative immunoturbidimetry, for adiponectin using quantitative enzyme-linked immunosorbent assay, for ferritin using quantitative chemiluminescent immunoassay, and for IL-2Ralpha using enzymatic immunoassay/high performance liquid chromatography.

81507

81507 **Fetal aneuploidy (trisomy 21, 18, and 13) DNA sequence analysis of selected regions using maternal plasma, algorithm reported as a risk score for each trisomy**

Non-invasive detection of fetal aneuploidy (trisomy 21, 18 and 13) can be accomplished by examining fetal DNA (shed from the placenta) circulating in maternal blood (plasma). Sequencing of fetal DNA can be accomplished using a number of techniques including shotgun sequencing, multiplex ligation-dependent probe amplification (MLPA) and digital polymerase chain reaction (digital PCR). The risk score for fetal aneuploidy using DNA analysis is more precise than the risk score devised from maternal age and maternal levels of human chorionic gonadotropin (hCG), unconjugated estriol, alpha-fetoprotein, inhibin A, or pregnancy-associated plasma protein A (PAPP-A), although these tests are often done first and subsequent DNA sequencing is then performed based on that initial score. Non-invasive screening decreases the need for more invasive diagnostic procedures (chorionic villus sampling and amniocentesis) that are associated with greater risk for maternal and fetal complications.

81508-81509

81508 **Fetal congenital abnormalities, biochemical assays of two proteins (PAPP-A, hCG [any form]), utilizing maternal serum, algorithm reported as a risk score**

81509 **Fetal congenital abnormalities, biochemical assays of three proteins (PAPP-A, hCG [any form], DIA), utilizing maternal serum, algorithm reported as a risk score**

A blood test is performed to measure maternal levels of specific proteins in pregnancy to determine the risk for certain chromosomal abnormalities including trisomy 18 and trisomy 21 (Down syndrome). In 81508, two proteins are measured – pregnancy-associated plasma protein (PAPP-A) and human chorionic gonadotropin (hCG). Test results are most sensitive when the sample is drawn between 10 weeks, 3 days and 13 weeks, 6 days of gestation. A blood sample is obtained by separately reportable venipuncture. Serum is tested using quantitative chemiluminescent immunoassay. In 81509, three proteins are measured – pregnancy-associated plasma protein (PAPP-A), human chorionic gonadotropin (hCG) and Inhibin A Dimer (DIA). Test results are most sensitive when the sample is drawn between 15 weeks, 0 days and 22 weeks, 6 days of gestation. A blood sample is obtained by separately reportable venipuncture. Serum is tested using quantitative chemiluminescent immunoassay.

81510-81512

81510 **Fetal congenital abnormalities, biochemical assays of three analytes (AFP, uE3, hCG [any form]), utilizing maternal serum, algorithm reported as a risk score**

81511 **Fetal congenital abnormalities, biochemical assays of four analytes (AFP, uE3, hCG [any form], DIA) utilizing maternal serum, algorithm reported as a risk score (may include additional results from previous biochemical testing)**

81512 **Fetal congenital abnormalities, biochemical assays of five analytes (AFP, uE3, total hCG, hyperglycosylated hCG, DIA) utilizing maternal serum, algorithm reported as a risk score**

A blood test is performed to measure maternal levels certain analytes in pregnancy to determine fetal risk for certain chromosomal abnormalities including trisomy 18, trisomy 21 (Down syndrome), open neural tube defect (ONTD, spinal bifida), pregnancy outcome (failure to carry to term or term gestation), preeclampsia and gestational trophoblastic disease. In 81510, three analytes are measured – alpha fetoprotein (AFP), estriol (uE3) and human chorionic gonadotropin (hCG). In 81511, four analytes are measured – alpha fetoprotein (AFP), estriol (uE3), human chorionic gonadotropin (hCG) and Inhibin A Dimer (DIA). In 81512, five analytes are measured – alpha fetoprotein (AFP), estriol (uE3), total

human chorionic gonadotropin (hCG), hyperglycosylated human chorionic gonadotropin (hCG-H) and Inhibin A Dimer (DIA). Test results are most sensitive when the sample is drawn between 14 weeks, 0 days and 24 weeks, 6 days of gestation. A blood sample is obtained by separately reportable venipuncture. Serum is tested using quantitative chemiluminescent immunoassay/electroluminescence assay.

81525

81525 **Oncology (colon), mRNA, gene expression profiling by real-time RT-PCR of 12 genes (7 content and 5 housekeeping), utilizing formalin-fixed paraffin-embedded tissue, algorithm reported as a recurrence score**

Gene expression profiling may be performed on colon cancer tissue sample(s) obtained from the patient during colonoscopy or surgical resection. Gene expression profiling examines how the coded information contained in a gene or group of genes is translated into cell proteins or mRNA by measuring which genes are turned on (producing mRNA or proteins) or turned off (not producing mRNA or proteins) in the sample. By examining the tumor cells, it is possible to create an algorithm based on the biology of the tumor to predict the likelihood of colon cancer recurrence and the benefits of adjunct treatment following surgery in patients with Stage II colon cancer. Formalin-fixed paraffin-embedded tumor tissue is tested for 12 genes (7 genes known to be related to colon cancer and 5 reference genes) using real-time polymerase chain reaction (RT-PCR) and the results are analyzed using a computer software program to produce an algorithm risk score for possible recurrence of colon cancer.

81528

81528 **Oncology (colorectal) screening, quantitative real-time target and signal amplification of 10 DNA markers (KRAS mutations, promoter methylation of NDRG4 and BMP3) and fecal hemoglobin, utilizing stool, algorithm reported as a positive or negative result**

A laboratory test is performed on a stool specimen to screen for colorectal cancer using quantitative real-time target and signal amplification of DNA markers and fecal hemoglobin. This screening tool is designed for asymptomatic patients between ages 50-85 who are at average risk for developing colorectal cancer. Colorectal epithelial cells containing DNA markers line the lumen of the bowel and are constantly shed in feces. By collecting a stool sample and selectively amplifying and enriching DNA target cells (KRAS, NDRG4, BMP3) and fecal hemoglobin, it is possible to identify molecular markers (altered DNA) shed by premalignant polyps and/or colorectal neoplasms. A stool sample is obtained by separately reportable procedure and tested for 10 DNA markers including KRAS mutations, promoter methylation of NDRG4 and BMP3, and fecal hemoglobin using a computer software program to generate a positive or negative algorithm result.

81535-81536

81535 **Oncology (gynecologic), live tumor cell culture and chemotherapeutic response by DAPI stain and morphology, predictive algorithm reported as a drug response score; first single drug or drug combination**

81536 **Oncology (gynecologic), live tumor cell culture and chemotherapeutic response by DAPI stain and morphology, predictive algorithm reported as a drug response score; each additional single drug or drug combination (List separately in addition to code for primary procedure)**

A laboratory test is performed on live gynecologic tumor cells to measure the response of chemotherapeutic agents on the cells using DAPI stain and morphology. These chemo-resistive and/or chemo-selective drug assays may be used to select or deselect the most appropriate chemotherapeutic regimens based on the unique morphological makeup of the tumor. Live cells are isolated from the tumor and established in an in vitro medium. The cells are incubated with chemotherapeutic agents for a prescribed period of time and then stained with DAPI (4', 6-diamidino-2-phenylindole) fluorescent stain. DAPI binds strongly to A-T rich segments of DNA and will stain dead cells more effectively than living cells, allowing the cells to be assessed for survival following exposure to tumor toxic drugs. A single drug or a combination of drugs may be tested and the predictive algorithm is reported as a drug response score. Code 81535 includes the first single drug or drug combination tested. Code 81536 is an adjunct code used with 81535 for each additional single drug or drug combination tested.

81539

● **81539** **Oncology (high-grade prostate cancer), biochemical assay of four proteins (Total PSA, Free PSA, Intact PSA, and human kallikrein-2 [hK2]), utilizing plasma or serum, prognostic algorithm reported as a probability score**

Total PSA (tPSA), Free PSA (fPSA), Intact PSA (iPSA) and human kallikrein-2 (hK2) in plasma or serum are assayed. Prostate specific antigen (PSA) is a glycoprotein enzyme belonging to the kallikrein family and secreted in the prostate gland by epithelial cells. Elevated PSA levels in plasma/serum may indicate benign prostatic hypertrophy, prostatitis, and possible malignancy. Human kallidrein-2 (hK2) is also secreted in the prostate gland by epithelial cells and elevated levels are more likely to be associated with malignant prostate tumors which may be aggressive and metastasize quickly, or never progress or cause no harm. A blood sample is obtained by separately reportable venipuncture. Serum/plasma is tested using electrochemiluminescence immunoassay. The results of the blood test are combined in an algorithm using the patient's age, absence or presence of prostate nodules on digital rectal exam (DRE), and prior negative biopsy results to generate a risk score for the probability of high grade prostate cancer (a Gleason score of ≥ 7) being found on biopsy. The probability score that is reported can assist the physician and patient in the decision to proceed with a prostate biopsy. This test is contraindicated in patients with a previous diagnosis of prostate cancer, DRE within 4 days, 5-alpha reductase inhibitor therapy, or treatment for symptomatic benign prostatic hypertrophy within 6 months.

81595

81595   Cardiology (heart transplant), mRNA, gene expression profiling by real-time quantitative PCR of 20 genes (11 content and 9 housekeeping), utilizing subfraction of peripheral blood, algorithm reported as a rejection risk score

Gene expression profiling may be performed on a peripheral blood sample to detect acute heart transplant rejection or the development of graft dysfunction. This test may be used as an adjunct to endomyocardial biopsy to adjust immunosuppressant drug dosage based on graft function and grade of acute cellular rejection. Gene expression profiling examines how the coded information contained in a gene or group of genes is translated into cell proteins or mRNA by measuring which genes are turned on (producing mRNA or proteins) or turned off (not producing mRNA or proteins) in the sample. A blood sample is obtained by separately reportable procedure and tested for 20 genes (11 genes known to relate to transplant rejection and 9 control genes) using real-time quantitative polymerase chain reaction (RT-PCR). The results are analyzed using a computer software program to produce an algorithm of the contribution of each gene in the panel and report it as a single rejection risk score number.

82009-82010

82009   Ketone body(s) (eg, acetone, acetoacetic acid, beta-hydroxybutyrate); qualitative

82010   Ketone body(s) (eg, acetone, acetoacetic acid, beta-hydroxybutyrate); quantitative

A blood test is performed for acetone, acetoacetic acid, beta-hydroxybutyrate or other ketone bodies. The qualitative test (82009) evaluates blood serum for the presence or absence of ketone bodies. A visual test is performed. Because visual tests show a spectrum of low to high levels which are based on color changes they are sometimes also referred to as semi-quantitative tests. The presence of ketone bodies in the blood are indicative of decreased carbohydrate utilization which is found in patients with diabetes mellitus; malnutrition, anorexia or other inadequate calorie intake; vomiting; and glycogen storage disease. The quantitative test (82010) measures the level of ketone bodies in blood serum. Quantitative testing is used to evaluate and manage diseases such as diabetic and alcoholic ketoacidosis either emergently or as a routine test. A blood sample is obtained by separately reportable venipuncture. Blood serum is then tested using gas chromatography.

82013

82013   Acetylcholinesterase

A blood test is performed to measure acetylcholinesterase levels. Acetylcholinesterase is an enzyme found in red blood cells. Elevated levels can result from organophosphate pesticide exposure. The test may be performed as routine screening or when exposure is suspected due to signs/symptoms. Levels may continue to be monitored to determine effectiveness or failure of treatment. A blood sample is obtained by separately reportable venipuncture. Whole blood is then tested using photometric analysis.

82016-82017

82016   Acylcarnitines; qualitative, each specimen

82017   Acylcarnitines; quantitative, each specimen

A blood test is for acylcarnitine. The qualitative test (82016) identifies the presence of absence of acylcarnitine in the blood. It is done routinely on infants as part of newborn screening to diagnose fatty acid beta-oxidation and organic aciduria disorders and may be performed at any age when symptoms of these disorders are present. A blood sample is obtained by separately reportable venipuncture or capillary draw. Plasma or whole blood is then tested using low injection analysis-tandem mass spectrometry. Report 82016 for each separate specimen obtained. The quantitative test (82017) is performed to measure acylcarnitines levels in the blood. The quantitative test is most often performed as follow up to a positive newborn screening qualitative test on whole blood or a positive plasma test on older patients. The quantitative test will be specified as Elevated Isolated C4 Acylcarnitine, Elevated Isolated C5 Acylcarnitine, or Elevations of C8, C6, C10 Acylcarnitine. A blood sample is obtained by separately reportable venipuncture or capillary draw. Plasma is then tested using Low Injection Analysis-Tandem Mass Spectrometry. Report 82017 for each separate specimen obtained.

82024

82024   Adrenocorticotropic hormone (ACTH)

A blood test is performed to measure adrenocorticotropic hormone (ACTH) levels. Adrenocortiotropic hormone (ACTH), also known as corticotropin is a polypeptide tropic hormone secreted from the anterior pituitary gland in response to biological stress. As part of the hypothalamic-pituitary-adrenal complex, it is responsible for increased production and release of corticosteroids including cortisol from the adrenal cortex. A blood sample is obtained by separately reportable venipuncture. The plasma is frozen and then tested using quantitative chemiluminescent immunoassay. Some synthetic ACTH preparations cannot be detected by this method.

82030

82030   Adenosine, 5-monophosphate, cyclic (cyclic AMP)

Blood or urine testing may be done to measure Adenosine, 5-monophosphate, cyclic (cyclic AMP) levels. Adenosine, 5-monophosphate is a nucleotide found on RNA as an ester of phosphoric acid and the nucleotide adenosine. Cyclic AMP (cAMP) is responsible for intracellular signaling and is created by the enzyme adenylate cyclase from ATP with regulation by the hormones adrenaline and glucagon. This test is most often used as a differential diagnosis for hypercalcemia and may also be used as an adjunctive test for parathyroid resistance. A blood sample is obtained by separately reportable venipuncture. The plasma is frozen and then tested using radioimmunoassay. The urine sample may be a 24 hour collection preserved with 10 ml 6M HCL or an unpreserved random sample (minimum 5 ml) with a notation of the total volume voided and the time interval. Urine may be tested using radioimmunoassay or high pressure liquid chromotography.

82040

82040   Albumin; serum, plasma or whole blood

A blood test is performed to measure albumin levels in serum, plasma, or whole blood. Albumin is a plasma protein responsible for regulating the colloidal osmotic pressure of blood. It is capable of binding water, electrolytes (sodium, potassium, calcium), fatty acids, hormones, bilirubin, and drugs/medications. Albumin levels are used to assess nutritional status. A blood sample is obtained by separately reportable venipuncture. The plasma, serum or whole blood is tested using spectrophotometry or quantitative nephelometry.

82042

82042   Albumin; urine or other source, quantitative, each specimen

A test on urine or other body fluids (except serum or cerebral spinal fluid) is performed to measure albumin levels. Albumin is a plasma protein responsible for regulating the colloidal osmotic pressure of blood. It is capable of binding water, electrolytes (sodium, potassium, calcium), fatty acids, hormones, bilirubin and drugs/medications. Albumin levels are used to assess nutritional status and renal functioning. A sample of urine or other body fluid is obtained and tested using quantitative nephelometry or spectrophotometry.

82043-82044

82043   Albumin; urine, microalbumin, quantitative

82044   Albumin; urine, microalbumin, semiquantitative (eg, reagent strip assay)

A test on urine is used to measure microalbumin levels and is routinely performed annually on diabetic patients with stable blood glucose levels to assess for early onset nephropathy. The quantitative test (82043), which measures the level of microalbumen in the urine, may be performed on a random urine sample, with a notation of total volume and voiding time or a 24 hour urine sample using immunoturbidimetric technique. The semi-quantitative test (82044) involves a chemical dipstick placed into the urine sample which reacts and changes color when albumin is present. This technique is called enzymatic colorimetric assay.

82045

82045   Albumin; ischemia modified

A blood test is performed to measure ischemia modified albumin levels. Ischemic albumin is a sensitivity marker for myocardial damage following a myocardial infarction or other ischemic cardiac event. A sample of blood is obtained by separately reportable procedure, such as venipuncture or percutaneous coronary intervention. Serum is tested using Albumin Cobalt Binding Test.

82055-82075

82075   Alcohol (ethanol), breath

Ethanol is a central nervous system depressant. Levels are obtained to document prior consumption or administration of the substance. In 82055, a blood or urine test is performed to measure alcohol (ethanol) levels. A sample of blood is obtained by separately reportable venipuncture and examined using gas liquid chromatography or enzymatic technique. Urine samples are tested using alcohol dehydrogenase or gas chromatography-flame ionization detection. In 82075, a breath test is performed to measure exhaled alcohol (ethanol) levels. Because ethanol is not digested after absorption from the gastrointestinal tract or chemically changed in the circulating blood, the concentration of alcohol in alveoli (lung) air can be correlated to blood alcohol content (BAC). The method for measuring alveoli alcohol can be chemical, infrared spectroscopy or fuel cell.

82085

82085   Aldolase

A blood test is performed to measure aldolase levels. Aldolase is an enzyme found predominately in muscle cells and is responsible for assisting in the conversion of glucose into usable energy. Blood levels may be monitored in patients with muscular dystrophy or other rare skeletal muscle conditions. Elevated levels are an indicator that muscle or liver damage has occurred. A sample of blood is obtained by separately reportable venipuncture. Serum is tested using enzymatic technique.

82088

82088   Aldosterone

A blood or urine test is performed to measure aldosterone levels. Aldosterone is a hormone produced in the adrenal cortex that controls blood volume and pressure by regulating sodium and potassium concentration in the blood. The production of aldosterone is regulated by renin and angiotension and separately reportable lab tests on these two proteins are often performed when testing for aldosterone levels. A sample of blood is obtained by separately reportable venipuncture, preferably between 10 am and noon, with the patient supine for 2 hours or upright for 2 hours. Serum is tested using radioimmunoassay. A 24 hour urine collection is obtained and a 10 ml sample is submitted for testing, noting the total volume voided and the collection time. Total volume is measured in a separately reportable procedure Urine is tested using radioimmunoassay.

82103-82104

82103   Alpha-1-antitrypsin; total
82104   Alpha-1-antitrypsin; phenotype

A blood test is performed to measure Alpha-1-antitrypsin (A1A) levels. Alpha-1-antitrypsin is a protein produced in the liver and released into the bloodstream. Alpha-1-antitrypsin is a serum protease inhibitor. Proteolytic enzymes from plasma are released onto the surface and into the tissue of body organs. The enzymes damage the organs in the absence of protease inhibitors like alpha-1-antitrypsin. The absence of alpha-1-antitrypsin is usually genetic. Alpha-1-antitrypsin is particularly important in protecting the lungs from elastase and testing is performed to help diagnose the cause of early onset emphysema. Levels may also be evaluated in patients with persistent jaundice or other symptoms of liver dysfunction. In 82103, total alpha-1-antitrypsin levels are measured. A sample of blood is obtained by separately reportable venipuncture. Serum is tested using immunoturbidimetric technique. In 82104, phenotype testing is performed. This test is typically performed when total alpha-1-antitrypsin levels are lower than normal. This test looks at the both the amount of type of alpha-1-antitrypsin in the blood and compares it with normal patterns. Identifying the homozygous and heterozygous phenotype of an Alpha-1-antitrypsin (A1A) deficiency aids in the treatment of the disease which usually manifests in infancy or childhood. A sample of blood is obtained by separately reportable venipuncture. Serum is tested using isoelectric focusing.

82105-82106

82105   Alpha-fetoprotein (AFP); serum
82106   Alpha-fetoprotein (AFP); amniotic fluid

Alpha-fetoprotein (AFP) is measured in serum (82105) or amniotic fluid (82106) during pregnancy to screen for neural tube defects such as spina bifida and anencephaly, chromosomal abnormalities such as Down syndrome (trisomy 21) or Edwards syndrome (trisomy 18), and omphalocele. AFP is a protein produced by the yolk sac of the fetus in early gestation and then later by the liver and gastrointestinal tract of the fetus. In 82105, a blood sample is obtained by separately reportable venipuncture between 14 and 22 weeks gestation. The blood (serum) test screens for high and low levels of AFP. High levels are associated with neural tube defects while low levels are associated with chromosomal abnormalities. In 82106, separately reportable amniocentesis is performed and an amniotic fluid sample is first obtained. The level of AFP in the amniotic fluid is then tested.

82107

82107   Alpha-fetoprotein (AFP); AFP-L3 fraction isoform and total AFP (including ratio)

This test measures the amount of L3 fraction isoform of alpha-fetoprotein (AFP) along with the total AFP and gives the results in a ratio. AFP-L3 has been shown to be a tumor marker for aggressive progression of hepatocellular carcinoma. AFP can be fractionated into three different glycoforms based on reactivity with a certain lectin. L3 reacts by binding strongly to the lectin. Liver cancer cells that express AFP-L3 glycoforms have a tendency to grow rapidly with early vascular invasion and metastasis. AFP-L3 is isolated by a liquid phase binding immunoassay and then quantified using chemical luminescence. Since the relationship of the total AFP to its L3 isoform is the clinically important determination, both are measured and the results are presented as a ratio of the amount of lectin reactive

AFP to total AFP, or the AFP-L3%. This is the standard measurement for quantifying the L3 isoform of AFP in the serum of high risk chronic liver disease patients. AFP-L3% ratios higher than 10% are indicative of early hepatocellular carcinoma.

82108

82108   Aluminum

A blood test is performed to measure aluminum levels. Aluminum is a member of the boron group of chemical elements and may be ingested orally in foods, nutritional supplements and medications. Symptoms of toxicity can include: encephalopathy, osteomalacia, aplastic bone disease, cardiac changes or arrhythmias and microcytic anemia. A blood sample is obtained by a separately reportable venipuncture. Blood serum is then tested using quantitative inductively coupled plasma mass spectrometry.

82120

82120   Amines, vaginal fluid, qualitative

A qualitative analysis of vaginal fluid amines is performed to test for bacterial vaginosis. The patient presents with complaints of vaginal discharge and odor. A swab of vaginal fluid is obtained and placed on the test media. A rapid colorimetric test using layered thin film technology is performed. The test detects the presence or absence of alkali volatilizable amines in vaginal fluid. The physician uses the test results in conjunction with clinical evaluation to diagnose or rule-out bacterial vaginosis as the cause of the vaginal discharge and odor.

82127-82128

82127   Amino acids; single, qualitative, each specimen
82128   Amino acids; multiple, qualitative, each specimen

A laboratory test is performed to identify the presence of a single amino acid (82127) or multiple amino acids (82128) in the blood or urine of an individual with a suspected inborn error of metabolism. Amino acids are the building blocks of proteins and an intermediate in metabolism, possessing a vast chemical versatility to catalyze reactions and control cellular activity. The clinical presentation of metabolic error disorders usually manifests in infancy or early childhood and depends on the specific amino acid involved. Common symptoms can include feeding problems, poor growth or failure to thrive, seizures, muscle weakness, renal or liver failure, developmental delays, and cognitive deficits. A blood sample is obtained by separately reportable venipuncture. A urine sample is obtained by voided specimen or catheterization. Serum/plasma and urine are tested using liquid chromatography-tandem mass spectrometry. A blood or urine sample is tested for a single amino acid. Code 82128 if the sample is tested for multiple amino acids. Code 82131 if the test measures the amount of an amino acid in the bloodstream.

82131

82131   Amino acids; single, quantitative, each specimen

A laboratory test is performed to measure the quantitative level of a single amino acid in the blood or urine of an individual with a suspected inborn error of metabolism. Amino acids are the building blocks of proteins and an intermediate in metabolism, possessing a vast chemical versatility to catalyze reactions and control cellular activity. The clinical presentation of metabolic error disorders usually manifests in infancy or early childhood and depends on the specific amino acid involved. Common symptoms can include feeding problems, poor growth or failure to thrive, seizures, muscle weakness, renal or liver failure, developmental delays, and cognitive deficits. Quantitative amino acid testing can be used to monitor treatment and dietary compliance in patients with phenylketonuria (PKU), a disorder of phenylalanine metabolism; cystinuria, a disorder of cystine metabolism which causes stones to form in the kidney and bladder; and Hartnup disease, a genetic disorder that inhibits the protein tryptophan from being absorbed by the intestines and then reabsorbed in the kidneys. A blood sample is obtained by separately reportable venipuncture. A urine sample is obtained by voided specimen or catheterization. Serum/plasma and urine are tested using quantitative liquid chromatography-tandem mass spectrometry.

82135

82135   Aminolevulinic acid, delta (ALA)

A urine test is performed to measure aminolevulinic acid, delta (ALA) levels. ALA is a compound found in the porphyrin synthesis pathway necessary for blood cell production. Elevated levels may indicate acute porphyria or hereditary tyrosinemia. ALA may be used as a photosensitizer for photodynamic therapy and to diagnose certain cancers. Alcohol ingestion must be avoided for 24 hours prior to the test. ALA levels can be abnormally elevated by alcohol, lead and other compounds. A random urine sample or 24-hour urine collection sample is obtained. Urine is then tested using quantitative ion exchange chromatography/spectrophotometry.

Pathology and Laboratory

82136-82139

82136 Amino acids, 2 to 5 amino acids, quantitative, each specimen
82139 Amino acids, 6 or more amino acids, quantitative, each specimen

A blood, urine or cerebral spinal fluid (CSF) sample is obtained to measure amino acid levels. Amino acids (AA) are molecules which contain an amine group, a carboxylic acid group and a side chain that varies to differentiate each molecule. Amino acids are the building blocks of protein (linear chains of amino acids) and are critical to metabolism and sustaining life. Symptoms that may indicate a problem with amino acid levels include: failure to thrive, persistent vomiting, neurological deterioration, hyperammonemia, extreme lethargy and metabolic acidosis. Medical conditions which warrant amino acid analysis include acute life threatening episodes and inborn errors of metabolism. The blood, urine or CSF specimen is then tested using ion exchange chromatography. A quantitative analysis measures the amount, level, or concentration of each specific amino acid being tested. The specific amino acids tested for are dependent on the condition being evaluated. For example, a cystinuria panel measures four amino acids, arginine, cystine, lysine, and ornithine. Use 82136 for quantitative analysis of 2-5 amino acids. Use 82139 for quantitative analysis of 6 or more amino acids. These codes are reported for each separate specimen tested.

82140

82140 Ammonia

A blood test is performed to measure ammonia levels. Ammonia is a by product of protein metabolism and is normally converted to urea by the liver and excreted via the kidney. Elevated ammonia levels may result from cirrhosis or hepatitis. Symptoms of elevated ammonia levels are confusion, tremors, excessive sleepiness or coma. Testing may be performed in disease states such as Reyes syndrome or liver failure. A blood sample is obtained by a separately reportable venipuncture or arterial access line. The specimen is then tested using colorimetry.

82143

82143 Amniotic fluid scan (spectrophotometric)

An amniotic fluid scan is performed using spectrophotometric methodology to test bilirubin levels. This test is performed to evaluate for suspected maternal-fetal blood incompatibility or hemolytic disease of the fetus. A separately reportable amniocentesis is performed to collect the amniotic fluid sample. A spectrophotometer is used to measure the intensity of light of a definite wavelength that is transmitted by a certain substance to provide a quantitative measure of the amount of that substance present in the solution. In this case, the amount of bilirubin in the amniotic fluid is measured.

82150

82150 Amylase

Laboratory testing for amylase may be performed on blood, urine and other body fluids. Amylase is an enzyme responsible for the break down of starches into sugar molecules (disaccharides and trisaccharides) and eventually to glucose for energy use by the cells. Amylase is produced in saliva and the pancreas. Abnormal amylase levels may result from pancreatic inflammation or trauma, perforated peptic ulcer, ovarian cyst (torsion), strangulation ileus, macroamylasemia, mumps viral infection and cystic fibrosis. A blood or body fluid sample is obtained. The sample is then tested using quantitative enzymatic methodology.

82154

82154 Androstanediol glucuronide

A blood test is performed to measure androstanediol glucuronide levels. Androstanediol glucuronide is a hormone produced by the liver, prostate and skin. It is a marker for peripheral androgen metabolism and action. Abnormal levels may be found in women with idiopathic hirsutism. A blood sample is obtained by separately reportable venipunture. The sample is then tested using quantitative radioimmunoassay (RIA) after hydrolysis of glucuronide and chromatography.

82157

82157 Androstenedione

A blood test is performed to measure androstenedione levels. Androstenedione is a steroid hormone produced by the adrenal gland. It is a precursor to the androgen hormone (testosterone) in males and estrogen hormones (esterone/estradiol) in females. The test is indicated for women with virilizing syndromes (females with male characteristics) and for suspected anabolic steroid abuse. A blood sample is obtained by separately reportable venipuncture. The sample is then tested using quantitative high performance liquid chromatography-tandem mass spectrometry.

82160

82160 Androsterone

A laboratory test is performed to monitor androsterone levels. Androsterone is an endogenous steroid hormone with weak androgen effects that helps to modulate GABA receptors and also has anticonvulsive properties. Androsterone may be elevated in patients with Cushing's syndrome. The patient should refrain from taking ACTH, steroids, and gonadotropins 48 hours prior to the test. A blood sample is obtained by separately reportable venipuncture. Serum/plasma is tested using radioimmunoassay.

82163

82163 Angiotensin II

A blood test is performed to measure angiotensin II. Angiotensin II is converted from angiotensin I by angiotensin I-converting enzyme (ACE). Angiotensin II functions as an endocrine, autocrine/paracrine and intracrine hormone, primarily acting on smooth muscle to raise blood pressure. A blood sample is obtained by separately reportable venipuncture. The plasma is then tested using immunoassay.

82164

82164 Angiotensin I - converting enzyme (ACE)

A blood test is performed to measure angiotensin I-converting enzyme (ACE). ACE is an enzyme produced by endothelial cells throughout the body (but especially in the capillary beds of the lungs) and may also be secreted by granulomas (immune/inflammatory tumor like masses). The test is indicated to diagnose and monitor sarcoidosis. A blood sample is obtained by separately reportable venipuncture. The serum is then tested using quantitative enzymatic methodology. Cerebral spinal fluid (CSF) may also be tested for ACE levels. A sample of CSF is obtained by separately reportable lumbar puncture (spinal tap). The sample is then tested using quantitative spectrophotometry.

82172

82172 Apolipoprotein, each

A blood test is performed to measure apolipoproteins. Apolipoproteins are made up of a protein molecule bound (encased) by a lipid. This allows the protein to circulate through the lymphatic and vascular systems without being altered. Apolipoprotein-A is found in high density liproproteins and Apolipoprotein-B is found in low density lipoproteins. They are synthesized in the liver and intestine. When expressed as a ratio, apolipoproteins estimate the relative risk for coronary artery disease (CAD). A fasting blood sample is obtained by separately reportable venipuncture. The sample is then tested using quantitative nephelometry. A ratio can then be determined by calculation. Report 82172 for qualitative analysis of each apolipoprotein (A and B) if both values are obtained.

82175

82175 Arsenic

Laboratory testing for arsenic may be performed on blood, urine, other body fluids, hair or nails. Arsenic is found in the environment and arsenic levels may be altered by the ingestion of shellfish or iodine containing medications and dietary or nutritional supplements. A blood sample is obtained by separately reportable venipunture. The sample is then tested for recent exposure by quantitative inductively coupled plasma-mass spectrometry. Alternatively, a urine, hair or nails may be tested for chronic exposure using quantitative high pressure liquid chromatography/quantitative inductively coupled plasma-mass spectrometry. Other body fluids are also tested by quantitative high pressure liquid chromatography/quantitative inductively coupled plasma-mass spectrometry.

82180

82180 Ascorbic acid (Vitamin C), blood

A blood test is performed to measure ascorbic acid (Vitamin C) levels. Ascorbic acid is a naturally occurring organic compound containing antioxidant properties. Absent or low levels of this nutrient may cause the disease scurvy. A blood test may be ordered to determine a deficiency of ascorbic acid in the body. A blood sample is obtained by separately reportable venipuncture. The sample is then tested using quantitative spectrophotometry.

82190

82190 Atomic absorption spectroscopy, each analyte

A laboratory test is performed using atomic absorption spectroscopy to measure the concentration of certain metals and metalloids in body fluid and tissue. Atomic absorption spectroscopy (ASS) uses the absorption of light (optical radiation) to measure free atoms in their gaseous state. Quantitative analysis using ASS can be used to determine exposure to chemical compounds that may be toxic to the human body. Whole blood, plasma, urine, saliva, semen, brain tissue, liver tissue, and muscle tissue may all undergo ASS for clinical testing.

Pathology and Laboratory

● New Code ▲ Revised Code

82232

82232   Beta-2 microglobulin

A laboratory test is performed to measure beta-2 microglobulin (B2M) levels. B2M is a small protein molecule found on the surface of cells, including B lymphocytes and tumor cells. The protein sheds into the blood and may also be found in urine and cerebral spinal fluid. B2M is not considered a differential test but does provide additional clinical information regarding disease progression. B2M testing may be ordered on patients with a diagnosis of multiple myeloma, lymphoma, multiple sclerosis, liver and kidney disease, chronic inflammatory disorders, HIV/AIDS, and CMV infections. A blood sample is obtained by separately reportable venipuncture. A cerebral spinal fluid (CSF) sample is obtained by separately reportable lumbar puncture. A urine sample is obtained by voided specimen or catheterization. The first urine specimen should be discarded, the patient given water to drink, and a second urine sample obtained within 1 hour for analysis. Serum/plasma and CSF are tested using quantitative immunoturbidimetry. Urine is tested using quantitative chemiluminescent immunoassay.

82239

82239   Bile acids; total

A laboratory test is performed to measure total bile acids. Bile acids are found in bile, a complex fluid that also contains water, electrolytes, cholesterol, phospholipids, and bilirubin. Bile acids are critical for digestion and absorption of fats and fat soluble vitamins. They also function as a hormone in the breakdown and synthesis of cholesterol. Serum levels of total bile acids will be elevated in liver disease including chronic and inactive hepatitis. A blood sample is obtained by separately reportable venipuncture. The patient should be fasting for at least 8 hours prior to the blood draw. Serum/plasma is tested using quantitative enzymatic method.

82240

82240   Bile acids; cholylglycine

A laboratory test is performed to measure bile acids, cholylglycine. Bile acids are found in bile, a complex fluid that also contains water, electrolytes, cholesterol, phospholipids, and bilirubin. Cholylglycine is a crystalline bile acid conjugated from cholic acid and glycine, and functions as a fat emulsifier. Elevated cholylglycine levels are a sensitive indicator of cholestasis and hepatic disease.

82247-82248

82247   Bilirubin; total
82248   Bilirubin; direct

A laboratory test is performed to measure total or direct bilirubin. Bilirubin is a pigmented waste product normally produced when red blood cells (RBCs) break down. Non-water soluble (unconjugated) bilirubin is carried on albumin to the liver where it attaches to sugar molecules to become conjugated. Conjugated (direct) bilirubin is water soluble and able to pass from the liver to the small intestine. Further breakdown of bilirubin occurs in the small intestine and it is eventually eliminated in the feces in the form of sterobilin. Total bilirubin is the sum of conjugated (direct) and unconjugated bilirubin. A test for either conjugated or direct bilirubin (82248) or total bilirubin (82247) may be ordered to diagnose and monitor liver disorders, hemolytic anemia, and newborn (physiologic) jaundice. A blood sample is obtained by separately reportable venipuncture or heel stick. Other body fluids, including cerebral spinal fluid, may be collected and tested for total bilirubin. Serum/plasma is tested using quantitative spectrophotometry.

82252

82252   Bilirubin; feces, qualitative

A laboratory test is performed to detect the presence of bilirubin in feces. Bilirubin is a pigmented waste product normally produced when red blood cells (RBCs) break down. Non-water soluble (unconjugated) bilirubin is carried on albumin to the liver where it attaches to sugar molecules to become conjugated. Conjugated (direct) bilirubin is water soluble and able to pass from the liver to the small intestine. Further breakdown of bilirubin occurs in the small intestine, and it is eventually eliminated in the feces in the form of sterobilin. A test for fecal bilirubin (sterobilin) may be ordered to diagnose and monitor liver disorders, including bile duct obstruction.

82261

82261   Biotinidase, each specimen

A laboratory test is performed to screen for biotinidase deficiency. Biotinidase is an enzyme found in the liver, kidney, and blood serum that cleaves biotin from biocytin. Biotin is a vitamin essential to fat, protein, and carbohydrate metabolism. Biotinidase deficiency is an inherited genetic disorder that prevents the body from reusing/recycling biotin. Symptoms usually present in infancy or early childhood and can include seizures, muscle weakness, decreased muscle tone (hyptotonia), developmental delays and respiratory problems. A blood sample is obtained by separately reportable venipuncture or heel stick. Serum/

plasma is tested using spectrophotometry. The patient sample should be paired with a control sample taken from a normal, healthy, non-biologically related individual.

82270-82272

82270   Blood, occult, by peroxidase activity (eg, guaiac), qualitative; feces, consecutive collected specimens with single determination, for colorectal neoplasm screening (ie, patient was provided 3 cards or single triple card for consecutive collection)
82271   Blood, occult, by peroxidase activity (eg, guaiac), qualitative; other sources
82272   Blood, occult, by peroxidase activity (eg, guaiac), qualitative, feces, 1-3 simultaneous determinations, performed for other than colorectal neoplasm screening

A fecal (stool) sample is obtained for colorectal neoplasm screening and tested for the presence of occult (hidden) blood by peroxidase activity. This test is also referred to as a fecal occult blood test (FOBT). Occult blood in a stool specimen is present in amounts too small to see with the naked eye, but becomes visible when chemical tests are performed. Guaiac is one type of chemical (reagent) test that can be performed to identify the presence of blood in the stool. If the test is performed in an office or hospital, the physician may obtain the sample during a rectal exam. If the test is performed at home, the patient is provided with a stool collection kit consisting of three cards or a single triple card. The patient obtains three consecutive stool specimens per the kit instructions. The stool specimens are then returned to the physician office or mailed to a laboratory. All three specimens are then tested using a chemical reagent for the presence of occult blood. A few drops of the chemical reagent are applied to each stool specimen. If blood is present, a color change will be detected on the card. Use 82271 for testing of samples other than stool. Use 82272 for testing of stool samples for a reason other than colorectal neoplasm screening.

82274

82274   Blood, occult, by fecal hemoglobin determination by immunoassay, qualitative, feces, 1-3 simultaneous determinations

A laboratory test is performed on fecal samples to determine the presence of occult blood using immunoassay method. This method isolates human hemoglobin by using goat antibodies to create an antigen-antibody reaction. Occult blood testing with immunoassay has a decreased rate of false positive/negative reactions to human foods and non-hemorrhagic fecal constituents which improves the detection of lower gastrointestinal bleeding. This test may be used to diagnose and monitor the presence of occult blood in the feces of patients with colon cancer and inflammatory bowel disease.

82286

82286   Bradykinin

A laboratory test is performed to measure bradykinin. Bradykinin (BK) is a peptide molecule that causes vasodilation, contraction of non-vascular smooth muscle in the bronchus and gut, increases vascular permeability, and synthesizes prostaglandins. Bradykinin is broken down by angiotensin-converting enzyme (ACE), aminopeptide P (APP) and carboxypeptidase N (CPN). Elevated levels of bradykinin may be present with hereditary angioedema and in patients who have tissue injury, chronic pain, or inflammatory disorders. A blood sample is obtained by separately reportable venipuncture. Serum/plasma is tested using enzyme-linked immunosorbent assay (ELISA).

82300

82300   Cadmium

A laboratory test is performed to measure cadmium. Cadmium is a transitional metal often encountered in the mining, smelting, and refining industries. Cadmium exposure can occur with inhalation of particles from the workplace or by smoking cigarettes. It can also be ingested in food crops grown in contaminated soil or water, or absorbed through the skin from jewelry containing high levels of the metal. Symptoms of cadmium exposure may include proteinuria, fever, headache, dyspnea, chest pain, sore throat, cough, conjunctivitis, and rhinitis. Cadmium toxicity can present with vomiting, diarrhea, abdominal pain and cramping. A blood sample is obtained by separately reportable venipuncture. A urine sample is obtained by voided specimen or catheterization (random or 24-hour timed collection). Blood and urine are tested using quantitative inductively coupled plasma-mass spectrometry.

82306

82306   Vitamin D; 25 hydroxy, includes fraction(s), if performed

Blood levels of 25-hydroxyvitamin D are used to primarily to determine whether a deficiency of Vitamin D or abnormal metabolism of calcium is the cause of bone weakness or malformation. Vitamin D is a fat soluble vitamin that is absorbed from the intestine like fat, and 25-hydroxyvitamin D levels are also evaluated in individuals with conditions or diseases that interfere with fat absorption, such as cystic fibrosis, Crohn's disease, or in patients who have undergone gastric bypass surgery. A blood sample is obtained. Levels of 25-hydroxyvitamin D3 and 25-hydroxyvitamin D2 are evaluated using chemiluminescent

Pathology and Laboratory

immunoassay. The test results may be the sum of Vitamin D3 and D2 or the results may include fractions of D3 and D2 as well as the sum of these values.

82308

82308   Calcitonin

A laboratory test is performed to measure calcitonin. Calcitonin, also known as thyrocalcitonin, is a hormone produced by the parafollicular cells (C-cells) in the thyroid gland. Calcitonin regulates blood calcium levels, and inhibits bone breakdown as well as tubular reabsorption of calcium and phosphorus in the kidney. The test may be ordered to diagnose and monitor medullary thyroid carcinoma (MTC), leukemia, and myeloproliferative disorders. It is also used to screen individuals at risk for multiple endocrine neoplasia type 2 (MEN2). A blood sample is obtained by separately reportable venipuncture. Serum/plasma is tested using quantitative chemiluminescent immunoassay.

82310

82310   Calcium; total

A blood sample is taken to measure the amount of total calcium. Calcium is one of the most important minerals in the body. About 99 percent of the calcium found the body is stored in the bones. The remaining one percent circulates in the blood. Calcium may be ionized (free) or attached (bound) to proteins. Free calcium is the calcium metabolically active in the body. Bound calcium is inactive. Total calcium is a measurement of the total amount of both free calcium and bound calcium circulating in the blood. Total calcium is measured to screen for or monitor a number of conditions, including those affecting the bones, heart, nerves, kidneys and teeth. Total calcium is measured using spectrophotometry.

82330

82330   Calcium; ionized

A blood sample is taken to measure the amount of ionized or free calcium. Ionized or free calcium is calcium that flows freely in the blood and is not attached to any proteins. Ionized calcium is metabolically active and available to support and regulate heart function, muscle contraction, central nervous system function, and blood clotting. Ionized calcium measurements may be obtained prior to major surgery, in critically ill patients, or when protein levels are abnormal. Ionized calcium is measured by ion selective electrode (ISE) or pH electrode methodology.

82331

82331   Calcium; after calcium infusion test

A laboratory test is performed to measure calcium blood levels following a calcium infusion test. Calcium is a mineral essential to bone health, heart function, muscle contraction, nerve signaling, and blood clotting. Most of the body's calcium is found in the bones. A very small percentage (1%) circulates in the blood with half that amount metabolically active, and the rest bound to albumin or complexed with phosphate. A calcium infusion test may be ordered for suspected gastrinoma or insulinoma with gastrin and insulin levels monitored before, during, and after the calcium infusion. A post infusion calcium level may be performed to monitor the patient for hypo- or hypercalcemia. A blood sample is obtained by separately reportable venipuncture. Serum/plasma is tested using quantitative spectrophotometry.

82340

82340   Calcium; urine quantitative, timed specimen

A laboratory test is performed to measure urine calcium levels. Calcium is a mineral essential to bone health, heart function, muscle contraction, nerve signaling, and blood clotting. Most of the body's calcium is found in the bones. A very small percentage (1%) circulates in the blood with half that amount metabolically active, and the rest bound to albumin or complexed with phosphate. Small amounts of calcium are normally excreted in urine. Urine calcium levels may be evaluated when a patient presents with abnormal serum calcium levels. Elevated urine calcium can differentially diagnose parathyroid disorders and familial hypocalciuric hypercalcemia (FHH). Intermittent monitoring of urine calcium levels may help direct treatment of these diseases. A random, timed or 24-hour urine sample is obtained by voided specimen or catheterization. Urine is tested using quantitative spectrophotometry.

82355-82360

82355   Calculus; qualitative analysis
82360   Calculus; quantitative analysis, chemical

A laboratory test is performed to analyze and record the characteristics of renal calculi. As the kidney filters blood and makes urine, chemicals can precipitate and form crystals. These crystals typically contain minerals, cysteine, or both. Kidney stones can obstruct urine and blood flow in the kidneys or dislodge and travel down the ureters, stretching, irritating, and damaging the ureteral walls. To analyze calculi, urine is caught in a clean container and strained though fine mesh. Calculi are collected in a container and brought to the lab. The collected calculi are washed and dried, then weighed and measured.

Observations are made regarding the qualitative (82355) characteristics of the stones—rough, smooth, horned, or waxy, and the stones are cut in half to check for a nucleus. If a nucleus is present, the nucleus and shell are divided and analyzed separately. After qualitative analysis of the stone(s) has been performed and recorded, if the stone does not appear to have a nucleus, the whole stone may be pulverized and a chemical analysis done to determine the composition of the calculi (82360). Calcium, magnesium, inorganic phosphate and oxalate are each measured and their levels are used to calculate the stones' composition in terms of calcium, oxalate, apatite, and magnesium ammonium phosphate.

82365-82370

82365   Calculus; infrared spectroscopy
82370   Calculus; X-ray diffraction

A laboratory test is performed to analyze the composition of renal calculi. As the kidney filters blood and makes urine, chemicals can precipitate and form crystals. These crystals typically contain minerals, cysteine, or both. Kidney stones can obstruct urine and blood flow in the kidneys or dislodge and travel down the ureters, stretching, irritating, and damaging the ureteral walls. To analyze calculi, urine is caught in a clean container and strained though fine mesh. Calculi are collected in a container and brought to the lab. Usually after qualitative analysis of the stone(s) has been performed and recorded separately, samples of the stones' surface, core, and cross section are taken and analyzed using infrared spectrometry in 82365 or the stone(s) are analyzed using roentgenogram (X-ray) diffraction to create a diffractogram in 82370. The sample is compared to a known database of possible stone composition materials and a determination of the calculi composition is then made.

82373

82373   Carbohydrate deficient transferrin

A blood sample is analyzed for carbohydrate deficient transferrin (CDT), which is a marker for chronic alcohol consumption. CDT is present in higher concentrations than normal in heavy consumers of alcohol. CDT may also be tested in patients with poorly controlled or uncontrolled diabetes mellitus to diagnose congenital glycosylation. A blood sample is obtained by separately reportable venipuncture. Blood serum is then tested using electrophoresis in patients with suspected chronic alcohol use in excess of 50 gm/day for longer than two weeks. Affinity chromatography/mass spectrometry is used when testing for congenital glycosylation.

82374

82374   Carbon dioxide (bicarbonate)

A blood sample is taken to measure the total carbon dioxide (CO_2) level. The total CO_2 level is composed of CO_2, bicarbonate (HCO_3-), and carbonic acid (H_2CO_3), with the primary constituent being bicarbonate. Bicarbonate is a negatively charged electrolyte that works in conjunction with other electrolytes, such as potassium, sodium, and chloride, to maintain proper acid-base balance and electrical neutrality at the cellular level. Bicarbonate is excreted and reabsorbed by the kidneys. Total CO_2 gives a rough estimate of bicarbonate concentration in the blood. CO_2 is measured by enzymatic methodology.

82375

82375   Carboxyhemoglobin; quantitative

A laboratory test is performed to measure carboxyhemoglobin (COHb) levels. COHb is a stable complex of carbon monoxide and hemoglobin that forms in red blood cells (RBCs). Trace levels will be present in all blood samples, with smokers having a somewhat higher than normal baseline level. Carbon monoxide easily displaces oxygen molecules in RBCs, making it difficult for the body to oxygenate vital organs when carbon monoxide or methylene chloride poisoning occurs. A blood sample is obtained by separately reportable venipuncture, heelstick, or arterial blood draw. Whole blood is tested for quantitative levels of COHb using spectrophotometry.

82376

82376   Carboxyhemoglobin; qualitative

A laboratory test is performed to assess the presence of carboxyhemoglobin (COHb), a stable complex of carbon monoxide and hemoglobin that forms in red blood cells (RBCs). Trace levels will be present in all blood samples, with smokers having a somewhat higher than normal baseline level. Carbon monoxide easily displaces oxygen molecules in RBCs, making it difficult for the body to oxygenate vital organs when carbon monoxide or methylene chloride poisoning occurs. A blood sample is obtained by separately reportable venipuncture, heelstick, or arterial blood draw. Whole blood is tested for COHb using colorimetry to detect for the presence (positive result) or absence (negative result) of carbon monoxide. A qualitative test is used as a quick diagnostic tool for suspected carbon monoxide exposure. A positive result is normally followed with quantitative testing to determine the level of carboxyhemoglobin.

● New Code   ▲ Revised Code

82378

82378   Carcinoembryonic antigen (CEA)

A laboratory test is obtained to measure carcinoembryonic antigen (CEA) levels in blood and body fluids. CEA is a protein normally present at high levels during fetal development but is low or absent after birth. Elevated levels of CEA may occur with colorectal, breast, lung, pancreatic, prostate, ovarian, and medullary thyroid cancers. CEA testing can help determine tumor size, stage, and metastasis. A baseline level is usually obtained following a cancer diagnosis. Serial testing is done to monitor treatment and response to therapy. Elevated levels of CEA have also been noted in smokers and in patients diagnosed with inflammatory disorders, cirrhosis, peptic ulcer, ulcerative colitis, rectal polyps, emphysema, and benign breast disease. CEA testing should not be used for screening in the general population. A blood sample is obtained by separately reportable venipuncture. Cerebral spinal fluid (CSF) is obtained by separately reportable lumbar puncture. Pleural and peritoneal fluids are obtained by needle aspiration. Serum/plasma and body fluids are tested using quantitative electrochemiluminescent immunoassay.

82379

82379   Carnitine (total and free), quantitative, each specimen

A laboratory test is obtained to measure free and total carnitine. Carnitine is a hydrophilic amino acid derivative produced in the liver and kidneys and absorbed from ingested meats and dairy. Carnitine is required for energy metabolism, specifically the breakdown of long chain fatty acids for use by the mitochondria. If long chain fatty acids are not available to the body for beta oxidation and energy production, ketones will not be available for use by the brain. Symptoms of carnitine deficiency include hypoglycemia (all available glucose is being used for energy by the cells), muscle weakness, anemia, heart and kidney problems. Newborns are screened for primary carnitine deficiency soon after birth. Secondary or acquired carnitine deficiency can develop as a result of type 2 diabetes, gastrointestinal disorders, familial cardiomyopathy, renal tubule disease, chronic renal failure, and prolonged treatment with steroids, antibiotics, anticonvulsants, and total parenteral nutrition (TPN). A blood sample is obtained by separately reportable venipuncture or heel stick. A urine sample is obtained by voided specimen or catheterization. Serum/plasma and urine are tested using tandem mass spectrometry.

82380

82380   Carotene

A blood test is performed to measure carotene levels. Carotene is a polyunsaturated hydrocarbon found in plants primarily as beta and alpha isomers. These compounds are often referred to as antioxidants and are an essential nutrient for the human body. Decreased levels may be related to an inadequate intake of dietary fats, the presence of intestinal parasites, certain fat malabsorption syndromes and diseases of the kidney, liver and pancreas. Some drugs/medications may prevent absorption of carotenes including: cholestyramine, alcohol, fat binding weight loss drugs and fiber supplements. Elevated levels may result from hypothyroidism, diabetes, myxedema, chronic nephritis and excessive vitamin intake. A blood sample is obtained by separately reportable venipuncture. Blood serum is tested for total carotene using quantitative spectrophotometry. Blood serum or plasma may be tested for fractionated carotene (alpha, beta, lutein and zeaxanthine) using qualitative high performance liquid chromotography.

82382-82384

82382   Catecholamines; total urine
82383   Catecholamines; blood
82384   Catecholamines; fractionated

A urine or blood test is performed to measure total or fractionated catecholamine levels. Catecholamines are hormones produced by nerve tissue (such as the brain) and adrenal glands. They include dopamine, norepinephrine and epinephrine (adrenaline). These hormones may be elevated when neuroendocrine tumors such as pheochromocytoma or neuroblastoma are present. Certain drugs may alter the test results. In 82382, a urine test is performed to measure total catecholamine levels. A urine sample is collected over 24 hours. The urine is tested using quantitative tandom mass spectrometry. In 82383, a blood sample is obtained by separately reportable venipuncture to measure total catecholamine levels, preferably with the patient calm and supine for 30 minutes prior to the blood draw. The blood sample is tested using quantitative high performance liquid chromatography. In 82384, a fractionated test is performed, which provides separate results for each of the three hormones, dopamine, norepinephrine and epinephrine (adrenaline). A blood sample is obtained by separately reportable venipuncture to measure fractionated catecholamine levels, preferably with the patient calm and supine for 30 minutes prior to the blood draw. Alternatively, a urine sample is collected over a 24 hour period to test for fractionated catecholamine levels. Blood is tested using quantitative high performance liquid chromatography. Urine is tested using quantitative tandom mass spectrometry.

82387

82387   Cathepsin-D

A blood test is performed to measure cathepsin-D levels. Cathepsin-D is a protein encoded by the CTSD gene and is part of the peptide A1 family with similarities to pepsin-A. Mutations of this gene have been linked to breast cancer and possibly Alzheimer's disease. It can be used as a tumor marker in individuals with breast cancer during and following treatment. A blood sample is obtained by separately reportable venipuncture. Serum is tested using fluorometric assay.

82390

82390   Ceruloplasmin

A blood test is performed to measure ceruloplasmin levels. Ceruloplasmin is a protein found in blood which carries copper molecules and also has a role in iron metabolism. This test is most often ordered in conjunction with other blood/urine copper tests to diagnose Wilson disease or a copper deficiency. A blood sample is obtained by separately reportable venipuncture. Serum or plasma is tested using quantitative immunoturbidimetric.

82397

82397   Chemiluminescent assay

Chemiluminescent assay is a variant of the standard enzyme-linked immunosorbent assay (ELISA) procedure and measures light emission resulting from a chemical reaction. The code 82397 is used in different types of testing such as for IgF binding protein-3 in suspected growth disorders; for leptin, a hormone that regulates fat storage in the cells; for vascular endothelial growth factor, a signal protein produced by cells to stimulate growth of new blood vessels; and for alpha subunit, pituitary glycoprotein hormones—to differentiate thyroid hormone resistance and thyrotropin-secreting pituitary hormone tumors, and delayed puberty disorders. A blood sample is obtained by separately reportable venipuncture. Serum/plasma is tested for a variety of particular factors, hormones, or proteins using chemiluminescent immunoassay.

82415

82415   Chloramphenicol

A blood test is performed to monitor therapeutic drug levels of chloramphenicol. Chloramphenicol is a broad spectrum antibiotic used to treat serious infections. It has been established that high levels of chloramphenicol are associated with bone marrow suppression, a side effect that is usually reversible, and aplastic anemia, a side effect that is often fatal. A blood sample is obtained by separately reportable venipuncture. Serum or plasma is tested using high performance liquid chromatography.

82435

82435   Chloride; blood

A blood sample is taken to measure chloride level. Chloride is a negatively charged electrolyte that works in conjunction with other electrolytes, such as potassium, sodium, and carbon dioxide (CO_2), to regulate fluid in the body and maintain proper acid-base balance. Chloride is found in all body fluids, but is concentrated in the blood. Chloride levels mirror sodium levels, increasing and decreasing in direct relationship to sodium, except when there is an acid-base imbalance. When an acid-base imbalance occurs, chloride acts as a buffer and chloride levels move independently of sodium. Chloride is measured to screen for or monitor electrolyte or acid-base balance. Chloride is measured by ion-selective electrode (ISE) methodology.

82436

82436   Chloride; urine

Chloride is a negatively charged molecule known as an electrolyte. It works with other electrolytes, such as potassium, salt (sodium), and carbon dioxide (CO_2), to help keep the proper balance of body fluids and maintain the body's acid-base balance. This test may be used to help determine the causes of hypokalemia, and to aid in the diagnosis of renal tubular acidosis. This test is performed by measuring the amount of chloride in a urine sample.

82438

82438   Chloride; other source

Chloride is a negatively charged molecule known as an electrolyte. It works with other electrolytes, such as potassium, salt (sodium), and carbon dioxide (CO_2), to help keep the proper balance of body fluids and maintain the body's acid-base balance. This test may be used to help determine the causes of hypokalemia, and to aid in the diagnosis of renal tubular acidosis. This test is performed by measuring the amount of chloride in a sample other than urine (e.g., blood).

Pathology and Laboratory

82441

82441   Chlorinated hydrocarbons, screen

A screening test for exposure to chlorinated hydrocarbons is performed on blood, urine or exhaled air from the lungs. Chlorinated hydrocarbons are chemical compounds made up of carbon, chlorine and hydrogen most often used as a pesticide to control vectors (disease carrying insects) or in solvents. Exposure usually occurs in occupational settings via inhalation of vaporous fumes or direct contact with skin.

82465

82465   Cholesterol, serum or whole blood, total

A laboratory test is performed to measure total cholesterol in serum or whole blood. Cholesterol is a waxy, fat-like steroid substance present in the cell membranes of all body tissues and organs. The majority of cholesterol is produced intrinsically by the body and a small amount is ingested from food sources. Cholesterol is an important component of hormones that regulate growth, development, and reproduction. It also forms bile acids that are necessary for digestion of food and nutrient absorption. Elevated cholesterol may be a risk factor for cardiovascular disease and stroke. Certain individuals may have a genetically inherited risk for elevated cholesterol. A blood sample is obtained by separately reportable venipuncture or fingerstick. Serum/plasma and whole blood are tested using quantitative enzymatic method.

82480

82480   Cholinesterase; serum

A blood test is performed to measure total serum cholinesterase levels. Cholinesterase is composed of two substances, acetylcholinesterase and pseudocholinesterase. Cholinesterase is an enzyme that assists with nervous system functioning. This test measures enzyme activity and is used to determine accidental exposure to organic phosphates (chemicals found in pesticides) and also to identify individuals who have an inherited pseudocholinesterase deficiency placing them at risk for prolonged paralysis when the drug succinylcholine is administered during surgery/anesthesia. Less commonly the test is performed to help diagnose liver disease. A blood sample is obtained by separately reportable venipuncture. Serum is tested using qualitative enzymatic methodology.

82482

82482   Cholinesterase; RBC

A blood test is performed to measure total cholinesterase levels in red blood cells (RBCs). Cholinesterase is composed of two substances, acetylcholinesterase and pseudocholinesterase. Cholinesterase is an enzyme that assists with nervous system functioning. This test measures enzyme activity and is used to determine accidental exposure to organic phosphates (chemicals found in pesticides) and also to identify individuals who have an inherited pseudocholinesterase deficiency placing them at risk for prolonged paralysis when the drug succinylcholine is administered during surgery/anesthesia. Less commonly the test is performed to help diagnose liver disease. A blood sample is obtained by separately reportable venipuncture. Red blood cells are tested using qualitative enzymatic methodology.

82485

82485   Chondroitin B sulfate, quantitative

A laboratory test is performed to measure chondroitin B sulfate. Chondroitin is made up of polysaccharides attached to amino acids (glycosaminoglycans, GAGs) that form porous gel-like structures in skin, cartilage, corneal tissue, and umbilical cord. This extracellular matrix provides mechanical support to tissue and allows diffusion of water soluble molecules and migration of cells. GAGs play a role in neurobiochemical activity, connective tissue homeostasis, coagulation, and cell growth and repair. Elevated levels of chondroitin B sulfate may correlate to the presence and typology (hard vs. soft) of atherosclerotic plaque.

82495

82495   Chromium

A blood or urine test is performed to measure chromium levels. Chromium in its trivalent form is a biologically active mineral necessary in trace amounts to maintain optimal health. Chromium in hexavalent form is a toxic waste product from industrial pollution. Lab tests may be used to assess nutritional status or to screen for exposure to toxic waste. Nutritional supplements, medications and iodine containing contrast media can alter test results. A blood sample is obtained by separately reportable venipuncture. Urine may be collected and saved over a 24 hour period or submitted as a single random sample. Serum and urine are both tested using quantitative inductively coupled plasma-mass spectrometry.

82507

82507   Citrate

A blood or urine test is performed to measure citrate (citric acid) levels. Citrate plays an important role in metabolism. A blood sample is obtained by separately reportable venipuncture. Urine may be collected over a 24 hour period or submitted as a single random sample. Serum is tested using spectrophotometry or enzymatic methodology. Urine is tested using quantitative enzymatic methodology.

82523

82523   Collagen cross links, any method

A blood or urine test is performed to measure levels of the collagen cross linked molecules N-Telopeptide and C-Telopeptide. N-Telopeptide is a peptide fragment from the protein matrix of bone and can be measured in both serum and urine. A baseline value is obtained prior to beginning treatment with bisphosphonates or hormone replacements in postmenopausal women or individuals with documented osteopenia. The test is repeated at 3 months and 6 months to evaluate response to therapy. C-Telopeptide is also a peptide fragment from the protein matrix of bone that can be measured in serum. The test is used to monitor therapeutic response to bisphosphonates or hormone replacement therapy in postmenopausal women and individuals with documented osteopenia. A blood sample is obtained by separately reportable venipuncture. Urine sample can be from a random or 24 hour collection. N-Telopeptide urine is tested using quantitative chemiluminescent immunoassay and serum is tested using quantitative enzyme-linked immunosorbent assay. C-Telopeptide serum is tested using quantitative electrochemiluminescent immunoassay.

82525

82525   Copper

Blood, urine or liver tissue is tested to determine copper levels. Copper is a mineral essential to many enzymes or enzymatic reactions in the body. Copper levels can be elevated in Wilson disease, pregnancy, illness/infection, stress and with ingestion of certain drugs (oral contraceptives, nutritional supplements). Decreased levels may be present with corticosteroid use, malnutrition or malabsorption syndromes. A blood sample is obtained by separately reportable venipuncture, liver sample by separately reportable liver biopsy, or urine sample from a 24 hour collection. Serum, liver and urine samples are tested using quantitative inductively coupled plasma-mass spectrometry.

82528

82528   Corticosterone

A laboratory test is performed to measure corticosterone. The glucocorticoid corticosterone is produced by the adrenal gland and is a precursor molecule to the mineralocorticoid aldosterone. Corticosterone secretion is influenced by the renin-angiotensin system and plays a role in brain function and metabolism. The majority of corticosterone is found circulating in the bloodstream; only small amounts are stored by the body. A blood sample is obtained by separately reportable venipuncture. Serum/plasma is tested using quantitative high performance liquid chromatography-tandem mass spectrometry.

82530-82533

82530   Cortisol; free
82533   Cortisol; total

Cortisol is a glucocorticoid (steroid hormone) produced by the adrenal gland in response to stress. The hormone causes an elevation in blood glucose levels, a decrease in immune system function and aids in the metabolism of fats, proteins and carbohydrates. The test may be used to diagnose Cushing syndrome (elevated cortisol levels) or Addison disease (decreased cortisol levels). In 82530, a urine test is performed to measure free cortisol (hydrocortisone) levels. A 24 hour or random urine sample is collected by separately reportable procedure. Urine is tested using quantitative liquid chromatography-tandom mass spectrometry. In 82533, a blood or saliva test is performed to measure total cortisol (hydrocortisone) levels. A blood sample is obtained by separately reportable venipuncture. Serum or plasma is tested using quantitative chemiluminescent immunoassay or quantitative liquid chromatography-tandom mass spectrometry. A saliva sample is obtained by separately reportable oral swab using a saliva collection device. Saliva is tested using quantitative enzyme immunoassay.

82540

82540   Creatine

A blood or urine test is performed to measure creatine levels. Creatine is a nitrogenous organic acid that can be manufactured by the body from amino acids. It is found primarily in muscle cells and is essential for cell metabolism and energy production. Test may be ordered to evaluate for inherited disorders of metabolism. A blood sample is obtained by separately reportable venipuncture or urine sample from random or timed collection. Serum, plasma and urine are tested using liquid chromatography/tandom mass spectrometry.

82542

82542   Column chromatography, includes mass spectrometry, if performed (eg, HPLC, LC, LC/MS, LC/MS-MS, GC, GC/MS-MS, GC/MS, HPLC/MS), non-drug analyte(s) not elsewhere specified, qualitative or quantitative, each specimen

Column chromatography/mass spectrometry is an analytical method that utilizes chromatography to separate chemical components during a stationary and mobile phase (gas or liquid), and then capture and measure the isolated molecule(s) when they fall, or elute, off the column by mass spectrometry. This procedure is done to determine the exact chemical structure of the components being analyzed. The technique is highly sensitive and selective, especially when multiple elements or intermediates are contained in a sample. Gas chromatography (GC) or high performance (pressure) liquid chromatography (HPLC) coupled with mass spectrometry (MS) is often used to detect compounds in blood or other body fluid and analyze it for chemical contamination. Code 82542 is used when quantifying the amount of a non-drug analyte present in a specific sample for which there is no other specified code.

82550-82554

82550   Creatine kinase (CK), (CPK); total
82552   Creatine kinase (CK), (CPK); isoenzymes
82553   Creatine kinase (CK), (CPK); MB fraction only
82554   Creatine kinase (CK), (CPK); isoforms

Creatine kinase (CK) also known as, creatine phosphokinase (CPK), is an enzyme found in the heart, brain, skeletal muscle and certain other tissue. The subtypes are known as CK-MM found primarily in skeletal and heart muscle, CK-MB found in heart muscle and CK-BB located in the brain. CK circulating in blood rarely contains CK-BB but is largely comprised of CK-MM or CK-MB. Levels may be elevated following heart muscle damage (heart attack/myocardial infarction) and skeletal muscle injury (trauma, vigorous exercise). Statin drugs that lower cholesterol level and alcohol intake may cause elevated CK blood levels. In 82550, a blood test is performed to measure total creatine kinase (CK) levels. A blood specimen is obtained by separately reportable venipuncture. Serum or plasma is tested using quantitative enzymatic methodology. In 82552, creatine kinase (CK) isoenzyme levels are measured. Testing for isoenzymes can help determine the exact location of muscle damage when total CK is elevated. A blood specimen is obtained by separately reportable venipuncture. Serum is tested using quantitative enzymatic methodology. In 82553, only creatine kinase (CK) MB fraction is measured. Testing for this isoenzyme can help identify heart muscle damage following a heart attack (myocardial infarction). A blood test is obtained by separately reportable venipuncture. Serum is tested using chemiluminescent immunoassay. In 82554, creatine kinase (CK) isoforms of the isoenzymes CK-MM and CK-MB are measured. Following their release, CK isoenzymes continue to break down into more distinct isoforms. The CK-MM contains at least three major isoform subtypes and CK-MB has at least two. Identifying isoform subtypes of the isoenzymes, can help identify and define the time as well as the location of muscle injury. A blood specimen is obtained by separately reportable venipuncture. Serum may be tested using a number of techniques including high resolution electrophoresis, isoelectric and chromatofocusing and liquid chromatography.

82565

82565   Creatinine; blood

A blood sample is taken to measure creatinine levels. Creatinine is a waste product produced by the muscles in the breakdown of creatine, which is a compound used by the muscles to create energy for contraction. The waste product, creatinine, is excreted by the kidneys and blood levels provide a good measurement of renal function. Creatinine may be checked to screen for or monitor treatment of renal disease. Creatinine levels may also be monitored in patients with acute or chronic illnesses that may impair renal function and in patients on medications that affect renal function. Creatinine is measured using spectrophotometry.

82570

82570   Creatinine; other source

A sample other than blood is taken to measure creatinine levels. Creatinine is a waste product produced by the muscles in the breakdown of creatine, which is a compound used by the muscles to create energy for contraction. The waste product, creatinine, is excreted by the kidneys and blood levels provide a good measurement of renal function. Creatinine may be checked to screen for or monitor treatment of renal disease. Creatinine levels may also be monitored in patients with acute or chronic illnesses that may impair renal function and in patients on medications that affect renal function.

82575

82575   Creatinine; clearance

A sample other than blood is taken to measure creatinine levels. Creatinine is a waste product produced by the muscles in the breakdown of creatine, which is a compound used by the muscles to create energy for contraction. The waste product, creatinine, is excreted by the kidneys and blood levels provide a good measurement of renal function. Creatinine may be checked to screen for or monitor treatment of renal disease. Creatinine levels may also be monitored in patients with acute or chronic illnesses that may impair renal function and in patients on medications that affect renal function.

82585

82585   Cryofibrinogen

A laboratory test is performed to measure cryofibrinogen. Cryofibrinogen is an abnormal protein that forms a precipitate when exposed to low temperatures, leading to a condition called cryofibrinogenemia (CFG). Primary CFG is a rare inherited genetic condition. Secondary CFG is the more common form and may develop in patients with non-Hodgkin's lymphoma, colorectal cancer, tuberculosis, herpes viral infection, streptococcal infection, Crohn's disease, systemic lupus erythematosus, and vasculitis. Symptoms are caused by vascular occlusion in areas of the body exposed to the cold and may include skin reactions such as itching, redness, swelling, and hives, purpura rash, skin lesions or ulcers, poor circulation, and phlebitis. Complications can include pulmonary embolism, stroke, myocardial infarctions, and gangrene. A blood sample is obtained by separately reportable venipuncture. The sample must be kept at 37° C until centrifuged for plasma cells. Plasma is tested using qualitative cold precipitation.

82595

82595   Cryoglobulin, qualitative or semi-quantitative (eg, cryocrit)

A blood sample is tested for cryoglobulins (cryocrit). Qualitative determination identifies the presence or absence of cryoglobulins while semi-quantitative determination provides an estimate of the amount. Cryoglobulins are associated with plasma cell and lymphoproliferative disorders, collagen vascular diseases, hepatitis C, infectious mononucleosis, and cytomegalovirus disease. A blood sample is obtained by separately reportable venipuncture. The sample is tested using cold precipitation and examined daily for 3-5 days for evidence of cryoglobulins.

82600

82600   Cyanide

A blood test is performed to measure cyanide levels. Cyanide is present in certain seeds/stone fruits, is produced by some bacteria, fungi and algae and is bound to sugar molecules in a number of plants. Cyanide may be ingested from these sources or inhaled as an atmospheric toxin produced when combustion of certain materials takes place. This test should not be performed on patients who are receiving nitroprusside therapy. The results will be inaccurate. A blood sample is obtained by separately reportable venipuncture. Blood is tested using spectrophotometry.

82607-82608

82607   Cyanocobalamin (Vitamin B-12)
82608   Cyanocobalamin (Vitamin B-12); unsaturated binding capacity

Cyanocobalamin is a vitamer of the B-12 vitamin family and plays an important role in metabolism, red blood cell production and nervous system function. In 82607 blood levels of cyanocobalamin are measured. Blood levels may be reduced with pernicious and other forms of anemia, and in individuals who follow a strict vegan diet, have chronic infections (such as HIV) and during pregnancy. A blood sample is obtained by separately reportable venipuncture. Serum is tested using quantitative chemiluminescent immunoassay. In 82608, a blood test is performed to measure cyanocobalamin unsaturated binding capacity. The unsaturated binding capacity of cyanocobalamin may be elevated in diseases such as myelocytic leukemia, polycythemia vera, some liver disorders and in Gaucher disease. Levels may be decreased with megaloblastic anemia from congenital transcobalamin II deficiency and from other causes. A blood sample is obtained by separately reportable venipuncture. Serum is tested using quantitative radioimmunassay.

82610

82610   Cystatin C

A blood sample is obtained to measure the Cystatin C level. Cystatin C, also referred to as cystatin 3 or CST 3, is a serum protein produced by all nucleated cells in the body, and has a low molecular mass that allows it to be filtered by the glomerular membrane in the kidneys. Cystatin C contained in the filtrate is then reabsorbed by the body and broken down. It is not returned to the blood. When glomerular filtration rate is impaired, Cystatin C levels in the blood increase, indicating decreased kidney function. Cystatin C measurement is used to evaluate glomerular filtration rate, screen for and monitor renal disease, and monitor treatment in patients with known renal disease. Cystatin C levels may also be used to predict survival following a heart attack with elevated levels indicating a poorer prognosis. Cystatin C is measured by nephelometry.

82615

82615   Cystine and homocystine, urine, qualitative

A laboratory test is performed to determine the presence of cystine and homocystine in urine. The amino acids lysine, ornithine, and arginine breakdown into cystine. When

Pathology and Laboratory

cystine fails to be reabsorbed in the kidney it can precipitate in the urine and form stones. Cystinuria is usually caused by an inherited genetic disorder. Homocystinuria may result from an inherited metabolic disorder of the amino acid methionine (cystathionine beta synthase deficiency), re-methylation defects, or vitamin B deficiencies (B2, B6, B9, B12). Symptoms of elevated homocystine can be multisystemic and include connective tissue and muscle disorders, central nervous system disorders, and cardiovascular problems. A urine sample is obtained by voided specimen or catheterization. Urine is tested for cystine and homocystine using spectrometry.

82626

82626   Dehydroepiandrosterone (DHEA)

A laboratory test is performed to measure dehydroepiandrosterone (DHEA). DHEA is a prohormone produced primarily in the adrenal glands from cholesterol. DHEA can also be produced in small amounts by the brain, ovaries, and testes. Elevated levels may indicate excess adrenal activity due to benign adrenal hyperplasia, malignant adrenal tumors, and polycystic ovarian syndrome. Symptoms can include ambiguous external genitalia, precocious puberty in boys, and virilization in girls. Adult women may present with increased body hair, menstrual irregularities, or infertility. Adult males are rarely symptomatic when they have elevated levels of DHEA. Low levels may interfere with bone formation, adipose and muscle tissue composition, insulin and glucose metabolism, and cause a loss of libido. A blood sample is obtained by separately reportable venipuncture. Serum/plasma is tested using quantitative high performance liquid chromatography-tandem mass spectrometry.

82627

82627   Dehydroepiandrosterone-sulfate (DHEA-S)

A laboratory test is performed to measure dehydroepiandrosterone-sulfate (DHEA-S). DHEA-S is the more stable form of DHEA, a prohormone produced in the adrenal glands from cholesterol and also manufactured in small amounts by the brain, ovaries, and testes. DHEA-S testing may be preferred by some practitioners because there is less diurnal variation when compared to DHEA, which normally peaks in the early morning. Elevated levels of DHEA/DHEA-S may indicate excess adrenal activity due to benign adrenal hyperplasia, malignant adrenal tumors, and polycystic ovarian syndrome. Symptoms can include ambiguous external genitalia, precocious puberty in boys, and virilization in girls. Adult women may present with increased body hair, menstrual irregularities, or infertility. Adult males are rarely symptomatic when they have elevated levels of DHEA. Low levels may interfere with bone formation, adipose and muscle tissue composition, insulin and glucose metabolism, and cause a loss of libido. A blood sample is obtained by separately reportable venipuncture. Serum/plasma is tested using quantitative electrochemiluminescent immunoassay.

82633

82633   Desoxycorticosterone, 11-

A laboratory test is performed to measure the level of 11-Desoxycorticosterone, a precursor compound of mature corticosteroids. The adrenal glands, ovaries, testes, and placenta produce corticosteroids and sex steroid hormones from cholesterol. At varies stages, enzyme reactions occur that can interrupt the synthesis of one or more of these hormones. Measuring sex hormone concentrations and precursor compounds (11-Desoxycorticosterone) of mature mineralocorticoid (aldosterone) and glucocorticoid (cortisol) steroids can aid in the diagnosis of congenital adrenal hyperplasia (CAH) and also identity the precise type. After diagnosis, the test is used to monitor the effects of steroid replacement therapy and other interventions. When ordering a laboratory test for 11-desoxycorticosterone, it is common to measure 11-deoxycortisol, corticosterone, 18-hydroxycorticosterone, cortisol, renin, aldosterone, and 17-hydroxyprogesterone as well. A blood sample is obtained by separately reportable venipuncture. Serum/plasma is tested using quantitative high performance liquid chromatography-tandem mass spectrometry.

82634

82634   Deoxycortisol, 11-

A blood test is performed to measure 11-desoxycortisol levels. Desoxycortisol is the immediate precursor to cortisol (hydrocortisone) a glucocorticoid steroid produced by the adrenal glands. The test may be ordered to evaluate adrenal function, including congenital adrenal hypoplasia. A blood sample is obtained by separately reportable venipuncture. Serum or plasma is tested using quantitative tandem mass spectrometry.

82638

82638   Dibucaine number

A blood test is performed to measure the dibucaine number (DN), which is the percent of pseudocholinesterase enzyme (PChE) activity inhibited by the drug dibucaine. The test is used to identify individuals with pseudocholinesterase deficiency who may be at increased risk of prolonged paralysis following succinylcholine administration. A blood sample is obtained by separately reportable venipuncture. Serum or plasma is tested using quantitative enzymatic methodology.

82652

82652   Vitamin D; 1, 25 dihydroxy, includes fraction(s), if performed

Blood levels of 1,25-dihydroxyvitamin D are measured when a patient has high levels of calcium in the blood to determine whether the patient has a disease, such as sarcoidosis or lymphoma, that might produce an excess of Vitamin D and abnormal metabolism of calcium. 1,25-dihydroxyvitamin D levels may also be evaluated to help diagnose or monitor disease of the parathyroid glands. A blood sample is obtained. Levels of 1,25-dihydroxyvitamin D are evaluated using radioimmunoassay. The test results may reflect total 1,25-dihydroxyvitamin D or the results may include the total vitamin D level and the fraction represented by 1,25-dihydroxyvitamin D.

82656

82656   Elastase, pancreatic (EL-1), fecal, qualitative or semi-quantitative

A laboratory test is performed to identify the presence of pancreatic elastase (EL-1) in feces or semi-quantify the amount. EL-1 is a glycoprotein digestive enzyme synthesized by the acinar cells of the pancreas and released into the intestine where it breaks down food, facilitates absorption of nutrients, and also combines with bile acids and neutral steroids to transport cholesterol. The fecal test for EL-1 can be used diagnostically to monitor pancreatic function in patients with cystic fibrosis (CF). It may also assist with the diagnosis or exclusion of pancreatic exocrine insufficiency caused by chronic pancreatitis, cystic fibrosis, pancreatic tumors, cholelithiasis, or diabetes mellitus. Pancreatic enzymes should be discontinued prior to the test. A sample of formed stool (feces) is collected in a clean container. Feces are tested using enzyme linked immunosorbent assay (ELISA).

82657

82657   Enzyme activity in blood cells, cultured cells, or tissue, not elsewhere specified; nonradioactive substrate, each specimen

A laboratory test is performed to monitor enzyme activity in blood cells, cultured cells, or tissue using a nonradioactive substrate. Many inherited genetic disorders are caused by the mutation of gene coding on enzyme proteins involved in the breakdown or transportation of normal body compounds or the activation or protection of body functions. Monitoring cells (blood, tissue) for enzyme activity can assist with the diagnosis of some genetic disorders. A blood sample is obtained by separately reportable venipuncture. Code 82657 can be used for the following: thiopurine methyltransferase in red blood cells by enzymatic/quantitative liquid chromotography-tandem mass spectrometry to screen individuals at increased risk for myelosuppression with standard doses of thiopurines; porphobilinogen (PBG) deaminase by quantitative enzymatic activity/fluorometry on whole blood to screen family members at risk for intermittent porphyria; alpha-galactosidase by quantitative fluorometry on serum to diagnose Fabry disease in males. Code 82657 is also used to examine small bowel tissue for disaccharidase using quantitative spectrophotometry. A tissue sample of the small bowel is obtained by separately reportable endoscopy.

82658

82658   Enzyme activity in blood cells, cultured cells, or tissue, not elsewhere specified; radioactive substrate, each specimen

A laboratory test is performed to monitor enzyme activity in blood cells, cultured cells, or tissue using a radioactive substrate. Many inherited genetic disorders are caused by the mutation of gene coding on enzyme proteins involved in the breakdown or transportation of normal body compounds or the activation or protection of body functions. Monitoring cells (blood, tissue) for enzyme activity can assist with the diagnosis of some genetic disorders. A blood sample is obtained by separately reportable venipuncture. Code 82658 can be used for test for leukocyte lysosomal enzymes in whole blood using enzyme activity to screen for lysosomal storage diseases. Lysosomal storage disorders are rare and cause an accumulation of undigested or partially digested macromolecules (fats, proteins, complex carbohydrates) in the cells. This can lead to dysfunction of body organs, connective tissue, eyes, and the central nervous system.

82664

82664   Electrophoretic technique, not elsewhere specified

A laboratory test is performed using electrophoretic technique. Electrophoresis is an analytical method for separating and characterizing certain molecules in blood and body fluid. These can include proteins, nucleic acids, and subcelluar particles such as viruses and small organelles. The particles in a sample will migrate and separate based on size and electrical charge to form a pattern of bands that are different widths and intensities. The code 82664 can be used for a chylomicron screen of body fluids which is tested using qualitative electrophoresis. Chylomicrons are small lipoprotein particles comprised of triglycerides, phospholipids, cholesterol, and protein that transport dietary fats from the intestines to other areas of the body.

82668

82668 Erythropoietin

A laboratory test is performed to measure the level of erythropoietin (EPO). EPO is a hormone produced primarily by the kidneys in response to low blood oxygen levels. The hormone is carried to the bone marrow where it stimulates stem cells to produce more red blood cells (RBCs). Serum levels of EPO can be affected by kidney damage or bone marrow disorders. A test for EPO may be used as an initial screening for polycythemia, to differentiate certain types of anemia, and to determine eligibility for erythropoietin therapy in patients with chronic renal failure. Elevated levels of EPO with corresponding low hematocrit (HCT) may indicate iron deficiency, or aplastic or hemolytic anemia. Elevated EPO with normal HCT may indicate renal transplant rejection, benign/malignant kidney tumors, or secondary polycythemia. Decreased levels of EPO may be found in hemochromatosis, while decreased levels with elevated HCT are present in polycythemia vera. Decreased levels of EPO with decreased HCT is found in HIV patients on AZT therapy. A blood sample is obtained my separately reportable venipuncture. Serum/plasma is tested using quantitative chemiluminescent immunoassay.

82670

82670 Estradiol

A laboratory test is performed to measure the amount of the hormone estradiol in the blood. Estradiol is the type of estrogen most often measured in non-pregnant women. Estradiol levels are measured to evaluate ovarian function and to diagnose the cause of precocious puberty in girls, amenorrhea in women, and gynecomastia in men. Estradiol is also measured to monitor follicle development in the ovaries of women undergoing in-vitro fertilization and hormone replacement therapy in post-menopausal women. The level in a pre-menopausal woman's blood varies throughout the menstrual cycle and drops to a very low but constant level after menopause. A blood sample is obtained by separately reportable venipuncture. Estradiol levels can be measured in plasma or serum. Chemoluminescent immunoassay is used for pre-menopausal women and tandem mass spectrometry is used for males, children, and post-menopausal women.

82671-82672

82671 Estrogens; fractionated
82672 Estrogens; total

A laboratory test is performed to measure the amount of fractionated (82671) or total (82672) estrogens in the blood. These tests measure estradiol, estriol, and estrone, the three most important estrogens. A blood sample is obtained by separately reportable venipuncture. Estrogens can be measured in plasma or serum. In 82671, the amounts of estradiol and estrone are measured and reported separately and the amount of total estrogen is calculated. Fractionated estrogens are tested to diagnose precocious or delayed puberty in girls and disorders of sex steroid metabolism, as well as to help assess bone mineral density, monitor hormone replacement therapy in post-menopausal women, evaluate hypogonadism and oligo-amenorrhea in women, and assess ovarian function, including follicle development for assisted reproduction (in-vitro fertilization). Estradiol is measured by chemoluminescent immunoassay for pre-menopausal women and tandem mass spectrometry for males, children, and post-menopausal women. Estrone is measured by tandem mass spectrometry, and then total estrogen is calculated. In 82672, the total amount of all three estrogens are measured together and reported as a single value. Total estrogens are used to diagnose estrogen-producing ovarian tumors in pre-menarche and post-menopausal females or to evaluate elevated estrogen levels in males. This test may also be used to establish time of ovulation and determine the optimal time for conception.

82677

82677 Estriol

A laboratory test is performed to measure the amount of estriol in the blood. Estriol is an estrogen hormone used to assess the risk of fetal abnormalities such as Down syndrome. Estriol levels are typically measured along with alpha-fetoprotein (AFP), human chorionic gonadotropin (hCG), and inhibin-A in a test called a maternal serum panel to screen for fetal abnormalities. A blood sample is obtained by separately reportable venipuncture. Estriol can be measured in plasma or serum. Estriol is measured by chemoluminescent immunoassay.

82679

82679 Estrone

A laboratory test is performed to measure the amount of estrone in the blood. Estrone is an estrogen hormone that is measured to help diagnose ovarian tumor, Turner's syndrome, and hypopituitarism in females. In males, it is used to help determine the cause of gynecomastia or detect estrogen-producing tumors. A blood sample is obtained by separately reportable venipuncture. Estrone can be measured in plasma or serum. Estrone is measured by mass spectrometry.

82693

82693 Ethylene glycol

A blood test is performed to measure ethylene glycol levels. Ethylene glycol is an organic compound commonly used as automotive antifreeze and ingestion of even small amounts can damage the brain, liver, kidneys, and lungs. It causes changes in body chemistry resulting in metabolic acidosis which can lead to shock, organ failure, or death. The test is performed when accidental or intentional poisoning by ethylene glycol is known or suspected. A blood sample is obtained by separately reportable venipuncture. Serum or plasma is tested using quantitative enzymatic assay.

82696

82696 Etiocholanolone

A laboratory test is performed to measure the level of etiocholanolone, an inactive androgenic ketosteroid metabolized from testosterone and androstenedione by 5-beta-reductase. Elevated levels of etiocholanolone may cause fever, immunostimulation, and leukocytosis. Etiocholanolone also has anticonvulsant effects on GABA receptors and acts as an endogenous modulator for seizure susceptibility. Individuals with androgenic alopecia (male pattern baldness) often have elevated levels of etiocholanolone in their urine. A blood sample is obtained by separately reportable venipuncture. Urine is collected by random voided specimen or catheterization.

82705

82705 Fat or lipids, feces; qualitative

A laboratory test is performed to detect the presence or absence of excess fat or lipids in feces. The body breaks down dietary fats in the intestine by utilizing pancreatic enzymes and bile. Neutral fats (monoglycerides, diglycerides, triglycerides) are broken into free fatty acids (split fats). Elevated neutral fats can result from impaired synthesis or secretion of pancreatic enzymes and/or bile. Elevated split fats may indicate impaired absorption of nutrients. Symptoms of excess fat in feces include persistent diarrhea, abdominal pain, and steatorrhea (fatty stools). A random 24 hour, 48 hour, or 72 hour stool sample is obtained. The sample should not be contaminated by urine, toilet water, or toilet paper. The fecal sample is tested using qualitative microscopy/stain.

82710-82715

82710 Fat or lipids, feces; quantitative
82715 Fat differential, feces, quantitative

A laboratory test is performed to measure the level of fat or lipids in feces. The body breaks down dietary fats in the intestine by utilizing pancreatic enzymes and bile. Neutral fats (monoglycerides, diglycerides, triglycerides) are broken into free fatty acids (split fats). Elevated neutral fats can result from impaired synthesis or secretion of pancreatic enzymes and/or bile. Elevated split fats may indicate impaired absorption of nutrients. Symptoms of excess fat in feces include persistent diarrhea, abdominal pain, and steatorrhea (fatty stools). A 24 hour, 48 hour, or 72 hour stool sample is obtained. The sample should not be contaminated by urine, toilet water, or toilet paper. The fecal sample is tested using nuclear magnetic resonance spectroscopy. In 82715, the sample is tested to quantify the differential fat composition contained in the sample, such as cholesterol, phospholipids, and triglycerides.

82725

82725 Fatty acids, nonesterified

A blood test is performed to measure nonesterified fatty acid levels, which are also referred to as free fatty acids. Blood lipids (fatty acids) may be free or bound to other molecules. Following ingestion, fat molecules are broken down in the digestive tract. Small molecules (short and medium chain fatty acids) are absorbed directly into the blood stream through intestinal capillaries. Larger (long chain fatty acids) are encapsulated by cholesterol and protein (lipoproteins) to become chylomicron, entering the lymphatic capillaries to bypass the liver and finally being deposited into the blood stream at the left subclavian vein. A fasting blood sample is obtained by separately reportable venipuncture. Serum is tested using quantitative spectrophotometry.

82726

82726 Very long chain fatty acids

A blood test is performed to measure very long chain fatty acid (VLCFA) levels. VLCFA are fat molecules with aliphatic tails greater than 22 carbons long. Following ingestion of fatty acids or the release of stored triglycerides from adipose (fat) tissue, fat molecules are used as fuel by the mitochondria (energy center of the cell) by producing adenosine triphosphate (ATP) through beta oxidation. Due to their size, VLCFA must first be broken down by perioxisomes before they are utilized as energy by the mitochondria. In individuals with certain adrenoleukodystrophy disorders, perioxisomes are not able to break down VLCFA leading to a build up in the blood. A blood sample is obtained by separately reportable venipuncture. Plasma is tested for VLCFA and branched chain fatty acids using liquid chromatography-tandem mass spectrometry.

● New Code ▲ Revised Code

Pathology and Laboratory

Pathology and Laboratory

82728

82728   Ferritin

A blood test is performed to measure ferritin levels. Ferritin is an intracellular protein that stores iron and releases it into circulation in a controlled manner to protect the body against iron overload and iron deficiency. Ferritin levels may be obtained to evaluate for elevated levels caused by excess storage diseases such as hemochromatosis and following multiple transfusions. Levels may also be obtained to evaluate for decreased levels due to iron deficiency. A blood sample is obtained by separately reportable venipuncture. Serum is tested using quantitative chemiluminescent immunoassay.

82731

82731   Fetal fibronectin, cervicovaginal secretions, semi-quantitative

A semi-quantitative test for fetal fibronectin is performed on cervicovaginal secretions. Fetal fibronectin (fFN) is a protein produced during pregnancy that serves as a biological glue attaching the fetal sac to the uterine lining. Fetal fibronectin is normally present in cervicovaginal secretions during the first 22 weeks of gestation. After 22 weeks, it is normally no longer present until one to three weeks before the onset of labor. Women with detectable levels of fetal fibronectin between weeks 24-34, along with symptoms of preterm labor, have an increased risk of preterm delivery. Cervicovaginal secretions are collected on a cotton swab and then tested for the presence or absence of fetal fibronectin.

82735

82735   Fluoride

A blood or urine test is performed to measure fluoride levels. Fluoride (fluorine) is a mineral found naturally in drinking water and food. Fluoride may be added to community drinking water and/or taken as a dietary supplement to decrease the incidence of tooth decay. Fluorine containing compounds may be present in pharmaceutical products, pesticides and toxic chemicals. A blood sample is obtained by separately reportable venipuncture. A urine sample is obtained from a random voided specimen. Blood is tested using quantitative ion chromatography. Urine is tested using ion specific electrode/colorimetry.

82746-82747

82746   Folic acid; serum
82747   Folic acid; RBC

A blood test is performed to measure folic acid (folate) levels in serum or red blood cells (RBC). Folic acid (folate) may also be referred to as Vitamin B9 and is essential for the growth, division and repair of cells, especially fetal growth during pregnancy and in early infancy. It is also necessary for the production of healthy red blood cells and to prevent anemia at all ages. The test may be used to diagnose anemia or certain neuropathies and to monitor the effectiveness of treatment for these conditions. A blood sample is obtained by separately reportable venipuncture. Use 82746 when serum is tested. Use 82747 when RBCs are tested. The amount of folic acid in red blood cells measures the level when the cell was made, up to 2 months earlier. Both tests are typically performed using quantitative chemiluminescent immunoassay.

82757

82757   Fructose, semen

Semen is tested to measure fructose levels. Fructose, an androgen dependent sugar, is produced in the seminal vesicles. The absence of fructose in seminal fluid may indicate obstruction of the seminal vesicles or ejaculatory duct or congenital absence of the vas deferens. A semen sample is obtained by ejaculation or other separately reportable procedure. Semen is tested using quantitative spectrophotometry.

82759

82759   Galactokinase, RBC

A blood test is performed to measure galactokinase levels. Galactokinase is an adenosine triphosphate (ATP) dependent enzyme in the galactokinase, homserine kinase, and mevalonite kinase (GHMP) family. GHMP kinase enzymes are needed to biosynthesize isoprenes and amino acides and to metabolize carbohydrates. Galactokinase is needed to metabolize the simple sugar galactose. A deficiency of galactokinase leads to galactosemia type 2 which manifests itself in infancy and can lead to the development of infantile cataracts. The condition is caused by a mutation in the GAL12 gene which is an inherited autosomal recessive disorder. A blood sample is obtained by separately reportable venipuncture. Whole blood/red blood cells are tested using quantitative radioisotopic methodology.

82760

82760   Galactose

A laboratory test is performed to measure the level of galactose, a simple sugar molecule which is part of lactose, a complex sugar commonly found in dairy products and infant formulas. Elevated levels of galactose in blood (galactosemia) or urine (galactosuria)

may result from an inherited genetic disorder of the enzyme Galactose-1-phosphate uridyltransferase. Testing for elevated galactose is useful for screening but should not be used as a definitive diagnosis for genetic disorders of galactose metabolism (GALK, GALT, GALE). Galactose levels may also be elevated with severe hepatitis, newborn biliary atresia, and, rarely, galactose intolerance. A blood sample is obtained by separately reportable venipuncture. Urine is collected by random voided specimen or catheterization. Plasma and urine are tested using kinetic spectrophotometry.

82775-82776

82775   Galactose-1-phosphate uridyl transferase; quantitative
82776   Galactose-1-phosphate uridyl transferase; screen

Galactose-1-phosphate uridyl transferase (GALT) is an enzyme responsible for converting dietary (ingested) galactose to glucose for energy use by the cells. The absence of this enzyme results in classic type galactosemia, a hereditary autosomal recessive gene disorder (mutation). In 82775, a quantitative analysis is performed to measure the amount of GALT in the blood A blood sample is obtained by separately reportable venipuncture. Blood is tested using enzymatic methodology. In 82776, a blood test is performed to screen for the presence of galactose-1-phosphate uridyl transferase (GALT). A GALT screening test is performed as part of a panel of tests to screen newborns for metabolic disorders.

82777

82777   Galectin-3

A blood test is performed to measure galectin-3 levels in patients identified with cardiac muscle injury. Galactin-3 is a protein which activates cells following cardiac injury. Elevated levels of Galectin-3 have been associated with excessive scarring and fibrosis which leads to changes in the shape and dimension of the heart (adverse remodeling) and chronic heart failure. A blood sample is obtained by separately reportable venipuncture. Serum or plasma is tested using enzyme-linked immunosorbent assay (ELISA).

82784-82787

82784   Gammaglobulin (immunoglobulin); IgA, IgD, IgG, IgM, each
82785   Gammaglobulin (immunoglobulin); IgE
82787   Gammaglobulin (immunoglobulin); immunoglobulin subclasses (eg, IgG1, 2, 3, or 4), each

A test is performed to measure immunoglobin levels in the blood or other body fluids, such as saliva or cerebral spinal fluid. Immunoglobins, also referred to as antibodies, are evaluated to help diagnose a variety of conditions including autoimmune diseases, allergies, or malignant neoplasms such as multiple myeloma or macroglobulinemia. In addition, immunoglobulin levels may be evaluated in patients with frequent infections to determine if there is a low level of immunoglobulin IgG. Immunoglobulins are also evaluated in patients with cancer or H. pylori infection to determine the effectiveness of treatment. There are five major types of antibodies. IgA antibodies are found in the nose, respiratory and digestive tracts, ears, eyes, and vagina. IgA protects the body surfaces from outside foreign substances. IgD is found in tissues lining the abdominal and thoracic cavity. IgE is found in the lungs, skin and mucous membranes and reacts to substances commonly associated with allergies, such as food, pollen, dander, dust, fungus spores, etc. High levels of IgE are associated with allergies. IgG is found in all body fluids and is important in fighting bacterial and viral infections. There are four subclasses of IgG, designated as IgG1, IgG2, IgG3, and IgG4. These different subclasses protect against different types of infection. For example IgG1 is particularly effective in protecting the body from viral proteins, whereas IgG2 is more effective against certain types of bacterial infections. Individuals may have selective IgG subclass deficiencies characterized by low levels of one or two IgG subclasses with normal total IgG. IgM is found in blood and lymph and is important in fighting infection. A blood specimen is obtained by separately reportable venipuncture, a CSF sample is obtained by separately reportable spinal puncture, or saliva is collected. The methodology used to test immunoglobulin levels is dependent on the type of specimen and the immunoglobulin being tested. Use 82784 to report each immunoglobulin IgA, IgD, IgG, or IgM determination. Use 82785, to report immunoglobulin IgE determination. Use 82787 to report each immunoglobulin subclass IgG1, IgG2, IgG3, or IgG4.

82800

82800   Gases, blood, pH only

A laboratory test is performed to measure blood pH—the level of hydrogen ions (H+) dissolved in the blood. To function optimally, the body will try to maintain a homeostatic acid-base balance (pH) of 7.35-7.45. When the pH falls below 7.35, the body is in a state of acidosis; above 7.45, the body is in a state of alkalosis. Regulation of the acid-base balance first involves plasma protein buffers which will accept some hydrogen ions in an attempt to maintain homeostasis. As the pH lowers, the respiratory rate will increase to blow off excess carbon dioxide (CO_2) via the lungs. Later, the kidneys and liver will increase circulating bicarbonate (HCO_3), a base that can accept H+ ions to help raise the blood pH. The most common cause of acidosis is a respiratory problem. The body retains carbon dioxide (CO_2) which dissolves in the blood to form a weak carbonic acid. Metabolic causes of acidosis can include diabetes and prolonged diarrhea. Alkalosis may have a respiratory origin (hyperventilation) or be metabolic as can occur with excessive vomiting. A blood sample is obtained by separately reportable venipuncture, heelstick, arterial, or umbilical cord draw.

82803

82803   Gases, blood, any combination of pH, pCO2, pO2, CO2, HCO3 (including calculated O2 saturation)

A laboratory test is performed to measure one or more components of blood gases. The homeostatic acid-base balance is measured as blood pH—the number of hydrogen ions (H+) dissolved in the blood. Partial pressure of carbon dioxide (pCO2) is the amount of carbon dioxide dissolved in the blood and reflects how well the lungs can move CO2 out of the body. Partial pressure of oxygen (pO2) is the level of oxygen dissolved in the blood and reflects the exchange of oxygen molecules in the alveoli. Bicarbonate (HCO3) is calculated from pH and pCO2 and is the metabolic component of acid-base balance reflecting the kidney's response to changes in pH. Oxygen saturation (O2 Sat) is the percent of hemoglobin that is carrying oxygen. Calculated O2 saturation uses a mathematical model to determine the percentage of hemoglobin that is carrying oxygen based on the level of pO2. Blood gas monitoring may be performed to evaluate lung function; detect an acid-base imbalance; monitor metabolic, respiratory, and kidney disorders; and evaluate the effectiveness of treatment. A blood sample is obtained by separately reportable venipuncture, heelstick, arterial, or umbilical cord draw.

82805

82805   Gases, blood, any combination of pH, pCO2, pO2, CO2, HCO3 (including calculated O2 saturation); with O2 saturation, by direct measurement, except pulse oximetry

A laboratory test is performed to measure one or more components of blood gases. The homeostatic acid-base balance is measured as blood pH—the number of hydrogen ions (H+) dissolved in the blood. Partial pressure of carbon dioxide (pCO2,) is the amount of carbon dioxide dissolved in the blood and reflects how well the lungs can move CO2 out of the body. Partial pressure of oxygen (pO2) is the level of oxygen dissolved in the blood and reflects the exchange of oxygen molecules in the alveoli. Bicarbonate (HCO3) is calculated from pH and pCO2 and is the metabolic component of acid-base balance reflecting the kidney's response to changes in pH. Oxygen saturation (O2 Sat) is the percentage of hemoglobin that is carrying oxygen. Direct measurement of O2 Sat is a more accurate value than calculated O2 Sat, especially in critically ill patients at risk for tissue hypoxia. O2 Sat by direct measurement is performed using a blood gas analyzer with CO-oximetry. Blood gas monitoring may be performed to evaluate lung function; detect an acid-base imbalance; monitor metabolic, respiratory, and kidney disorders; and evaluate the effectiveness of treatment. A blood sample is obtained by separately reportable venipuncture, heelstick, arterial, or umbilical cord draw.

82810

82810   Gases, blood, O2 saturation only, by direct measurement, except pulse oximetry

A laboratory test is performed to measure blood oxygen saturation (O2 Sat). Oxygen saturation is the percentage of hemoglobin that is carrying oxygen. Direct measurement of O2 Sat is performed using a blood gas analyzer with CO-oximetry. Measurement of blood oxygen saturation may be done to correlate the reading of an external monitoring device (pulse oximeter) or to determine oxygen saturation in critically ill patients with poor tissue perfusion. A blood sample is obtained by separately reportable venipuncture, heelstick, arterial, or umbilical cord draw.

82820

82820   Hemoglobin-oxygen affinity (pO2 for 50% hemoglobin saturation with oxygen)

A blood test is performed to measure hemoglobin-oxygen affinity (pO2 for 50% hemoglobin saturation with oxygen) levels. The affinity of hemoglobin and oxygen measures how easily oxygen molecules can attach to hemoglobin and then be released back into body fluids. Mutations of globin genes can cause altered hemoglobin function which may manifest as an increased or decreased affinity for oxygen. Hemoglobin variants with high oxygen affinity deliver less oxygen to the peripheral tissues leading to hypoxia and increased erythropoietin production. This results in benign hereditary polycythemia. Low oxygen affinity variants are related to anemia and cyanosis. The test is performed by determining the oxygen dissociation curve (ODC) and P50 value (partial pressure of oxygen where hemoglobin is 50 percent oxygenated). The sample to be tested must be accompanied by a control sample from a non-smoking, biologically unrelated individual. A blood sample is obtained by separately reportable venipuncture. Blood is tested using Clark electrode to evaluate oxygen partial pressure and spectrophotometry to measure the degree of oxygen saturation of hemoglobin. A full oxygen dissociation curve is generated using multiple instantaneous measurements from an oxygen sensor. P50 is defined as the partial pressure of oxygen where hemoglobin is 50 percent oxygenated.

82930

82930   Gastric acid analysis, includes pH if performed, each specimen

A sample of stomach contents is obtained in a separately reportable procedure and gastric acid analysis is performed. Gastric acid is composed primarily of hydrochloric acid which is secreted by the parietal cells. This test is performed to identify hypersecretion or hyposecretion. Increased secretion can cause gastric ulcers or damage to the esophagus due to gastroesophageal reflux. Reduced secretion can be indicative of conditions such as pernicious anemia, atrophic gastritis, or Menetrier's disease. Gastric acid analysis is typically performed both without and with stimulation. Multiple timed samples may be obtained without stimulation to evaluate basal acid output. Following separately reportable administration of medication that stimulates gastric secretion, additional samples may be obtained. Each sample is then evaluated using titration assay for analysis of volume, color, hydrogen ion concentration, and pH. Analysis of each specimen is reported separately.

82938

82938   Gastrin after secretin stimulation

A blood test is performed to measure gastrin levels after an injection of the digestive hormone secretin. Gastrin is a hormone produced by G-cells in the lining of the stomach. Gastrin is released in response to food ingestion which then triggers the release of gastric acid. It also has a mild effect on the pancreas to release digestive enzyme, the liver to release bile and the intestines to increase motility. The test may be performed to diagnose tumors of the pancreas and small intestine, G-cell hyperplasia, pernicious anemia and the cause of recurrent peptic ulcers. A blood sample is obtained by separately reportable venipuncture at the time of injection and 5, 10, 15 and 30 minutes post injection. Serum is tested using quantitative chemiluminescent immunoassay.

82941

82941   Gastrin

A blood test is performed to measure gastrin levels. Gastrin is a hormone produced by G-cells in the lining of the stomach. Gastrin is released in response to food ingestion which triggers the release of gastric acid. It also has a mild effect on the pancreas to release digestive enzymes, the liver to release bile and the intestines to increase motility. A blood sample is obtained by separately reportable venipuncture. Serum is tested using quantitative chemiluminescent immunoassay.

82943

82943   Glucagon

A laboratory test is performed to measure the level of glucagon, a hormone produced by the pancreas. Glucagon raises blood sugar levels by stimulating the liver to release its glycogen stores (glycogenolysis). This test may be ordered to evaluate and monitor glycogonoma and other glucagon producing tumors. A blood sample is obtained by separately reportable venipuncture. Plasma is tested using qualitative radioimmunoassay.

82945

82945   Glucose, body fluid, other than blood

A sample of body fluid other than blood is tested for glucose. Body fluids that may be tested include pericardial, peritoneal, pleural, or synovial fluid. Decreased glucose concentration in these body fluids is typically associated with septic or inflammatory processes. In the case of pleural effusion, low glucose is associated with empyema, tuberculosis, malignant neoplasm, and rheumatoid effusion. Specimen is collected by separately reportable pericardiocentesis, thoracentesis, peritoneocentesis, or aspiration of synovial fluid. The body fluid is tested using enzymatic methodology.

82946

82946   Glucagon tolerance test

A laboratory test is performed to measure glucose and lactate levels following the administration of glucagon. Glucagon is a hormone produced by the pancreas that raises blood sugar levels by stimulating the liver to release its glycogen stores (glycogenolysis). The glucagon tolerance test may be used to differentiate or diagnose glycogen storage diseases (von Gierke's disease, Cori's disease). The patient should fast for a minimum of 14 hours prior to the start of the test. An intravenous (IV) line may be placed by separately reportable procedure. A blood sample is obtained for glucose and lactate levels from the IV line or by separately reportable venipuncture. Glucagon is administered via IV push or intramuscularly (IM). Blood samples are drawn at 30, 60, 90, and 120 minutes post injection for glucose and lactate levels by separately reportable venipuncture. Serum/plasma is tested for glucose and lactate using quantitative enzymatic method.

82947-82948

82947   Glucose; quantitative, blood (except reagent strip)
82948   Glucose; blood, reagent strip

A blood sample is obtained to measure total (quantitative) blood glucose level. Glucose is a simple sugar that is the main source of energy for the body. Carbohydrates are broken

Pathology and Laboratory

down into simple sugars, primarily glucose, absorbed by the intestine, and circulated in the blood. Insulin, a hormone produced by the pancreas, regulates glucose level in the blood and transports glucose to cells in other tissues and organs. When more glucose is available in the blood than is required, it is converted to glycogen and stored in the liver or converted to fat and stored in adipose (fat) tissue. If the glucose/insulin metabolic process is working properly, blood glucose will remain at a fairly constant, healthy level. Glucose is measured to determine whether the glucose/insulin metabolic process is functioning properly. It is used to monitor glucose levels and determine whether they are too low (hypoglycemia) or too high (hyperglycemia) as well as test for diabetes and monitor blood sugar control in diabetics. Use 82947 for quantitative blood glucose determination by enzymatic methodology or any method other than reagent strip. Use 82948 for blood glucose determination by reagent strip. A drop of blood is placed on a reagent strip, which is then compared to a calibrated color scale and a visual determination is made as to the amount of glucose present in the specimen.

82950

82950   Glucose; post glucose dose (includes glucose)

A laboratory test is performed to measure the level of glucose, a simple sugar molecule that provides energy to cells. Glucose is ingested in many different foods and can also be synthesized from glycogen stores in the liver and muscle tissue. The pancreatic hormones insulin and glucagon help to regulate blood glucose levels (BGL). A post load, BGL is routinely monitored during pregnancy, usually between 24-28 weeks gestation. Hormones produced by the placenta can cause impaired glucose metabolism in the mother leading to elevated maternal BGL and overnutrition/excess growth of the baby. The patient does not need to be fasting for this test. A 50 g oral dose of concentrated glucose (Glucola) is given to the patient. A blood sample is obtained by separately reportable venipuncture 60 minutes post ingestion. Plasma is tested using quantitative enzymatic method.

82951-82952

82951   Glucose; tolerance test (GTT), 3 specimens (includes glucose)
82952   Glucose; tolerance test, each additional beyond 3 specimens (List separately in addition to code for primary procedure)

A laboratory test is performed to measure glucose, a simple sugar molecule that provides energy to cells. Glucose is ingested in many different foods and can also be synthesized from glycogen stores in the liver and muscle tissue. The pancreatic hormones insulin and glucagon help to regulate blood glucose levels (BGL). A glucose tolerance test (GTT) may be ordered when a patient has a positive glucose screening test to diagnose gestational diabetes, diabetes mellitus, or impaired glucose tolerance and may also be used to test for lactose intolerance and malabsorption disorders. The patient should fast for a minimum of 8 hours prior to the test. A blood sample is obtained by separately reportable venipuncture for a baseline blood glucose level. A 75 g (100 g if the patient is pregnant) oral dose of concentrated glucose (Glucola) is given to the patient. A blood sample is obtained by separately reportable venipuncture at 60, 120, and 180 minutes post ingestion. Plasma is tested using quantitative enzymatic method. When testing for lactose intolerance and malabsorption disorders, a baseline blood glucose level is obtained followed by a 50 g oral dose of concentrated glucose (Glucola). Blood samples are obtained at 30, 60, 120, and 180 minutes post ingestion and plasma is tested for glucose levels using quantitative enzymatic method. The first 3 blood samples are reported using code 82951; additional samples are reported using code 82952.

82955-82960

82955   Glucose-6-phosphate dehydrogenase (G6PD); quantitative
82960   Glucose-6-phosphate dehydrogenase (G6PD); screen

Glucose-6-phosphate dehydrogenase (G6PD) is an enzyme important in red blood cell metabolism. Genetic mutations on the X chromosome may lead to a reduction of the G6PD enzyme which can then cause abnormal red blood cell breakdown (hemolysis). Neonates with G6PD deficiency may have prolonged neonatal jaundice. G6PD deficiency can cause non-immune hemolytic anemia and/or crisis in response to infection or other illness or exposure to certain foods (fava beans), chemicals or drugs. In 82955, a blood sample is obtained to measure the amount of G6PD in the blood. Blood is tested using quantitative enzymatic methodology. In 82960, a blood test is performed to screen for the presence of G6PD in the blood. Screening is performed by Beutler fluorescent spot test.

82962

82962   Glucose, blood by glucose monitoring device(s) cleared by the FDA specifically for home use

A portable testing device called a glucometer is used at the patient's home or a physician's office to monitor glucose levels in the the blood. Glucose is a monosaccharide (single sugar) used for energy by the body. Certain diseases, such as diabetes, and medications may cause glucose levels to be abnormally high or low. A blood sample is obtained by fingerstick and placed on a test strip. Most commercial glucometers use a chemically treated test strip that produces a small electric current when blood is introduced. The strength of the electrical charge is dependent on the level of glucose in the sample. The

glucose level is displayed on the monitoring device in a numeric measurement as mg/dL. This code is only reported when the physician or other healthcare professional uses this type of device in the office or other setting to check glucose levels, not when the patient self-administers the test.

82963

82963   Glucosidase, beta

A laboratory test is performed to measure the level of beta-glucosidase, an enzyme required for carbohydrate metabolism. Absent or deficient beta-glucosidase may be found in Gaucher's disease, a lysosomal storage disorder. Further genetic studies should be performed when the results of beta-glucosidase testing are abnormal. A blood sample is obtained by separately reportable venipuncture. Leukocytes are tested using fluorometry.

82965

82965   Glutamate dehydrogenase

A laboratory test is performed to measure the level of glutamate dehydrogenase (GLDH). GLDH is a mitochondrial enzyme necessary for carbon-nitrogen (urea) metabolism. A GLDH level may be ordered as a differential tool when other liver function tests are abnormal. Elevated levels of GLDH are present in hepatocytic necrosis due to toxic or hypoxic liver damage, but will not elevate with inflammatory hepatitis. A blood sample is obtained by separately reportable venipuncture. Serum is tested using spectrophotometry.

82977

82977   Glutamyltransferase, gamma (GGT)

A blood test is performed to measure gamma glutamyltransferase (GGT) levels. GGT is an enzyme that assists with the transfer of amino acids across cell membranes, including cells found in the liver, kidney, pancreas, heart, brain, and seminal vesicles. GGT levels are used as a diagnostic marker for certain diseases of the liver, bile ducts, and pancreas. A blood sample is obtained by separately reportable venipuncture. Serum or plasma is tested using quantitative enzymatic methodology.

82978

82978   Glutathione

A laboratory test is performed to measure glutathione. Glutathione is an important antioxidant easily synthesized by the body from the amino acids cysteine, glutamine, and glycine. The enzyme glutamine synthase is required for this process and glutathione levels can be affected when a mutation occurs on certain genes (GSTM1, GSTP1). Testing for glutathione in patients with chronic diseases, immune system dysfunction, and myopathies or neurological disorders may be helpful in determining a genetically inherited cause for illness. A blood sample is obtained by separately reportable venipuncture. Whole blood is tested using quantitative kinetic.

82985

82985   Glycated protein

A blood test is performed to measure glycated protein which is a compound formed when glucose molecules combine with proteins. This test is not specific for one type of glycated protein and may be used for evaluation of glycated albumin, fructosamine, alpha 1 acid glycoprotein (A1AG) (AGP) or other glycated proteins. Glycated albumin or fructosamine testing is performed on a diabetic patient to monitor blood glucose levels over time and to determine whether changes in the treatment plan have been effective. This test is performed to evaluate average blood glucose levels over the previous 2-3 weeks. An increased value of glycated albumin or fructosamine indicates that average glucose levels over the previous 2-3 weeks have also been elevated. This code is also used for evaluation of A1AG levels. A1AG is an acute-phase protein secreted by the liver that increases in concentration when inflammation is present in the body. An elevated serum level of acute-phase inflammatory markers such as A1AG is associated with an increased risk of cardiovascular disease. A blood sample is obtained by separately reportable venipuncture. A test for glycated albumin is performed on serum or plasma using quantitative boronate affinity chromatography/immunoturbidimetric. To test for fructosamine in serum or plasma, quantitative spectrophotometry is used. Ascorbic acid (Vitamin C) can influence the results of fructosamine testing and should not be taken 24 hours prior to the blood draw. A1AG is measured in serum using quantitative nephelometry.

83001-83002

83001   Gonadotropin; follicle stimulating hormone (FSH)
83002   Gonadotropin; luteinizing hormone (LH)

A blood or urine sample is tested for the presence of follicle stimulating hormone (FSH) (83001) or luteinizing hormone (LH) (83002). Both of these hormones are gonadotropins— hormones produced by the pituitary gland that promote growth and function of the gonads (sex organs). Gonadotropins are essential for egg and sperm development and are also responsible for development of secondary female and male sex characteristics including voice, muscle, hair, and breast development. Each gonadotropin serves a very specific function. In females, LH and FSH work together to stimulate development of the graafian follicle and ovulation. In males, LH stimulates the production of testosterone while FSH promotes sperm formation. Serum FSH and LH levels are obtained together with other tests to work up infertility in both men and women. Serum FSH and LH levels are also used to investigate menstrual irregularities, help diagnose disorders of the pituitary gland or diseases of the ovaries or testes, and to diagnose delayed or precocious puberty. Urine LH levels are performed to detect a rise in LH associated with ovulation. Both FSH and LH serum tests are performed using electrochemiluminescent immunoassay.

83003

83003   Growth hormone, human (HGH) (somatotropin)

A blood test is performed to measure human growth hormone (HGH) or somatotropin. HGH is produced by the pituitary gland and released in bursts throughout the day. Random levels are not clinically significant and general screening for this hormone is not routinely done. Testing is most often performed when there is evidence of delayed or excessive growth in children and/or young adults. A blood sample is obtained by separately reportable venipuncture. Serum or plasma is tested using quantitative chemiluminescent immunoassay.

83009

83009   Helicobacter pylori, blood test analysis for urease activity, non-radioactive isotope (eg, C-13)

A laboratory test is performed to measure blood urease activity using a non-radioactive isotope (C-13). The blood urease test may be used to diagnose Helicobacter pylori infection in patients with chronic active gastritis, duodenal ulcer, or nonulcerative dyspepsia. H. pylori is a bacterium found in the stomach. It burrows into the gastric mucosa to reach the less acidic epithelial cells and produces an enzyme called urease that further enables it to survive in an acidic environment. The bacterium causes inflammation followed by an immune response. A baseline blood sample is collected by separately reportable venipuncture and a second blood sample is collected following oral ingestion of C-13. In the presence of gastric H. pylori, (13) C-urea will produce (13) CO2 which is absorbed by the blood and later exhaled in the breath.

83010-83012

83010   Haptoglobin; quantitative
83012   Haptoglobin; phenotypes

Haptoglobin (Hp) is a protein encoded by the HP gene. It binds with free plasma hemoglobin which is then filtered and removed from the blood by the spleen. The removal of free hemoglobin prevents kidney damage and iron loss. The test is most often used to screen for or monitor intravascular hemolytic anemia including transfusion reactions, autoimmune hemolytic anemia and acute inflammatory reactions. In 83010, a blood test is performed to measure the haptoglobin (Hp) level. A blood sample is obtained by separately reportable venipuncture. Serum or plasma is tested using quantitative immunoturbidimetric. In 83012, haptoglobin phenotypes are identified. There are 3 haptoglobin phenotypes; Hp 1-1 which is the most active in binding free hemoglobin and suppressing inflammatory responses, Hp 2-1 which shows moderate activity in response to free hemoglobin and inflammation and Hp 2-2 which shows very little activity. There are also some additional very rare haptoglobin phenotypes. The various haptoglobin phenotypes are associated with different clinical conditions and testing for the specific phenotype may be performed to identify susceptibility to certain conditions.

83013-83014

83013   Helicobacter pylori; breath test analysis for urease activity, non-radioactive isotope (eg, C-13)
83014   Helicobacter pylori; drug administration

A laboratory test is performed to measure exhaled breath for urease activity. This test may be used to diagnose and monitor Helicobacter pylori infection in patients with chronic active gastritis, duodenal ulcer, or nonulcerative dyspepsia. H. pylori is a bacterium found in the stomach. It burrows into the gastric mucosa to reach the less acidic epithelial cells and produces an enzyme called urease that further enables it to survive in an acidic environment. The bacterium causes inflammation followed by an immune response. A baseline breath sample is collected from the patient followed by the oral ingestion of a capsule or solution of reconstituted Pranactin-Citric containing 75 mg of (13) C-urea which decomposes to (13) CO2 and NH4 in the stomach. A second breath sample is collected 13-18 minutes following the ingestion of Pranactin-Citric. In the presence of gastric H. pylori, (13) C-urea will produce (13) CO2 which is absorbed by the blood and exhaled in the breath. Exhaled breath is tested using quantitative infrared spectrophotometry. Code 83013 is used for the analysis of the breath sample and includes medication and test supplies. Code 83014 is used for administration of the medication and collection of the breath sample.

83015-83018

▲ **83015   Heavy metal (eg, arsenic, barium, beryllium, bismuth, antimony, mercury); qualitative, any number of analytes**
▲ **83018   Heavy metal (eg, arsenic, barium, beryllium, bismuth, antimony, mercury); quantitative, each, not elsewhere specified**

Heavy metals occur naturally in the ecosystem and may include any element that exhibits some metallic properties. They are often present in the form of environmental pollution especially fuel waste, and toxic exposure, such as alloy production and manufacturing. In order to function optimally, the human body may have a biological need for certain heavy metals in very small amounts. Other heavy metals, to much accumulation, are toxic to the body. In 83015, a laboratory test is performed to qualify the presence of a specific heavy metal(s) in any number of analytes. This test may be performed when there has been a known exposure such as in the workplace or during an environmental disaster. It may also be carried out when there are symptoms suggestive of an exposure such as anemia, neurological changes, brain dysfunction, kidney or liver damage, or fetal loss. Samples of blood, urine, hair, fingernails, or other body tissue may be tested. In 83018, a quantitative analysis is performed to determine the amount of each heavy metal, not elsewhere specified, present in a laboratory specimen. The testing methodology depends on the specific heavy metal being evaluated.

83020-83021

83020   Hemoglobin fractionation and quantitation; electrophoresis (eg, A2, S, C, and/or F)
83021   Hemoglobin fractionation and quantitation; chromatography (eg, A2, S, C, and/or F)

A blood test is performed to identify and measure hemoglobin (Hb) variants on red blood cells (RBCs). Hemoglobin is the protein molecule responsible for transporting oxygen on RBCs. Normal adult hemoglobin (HbA) is most common and is characterized by 2 alpha and 2 beta chains. A normal variant of HbA is HbA2, with 2 alpha chains and 2 delta chains. The presences of delta chains may indicate delta thalassemia trait or disease. HbC, is an abnormal hemoglobin with a substitution of lysine for glutamic acid in position 6 of the Beta globulin chain, it can cause mild hemolytic anemia with homozygous pairing of the gene mutation. HbF represents fetal hemoglobin and is made up of 2 alpha and 2 gamma chains. Fetal hemoglobin is present during the 2nd and 3rd trimesters of pregnancy and may be found normally in infants up to 6 months of age. The gamma chains allow oxygen to bind more readily, ensuring the fetus receives adequate oxygen supplies from the mother. Fetal hemoglobin may be reactivated in adults using hydroxyurea and recombinant erythropoietin to treat sickle cell disease. HbS arises from the substitution of valine for glutamic acid in position 6 of the Beta globulin chain. This gene mutation causes sickle cell trait or disease. A blood sample is obtained by separately reportable venipuncture. In 83020, whole blood is tested using high performance liquid electrophoresis to determine the types and quantities of hemoglobin variants HbA2, HbC, HbS and/or HbF. In 83021, whole blood is tested using high performance liquid chromatography.

83026

83026   Hemoglobin; by copper sulfate method, non-automated

A blood test is performed to determine if hemoglobin levels are above or below 12.5 g/dl. Hemoglobin is the protein molecule responsible for transporting oxygen on red blood cells (RBCs). The assessment of hemoglobin levels by non-automated copper sulfate method is most often performed as a quick screening to determine if someone can be a blood donor. A drop of blood is obtained from a fingerstick and collected in a capillary tube. The blood droplet is placed in a clear test tube containing copper sulfate solution. If the droplet sinks quickly it can be safely assumed the hemoglobin level of the sample is >12.5 g/dl. and a blood donation can be made. A blood droplet that floats or sinks slowly in the solution may indicate a hemoglobin level <12.5 g/dl. and a more precise separately reportable test is typically performed.

83030

83030   Hemoglobin; F (fetal), chemical

A laboratory test is performed to measure fetal hemoglobin (Hemoglobin F, HbF). Hemoglobin is the oxygen carrying molecule attached to red blood cells (RBCs), and fetal hemoglobin has a greater oxygen binding ability than adult hemoglobin. Hemoglobin F is present during fetal development starting at approximately 10 weeks gestation and continues for 6 months after birth. Hemoglobin F may persist in children with thalassemia disorders and may be pharmacologically reactivated in adults using hydroxyurea and recombinant erythropoietin to treat sickle cell disease. A serum test for hemoglobin F may be used to evaluate and diagnose hemolytic anemia, hereditary persistence of fetal hemoglobin, thalassemia, sickle cell disease, and to evaluate the need for additional doses of Rh-immune globulin in an Rh-negative mother who has given birth to an Rh-positive infant. A blood sample is obtained by separately reportable venipuncture. Blood may be tested using high performance liquid chromatography, flow cytometry, or mixed field agglutination.

83033

83033   Hemoglobin; F (fetal), qualitative

A laboratory test is performed to identify fetal hemoglobin (Hemoglobin F, HbF) in gastric or stool samples and in amniotic fluid. Hemoglobin is the oxygen carrying molecule attached to red blood cells (RBCs), and fetal hemoglobin has a greater oxygen binding ability than adult hemoglobin. Hemoglobin F is present during fetal development starting at approximately 10 weeks gestation and continues for 6 months after birth. A qualitative test for hemoglobin F may be performed on gastric or stool specimens from an infant to determine the source of gastrointestinal blood (maternal vs. infant). Qualitative fetal hemogloblin testing may be done in conjunction with testing for alpha fetoprotein (AFP) and acetylcholinesterase to validate elevated levels of AFP in amniotic fluid.

83036-83037

83036   Hemoglobin; glycosylated (A1C)
83037   Hemoglobin; glycosylated (A1C) by device cleared by FDA for home use

A blood test is performed to measure glycosylated hemoglobin (HbA1C) levels. Plasma glucose binds to hemoglobin and the HbA1C test measures the average plasma glucose concentration over the life of red blood cells (approximately 90-120 days). HbA1C levels may be used as a diagnostic reference for patients with suspected diabetes mellitus (DM) and to monitor blood glucose control in patients with known DM. HbA1C levels should be monitored at least every 6 months in patients with DM and more frequently when the level is >7.0%. In 83036, a blood sample is obtained by separately reportable venipuncture. Whole blood is tested using quantitative high performance liquid chromatography/boronate affinity. In 83037, the HbA1C test is performed using a FDA approved testing device for home use. A capillary or venous blood sample is obtained. A drop of blood is placed in buffer solution and shaken to lyse the red blood cells. The sample is then transferred to the testing device where the HbAlC levels are measured and results displayed on the device.

83045-83050

83045   Hemoglobin; methemoglobin, qualitative
83050   Hemoglobin; methemoglobin, quantitative

Methemoglobin is an oxygen carrying metalloprotein hemoglobin in which the iron of the heme group is in the oxidized ferric state instead of the reduced ferrous state. The heme group is not able to release bound oxygen. Approximately 1-2% of all hemoglobin in the human body is in the methemoglobin form. Larger amounts may be inherited (rare) but are more often acquired as a result of exposure to drugs or toxins. A blood sample is obtained by separately reportable venipuncture. Use 83045 when the specimen is tested for the presence of methemoglobin. Use 83050 when the amount of methemoglobin in the blood is determined.

83051

83051   Hemoglobin; plasma

A blood test is performed to measure plasma hemoglobin levels. Hemoglobin is normally found inside erythrocytes (red blood cells). Intravascular hemolysis due to hereditary, acquired, or iatrogenic conditions can occur, causing hemoglobin to be released from erythrocytes into the surrounding plasma. Protective hemoglobin scavenging mechanisms will then take place but once these mechanisms have been saturated, free hemoglobin levels increase to measurable levels in the plasma. A blood sample is obtained by separately reportable venipuncture. Plasma is tested using quantitative spectrophotometry.

83055-83060

83060   Hemoglobin; sulfhemoglobin, quantitative

Sulfhemoglobinemia is a rare condition that occurs when sulfur atoms incorporate into the hemoglobin molecule. The red blood cells are then incapable of binding and carrying oxygen. This very rare condition usually results from an overdose of medication containing sulfonamides or occupational exposure to sulfur compounds. A blood sample is obtained by separately reportable venipuncture. In 83055, a qualitative blood test is performed to determine whether sulfhemoglobin is present. In 83060, a blood test is performed to measure sulfhemoglobin levels in whole blood. Whole blood is tested using spectrophotometry.

83065

83065   Hemoglobin; thermolabile

A blood sample is drawn and subjected to heat, which effectively kills the globin in the blood sample for further study.

83068

83068   Hemoglobin; unstable, screen

A blood test is performed to identify unstable hemoglobin molecules. Unstable hemoglobin is caused by an inherited genetic mutation of the globin gene. It is a rare, usually autosomal dominate disorder which causes an alteration in the solubility of hemoglobin

due to amino acid residue oxidation in globin chains. The test is performed when there is unexplained hemolytic anemia and other hemolytic disorders such as sickle hemoglobin, fetal hemoglobin and methemoglobin disorders have been ruled out. Test results on infants (age 6 months and younger) are considered to be unreliable. A blood sample is obtained by separately reportable venipuncture. Whole blood is tested using visual identification of hemoglobin precipitates.

83069

83069   Hemoglobin; urine

A laboratory test is performed to measure free hemoglobin in urine. Hemoglobin is the oxygen carrying molecule attached to red blood cells (RBCs). Hemoglobinuria may present with RBCs in the form of gross hematuria, or it may be detectable only microscopically. Hemoglobinuria with RBCs occurs most commonly as a result of direct bleeding in the urinary tract. Hemoglobinuria without RBCs usually indicates a rapid rise in free hemoglobin levels, which are elevated in the blood and the kidneys then try to excrete it. The condition may be caused by kidney infection, inflammation, or tumor, severe burns, malaria, hemolytic urea syndrome, sickle cell disease, transfusion reactions, thrombocytic purpura, and hemolytic anemia. A urine sample is obtained from the patient by random void or catheterization. Urine is tested using quantitative spectrophotometry.

83070

83070   Hemosiderin, qualitative

Hemosiderin is an insoluble iron-containing protein present inside of cells, most commonly found in macrophages. They are a marker for intravascular hemorrhage. Hemosiderin appears in urine when free hemoglobin levels are elevated in the blood and the kidney then tries to excrete it. A random urine or first morning voided specimen are obtained and a qualitative test is performed to identify the presence of hemosiderin using a methodology such as semi-quantitative microscopic stain.

83080

83080   b-Hexosaminidase, each assay

A blood test is performed to measure b-Hexosaminidase levels on serum and leukocytes. Hexosaminidase is an enzyme involved in hydrolysis of hexosamine. The enzyme has three (3) functional lysosomal forms (A, B, S). Hex A is the deficient enzyme in Tay-Sachs disease and other variants. Total deficiency, Hex A plus Hex B is present in Sandhoff disease and variants. Hex S is a minor component and does not factor into Sandhoff disease. A blood sample is obtained by separately reportable venipuncture. Serum is tested using heat inactivation/fluorometric/automated. Leukocytes are tested using heat inactivation/fluorometric/semiautomated. Report code 83080 for each assay performed.

83088

83088   Histamine

A blood or urine test is performed to measure histamine levels. Histamine is a nitrogen compound produced by basophiles and mast cells and is involved in the local immune response to foreign pathogens. Histamine also regulates the physiological function of the stomach and intestines and acts as a neurotransmitter. A blood sample is obtained by separately reportable venipuncture. A urine sample may be from a random void or 24 hour specimen collection. Plasma and whole blood are tested using quantitative enzyme-linked immunosorbent assay. Urine is tested using quantitative enzyme immunoassay.

83090

83090   Homocysteine

A blood test is performed to measure homocysteine levels. Homocysteine is a non-protein homologue of the amino acid cysteine. It is biosynthesized in the body by a multi-step process from methionine. Elevated levels of homocysteine are a risk factor for cardiovascular disease. Other conditions that may cause elevated homocysteine levels include: Vitamin B deficiency, intense (prolonged) exercise, alcoholism, genetically inherited diseases. A blood sample is obtained by separately reportable venipuncture. Serum or plasma is tested using quantitative enzymatic technique.

83150

83150   Homovanillic acid (HVA)

A test is performed on urine to measure homovanillic acid (HVA) levels. HVA is catecholamine metabolite that may be elevated in response to metabolic stress and in the presence of a neuroblastoma or malignant pheochromocytoma. Other factors that my raise HVA levels are: hypertension, anxiety, intense physical activity and many prescription and OTC drugs. Levels may be markedly decreased in smokers. A random voided or 24 hour urine specimen is obtained. Urine is tested using quantitative high performance liquid chromatography.

Pathology and Laboratory

● New Code   ▲ Revised Code   CPT © 2016 American Medical Association. All Rights Reserved.

83491

83491   Hydroxycorticosteroids, 17- (17-OHCS)

A blood or urine test is performed to measure 17-hydroxycorticosteroids (17-OHCS) levels. 17-OHCS is an inactive product that forms when the hormone cortisol, is broken down by the liver and other body tissue. High levels can indicate Cushing's syndrome. 17-OHCS levels may vary significantly at different times of the day. The ideal time to collect a sample for testing is between 6 am and 11 am. The following drugs/medications may increase the blood and/or urine levels: estrogen, dexamethasone, antibiotics such as ampicillin and gentamycin. A blood sample is obtained by separately reportable venipuncture. Serum or plasma is tested using quantitative high performance liquid chromatography-tandem mass spectrometry. A random voided or 24 hour urine specimen is tested using quantitative phenylhydrazine-sulfuric acid reaction (Porter-Silber test).

83497

83497   Hydroxyindolacetic acid, 5-(HIAA)

A urine test is performed to measure 5-hydroxyindolacetic acid (5-HIAA). 5-HIAA is a metabolite of serotonin, a monoamine neurotransmitter derived from tryptophan. Levels of 5-HIAA may be elevated in patients with tumors (especially of the small intestine), kidney disease/dysfunction, small bowel resection and autism spectrum disorders. Certain drugs/medications that alter serotonin levels and foods rich in serotonin may alter the test results. These foods/drugs should be avoided for 72 hours prior to and during the collection of the urine sample. A random voided or 24 hour urine specimen is tested using quantitative high performance liquid chromatography.

83498

83498   Hydroxyprogesterone, 17-d

A blood or urine test is performed to measure 17-hydroxyprogesterone (17-OHP). 17-OHP is a naturally occurring progesterone produced primarily in the adrenal glands and corpus luteum of the ovary. Levels may be increased in infants with congenital adrenal hyperplasia and this test is included in newborn screening panels. In adults, levels may also be influenced by the presence of adrenal and ovarian tumors, polycystic ovarian syndrome (PCOS) and pregnancy (3rd trimester). A blood test is obtained by separately reportable venipuncture. Infants may have blood drawn by heelstick/capillary method. Serum or plasma is tested using quantitative high performance liquid chromatography-tandem mass spectrometry or quantitative radioimmunoassay. Alternatively, a 24 hour urine specimen may be collected and tested using radioimmunoassay.

83499

83499   Hydroxyprogesterone, 20-

A laboratory test is performed to measure the level of 20-alpha (20α) hydroxyprogesterone, an inactive form of the hormone progesterone. 20α-hydroxyprogesterone is catalyzed from progesterone by the enzyme 20α hydroxysteroid dehydrogenase (20α-HSD). Progesterone is essential for conception and the maintenance of pregnancy. An imbalance of active progesterone and 20α hydroxyprogesterone may cause infertility, miscarriage, and/or preterm labor. A blood sample is obtained by separately reportable venipuncture. Serum is tested using radioimmune assay.

83500-83505

83500   Hydroxyproline; free
83505   Hydroxyproline; total

Hydroxyproline is a non-protein amino acid found primarily in collagen protein. Hydroxyproline is a non-protein amino acid found primarily in collagen protein. Levels may be elevated in Paget's disease, bone metastatic cancer, hyperparathyroidism, osteoporosis, glucocorticoid excess. Test may be used as a non-specific marker for bone resorption although newer tests are available. The ingestion of collagen may alter test results. In 83500, free hydroxyproline in the blood is measured. A blood specimen is obtained by separately reportable venipuncture and quantitative analysis performed on blood plasma or serum by high performance liquid chromatography. Alternatively, a urine test may performed to measure free hydroxyproline levels. Patients should be on a collagen free diet for 72 hours prior to the collection of urine. A 24 hour urine specimen is collected and tested using colorimetric methodology. In 83505, total hydroxyproline in the urine is evaluated. Patients should be on a collagen free diet for 72 hours prior to the collection of urine. A 24 hour urine specimen is collected and tested using ion exchange chromatography or high performance liquid chromatography.

83516-83518

83516   Immunoassay for analyte other than infectious agent antibody or infectious agent antigen; qualitative or semiquantitative, multiple step method
83518   Immunoassay for analyte other than infectious agent antibody or infectious agent antigen; qualitative or semiquantitative, single step method (eg, reagent strip)

An immunoassay is performed to detect a chemical substance (analyte) other than an antigen or antibody produced by the body in response to an infectious agent. There are dozens of immunoassays for non-infectious antigens and antibodies that are reported with these codes. Examples of non-infectious diseases and disorders that may be worked up using these tests include: celiac disease, motor and sensory neuropathy, Crohn's disease or other inflammatory bowel disease, liver disease, thyroid disease. Examples of specific antigens and antibodies reported with these codes include: Asialo IgG and IgM, ganglioside IgG and IgM, gliadin IgA and IgG. Codes are reported for each immunoglobin class or subclass tested using this technique, so for example when testing for gliadin IgA and IgG by immunoassay, the code would be reported twice. Qualitative or semiquantitative testing is performed. Qualitative tests detect only the presence or absence of the specific substance. Semiquantitative tests provide a rough estimate of the amount of the substance being tested. Use 83516 for qualitative or semiquantitative immunoassay using a multistep method. Use 83518 for a single step method such as a reagent strip test.

83519-83520

83519   Immunoassay for analyte other than infectious agent antibody or infectious agent antigen; quantitative, by radioimmunoassay (eg, RIA)
83520   Immunoassay for analyte other than infectious agent antibody or infectious agent antigen; quantitative, not otherwise specified

A quantitative immunoassay is performed to detect a chemical substance (analyte) other than an antigen or antibody produced by the body in response to an infectious agent. There are dozens of immunoassays for non-infectious antigens and antibodies that are reported with these codes. Examples of non-infectious diseases and disorders that may be worked up using these tests include: myasthenia gravis, pancreatic disease, parathyroid disease as well as many other diseases and conditions. Examples of specific substances reported with these codes include: neuronal antibodies, cytokine production, vascular endothelial growth factor and many others. Quantitative testing measures the exact amount or level of the substance in the test sample. Use 83519 for quantitative radioimmunoassay (RIA) testing method. RIA uses radioisotope labeled antigens or other radioisotope labeled substances along with unlabeled substances to bind the specific antigen or substance being tested. Binding of the substance to the radiolabeled antigen or other substance allows the substance to be measured (quantified). RIA allows the measurement of minute quantities of enzymes, hormones or other substances. Use 83520 for any quantitative testing method other than radioimmunoassay. Codes are reported for each substance class or subclass tested using this technique, so for example when testing for interleukin 4, 5, 10, and 13 by multi-analyte fluorescence detection, the code 83520 would be reported four times.

83525-83527

83525   Insulin; total
83527   Insulin; free

Insulin is a hormone produced by the pancreas. It helps the body to utilize circulating blood glucose for energy and stores excess glucose as glycogen in liver and muscle cells. A blood sample is obtained by separately reportable venipuncture. Specimen may be taken at a random time, when the patient fasting and/or at timed intervals (30, 60, 90, 120 minutes) following a 75 gram glucose challenge. In 83525, a blood test is performed to measure total insulin levels. Serum or plasma is tested using quantitative chemiluminescent immunoassay. In 83527, a blood test is performed to measure free insulin levels. Patient should be fasting. Serum or plasma is tested using quantitative ultrafiltration.

83528

83528   Intrinsic factor

A laboratory test is performed to measure the level of intrinsic factor (IF). Intrinsic factor is a glycoprotein produced by parietal cells in the stomach and necessary for absorption of vitamin B12 (cobalamin) in the intestine. The production of IF may be affected by autoimmune disorders that target intrinsic factor and/or parietal cells; atropic gastritis that damages parietal cells; bariatric surgery; gastric tumors; and congenital deficiencies of intrinsic factor caused by a mutation in the GIF gene on chromosome 11. A deficiency of intrinsic factor can lead to megaloblastic anemia, autoimmune pernicious anemia, and with congenital deficiency, a failure to thrive as well as neurological abnormalities. Gastric aspirate may be tested for intrinsic factor using the charcoal method of immunoassay.

83540

83540   Iron

A blood, urine or liver test is performed to measure iron levels. Iron (Fe) is an essential element that circulates in the blood attached to the protein transferrin. Iron is necessary component of hemoglobin, found in red blood cells (RBCs) and myoglobin found in muscle cells. Low iron levels may cause a decrease in red blood cells and iron deficiency anemia. High iron levels may be caused by excessive intake of iron supplements or a hereditary genetic condition such as hemochromatosis from a mutation of the RGMc gene or HAMP gene. A blood sample is obtained by separately reportable venipuncture. Serum or plasma is tested using quantitative spectrophotometry. A random voided or 24 hour urine specimen is obtained and tested using quantitative inductively coupled plasma/emission spectrometry. Patient should wait 2-4 days after receiving iodine or gadolinium contrast media to collect a urine specimen. A liver sample is obtained by a separately reportable procedure. Liver tissue is tested using quantitative inductively coupled plasma-mass spectrometry.

83550

83550   Iron binding capacity

A blood test is performed to measure the iron binding capacity of transferrin. Transferrin, a protein found in circulating blood is responsible for carrying iron molecules. This test measures the ability of transferrin to carry iron. A blood sample is obtained by separately reportable venipuncture. Serum or plasma is tested using quantitative spectrophotometry/calculation.

83570

83570   Isocitric dehydrogenase (IDH)

A laboratory test is performed to measure the level of isocitric dehydrogenase (IDH). Isocitric dehydrogenase is an enzyme that catalyzes the oxidative decarboxylation of isocitrate to form alpha-ketoglutarate (α-ketoglutarate) and carbon dioxide ($CO2$). The process takes place in the citric acid cycle with the conversion of NAD(P)+ to NAD(P)H within the cytosol, mitochondria, and peroxisomes. This crossroad reaction of cellular metabolism is fundamental in lipid synthesis, oxygen sensing and signal transduction, oxidative respiration, and for cellular defense against oxidative stress. Mutations of IDH have been identified in human cancers including gliomas and acute myeloid leukemia.

83582

83582   Ketogenic steroids, fractionation

A laboratory test is performed to measure fractionated ketogenic steroids. A ketogenic steroid is any corticosteroid and its metabolites that contain an hydroxyl group and a short carbon chain on the steroid nucleus. These include adrenal synthesized cortisol, cortisone 11-desoxycortisol, deoxycorticosterone, and their tetrahydroderivatives. Ketogenic steroid levels may be elevated in adrenal hyperplasia with precocious puberty, Cushing syndrome, obesity, and pathological stress conditions such as acute illness or infection, surgery, and burns. Ketogenic steroid levels may be decreased in Addison's disease, adrenocorticotropic hormone (ACTH) deficiency, and hypopituitarism.

83586-83593

83586   Ketosteroids, 17- (17-KS); total
83593   Ketosteroids, 17- (17-KS); fractionation

A laboratory test is performed to measure total 17-ketosteroid (17-KS) in urine. 17-KS is a ketogenic steroid that contains an hydroxyl group and a short carbon chain at the 17 position on the steroid nucleus. It can be synthesized from the adrenal hormones cortisol, cortisone 11-desoxycortisol, deoxycorticosterone, and their tetrahydroderivatives. 17-KS may be elevated in adrenal hyperplasia with precocious puberty, Cushing syndrome, obesity, and pathological stress conditions such as acute illness or infection, surgery, and burns. 17-KS may be decreased in Addison's disease, adrenocorticotropic hormone (ACTH) deficiency, and hypopituitarism. A 24-hour urine sample is obtained and tested using quantitative spectrophotometry. Use 83593 for measuring fractionated 17-ketosteroid (17-KS).

83605

83605   Lactate (lactic acid)

A blood or body fluid test is performed to measure lactate (lactic acid) levels. Lactic acid is produced primarily by muscle tissue and red blood cells in the body. Elevated levels may be caused by strenuous exercise, heart failure, severe infection (sepsis), shock states (cardiogenic, hypovolemic) and liver disease. A blood sample is obtained by separately reportable venipuncture. Cerebral spinal fluid (CSF) is obtained by lumbar puncture (spinal tap). Other body fluids may also be collected and tested. Plasma, CSF, and other body fluids are tested using enzymatic methodology.

83615

83615   Lactate dehydrogenase (LD), (LDH)

A blood or body fluid test is performed to measure lactate dehydrogenase (LD) (LDH) levels. LDH is an enzyme present in red blood cells (RBCs) and in the tissue of heart, liver, pancreas, kidney, skeletal muscle, brain and lungs. LDH levels are used as a marker for tissue and RBC damage. Elevated blood levels can be caused by stroke, myocardial infarction, liver disease, pancreatitis, muscular dystrophy, infectious mononucleosis,

hemolytic anemia and tumors/cancers such as lymphoma. Elevated cerebral spinal fluid (CSF) levels are usually indicative of bacterial meningitis. LDH levels in pleural and/or pericardial fluid can indicate if the effusion is an exudate, caused by an infection or a transudate caused by fluid pressure problem. A blood sample is obtained by separately reportable venipuncture. Cerebral spinal fluid is obtained by separately reportable lumbar puncture (spinal tap). Pericardial fluid is obtained by separately reportable pericardiocentesis. Fluid from a pleural effusion is obtained by separately reportable thoracentesis. Serum or plasma and all body fluids are tested using quantitative enzymatic methodology.

83625

83625   Lactate dehydrogenase (LD), (LDH); isoenzymes, separation and quantitation

A blood test is performed to measure lactate dehydrogenase (LD) (LDH) isoenzyme levels. LDH is an enzyme present in red blood cells (RBCs) and in the tissue of heart, liver, pancreas, kidney, skeletal muscle, brain and lungs. LDH is present in five forms, which differ slightly in structure and these five forms are found primarily in specific organs. Testing for specific LDH isoenzyme levels can determine the location of damaged tissue. LDH-1 is found primarily in heart muscle and red blood cells; LDH-2 in white blood cells; LDH-3 in the lung; LDH-4 in the kidney, placenta, and pancreas; and LDH-5 in the liver and skeletal muscle. A blood sample is obtained by separately reportable venipuncture. Serum is tested using quantitative enzymatic methodology/electrophoresis. Each LDH isoenzyme is separated and quantified individually.

83630-83631

83630   Lactoferrin, fecal; qualitative
83631   Lactoferrin, fecal; quantitative

Lactoferrin (LF) is the iron binding glycoprotein component of neutrophilic granules in white blood cells (WBCs). In 83630, a test is performed on feces to identify the presence of lactoferrin. The presence of WBCs in feces is a marker for inflammatory diarrhea caused by bacteria, ulcerative colitis or Crohn's disease. A stool sample is collected after a bowel movement and tested using qualitative enzyme-linked immunosorbent assay (ELISA). In 83631, a quantitative test is performed to measure the concentration of lactoferrin present in the stool sample. The test is used as a diagnostic aid to differentiate between inflammatory and noninflammatory types of bowel disease and can also be used to assess response to treatment in patients with inflammatory bowel disease. This test is performed using quantitative ELISA.

83632

83632   Lactogen, human placental (HPL) human chorionic somatomammotropin

A blood test is performed to measure human placental lactogen (HPL) levels. HPL, also referred to as human chorionic somatomammotropin is a polypeptide placental hormone that modifies the maternal metabolic state to ensure fetal nutrition. Maternal levels rise in relation to fetal and placental growth and are highest in the last trimester of pregnancy. HPL levels may be used as an indicator of fetal well being. A blood sample is obtained by separately reportable venipuncture. Serum is tested using enzyme immunoassay.

83633

83633   Lactose, urine, qualitative

A laboratory test is performed to detect the presence of lactose in urine and to measure the amount. Lactose is a disaccharide sugar found in milk. It is broken down in the digestive tract to glucose and galactose by the enzyme lactase. Urine lactose (lactosuria) may be a normal finding in late pregnancy and during lactation, especially when milk flow is prevented. Lactosuria may also be present in newborn infants as a transient condition without gastrointestinal symptoms. The condition is usually caused by lactose intolerance, a gastrogenic disorder that makes the gastric mucosa abnormally permeable to the sugar molecule which is not broken down. Lactose is absorbed into the blood and excreted in urine. A urine sample is obtained by random void or catheterization and tested qualitatively for lactose using chromatography.

83655

83655   Lead

A test is performed on blood, urine, hair or nails to measure lead levels. Lead is a heavy metal that can accumulate in soft tissue and bone causing damage to the nervous system and brain. Tests are performed to determine exposure and evaluate treatment. A blood sample is obtained by separately reportable venipuncture or capillary (heelstick) draw and whole blood is tested; a random voided or 24 hour urine specimen is obtained and tested; hair samples are obtained from scalp, axilla, pubic or face; or nail clippings are obtained from all 10 fingernails and toenails. All types of specimens are tested for lead using quantitative inductively coupled plasma-mass spectrometry.

83661

83661   Fetal lung maturity assessment; lecithin sphingomyelin (L/S) ratio

A fetal lung maturity assessment is performed by lecithin sphingomyelin (L/S) ratio. This test is performed before delivery on amniotic fluid to evaluate lung maturity and determine the probability of neonatal respiratory distress syndrome (RDS), also called hyaline membrane disease, developing after delivery. The test helps determine whether an attempt should be made to suppress premature labor or whether the lungs are mature enough to allow the delivery to progress. Another indication for the test is to determine whether the lungs are mature enough to allow induction of labor in patients with complications affecting the health of the mother and/or fetus. A separately reportable amniotic fluid sample is obtained. The lecithin sphingomyelin (L/S) ratio is determined. Pulmonary surfactant contains lecithin. The amount of lecithin synthesized in the lung increases as the lung matures and begins to produce surfactant. The amount of amniotic fluid and the amount of lecithin in it can vary. So, the amount of lecithin is compared to the amount of sphingomyelin, a non-pulmonary lipid, which remains relatively constant in the amniotic fluid. The result is expressed as a lecithin to sphingomyelin (L/S) ratio. L/S is tested by thin layer chromatography. L/S ratios greater than 2 indicate low risk of RDS.

83662-83664

83662   Fetal lung maturity assessment; foam stability test
83663   Fetal lung maturity assessment; fluorescence polarization
83664   Fetal lung maturity assessment; lamellar body density

A fetal lung maturity assessment is performed by foam stability test (83662), fluorescence polarization (83663), or lamellar body density (83664). These tests are performed before delivery on amniotic fluid to evaluate lung maturity and determine the probability of neonatal respiratory distress syndrome (RDS), also called hyaline membrane disease, developing after delivery. The tests help determine whether an attempt should be made to suppress premature labor or whether the lungs are mature enough to allow the delivery to progress. Another indication for the test is to determine whether the lungs are mature enough to allow induction of labor in patients with complications affecting the health of the mother and/or fetus. A separately reportable amniotic fluid sample is obtained. In 83662, foam stability index (FSI) is used to measure surfactant function in amniotic fluid. A kit containing test wells with a predispensed volume of ethanol is used. Amniotic fluid (0.5 ml) is added to the test wells. The amniotic fluid/ethanol mixture is shaken and the FSI value is read. The FSI value is represented by the ring of stable foam that results from the shaking process in the well with the highest value. In 83663, fluorescence polarization is used to test for lung maturity using an automated fluorescence polarimeter which detects the capacity of complex lipid molecules (lecithin/sphingomyelin) to retain molecular orientation when irradiated with ultraviolet light. Using this method, the relative concentration of lecithin and sphingomyelin is determined. Fluorescence polarization can also determine the surfactant to albumin ratio (SAR). A ratio of 50-70 mg of surfactant per gram of albumin is indicative of lung maturity. In 83664, fetal lung maturity is evaluated using lamellar body density. Lamellar bodies store surfactant. A small amount of amniotic fluid (less than 1 ml) is used. The number/volume of lamellar bodies in amniotic fluid is estimated using light scatter at a specific wave length or counted using the platelet channel of an automated hematology cell counting instrument. A count greater than 30,000/αl is indicative of lung maturity.

83670

83670   Leucine aminopeptidase (LAP)

A blood test is performed to measure leucine aminopeptidase (LAP) levels. LAP is a protein enzyme found in the liver and small intestine and is responsible for cell maintenance. Elevated LAP levels can indicate liver damage from conditions such as hepatitis, cirrhosis, tumors. Elevated levels may be a normal finding in the third trimester of pregnancy. A blood sample is obtained by separately reportable venipuncture. Serum is tested using quantitative spectrophotometry.

83690

83690   Lipase

A test is performed on blood and body fluids to measure lipase levels. Lipase is an enzyme released by the pancreas into the small intestine and is essential for the digestion of dietary fats. Elevated levels may result from small bowel obstruction, celiac disease, cholecystitis, duodenal ulcer, severe gastroenteritis, macrolipasemia, pancreatitis and pancreatic tumors. The test may be ordered when there is a family history of lipoprotein lipase deficiency. A blood sample is obtained by separately reportable venipuncture. Other body fluids collected by other methods. Blood and other body fluids are tested using quantitative enzymatic methodology.

83695

83695   Lipoprotein (a)

A blood test is performed to measure lipoprotein (a) levels. Abbreviated as Lp (a), lipoprotein (a) is LDL cholesterol bound to the protein, apolipoprotein (a). Lp (a) levels are genetically determined and remain fairly constant over an individuals lifetime. This test

may be used as a risk marker for cardiovascular disease. Elevated levels may result from depleted estrogen, familial hypercholesterolemia, hypothyroidism, diabetes and kidney disease. A blood sample is obtained by separately reportable venipuncture. Serum or plasma is tested using quantitative immunoturbidimetry.

83698

83698   Lipoprotein-associated phospholipase A2 (Lp-PLA2)

This code reports a test for lipoprotein-associated phospholipase A2, or Lp-PLA2, which is being used as an inflammatory risk marker for cardiovascular disease. Lp-PLA2 is an enzyme circulating in the blood that attaches to particles of LDL cholesterol in the bloodstream. When these particles adhere to arterial walls, oxidation takes place, and the oxidized LDL become susceptible to enzymatic attack. This promotes inflammatory molecules that trigger the atherosclerotic process by helping to build up fatty deposits of plaque in the arteries and also attract and bind to monocytes, large white blood cells which become macrophages that increase the amount of plaque build-up. Studies show inflammation has a role in cardiovascular disease and Lp-PLA2 is currently considered a risk marker as it has been linked to the atherosclerotic process. Higher levels have been shown to be a predictive factor in future events independent of other traditional risk factors. Lp-PLA2 is measured through a simple blood test using the enzyme linked immunosorbent assay, or ELISA test technique. This is also called the PLAC test and the values are measured in ng/mL. The average female value is 174, while the average male value is 251 ng/mL.

83700-83704

83700   Lipoprotein, blood; electrophoretic separation and quantitation
83701   Lipoprotein, blood; high resolution fractionation and quantitation of lipoproteins including lipoprotein subclasses when performed (eg, electrophoresis, ultracentrifugation)
83704   Lipoprotein, blood; quantitation of lipoprotein particle numbers and lipoprotein particle subclasses (eg, by nuclear magnetic resonance spectroscopy)

A blood test is performed to measure lipoprotein levels. Lipoproteins are biochemical structures containing lipid (fat) molecules bound to protein. Lipoproteins are transported throughout the body by circulating blood. Lipoproteins vary in size from large and less dense (fat>protein) to small and more dense (protein >fat). They may be of exogenous origin (dietary fats) or endogenous (formed in the liver). A blood sample is obtained by separately reportable venipuncture. In 83700, lipoproteins in the blood are separated using electrophoresis. Electrophoresis uses an electrical field to separate lipoprotein molecules which are then stained and quantified using a densitometer. In 83701, high resolution fractionation and quantitation of lipoproteins including separation and quantitation of lipoprotein subclasses as needed is performed using a technique such as quantitative electrophoresis or ultracentrifugation. If ultracentrifugation is performed, the lipoproteins are separated based on their hydrated densities. Salts are used to fractionate the lipoproteins and the specimen is then spun (centrifuged) which separates the very low density and low density lipoproteins from high density lipoproteins. The amount of each type is then quantified. In 83704, nuclear magnetic resonance (NMR) spectroscopy for quantitation of lipoprotein particle numbers and lipoprotein particle subclasses is performed. NMR spectroscopy detects lipoprotein particles of different sizes which allows quantitation of lipoprotein subclasses. Knowing the exact amounts of each subclass particle is helpful in assessing and managing patients with elevated triglyceride levels and also with managing cardiovascular disease risk in patients with diabetes.

83718-83721

83718   Lipoprotein, direct measurement; high density cholesterol (HDL cholesterol)
83719   Lipoprotein, direct measurement; VLDL cholesterol
83721   Lipoprotein, direct measurement; LDL cholesterol

A blood test is performed to measure lipoprotein levels. Lipoproteins are biochemical structures containing lipid (fat) molecules bound to protein and are transported throughout the body by circulating blood. Lipoproteins vary in size from large and less dense (fat>protein) to small and more dense (protein >fat). They may be of exogenous origin (dietary fats) or endogenous, formed in the liver. Direct measurement of lipoproteins involves use of a specific laboratory test for high density or low density lipoproteins rather than calculating the levels by using the results of tests for total cholesterol, high density lipoproteins, and triglycerides. A blood sample is obtained by separately reportable venipuncture. In 83718, serum/plasma is tested for high density lipoproteins (HDL) by detergent solubilization/enzymatic methodology. In 83719, very low density lipoproteins (VLDL) are measured. In 83721, serum/plasma is tested for low density lipoprotein (LDL) cholesterol by quantitative detergent solubilization/enzymatic methodology.

83727

83727   Luteinizing releasing factor (LRH)

A blood sample is tested to measure levels of luteinizing releasing factor (LRF), also referred to as luteinizing releasing hormone (LRH). LRH is a hormone produced by the

CPT © 2016 American Medical Association. All Rights Reserved.

● New Code   ▲ Revised Code

Pathology and Laboratory

hypothalamus that stimulates the pituitary gland to release follicle stimulating hormone (FSH) and luteinizing hormone (LH). Luteinizing releasing factor is tested to evaluate delayed puberty, particularly in males, and menstrual disorders, fertility problems, hirsutism, and virilization in females. After injection with gonadotropin releasing hormone, multiple blood samples are obtained at 15 minute intervals over a 1-2 hour period to determine whether the pituitary gland is responding normally to gonadotropin releasing hormone.

83735

83735   Magnesium

A blood, urine or fecal test is performed to measure magnesium levels. Magnesium is an essential dietary mineral responsible for enzyme function, energy production and contraction and relaxation of muscle fibers. Decreased levels may result from severe burns, metabolic disorders, certain medications and low blood calcium levels. A blood sample is obtained by separately reportable venipuncture. Red blood cells (RBCs) are tested using quantitative inductively coupled plasma-mass spectrometry. Serum/plasma is tested using quantitative spectrophotometry. A 24 hour voided urine specimen is tested using quantitative spectrophotometry. A random or 24 hour fecal sample is tested using quantitative spectrophotometry.

83775

83775   Malate dehydrogenase

A laboratory test is performed to measure malate dehydrogenase (MDH), a nucleotide binding protein enzyme with several isoforms differing in subcellular location and function. MDH reversibly catalyzes the oxidation of malate to oxaloacetate by reduction of NAD+ to NADH during the citric acid cycle and along other metabolic pathways primarily in the mitochondria and cytosol. MDH is also involved with glucose synthesis (gluconeogenesis). Sample is tested using spectrophotometry.

83785

83785   Manganese

A blood or urine test is performed to measure manganese levels. Manganese is a trace mineral found in bone, liver, pancreas and kidney tissue. It cofactors with enzymes to detoxify free radicals and is necessary to form bone and connective tissue, (blood) clotting factors and sex hormones. Manganese also assists with fat and carbohydrate metabolism, regulation of blood glucose levels and in the function of brain and nerve cells. A blood sample is obtained by separately reportable venipuncture. Urine may be a random void or 24 hour specimen. Serum, whole blood and urine are tested using quantitative inductively coupled plasma-mass spectrometry.

83789

83789   Mass spectrometry and tandem mass spectrometry (eg, MS, MS/MS, MALDI, MS-TOF, QTOF), non-drug analyte(s) not elsewhere specified, qualitative or quantitative, each specimen

Mass spectrometry (MS) and tandem mass spectrometry (MS/MS) is an analytical technique used to detect molecules by measuring their weight electronically and displaying the results as a mass spectrum graph. The graph shows all molecules present (qualitative result) and the amount of each individual molecule (quantitative result) in the sample. The testing sample can be liquid, solid, or gas and may go through a single step phase (MS) or multiple steps with fragmentation occurring between the stages (MS/MS). Matrix-assisted laser desorption/ionization (MALDI) is a technique used on thin tissue samples for mass spectrometry imaging in which the sample is embedded or mixed in a matrix material that absorbs the laser irradiation wavelength and ionizes the analyte for mass spectrum recording. Mass spectrometry time-of-flight (MS-TOF) technique accelerates ions through an electric field of selected strength, resulting in the same kinetic energy for all ions with the same charge. The velocity depends upon the mass-to-charge ratio, which is then determined by the timed measurement for the ion particle to reach a detector at a known distance under the set experimental parameters. These techniques can be applied in many areas including biochemistry to measure proteins, peptides, sugars, oligonucleotides and even larger organic molecules; in the pharmaceutical industry for drug discovery, combinational chemistry, pharmacokinetics, and drug metabolism; and in clinical medicine for newborn screening and drug testing. Code 83789 is used to report qualitative or quantitative testing for non-drug analytes not elsewhere listed.

83825

83825   Mercury, quantitative

A test is performed on blood, urine, hair, fingernails and other body tissues to determine mercury levels. Mercury is a heavy metal that may be toxic to the body in large amounts. Individuals may come in contact with mercury by ingesting certain foods (fish), in dental amalgams (fillings), as a preservative in some vaccines (thimerosal) or in the workplace as an occupational exposure. A blood sample is obtained by separately reportable venipuncture. Whole blood is tested using quantitative atomic absorption/quantitative inductively coupled plasma-mass spectrometry. A random voided or 24 hour urine

specimen is obtained and tested using quantitative inductively coupled plasma-mass spectrometry. Scalp hair, fingernail clippings and body tissue samples are tested using inductively coupled plasma/mass spectrometry.

83835

83835   Metanephrines

A blood or urine test is performed to measure metanephrine levels. Metanephrine is a metabolite of epinephrine. Levels may be elevated by neuroendocrine tumors (pheochromocytomas), intense physical exercise, physiologic stress such as a life threatening illness and drug ingestion (epinephrine, caffeine, alcohol). A blood sample is obtained by separately reportable venipuncture. Plasma is tested using quantitative liquid chromatography-tandem mass spectrometry. Random voided or 24 hour urine specimen is tested using quantitative high performance liquid chromatography-tandem mass spectrometry.

83857

83857   Methemalbumin

A blood test is performed to measure methemalbumin levels. Methemalbumin is an abnormal albumin complex comprised of albumin and heme molecules. It occurs with hemolytic and hemorrhagic blood disorders, giving plasma an unusual brown pigment. A blood sample is obtained by separately reportable venipuncture. Serum/plasma is tested using spectrophotometry.

83861

83861   Microfluidic analysis utilizing an integrated collection and analysis device, tear osmolarity

Microfluidic analysis of tear osmolarity is performed to evaluate dry eye disease. Hyperosmolarity is a condition in which the quantity or quality of secreted tears is compromised and this condition is a primary indicator of dry eye disease. Tears perform essential functions such as maintaining eye surface integrity, protecting against infection, and preserving visual acuity. When the quantity or quality of the tears secreted is disrupted, deficient, or absent, damage to the ocular surface can occur including eye infections, dessication of the corneal epithelium, and ulceration or perforation of the cornea. A sample of tear film is collected from each eye using an integrated collection and analysis device. The tear film sample from one eye is placed in the analysis device which evaluates a predetermined set of criteria related to the tear film and displays the osmolarity measurement on a display panel. This is repeated with the sample from the second eye. The osmolarity measurement of the eye with the highest level of hyperosmolarity is used to determine whether the patient has normal osmolarity or whether dry eye disease is present. The measurement determines the degree of dry eye disease which is classified as mild, moderate, or severe.

83864

83864   Mucopolysaccharides, acid, quantitative

An acid mucopolysaccaride test is performed on a urine sample. Mucopolysaccharides, also known as glycosaminoglycans, are long chain sugar molecules found in bone, connective tissue, and joint fluid. Genetically inherited metabolic syndromes (such as Hunter, Hurler, Sanfilippo, Scheie, Morquio) lack an enzyme that breaks down sugar molecule chains which leads to mucopolysaccharidosis (MPS). In 83864, a quantitative test is performed on a urine sample to measure acid mucopolysaccharide levels. Quantitative testing is typically performed to monitor glycosaminoglycans (GAGs) in patients previously diagnosed with MPS. A urine specimen (first morning void preferred) is obtained. Alternatively, a 24-hour urine specimen may be used. The test is performed by spectrophotometry.

83872

83872   Mucin, synovial fluid (Ropes test)

Ropes test or mucin clot test is performed on synovial fluid. The test is used to determine inflammatory damage to hyalurinic polymers present in synovial (joint) fluid. Fluid is aspirated from affected joint(s) in a separately reportable procedure and a few drops are dispersed into acetic acid. The fluid will form a solid clot if no inflammation or mild inflammation is present (osteoarthritis, trauma, hemophilic arthritis). A soft clot with slightly turbid solution will be present with inflammatory conditions such as subacute or chronic systemic lupus erythematosis (SLE) and rheumatoid arthritis. Turbid solution with a crumbling clot or no clot is found with septic and acute crystalline (gouty) arthritis.

83873

83873   Myelin basic protein, cerebrospinal fluid

A test is performed on cerebral spinal fluid (CSF) to measure myelin basic protein (MBP) levels. MBP is a protective covering on nerve cells. When the protein breaks down, levels become elevated in cerebrospinal fluid. The most common cause of breakdown is multiple sclerosis (MS). Other causes include: central nervous system (CNS) trauma, infection or bleeding, encephalopathies and stroke. A sample of CSF is obtained by separately reportable lumbar puncture (spinal tap). Fluid is tested using quantitative enzyme-linked immunosorbent assay.

83874

83874   Myoglobin

A blood or urine test is performed to measure myoglobin levels. Myoglobin is an iron/oxygen binding protein found in muscle tissue. Levels may be elevated in blood and urine following muscle injury, myocardial infarction or extreme exercise. Elevated myoglobin is toxic to the renal tubules and may cause acute renal failure. A blood sample is obtained by separately reportable venipuncture. Urine may be obtained from a random voided sample or 24 hour specimen. Serum/plasma and urine are tested using quantitative electrochemiluminescent immunoassay.

83876

83876   Myeloperoxidase (MPO)

A blood sample is obtained by separately reportable venipuncture to determine the level of myeloperoxidase (MPO), also referred to as cardio-MPO. Myeloperoxidase is a biomarker that can be used to identify patients at risk for myocardial infarction and those in need of cardiac revascularization procedures. An enzyme-linked immunosorbent assay (ELISA) is performed to quantitate the level of myeloperoxidase in the blood plasma. Patients presenting with chest pain with elevated levels of circulating myeloperoxidase are at risk for a major cardiac event.

83880

83880   Natriuretic peptide

The level of the natriuretic peptide in the blood is measured to evaluate heart failure and to differentiate symptoms that might be indicative of heart failure from other disorders that cause similar symptoms. A separately reportable venipuncture is performed and whole blood or plasma collected using EDTA as an anticoagulant. An automated immunoassay is performed using murine monoclonal and polyclonal antibodies against natriuretic peptide. The antibodies are labeled with a fluorescent dye and immobilized on the solid phase. The specimen is placed in the sample chamber and the analysis is run. The physician reviews the results and uses them to make diagnosis and treatment decisions.

83883

83883   Nephelometry, each analyte not elsewhere specified

Nephelometry is a technique used in immunology to determine levels of certain proteins (globulins). It measures light passed through a sample at an angle. Examples of tests performed on blood or urine using quantitative nephelometry and not having a more specific code include: Kappa/Lambda Quantitative Free Light Chains with ratio-serum used to diagnose and monitor plasma cell disorders such as relapsing/evolving myeloma or primary amyloidosis; Alpha-1-Microglobulin-urine (random void or 24 hour collection) to identify renal tubular injury or dysfunction; Alpha-1-Macroglobulin-serum used to diagnose nephrotic syndrome or pancreatitis; Retinol Binding Protein-serum useful in determining Vitamin A deficiencies and the nutritional health of an individual. Report this code for each analyte tested using nephelometry when the analyte does not have a more specific code.

83885

83885   Nickel

A blood or urine test is performed to measure nickel levels. Nickel is a metal which is toxic to the human body and may be present as a pollutant in food, water and the air. A blood sample is obtained by separately reportable venipuncture. Urine may be obtained from a random voided sample or 24 hour specimen. Serum and urine are tested using quantitative inductively coupled plasma-mass spectrometry.

83915

83915   Nucleotidase 5'-

A blood test is performed to measure 5'-nucleotidase (5'-NT) levels. 5'-NT is a protein enzyme produced by the liver. Levels may be elevated in patients with cholestasis, liver disease/damage, hepatitis or liver tumors. A blood sample is obtained by separately reportable venipuncture. Serum is tested using quantitative enzymatic methodology.

83916

83916   Oligoclonal immune (oligoclonal bands)

Oligoclonal bands are protein fragments secreted by plasma cells. This test requires two separate specimens, cerebral spinal fluid (CSF) and blood. CSF is obtained by separately reportable lumbar puncture. Blood is obtained by separately reportable venipuncture. CSF and serum are examined to find the ratio of bands between the two specimen sources. An elevated ratio of bands in CSF may be diagnostic for the following conditions: multiple sclerosis, Lyme disease, Devic's disease, systemic lupus erythematosus, neurosarcoidosis, subacute sclerosing panencephalitis, subarachnoid hemorrhage, syphilis, primary central

nervous system lymphoma, Sjogren's syndrome and Guillain-Barre syndrome. Serum and CSF are tested using qualitative isoelectric focusing/immunofixation.

83918-83921

83918   Organic acids; total, quantitative, each specimen
83919   Organic acids; qualitative, each specimen
83921   Organic acid, single, quantitative

An analysis of organic acids is performed. Organic acids are biochemical by-products of metabolic processes that normally break down to carbon dioxide and water. However, in individuals with organic acid disorders, some proteins do not break down properly, resulting in a number of health problems from nutrient deficiencies to metabolic crisis. Organic acid disorders are autosomal recessive inherited disorders that affect both males and females. Symptoms and treatment vary depending on the specific organic acid disorder. Some of the more common organic acids tested include: 2,4 dichlorphrenoxyacetic acid, formic acid, glutaric acid (indicative of glutaric acidemia type 1 caused by the inability to break down lysine and tryptophan in food), hippuric acid, homgentisic acid, methylhippuric acid, methylmalonic acid (indicative of vitamin B12 deficiency), orotic acid, and trichlorocetic acid. Testing may be performed on blood or urine. If blood is used, a separately reportable venipuncture is performed. Methodology is dependent on both the type of specimen and the organic acid being tested. In 83918, a quantitative total analysis of multiple organic acids is performed. This test measures the amount of multiple organic acids in the blood or urine. Each specimen tested is reported separately. In 83919, a qualitative analysis for organic acids is performed. A qualitative test identifies the presence or absence of organic acids in the specimen but does not provide a measurement of the amount. Each specimen tested is reported separately. In 83921, a quantitative analysis of a single organic acid is performed. This test measures the amount of a single organic acid in blood or urine.

83930-83935

83930   Osmolality; blood
83935   Osmolality; urine

Osmolality of blood (83930) or urine (83935) is tested. Osmolality refers to the number of solutes present in blood (plasma or serum) or urine. Osmotically active particles include sodium, chloride, potassium, urea, and glucose. Osmolality is tested using freezing point methodology or vapor pressure osmometer. The higher the concentration of solutes, the lower the freezing point as compared to water. In 83930, a blood specimen is obtained by separately reportable venipuncture. Blood (serum, plasma) osmolality is tested to investigate hyponatremia (low levels of sodium in the blood), identify toxins, and monitor drug therapies. In 83935, a random urine specimen is obtained. Urine osmolality is tested to help evaluate fluid balance or to assess kidney function as demonstrated by the ability to produce and concentrate urine. Often both urine and blood osmolality is measured to determine the ratio of urine osmolality to serum osmolality.

83937

83937   Osteocalcin (bone g1a protein)

A blood test is performed to measure osteocalcin (bone g1a protein) levels, a non-collagen protein produced by osteoblasts. It may be used as a marker for bone turnover and to monitor effectiveness of drug therapy in patients with osteopenia/osteoporosis. Levels may be elevated in conditions such as Paget's disease, bone cancer, fractures, acromegaly, primary hyperparathyroidism, hyperthyroidism and renal osteodystrophy. Levels may be decreased with hypoparathyroidism, hypothyroidism and deficiencies of growth hormone. A blood sample is obtained by separately reportable venipuncture. Serum/plasma is tested using quantitative electrochemiluminescent immunoassay.

83945

83945   Oxalate

A blood or urine test is performed to measure oxalate levels. Oxalate has a conjugate base of oxalic acid which freely binds with calcium and magnesium to form an oxalate compound. A blood sample is obtained by separately reportable venipuncture and tested using enzymatic assay. Urine from a 24 hour collection is tested using quantitative spectrometry.

83950

83950   Oncoprotein; HER-2/neu

The HER-2/neu oncoprotein is a cell surface growth factor receptor responsible for regulating normal cell division and growth. The protein is expressed on the membrane of some epithelial cells. When the cell nucleus contains an increased number of HER-2/neu proto-oncogenes that encode for this oncoprotein, it causes overexpression, resulting in higher cell growth rates and mutation leading to cell transformation and cancer. Immunohistochemistry methods apply antibodies that bind to the specific target protein. A staining process is then used to detect and visualize the amount of HER-2/neu oncoprotein present on the cell membrane and to evaluate for overexpression.

Pathology and Laboratory

83951

83951   Oncoprotein; des-gamma-carboxy-prothrombin (DCP)

A blood sample is obtained by separately reportable venipuncture to determine the blood serum level of the oncoprotein des-gamma-carboxy-prothrombin (DCP). Oncoproteins are proteins encoded with an oncogene. They are normally involved with cell growth but may also be indicative of a malignant process. Elevated levels of the oncoprotein DCP in patients with chronic liver disease indicate that the patient may be at risk for the development of hepatocellular cancer. The blood serum is exposed to two labeled monoclonal antibodies, one being a monoclonal antibody for prothrombin and the other for DCP. Anion exchange chromatography is used to separate the oncoprotein DCP from the prothrombin and from the unbound enzyme labeled monoclonal antibody. The peroxidase enzyme activity is measured using fluorescence. The concentration of DCP is then calculated using calibrators and reported in nannograms per milliliter.

83970

83970   Parathormone (parathyroid hormone)

A blood or tissue test is performed to measure parathormone (parathyroid hormone, parathyrin) levels. Parathyroid hormone (PTH) is produced by chief cells in the parathyroid gland. The hormone helps to regulate blood calcium levels, absorption/excretion of phosphate by the kidneys and in Vitamin D synthesis in the body. Elevated levels (hyperparathyroidism) may be caused by parathyroid gland tumors or chronic renal failure. Decreased levels (hypoparathyroidism) may result from inadvertent removal (during thyroid gland surgery), autoimmune disorders or genetic inborn errors of metabolism. A blood sample is obtained by separately reportable venipuncture. Parathyroid gland tissue is obtained by separately reportable fine needle aspirate. Serum/plasma or tissue sample are tested using quantitative electrochemiluminescent immunoassay. Plasma is tested for parathyroid hormone, CAP (Cyclase Activating Parathyroid Hormone) using immunoradiometric assay.

83986-83987

83986   pH; body fluid, not otherwise specified
83987   pH; exhaled breath condensate

A test is performed to determine pH concentration, which is a measurement of the level of hydrogen ion (H+). The pH level indicates whether the substance being tested has the appropriate acid/base balance. A lower than normal pH indicates that the specimen is too acidic (acidosis), while a higher than normal pH indicates that the specimen is too alkaline (alkalosis). Use 83986 to report pH of body fluid that does not have a more specific code, such as urine and cerebral spinal fluid. The methodology depends on the body fluid being tested and includes pH reagent, meter, or electrode testing. Use 83987 to report pH of exhaled breath condensate, which is tested to help diagnose inflammatory lung diseases and to evaluate response to treatment. A device is used to collect exhaled air. One device uses a tube with a one-way valve that directs the exhaled air into a collection chamber where the moisture in the breath condenses. The droplets are collected and a pH meter or probe is used to evaluate the acid/base balance.

83992

83992   Phencyclidine (PCP)

A test is performed on blood, urine or meconium stool to measure phencyclidine (PCP) levels. PCP is a neurotoxic dissociative anesthetic drug, often ingested by recreational drug abusers for its hallucinogenic effects. A blood sample is obtained by separately reportable venipuncture, urine specimen by random void or meconium stool collected from the diaper of a newborn infant. Serum/plasma, urine and meconium are all tested using quantitative gas chromotography-mass spectrometry.

83993

83993   Calprotectin, fecal

A random stool sample is obtained to measure calprotectin level. Calprotectin is a calcium binding protein found in abundance in neutrophils. Neutrophil influx into the bowel lumen occurs during inflammation. An elevated calprotectin level in feces is an indicator of inflammatory disease of the gastrointestinal tract, including Crohn's disease and ulcerative colitis. The measurement may be used as one indicator to differentiate inflammatory bowel disease from functional bowel disease. The test is performed using enzyme linked immunosorbent assay (ELISA) technique.

84030

84030   Phenylalanine (PKU), blood

Phenylalanine is an amino acid found in most foods that contain protein. A blood test is performed, usually as part of a Newborn Screening Panel, to determine if there is a genetic mutation of the hepatic enzyme, phenylalanine hydroxylase (PAH) making it nonfunctional. If the enzyme is not functional, phenylalanine will not break down into tyrosine. Phenylalanine builds up in the blood, causing damage to the brain and nervous system. Eventually phenylalanine is converted into phenylpyruvate (phenylketone) and

excreted in the urine. Testing methods may include: bacterial inhibition assay (Guthrie test), fluorometric or photometric immunoassay or measurement of amino acids using tandem mass spectrometry.

84035

84035   Phenylketones, qualitative

Phenylketones are found in urine, often as a result of an inherited genetic disorder causing the enzyme, phenylalanine hydroxylase (PAH) to be nonfunctional. Without this enzyme, phenylalanine builds up in the blood and is eventually converted to phenylketones, processed through the kidneys and excreted in urine. Testing for the presence of phenylketones in urine is useful to diagnose and treat phenylketonuria.

84060

84060   Phosphatase, acid; total

A blood test is performed to measure acid phosphatase levels. Acid phosphatase is a type of enzyme stored in the form of lysosomes in many different body organs. The function of these enzymes is to fuse endosomes during digestion to create an acidic pH environment. A blood sample is obtained by separately reportable venipuncture. Serum is tested using quantitative enzymatic methodology.

84061

84061   Phosphatase, acid; forensic examination

Acid phosphatase mapping is an inexpensive and reliable method of identifying semen on swabs collected from sexual assault victims and fluid stains found on clothing and bedding. Prostatic acid phosphatase (PAP) is an enzyme specific to the prostate and is present is seminal fluid. Forensic testing for the presence of semen may be performed using a modified Fishman or Lerner method or by isoenzyme technique.

84066

84066   Phosphatase, acid; prostatic

A blood test is performed to measure prostatic acid phosphatase (PAP) levels. PAP is an enzyme specific to the prostate and is present in seminal fluid. The enzyme fuses endosomes to create an acidic pH environment. Levels may be elevated in patients with benign prostatic hyperplasia (BPH), prostate cancer, infection or infarction and in Paget's or Gaucher's disease. Prostate manipulation such as biopsy or massage may elevate PAP levels for 24-48 hours following the procedure. The test for PAP is not useful in screening but may be helpful in predicting disease recurrence and to monitor response to treatment. A blood sample is obtained by separately reportable venipuncture. Serum is tested using quantitative chemiluminescent immunoassay.

84075-84080

84075   Phosphatase, alkaline
84078   Phosphatase, alkaline; heat stable (total not included)
84080   Phosphatase, alkaline; isoenzymes

A blood test is performed to measure alkaline phosphatase (ALP) levels. ALP is a hydrolase enzyme that removes the phosphate group from molecules and is found abundantly in the liver, bile ducts, kidney, bone and placenta. Elevated levels may be associated with bile duct obstruction, Paget's disease and seminomas. Levels may be decreased in hypophosphatasia (an autosomal recessive genetic disease), Wilson's disease, certain types of anemia/leukemia, in postmenopausal women on estrogen therapy for osteoporosis and in women taking oral contraceptives, in men following cardiac surgery and with malnutrition or hypothyroidism, and in children with achondroplasia, cretinism or severe enteritis. A blood sample is obtained by separately reportable venipuncture. In 84075, total alkaline phosphatase is measured. Serum/plasma is tested using quantitative enzymatic methodology. In 84078, heat stable alkaline phosphatase is measured. Placental alkaline phosphatase (ALPP or Regan isoenzyme) has been identified as the most heat stable. In 84080, alkaline phosphatase isoenzyme levels are measured. Isoenzymes are classified as ALPI (intestine), ALPL (non-specific, liver/bone/kidney) and ALPP (placental). Serum/plasma is tested using quantitative heat inactivation/enzymatic technique.

84081

84081   Phosphatidylglycerol

Fetal lung maturity is assessed by testing for phosphatidylglycerol (PG). PG is a lipid that is detectable in amniotic fluid only when the lungs are mature. This test is performed on amniotic fluid before delivery in order to evaluate lung maturity and determine the probability of neonatal respiratory distress syndrome (RDS), also called hyaline membrane disease, developing after delivery. This test is performed in order to determine whether to suppress premature labor or whether the lungs are mature enough to allow the delivery to progress. Another indication is to determine whether fetal lungs are mature enough to allow induction of labor in patients with complications affecting the health of the mother and/or fetus. A separately reportable amniotic fluid sample is obtained. PG assay is performed by latex agglutination. If PG is present in the amniotic fluid, neonatal RDS risk is low.

84085

84085 Phosphogluconate, 6-, dehydrogenase, RBC

A blood sample is taken and the levels of 6PGD are measured. 6-phosphogluconate dehydrogenase (6PGD) is an enzyme in the pentose phosphate pathway, catalyzing 6-phosphogluconate to ribulose 5-phosphate. This enzyme is especially important in red blood cell (RBC) metabolism. A genetic deficiency of the enzyme (6PGD) may lead to episodic hemolytic events during times of stress.

84087

84087 Phosphohexose isomerase

Phosphohexose isomerase, also called glucose-6-phosphate isomerase, is an enzyme that catalyzes the conversion of glucose-6-phosphate into fructose-6-phosphate in the 2nd stage of glycolosis. This enzyme is encoded by the GPI gene. Defects in the gene cause nonspherocytic hemolytic anemia, and in cases of severe deficiency, hydrops fetalis.

84100-84105

84100 Phosphorus inorganic (phosphate)
84105 Phosphorus inorganic (phosphate); urine

A blood or urine test is performed to measure inorganic phosphorus (phosphate) levels. Phosphate is an intracellular anion, found primarily in bone and soft tissue. It plays an important role in cellular energy (nerve and muscle function) and the building/repair of bone and teeth. Decreased levels are most often caused by malnutrition and lead to muscle and neurological dysfunction. Elevated levels may be due to kidney or parathyroid gland problems. In 84100, a blood sample is obtained by separately reportable venipuncture. Serum/plasma is tested using quantitative spectrophotometry. In 84105, a 24-hour or random urine sample is obtained. Urine is tested using quantitative spectrophotometry.

84106-84110

84106 Porphobilinogen, urine; qualitative
84110 Porphobilinogen, urine; quantitative

Porphobilinogen (PBG) is one of several types of porphyrins found in the body. Normally, the body breaks down PBG and other porphyrins into heme, an important component of hemoglobin. If this process is impaired, porphyrins such as PBG can build up in the body. PBG testing is performed to help diagnosis porphyria which is an inherited metabolic disorder involving a deficiency of enzymes in the heme synthesis pathway. Porphyrins are excreted in urine so urine. In 84106, urine is tested to determine the presence of PBG. To obtain qualitative results, urine is most often tested using the Watson-Schwartz test. In 84110, the amount of PBG in the urine is measured. A 24-hour urine sample is obtained. Alternatively, a random sample may also be used during acute symptomatic periods. Urine is tested using quantitative ion exchange chromatography/spectrophotometry.

84112

84112 Evaluation of cervicovaginal fluid for specific amniotic fluid protein(s) (eg, placental alpha microglobulin-1 [PAMG-1], placental protein 12 [PP12], alpha-fetoprotein), qualitative, each specimen

Evaluation of cervicovaginal fluid for specific amniotic fluid proteins is performed when premature rupture of membranes is suspected. Certain proteins are found at high concentrations in amniotic fluid but at very low concentrations in cervicovaginal secretions. Placental alpha microglobulin-1 (PAMG-1) is synthesized in the fetal liver and yolk sac and reaches high levels in the amniotic fluid during the second and third trimesters. Placental protein 12 (PP12) is synthesized by the placental decidua and reaches peak concentrations in the amniotic fluid during the first trimester and stays elevated until delivery. AFP is a protein produced by the yolk sac of the fetus in early gestation and then later by the liver and gastrointestinal tract of the fetus. Test kits are now available that test for one or more of the proteins. The cervix and vagina are swabbed. Cervicovaginal secretions are tested using immunoassay and a series of monoclonal and/or polyclonal antibodies to one or more of these proteins. Test kit instructions are followed to determine whether elevated levels of one or more of the specific proteins are present in cervicovaginal fluid, which may indicate premature rupture of membranes.

84119-84120

84119 Porphyrins, urine; qualitative
84120 Porphyrins, urine; quantitation and fractionation

A urine test is performed to determine the presence of porphyrin in 84119 and to measure porphyrin levels in 84120. Elevated levels may be diagnostic for lead poisoning, liver disease, or porphyria, an inherited metabolic disorder involving a deficiency of enzymes in the heme synthesis pathway. Heme is a component of red blood cells and muscle cells. Porphyrins help form many important substances for the body, including hemoglobin. A quantitation and fractionation test (84120) is often ordered in conjunction with urine porphobilinogen (84106). A 24-hour urine sample is obtained. A random sample may

also be used during acute symptomatic periods. Urine is tested using quantitative high performance liquid chromatography.

84126

84126 Porphyrins, feces, quantitative

A test on feces is performed to measure porphyrin levels. Elevated levels may be diagnostic for lead poisoning, liver disease, or porphyria, an inherited metabolic disorder involving a deficiency of enzymes in the heme synthesis pathway. A definitive diagnosis of porphyria often requires a total determination of porphyria in urine, feces, and blood. Porphyrins help form many important substances for the body, including hemoglobin. A random stool (feces) sample is obtained and tested using quantitative high performance liquid chromatography. HemoQuant may also be reported using 84126 in which the stool sample is tested using fluorescence quantitation.

84132

84132 Potassium; serum, plasma or whole blood

A blood sample is obtained to measure potassium level. Potassium is a positively charged electrolyte that works in conjunction with other electrolytes, such as sodium, chloride, and carbon dioxide (CO_2), to regulate body fluid, stimulate muscle contraction, and maintain proper acid-base balance. Potassium is found in all body fluids but mostly stored within cells, not in extracellular fluids, blood serum, or plasma. Small fluctuations in blood potassium, either too high (hyperkalemia) or too low (hypokalemia), can have serious, even life-threatening, consequences. Potassium level is used to screen for and monitor renal disease; monitor patients on certain medications, such as diuretics, as well as patients with acute and chronic conditions, such as dehydration or endocrine disorders. Because blood potassium affects heart rhythm and respiratory rate, it is routinely checked prior to major surgical procedures. Potassium is measured by ion-selective electrode (ISE) methodology.

84133

84133 Potassium; urine

A urine test is performed to measure potassium levels. Potassium is a chemical element essential for proper functioning of the heart, kidneys, intestine, muscles, and nerves. Levels may be elevated in kidney disease, Cushing's syndrome, hyperaldosteronism, eating disorders, diabetic/metabolic acidosis, hypomagnesemia, and with the use of certain diuretics. Decreased levels may be caused by adrenal gland insufficiency, hypoaldosteronism, and medications such as beta blockers, lithium, and NSAIDs. A 24-hour or random urine sample is obtained. Urine is tested using quantitative ion-selective electrode.

84134

84134 Prealbumin

A blood test is performed to measure prealbumin levels. Prealbumin, also referred to as transthyretin (TTR) is found in serum and cerebral spinal fluid (CSF). It is responsible for transporting thyroxin and retinol binding protein carried on retinol. The test may be ordered to detect protein-calorie malnutrition in chronically or critically ill individuals. Levels may be elevated with the use of high dose corticosteroids or non-steroidal anti-inflammatory drugs (NSAIDs), adrenal gland disorders, Hodgkin's disease, and kidney failure. Decreased levels may be caused by hyperthyroidism, liver disease, severe infection, inflammatory diseases, and certain digestive disorders. A blood sample is obtained by separately reportable venipuncture. Serum/plasma is tested using immunoturbidimetric method.

84135

84135 Pregnanediol

Pregnanediol is an inactive bi-product of progesterone breakdown. The measurement of pregnanediol in urine can be useful in determining progesterone levels in the body. This test may be used at home for ovulation detection. Levels may be altered by ACTH (causing an increase in levels), oral contraceptives, or replacement hormones (causing a decrease in levels). Elevated levels may also result from ovarian cysts or tumors, adrenocortical hyperplasia, and hyperadrenocorticism. Levels may be decreased in cases of amenorrhea, ovarian failure, fetal death, and preeclampsia.

84138

84138 Pregnanetriol

Pregnanetriol is a steroid metabolite of 17-hydroxyprogesterone and is excreted in urine. It is a precursor to the biosynthesis of cortisol. Elevated levels can result from disorders of the adrenal cortex, such as adrenal hyperplasia or adrenogenital syndrome. The test is performed on a 24-hr urine collection (2.1-5 mL) using gas chromatography mass spectrophotometry.

Pathology and Laboratory

84140

84140   Pregnenolone

A blood test is performed to measure pregnenolone levels. Pregnenolone is a precursor hormone to progesterone, androgen, estrogen, mineralocorticoids, and glucocorticoids and is synthesized from cholesterol. A blood sample is obtained by separately reportable venipuncture. Serum/plasma is tested using quantitative high performance liquid chromatography-tandem mass spectrometry.

84143

84143   17-hydroxypregnenolone

A blood test is performed to measure 17-hydroxypregnenolone levels. This complex molecule is a C-21 steroid formed by hydroxylation of pregnenolone and catalyzed by enzymes located in the adrenal glands and gonads. Peak levels are attained by the end of puberty and then decline. Levels will elevate during pregnancy. This test is used to aid in the diagnosis of congenital adrenal hyperplasia and to evaluate women with evidence of hirsutism and infertility. A blood sample is obtained by separately reportable venipuncture. Serum/plasma is tested using quantitative high performance liquid chromatography-tandem mass spectrometry.

84144

84144   Progesterone

A blood test is performed to measure progesterone levels to confirm ovulation or to assess corpus luteum function. Progesterone belongs to a class of steroid hormones called progestogens and is produced by the corpus luteum following ovulation, by the placenta during pregnancy, and by the adrenal glands. It is also stored in fat cells. A blood sample is obtained by separately reportable venipuncture. Serum is tested using chemiluminescent immunoassay.

84145

84145   Procalcitonin (PCT)

Procalcitonin is a highly specific marker for early detection and therapeutic monitoring of clinically relevant bacterial infection or sepsis. Elevated procalcitonin levels in blood serum are an indication of both the presence and severity of bacterial infection or sepsis. This test allows the physician to differentiate between bacterial infections and viral infection or other nonbacterial inflammation. A blood sample is obtained by separately reportable venipuncture. Immunofluorescence is used to determine serum concentrations of procalcitonin.

84146

84146   Prolactin

A blood test is performed to measure prolactin levels. Prolactin is a hormone produced by the pituitary gland. Normal variations in prolactin levels occur during the day and night. Normal elevations occur during pregnancy, lactation (breast feeding), and times of physical or emotional stress. Abnormal elevations can occur with kidney and liver disease, hypothyroidism, and pituitary gland tumors (prolactinomas). Decreased levels may result from pituitary gland damage. This test may be ordered to evaluate nipple discharge, infertility, and erectile dysfunction. This code may be used to report prolactin, prolactin macroadenoma (dilution study) for patients with prolactin secreting tumors, and thyroid releasing hormone stimulation of Prolactin at 0, 30, 60, 90 minutes. A blood sample is obtained by separately reportable venipuncture. Serum/plasma is tested using quantitative chemiluminescent immunoassay.

84150

84150   Prostaglandin, each

Prostaglandins are autocrine/paracrine hormones produced throughout the body from essential fatty acids. Prostaglandins can activate the inflammatory response, produce pain and fever, cause platelets to aggregate and form blood clots, induce labor in pregnant women, inhibit acid secretion, increase mucus production in the digestive tract, increase blood flow to the kidneys, and constrict bronchi. There are three identified prostaglandins: Prostacyclin I 2, Prostaglandin E 2, and Prostaglandin F 2 alpha.

84152-84154

84152   Prostate specific antigen (PSA); complexed (direct measurement)
84153   Prostate specific antigen (PSA); total
84154   Prostate specific antigen (PSA); free

Prostate specific antigen (PSA) is measured. PSA is a protein produced by normal prostate cells found in serum and exists in both free form and complexed with other proteins. In 84152, complexed PSA is measured by direct measurement. A higher level of complexed PSA is suggestive of prostate cancer and is a better indicator of malignancy than total PSA. In 84153, total PSA is measured ad the total amount of both free and complexed forms. Total PSA levels are higher in men with benign prostatic hyperplasia (BPH), acute bacterial prostatitis, or prostate cancer. Total PSA is used to screen for prostate cancer and evaluate

the response to treatment in those with prostate cancer, but cannot be used by itself to definitively diagnose prostate cancer. In 84154, free PSA is measured, often in conjunction with total PSA, to provide an indirect measurement of complexed PSA.

84155

84155   Protein, total, except by refractometry; serum, plasma or whole blood

A blood test is performed to measure total protein levels. Total protein is often reported as a ratio of albumin to globulin (A/G ratio), and normal results will show albumin slightly greater than globulin. The test may be used to monitor nutritional status or diagnose kidney and liver disease. Elevated levels can indicate chronic inflammation, viral hepatitis, HIV infection, and multiple myeloma. Levels that are decreased may result from malnutrition or malabsorption syndromes such as celiac disease or inflammatory bowel disease. A blood sample is obtained by separately reportable venipuncture. Serum, plasma, or whole blood may be tested using quantitative spectrophotometry.

84156

84156   Protein, total, except by refractometry; urine

A urine test is performed to measure total protein levels. Protein is not normally found in urine and usually indicates damage or disease in the kidneys. Elevated levels are often present in patients with diabetes, hypertension, and multiple myeloma. A 24-hour or random urine sample is obtained and tested using quantitative spectrophotometry.

84157

84157   Protein, total, except by refractometry; other source (eg, synovial fluid, cerebrospinal fluid)

A test is performed on body fluids other than blood or urine, such as cerebral spinal fluid or synovial fluid, in order to measure total protein levels. Elevated protein levels in cerebral spinal fluid (CSF) may be caused by tumors, bleeding, inflammation, or injury in the brain or central nervous system. A decrease in protein levels may result from a rapid turnover/ replacement of cerebral spinal fluid. An elevated level of total protein in synovial fluid is most often caused by inflammation. CSF is obtained by separately reportable lumbar puncture (spinal tap), while synovial fluid is obtained by arthrocentesis from the affected joint. All body fluids are tested using reflectance spectrophotometry.

84160

84160   Protein, total, by refractometry, any source

Total protein levels may be measured in any fluid or liquid substances of the body including urine, serum, cerebral spinal fluid, and synovial fluid using refractometry. A sample of blood, urine, amniotic fluid, or serum is obtained and the patient's level of protein is measured. The total protein level determines the overall nutritional level of the patient.

84163

84163   Pregnancy-associated plasma protein-A (PAPP-A)

A blood sample is obtained to evaluate the level of pregnancy-associated plasma protein-A (PAPP-A). This test is used primarily as a screening test during pregnancy. Women with low levels of PAPP-A between 8 to 14 weeks of gestation are at higher risk for intrauterine growth restriction, trisomy 18 and 21, premature delivery, preeclampsia, and stillbirth. The test requires that a separately reportable nuchal translucency (NT) measurement be performed using ultrasonagraphy prior to the PAPP-A test. Information collected at the time of the ultrasonography and required for PAPP-A includes fetal crown-rump length measurement in cm, date of ultrasound, patient's date of birth, current weight, due date, number of fetuses present, patient's race, any history of previous pregnancy with chromosome abnormality. If the pregnancy is the result of an egg donor, the age of the donor is required. PAPP-A levels are then tested using enzyme-linked immunosorbent assay and risk for the listed complications evaluated.

84165

84165   Protein; electrophoretic fractionation and quantitation, serum

A blood test is performed to measure protein levels in serum. This test is often performed in conjunction with total protein (84155) to detect pathophysiologic states such as inflammation, gammopathies, and dysproteinemias. There are more sensitive tests available to detect these and similar disorders. A blood sample is obtained by separately reportable venipuncture. Serum is tested using electrophoretic fractionation and quantitation.

84166

84166   Protein; electrophoretic fractionation and quantitation, other fluids with concentration (eg, urine, CSF)

A test is performed on body fluids with concentration, such as cerebral spinal fluid or urine, to measure protein levels. Elevated protein levels in cerebral spinal fluid (CSF) may be caused by central nervous system tumors or neurological illness. Elevated protein levels in urine may indicate kidney disease or damage. There are more sensitive tests available to detect these and similar disorders. CSF is obtained by separately reportable lumbar puncture (spinal tap), while urine is obtained from a 24-hour specimen. Body fluids are tested for fractionation and quantitation using quantitative electrophoresis.

84181-84182

84181   Protein; Western Blot, with interpretation and report, blood or other body fluid

84182   Protein; Western Blot, with interpretation and report, blood or other body fluid, immunological probe for band identification, each

Western Blot, or protein immunoblot, is an analytical technique used to detect specific proteins in body tissues or fluids. 84181 and 84182 are performed on blood or other body fluids. Proteins are separated using gel electrophoresis and transferred to a nitrocellulose or PVDF membrane where they can then be detected and identified using target specific protein antibodies. Interpretation and report is included in these codes. Code 84182 employs the use of an immunological probe for identification and is reported for each probe.

84202

84202   Protoporphyrin, RBC; quantitative

A blood test is performed to measure protoporphyrin levels in red blood cells. Protoporphyrins are biochemical carrier molecules that accumulate in patients with genetic disorders of the heme biosynthesis pathway and in individuals exposed to lead. This code may be used to report zinc protoporphyrins or erythrocyte porphyrin levels. Elevated levels of zinc protoporphyrins may be present in patients with certain types of anemia (iron deficiency, sickle cell, sideroblastic), lead poisoning, and vanadium exposure. Erythrocyte porphyrin elevation may result from erythropoietic protoporphyria, zinc coproporphyrin, iron deficiency, anemia in chronic disease, or chronic lead poisoning. A blood sample is obtained by separately reportable venipuncture. Whole blood is tested for zinc protoporphyrin using quantitative hematofluorometry. Whole blood is tested for erythrocyte porphyrin using quantitative extraction/fluorometry.

84203

84203   Protoporphyrin, RBC; screen

A blood test is performed to detect the presence of protoporphyrin in whole blood. Protoporphyrins are biochemical carrier molecules that accumulate in patients with genetic disorders of the heme biosynthesis pathway and in individuals exposed to lead. Iron deficiency anemia is the most common cause of increased RBC protoporphyrin which is also characteristic of erythropoietic protoporphyria (EPP) and of porphyrias caused by heavy metals, solvents, and medications. When total RBC porphyrins are elevated, the test may be performed to differentiate iron-deficiency anemia from other causes of elevated porphyrin levels.

84206

84206   Proinsulin

A blood test is performed to measure proinsulin levels. Proinsulin is a hormone precursor to insulin produced by beta cells in the pancreas, specifically in an area called the Islets of Langerhans. A blood sample is obtained by separately reportable venipuncture. Serum is tested using qualitative enzyme-linked immunosorbent assay. This test is often performed to measure stages of pre-diabetes and progression toward type 2 diabetes mellitus. Elevated proinsulin levels may also be present in patients with benign or malignant B-cell tumors of the pancreas, renal failure, cirrhosis, or hyperthyroidism.

84207

84207   Pyridoxal phosphate (Vitamin B-6)

A blood test is performed to measure pyridoxal 5-phosphate (Vitamin B6) levels. This active form of Vitamin B6 functions as a co-enzyme for many reactions in the body. It is involved in amino acid and lipid metabolism, gluconeogenesis, neurotransmitter and histamine synthesis, hemoglobin synthesis and function, and gene expression. The level of pyridoxal 5-phosphate present in the body is a reliable measurement of Vitamin B6 nutritional status. A blood sample is obtained by separately reportable venipuncture. Serum/plasma is tested using quantitative high performance liquid chromatography.

84210

84210   Pyruvate

A test is performed on blood and cerebral spinal fluid (CSF) to measure pyruvate (pyruvic acid) levels. Pyruvic acid is a simple alpha-keto acid that supplies energy to cells during the citric acid cycle, and is active in both aerobic and anaerobic metabolism. Blood and CSF samples are collected and tested at the same time, often in conjunction with a test for lactate to diagnose mitochondrial metabolic disorders. A blood sample is obtained by separately reportable venipuncture, while CSF is obtained by separately reportable lumbar puncture (spinal tap). Whole blood and CSF are tested using quantitative enzymatic method.

84220

84220   Pyruvate kinase

A blood test is performed to measure pyruvate kinase levels. Pyruvate kinase is an enzyme involved in glycolysis. A genetic defect may lead to a deficiency of pyruvate kinase which slows gluconeogenesis in erythrocytes and leads to hemolytic anemia. A blood sample is obtained by separately reportable venipuncture. Whole blood is tested using quantitative enzymatic method.

84228

84228   Quinine

A blood or urine test is performed to measure quinine levels. Quinine is found naturally in the bark of cinchona trees and used commercially in the beverage of Tonic Water. It may be prescribed to treat malaria, systemic lupus erythematosus (SLE), arthritis, and nocturnal leg cramps. It also has anti-pyretic (fever reducing) and anti-inflammatory properties. A blood sample is obtained by separately reportable venipuncture. Urine sample is obtained by random void. Serum/plasma and urine are tested using high performance liquid chromatography/tandem mass spectrometry.

84233-84234

84233   Receptor assay; estrogen

84234   Receptor assay; progesterone

A receptor assay is performed to determine whether a tumor displays hormone receptors and will therefore likely respond to hormone therapy. In 84233, an estrogen receptor assay is performed on breast cancer cells to see if estrogen receptors are present. Normal breast cells and some breast cancer cells are stimulated by estrogen. The receptors are molecules that allow estrogen circulating in the blood to bind to the normal and/or cancerous breast cells and deliver information relating to growth and reproduction. Breast cancer cells that are estrogen receptor negative do not have these receptors and therefore will not respond well to hormone therapy as treatment. Breast cancer cells that are estrogen receptor positive do have estrogen receptors and will respond well to hormone therapy, which might include the use of anti-estrogen drugs and/or the removal of the ovaries. In 84234, a progesterone receptor assay is performed on breast cancer tissue to see if progesterone receptors are present and whether the breast cancer depends on progesterone for growth. Progesterone receptor negative breast cancer is unlikely to respond to hormone therapy whereas progesterone receptor positive breast cancer can be treated with hormones.

84235-84238

84235   Receptor assay; endocrine, other than estrogen or progesterone (specify hormone)

84238   Receptor assay; non-endocrine (specify receptor)

A receptor assay is performed to determine whether a tumor displays hormone receptors and will therefore likely respond to hormone therapy. In 84235, an endocrine receptor assay for a hormone other than estrogen or progesterone is performed on tumor cells to see if endocrine receptors are present for the hormone being tested. Normal cells and some cancer cells are stimulated in their growth by certain hormones. Receptors are molecules that allow a specific substance, e.g. hormone, circulating in the blood to bind to the normal and/or cancerous cells and deliver information relating to growth and reproduction. Cancer cells that are receptor negative for the hormone being tested do not have these receptors and therefore will not respond well to hormone therapy. Cancer cells that are receptor positive for the hormone being tested do have receptors and will respond well to hormone therapy. In 84238, a non-endocrine receptor assay is performed on cancer tissue to see if the specific non-endocrine receptors are present on tumor cells or not and whether the cancer depends on the non-endocrine hormones for growth. Receptor negative cancer is unlikely to respond to certain therapies whereas non-endocrine receptor positive cancer can be treated with therapies directed at the non-endocrine receptor.

84244

84244   Renin

A blood test is performed to measure renin levels. Renin is an enzyme released by the kidney in response to decreased sodium levels or blood volume, working with angiotensin and aldosterone to regulate mean arterial pressure. Levels may be elevated in Addison's Disease, cirrhosis, congestive heart failure, dehydration, hemorrhage, hypertension, hypokalemia, nephrotic syndrome, and renal tumors. Decreased levels may be caused by ADH therapy, hyperaldosteronism, steroid use, or sodium sensitive hypertension. This test is often ordered in conjunction with Aldosterone (82088). A blood sample is obtained by separately reportable venipuncture. Plasma is tested for direct renin using quantitative immunoradiometric assay and for plasma renin activity using quantitative radioimmunoassay.

Pathology and Laboratory

84252

84252   Riboflavin (Vitamin B-2)

A blood test is performed to measure riboflavin (Vitamin B2) levels. Daily intake of this micronutrient is necessary for body growth and red blood cell (RBC) production. It is active in the metabolism of fats, proteins, carbohydrates, and ketone bodies. Decreased levels may result in anemia. A blood sample is obtained by separately reportable venipuncture. Plasma is tested using quantitative high performance liquid chromatography.

84255

84255   Selenium

A blood or urine test is performed to measure selenium levels. Selenium is a trace mineral essential to the body to maintain optimum health. It is found abundantly in plants and seafood in most areas of the world. Deficiency of this mineral may lead to heart disease, thyroid problems, and a weak immune system. Diseases identified with selenium deficiency include Keshan, Kashin-Beck, and Myxedematous Endemic Cretinism. A blood sample is obtained by separately reportable venipuncture. Urine sample is obtained from a 24-hour collection. Serum/plasma or urine are tested using quantitative inductively coupled plasma-mass spectrometry.

84260

84260   Serotonin

A blood test is performed to measure serotonin levels. Serotonin is a monoamine neurotransmitter derived from tryptophan. Most serotonin is produced by the intestine where it regulates motility. It moves out of intestinal cells into the blood and is carried on platelets, helping to regulate hemostasis and blood clotting. The central nervous system (CNS) also produces a small amount of serotonin which helps to regulate mood, appetite, and sleep. Elevated levels may be found with intestinal obstruction, metastatic abdominal cancer, myocardial infarction, cystic fibrosis, dumping syndrome, and non-tropical sprue. Serotonin levels may be affected by certain medications if used within 72 hours of the blood test: lithium, MAO inhibitors, methyldopa, morphine, and reserpine. A blood sample is obtained by separately reportable venipuncture. Whole blood or serum is tested using quantitative high performance liquid chromatography.

84270

84270   Sex hormone binding globulin (SHBG)

A blood test is performed to measure sex hormone binding globulin (SHBG) levels. SHBG is a glycoprotein that binds testosterone and estradiol. The measurement of SHBG levels is usually performed in conjunction with a test for total testosterone (84403). Low levels of SHBG in men usually correspond with decreased testosterone levels which may cause infertility and erectile dysfunction. Women with elevated levels may have amenorrhea, infertility, acne, hirsutism, and polycystic ovarian syndrome. A blood sample is obtained by separately reportable venipuncture. Serum/plasma is tested using quantitative electrochemiluminescent immunoassay.

84275

84275   Sialic acid

A blood test is performed to measure sialic acid levels. Sialic acid, also known as N-Acetylneuraminic acid, is a derivative of the monosaccharide neuraminic acid produced when certain proteins and fats are metabolized. Levels may be elevated in patients with sialic acid storage diseases caused by an autosomal recessive genetic mutation. A blood sample is obtained by separately reportable venipuncture. Serum is tested for lipid associated sialic acid using quantitative spectrophotometry.

84285

84285   Silica

A blood or urine test is performed to measure silica levels. Silica is normally found in the body bound to protein and lipids. It is a constituent of collagen, maintaining the elasticity of skin and the strength of bone. Levels may be elevated from workplace exposure of inhaled particles causing silicosis, lung cancer, pulmonary tuberculosis, chronic airway diseases, autoimmune disorders, and chronic renal failure. A blood sample is obtained by separately reportable venipuncture. Urine is obtained from a random void. Serum/plasma is tested using quantitative inductively coupled plasma/atomic emission spectrometry. Urine is tested using quantitative inductively coupled plasma/optical emission spectrometry. The use of gadolinium contrast media within 48 hours of collecting a urine sample may alter test results.

84295

84295   Sodium; serum, plasma or whole blood

A blood sample is obtained to measure sodium level. Sodium is a positively charged electrolyte that works in conjunction with other electrolytes, such as potassium, chloride, and carbon dioxide (CO2), to regulate fluid in the body and maintain proper acid-base balance. Sodium is an essential mineral in the body, necessary for maintaining normal metabolic processes, fluid levels, and vascular pressure. Sodium level is used to screen for and monitor elevated blood sodium (hypernatremia), low blood sodium (hyponatremia), and electrolyte imbalances. Sodium may be monitored in patients on certain medications, such as diuretics, that can cause electrolyte imbalance. Sodium is measured by ion-selective electrode (ISE) methodology.

84300

84300   Sodium; urine

A urine sample is obtained to measure sodium level. Sodium is a positively charged electrolyte that works in conjunction with other electrolytes, such as potassium, chloride, and carbon dioxide (CO2), to regulate fluid in the body and maintain proper acid-base balance. Sodium is an essential mineral in the body, necessary for maintaining normal metabolic processes, fluid levels, and vascular pressure. Sodium level is used to screen for and monitor elevated blood sodium (hypernatremia), low blood sodium (hyponatremia), and electrolyte imbalances. Sodium may be monitored in patients on certain medications, such as diuretics, that can cause electrolyte imbalance.

84302

84302   Sodium; other source

A sample other than urine, blood, plasma, or serum is obtained to measure sodium level. Sodium is a positively charged electrolyte that works in conjunction with other electrolytes, such as potassium, chloride, and carbon dioxide (CO2), to regulate fluid in the body and maintain proper acid-base balance. Sodium is an essential mineral in the body, necessary for maintaining normal metabolic processes, fluid levels, and vascular pressure. Sodium level is used to screen for and monitor elevated blood sodium (hypernatremia), low blood sodium (hyponatremia), and electrolyte imbalances. Sodium may be monitored in patients on certain medications, such as diuretics, that can cause electrolyte imbalance.

84305

84305   Somatomedin

A blood test is performed to measure somatomedin (Insulin-Like Growth Factor-1 or IGF1) levels. IGF1, produced by liver and muscle cells, is a growth factor stimulated by somatotropin (human growth hormone or hGh) and promotes cell growth and division. Somatotropin levels vary throughout the day, so testing for somatomedin, which stays constant, is useful in evaluating the production of hGh by the pituitary gland. Low levels may indicate malnutrition, short stature, and delayed puberty. Elevated levels may be present with gigantism. A blood sample is obtained by separately reportable venipuncture. Serum is tested using quantitative chemiluminescent immunoassay.

84307

84307   Somatostatin

A blood test is performed to measure somatostatin levels. Somatostatin (growth hormone-inhibiting hormone, GHIH, or somatotropin release-inhibiting factor, SRIF) is an inhibitory hormone produced in the stomach, intestine, delta cells of the pancreas, and the brain. It regulates the endocrine system and affects neurotransmission and cell proliferation by inhibiting the release of secondary hormones including thyroid stimulating hormone, growth hormone, and numerous gastrointestinal hormones. A blood sample is obtained by separately reportable venipuncture. Plasma is tested using quantitative extraction/radioimmunoassay.

84311

84311   Spectrophotometry, analyte not elsewhere specified

Spectrophotometry is an analytical technique that detects molecules by measuring the amount of light that is absorbed. The use of spectrophotometry is widespread, including in the areas of chemistry and biochemistry, physics, material and chemical engineering, and clinical diagnostics. Code 84311 is used for quantitative analysis of blood and body fluid for cholesterol, phospholipids, hemoglobin, porphyrins, adenosine deaminase, aromatic primary amines, arylsulfatase A, chymotrypsin, and bilirubin.

84315

84315   Specific gravity (except urine)

Specific gravity measures the ratio of density. A particle with a specific gravity equal to 1 is neutrally buoyant in water. If the specific gravity increases, the particle becomes >1, denser, and sinks in water. When the specific gravity decreases, the particle becomes <1, less dense, and floats in water. Determining the specific gravity of a body fluid can help distinguish between transudative and exudative fluids—the specific gravity is greater in exudates than in transudates. Transudate fluids occur in association with conditions such as heart failure and cirrhosis, while exudative fluids develop as a result of inflammation or disorders such as tuberculosis, pneumonia, or cancer.

84375

84375   Sugars, chromatographic, TLC or paper chromatography

Sugar molecules may be simple (monosaccharides) such as ribose and glucose, or complex (oligosaccharides, polysaccharides) with polymers of simple sugars held together by glycosidic bonds. Thin layer chromatography technique is used to separate components of a mixture using a thin stationary phase supported by inert backing. Individual compounds will appear as spots separated vertically. Paper chromatography follows the basic principle of chromatography and is one of the easiest chromatographic methods. It only requires small samples and is very useful in testing and diagnostics. Paper chromatography is also often used to detect the presence of alcohol or chemicals in blood.

84376-84377

84376   Sugars (mono-, di-, and oligosaccharides); single qualitative, each specimen
84377   Sugars (mono-, di-, and oligosaccharides); multiple qualitative, each specimen

A laboratory test is performed to measure sugar in blood, body fluids, or excrement. Sugar molecules can contain a single (monosaccharide) carbohydrate such as glucose, fructose, or galactose; or they can be comprised of two carbohydrates (disaccharides) in the form of sucrose (fructose, glucose), lactose (glucose, galactose), and maltose (glucose, glucose). The body oxides simple sugar molecules to use as energy. Oligosaccharides are polymers typically containing 3-10 simple sugars that can link to proteins and lipids to form glycans. Oligosaccharides are a natural component of plant fiber (starch, cellulose) and function as prebiotics supporting bacteria in the large intestine to produce short chain fatty acids (SCFAs) and certain B vitamins. This test may be used to screen for carbohydrate malabsorption disorders and detect lysosomal storage diseases such as mannosidosis, fucosidosis, GM1 gangliosidosis, and sialic acid storage disease. Code 84376 is used for qualitative analysis of a single substance and may be applied when testing for reducing substances in fecal samples using colorimetry. Code 84377 is used when qualitatively testing for multiple sugar molecules in a sample and may be applied when testing for oligosaccharides in urine by thin layer chromatography.

84378-84379

84378   Sugars (mono-, di-, and oligosaccharides); single quantitative, each specimen
84379   Sugars (mono-, di-, and oligosaccharides); multiple quantitative, each specimen

A laboratory test is performed to measure sugar in blood, body fluids, or excrement. Sugar molecules can contain a single (monosaccharide) carbohydrate such as glucose, fructose, or galactose; or they can be comprised of two carbohydrates (disaccharides) in the form of sucrose (fructose, glucose), lactose (glucose, galactose), and maltose (glucose, glucose). The body oxides simple sugar molecules to use as energy. Oligosaccharides are polymers typically containing 3-10 simple sugars that can link to proteins and lipids to form glycans. Oligosaccharides are a natural component of plant fiber (starch, cellulose) and function as prebiotics supporting bacteria in the large intestine to produce short chain fatty acids (SCFAs) and certain B vitamins. This test may be used to screen for carbohydrate malabsorption disorders and detect lysosomal storage diseases such as mannosidosis, fucosidosis, GM1 gangliosidosis, and sialic acid storage disease. Code 84378 is used for quantitative analysis of a single sugar and can be applied when testing galactose-1-phosphate on red blood cells by gas chromatography-mass spectrometry and 1,5 anhydroglucitol in serum/plasma by quantitative enzymatic method. Code 84379 is used when quantitatively testing the amount of multiple sugar molecules in a sample.

84392

84392   Sulfate, urine

A test is performed on urine to measure sulfate levels. This test can assess an individual's protein intake and nutritional status. Protein from animal sources (meat, fish, poultry) contain the sulfur-rich amino acids, methionine and cysteine. High levels of animal protein increase sulfur and calcium excretion in the urine, raising the risk of renal calculi (kidney stone) formation. Urine sulfates also impact buffering and hydrogen ion exchange to modulate the supersaturation of uric acid. A 24-hour urine collection is obtained and tested using quantitative spectrophotometry.

84402

84402   Testosterone; free

A blood test is performed to measure free testosterone levels. Testosterone is an androgen hormone secreted in the testes of men, ovaries of women, and the adrenal glands of both sexes. Testosterone helps promote protein synthesis and supports the growth of cells and tissue. This test is often performed in conjunction with sex hormone binding globulin (84270). A blood sample is obtained by separately reportable venipuncture. Serum/plasma of adult males is tested using quantitative electrochemiluminescent immunoassay with the value derived from a mathematical expression using sex hormone binding globulin (SHBG). Serum/plasma of adult males may also be tested using quantitative equilibrium dialysis/high performance liquid chromatography-tandem mass spectrometry. Serum/

plasma of children and adult females is tested using quantitative high performance liquid chromatography-tandem mass spectrometry/electrochemiluminescent immunoassay with the value also derived from a mathematical expression using sex hormone binding globulin (SHBG).

84403

84403   Testosterone; total

A blood or urine test is performed to measure total testosterone levels. Testosterone is an androgen hormone secreted in the testes of men, ovaries of women, and the adrenal glands of both sexes. Testosterone helps promote protein synthesis and supports the growth of cells and tissue. This test is often performed in conjunction with sex hormone binding globulin (84270). A blood sample is obtained by separately reportable venipuncture. Urine is obtained from a 24-hour specimen collection. Serum/plasma of adult males is tested using quantitative electrochemiluminescent immunoassay. Serum/plasma of children and adult females is tested using quantitative high performance liquid chromatography-tandem mass spectrometry. Urine is tested using quantitative gas chromatography mass spectrometry.

84410

● **84410   Testosterone; bioavailable, direct measurement (eg, differential precipitation)**

A laboratory test is performed to measure bioavailable testosterone in serum. Testosterone is an androgen hormone secreted by both males and females. The majority of circulating testosterone is tightly bound to sex hormone binding globulin (SHBG) and biologically inactive. Free and albumin bound testosterone are active, bioavailable compounds. This test may be used to diagnose androgen deficiency in males when total testosterone is at the lower limits of normal and/or for suspected alteration of SHBG due to aging, obesity, or ingestion of certain medications. The test may also be used to diagnose hyperandrogenism in women who present with amenorrhea, hirsutism, polycystic ovarian syndrome (PCOS), and/or virilization. A blood sample is obtained by separately reportable venipuncture. The serum concentration of free testosterone is measured by differential precipitation of SHBG and ammonium sulfate following equilibration of the serum specimen tracer amounts of tritium-labeled testosterone.

84425

84425   Thiamine (Vitamin B-1)

A blood test is performed to measure thiamine (Vitamin B1) levels. Thiamine is essential for muscle and nerve function and helps cells convert carbohydrates into energy. Decreased levels are found with alcohol abuse, beriberi, Korsakoff's psychosis, Wernicke's encephalopathy and Wernicke-Korsakoff syndrome. A blood sample is obtained by separately reportable venipuncture. Plasma is tested for total thiamine, thiamine, and thiamine monophosphate using quantitative high performance liquid chromatography. Whole blood is tested for thiamine diphosphate using quantitative high performance liquid chromatography.

84430

84430   Thiocyanate

A test is performed on blood or urine to measure thiocyanate levels. Thiocyanate (rhodanide) is important for the human host defense system and is produced by the body with the metabolism of cysteine and the detoxification of cyanide. Levels may be elevated in individuals who use tobacco products, inhale environmental smoke, or in patients receiving the drug nitroprusside. Levels may be decreased in diseases such as cystic fibrosis. A blood sample is obtained by separately reportable venipuncture. Urine is obtained by random void or 24-hour specimen collection. Serum/plasma and urine are tested using quantitative colorimetry.

84431

84431   Thromboxane metabolite(s), including thromboxane if performed, urine

Thromboxane is a substance produced by platelets that causes blood clotting and constriction of blood vessels. There are two thromboxanes. Thromboxane A2 is active but very unstable. Thromboxane B2 is a metabolite of A2 and is inactive. Excretion of thomboxane B2 metabolites in the urine are used to evaluate a number of disease states, such as liver disease, inflammatory disease of the lungs, organ rejection in transplant patients, as well as other conditions. Typically a 24-hour urine sample is collected. The specimen is then tested for the presence of thromboxane B2 metabolites. The specimen may also be tested for the presence of thromboxane A2.

84432

84432   Thyroglobulin

A test is performed on blood or fine needle aspirate fluid to measure thyroglobulin (Tg) levels. Tg is a protein produced by and used within the thyroid gland. It is the protein building block for the two thyroid hormones, thyroxine (T4) and triiodothyronine (T3). Elevated blood levels may result from papillary or follicular thyroid cancer or Hashimoto's thyroiditis (Grave's disease). This test is often ordered in conjunction with thyroglobulin antibody, TgAb (86800). The presence of TgAb can interfere with the results of Tg testing. A blood sample is obtained by separately reportable venipuncture. Samples of thyroid cells are obtained by separately reportable fine needle aspiration (FNA). Serum/plasma and FNA fluid are tested using quantitative chemiluminescent immunoassay.

84436-84439

84436 Thyroxine; total
84437 Thyroxine; requiring elution (eg, neonatal)
84439 Thyroxine; free

A blood sample is obtained and levels of total thyroxin (84436), thyroxine requiring elution as for testing in neonates (84437), or free thyroxine (84439) are evaluated. Thyroxine, also referred to as T4, is tested to determine whether the thyroid is functioning properly and is used to aid in the diagnosis of overactive (hyperthyroidism) or underactive (hypothyroidism) thyroid function. In 84436, total thyroxine levels are evaluated. Total thyroxine measures the total amount of both bound and unbound (free) thyroxine in the blood. In 84437, a thyroxine level requiring elution is performed. This test is typically performed on neonates using cord blood to diagnose congenital hypothyroidism. In 84439, free thyroxine levels are tested. Free thyroxine is the amount of active thyroxine in the blood. Free thyroxine levels are considered to be a more accurate indicator of thyroid function. All thyroxine tests use electrochemiluminescent immunoassay methodology.

84442

84442 Thyroxine binding globulin (TBG)

A blood test is obtained to determine the amount of thyroxine binding globulin (TBG). TBG is one of three proteins that bind to thyroid hormones T3 and T4. The other two proteins that bind to thyroid hormones are transthyretin and albumin. Bound thyroid hormones are not active and do not affect the overall health of the individual, because the levels of active free thyroid hormones are not affected. In some individuals with an inherited or acquired variation in the concentration of TBG and the other thyroid binding proteins, high or low levels of total thyroid hormones T3 and T4 may be found in the blood. Measurement of TBG can aid the physician in determining whether the patient has an underactive or overactive thyroid disorder which requires treatment or just a variation in the amount of TBG. This test is performed by chemiluminescent immunoassay methodology.

84443

84443 Thyroid stimulating hormone (TSH)

A blood test is performed to determine levels of thyroid stimulating hormone (TSH). TSH is produced in the pituitary and helps to regulate two other thyroid hormones, triiodothyronine (T3) and thyroxin (T4), which in turn help regulate the body's metabolic processes. TSH levels are tested to determine whether the thyroid is functioning properly. Patients with symptoms of weight gain, tiredness, dry skin, constipation, or menstrual irregularities may have an underactive thyroid (hypothyroidism). Patients with symptoms of weight loss, rapid heart rate, nervousness, diarrhea, feeling of being too hot, or menstrual irregularities may have an overactive thyroid (hypothyroidism). TSH levels are also periodically tested in individuals on thyroid medications. The test is performed by electrochemiluminescent immunoassay.

84445

84445 Thyroid stimulating immune globulins (TSI)

A blood sample is obtained to evaluate levels of thyroid stimulating immune globulins (TSI). This test is performed to identify overactive thyroid disease (hyperthyroidism) as seen in Grave's disease, Hashimoto's thyroiditis, and toxic multinodular goiter. TSIs are autoantibodies produced by the immune system that bind to the surface of follicular cells in the thyroid gland. TSIs then mimic the action of thyroid stimulating hormone, causing excessive production and secretion of thyroid hormones. This test is performed by bioassay and chemiluminescence methodology.

84446

84446 Tocopherol alpha (Vitamin E)

A blood test is performed to measure tocopherol alpha (Vitamin E) levels. Tocopherol alpha is the form of Vitamin E most readily absorbed and accumulated by human cells and tissue. Elevated levels may have an anticoagulant affect and cause bleeding disorders. Decreased levels may cause neuromuscular problems. A blood sample is obtained by separately reportable venipuncture. Serum/plasma is tested using quantitative high performance liquid chromatography.

84449

84449 Transcortin (cortisol binding globulin)

A blood test is performed to measure transcortin (cortisol binding globulin, CBG) levels. Transcortin is an alpha globulin that binds the steroid hormones cortisol, progesterone, aldosterone, and 11-Deoxycorticosteroid. It is produced by the liver and regulated by the hormone estrogen. Normal elevations occur during pregnancy. Decreased levels may

be caused by liver disorders such as cirrhosis. A blood sample is obtained by separately reportable venipuncture. Serum is tested using radioimmunoassay.

84450

84450 Transferase; aspartate amino (AST) (SGOT)

A blood test is performed to measure aspartate aminotransferase (AST) levels. This enzyme was previously referred to as serum glutamic oxaloacetic transaminase (SGOT). AST is an enzyme found primarily in liver and muscle cells. Elevated levels may result from liver disease or damage such as hepatitis, cirrhosis, ischemia, drug toxicity, and/or muscle damage, especially cardiac muscle (myocardial infarction). This test is often ordered in conjunction with alanine transferase, ALT (84460) or other liver function tests (LFTs) to diagnose disease and monitor individuals taking cholesterol lowering medications. A blood sample is obtained by separately reportable venipuncture. Serum/plasma is tested using quantitative enzymatic method.

84460

84460 Transferase; alanine amino (ALT) (SGPT)

A blood test is performed to measure alanine aminotransferase (ALT) levels. This enzyme was previously referred to as serum glutamic pyruvic transaminase (SGPT). ALT is an enzyme found primarily in liver and muscle cells. Elevated levels may result from liver disease or damage such as hepatitis, cirrhosis, ischemia, drug toxicity, and/or muscle damage, especially cardiac muscle (myocardial infarction). This test is often ordered in conjunction with aspartate transferase, AST (84450) or other liver function tests (LFTs) to diagnose disease and monitor individuals taking cholesterol lowering medications. A blood sample is obtained by separately reportable venipuncture. Serum/plasma is tested using quantitative enzymatic method.

84466

84466 Transferrin

A blood test is performed to measure transferrin levels. Transferrin is a glycoprotein produced primarily by the liver and released into blood plasma to bind and carry iron molecules. Levels may be decreased in cases of liver disease, certain anemic or inflammatory conditions, and malnutrition. Increased levels may result from iron overload diseases such as hemochromatosis. A blood sample is obtained by separately reportable venipuncture. Serum/plasma is tested using quantitative immunoturbidometry.

84478

84478 Triglycerides

A test is performed on blood or body fluids to measure triglyceride levels. Triglycerides contain glycerol and 3 fatty acid molecules and are a component of very low density lipoproteins (VLDL) found in blood and chylomicrons (cholesterol, protein, triglycerides) found in lymphatic fluid. They provide an energy source during metabolism and carry any unused dietary fats or calories to the liver and fat cells where they can be stored. Elevated levels may reflect recent carbohydrate and/or fat consumption. Blood samples should be obtained with the patient fasting for 12 hours. A blood sample is obtained by separately reportable venipuncture. Body (lymphatic) fluid is obtained by needle aspiration or incision/drainage of pooled fluid. Serum/plasma and body fluids are tested using quantitative enzymatic methods.

84479

84479 Thyroid hormone (T3 or T4) uptake or thyroid hormone binding ratio (THBR)

A blood sample is obtained to determine T3 (triiodothyronine) or T4 (thyroxine) thyroid hormone uptake, also referred to as thyroid hormone binding ratio (THBR). Three proteins including thyroid binding globulin (TBG), transthyretin, and albumin bind thyroid hormones rendering them inactive. Thyroid hormone uptake on T3 or T4 is presented as a ratio of the solid matrix uptake and the serum uptake. Calculation of THBR helps the physician determine whether the patient has a potential binding protein abnormality. This test is performed by electrochemiluminescent immunoassay.

84480-84482

84480 Triiodothyronine T3; total (TT-3)
84481 Triiodothyronine T3; free
84482 Triiodothyronine T3; reverse

A blood sample is tested to determine levels of total triiodothyronine (T3) (84480), free T3 (84481), or reverse T3. T3 is a hormone made by the thyroid gland that affects almost every metabolic process including body temperature, growth, and heart rate. T3 can either be produced by the thyroid or synthesized by the body from T4. Approximately 95% of T3 is bound to proteins in the blood and is inactive. The remaining 5% is free and active. T3 tests are used to help determine whether the thyroid is functioning properly, to diagnose hyperthyroidism, and to monitor patients with known thyroid disorders. In 84480, total T3, which reflects the amount of both bound and free T3, is measured. In 84481, only the active free T3 is measured. Total and free T3 are evaluated using electrochemiluminescent immunoassay. In 84482, reverse T3 is measured. If the thyroid does not produce enough

T3 or not enough is synthesized from T4, an inactive form of T3, referred to as reverse T3 or rT3, may be produced. Elevated levels of rT3 may be indicative of a thyroid disorder. Radioimmunoassay is used to evaluate rT3 levels.

84484

84484   Troponin, quantitative

A blood test is performed to measure troponin levels. Troponins are regulatory proteins that facilitate contraction of skeletal and smooth muscle by forming calcium bonds. Troponin T binds to tropomyocin to form a complex. Tropocin I binds to actin and holds the Troponin T-Tropomyocin complex together. Elevation of troponins, coupled with cardiac symptoms such as chest pain are considered diagnostic for cardiac injury. This test is commonly ordered in the Emergency Department when a patient presents with possible myocardial infarction, and is then repeated at 6 hour intervals. It may be ordered with other tests that assess cardiac biomarkers such as CK, CK-MB, and myoglobin. A blood sample is obtained by separately reportable venipuncture. Serum/plasma is tested for Troponin T using quantitative electrochemiluminescent immunoassay. Serum is tested for Troponin I using chemiluminescent immunoassay.

84485

84485   Trypsin; duodenal fluid

Trypsin is a serine protease produced by the pancreas as inactive zymogen trypsinogen. This inactive molecule enters the duodenum via the pancreatic duct where the enzyme enteropeptidase activates it into trypsin. Ingested proteins are hydrolysed by trypsin into smaller amino acid molecules , then absorbed and digested. The measurement of trypsin levels in duodenal juices can be used as a test of pancreatic function. Severely reduced trypsin levels in duodenal fluid occurs with chronic pancreatitis and carcinoma of the head of the pancreas. Less severely reduced trypsin levels occur with diabetic glucose intolerance and obstruction of the common bile duct.

84488-84490

84488   Trypsin; feces, qualitative
84490   Trypsin; feces, quantitative, 24-hour collection

A test is performed to measure fecal trypsin titers. Trypsin is a serine protease produced by the pancreas as inactive zymogen trypsinogen. This inactive molecule enters the duodenum via the pancreatic duct where the enzyme enteropeptidase activates it into trypsin. Ingested proteins are hydrolysed by trypsin into smaller amino acid molecules, then absorbed and digested. This test may be used to determine exocrine pancreatic function. When the pancreas is not producing enough trypsin, decreased levels can be seen in a stool sample. This is often due to chronic pancreatitis. A random stool specimen is obtained in 84488 and tested using semi-quantitative film digestion. The test for fecal trypsin is also performed on symptomatic newborns and infants as a screening tool for cystic fibrosis, because mucous plugs can form in the pancreatic ducts with cystic fibrosis that block the flow of trypsinogen into the small intestine. Use 84490 for a quantitative fecal test of trypsin.

84510

84510   Tyrosine

A blood test is performed to measure tyrosine levels. Tyrosine is a nonessential amino acid that can be derived from phenylalanine and is necessary to the body in forming neurotransmitters such dopamine, epinephrine, and nor-epinephrine. It also assists in the function of adrenal, thyroid, and pituitary glands. Levels may be decreased in individuals with the genetic disorder phenylketonuria, because the body does not synthesize the protein phenylalanine. A blood sample is obtained by separately reportable venipuncture. Plasma is tested using ion exchange chromatography.

84512

84512   Troponin, qualitative

Troponins are regulatory proteins that facilitate contraction of skeletal and smooth muscle by forming calcium bonds. Troponin T binds to tropomyocin to form a complex. Tropocin I binds to actin and holds the Troponin T-Tropomyocin complex together. Elevation of troponins, coupled with cardiac symptoms (chest pain), are considered diagnostic for cardiac injury. This test is commonly ordered in the Emergency Department when a patient presents with possible myocardial infarction, and then repeated at 6 hour intervals. It may be ordered with other tests that assess cardiac biomarkers such as CK, CK-MB, and myoglobin. A blood sample is obtained by separately reportable venipuncture and serum/plasma is tested for the presence of Troponin T.

84520

84520   Urea nitrogen; quantitative

A blood sample is obtained to measure total (quantitative) urea nitrogen (BUN) level. Urea is a waste product produced in the liver by the breakdown of protein from a sequence of chemical reactions referred to as the urea or Krebs-Henseleit cycle. Urea then enters the bloodstream, is taken up by the kidneys and excreted in the urine. Blood BUN is measured

to evaluate renal function, to monitor patients with renal disease, and to evaluate effectiveness of dialysis. BUN may also be measured in patients with acute or chronic illnesses that affect renal function. BUN is measured using spectrophotometry.

84525-84545

84525   Urea nitrogen; semiquantitative (eg, reagent strip test)
84540   Urea nitrogen, urine
84545   Urea nitrogen, clearance

A blood sample is obtained to measure total (quantitative) blood urea nitrogen (BUN) level. Urea is a waste product made in the liver by the breakdown of protein through a sequence of chemical reactions referred to as the urea or Krebs-Henseleit cycle. Urea enters the bloodstream, is taken up by the kidneys, and excreted in the urine. BUN is measured to evaluate renal function, monitor current renal disease, and evaluate the effectiveness of dialysis. BUN may also be measured in patients with acute or chronic illnesses that affect renal function. In 84525, the test is performed with a reagent strip, which reacts with a urine sample. In 84540, only the BUN is performed. In 84545, a urine sample is collected over a 24-hour period.

84550

84550   Uric acid; blood

A blood test is performed to measure uric acid levels. Uric acid forms from the natural breakdown of body cells and the food we ingest. Uric acid is normally filtered by the kidneys and excreted in urine. Elevated blood levels may result from kidney disease, certain cancers and/or cancer therapies, hemolytic or sickle cell anemia, heart failure, cirrhosis, lead poisoning, and low levels of thyroid or parathyroid hormones. Levels may be decreased in Wilson's disease, poor dietary intake of protein, and with the use of certain drugs. A blood sample is obtained by separately reportable venipuncture. Serum/plasma is tested using quantitative spectrophotometry.

84560

84560   Uric acid; other source

A test is performed on urine or synovial (joint) fluid to measure uric acid levels. Uric acid forms from the natural breakdown of body cells and the food we ingest. It is normally filtered by the kidneys and excreted in urine. Elevated levels may result from kidney disease, certain cancers and/or cancer therapies, hemolytic or sickle cell anemia, heart failure, cirrhosis, a diet high in purine, lead poisoning, and low levels of thyroid or parathyroid hormones. Levels may be decreased with gout, folic acid deficiency, and certain medications. A 24-hour or random urine specimen is obtained and tested using quantitative spectrophotometry. Uric acid found in synovial fluid is usually in the form of monosodium urate crystals. The joints most commonly affected are in the feet and legs. Synovial fluid is aspirated from the affected joint(s) by separately reportable arthrocentesis and tested using quantitative spectrophotometry.

84577

84577   Urobilinogen, feces, quantitative

Urobilinogen is a product of bilirubin reduction. It is formed in the intestines by bacterial action on stercobilinogen which is reduced and oxidized to stercobilin. This is what gives feces a brown color. Levels may be decreased with biliary obstruction or the intake of certain antibiotics that destroy bacteria.

84578-84583

84578   Urobilinogen, urine; qualitative
84580   Urobilinogen, urine; quantitative, timed specimen
84583   Urobilinogen, urine; semiquantitative

Urobilinogen is a product of bilirubin reduction which takes place in the intestine. A small amount is reabsorbed from the intestine and circulated via blood to the kidneys for filtration. This is called the enterohepatic urobilinogen cycle. Elevated levels in urine may result from biliary obstruction; hepatic infection, poisoning, or inflammation; and from hemolytic anemia. Elevated levels may also occur in the presence of a large hematoma that the body must absorb. Levels may be deceased with congenital enzymatic jaundice and in the presence of urine acidifying drugs. Use 84578 for qualitative evaluation; 84580 for quantitative, timed specimen urobilinogen evaluation; and 84583 for a semiquantitative evaluation.

84585

84585   Vanillylmandelic acid (VMA), urine

A urine test is performed to measure vanillylmandelic acid (VMA) levels. VMA is a metabolite of the catecholamine hormones, epinephrine and norepinephrine, produced by the adrenal glands. Small fluctuation in levels is common, with mildly elevated levels resulting from hypertension, anxiety, exercise, certain over the counter (OTC) medications, and herbs. Higher levels may indicate neuroendocrine tumors such as neuroblastoma or pheochromocytoma. This test may be used to diagnose disorders and monitor the

Pathology and Laboratory

effectiveness of treatment. A 24-hour or random urine specimen is obtained and tested using quantitative high performance liquid chromatography.

84586

84586   Vasoactive intestinal peptide (VIP)

A blood test is performed to measure vasoactive intestinal peptide (VIP) levels. VIP is a hormone produced by the pancreas that stimulates heart contractions; causes vasodilation to lower arterial blood pressure; relaxes smooth muscles of the trachea, stomach, and gall bladder; and increases glycogenolysis. Levels may be elevated with VIPoma, a rare type of cancer in the islet cells of the pancreas. A blood sample is obtained by separately reportable venipuncture. Plasma is tested using quantitative radioimmunoassay.

84588

84588   Vasopressin (antidiuretic hormone, ADH)

A blood test is performed to measure arginine vasopressin hormone (antidiuretic hormone, ADH) levels. ADH is a neurohypophyseal hormone that regulates water, glucose, and sodium levels in the blood. It is synthesized by the hypothalamus and stored in the posterior pituitary gland. ADH is released in response to dehydration causing the kidney to conserve water and concentrate urine volume. The hormone also increases peripheral vascular resistance which causes an elevation in blood pressure from vasoconstriction. A blood sample is obtained by separately reportable venipuncture. Plasma is tested using quantitative radioimmunoassay.

84590

84590   Vitamin A

A blood test is performed to measure vitamin A (retinol) levels. Retinol is the storage form of vitamin A found in the body. It produces the pigment found in the eye (retina) and is necessary for the maintenance of healthy eyes, skin, teeth, mucous membranes, and soft tissue. Decreased levels may contribute to infections and vision problems, even blindness. Levels may be elevated with renal compromise (kidney disease) and certain drug interactions. A blood sample is obtained by separately reportable venipuncture. Serum/plasma is tested using quantitative high performance liquid chromatography.

84591

84591   Vitamin, not otherwise specified

A specimen is tested to determine the levels of a vitamin not specifically listed in any other code. Vitamins that are reported with this code include biotin and niacin. A blood sample is obtained by separately reportable venipuncture. The levels of the vitamin are then determined using high performance liquid chromatography or other methodology.

84597

84597   Vitamin K

A blood test is performed to measure vitamin K levels. Vitamin K is necessary for proper blood clotting (coagulation) and can be absorbed by the body during digestion of certain foods and also produced by bacteria in the intestines. Decreased levels may result from certain malabsorption syndromes and antibiotic use. A blood sample is obtained by separately reportable venipuncture. Serum is tested using quantitative high performance liquid chromatography.

84600

84600   Volatiles (eg, acetic anhydride, diethylether)

Volatiles are chemical elements and compounds with low boiling points. Elevated levels found in the body are often associated with workplace exposure. The sample used and the testing method employed vary according to the chemical compound being test for, such as phenol (carbolic acid), acetic anhydride, aromatic solvents like toluene, xylene, and benzene, naphthalene and other aromatic hydrocarbons, oxygenated volatiles, acetone, propylene glycol, creosols, ether, and other inhalants.

84620

84620   Xylose absorption test, blood and/or urine

Blood and urine are tested to measure xylose absorption. This test is used to evaluate the absorption of carbohydrates from the proximal small intestine. It is performed by obtaining a fasting serum level followed by administration of a 5g or 25g dose of xylose in adults (dose is based upon weight in a child). At 2 hours, a second serum level is drawn, and urine collection continues for 5 hours following the xylose dose. Decreased levels may be caused by malabsorption syndromes such as celiac disease, Crohn's disease, or Whipple disease, intestinal inflammatory disorders, short bowel syndrome, or parasitic infections including giardia and hookworm. A blood sample is obtained by separately reportable venipuncture. Urine collection is by normal void. Serum and urine are tested using quantitative spectrophotometry.

84630

84630   Zinc

A blood or urine test is performed to measure zinc levels. Zinc is a mineral, essential for growth and development. Prolonged undernourishment of zinc can lead to growth retardation, delayed puberty, diarrhea, and increased susceptibility to infection. Decreased levels may result from malnutrition, infection, inflammation, stress, pregnancy, and oral contraceptive use. Levels may be elevated during prolonged fasting states and overdose of oral supplements. A blood sample is obtained by separately reportable venipuncture, urine is obtained from 24-hour collection or random urine sample. Whole blood is tested using quantitative flame atomic absorption spectroscopy. Serum and urine are tested using quantitative inductively coupled plasma mass spectrometry.

84681

84681   C-peptide

A blood or urine test is performed to measure C-peptide levels. This test can monitor insulin production and help determine the cause of low blood glucose levels. It may be ordered to determine residual beta cell function in patients with newly diagnosed diabetes and metabolic syndrome or to monitor and test for insulinomas (tumors in the islet cells of the pancreas). Levels may be elevated with endogenous insulin production, insulinomas, hypokalemia, pregnancy, Cushing syndrome, and renal failure. Low levels may be caused by low beta cell function. A blood sample is obtained by separately reportable venipuncture. Urine sample is from a 24-hour collection. Serum and urine are tested using quantitative chemiluminescent immunoassay.

84702-84703

84702   Gonadotropin, chorionic (hCG); quantitative
84703   Gonadotropin, chorionic (hCG); qualitative

A specimen is tested for chorionic gonadotropin (hCG). In 84702, a blood specimen is obtained by separately reportable venipuncture and a quantitative analysis of chorionic gonadotropin is performed. Quantitative analysis measures the amount of the hormone present in the blood and is used to help diagnose an ectopic pregnancy, monitor a pregnancy for threatened or missed abortion, or following a spontaneous abortion. It may also be used to diagnose trophoblastic disease (hydatidiform mole) or germ cell tumors of the testes or ovaries, monitor the effectiveness of treatment, or the recurrence of these conditions. In 84703, a qualitative test is performed to test for the presence of absence of hCG only. This test may be performed on blood or urine. Qualitative hCG testing is performed to confirm pregnancy.

84704

84704   Gonadotropin, chorionic (hCG); free beta chain

A blood sample is obtained to measure free beta chain human chorionic gonadotropin (hCG) level. Human chorionic gonadotropin is a glycoprotein secreted by the trophoblast cells of the placenta. It contains two subunits, alpha hCG and beta hCG. Elevated levels of both subunits are present in the blood during pregnancy. Significant elevation of free beta chain hCG during the first trimester is a specific and sensitive diagnostic marker for gestational trophoblastic neoplasms, including hydatidiform mole and choriocarcinoma, as well as Down syndrome, trisomy 18, and neural tube defects. The test is performed using a two-step process involving two monoclonal antibodies of high affinity in an immunoradiometric assay (IRMA) system.

84830

84830   Ovulation tests, by visual color comparison methods for human luteinizing hormone

An ovulation test for human luteinizing hormone (LH) is performed by visual color comparison methods. Luteinizing hormone is present only in small quantities until mid-cycle when an LH surge occurs that precedes ovulation by one to two days. This test is performed to detect the LH surge so that the most likely time for conception can be determined. The test should be performed between 11 am and 8 pm as LH is at its highest levels during this time of day. A test kit is used. A urine sample is obtained. A test strip is dipped into the urine. The test strip will change color and is then visually compared to a color chart to determine if LH levels are increased and the LH surge has occurred.

85002

85002   Bleeding time

A test is performed to determine bleeding time. A laboratory test for platelet count may be ordered prior to the bleeding time test. A blood pressure cuff is placed on the upper arm and inflated to 20-40 mmHg. Two small cuts are made on the lower arm using a lancet or Surgicutt bleeding device. The time is noted and the blood pressure cuff is deflated. Blotting paper is touched to the cuts every 30 seconds until the bleeding stops completely. The time is again noted. Bleeding time is a coagulation test used to measure platelet function and the integrity of blood vessel walls.

Pathology and Laboratory

85004

85004   Blood count; automated differential WBC count

A WBC is a count of the number of white blood cells (leukocytes) in a specific volume of blood. This test is performed to evaluate overall health and can help the physician evaluate conditions such as infection, allergy, systemic illness, inflammation, and leukemia. There are five types of WBCs, neutrophils, eosinophils, basophils, monocytes, and lymphocytes. In an automated WBC count each of the five types are counted separately using an electronic cell counter or an image analysis instrument.

85007-85008

85007   Blood count; blood smear, microscopic examination with manual differential WBC count

85008   Blood count; blood smear, microscopic examination without manual differential WBC count

A blood smear is performed with microscopic examination with or without a manual differential WBC count. A blood smear is typically performed following an automated test that indicates the presence of abnormal or immature blood cells. It may also be performed when the physician suspects a condition that affects blood cell production, such as anemia. A blood sample is obtained by separately reportable venipuncture. A blood smear is prepared and examined under a microscope by a technician for immature or abnormal cells. In 85007, the test is performed with a manual differential white blood cell (WBC) count. The technician examines and counts each of the five types of WBCs separately. Neutrophils comprise the majority of WBCs in healthy adults and are differentiated by cytoplasm with pink or purple granules. Eosinophils normally comprise 1-3% of total WBCs and are differentiated in stained smears by their large, red-orange granules. Elevated levels of eosinophils may indicate allergy or parasitic infection. Basophils normally comprise only 1% of total WBCs and are differentiated by their large black granules. Elevated levels of basophils may be indicative of certain leukemias, varicella (chicken pox) infection, or ulcerative colitis. Monocytes are the largest WBCs and act as scavengers to ingest (phagocytize) cellular debris, bacteria, and other particles. Lymphocytes produce antibodies (immunoglobulins) and are differentiated by their homogenous cytoplasm and smooth, round nucleus. In 85008, the blood smear is performed without manual differential WBC count.

85009

85009   Blood count; manual differential WBC count, buffy coat

A manual white blood cell (WBC) count is estimated using a rapid technique referred to as buffy coat. A blood sample is obtained by separately reportable venipuncture. The blood specimen is placed in a microhematocrit tube and centrifuged (spun) to separate the WBCs which appear as a thin layer of white cells between the RBCs and plasma. This thin layer is called the buffy coat and is used to estimate whether WBC count is higher than normal. The technician then performs a manual differential WBC count, which involves identifying and counting each of the five types of WBCs separately. Neutrophils comprise the majority of WBCs in healthy adults and are differentiated by cytoplasm with pink or purple granules. Eosinophils normally comprise 1-3% of total WBCs and are differentiated in stained smears by their large, red-orange granules. Elevated levels of eosinophils may indicate allergy or parasitic infection. Basophils normally comprise only 1% of total WBCs and are differentiated by their large black granules. Elevated levels of basophils may be indicative of certain leukemias, varicella (chicken pox) infection, or ulcerative colitis. Monocytes are the largest WBCs and act as scavengers to ingest (phagocytize) cellular debris, bacteria, and other particles. Lymphocytes produce antibodies (immunoglobulins) and are differentiated by their homogenous cytoplasm and smooth, round nucleus.

85013-85014

85013   Blood count; spun microhematocrit

85014   Blood count; hematocrit (Hct)

A blood test is performed to determine hematocrit (Hct). Hematocrit refers to the volume of red blood cells (erythrocytes) in a given volume of blood and is usually expressed as a percentage of total blood volume. A blood sample is obtained by separately reportable venipuncture or finger, heel, or ear stick. In 85013, the blood sample is collected in a microhematocrit tube which is centrifuged (spun) to separate the WBCs and plasma from the RBCs. The Hct (volume of RBCs) is then calculated and expressed as a percentage of total blood volume (RBCs + WBCs + plasma). In 85014, Hct is calculated using an electronic cell counter.

85018

85018   Blood count; hemoglobin (Hgb)

A blood test is performed to determine hemoglobin (Hgb) which is a measurement of the amount of oxygen-carrying protein in the blood. Hgb is measured to determine the severity of anemia or polycythemia, monitor response to treatment for these conditions, or determine the need for blood transfusion. A blood sample is collected by separately reportable venipuncture or finger, heel, or ear stick. The sample may be sent to the lab or a rapid testing system may be used in the physician's office. Systems consist of a portable

photometer and pipettes that contain reagent. The pipette is used to collect the blood sample from a capillary stick and the blood is automatically mixed with the reagent in the pipette. The photometer is then used to read the result which is displayed on the photometer device.

85025-85027

85025   Blood count; complete (CBC), automated (Hgb, Hct, RBC, WBC and platelet count) and automated differential WBC count

85027   Blood count; complete (CBC), automated (Hgb, Hct, RBC, WBC and platelet count)

An automated complete blood count (CBC) is performed with or without automated differential white blood cell (WBC) count. A CBC is used as a screening test to evaluate overall health and symptoms such as fatigue, bruising, bleeding, and inflammation, or to help diagnose infection. A CBC includes measurement of hemoglobin (Hgb) and hematocrit (Hct), red blood cell (RBC) count, white blood cell (WBC) count with or without differential, and platelet count. Hgb measures the amount of oxygen-carrying protein in the blood. Hct refers to the volume of red blood cells (erythrocytes) in a given volume of blood and is usually expressed as a percentage of total blood volume. RBC count is the number of red blood cells (erythrocytes) in a specific volume of blood. WBC count is the number of white blood cells (leukocytes) in a specific volume of blood. There are five types of WBCs: neutrophils, eosinophils, basophils, monocytes, and lymphocytes. If a differential is performed, each of the five types is counted separately. Platelet count is the number of platelets (thrombocytes) in the blood. Platelets are responsible for blood clotting. The CBC is performed with an automated blood cell counting instrument that can also be programmed to provide an automated WBC differential count. Use 85025 for CBC with automated differential WBC count or 85027 for CBC without differential WBC count.

85032

85032   Blood count; manual cell count (erythrocyte, leukocyte, or platelet) each

A manual blood cell count of red blood cells (RBCs/erythrocytes), white blood cells (WBCs/leukocytes), or platelets (thrombocytes) is performed. A blood sample is obtained. A capillary pipette and hemocytometer may be used to obtain the sample. Manual erythrocyte count is performed by placing the hemocytometer on the microscope stage. The central area is ruled off into 25 squares. Erythrocytes in the four corner squares and the middle square are then counted. The number of erythrocytes in each square should not vary by more than 10 cells. The erythrocyte count is calculated by averaging the number of erythrocytes in the squares counted. Leukocytes and platelets are counted in the same manner except that the hemocytometer is divided into nine squares, and cells in all nine squares are counted and then averaged. Report 85032 for each type of blood cell (erythrocyte, leukocyte, or platelet) counted.

85041

85041   Blood count; red blood cell (RBC), automated

An automated red blood cell (RBC) count is performed to evaluate any decrease or increase in the number of RBCs in a specific volume of blood. RBC count may be performed as part of a general health screen or prior to a surgical procedure. It may also be performed to monitor patients undergoing chemotherapy or radiation therapy, or to monitor and evaluate response to treatment in patients with bleeding disorders, chronic anemia, or polycythemia. The RBC count is performed with an automated blood cell counting instrument.

85044

85044   Blood count; reticulocyte, manual

A manual reticulocyte count is performed. Reticulocytes are new red blood cells (RBCs) that circulate in the peripheral blood for 1-2 days before losing sufficient RNA to become mature RBCs. A reticulocyte count may be performed when a blood test shows decreased RBCs and/or decreased hemoglobin or hematocrit measurements. The test can help determine if the bone marrow is responding to the body's need for RBCs. Indications for monitoring reticulocytes include vitamin B12 or folate deficiency, kidney disease, chemotherapy, bone marrow transplant, and treatment with erythropoietin or darbopoietin. A blood sample is obtained. The blood is placed in a tube with new methylene blue and a blood film is prepared. The film is placed under a microscope and reticulocytes are manually counted.

85045-85046

85045   Blood count; reticulocyte, automated

85046   Blood count; reticulocytes, automated, including 1 or more cellular parameters (eg, reticulocyte hemoglobin content [CHr], immature reticulocyte fraction [IRF], reticulocyte volume [MRV], RNA content), direct measurement

An automated reticulocyte count is performed. Reticulocytes are new red blood cells (RBCs) that circulate in the peripheral blood for 1-2 days before losing sufficient RNA to become mature RBCs. A reticulocyte count may be performed when a blood test shows

● New Code   ▲ Revised Code

Pathology and Laboratory

decreased RBCs and/or decreased hemoglobin or hematocrit measurements. The test can help determine if the bone marrow is responding to the body's need for RBCs. Indications for monitoring reticulocytes include vitamin B12 or folate deficiency, kidney disease, chemotherapy, bone marrow transplant, and treatment with erythropoietin or darbopoietin. A blood sample is obtained. A reticulocyte count is performed with an automated blood cell counting instrument. Automated reticulocyte count performed alone is reported with 85045. When automated reticulocyte count is performed with direct measurement of one or more cellular parameters, such as reticulocyte hemoglobin content (CHr), immature reticulocyte fraction (IRF), mean reticulocyte volume (MRV), or RNA content, 85046 is reported. CHr measures the amount of hemoglobin in reticulocytes, which is an indicator of iron utilization for RBC production, and is used to diagnosis iron deficiency. IRF is used to determine whether reticulocytes are being released prematurely and to quantify the proportion of immature reticulocytes. Premature release occurs during periods of high demand for RBCs in chronic kidney disease, following chemotherapy or bone marrow transplant, or in patients with AIDs or malignant disease, as well as other conditions. IRF is calculated as a ratio of immature reticulocytes to the total number of reticulocytes (both immature and mature). MRV looks at the total volume of reticulytes compared to total red blood cells and is used to evaluate iron utilization. RNA content is evaluated to determine the maturity of circulating reticulocytes.

85048

85048   Blood count; leukocyte (WBC), automated

An automated white blood cell (WBC/leukocyte) count is performed to evaluate any decrease or increase in the number of leukocytes in a specific volume of blood. Leukocyte count may be performed to monitor conditions such as HIV and AIDs, or to monitor medical therapies such as chemotherapy or radiation therapy that weaken the immune system and cause a decrease in WBCs. It may also be performed to screen for elevated levels found with bacterial infections, inflammation, leukemia, or trauma. The leukocyte count is performed with an automated blood cell counting instrument.

85049

85049   Blood count; platelet, automated

An automated platelet count is performed. Platelets, also referred to as thrombocytes, are responsible for blood clotting. A platelet count is performed to diagnose a bleeding disorder, such as Von Willebrand's disease, or bone marrow diseases, such as leukemia or other blood cancers. Platelet levels may also be monitored in patients who have undergone bone marrow transplant, who are receiving chemotherapy, or who have chronic kidney disease or autoimmune disorders. Platelets are counted electronically using an automated device.

85055

85055   Reticulated platelet assay

A laboratory test is performed to monitor reticulated platelet activity. Platelets are tiny cells that circulate in the blood, binding together to form clots when blood vessels are damaged. Platelets are manufactured in the bone marrow, and reticulated platelets are newly formed and immature. Thrombocytopenia is a common hematological abnormality associated with severe bleeding. Diagnostic tests to determine pathogenesis of thrombocytopenia usually require a sample of bone marrow through an invasive and uncomfortable procedure. The reticulated platelet assay is a simple and much less invasive procedure that reflects the rate of thrombopoiesis in the bone marrow. The ratio of immature platelet fraction (IPF) will be low when production is suppressed (thrombocytopenia due to chemotherapy) and increased when thrombocytopenia is caused by destruction of platelets (idiopathic thrombocytopenia purpura). The IPF ratio may also help predict platelet recovery following peripheral blood hematopoietic progenitor cell (HPC) transplant. Persistent low IPF suggests failure of thrombopoietic recovery. A blood sample is obtained by separately reportable venipuncture. Whole blood is tested using flow cytometry.

85060

85060   Blood smear, peripheral, interpretation by physician with written report

A laboratory test is performed by a physician to examine, interpret, and submit a written report of a peripheral blood smear. This test is usually ordered when an automated complete blood count (CBC) is abnormal. A drop of blood is placed on a glass slide, spread thinly and fixed in place with a special stain. The slide is then placed under a microscope and the cells are counted and examined for size, shape, and appearance. Characteristics of red blood cells (RBC, erythrocytes), white blood cells (WBC, leukocytes) and platelets (thrombocytes) can diagnose a number of diseases and deficiencies involving blood production, function, and cell destruction. Cell production and maturity may be monitored using a blood smear in patients with anemia, myeloproliferative disorders, bone marrow disease, leukemia, and hemoglobin variant conditions such as sickle cell disease and thalassemia, and during cancer treatment with chemotherapy or radiation. A blood sample is obtained by separately reportable venipuncture, finger, ear, or heel stick. Whole blood is examined using stain and microscope.

85097

85097   Bone marrow, smear interpretation

A laboratory test is performed by a physician or technician to examine, interpret, and submit a written report of a bone marrow smear. Bone marrow is a sponge like tissue filled with a fluid that contains hematopoetic stem cells which produce red blood cells (RBC, erythrocytes), white blood cells (WBC, leukocytes) and platelets (thrombocytes). Bone marrow also contains iron, vitamin B12, folate, and fat. An automated complete blood count (CBC) and/or peripheral blood smear may be ordered at the same time and used for comparison. Bone marrow aspirate, core or clot, or a section from flow cytometry is placed on a glass slide, spread thinly, and fixed in place with a special stain. The slide is then placed under a microscope and the cells are counted and examined for size, shape, and appearance. The myeloid (WBC precursor) to erythroid (RBC precursor) ratio is determined along with a differential count and maturation level of the total WBC, RBC, and platelets. Abnormal cells are characterized, and the cellularity of the sample and structure of the marrow are reported, if present in the sample. A bone marrow smear may be performed to diagnose, stage, and/or monitor treatment of leukemia, anemia, thrombocytopenia, myelodysplastic disorders, lymphoma, myeloma, and other cancers. A bone marrow sample is obtained by separately reportable procedure and examined using stain and microscope.

85130

85130   Chromogenic substrate assay

Chromogenic substrate assay is an analytical technique used to determine enzyme activity. The intensity of color produced after a chromogenic-linked substrate is added to body tissue or fluid shows the relative activity of the factor being observed. This technique is widely used when testing anti-thrombotic drugs (heparin), the anticoagulant proteins, antithrombin (AT) or Protein C (PC), and other components of the fibrinolytic system. A blood sample is obtained by separately reportable venipuncture. Plasma may be tested for heparin cofactor II using quantitative chromogenic substrate assay.

85170

85170   Clot retraction

A laboratory test is performed to measure the amount of time it takes for a sample of whole blood to clot in a test tube. This test gives an overall indication of platelet function, from adhesion to aggregation, and finally retraction. In response to injury, collagen in the endothelium of the blood vessel is exposed and triggers the conversion of fibrinogen to fibrin. Platelets trapped by the fibrin form a thrombus. Integrin $\alpha IIb\alpha 3$ which is bound to fibrin contracts the platelet's actin-myosin cytoskeleton pulling the clot in and expelling excess fluid. The retraction of the clot clears the obstructed blood vessel renewing blood flow. Normal clot retraction time is 0-120 minutes. Increased clot retraction time may indicate an abnormality sometime after Integrin $\alpha IIb\alpha 3$ interacts with fibrin. This could be due to an acquired or hereditary platelet disorder (Glanzmann thrombasthenia), the use of anti-platelet medications, decreased platelet or fibrinogen levels, or increased red blood cells. Decreased clot retraction time may indicate a tendency toward thrombosis formation. A blood sample is obtained by separately reportable venipuncture. There are two methods for conducting this test. With the first method, the test tube is set up next to a camera. Photographs are taken initially and every 30 minutes until the clot is noted to be completely retracted by a human observer. With the second method, a metal rod coated with platelet rich plasma is inserted into a vial containing a measured sample of whole blood. After the clot forms on the rod, the rod and clot are removed and the amount of serum is measured. The patient sample is always tested with a control sample.

85175

85175   Clot lysis time, whole blood dilution

A laboratory test for clot lysis time using whole blood dilution is performed to assess the overall activity of the fibrinolytic system. Fibrin breakdown in a blood clot is activated by the plasmin serine protease pathway. Elevated activity can cause an increase in bleeding tendency (hemorrhage) while decreased activity leads to thrombosis formation (blood clots). Whole blood is collected in a test tube and clotted by adding thrombin. The sample is incubated at 37° C and the release of erythrocytes from the clot is observed and counted at 30 minute intervals. Exogenous TPA, activated Protein C, or anti-PAI antibodies may be added to the test tube to speed up the clot lysis reaction. This test may be used to diagnose and monitor atherosclerosis associated diseases, survey coagulation status of liver transplants, and during/after cardiovascular surgery.

85210

85210   Clotting; factor II, prothrombin, specific

A laboratory test is performed to measure factor II (prothrombin) activity. Prothrombin is a vitamin K-dependent proenzyme produced in the liver which proteolytically cleaves to form thrombin, a necessary component of the coagulation cascade. Prothrombin deficiency may be an inherited genetic disorder or caused by liver disease, vitamin K deficiency, anticoagulant therapy, or an autoimmune disorder. Symptoms of prothrombin deficiency include bruising, nose bleeds, soft tissue hemorrhage, and excessive postsurgical or menstrual bleeding. Elevated levels of prothrombin may be due to a mutation of prothrombin 20210a which leads to excessive clotting and increased risk of thrombus formation. The test for prothrombin activity may be ordered when a patient has abnormal bleeding time tests (PT, PTT) or a family history of coagulation factor deficiencies, as well as to monitor the severity of the factor defect and effectiveness of treatment. A blood sample is obtained by separately reportable venipuncture. Platelet-poor plasma is tested using prothrombin clot-based assay.

85220

85220   Clotting; factor V (AcG or proaccelerin), labile factor

A laboratory test is performed to measure factor V (AcG, proaccelerin) labile factor activity. Factor V is a vitamin K-dependent protein produced in the liver and endothelium, and by megakaryocytes and platelets. Factor V is not an active enzyme but does function as a co-factor activated by thrombin in the coagulation cascade. Inherited Factor V deficiency is a rare genetic disorder that causes a mild form of hemophilia (Owren hemophilia). The deficiency is more often acquired and may be due to liver disease, autoimmune disorders, cancer and myeloproliferative diseases, intravascular coagulation disorders (DIC), secondary fibrinolysis, and medications. Symptoms of Factor V deficiency include bruising, nose bleeds, soft tissue hemorrhage, and excessive postsurgical or menstrual bleeding. Elevated levels of Factor V (Leiden) is caused by a genetic mutation which leads to hypercoagulability and venous thrombosis. The test for factor V activity may be ordered when a patient has abnormal bleeding time tests (PT, PTT) or a family history of coagulation factor deficiencies, as well as to monitor the severity of the factor defect and effectiveness of treatment. A blood sample is obtained by separately reportable venipuncture. Platelet-poor plasma is tested using prothrombin clot-based assay.

85230

85230   Clotting; factor VII (proconvertin, stable factor)

A laboratory test is performed to measure factor VII (proconvertin) stable factor activity. Factor VII is a vitamin K-dependent protein enzyme of the serine protease class. Factor VII initiates coagulation in conjunction with Factor III (tissue factor). Inherited Factor VII deficiency is a rare genetic occurrence that causes a hemophilia-like bleeding disorder. The deficiency is more often acquired due to vitamin K deficiency, bile duct obstruction, liver disease, or anticoagulant therapy. Symptoms of Factor VII deficiency include bruising, nose bleeds, soft tissue or joint hemorrhage, and excessive postsurgical or menstrual bleeding. The test for factor VII activity may be ordered when a patient has abnormal bleeding time tests (PT, PTT) or a family history of coagulation factor deficiencies, as well as to monitor the severity of the factor defect and effectiveness of treatment. A blood sample is obtained by separately reportable venipuncture. Platelet-poor plasma is tested using prothrombin clot based assay.

85240

85240   Clotting; factor VIII (AHG), 1-stage

Hemophilia A, also known as clotting factor VIII deficiency or classic hemophilia, is the most common type of hemophilia. Hemophilia A is an inherited disorder in which factor VIII, a protein needed to form blood clots, is missing or reduced. This test is used to detect factor VIII deficiency due to hemophilia A or an acquired deficiency caused by liver disease or disseminated intravascular coagulopathy (DIC). A blood sample is obtained. A one stage clotting test is performed to evaluate factor VIII activity by comparing dilutions of the patient sample to a known set of standard dilutions. The results are expressed as a percentage.

85244

85244   Clotting; factor VIII related antigen

A laboratory test is performed to measure factor VIII related antigen. Factor VIII (antihemophilic factor) is a protein necessary for blood clotting. Deficiency of factor VIII is usually an inherited genetic condition that leads to Hemophilia A, or classic hemophilia. As an X-linked genetic mutation, the condition affects males much more often than females with the severe form (<1% Factor VIII) occurring in 60% of cases, the moderate form (1-5% Factor VIII) in 15% of cases, and the mild form (6-30% Factor VIII) seen in 25% of patients with the disorder. Bleeding in mild disease will only occur with severe injury or trauma while in the moderate form, bleeding may also occasionally happen spontaneously in the joints and soft tissues. Individuals with severe factor VIII deficiency are at risk for spontaneous bleeding at all times. The test for factor VIII related antigen may be used to assess factor VIII replacement therapy, determine carrier status, or to distinguish patients who may be cross-reactive positive (CRP). A blood sample is obtained by separately reportable venipuncture and tested using immunoassay.

85245

85245   Clotting; factor VIII, VW factor, ristocetin cofactor

A laboratory test is performed to measure factor VIII, VW factor, ristocetin cofactor. Factor VIII (antihemophilic factor) and von Willebrand factor (VWF) complex together to form a unique plasma glycoprotein. VWF is the carrier protein for coagulation factor VIII, stabilizing its procoagulant activity. VWF is found in two forms, one circulates freely in plasma and the

other is bound to alpha granules of circulating platelets. Plasma VWF is synthesized and released by vascular endothelial cells. Platelet VWF is synthesized by bone marrow and megakaryocytes. The test for ristocetin cofactor can determine VWF activity and its ability to form blood clots in response to injury and may be ordered as part of an initial work up for von Willebrand disease. A blood sample is obtained by separately reportable venipuncture. Platelet-poor plasma is tested using platelet agglutination.

85246

85246   Clotting; factor VIII, VW factor antigen

A laboratory test is performed to measure factor VIII, VW factor antigen. Factor VIII (antihemophilic factor) and von Willebrand factor (VWF) complex together to form a unique plasma glycoprotein. VWF is the carrier protein for coagulation factor VIII, stabilizing its procoagulant activity. VWF is found in two forms, one circulates freely in plasma and the other is bound to alpha granules of circulating platelets. Plasma VWF is synthesized and released by vascular endothelial cells. Platelet VWF is synthesized by bone marrow and megakaryocytes. The test for VW factor antigen measures the mass of the antigen present but does not indicate VWF activity or functionality. Decreased levels of VWF antigen may be an inherited disorder caused by congenital von Willebrand disease or it can be acquired due to monoclonal gammopathies, lymphoproliferative disorders, autoimmune disease, or hypothyroidism. Conditions that cause elevated levels of VWF antigen include pregnancy and/or estrogen use, acute phase inflammation, exercise and stress, liver disease, vasculitis, and thrombocytopenic purpura hemolytic uremic syndrome. The test for VWF antigen may be ordered as part of an initial work-up for von Willebrand disease. A blood sample is obtained by separately reportable venipuncture. Platelet-poor plasma is tested using microlatex particle-mediated immunoassay.

85247

85247   Clotting; factor VIII, von Willebrand factor, multimetric analysis

A laboratory test for multimetric analysis of factor VIII, von Willebrand factor is performed. Factor VIII (antihemophilic factor) and von Willebrand factor (VWF) complex together to form a unique plasma glycoprotein. VWF is the carrier protein for coagulation factor VIII, stabilizing its procoagulant activity. VWF is found in two forms, one circulates freely in plasma and the other is bound to alpha granules of circulating platelets. Plasma VWF is synthesized and released by vascular endothelial cells. Platelet VWF is synthesized by bone marrow and megakaryocytes. The multimetric analysis test includes factor VIII, activity; VWF, activity; and VWF, ristocetin cofactor. The multimetric analysis is ordered when inherited von Willebrand disease is highly suspected . A blood sample is obtained by separately reportable venipuncture. Platelet-poor plasma is tested using electrophoresis/western blot/clotting/microlatex particle-mediated immunoassay/platelet agglutination.

85250

85250   Clotting; factor IX (PTC or Christmas)

A laboratory test is performed to measure clotting factor IX (PTC, Christmas) activity. Factor IX is a vitamin K dependent protein necessary for blood clotting. It circulates in plasma as an inactive zymogen and is activated to a serine protease when the clotting cascade takes place. Deficiency of factor IX is usually an inherited genetic condition that leads to Hemophilia B (Christmas disease). As an X-linked genetic mutation, the condition affects males more often than females with the severe form (<1% Factor IX) occurring in 60% of cases; the moderate form (1-5% Factor IX) in 15% of cases; and the mild form (6-30% Factor IX) seen in 25% of patients with the disorder. Bleeding in all forms of the disease will occur with severe injury or trauma while in the moderate form, bleeding may be induced by only mild to moderate injury and occasionally will occur spontaneously in the joints and soft tissue. Individuals with severe factor IX deficiency are at risk for spontaneous bleeding at all times. A rare genetic mutation can also cause elevated levels of factor IX which predisposes the individual to hypercoagulation and thrombus formation. This test may be used to diagnose factor IX deficiency, monitor replacement therapy, investigate abnormal bleeding time tests (PT, PTT), or assess the impact of liver disease on hemostasis. A blood sample is obtained by separately reportable venipuncture. Platelet-poor plasma is tested using activated partial thromboplastin clot-based immunoassay.

85260

85260   Clotting; factor X (Stuart-Prower)

A laboratory test is performed to measure clotting factor X (Stuart-Prower) activity. Factor X is a vitamin K dependent serine protease and is the first enzyme to be activated in the clotting cascade. A deficiency of factor X is rare and may be due to an inherited genetic disorder or result from vitamin K deficiency, systemic amyloidosis, severe liver disease, or anticoagulant therapy. Symptoms can include bruising, nose bleeds, hematuria, heavy menstrual bleeding, and soft tissue or joint hemorrhage. This test may be ordered to diagnose factor X deficiency (congenital or acquired), investigate abnormal bleeding time tests (PT, PTT), or to assess the impact of liver disease on hemostasis. A blood sample is obtained by separately reportable venipuncture. Platelet-poor plasma is tested using prothrombin clot-based assay.

Pathology and Laboratory

85270

85270   Clotting; factor XI (PTA)

A laboratory test is performed to measure clotting factor XI activity. Factor XI may also be referred to as plasma thromboplastin antecedent (PTA), and a deficiency causes hemophilia C or Rosenthal syndrome. Factor XI is a zymogen activated by factor XIIa or thrombin to form a trypsin-like serine protease that activates other factors and enzymes in the clotting cascade. It circulates in two forms, platelet and plasma. Platelet factor XI is produced by megakaryocytes, and plasma factor XI is synthesized in the liver. A deficiency of factor XI is most often caused by an inherited genetic disorder affecting both males and females, but has also been (rarely) observed in patients with lupus erythematosus. Manifestations of the disorder do not correlate with measurable levels of factor XI and can be inconsistent for each individual. Bleeding may be immediate or delayed and heavy menstrual bleeding is reported by the majority of women with the condition. Many individuals with factor XI deficiency will have no bleeding symptoms and the condition is diagnosed after an abnormal laboratory test for bleeding time (aPTT) is uncovered. This test may be used to diagnose factor XI deficiency and to investigate the cause of an abnormal aPTT. A blood sample is obtained by separately reportable venipuncture. Platelet-poor plasma is tested using activated partial thromboplastin clot-based assay.

85280

85280   Clotting; factor XII (Hageman)

A laboratory test is performed to measure factor XII (Hageman) activity. Factor XII is a plasma transglutaminase that catalyzes the last step of the clotting cascade, allowing fibrin to form a solid structure and binding fibronectin, α2-plasmin inhibitor, and collagen to the fibrin plug at the wound site. It also facilitates the fibrin-fibronectin cross-linking at the site of placental implantation. A deficiency of factor XII is a rare inherited genetic disorder characterized by severe bleeding that affects males and females equally. It may occasionally manifest as an acquired condition due to hepatic failure, inflammatory bowel disease, or myeloid leukemia. Eighty percent of infants with a congenital factor XII deficiency will have umbilical stump bleeding. Central nervous system bleeding in an infant following a normal birth, or in a person of any age with very mild head trauma is not uncommon. Women with the disorder have a high incidence of spontaneous abortion. Other symptoms can include soft tissue or joint bleeding and delayed wound healing. This test may be used to diagnose factor XII deficiency or determine the cause of prolonged activated thromboplastin time (aPTT). A blood sample is obtained by separately reportable venipuncture. Platelet-poor plasma is tested using activated partial thromboplastin clot-based assay.

85290

85290   Clotting; factor XIII (fibrin stabilizing)

A laboratory test is performed to measure clotting factor XIII (fibrin stabilizing) activity. Factor XIII is necessary for clot preservation, wound repair, and healing. A deficiency can cause defects in fibrin cross-linking leading to early spontaneous miscarriage or heavy menstrual bleeding in women, umbilical stump bleeding in infants, central nervous system bleeding following mild head trauma in children or spontaneously in adults, and bruising and soft tissue bleeding of the gums, muscles, and joints. Factor XIII deficiency is usually caused by a rare inherited genetic disorder but may occur when auto-antibodies are triggered by isoniazide drug therapy. This test is most often ordered to confirm factor XIII deficiency when a qualitative test is positive and to monitor treatment in patients with known deficiency. The test can also be used to evaluate patients with symptoms of abnormal bleeding when bleeding time tests (PT, PTT) and platelet levels are normal. A blood sample is obtained by separately reportable venipuncture. Platelet-poor plasma is tested using chromogenic assay.

85291

85291   Clotting; factor XIII (fibrin stabilizing), screen solubility

A laboratory test is performed to screen for clotting factor XIII (fibrin stabilizing) solubility. Factor XIII is necessary for clot preservation, wound repair, and healing. A deficiency can cause defects in fibrin cross-linking leading to early spontaneous miscarriage or heavy menstrual bleeding in women, umbilical stump bleeding in infants, central nervous system bleeding following mild head trauma in children or spontaneously in adults, and bruising and soft tissue bleeding of the gums, muscles, and joints. Factor XIII deficiency is usually caused by a rare inherited genetic disorder but may occur when auto-antibodies are triggered by isoniazide drug therapy. This qualitative test is usually ordered as an initial screen for factor XIII deficiency. If the results are positive, a quantitative test (85290) should be done. A blood sample is obtained by separately reportable venipuncture. Platelet-poor plasma is tested using qualitative solubility.

85292

85292   Clotting; prekallikrein assay (Fletcher factor assay)

A laboratory test is performed to measure prekallikrein (Fletcher factor) activity. Prekallikrein is a serine protease coagulation protein that is activated to kallikrein by factor XII (Hageman) along the intrinsic pathway in the clotting cascade. A deficiency of

prekallikrein factor rarely causes spontaneous or excessive bleeding and is most often diagnosed when a patient has an abnormal bleeding time test (PTT, aPTT). The deficiency is usually caused by a rare inherited genetic disorder but may be acquired in patients with liver disease, disseminated intravascular coagulation (DIC), and severe infection or sepsis. A blood sample is obtained by separately reportable venipuncture. Platelet-poor plasma is tested using clotting activity assay.

85293

85293   Clotting; high molecular weight kininogen assay (Fitzgerald factor assay)

A laboratory test is performed to measure high molecular weight kininogen (HMWK, Fitzgerald factor) activity. HMWK is produced by the liver and circulates as an inactive plasma protein until it adheres to injured epithelium and binds with prekallikrein and factor XI activating factor XIIa along the intrinsic pathway in the clotting cascade. A deficiency of HMWK rarely causes spontaneous or excessive bleeding and is most often diagnosed when a patient has an abnormal bleeding time test (PTT). The deficiency is usually caused by a rare inherited genetic disorder but may be acquired in patients with liver disease or disseminated intravascular coagulation (DIC). A blood sample is obtained by separately reportable venipuncture. Plasma is tested using clotting activity assay.

85300-85301

85300   Clotting inhibitors or anticoagulants; antithrombin III, activity
85301   Clotting inhibitors or anticoagulants; antithrombin III, antigen assay

A diluted blood sample is mixed with antithrombin-deficient plasma containing intrinsic coagulation enzymes, an AT augmenting compound (e.g., heparin), a phospholipid and an activator of the contact phase of the intrinsic coagulation pathway. Following addition of calcium ions, coagulation time is measured and compared to a reference standard to determine the level of activity in the sample. In 85301, the method consists of adding serum to a thrombin solution and measuring, after a fixed incubation time, the residual thrombin activity on the plasma.

85302-85303

85302   Clotting inhibitors or anticoagulants; protein C, antigen
85303   Clotting inhibitors or anticoagulants; protein C, activity

Protein C is a natural anticoagulant, deficiencies of which have been found in patients with recurrent thrombosis and warfarin-induced skin necrosis. A blood sample is diluted and sodium citrate or citric acid is added. It is then incubated in microwells coated with antibody specific for human Protein C. During an incubation period, the sample of Protein C from the patient is allowed to bind to the surface. Horseradish peroxidase (HRP) conjugated anti-human Protein C detection antibody is added. After washing to remove unbound conjugate, a chromogenic substrate is added, resulting in a soluble colored product that is measured. In 85303, protein C activity is measured. The protein C activity assay is ordered to determine if a patient has a decrease in coagulation control protein C, which increases the patient's risk for venous thromboembolism.

85305

85305   Clotting inhibitors or anticoagulants; protein S, total

A laboratory test is performed to measure total protein S, a vitamin K dependent single chain glycoprotein that circulates in free and bound states in plasma. Protein S functions as a non-enzyme cofactor for the activation of the coagulation protein, activated protein C (APC). Protein S deficiency is usually caused by a rare inherited genetic disorder but can also be acquired with liver disease, vitamin K deficiency, disseminated intravascular coagulation (DIC), pregnancy, and inflammatory syndromes. The condition is characterized by increased blood clotting, recurrent venous thrombosis, and/or embolism. Women with the deficiency are at increased risk for fetal loss. The test for total protein S is usually used to subtype a known deficiency. Type I deficiency will have low levels of free and total protein S, Type III will have a decrease in only free protein S. In Type II, antigenic levels are normal but cofactor activity is decreased. The patient should refrain from taking the anticoagulant warfarin or coumadin for 2 weeks prior to the test. A blood sample is obtained by separately reportable venipuncture. Platelet-poor plasma is tested using microlatex particle-mediated immunoassay.

85306

85306   Clotting inhibitors or anticoagulants; protein S, free

A laboratory test is performed to measure free protein S, a vitamin K dependent single chain glycoprotein that circulates in free and bound states in plasma. Protein S functions as a non-enzyme cofactor for the activation of the coagulation protein, activated protein C (APC). Protein S deficiency is usually caused by a rare inherited genetic disorder but can also be acquired with liver disease, vitamin K deficiency, disseminated intravascular coagulation (DIC), pregnancy, and inflammatory syndromes. The condition is characterized by increased blood clotting, recurrent venous thrombosis, and/or embolism. Women with the deficiency are at increased risk for fetal loss. The test for free protein S is usually used to screen an individual for a deficiency. A positive result should be reflexed to include a test for total protein S in order to subtype the disorder. Type I deficiency will have low levels of free and total protein S; Type III will have a decrease in only free protein S. In Type II, antigenic levels are normal but cofactor activity is decreased. The patient should refrain from taking the anticoagulant warfarin or coumadin for 2 weeks prior to the test. A blood sample is obtained by separately reportable venipuncture. Platelet-poor plasma is tested using microlatex particle-mediated immunoassay.

85307

85307   Activated Protein C (APC) resistance assay

An Activated Protein C (APC) resistance assay is performed on patients with unexplained venous thromboembolism to determine whether the cause is a single point mutation of the Factor V gene referred to as Factor V Leiden. There are two variations on this test. A dilution of the specimen to be tested from the patient and a control specimen with Factor V deficient plasma are made. Activated Protein C is then added. If APC resistance is not present, the addition of APC will result in a two-fold prolongation of activated partial thromboplastin time (aPTT). If mutated Factor V is present, the aPTT will be prolonged, but not as much as with normal plasma. The results are normalized by comparing the results of the patient specimen and the control specimen. A ratio of aPTT with APC to aPTT without APC is computed for both the specimen and the control. If a mutation of Factor V is not present, the patient ratio and normalized ratio will be approximately the same. If a mutation is present, the patient ratio will be lower than the control.

85335

85335   Factor inhibitor test

A laboratory test is performed to measure factor inhibitor activity. Inhibitor factors are IgG antibodies which develop against clotting factors and can lead to clotting factor concentrate failure, bleeding episodes, and life threatening hemorrhage. They are most often observed in patients with factor VIII (hemophilia A) or factor IX (hemophilia B) deficiencies who receive clotting factor concentrate to treat their hemolytic disorder. Inhibitor factor antibodies may also develop in elderly patients with no history of hemophilia, in postpartum women, and in patients with other autoimmune disorders. A blood sample is obtained by separately reportable venipuncture. Platelet-poor plasma is tested using clot-based assay.

85337

85337   Thrombomodulin

A laboratory test is performed to measure thrombomodulin, a glycoprotein located on the surface of endothelial cells. Thrombomodulin serves as a cofactor for thrombin to activate protein C and initiate an essential anticoagulant pathway. It may also serve to down-regulate thrombin formation and limit the inflammatory response. Elevated levels of thrombomodulin may be present with vascular damage, acute infections, sepsis, and inflammatory conditions. A blood sample is obtained by separately reportable venipuncture and tested for thrombomodulin using enzyme-linked immunosorbent assay.

85345

85345   Coagulation time; Lee and White

A laboratory test is performed to measure coagulation time using Lee-White method. Coagulation time measures the number of minutes it takes a sample of blood to form a clot and may be used to assess platelet function. The Lee-White coagulation test requires human observation of 3 test tubes containing one patient's whole blood sample and timing with a stop watch the clot formation in each of the tubes. The number of minutes it takes each tube to form a clot is averaged to determine the coagulation time. This test is nonspecific and less accurate than other available coagulation time tests. It has largely been replaced with automated tests such as prothrombin time (PT) or activated partial thromboplastin time (PTT, aPTT).

85347

85347   Coagulation time; activated

A laboratory test is performed to measure coagulation time using activated (ACT) method. Coagulation time measures the number of minutes it takes a sample of blood to form a clot and may be used to assess platelet function. The activated coagulation test measures blood clotting time following exposure to an intrinsic pathway activator (kaolin, celite, diatomaceous earth). This test may be performed manually when clinically indicated before, during, and immediately following procedures that require intense anticoagulation with heparin. These can include cardiac bypass surgery, angioplasty, extra-corporeal membrane oxygenation (ECMO), thrombolysis, and dialysis. The manual ACT test has largely been replaced by automated machines that use rapid diagnostic instrumentation with the capability to assess multiple clotting assays (PT, PTT, thrombin, fibrinogen) on a single blood sample.

85348

85348   Coagulation time; other methods

A laboratory test is performed to measure coagulation time. Coagulation time is the number of minutes it takes a sample of blood to form a clot and may be used to assess platelet function. Code 85348 can be used when the procedure for evaluating the coagulation time has not been specified as Lee-White, activated, or another definitive coagulation time testing method that has a specific code.

85360

85360   Euglobulin lysis

A laboratory test is performed to measure euglobulin clot lysis time (ECLT). The fibrinolytic activity in plasma can provide an overall assessment of the fibrin clotting system and is helpful for monitoring patients receiving streptokinase therapy. A blood sample is obtained by separately reportable venipuncture. The whole blood sample is mixed with trisodium citrate as an anticoagulant and chilled. The sample is centrifuged, the plasma is extracted and diluted with acetic acid, then incubated for 15 minutes on ice. The precipitate that forms (euglobulin fraction of plasma) contains plasminogen, plasminogen activators (t-PA), and fibrinogen. The sample is centrifuged again and the precipitate is collected and dissolved in a buffer. The sample is clotted with thrombin and inspected for clot lysis at 15 minute intervals. A control sample should always be tested with the patient sample.

85362

85362   Fibrin(ogen) degradation (split) products (FDP) (FSP); agglutination slide, semiquantitative

A laboratory test is performed to measure semiquantitative fibrin(ogen) degradation (split) products (FDP) (FSP) using agglutination slide. FDP (FSP) are fragments of dissolved or disintegrating fibrin released when a clot is broken down by the enzyme plasmin. This test can detect the presence of large amounts of FDP (FSP) but does not differentiate clot fibrinolysis from the degradation of intact fibrinogen (fibrinogenolysis). Serum and plasma will both contain FDP (FSP); however, serum testing is not recommended for assessing FDP or coagulopathies, such as disseminated intravascular coagulation (DIC). Plasma testing provides a more reliable measure of FDP and the D-dimer test should be used for coagulopathies. Elevated levels of FDP (FSP) can occur with DIC, thromboembolitic events, acute myocardial infarction, preeclampsia, renal failure, sepsis/shock, post-operative status, and with strenuous exercise. A blood sample is obtained by separately reportable venipuncture. Serum/plasma is tested using latex agglutination.

85366

85366   Fibrin(ogen) degradation (split) products (FDP) (FSP); paracoagulation

A laboratory test is performed to measure fibrin(ogen) degradation (split) products (FDP) (FSP) using paracoagulation. FDP (FSP) are fragments of dissolved or disintegrating fibrin released when a clot is broken down by the enzyme plasmin. This test evaluates soluble intermediates of fibrinogen-fibrin conversion by using erythrocytes coated with fibrin monomers. The soluble fibrin monomer complex (SFMC) is a sensitive marker for hypercoagulation. This test may be used to diagnose and monitor disseminated intravascular coagulation. A blood sample is obtained by separately reportable venipuncture. Platelet-poor plasma is tested using qualitative hemagglutination.

85370

85370   Fibrin(ogen) degradation (split) products (FDP) (FSP); quantitative

A laboratory test is performed to measure the quantitative level of fibrin(ogen) degradation (split) products (FDP) (FSP) present in blood. FDP (FSP) are fragments of dissolved or disintegrating fibrin released when a clot is broken down by the enzyme plasmin. Elevated levels of FDP (FSP) can occur with disseminated intravascular coagulation, thromboembolitic events, acute myocardial infarction, preeclampsia, renal failure, sepsis/shock, post-operative status, and with strenuous exercise. A blood sample is obtained by separately reportable venipuncture and tested using enzyme-linked immunosorbent assay.

85378-85380

85378   Fibrin degradation products, D-dimer; qualitative or semiquantitative
85379   Fibrin degradation products, D-dimer; quantitative
85380   Fibrin degradation products, D-dimer; ultrasensitive (eg, for evaluation for venous thromboembolism), qualitative or semiquantitative

D-dimer testing for fibrin degradation products is performed to help rule out the presence of a thrombus. D-dimer tests are also used to rule-out hypercoagulability. D-dimer has a negative predictive value for these conditions which means that a negative result indicates that there is not an elevated level of fibrin degradation products present in the specimen. A positive result indicates an abnormally high level of fibrin degradation products which may be indicative of a thrombus. It is used to help diagnosis deep vein thrombophlebitis, pulmonary embolus, and stroke. The test is also used to evaluate for hypercoagulability which predisposes the patient to blood clots and to help diagnose disseminated intravascular coagulation (DIC) and monitor the effectiveness of DIC treatment. In 85379, a quantitative test is performed which provides the level of fibrin degradation products in the specimen. In 85378 and 85380, D-dimer qualitative and semiquantitative testing for fibrin degradation products is performed. Use 85378 for standard less sensitive testing methodology that detects the presence of fibrin degradation products and provides a

● New Code   ▲ Revised Code

Pathology and Laboratory

rough estimate of the level. Use 85380 for ultrasensitive tests that provided rapid, highly accurate results due to the high sensitivity of the test.

85384-85385

85384   Fibrinogen; activity
85385   Fibrinogen; antigen

A laboratory test is performed to measure fibrinogen activity. Fibrinogen is a protein coagulation factor (factor I) produced by the liver and essential for blood clot formation. At the end of the clotting cascade, soluble fibrinogen converts to insoluble fibrin threads to stabilize the injury site and stop bleeding. The test for fibrinogen activity (85384) measures the functionality of circulating fibrinogen. This test may be done together with a fibrinogen antigen test (85385), which measures the level of circulating fibrinogen. These tests are used to detect and monitor the level of fibrinogen circulating in the blood as well as its ability to function properly. These tests can be used to investigate unusual bleeding or thrombotic episodes, abnormal bleeding time tests (PT, PTT), or when there is a family history of hereditary fibrinogen deficiency. The tests are sometimes used to assess an individual's risk of developing cardiovascular disease. A blood sample is obtained by separately reportable venipuncture. Platelet-poor plasma is tested using electromagnetic mechanical clot detection.

85390

85390   Fibrinolysins or coagulopathy screen, interpretation and report

A written report specific to fibrin or coagulation studies is made by a pathologist or other similarly qualified professional from a hospital or independent testing laboratory. The request for an interpretive report may come from the attending physician or be a standing order of the hospital/care facility. The report should contain patient specific diagnostic information, treatment strategies, and future testing options.

85396

85396   Coagulation/fibrinolysis assay, whole blood (eg, viscoelastic clot assessment), including use of any pharmacologic additive(s), as indicated, including interpretation and written report, per day

A laboratory test is performed on whole blood for coagulation/fibrinolysis assay using pharmacologic additives and includes a written interpretive report. This test provides a global assessment of the patient's hemorrhage or thrombotic risk by measuring multiple elements involved in the clotting cascade. The rate of clot formation, and the strength and stability of the clot can be assessed from fibrin formation, platelet function, and fibrinolytic activity. The whole blood assay gives a broad view of hemostatic imbalance in patients with acute bleeding or major trauma and can be used to direct appropriate transfusion support. A blood sample is obtained by separately reportable venipuncture, arterial or central line draw. Whole blood is tested with the addition of thromboelastogram (TEG) plain kaolin and heparinase. A written report specific to the assay is made by a pathologist or other similarly qualified professional from a hospital or independent testing laboratory. The report should contain patient specific diagnostic information, treatment strategies, and future testing options.

85397

85397   Coagulation and fibrinolysis, functional activity, not otherwise specified (eg, ADAMTS-13), each analyte

A blood sample is obtained by separately reportable venipuncture to evaluate coagulation and fibrinolysis functional activity for ADAMTS-13 or other analytes that do not have a more specific code. Coagulation refers to the ability of the blood to clot, while fibrinolysis refers to the dissolution or breakdown of fibrin in blood clots. The presence of certain human autoantibodies in serum and plasma can inhibit analyte activity and affect blood clot formation and breakdown of fibrin, which can result in coagulation disorders. ADAMTS-13 is one such analyte. The presence of human autoantibodies (IgG) in serum or plasma against ADAMTS-13 may be one cause of thrombotic thrombocytopenic purpura (TTP). Testing for the presence of the analyte ADAMTS-13 is performed by enzyme-linked immunosorbent assay (ELISA). The assay measures the functional activity of the protease ADAMTS-13. Testing for other analytes or other proteins (proteases) that participate in the coagulation and fibrinolysis process may use other types of assays. Report code 85397 for each analyte tested.

85400

85400   Fibrinolytic factors and inhibitors; plasmin

A laboratory test is performed to measure plasmin activity. Plasmin is a serine protease enzyme produced by the liver. It is released as plasminogen which circulates in the blood in inactive form until binding to a clot or cell surface. Plasminogen is activated to plasmin by tissue plasminogen activator (tPA), urokinase plasminogen activator (uPA), kallikrein and factor XII (Hageman). Activated plasmin breaks down plasma proteins including fibrin clots (fibrinolysis), activates collagenases, and weakens the wall of Graafian follicles to facilitate ovulation. Plasmin has an integral role in wound healing, liver repair, and liver

homeostasis. A blood sample is obtained by separately reportable venipuncture and tested using fluorimetry.

85410

85410   Fibrinolytic factors and inhibitors; alpha-2 antiplasmin

A laboratory test is performed to measure alpha-2-antiplasmin activity. Alpha-2-antiplasmin is a serine protease inhibitor responsible for inactivating plasmin, an enzyme that breaks down plasma proteins including fibrin clots. This test may be used to diagnose congenital alpha-2-plasmin inhibitor deficiency, assess patients with disseminated intravascular coagulation (DIC), fibrinolysis, or liver disease and monitor the effects of fibrinolytic or antifibrinolytic therapy. A blood sample is obtained by separately reportable venipuncture. Platelet-poor plasma is tested using chromogenic assay.

85415

85415   Fibrinolytic factors and inhibitors; plasminogen activator

A laboratory test is performed to measure plasminogen activator, a serine protease inhibitor produced by endothelial cells and adipose tissue (PAI-I) and also by the placenta (PAI-2). Plasminogen activator targets tissue plasminogen activator (tPA) and urokinase plasminogen activator (uPA) to down regulate fibrinolysis. An inherited genetic disorder can cause a deficiency of PAI-1 characterized by delayed mild to moderate bleeding typically following trauma or surgery. Elevated levels of PAI-I may be due to certain cancers (breast, gastric, lung, cervical), obesity, metabolic syndrome, and inflammatory disorders. A blood sample is obtained by separately reportable venipuncture. Platelet-poor plasma is tested for plasminogen activator inhibitor I activity by bioimmunoassay and tested for tissue plasminogen activator antigen by enzyme-linked immunosorbent assay.

85420

85420   Fibrinolytic factors and inhibitors; plasminogen, except antigenic assay

A laboratory test is performed to measure plasminogen activity. Plasminogen is produced by the liver and circulates in the blood as an inactive form until binding to a clot or cell surface. Plasminogen is activated to plasmin by tissue plasminogen activator (tPA), urokinase plasminogen activator (uPA), kallikrein, and factor XII (Hageman). Decreased levels of plasminogen can be caused by an inherited genetic disorder or acquired with disseminated intravascular coagulation (DIC), liver disease, thrombolytic therapy, or L-asparaginase drug use. Elevated levels have been linked to anabolic steroid use, hypothyroidism, hormone contraceptives, infection, inflammation, trauma, and pregnancy. This test measures the functional activity of plasminogen and can be used to evaluate patients with incidental or recurrent thromboembolytic events, a family history of arterial or venous thrombophilia, or ligneous conjunctiva. If plasminogen activity is abnormal, a test for plasminogen antigen (85421) may be performed to further evaluate a genetic disorder. A blood sample is obtained by separately reportable venipuncture. Platelet-poor plasma is tested using chromogenic assay.

85421

85421   Fibrinolytic factors and inhibitors; plasminogen, antigenic assay

A laboratory test is performed to measure plasminogen antigen. Plasminogen is produced by the liver and circulates in the blood as an inactive form until binding to a clot or cell surface. Plasminogen is activated to plasmin by tissue plasminogen activator (tPA), urokinase plasminogen activator (uPA), kallikrein, and factor XII (Hageman). This test can be used to evaluate a patient for the inherited genetic deficiency disorder hypoplasminogenemia (Type I deficiency) or dysplasminogenemia (Type 2 deficiency). Type I is a systemic disorder of impaired extracellular fibrinolysis which leads to the formation of fibrin-rich pseudomembranous lesions during wound healing. Manifestation is most common on the conjunctiva (ligneous conjunctiva). There is a parallel decrease in immunoreaction and functional activity in Type I deficiency but no increased risk factor for thrombophilia. In Type 2 deficiency, there is a normal or very slight decrease in circulating plasminogen levels but functional activity is markedly diminished. A blood sample is obtained by separately reportable venipuncture. Serum/plasma or cultured cells are tested using enzyme-linked immunosorbent assay.

85441

85441   Heinz bodies; direct

A laboratory test is performed to measure Heinz bodies, denatured hemoglobin that can be found inside red blood cells (RBCs). Heinz bodies may form when hemoglobin is damaged by oxidating drugs, aniline derived drugs, certain enzyme deficiency syndromes (NADPH, G-6-PD, alpha thalassemia) or with unstable hemoglobin (Hemoglobin H, Zurich, Koln, Seattle, Gun Hill). This test may be used to evaluate hemolytic anemia with RBC enzyme deficiencies, or be part of a work-up when "bite cells" are present on a routine blood smear. Bite cells are formed when hemoglobin is removed and its membrane damaged by splenic macrophages. A blood sample is obtained by separately reportable venipuncture. Whole blood is tested using Supravital Stain and direct visualization of cells under a microscope.

Pathology and Laboratory

85445

85445   Heinz bodies; induced, acetyl phenylhydrazine

A laboratory test is performed to measure Heinz bodies, denatured hemoglobin that can be found inside red blood cells (RBCs). Heinz bodies may form when hemoglobin is damaged by oxidating drugs, aniline derived drugs, certain enzyme deficiency syndromes (NADPH, G-6-PD, alpha thalassemia) or with unstable hemoglobin (hemoglobin H, Zurich, Koln, Seattle, Gun Hill). This test may be used to evaluate hemolytic anemias with RBC enzyme deficiencies, or be part of a work-up when "bite cells" are present on a routine blood smear. Bite cells are formed when hemoglobin is removed and its membrane damaged by splenic macrophages. Observation of induced Heinz bodies can assist with diagnosing oxidative chemical ingestion, G-6-PD deficiency, alpha thalassemia, and certain unstable hemoglobin conditions. A blood sample is obtained by separately reportable venipuncture. Acetyl phenylhydrazine is added to whole blood to increase Heinz body production and the sample is examined using Supravital Stain and direct visualization of cells under a microscope.

85460

85460   Hemoglobin or RBCs, fetal, for fetomaternal hemorrhage; differential lysis (Kleihauer-Betke)

A laboratory test is performed to measure the percentage of fetal hemoglobin in maternal blood. This acid elution test eliminates maternal hemoglobin while fetal hemoglobin remains stable and accepts a stain. Fetal blood can mix with maternal blood in fetomaternal hemorrhage (FMH) during pregnancy and/or delivery. In the case of an Rh-negative woman who is pregnant with an Rh-positive fetus, the transfer of fetal cells may cause maternal Rh immunization and affect future pregnancies. Quantifying the extent of FMH can help determine the dose of Rh immune globulin (RhoGAM) to be administered to a woman postpartum or following a (preterm) fetal loss. A blood sample is obtained by separately reportable venipuncture. Whole blood is tested using semi-quantitative acid elution eosin stain/microscopy.

85461

85461   Hemoglobin or RBCs, fetal, for fetomaternal hemorrhage; rosette

A laboratory test is performed to measure fetal hemoglobin in maternal blood. This qualitative screening test may be ordered when a larger than expected fetomaternal hemorrhage (FMH) has occurred. Fetal blood can mix with maternal blood during pregnancy and/or delivery. In the case of an Rh-negative woman who is pregnant with an Rh-positive fetus, the transfer of fetal cells may cause maternal Rh immunization and affect future pregnancies. A positive qualitative screening test should be followed by a quantitative test (85460) to determine the dose of Rh immune globulin (RhoGAM) to be administered to a woman postpartum or following a (preterm) fetal loss. A blood sample is obtained by separately reportable venipuncture. Whole blood is tested using red blood cell rosetting.

85475

85475   Hemolysin, acid

A laboratory test is performed using acid hemolysis (Ham test) to observe the condition and fragility of red blood cells (RBCs) following the addition of a mild acid solution to the blood sample. The Ham test may be used to diagnose acquired or inherited blood disorders including dyserythropoietic anemia type II. Dyserythropoietic anemia type II is characterized by ineffective erythropoiesis leading to anemia with distinctive morphologic abnormalities of bone marrow erythrocytes. A blood sample is obtained by separately reportable venipuncture. Serum and whole blood are tested using complement lysis and visual identification.

85520

85520   Heparin assay

A laboratory test is performed to measure plasma unfractionated heparin (UH) and/or low molecular weight heparin (LMWH) antibodies (Heparin Anti-Xa). Heparin is an anti-coagulant used to prevent or treat blood clots. Antibodies may form when heparin combines with a substance on platelets called platelet factor 4 (PF4) creating a heparin-PF4 complex. The immune system identifies this complex as foreign and produces antibodies. The antibodies activate platelet production triggering more PF4 which can lead to a condition called immune-mediated heparin-induced thrombocytopenia (HIT type II) characterized by the presence of HIT antibody, low platelet count, and excessive clotting. A blood sample is obtained by separately reportable venipuncture. Platelet-poor plasma is tested using chromogenic assay.

85525

85525   Heparin neutralization

A laboratory test is performed to measure clotting time with heparin neutralization of the sample. This is one of many tests (PTT, LA-PTT, DRVVT) usually ordered sequentially to evaluate a prolonged partial thromboplastin time (PTT). It may be useful for ruling out

heparin contamination in abnormal coagulation tests (PT, PTT, TT, factor assays) or to evaluate liver function in patients receiving heparin therapy. The technique can also be performed prior to coagulation studies to remove heparin in a blood sample drawn from a heparinized central line. A blood sample is obtained by separately reportable venipuncture or central line draw. Plasma is tested prior to and after the addition of heparinase, an enzyme that degrades unfractionated heparin (UF) and low molecular weight heparin (LMWH).

85530

85530   Heparin-protamine tolerance test

A laboratory test is performed to measure heparin-protamine tolerance. Heparin is an anti-coagulant used to prevent or treat blood clots. Protamine is a drug that binds to heparin reversing its anti-coagulant effects. This test may be used to assess heparin therapy.

85536

85536   Iron stain, peripheral blood

A laboratory test is performed to identify iron stores in a peripheral blood smear. This test is more commonly used to assess bone marrow but may be performed on peripheral blood when Pappenheimer bodies (siderotic granules) are highly suspected. This information can aid in the diagnosis of sideroblastic anemia. A blood sample is obtained by separately reportable venipuncture. Whole blood is smeared on a glass slide, stained with Perl's Prussion Blue, and examined under a microscope for cytochemical demonstration of iron-bearing pigment.

85540

85540   Leukocyte alkaline phosphatase with count

A laboratory test is performed to measure leukocyte alkaline phosphatase (LAP), an enzyme in white blood cells (WBCs), or leukocytes. This test has largely been replaced by more advanced techniques but may still be used to differentially diagnose chronic granulocytic leukemia from leukemoid reaction (elevated WBCs not caused by infection or malignancy) and to evaluate patients with polycythemia vera, myelofibrosis, aplastic anemia, pernicious anemia, and essential thrombocytopenia. A blood sample is obtained by separately reportable venipuncture. Whole blood is examined under a microscope using enzyme assay and/or cytochemical stain.

85547

85547   Mechanical fragility, RBC

A laboratory test is performed to measure the mechanical fragility of red blood cells (RBCs). RBC fragility is the propensity of blood cells to hemolyze, or rupture, when placed under stress. It is difficult to standardize a test for mechanical, shear stress fragility but it is usually performed by placing a sample of whole blood into a test tube containing glass beads. The test tube is vigorously agitated and the sample tested for hemoglobin to determine the extent of RBC damage. This can be a critical variable when assessing damage to cells during dialysis, intra-operative auto-transfusion, or other procedures that utilize pumps, valves, cannulas, or gas exchange devices. Stored blood products may also be subject to mechanical stress and damage to RBCs.

85549

85549   Muramidase

A laboratory test is performed to measure muramidase, a bacterolytic enzyme which is part of the innate immune system. Muramidase is found abundantly in tears, saliva, mucus, human breast milk, and cytoplasmic granules of polymorphonuclear neutrophils. The serum level of muramidase may rise with degradation of polymorphonuclear neutrophil in benign conditions such as infection and inflammation or malignant diseases including acute or chronic granulocytic or monocytic leukemias (FAB-M4, CMML, CML). Serum and urine levels may be elevated with severe renal insufficiency, renal transplant rejection, and urinary tract infections. A blood sample is obtained by separately reportable venipuncture; urine sample by random void or catheterization. Tears and cerebrospinal fluid may also be collected and tested for muramidase levels. Serum, urine, tears, and cerebrospinal fluid are all tested using quantitative radial immunodiffusion.

85555-85557

85555   Osmotic fragility, RBC; unincubated
85557   Osmotic fragility, RBC; incubated

A laboratory test is performed to measure the osmotic fragility of red blood cells (RBCs). RBC fragility is the propensity of blood cells to hemolyze, or rupture, when placed under stress. The test for osmotic fragility bathes RBCs in hypotonic saline causing fluid to enter the cells and rupture when filled to capacity. This test may be used to evaluate patients with suspected hereditary spherocytic hemolytic anemia. Spherocytic RBCs have a decreased ability to expand and will rupture under milder hypotonic conditions. Abnormal results from an unincubated test will be magnified when the specimen is heated for an incubated test. Results are considered to be positive for osmotic fragility when RBC lysis is noted in 3 or more concentrations of NaCl–0.50 g/dl, 0.60 g/dl, 0.65 g/dl,

Pathology and Laboratory

                       ● New Code   ▲ Revised Code

0.75 g/dl. Increased fragility may be present with immunohemolytic anemia, recent blood transfusion, and hemolytic disorders such as congenital nonspherocytic hemolytic anemia caused by G-6-PD or pyruvate kinase deficiency. Decreased fragility may be noted post splenectomy and in patients with chronic liver disease, iron deficiency anemia, thalassemia, hyponatremia, polycythemia vera, and sickle cell disease. A blood sample is obtained by separately reportable venipuncture. Whole blood is tested using spectrophotometry or osmotic lysis-flow cytometry.

85576

85576   Platelet, aggregation (in vitro), each agent

A laboratory test is performed to measure platelet aggregation, the ability of platelets to clump together and form a blood clot. In vitro aggregation adds known platelet activators such as ADP, arachidonic acid, thrombin, epinephrine, or ristocetin to whole blood samples and monitors the platelet response. This test may be used to screen at risk patients prior to surgery, monitor platelet function during surgery, detect aspirin resistance, diagnose and evaluate excessive bruising/bleeding disorders, and monitor effectiveness of anti-platelet therapy. Ristocetin activator testing may help subtype von Willebrand syndrome. A blood sample is obtained by separately reportable venipuncture. Whole blood is tested using aggregation, quantitative aggregation, or light transmission aggregometry.

85597

85597   Phospholipid neutralization; platelet

This test may also be referred to as an anti-phospholipid antibody test and is used to test for lupus anticoagulants (LA). LA are a group of heterogenous antibodies directed against phospholipid protein complexes. LA in the blood prolongs the clotting time. When a lysed platelet phospholipid is added, LA present are neutralized which shortens clotting time. Lysed platelet phospholipid neutralization is performed using photo optical clot detection. Clotting time with and without lysed platelet phospholipid is compared and increased clotting time without the lysed platelet phospholipid is indicative of the presence of LA. A positive test may be indicative of systemic lupus erythematosis (SLE). However, the majority of individuals with positive tests do not have SLE. The test is more often performed to help determine the cause of otherwise unexplained thrombosis, recurrent fetal loss, thrombocytopenia, or prolonged PTT test.

85598

85598   Phospholipid neutralization; hexagonal phospholipid

A hexagonal phospholipid neutralization assay is used to test for lupus anticoagulants (LA). LA are a group of heterogenous antibodies directed against phospholipid protein complexes. LA in the blood prolongs the clotting time. When a hexagonal phospholipid source is added, LA present are neutralized which shortens the clotting time. Hexagonal phospholipid neutralization is performed using a two-part aPTT-based assay that is performed with and without hexagonal phase phosphatidyl-ethanolamine (HPE) using a LA sensitive reagent. Clotting time of the two assays is compared. If the clotting time of the assay without HPE is greater than the clotting time of assay with HPE by 8 seconds or more, the specimen is positive for LA. A positive test may be indicative of systemic lupus erythematosis (SLE). However, the majority of individuals with positive tests do not have SLE. The test is more often performed on patients with a history of spontaneous abortion, thrombosis, or infection as the persistent presence of LA in human plasma increases the risk for these conditions, particularly the risk for arterial and venous thrombosis.

85610-85611

85610   Prothrombin time
85611   Prothrombin time; substitution, plasma fractions, each

Prothrombin time (PT) measures how long it takes for blood to clot. Prothrombin, also called factor II, is one of the clotting factors made by the liver and adequate levels of vitamin K are needed for the liver to produce sufficient prothrombin. Prothrombin time is used to help identify the cause of abnormal bleeding or bruising; to check whether blood thinning medication, such as warfarin (Coumadin), is working; to check for low levels of blood clotting factors I, II, V, VII, and X; to check for low levels of vitamin K; to check liver function, to see how quickly the body is using up its clotting factors. The test is performed using electromagnetic mechanical clot detection. If prothrombin time is elevated and the patient is not on a blood thinning medication, a second prothrombin time using substitution plasma fractions (85611), also referred to as a prothrombin time mixing study, may be performed. This is performed by mixing patient plasma with normal plasma using a 1:1 mix. The mixture is incubated and the clotting time is again measured. If the result does not correct, it may be indicative that the patient has an inhibitor, such as lupus anticoagulant. If the result does correct, the patient may have a coagulation factor deficiency. Code 85611 is reported for each prothrombin time mixing study performed.

85612-85613

85612   Russell viper venom time (includes venom); undiluted
85613   Russell viper venom time (includes venom); diluted

A blood sample is obtained and Russell viper venom time (RVVT) measured. In 85612, an undiluted RVVT test is performed to detect a deficiency of certain blood clotting factors. Undiluted Russell viper venom is used as an activating agent (reagent). Clotting time is measured. In 85613, a diluted RVVT, also referred to as dRVVT, is performed to detect the presence lupus anticoagulants in plasma. Lupus anticoagulants are nonspecific clotting inhibitors. The test is performed using a low phospholipid reagent consisting of Russell viper venom with excess calcium that is mixed with the patient plasma. The dRVVT reagent is diluted to ensure a low phospholipid concentration and increase the sensitivity for lupus anticoagulant. The clotting time is then measured photo-optically.

85635

85635   Reptilase test

A Reptilase test is performed to measure clotting time. A reptilase test is typically performed as a follow-up to a thrombin time test to confirm the presence of heparin as the cause of prolonged clotting time. If heparin is present, the reptilase clotting time is normal. If the reptilase clotting time is prolonged, it may indicate a fibrinogen deficiency, abnormal fibrinogen due to liver disease, or the presence lupus anticoagulants in plasma. The test is performed by adding reptilase to citrated blood plasma and measuring the rate of fibrin clot formation.

85651-85652

85651   Sedimentation rate, erythrocyte; non-automated
85652   Sedimentation rate, erythrocyte; automated

A blood sample is obtained and a nonautomated erythrocyte sedimentation rate (ESR) performed. This test may also be referred to as a Westergren ESR. ESR is a non-specific test used to identify conditions associated with acute and chronic inflammation such as infection, cancer, and autoimmune diseases. ESR is typically used in conjunction with other tests that can more specifically identify the cause of the inflammatory process. The blood sample is anti-coagulated and placed in a tall thin tube. The distance erythrocytes (red blood cells) have fallen in one hour in a vertical column under the influence of gravity is then measured. In 85652, an automated ESR is performed. The blood sample is anti-coagulated, aspirated, and put into the automated system. An automated sedimentation rate reading is provided after the required sedimentation time has elapsed. There are a number of different automated systems available and the technique varies slightly depending on the automated system used.

85660

85660   Sickling of RBC, reduction

A blood sample is tested for hemoglobin S, also referred to as HbS or HgbS, an abnormal hemoglobin variant. This test is referred to as a sickling of RBC reduction test or more commonly as an HbS solubility test. The test is performed to screen for sickle cell anemia, an inherited disorder that causes red blood cells (RBC) to change from the normal round disc shape to a crescent or sickle shape and primarily affects people of African ancestry, but also occurs in people of Mediterranean and Middle Eastern descent. The sickled RBCs do not flow smoothly through the body and do not transport oxygen effectively. Sickled RBCs also have a lifespan of only 10-20 days as compared to the normal 120 days. Individuals with sickle cell anemia can become anemic due to the shortened RBC lifespan, and can also suffer painful episodes from a number of complications when the sickled RBCs obstruct small blood vessels. The HbS solubility test is performed by adding a chemical to the blood sample that reduces the amount of oxygen it carries. The reduction in oxygen causes hemoglobin S related polymers to form and affected RBCs to sickle. This test will detect even small amounts of hemoglobin S and is used to screen for sickle cell trait (individuals with only one sickle cell gene) as well as sickle cell anemia (individuals with two sickle cell genes).

85670-85675

85670   Thrombin time; plasma
85675   Thrombin time; titer

A blood sample is tested for plasma thrombin time. This test is also referred to as a thrombin clotting time (TCT) test. TCT is used to diagnose fibrinogen deficiency due to congenital or acquired conditions. Congenital conditions causing fibrinogen deficiency include afibrinogenemia, hypofibrinogenemia, and dysfibrinogenemia. Acquired conditions include liver or renal disease, disseminated intravascular coagulation (DIC), amyloidosis, malignancy, and anticoagulant drug therapy. The test is performed by mixing the blood sample with human thrombin and measuring clotting time photometrically. In 85675, a thrombin time titer is measured.

Pathology and Laboratory

85705

85705   Thromboplastin inhibition, tissue

A tissue thromboplastin inhibition (TTI) test is performed on a blood specimen to qualitatively detect the presence of lupus anticoagulants (LA) in plasma. LA are a group of antibodies that cause a variety of clinical and laboratory effects. LA are often discovered accidently when a prolonged activated partial thromboplastin time (APTT) is identified. The presence of lupus anticoagulants may be due to an autoimmune disease, such as systemic lupus erythematosus (SLE). Other causes of LA include inflammatory bowel disease, infection, or malignant neoplasm. Lupus anticoagulants may also be found in individuals on certain medications. LA may cause recurrent thromboses, multiple spontaneous miscarriages, migraine headaches, stroke, or bleeding disorders. However, the majority of individuals with LA have no clinical symptoms. This test is typically performed to identify the cause of increased clotting time as due to the presence of lupus anticoagulants. The test is performed by diluting the blood specimen to increase sensitivity to inhibitors. Methodology is photometric or automated enzyme immunoassay (EIA).

85730-85732

85730   Thromboplastin time, partial (PTT); plasma or whole blood
85732   Thromboplastin time, partial (PTT); substitution, plasma fractions, each

This test may also be referred to as an activated PTT or aPTT. PTT may be performed to diagnose the cause of bleeding or as a screening test prior to surgery to rule-out coagulation defects. A silica and synthetic phospholipid PTT reagent is mixed with the patient plasma. The silica provides a negatively-charged particulate surface that activates the contact pathway for coagulation. Clot formation is initiated by adding calcium chloride to the mixture. Clotting time is measured photo-optically. If PTT is elevated and the patient is not on a blood thinning medication, a second PTT using substitution plasma fractions (85732), also referred to as a PTT mixing study, may be performed. This is performed by mixing patient plasma with normal plasma using a 1:1 mix. The mixture is incubated and the clotting time is again measured. If the result does not correct, it may be indicative that the patient has an inhibitor, such as lupus anticoagulant. If the result does correct, the patient may have a coagulation factor deficiency. Code 85732 is reported for each PTT mixing study performed.

85810

85810   Viscosity

A blood sample is tested to determine its viscosity. Viscosity is a property of fluid that describes the resistance of flow due to a shearing force. When applied to blood, viscosity describes the internal friction between the blood and the wall of the vessel. Viscosity varies based on hematocrit, temperature, and flow rate. Blood viscosity may be tested in patients with cardiac or blood conditions, such as ischemic heart disease, stroke, sickle cell anemia, or polycythemia, where an increase in blood viscosity is associated with adverse events. The test may be performed on whole blood or serum and is performed by cone-plate viscometer.

86000

86000   Agglutinins, febrile (eg, Brucella, Francisella, Murine typhus, Q fever, Rocky Mountain spotted fever, scrub typhus), each antigen

A blood sample is tested for the presence of agglutinating antibodies against one or more febrile antigens. The test is used to evaluate for the presence of a cryptic infection, that is, an infection caused by a pathogen that has not yet been identified. Testing is often done for multiple possible pathogens and when done for multiple pathogens, the test may be referred to as a febrile agglutination profile. When testing for opportunistic infection by Proteus vulgaris, the test may be referred to as a Weil Felix test. Some of the more common pathogens tested include: Brucella, Francisella, Murine typhus, Q fever, Rocky Mountain spotted fever, and scrub typhus. This test may also be used to identify some Salmonella groups including Salmonella group D 'O' (somatic) antigen, Salmonella groups A, B, and D 'H' (flagellar) antigen, as well as some Proteus vulgaris strains including OX-2, OX-K, and OX-19 antigens. Testing is by direct agglutination (DA). Code 86000 is reported for each antigen.

86001

86001   Allergen specific IgG quantitative or semiquantitative, each allergen

A blood sample is obtained to test for one or more allergen specific IgG immunoglobulins using quantitative or semiquantitative technique. Allergy tests that use blood are also referred to as in vitro tests and differ from skin (in vivo) tests. The test is used to identify a wide variety of IgG immunoglobulins, also referred to antibodies, associated with allergic reactions to foods or venoms. The test may be referred to as a food allergy panel when testing for sensitivity to multiple foods or a stinging insect allergy profile when testing for multiple venoms. Code 86001 is reported for each antigen.

86003-86005

86003   Allergen specific IgE; quantitative or semiquantitative, each allergen
86005   Allergen specific IgE; qualitative, multiallergen screen (dipstick, paddle, or disk)

This test may also be referred to as a radioallergosorbent test (RAST). Allergy tests that use blood are also referred to as in vitro tests and differ from skin (in vivo) tests. Most allergy tests are quantitative or semiquantitative which means that the test provides IgE units of measurement which are then interpreted using a scoring system. The test is used to identify a wide variety of IgE immunoglobulins, also referred to antibodies, that are associated with allergy symptoms and allergic reactions to foods, animal dander, dust (dust mites), molds, grasses, trees, weeds, and insects. New technologies associated with allergy testing provide high binding capacity of allergen proteins including those present at very low levels and so can more readily identify specific allergies. Multiple respiratory, food, or environmental allergens, specific to a region (state/geographic location) or population (adult/child) are typically tested for in an allergy panel or profile. Panels or profiles can contain a dozen or more common allergens. Types of panels or profiles include upper respiratory allergy profile, adult food allergy profile, child food allergy profile, or child environmental allergy profile. Code 86003 is reported for each allergen tested using a quantitative or semiquantitative technique. Code 86005 is reported when a qualitative multiallergen screen is performed using a dipstick, paddle or disc. Qualitative allergen screening tests identify only the presence or absence of the allergen specific IgE being tested, but do not provide IgE units of measurement or an allergy score.

86021-86023

86021   Antibody identification; leukocyte antibodies
86022   Antibody identification; platelet antibodies
86023   Antibody identification; platelet associated immunoglobulin assay

Leukocytes are white blood cells that are further categorized as lymphocytes, neutrophils, eosinophils, macrophages, and mast cells. White blood cells attack bacteria and help the body fight infection. Leukocyte antibodies are immunoglobulin molecules that attack and destroy white blood cells. This test is used to identify specific types of leukocyte antibodies that cause conditions such as autoimmune disorders, miscarriage, and tissue and organ transplant rejection. The test may be referred to as anti-leukocyte antibody identification or by the specific type of white blood cell being identified or by the specific antibody, such as lymphocyte antibody identification, anti-neutrophil antibody detection, or OKT3 antibody detection. This test is typically performed by flow cytometry. In 86022, a blood sample is obtained for platelet antibody identification. This test is the primary test used for detection of platelet-specific antibodies and can detect both alloantibodies and autoantibodies. This test is used in conjunction with clinical information and other blood tests to identify a number of conditions including neonatal alloimmune thrombocytopenia (NATP) and post-transfusion purpura (PTP). The test is performed by enzyme-linked immunosorbent assay (ELISA) and is designed to detect antibodies to platelet glycoproteins and Class I human leukocyte antigens (HLA) Class I antigens. In 86023, a blood sample is obtained to identify platelet associated immuglobulins (antibodies) by direct assay. The test is used to identify excess IgG and/or IgM platelet associated immunoglobulin. An increase in platelet associated immunoglobulins is indicative of thrombocytopenia of immune origin, while the absence of excess antibodies is indicative of thrombocytopenia of nonimmune origin. The test is performed by flow cytometry. Code 86023 is reported once for the IgG assay and once for the IgM assay.

86038-86039

86038   Antinuclear antibodies (ANA)
86039   Antinuclear antibodies (ANA); titer

A blood sample is obtained to screen for the presence of antinuclear antibodies (ANA) (86038) or to measure the concentration of antinuclear antibody in the blood, which is referred to as an ANA titer (86039). Antinuclear antibodies are auto-antibodies that bind to structures within the nucleus of cells. Auto-antibodies are a type of antibody that is directed against the body's own tissues. The presence and concentration of antinuclear antibodies may indicate one of several autoimmune disorders that cause inflammation of body tissues including systemic lupus erythematosus, Sjorgren's syndrome, rheumatoid arthritis, polymyositis, scleroderma, Hashimoto's thyroiditis, juvenile diabetes mellitus, Addison disease, vitiligo, pernicious anemia, glumerulonephritis, and pulmonary fibrosis. When testing for antinuclear antibodies, the specimen is typically screened first (86038) using an enzyme-linked immunosorbent assay (ELISA) If the screening test is positive, that is if antinuclear antibodies are detected, a titer (86039) is then obtained. An antinuclear antibody titer is performed by diluting the blood sample with increasing amounts of a saline solution and retesting until antinuclear antibodies are no longer detectable. ANA titer is expressed as 1:10, 1:20, 1:40, 1:80, etc, with the 1 indicating 1 part blood and the second number indicating the parts of saline solution. A higher second number indicates a higher concentration of antinuclear antibodies in the blood.

Pathology and Laboratory

86060-86063

86060   **Antistreptolysin 0; titer**
86063   **Antistreptolysin 0; screen**

A blood sample is obtained to screen for the presence antistreptolysin O (ASO) antibodies (86063) or to measure the concentration of ASO antibodies, also referred to as an ASO titer (86060). ASO antibodies are produced by Group A Streptococcus bacteria and the presence of ASO antibodies in the blood may indicate an active streptococcal infection, bacterial endocarditis, post-streptococcal glumerolunephritis, rheumatic fever, or scarlet fever. There are a number of different methods used for ASO screens and titers, including nephelometry and latex immunoturbidimetry. In 86060, the results are typically expressed as the number of Todd units per milliliter with higher Todd units indicating a higher level of antibody in the blood. In 86063, only the presence or absence of ASO antibodies is indicated.

86077-86079

86077   **Blood bank physician services; difficult cross match and/or evaluation of irregular antibody(s), interpretation and written report**
86078   **Blood bank physician services; investigation of transfusion reaction including suspicion of transmissible disease, interpretation and written report**
86079   **Blood bank physician services; authorization for deviation from standard blood banking procedures (eg, use of outdated blood, transfusion of Rh incompatible units), with written report**

The physician analyzes a batch of donated blood that is going to be infused into a patient. The physician determines issues involving matching the blood type or identifying any unusual antibodies in the bloodstream, or in the donated blood. The physician presents his or her findings in a written report. Code 86078 if the physician investigates an unusual occurrence after the donated blood has been infused, such as the possibility of the patient contracting a disease from the donated blood. Code 86079 in which the physician authorizes the infusion of donated blood that has exceeded its shelf life, is of the wrong blood type, or other situations in which there is a deviation from normal blood bank procedure.

86140

86140   **C-reactive protein**

A blood test is performed to measure C-reactive protein (CRP) levels. This standard test has a wide value range. CRP is an acute phase protein, synthesized by the liver and released in response to inflammation and infection. The test is not diagnostic for any specific disease or condition but can be used as a marker to monitor the body's response to treatment(s) or to evaluate the need for further testing. Elevation of CRP levels may be found during pregnancy, with the use of oral contraceptives, or hormone replacement therapy. Diseases/conditions that cause an elevation of CRP include: lymphoma, arteritis/vasculitis, osteomyelitis, inflammatory bowel disease, rheumatoid arthritis, pelvic inflammatory disease (PID), systemic lupus erythematosus (SLE), acute infections, burns, surgical procedures, and organ transplants. A blood sample is obtained by separately reportable venipuncture. Serum in neonates is tested using immunoassay. Serum/plasma in all other patients is tested using quantitative immunoturbidimetric method.

86141

86141   **C-reactive protein; high sensitivity (hsCRP)**

A blood test is performed to measure high sensitivity C-reactive protein (hsCRP) levels. This test measures a narrow range of low CRP concentrations and is useful for determining risk of cardiovascular disease, stroke, myocardial infarction, and peripheral vascular disease in healthy individuals. CRP (including hsCRP) is an acute phase protein, synthesized by the liver and released in response to inflammation and infection. Levels of hsCRP may be decreased with the use of nonsteroidal anti-inflammatory drugs (NSAIDs) and statins. Levels may be increased following illness or tissue injury, with certain infectious diseases or inflammatory conditions, or with the use of hormone replacement therapy. This test is usually ordered in conjunction with a lipid panel or other cardiac risk assessment tests. A blood sample is obtained by separately reportable venipuncture. Serum/plasma is tested using quantitative immunoturbidimetric method.

86146

86146   **Beta 2 Glycoprotein I antibody, each**

A blood sample is tested for the presence of Beta 2 Glycoprotein 1 antibodies, which are a heterogeneous group of autoantibodies associated with antiphospholipid syndrome (APS). APS may be suspected in patients with recurrent venous or arterial thrombosis and/or fetal losses. If the patient has APS, laboratory tests will show persistently elevated levels of anti-beta-2 glycoprotein I antibodies (IgG or IgM) in serum or plasma. Blood tests for APS are typically performed on two occasions at least twelve weeks apart. Tests for both IgG and IgM antibodies may be performed and each is reported separately.

86147

86147   **Cardiolipin (phospholipid) antibody, each Ig class**

A blood sample is tested for the presence of cardiolipin (phospholipid) antibodies, each Ig class (IgA, IgG, IgM). Tests for cardiolipin antibodies may be performed in patients with unexplained venous or arterial thrombosis, thrombocytopenia, and/or fetal losses. If one or more classes of cardiolipin antibodies are detected, the test is typically repeated about six weeks later to determine whether the presence of the antibodies is persistent or temporary. Low or moderate levels of cardiolipin antibodies are often temporarily present due to infection or taking certain drugs. Persistent higher levels indicate that the cardiolipin antibodies may be the reason for thrombosis, thrombocytopenia, or fetal losses. Tests for IgA, IgG, and IgM antibodies may be performed and each is reported separately.

86148

86148   **Anti-phosphatidylserine (phospholipid) antibody**

A blood test is performed to measure anti-phosphatidylserine (phospholipid) antibody levels. These antibodies (IgG, IgM, IgA) are present in the membrane of endothelial cells and platelets and are an essential part of the coagulation (blood clotting) cascade. Elevated levels may be clinically significant in individuals who have had unexplained thrombotic events, swelling and pain in extremities or joints, headaches, respiratory distress, recurrent fetal loss, thrombocytopenia, or elevated PTT. A negative test result may indicate that the antibody is not present at that exact time and the test should be repeated if symptoms persist. A positive result to one or more antibodies may be relevant when symptoms are present and should be repeated in 8-10 weeks to determine if the elevation is persistent or temporary. A blood sample is obtained by separately reportable venipuncture. Serum is tested using semi-quantitative enzyme-linked immunosorbent assay.

86152-86153

86152   **Cell enumeration using immunologic selection and identification in fluid specimen (eg, circulating tumor cells in blood)**
86153   **Cell enumeration using immunologic selection and identification in fluid specimen (eg, circulating tumor cells in blood); physician interpretation and report, when required**

A test is performed on blood or other body fluids to identify the presence of circulating tumor cells in patients diagnosed with cancer. The spread of cancer (metastatic disease) occurs by dissemination and deposition of tumor cells to other organs via the circulating system (blood, bone marrow, lymphatic). The presence of tumor cells in body fluid can help determine the disease prognosis and course of treatment for many cancers including: breast, colorectal, prostate, renal, bladder and non-small cell lung. The presence of cells usually correlates to a lower survival rate. A blood sample is obtained by separately reportable venipuncture, bone marrow sample by bone marrow biopsy, lymph fluid by other method. Blood may be tested using cell search method with a positive result if 5 or more cells are found or by morphological appearance which is a technique that requires microscopic identification by visualizing the cell. A physician interpretation and report may be necessary and appropriate with these tests. Use 86152 for the cell enumeration test and 86153 for any required physician interpretation and report.

86155

86155   **Chemotaxis assay, specify method**

A blood sample is drawn and the response of white blood cells to an injured or diseased area of the body is monitored. One of a variety of methods can be used, and must be specified. Chemotaxis assay measures cell migration and is useful when evaluating immune function and cancer progression. Qualitative tests may involve the use of aggregation or T-maze adaptations for microplates. A semi-quantitative test overlays cells in a test substrate and records the change in opalescence.

86156-86157

86156   **Cold agglutinin; screen**
86157   **Cold agglutinin; titer**

Cold agglutinins are antibodies released by the immune system in response to infection. Elevated cold agglutinin levels cause red blood cells (RBCs) to clump (agglutinate) at low body temperatures and may eventually damage or destroy the cells. This can lead to a condition called autoimmune hemolytic anemia. Use 86156 for a screening test for the presence of cold agglutinin antibodies. Use 86157 when a blood test is performed to measure cold agglutinin titers. Elevated titers may be found with mononucleosis, HIV, lymphoma and chronic lymphoid leukemia, and atypical pneumonia due to mycoplasma, influenza A or B, parainfluenza, and adenoviruses. Abnormally low titers may result from malaria, peripheral vascular disease, and common respiratory disorders. A blood sample is obtained by separately reportable venipuncture. Serum is tested using semi-quantitative hemagglutination.

   ● New Code   ▲ Revised Code

Pathology and Laboratory

86160

86160   Complement; antigen, each component

A blood test is performed to measure complement antigen levels. Complement factors help to clear immune complexes from the blood. Proteins are activated in response to the immune complex and generate peptides that bind the complexes and complement receptors. The cell membrane breaks apart and an attack complex is formed. A blood sample is obtained by separately reportable venipuncture. Complements are tested in serum or plasma samples, using specified methods, particularly quantitative radial immunodiffusion. Report 86160 for each complement component tested: 2-9 (2 being the most common inherited complement deficiency), 3A (the most abundant of all complement components), 4A, and 1Q; complement factor B and Bb; and C1-esterase inhibitor.

86161

86161   Complement; functional activity, each component

A blood test is performed to measure complement functional activity. Complement factors help to clear immune complexes from the blood. The complement cascade of the membrane attack complex (MAC) provides the body with an innate and adaptive immune response by attaching to the cell membrane causing the cell to split open and/or form pores. Individuals with low functional activity levels have higher rates of infections. A blood sample is obtained by separately reportable venipuncture and complement functional activity is tested using specified methods, mainly quantitative hemolytic assay. Report 86161 for each complement functional activity tested: 1, 6, 7, 8, 9, and C1-esterase inhibitor functional activity.

86162

86162   Complement; total hemolytic (CH50)

A blood test is performed to measure total hemolytic complement (CH50, AH50) activity. Code 86162 may be used for the complement activity enzyme immunoassay, a test that can help identify abnormalities or deficiencies in the complement system that may be contributing to infectious diseases or inflammatory conditions such as SLE, RA, and vasculitis, and for the complement activity alternative pathway test, which also screens functional activity of the complement system. Abnormal results may indicate an inherited or acquired functional defect in one or more of the individual components of the system. A blood sample is obtained by separately reportable venipuncture. For the complement activity enzyme test, serum is tested using semiquantitative enzyme-linked immunosorbent assay. For the alternative pathway test, serum is tested using semiquantitative radial immunodiffusion.

86171

86171   Complement fixation tests, each antigen

A blood test is performed to measure complement fixation. Complement fixation is an immunological test that can be used to identify specific antigens or antibodies in serum. It is reported for each antigen test, but has largely been replaced by methods such as ELISA and PCR. Code 86171 is used to test for total Neisseria Gonorrhoea antibodies. This titer may be elevated with past or current infections. A blood sample is obtained by separately reportable venipuncture. Serum is tested using semiquantitative complement fixation.

86185

86185   Counterimmunoelectrophoresis, each antigen

Counterimmunoelectrophoresis (CIEP) is a laboratory technique that propels oppositely charged antigens and antibodies toward each other by adding an electrical charge to the diffusion medium. This technique can detect the migration and binding of very low concentrations of antigens/antibodies in a short amount of time. It has been used successfully to measure antigens such as hepatitis (HAA), influenza, pneumococcus, rabies, Group B coxsackie virus, and cytomegalovirus (CMV). Report 86185 for each antigen tested.

86200

86200   Cyclic citrullinated peptide (CCP), antibody

A blood test is performed to measure cyclic citrullinated peptide (CCP) antibody levels. CCP is a serum marker for rheumatoid arthritis, a chronic inflammatory disorder of the synovial membrane. This test may show positive results before clinical signs of the disease are manifested. The test for CCP is often ordered in conjunction with a test for rheumatoid factor (86431). A blood sample is obtained by separately reportable venipuncture. Serum is tested using semiquantitative enzyme-linked immunosorbent assay.

86215

86215   Deoxyribonuclease, antibody

A blood test is performed to measure deoxyribonuclease (DNase) antibody titers. DNase antibodies are enzymes produced by some strains of beta hemolytic streptococcus. This test may be helpful in diagnosing streptococcal infections when ASO titers are not elevated. DNase antibodies rise more slowly than ASO and remain elevated longer so this test may

be diagnostic with suspected Sydenham's chorea, post streptococcal rheumatic fever, or glomerulonephritis. A blood sample is obtained by separately reportable venipuncture. Serum is tested using quantitative nephelometry.

86225

86225   Deoxyribonucleic acid (DNA) antibody; native or double stranded

A laboratory test is performed to measure native or double stranded deoxyribonucleic acid (DNA) antibody, IgG. The presence of DNA antibody is often associated with systemic lupus erythematosus (SLE). This test may be used as a secondary screening test for SLE when the test for anti-nuclear antibodies is positive, or to monitor disease activity in patients with previously diagnosed SLE. The high avidity test is very specific to SLE with renal involvement (lupus nephritis) making it less sensitive to detecting DNA antibody than the low affinity test. A blood sample is obtained by separately reportable venipuncture. Serum is tested using qualitative enzyme linked immunosorbent assay.

86226

86226   Deoxyribonucleic acid (DNA) antibody; single stranded

A laboratory test is performed to measure single stranded deoxyribonucleic acid (DNA) antibody, IgG. Elevated levels of single stranded DNA antibody may occur during active and inactive phases of systemic lupus erythematosus (SLE) and with infectious mononucleosis, autoimmune hepatitis, acute and chronic myeloid leukemia, acute lymphatic leukemia, juvenile rheumatoid arthritis, and drug induced SLE. Because some double stranded DNA can be detected with single stranded DNA, a separate test for double stranded DNA, reported with 86225, is usually preformed in conjunction with 86226 to calculate the ratio of double stranded DNA IgG to single stranded DNA IgG and differentiate a diagnosis of SLE from other disorders. A blood sample is obtained by separately reportable venipuncture. Serum is tested using semi-quantitative enzyme-linked immunosorbent assay.

86235

86235   Extractable nuclear antigen, antibody to, any method (eg, nRNP, SS-A, SS-B, Sm, RNP, Sc170, J01), each antibody

A blood test is performed to measure extractable nuclear antigen or antibody to it. One or more of these antibodies are typically elevated in autoimmune diseases such as Sjogren Syndrome, polymyositis, systemic lupus erythematosus, and progressive systemic sclerosis. Many are included in comprehensive panels that screen for multiple antibodies at one time. A blood sample is obtained by separately reportable venipuncture and tested by any method, particularly semiquantitative multi-analyte fluorescent detection. Report once for each antibody, such as: SSA (Ro) (ENA) Antibody, IgG; Jo-1 Antibody, IgG; scleroderma (Scl-70) (ENA) Antibody, IgG; Smith (ENA) Antibody, IgG; SSB (La) (ENA) Antibody, IgG; and RNP (U1) (Ribonucleic Protein) (ENA) Antibody, IgG.

86243

86243   Fc receptor

Fc receptor testing is done to detect these particular proteins that help protect the immune system and are found on the surface of cells such as natural killer cells, macrophages, neutrophils, and mast cells. Fc receptors bind to antibodies that are attached to infecting cells or pathogens. This stimulates phagocytic or cytotoxic destruction of microbes. There are three types of Fc receptors. Fc-gamma belongs to the immunoglobulin superfamily which induces phagocytosis of coated (opsonized) microbes. Fc-alpha is found on the surface of white blood cells including neutrophils, eosinophils, monocytes, some macrophages (including Kupffer cells), and dendritic cells. Fc-epsilon, high affinity receptors are found on epidermal Langerhans cells, eosinophils, mast cells, and basophils. They are active in the allergic response and are also found on antigen-presenting cells that produce cytokines. Fc-epsilon, low affinity controls B cell growth and blocks IgE binding of eosinophils, monocytes, and basophils.

86255-86256

86255   Fluorescent noninfectious agent antibody; screen, each antibody
86256   Fluorescent noninfectious agent antibody; titer, each antibody

These codes report fluorescent technique to screen for the presence of antibodies to noninfectious agents (86255), usually performed first, and to get a titer count (86256) if antibodies are present or elevated. These tests are performed on a blood sample or cerebral spinal fluid (CSF) obtained by separately reportable venipuncture or lumbar puncture (spinal tap). The antibodies tested for in these screenings indicate conditions and/or the risk of developing conditions that are not contracted by an infectious process, such as celiac disease, premature ovarian failure, myasthenia gravis, other autoimmune disorders, exposure to environmental toxins that result in autoimmune disease, cancers, graft vs. host disease following transplant, and myocardial infarction and other cardiac injury. These antibody screenings and titers may also be used as a marker to monitor the effectiveness of immunosuppressant therapy.

Pathology and Laboratory

86277

86277   Growth hormone, human (HGH), antibody

A blood test is performed to measure human growth hormone antibody levels. Individuals treated with recombinant human growth hormone (rhGH) may develop antibodies which neutralize the circulating growth hormone and inhibit its effects. This test may be ordered at regular intervals to monitor individuals during treatment with rhGH. A blood sample is obtained by separately reportable venipuncture. Serum is tested using radiobinding assay.

86280

86280   Hemagglutination inhibition test (HAI)

Hemagglutination inhibition (HAI) test is a method of identifying a virus or bacteria. The test is relatively simple, fast, and very accurate. Surface proteins on some viruses and many bacteria cause them to stick together (agglutinate) to circulating red blood cells, forming a lattice-like structure. The test identifies the presence of a specific antigen or quantitates an antibody by mixing a fixed amount of antibodies to the antigen in question with a fixed amount of red blood cells coated with the antigen. If the sample contains the antigen in question, the soluble antigen will compete with that coated on the red blood cells for binding to the introduced antibodies, thereby inhibiting the agglutination to the red blood cells.

86294

86294   Immunoassay for tumor antigen, qualitative or semiquantitative (eg, bladder tumor antigen)

A qualitative or semi-quantitative immunoassay for tumor antigen, such as bladder tumor antigen, is performed. Tumor antigens, also referred to as tumor markers, are indicators that a malignant neoplasm may be present. Significant circulating levels found in serum are associated with malignancy. In the case of bladder tumor antigen (BTA), a latex agglutination assay is used to determine the presence or absence of BTA in urine. The presence of BTA in the urine is not a definitive test for bladder tumor since other conditions, such as renal stones, nephritis, renal cancer, urinary tract infection, cystitis, or recent trauma to the bladder or kidneys can cause a positive result. A positive test for BTA indicates the need for further testing to determine whether a bladder tumor is present.

86300

86300   Immunoassay for tumor antigen, quantitative; CA 15-3 (27.29)

A quantitative immunoassay for tumor antigen CA 15-3 or CA 27.29 is performed. Tumor antigens, also referred to as tumor markers, are indicators that a malignant neoplasm may be present. Significant circulating levels found in serum are often associated with malignancy. Tumor antigens CA 15-3 and CA 27.29 are used to monitor response to treatment in patients with Stage II and III breast cancer. CA 15-3 uses an electrochemiluminescent immunoassay test kit and CA 27.29 uses a chemiluminescent immunoassay test kit. Periodic tumor antigen testing is used in conjunction with other clinical methods to monitor progression or regression of breast cancer.

86301

86301   Immunoassay for tumor antigen, quantitative; CA 19-9

A quantitative immunoassay for tumor antigen CA 19-9 is performed. Tumor antigens, also referred to as tumor markers, are indicators that a malignant neoplasm may be present. Significant circulating levels found in serum are often associated with malignancy. Tumor antigen CA 19-9 is used to monitor response to treatment in patients with an established diagnosis of pancreatic, colorectal, gastric, or biliary cancer. The test may be performed on body fluids or blood. If body fluid is used, the source should be identified. CA 19-9 uses an electrochemiluminescent immunoassay test kit. Periodic tumor antigen testing is used in conjunction with other clinical methods to monitor progression or regression of the malignancy.

86304

86304   Immunoassay for tumor antigen, quantitative; CA 125

A quantitative immunoassay for tumor antigen CA 125 is performed. Tumor antigens, also referred to as tumor markers, are indicators that a malignant neoplasm may be present. Significant circulating levels found in serum are often associated with malignancy. Tumor antigen CA 125 is used in patients with a documented ovarian mass to help determine whether the mass is benign or malignant. It is also used to monitor response to treatment in patients with an established diagnosis of ovarian, fallopian tube, or endometrial cancer. CA 125 uses an electrochemiluminescent immunoassay test kit. Periodic tumor antigen testing is used in conjunction with other clinical methods to monitor progression or regression of the malignancy.

86305

86305   Human epididymis protein 4 (HE4)

Human epididymis protein 4 (HE4) is a glycoprotein that is elevated in patients with serous and endometroid ovarian cancer and some clear cell ovarian cancers. HE4 levels are obtained to screen for ovarian cancer in patients presenting with symptoms that could be indicative of ovarian cancer and patients with a family history of ovarian cancer. Elevated HE4 is considered to be a serologic marker for ovarian cancer. A blood sample is obtained. Analyte-specific reagents are used to detect elevated levels of HE4 in blood serum.

86308-86309

86308   Heterophile antibodies; screening
86309   Heterophile antibodies; titer

A blood test is performed to screen for heterophile antibodies (86308) which may be present when an individual has contracted the Epstein-Barr virus (EBV). EBV is the causative virus of infectious mononucleosis (IM). To screen for heterophile antibodies, the test is referred to as Infectious Mononucleosis Slide Test by LA. The test is usually ordered when a patient has symptoms suggestive of IM including fever, headache, sore throat, swollen glands, fatigue/weakness, enlarged liver/spleen, abdominal pain or rash. The test may be negative in the early stages of the infection and should be repeated if symptoms persist. Infants and young children do not make heterophile antibodies and this test will be negative even with documented EBV infection. A blood sample is obtained by separately reportable venipuncture. Serum/plasma is tested using semiquantitative latex agglutination. When the test is performed to measure the amount of heterophile antibody titers present after the Infectious Mononucleosis Slide Test by LA is positive, report 86309.

86310

86310   Heterophile antibodies; titers after absorption with beef cells and guinea pig kidney

Heterophile antibodies are typically elevated with infectious mononucleosis (IM). Titers for this antibody rise during the first 2-3 weeks of illness and then start to decline, disappearing in 8-12 weeks following the onset of symptoms. The original Paul-Bunnell test added the Davidsohn differential test (Paul-Bunnell-Davidsohn test) and examined serum containing IM antibodies added to guinea pig kidney cells. The IM antibodies were not absorbed by the kidney cells but do react with beef (ox) red blood cells by agglutinating. This indicates the titer level in the serum sample that is positive for IM.

86316

86316   Immunoassay for tumor antigen, other antigen, quantitative (eg, CA 50, 72-4, 549), each

A quantitative immunoassay for tumor antigen not specified elsewhere is performed. Tumor antigens, also referred to as tumor markers, are indicators that a malignant neoplasm may be present. Significant circulating levels found in serum are often associated with malignancy. Examples of tumor antigens reported with 86316 include CA 50, CA 72-4, and CA 549. Tumor antigen CA 50 is found in gastrointestinal cancers, including pancreatic, gastric, colorectal, and hepatic carcinomas. CA 72-4 is used to test for gastrointestinal and breast cancer. CA 549 is used for patients with breast cancer. A variety of immunoassay techniques is used to test for these and other tumor antigens. CA 50, CA 72-4, and CA 549 use monoclonal antibodies and radioimmunoassay technique. Another tumor antigen also reported with this code, soluble mesothelin related peptides, is tested using enzyme linked immunosorbent assay to help manage treatment of patients with mesothelioma. Other tumor antigens use enzyme immunoassay, chemiluminescent immunoassay, or other methods. Periodic tumor antigen testing is used in conjunction with other clinical methods to monitor progression or regression of the malignancy.

86317-86318

86317   Immunoassay for infectious agent antibody, quantitative, not otherwise specified
86318   Immunoassay for infectious agent antibody, qualitative or semiquantitative, single step method (eg, reagent strip)

Code 86317 is reported for infectious agents that are screened or tested for using antibody immunoassay by various specified methods. In 86317, a blood test is performed to measure antibody levels quantitatively, such as Toxoplasma gondii (T. gondii) antibody levels, tetanus antibody levels, Streptococcus pneumoniae antibodies (14 serotypes), rubella antibodies, Hepatitis B surface antibody levels, Haemophilus influenzae B antibody levels, and diphtheria antibody, often using quantitative multi-analyte fluorescent detection. Report 86318 for qualitative or semiquantitative immunoassay done to identify an infectious agent antibody by single step method using dipstick or reagent strip methodology. Results by this method are usually obtained within 5 minutes. Antibodies typically screened for in this way include Helicobactor pylori (H. pylori), influenza type A and B, infectious mononucleosis (IM), Respiratory Syncytial Virus (RSV), and Group A Streptococcus.

● New Code   ▲ Revised Code   CPT © 2016 American Medical Association. All Rights Reserved.   © 2017 DecisionHealth

86320-86325

86320   Immunoelectrophoresis; serum
86325   Immunoelectrophoresis; other fluids (eg, urine, cerebrospinal fluid) with concentration

Immunoelectrophoresis is a method of separating and characterizing proteins based on their reaction with antibodies. There are a number of variations using one-dimensional and two-dimensional methods. All variations test for immunoglobulins (proteins) functioning as antibodies. The serum test (86320) is most often done to check the levels of abnormal immunoglobulins that include monoclonal immunoglobulins typically associated with multiple myeloma, chronic lymphocytic leukemia, Waldenstrom's macroglobulinemia, amyloidosis, and lymphoma. This test has been largely replaced by another test method called immunofixation. Report 86325 for immunoelectrophoresis done on other body fluids such as cerebral spinal fluid, synovial fluid, and urine.

86327

86327   Immunoelectrophoresis; crossed (2-dimensional assay)

Immunoelectrophoresis, crossed or two-dimensional, is a combination of conventional electrophoretic separation and electroimmunodiffusion. Electrophoresis is first carried out and then the strip is placed on a slide with an antibody containing agarose solution. This is allowed to solidify and electrophoresis is again performed at a right angle to the original separation.

86329

86329   Immunodiffusion; not elsewhere specified

A blood test is performed to measure teichoic acid antibody (TAA) levels. Elevated TAA levels may indicate a recent staphylococcal infection such as endocarditis or bacteremia with metastatic foci of abscesses due to delayed treatment. A positive TAA test may be used to confirm specific bacteriological disease earlier than a culture. This test is especially useful when the culture is difficult to obtain from sites such as the lung (pneumonia), bone (osteomyelitis) or deep tissue abscesses. A blood sample is obtained by separately reportable venipuncture. Serum is tested using semiquantitative immunodiffusion.

86331

86331   Immunodiffusion; gel diffusion, qualitative (Ouchterlony), each antigen or antibody

A blood test is performed to measure precipitation antibodies associated with hypersensitivity pneumonitis. The following are included with the Hypersensitivity Pneumonitis I test: Aspergillus fumigatus #1 and #6, Aureobasidium pullulans, Pigeon serum, Micropolyspora faeni, Thermoactinomyces vulgaris #1. The following are included with the Hypersensitivity Pneumonitis II test: Aspergillus fumigatus #2 and #3, Aspergillus flavus, Saccharomospora viridis, Thermoactinomyces candidus, and Thermoactinomyces sacchari. Precipitation antibodies are usually identified with active cases of hypersensitivity pneumonitis but may also be present in asymptomatic individuals. A positive test is helpful when diagnosing someone who also has a positive history and clinical evidence of hypersensitivity pneumonitis but a negative test does not rule out the condition. A blood sample is obtained by separately reportable venipuncture. Serum is tested using qualitative immunodiffusion.

86332

86332   Immune complex assay

A laboratory test is performed to measure circulating immune cells using an immune complex assay. Circulating immune cells are formed by the interaction of antibodies and antigens. In a normal immune response, the clearance of circulating immune cells takes place rapidly through the reticuloendothelial system. When this system contains inflammation-mediated tissue, it may take longer to clear the immune cells, allowing them to remain in the circulatory system. The immune complex assay may be used to detect circulating immune cells that bind to complement receptors on certain cells called Raji cells. Further quantitative analysis can assist with staging immunological disorders. Elevated levels of circulating immune cells have been associated with autoimmune disorders such as systemic lupus erythematosus, rheumatoid arthritis, vasculitis, sarcoidosis, and glomerulonephritis; infectious diseases such as Lyme disease and HIV; and with some malignancies. Circulating immune cells may also be detected without evidence of underlying pathology. A blood sample is obtained by separately reportable venipuncture and tested.

86334-86335

86334   Immunofixation electrophoresis; serum
86335   Immunofixation electrophoresis; other fluids with concentration (eg, urine, CSF)

A blood test is performed to identify the presence of abnormal proteins; the absence of normal proteins; and high or low levels of certain groups of proteins using immunofixation electrophoresis (IFE). This is helpful in identifying inflammatory conditions, autoimmune diseases, acute or chronic infections, kidney and liver disorders, protein-losing conditions, and multiple myeloma. The results from this test should be correlated with results from tests that measure quantitative immunoglobulin levels and other clinical/laboratory data. In 86334, a blood sample is obtained by separately reportable venipuncture and serum is tested using qualitative immunofixation electrophoresis (IFE) to help identify disease states and monitor treatment or the course of a disease. In 86335, the test is performed on urine, CSF, or other body fluids. Code 86335 is often used for identifying Beta-2 Transferrin, usually performed in conjunction with serum IFE (86334) because Beta-2 transferrin is not normally found in serum, when tested using IFE. The presence of Beta-2 Transferrin is considered to be diagnostic for the presence of a cerebral spinal fluid leak.

86336

86336   Inhibin A

A blood test is performed to measure inhibin A levels. Inhibin A, a heterodimeric protein hormone, is secreted by granulose cells in the female ovary and Sertoli cells in the male testis. It is also produced by the placenta during pregnancy. A normal fluctuation/elevation of this hormone may be present during specific times in the female menstrual cycle and with pregnancy. Abnormal elevation can occur with ovarian tumors (granulose cell and epithelial mucinous-type), congenital abnormalities in the fetus (Down Syndrome), or a pregnancy complicated by preeclampsia. When diagnosing fetal or pregnancy related problems, the test is usually performed in conjunction with AFT (82105), hCG (84702), and Estriol (82677). A blood sample is obtained by separately reportable venipuncture. Serum is tested using quantitative chemiluninescent immunotherapy.

86337

86337   Insulin antibodies

A blood test is performed to measure insulin antibody levels. Insulin antibodies may include human serum autoantibodies to endogenous insulin, antibodies to exogenous insulin, or antibodies to injected insulin synthesized from animals (pork, beef), recombinant DNA, or analogue technology. This test may be used to identify individuals at risk for developing type 1 diabetes mellitus; to differentiate between latent autoimmune diabetes of adults (LADA) and type 2 or gestational diabetes; and to monitor the clinical progression of type 1 diabetes mellitus. A blood sample is obtained by separately reportable venipuncture and serum is tested using quantitative radioimmunoassay.

86340

86340   Intrinsic factor antibodies

A blood test is performed to identify the presence of intrinsic factor blocking antibodies (IFBA). Intrinsic factor is produced in the stomach. It binds to free vitamin B12, carries it to receptors on the ileal mucosa, and then facilitates absorption in the small intestine. An absence of intrinsic factor may lead to pernicious anemia (PA). IFBA are found in 50% of individuals with PA but may also be present with autoimmune thyroid disease, type 1 diabetes mellitus, and rheumatoid arthritis. A blood sample is obtained by separately reportable venipuncture. Serum is tested using qualitative enzyme-linked immunosorbent assay.

86341

86341   Islet cell antibody

A blood test is performed to identify the presence of islet cell antibodies (ICA). Islet cells are located in the pancreas and produce hormones such as insulin, glucagon, somatomammotropin, and pancreatic polypeptides. ICA may be associated with type 1 diabetes mellitus, an autoimmune endocrine disorder. This test may be used to identify individuals at risk for developing type 1 diabetes or to differentiate between latent autoimmune diabetes of adults (LADA) and type 2 or gestational diabetes. A blood sample is obtained by separately reportable venipuncture. Serum is tested for IA-2 antibody using semiquantitative radioimmunoassay. Serum is tested for islet cell antibody, IgG using quantitative indirect fluorescent antibody.

86343

86343   Leukocyte histamine release test (LHR)

Leukocyte histamine release test measures the amount of histamine released from peripheral blood leukocytes after varied concentrations of an allergen extract is introduced. If the individual has a hypersensitivity to a specific allergen, histamine will be released from the leukocytes. Only a limited number of allergens can be introduced into a single sample of blood and there is some variability in the ability to measure the histamine. This test may still be considered as investigational by many policies.

86344

86344   Leukocyte phagocytosis

Leukocytes are produced and stored in lymphoid organs and clumps of tissue throughout the body. They circulate in lymphatic channels and blood, identifying and destroying invading organisms. One type of leukocyte found in blood that targets bacteria is the neutrophil. The phagocyte test determines quantitatively the ingestion activity of bacteria

Pathology and Laboratory

by measuring the percentage of neutrophils that have ingested bacteria and the number of bacteria per cell. A whole blood sample is used and incubated with labeled E.coli bacteria. The phagocytosis process is stopped and a quenching solution is added that will differentiate between attachment and internalization of the bacteria by quelling the fluorescence of surface bound bacteria and leaving the fluorescence of internalized bacteria only. A lysing solution is added which removes red blood cells and fixes the leukocytes. The sample is washed; a DNA staining solution is added to exclude nontarget aggregates; and flow cytometry analysis in then done on the sample.

86352

86352   Cellular function assay involving stimulation (eg, mitogen or antigen) and detection of biomarker (eg, ATP)

Cellular function assay is performed using a live cell culture. The cells are then stimulated using a mitogen or antigen to provoke a cellular response. The cell culture is evaluated using an assay, such as a chemilumescent assay, for the presence and/or level of a biomarker such as adenosine triphosphate (ATP). The presence and/or level of the biomarker is an indicator of cell function.

86353

86353   Lymphocyte transformation, mitogen (phytomitogen) or antigen induced blastogenesis

A blood test is performed to measure lymphocyte transformation, mitogen (phytomitogen) or antigen induced blastogenesis. This test may be used to assess T-cell function in patients with impaired immunity related to immunosuppressive drug therapy following organ transplant or disease related or iatrogenic immune deficiency syndromes. The test may also be used to monitor response of T-cells following bone marrow or stem cell transplant. This code may be used for lymphocyte antigen proliferation and lymphocyte mitogen proliferations. A blood sample is obtained by separately reportable venipuncture. Whole blood is tested using cell culture.

86355

86355   B cells, total count

A blood test is performed to measure total B-cell count. This test is used to assess immune function and is most often performed in conjunction with all or some of the following tests: 86357 (NK cells, total count), 86359 (T-cells, total count), 86360 (absolute CD4 & CD8 counts w/ratio) and 86356 (CD4, CD45RA, CD45RO, CD2, HLA-DR). Elevated levels of B lymphocytes may be present with chronic lymphocytic leukemia, multiple myeloma, Waldenstrom's macroglobinemia, and DiGeorge syndrome. Decreased levels may be found with acute lymphocytic leukemia and congenital immunoglobulin deficiency syndrome. A blood sample is obtained my separately reportable venipuncture. Whole blood is tested using quantitative flow cytometry.

86356

86356   Mononuclear cell antigen, quantitative (eg, flow cytometry), not otherwise specified, each antigen

A quantitative mononuclear cell antigen test is performed using flow cytometry on an antigen without a more specific code. Mononuclear cells are harvested from heparinized whole blood. The mononuclear fraction is diluted and paired aliquots are incubated using monoclonal antibodies. The samples and control specimens are then analyzed using flow cytometry. This code should be reported for each antigen tested.

86357

86357   Natural killer (NK) cells, total count

A blood test is performed to measure total natural killer (NK) cell count. NK cells are large granular lymphocytes that make up a major component of the immune system. This test is used to assess immune function and is often performed in conjunction with all or some of the following tests: 86355 (B-Cells, total count), 86359 (T-cells, total count), 86360 (absolute CD4 & CD8 counts w/ratio) and 86356 (CD4, CD45RA, CD45RO, CD2, HLA-DR). A blood sample is obtained by separately reportable venipuncture. Whole blood is tested using quantitative flow cytometry.

86359

86359   T cells; total count

A blood test is performed to measure total T-cell count. T-cells are a type of lymphocyte (white blood cell) with a central role in cell mediated immunity. This test is used to assess immune function and is usually ordered in conjunction with other tests. Elevated T-cell levels may be present with infectious mononucleosis, acute lymphocytic leukemia, and multiple myeloma. Decreased levels may be found with congenital T-cell deficiency, Wiskott-Aldrich syndrome, or AIDS. Whole blood is tested using quantitative flow cytometry.

86360

86360   T cells; absolute CD4 and CD8 count, including ratio

A blood test is performed to measure T-cell absolute CD4 and CD8 count, including ratio. T-cells are a type of lymphocyte with a central role in cell mediated immunity. CD4 cells are most commonly identified as helper T-cells and CD8 as suppressor T-cells. This test is used to assess immune function and is used mainly for HIV patients. Since the HIV virus attacks CD4 cells and uses them to make more copies of the virus, an absolute CD4 count or ratio compared to the CD8 count is very useful for tracking the progression of the disease. This test is also useful in diagnosing and monitoring other conditions, such as lymphoma, post-transplant status, and DiGeorge Syndrome. A blood sample is obtained by separately reportable venipuncture. Whole blood is tested using quantitative flow cytometry.

86361

86361   T cells; absolute CD4 count

A blood test is performed to measure T-cell absolute CD4 count. T-cells are a type of lymphocyte with a central role in cell mediated immunity. Since the HIV virus attacks CD4 cells in particular and uses them to make more copies of the virus, an absolute CD4 count is used to categorize HIV infections according to CDC guidelines and to establish decision points for beginning treatment in asymptomatic patients or changing current antiviral treatment, as well as for monitoring response to treatment. When monitoring an individual with known HIV infection, it is recommended that this test be performed every 3-6 months. A blood sample is obtained by separately reportable venipuncture. T-cell Absolute CD4 Count or Lymphocyte Subset Panel 1 CD4 Absolute Count Only are tested using quantitative flow cytometry. An HIV infected person with a CD4 count below 200 is considered by the CDC to have AIDS, regardless of signs or symptoms and treatment is undertaken.

86367

86367   Stem cells (ie, CD34), total count

A laboratory test is performed to measure CD34 stem cells. The CD34 molecule is a cell surface glycoprotein that mediates the attachment of stem cells to bone marrow extracellular matrix or directly to stromal cells. It is also required for T cells to enter the lymph nodes. Monoclonal antibodies are used to quantify and purify hematopoietic progenitor stem cells. The CD34 count is important information for patients preparing to undergo autologous or allogenic stem cell transplant. A blood sample is obtained by separately reportable venipuncture. Whole blood is tested using multi-colored immunofluorescence and flow cytometry.

86376

86376   Microsomal antibodies (eg, thyroid or liver-kidney), each

A blood test is performed to identify the presence of microsomal antibodies (thyroid or liver-kidney). Microsomes are located inside of cells in the thyroid, liver, and kidney. When these cells are damaged, microsomes are released, and the body produces antibodies to the microsomes in response to the damage. A blood sample is obtained by separately reportable venipuncture and tested for the presence of the microsomal antibodies. For the thyroid, the test is done to confirm thyroid problems, such as Hashimoto's thyroiditis, cancer, or nontoxic nodular goiter. For liver-kidney microsome antibody, semiquantitative indirect fluorescence or semiquantitative enzyme-linked immunosorbent assay is done to determine cell damage, such as with autoimmune hepatitis type 2 (AIH-2).

86378

86378   Migration inhibitory factor test (MIF)

A laboratory test is performed to measure migration inhibitory factor (MIF). MIF is a macrophage that functions as an inflammatory cytokine binding to immune cells like CD74 and others to trigger an acute immune response. It is released by white blood cells after stimulation from bacterial antigens or glucocorticoids and by the anterior pituitary gland when activated by trauma. This test measures the production of lymphocytes following stimulation with common antigens such as streptokinase-streptodornase, candida antigen, PPD, concanavalin A, phytohemagglutinin, and poke weed and can help determine immune competence and delayed-type hypersensitivity reactions. Low or absent MIF may occur with immunodeficiency syndromes such as AIDS, DiGeorge, or Wiskott-Aldrich syndrome.

86382

86382   Neutralization test, viral

A laboratory test is performed to measure viral neutralization. This test may be used to determine the presence of neutralizing antibodies toward a specific virus like polio or rabies. The presence of antibodies may imply immunity to a virus, or the functionality of the antibody as it complexes with a live virus and clears it so further infection is neutralized. The rapid fluorescent focus inhibition test (RFFIT) is ordered for rabies testing using code 86382. RFFIT is performed 14-21 days following completion of an initial series of rabies vaccine and possibly after receiving a booster dose. Individuals who are at continuous risk for rabies exposure may have this test performed every 6 months and those with frequent risk, tested every two years. A blood sample is obtained by separately reportable venipuncture and tested using culture/neutralization.

86384

86384   Nitroblue tetrazolium dye test (NTD)

Nitroblue tetrazolium dye test is useful for screening an individual for chronic granulomatous disease (CGD). CGD is a heterogenous disorder where phagocytes fail to kill ingested micro-organisms which leads to severe, recurrent pyogenic infections. This test observes if certain immune system cells can change the colorless chemical to a deep blue color. When an individual has CGD, the white blood cells will fail to turn blue when exposed to nitroblue tetrazolium.

86386

86386   Nuclear Matrix Protein 22 (NMP22), qualitative

A screening test for Nuclear Matrix Protein 22 (NMP22) is performed in a patient with hematuria to help differentiate hematuria due to bladder cancer from hematuria due to other causes. NMP22 is a protein found in the cell nucleus. Malignant neoplasms of the bladder increase the intracellular levels of NMP22 and cause shedding of the protein into the urine. A urine sample is obtained. A test kit specific to NMP22 is then used to identify the presence or absence of NMP22 in the urine and to estimate the concentration of the protein. A level of NMP22 greater than 7 is suggestive of bladder malignancy.

86403-86406

86403   Particle agglutination; screen, each antibody
86406   Particle agglutination; titer, each antibody

Particle agglutination tests are ordered to evaluate infection status and to identify certain viruses and bacteria, such as measles virus infection, streptococcal infection, or Treponema pallidum infection (syphilis). Code 86403 is reported for each separate antibody screened. When the screen is positive, code 86406 is reported for titer levels done on each antibody. A blood sample is obtained by separately reportable venipuncture and serum/plasma is tested using several different methods, such as semiquantitative hemagglutination, fluorescent enzyme assay and light flow cytometry.

86430-86431

86430   Rheumatoid factor; qualitative
86431   Rheumatoid factor; quantitative

A blood test is performed to measure qualitative (86430) or quantitative (86431) levels of rheumatoid factor. Elevated levels of rheumatoid factor (IgM, IgG, IgA) may be found with rheumatoid arthritis, hepatitis C, Sjogren syndrome, and other chronic infections. A blood sample is obtained by separately reportable venipuncture. Serum is tested using semiquantitative enzyme-linked immunosorbent assay.

86480-86481

86480   Tuberculosis test, cell mediated immunity antigen response measurement; gamma interferon
86481   Tuberculosis test, cell mediated immunity antigen response measurement; enumeration of gamma interferon-producing T-cells in cell suspension

This test is performed on individuals suspected of having or being at high risk for Mycobacterium tuberculosis (TB) infection. This test measures cell mediated immunity (CMI) antigen response to stimulation with TB-specific proteins. Two proteins, early-secreted antigenic target 6-kDa protein (ESAT-6) and culture filtrate protein (CFP-10), are used in CMI antigen response tests for TB. Individuals with TB infection have lymphocytes in their blood that recognize these proteins. A blood sample is obtained by separately reportable venipuncture. The blood sample is stimulated with ESAT-6 and CFP-10. If the blood sample reacts to these proteins, which is indicated by the secretion of cytokine interferon gamma, the test is positive for TB. Cytokines are hormone-like proteins secreted by cells that regulate the intensity and duration of immune response. Both the presence and amount of cytokine interferon gamma present in the blood sample are used for diagnosis of TB. Use 86480 when blood is tested for gamma interferon CMI antigen response; use 86481 when gamma interferon-producing T-cells in a cell suspension are quantified.

86485

86485   Skin test; candida

A candida skin test is often used as an anergy control to provide a basis when interpreting a delayed type hypersensitivity response to tuberculin skin testing in patient's whose cellular immunity is compromised (anergy). Compromised patients can register a false negative during TB testing, which makes diagnosis difficult. However, in most individuals, exposure to candida will produce a positive response if the immune system is functioning properly. The positive response of an individual to candida allows a compromised immune system to be ruled out as a possible factor in persons whose reaction toward a PPD skin test was evaluated as negative.

86486

86486   Skin test; unlisted antigen, each

A skin test for an unlisted antigen is performed. An antigen is a substance that causes a reaction, such as sensitivity or immune response, when it comes into contact with cells that have been sensitized to it. An antigen without a more specific skin test code is introduced just under the skin. This produces a discrete pale elevation of the skin called a wheal. The wheal is quickly absorbed. If an individual has antibodies to the antigen, localized swelling and/or itching will occur at the site of the injection. The test injection site is checked (read) 48 to 72 hours following injection. Any raised or hardened area is noted and the extent of the reaction is measured and recorded.

86490

86490   Skin test; coccidioidomycosis

Coccidioidomycosis is caused by a soil fungus native to areas of Southern California, Southwestern United States, Northwestern Mexico, and scattered areas of Central and South America. Skin testing is performed to assess cellular immune response in those who have been in contact with the fungus. A positive skin test result may indicate active infection or a past history of exposure. The fungus is introduced into the skin by pinprick, and the site is examined at intervals for the reaction.

86510

86510   Skin test; histoplasmosis

Histoplasmosis is caused by a fungus that grows in soil contaminated by bat or bird droppings and is endemic to Central and Eastern United States and caves in Eastern Africa. Skin testing is performed to assess cellular immune response in those who have been in contact with the fungus. A positive skin test result may indicate active infection or a past history of exposure. The fungus is introduced into the skin by pinprick, and the site is examined at intervals for the reaction.

86580

86580   Skin test; tuberculosis, intradermal

Tuberculosis is caused by a bacterium endemic to all areas of the world. Skin testing is performed to assess cellular immune response in those who have been in contact with the bacterium. Tuberculin purified protein derivative (PPD) is injected into the surface layers of skin. Forty-eight to 72 hours after administration, the size of the reaction is measured and recorded. A positive skin test result may indicate active infection, a past history of exposure, or having received the BCG vaccine.

86590

86590   Streptokinase, antibody

A blood test is performed to measure streptokinase antibody. Streptokinase is an enzyme produced by certain stains of the streptococcus bacteria which liquefies blood clots by converting plasminogen to plasmin. Streptokinase antibodies may cause resistance to the anticoagulant function of the enzyme leading to suboptimal thrombolytic therapy. A blood sample is obtained by separately reportable venipuncture and tested using rapid latex-bead assay or enzyme immunoassay.

86592-86593

86592   Syphilis test, non-treponemal antibody; qualitative (eg, VDRL, RPR, ART)
86593   Syphilis test, non-treponemal antibody; quantitative

A test for syphilis is performed. Syphilis is a sexually-transmitted disease (STD) caused by the bacterium Treponema pallidum. During the primary stage, a sore called a chancre appears at the site where the syphilis bacterium entered the body. The chancre resolves without treatment in 3-6 weeks but the patient remains infected. Without treatment, the infection will progress to a secondary stage in which a skin rash and mucous membrane lesions appear. The most common site of the rash is the palms of the hands and soles of the feet. Other symptoms during the secondary stage include fever, swollen lymph nodes, sore throat, hair loss, headaches, weight loss, muscle aches, and fatigue. Symptoms of secondary syphilis also resolve spontaneously but the patient remains infected. The patient then enters the late or latent stage of the disease. Symptoms of this stage may not appear for 10-20 years. Symptoms of late stage syphilis include difficulty coordinating muscle movements, paralysis, numbness, gradual blindness, and dementia. These symptoms occur as the disease damages internal organs including the brain, nerves, eyes, heart, blood vessels, liver, bones, and joints. Of particular concern is undiagnosed syphilis infection during pregnancy as the infection can be passed to the baby in utero. This increases the risk of stillbirth or death shortly after birth. Untreated infants who survive often experience developmental delays or seizures. In 86592, a qualitative syphilis test, such as the venereal disease research laboratory (VDRL) test, rapid plasma reagin (RPR) test, or automated reagin test (ART). The VDRL, RPR, ART are nontreponemal tests that measure antibody response to lipoidal antigen from T. pallidum and/or antibody interaction with host tissues. If a screening test is positive and the result is confirmed with a second confirmatory test, quantitative testing is then performed to determine disease activity and monitor response

Pathology and Laboratory

to treatment. Quantitative testing may be performed by enzyme linked immunosorbent assay (ELISA). Use 86593 for quantitative testing. Both qualitative and quantitative tests can be performed on blood, or in the case of suspected central nervous system involvement, the test may be performed on cerebral spinal fluid (CSF).

86602

86602   Antibody; actinomyces

A specimen is tested for antibodies to actinomyces. There are six actinomyces organisms that cause infection, including A. Israeli, A. gerencseriae, A. naeslundii, A. odontolyticus, A. viscosus, A. meyer, and Propionibacterium propionicum. Actinomyces organisms cause subacute or chronic bacterial infection characterized by dense granulomatous inflammation with multiple abscesses and draining fistulas containing sulphur granules. Common infection sites include oral/cervicofacial (lumpy jaw), thoracic, abdominal, and the pelvic are in women. IgG testing is performed to diagnose a current or past infection, and IgM testing is performed to identify a current infection with a specific actinomyces organism. If both IgG and IgM testing is performed, the test for each immunoglobulin class should be reported separately. This is not a commonly performed test for actinomyces, which is more commonly diagnosed by culture and gram stain.

86603

86603   Antibody; adenovirus

A blood sample is tested for antibodies to adenovirus. Adenoviruses cause upper respiratory infections with symptoms including the common cold, pneumonia, croup, and bronchitis; gastroenteritis; conjunctivitis; cystitis; and rash. Acute respiratory disease (ARD) can also result from infection with adenoviruses, which are most commonly identified by enzyme-linked immunosorbent assay (ELISA) methodology. IgG testing is performed to diagnose a current or past infection, and IgM testing is performed to identify a current infection with a specific adenovirus organism. If both IgG and IgM testing is performed, the test for each immunoglobulin class should be reported separately.

86606

86606   Antibody; Aspergillus

A blood or cerebral spinal fluid sample is tested for antibodies to Aspergillus, a fungus found in soil, on plants, decaying plant material, dust, building materials, and some food items. There are several different Aspergillus fungi. The most common is A. fumigatus and A. flavus. Aspergillus infection can cause allergic bronchopulmonary disease with symptoms of wheezing and coughing but without tissue damage. However, severe infections can invade and destroy tissue and this is called invasive aspergillosis. Immunocompromised individuals are at risk for developing invasive aspergillosis which affects primarily the lungs but can also affect other organs including the central nervous system. There are several methods available to test for Aspergillus infection including complement fixation, immunodiffusion, or enzyme-linked immunosorbent assay (ELISA). Tests for Aspergillus generally measure IgG antibodies only. However, multiple methodologies may be used to isolate the antibody, such as immunodiffusion and complement fixation and each methodology is reported separately.

86609

86609   Antibody; bacterium, not elsewhere specified

A blood sample is tested for antibodies to bacteria not specified in any other code. Some of the commonly tested antibodies reported with this code include listeria, mycobacterium tuberculosis, and toxic shock syndrome antibody. A humoral immunity panel which tests for multiple organisms in patients with chronic and recurrent infections also includes tests for bacteria not listed in other codes. Methodology depends on the antibody being tested. Listeria uses complement fixation. Mycobacterium tuberculosis uses enzyme-linked immunosorbent assay (ELISA). Toxic shock syndrome uses multi-analyte immunodetection (MAID). IgG antibody is the most common antibody class tested. This code may be reported multiple times depending on how many organisms are tested, the number of antibody classes (IgG, IgM), and the different methodologies used for each organism.

86611

86611   Antibody; Bartonella

A blood sample is tested for antibodies to Bartonella, a bacteria that causes fever, chills, headaches, and progressive anemia in the acute phase and musculoskeletal pain and lesions on the skin and mucous membranes in the chronic phase. In the acute phase, it can also invade the central nervous system causing meningoencephalitis with seizures and paralysis, sometimes leading to death. B. henselae is the most common form found in the United States. In patients with HIV infection, B. henselae may present as skin lesions similar in appearance to Kaposi's sarcoma. B. henselae is also the organism that causes cat-scratch disease, a localized infection that causes fever, headache, loss of appetite, and regionalized lymphadenopathy. There are several methods available to test for Bartonella infection including indirect hemagglutination (IHA), indirect fluorescent antibody (IFA), or enzyme-linked immunosorbent assay (ELISA). IgG testing is performed to diagnose a current or past infection, and IgM testing is performed to identify a current infection with

a specific Bartonella organism. If both IgG and IgM testing is performed, the test for each immunoglobulin class should be reported separately.

86612

86612   Antibody; Blastomyces

A blood or cerebral spinal fluid sample is tested for antibodies to Blastomyces. Blastomycosis dermatitidis is a fungus found in soil that causes infection when it is inhaled. Acute infection can cause flu-like symptoms of fever, chills, myalgia, headache, and cough. More severe acute infection may present with productive cough and symptoms similar to bacterial pneumonia. Chronic illness presents with low grade fever, productive cough, night sweats, and weight loss. Immunocompromised individuals are at risk for developing disseminated blastomycosis which affects other organs including the central nervous system. There are several methods available to test for Blastomyces infection including complement fixation and immunodiffusion.

86615

86615   Antibody; Bordetella

A laboratory test is performed to measure Bordetella antibody. Bordetella pertussis is the bacterium that causes whooping cough. A culture is used for diagnosing an infection. Antibody testing for Bordetella may be used to monitor the body's response to pertussis infection. IgG antibodies will be present in vaccinated individuals and newborns or infants with placental transfer of antibodies. Levels may be elevated after a recent active infection. A rise in IgA and IgM antibodies is usually associated with active infection and is considered to be more diagnostic for whooping cough (pertussis). A blood sample is obtained by separately reportable venipuncture. Serum is tested using semi-quantitative enzyme-linked immunosorbent assay and qualitative immunoblot.

86617

86617   Antibody; Borrelia burgdorferi (Lyme disease) confirmatory test (eg, Western Blot or immunoblot)

A laboratory test is performed to confirm the presence of Borrelia burgdorferi (Lyme disease) antibodies in serum and/or cerebral spinal fluid (CSF). This test may be ordered when a patient has symptoms of Lyme disease infection and an ELISA test is positive or equivocal for the B. burgdorferi antibodies. IgM antibodies will begin to rise 2-3 weeks after exposure to the bacterium, reaching maximum concentration by 6 weeks before declining. IgG antibodies take several weeks to elevate and may not reach maximum concentration for 4-6 months. Levels of IgG can remain elevated for many years after the initial infection. A blood sample is obtained by separately reportable venipuncture; cerebrospinal fluid by separately reportable lumbar puncture. Serum and CSF are tested using quantitative western blot or immunoblot.

86618

86618   Antibody; Borrelia burgdorferi (Lyme disease)

A laboratory test is performed to measure Borrelia burgdorferi (Lyme disease) antibodies in serum and/or cerebral spinal fluid (CSF). This test is used for first line screening when a patient has symptoms of Lyme disease infection and lives or has visited an area endemic to black legged ticks. It is most reliable when performed within four weeks of a tick bite and the appearance of erythema migrans (bull's eye) rash. The presence of C6 peptide antibodies to B. burgdorferi is considered a stand-alone diagnostic test for Lyme disease. IgM antibodies will be positive within 2-3 weeks of exposure and may also be used to diagnose early disease. IgG antibodies rise with early exposure but do not peak until 4-6 months after the initial infection. A positive test for C6 peptide antibodies is often followed with screening for IgG and IgM antibodies. Positive or equivocal test results for C6 peptide, IgM and IgG antibodies should always be reflexed for a Western Blot or immunoblot confirmation test. A blood sample is obtained by separately reportable venipuncture; CSF by separately reportable lumbar puncture. Serum and CSF are tested using semi-quantitative enzyme-linked immunosorbent assay (ELISA).

86619

86619   Antibody; Borrelia (relapsing fever)

A laboratory test is performed to measure Borrelia (relapsing fever) antibody. The Borrelia spirochetes which cause relapsing fever may be tick borne (TBRF) or louse borne (LBRF). Tick borne disease is found in the western United States usually in rodent infested mountainous cabins. Louse borne disease is generally restricted to refugee populations in underdeveloped areas of the world. Relapsing fever is characterized by fever, chills, headache, muscle and joint pain, nausea, and possibly a rash. The onset of symptoms typically occurs 5-15 days after a tick or louse bite and will continue for 2-9 days. After a spontaneous remission, the cycle of symptoms will be repeated until the patient is treated with antibiotics. A blood sample is obtained by separately reportable venipuncture. Serum is tested using semi-quantitative immunofluorescence assay/indirect fluorescent antibody.

86622

86622   Antibody; Brucella

A laboratory test is performed to measure Brucella antibody. The Brucella bacteria is found primarily in animals but may infect humans who eat or drink unpasteurized, raw dairy products. Infection can also occur via inhalation or skin contact as might occur with veterinarians, hunters, laboratory personnel, and meatpacking or slaughterhouse workers. Symptoms typically occur 2-4 weeks following exposure and may include fever, sweats, headache, muscle and joint pain, and fatigue. A positive Brucella antibody titer is suggestive of burcellosis infection when clinical symptoms are present and there is a history of possible exposure. A blood sample is obtained by separately reportable venipuncture. Serum is tested using semi-quantitative agglutination.

86625

86625   Antibody; Campylobacter

A laboratory test is performed to measure Campylobacter antibody. Campylobacter is a spiral shaped bacteria that can infect humans and animals causing gastrointestinal symptoms including diarrhea (often bloody), nausea and vomiting, abdominal pain, and fever. Outbreaks are more common in summer and tend to be isolated and sporadic. Ingesting raw or undercooked meat and poultry or foods contaminated by them is the most common source of infection. Unpasteurized dairy products, contaminated drinking water, or contact with infected household pets may also lead to infection in humans. A positive titer for Campylobacter jejuni IgG antibodies is suggestive for current or past infection with the bacteria. A blood sample is obtained by separately reportable venipuncture. Serum is tested using semi-quantitative indirect fluorescent antibody.

86628

86628   Antibody; Candida

A blood sample is tested for antibodies to Candida, a fungus normally present on the skin and in mucous membranes such as the vagina, mouth, or rectum. Candida becomes an infectious agent only when a change in body chemistry allows the fungus to grow out of control and is referred to as Candidiasis moniliasis. Individuals on antibiotics and those who are immunocompromised are susceptible to Candida infection as are infants. Typically, the infection is localized in the mouth, skin, nails, or vagina; less commonly, the esophagus and gastrointestinal tract are affected. However, Candida can also infect the blood and cause damage to the kidneys, heart, lungs, eyes, or brain. There are several methods available to test for Candida infection including immunodiffusion and enzyme-linked immunosorbent assay (ELISA). Tests for Candida by ELISA generally measure IgA, IgG, and IgM antibodies and each immunoglobulin class (IgA, IgG, and/or IgM) tested is reported separately.

86631-86632

86631   Antibody; Chlamydia
86632   Antibody; Chlamydia, IgM

A blood sample is tested for antibodies to Chlamydia, a group of bacteria that cause a variety of infections. The most common infection is C. trachomatis, a sexually transmitted disease (STD) that often produces no symptoms, but can cause irreversible damage to the female reproductive tract resulting in infertility. In men, symptoms include burning and itching of the urethra, but men rarely suffer reproductive damage from the infection. Another species, C. pneumoniae, causes upper respiratory infection, including pneumonia, bronchitis, rhinitis, and pharyngitis. A third species, C. psittaci, primarily affects birds but humans can acquire the disease by handling or being exposed to infected birds. C. psittaci causes flu-like symptoms. There are several methods available to test for Chlaymida antibodies including indirect fluorescent antibody and enzyme-linked immunosorbent assay (ELISA). Use 86631 for screening tests for all chlamydial species and tests for IgG antibodies. Use 86632 for IgM antibodies. Each species and each immunoglobulin class (IgG, IgM) tested is reported separately.

86635

86635   Antibody; Coccidioides

A laboratory test is performed to measure Coccidioides antibody. Coccidioides is a fungus found in soil, particularly in the Southwestern United States, parts of Mexico, and Central and South America, that can infect humans who breathe in airborne spores causing a flu-like illness known as coccidioidomycosis, or Valley Fever). The incubation period is 1-3 weeks and many individuals will have no signs or symptoms of illness. When symptoms do manifest, they usually include fever, fatigue, cough, headache, night sweats, muscle and joint pain and sometimes a rash on the upper body and legs. Positive antibody titers may indicate a past or present infection. Coccidioides IgM antibodies will be present by the 2nd week of infection and usually disappear by 4 months. However, they may reappear with relapse or persist with disseminated infection. IgG antibodies appear by the 3rd week of infection and can remain elevated for many years. A blood sample is obtained by separately reportable venipuncture. Serum is tested for Coccidioides antibodies (IgM, IgG) using semi-quantitative complement fixation, or semi-quantitative enzyme-

linked immunosorbent assay, and Coccidioides immitis antibodies using qualitative immunodiffusion.

86638

86638   Antibody; Coxiella burnetii (Q fever)

A laboratory test is performed to measure Coxiella burnetii (Q fever) antibody. C. burnetii is a bacterium found worldwide in animals and may cause acute or chronic infection in humans. The bacteria is commonly shed in the milk, urine, feces, and amniotic fluid of infected animals and can then be inhaled in barnyard dust, ingested in unpasteurized milk and dairy products, or transmitted via tick bite to humans. Onset of acute symptoms typically occurs 2-3 weeks following exposure and may include fever, malaise, chills, night sweats, cough, muscle aches, nausea and vomiting, diarrhea, or abdominal pain. If left untreated, chronic symptoms may develop including endocarditis, aortic aneurysm, and infection of the liver, bones, or reproductive organs (testes). A post Q Fever fatigue syndrome has also been reported. A positive Phase I titer usually indicates chronic or convalescent phase infection. A positive Phase II titer is more indicative of exposure to the C. burnetii bacteria at some time prior to the specimen collection. A blood sample is obtained by separately reportable venipuncture. Serum is tested for IgG antibodies using semi-quantitative indirect fluorescence, and for IgG and IgM antibodies using immunofluorescence assay.

86641

86641   Antibody; Cryptococcus

A laboratory test is performed to measure Cryptococcus neoformans antibody. C. neoformans is an encapsulated fungus commonly found in bird droppings. Immune compromised individuals are very susceptible to infection with this organism. It usually infects humans via the respiratory tract, causing pneumonia and extra-pulmonary tissue infection. From the lungs, the fungus migrates to the brain and causes acute, subacute, or chronic meningoencephalitis. Another symptom of the disease is lesions of the bone and skin. A blood sample is obtained by separately reportable venipuncture. Serum is tested using agglutination or indirect ELISA.

86644-86645

86644   Antibody; cytomegalovirus (CMV)
86645   Antibody; cytomegalovirus (CMV), IgM

A blood sample is tested for antibodies to cytomegalovirus (CMV) which is part of the herpes virus group of infections. It is transmitted by direct contact with body fluids, including breast milk, and sexual contact. In healthy adults, CMV produces symptoms resembling those of mononucleosis. CMV can cause birth defects in newborns if the mother is infected during pregnancy. Individuals with compromised immune systems, including those with acquired immune deficiency syndrome (AIDS) or patients with malignancies are at risk for development of chorioretinitis, gastrointestinal disorders, pneumonitis, or central nervous system disease related to CMV. In 86644, total (IgG and IgM) or IgG CMV antibodies are identified by solid phase agglutination or chemiluminescent immunoassay. Total CMV antibodies are tested to screen for a past or present infection. IgG antibodies typically indicate a past infection but may also be present with a current infection. In 86645, IgM antibodies are identified which may indicate a present or recent infection, although IgM antibodies may persist for up to 12 months. IgM is tested by enzyme linked immunosorbent assay (ELISA).

86648

86648   Antibody; Diphtheria

A laboratory test is performed to measure Diphtheria antibody. Diphtheria is an acute, contagious disease caused by the Corynebacterium diphtheriae bacteria. This bacteria produces an exotoxin from which the patient develops fibrinous pseudomembranes in respiratory, myocardial, and/or neural tissue. The test for Diphtheria antibodies measures IgG Subclass I and may be used to determine an individual's protective antibody level pre/post vaccination, assess immunity status during a community outbreak, or evaluate for antibody deficiencies in patients with recurrent infections. A blood sample is obtained by separately reportable venipuncture. Serum is tested using enzyme immunoassay.

86651

86651   Antibody; encephalitis, California (La Crosse)

A laboratory test is performed to measure California (La Crosse) encephalitis antibody in blood or cerebral spinal fluid (CSF). This mosquito borne bunyaviridae virus causes a mild illness seen typically in children during the late summer. Symptoms of stiff neck and lethargy usually manifest about a week after exposure and may last up to 10 days. Seizures may also accompany acute infection and/or be sequelae of the disease. A positive titer for IgG antibodies is suggestive of current or past infection. A positive titer for IgM antibodies with clinical suspicion of California (La Crosse) viral infection is suggestive of current or recent infection. A blood sample is obtained by separately reportable venipuncture; CSF by separately reportable lumbar puncture. Serum and CSF are tested using semi-quantitative indirect fluorescent antibody.

86652

86652   Antibody; encephalitis, Eastern equine

A laboratory test is performed to measure Eastern equine encephalitis (EEE) antibody in serum and/or cerebrospinal fluid (CSF). EEE falls within the alphavirus group of arboviruses transmitted through mosquitoes and wild birds in the Eastern and Gulf states. It has a low prevalence in human populations with peak outbreaks occurring in summer and early fall. Symptoms are typically mild and include headache and fever. Central nervous system symptoms occur in a minority of infected persons. Children usually manifest more severe signs and symptoms of the disease. IgG antibody titers may be positive with current or past EEE infection; IgM antibodies with current or recent EEE infection. Both of these antibodies may show cross reactivity with Western equine encephalitis (WEE) infection. Travel history as well as medical and epidemiological data should be considered in symptomatic patients if the virus has not been isolated. A blood sample is obtained by separately reportable venipuncture; CSF is obtained by separately reportable lumbar puncture. Serum and CSF are tested using semi-quantitative indirect fluorescent antibody or immunofluorescent assay.

86653

86653   Antibody; encephalitis, St. Louis

A laboratory test is performed to measure St. Louis encephalitis antibody in serum and/or cerebrospinal fluid (CSF). St. Louis encephalitis is a mosquito borne disease common in the Western United States, Texas, Ohio-Mississippi Valley, and Florida with peak outbreaks occurring in summer and autumn. Early symptoms include fever, chills, headache, and malaise, with sleepiness, nausea, sore throat, and cough sometimes reported. Central nervous system symptoms occur 1-4 days later and may last for months or years. CNS symptoms are more common in elderly patients and can include irritability, sleepiness, depression, and memory loss. IgG antibody titers may be positive with current or past infection; IgM antibodies with current or recent infection. Travel history as well as medical and epidemiological data should be considered in symptomatic patients if the virus has not been isolated. A blood sample is obtained by separately reportable venipuncture; CSF is obtained by separately reportable lumbar puncture. Serum and CSF are tested using semi-quantitative indirect fluorescent antibody or immunofluorescent assay.

86654

86654   Antibody; encephalitis, Western equine

A laboratory test is performed to measure Western equine encephalitis (WEE) antibody in serum and/or cerebrospinal fluid (CSF). WEE is found throughout the United States and Canada with outbreaks occurring most commonly in the Western states and provinces. Sudden onset of headache and fever often followed by photophobia, malaise, abdominal pain, nausea and vomiting, sore throat, and respiratory problems are typical symptoms of WEE. The headache may intensify over a few days with drowsiness, restlessness, and possible coma occurring. Infants and children are especially susceptible to central nervous system disease with this infection and recovery can take months to years. IgG antibody titers may be positive with current or past WEE infection; IgM antibodies with current or recent WEE infection. Both of these antibodies may show cross reactivity with Eastern equine encephalitis (EEE) infection. Travel history as well as medical and epidemiological data should be considered in symptomatic patients if the virus has not been isolated. A blood sample is obtained by separately reportable venipuncture; CSF is obtained by separately reportable lumbar puncture. Serum and CSF are tested using semi-quantitative indirect fluorescent antibody or immunofluorescent assay.

86658

86658   Antibody; enterovirus (eg, coxsackie, echo, polio)

A laboratory test is performed to measure enterovirus antibodies (coxsackie, echo, polio) in serum and/or cerebrospinal fluid (CSF). Coxsackie virus, enteric cytopathic human orphan (ECHO) virus, and poliovirus are all members of the picornaviridae family of enteroviruses. Coxsackie virus has two groups, A and B, with 24 subtypes within these groups. Coxsackie virus A causes a blister like herpangina infection of the hand, foot, and mouth and may also cause conjunctivitis. Coxsackie virus B infection usually causes epidemic pleurodynia, characterized by fever, headache, and pleural and gastrointestinal pain. Both infections can lead to meningitis, myocarditis, and pericarditis. Echovirus causes an acute febrile illness and may be accompanied by a skin rash. The echovirus has been implicated in meningitis and myositis, followed by weak paralytic symptoms. Poliovirus has 3 identified serotypes, all extremely infectious, causing gastrointestinal symptoms, fever, headache, and sore throat, followed by central nervous system infection with muscle pain, spasms, and paralysis. A blood sample is obtained by separately reportable venipuncture; cerebrospinal fluid (CSF) by separately reportable lumbar puncture. CSF is tested for Coxsackie virus A and B and Echovirus using compliment fixation and should be measured with serum to determine antibody ratios. Serum is tested for Coxsackievirus B, Echovirus, and Poliovirus using semi-quantitative serum neutralization. Cross reactivity among the enteroviruses may occur. The virus with the highest titer usually indicates the infecting serotype.

86663-86665

86663   Antibody; Epstein-Barr (EB) virus, early antigen (EA)
86664   Antibody; Epstein-Barr (EB) virus, nuclear antigen (EBNA)
86665   Antibody; Epstein-Barr (EB) virus, viral capsid (VCA)

A laboratory test is performed to measure Epstein-Barr virus (EBV) antibodies. EBV causes infectious mononucleosis, a common infection in children and young adults. The disease is typically mild and self limiting characterized by fever, fatigue, sore throat, swollen lymph nodes, and sometimes an enlarged spleen. The virus is spread through saliva during active disease and remains present in body lymphocytes for life, sometimes reactivating without symptoms. An X-linked lymphoproliferative syndrome in males and certain cancers such as Burkitt's lymphoma, Hodgkin's lymphoma, and nasopharyngeal carcinoma, are also associated with EBV infection. In 86663, the early antigen (EA) IgG antibody test is done to aid in diagnosing an acute EBV infection or reactivation, but should not be considered a stand-alone test for the disease. In 86664, the EBV nuclear antigen (EBNA) IgG antibody test is done and in 86665, the EBV viral capsid antigen (VCA) test for IgG and IgM antibodies is done. Both tests can be used to document past exposure to the EBV and to diagnose primary EBV infectious mononucleosis in conjunction with other tests; however, the EBV viral capsid antigen (VCA) test for IgA antibody cannot be used to diagnose EBV infectious mononucleosis, but may aid with detection and prognosis of nasopharyngeal carcinoma. A blood sample is obtained by separately reportable venipuncture. Serum is tested using semi-quantitative chemiluminescent immunoassay.

86666

86666   Antibody; Ehrlichia

A blood sample is tested for antibodies to Ehrlichia, a genus of organisms that cause bacterial diseases in humans and animals, and is transmitted by the bite of an infected tick. There are four Ehrlichia species known to cause disease in humans and are transmitted by the bite of a tick, namely Amblyomma americanum (lone star tick) and blacklegged ticks, Ixodes scapularis (Northeasten US), Ixodes pacificus (Western US), and Ixodes ricinus (Europe). Infection causes fever, headache, fatigue, and muscle aches. Indirect hemagglutination (IHA) methodology is commonly used to test for Ehrlichia antibodies. IgG testing is performed to diagnose a current or past infection, and IgM testing is performed to identify a current infection with a specific Ehrlichia organism. If both IgG and IgM testing is performed, the test for each immunoglobulin class should be reported separately.

86668

86668   Antibody; Francisella tularensis

A laboratory test is performed to measure Francisella tularensis antibody. The F. tularensis bacterium is found across the continental United States and can infect both animals and humans. It may be transmitted by tick and deer fly bites, skin contact with an infected animal, ingesting contaminated water, inhalation of contaminated dust, or by laboratory exposure. Symptoms include skin ulcer, enlarged lymph nodes, sore throat, mouth sores in oral contact, and pneumonia with inhalation. Elevated IgG antibodies may indicate a current or past exposure, while elevated IgM antibodies are more indicative of a current or recent exposure. A blood sample is obtained by separately reportable venipuncture. Serum/plasma is tested using semi-quantitative enzyme-linked immunosorbent assay. There may be cross reactivity with Brucella, Yersinia, and Proteus OX19 antibodies.

86671

86671   Antibody; fungus, not elsewhere specified

A laboratory test is performed to measure fungus antibodies, not elsewhere specified. A blood sample is obtained by separately reportable venipuncture. Code 86671 may be applied when testing serum for Saccharomyces cerevisiae antibodies IgG and IgA using semi-quantitative enzyme-linked immunosorbent assay. This test can aid in differentiating ulcerative colitis and Crohn's disease in patients exhibiting clinical features of inflammatory bowel disease. Code 86671 is also used to test for Trichophyton rubrum IgG antibodies in serum by quantitative immunocap fluorescent enzyme immunoassay, for Strachybotrys chartorum/atra antibodies using quantitative fluorescent enzyme immunoassay and Sporothrix antibody using quantitative latex agglutination.

86674

86674   Antibody; Giardia lamblia

A laboratory test is performed to measure Giardia lamblia antibodies. G. lamblia is a microscopic parasite found worldwide in soil, food, and water. It is transmitted via infected feces from humans and animals. The organism causes an intestinal infection characterized by abdominal cramps, bloating, diarrhea, and weight loss with continued infection. Elevated IgM antibodies or a marked (four-fold) rise in IgG/IgA antibody titers between acute and convalescent sera would suggest recent or current giardia infection. A positive IgG/IgA antibody titer without measurable IgM antibodies is more indicative of past infection. A blood sample is obtained my separately reportable venipuncture. Serum is tested for IgG/IgA/IgM antibodies using semi-quantitative enzyme-linked immunosorbent assay.

86677

86677   Antibody; Helicobacter pylori

A laboratory test is performed to measure Helicobacter pylori antibodies. H. pylori is a bacterium found in contaminated food and water and may be spread person to person. The organism causes chronic inflammation of the gastrointestinal mucosa, primarily in the stomach and duodenum, which leads to erosion or ulcer formation. The seroconversion of IgA and IgG antibodies will occur together within about 60 days of exposure. Elevated titers to both IgA and IgG antibodies in the presence of symptoms may represent an active H. pylori infection. The antibody test should be confirmed with bacterial isolation or other diagnostic tests such as H. pylori breath test, or fecal antigen by EIA. It is also possible to test for IgM antibodies, however the clinical usefulness of this measurement has not been clearly established. A blood sample is obtained by separately reportable venipuncture. Serum is tested for IgA/IgG antibodies using semi-quantitative enzyme immunoassay and for IgM antibodies using semi-quantitative enzyme-linked immunosorbent assay.

86682

86682   Antibody; helminth, not elsewhere specified

A laboratory test is performed to measure helminth antibodies, not elsewhere specified. Helminth or parasitic worms are numerous and code 86682 may be applied when testing for IgG antibodies in serum to the following: Cysticercosis, Toxocara, Schistosoma, Strongyloides, Filaria, and Echinococcus. Cysticercosis is a parasitic infection of the brain, muscle, or other tissue caused by the tapeworm Taenia solium, that infects humans who ingest the larvae. Toxocara are round worms found primarily in dogs and cats that invades the intestine of the host animal and is shed in their feces. Human infection is often asymptomatic but may present with vision loss, eye inflammation, and retinal damage, or liver and central nervous system symptoms causing fever, fatigue, cough, wheezing, or abdominal pain. The schistosoma parasite is not found in the United States but is endemic in other areas of the world. The larvae breed in freshwater snails where water has been contaminated. The parasite enters the body through skin penetration causing a rash and/or itching at the site followed later by fever, chills, cough, and muscle aches. The worm migrates to the liver and bladder causing inflammation and scarring. Filaria is a thread-like worm that can infect humans through the bite of tropical mosquitoes. The parasite migrates to lymphatic tissue causing lymphedema. Echinococcus is a tiny parasitic tapeworm carried by dogs, sheep, cattle, goats, and pigs that can cause cystic disease in humans in the lungs, liver, and other organs.

86684

86684   Antibody; Haemophilus influenza

A laboratory test is performed to measure Haemophilus influenzae type B (HIB) IgG antibodies. This test may be used to assess the immune status of a patient against HIB following vaccination and can aid in the evaluation of immunodeficiency response syndromes. H. influenzae is an encapsulated bacterium capable of causing severe infection, especially in children under the age of 5 years. There are six identified types (A-F) and other nontypeable strains. H. influenza, type B is the most common, causing diseases that include meningitis, bacteremia, cellulitis, epiglottitis, pneumonia, and septic arthritis. A blood sample is obtained by separately reportable venipuncture. Serum is tested using enzyme-linked immunosorbent assay.

86687-86689

86687   Antibody; HTLV-I
86688   Antibody; HTLV-II
86689   Antibody; HTLV or HIV antibody, confirmatory test (eg, Western Blot)

A blood sample is tested for antibodies to human T-lymphotropic virus type I (HTLV-1) (86687) or human T-lymphotropic type II (HTLV-II) (86688), or a confirmatory test is performed for HTLV-I, HTLV-II, or human immunodeficiency virus I or II (HIV-I, HIV-II) (86689). HTLV and HIV virus infections are sexually transmitted diseases that can also be transmitted from unscreened blood, shared needles, from mother to child in utero, or by breast feeding. HTLV-I and HTLV-II cause disorders of bone marrow and blood cells derived from bone marrow. HTLV-I also causes adult T-cell leukemia. Human immunodeficiency virus (HIV) attacks the immune system by destroying T cells or CD4 cells, which are a type of white blood cell. This hampers the body's ability to fight infection. Acquired immunodeficiency syndrome (AIDS) is the final stage of HIV infection. HTLV-I and HTLV-II antibody tests are performed by enzyme immunosorbent assay (EIA) using test kits designed to detect antibodies to these viruses in human serum or plasma. If the EIA test is positive, a confirmatory test for HTLV-I or HTLV-II is performed by immunoblot or Western blot, reported with 86689. Confirmatory antibody testing for HIV-I and HIV-II viruses performed by Western Blot is also reported with 86689. Western blot is an immunoassay test method that detects specific proteins, in this case HTLV-I, HTLV-II, HIV-I or HIV-II, in blood. The test is performed by placing multiple samples and a control containing the HIV-I or HIV-II protein side-by-side in separate lanes on a spot at one end of a layer of gel. An electrical current is then passed through the layer of gel, causing the sample proteins to move across the gel, separating them by size and shape. The samples and control are then transferred (blotted) onto a thin membrane. The patient sample is added to the blot

and antibodies to HTLV-I, HTLV-II, HIV-I or HIV-II, if present, bind to the proteins on the membrane. Labelled or tagged antibodies are then used to detect the virus. The results are then compared with the known negative and positive control samples in the other lanes.

86692

86692   Antibody; hepatitis, delta agent

A laboratory test is performed to measure hepatitis delta agent (HDV) total and/or IgM antibodies. Hepatitis delta is an RNA virus unrelated to Hepatitis A, B, or C. It is considered to be a sub or incomplete virus because it requires the presence of Hepatitis B virus (HBV) to replicate. HDV is a blood borne pathogen that may be contracted at the same time as HBV (co-infection) or later to cause a super-infection. Individuals with HDV/HBV infection have a greater chance of developing liver cirrhosis, liver failure, and liver cancer. A positive titer for total HDV antibodies may indicate acute or chronic HDV infection. Measuring IgM antibodies alone can help distinguish active replication that takes place during acute infection and reactivation of chronic infection. A blood sample is obtained by separately reportable venipuncture. Serum is tested for total antibodies using qualitative enzyme immunoassay and IgM antibodies using enzyme immunoassay.

86694-86696

86694   Antibody; herpes simplex, non-specific type test
86695   Antibody; herpes simplex, type 1
86696   Antibody; herpes simplex, type 2

A blood or cerebral spinal fluid sample is tested for antibodies to the herpes simplex virus (HSV). HSV is spread by direct contact. The primary infection typically presents with an area of ulceration in the skin or mucous membrane. Following the primary infection, the virus enters a latent phase and is reactivated in response to other illnesses, infection, and stress. Neonates and immunocompromised individuals are at risk for developing ocular or central nervous system infection. There are several methods available to test for HSV infection including indirect hemagglutination (IHA), chemiluminescent immunoassay, or enzyme-linked immunosorbent assay (ELISA). IgG and IgM testing is performed to diagnose HSV infection. If both IgG and IgM testing is performed, the test for each immunoglobulin class should be reported separately. Use 86694 when a non-specific type HSV test is performed. Use 86695 when the test is specific for HSV type 1 or 86696 when the test is specific for HSV type II. These codes are also used to report HSV type 1 and/or type 2 glycoprotein G-specific antibody IgG and/or IgM.

86698

86698   Antibody; histoplasma

A laboratory test is performed to measure Histoplasma antibodies in serum and/or cerebrospinal fluid (CSF). Histoplasma, most commonly, capsulatum, is a fungus that contaminates soil typically from bird or bat droppings. The fungal spores are inhaled causing a largely asymptomatic and self limiting infection in the lungs. In young children and/or immune compromised individuals, the infection may lead to chronic cavitary pulmonary disease, disseminated histoplasmosis, or meningitis. Symptoms can include fever, chest pain, dry cough, and joint pain. A blood sample is obtained by separately reportable venipuncture; CSF by separately reportable lumbar puncture. Serum can be tested using qualitative immunodiffusion, serum and CSF using semi-quantitative complement fixation.

86701-86703

86701   Antibody; HIV-1
86702   Antibody; HIV-2
86703   Antibody; HIV-1 and HIV-2, single result

HIV virus infections are sexually transmitted diseases that can also be transmitted from unscreened blood and shared needles, from mother to child in utero, or by breast feeding. HIV attacks the immune system by destroying T cells or CD4 cells, which are types of white blood cells. This hampers the body's ability to fight infection. AIDS is the final stage of HIV infection. A blood sample is obtained and tested for HIV-1 and/or HIV-2 antibodies. This is a qualitative test to identify the presence or absence of antibodies to HIV-1 and/or HIV-2. Use 86701 to report antibody screening for HIV-1 performed by qualitative chemiluminescent immunoassay. Use 86702 to report antibody screening for HIV-2 performed by qualitative enzyme immunoassay. Use 86703 to report antibody screening for both HIV-1 and HIV-2 in a single test result using qualitative chemiluminescent immunoassay.

86704-86705

86704   Hepatitis B core antibody (HBcAb); total
86705   Hepatitis B core antibody (HBcAb); IgM antibody

A blood sample is tested for hepatitis B core antibody (HBcAB). Hepatitis B is an inflammation of the liver caused by the hepatitis B virus (HBV) and has an acute and chronic phase. The core antibody is produced during and after an acute HBV infection, even in individuals who have cleared the virus without developing a chronic infection, and also during the chronic phase. In 86704, total HBcAB is tested using chemiluminescent assay. Both IgG and IgM antibodies are identified in a single test that does not differentiate between the two. Since IgM antibody is found in the initial phase of the infection and IgG in the later phase, this test is not specific to the acute or chronic phase of the infection. In 86705, testing is specific for IgM antibody to HBcAB and is used to diagnose an acute infection.

86706

86706   Hepatitis B surface antibody (HBsAb)

A blood sample is tested for hepatitis B surface antibody (HBsAB). Hepatitis B is an inflammation of the liver caused by the hepatitis B virus (HBV). HBsAB testing is performed to identify previous exposure to HBV without current acute or chronic infection, to determine the need for vaccination, and whether or not a previously administered vaccination has been successful. Individuals with a positive HBsAB test have been exposed to the virus but no longer carry an active form of the virus, cannot pass it on to others, and are immune from future HBV infection. HBsAB is tested using chemiluminescent assay.

86707

86707   Hepatitis Be antibody (HBeAb)

A laboratory test is performed to measure Hepatitis Be-antibodies (HBeAb). This antibody is produced by the body in response to the Hepatitis Be-antigen and may remain elevated for several years following recovery from an acute HBV infection. Measurement of HBeAb levels may help to determine the infectivity of HBV carriers, monitor the infection status of patients with chronic HBV infection, and/or monitor the immune response of patients with chronic HBV infection receiving antiviral therapy. HBV carriers and persons with chronic HBV infection who have positive HBeAb titers but are negative for HBV DNA in their sera are generally considered to have viral inactivity and low infectivity. Positive HBV DNA in sera is more indicative of active viral replication with a higher likelihood for infecting others. A blood sample is obtained by separately reportable venipuncture. Serum is tested using qualitative enzyme immunoassay.

86708-86709

86708   Hepatitis A antibody (HAAb)
86709   Hepatitis A antibody (HAAb); IgM antibody

A blood sample is tested for hepatitis A antibody (HAAb). Hepatitis A is an acute inflammation of the liver caused by the hepatitis A virus (HAV). The liver becomes inflamed during the acute infectious phase but then heals completely before becoming chronic. The patient develops a lifelong immunity to HAV. In 86708, HAAb is tested using enzyme immunoassay. Both IgG and IgM antibodies may be identified in the single test without differentiating between the type of antibody detected. This test is used primarily to determine the response to a previous hepatitis A vaccine and whether the patient has immunity to hepatitis A. In 86709, testing is specific for IgM antibody to HAAb and is used to diagnose a current, acute infection.

86710

86710   Antibody; influenza virus

A laboratory test is performed to measure influenza (A, B) antibodies. Influenza is usually a mild upper respiratory illness that may lead to lower respiratory pneumonia. Influenza type A can be particularly serious in children under the age of 2 years causing croup, bronchitis, pneumonia, and precipitating asthmatic episodes and chronic pulmonary complications. Type A influenza has been noted to respond to the antiviral medication amantidine. Influenza type B is less severe than type A and outbreaks are more localized. Type B does not respond to antiviral therapy. Testing for antibodies is helpful when the organism cannot be successfully isolated. Elevated IgA antibodies in both types of influenza suggest current or past infection; elevated IgM antibodies suggest current or recent infection. A blood sample is obtained by separately reportable venipuncture. Serum is tested using semi-quantitative enzyme-linked immunosorbent assay.

86711

86711   Antibody; JC (John Cunningham) virus

A blood test is performed to detect antibodies to the John Cunningham polyomavirus (JCV). JCV is a virus that commonly infects during childhood and then lies latent in the kidneys and gastrointestinal tract, causing no problems in healthy individuals. JCV can activate when the immune system becomes weakened due to HIV, certain cancers, systemic lupus erythematosis and drugs prescribed to prevent organ rejection or to treat multiple sclerosis and Crohn's disease. Once activated, an individual is at increased risk for developing progressive multifocal leukoencephalopathy (PML) which destroys myelin in brain and nerve cells. A blood sample is obtained by separately reportable venipuncture. Serum or plasma is tested using enzyme-linked immunosorbent assay (ELISA).

86713

86713   Antibody; Legionella

A laboratory test is performed to measure Legionella antibodies. Legionella is a bacteria found naturally in the environment, usually in water. Hot tubs, hot water tanks, swamp

coolers, large plumbing systems, and decorative fountains can all harbor the organism. Humans may exhibit pneumonia or a flu-like illness after inhaling mist or vapor containing the bacteria. There are 6 antibody serotypes identifiable with testing. Type 1 is most common and is often tested for alone. IgM and IgG antibodies develop concurrently and IgM results will remain elevated as long as the IgG response is active. Testing should include both IgM and IgG antibodies for accurate clinical interpretation. A blood sample is obtained by separately reportable venipuncture. Serum is tested using semi-quantitative indirect fluorescent antibody.

86717

86717   Antibody; Leishmania

A laboratory test is performed to measure Leishmania antibodies. Leishmania is a parasite endemic to the tropics, subtropics, and Southern Europe transmitted by the bite of a sand fly. The organism can cause cutaneous or visceral disease. The cutaneous form is characterized by skin sores or ulcers that may scab or crust over and is often accompanied by swollen lymph nodes. In the visceral form, the parasite invades the liver, spleen, and/or bone marrow. The disease can be entirely asymptomatic or the patient may present with fever, weight loss, enlarged spleen/liver, anemia, leukopenia, or thrombocytopenia. A positive IgG antibody titer suggests current or past infection. A blood sample is obtained by separately reportable venipuncture. Serum is tested using semi-quantitative immunoassay.

86720

86720   Antibody; Leptospira

A laboratory test is performed to measure Leptospira antibodies. Leptospira is a spirochete bacteria found worldwide that infects humans and animals. It is largely an occupational disease because it is spread via direct contact with the mucous membranes of an infected animal or soil contaminated with the urine of a chronic carrier animal. Farm/agriculture/fish industry workers, veterinarians, pet shop employees, and slaughterhouse/meat handlers are at increased risk for the infection; however, recreational contact is also possible with water sports and hiking. The disease can manifest in two forms—anicteric and icteric (Weils disease). The anicteric form is a self limiting, mild flu-like illness with sudden onset of symptoms including headache, fever, muscle pain, sore throat, cough, conjunctivitis, and rash. The icteric form is more severe, presenting with fever, jaundice, renal failure, and hemorrhage and may affect other organs including the heart and lungs, and the central nervous system. A blood sample is obtained by separately reportable venipuncture. Serum is tested for total antibodies using semi-quantitative indirect hemagglutination and IgM antibodies using qualitative immunoblot.

86723

86723   Antibody; Listeria monocytogenes

A laboratory test is performed to measure Listeria monocytogenes antibodies in blood and cerebrospinal fluid (CSF). L. monocytogenes is a bacterium found in soil and water and may contaminate raw fruits and vegetables, milk, and meat during processing. The organism can survive refrigeration and freezing. It usually causes a mild gastrointestinal illness but children, the elderly, and immunocompromised individuals are at risk for more severe illness with symptoms that include fever, muscle pain, nausea, diarrhea, headache, stiff neck, confusion, balance loss, and seizures. The L. monocytogenes bacteria are able to cross the placenta making a pregnant woman and her unborn baby especially vulnerable. A blood sample is obtained by separately reportable venipuncture; CSF by separately reportable lumbar puncture. Serum and CSF are tested using semi-quantitative complement fixation.

86727

86727   Antibody; lymphocytic choriomeningitis

A laboratory test is performed to measure lymphocytic choriomeningitis virus (LCMV) antibodies in blood and/or cerebrospinal fluid. LCMV is a rodent borne arenaviridae virus that can infect humans who come in contact with fresh urine, droppings, saliva, or nesting materials of house mice and possibly pet rodents such as hamsters. Transmission of the virus to humans occurs via broken skin, through the mouth, nose, and eyes or from an animal bite. The virus is not spread person to person but it can pass to an unborn baby via placental transfer. A biphasic illness is common with LCMV and presents with fever, malaise, decreased appetite, headache, muscle pain, nausea, and/or vomiting in the first phase followed by central nervous system (CNS) symptoms in the second phase including fever, stiff neck, headache, drowsiness, confusion, sensory-motor abnormalities, or a combination of both. The illness does not have a chronic state and the patient usually recovers once the body completely eliminates the virus. A positive LCMV titer suggests current or past infection. A blood sample is obtained by separately reportable venipuncture; CSF by separately reportable lumbar puncture. Serum and CSF are tested for IgG/IgM antibodies using semi-quantitative indirect fluorescent antibody.

86729

86729   Antibody; lymphogranuloma venereum

A blood sample is tested for antibodies to lymphogranuloma venereum (LGV). LGV is a sexually transmitted disease caused by Chlamydia trachomatis serovars (strains) L1, L2, and L3. The organism gains access to the lymph system through breaks in the skin or by crossing through mucous membranes. It then travels through the lymph system to the regional lymph nodes where the organism multiples. LGV has three stages: the primary stage occurs at the site of infection and appears as a painless herpetiform ulceration. The secondary stage is marked by painful lymphangitis in regional lymph nodes. In heterosexual men, the inguinal lymph nodes are primarily affected. In homosexual men, the perirectal nodes may also be affected. In women, the pelvic, inguinal, and perirectal lymph nodes may be involved. The third stage is characterized by anogenitorectal syndrome, including perirectal strictures and elephantiasis of genitals. LGV antibody tests are performed by microimmunofluorescence. Tests for each serovar or strain may be required and the code may be reported multiple times.

86732

86732   Antibody; mucormycosis

A laboratory test is performed to measure mucormycotina antibodies. The mucormycotina fungi are found abundantly in soil and decaying organic matter of leaves, wood, fruit, and bread, and can cause a rare but life threatening infection called mucormycosis. The organism enters the body via inhalation or through broken skin. The disease can manifest in 5 different ways—pulmonary, rhinocerebral, gastrointestinal, cutaneous, and central nervous system disease. Symptoms include fever, headache, facial pain, periorbital cellulitis, and cough. With cutaneous disease, blisters, ulcers, redness, and swelling may be present. Individuals with uncontrolled diabetes mellitus and those who are immunocompromised are at greatest risk for infection. Antibodies have been successfully detected using enzyme-linked immunosorbent assay, immunoblot, and immunodiffusion.

86735

86735   Antibody; mumps

A laboratory test is performed to measure mumps virus antibodies in blood and/or cerebral spinal fluid (CSF). The mumps virus causes a very contagious illness characterized by fever, headache, muscle aches, fatigue, decreased appetite, and swollen parotid (salivary) glands. The mode of transmission is largely airborne via respiratory droplets in saliva and mucus but the virus may also be contracted by sharing food, beverages, and eating utensils with an infected person. A positive IgM antibody titer suggests current or recent infection or immunization; however, low levels of IgM may occasionally persist for more than 12 months post infection or immunization. A positive IgG antibody titer suggests current or past exposure or immunization to mumps virus. A blood sample is obtained by separately reportable venipuncture; CSF by separately reportable lumbar puncture. Serum and CSF are tested for IgM antibodies using semi-quantitative enzyme-linked immunosorbent assay and IgG antibodies using semi-quantitative chemiluminescent immunoassay.

86738

86738   Antibody; mycoplasma

A laboratory test is performed to measure mycoplasma antibodies. Mycoplasma is the smallest free living organism and lacks a cell wall. M. pneumoniae is commonly found in the mucosa of the throat, respiratory tract, and genitourinary system. It is often identified as the infective agent in "atypical" pneumonia, a mild, self-limiting illness characterized by bronchitis, runny nose, and cough. Infants and immunocompromised individuals are at risk for more severe infection. The mycoplasma organism is difficult to culture and antibody testing may be used to identify it as the probable cause of an illness. A positive IgM antibody titer suggests current or recent infection. A positive IgG antibody titer is present in over 50% of all serum samples and suggests past exposure. IgA antibody titers may be tested for in conjunction with IgM and IgG. A blood sample is obtained by separately reportable venipuncture. Serum is tested for IgM/IgG/IgA antibodies using semi-quantitative enzyme-linked immunosorbent assay.

86741

86741   Antibody; Neisseria meningitidis

A laboratory test is performed to measure Neisseria meningitidis antibodies. N. meningitidis is a bacteria linked to a severe infection of the central nervous system and blood stream. N. meningitidis is a very contagious disease transmitted via respiratory droplets in saliva and mucus. Onset of symptoms is sudden and may include fever, headache, stiff neck, nausea and vomiting, skin rash, sensitivity to light, and confusion. This test for IgG antibodies includes serogroups A, C, W-135, and Y and may be used to measure the immune response to vaccination and help assess an individual with suspected immune deficiency. The test is not used to diagnose acute infection or serotype. A blood sample is obtained by separately reportable venipuncture. Serum is tested using quantitative multiplex bead assay.

86744

86744   Antibody; Nocardia

A laboratory test is performed to measure Nocardia antibodies. The Norcardia species are aerobic actinomycetes commonly found in soil. The species most often identified with human infection is N. asteroides and may cause acute, subacute, or chronic disease in both immune competent and immune compromised individuals. Local infection of the skin is most common when the immune system is healthy and disseminated infection as pneumonia, sepsis, brain abscess, eye infection, and joint infection is more likely to occur with immune deficiency. Serum may be tested for IgG antibodies using complement fixation, enzyme immunoassay, or immunoblot.

86747

86747   Antibody; parvovirus

A laboratory test is performed to measure parvovirus B19 antibodies. Parvovirus B19 causes a mild rash illness called Fifth disease (Erythema infectiosum) characterized by fever, runny nose, and headache followed by a "slapped cheek" facial rash and an often itchy, lace-like body rash. Adults and some children may also experience pain and swelling in their joints. The virus is transmitted via respiratory droplets and may be passed to an unborn baby through placental transfer. A positive IgM antibody titer suggests current or recent infection with parvovirus B19; however, IgM antibodies may occasionally persist for more than 12 months post infection. A positive IgG antibody titer suggests current or past infection with the virus. A blood sample is obtained by separately reportable venipuncture. Serum is tested using semi-quantitative enzyme-linked immunosorbent assay.

86750

86750   Antibody; Plasmodium (malaria)

A laboratory test is performed to measure Plasmodium antibodies. Plasmodium, a parasite transmitted by mosquitoes, causes malaria. There are four species known to infect humans. P. vivax and P. ovale can cause relapsing disease in which symptoms continue cyclically for months or years while the parasite remains dormant in the liver. P. malariae and P. falciparum cause acute illness but are not non-relapsing. P. falciparum may cause a severe, life threatening illness if the parasite invades the brain, kidney, or lungs leading to organ failure. Symptoms of malaria include fever, chills, sweats, headache, body aches, and malaise. In severe disease, the symptoms may progress to nausea and vomiting, diarrhea, anemia, jaundice, enlarged liver and/or spleen, seizures, and coma. A positive antibody titer will establish evidence of past exposure to any of the four species but should not be used to diagnose an acute infection. A blood sample is obtained by separately reportable venipuncture. Serum is tested using semi-quantitative enzyme-linked immunosorbent assay.

86753

86753   Antibody; protozoa, not elsewhere specified

A laboratory test is performed to measure antibodies to protozoa, not elsewhere specified. This code may be used to test blood serum for IgG antibodies against the following parasites: Entamoeba histolytica, Trypanosoma cruzi, Babesia microti, and Babesia duncani. Positive antibody titers suggest current or past infection. The E. histolytica parasite is most often found in tropical areas with poor sanitation and is transmitted by infected feces. It usually causes only a mild gastrointestinal illness with diarrhea, upset stomach, and abdominal cramps but can cause amebic dysentery with fever and bloody diarrhea, liver abscess, or infection of the brain and lungs. The T. cruzi parasite causes trypanosomiasis, known as Chagas disease, which is transmitted to animals and humans in the feces of insect vectors through mucous membranes or breaks in the skin. The parasite is found throughout the Americas mainly in impoverished rural areas. Chagas disease has an acute stage with symptoms that can include fever, fatigue, body aches, headache, vomiting, diarrhea, and enlarged liver, spleen, or lymph nodes and a chronic stage that may remain silent for decades or manifest with cardiomyopathy, heart failure, arrhythmias, enlarged esophagus, or colon. The B. microti parasite is transmitted by the black legged deer tick in Northeastern and Upper Midwestern areas of the United States. The parasite invades red blood cells causing a mild flu-like illness and is often accompanied by hemolytic anemia. Severe infection may occur in the elderly and immunocompromised. Babesia duncani is a tick borne parasite most often found in the Pacific coast areas of the United States.

86756

86756   Antibody; respiratory syncytial virus

A laboratory test is performed to measure respiratory syncytial virus (RSV) antibodies. RSV is endemic in the United States from late fall though spring causing an illness characterized by runny nose, congestion, and cough. The disease may be quite severe in infants and includes bronchitis and pneumonia. A positive IgG/IgM antibody titer suggests current or past infection. A blood sample is obtained by separately reportable venipuncture. Serum is tested using immunofluorescence.

Pathology and Laboratory

86757

86757   Antibody; Rickettsia

A blood sample is tested for antibodies to Rickettsia. There are two rickettsial organisms that are tested for in the United States: R. rickettsii and R. typhus. R. rickettsii is transmitted by the bite of an infected tick and causes Rocky Mountain spotted fever. Infection initially causes fever, headache, fatigue, nausea, and muscle aches followed by rash, and abdominal and joint pain. R. typhus is transmitted by the bite of an infected body louse (epidemic typhus), flea (murine typhus), or mite (scrub typhus). Infection causes acute febrile illness. Indirect fluorescent antibody (IFA) and enzyme-linked immunosorbent assay (ELISA) methodologies are commonly used to test for Rickettsia antibodies. IgG testing is performed to diagnose a current or past infection, and IgM testing is performed to identify a current infection with a specific Rickettsia organism. If both IgG and IgM testing is performed, the test for each immunoglobulin class should be reported separately.

86759

86759   Antibody; rotavirus

A laboratory test is performed to measure rotavirus antibodies. Rotavirus causes a gastrointestinal illness in infants and young children characterized by diarrhea, vomiting, fever, and abdominal pain. Symptoms may lead to dehydration and require the patient to be hospitalized for treatment. A positive IgM antibody titer suggests recent infection. A positive IgG titer is suggestive of past infection; however, in infants it may represent passive receipt of maternal antibodies. A positive IgA antibody titer is most often observed during the convalescent phase following infection. A blood sample is obtained by separately reportable venipuncture. Serum is tested for IgG/IgM/IgA antibodies using indirect enzyme immunoassay.

86762

86762   Antibody; rubella

A blood sample is tested for antibodies to rubella which causes German measles. This test is performed in pregnant women because a current rubella infection can cause fetal anomalies during the first trimester. Chemiluminscent immunoassay methodology is commonly used to test for rubella antibodies. IgG testing is performed to diagnose a current or past infection, and IgM testing is performed to identify a current infection. If both IgG and IgM testing is performed the test for each immunoglobulin class should be reported separately.

86765

86765   Antibody; rubeola

A laboratory test is performed to measure rubeola antibodies in serum and cerebrospinal fluid (CSF). Rubeola, a highly contagious viral infection transmitted via respiratory droplets, causes measles. Symptoms include fever, runny nose, cough, and body rash. Complications include otitis and pneumonia. Infants and children under 5 years of age, and adults over the age of 20, are at greater risk for severe disease and/or complications. A positive IgM antibody titer suggests current or recent infection or immunization but low levels of IgM may persist for more than 12 months following infection or immunization. A positive IgG antibody titer suggests current or past exposure or immunization. A blood sample is obtained by separately reportable venipuncture; CSF by separately reportable lumbar puncture. Serum and CSF are tested for IgM antibodies using semi-quantitative enzyme-linked immunosorbent assay and IgG antibodies using semi-quantitative chemiluminescent immunoassay.

86768

86768   Antibody; Salmonella

A laboratory test is performed to measure Salmonella typhi antibodies. S. typhi is the bacterium that causes typhoid fever. This human host disease is transmitted through feces. An individual may carry and shed the bacterium without symptoms, infecting others through contaminated food and beverages. Typhoid fever may also be contracted when sewage contaminates water and food supplies. Symptoms of the disease can include high fever, weakness, abdominal pain, headache, loss of appetite, and body rash. The test for salmonella antibodies includes S. typhi H type A, B, D and O type D and VI. A positive result indicates past exposure via infection or vaccination to S. paratyphi. This test is not used to confirm an acute infection of salmonellosis. A blood sample is obtained by separately reportable venipuncture. Serum is tested using qualitative immunoblot.

86771

86771   Antibody; Shigella

A laboratory test is performed to measure Shigella antibodies. The Shigella bacterium invades the intestinal lining causing inflammation and acute dysentery. Symptoms include abdominal pain, fever, loss of appetite, vomiting, and bloody diarrhea. The organism is transmitted via fecal-oral route and is capable of contaminating water and a wide variety of foods. Blood and feces can be tested for antibodies using Western Blot or enzyme-linked immunosorbent assay.

86774

86774   Antibody; tetanus

A laboratory test is performed to measure tetanus antibodies. The Clostridium tetani bacterium is most often introduced into the body through a puncture wound or break in the skin. C. tetani produces a toxin called tetanospasmin that causes tetanus, a serious disease characterized by severe muscle spasms and rigidity especially in the jaw and neck, producing lockjaw. The test for tetanus toxoid IgG antibodies may be used to monitor vaccine response or evaluate for immune deficiency syndromes. A blood sample is obtained by separately reportable venipuncture. Serum is tested using enzyme-linked immunosorbent assay.

86777-86778

86777   Antibody; Toxoplasma
86778   Antibody; Toxoplasma, IgM

A laboratory test to identify antibodies to toxoplasma is performed. Toxoplasma gondii is a parasite that infects a number of animals. Toxoplasma infection is caused by eating undercooked or raw meats from infected animals and also from the feces of infected cats. Toxoplasmosis is generally a mild disease that resolves without treatment, but can cause blindness and brain damage of the fetus in pregnant women and life threatening illness in immunocompromised individuals. Testing is typically performed using a blood sample, but cerebral spinal fluid (CSF) may also be tested. In 86777, total (IgG and IgM) or IgG toxoplasma antibodies are identified by enzyme linked immunosorbent assay (ELISA) or chemiluminescent immunoassay. Total toxoplasma antibodies are tested to screen for a past or present infection. IgG antibodies typically indicate a past infection but may also be present with a current infection. In 86778, IgM antibodies are identified which are indicative of a present or recent infection. IgM is tested by chemiluminescent immunoassay.

86780

86780   Antibody; Treponema pallidum

An antibody test for Treponema pallidum, the causative agent of syphilis, is performed using a technique such as fluorescent treponemal antibody absorption (FTA-ABS), T. pallidum particle agglutination (TP-PA), or indirect fluroescent antibody (IFA). Syphilis is a sexually transmitted disease (STD). During the primary stage of syphilis, a sore called a chancre appears at the site where the syphilis bacterium entered the body. The chancre resolves without treatment in three to six weeks but the patient remains infected and without treatment the infection will progress to a secondary stage. During the second stage, a skin rash and mucous membrane lesions appear. The most common site of the rash is the palms of the hands and soles of the feet. Other symptoms during the secondary stage include fever, swollen lymph nodes, sore throat, hair loss, headaches, weight loss, muscle aches, and fatigue. Symptoms of secondary syphilis also resolve spontaneously but the patient remains infected. The patient then enters the late or latent stage of the disease and symptoms of this stage may not appear for 10-20 years. Symptoms of late stage syphilis include difficulty coordinating muscle movements, paralysis, numbness, gradual blindness, and dementia. These symptoms occur as the disease damages internal organs including the brain, nerves, eyes, heart, blood vessels, liver, bones, and joints. Of particular concern is undiagnosed syphilis infection during pregnancy as the infection can be passed to the baby in utero. This increases the risk of stillbirth or of a live born infant dying shortly after birth. Untreated infants who survive often experience developmental delays or seizures. The FTA-ABS and IFA tests can be performed on blood or cerebral spinal fluid (CSF) samples. TP-PA is used only on blood samples.

86784

86784   Antibody; Trichinella

A laboratory test is performed to measure Trichinella antibodies. Trichinella is a parasitic worm that may infect humans who eat raw or undercooked meat. Animals capable of harboring and transmitting trichinella include domestic pigs, wild boar, wild cats, foxes, dogs, horses, seals, and walruses. The meat of these animals may contain larvae (cysts) from the worm which hatch in the intestine and travel through the blood stream to the muscles. Symptoms of infection include headache, fever, chills, cough, face and eye swelling, and muscle and joint pain. In severe infection, muscle coordination may be affected and heart and lung problems can arise. A blood sample is obtained by separately reportable venipuncture. Serum is tested using enzyme-linked immunosorbent assay.

86787

86787   Antibody; varicella-zoster

A laboratory test is performed to measure varicella-zoster antibodies in blood and/or cerebrospinal fluid (CSF). The varicella-zoster virus is transmitted via respiratory droplets and enters the body through the nose, mouth, or conjunctiva. The virus causes the primary infection of chicken pox characterized by fever, malaise, and an itchy macular rash that progresses to a papule stage and finally forms vesicular lesions that crust and scab over. The virus may then enter a dormant phase in sensory nerve ganglia and emerge later as the latent disease shingles, characterized by skin paresthesia, pain, and unilateral vesicular eruption along sensory nerves in the trunk or the 5th cranial nerve. A positive IgM antibody titer suggests current or recent infection; however, IgM antibodies may occasionally remain elevated for more than 12 months following infection. A positive IgG antibody titer is suggestive of current or past infection. A blood sample is obtained by separately reportable venipuncture; CSF by separately reportable lumbar puncture. Serum and CSF are tested for IgM antibodies using semi-quantitative enzyme-linked immunosorbent assay and IgG antibodies using semi-quantititiave chemiluminescent immunoassay.

86788-86789

86788   Antibody; West Nile virus, IgM
86789   Antibody; West Nile virus

These codes report antibody titer tests for West Nile virus-specific immunoglobulin M (IgM) (86788) and West Nile virus (86789). Testing for antibody to West Nile virus is done with blood serum or cerebrospinal fluid samples collected between 8-21 days of symptom onset. Serum is normally tested using samples taken at least two weeks apart in the acute and convalescent phase for confirmation. The most specific test is for IgM antibody in CSF detected by MAC-ELISA method (IgM antibody capture enzyme linked immunosorbent assay). Since the IgM antibody does not cross an intact blood-brain barrier, its presence in CSF is confirmative. Plaque-reduction neutralizing tests for West Nile virus antibody titer in both serum or CSF paired samples timed at least two weeks apart are another possibility for testing with a four-fold serial increase confirming West Nile.

86800

86800   Thyroglobulin antibody

A laboratory test is performed to measure thyroglobulin antibodies. Thyroglobulin (Tg) is a thyroid-specific protein actively involved in the synthesis, storage, and release of thyroid hormone. Tg is not normally found in systemic circulation but may leak into the bloodstream when thyroid follicles are destroyed by inflammation, hemorrhage, or rapid disordered growth. Once Tg travels beyond the thyroid gland, auto-antibodies can form and target the protein. The Tg antibody test may be used alone or with adjunct tests to diagnose autoimmune thyroid disease or to evaluate possibly unreliable Tg results in patients with follicular-cell derived thyroid carcinoma. A blood sample is obtained by separately reportable venipuncture. Serum is tested using quantitative chemiluminescent immunoassay.

86803-86804

86803   Hepatitis C antibody
86804   Hepatitis C antibody; confirmatory test (eg, immunoblot)

A laboratory test is performed to measure Hepatitis C virus (HCV) antibodies. Hepatitis C causes acute or chronic liver inflammation and may be transmitted via blood transfusion, needle sticks or sharing of needles in occupational situations or recreational drug use, unprotected sex, placental transfer during pregnancy, or sharing personal items such as a razor or toothbrush. The test reported with 86803 is used to screen individuals at risk for infection with HCV. A blood sample is obtained by separately reportable venipuncture. Serum is tested using qualitative chemiluminescent immunoassay. Antibodies toward HCV may not start to elevate until 2 months after exposure, so a negative test screening should be repeated if there is a strong suspicion of HCV infection. A positive antibody screen result should be confirmed with further testing, reported with 86804, when blood serum is tested using recombinant immunoblot assay.

86805-86806

86805   Lymphocytotoxicity assay, visual crossmatch; with titration
86806   Lymphocytotoxicity assay, visual crossmatch; without titration

A laboratory test is performed to measure the lymphocytotoxicity of recipient and donor blood to identify transplant patients at risk for antibody mediated damage to organ or tissue grafts. This test may be used for solid organ transplants such as kidney, heart, and lung, and on patients being considered for refractory platelet and/or bone marrow transplant who possibly have human leukocyte antigen (HLA) antibodies. HLAs are integral cell membrane glycoproteins linked to the immune system. The presence of HLAs may be a barrier to successful organ and tissue transplant. Lymphocytotoxicity assay with visual crossmatch uses a complement-dependent method to identify IgG antibodies to Class I HLA (-A, -B, -C) in nucleated cells and Class II HLA (-DR, -DQ, -DP) expressed on B-cells, monocytes, macrohages, dendrite and activated T-cells. A patient with a positive crossmatch is at increased risk for graft/transplant rejection. Use 86805 when a titration process is used to add a known volume of one solution, the titrant, to a specific quantity of the analyte solution being tested in order to facilitate a reaction and determine the concentration of antibodies present.

86807-86808

86807   Serum screening for cytotoxic percent reactive antibody (PRA); standard method
86808   Serum screening for cytotoxic percent reactive antibody (PRA); quick method

A laboratory test is performed to screen for cytotoxic percent reactive antibody (PRA) in serum. This test is performed prior to organ transplant to evaluate human leukocyte antigen (HLA) antibodies that may be present in the organ recipient that could lead to an immune response or hyperacute rejection to the transplanted organ. HLAs are highly reactive glycoproteins carried on the surface of cell membranes and may be a barrier to successful organ and tissue transplant. Class I antigens directly activate killer T-cells, while Class II antigens activate helper T-4 cells, macrophages, and B-cells. The serum of the recipient is mixed with combined leukocytes from a pool of donors and tested using flow cytometry, enzyme-linked immunosorbent assay (ELISA), complement-dependent cytotoxicity, or anti-human globulin augmentation to find the percentage of reactions within the sample panel. The greater the percentage of reaction that occurs, the higher the patient's risk for organ rejection becomes. Use 86806 when a quick method is performed to screen for cytotoxic PRA.

86812-86813

86812   HLA typing; A, B, or C (eg, A10, B7, B27), single antigen
86813   HLA typing; A, B, or C, multiple antigens

Human leukocyte antigen (HLA) typing is performed on A, B, or C antigens. Testing for specific HLA alleles is performed to identify individuals with susceptibility to a particular disease and to determine tissue compatibility of a potential stem cell, bone marrow, or solid organ transplant donor with the intended transplant recipient, and to determine eligibility for certain vaccine or immunotherapy procedures. Another use of HLA typing is to determine platelet compatibility and improve platelet survival following transfusion. HLA antigens are divided into Class I and Class II alleles. Current tests available for potential susceptibility for disease include HLA-B27 DNA typing for ankylosing spondylitis and related diseases. Tests for Class I HLA-A DNA typing, HLA-B DNA typing, and HLA-C DNA typing are used to identify susceptibility to other autoimmune disorders and to determine tissue compatibility between potential donors and recipients. Use 86812 when typing a single antigen and 86813 when multiple HLA antigens are typed.

86816-86817

86816   HLA typing; DR/DQ, single antigen
86817   HLA typing; DR/DQ, multiple antigens

Human leukocyte antigen (HLA) typing is performed on DR/DQ antigens. Testing for specific HLA alleles is performed to identify individuals with susceptibility to a particular disease and to determine tissue compatibility of a potential stem cell, bone marrow, or solid organ transplant donor with the intended transplant recipient. HLA antigens are divided into Class I and Class II alleles. Current tests available for potential susceptibility for disease include HLA-DQ2 and HLA-DQ8 typing for celiac disease in symptomatic patients or patients with a family history of celiac disease. Other tests are HLA-DR15 and HLA DQ6 which help differentiate narcolepsy from other sleep disorders. Tests for Class II HLA-DR DNA typing and HLA-DQ DNA typing are used to identify susceptibility to other autoimmune disorders and to determine tissue compatibility between potential donors and recipients. Use 86816 when typing a single antigen and 86817 when multiple HLA antigens are typed.

86821-86822

86821   HLA typing; lymphocyte culture, mixed (MLC)
86822   HLA typing; lymphocyte culture, primed (PLC)

Human leukocyte antigen (HLA) typing is performed using a lymphocyte culture that is mixed or primed. Testing for specific HLA alleles is performed to identify individuals with susceptibility to a particular disease and to determine tissue compatibility of a potential stem cell, bone marrow, or solid organ transplant donor with the intended transplant recipient. HLA antigens are divided into Class I and Class II alleles. Mixed lymphocyte culture (MLC) uses cells that are homozygous for the HLA antigens as the stimulators and the test cells as the responders. Cells that respond to the stimulator differ and are not compatible, whereas cells that do not respond are the same and are compatible. Primed lymphocyte culture (PLC) uses primed lymphocyte typing (PLT) reagents as the responder and the cells to be tested as the stimulator. Using a syringe, the PLT responder cells are placed on microtiter plates along with the stimulator cells. The plates are sealed and incubated for 48 hours. Thymidine is then added and the plates are incubated for another 16 hours. The cultures are harvested and dried on glass fiber filter paper. When dried, each filter spot is placed in a separate tube in scintillation fluid. The tubes are then placed in a scintillation counter. PLT results are then interpreted. Use 86821 for HLA typing using mixed lymphocyte culture and 86822 for HLA typing using primed lymphocyte culture.

86825-86826

86825   Human leukocyte antigen (HLA) crossmatch, non-cytotoxic (eg, using flow cytometry); first serum sample or dilution

86826   Human leukocyte antigen (HLA) crossmatch, non-cytotoxic (eg, using flow cytometry); each additional serum sample or sample dilution (List separately in addition to primary procedure)

Human leukocyte antigens (HLA) are protein molecules that are on the surface of most body cells. HLAs recognize foreign cells and so are important indicators of compatibility in transplant procedures. While there are hundreds of different HLA molecules only six are looked for in transplant crossmatch procedures. HLAs are crossmatched by first determining which HLA markers are present in the recipient and donor. This is called typing the HLAs and is performed in a separate procedure. Ideally the donor will have the exact same HLAs. However, if the donor does not have the same HLAs it is still possible to perform the transplant procedure if the recipient has not developed antibodies to the donors HLAs. If the recipient has developed antibodies against any of the donor HLA markers, the antibodies will attack the transplanted cells, tissue, or organ. A blood sample is obtained from both the donor and recipient. The donor cells are then mixed with the recipient serum and observed for evidence of a negative or positive reaction using a noncytotoxic methodology such as flow cytometry. A negative reaction indicates that the recipient does not have antibodies to the donor HLAs and the transplant procedure can be performed. A positive reaction indicates that the recipient does have antibodies to the donor HLA and that a transplant cannot be performed. Use 86825 for the first sample or dilution. Use 86826 for each additional serum sample or sample dilution

86828-86829

86828   Antibody to human leukocyte antigens (HLA), solid phase assays (eg, microspheres or beads, ELISA, flow cytometry); qualitative assessment of the presence or absence of antibody(ies) to HLA Class I and Class II HLA antigens

86829   Antibody to human leukocyte antigens (HLA), solid phase assays (eg, microspheres or beads, ELISA, Flow cytometry); qualitative assessment of the presence or absence of antibody(ies) to HLA Class I or Class II HLA antigens

The human leukocyte antigen (HLA) system forms part of the major histocompatibility complex (MHC). The MHC is responsible for self-recognition which means that it identifies the specific characteristics of an individual's cells and tissues and defends the body against foreign substances including microorganisms and nonself cells and tissues. HLAs are comprised of two classes, Class I and Class II. In 86828, a test is performed to determine the presence and characteristics of human leukocyte antigen (HLA) alloantibodies and predict the risk of immunological response to organ transplant. A qualitative assessment of the presence or absence of antibodies to both HLA Class I and HLA Class II antigens. The test is usually performed using enzyme-linked immunosorbent assay (ELISA) on fluorescent beads implanted with HLA molecules that can then be detected by conventional flow cytometry or in conjunction with luminex instrumentation. In 86829, the presence or absence of antibodies to either HLA Class I or HLA Class II antigens is assessed. This test is most often used when the test is a follow-up for a patient who has been classified with Class I HLA or Class II HLA antibodies.

86830-86831

86830   Antibody to human leukocyte antigens (HLA), solid phase assays (eg, microspheres or beads, ELISA, Flow cytometry); antibody identification by qualitative panel using complete HLA phenotypes, HLA Class I

86831   Antibody to human leukocyte antigens (HLA), solid phase assays (eg, microspheres or beads, ELISA, Flow cytometry); antibody identification by qualitative panel using complete HLA phenotypes, HLA Class II

The human leukocyte antigen (HLA) system forms part of the major histocompatibility complex (MHC). The MHC is responsible for self-recognition which means that it identifies the specific characteristics of an individual's cells and tissues and defends the body against foreign substances including microorganisms and nonself cells and tissues. HLAs are comprised of two classes, Class I and Class II. These tests are performed to determine the presence and characteristics of human leukocyte antigen (HLA) alloantibodies and predict the risk of immunological response to organ transplant using complete HLA phenotypes for HLA Class I or HLA Class II. Use 86830 when a complete panel of Class I HLA phenotypes is used to identify as many as 80 antibodies using 50 or more bead array. Use 86831 when a complete panel of Class II HLA phenotypes are used to identify antibodies to about 40 antigens using 30 or more bead array. Testing for Class I or Class II HLA phenotypes is usually performed using enzyme-linked immunosorbent assay (ELISA) on fluorescent beads implanted with HLA molecules that can then be detected by conventional flow cytometry or in conjunction with Luminex instrumentation.

86832-86833

86832   Antibody to human leukocyte antigens (HLA), solid phase assays (eg, microspheres or beads, ELISA, Flow cytometry); high definition qualitative panel for identification of antibody specificities (eg, individual antigen per bead methodology), HLA Class I

86833   Antibody to human leukocyte antigens (HLA), solid phase assays (eg, microspheres or beads, ELISA, Flow cytometry); high definition qualitative panel for identification of antibody specificities (eg, individual antigen per bead methodology), HLA Class II

The human leukocyte antigen (HLA) system forms part of the major histocompatibility complex (MHC). The MHC is responsible for self-recognition which means that it identifies the specific characteristics of an individual's cells and tissues and defends the body against foreign substances including microorganisms and nonself cells and tissues. HLAs are comprised of two classes, Class I and Class II. These tests are performed to determine the presence and characteristics of human leukocyte antigen (HLA) alloantibodies and predict the risk of immunological response to organ transplant using a high definition qualitative panel for identification of antibody specificities. The test is usually performed using enzyme-linked immunosorbent assay (ELISA) on fluorescent beads implanted with HLA molecules that can then be detected by conventional flow cytometry or in conjunction with Luminex instrumentation. Use code 86832 when a complete panel of cloned Class I HLA antigens is used to identify antibody specificities to as many as 80 HLA A/B/C antigens using up to 98 beads in the array. Use code 86833 when a complete panel of cloned Class II HLA antigens are used to identify antibody specificities to individual HLA DRB1/3/4/5, DQA1, DQB1, DPA1, DPB1 antigens using up to 98 beads in the array.

86834-86835

86834   Antibody to human leukocyte antigens (HLA), solid phase assays (eg, microspheres or beads, ELISA, Flow cytometry); semi-quantitative panel (eg, titer), HLA Class I

86835   Antibody to human leukocyte antigens (HLA), solid phase assays (eg, microspheres or beads, ELISA, Flow cytometry); semi-quantitative panel (eg, titer), HLA Class II

The human leukocyte antigen (HLA) system forms part of the major histocompatibility complex (MHC). The MHC is responsible for self-recognition which means that it identifies the specific characteristics of an individual's cells and tissues and defends the body against foreign substances including microorganisms and nonself cells and tissues. HLAs are comprised of two classes, Class I and Class II. HLA semi-quantitative analysis with titer is performed to monitor pre-transplant desensitization protocols for potential transplant recipients who are sensitized or to monitor treatment of antibody mediated rejection post transplant. These tests are usually performed using enzyme-linked immunosorbent assay (ELISA) on fluorescent beads implanted with HLA molecules that can then be detected by conventional flow cytometry or in conjunction with Luminex instrumentation. Use code 86834 for a semi-quantitative panel with titer for HLA Class I. Use 86835 for semi-quantitative panel with titer for HLA Class II.

86850

86850   Antibody screen, RBC, each serum technique

A blood sample is tested for antibodies directed against red blood cell (RBC) antigens other than A and B antigens. This test may also be referred to as an indirect antiglobulin test (IAT). This test is performed as part of a blood typing and screening test when it is anticipated that a blood transfusion might be required. If an antibody is detected, then separately reportable antibody identification is performed to identify the specific antibodies present. The test may be performed using IAT methodology or another serum technique such as solid phase. If multiple serum techniques are used, each reported separately.

86860

86860   Antibody elution (RBC), each elution

A laboratory test is performed to measure red blood cell (RBC) antibody elution. This test may be ordered when an antibody screening test detects IgG and/or complement fragments (direct anti-globulins) on the surface of RBCs. These antibodies may cause transfusion reactions or lead to hemolytic disease in a newborn. The elution test can identify specific antibodies and assist in transfusing the most compatible blood products possible. It may also be ordered post transfusion when a reaction has occurred. A blood sample is obtained by separately reportable venipuncture. Whole blood is tested using hemagglutination.

86870

86870   Antibody identification, RBC antibodies, each panel for each serum technique

A laboratory test is performed to identify specific red blood cell (RBC) antibodies. This test may be ordered when an antibody screening test, such as 86850, detects IgG and/or complement fragments (direct anti-globulins) on the surface of RBCs. It is used to monitor

● New Code   ▲ Revised Code   © 2017 DecisionHealth

antibody levels during pregnancy and assess the risk of hemolytic disease in a newborn. Maternal IgG alloantibodies to RBC antigens have the ability to cross the placenta. An antigen-antibody reaction may cause RBC hemolysis in the fetus resulting in harmful and/or fatal fetal anemia and hyperbilirubinemia. A blood sample is obtained by separately reportable venipuncture. Serum is tested using hemagglutination.

86880

86880   Antihuman globulin test (Coombs test); direct, each antiserum

A laboratory test is performed to measure antihuman globulin by direct antihuman globulin test (Coombs test) method. This test may be performed when an antibody screening test for anti-globulins is positive or when a patient presents with hemolytic anemia. Hemolytic anemia occurs when red blood cells are destroyed prematurely due to antibodies attached to the cells. Symptoms of hemolytic anemia may include pale skin, fatigue, weakness, and dizziness. Hemolytic anemia can result from autoimmune diseases such as systemic lupus erythematous, malignant conditions like lymphoma or chronic lymphocytic leukemia, infections such as mycoplasma pneumonia and infectious mononucleosis, or even medications like penicillin, as well as transfusion reactions. Infants exposed to maternal antibodies in utero may be born with hemolytic disease of the newborn. A blood sample is obtained by separately reportable venipuncture. Serum is tested using hemagglutination.

86885-86886

86885   Antihuman globulin test (Coombs test); indirect, qualitative, each reagent red cell

86886   Antihuman globulin test (Coombs test); indirect, each antibody titer

An indirect antihuman globulin (Coombs) test is done to detect clinically significant antibodies in the blood. Some red cells are coated with complement or IgG antibodies and do not agglutinate when centrifuged. This is also referred to as IgG or complement sensitization. Another antibody that reacts with the IgG or complement must be introduced to allow agglutination to occur. Indirect antihuman globulin tests are performed on in vitro specimens. The specimen is incubated at 37 degrees Centigrade, allowing the antibodies in the serum to react with the cells in vitro. The cells are then washed and an antiglobulin reagent is used to detect antibody coating of the cells. The cells are centrifuged and the test is read. Use 86885 for qualitative testing performed on each reagent red cell. Red cell antigen testing involves using the patient's red cells plus a reagent antiserum. The patient's cells are the unknown antigen and the reagent antiserum is the known antibody. The patient's blood is tested to determine the presence of clinically significant antibodies, usually prior to a blood transfusion. The qualitative test will determine the presence of antibodies but not the quantity of antibodies. If antibodies are detected, other tests will be performed to identify the specific antibody(s). Report 86885 for each reagent red cell test to identify antibodies. Use 86886 for each antibody titer. An antibody identified on a previous test is analyzed to determine the strength or potency of the antibody. Report 86886 for each antibody titer performed.

86890-86891

86890   Autologous blood or component, collection processing and storage; predeposited

86891   Autologous blood or component, collection processing and storage; intra- or postoperative salvage

A laboratory procedure is performed to collect, process, and store autologous whole blood or blood component (red blood cells, leukocytes, platelets) prior to patient need. The blood/blood product is labeled for the specific patient and is not subject to screening or tests necessary for general blood supply use. An individual may donate as early as 42 days prior to their scheduled procedure and may continue to donate weekly if they are hemodynamically stable. The use of autologous blood products can decrease the risk of transfusion reaction and transmission of infectious diseases. Use 86891 is collection processing and storage of whole blood or blood components is done intra-operatively or post-operatively. Blood/blood components are collected from a wound, body cavity, or drainage tube into a reservoir until sufficient volume has been obtained. The salvaged blood/blood component is pumped through a centrifuge, concentrated, and washed with isotonic solution (usually saline), and then pumped into a transfusion bag for immediate or later transfusion back into the patient.

86900-86901

86900   Blood typing, serologic; ABO

86901   Blood typing, serologic; Rh (D)

A blood specimen is tested to determine blood type (ABO) (86900) or Rh(D) (86901). In 86900, blood is grouped using an ABO blood typing system which identifies four blood types: type A, B, AB, or O. The blood sample is mixed with antibodies against Type A and B blood and then checked to determine if the blood cells agglutinate, or stick together. Type A blood has anti-B antibodies; type B blood has anti-A antibodies; type O blood has antibodies to both A and B; and type AB blood does not have anti-A or anti-B antibodies. Type A blood agglutinates when type B antibodies are introduced. Type B blood agglutinates when type A antibodies are introduced. Type O blood agglutinates when type A or B

antibodies are introduced. Type AB blood does not agglutinate when type A or B antibodies are introduced. The blood is then back typed. Blood serum is mixed with blood that is known to be type A or B. In 86901, blood is tested for Rh factor, which is an antigen on red blood cells. Blood is Rh+ if the antigen is present or Rh- if the antigen is absent. Blood is tested by mixing the blood sample with antibodies against Rh factor and then checking for agglutination. If agglutination occurs, the blood is Rh+. If the blood does not agglutinate, it is Rh-.

86902

86902   Blood typing, serologic; antigen testing of donor blood using reagent serum, each antigen test

Blood typing is performed to determine the compatibility of donor blood with that of the intended recipient. This test is used to identify the presence or absence of specific antibodies in the donor blood. Reagent serum is blood serum containing a specific known antigen. The reagent serum is added to donor blood to identify whether the donor blood has antibodies to the antigen. If the donor blood has antibodies to the antigen, a positive response is elicited which is usually indicated by blood agglutination, or clotting. The reagent serum is added to the donor blood and the donor blood response is observed to determine whether the blood is sensitive to the specific antigen. Sensitivity to the antigen is noted in the test result as positive or negative. Use 86902 for each antigen tested.

86904

86904   Blood typing, serologic; antigen screening for compatible unit using patient serum, per unit screened

Units of donated blood are screened prior to a blood transfusion to make sure they are compatible with the recipient's blood type. The antibodies in the donated blood are identified. In emergency situations, there may not be time to perform an antibody test. In this case, use 86904 for a serum test.

86910

86910   Blood typing, for paternity testing, per individual; ABO, Rh and MN

A blood sample is drawn from a male and a child to determine if the male is the father of the child. Blood antibodies are identified and compared, resulting in a statistical probability of the male being the child's father. Code 86911 if the test results are inconclusive and further testing is performed.

86911

86911   Blood typing, for paternity testing, per individual; each additional antigen system

A blood sample is drawn from a male and a child to determine if the male is the father of the child. Blood antibodies are identified and compared, resulting in a statistical probability of the male being the child's father. Code 86911 if the test results are inconclusive and further testing is performed.

86920

86920   Compatibility test each unit; immediate spin technique

A unit of blood that is going to be transfused into a patient is checked for compatibility with the patient's blood type (A, B, O, or AB). Code 86921 if the samples are incubated before they are tested, and 86922 if antibodies are identified in the patient's bloodstream, requiring a final test to make sure the donor blood is compatible.

86921

86921   Compatibility test each unit; incubation technique

A unit of blood that is going to be transfused into a patient is checked for compatibility with the patient's blood type (A, B, O, or AB). Code 86921 if the samples are incubated before they are tested, and 86922 if antibodies are identified in the patient's bloodstream, requiring a final test to make sure the donor blood is compatible.

86922

86922   Compatibility test each unit; antiglobulin technique

A unit of blood that is going to be transfused into a patient is checked for compatibility with the patient's blood type (A, B, O, or AB). Code 86921 if the samples are incubated before they are tested, and 86922 if antibodies are identified in the patient's bloodstream, requiring a final test to make sure the donor blood is compatible.

86940-86941

86940   Hemolysins and agglutinins; auto, screen, each

86941   Hemolysins and agglutinins; incubated

A unit of blood is screened before transfusion for hemolysins and cold agglutinins. Hemolysins are toxic agents that destroy red blood cells, and cold agglutinins may make it hard to identify antigens that may cause problems after the transfusion. Code 86941 if the sample is incubated during the test.

Pathology and Laboratory

86965

86965   Pooling of platelets or other blood products

Platelets or other blood products are taken from different sources of units of blood are pooled together so that a patient can be given a concentrated dose of platelets or other blood products.

86970

86970   Pretreatment of RBCs for use in RBC antibody detection, identification, and/or compatibility testing; incubation with chemical agents or drugs, each

After a blood sample has tested positive for an antibody to a drug, a test is performed by taking red blood cells and incubating them in the suspected drug and analyzing the reaction. This allows the physician to determine if the drug is present in the bloodstream. Code 86971 if the sample is treated with enzymes prior to examination. Code 86972 if the components of the blood are separated before the test is performed.

86971

86971   Pretreatment of RBCs for use in RBC antibody detection, identification, and/or compatibility testing; incubation with enzymes, each

After a blood sample has tested positive for an antibody to a drug, a test is performed by taking red blood cells and incubating them in the suspected drug and analyzing the reaction. This allows the physician to determine if the drug is present in the bloodstream. Code 86971 if the sample is treated with enzymes prior to examination. Code 86972 if the components of the blood are separated before the test is performed.

86972

86972   Pretreatment of RBCs for use in RBC antibody detection, identification, and/or compatibility testing; by density gradient separation

After a blood sample has tested positive for an antibody to a drug, a test is performed by taking red blood cells and incubating them in the suspected drug and analyzing the reaction. This allows the physician to determine if the drug is present in the bloodstream. Code 86971 if the sample is treated with enzymes prior to examination. Code 86972 if the components of the blood are separated before the test is performed.

86975

86975   Pretreatment of serum for use in RBC antibody identification; incubation with drugs, each

A blood sample is treated with special antigens by adding red blood cells with the antigens already attached to a serum made from the blood sample. Code 86976 if the sample is diluted before the red blood cells are added. Code 86977 if an inhibitor is added to the serum to neutralize a drug present in the sample. Code 86978 if red blood cells and blood serum are incubated together before the test is performed.

86976

86976   Pretreatment of serum for use in RBC antibody identification; by dilution

A blood sample is treated with special antigens by adding red blood cells with the antigens already attached to a serum made from the blood sample. Code 86976 if the sample is diluted before the red blood cells are added. Code 86977 if an inhibitor is added to the serum to neutralize a drug present in the sample. Code 86978 if red blood cells and blood serum are incubated together before the test is performed.

86977

86977   Pretreatment of serum for use in RBC antibody identification; incubation with inhibitors, each

A blood sample is treated with special antigens by adding red blood cells with the antigens already attached to a serum made from the blood sample. Code 86976 if the sample is diluted before the red blood cells are added. Code 86977 if an inhibitor is added to the serum to neutralize a drug present in the sample. Code 86978 if red blood cells and blood serum are incubated together before the test is performed.

86978

86978   Pretreatment of serum for use in RBC antibody identification; by differential red cell absorption using patient RBCs or RBCs of known phenotype, each absorption

A blood sample is treated with special antigens by adding red blood cells with the antigens already attached to a serum made from the blood sample. Code 86976 if the sample is diluted before the red blood cells are added. Code 86977 if an inhibitor is added to the serum to neutralize a drug present in the sample. Code 86978 if red blood cells and blood serum are incubated together before the test is performed.

86985

86985   Splitting of blood or blood products, each unit

A unit of blood or a blood product such as platelets is split into smaller units so that it can be infused into child or another patient where the full amount of blood in the unit would be too much.

87071

87071   Culture, bacterial; quantitative, aerobic with isolation and presumptive identification of isolates, any source except urine, blood or stool

A tissue sample besides blood, urine, or stool is collected and placed in a medium conducive to the growth of bacteria. The culture is examined for the growth of bacteria, and the amount of any bacteria in the medium is measured. Code 87073 if the the test looks for bacteria that can survive without oxygen.

87073

87073   Culture, bacterial; quantitative, anaerobic with isolation and presumptive identification of isolates, any source except urine, blood or stool

A tissue sample besides blood, urine, or stool is collected and placed in a medium conducive to the growth of bacteria. The culture is examined for the growth of bacteria, and the amount of any bacteria in the medium is measured. Code 87073 if the the test looks for bacteria that can survive without oxygen.

87081-87084

87081   Culture, presumptive, pathogenic organisms, screening only
87084   Culture, presumptive, pathogenic organisms, screening only; with colony estimation from density chart

This test is performed when a specific pathogen is suspected. A blood sample is taken and placed in a medium conducive to the growth of the suspected pathogen. Any colonies that grow in the medium are then examined. Code 87084 if the amount of pathogenic material in the colony is estimated at using a reference chart.

87110

87110   Culture, chlamydia, any source

A Chlamydia culture is performed on a tissue or cell sample from any source. Chlamydia is a group of bacteria that cause a variety of infections. The most common infection is C. trachomatis, which is a sexually transmitted disease (STD) that often produces no symptoms, but can cause irreversible damage to the female reproductive tract, resulting in infertility. In men, symptoms include burning and itching of the urethra, but men rarely suffer reproductive damage from the infection. The specimen may be obtained from the cervix, urethra, rectum, eye, nose, or throat. Excess mucous or secretions are removed from the infected site using a swab. A second swab is then used to obtain the specimen culture, taking care to obtain adequate numbers of columnar epithelial cells. The swabs are placed in viral chlamydial transport medium. Specimens are then inoculated onto tissue culture cells with trachomatis specific antibodies and incubated. Immunofluorescence is then used to identify whether the patient has a Chlamydia infection.

87149-87150

87149   Culture, typing; identification by nucleic acid (DNA or RNA) probe, direct probe technique, per culture or isolate, each organism probed
87150   Culture, typing; identification by nucleic acid (DNA or RNA) probe, amplified probe technique, per culture or isolate, each organism probed

A microorganism, such as a bacteria, virus, fungus, or parasite is definitively identified to the genus or species level from a culture of the microorganism using nucleic acid probe technique. Culture for presumptive identification is performed first in a separately reportable procedure. Once a presumptive identification of the microorganism is accomplished additional cultures are used to more specifically identify the organism. Following culture of the organism, a direct or amplified probe technique is used to more specifically identify the organism. In 87149, a direct probe technique is used. Lysate is used to rupture the cells and release nucleic acids (DNA, RNA). The lysate is placed in a sample well and the cultured organism is placed on a test slide. The test slide is dipped in the lysate and incubated robotically. A DNA or RNA probe for a specific organism is then placed in the test well. The probe consists of laboratory-prepared, complementary strands of the target nucleic acid for a specific genus or species of the organism. If the cultured cells contain complementary strands of DNA or RNA, the probe will bind with the nucleic acids from the cells in the culture forming a double-stranded complex or hybrid. Binding of the probe with the cultured organism indicates that the genus or species being tested is present in the culture. Binding is often indicated using probes that are labeled with chemical fluorescence and a positive result is indicated by a change in color. Report a direct probe for each culture or isolate probed using this technique and for each organism probed. In 87150, an amplification technique, such as polymerase chain reaction (PCR) is used to create copies of the nucleic acids. Amplification is used when it is suspected that there are low levels of the suspected microorganism in the specimen that would not be detected using a direct probe. The organism nucleic acids are then detected using a variety

Pathology and Laboratory

of techniques. Report an amplified probe for each culture or isolate probed using this technique and for each organism probed.

87152

87152   Culture, typing; identification by pulse field gel typing

A blood sample is placed in a solution conducive to the growth of bacteria. Any bacteria harvested from the sample are placed in a special gel that is run through a machine that identifies DNA molecules in the colony to identify the bacteria.

87153

87153   Culture, typing; identification by nucleic acid sequencing method, each isolate (eg, sequencing of the 16S rRNA gene)

Nucleic acids (DNA, RNA) may be analyzed to determine the sequence of nucleotide bases. Sequencing is performed to rapidly differentiate similar organisms. One application is to rapidly identify Bacillus anthracis (anthrax) from other closely related spore-forming Bacillus such as B. cereus and B. thuringiensis. Automated sequencing systems and DNA alignment software has been developed to perform the sequencing procedure. The DNA is first amplified using a technique such as polymerase chain reaction (PCR). The amplified DNA is then sequenced using primers. Sequencing of the 16s rRNA gene found in anthrax requires the use of 16 primers. A sequencing kit is used. The sequencing products are first purified using special equipment. An automated DNA sequencing system is then used to sequence the DNA. The length of sequences may differ based on each different primer used. An inner fragment of the sequenced DNA is then analyzed for each primer used. The specific organism is identified. Sequencing also allows identification of new or novel types of the organism to be identified.

87164-87166

87164   Dark field examination, any source (eg, penile, vaginal, oral, skin); includes specimen collection

87166   Dark field examination, any source (eg, penile, vaginal, oral, skin); without collection

A dark field examination, also called dark field microscopy, is performed on a specimen from any source including penile, vaginal, oral, skin, or lymph node. This test is performed to identify microorganisms that are easily visible against a dark background, such as Treponema pallidum spirochetes that cause syphilis. If the sample is from a lymph node, lymph node aspiration biopsy is first performed. If the sample is obtained from an ulcerative lesion on the skin or mucous membrane, the lesion is first cleaned and abraded with gauze, then squeezed to obtain a drop of serous transudate which is placed on a glass slide and covered with a cover slip. The slide is then examined using a microscope with a dark-field condenser or with a phase contrast microscope for the presence or absence of motile spirochetes. Use 87164 for the dark field examination including specimen collection. Use 87166 when the lab that performs the test is not responsible for collecting the specimen.

87181-87190

87190   Susceptibility studies, antimicrobial agent; mycobacteria, proportion method, each agent

87181   Susceptibility studies, antimicrobial agent; agar dilution method, per agent (eg, antibiotic gradient strip)

87184   Susceptibility studies, antimicrobial agent; disk method, per plate (12 or fewer agents)

87185   Susceptibility studies, antimicrobial agent; enzyme detection (eg, beta lactamase), per enzyme

87186   Susceptibility studies, antimicrobial agent; microdilution or agar dilution (minimum inhibitory concentration [MIC] or breakpoint), each multi-antimicrobial, per plate

87187   Susceptibility studies, antimicrobial agent; microdilution or agar dilution, minimum lethal concentration (MLC), each plate (List separately in addition to code for primary procedure)

87188   Susceptibility studies, antimicrobial agent; macrobroth dilution method, each agent

A study is performed to determine the effectiveness of a specific antibiotic agent to a specific bacteria. The test is performed in an agar solution. Code 87184 if the bacteria is put on a disc along with the antibiotic solution and observed. Code 87185 if the test determines if the bacteria releases enzymes that counteract the antibiotic. Code 87186 if the bacteria is placed on a plate and impregnated with an antibiotic to determine the minimum amount of antibiotic that is required to kill the bacteria. Add 87187 if the test measures how much the antibiotic can be diluted in order to be effective. Code 87188 if macrobroth dilution is used to measure the effectiveness of the antibiotic. Code 87190 if the test is performed on a mycobacteria, such as tuberculosis.

87205-87210

87205   Smear, primary source with interpretation; Gram or Giemsa stain for bacteria, fungi, or cell types

87206   Smear, primary source with interpretation; fluorescent and/or acid fast stain for bacteria, fungi, parasites, viruses or cell types

87207   Smear, primary source with interpretation; special stain for inclusion bodies or parasites (eg, malaria, coccidia, microsporidia, trypanosomes, herpes viruses)

87210   Smear, primary source with interpretation; wet mount for infectious agents (eg, saline, India ink, KOH preps)

A body fluid sample is smeared on a slide and examined under a microscope to identify any bacteria, fungi, or other structures in the sample. Code 87206 if the slide is prepared with acid or a fluorescent dye. Code 87207 for a special stain that looks for inclusion bodies or parasitic organisms. Code 87209 for a special stain for inclusion bodies or parasites (e.g., malaria, coccidia, microsporidia, trypanosomes, herpes virus). Code 87210 if the sample is mounted on a wet slide and dyed to observe any bacteria that are moving.

87209

87209   Smear, primary source with interpretation; complex special stain (eg, trichrome, iron hemotoxylin) for ova and parasites

A body fluid sample is smeared on a slide and examined under a microscope to identify any bacteria, fungi, or other structures in the sample. Code 87206 if the slide is prepared with acid or a fluorescent dye. Code 87207 for a special stain that looks for inclusion bodies or parasitic organisms. Code 87209 for a special stain for inclusion bodies or parasites (e.g., malaria, coccidia, microsporidia, trypanosomes, herpes virus). Code 87210 if the sample is mounted on a wet slide and dyed to observe any bacteria that are moving.

87220

87220   Tissue examination by KOH slide of samples from skin, hair, or nails for fungi or ectoparasite ova or mites (eg, scabies)

A sample of hair, skin, or nails is examined on a wet slide with or without fluorescent dye and examined under a microscope for the presence of fungi, parasite eggs, or mites. Mites are small parasitic insects.

87270

87270   Infectious agent antigen detection by immunofluorescent technique; Chlamydia trachomatis

A specimen is tested for Chlamydia trachomatis using C. trachomatis antigen detection by immunofluroescent technique. C. trachomatis is a sexually transmitted disease (STD) that often produces no symptoms, but can cause irreversible damage to the female reproductive tract, resulting in infertility. In men, symptoms include burning and itching of the urethra, but men rarely suffer reproductive damage from the infection. Immunofluorescent antigen detection for C. trachomatis is performed by direct fluorescent antibody (DFA) technique. A genital, rectal, ocular, or nasopharyngeal swab is obtained. Reagent for C. trachomatis is then applied to the specimen and incubated for 15-30 min at body temperature in a humid environment to allow the antigen-antibody reaction to occur. The specimen is washed to remove unbound conjugate and then dried and mounted. A fluorescence microscope fitted with the appropriate fluorescent light source and barrier filters is then used to examine the specimen for antigen-antibody binding. Binding appears as bright green or orange-yellow objects when viewed under the microscope which indicates a positive test result.

87273-87274

87273   Infectious agent antigen detection by immunofluorescent technique; Herpes simplex virus type 2

87274   Infectious agent antigen detection by immunofluorescent technique; Herpes simplex virus type 1

A blood sample is tested for Herpes simplex virus (HSV) using HSV antigen detection by immunofluroescent technique. HSV is spread by direct contact and the primary infection typically presents with an area of ulceration in the skin or mucous membrane. Following the primary infection, the virus enters a latent phase and is reactivated in response to other illnesses, infection, or stress. Neonates and immunocompromised individuals are at risk for developing ocular or central nervous system infection. There are two types of HSV referred to as type 1 and type 2. Type 1 typically causes oral herpes, also referred to as cold sores, but can also cause genital infections. Type 2 typically causes genital herpes. Immunofluorescent antigen detection for HSV is performed by direct fluorescent antibody (DFA) technique. A blood sample is obtained. Reagent for HSV is then applied to the specimen and incubated for 15-30 min at body temperature in a humid environment to allow the antigen-antibody reaction to occur. The specimen is washed to remove unbound conjugate and then dried and mounted. A fluorescence microscope fitted with the appropriate fluorescent light source and barrier filters is then used to examine the specimen for antigen-antibody binding. Binding appears as bright green or orange-yellow

Pathology and Laboratory

objects when viewed under the microscope and indicates a positive test result. Use 87273 for HSV type 2 and 87274 for HSV type 1.

87285

87285   Infectious agent antigen detection by immunofluorescent technique; Treponema pallidum

A test for Treponema pallidum, the causative agent of syphilis, is performed using T. pallidum antigen detection by immunofluorescent technique. Syphilis is a sexually transmitted disease (STD). This test uses cells or tissues from a suspicious lesion to test for primary syphilis, or less commonly, tissue from the umbilical cord is used if there is concern about congenital syphilis. During the primary stage of syphilis, a sore called a chancre appears at the site where the syphilis bacteria entered the body. Undiagnosed syphilis infection during pregnancy can be passed to the baby in utero, increasing the risk of stillbirth or death shortly after birth. Untreated infants who survive often experience developmental delays or seizures. Immunofluorescent antigen detection for T. pallidum is performed by direct fluorescent antibody (DFA) technique. The suspicious lesion (chancre) is scraped to obtain a specimen. Reagent for T. pallidum is then applied to the specimen and incubated for 15-30 min at body temperature in a humid environment to allow the antigen-antibody reaction to occur. The specimen is washed to remove unbound conjugate and then dried and mounted. A fluorescence microscope fitted with the appropriate fluorescent light source and barrier filters is then used to examine the specimen for antigen-antibody binding. Binding appears as bright green or orange-yellow objects when viewed under the microscope and indicates a positive test result.

87305

87305   Infectious agent antigen detection by immunoassay technique, (eg, enzyme immunoassay [EIA], enzyme-linked immunosorbent assay [ELISA], immunochemiluminometric assay [IMCA]) qualitative or semiquantitative, multiple-step method; Aspergillus

This code reports a multiple-step, immunoassay technique test such as enzyme immunoassay (EIA), enzyme-linked immunosorbent assay (ELISA), and immunochemiluminometric assay (IMCA) for the qualitative or semiquantitative detection of IgG antibodies in blood serum or plasma against the Aspergillus species, commonly A. fumigatus, which occurs in hay, grain, rotten plants, and bird feces. This invasive fungal infection is generally airborne and occurs in damaged tissue or immunosuppressed patients and can cause chronic lung, eye, and sinus infections. For enzyme immunoassay, immobilized Aspergillus antigen is first bound to microtiter plates or strips. A sample of the patient's serum is placed onto the microtiter plate and binding between the IgG antibodies in serum and the immobilized antigen takes place. After incubation, the plate is washed with solution to remove the unbound matter. An anti-human-IgG peroxidase (enzyme) conjugate is then added, incubated, and washed again. The substrate is again incubated, developing a blue dye in the plate. Color development is stopped by a solution that turns the dye yellow. ELISA also detects very small quantities of the antigen when bound to its specific antibody in a sample by adding a secondary, enzyme-labeled antibody to detect its presence. A chromogenic reaction of the enzyme produces a visible color change or fluorescence. Qualitative and semi-quantitative measures are assessed by the colorimetric reading as the concentration of Aspergillus antibodies is proportional to the intensity of the color. Immunochemiluminometric assay uses the reaction of antibodies labeled with a chemiluminescent substance to identify and quantify the bound antigen-antibody complex by light emission.

87320

87320   Infectious agent antigen detection by immunoassay technique, (eg, enzyme immunoassay [EIA], enzyme-linked immunosorbent assay [ELISA], immunochemiluminometric assay [IMCA]) qualitative or semiquantitative, multiple-step method; Chlamydia trachomatis

A specimen is tested for Chlamydia trachomatis using antigen detection by immunoassay technique such as enzyme immunoassay (EIA), enzyme-linked immunosorbent assay (ELISA), and immunochemiluminometric assay (IMCA). Chlamydia is a sexually transmitted disease that often produces no symptoms, but can cause irreversible damage to the female reproductive tract, resulting in infertility. In men, symptoms include burning and itching of the urethra, although men rarely suffer reproductive damage. A cervical, urethral, or rectal swab is obtained and the sample is tested. Both EIA and ELISA detect very small quantities of the antigen when bound to its specific antibody in a sample by adding a secondary, enzyme-labeled antibody to detect its presence. A chromogenic reaction of the enzyme produces a visible color change or fluorescence. Qualitative and semi-quantitative measures are assessed by the colorimetric reading. Immunochemiluminometric assay uses the reaction of antibodies labeled with a chemiluminescent substance to identify and quantify the bound antigen-antibody complex by light emission.

87324

87324   Infectious agent antigen detection by immunoassay technique, (eg, enzyme immunoassay [EIA], enzyme-linked immunosorbent assay [ELISA], immunochemiluminometric assay [IMCA]) qualitative or semiquantitative, multiple-step method; Clostridium difficile toxin(s)

A laboratory test is performed to detect Clostridium difficile toxin antigen in a fecal sample by immunoassay technique such as enzyme immunoassay (EIA), enzyme-linked immunosorbent assay (ELISA), and immunochemiluminometric assay (IMCA). Clostridium difficile is a bacterium found in the colon that releases toxins if present in large enough amounts, causing serious enteric disease. C. difficile is the most common cause of bacterial diarrhea in hospitalized patients and is also associated with antimicrobial drug therapy. A fecal sample is obtained and placed in a fixative or sent fresh to the laboratory for processing. Both EIA and ELISA detect very small quantities of the antigen when bound to its specific antibody in a sample by adding a secondary, enzyme-labeled antibody to detect its presence. A chromogenic reaction of the enzyme produces a visible color change or fluorescence. Qualitative and semi-quantitative measures are assessed by the colorimetric reading. Immunochemiluminometric assay uses the reaction of antibodies labeled with a chemiluminescent substance to identify and quantify the bound antigen-antibody complex by light emission.

87327

87327   Infectious agent antigen detection by immunoassay technique, (eg, enzyme immunoassay [EIA], enzyme-linked immunosorbent assay [ELISA], immunochemiluminometric assay [IMCA]) qualitative or semiquantitative, multiple-step method; Cryptococcus neoformans

A laboratory test is performed to detect Cryptococcus neoformans antigen in a sample by immunoassay technique such as enzyme immunoassay (EIA), enzyme-linked immunosorbent assay (ELISA), and immunochemiluminometric assay (IMCA). Cryptococcus neoformans is an encapsulated yeastlike fungus in the environment that can cause infections in many parts of the body after breathing in the microscopic fungus, particularly of the lungs and central nervous system in those who are immunocompromised. A sample such as cerebrospinal fluid is obtained and placed in a fixative or sent fresh to the laboratory for processing. Both EIA and ELISA detect very small quantities of the antigen when bound to its specific antibody in a sample by adding a secondary, enzyme-labeled antibody to detect its presence. A chromogenic reaction of the enzyme produces a visible color change or fluorescence. Qualitative and semi-quantitative measures are assessed by the colorimetric reading. Immunochemiluminometric assay uses the reaction of antibodies labeled with a chemiluminescent substance to identify and quantify the bound antigen-antibody complex by light emission.

87328

87328   Infectious agent antigen detection by immunoassay technique, (eg, enzyme immunoassay [EIA], enzyme-linked immunosorbent assay [ELISA], immunochemiluminometric assay [IMCA]) qualitative or semiquantitative, multiple-step method; cryptosporidium

A laboratory test is performed to detect cryptosporidium antigen in a fecal sample by immunoassay technique such as enzyme immunoassay (EIA), enzyme-linked immunosorbent assay (ELISA), and immunochemiluminometric assay (IMCA). Cryptosporidium is a one-celled, microscopic parasite causing the diarrheal disease, cryptosporidiosis. The parasites burrow into the intestinal walls and are shed later in feces, producing watery diarrhea, dehydration, lack of appetite, weight loss, and stomach cramps that can last up to a couple of weeks and repeat sporadically even longer. A fecal sample is obtained and placed in a fixative or sent fresh to the laboratory for processing. Both EIA and ELISA detect very small quantities of the antigen when bound to its specific antibody in a sample by adding a secondary, enzyme-labeled antibody to detect its presence. A chromogenic reaction of the enzyme produces a visible color change or fluorescence. Qualitative and semi-quantitative measures are assessed by the colorimetric reading. Immunochemiluminometric assay uses the reaction of antibodies labeled with a chemiluminescent substance to identify and quantify the bound antigen-antibody complex by light emission.

87329

87329   Infectious agent antigen detection by immunoassay technique, (eg, enzyme immunoassay [EIA], enzyme-linked immunosorbent assay [ELISA], immunochemiluminometric assay [IMCA]) qualitative or semiquantitative, multiple-step method; giardia

A laboratory test is performed to detect giardia antigen in a fecal sample by immunoassay technique such as enzyme immunoassay (EIA), enzyme-linked immunosorbent assay (ELISA), and immunochemiluminometric assay (IMCA). Giardia is a protozoan found in contaminated food and water that causes diarrhea, gastrointestinal symptoms, and weight loss when ingested. A fecal sample is obtained and placed in formalin or sent fresh to the laboratory for processing. Both EIA and ELISA detect very small quantities of the antigen when bound to its specific antibody in a sample by adding a secondary, enzyme-labeled antibody to detect its presence. A chromogenic reaction of the enzyme produces a visible color change or fluorescence. Qualitative and semi-quantitative measures are assessed by the colorimetric reading. Immunochemiluminometric assay uses the reaction of antibodies labeled with a chemiluminescent substance to identify and quantify the bound antigen-antibody complex by light emission.

87332

> 87332   Infectious agent antigen detection by immunoassay technique, (eg, enzyme immunoassay [EIA], enzyme-linked immunosorbent assay [ELISA], immunochemiluminometric assay [IMCA]) qualitative or semiquantitative, multiple-step method; cytomegalovirus

A laboratory test is performed to detect cytomegalovirus antigen in a sample by immunoassay technique such as enzyme immunoassay (EIA), enzyme-linked immunosorbent assay (ELISA), and immunochemiluminometric assay (IMCA). Cytomegalovirus (CMV) is a herpes family virus that can infect almost anyone, but is dangerous to newborns and those who are immunocompromised. CMV causes congenital infection in an infant who acquires it from the birth canal during delivery. Infected babies may have symptoms of low birth weight, jaundice, splotchy skin, hepatosplenomegaly, seizures, microcephaly and developmental delays, hearing loss, or visual impairment. In affected, healthy adults, the virus may resemble mononucleosis, with fatigue, fever, and muscle aches. In those with weakened immune systems, signs and symptoms can include pneumonia, hepatitis, encephalitis, seizures, fever, gastrointestinal ulcers, visual impairment, and even coma. A blood or amniotic fluid sample is obtained and placed in a fixative or sent fresh to the laboratory for processing. Both EIA and ELISA detect very small quantities of the antigen when bound to its specific antibody in a sample by adding a secondary, enzyme-labeled antibody to detect its presence. A chromogenic reaction of the enzyme produces a visible color change or fluorescence. Qualitative and semi-quantitative measures are assessed by the colorimetric reading. Immunochemiluminometric assay uses the reaction of antibodies labeled with a chemiluminescent substance to identify and quantify the bound antigen-antibody complex by light emission.

87335

> 87335   Infectious agent antigen detection by immunoassay technique, (eg, enzyme immunoassay [EIA], enzyme-linked immunosorbent assay [ELISA], immunochemiluminometric assay [IMCA]) qualitative or semiquantitative, multiple-step method; Escherichia coli O157

A laboratory test is performed on a fecal sample to detect Escherichia coli O157 antigen by immunoassay technique such as enzyme immunoassay (EIA), enzyme-linked immunosorbent assay (ELISA), and immunochemiluminometric assay (IMCA). E. coli O157 is a Shiga-like toxin producing bacteria associated with hemorrhagic colitis and hemolytic uremic syndrome. Symptoms include fever, nausea/vomiting, abdominal cramps, and bloody diarrhea. The pathogen infects humans via contaminated food and water and can be passed person to person by contaminated feces. Both EIA and ELISA detect very small quantities of the antigen when bound to its specific antibody in a sample by adding a secondary, enzyme-labeled antibody to detect its presence. A chromogenic reaction of the enzyme produces a visible color change or fluorescence. Qualitative and semi-quantitative measures are assessed by the colorimetric reading. Immunochemiluminometric assay uses the reaction of antibodies labeled with a chemiluminescent substance to identify and quantify the bound antigen-antibody complex by light emission.

87336-87337

> 87336   Infectious agent antigen detection by immunoassay technique, (eg, enzyme immunoassay [EIA], enzyme-linked immunosorbent assay [ELISA], immunochemiluminometric assay [IMCA]) qualitative or semiquantitative, multiple-step method; Entamoeba histolytica dispar group
>
> 87337   Infectious agent antigen detection by immunoassay technique, (eg, enzyme immunoassay [EIA], enzyme-linked immunosorbent assay [ELISA], immunochemiluminometric assay [IMCA]) qualitative or semiquantitative, multiple-step method; Entamoeba histolytica group

A laboratory test is performed a stool sample to detect Entamoeba histolytica group antigen (87337) or E. histolytica dispar group antigen (87336) in feces by immunoassay technique. E. histolytica is a parasite that can cause liver abscesses, intestinal inflammation, peritonitis, and acute colitis, including toxic megacolon. The parasite may be transmitted sexually or ingested via contaminated food and water, and has two morphologic forms: a hardy, tetranucleated, infective cyst and a fragile, potentially pathogenic trophozoite. E. histolytica dispar group is considered to be non-invasive and non-pathogenic, but may occasionally cause diarrheal illness. E. histolytica group is invasive and pathogenic and more often associated with acute illness. Both enzyme immunoassay and enzyme-linked immunosorbent assay techniques detect very small quantities of the antigen when bound to its specific antibody in a sample by adding a secondary, enzyme-labeled antibody to detect its presence. A chromogenic reaction of the enzyme produces a visible color change or fluorescence. Qualitative and semi-quantitative measures are assessed by the colorimetric reading. Immunochemiluminometric assay uses the reaction of antibodies labeled with a chemiluminescent substance to identify and quantify the bound antigen-antibody complex by light emission.

87338-87339

> 87338   Infectious agent antigen detection by immunoassay technique, (eg, enzyme immunoassay [EIA], enzyme-linked immunosorbent assay [ELISA], immunochemiluminometric assay [IMCA]) qualitative or semiquantitative, multiple-step method; Helicobacter pylori, stool
>
> 87339   Infectious agent antigen detection by immunoassay technique, (eg, enzyme immunoassay [EIA], enzyme-linked immunosorbent assay [ELISA], immunochemiluminometric assay [IMCA]) qualitative or semiquantitative, multiple-step method; Helicobacter pylori

A laboratory test is performed to detect Helicobactor pylori antigen in a stool sample (87338) or other tissue sources, except blood and breath samples (87339) by immunoassay technique for initial diagnosis, therapeutic monitoring, and eradication confirmation. H. pylori is a gram negative rod bacteria that infects the lining of the stomach and/or duodenum and is linked to development of gastritis, peptic ulcer disease (PUD), gastric adenocarcinoma, and possibly low-grade gastric lymphoma. The bacteria are transmitted person to person or via contaminated food and water. Symptoms may include abdominal pain, bloating, nausea/vomiting, loss of appetite, and weight loss. Both enzyme immunoassay and enzyme-linked immunosorbent assay techniques detect very small quantities of the antigen when bound to its specific antibody in a sample by adding a secondary, enzyme-labeled antibody to detect its presence. A chromogenic reaction of the enzyme produces a visible color change or fluorescence. Qualitative and semi-quantitative measures are assessed by the colorimetric reading. Immunochemiluminometric assay uses the reaction of antibodies labeled with a chemiluminescent substance to identify and quantify the bound antigen-antibody complex by light emission.

87340

> 87340   Infectious agent antigen detection by immunoassay technique, (eg, enzyme immunoassay [EIA], enzyme-linked immunosorbent assay [ELISA], immunochemiluminometric assay [IMCA]) qualitative or semiquantitative, multiple-step method; hepatitis B surface antigen (HBsAg)

A laboratory test is performed to detect hepatitis B surface antigen (HBsAg) in a blood sample by immunoassay technique such as enzyme immunoassay (EIA), enzyme-linked immunosorbent assay (ELISA), and immunochemiluminometric assay (IMCA). HBsAg is a protein produced by the hepatitis B virus (HBV) that infects the liver, and is the earliest indicator of an acute HBV infection. This antigen is also present in individuals with chronic HBV infection. Both EIA and ELISA detect very small quantities of the antigen when bound to its specific antibody in a sample by adding a secondary, enzyme-labeled antibody to detect its presence. A chromogenic reaction of the enzyme produces a visible color change or fluorescence. Qualitative and semi-quantitative measures are assessed by the colorimetric reading. Immunochemiluminometric assay uses the reaction of antibodies labeled with a chemiluminescent substance to identify and quantify the bound antigen-antibody complex by light emission.

87341-87350

> 87341   Infectious agent antigen detection by immunoassay technique, (eg, enzyme immunoassay [EIA], enzyme-linked immunosorbent assay [ELISA], immunochemiluminometric assay [IMCA]) qualitative or semiquantitative, multiple-step method; hepatitis B surface antigen (HBsAg) neutralization
>
> 87350   Infectious agent antigen detection by immunoassay technique, (eg, enzyme immunoassay [EIA], enzyme-linked immunosorbent assay [ELISA], immunochemiluminometric assay [IMCA]) qualitative or semiquantitative, multiple-step method; hepatitis Be antigen (HBeAg)

A laboratory test is performed to detect hepatitis B surface antigen (HBsAg) neutralization (87341) or hepatitis Be antigen (HBeAg) (87350) in serum or plasma by immunoassay technique. HBsAg is a protein produced by the hepatitis B virus (HBV) that infects the liver. An individual with chronic HBV infection has an increased risk of developing cirrhosis and hepatocellular carcinoma. HBV may be transmitted in blood and body fluids between sexual partners, from mother to infant, and through contaminated objects such as needles, razors, and toothbrushes. The virus may cause fever, fatigue, abdominal pain, weight loss, nausea/vomiting, and joint pain or it may be asymptomatic. Both enzyme immunoassay and enzyme-linked immunosorbent assay techniques detect very small quantities of the antigen when bound to its specific antibody in a sample by adding a secondary, enzyme-labeled antibody to detect its presence. A chromogenic reaction of the enzyme produces a visible color change or fluorescence. Qualitative and semi-quantitative measures are assessed by the colorimetric reading. Immunochemiluminometric assay uses the reaction of antibodies labeled with a chemiluminescent substance to identify and quantify the bound antigen-antibody complex by light emission. The HBsAg neutralization test is used to confirm a positive HBsAg test. The Hepatitis Be antigen (HBeAg) test is used to monitor an active HBV infection and response to therapy.

Pathology and Laboratory

87380

87380 **Infectious agent antigen detection by immunoassay technique, (eg, enzyme immunoassay [EIA], enzyme-linked immunosorbent assay [ELISA], immunochemiluminometric assay [IMCA]) qualitative or semiquantitative, multiple-step method; hepatitis, delta agent**

A laboratory test is performed to detect antigen to the hepatitis delta agent in a blood sample by immunoassay technique such as enzyme immunoassay (EIA), enzyme-linked immunosorbent assay (ELISA), and immunochemiluminometric assay (IMCA). Delta agent, also known as hepatitis D virus (HDV) only occurs in people who carry the hepatitis B virus. The delta agent is a defective RNA virus not structurally related to the hepatitis A, B, and C viruses and requires HBV for its own replication. HDV causes serious, worsening liver disease in those with acute or chronic hepatitis B that can lead to fulminant acute hepatitis, cirrhosis, and hepatocellular carcinoma. A blood sample is obtained and placed in a fixative or sent fresh to the laboratory for processing. Both EIA and ELISA detect very small quantities of the antigen when bound to its specific antibody in a sample by adding a secondary, enzyme-labeled antibody to detect its presence. A chromogenic reaction of the enzyme produces a visible color change or fluorescence. Qualitative and semi-quantitative measures are assessed by the colorimetric reading. Immunochemiluminometric assay uses the reaction of antibodies labeled with a chemiluminescent substance to identify and quantify the bound antigen-antibody complex by light emission.

87385

87385 **Infectious agent antigen detection by immunoassay technique, (eg, enzyme immunoassay [EIA], enzyme-linked immunosorbent assay [ELISA], immunochemiluminometric assay [IMCA]) qualitative or semiquantitative, multiple-step method; Histoplasma capsulatum**

A laboratory test is performed to detect Histoplasma capsulatum antigen in a sample by immunoassay technique such as enzyme immunoassay (EIA), enzyme-linked immunosorbent assay (ELISA), and immunochemiluminometric assay (IMCA). Histoplasma capsulatum is a fungus in the environment, particularly soil laden with bat or bird droppings. Breathing in the spores does not always cause disease, but may produce cough, fever, and fatigue generally or more severe disease in those with compromised immune systems when it spreads from the lungs to other organs. A blood or respiratory secretion sample is obtained and placed in a fixative or sent fresh to the laboratory for processing. Both EIA and ELISA detect very small quantities of the antigen when bound to its specific antibody in a sample by adding a secondary, enzyme-labeled antibody to detect its presence. A chromogenic reaction of the enzyme produces a visible color change or fluorescence. Qualitative and semi-quantitative measures are assessed by the colorimetric reading. Immunochemiluminometric assay uses the reaction of antibodies labeled with a chemiluminescent substance to identify and quantify the bound antigen-antibody complex by light emission.

87389-87391

87389 **Infectious agent antigen detection by immunoassay technique, (eg, enzyme immunoassay [EIA], enzyme-linked immunosorbent assay [ELISA], immunochemiluminometric assay [IMCA]) qualitative or semiquantitative, multiple-step method; HIV-1 antigen(s), with HIV-1 and HIV-2 antibodies, single result**

87390 **Infectious agent antigen detection by immunoassay technique, (eg, enzyme immunoassay [EIA], enzyme-linked immunosorbent assay [ELISA], immunochemiluminometric assay [IMCA]) qualitative or semiquantitative, multiple-step method; HIV-1**

87391 **Infectious agent antigen detection by immunoassay technique, (eg, enzyme immunoassay [EIA], enzyme-linked immunosorbent assay [ELISA], immunochemiluminometric assay [IMCA]) qualitative or semiquantitative, multiple-step method; HIV-2**

A blood or saliva sample is tested for human immunodeficiency virus (HIV) antigen by multiple-step, immunoassay technique test such as enzyme immunoassay (EIA), enzyme-linked immunosorbent assay (ELISA), and immunochemiluminometric assay (IMCA). HIV virus infections are sexually transmitted diseases that can also be transmitted from unscreened blood and shared needles, from mother to child in utero, or by breast feeding. HIV attacks the immune system by destroying T cells or CD4 cells, types of white blood cells. This hampers the body's ability to fight infection. AIDS is the final stage of HIV infection. A blood or saliva sample is obtained and placed in a fixative or sent fresh to the laboratory for processing. Both EIA and ELISA detect very small quantities of the antigen when bound to its specific antibody in a sample by adding a secondary, enzyme-labeled antibody to detect its presence. A chromogenic reaction of the enzyme produces a visible color change or fluorescence. Qualitative and semi-quantitative measures are assessed by the colorimetric reading. Immunochemiluminometric assay uses the reaction of antibodies labeled with a chemiluminescent substance to identify and quantify the bound antigen-antibody complex by light emission. Use 87389 when testing for HIV-1 antigen(s), with HIV-1 and HIV-2 antibodies, single result. Use 87390 when testing for HIV-I alone. Use 87391 for HIV-II alone.

87400

87400 **Infectious agent antigen detection by immunoassay technique, (eg, enzyme immunoassay [EIA], enzyme-linked immunosorbent assay [ELISA], immunochemiluminometric assay [IMCA]) qualitative or semiquantitative, multiple-step method; Influenza, A or B, each**

A laboratory test is performed to detect Influenza A or B antigen in a sample by immunoassay technique such as enzyme immunoassay (EIA), enzyme-linked immunosorbent assay (ELISA), and immunochemiluminometric assay (IMCA). Influenza A or B are viruses which cause the flu. Symptoms depend upon the particular virus and include normal flu-like symptoms to pneumonia and other severe respiratory diseases and manifestations. Type B is specific to humans while type A commonly infects animals, such as swine and birds, and is communicated to humans. A blood or respiratory secretion sample is obtained and placed in a fixative or sent fresh to the laboratory for processing. Both EIA and ELISA detect very small quantities of the antigen when bound to its specific antibody in a sample by adding a secondary, enzyme-labeled antibody to detect its presence. A chromogenic reaction of the enzyme produces a visible color change or fluorescence. Qualitative and semi-quantitative measures are assessed by the colorimetric reading. Immunochemiluminometric assay uses the reaction of antibodies labeled with a chemiluminescent substance to identify and quantify the bound antigen-antibody complex by light emission.

87420

87420 **Infectious agent antigen detection by immunoassay technique, (eg, enzyme immunoassay [EIA], enzyme-linked immunosorbent assay [ELISA], immunochemiluminometric assay [IMCA]) qualitative or semiquantitative, multiple-step method; respiratory syncytial virus**

A laboratory test is performed to detect respiratory syncytial virus antigen in a sample by immunoassay technique such as enzyme immunoassay (EIA), enzyme-linked immunosorbent assay (ELISA), and immunochemiluminometric assay (IMCA). Respiratory syncytial virus is a very common virus that infects most children by age 2 and causes mild cold symptoms in healthy persons but can be severe in young babies causing pneumonia or bronchiolitis and difficulty breathing. A blood or respiratory secretion sample is obtained and placed in a fixative or sent fresh to the laboratory for processing. Both EIA and ELISA detect very small quantities of the antigen when bound to its specific antibody in a sample by adding a secondary, enzyme-labeled antibody to detect its presence. A chromogenic reaction of the enzyme produces a visible color change or fluorescence. Qualitative and semi-quantitative measures are assessed by the colorimetric reading. Immunochemiluminometric assay uses the reaction of antibodies labeled with a chemiluminescent substance to identify and quantify the bound antigen-antibody complex by light emission.

87425

87425 **Infectious agent antigen detection by immunoassay technique, (eg, enzyme immunoassay [EIA], enzyme-linked immunosorbent assay [ELISA], immunochemiluminometric assay [IMCA]) qualitative or semiquantitative, multiple-step method; rotavirus**

A laboratory test is performed to detect rotavirus antigen in a sample by immunoassay technique such as enzyme immunoassay (EIA), enzyme-linked immunosorbent assay (ELISA), and immunochemiluminometric assay (IMCA). Rotavirus is actually a group of wheel-shaped viruses that commonly infect the intestines. Rotaviral enteritis is most often seen in infants and young children, causing severe diarrhea with copious amounts of watery stool resulting in dehydration, abdominal cramps, anorexia, low-grade fever, vomiting, and significantly decreased urine output with loss of electrolytes. A fecal sample is obtained and placed in a fixative or sent fresh to the laboratory for processing. Both EIA and ELISA detect very small quantities of the antigen when bound to its specific antibody in a sample by adding a secondary, enzyme-labeled antibody to detect its presence. A chromogenic reaction of the enzyme produces a visible color change or fluorescence. Qualitative and semi-quantitative measures are assessed by the colorimetric reading. Immunochemiluminometric assay uses the reaction of antibodies labeled with a chemiluminescent substance to identify and quantify the bound antigen-antibody complex by light emission.

87427

87427 **Infectious agent antigen detection by immunoassay technique, (eg, enzyme immunoassay [EIA], enzyme-linked immunosorbent assay [ELISA], immunochemiluminometric assay [IMCA]) qualitative or semiquantitative, multiple-step method; Shiga-like toxin**

A laboratory test is performed on a cultured fecal sample in which E.coli is isolated to detect Shiga-like toxin antigen by immunoassay technique. Shiga-like toxin is produced by certain stains of the Escherichia coli bacteria including E. coli O157, E. coli O26, E. coli O111, and E. coli O103. The pathogen infects humans via contaminated food and water and may be passed from person to person in contaminated feces. Infection can lead to hemorrhaging colitis and hemolytic uremic syndrome. Both enzyme immunoassay and enzyme-linked immunosorbent assay techniques detect very small quantities of the antigen when bound to its specific antibody in a sample by adding a secondary, enzyme-labeled antibody to detect its presence. A chromogenic reaction of the enzyme produces a visible color change or fluorescence. Qualitative and semi-quantitative measures are assessed by the colorimetric reading. Immunochemiluminometric assay uses the reaction of antibodies labeled with a chemiluminescent substance to identify and quantify the bound antigen-antibody complex by light emission.

87430

87430   Infectious agent antigen detection by immunoassay technique, (eg, enzyme immunoassay [EIA], enzyme-linked immunosorbent assay [ELISA], immunochemiluminometric assay [IMCA]) qualitative or semiquantitative, multiple-step method; Streptococcus, group A

A laboratory test is performed to detect streptococcus, group A, or S. pyogenes, antigen in a sample by immunoassay technique such as enzyme immunoassay (EIA), enzyme-linked immunosorbent assay (ELISA), and immunochemiluminometric assay (IMCA). Group A Streptococcus is the bacteria that causes strep throat, rheumatic fever, and scarlet fever as well as streptococcal sepsis. Sepsis caused by Group A streptococcus is spread from the nasopharynx into the systemic circulation and is also a common strain contracted in hospitals. The sample obtained is placed in a fixative or sent fresh to the laboratory for processing. Both EIA and ELISA detect very small quantities of the antigen when bound to its specific antibody in a sample by adding a secondary, enzyme-labeled antibody to detect its presence. A chromogenic reaction of the enzyme produces a visible color change or fluorescence. Qualitative and semi-quantitative measures are assessed by the colorimetric reading. Immunochemiluminometric assay uses the reaction of antibodies labeled with a chemiluminescent substance to identify and quantify the bound antigen-antibody complex by light emission.

87449-87451

87449   Infectious agent antigen detection by immunoassay technique, (eg, enzyme immunoassay [EIA], enzyme-linked immunosorbent assay [ELISA], immunochemiluminometric assay [IMCA]), qualitative or semiquantitative; multiple-step method, not otherwise specified, each organism

87450   Infectious agent antigen detection by immunoassay technique, (eg, enzyme immunoassay [EIA], enzyme-linked immunosorbent assay [ELISA], immunochemiluminometric assay [IMCA]), qualitative or semiquantitative; single step method, not otherwise specified, each organism

87451   Infectious agent antigen detection by immunoassay technique, (eg, enzyme immunoassay [EIA], enzyme-linked immunosorbent assay [ELISA], immunochemiluminometric assay [IMCA]), qualitative or semiquantitative; multiple step method, polyvalent for multiple organisms, each polyvalent antiserum

An enzyme immunoassay test is performed to detect an infectious agent. The test examines the chemical bond between an antibody or antigen and an enzyme to identify the infectious agent. This multiple-step test looks for an organism not specified in any other code. Code 87450 for a single-step test. Code 87451 for a multiple step test that looks for more than one organism.

87480-87482

87480   Infectious agent detection by nucleic acid (DNA or RNA); Candida species, direct probe technique

87481   Infectious agent detection by nucleic acid (DNA or RNA); Candida species, amplified probe technique

87482   Infectious agent detection by nucleic acid (DNA or RNA); Candida species, quantification

Infectious agent antibody detection by nucleic acid technique (RNA or DNA) is used to identify Candida infection using direct probe (87480), amplified probe (87481), or quantification (87482) of the amplified probe. Candida is a fungus normally present on the skin and in mucous membranes such as the vagina, mouth, or rectum. Candida becomes an infectious agent only when a change in body chemistry allows the fungus to grow out of control and is referred to as Candidiasis moniliasis. Individuals on antibiotics and those who are immunocompromised are susceptible to Candida infection as are infants. Candidiasis moniliasis affects the mouth, skin, nails, or vagina. Less commonly, the esophagus or gastrointestinal tract is affected. Nucleic acid tests are typically performed only for vaginal infection. Some types of nucleic acid tests are rapid tests that may be performed in the physician office using a test kit. In 87480, a vaginal swab is obtained and incubated with lysate to rupture all cells and release nucleic acids. The lysate is placed in the sample well and the test slide is dipped and incubated robotically. The Candida specific probe is attached to a stationary microparticle bead in the test well. The bead captures the target DNA sequence and holds it on the slide. The slide is washed to remove cellular debris and unbound nucleic acids. A second probe containing a color development substrate is added. The slide is again washed and an enzyme is added to catalyze the color substrate. If Candida is present, the bead will turn blue indicating a positive result. If Candida is not present, no color change occurs. In 87481, an amplification technique, such as polymerase chain reaction (PCR) is used to create copies of the Candida nucleic

acids. Amplification is used when it is suspected that there are low levels of the targeted microorganism in the specimen that would not be detected using a direct probe. The Candida nucleic acids are then detected using a variety of techniques. In 87482, the amplified product is quantified to provide an assessment of how many Candida organisms are present. Quantification may be used to evaluate the severity of the infection and response to treatment.

87490-87492

87490   Infectious agent detection by nucleic acid (DNA or RNA); Chlamydia trachomatis, direct probe technique

87491   Infectious agent detection by nucleic acid (DNA or RNA); Chlamydia trachomatis, amplified probe technique

87492   Infectious agent detection by nucleic acid (DNA or RNA); Chlamydia trachomatis, quantification

Infectious agent antibody detection by nucleic acid technique (DNA or RNA) is used to identify Chlamydia trachomatis infection using direct probe (87490), amplified probe (87491), or quantification (87492) of the amplified probe. C. trachomatis infection is a sexually transmitted disease (STD) that often produces no symptoms, but can cause irreversible damage to the female reproductive tract, resulting in infertility. In men, symptoms include burning and itching of the urethra, but men rarely suffer reproductive damage from the infection. Some types of nucleic acid tests are rapid tests that may be performed in the physician office using a test kit. A swab is used to obtain a specimen from the cervix, male urethra, or eye. In 87490, the exact methodology is dependent on the test kit used as there are several manufacturers. One test kit uses a nucleic acid hybridization method. A single stranded chemiluminescent DNA probe is used that is complementary to the ribosomal RNA of the Chlamydia organism. Lysate is used to rupture cells and release nucleic acids. The ribosomal RNA from the Chlamydia organism then combines with the labeled DNA probe to form a stable DNA:RNA hybrid. The presence of DNA:RNA hybrids is then detected using a luminometer. In 87491, an amplification technique, such as polymerase chain reaction (PCR), is used to create copies of the Chlamydia nucleic acids. Amplification is used when it is suspected that there are low levels of the targeted microorganism in the specimen that would not be detected using a direct probe. The Chlamydia nucleic acid is then detected using a variety of techniques. In 87492, the amplified product is quantified to provide an assessment of how many Chlamydia organisms are present. Quantification may be used to evaluate the severity of the infection and response to treatment.

87493

87493   Infectious agent detection by nucleic acid (DNA or RNA); Clostridium difficile, toxin gene(s), amplified probe technique

Clostridium difficile is a bacterium that causes diarrhea. Most infected individuals have a mild illness that resolves without treatment or with antibiotics. However, C. difficile can produce toxins that attack the lining of the intestine causing inflammation of the intestinal lining (colitis) and in some cases sepsis. Detection of C. difficile toxin genes is performed using an amplified nucleic acid (DNA, RNA) probe technique, such as polymerase chain reaction (PCR) which is used to create copies of the nucleic acids. Amplification is used when there are low levels of the suspected microorganism in the specimen that would not be detected using a direct probe. Amplification is an enzymatic process that replicates target sequences or positions in the specimen DNA or RNA. Primers are artificial short strands of DNA or RNA that are complementary to the beginning or end of the target DNA or RNA fragment to be amplified. The primer adheres to the target DNA or RNA at these points. The polymerase enzyme copies the region and builds the new DNA or RNA. The amplified DNA or RNA is then tested using a probe that consists of laboratory-prepared, complementary strands of C. difficile. If the specimen contains complementary strands of DNA or RNA, the probe will bind with the specimen DNA forming a double-stranded complex or hybrid. Binding of the probe indicates that the organism is present in the specimen (positive result) which is typically indicated by a change in color.

87498

87498   Infectious agent detection by nucleic acid (DNA or RNA); enterovirus, amplified probe technique, includes reverse transcription when performed

An enterovirus is one that preferentially lives in the intestinal tract and can cause an array of disease symptoms. Nucleic acid detection for diagnostic purposes is a useful alternative to culturing. DNA or RNA probing detects much lower levels of the infectious agent, sometimes even the presence of a single organism. Probing involves identifying the infectious agent's nucleic acid (DNA or RNA) by releasing it from the cell and extracting it through nucleic acid hybridization using a probe. The probe consists of laboratory-prepared, complimentary strands of nucleic acid, often labeled with chemical fluorescence, specifically designed to align and bind with the target nucleic acid to form stable, double-stranded complexes or hybrids. Amplified probing provides greater sensitivity for more direct, qualitative detection by using techniques such as reverse transcription polymerase chain reaction (RT-PCR) to enzymatically replicate certain target sequences or positions in the nucleic acid which allows exponential amplification of the original target nucleic acid. An amplification primer is used in addition to the probe. Primers are artificial, short strands

Pathology and Laboratory

of nucleic acid complementary to the beginning or end of the nucleic acid fragment to be amplified. The primer adheres to the target nucleic acid at these points. The polymerase enzyme copies the region and builds the new nucleic acid.

87500

87500   Infectious agent detection by nucleic acid (DNA or RNA); vancomycin resistance (eg, enterococcus species van A, van B), amplified probe technique

An amplified probe technique is used to identify vancomycin resistant infectious agents, such as enterococcus species van A and van B. Vancomycin is a strong antibiotic used to treat gram positive bacterial infections. However, vancomycin resistant enterococci are becoming increasingly common. Vancomycin resistant enterococci can be detected by nucleic acid (DNA or RNA) amplified probe technique that identifies the presence of the vancomycin resistant gene in the bacteria. A specimen is obtained and the bacteria isolated. Cells contained in the specimen are treated to expose single-stranded target nucleic acid molecules that react with a probe nucleic acid sequence that allows the target and the probe strands to hybridize to each other. The target and the probe form a double-stranded, target-probe complex. Then, an enzyme molecule cleaves the link of the target-probe complex and one or more fragments of the nucleic acid probe are released. If cleaved portions of the nucleic acid probe are produced, the bacterium causing the infection is vancomycin resistant. Nucleic acid probes also identify the genotype A or B.

87501-87503

87501   Infectious agent detection by nucleic acid (DNA or RNA); influenza virus, includes reverse transcription, when performed, and amplified probe technique, each type or subtype

87502   Infectious agent detection by nucleic acid (DNA or RNA); influenza virus, for multiple types or sub-types, includes multiplex reverse transcription, when performed, and multiplex amplified probe technique, first 2 types or sub-types

87503   Infectious agent detection by nucleic acid (DNA or RNA); influenza virus, for multiple types or sub-types, includes multiplex reverse transcription, when performed, and multiplex amplified probe technique, each additional influenza virus type or sub-type beyond 2 (List separately in addition to code for primary procedure)

This test allows the specific type or subtype of influenza present in the sample to be identified. There are two main types of influenza, type A and type B. Within these two types are subtypes. Examples of type A subtypes include H1N1, H3N2, and H5N1. Nucleic acid detection of specific types and subtypes of the influenza virus involves identification by releasing DNA or RNA from the blood or other cells in the laboratory specimen and extracting the specific type or subtype of influenza using reverse transcription, when performed, and an amplified probe. Using reverse transcription polymerase chain reaction (RT-PCR), DNA or RNA from specific strains of influenza type A, such as H1N1, H3N2, and H5N1, and influenza type B are extracted and amplified. The amplified DNA or RNA fragments are sized and analyzed for the specific types or subtypes. Use 87501 for each single type or subtype of the influenza virus. Use 87502 for multiplex testing for the first two types or subtypes tested, and code 87503 for multiplex testing for each additional influenza type or subtype beyond the first two.

87505-87507

87505   Infectious agent detection by nucleic acid (DNA or RNA); gastrointestinal pathogen (eg, Clostridium difficile, E. coli, Salmonella, Shigella, norovirus, Giardia), includes multiplex reverse transcription, when performed, and multiplex amplified probe technique, multiple types or subtypes, 3-5 targets

87506   Infectious agent detection by nucleic acid (DNA or RNA); gastrointestinal pathogen (eg, Clostridium difficile, E. coli, Salmonella, Shigella, norovirus, Giardia), includes multiplex reverse transcription, when performed, and multiplex amplified probe technique, multiple types or subtypes, 6-11 targets

87507   Infectious agent detection by nucleic acid (DNA or RNA); gastrointestinal pathogen (eg, Clostridium difficile, E. coli, Salmonella, Shigella, norovirus, Giardia), includes multiplex reverse transcription, when performed, and multiplex amplified probe technique, multiple types or subtypes, 12-25 targets

Gastrointestinal (GI) pathogens cause diarrheal disease which is the leading cause of malnutrition in children under the age of 5 years and the 2nd leading cause of death. Simultaneous qualitative detection of pathogenic viruses, bacteria, and parasites can be made from fecal specimens of patients with signs and symptoms of infectious colitis or gastroenteritis. The fecal sample is placed in a culture medium and the nucleic acid (DNA and RNA) targets are amplified using polymerase chain reaction (PCR) or reverse transcription and analyzed using technology such as Luminex x TAG that detects the absence or presence of each pathogen in the sample. Pathogens can include types and subtypes of Clostridium difficile, Escherichia coli, Campylobacter, Salmonella, Shigella, norovirus, Rotavirus, Giardia, and Cryptosporidium. Code 87505 is used for a panel with

3-5 pathogenic targets. Code 87506 is used for a panel with 6-11 pathogenic targets. Code 87507 is used for a panel with 12-25 pathogenic targets.

87510-87512

87510   Infectious agent detection by nucleic acid (DNA or RNA); Gardnerella vaginalis, direct probe technique

87511   Infectious agent detection by nucleic acid (DNA or RNA); Gardnerella vaginalis, amplified probe technique

87512   Infectious agent detection by nucleic acid (DNA or RNA); Gardnerella vaginalis, quantification

Infectious agent antibody detection by nucleic acid technique (RNA or DNA) is used to identify Gardnerella vaginalis using direct probe (87510), amplified probe (87511), or quantification (87512) of the amplified probe. Gardnerella is a bacterial infection of the female genital tract also referred to as bacterial vaginosis. Some types of nucleic acid tests are rapid tests that may be performed in the physician office using a test kit. In 87510, a vaginal swab is obtained and incubated with lysate to rupture all cells and release nucleic acids. The lysate is placed in the sample well and the test slide is dipped and incubated robotically. The Gardnerella specific probe is attached to a stationary microparticle bead in the test well. The bead captures the target DNA sequence and holds it on the slide. The slide is washed to remove cellular debris and unbound nucleic acids. A second probe containing a color development substrate is added. The slide is again washed and an enzyme is added to catalyze the color substrate. If Gardnerella is present, the bead will change color indicating a positive result. If Gardnerella is not present, no color change occurs. In 87511, an amplification technique, such as polymerase chain reaction (PCR) is used to create copies of the Gardnerella nucleic acids. Amplification is used when it is suspected that there are low levels of the targeted microorganism in the specimen that would not be detected using a direct probe. The Gardnerella nucleic acids are then detected using a variety of techniques. In 87512, the amplified product is quantified to provide an assessment of how many Gardnerella organisms are present. Quantification may be used to evaluate the severity of the infection and response to treatment.

87520-87522

87520   Infectious agent detection by nucleic acid (DNA or RNA); hepatitis C, direct probe technique

87521   Infectious agent detection by nucleic acid (DNA or RNA); hepatitis C, amplified probe technique, includes reverse transcription when performed

87522   Infectious agent detection by nucleic acid (DNA or RNA); hepatitis C, quantification, includes reverse transcription when performed

The hepatitis C virus (HCV) causes inflammation of the liver. Individuals infected with HCV often develop chronic hepatitis C which can lead to cirrhosis and liver cancer. Nucleic acid detection of HCV is performed to evaluate whether a patient has an ongoing or chronic HCV infection. DNA or RNA probing detects much lower levels of the infectious agent, sometimes even the presence of a single organism. Probing involves identifying the infectious agent's nucleic acid (DNA or RNA) by releasing it from the cell and extracting it through nucleic acid hybridization using a probe. A direct probe (87520) consists of laboratory-prepared, complimentary strands of nucleic acid, often labeled with chemical fluorescence, specifically designed to align and bind with the target nucleic acid to form stable, double-stranded complexes or hybrids. Amplified probing (87521) provides greater sensitivity for more direct, qualitative detection by using techniques such as reverse transcription polymerase chain reaction (RT-PCR) to enzymatically replicate certain target sequences or positions in the nucleic acid which allows exponential amplification of the original target nucleic acid. An amplification primer is used in addition to the probe. Primers are artificial, short strands of nucleic acid complementary to the beginning or end of the nucleic acid fragment to be amplified. The primer adheres to the target nucleic acid at these points. The polymerase enzyme copies the region and builds the new nucleic acid. Following amplification, the amount of the infectious agent in the sample may be evaluated using reverse transcription and quantification (87522). Quantification is performed to evaluate the severity of the infection and response to treatment.

87528-87530

87528   Infectious agent detection by nucleic acid (DNA or RNA); Herpes simplex virus, direct probe technique

87529   Infectious agent detection by nucleic acid (DNA or RNA); Herpes simplex virus, amplified probe technique

87530   Infectious agent detection by nucleic acid (DNA or RNA); Herpes simplex virus, quantification

Infectious agent antibody detection by nucleic acid technique (RNA or DNA) is used to identify Herpes simplex virus (HSV) using direct probe (87528), or amplified probe (87529, or quantification (87530) of the amplified probe. HSV is spread by direct contact and the primary infection typically presents with an area of ulceration in the skin or mucous membrane. Following the primary infection, the virus enters a latent phase and is reactivated in response to other illnesses, infection, or stress. Neonates and immunocompromised individuals are at risk for developing ocular or central nervous system infection. There are two types of HSV: type 1 and type 2. Type 1 typically causes oral herpes, also referred to as cold sores, but can also cause genital infections. Type 2 typically causes genital herpes. A specimen is obtained from an oral or genital lesion, from vitreous of the eye, or from a blood sample. In 87528, the specimen is incubated with lysate to rupture all cells and release nucleic acids. The lysate is placed in the sample well and the test slide is dipped and incubated. Probes specific for HSV-1 and/or HSV-2 are introduced. The slide is washed to remove cellular debris and unbound nucleic acids. A second probe containing a color development substrate is added. The slide is again washed and an enzyme is added to catalyze the color substrate. A luminometer is used to determine whether HSV-1 or HSV-2 is present. In 87529, an amplification technique, such as polymerase chain reaction (PCR) is used to create copies of the HSV-1 and/or HSV-2 nucleic acids. Amplification is used when it is suspected that there are low levels of the targeted microorganism in the specimen that would not be detected using a direct probe. The HSV-1 and/or HSV-2 nucleic acids are then detected using a variety of techniques. In 87530, the amplified product is quantified to provide an assessment of how many HSV-1 and/or HSV-2 organisms are present. Quantification may be used to evaluate the severity of the infection and response to treatment. If the specimen is tested for both HSV-1 and HSV-2, the code for the direct or amplified probe is reported for each serotype as is the quantification procedure if quantification is also performed.

87534-87536

87534   Infectious agent detection by nucleic acid (DNA or RNA); HIV-1, direct probe technique
87535   Infectious agent detection by nucleic acid (DNA or RNA); HIV-1, amplified probe technique, includes reverse transcription when performed
87536   Infectious agent detection by nucleic acid (DNA or RNA); HIV-1, quantification, includes reverse transcription when performed

Infectious agent antibody detection by nucleic acid technique (RNA or DNA) is used to identify HIV-1 using direct probe (87534), amplified probe (87535), or quantification (87536) of the amplified probe. HIV virus infections are sexually transmitted diseases that can also be transmitted from unscreened blood, shared needles, from mother to child in utero, or by breast feeding. HIV attacks the immune system by destroying T-cells or CD4 cells, which are types of white blood cell. This hampers the body's ability to fight infection. Acquired immunodeficiency syndrome (AIDS) is the final stage of HIV infection. There are two HIV serotypes (HIV-1, HIV-2). These tests are performed to identify HIV-1. A blood sample is obtained. In 87534, a direct probe is performed. Direct probes are rarely used as they require culture of the specimen. In 87535, an amplification technique, such as reverse transcription polymerase chain reaction (RT-PCR) is used to create copies of the HIV-1 nucleic acids. Amplification is used when there may be such low levels of the suspected microorganism in the specimen that it would not be detected using a direct probe. The HIV-1 nucleic acids are then detected using a variety of techniques. Test kits that may be used have three components: the specimen collection and preparation component, an amplification component, and a detection component. Red blood cells are selectively lysed leaving leukocytes intact. The leukocytes are pelleted and then washed several times. DNA is extracted from the pellet. Proviral HIV-1 DNA is then amplified. The detection component is then used to determine whether HIV-1 DNA is present in the specimen. In 87536, the amount of the infectious agent in the sample is evaluated following amplification. Using reverse transcription and quantification techniques the HIV-1 viral load is determined. Quantification of HIV-1 is typically performed to evaluate response to treatment.

87537-87539

87537   Infectious agent detection by nucleic acid (DNA or RNA); HIV-2, direct probe technique
87538   Infectious agent detection by nucleic acid (DNA or RNA); HIV-2, amplified probe technique, includes reverse transcription when performed
87539   Infectious agent detection by nucleic acid (DNA or RNA); HIV-2, quantification, includes reverse transcription when performed

Infectious agent antibody detection by nucleic acid technique (RNA or DNA) is used to identify HIV-2 using direct probe (87537), amplified probe (87538), or quantification (87539) of the amplified probe. HIV virus infections are sexually transmitted diseases that can also be transmitted from unscreened blood, shared needles, from mother to child in utero, or by breast feeding. HIV attacks the immune system by destroying T-cells or CD4 cells, which are types of white blood cell. This hampers the body's ability to fight infection. Acquired immunodeficiency syndrome (AIDS) is the final stage of HIV infection. There are two HIV serotypes (HIV-1, HIV-2). These tests are performed to identify HIV-2. A blood sample is obtained. In 87537, a direct probe is performed. Direct probes are rarely used as they require culture of the specimen. In 87538, an amplification technique, such as reverse transcription polymerase chain reaction (RT-PCR) is used to create copies of the HIV-2 nucleic acids. Amplification is used when there may be such low levels of the suspected microorganism in the specimen that it would not be detected using a direct probe. The HIV-2 nucleic acids are then detected using a variety of techniques. Test kits that may be used have three components: the specimen collection and preparation component, an amplification component, and a detection component. Red blood cells are selectively lysed leaving leukocytes intact. The leukocytes are pelleted and then washed several times. DNA is extracted from the pellet. Proviral HIV-2 DNA is then amplified. The detection component

is then used to determine whether HIV-2 DNA is present in the specimen. In 87539, the amount of the infectious agent in the sample is evaluated following amplification. Using reverse transcription and quantification techniques the HIV-2 viral load is determined. Quantification of HIV-2 is typically performed to evaluate response to treatment.

87590-87592

87590   Infectious agent detection by nucleic acid (DNA or RNA); Neisseria gonorrhoeae, direct probe technique
87591   Infectious agent detection by nucleic acid (DNA or RNA); Neisseria gonorrhoeae, amplified probe technique
87592   Infectious agent detection by nucleic acid (DNA or RNA); Neisseria gonorrhoeae, quantification

Neisseria gonorrhoeae (N. gonorrhoeae) causes gonorrhea, a sexually transmitted disease (STD), that is spread through direct contact and can infect the reproductive tract, mouth, throat, eyes, and anus. N. gonorrhoeae often causes no symptoms in women, but can cause irreversible damage to the reproductive tract of women which can result in infertility. In men, symptoms include burning, itching, and discharge of the urethra, but men rarely suffer reproductive damage from the infection. Some types of nucleic acid tests are rapid tests that may be performed in the physician office using a test kit. A swab is used to obtain a specimen from the cervix, male urethra, mouth, throat, or eye. In 87590, the exact methodology is dependent on the test kit used as there are several manufacturers. One test kit uses a nucleic acid hybridization method. A single stranded chemiluminescent DNA probe is used that is complementary to the ribosomal RNA of the N. gonorrhoeae organism. Lysate is used to rupture cells and release nucleic acids. The ribosomal RNA from the organism then combines with the labeled DNA probe to form a stable DNA:RNA hybrid. The presence of DNA:RNA hybrids is then detected using a luminometer. In 87591, an amplification technique, such as polymerase chain reaction (PCR) or transcription mediated amplification (TMA) is used to create copies of the N. gonorrhoeae nucleic acids. Amplification is used when there may be low levels of the suspected microorganism in the specimen that would not be detected using a direct probe. The N. gonorrhoeae nucleic acid is then detected using a variety of techniques. In 87592, the amplified product is quantified to provide an assessment of how many N. gonorrhoeae organisms are present. Quantification may be used to evaluate severity of infection and response to treatment.

87623-87625

87623   Infectious agent detection by nucleic acid (DNA or RNA); Human Papillomavirus (HPV), low-risk types (eg, 6, 11, 42, 43, 44)
87624   Infectious agent detection by nucleic acid (DNA or RNA); Human Papillomavirus (HPV), high-risk types (eg, 16, 18, 31, 33, 35, 39, 45, 51, 52, 56, 58, 59, 68)
87625   Infectious agent detection by nucleic acid (DNA or RNA); Human Papillomavirus (HPV), types 16 and 18 only, includes type 45, if performed

Human papillomavirus (HPV) invades skin and mucosal epithelia causing site specific clinical and subclinical infection. There are more than 100 types of HVP known to cause infection in humans, and 40 types can be found predominately in the anogenital tract. High risk oncogenic HPV types are frequently detected in high-grade squamous intraepithelial lesions (HSIL) and invasive cancers. Low risk HPV types are associated with acuminate condylomas of the genitals and low-grade squamous intraepithelial lesions (LSIL) of the cervix. Infectious agent detection by nucleic acid (DNA or RNA) for HPV is now considered routine in the management of cervical disease in women. Exfoliated cervical cells are collected using a cytobrush, swab, or plastic spatula and re-suspended in a liquid transport medium. The cell sample is treated with sodium hydroxide to denature the DNA and then hybridized in a solution with two mixtures of non-isotope single-stranded RNA probes. One probe detects 5 low risk HPV types and the other probe detects 13 high risk HPV types. The hybridized products are transferred to a microplate with antibody coated wells that will specifically recognize the HPV DNA/RNA hybrids. An alkaline phosphatase-labeled monoclonal antibody against the DNA/RNA hybrids is added along with a chemiluminescent substrate and the light produced is measured with an aluminometer to give the ratio of reactivity. Code 87623 is used when testing for low risk HPV types (6, 11, 42, 43 and 44). Code 87624 is used when testing for high risk HPV types (16, 18, 31, 33, 35, 39, 45, 51, 52, 56, 58, 59 and 68). Code 87624 is also the default code used when both low and high-risk types are tested within a single assay. Code 87625 is used when testing for HPV types 16 and 18 only, and includes type 45 also, if performed.

87631-87633

87631 Infectious agent detection by nucleic acid (DNA or RNA); respiratory virus (eg, adenovirus, influenza virus, coronavirus, metapneumovirus, parainfluenza virus, respiratory syncytial virus, rhinovirus), includes multiplex reverse transcription, when performed, and multiplex amplified probe technique, multiple types or subtypes, 3-5 targets

87632 Infectious agent detection by nucleic acid (DNA or RNA); respiratory virus (eg, adenovirus, influenza virus, coronavirus, metapneumovirus, parainfluenza virus, respiratory syncytial virus, rhinovirus), includes multiplex reverse transcription, when performed, and multiplex amplified probe technique, multiple types or subtypes, 6-11 targets

87633 Infectious agent detection by nucleic acid (DNA or RNA); respiratory virus (eg, adenovirus, influenza virus, coronavirus, metapneumovirus, parainfluenza virus, respiratory syncytial virus, rhinovirus), includes multiplex reverse transcription, when performed, and multiplex amplified probe technique, multiple types or subtypes, 12-25 targets

A test is performed on a respiratory specimen obtained by bronchoalveolar lavage, nasal wash, nasopharyngeal swab, or pleural fluid aspiration to identify specific types or subtypes of certain respiratory viral infections which may include adenovirus, influenza virus, coronavirus, metapneumovirus, parainfluenza virus, respiratory syncytial virus (RSV), and/or rhinovirus. The specimen is tested using DNA or RNA multiplex reverse transcription and amplification probe technique. Using multiplex reverse transcription polymerase chain reaction (RT-PCR), DNA or RNA from multiple types or subtypes of specific respiratory viruses is extracted and amplified. The amplified DNA or RNA fragments are sized and analyzed for the specific types or subtypes. Use 87631 for 3-5 targets (types or subtypes) of the specific respiratory viruses. Use 87632 for 6-11 targets. Use 87633 for 12-25 targets.

87640-87641

87640 Infectious agent detection by nucleic acid (DNA or RNA); Staphylococcus aureus, amplified probe technique

87641 Infectious agent detection by nucleic acid (DNA or RNA); Staphylococcus aureus, methicillin resistant, amplified probe technique

These codes report amplified probe technique detection of Staphylococcus aureus infection (87640) or methicillin resistant Staphylococcus aureus infection by DNA or RNA (87641). Nucleic acid detection for diagnostic purposes is a useful alternative to culturing. DNA probing also detects much lower levels of the infectious agent, sometimes even the presence of a single organism. Probing involves identifying the infectious agent DNA or RNA by releasing it from the cell and extracting it through nucleic acid hybridization using a probe. The probe consists of laboratory-prepared, complimentary strands of nucleic acid, often labeled with chemical fluorescence, specifically designed to align and bind with the target DNA to form stable, double-stranded complexes or hybrids. Amplified probing provides greater sensitivity for more direct, qualitative detection by using techniques such as polymerase chain reaction to enzymatically replicate certain target sequences or positions in the DNA to amplify it exponentially. An amplification primer is used in addition to the probe. Primers are artificial, short strands of DNA complementary to the beginning or end of the DNA fragment to be amplified. The primer adheres to the target DNA at these points. The polymerase enzyme copies the region and builds the new DNA.

87653

87653 Infectious agent detection by nucleic acid (DNA or RNA); Streptococcus, group B, amplified probe technique

Nucleic acid detection for diagnostic purposes is a useful alternative to culturing. DNA probing also detects much lower levels of the infectious agent, sometimes even the presence of a single organism. Probing involves identifying the infectious agent DNA or RNA by releasing it from the cell and extracting it through nucleic acid hybridization using a probe. The probe consists of laboratory-prepared, complimentary strands of nucleic acid, often labeled with chemical fluorescence, specifically designed to align and bind with the target DNA to form stable, double-stranded complexes or hybrids. Amplified probing provides greater sensitivity for more direct, qualitative detection by using techniques such as polymerase chain reaction to enzymatically replicate certain target sequences or positions in the DNA to amplify it exponentially. An amplification primer is used in addition to the probe. Primers are artificial, short strands of DNA complementary to the beginning or end of the DNA fragment to be amplified. The primer adheres to the target DNA at these points. The polymerase enzyme copies the region and builds the new DNA.

87660

87660 Infectious agent detection by nucleic acid (DNA or RNA); Trichomonas vaginalis, direct probe technique

Trichomonas vaginalis (T. vaginalis) is a single celled protozoan parasite that causes trichomoniasis. Trichomoniasis is a sexually transmitted disease (STD) that causes vaginal itching, burning and discharge as well as discomfort during intercourse and painful urination. Some types of nucleic acid tests are rapid tests that may be performed in the physician office using a test kit. A vaginal swab is obtained and incubated with lysate

to rupture all cells and release nucleic acids. The lysate is placed in the sample well and the test slide is dipped and incubated robotically. The T. vaginalis specific probe is attached to a stationary microparticle bead in the test well. The bead captures the target DNA sequence and holds it on the slide. The slide is washed to remove cellular debris and unbound nucleic acids. A second probe containing a color development substrate is added. The slide is again washed and an enzyme added to catalyze the color substrate. If T. vaginalis is present, the bead will change color indicating a positive result. If it is not present no color change occurs.

87661

87661 Infectious agent detection by nucleic acid (DNA or RNA); Trichomonas vaginalis, amplified probe technique

Trichomonas vaginalis is a single cell protozoan that commonly causes vaginitis. The organism is sexually transmitted and can infect both the urethra and vagina. Rapid direct identification of Trichomonas by nucleic acid (DNA or RNA) can be accomplished using amplified probe technique on the patient sample and can definitively diagnose trichomonas vaginalis infection even in the presence of other organisms and host DNA. A vaginal swab is obtained and incubated with lysate to rupture all cells and release nucleic acids. The technique depends on the recognition of a specific nucleotide sequence present in the clinical sample using a radiolabeled or nonisotopically labeled DNA probe. The probe consists of laboratory-prepared, complimentary strands of nucleic acid often labeled with chemical fluorescence, specifically designed to align and bind with the target DNA to form stable, double-stranded complexes or hybrids. Amplified probing provides greater sensitivity for more direct qualitative detection by using techniques such as polymerase chain reaction to enzymatically replicate certain target sequences or positions in the DNA to amplify it exponentially. An amplification primer is used in addition to the probe. Primers are artificial, short strands of DNA complementary to the beginning or end of the DNA fragment to be amplified. The primer adheres to the target DNA at these points. The polymerase enzyme copies the region and builds the new DNA.

87802

87802 Infectious agent antigen detection by immunoassay with direct optical observation; Streptococcus, group B

Strep B causes life-threatening infections in newborns, including pneumonia, meningitis, and sepsis. It can also cause serious infections, such as sepsis, urinary tract infections, skin infections, and pneumonia in pregnant women, the elderly and immunocompromised individuals. This test is used to screen for Strep B during pregnancy. A specimen is obtained by swabbing the cervix and the lower third of the vagina. A rapid test kit is used to detect Strep B antigens and the exact procedure will depend on the test manufacturer. This is a description of the basic process. The first of several reagents is introduced into antigen extraction tube followed by the swab containing the specimen which is used to mix the solution. A second reagent is added and mixed with the swab. The swab is left in the solution for several minutes. The swab is then removed and a third reagent introduced. A pipette is used to transfer the solution in the specimen tube to test device. The surface is washed with a fourth reagent. A drop of substrate is applied and then washed. The device is then examined under bright light. If the test is positive both a control spot and the test spot will change color.

87803

87803 Infectious agent antigen detection by immunoassay with direct optical observation; Clostridium difficile toxin A

Clostridium difficile toxin (C. difficile) is a spore-forming, gram-positive, anaerobic bacillus that produces two exotoxins, toxin A and B. C. difficile testing is performed on patients on antibiotics with suspected antibiotic-associated diarrhea. C. difficile can cause pseudomenbranous colitis, toxic megacolon, perforations of the colon, and sepsis. A fecal specimen is obtained. A test kit is used to perform rapid chromatographic immunoassay to test for the presence of C. difficile Toxin A in the stool sample. The kit uses a series of reagents that detect the C. difficile antigen. Presence of the toxin is identified by observing a color change on the test strip or other testing platform. If the toxin is present, a test line or dot will change color as will a second control line or dot.

87804

87804 Infectious agent antigen detection by immunoassay with direct optical observation; Influenza

A quick test to detect influenza (Type A or B) by immunoassay with direct optical observation is performed. It is a rapid, qualitative test performed using lateral flow immunoassay. Influenza is an acute, highly contagious, viral upper respiratory infection. There are three types of influenza viruses delineated as Type A, B, or C with Type A being the most severe and prevalent type. Type B is generally less severe. Type C is the least common and is not associated with large human epidemics. Type A and B can both be detected by a rapid test. A nasal or nasopharyngeal swab is obtained. Alternatively nasal wash or aspirate may be used. The specimen is placed in a tube containting an extraction reagent that disrupts the virus particles in the specimen and exposes viral nucleoproteins. A test strip is then inserted into the tube. If the influenza virus being tested (Type A or B) is present, a line on the test strip will change color along with a control line. If the specimen is tested for both Type A and B, report 87804 twice.

87806

87806 **Infectious agent antigen detection by immunoassay with direct optical observation; HIV-1 antigen(s), with HIV-1 and HIV-2 antibodies**

Human immunodeficiency virus (HIV) is a retrovirus that affects the immune system by destroying CD4+ positive T-cells. The virus is spread by sexual contact, exposure to blood or blood products and from infected mother to her fetus/neonate during the perinatal period. HIV type 1 (HIV-1) is the major etiologic agent for acquired immune deficiency syndrome (AIDS) worldwide, while HIV type 2 (HIV-2) is primarily found in West Africa. HIV antigen can be found in serum, plasma, and whole blood 12-26 days after infection. HIV antibodies appear 20-45 days after infection. HIV-1 p24 antigen and HIV-1, HIV-2 antibodies can be detected with a rapid, immunochromatographic test utilizing immunoassay and direct optical observation in the point of care setting (clinic, physician office). This screening test is used primarily for at risk, asymptomatic individuals. The commercial test strip (Alere Determine) is opened and the sample is applied. When testing serum/plasma, a second step is not necessary. When using whole blood, a drop of buffering solution is applied. The test strip has both a control zone and a patient section. The control will show a red line in the middle of the test zone with both a negative and positive patient result. A positive patient result will have a red line in the middle of the patient test section, a negative patient result will not.

87807

87807 **Infectious agent antigen detection by immunoassay with direct optical observation; respiratory syncytial virus**

Respiratory syncytial virus (RSV) causes an acute, highly contagious infection of the respiratory tract that may include bronchiolitis and pneumonia requiring hospitalization particularly in children under the age of one. This test is a rapid, qualitative dipstick immunoassay that detects RSV antigen from a nasopharyngeal swab or aspirate. The specimen is placed in a tube containing a reagent that extracts the RSV antigen. The dipstick is then placed in the tube where RSV antigen will react with the reagents in the test strip. If the specimen contains RSV antigen the test line on the dipstick will change color as will a second control line indicating a positive result.

87808

87808 **Infectious agent antigen detection by immunoassay with direct optical observation; Trichomonas vaginalis**

Trichomonas vaginalis is a protozoan parasite with four flagella found in the genital tract and is the most common type of non-viral sexually transmitted disease, which may be asymptomatic when present, but leads to increase risks for HIV infection and cervical neoplasia. The enzyme immunoassay test is performed on the clinical sample, often a vaginal swabbing. The sample is placed onto a microtiter plate which has been coated with antibodies to Trichomonas vaginalis. After incubation, the antigen is captured within the antibody-antigen binding complex that forms. After washing, the antigen in the complex is probed by incubating with an enzyme conjugated form of anti-T. vaginalis antigen. The sample is washed again and an enzyme substrate and chromogenic reagent are added. Incubation is halted by adding an acid, which also changes the amount of color produced by the chromogenic agent. The amount of T. vaginalis present in the sample is proportional to the optical density measured in a photometer.

87809

87809 **Infectious agent antigen detection by immunoassay with direct optical observation; adenovirus**

Infectious agent antigen detection of adenovirus is performed by immunoassay with direct optical observation. Adenoviral infections are caused by a group of viruses that can infect the membranes of the respiratory tract, eyes, intestines, and urinary tract. This code reports a rapid detection technique for adenovirus infections of the eye. The lower eyelid is pulled back to expose the inner fornix. A sample collection pad provided with the rapid test kit is dabbed on the inside of the lower eyelid until it is saturated. The pad is then processed per the rapid test kit instructions by placing it in a buffer solution for the specified amount of time, waiting for the results to develop, and then reading the results to determine the presence of adenovirus eye infection.

87810

87810 **Infectious agent antigen detection by immunoassay with direct optical observation; Chlamydia trachomatis**

A direct optical test to detect Chlamydia trachomatis is a rapid, qualitative test performed using lateral flow immunoassay. C. trachomati is a sexually transmitted disease (STD) that often causes no symptoms, but that can cause irreversible damage to the reproductive tract of women which can result in infertility. In men, symptoms include burning and itching of the urethra, but men rarely suffer reproductive damage from the infection. This type of quick test is typically performed on women. The exocervix is swabbed to remove

excess mucous. A second swab or cytology brush is then used to obtain columnar or cuboidal cells, the main reservoir of Chlamydia organisms, from the endocervical canal. The specimen is placed in a tube containing a reagent and incubated for a few minutes. A second reagent is then added and incubated. A sample is extracted from the test tube and added to a test cassette. If the sample contains C. trachomatis antigen the test line will change color as will a second control line.

87850

87850 **Infectious agent antigen detection by immunoassay with direct optical observation; Neisseria gonorrhoeae**

N. gonorrhoeae causes gonorrhea, a sexually transmitted disease (STD), that is spread through direct contact and can infect the reproductive tract, mouth, throat, eyes , and anus. N. gonorrhoeae often causes no symptoms in women, but that can cause irreversible damage to the reproductive tract of women which can result in infertility. In men, symptoms include burning, itching, and discharge of the urethra, but men rarely suffer reproductive damage from the infection. A swab is used to obtain a specimen from the cervix, male urethra, mouth, throat, or eye. Alternatively a urine sample may be obtained. This test is a rapid, qualitative sandwich immunoassay that detects gonorrhea antigen in the specimen. The specimen is placed in a tube containing a reagent that extracts the gonorrhea antigen. Monoclonal and polyclonal antibodies are then used to identify N. gonorrhoeae. If the sample contains the antigen the test strip, line or dot will change color as will a second control strip, line or dot indicating a positive result.

87880

87880 **Infectious agent antigen detection by immunoassay with direct optical observation; Streptococcus, group A**

A direct optical test to detect Streptococcus Group A (Strep A) by immunoassay is a rapid, qualitative test performed using lateral flow immunoassay. Strep A causes acute upper respiratory infection with the most common symptoms being pharyngitis (sore throat) and fever. If left untreated serious complications can occur including rheumatic fever and glomerulonephritis. This type of test is a rapid, qualitative test performed using lateral flow immunoassay. A throat swab is obtained. Two reagents are added to extract Strep A antigen from the specimen. A dipstick is added to the extracted sample. If Strep A antigen is present the test line and a control line will change color indicating a positive test. Another method uses a throat swab specimen inserted into a test cassette. Antigen extraction solutions are then mixed in a separate chamber of the tube and added to the swab chamber. If Strep A is present, a test line will change color as will a second control line.

87901

87901 **Infectious agent genotype analysis by nucleic acid (DNA or RNA); HIV-1, reverse transcriptase and protease regions**

This test is used to analyze and identify mutations in HIV-1 genes that cause resistance to 19 commonly prescribed reverse transcriptase and protease inhibitors, which are types of medications used to treat HIV-1. Human immunodeficiency virus (HIV) attacks the immune system by destroying T cells or CD4 cells which are a type of white blood cell. This hampers the ability of the body to fight infection. HIV is the virus that causes acquired immunodeficiency syndrome (AIDS) and AIDS is the final stage of HIV infection. HIV is an RNA virus with a high replication rate. The reverse transcription enzyme required for replication can cause mutations and some of these mutations result in resistance to anti-viral drugs. Initial drug therapy for HIV typically uses a combination of anti-retrovirals with different mechanisms of action to reduce the viral load and help prevent mutations that cause drug resistance. This is referred to as highly active anti-retroviral therapy (HAART). When initial drug therapy fails, a genotype analysis is performed using reverse transcriptase and protease genes to detect known mutations that cause drug resistance. Genotyping is a very complex test that uses a blood sample to evaluate HIV-1 for the presence of specific nucleic acid sequences. Three steps are required. First, one or more very specific nucleic acid sequences are amplified using a technique such as polymerase chain reaction (PCR). Next, the amplified product is purified and further molecular analysis is performed. Then, the amplified sequence is compared to known sequences that confer known drug resistance. This information is used to develop a drug regimen that will better control the HIV infection.

87902

87902 **Infectious agent genotype analysis by nucleic acid (DNA or RNA); Hepatitis C virus**

Infectious agent genotype analysis by nucleic acid (DNA or RNA) for Hepatitis C is performed by reverse transcriptase and protease. The Hepatitis C virus (HCV) causes an acute inflammation of the liver that can become chronic, causing impairment of liver function, cirrhosis, and liver cancer. HCV has six major genotypes with more than 90 subtypes that vary in their response to antiviral therapy. Genotype 1 is associated with 70% of the cases in the United States and has a relatively poor response to drug therapy. Genotype 1 is also associated with a higher incidence of liver cancer. Genotyping of HCV is used to determine the specific genotype so that the most effective treatment plan can be developed. Genotyping is a very complex test that uses a blood sample to evaluate

● New Code   ▲ Revised Code

Pathology and Laboratory

HCV for the presence of specific nucleic acid sequences. Three steps are required. First, one or more very specific nucleic acid sequences are amplified using a technique such as polymerase chain reaction (PCR). Next, the amplified product is purified and further molecular analysis is performed. Then, the amplified sequence is compared to known sequences to determine the specific HCV genotype.

87903-87904

87903   **Infectious agent phenotype analysis by nucleic acid (DNA or RNA) with drug resistance tissue culture analysis, HIV 1; first through 10 drugs tested**

87904   **Infectious agent phenotype analysis by nucleic acid (DNA or RNA) with drug resistance tissue culture analysis, HIV 1; each additional drug tested (List separately in addition to code for primary procedure)**

Infectious agent phenotype analysis by nucleic acid (DNA or RNA) for HIV I is performed with drug resistance tissue culture analysis for HIV I. Human immunodeficiency virus (HIV) attacks the immune system by destroying T cells or CD4 cells which are a type of white blood cell. This hampers the ability of the body to fight infection. HIV is the virus that causes acquired immunodeficiency syndrome (AIDS) and AIDS is the final stage of HIV infection. Phenotyping is typically performed on a blood sample but a tissue sample may also be used. The blood or tissue is cultured and tested for drug resistance using multiple anti-retroviral drugs and different concentrations of these drugs. This is an extremely complicated test requiring high labor inputs and skilled clinicians to perform and accurately interpret the results. Use 87903 for the first ten drugs tested and 87904 for each additional drug.

87905

87905   **Infectious agent enzymatic activity other than virus (eg, sialidase activity in vaginal fluid)**

A body fluid specimen is obtained, such as a vaginal swab for vaginal fluid, to test for infectious agent enzymatic activity other than that due to viral infection, such as sialidase activity. Sialidases are enzymes that enhance the ability of microorganisms to invade and destroy tissue. Elevated levels of sialidase activity in vaginal fluid may be an indication of bacterial vaginosis. To test for sialidase, the lower third of the vaginal wall is swabbed. The swab is rotated for 10 to 20 seconds to collect a sufficient amount of fluid and then placed in a tube, which is capped. A chromogenic enzyme activity test is performed to identify the presence of sialidase activity. Code 87905 may be used to report other enzymatic activity tests for infectious agents other than viruses in other body fluids.

87906

87906   **Infectious agent genotype analysis by nucleic acid (DNA or RNA); HIV-1, other region (eg, integrase, fusion)**

This test is used to analyze and identify mutations in HIV-1 genes that cause resistance to certain drug regimens other than reverse transcriptase and protease inhibitors, such as mutations to the HIV-1 integrase gene which indicates that the infection is resistant to HIV integrase inhibitor drugs, including raltegravir and eltigravir. Human immunodeficiency virus (HIV) attacks the immune system by destroying T cells or CD4 cells which are a type of white blood cell. This hampers the ability of the body to fight infection. HIV is the virus that causes acquired immunodeficiency syndrome (AIDS) and AIDS is the final stage of HIV infection. HIV is an RNA virus with a high replication rate. The reverse transcription enzyme required for replication can cause mutations and some of these mutations result in resistance to anti-viral drugs. Initial drug therapy for HIV typically uses a combination of anti-retrovirals with different mechanisms of action to reduce the viral load and help prevent mutations that cause drug resistance. This is referred to as highly active anti-retroviral therapy (HAART). When initial drug therapy fails, a genotype analysis is performed. Genotyping is a very complex test that uses a blood sample to evaluate HIV-1 for the presence of specific nucleic acid sequences. Three steps are required. First, one or more very specific nucleic acid sequences are amplified using a technique such as polymerase chain reaction (PCR). Next, the amplified product is purified and further molecular analysis is performed. Then, the amplified sequence is compared to known sequences that confer known drug resistance. This information is used to develop a drug regimen that will better control the HIV infection.

87910

87910   **Infectious agent genotype analysis by nucleic acid (DNA or RNA); cytomegalovirus**

A blood test is performed to identify the specific cytomegalovirus (CMV) genotype in a patient who tests positive for CMV infection. CMV is a common infection that rarely causes symptoms in healthy individuals. When the immune system is impaired (e.g., transplant recipients, HIV), the virus can multiply and cause acute infection. Genotyping amplifies and increases targeted DNA to permit detection. Identification of the specific genotype can provide prognostic information and identify antiviral treatment choices. A blood sample is obtained by separately reportable venipuncture. Serum or plasma is tested using polymerase chain reaction/sequencing.

87912

87912   **Infectious agent genotype analysis by nucleic acid (DNA or RNA); Hepatitis B virus**

A blood test is performed to identify the specific hepatitis B virus (HBV) genotype in patients who test positive for HBV. HBV is an infection that can damage the liver and may lead to liver cancer. Genotyping amplifies and increases targeted DNA to permit detection. Identification of the specific genotype can provide prognostic information and identify antiviral treatment choices. A blood sample is obtained by separately reportable venipuncture. Serum or plasma is tested using polymerase chain reaction/sequencing.

88025

88025   **Necropsy (autopsy), gross and microscopic; with brain**

An autopsy is performed on a corpse by a physician or other medical professional. The body is opened and internal organs are removed and studied. Tissue samples from organs or other body parts may be microscopically examined and/or subjected to laboratory tests. The brain is examined, and portions of it may be studied under a microscope and/or be subjected to lab tests.

88027

88027   **Necropsy (autopsy), gross and microscopic; with brain and spinal cord**

An autopsy is performed on a corpse by a physician or other medical professional. The body is opened and internal organs are removed and studied. Tissue samples from organs or other body parts may be microscopically examined and/or subjected to laboratory tests. The brain and spinal cord are examined, and portions of them may be studied under a microscope and/or be subjected to lab tests.

88028

88028   **Necropsy (autopsy), gross and microscopic; infant with brain**

An autopsy is performed on the corpse of an infant by a physician or other medical professional. The body is opened and internal organs are removed and studied. Tissue samples from organs or other body parts may be microscopically examined and/or subjected to laboratory tests. The brain is examined, and portions of it may be studied under a microscope and/or be subjected to lab tests.

88029

88029   **Necropsy (autopsy), gross and microscopic; stillborn or newborn with brain**

An autopsy is performed on the corpse of a stillborn or newborn infant by a physician or other medical professional. The body is opened and internal organs are removed and studied. Tissue samples from organs or other body parts may be microscopically examined and/or subjected to laboratory tests. The brain is examined, and portions of it may be studied under a microscope and/or be subjected to lab tests.

88037

88037   **Necropsy (autopsy), limited, gross and/or microscopic; single organ**

An autopsy is performed on a corpse by a physician or other medical professional. The body is opened and a single organ is removed and studied. Tissue samples from the organ may be microscopically examined and/or subjected to laboratory tests.

88040

88040   **Necropsy (autopsy); forensic examination**

An autopsy is performed by a coroner or other medical professional. The body is opened and internal organs are removed and studied. Tissue samples from organs or other body parts may be microscopically examined and/or subjected to laboratory tests. This code denotes an autopsy performed to aid in a criminal investigation. Code 88045 if a coroner is called upon to perform the autopsy and/or provide a death certificate.

88045

88045   **Necropsy (autopsy); coroner's call**

An autopsy is performed by a coroner or other medical professional. The body is opened and internal organs are removed and studied. Tissue samples from organs or other body parts may be microscopically examined and/or subjected to laboratory tests. This code denotes an autopsy performed to aid in a criminal investigation. Code 88045 if a coroner is called upon to perform the autopsy and/or provide a death certificate.

88120-88121

88121 Cytopathology, in situ hybridization (eg, FISH), urinary tract specimen with morphometric analysis, 3-5 molecular probes, each specimen; using computer-assisted technology

88120 Cytopathology, in situ hybridization (eg, FISH), urinary tract specimen with morphometric analysis, 3-5 molecular probes, each specimen; manual

A specimen containing cells from the urinary tract, such as a urine sample or bladder irrigation (washing) specimen, is tested for the presence of abnormal cells using an in situ hybridization technique such as fluorescence in situ hybridization (FISH). This test evaluates exfoliated urothelial cells for genetic alterations indicative of urinary tract cancer. The test involves the use of multiple (3-5) DNA probes that identify chromosome changes in specific regions of specific chromosomes that are indicative of a urinary tract cancer. A DNA probe is labeled with fluorescent dye and applied to cells in which the nuclei are in interphase. The probe binds to its complementary sequence and labels a specific chromosome which is then visualized under fluorescent microscope. Nuclei exhibiting chromosomal changes indicative of urothelial cancer fluoresce when viewed under the fluorescent microscope. Use 88120 for a manual test. Use 88121 when computer-assisted technology is used to evaluate the specimen. Report these codes for each specimen tested using manual or computer-assisted technology.

88130-88140

88130 Sex chromatin identification; Barr bodies

88140 Sex chromatin identification; peripheral blood smear, polymorphonuclear drumsticks

In 88130, a buccal smear is obtained and X-chromatin is identified by staining interphase cells with orcein. X-chromosomes appear as a dark body also referred to as a Barr body. The number of Barr bodies in the cell relates to the number of X-chromosomes in the cell. The number of X chromosomes in the cell is equal to the number of inactivated X-chromosomes in the cell minus one. XY males have no Barr bodies. XX females have one Barr body. XXX females have two Barr bodies. In 88140, a peripheral blood sample is obtained. An X-chromosome specific nucleic acid probe is used to identify X-chromosomes in leukocyte nuclei. Following in situ hybridization of the smear, the specimen is examined for drumstick-like structures in the polymorphonuclear leukocytes which are present only in females.

88141

88141 Cytopathology, cervical or vaginal (any reporting system), requiring interpretation by physician

Cytopathology examination is performed to determine whether there are any changes within the cell structure itself that would indicate disease. This test can detect changes such as cervical dysplasia and in situ carcinoma, so that monitoring and treatment can be provided before these conditions progress to invasive malignant disease. This test is also referred to as a Papanicolaou (PAP) smear. A pathologist reviews the PAP smear findings after a PAP smear evaluated by any type reporting system has been determined to have changes in cell structure requiring physician interpretation. If the findings are abnormal, the pathologist may recommend another PAP smear during a shorter time interval than usual or the performance of additional tests such as colposcopy, endocervical curettage or biopsy.

88142-88143

88142 Cytopathology, cervical or vaginal (any reporting system), collected in preservative fluid, automated thin layer preparation; manual screening under physician supervision

88143 Cytopathology, cervical or vaginal (any reporting system), collected in preservative fluid, automated thin layer preparation; with manual screening and rescreening under physician supervision

Cytopathology examination is performed to determine whether there are any changes within the cell structure itself that would indicate disease. This test can detect changes such as cervical dysplasia and in situ carcinoma, so that monitoring and treatment can be provided before these conditions progress to invasive malignant disease. This test is also referred to as a Papanicolaou (PAP) smear. Cells are collected from the endocervix using a special stick or brush. The specimen is placed in preservative fluid and sent to the laboratory. At the laboratory the liquid cell suspension is centrifuged to remove debris and reduce the cervical cells so that the cells can be retrieved. The cells are then prepared using an automated system that stains and transfers cells to slides and coverslips the slides. The slides are then examined under a microscope. In 88142, the manual screening is performed by a trained technician under physician (pathologist) supervision. In 88143, the manual screening is performed by a trained technician and is then manually rescreened under physician (pathologist) supervision. Manual rescreening involves a complete reassessment of the entire slide, which may be performed by a second technician. Findings are communicated to the treating physician. If the findings are abnormal, the pathologist may recommend another PAP smear during a shorter time interval than usual or the performance of additional tests such as colposcopy, endocervical curettage or biopsy.

88147-88148

88147 Cytopathology smears, cervical or vaginal; screening by automated system under physician supervision

88148 Cytopathology smears, cervical or vaginal; screening by automated system with manual rescreening under physician supervision

Cytopathology examination is performed to determine whether there are any changes within the cell structure itself that would indicate disease. This test can detect changes such as cervical dysplasia and in situ carcinoma, so that monitoring and treatment can be provided before these conditions progress to invasive malignant disease. This test is also referred to as a Papanicolaou (PAP) smear. Cells are collected from the endocervix using a special stick or brush. The specimen is placed on a slide, prepared, and coverslipped. Using an automated microscope, a full color camera, and high-speed image processing computer, the automated system screens slides for evidence of abnormalities. Abnormal cells or cell clusters are then pinpointed and these images stored in the computer. In 88147, a technician evaluates the automated results under physician supervision. In 88148, a technician evaluates the automated screening and then manually rescreens the PAP smear using a microscope under physician (pathologist) supervision. Manual rescreening involves a complete reassessment of the entire slide. Findings are communicated to the treating physician. If the findings are abnormal, the pathologist may recommend another PAP smear during a shorter time interval than usual or the performance of additional tests such as colposcopy, endocervical curettage or biopsy.

88150-88154

88150 Cytopathology, slides, cervical or vaginal; manual screening under physician supervision

88152 Cytopathology, slides, cervical or vaginal; with manual screening and computer-assisted rescreening under physician supervision

88153 Cytopathology, slides, cervical or vaginal; with manual screening and rescreening under physician supervision

88154 Cytopathology, slides, cervical or vaginal; with manual screening and computer-assisted rescreening using cell selection and review under physician supervision

This test is also referred to as a Papanicolaou (PAP) smear. These codes are used for conventional PAP smears that are examined using a non-Bethesda reporting system, such as the class system, the dysplasia system or the cervical intraepithelial neoplasia (CIN) system. PAP smears are used to determine whether there are any changes within the cell structure itself that would indicate disease. This test can detect changes such as cervical dysplasia and in situ carcinoma, so that monitoring and treatment can be provided before these conditions progress to invasive malignant disease. Cells are collected from the endocervix using a special stick or brush. The specimen is smeared on a slide, fixed using a spray or immersion, and coverslipped. The slide is sent to a cytology laboratory where it is stained. Using a microscope, a trained technician then screens the slide for evidence of abnormalities. Abnormal cells or cell clusters are pinpointed. In 88150, a single screening is performed by the technician under physician supervision. In 88152, a technician performs a manual screening using a microscope. The PAP smear is then rescreened using a computer. The computer is programmed to recognize suspicious single cells as well as abnormal cell structures. The technician then reviews the computer-assisted findings, compares these findings with the manual findings, and interprets the two screenings. In 88153, a technician manually screens the PAP smear using a microscope and then a manual rescreening is performed. Manual rescreening involves a complete reassessment of the entire slide, which may be performed by a second technician. In 88154, a technician performs a manual screening using a microscope. The PAP smear is then rescreened using a computer as described in 88152. Suspicious single cells and cell clusters are pinpointed for review by the technician. The technician then reviews the computer-assisted findings, carefully reviews pinpointed abnormalities, compares these findings with the manual findings, and interprets the two screenings. The PAP smear may be referred to a physician (pathologist) for separately reportable review and interpretation. Findings are communicated to the treating physician. If the findings are abnormal, the pathologist may recommend another PAP smear during a shorter time interval than usual or the performance of additional tests such as colposcopy, endocervical curettage or biopsy.

88155

88155 Cytopathology, slides, cervical or vaginal, definitive hormonal evaluation (eg, maturation index, karyopyknotic index, estrogenic index) (List separately in addition to code[s] for other technical and interpretation services)

A cervical or vaginal cell sample is obtained using a stick or brush. The cell sample is then smeared on a slide and the slide is coverslipped. A cytologic definitive hormonal evaluation involves examination of cervical or vaginal cells to identify any hormonal imbalances, such as those that might contribute to infertility. Cytologic hormone analysis is performed by identifying the degree of maturation of squamous epithelium, which is dependent on steroid hormones such as estrogen. Estrogen receptors are present in squamous epithelium of cervical and vaginal cells, especially in the basal cells. These estrogen receptors are expressed more strongly during the proliferative phase of the cell cycle than during the

Pathology and Laboratory

secretory phase. This results in changes in epithelial maturation, which can be seen in cells when they are examined under a microscope. A quantitative analysis of variations in the degree of maturation in these cells can be calculated. The maturation index (MI) reflects the relationship of parabasal cells to intermediate cells to superficial cells. The MI reflects the hormonal status of the woman being tested with normal levels for menstruating women at the time of ovulation being 0:35:65 and that of postmenopausal women being 90:10:0. The karyopyknotic index (KI) reflects the relationship of superficial squamous cells with pyknotic nuclei to all mature squamous cells. This index is used to detect ovulation as the KI is highest at this time. The estrogenic index may be used to evaluate the effectiveness of estrogen therapy on postmenopausal women.

88164-88167

88164　Cytopathology, slides, cervical or vaginal (the Bethesda System); manual screening under physician supervision

88165　Cytopathology, slides, cervical or vaginal (the Bethesda System); with manual screening and rescreening under physician supervision

88166　Cytopathology, slides, cervical or vaginal (the Bethesda System); with manual screening and computer-assisted rescreening under physician supervision

88167　Cytopathology, slides, cervical or vaginal (the Bethesda System); with manual screening and computer-assisted rescreening using cell selection and review under physician supervision

This test is also referred to as a Papanicolaou (PAP) smear. These codes report conventional PAP smears using the Bethesda reporting system, which is the most commonly used reporting system in the United States. The Bethesda system reports the following: adequacy of the PAP smear, evidence of infection, benign cellular changes, atypical squamous cell changes undetermined significance (ASCUS) favor benign or atypical glandular cell changes undetermined significance (AGCUS) favor benign, ASCUS or AGCUS favor dysplasia, or squamous intraepithelial lesions (SIL). Squamous intraepithelial lesions are then classified as low grade (LGSIL), high grade (HGSIL), or carcinoma. Cells are collected from the endocervix using a special stick or brush. The specimen is smeared on a slide, fixed using a spray or immersion, and coverslipped. The slide is sent to a cytology laboratory for where it is stained. Using a microscope, a trained technician then screens the slide for evidence of abnormalities. Abnormal cells or cell clusters are pinpointed. In 88164, a single screening is performed by the technician under physician supervision. In 88165, a technician performs a manual screening using a microscope. The PAP smear is then rescreened using a computer. The computer is programmed to recognize suspicious single cells as well as abnormal cell structures. The technician reviews the computer-assisted findings, compares these findings with the manual findings, and interprets the two screenings. In 88166, a technician manually screens the PAP smear using a microscope and then a manual rescreening is performed. Manual rescreening involves a complete reassessment of the entire slide, which may be performed by a second technician. In 88167, a technician performs a manual screening using a microscope. The PAP smear is then rescreened using a computer as described in 88165. Suspicious single cells and cell clusters are pinpointed for review by the technician. The technician then reviews the computer-assisted findings, carefully reviews pinpointed abnormalities, compares these findings with the manual findings, and interprets the two screenings. The PAP smear may be referred to a physician (pathologist) for separately reportable review and interpretation. Findings are communicated to the treating physician. If the findings are abnormal, the pathologist may recommend another PAP smear during a shorter time interval than usual or the performance of additional tests such as colposcopy, endocervical curettage or biopsy.

88172-88173

88172　Cytopathology, evaluation of fine needle aspirate; immediate cytohistologic study to determine adequacy for diagnosis, first evaluation episode, each site

88173　Cytopathology, evaluation of fine needle aspirate; interpretation and report

A separately reportable fine needle aspiration is performed to obtain fluid or tissue. The cells are placed on a slide at which time the cells form clusters of approximately 10 cells each. A smear is then created by laying another slide on top. Stains are used to enhance cellular detail as needed. The cells are then examined for evidence of disease, such as malignancy. In 88172, an immediate cytohistologic study is performed to determine the adequacy of the specimen. The physician examines the specimen under a microscope to determine whether the cell sample contains a sufficient number of cells for evaluation and diagnosis. Diagnostic accuracy increases when there are six or more cell clusters available for review. If an inadequate number of cells are present, the aspiration procedure may be repeated. Report this for the first evaluation episode for each site from which separate specimens are obtained. In 88173, a cell sample with an adequate number of cells is examined for definitive diagnosis. The cells are examined under a microscope for evidence of malignancy or other disease. The physician provides an interpretation which describes the characteristics of the cells in the sample and will typically indicate whether the cells are clearly benign, clearly malignant, or indeterminate—meaning no definitive diagnosis can be made. A written report is provided.

88174-88175

88174　Cytopathology, cervical or vaginal (any reporting system), collected in preservative fluid, automated thin layer preparation; screening by automated system, under physician supervision

88175　Cytopathology, cervical or vaginal (any reporting system), collected in preservative fluid, automated thin layer preparation; with screening by automated system and manual rescreening or review, under physician supervision

Cytopathology examination is performed to determine whether there are any changes within the cell structure itself that would indicate disease. This test can detect changes such as cervical dysplasia and in situ carcinoma, so that monitoring and treatment can be provided before these conditions progress to invasive malignant disease. This test is also referred to as a Papanicolaou (PAP) smear. Cells are collected from the endocervix using a special stick or brush. The specimen is placed in preservative fluid and sent to the laboratory. At the laboratory the liquid cell suspension is centrifuged to remove debris and reduce the cervical cells so that the cells can be retrieved. The cells are then prepared using an automated system that stains and transfers cells to slides and coverslips the slides. The automated system screens and interprets the prepared smears. In 88174, the automated screening is reviewed by a trained technician under physician (pathologist) supervision. In 88175, a technician evaluates the automated screening and then manually rescreens the PAP smear using a microscope under physician (pathologist) supervision. Manual rescreening involves a complete reassessment of the entire slide. If the findings are abnormal, the pathologist may recommend another PAP smear during a shorter time interval than usual or the performance of additional tests such as colposcopy, endocervical curettage or biopsy.

88177

88177　Cytopathology, evaluation of fine needle aspirate; immediate cytohistologic study to determine adequacy for diagnosis, each separate additional evaluation episode, same site (List separately in addition to code for primary procedure)

A separately reportable fine needle aspiration is performed to obtain fluid or tissue. Following a separately reportable initial evaluation episode, one or more additional cytohistologic studies are performed on a specimen from the same site to determine the adequacy of the specimen. The cells are placed on a slide at which time the cells form clusters of approximately 10 cells each. A smear is then created by laying another slide on top. Stains are used to enhance cellular detail as needed. The cells are then examined for evidence of disease, such as malignancy. The physician examines the specimen under a microscope to determine whether the cell sample contains a sufficient number of cells for evaluation and diagnosis. Diagnostic accuracy increases when there are six or more cell clusters available for review. If an inadequate number of cells are present, the aspiration procedure may be repeated. Report 88177 for each additional separate evaluation episode performed on a specimen from the same site following the initial evaluation episode.

88230-88235

88230　Tissue culture for non-neoplastic disorders; lymphocyte

88233　Tissue culture for non-neoplastic disorders; skin or other solid tissue biopsy

88235　Tissue culture for non-neoplastic disorders; amniotic fluid or chorionic villus cells

A tissue culture is obtained so that a separately reportable chromosome analysis for non-neoplastic disorders can be performed. Non-neoplastic disorders include sister chromatid exchange (SCE), breakage syndromes, trisomies, mosaicism, as well as other genetic conditions that cause congenital or other anomalies. In 88230, lymphocytes are cultured. A peripheral blood sample is obtained and lymphocytes (white blood cells) are separated from other blood constituents. The lymphocytes are cultured and stimulated to divide using an aspecific antigen such as phytohaemoagglutinin. A spindle inhibitor is then added to block cells in metaphase from a second mitosis. This ensures that the specimen will have a sufficient number of mitotic cells for analysis. Depending on the specific chromosome analysis being performed, different stains or chemicals may be added to the tissue culture. In 88233, skin or other solid tissue is biopsied and the skin or solid tissue is cultured to promote cell growth in a manner similar to that described in 88230. In 88235, amniotic fluid or chorionic villus cells are cultured. A separately reportable amniocentesis or chorionic villus sampling (CVS) is performed. The amniotic fluid is collected using special syringes and placed in screw top tubes. Alternatively, a CVS specimen may be obtained and a stereomicroscope and sterile gloves used to remove any blood clots before placing the specimen in screw top tubes. The amniotic fluid or CVS is then transported to the lab in culture medium where the cells are cultured for use in a genetic testing (chromosome analysis) procedure.

88245-88249

88245 Chromosome analysis for breakage syndromes; baseline Sister Chromatid Exchange (SCE), 20-25 cells

88248 Chromosome analysis for breakage syndromes; baseline breakage, score 50-100 cells, count 20 cells, 2 karyotypes (eg, for ataxia telangiectasia, Fanconi anemia, fragile X)

88249 Chromosome analysis for breakage syndromes; score 100 cells, clastogen stress (eg, diepoxybutane, mitomycin C, ionizing radiation, UV radiation)

A chromosome analysis is performed for breakage syndromes. In 88245, Sister Chromatid Exchange (SCE) test is performed. Sister chromatids are those derived from the same chromosomes during cell replication. Exchanges between sister chromatids are rare. However, exposure to certain chemicals and infective agents as well as some physiological disorders is associated with an increased frequency of SCE. The test is performed using peripheral blood lymphocytes that are cultured in a separately reportable procedure and stimulated to divide using an aspecific antigen such as phytohaemoagglutinin. A spindle inhibitor is then added to block cells in metaphase from a second mitosis. This ensures that the specimen will have a sufficient number of mitotic cells for analysis. Bromo-deoxy-uridine (BrdU) is then added to the culture medium for the duration of two complete cell cycles. BrdU allows for differential staining of both chromatids. Chromatids in which only one strand of DNA is incorporated show dark Giemsa staining whereas those with two substituted strands stain less darkly. If an exchange occurred, dark staining is seen on one arm of the chromosome. Chromosomes with exchanges are called harlequin chromosomes. In 88248, lymphocytes are cultured in a separately reportable procedure and special techniques used to produce elongated or prometaphase chromosomes so that specific breakage syndromes, such as ataxia telangiectasia, Fanconi anemia, or fragile X, can be identified. The technique is similar to that described above except that 50-100 cells are scored, 20 cells are counted, and two karyotyping procedures performed. Karyotyping is an evaluation of the size, shape, and number of chromosomes in the cell samples. Banding is a chromosome staining technique used to identify individual chromosomes that produce characteristic bands. Giemsa banding is a complex process that involves acetic acid fixation, air drying, denaturing of chromosomes by proteolytic enzymes or other technique, and Giemsa staining. Alternatively, chromosome banding may be performed using fluorochrome and Q-banding stain. Any extra, missing, or abnormal positions of chromosome pieces are identified. Two karyotypes are present in some individuals with some chromosomal abnormalities. This means that some cells have a normal 46XX or 46XY chromosome count, while other cells have breakage with translocation or trisomies. In 88249, 100 cells are scored and a clastogen stress test is performed. In some patients with symptoms of a breakage syndrome, spontaneous chromosome breakage is not demonstrated when chromosome analysis is performed for breakage syndromes. However, stressing cells with chemical agents or radiation often allows detection of the breakage syndrome as well as identification of the specific breakage syndrome genotype. For example, clastogen stress test helps detect Franconi anemia homozygotes and heterozygotes (expressed as fa/fa, Fa/fa, FA/FA).

88261-88264

88261 Chromosome analysis; count 5 cells, 1 karyotype, with banding

88262 Chromosome analysis; count 15-20 cells, 2 karyotypes, with banding

88263 Chromosome analysis; count 45 cells for mosaicism, 2 karyotypes, with banding

88264 Chromosome analysis; analyze 20-25 cells

All tests are performed using using peripheral blood lymphocytes, skin or solid tissue that is cultured in a separately reportable procedure. In 88261, five cells are identified and a single karyotype analysis performed with banding. Karyotyping is an evaluation of the size, shape, and number of chromosomes in the cell samples. Banding is a chromosome staining technique used to identify individual chromosomes that produce characteristic bands. Giemsa banding is a complex process that involves acetic acid fixation, air drying, denaturing of chromosomes by proteolytic enzymes or other technique, and Giemsa staining. Alternatively, chromosome banding may be performed using fluorochrome and Q-banding stain. Any extra, missing, or abnormal positions of chromosome pieces are identified. Normal karyotypes are 46 XX (female) and 46 XY (male). In 88262, 15-20 cells are identified and two karyotypes are analyzed with banding. Two karyotypes are present in some individuals with some chromosomal abnormalities. This means that some cells have a normal 46XX or 46XY chromosome count, while other cells have chromosome abnormalities. In 88263, 45 cells are identified and analyzed for mosaicism, which includes analysis of two karyotypes with banding. When cells divide, they can undergo changes that result in some cells having a normal chromosome count while other cells have an extra chromosome known as a trisomy. The term for this is mosaicism or trisomy mosaicism. Even though not all the cells are affected in trisomy mosaicism when certain chromosomes are affected, including chromosomes 9, 14, and 22, the abnormality in some of the cells can cause a variety of conditions, including mental retardation, congenital heart defects, abnormalities of skull and facial bones, other abnormalities of the musculoskeletal system, urogenital anomalies, as well as other conditions. The extent of abnormality can vary significantly from one individual to another depending on how many of the cells are affected. Chromosome analysis is the only method of definitively diagnosing

mosaicism. Because not all cells are affected, 45 cells are required for this analysis. In 88264, chromosome analysis is performed on 20-25 cells without karyotyping.

88267

88267 Chromosome analysis, amniotic fluid or chorionic villus, count 15 cells, 1 karyotype, with banding

Chromosome analysis may be performed due to advanced maternal age, abnormal prenatal ultrasound findings, abnormal maternal blood screen results, previous child with a chromosome abnormality, known familial chromosome rearrangement, or known familial genetic disorder. A separately reportable amniocentesis or CVS is performed. The amniotic fluid is collected using special syringes and placed in screw top tubes. Alternatively, a CVS specimen may be obtained and a stereomicroscope and sterile gloves used to remove any blood clots before placing the specimen in screw top tubes. The amniotic fluid or CVS is then transported to the lab where fifteen cells are identified and direct analysis performed. Karyotyping is an evaluation of the size, shape, and number of chromosomes in the cell samples. Banding is a chromosome staining technique used to identify individual chromosomes that produce characteristic bands. Giemsa banding is a complex process that involves acetic acid fixation, air drying, denaturing of chromosomes by proteolytic enzymes or other technique, and Giemsa staining. Alternatively, chromosome banding may be performed using fluorochrome and Q-banding stain. Any extra, missing, or abnormal positions of chromosome pieces are identified. Normal karyotypes are 46 XX (female) and 46 XY (male).

88269

88269 Chromosome analysis, in situ for amniotic fluid cells, count cells from 6-12 colonies, 1 karyotype, with banding

Chromosome analysis may be performed due to advanced maternal age, abnormal prenatal ultrasound findings, abnormal maternal blood screen results, previous child with a chromosome anomaly, known familial chromosome rearrangement, or known familial genetic disorder. A separately reportable amniocentesis is performed. The amniotic fluid is collected using special syringes and placed in screw top tubes with tissue culture transport medium and transported to the lab. The cells are cultured and prepared for band chromosome analysis. Six to twelve colonies are cultured in one or more different culture mediums. The cells in these colonies are counted and one karyotyping performed. Karyotyping is an evaluation of the size, shape, and number of chromosomes in the cell samples. Banding is a chromosome staining technique used to identify individual chromosomes that produce characteristic bands. Giemsa banding is a complex process that involves acetic acid fixation, air drying, denaturing of chromosomes by proteolytic enzymes or other technique, and Giemsa staining. Alternatively, chromosome banding may be performed using fluorochrome and Q-banding stain. Any extra, missing, or abnormal positions of chromosome pieces are identified. Normal karyotypes are 46 XX (female) and 46 XY (male).

88300

88300 Level I - Surgical pathology, gross examination only

Tissue removed during a surgical procedure, such as a biopsy, excision, or resection, is examined macroscopically in a gross or visual examination.

88302-88309

88302 Level II - Surgical pathology, gross and microscopic examination Appendix, incidental Fallopian tube, sterilization Fingers/toes, amputation, traumatic Foreskin, newborn Hernia sac, any location Hydrocele sac Nerve Skin, plastic repair Sympathetic ganglion Testis, castration Vaginal mucosa, incidental Vas deferens, sterilization

88304 Level III - Surgical pathology, gross and microscopic examination Abortion, induced Abscess Aneurysm - arterial/ventricular Anus, tag Appendix, other than incidental Artery, atheromatous plaque Bartholin's gland cyst Bone fragment(s), other than pathologic fracture Bursa/synovial cyst Carpal tunnel tissue Cartilage, shavings Cholesteatoma Colon, colostomy stoma Conjunctiva - biopsy/pterygium Cornea Diverticulum - esophagus/small intestine Dupuytren's contracture tissue Femoral head, other than fracture Fissure/fistula Foreskin, other than newborn Gallbladder Ganglion cyst Hematoma Hemorrhoids Hydatid of Morgagni Intervertebral disc Joint, loose body Meniscus Mucocele, salivary Neuroma - Morton's/traumatic Pilonidal cyst/sinus Polyps, inflammatory - nasal/sinusoidal Skin - cyst/tag/debridement Soft tissue, debridement Soft tissue, lipoma Spermatocele Tendon/tendon sheath Testicular appendage Thrombus or embolus Tonsil and/or adenoids Varicocele Vas deferens, other than sterilization Vein, varicosity

88305 Level IV - Surgical pathology, gross and microscopic examination Abortion - spontaneous/missed Artery, biopsy Bone marrow, biopsy Bone exostosis Brain/meninges, other than for tumor resection Breast, biopsy, not requiring microscopic evaluation of surgical margins Breast, reduction mammoplasty Bronchus, biopsy Cell block, any source Cervix, biopsy Colon, biopsy Duodenum, biopsy Endocervix, curettings/biopsy

Endometrium, curettings/biopsy Esophagus, biopsy Extremity, amputation, traumatic Fallopian tube, biopsy Fallopian tube, ectopic pregnancy Femoral head, fracture Fingers/toes, amputation, non-traumatic Gingiva/oral mucosa, biopsy Heart valve Joint, resection Kidney, biopsy Larynx, biopsy Leiomyoma(s), uterine myomectomy - without uterus Lip, biopsy/wedge resection Lung, transbronchial biopsy Lymph node, biopsy Muscle, biopsy Nasal mucosa, biopsy Nasopharynx/oropharynx, biopsy Nerve, biopsy Odontogenic/dental cyst Omentum, biopsy Ovary with or without tube, non-neoplastic Ovary, biopsy/wedge resection Parathyroid gland Peritoneum, biopsy Pituitary tumor Placenta, other than third trimester Pleura/pericardium - biopsy/tissue Polyp, cervical/endometrial Polyp, colorectal Polyp, stomach/small intestine Prostate, needle biopsy Prostate, TUR Salivary gland, biopsy Sinus, paranasal biopsy Skin, other than cyst/tag/debridement/plastic repair Small intestine, biopsy Soft tissue, other than tumor/mass/lipoma/debridement Spleen Stomach, biopsy Synovium Testis, other than tumor/biopsy/castration Thyroglossal duct/brachial cleft cyst Tongue, biopsy Tonsil, biopsy Trachea, biopsy Ureter, biopsy Urethra, biopsy Urinary bladder, biopsy Uterus, with or without tubes and ovaries, for prolapse Vagina, biopsy Vulva/labia, biopsy

88307   Level V - Surgical pathology, gross and microscopic examination Adrenal, resection Bone - biopsy/curettings Bone fragment(s), pathologic fracture Brain, biopsy Brain/meninges, tumor resection Breast, excision of lesion, requiring microscopic evaluation of surgical margins Breast, mastectomy - partial/simple Cervix, conization Colon, segmental resection, other than for tumor Extremity, amputation, non-traumatic Eye, enucleation Kidney, partial/total nephrectomy Larynx, partial/total resection Liver, biopsy - needle/wedge Liver, partial resection Lung, wedge biopsy Lymph nodes, regional resection Mediastinum, mass Myocardium, biopsy Odontogenic tumor Ovary with or without tube, neoplastic Pancreas, biopsy Placenta, third trimester Prostate, except radical resection Salivary gland Sentinel lymph node Small intestine, resection, other than for tumor Soft tissue mass (except lipoma) - biopsy/simple excision Stomach - subtotal/total resection, other than for tumor Testis, biopsy Thymus, tumor Thyroid, total/lobe Ureter, resection Urinary bladder, TUR Uterus, with or without tubes and ovaries, other than neoplastic/prolapse

88309   Level VI - Surgical pathology, gross and microscopic examination Bone resection Breast, mastectomy - with regional lymph nodes Colon, segmental resection for tumor Colon, total resection Esophagus, partial/total resection Extremity, disarticulation Fetus, with dissection Larynx, partial/total resection - with regional lymph nodes Lung - total/lobe/segment resection Pancreas, total/subtotal resection Prostate, radical resection Small intestine, resection for tumor Soft tissue tumor, extensive resection Stomach - subtotal/total resection for tumor Testis, tumor Tongue/tonsil -resection for tumor Urinary bladder, partial/total resection Uterus, with or without tubes and ovaries, neoplastic Vulva, total/subtotal resection

Tissue removed during a surgical procedure, such as a biopsy, excision, or resection, is examined macroscopically (gross or visual examination) and then under a microscope. The cells, tissues, or organ are transported from the surgical suite to the pathologist. The pathologist first visually examines the specimen and notes any defining characteristics. The specimen is then prepared for microscopic evaluation. The physician carefully analyzes the specimens to help establish a diagnosis, identify the presence or absence of malignant neoplasm, identify the exact type malignancy if present, examine the margins of the specimen to determine whether or not the entire diseased area was removed. A written report of findings is then prepared and a copy sent to the treating physician. Pathology services are reported based on the type of tissue examined, whether or not the tissue is expected to be normal or diseased, the difficulty of the pathology exam, and the time required to complete the exam. Use 88302 for a Level II pathology examination; 88304 for a Level III exam; 88305 for a Level IV exam; 88307 for a Level V exam; and 88309 for a Level VI exam.

88311

88311   Decalcification procedure (List separately in addition to code for surgical pathology examination)

A surgical or other specimen containing calcium, such as bone, bone marrow, or other calcified tissue is treated to remove the calcium. The specimen is first placed in an acid solution to remove the calcium. Ion exchange is then performed by bathing the specimen in another solution that removes calcium ions. The decalcified specimen is then prepared for examination.

88312-88313

88312   Special stain including interpretation and report; Group I for microorganisms (eg, acid fast, methenamine silver)
88313   Special stain including interpretation and report; Group II, all other (eg, iron, trichrome), except stain for microorganisms, stains for enzyme constituents, or immunocytochemistry and immunohistochemistry

Special staining techniques are sometimes required to visualize microorganisms or cell and tissue structures. Staining is composed of a number of steps beginning with fixation of the specimen using a fixative or by freezing to prevent damage to the internal structure of the organism, cell, or tissue. If tissue is being evaluated, the tissue must be prepared for slicing and then sliced into very thin sections using a vibrotome. The specimen is then treated with a variety of reagents, solutions, and stains designed to highlight specific features or components of the microorganism, cell, or tissue. The specimen is then examined under a microscope. The staining results are interpreted and a written report of findings is provided. Use code 88312 for Group I special stains for microorganisms; use 88313 for Group II special stains for all other specimens excluding stains for microorganisms, stains for enzyme constituents, and immunohistochemistry.

88314

88314   Special stain including interpretation and report; histochemical stain on frozen tissue block (List separately in addition to code for primary procedure)

Histochemical staining of tissue involves the use of one or more stains that add color to the tissue components making it easier to evaluate the tissue and cell structure. Frozen blocks are used because freezing stabilizes the internal structure of the tissue and prevents cell lysis. The tissue may be embedded in epoxy resin so that it can be sliced into thin sections. A vibrotome is used to slice the tissue, which may be treated with a variety of reagents or solutions prior to staining. The tissue is stained. Two examples of histochemical staining techniques are Golgi silver impregnation staining and Nissl staining using cresyl violet. The specimen is examined under a microscope. The staining results are interpreted and a written report of findings is provided. Use 88314 for each tissue block examined using histochemical stains.

88319

88319   Special stain including interpretation and report; Group III, for enzyme constituents

Special stains of blood, bone marrow, or tissue are performed to identify enzyme constituents. Cytochemical stains for enzyme constituents are used to aid in identification of abnormal cells and to provide additional diagnostic information about normal appearing cells. Staining of blood or bone marrow, or organ imprints for enzyme constituents is performed using a fresh specimen that is smeared onto a slide. A fixative is applied to adhere the specimen to the slide. The slide is then washed and the staining reagent is applied. The slide is washed again and additional counterstaining is performed as needed to enhance detail. A control sample of normal cells is also stained at the same time for quality control purposes. The presence or absence of enzyme activity for the specific enzyme being tested is represented by the presence or absence and relative intensity of the stain in various constituents of blood, bone marrow, or tissue cells. Examples of some types of stains for enzyme constituents include tartrate resistant acid phosphatase stain, myeloperoxidase (MPO) stain, and chloracetate esterase stain.

88321-88323

88321   Consultation and report on referred slides prepared elsewhere
88323   Consultation and report on referred material requiring preparation of slides

Use code 88321 when the physician provides consultative advice and prepares a report on slides that were prepared elsewhere, outside of the physician's office. In 88323, the physician provides consultative advice and prepares a report on a tissue or cell sample that was collected elsewhere and sent to the physician's office, which then requires slide preparation by the physician's office.

88331-88332

88331   Pathology consultation during surgery; first tissue block, with frozen section(s), single specimen
88332   Pathology consultation during surgery; each additional tissue block with frozen section(s) (List separately in addition to code for primary procedure)

The pathologist examines a tissue block at the request of the surgeon during the course of the surgical procedure to identify the presence or absence of disease or malignancy and/or to determine whether the surgical margins are free of disease or malignancy. A tissue block is a sample of tissue submitted as a single specimen that has been prepared for examination. A gross examination of the tissue block is performed. The tissue block is then flash frozen and cut into thin sections and each frozen section is examined microscopically. The pathologist provides an initial verbal report of findings including the presence or absence of neoplasm or other disease, the extent of involvement, the presence or absence of clean margins, and any other clinically significant characteristics of the tissue sample.

A written report is also provided and placed in the medical record. Use 88331 for the first tissue block and all frozen sections from the first tissue block. Use 88332 for each additional tissue block with frozen sections.

88333-88334

88333 Pathology consultation during surgery; cytologic examination (eg, touch prep, squash prep), initial site

88334 Pathology consultation during surgery; cytologic examination (eg, touch prep, squash prep), each additional site (List separately in addition to code for primary procedure)

The pathologist performs an intraoperative cytologic examination at the request of the surgeon to identify the presence or absence of disease or malignancy. To perform intraoperative touch prep cytologic examination, the margin of the tissue sample is touched against a glass slide. Cells from the tissue sample stick to the slide. The slide is then prepared by air drying, stained, and examined under a microscope. To perform intraoperative squash prep cytologic examination, a scalpel is used to slice off 1-2 mm from a tissue specimen, which is placed in a smear slide. The specimen is covered and crushed with another slide using just enough pressure to create a thin film from the tissue. The specimen is fixed, stained, and examined under a microscope. The pathologist provides an initial verbal report of findings including the presence or absence of abnormal or malignant cells and any other clinically significant characteristics of the cell sample. A written report is also provided and placed in the medical record. Use 88333 for examination of the cells from the initial site. Use 88334 for examination of cells from each additional site.

88341-88344

88341 Immunohistochemistry or immunocytochemistry, per specimen; each additional single antibody stain procedure (List separately in addition to code for primary procedure)

88342 Immunohistochemistry or immunocytochemistry, per specimen; initial single antibody stain procedure

88344 Immunohistochemistry or immunocytochemistry, per specimen; each multiplex antibody stain procedure

Immunohistochemistry or immunocytochemistry identifies a certain antigen by using an antibody specific to that antigen when examining cells contained in a specimen such as a tissue block, brushed cell samples, blood smear, or fine needle biopsy (FNB). The specimen is prepped for histological or cytological examination on a glass slide that has been fixed with a commercially available antibody. Enzymes and/or special stains are then applied to the specimen slide. The characteristic changes to the cells in the sample can help determine the antigenic profile of morphologically undifferentiated cells, and aid in the diagnosis of malignant neoplasms. The prepped slide specimen may be used to identify a single antibody or multiple antibodies. Use code 88342 for the first identifiable single antibody per slide/stain procedure. Use code 88341 for each additional single antibody. Use code 88344 when multiple separately identifiable antibodies are applied to the same slide/stain specimen.

88360

88360 Morphometric analysis, tumor immunohistochemistry (eg, Her-2/neu, estrogen receptor/progesterone receptor), quantitative or semiquantitative, per specimen, each single antibody stain procedure; manual

Morphometric analysis to check for tumor immunohistochemistry (i.e. the body's resistance to tumors) by studying a tissue sample as various antibodies are administered. Use this code for manual observation.

88361

88361 Morphometric analysis, tumor immunohistochemistry (eg, Her-2/neu, estrogen receptor/progesterone receptor), quantitative or semiquantitative, per specimen, each single antibody stain procedure; using computer-assisted technology

Morphometric analysis to check for tumor immunohistochemistry (i.e. the body's resistance to tumors) by studying a tissue sample as various antibodies are administered. Use this code for computer-assisted observation.

88363

88363 Examination and selection of retrieved archival (ie, previously diagnosed) tissue(s) for molecular analysis (eg, KRAS mutational analysis)

A tissue sample that has already been examined with a diagnosis made based on the earlier examination, is retrieved and additional molecular analysis is performed. This procedure is performed to obtain additional information regarding a neoplasm or other disease process to aid in development of a treatment regimen. Molecular analysis involves tests to examine chromosomes, chromosome mutations, genes, and gene mutations that contribute to disease states and affect treatment outcomes. For example, KRAS mutational analysis is used in patients with certain types of malignancies to identify mutations in the

KRAS gene that are associated with a poor prognosis or limited response to treatments targeting the epidermal growth factor receptor (EGFR) pathway (a series of complex signals involved in the development and growth of cancer).

88364-88366

88364 In situ hybridization (eg, FISH), per specimen; each additional single probe stain procedure (List separately in addition to code for primary procedure)

88365 In situ hybridization (eg, FISH), per specimen; initial single probe stain procedure

88366 In situ hybridization (eg, FISH), per specimen; each multiplex probe stain procedure

In situ hybridization (FISH) is a technique that localizes specific nucleic acid (DNA and RNA) targets within fixed tissue or cells to obtain temporal/spatial information of gene expression and genetic coding. This information can aide in understanding the organization, regulation, and function of genes. The sample cells or tissue are treated to fix in place the target transcripts. The DNA/RNA probe hybridizes (binds) to the target sequence at an elevated temperature and the excess probe is washed away. The remaining DNA/RNA target(s) is then stained with spectrally distinct fluorophone labels to enable visualization under fluorescent microscopy (FISH). DNA-FISH can show gene presence, copy number and location and is used for gene mutation analysis. RNA-FISH can show gene expression, RNA temporal and spatial localization. The FISH technique has the capability to use multiple targets/probes simultaneously to visualize co-locations within a single specimen. Code 88365 is used for the initial single probe stain per specimen. Code 88364 is reported for each additional single probe stain, and code 88366 is reported when multiple probes are used in the same stain procedure.

88367

88367 Morphometric analysis, in situ hybridization (quantitative or semi-quantitative), using computer-assisted technology, per specimen; initial single probe stain procedure

Morphometric analysis, in situ hybridization (quantitative or semi-quantitative) is a fluorescent tagging technique used by pathologists or geneticists to visualize specific genes or portions of genes. The technique allows for the detection, identification, interpretation, and analysis of certain genetic abnormalities like translocation, deletion, duplication, amplification, and inversion on chromosomes, hematologic cells, and/or solid tumor cancers. This information can help determine patient eligibility for certain treatments, plan a treatment course, and monitor response to treatment. Cells are fixed to the surface of a slide and treated to denature the DNA into a single strand. A short sequence (probe) of single stranded DNA that matches a portion of the target gene(s) is tagged with one or more fluorescent labels and applied to the slide. The slide DNA is allowed to hybridize (bind) to the probe DNA and the slide is washed to remove the excess. The slide is then read using computer assisted technology to determine if genetic abnormalities are present in the specimen. Use this code for the initial single probe stain performed.

88368-88369

88368 Morphometric analysis, in situ hybridization (quantitative or semi-quantitative), manual, per specimen; initial single probe stain procedure

88369 Morphometric analysis, in situ hybridization (quantitative or semi-quantitative), manual, per specimen; each additional single probe stain procedure (List separately in addition to code for primary procedure)

Morphometric analysis, in situ hybridization (quantitative or semi-quantitative) is a fluorescent tagging technique used by pathologists or geneticists to visualize specific genes or portions of genes. The technique allows for the detection, identification, interpretation and analysis of certain genetic abnormalities like translocation, deletion, duplication, amplification, and inversion on chromosomes, hematologic cells, and/or solid tumor cancers. This information can help determine patient eligibility for certain treatments, plan a treatment course, and monitor response to treatment. Cells are fixed to the surface of a slide and treated to denature the DNA into a single strand. A short sequence (probe) of single stranded DNA that matches a portion of the target gene(s) is tagged with one or more fluorescent labels and applied to the slide. The slide DNA is allowed to hybridize (bind) to the probe DNA and the slide is washed to remove the excess. The slide is then viewed manually under a microscope to determine if genetic abnormalities are present. Use 88368 for the initial single probe stain performed and 88369 for each additional single probe stain procedure.

Pathology and Laboratory

88373-88374

88373 Morphometric analysis, in situ hybridization (quantitative or semi-quantitative), using computer-assisted technology, per specimen; each additional single probe stain procedure (List separately in addition to code for primary procedure)

88374 Morphometric analysis, in situ hybridization (quantitative or semi-quantitative), using computer-assisted technology, per specimen; each multiplex probe stain procedure

Morphometric analysis, in situ hybridization (quantitative or semi-quantitative) is a fluorescent tagging technique used by pathologists or geneticists to visualize specific genes or portions of genes. The technique allows for the detection, identification, interpretation, and analysis of certain genetic abnormalities like translocation, deletion, duplication, amplification, and inversion on chromosomes, hematologic cells, and/or solid tumor cancers. This information can help determine patient eligibility for certain treatments, plan a treatment course, and monitor response to treatment. Cells are fixed to the surface of a slide and treated to denature the DNA into a single strand. A short sequence (probe) of single stranded DNA that matches a portion of the target gene(s) is tagged with one or more fluorescent labels and applied to the slide. The slide DNA is allowed to hybridize (bind) to the probe DNA and the slide is washed to remove the excess. The slide is then read using computer assisted technology to determine if genetic abnormalities are present. Code 88373 is used together with 88367 to report each addition single probe stain procedure. Code 88374 is reported when multiple probes are used simultaneously in the same stain procedure.

88375

88375 Optical endomicroscopic image(s), interpretation and report, real-time or referred, each endoscopic session

Optical endomicroscopy provides in vivo visualization and characterization of the mucosal tissue and pathophysiological processes at the microscopic level. Separately reportable endoscopy is performed and optical endomicroscopic images are obtained. The images are submitted for histological evaluation which may be performed in real time as the endoscopic procedure is being performed or at a later time. Each optical slice is reviewed for histological changes and these changes are characterized in a written report. Code 88375 is reported once per endoscopic session regardless of the number of optical slices submitted for histological evaluation.

88377

88377 Morphometric analysis, in situ hybridization (quantitative or semi-quantitative), manual, per specimen; each multiplex probe stain procedure

Morphometric analysis, in situ hybridization (quantitative or semi-quantitative) is a fluorescent tagging technique used by pathologists or geneticists to visualize specific genes or portions of genes. The technique allows for the detection, identification, interpretation and analysis of certain genetic abnormalities like translocation, deletion, duplication, amplification, and inversion on chromosomes, hematologic cells, and/or solid tumor cancers. This information can help determine patient eligibility for certain treatments, plan a treatment course, and monitor response to treatment. Cells are fixed to the surface of a slide and treated to denature the DNA into a single strand. Multiple short sequences (probes) of single stranded DNA that match a portion of the target gene(s) are tagged with one or more fluorescent labels and applied to the slide. The slide DNA is allowed to hybridize (bind) to the probe DNA and the slide is washed to remove the excess. The slide is then viewed manually under a microscope to determine if genetic abnormalities are present.

88380-88381

88380 Microdissection (ie, sample preparation of microscopically identified target); laser capture

88381 Microdissection (ie, sample preparation of microscopically identified target); manual

Microdissection of a tissue sample is performed by laser capture in 88380, following separately reportable preparation of microscopically identified target tissue. Stained sections of a single tissue block are compared and abnormal or neoplastic tissue is identified. The pathologist separates individual abnormal or neoplastic cells from normal tissue using laser capture microdissection, which may be followed by additional separately reportable special stains and molecular analysis to classify the abnormal or neoplastic cells for determining an optimal treatment regimen. Use 88381 for manual microdissection. Manual separation of abnormal or neoplastic tissue from normal tissue is performed under a dissecting microscope using a razor blade or scalpel.

88387-88388

88387 Macroscopic examination, dissection, and preparation of tissue for non-microscopic analytical studies (eg, nucleic acid-based molecular studies); each tissue preparation (eg, a single lymph node)

88388 Macroscopic examination, dissection, and preparation of tissue for non-microscopic analytical studies (eg, nucleic acid-based molecular studies); in conjunction with a touch imprint, intraoperative consultation, or frozen section, each tissue preparation (eg, a single lymph node) (List separately in addition to code for primary procedure)

The tissue sample is visually examined and definitive characteristics noted. The tissue is dissected and evaluated. The tissue is then prepared by either fixing the tissue using an aldehyde or alcohol fixator or freezing the tissue. The tissue is embedded in paraffin or resin and sliced into sections for use in non-microscopic analytical studies such as nucleic acid-based molecular studies. These types of studies are performed on individuals with certain diseases caused by genetic mutations and on malignant neoplasms. A variety of molecular studies may be performed depending on the patient's diagnosis or suspected disease. Following completion of the studies, the physician interprets the results and provides a written report of findings. Use 88387 for each tissue preparation performed alone; use 88388 for each tissue preparation performed in conjunction with a touch imprint, intraoperative consultation or frozen

88720

88720 Bilirubin, total, transcutaneous

A total transcutaneous bilirubin (TcB) test is performed. This is a simple, noninvasive test performed with a bilirubin analyzer device that measures total bilirubin levels through the skin. This is an alternative to subcutaneous bilirubin tests, such as the traditional heel stick for total serum bilirubin. The bilirubin analyzer device is turned on and initialized. The device then performs a self-test to ensure that it is working properly. The device is calibrated and the tester presses the tip of the handheld device against the patient's forehead or sternum. Light from the analyzer device is reflected from the patient's skin. Known characteristics of major skin components that affect spectral reflectance, such as collagen, melanin, hemoglobin, and bilirubin, are evaluated using the principle of spectral subtraction. The device measures the total bilirubin concentration, derived by spectral subtraction of the other major skin components. The device is then lifted away from the skin to complete the first measurement. A series of five measurements are typically performed. Following the fifth measurement, the total bilirubin level is calculated and displayed by the device.

88738

88738 Hemoglobin (Hgb), quantitative, transcutaneous

Using a handheld device, the level of circulating hemoglobin is measured transcutaneously using noninvasive white light spectroscopy. A probe that emits the white light is placed on the skin, usually the forearm. The light travels through the skin tissue and hemoglobin absorbs some of the light. The rest is reflected back and collected by the device. The device provides a measurement of hemoglobin in the blood by calculating the difference between the amount of emitted light and the amount of light that is reflected back. The hemoglobin value is recorded in the patient's medical record.

88740-88741

88740 Hemoglobin, quantitative, transcutaneous, per day; carboxyhemoglobin

88741 Hemoglobin, quantitative, transcutaneous, per day; methemoglobin

A quantitative transcutaneous hemoglobin test for carboxyhemoglobin (88740) or methemoglobin (88741) is performed. Carboxyhemoglobin is a stable union of carbon monoxide with hemoglobin that occurs with carbon monoxide inhalation. The formation of carboxyhemoglobin prevents the normal transfer of carbon dioxide and oxygen in the blood. High levels of carboxyhemoglobin are referred to as carbon monoxide poisoning or asphyxiation and may result in death. Methemoglobin is a form of hemoglobin that cannot carry oxygen. Normally, only 1-2 percent of total hemoglobin is methemoglobin. A higher percentage may be present in patients with certain genetic conditions or in those with exposure to certain toxins. The term methemoglobinemia refers to higher levels of methomoglobin that cause health problems. A simple, noninvasive test is performed with an eight-wavelength pulse oxymeter to measure carboxyhemoglobin or methemoglobin transcutaneously. The measurement sensor is attached to the patient's finger and the levels of either carboxyhemoglobin or methemoglobin are measured on a per day basis.

89230

89230 Sweat collection by iontophoresis

Sweat collection by iontophoresis or the introduction of certain medication (usually pilocarpine) into the skin with patches stimulated with an electrical current. The medication causes sweating, which is collected and tested to diagnose certain disorders (e.g. cystic fibrosis).

● New Code ▲ Revised Code

89250-89251

89250 Culture of oocyte(s)/embryo(s), less than 4 days
89251 Culture of oocyte(s)/embryo(s), less than 4 days; with co-culture of oocyte(s)/embryos

Following separately reportable retrieval of ova by laparoscopic or other technique, the oocytes (eggs)/embryos (fertilized eggs) are identified, isolated, placed in culture , and incubated for one to three days under carefully controlled conditions to maintain viability and functionality prior to implantation in the uterus. If the oocytes are not fully mature they are placed in the culture medium and allowed to mature. If the oocytes are mature, they are fertilized in a separately reportable insemination procedure and the embryos are then carefully monitored for less than four days while the embryo develops. In 89250, standard culturing techniques are used. In 89251 co-culturing techniques are used. Co-culture involves culture of oocytes/embryos with oviductal, uterine, granulose, or other substrate cells. The procedure includes isolation of the substrate cells, which are examined microscopically and cytochemically. The substrate cells are plated and co-cultured with the oocytes/embryos. Typically co-culture techniques are used when ten or more oocytes are harvested. The typical patient has eight or fewer mature oocytes available for microfertilization and additional work including co-culture is required when more than ten mature oocytes are available.

89253

89253 Assisted embryo hatching, microtechniques (any method)

This procedure is also referred to as assisted hatching (AH) or assisted zygote hatching (AZH). The embryo must break free of the zona pellucida, which is the outer shell of the embryo, to facilitate implantation in the uterine lining. Indications for AH include: age, women age 38 or over often have a more rigid zona pellucida; poor egg quantity and quality; poor embryo quality which includes embryos showing excessive fragmentation or slow rates of cell division; identification of thick zona pellucida; or previous in vitro fertilization failures. The embryo is placed under a microscope and held stationary with a specialized holding pipette. A very small hollow needle is then placed against the zona pellucida of the embryo and an acidic solution expelled. The acidic solution digests the zona pellucida making a small hole where the solution was expelled. The embryo is then washed and returned to the culture medium until the embryo transfer procedure is performed.

89254

89254 Oocyte identification from follicular fluid

Follicular aspirates are collected in a separately reportable procedure and placed in a test tube. The contents of the test tube are then placed in a very thin layer in several Petri dishes. Each Petri dish is examined for the presence of oocytes (eggs) under a stereo dissecting microscope with an illuminated base and heated stage. When an oocyte is found, the stage of maturation is determined and condition of the surrounding coronal and cumulus cells evaluated. The presence of a single polar body indicates maturity of the oocyte. The process is continued until all oocytes have been identified, isolated, and examined.

89255

89255 Preparation of embryo for transfer (any method)

Embryos are typically transferred to the uterus on either day three or five. The embryologist carefully examines the embryos and identifies those that are healthiest. Two to four embryos are then placed in a small amount of fluid and transferred with the fluid to a catheter. A separately reportable procedure is then performed to insert the catheter through the cervix and into the uterus where the embryos and fluid are released in the upper part of the uterus.

89258-89259

89258 Cryopreservation; embryo(s)
89259 Cryopreservation; sperm

In 89258, a fertilized egg is frozen for future use. Embryos are placed in a freezing solution that contains a cryoprotectant. Cryoprotectants enable the embryo to be frozen into a solid without any ice crystal formation. A rapid freezing technique called vitrification is then used to freeze and preserve the embryos. Embryos may be frozen at the pronuclear (one cell) stage, or at any stage up to and including the blastocyst stage which occurs approximately 5-7 days following fertilization. The frozen embryos are then placed in storage for future use. In 89259, sperm are frozen for future use. Ejaculate containing sperm and semen is placed in one or more individual vials and cryoprotectants are added. The vials are slowly cooled, frozen, placed in liquid nitrogen tanks, and stored for future use.

89260-89261

89260 Sperm isolation; simple prep (eg, sperm wash and swim-up) for insemination or diagnosis with semen analysis
89261 Sperm isolation; complex prep (eg, Percoll gradient, albumin gradient) for insemination or diagnosis with semen analysis

Sperm are isolated for use in an assisted reproductive procedure or for diagnostic purposes. A semen analysis is performed first. Semen analysis includes an evaluation for the presence and motility of sperm. The total density of sperm per millimeter of semen is calculated and then the motile density is calculated. Motile density evaluates the number of sperm showing good forward motion. Semen analysis may also include an evaluation of volume and differential. Volume refers to the total volume of semen in a single ejaculation. Differential is an evaluation of the number of sperm that appear normal when examined under a microscope. Following semen analysis the sperm are isolated. In 89260, a sample of unsorted spermatozoa is placed in the bottom of a laboratory test tube containing sperm wash medium. The tube is then placed in an upright position and allowed to stand for 30-60 minutes while maintaining a constant temperature of 37 degrees C. During this 30-60 minute period viable, motile sperm will swim up to the top of the tube. In 89261, a test tube is prepared with a solution of 90% Percoll or albumin gradient on the bottom half of the tube and a second solution on the top half containing a 45% Percoll or albumin gradient solution. Unsorted spermatozoa are then placed on top of the 45% solution. The test tube is centrifuged for 30 minutes while maintaining a temperature of 25 degrees C. Following the centrifugation process nonviable sperm remain suspended in the 45% solution while viable sperm fall to the bottom of the tube. Following sperm wash and swim up or Percoll gradient sperm isolation, the viable sperm are removed for further diagnostic analysis or prepared for a separately reportable artificial insemination procedure.

89264

89264 Sperm identification from testis tissue, fresh or cryopreserved

Fresh or frozen sperm retrieved from testis tissue by a separately reportable aspiration or biopsy procedure are identified in the embryology lab. Prior to transport to the lab the tissue is minced into very small segments and placed in a tube containing yolk test buffer. At the embryology lab the tissue samples are carefully examined under a microscope for the presence of viable sperm. Identification of sperm in testis tissue can be a time consuming and tedious procedure. Once sperm are identified, they are prepared for use in a separately reportable assisted reproduction procedure. Frozen testis tissue is thawed and then examined in the embryology lab to identify viable sperm using the same techniques as those described for fresh testicular tissue.

89268

89268 Insemination of oocytes

Oocytes are inseminated in a culture dish. Oocytes and spermatozoa are first examined microscopically to determine their viability and functionality. Petri dishes are prepared with mineral oil. Spermatozoa isolated from seminal plasma are then suspended in fluid. A drop of fluid containing spermatozoa is placed in a Petri dish. An oocyte is placed in the drop of fluid containing the spermatozoa. The culture dishes are incubated and carefully monitored for 24 hours. Following incubation the oocyte is examined to determine whether fertilization has occurred.

89272

89272 Extended culture of oocyte(s)/embryo(s), 4-7 days

Following separately reportable culture for the first three days, the oocytes/embryos are maintained in culture medium for another four to seven days. This allows development of an embryo to eight cells which is the blastocyst stage.

89280-89281

89280 Assisted oocyte fertilization, microtechnique; less than or equal to 10 oocytes
89281 Assisted oocyte fertilization, microtechnique; greater than 10 oocytes

Assisted oocyte fertilization involves introduction of a single spermatozoon into the interior of a mature oocyte. This procedure is typically performed when the man has an extremely low sperm count or a large number of immotile sperm. The ova are first stripped of the outer layers including the granulosa, cumulus oophorus, and corona radiate either mechanically or with the use of enzymes. The oocyte is examined microscopically to ensure maturity, which can be verified by identification of an extruded first polar body. Spermatozoa are examined microscopically and then isolated from seminal fluid, testicular tissue, epididymal fluid, or urine. Micro-mechanical assisted fertilization is then performed under high power magnification. A single sperm is identified and grasped by the tail using a injection pipette. The oocyte is grasped by a holding pipette and the single sperm is injected into the cytoplasm of the oocy;te. The oocyte is examined to ensure that the zona pelluicida and oolemma has been breached and also that the oocyte has not degenerated during the fertilization procedure. The oocyte is examined approximately 24 hours later to ensure fertilization has occurred. Use 89280 for assisted fertilization of ten or fewer oocytes or 89281 greater than ten oocytes.

Pathology and Laboratory

89290-89291

89290   Biopsy, oocyte polar body or embryo blastomere, microtechnique (for pre-implantation genetic diagnosis); less than or equal to 5 embryos

89291   Biopsy, oocyte polar body or embryo blastomere, microtechnique (for pre-implantation genetic diagnosis); greater than 5 embryos

This procedure is performed to identify genetically normal oocytes or embryos for patients who are known carriers of certain genetic diseases. If genetic testing is performed on an oocyte it is first examined microscopically for maturity prior to polar body biopsy. If the testing is performed on an embryo it also examined to determine embryo viability. The oocyte or embryo is then grasped using a holding pipette while being viewed under a microscope. A small hole is made in the oocyte or embryo using either a mechanical or enzymatic technique. A biopsy pipette is then used to remove one or two polar bodies or blastomeres are removed for separately reportable genetic analysis. Use 89290 for biopsy of five or fewer oocytes or embryos. Use 89291 for more than five oocytes/embryos.

89300

89300   Semen analysis; presence and/or motility of sperm including Huhner test (post coital)

The postcoital test evaluates how the woman's cervical mucus interacts with her partner's sperm at the time of ovulation. When separately reportable laboratory testing indicates that ovulation is about to occur, the couple is instructed to have intercourse after a two day period of abstinence and present to the physician's office six to ten hours later for testing. A small drop of mucus is removed from the endocervix and examined under the microscope. The presence of sperm in the mucus and the movement of sperm are evaluated. A favorable postcoital test result shows large numbers of active sperm in the mucus with good forward motion through the mucus. An unfavorable postcoital test result does not show large numbers of sperm and/or sperm are not active with good forward motion.

89310-89320

89310   Semen analysis; motility and count (not including Huhner test)

89320   Semen analysis; volume, count, motility, and differential

A semen analysis to evaluate the presence and/or motility of sperm is performed. The total density of sperm per milliliter of semen is calculated with a normal sperm count being 20 million per milliliter or above. The motile density is then evaluated. Motile density evaluates the number of active sperm showing good forward motion that would be capable of moving from the site of sperm deposition to the site of fertilization. A normal motility count is eight million per milliliter or higher. Use 89320 when motility and count as described above is performed with an evaluation of volume and differential. Volume evaluates the total volume of semen in a single ejaculation. Differential is an evaluation of the number of sperm that appear normal when viewed under the microscope.

89321

89321   Semen analysis; sperm presence and motility of sperm, if performed

A semen analysis is performed to identify the presence of sperm. This test is typically performed following vasectomy to verify that the sterilization procedure was successful. A successful vasectomy result shows no sperm present in the semen. If sperm are present, the motility (movement) of sperm may be evaluated.

89322

89322   Semen analysis; volume, count, motility, and differential using strict morphologic criteria (eg, Kruger)

A semen analysis is performed to evaluate the volume of semen in a single ejaculation, the number of sperm present per milliliter, the motility (movement) of sperm, and the differential number of sperm that are normal using strict morphologic criteria. The total volume of semen in a single ejaculation is measured. The total density of sperm per milliliter of semen is calculated with a normal sperm count being 20 million per milliliter or above. The motile density is then evaluated for the number of active sperm, showing good forward motion, capable of moving from the site of sperm deposition to the site of fertilization. A normal motility count is eight million per milliliter or higher. Next, a differential using strict morphologic criteria is performed. A stained slide is prepared and several hundred individual sperm are evaluated. Each sperm is carefully inspected and any abnormalities in structure of the head, neck, or tail are noted. This detailed morphologic exam allows greater accuracy in the determination of the number of normal versus abnormal sperm present.

89325

89325   Sperm antibodies

This test is also referred to as an antisperm antibody test. Semen can cause an immune system response in either the man or woman in which antibodies damage or kill sperm causing a type of infertility referred to as immunologic infertility. Sperm antibodies, which are proteins, may be present in blood, vaginal fluids or semen. These antibodies attack

the sperm, which are seen as a foreign substance. Men may develop sperm antibodies following infection, traumatic injury or surgery, such as biopsy or vasectomy, on the testicle. The majority of men with fertility problems following successful vasectomy reversal have immunologic infertility. A women can also develop antibodies to her partner's semen or sperm. An immunobead test (IBT) is performed to detect sperm-bound antibodies. Typically both IgA and IgG antibody tests are performed and 89325 is reported separately for each immunoglobulin class.

89329

89329   Sperm evaluation; hamster penetration test

Fertilization is dependent on fusion of the sperm with the vitelline membrane of the oocyte. In order to accomplish fusion the plasma membrane of the equatorial segment of the sperm head must undergo changes to allow fusion. The hamster penetration test is used to determine whether the sperm being tested are able to undergo the necessary changes to fertilize an egg. The zona pellucida layer is removed from the hamster egg. This is the species-specific barrier to penetration but not fertilization of the hamster ova. The oocytes are then exposed to the human sperm of the man being evaluated and the eggs and sperm are monitored to determine whether penetration has occurred. If the sperm being tested are unable to penetrate the hamster oocytes, then additional testing is indicated. However, this test yields a high number of false positives and negatives. The test cannot provide definitive results but only an indicator as to whether or not the sperm being tested will be able to fertilize a human egg.

89330

89330   Sperm evaluation; cervical mucus penetration test, with or without spinnbarkeit test

This test may also be referred to as a post-coital test, Huhner test, or Sim-Huhner test. This test evaluates the woman's cervical mucus at the time of ovulation and how her mucus interacts with her partner's sperm. Sexual intercourse is avoided for at least two days prior to ovulation. Following other separately reportable tests to detect impending ovulation, the couple then has intercourse and presents to the physician office 6-10 hours later. A small drop of mucus is aspirated from the endocervix and the mucus is then examined under a microscope. A spinnbarkeit test, which evaluates the consistency of the mucus may be performed. Mucus should be thin and elastic. Sperm within the drop of mucus are evaluated for number as well as forward motility.

89331

89331   Sperm evaluation, for retrograde ejaculation, urine (sperm concentration, motility, and morphology, as indicated)

A urine specimen is obtained to evaluate sperm concentration, motility, and morphology in a patient with suspected retrograde ejaculation. Retrograde ejaculation is a condition in which semen enters the bladder during ejaculation rather than being discharged through the urethra and is relativelyuncommon. Diabetes, some medications, or previous urinary tract procedures increase the risk of developing retrograde ejaculation. Medication is administered to increase the alkalinity of the urine. Following sexual climax, a urine specimen is obtained. The number, or concentration, of sperm in the urine is evaluated. Motility is then evaluated to determine the number of active sperm showing good forward motion. A morphological examination of the sperm may also be performed to determine the number of normal to abnormal sperm.

89335

89335   Cryopreservation, reproductive tissue, testicular

Testicular reproductive tissue is cryopreserved for use in a future assisted reproduction procedure or for future reimplantation in boys or men undergoing cancer treatment that might render them permanently infertile. Testicular tissue may be cryopreserved intact or minced. The tissue is moved through a series of cryoprotectant solutions of increasing concentration. It is placed in special storage straws or vials and then gradually cooled and frozen to -270 degrees C. The procedure is carefully monitored to ensure that the proper controlled freezing rate is maintained and that all instruments are functioning properly.

Pathology and Laboratory

89337

89337   Cryopreservation, mature oocyte(s)

Cryopreservation of mature oocytes may be used to preserve or enhance reproductive potential in women who are at risk for primary ovarian insufficiency or failure. This can include women who are being treated with chemotherapeutic drugs or undergoing pelvic radiotherapy for cancer or other serious medical conditions, and those with certain genetic/chromosomal abnormalities such as fragile X premutation and mosaicism for monosomy X. Mature oocytes are retrieved after superovulation and immersed in a highly concentrated cryopreservative, such as glycerol, propanediol, ethylene glycol, or dimethyl sulfate. The oocytes then undergo ultra-rapid cooling, known as vitrification, using liquid nitrogen to solidify the cell. Cryopreservation stops all biologic activity, preserving the cell for future use.

89342-89346

89342   Storage (per year); embryo(s)
89343   Storage (per year); sperm/semen
89344   Storage (per year); reproductive tissue, testicular/ovarian
89346   Storage (per year); oocyte(s)

Embryos, sperm/semen, testicular/ovarian reproductive tissue, or oocytes are stored for use in a future assisted reproductive procedure. Embryos, reproductive tissue, or cells are stored in the vapor phase or submerged under liquid nitrogen and maintained at a constant temperature of -270 degrees C. Liquid nitrogen levels and other storage conditions are checked at predetermined intervals to ensure that the necessary storage temperature is maintained. The embryos, sperm/semen, testicular/ovarian reproductive tissue, or oocytes are stored for as long as the storage protocol requires. Use 89342 for storage of embryos, 89343 for storage of sperm/semen, 89344 for storage of testicular or ovarian reproductive tissue, and 89346 for oocytes.

89352-89356

89352   Thawing of cryopreserved; embryo(s)
89353   Thawing of cryopreserved; sperm/semen, each aliquot
89354   Thawing of cryopreserved; reproductive tissue, testicular/ovarian
89356   Thawing of cryopreserved; oocytes, each aliquot

Cryopreserved embryos, sperm/semen, testicular/ovarian reproductive tissue, or oocytes are thawed for use in an assisted reproductive procedure. In 89352, the cryopreserved embryos are removed from storage and warmed using one of several techniques including a controlled rate thawing chamber, water bath, or room temperature. Following thawing, the cryoprotectant is removed using a series of culture mediums that contain decreasing concentration of cryoprotectant. Once the cryoprotectant has been removed, the embryos are placed in a culture medium and then incubated for up to 24 hours to determine whether the embryos resume development or exhibit cell division. In 89353, the cryopreserved sperm or semen is thawed and warmed. Cryoprotectant is removed by washing or density gradiant centrifugation techniques. The washed sperm are placed in culture medium and incubated prior to performing a separately reportable assisted reproductive procedure. In 89354, testicular or ovarian reproductive tissue is thawed and warmed. Cryoprotectant is removed by the same technique used for embryos. The reproductive tissue is placed in culture medium and incubated for up to 48 hours. Viability of the tissue is then evaluated. Separately reportable assisted reproductive procedures including preparation of the reproductive tissue is then performed. In 89356, oocytes are thawed and warmed. Cryoprotectant is removed using the same technique as for embryos. The oocytes are placed in culture medium and incubated for up to 48 hours. Viability is evaluated. Separately reportable assisted reproductive procedures are then performed.

Pathology and Laboratory

● New Code   ▲ Revised Code

Medicine

90281-90283

90281   Immune globulin (Ig), human, for intramuscular use
90283   Immune globulin (IgIV), human, for intravenous use

Immune globulins are immunizing agents that confer effective, short-term, passive immunity as the antibodies circulate through the body. The recipient's own immune system is not stimulated to produce more of its own antibodies, making it passive protection. This passive form of immunity is achieved by giving injections/infusions of human immune globulin as a concentrated solution of antibodies pooled from the blood of many donors. Code 90281 reports human immune globulin (Ig) that is given intramuscularly; 90283 reports intravenous immune globulin (IgIV). These codes report only the product (immune globulin) used.

90284

90284   Immune globulin (SCIg), human, for use in subcutaneous infusions, 100 mg, each

Immune globulins are immunizing agents that confer effective, short-term, passive immunity as the antibodies circulate through the body. The recipient's own immune system is not stimulated to produce more of its own antibodies, making it passive protection. This passive form of immunity is achieved by giving injections/infusions of human immune globulin as a concentrated solution of antibodies pooled from the blood of many donors. SCIg helps to prevent or reduce the severity of certain infections in patients who are at risk. It is also used to treat immune system problems, thrombocytopenia, and Kawasaki syndrome. Code 90284 reports human immune globulin (Ig) that is infused subcutaneously per each 100 mg and reports only the product (immune globulin) used.

90287

90287   Botulinum antitoxin, equine, any route

Equine botulinum antitoxin is an immunizing agent that confers effective passive immunity to the recipient as it circulates through the body. The antitoxin is derived from the blood serum of horses that have been immunized. The antibodies received through the horse serum are able to neutralize toxins produced by the Botulinum bacteria and are delivered by any route. This code reports only the product (antitoxin) used.

90288

90288   Botulism immune globulin, human, for intravenous use

The botulism immune globulin is an immunizing agent that confers effective, short-term, passive immunity as the antibodies circulate through the body. The recipient's own immune system is not stimulated to produce more of its own antibodies, making it passive protection. This passive form of immunity protects the recipient against botulism and is derived from pooled donor blood from those who have already developed antibodies. This code reports human botulism immune globulin for intravenous use and reports only the product (immune globulin) used.

90291

90291   Cytomegalovirus immune globulin (CMV-IgIV), human, for intravenous use

The human cytomegalovirus immune globulin is an immunizing agent in the form of a concentrated solution of antibodies that confers effective, short-term, passive immunity as the antibodies circulate through the body. The recipient's own immune system is not stimulated to produce more of its own antibodies, making it passive protection. This passive form of immunity protects the exposed recipient against the cytomegalovirus and is derived from the pooled blood of many donors who have already developed antibodies. This code reports human cytomegalovirus immune globulin for intravenous use (CMV-IgIV) and reports only the product (immune globulin) used.

90296

90296   Diphtheria antitoxin, equine, any route

Equine diptheria antitoxin is an immunizing agent that confers effective passive immunity to the recipient as it circulates through the body. The antitoxin is derived from the blood serum of horses that have been immunized and developed antibodies. The antibodies received through the horse serum are able to neutralize toxins produced by the diphtheria bacteria and are delivered by any route. This code reports only the product (antitoxin) used.

90371

90371   Hepatitis B immune globulin (HBIg), human, for intramuscular use

The hepatitis B immune globulin is an immunizing agent in the form of a concentrated solution of antibodies that confers effective, short-term, passive immunity as the antibodies circulate through the body. The recipient's own immune system is not stimulated to produce more of its own antibodies, making it passive protection. This passive form of immunity protects the recipient against hepatitis B and is derived from the pooled blood of many donors who have already developed antibodies. This code reports human hepatitis B immune globulin for intramuscular use (HBIg) and reports only the product (immune globulin) used.

90375-90376

90375   Rabies immune globulin (RIg), human, for intramuscular and/or subcutaneous use
90376   Rabies immune globulin, heat-treated (RIg-HT), human, for intramuscular and/or subcutaneous use

The rabies immune globulin is an immunizing agent in the form of a concentrated solution of antibodies that confers effective, short-term, passive immunity as the antibodies circulate through the body. The recipient's own immune system is not stimulated to produce more of its own antibodies, making it passive protection. This passive form of immunity protects the exposed recipient against rabies and is derived from pooled donor blood from those who have already developed antibodies. These codes report human rabies immune globulin for intramuscular or subcutaneous use (RIg). These codes report only the product (immune globulin) used. Report code 90376 when using human rabies immune globulin (RIg-HT) that has undergone an additional heat treating process of 58-60 degrees Celsius for 10 hours to inactivate viruses and reduce the risk of blood-borne viral transmission.

90378

90378   Respiratory syncytial virus, monoclonal antibody, recombinant, for intramuscular use, 50 mg, each

The respiratory syncytial virus (RSV) recombinant monoclonal antibody is an immunizing agent that confers effective, short-term, passive immunity to RSV by providing RSV-neutralizing antibody to the patient. Monoclonal antibodies are produced by recombinant DNA technology using murine and human antibody sequences. RSV recombinant monoclonal antibody is administered via an intramuscular injection on a monthly basis to high risk infants including premature infants, infants that have conditions that affect pulmonary function, and infants that have congenital heart disease. Dosage is dependent on weight. Report code 90378 for each 50 mg dose of RSV recombinant monoclonal antibody for intramuscular administration. This code reports only the recombinant globulin product.

90384-90386

90384   Rho(D) immune globulin (RhIg), human, full-dose, for intramuscular use
90385   Rho(D) immune globulin (RhIg), human, mini-dose, for intramuscular use
90386   Rho(D) immune globulin (RhIgIV), human, for intravenous use

The Rho(D) immune globulin is an immunizing agent in the form of a concentrated solution of antibodies that confers effective, short-term, passive immunity as the antibodies circulate through the body. The recipient's own immune system is not stimulated to produce more of its own antibodies, making it passive protection. This passive form of immunity protects the recipient against blood reactions between red blood cells that are positive for Rh surface antigens and red blood cells that are negative for Rh surface antigens, such as may occur between mother and baby. The immune globulin is derived from the pooled blood of many donors. Code 90384 reports a full dose of human Rho(D) immune globulin for intramuscular use (RhIg), and code 90385 reports a mini dose. Code 90386 reports human Rho(D) immune globulin for intravenous use (RhIgIV). These codes report only the product (immune globulin) used.

90389

90389   Tetanus immune globulin (TIg), human, for intramuscular use

The tetanus immune globulin is an immunizing agent in the form of a concentrated solution of antibodies that confers effective, short-term, passive immunity as the antibodies circulate through the body. The recipient's own immune system is not stimulated to produce more of its own antibodies, making it passive protection. This passive form of immunity protects the recipient against tetanus and is derived from the pooled blood of many donors who have already developed antibodies. This code reports human tetanus immune globulin for intramuscular use (TIg). This code reports only the product (immune globulin) used.

© 2017 DecisionHealth   CPT © 2016 American Medical Association. All Rights Reserved.   ● New Code   ▲ Revised Code   **635**

90393

90393   Vaccinia immune globulin, human, for intramuscular use

The vaccinia immune globulin is an immunizing agent in the form of a concentrated solution of antibodies that confers effective, short-term, passive immunity as the antibodies circulate through the body. The recipient's own immune system is not stimulated to produce more of its own antibodies, making it passive protection. This passive form of immunity protects the recipient against the vaccinia virus and is derived from the pooled blood of many donors who have already developed antibodies. The vaccinia virus is the live virus used in the smallpox vaccine and can cause rash, fever, headache, bodyaches, or more severe systemic complications when the virus is spread from an unhealed vaccination site. This code reports human vaccinia immune globulin for intramuscular use. This code reports only the product (immune globulin) used.

90396

90396   Varicella-zoster immune globulin, human, for intramuscular use

The varicella-zoster immune globulin is an immunizing agent in the form of a concentrated solution of antibodies that confers effective, short-term, passive immunity as the antibodies circulate through the body. The recipient's own immune system is not stimulated to produce more of its own antibodies, making it passive protection. This passive form of immunity protects the recipient against the varicella-zoster virus that causes chickenpox and is derived from the pooled blood of many donors who have already developed antibodies. This code reports human varicella-zoster immune globulin for intramuscular use. This code reports only the product (immune globulin) used.

90460-90461

90460   Immunization administration through 18 years of age via any route of administration, with counseling by physician or other qualified health care professional; first or only component of each vaccine or toxoid administered

90461   Immunization administration through 18 years of age via any route of administration, with counseling by physician or other qualified health care professional; each additional vaccine or toxoid component administered (List separately in addition to code for primary procedure)

During a face-to-face encounter with a physician or other qualified health care professional, such as a physician assistant or nurse practitioner, the patient, parent, or other family member is provided with information about the vaccine and/or toxoid to be administered. Information includes the indications for the vaccine and/or toxoid, whether the vaccine/toxoid is administered in a single dose or whether a multiple dose schedule must be followed, possible side effects, and which side effects require medical follow-up. Any questions about the vaccine and/or toxoid are answered. The vaccine or a combination vaccine/toxoid is administered. Possible routes of administration include percutaneous, intradermal, subcutaneous, intramuscular, intranasal, or oral. Use 90460 for the first or only component of each vaccine/toxoid administered to a patient 18 years of age or younger via any route of administration. Use 90461 for each additional vaccine/toxoid component administered.

90471-90472

90471   Immunization administration (includes percutaneous, intradermal, subcutaneous, or intramuscular injections); 1 vaccine (single or combination vaccine/toxoid)

90472   Immunization administration (includes percutaneous, intradermal, subcutaneous, or intramuscular injections); each additional vaccine (single or combination vaccine/toxoid) (List separately in addition to code for primary procedure)

A single vaccine or a combination vaccine/toxoid is administered by injection to a patient over age 18 with or without a face-to-face encounter with the physician or other health care professional. These codes are also used when a vaccine/toxoid is given to a patient age 18 or younger without any face-to-face counseling by the physician or other health care professional. Routes of administration include percutaneous, intradermal, subcutaneous, or intramuscular. Use 90471 for the first injection. Use 90472 for each additional injection during the same encounter.

90473-90474

90473   Immunization administration by intranasal or oral route; 1 vaccine (single or combination vaccine/toxoid)

90474   Immunization administration by intranasal or oral route; each additional vaccine (single or combination vaccine/toxoid) (List separately in addition to code for primary procedure)

A single vaccine or a combination vaccine/toxoid is administered by oral or intranasal route to a patient over age 18 with or without a face-to-face encounter with the physician or other health care professional. These codes are also used when a vaccine/toxoid is given to a patient age 18 or younger without face-to-face counseling by the physician or other

health care professional. Use 90473 for the first vaccine/toxoid administered. Use 90474 for each additional vaccine/toxoid administered during the same encounter.

90476-90477

90476   Adenovirus vaccine, type 4, live, for oral use

90477   Adenovirus vaccine, type 7, live, for oral use

Unlike immune globulins which provide short-term, passive immunity, a vaccine provides active, long-term immunity by exposing the recipient's immune system to altered versions of specific viruses or bacteria that induce the immune system to produce its own antibodies against the invading micro-organism. The body then remembers how to make antibodies when exposed to the antigen again. Adenoviruses commonly cause respiratory illness, ranging from the common cold to croup, bronchitis, and pneumonia. Adenoviruses also cause various other illnesses such as conjunctivitis, cystitis, and gastroenteritis, depending on the serotype and location of infection. These codes report live adenovirus vaccine for oral use. Code 90476 is for type 4 and 90477 is for type 7. These codes report only the product (vaccine) used.

90581

90581   Anthrax vaccine, for subcutaneous or intramuscular use

Unlike immune globulins which provide short-term, passive immunity, a vaccine provides active, long-term immunity by exposing the recipient's immune system to altered versions of specific viruses or bacteria that induce the immune system to produce its own antibodies against the invading micro-organism. The body then remembers how to make antibodies when exposed to the antigen again. Anthrax is caused by the bacteria, Bacillus anthracis, and its spores. The inhaled form is fatal and causes pneumonia. The cutaneous form is more common for humans. This code reports an anthrax vaccine for subcutaneous or intramuscular use. This code reports only the product (vaccine) used.

90585-90586

90585   Bacillus Calmette-Guerin vaccine (BCG) for tuberculosis, live, for percutaneous use

90586   Bacillus Calmette-Guerin vaccine (BCG) for bladder cancer, live, for intravesical use

Unlike immune globulins which provide short-term, passive immunity, a vaccine provides active, long-term immunity by exposing the recipient's immune system to altered versions of specific viruses or bacteria that induce the immune system to produce its own antibodies against the invading micro-organism. The body then remembers how to make antibodies when exposed to the antigen again. The Bacillus Calmette-Guerin vaccine (BCG) is used against human tuberculosis. The vaccine is prepared from a live, weakened strain of the bovine tuberculosis, Mycobacterium bovis. The live virus is attenuated, or weakened, by being cultured in a specific artificial medium for years, until the strain is nonvirulent to humans. The BCG vaccine is also used to treat bladder cancer, although the way it works against cancer is not fully known. Code 90585 reports the live Bacillus Calmette-Guerin vaccine (BCG) against tuberculsosis for percutaneous injection. Use code 90586 if the live BCG vaccine is instilled through a catheter into the bladder to treat bladder cancer. These codes report only the product (vaccine) used.

90625

90625   Cholera vaccine, live, adult dosage, 1 dose schedule, for oral use

Unlike immune globulins which provide short-term, passive immunity, a vaccine provides active, long-term immunity by exposing the recipient's immune system to altered versions of specific viruses or bacteria that induce the immune system to produce its own antibodies against the invading micro-organism. The body then remembers how to make antibodies when exposed to the antigen again. This code reports an oral use, live, adult dose vaccine to protect against cholera, an acute diarrheal infection caused by the Vibrio Cholerae bacterium, not common in industrialized nations but still common in sub-Saharan Africa and the Indian subcontinent. Some cases cause such severe diarrhea and vomiting that cramping, dehydration, and shock can lead to death within hours. This code reports only the product (vaccine) used.

90630

90630   Influenza virus vaccine, quadrivalent (IIV4), split virus, preservative free, for intradermal use

A quadrivalent, split virus, preservative-free influenza vaccine product for intradermal use is provided. Unlike immune globulins which provide short-term, passive immunity, a vaccine provides active, long-term immunity by exposing the recipient's immune system to altered versions of specific viruses or bacteria that induce the immune system to produce its own antibodies against the invading micro-organism. The body then remembers how to make antibodies when exposed to the antigen again. A preservative-free formulation does not contain the preservative thimerosal, or contains only trace amounts, and is either thimerosal-free or thimerosal-reduced. The FDA considers both to be preservative-free and both are labeled as such. This vaccine is administered by intradermal injection, which is reported separately. Influenza vaccine is developed in embryonated chicken eggs. Fluid containing the virus is then harvested and inactivated with formaldehyde. The influenza virus is concentrated and purified, followed by chemical disruption to create a split virus and further purification. Quadrivalent influenza vaccines are formulated to protect against four different influenza viruses, which include two different influenza type A strains and two influenza type B strains.

90632-90636

90632   Hepatitis A vaccine (HepA), adult dosage, for intramuscular use
90633   Hepatitis A vaccine (HepA), pediatric/adolescent dosage-2 dose schedule, for intramuscular use
90634   Hepatitis A vaccine (HepA), pediatric/adolescent dosage-3 dose schedule, for intramuscular use
90636   Hepatitis A and hepatitis B vaccine (HepA-HepB), adult dosage, for intramuscular use

Unlike immune globulins which provide short-term, passive immunity, a vaccine provides active, long-term immunity by exposing the recipient's immune system to altered versions of specific viruses or bacteria that induce the immune system to produce its own antibodies against the invading micro-organism. The body then remembers how to make antibodies when exposed to the antigen again. The hepatitis A vaccine (HepA) provides long-term protection against the serious liver disease that can result in hospitalization and even death. The hepatitis B vaccine also provides protection against the consequences of hepatocellular carcinoma. The vaccine may be prepared from blood plasma of asymptomatic carriers or synthesized using recombinant technology, in which a plasmid containing the gene for hepatitis is inserted into common baker's yeast, then purified by lysing the yeast and separating out the yeast components. These codes report hepatitis vaccines for intramuscular use. Use code 90632 for HepA, adult dosage; 90633 for HepA pediatric/adolescent dosage over a 2-dose schedule; and 90634 for HepA pediatric/adolescent dosage over a 3-dose schedule. Code 90636 is for HepA-HepB adult dosage vaccine. These codes report only the product (vaccine) used.

90644

▲ **90644**   Meningococcal conjugate vaccine, serogroups C & Y and Haemophilus influenzae type b vaccine (Hib-MenCY), 4 dose schedule, when administered to children 6 weeks-18 months of age, for intramuscular use

This code reports a combination vaccine used to prevent meningococcal disease for serogroups C and Y and Haemophilus influenzae type b (Hib-MenCY). Meningococcal disease is caused by Neisseria meningitides, an infection spread by respiratory tract secretions that can cause septicemia or meningitis. There are 13 different subtypes and this vaccine provides protection against the C and Y subtypes. Hib infection can cause pneumonia, epiglottitis, infection of the joints and bones, and meningitis. This vaccine is formulated for children age 6 weeks -18 months. This code reports supply of the combination vaccine only. An administration code is reported additionally for the intramuscular injection.

90647-90648

90647   Haemophilus influenzae type b vaccine (Hib), PRP-OMP conjugate, 3 dose schedule, for intramuscular use
90648   Haemophilus influenzae type b vaccine (Hib), PRP-T conjugate, 4 dose schedule, for intramuscular use

Unlike immune globulins which provide short-term, passive immunity, a vaccine provides active, long-term immunity by exposing the recipient's immune system to altered versions of specific viruses or bacteria that induce the immune system to produce its own antibodies against the invading micro-organism. The body then remembers how to make antibodies when exposed to the antigen again. Haemophilus influenzae type b (Hib) is a serious disease affected children under 5. Bacteria in the lungs or bloodstream causes pneumonia, serious throat swelling, infection of the joints and bones, and meningitis with possible brain damage and deafness. These codes report a conjugate Hib vaccine for intramuscular use. Code 90647 reports PRP-OMP conjugate 3-dose schedule and 90648 reports PRP-T conjugate 4-dose schedule. These codes report only the product (vaccine) used.

90649-90651

90649   Human Papillomavirus vaccine, types 6, 11, 16, 18, quadrivalent (4vHPV), 3 dose schedule, for intramuscular use
90650   Human Papillomavirus vaccine, types 16, 18, bivalent (2vHPV), 3 dose schedule, for intramuscular use
90651   Human Papillomavirus vaccine types 6, 11, 16, 18, 31, 33, 45, 52, 58, nonavalent (9vHPV), 3 dose schedule, for intramuscular use

A human papillomavirus (HPV) vaccine is provided for intramuscular injection over a three-dose schedule. Unlike immune globulins, which provide short-term, passive immunity, a vaccine provides long-term immunity by exposing the recipient's immune system to an altered version of specific viruses or bacteria that induce the immune system to produce its own antibodies against the invading microorganism. The body then remembers how to make antibodies when exposed to the antigen at a later time. The human papilloma viruses are, in actuality, a group of more than 100 viruses. Some cause warts or benign tumors,

while certain high-risk strains have been shown to cause cervical cancer. The vaccine can effectively prevent infection from the virus and its long-term consequences of cancer if it is administered before the individual is infected. Code 90649 reports the supply only of the quadrivalent (4vHPV) vaccine against types 6, 11, 16, and 18. Code 90650 reports supply of the bivalent (2vHPV) vaccine against types 16 and 18, which are the strains that cause the greatest percentage of cervical cancer. Code 90651 reports supply of the nonavalent (9vHPV) vaccine against a multitude of nine other common HPV types also found in cancers worldwide.

90653

90653   Influenza vaccine, inactivated (IIV), subunit, adjuvanted, for intramuscular use

Unlike immune globulins which provide short-term, passive immunity, a vaccine provides active, long-term immunity by exposing the recipient's immune system to altered versions of specific viruses or bacteria that induce the immune system to produce its own antibodies against the invading micro-organism. The body then remembers how to make antibodies when exposed to the antigen again. Influenza vaccine is developed in embryonated chicken eggs. Fluid containing the virus is harvested and inactivated with formaldehyde. Subunit influenza vaccines include only the antigens that best stimulate the immune system which requires identification and isolation of the essential antigens. The essential antigens can be obtained by growing the microbe in the laboratory and then using chemicals to separate and obtain the essential antigens. Alternatively, the essential antigens can be produced using recombinant DNA technology. Once the subunit vaccine has been manufactured, an adjuvant is added. An adjuvant is a substance that helps stimulate the body's immune response. This inactivated influenza vaccine (IIV) is administered by intramuscular injection, which is reported separately.

90654

90654   Influenza virus vaccine, trivalent (IIV3), split virus, preservative-free, for intradermal use

A trivalent, split virus, preservative-free influenza vaccine product for intradermal use is provided. Unlike immune globulins which provide short-term, passive immunity, a vaccine provides active, long-term immunity by exposing the recipient's immune system to altered versions of specific viruses or bacteria that induce the immune system to produce its own antibodies against the invading micro-organism. The body then remembers how to make antibodies when exposed to the antigen again. A preservative-free formulation does not contain the preservative thimerosal, or contains only trace amounts, and is either thimerosal-free or thimerosal-reduced. The FDA considers both to be preservative-free and both are labeled as such. This vaccine is administered by intramuscular injection, which is reported separately. Influenza vaccine is developed in embryonated chicken eggs. Fluid containing the virus is then harvested and inactivated with formaldehyde. The influenza virus is concentrated and purified, followed by chemical disruption to create a split virus and further purification. Trivalent influenza vaccines are formulated with three influenza viruses, which include two different influenza type A strains and one influenza type B strain. This code reports only the product (vaccine) used. Report the intradermal injection separately.

90655-90656

▲ **90655**   Influenza virus vaccine, trivalent (IIV3), split virus, preservative free, 0.25 mL dosage, for intramuscular use
▲ **90656**   Influenza virus vaccine, trivalent (IIV3), split virus, preservative free, 0.5 mL dosage, for intramuscular use

A trivalent, split virus, preservative-free influenza vaccine (IIV3) product for intramuscular use is provided. Unlike immune globulins which provide short-term, passive immunity, a vaccine provides active, long-term immunity by exposing the recipient's immune system to altered versions of specific viruses or bacteria that induce the immune system to produce its own antibodies against the invading micro-organism. The body then remembers how to make antibodies when exposed to the antigen again. A preservative-free formulation does not contain the preservative thimerosal, or contains only trace amounts, and is either thimerosal-free or thimerosal-reduced. The FDA considers both to be preservative-free and both are labeled as such. This vaccine is administered by intramuscular injection, which is reported separately. Influenza vaccine is developed in embryonated chicken eggs. Fluid containing the virus is then harvested and inactivated with formaldehyde. The influenza virus is concentrated and purified, followed by chemical disruption to create a split virus and further purification. Trivalent influenza vaccines are formulated for protection against 3 influenza viruses, which include two different influenza type A strains and one influenza type B strain. Report code 90655 for a 0.25 mL dosage of the vaccine to be administered intramuscularly and code 90656 for a 0.5 mL dosage. These codes report only the product (vaccine) used. Report the intramuscular injection separately.

Medicine

90657-90658

▲ **90657**   **Influenza virus vaccine, trivalent (IIV3), split virus, 0.25 mL dosage, for intramuscular use**

▲ **90658**   **Influenza virus vaccine, trivalent (IIV3), split virus, 0.5 mL dosage, for intramuscular use**

A trivalent, split virus, influenza vaccine (IIV3) product for intramuscular use is provided. Unlike immune globulins which provide short-term, passive immunity, a vaccine provides active, long-term immunity by exposing the recipient's immune system to altered versions of specific viruses or bacteria that induce the immune system to produce its own antibodies against the invading micro-organism. The body then remembers how to make antibodies when exposed to the antigen again. An influenza split-virus vaccine containing the preservative thimerosal is developed in embryonated chicken eggs. Fluid containing the virus is then harvested and inactivated with formaldehyde. The influenza virus is concentrated and purified followed by chemical disruption to create a split virus and further purification. Trivalent influenza vaccines are formulated with three influenza viruses, which include two different influenza type A strains and one influenza type B strain. Report 90657 for a 0.25mL vaccine dosage to be administered intramuscularly and 90658 for a 0.5mL doage. These codes report only the product (vaccine) used. Report the intramuscular injection separately.

90660

90660   **Influenza virus vaccine, trivalent, live (LAIV3), for intranasal use**

A trivalent live influenza virus vaccine (LAIV3) for intranasal use is provided. Unlike immune globulins which provide short-term, passive immunity, a vaccine provides active, long-term immunity by exposing the recipient's immune system to altered versions of specific viruses or bacteria that induce the immune system to produce its own antibodies against the invading micro-organism. The body then remembers how to make antibodies when exposed to the antigen again. The intranasal influenza virus vaccine is a live attenuated (LAIV) vaccine. LAIV contains the live influenza virus, although the virus is weakened (attenuated). When introduced into the nose as a nasal spray, LAIV stimulates the production of antibodies to the influenza virus by the body's immune system. Because LAIV is cold-adapted and temperature sensitive, the influenza virus grows only in the nose and throat without spreading to the upper respiratory tract where body temperature is higher. Trivalent influenza vaccines are formulated with three influenza viruses, which include two different influenza type A strains and one influenza type B strain. This influenza vaccine is administered as a nasal spray. This code reports only the product (vaccine). Report the intranasal administration separately.

90661

▲ **90661**   **Influenza virus vaccine, trivalent (ccIIV3), derived from cell cultures, subunit, preservative and antibiotic free, 0.5 mL dosage, for intramuscular use**

Unlike immune globulins which provide short-term, passive immunity, a vaccine provides active, long-term immunity by exposing the recipient's immune system to altered versions of specific viruses or bacteria that induce the immune system to produce its own antibodies against the invading micro-organism. The body then remembers how to make antibodies when exposed to the antigen again. A preservative and antibiotic-free influenza virus vaccine derived from cell cultures (ccIIV3) is different from other influenza vaccine formulations in that it is produced from cell cultures in master and working cell banks in a sterile, controlled environment. Influenza vaccine produced in this manner does not require embryonated eggs, antibiotics, or preservatives, and is a non-allergenic, preservative-free, antibiotic-free formulation. Trivalent influenza vaccines are formulated with three influenza viruses, which include two different influenza type A strains and one influenza type B strain. Code 90661 reports a 0.5mL dosage of a trivalent, preservative and antibiotic-free, influenza virus vaccine derived from cell cultures to be administered intramuscularly. This code reports only the product (vaccine) used.

90662

90662   **Influenza virus vaccine (IIV), split virus, preservative free, enhanced immunogenicity via increased antigen content, for intramuscular use**

Unlike immune globulins which provide short-term, passive immunity, a vaccine provides active, long-term immunity by exposing the recipient's immune system to altered versions of specific viruses or bacteria that induce the immune system to produce its own antibodies against the invading micro-organism. The body then remembers how to make antibodies when exposed to the antigen again. A preservative free, split-virus influenza vaccine with increased antigen content for enhanced immunogenicity has significantly more hemagglutinin per influenza strain in each vaccine and provides an improved immune response. The preservative-free formulation does not contain the preservative thimerosal, or contains only trace amounts, and is either thimerosal-free or thimerosal-reduced. The FDA considers both to be preservative-free and both are labeled as such. Like other split-virus influenza vaccines, this formulation is developed in embryonated chicken eggs. The fluid containing the virus is harvested and inactivated with formaldehyde. The influenza virus is concentrated using a technique that increases antigen content and purified. This is followed by chemical disruption to create a split virus and further purification. The

enhanced immunogenicity split-virus influenza vaccine is indicated for use in the elderly where immune responsiveness is reduced. A preservative-free, enhanced immunogenicty, split-virus influenza vaccine is administered by intramuscular injection, which is reported separately. This code reports only the product (vaccine) used.

90664

90664   **Influenza virus vaccine, live (LAIV), pandemic formulation, for intranasal use**

The intranasal vaccine for the influenza virus is a live attenuated influenza virus (LAIV) vaccine meaning it contains the live influenza virus, although in a weakened state (attenuated). Pandemic vaccine formulations may differ from interpandemic strains and may have different additives (adjuvants) to enhance the antigen content, as well as different dosages. An influenza pandemic occurs when a new influenza strain appears and spreads in the human population. Individuals have little or no immunity to this new strain and so there may be widespread severe illness (morbidity) and death (mortality) associated with the outbreak. When introduced into the nose as a nasal spray, LAIV stimulates the production of antibodies to the influenza virus by the body's immune system. Because LAIV is cold-adapted and temperature sensitive, the influenza virus grows only in the nose and throat without spreading to the upper respiratory tract where body temperature is higher. Use this code for the vaccine product. Report the intranasal administration separately.

90666-90668

90666   **Influenza virus vaccine (IIV), pandemic formulation, split virus, preservative free, for intramuscular use**

90667   **Influenza virus vaccine (IIV), pandemic formulation, split virus, adjuvanted, for intramuscular use**

90668   **Influenza virus vaccine (IIV), pandemic formulation, split virus, for intramuscular use**

There are two main types of influenza, Type A and Type B. Within these types are subtypes. Examples of subtypes of influenza Type A include H1N1, H3N2, and H5N1. Pandemic influenza vaccine formulations may differ from those for interpandemic strains, have different additives (adjuvants), and be administered in different dosages. An influenza pandemic occurs when a new influenza strain appears and spreads in the human population. Individuals have little or no immunity to this new strain and so there may be widespread severe illness (morbidity) and death (mortality) associated with the outbreak. Like other split-virus influenza vaccines, the pandemic formulation is developed in embryonated chicken eggs. The fluid containing the virus is harvested and inactivated with formaldehyde. The influenza virus is concentrated using a technique that increases antigen content and then purified. This is followed by chemical disruption to create a split virus and further purification. All of the split virus vaccines for pandemic influenza are administered via separately reportable intramuscular injection. Use 90666 for a pandemic-type, split, preservative-free, influenza virus vaccine. The preservative-free formulation does not contain the preservative thimerosal or contains only trace amounts. The former may be referred to as thimerosal-free and the latter as thimerosal-reduced. The FDA considers both to be preservative-free and both are labeled as such. Use 90667 for a pandemic-type, split, adjuvanted influenza virus vaccine. Adjuvanted vaccines have additives that enhance the antigen content. Influenza vaccines with increased antigen content for enhanced immunogenicity have significantly more hemagglutinin per influenza strain in each vaccine and provide an improved immune response. The adjuvanted split-virus influenza vaccine is indicated for use in the elderly and other individuals with reduced immune responsiveness. Use 90668 for all other pandemic-type, influenza vaccine products not described as either preservative-free or adjuvanted.

90670

90670   **Pneumococcal conjugate vaccine, 13 valent (PCV13), for intramuscular use**

Unlike immune globulins which provide short-term, passive immunity, a vaccine provides active, long-term immunity by exposing the recipient's immune system to altered versions of specific viruses or bacteria that induce the immune system to produce its own antibodies against invading microorganisms. The body then remembers how to make antibodies when exposed to the antigen again. Pneumococcal bacteria can exist in the nose and throat without causing disease, but when the bacteria invade the body, they can cause pneumococcal pneumonia, bacteremia, and meningitis. Children under 5, the elderly and immune suppressed individuals are most susceptible. The vaccine is administered by separately reportable intramuscular injection. Pneumococcal conjugate vaccines are differentiated by the number of different serotypes of the pneumococcal bacterium that are covered by the vaccine. Code 90670 reports a 13 valent pneumococcal conjugate vaccine (PCV13) that covers the serotypes designated as 4, 6B, 9V, 14, 18C, 19F, 23F, and 1, 3, 5, 6A, 7F, and 19A.

90672

90672   **Influenza virus vaccine, quadrivalent, live (LAIV4), for intranasal use**

Unlike immune globulins which provide short-term, passive immunity, a vaccine provides active, long-term immunity by exposing the recipient's immune system to altered versions of

Medicine

specific viruses or bacteria that induce the immune system to produce its own antibodies against the invading micro-organism. The body then remembers how to make antibodies when exposed to the antigen again. The quadrivalent intranasal influenza virus vaccine is a live attenuated vaccine (LAIV4). LAIV4 contains the live influenza virus, although the virus is weakened (attenuated). A quadrivalent vaccine contains two influenza A and two influenza B viruses. When introduced into the nose as a nasal spray, LAIV4 stimulates the production of antibodies to the influenza virus by the body's immune system. Because LAIV4 is cold-adapted and temperature sensitive, the influenza virus grows only in the nose and throat without spreading to the upper respiratory tract where body temperature is higher. This code reports only the product (vaccine) used. Report the intranasal administration separately.

90673

90673   Influenza virus vaccine, trivalent (RIV3), derived from recombinant DNA, hemagglutinin (HA) protein only, preservative and antibiotic free, for intramuscular use

Influenza virus vaccine, trivalent (Flublok) is an influenza vaccine (RIV3) produced without the use of influenza virus or eggs. It is manufactured using an insect virus (baculovirus) expression system and recombinant DNA technology to produce the influenza virus protein, hemagglutinin (HA). This new technology can facilitate a faster start up and larger produced quantity in the event of pandemic influenza infection. Trivalent vaccines contain three, full strength, recombinant HA proteins that help protect against two strains of Influenza A and one strain of Influenza B. The vaccine is injected intramuscularly. Administration of the vaccine is reported separately.

90674

● 90674   Influenza virus vaccine, quadrivalent (ccIIV4), derived from cell cultures, subunit, preservative and antibiotic free, 0.5 mL dosage, for intramuscular use

Unlike immune globulins which provide short-term, passive immunity, a vaccine provides active, long-term immunity by exposing the recipient's immune system to altered versions of specific viruses or bacteria that induce the immune system to produce its own antibodies against the invading micro-organism. The body then remembers how to make antibodies when exposed to the antigen again. A preservative and antibiotic-free influenza virus vaccine derived from cell cultures (ccIIV3) is different from other influenza vaccine formulations in that it is produced from cell cultures in master and working cell banks in a sterile, controlled environment. Influenza vaccine produced in this manner does not require embryonated eggs, antibiotics, or preservatives, and is a non-allergenic, preservative-free, antibiotic-free formulation. Quadrivalent influenza vaccines are formulated with four influenza viruses, which include two different influenza type A strains and two influenza type B strains. Code 90674 reports a 0.5mL dosage of a quadrivalent, preservative and antibiotic-free, influenza virus vaccine derived from cell cultures to be administered intramuscularly. This code reports only the product (vaccine) used.

90675-90676

90675   Rabies vaccine, for intramuscular use
90676   Rabies vaccine, for intradermal use

Unlike immune globulins which provide short-term, passive immunity, a vaccine provides active, long-term immunity by exposing the recipient's immune system to altered versions of specific viruses or bacteria that induce the immune system to produce its own antibodies against the invading micro-organism. The body then remembers how to make antibodies when exposed to the antigen again. These codes report vaccines to protect against rabies. Use 90675 for intramuscular use and 90676 for intradermal use. These codes report only the product (vaccine) used.

90680

90680   Rotavirus vaccine, pentavalent (RV5), 3 dose schedule, live, for oral use

Unlike immune globulins which provide short-term, passive immunity, a vaccine provides active, long-term immunity by exposing the recipient's immune system to altered versions of specific viruses or bacteria that induce the immune system to produce its own antibodies against the invading micro-organism. The body then remembers how to make antibodies when exposed to the antigen again. Rotavirus disease is highly contagious and affects almost every child in the U.S. by the age of 5. It causes repeated episode of vomiting and severe diarrhea that can lead to hospitalization. The live, pentavalent Rotavirus vaccine (RV5) contains the actual virus and is prepared for oral use in a 3-dose schedule. This code reports only the product (vaccine) used.

90681

90681   Rotavirus vaccine, human, attenuated (RV1), 2 dose schedule, live, for oral use

A live attenuated human rotavirus vaccine (RV1) is provided for oral use in a two dose schedule. Unlike immune globulins which provide short-term, passive immunity, a vaccine provides long-term immunity by exposing the recipient's immune system to an altered

version of specific viruses or bacteria that induce the immune system to produce its own antibodies against the invading microorganism. The body then remembers how to make antibodies when exposed to the antigen at a later time. Rotavirus disease is highly contagious and affects almost every child in the U.S. by the age of 5. It causes repeated episodes of vomiting and severe diarrhea that can lead to hospitalization. The live attenuated rotavirus vaccine contains a weakened strain of the live virus that is prepared for oral use. This code reports the supply only (oral administration is not included) of the vaccine.

90685-90686

▲ 90685   Influenza virus vaccine, quadrivalent (IIV4), split virus, preservative free, 0.25 mL dosage, for intramuscular use
▲ 90686   Influenza virus vaccine, quadrivalent (IIV4), split virus, preservative free, 0.5 mL dosage, for intramuscular use

A quadrivalent, split virus, preservative-free influenza vaccine (IIV4) product for intramuscular use is provided. Unlike immune globulins which provide short-term, passive immunity, a vaccine provides active, long-term immunity by exposing the recipient's immune system to altered versions of specific viruses or bacteria that induce the immune system to produce its own antibodies against the invading micro-organism. The body then remembers how to make antibodies when exposed to the antigen again. A preservative-free formulation does not contain the preservative thimerosal, or contains only trace amounts, and is either thimerosal-free or thimerosal-reduced. The FDA considers both to be preservative-free and both are labeled as such. This vaccine is administered by intramuscular injection, which is reported separately. Influenza vaccine is developed in embryonated chicken eggs. Fluid containing the virus is then harvested and inactivated with formaldehyde. The influenza virus is concentrated and purified, followed by chemical disruption to create a split virus and further purification. Quadrivalent influenza vaccines are formulated for protection against 4 influenza viruses, which include two different influenza type A strains and two influenza type B strains. Report code 90685 for a 0.25 mL dosage of the vaccine to be administered intramuscularly and code 90686 for a 0.5 mL dosage. These codes report only the product (vaccine) used. Report the intramuscular injection separately.

90687-90688

▲ 90687   Influenza virus vaccine, quadrivalent (IIV4), split virus, 0.25 mL dosage, for intramuscular use
▲ 90688   Influenza virus vaccine, quadrivalent (IIV4), split virus, 0.5 mL dosage, for intramuscular use

A quadrivalent, split virus influenza vaccine (IIV4) product for intramuscular use is provided. Unlike immune globulins which provide short-term, passive immunity, a vaccine provides active, long-term immunity by exposing the recipient's immune system to altered versions of specific viruses or bacteria that induce the immune system to produce its own antibodies against the invading micro-organism. The body then remembers how to make antibodies when exposed to the antigen again. This vaccine is administered by intramuscular injection, which is reported separately. Influenza vaccine is developed in embryonated chicken eggs. Fluid containing the virus is then harvested and inactivated with formaldehyde. The influenza virus is concentrated and purified, followed by chemical disruption to create a split virus and further purification. Quadrivalent influenza vaccines are formulated for protection against 4 influenza viruses, which include two different influenza type A strains and two influenza type B strains. Report code 90687 for a 0.25 mL dosage of the vaccine to be administered intramuscularly and code 90688 for a 0.5 mL dosage. These codes report only the product (vaccine) used. Report the intramuscular injection separately.

90690-90691

90690   Typhoid vaccine, live, oral
90691   Typhoid vaccine, Vi capsular polysaccharide (ViCPs), for intramuscular use

Unlike immune globulins which provide short-term, passive immunity, a vaccine provides active, long-term immunity by exposing the recipient's immune system to altered versions of specific viruses or bacteria that induce the immune system to produce its own antibodies against the invading micro-organism. The body then remembers how to make antibodies when exposed to the antigen again. Typhoid is caused by Salmonella typhi, causing high fever, rash, and diarrhea. It is spread by contaminated food, water, and milk. These codes report different preparations of vaccines that provide protection against typhoid infection. Use code 90690 for an oral vaccine that contains the live, actual virus. Use code 90691 for Vi capsular polysaccharide (ViCPs) vaccine for intramuscular injection. These codes report only the product (vaccine) used.

90696

90696   Diphtheria, tetanus toxoids, acellular pertussis vaccine and poliovirus vaccine, inactivated (DTaP-IPV), when administered to children 4 through 6 years of age, for intramuscular use

A combination vaccine for diphtheria, tetanus toxoids, acellular pertussis (DTaP), and inactivated poliovirus (IPV) is provided for intramuscular administration to children aged 4 through 6. Unlike immune globulins, which provide short-term, passive immunity, a

Medicine

vaccine provides long-term immunity by exposing the recipient's immune system to an altered version of specific viruses or bacteria that induce the immune system to produce its own antibodies against the invading microorganism. The body then remembers how to make antibodies when exposed to the antigen at a later time. The vaccine prevents diphtheria, tetanus, pertussis, and poliomyelitis. Diphtheria is a potent toxin that causes severe inflammation and coating of the mucous membranes of the pharynx, nose, and tracheobronchial tree with thick fibrinous exudates. Tetanus is a neurotropic toxin that causes painful tonic contraction of muscles. Pertussis, also referred to as whooping cough, is an acute infection of the upper respiratory tract characterized by inflammation and spasmodic coughing. The acellular pertussis vaccine contains purified antigenic components of the infectious agent, Bordetella pertussis, which is less likely to cause adverse reactions than the whole-cell pertussis vaccine. Poliovirus is a viral infection that causes inflammation of the gray matter of the brain and spinal cord. Vaccine-associated paralytic poliomyelitis was a rare complication of oral poliovirus vaccines. Inactivated poliovirus cannot cause this complication and is now the preferred form of the vaccine, even though it must be administered by injection. This code reports the supply only (intramuscular injection is not included) of the combined vaccine/toxoid.

90698

90698   Diphtheria, tetanus toxoids, acellular pertussis vaccine, haemophilus influenzae type b, and inactivated poliovirus vaccine, (DTaP-IPV/Hib), for intramuscular use

Toxoids provide long lasting immunity by stimulating the body's own defense system to make antibodies that destroy specific toxins produced by bacteria. Vaccines also provide active, long-term immunity by exposing the recipient's immune system to altered versions of specific viruses or bacteria that induce the immune system to produce its own antibodies against the invading micro-organism. The body then remembers how to make antibodies when exposed to these same agents again. This code is for an immunization supply of toxoids against diphtheria and tetanus, and acellular, (synthetic or more purified) pertussis vaccine combined with Haemophilus influenzae type B (Hib) and inactivated poliovirus vaccine (DTap-IPV/Hib) for intramuscular injection. This code reports only the product (toxoid/vaccine) used.

90700

90700   Diphtheria, tetanus toxoids, and acellular pertussis vaccine (DTaP), when administered to individuals younger than 7 years, for intramuscular use

Toxoids provide long lasting immunity by stimulating the body's own defense system to make antibodies that destroy specific toxins produced by bacteria. Vaccines also provide active, long-term immunity by exposing the recipient's immune system to altered versions of specific viruses or bacteria that induce the immune system to produce its own antibodies against the invading micro-organism. The body then remembers how to make antibodies when exposed to these same agents again. Code 90700 reports intramuscular immunization supply of toxoids against diphtheria and tetanus, and acellular pertussis vaccine (DTaP) for patients under 7 years. The acellular pertussis component is a synthetic, or more purified form of pertussis, that produces fewer side effects. This code reports only the product (toxoid/vaccine) used.

90702

90702   Diphtheria and tetanus toxoids adsorbed (DT) when administered to individuals younger than 7 years, for intramuscular use

Toxoids provide long lasting immunity by stimulating the body's own defense system to make antibodies that destroy specific toxins produced by bacteria. The toxoid vaccine is an inactivated poison, called a toxin, produced by culturing the bacteria in a liquid medium, then purifying and inactivating the poison produced by the bacteria. Since toxoids are not a live vaccine, booster doses are recommended because immunity will decline over time. Code 90702 reports diphtheria and tetanus toxoids (DT) adsorbed for intramuscular use in patients younger than 7 years. This code reports only the product (toxoid) used.

90707-90710

90707   Measles, mumps and rubella virus vaccine (MMR), live, for subcutaneous use

90710   Measles, mumps, rubella, and varicella vaccine (MMRV), live, for subcutaneous use

Unlike immune globulins which provide short-term, passive immunity, a vaccine provides active, long-term immunity by exposing the recipient's immune system to altered versions of specific viruses or bacteria that induce the immune system to produce its own antibodies against the invading micro-organism. The body then remembers how to make antibodies when exposed to the antigen again. These codes report vaccines containing the live virus for measles, mumps, and rubella for subcutaneous use. The live virus has been attenuated, or weakened, so that it still triggers the immune response to build antibodies against it without being virulent enough to cause the disease. Code 90707 reports a live virus vaccine for the combination of measles, mumps, and rubella together (MMR), and 90710 reports a live viral vaccine against measles, mumps, rubella, and the varicella virus (MMRV). These codes report only the product (vaccine) used.

90713

90713   Poliovirus vaccine, inactivated (IPV), for subcutaneous or intramuscular use

Unlike immune globulins which provide short-term, passive immunity, a vaccine provides active, long-term immunity by exposing the recipient's immune system to altered versions of specific viruses or bacteria that induce the immune system to produce its own antibodies against the invading micro-organism. The body then remembers how to make antibodies when exposed to the antigen again. Code 90713 reports an inactivated poliovirus vaccine (IPV) for subcutaneous or intramuscular use. This code reports only the product (vaccine) used.

90714-90717

90714   Tetanus and diphtheria toxoids adsorbed (Td), preservative free, when administered to individuals 7 years or older, for intramuscular use

90715   Tetanus, diphtheria toxoids and acellular pertussis vaccine (Tdap), when administered to individuals 7 years or older, for intramuscular use

90716   Varicella virus vaccine (VAR), live, for subcutaneous use

90717   Yellow fever vaccine, live, for subcutaneous use

Toxoids provide long lasting immunity by stimulating the body's own defense system to make antibodies that destroy specific toxins produced by bacteria. Vaccines also provide active, long-term immunity by exposing the recipient's immune system to altered versions of specific viruses or bacteria that induce the immune system to produce its own antibodies against the invading micro-organism. The body then remembers how to make antibodies when exposed to these same agents again. The toxoid vaccine is an inactivated poison, called a toxin, produced by culturing the bacteria in a liquid medium, then purifying and inactivating the poison produced by the bacteria. Since toxoids are not a live vaccine, booster doses are recommended because immunity will decline over time. These tetanus toxoid combinations are formulations for adults and those over 7 years of age, given by intramuscular injection. Code 90715 reports supply of tetanus toxoid combined with diphtheria toxoid and acellular pertussis vaccine (Tdap). The acellular pertussis component is a synthetic, or more purified form of pertussis, that produces fewer side effects. Code 90714 reports preservative free tetanus and diphtheria toxoids (Td) adsorbed. These codes report only the product (toxoid/vaccine) used. Code 90717 is the subcutaneous use vaccine against yellow fever, more commonly used when traveling abroad, especially to South America and sub-Saharan Africa; code 90716 reports the subcutaneous use vaccine against the varicella virus (VAR).

90723

90723   Diphtheria, tetanus toxoids, acellular pertussis vaccine, hepatitis B, and inactivated poliovirus vaccine (DTaP-HepB-IPV), for intramuscular use

Diptheria, tetanus, and pertussis vaccines are supplied in differing combinations for intramuscular use. Toxoids provide long lasting immunity by stimulating the body's own defense system to make antibodies that destroy specific toxins produced by bacteria. Vaccines also provide active, long-term immunity by exposing the recipient's immune system to altered versions of specific viruses or bacteria that induce the immune system to produce its own antibodies against the invading micro-organism. The body then remembers how to make antibodies when exposed to these same agents again. The toxoid is an inactivated poison, called a toxin, produced by culturing the bacteria in a liquid medium, then purifying and inactivating the poison produced by the bacteria. The acellular pertussis component is a synthetic, or more purified form of pertussis that produces fewer side effects. Code 90723 reports intramuscular diphtheria and tetanus toxoids, acellular pertussis, hepatitis B, and inactivated poliovirus vaccine (DTaP-HepB-IPV). This code reports only the product (toxoid/vaccine) used.

90732

90732   Pneumococcal polysaccharide vaccine, 23-valent (PPSV23), adult or immunosuppressed patient dosage, when administered to individuals 2 years or older, for subcutaneous or intramuscular use

Unlike immune globulins which provide short-term, passive immunity, a vaccine provides active, long-term immunity by exposing the recipient's immune system to altered versions of specific viruses or bacteria that induce the immune system to produce its own antibodies against the invading micro-organism. The body then remembers how to make antibodies when exposed to the antigen again. The pneumococcal bacteria exist in many people's noses and throats without causing disease, but when it invades the body, it can cause pneumococcal pneumonia, bacteremia, and meningitis. Children under five, the elderly, and the immune suppressed are most susceptible. Pneumococcal disease is the leading cause of death from vaccine-preventable disease in the U.S. This code reports a polysaccharide, 23-valent pneumococcal vaccine (PPSV23) for adults or immunosuppressed over two years old, given either subcutaneously or intramuscularly. This code reports only the product (vaccine) used.

Medicine

90733-90734

90733   Meningococcal polysaccharide vaccine, serogroups A, C, Y, W-135, quadrivalent (MPSV4), for subcutaneous use

90734   Meningococcal conjugate vaccine, serogroups A, C, Y and W-135, quadrivalent (MenACWY), for intramuscular use

Unlike immune globulins which provide short-term, passive immunity, a vaccine provides active, long-term immunity by exposing the recipient's immune system to altered versions of specific viruses or bacteria that induce the immune system to produce its own antibodies against the invading micro-organism. The body then remembers how to make antibodies when exposed to the antigen again. These codes report different vaccines against meningococcal disease, a serious illness caused by Neisseria meningitidis, transferred by respiratory or throat secretions, and causing septicemia or meningitis which can lead to shock, coma, and death, or permanent hearing loss or brain damage. There are 13 different subtypes of meningococcus, and five cause invasive disease: A,B,C,Y, and W-135. Code 90733 reports quadrivalent meningococcal polysaccharide vaccine of serogroups A,C,Y, and W-135 (MPSV4) for subcutaneous use. The polysaccharide vaccine is for persons 2 years and older, and is made from the outer polysaccharide sugar capsule or coat of the bacteria and does not contain live virus. This is given into the fat of the arm. Code 90734 reports a quadrivalent meningococcal conjugate vaccine that protects against serogroups A,C,Y, and W-135 (MenACWY) with better, longer-lasting protection than the MPSV4. The MenACWY vaccine contains the capsular polysaccharide antigens from all four serogroups individually conjugated to diphtheria toxoid protein. It is given intramuscularly. No vaccine prevents against subtype B. These codes report only the product (vaccine) used.

90736

90736   Zoster (shingles) vaccine (HZV), live, for subcutaneous injection

Unlike immune globulins which provide short-term, passive immunity, a vaccine provides active, long-term immunity by exposing the recipient's immune system to altered versions of specific viruses or bacteria that induce the immune system to produce its own antibodies against the invading micro-organism. The body then remembers how to make antibodies when exposed to the antigen again. This code reports a live virus vaccine for subcutaneous use against the zoster virus alone (HZV), which is the latent, reactivated form of the varicella virus that initially causes chicken pox. The zoster virus causes shingles in an individual who has previously had chicken pox when the virus is reactivated in the body, by stress or decreased immunity. This code reports only the product (vaccine) used.

90738

90738   Japanese encephalitis virus vaccine, inactivated, for intramuscular use

An inactivated vaccine for the Japanese encephalitis virus is provided for intramuscular administration. Unlike immune globulins which provide short-term, passive immunity, a vaccine provides long-term immunity by exposing the recipient's immune system to an altered version of specific viruses or bacteria that induce the immune system to produce its own antibodies against the invading microorganism. The body then remembers how to make antibodies when exposed to the antigen at a later time. The Japanese encephalitis (JE) virus causes inflammation (swelling) of the brain. The disease is found in certain rural regions of Asia and is spread through the bite of infected mosquitoes. The vaccine is recommended for people who live or travel in these regions. This code reports the supply only (intramuscular injection is not included) of the vaccine.

90739-90747

90739   Hepatitis B vaccine, adult dosage (2 dose schedule), for intramuscular use

90740   Hepatitis B vaccine (HepB), dialysis or immunosuppressed patient dosage, 3 dose schedule, for intramuscular use

90743   Hepatitis B vaccine (HepB), adolescent, 2 dose schedule, for intramuscular use

90744   Hepatitis B vaccine (HepB), pediatric/adolescent dosage, 3 dose schedule, for intramuscular use

90746   Hepatitis B vaccine (HepB), adult dosage, 3 dose schedule, for intramuscular use

90747   Hepatitis B vaccine (HepB), dialysis or immunosuppressed patient dosage, 4 dose schedule, for intramuscular use

Unlike immune globulins which provide short-term, passive immunity, a vaccine provides active, long-term immunity by exposing the recipient's immune system to altered versions of specific viruses or bacteria that induce the immune system to produce its own antibodies against the invading micro-organism. The body then remembers how to make antibodies when exposed to the antigen again. The hepatitis B vaccine provides long-term protection against the chronic, serious liver disease that can result in hospitalization and even death. It also provides protection against the disease's long-term consequences of hepatocellular carcinoma and is therefore one of the first cancer vaccines in use. The vaccine may be prepared from blood plasma of asymptomatic carriers or synthesized using recombinant technology, in which a plasmid containing the gene for hepatitis is inserted into common baker's yeast, and then purified by lysing the yeast and separating out the yeast components. These codes report only the hepatitis B vaccine product (HepB) for

intramuscular use. The injection is reported separately. Code 90739 reports adult dosage in a 2-dose schedule. Code 90740 reports dosage for dialysis or immunosuppressed patients in a 3-dose schedule. Code 90743 reports an adolescent 2-dose schedule. Code 90744 reports a pediatric/adolescent dosage for a 3-dose schedule. Code 90746 reports an adult 3-dose shedule dosage. Code 90747 reports dosage for dialysis or immunosuppressed patients in a 4-dose schedule.

90748

90748   Hepatitis B and Haemophilus influenzae type b vaccine (Hib-HepB), for intramuscular use

A combination vaccine for hepatitis B and Haemophilus influenzae type b (Hib-HepB) is provided. Unlike immune globulins which provide short-term, passive immunity, a vaccine provides active, long-term immunity by exposing the recipient's immune system to altered versions of specific viruses or bacteria that induce the immune system to produce its own antibodies against the invading micro-organism. The body then remembers how to make antibodies when exposed to the antigen again. The hepatitis B component of the vaccine provides long-term protection against the chronic, serious liver disease that can result in hospitalization and even death. It also provides protection against the disease's long-term consequences of hepatocellular carcinoma and is therefore one of the first cancer vaccines in use. The vaccine may be prepared from blood plasma of asymptomatic carriers or synthesized using recombinant technology, in which a plasmid containing the gene for hepatitis is inserted into common baker's yeast, then purified by lysing the yeast and separating out the yeast components. The Haemophilus influenzae type b (Hib) component of the vaccine provides long-term protection against Hib. Hib is a serious disease affecting children under age 5 which can cause pneumonia, serious throat swelling, infection of the joints and bones, and meningitis with possible brain damage and deafness. The Hib-HepB vaccine is administered intramuscularly which is reported separately.

90785

90785   Interactive complexity (List separately in addition to the code for primary procedure)

During a separately reportable psychiatric service, treatment is provided to a patient where factors related to difficulty in communication increase the complexity of the encounter. The difficulty may be due to communication issues on the part of the patient, such as a young child's or a developmentally or mentally impaired individual's inability to communicate with the provider. Communication difficulties may occur when there are other individuals involved in the patient's care such as parents or guardians, state agencies, court officers, or schools. Communication difficulties may also occur due to language barriers or the need to use an interpreter. The provider may report code 90785 for interactive complexity as an add-on service with codes for psychiatric evaluation, individual psychotherapy with or without an evaluation and management service, or group psychotherapy. Reporting code 90785 requires documentation of at least one complicating communication factor, such as maladaptive communication on the part of the patient or parent/guardian; caregiver issues related to emotions or behavior that adversely affect the treatment of the patient; mandated third party involvement (state agency, court, school); language barriers requiring the use of play equipment or other communication devices, interpreters, or translators; or lack of expressive language communication skills, including a child who has not yet developed these skills or an older person who has lost these skills due to illness or aging.

90791-90792

90791   Psychiatric diagnostic evaluation

90792   Psychiatric diagnostic evaluation with medical services

Code 90791 reports a psychiatric diagnostic interview exam including a complete medical and psychiatric history, a mental status exam, ordering of laboratory and other diagnostic studies with interpretation, and communication with other sources or informants. The psychiatrist then establishes a tentative diagnosis and determines the patient's capacity to benefit from psychotherapy treatment. The patient's condition will determine the extent of the mental status exam needed during the diagnostic interview. In determining mental status, the doctor looks for symptoms of psychopathology in appearance, attitude, behavior, speech, stream of talk, emotional reactions, mood, and content of thoughts, perceptions, and sometimes cognition. The diagnostic interview exam is done when the provider first sees a patient, but may also be utilized again for a new episode of illness, or for re-admission as an inpatient due to underlying complications. When a psychiatric diagnostic evaluation is performed alone, report code 90791. When medical services are provided in conjunction with the psychiatric diagnostic evaluation, report code 90792.

90832-90833

▲ 90832   Psychotherapy, 30 minutes with patient

▲ 90833   Psychotherapy, 30 minutes with patient when performed with an evaluation and management service (List separately in addition to the code for primary procedure)

Individual psychotherapy is provided to a patient utilizing reeducation, support and reassurance, insight discussions, and occasionally medication to affect behavior-

Medicine

modification through self-understanding, or to evaluate and improve family relationship dynamics as they relate to the patient's condition. If psychotherapy alone is provided, report 90832 for 30 minutes, 90834 for 45 minutes, and 90837 for 60 minutes. If medical evaluation and management services are performed with the psychotherapy, report code 90833 for 30 minutes, 90836 for 45 minutes, and 90838 for 60 minutes.

90834-90836

▲ **90834   Psychotherapy, 45 minutes with patient**

Individual psychotherapy is provided to a patient utilizing reeducation, support and reassurance, insight discussions, and occasionally medication to affect behavior-modification through self-understanding, or to evaluate and improve family relationship dynamics as they relate to the patient's condition. If psychotherapy alone is provided, report 90832 for 30 minutes, 90834 for 45 minutes, and 90837 for 60 minutes. If medical evaluation and management services are performed with the psychotherapy, report code 90833 for 30 minutes, 90836 for 45 minutes, and 90838 for 60 minutes.

90837-90838

▲ **90837   Psychotherapy, 60 minutes with patient**
▲ **90838   Psychotherapy, 60 minutes with patient when performed with an evaluation and management service (List separately in addition to the code for primary procedure)**

Individual psychotherapy is provided to a patient utilizing reeducation, support and reassurance, insight discussions, and occasionally medication to affect behavior-modification through self-understanding, or to evaluate and improve family relationship dynamics as they relate to the patient's condition. If psychotherapy alone is provided, report 90832 for 30 minutes, 90834 for 45 minutes, and 90837 for 60 minutes. If medical evaluation and management services are performed with the psychotherapy, report code 90833 for 30 minutes, 90836 for 45 minutes, and 90838 for 60 minutes.

90839-90840

90839   Psychotherapy for crisis; first 60 minutes
90840   Psychotherapy for crisis; each additional 30 minutes (List separately in addition to code for primary service)

A mental health crisis occurs when the patient feels overwhelmed or unable to cope with a situation or event. Psychotherapy for crisis provides immediate, short-term help to patients who experience a situation or event that produces emotional, mental, and behavioral distress. Psychotherapy is focused on the immediate situation, minimizing the stress of the event, providing emotional support and developing coping strategies to deal with the crisis. Therapy may also include reassurance and psychotropic medications aimed at decreasing the patient's anxiety and improving coping abilities. Code 90839 is reported for the first 60 minutes of psychotherapy for the crisis. Code 90840 is reported for each additional 30 minutes of psychotherapy for the crisis.

90845

90845   Psychoanalysis \

Psychoanalysis is a treatment modality that explores how unconscious factors affect the patient's current relationships, thought patterns, emotions, and behavior. The patient typically meets with the psychoanalyst multiple times a week. Therapy is conducted with the patient lying on a couch. The patient is encouraged to talk as freely and openly as possible about whatever is on his/her mind. The psychoanalyst listens and helps the patient identify patterns of thought, emotions, and behavior that are affecting his/her current relationships and life situation. These patterns are then traced back to their origins and analyzed to determine how they have changed over time. Exposing unconscious factors that are affecting the patient can help the patient understand the underlying causes of thought patterns, emotions, and behavior and how these are currently affecting the patient's life. Exposing unconscious factors can also help the patient learn to cope more effectively with his/her current life situation.

90846-90847

▲ **90846   Family psychotherapy (without the patient present), 50 minutes**
▲ **90847   Family psychotherapy (conjoint psychotherapy) (with patient present), 50 minutes**

Family psychotherapy is performed to help family members improve communication skills and their understanding of each other so they can cope better with stress, anger, and grief, and work to resolve any interpersonal conflicts. Family therapy may involve all family members, only those who are experiencing difficulties, or only those who are willing and able to participate. Sometimes family therapy is needed when a family member has a mental health condition, addiction, or a physical illness, and the entire family needs assistance in coping with these challenges. Therapy examines the family's interactions, communication skills, and ability to work together to solve problems. Family roles may be explored, rules and discipline issues discussed, and individual behavior patterns evaluated. Sources of stress, anger, grief, and conflict are also explored. The therapist works with the family to help identify challenges, improve family coping skills, and change patterns

of behavior. The therapist may then suggest changes in how individuals interact and help family members develop more constructive patterns of communication and behavior. Use 90846 for 50 minutes of family psychotherapy when a specific family member, the patient, is experiencing personal challenges and is not present . Use code 90847 for 50 minutes of conjoint family psychotherapy with the patient present.

90849

90849   Multiple-family group psychotherapy

Multiple-family group psychotherapy involves working with several families who are experiencing similar stressors in a group therapy session. These families may have a member who has a similar developmental or mental disorder, addition problem, or life-altering medical condition. They may be families who have children or other family members with similar behavioral or emotional disorders or families that have experienced domestic violence or sexual abuse. The therapist works with the multiple family group, facilitating discussion related to their shared challenges, encouraging participants to share their experiences, failures, and successes in dealing with their common challenges. Participants are encouraged to discuss their coping mechanisms or behaviors that may be problematic. The group may then discuss alternate methods of coping that other families have used or may share how they dealt with a similar situation or problem. The group or therapist may suggest new ways of responding to a similar situation or may suggest activities or exercises to be practiced at home in an effort to help change behaviors or coping mechanisms that are counter-productive. Therapy sessions typically last between 1-2 hours.

90853

90853   Group psychotherapy (other than of a multiple-family group)

Group psychotherapy involves a therapist working with several individuals who are experiencing similar stressors simultaneously, such as a divorce or job loss, a difficult medical condition or mental disorder, like cancer or depression, or suffering from chemical or substance addiction. Individuals may also be members of a family with addicts. The therapist works with the group, facilitating discussion related to their shared challenges, encouraging participants to share their experiences, failures, and successes in dealing with their common challenges. Participants are encouraged to discuss their coping mechanisms or behaviors that may be problematic. The group may then discuss alternate methods of coping that they have used or may share how they dealt with a similar situation or problem. The group or therapist may suggest new ways of responding to a similar situation or may suggest activities or exercises to be practiced at home in an effort to help change behaviors or coping mechanisms that are counter-productive. Therapy sessions typically last between 1-2 hours.

90863

90863   Pharmacologic management, including prescription and review of medication, when performed with psychotherapy services (List separately in addition to the code for primary procedure)

Management of psychotropic medications is often required in order to ensure that the prescribed medication is achieving the desired results. In addition, many psychotropic drugs have side effects that must be monitored. In each session, the interval history and mental status examination of the patient focus on response to medication and a review of side effects. The physician queries the patient about the perceived effectiveness of the medication and any side effects. Separately reportable laboratory tests may be performed to evaluate blood levels of the medication or to screen for adverse effects. The physician may then increase or decrease the dosage of a medication. The physician may discontinue the use of a drug which may require weaning the patient off the drug to avoid adverse effects. A new medication may be prescribed to replace an ineffective medication or one that is causing adverse effects. A new medication may be added to the treatment regimen in an effort to obtain better management of the mental health problem being treated. Code 90863 is an add-on code that is reported when pharmacologic management is provided in with psychotherapy services.

90865

90865   Narcosynthesis for psychiatric diagnostic and therapeutic purposes (eg, sodium amobarbital (Amytal) interview)

Narcosynthesis involves intravenous administration of a sedative such as amobarbital (Amytal), thiopental (Pentothal), or pentobarbital (Nembutal) for psychiatric diagnostic and/or therapeutic purposes. An intravenous line is placed and a 5% solution of the selected sedative is administered at a rate of 25-50 mg per minute up to a total dose of 200-500 mg. The physician talks with the patient while administrating the sedative and halts the administration temporarily when the desired level of sedation is achieved as evidenced by physical signs such as lateral nystagmus for light sedation or slurred speech for deeper sedation. Intravenous administration of the drug is then resumed as a rate that will maintain the desired level of sedation. The patient experiences a relaxed, sleepy state. While in this state, patients with certain conditions may become more talkative, uninhibited, and spontaneous and this may be helpful in diagnosing the mental disorder. In addition, the calming effect of sedatives during narcosynthesis may also have therapeutic effects, such as assisting the patient in recalling and coping with traumatic images or memories.

90867-90869

90867 **Therapeutic repetitive transcranial magnetic stimulation (TMS) treatment; initial, including cortical mapping, motor threshold determination, delivery and management**

90868 **Therapeutic repetitive transcranial magnetic stimulation (TMS) treatment; subsequent delivery and management, per session**

90869 **Therapeutic repetitive transcranial magnetic stimulation (TMS) treatment; subsequent motor threshold re-determination with delivery and management**

Repetitive transcranial magnetic stimulation (rTMS) is used primarily to treat depression in individuals who have not responded to other treatment modalities. rTMS may also be used as a treatment for anxiety, obsessive compulsive disorder, auditory hallucinations, and migraines. In these disorders, one part of the brain is overactive or sluggish. For example, the left prefrontal cortex is less active in people with depression. The procedure involves the use of magnetic fields to stimulate nerve cells in the region of the brain associated with the mood or other disorder. A large electromagnetic coil is placed against the scalp over the appropriate region of the brain. The electromagnetic coil delivers painless electric currents that stimulate the nerve cells. This therapy alters the brain's biochemistry, the firing patterns of neurons in the cortex, and the levels of neurotransmitters like serotonin. In 90867, in an initial planning, treatment, and management session, the physician determines the best sites on the forehead for placement of the magnets, the optimal rate of stimulating pulses, and the optimal dose of magnetic energy for treatment. The electromagnetic coil is placed against the forehead and switched on and off at a rate of up to 10 times per second. When the device is on, it delivers stimulating pulses that result in a tapping or clicking sound and a tapping sensation on the head. During the mapping process, the optimal site is identified by moving the electromagnetic coils and the optimal rate of the pulses is determined by varying the pulse rate. The physician then determines the optimal dose. The energy delivered is increased until the fingers or hands twitch to determine the motor threshold. Once the motor threshold has been determined, the physician calculates the optimal dose. During the course of treatment, the optimal dose may be adjusted depending on the response to treatment and side effects. Use 90868 for each subsequent delivery and management session when motor threshold does not require adjustment. During each subsequent treatment session, the magnets are placed on the head and the optimal level and duration of stimulation is delivered. Use 90869 for each subsequent delivery and management session requiring motor threshold re-determination. During each subsequent treatment session following re-determination of motor threshold, the magnets are placed on the head and the optimal level and duration of stimulation is delivered.

90870

90870 **Electroconvulsive therapy (includes necessary monitoring)**

Electric currents are passed through the brain in electroconvulsive therapy (ECT) to deliberately trigger a brief seizure and cause chemical aspects of brain function to change. These chemical changes build on one another and help reduce the symptoms of severe depression and other mental illness such as schizophrenia, mania, and catatonia. ECT is done under general anesthesia. Electrode pads are placed on the patient's head, either unilaterally or bilaterally to receive the electric currents. Anesthesia and a muscle relaxant are given intravenously and a blood pressure cuff is placed around the ankle or forearm to prevent paralysis of those particular muscles. The physician sends a small amount of current through the electrodes to produce a seizure that lasts 30-60 seconds, and monitors the seizure by watching the movement in the cuffed hand or foot and the dramatic increase in brain activity on the EEG. Most people notice improvement after two or three treatments. ECT is more effective with multiple treatments.

90875-90876

90875 **Individual psychophysiological therapy incorporating biofeedback training by any modality (face-to-face with the patient), with psychotherapy (eg, insight oriented, behavior modifying or supportive psychotherapy); 30 minutes**

90876 **Individual psychophysiological therapy incorporating biofeedback training by any modality (face-to-face with the patient), with psychotherapy (eg, insight oriented, behavior modifying or supportive psychotherapy); 45 minutes**

Psychophysiological therapy using both biofeedback training and psychotherapy is provided in an individual, face-to-face setting. Psychophysiological therapy is designed to help individuals cope with stressors that cause anxiety disorders, chronic pain, and somatic symptoms. Biofeedback uses electronic sensory monitoring and feedback to help the patient achieve control over autonomic nervous system function. The biofeedback system monitors skin conductance (sweating), muscle tension, skin temperature and heart rate. Psychotherapy uses reeducation, support and reassurance, insight discussions, and

occasionally medication to affect behavior-modification through self-understanding. Use code 90875 for a 30 minute session and 90876 for a 45 minute session.

90880

90880 **Hypnotherapy**

Hypnotherapy is derived from the Greek term hypnos, meaning sleep. The aim of hypnotherapy is to reach an altered state of consciousness in which the conscious mind is relaxed, and the unconscious mind is more accessible. This state is used to explore memories, answer questions, and suggest specific goals, impressions, or new behaviors. Techniques for inducing an altered state of consciousness vary. There is no universally accepted standard. Sessions may vary from a single, brief encounter to longer, regularly scheduled appointments. Group sessions may also be done. Hypnotherapy is used in a multitude of applications to treat a wide variety of conditions and/or relieve symptoms. Examples for the use of hypnotherapy include anxiety, pain, psychosomatic disorders, headache, depression, bed-wetting, eating disorders, addictions, ulcers, erectile dysfunction, fibromyalgia, gastric disorders, insomnia, labor pain, and post-surgical recovery.

90882

90882 **Environmental intervention for medical management purposes on a psychiatric patient's behalf with agencies, employers, or institutions**

A psychiatrist or other mental health professional is called upon to intervene in a psychiatric patient's environment for any reason that helps manage the patient from a medical standpoint. This intervention takes place with the psychiatrist or mental health professional personally intervening with specific agencies, work places, or institutions with which the patient is engaged. For instance, the psychiatrist or mental health professional may appear in person at the patient's place of work to present information to the employer regarding the kind of work, or type of shift that may be inappropriate for that particular patient to attempt to perform. A psychiatrist or mental health professional may go to a child's school and be present in the classroom to aid in the management or treatment of a phobia-based condition.

90885

90885 **Psychiatric evaluation of hospital records, other psychiatric reports, psychometric and/or projective tests, and other accumulated data for medical diagnostic purposes**

The psychiatrist or other mental health professional performs an evaluation of hospital records, other psychiatric reports, results of psychometric tests or other evaluations, and other types of accumulated data on the patient for the purpose of making a medical diagnosis. Records could be from inpatient or outpatient hospitalization, drug or alcohol rehabilitation programs or facilities, initial diagnostic interview examinations, group therapy sessions, or any other form or type of data collected on the patient for diagnostic purposes, or during treatment or medical management of specific condition(s).

90887

90887 **Interpretation or explanation of results of psychiatric, other medical examinations and procedures, or other accumulated data to family or other responsible persons, or advising them how to assist patient**

The physician meets with family members or other persons involved in the care of a patient with a mental or behavioral condition. The mental or behavioral condition is explained to the family, caregiver, and other individuals involved in the patient's care and their questions are answered. Any diagnostic tests that have been performed are explained. Treatment alternatives may be discussed and the current treatment plan will be described which may include the use of inpatient care, partial hospitalization, or outpatient care. Medications are discussed including dose, desired therapeutic effects, and side effects. Any planned procedures to help treat the condition are explained. The individuals involved in the patient's care may also be advised on what they can do to help the patient with their medical needs and activities of daily living.

90889

90889 **Preparation of report of patient's psychiatric status, history, treatment, or progress (other than for legal or consultative purposes) for other individuals, agencies, or insurance carriers**

A comprehensive report is prepared for a patient undergoing psychiatric treatment and is provided to other individual's, agencies or insurance carriers after appropriate written patient consent is obtained. The report provides information related to the patient's psychiatric status and includes pertinent historical and current information on the treatment provided and the patient's progress. Note that this code is not reported when the report is for legal purposes or is related to consultative services.

Medicine

90901

90901   Biofeedback training by any modality

Biofeedback training is provided to help a patient learn to control automatic bodily responses. While biofeedback cannot cure disease, it can help patients learn to control physical responses that influence their health. Biofeedback is used by a variety of specialists to treat physical conditions, such as migraine headaches and other types of pain, digestive system disorders, high or low blood pressure, cardiac arrhythmias, Raynaud's disease, epilepsy, paralysis due to stroke, or cerebral palsy. Biofeedback includes identification of triggers that bring on symptoms and the use of relaxation techniques to help control symptoms. A clinician places electrical sensors on different parts of the body that monitor muscle tension, increased heart rate, temperature, or other physiologic signs. The sensors are attached to a biofeedback machine that provides cues such as a beeping sound or flashing light to indicate physiologic changes, such as increased muscle tension or heart rate, changes in temperature or other physiological responses. The patient then responds by concentrating on reducing muscle tension, slowing heart rate, modifying temperature, or providing another appropriate response to the biofeedback information. A typical biofeedback training session lasts from 30 to 60 minutes. The patient is also required to practice biofeedback methods at home on a day-to-day basis to help modify and control physiological responses.

90911

90911   Biofeedback training, perineal muscles, anorectal or urethral sphincter, including EMG and/or manometry

Biofeedback training involving the perineal muscles, anorectal or urethral sphincter is provided for conditions such as urinary retention or incontinence or fecal incontinence or constipation. This type of biofeedback training includes the use of electromyography (EMG) or manometry. Anorectal biofeedback is performed using a manometer probe with multiple microsensors and a balloon or a water perfused probe with side holes in the rectum. These devices provide a visual or auditory display of muscle activity in the abdomen, rectum, pelvic floor, and anal sphincter and are able to alert the patient to dyssynergic (uncoordinated) muscle activity preventing normal defecation. The patient uses neuromuscular conditioning techniques to improve anorectal muscle coordination. Biofeedback training for bladder sphincter dyssynergia is performed using exercises to tense and relax pelvic muscles. The patient also practices relaxation of pelvic muscles during voiding. A biofeedback device that uses a recording of urinary flow and EMG with a visual display is also used to alert the patient to changes in pelvic floor and urethral sphincter tension. The patient then uses these biofeedback techniques to help coordinate the pelvic floor muscles and improve urethral sphincter control.

90935-90937

90935   Hemodialysis procedure with single evaluation by a physician or other qualified health care professional
90937   Hemodialysis procedure requiring repeated evaluation(s) with or without substantial revision of dialysis prescription

A nurse or technician inserts two needles into a previously created vascular access site. The vascular access site may be a surgically created internal fistula or shunt, an internal graft, or less commonly a central venous catheter. Each needle is attached to a separate piece of flexible plastic tubing that is connected to the dialysis machine. One tube removes blood from the body. The blood is circulated through the dialysis machine and then returned to the body through the second tube. The blood circulating through the dialysis machine passes on one side of a membrane and dialysis fluid passes on the other. The wastes and excess fluid pass from the blood through the membrane and into the dialysis fluid. These wastes are discarded with the dialysis fluid. The cleansed blood is returned to the bloodstream through the second tube. The hemodialysis procedure includes all evaluation and management services performed on the date of the dialysis procedure that are related to the patient's renal disease. Code 90935 is used when a single evaluation and management service is performed on the date of the hemodialysis procedure. Code 90937 is used when repeated evaluation and management services are required during the course of the hemodialysis procedure.

90940

90940   Hemodialysis access flow study to determine blood flow in grafts and arteriovenous fistulae by an indicator method

A hemodialysis access flow study is performed to determine blood flow in grafts and arteriovenous (AV) fistulae using an indicator method. Monitoring of AV graft patency using an indicator method provides early detection of stenosis, reduces graft thrombosis, and can extend the life of the graft. The physician or trained staff member performs the procedure during a regularly scheduled hemodialysis session. Two ultrasound sensors are clipped onto hemodialysis tubing blood lines, one sensor on the tube receiving the blood from the body and another one on the tube returning the cleansed blood from the dialyzer. These sensors transmit minute levels of ultrasound through the tubing wall into the blood stream. An isotonic saline solution is injected into the blood to dilute it and reduce the ultrasound velocity. As the saline bolus passes through the tubing, two sensors measure

changes in the ultrasound characteristics of the blood in the tubes of the extracorporeal circuit. These measurements are evaluated and used to identify any blood flow problems. Hook-up, measurement, and disconnection from the monitoring device are included.

90945-90947

90945   Dialysis procedure other than hemodialysis (eg, peritoneal dialysis, hemofiltration, or other continuous renal replacement therapies), with single evaluation by a physician or other qualified health care professional
90947   Dialysis procedure other than hemodialysis (eg, peritoneal dialysis, hemofiltration, or other continuous renal replacement therapies) requiring repeated evaluations by a physician or other qualified health care professional, with or without substantial revision of dialysis prescription

A dialysis procedure other than hemodialysis with related evaluation services is performed. Types of dialysis procedures performed include peritoneal dialysis, hemofiltration, or other continuous renal replacement therapies. Peritoneal dialysis, hemofiltration, and other continuous renal replacement therapies filter blood continuously without interruption. If peritoneal dialysis is performed, a nurse or technician instills dialysis fluid through a previously placed abdominal catheter. The dialysis solution contains the sugar dextrose, which pulls wastes and extra fluid out of the blood through the peritoneal membrane and into the abdominal cavity. The dialysis fluid remains in the abdominal cavity for a period of four to six hours after which the dialysis solution along with the wastes and excess fluid is removed from the abdomen through the catheter. This process of filling and draining the abdomen may be repeated several times during the day. Hemofiltration may be performed by an arteriovenous or venovenous procedure. In an arteriovenous procedure, the femoral artery is cannulated. Arterial pressure forces blood through a filter into the femoral vein. Water and soluble waste products filter from the blood through a permeable membrane and are discarded. The cleansed blood is returned to the body with replacement fluid of physiologically balanced water and electrolytes. The procedure for venovenous filtration is similar. A double lumen catheter is placed in the femoral, subclavian, or internal jugular vein. A pump is used to push blood from the vein through the dialysis circuit. The cleansed blood is then pushed back into the same vein. Code 90945 is used when a single evaluation and management service is performed on the date of the peritoneal dialysis, hemofiltration, or other continuous renal replacement therapy. Code 90947 is used when repeated evaluation and management services are required during the course of the peritoneal dialysis procedure, hemofiltration procedure, or other continuous renal replacement therapy procedure.

90951-90953

90951   End-stage renal disease (ESRD) related services monthly, for patients younger than 2 years of age to include monitoring for the adequacy of nutrition, assessment of growth and development, and counseling of parents; with 4 or more face-to-face visits by a physician or other qualified health care professional per month
90952   End-stage renal disease (ESRD) related services monthly, for patients younger than 2 years of age to include monitoring for the adequacy of nutrition, assessment of growth and development, and counseling of parents; with 2-3 face-to-face visits by a physician or other qualified health care professional per month
90953   End-stage renal disease (ESRD) related services monthly, for patients younger than 2 years of age to include monitoring for the adequacy of nutrition, assessment of growth and development, and counseling of parents; with 1 face-to-face visit by a physician or other qualified health care professional per month

End-stage renal disease (ESRD) related services are provided per one full month in an outpatient setting, including monitoring of the adequacy of nutrition, assessment of growth and development, and counseling of parents for services provided to a child younger than 2 years of age. The physician or other qualified health care professional establishes the dialyzing cycle, performs outpatient evaluation and management services related to the dialysis services, and provides oversight and management of the patient during the dialysis services as well as telephone follow-up as needed for the entire month. The patient is examined on a routine basis for existing and potential medical problems. The patient is seen as needed when new symptoms or problems develop. The physician or other qualified health care professional ensures that dialysis services are being provided as prescribed and makes adjustments to the dialysis prescription as needed, including monitoring the patient's weight, making recommendations regarding diet and fluid intake, and prescribing special renal supplement formula as needed. Laboratory data are reviewed. Medications and nutritional supplements are monitored, and changes are made as needed. Interventions for delays in growth or development are initiated as needed, which may include injection of growth hormones. Social development is monitored and any behavioral or school problems are also addressed. The physician or other health care professional counsels the parents and caregivers and responds to their questions and concerns. These ESRD services are included in one code, which is reported only once per month based on the number of face-to-face visits provided each month. Code 90951 is for four or more face-to-face visits per month; code 90952 is for two to three face-to-face visits per month; and code 90953 reports one face-to-face visit per month.

90954-90956

90954 End-stage renal disease (ESRD) related services monthly, for patients 2-11 years of age to include monitoring for the adequacy of nutrition, assessment of growth and development, and counseling of parents; with 4 or more face-to-face visits by a physician or other qualified health care professional per month

90955 End-stage renal disease (ESRD) related services monthly, for patients 2-11 years of age to include monitoring for the adequacy of nutrition, assessment of growth and development, and counseling of parents; with 2-3 face-to-face visits by a physician or other qualified health care professional per month

90956 End-stage renal disease (ESRD) related services monthly, for patients 2-11 years of age to include monitoring for the adequacy of nutrition, assessment of growth and development, and counseling of parents; with 1 face-to-face visit by a physician or other qualified health care professional per month

End-stage renal disease (ESRD) related services are provided per one full month in an outpatient setting, including monitoring of the adequacy of nutrition, assessment of growth and development, and counseling of parents for services provided to children aged 2 through 11 years. The physician or other qualified health care professional establishes the dialyzing cycle, performs outpatient evaluation and management services related to the dialysis services, and provides oversight and management of the patient during the dialysis service as well as telephone follow-up as needed for the entire month. The patient is examined on a routine basis for existing and potential medical problems. The patient is seen as needed when new symptoms or problems develop. The physician or other qualified health care professional ensures that dialysis services are being provided as prescribed and makes adjustments to the dialysis prescription as needed, including monitoring the patient's weight, making recommendations regarding diet and fluid intake, and prescribing special renal supplement formula as needed. Laboratory data are reviewed. Medications and nutritional supplements are monitored, and changes are made as needed. Interventions for delays in growth or development are initiated as needed, which may include injection of growth hormones. Social development is monitored and any behavioral or school problems are also addressed. The physician or other qualified health care professional counsels the parents and caregivers and responds to their questions and concerns. These ESRD services are included in one code, which is reported only once per month based on the number of face-to-face visits provided each month. Code 90954 is for four or more face-to-face visits per month; code 90955 is for two to three face-to-face visits per month; and code 90956 reports one face-to-face visit per month.

90957-90959

90957 End-stage renal disease (ESRD) related services monthly, for patients 12-19 years of age to include monitoring for the adequacy of nutrition, assessment of growth and development, and counseling of parents; with 4 or more face-to-face visits by a physician or other qualified health care professional per month

90958 End-stage renal disease (ESRD) related services monthly, for patients 12-19 years of age to include monitoring for the adequacy of nutrition, assessment of growth and development, and counseling of parents; with 2-3 face-to-face visits by a physician or other qualified health care professional per month

90959 End-stage renal disease (ESRD) related services monthly, for patients 12-19 years of age to include monitoring for the adequacy of nutrition, assessment of growth and development, and counseling of parents; with 1 face-to-face visit by a physician or other qualified health care professional per month

End-stage renal disease (ESRD) related services are provided per one full month in an outpatient setting, including monitoring of the adequacy of nutrition, assessment of growth and development, and counseling of parents for services provided to a child aged 12-19 years. The physician or other qualified health care professional establishes the dialyzing cycle, performs outpatient evaluation and management services related to the dialysis services, and provides oversight and management of the patient during the dialysis services as well as telephone follow-up as needed for the entire month. The patient is examined on a routine basis for existing and potential medical problems, and is seen as needed when new symptoms or problems develop. The physician or other qualified health care professional ensures that dialysis services are being provided as prescribed and makes adjustments to the dialysis prescription as needed, including monitoring the patient's weight, making recommendations regarding diet and fluid intake, and prescribing special renal supplement formula as needed. Laboratory data are reviewed. Medications and nutritional supplements are monitored, and changes are made as needed. Interventions for delays in growth or development are initiated as needed, which may include injection of growth hormones. Social development is monitored and any behavioral or school problems are also addressed. The physician or other qualified health care professional counsels the parents and caregivers and responds to their questions and concerns. These ESRD services are included in one code, and reported only once per month based on the number of face-to-face visits. Code 90957 is for 4 or more face-to-face visits per month; code 90958

is for 2-3 face-to-face visits per month; and code 90959 reports one face-to-face visit per month.

90960-90962

90960 End-stage renal disease (ESRD) related services monthly, for patients 20 years of age and older; with 4 or more face-to-face visits by a physician or other qualified health care professional per month

90961 End-stage renal disease (ESRD) related services monthly, for patients 20 years of age and older; with 2-3 face-to-face visits by a physician or other qualified health care professional per month

90962 End-stage renal disease (ESRD) related services monthly, for patients 20 years of age and older; with 1 face-to-face visit by a physician or other qualified health care professional per month

End-stage renal disease (ESRD) related services are provided per one full month in an outpatient setting to a patient 20 years of age and older. The physician or other qualified health care professional establishes the dialyzing cycle, performs outpatient evaluation and management services related to the dialysis services, and provides oversight and management of the patient during the dialysis service as well as telephone follow-up as needed for the entire month. The patient is examined on a routine basis for existing and potential medical problems, and is seen as needed when new symptoms or problems develop. The physician or other qualified health care professional ensures that dialysis services are being provided as prescribed and makes adjustments to the dialysis prescription as needed. Laboratory data are reviewed. Medications and nutritional supplements are monitored, and changes are made as needed. The physician or other qualified health care professional also establishes, monitors, and coordinates care, which may include social service interventions, nutritional support, kidney transplant planning, and services provided by other medical and/or surgical specialists. These ESRD services are included in one code, which is reported only once per month based on the number of face-to-face visits. Code 90960 is for 4 or more face-to-face visits per month; code 90961 is for 2-3 face-to-face visits per month; and code 90962 reports one face-to-face visit per month.

90963-90965

90963 End-stage renal disease (ESRD) related services for home dialysis per full month, for patients younger than 2 years of age to include monitoring for the adequacy of nutrition, assessment of growth and development, and counseling of parents

90964 End-stage renal disease (ESRD) related services for home dialysis per full month, for patients 2-11 years of age to include monitoring for the adequacy of nutrition, assessment of growth and development, and counseling of parents

90965 End-stage renal disease (ESRD) related services for home dialysis per full month, for patients 12-19 years of age to include monitoring for the adequacy of nutrition, assessment of growth and development, and counseling of parents

End-stage renal disease (ESRD) related services are provided for one full month for home dialysis, including monitoring of the adequacy of nutrition, assessment of growth and development, and counseling of parents for services provided to a child. The physician establishes the dialyzing cycle, performs outpatient evaluation and management services related to the home dialysis services, and provides oversight and management of the patient during the dialysis as well as telephone follow-up as needed for the entire month. The physician examines the patient on a routine basis for existing and potential medical problems. The patient is seen as needed when new symptoms or problems develop. The physician ensures that dialysis services are being provided in the home as prescribed and makes adjustments to the dialysis prescription as needed. The physician monitors the patient's weight and makes recommendations regarding the patient's diet and fluid intake and prescribes special renal supplement formula as needed. Laboratory data are reviewed. Medications and nutritional supplements are monitored, and changes are made as needed. The physician initiates the necessary interventions for delays in growth or development, which may include injection of growth hormones. The physician reviews social development and monitors any behavioral or school problems, making referrals and intervening as needed. The physician counsels the parents and caregivers and responds to their questions and concerns. These ESRD-related services for home dialysis are included in one code, which is reported only once per month and are age-specific. Code 90963 is reported for patients younger than 2 years of age; code 90964 is for patients 2-11 years old; and code 90965 is for patients aged 12-19.

90966

90966 End-stage renal disease (ESRD) related services for home dialysis per full month, for patients 20 years of age and older

End-stage renal disease (ESRD) related services are provided for one full month for home dialysis for patients 20 years of age and older. The physician establishes the dialyzing cycle, performs outpatient evaluation and management services related to the home dialysis services, and provides oversight and management of the patient during the dialysis

Medicine

as well as telephone follow-up as needed for the entire month. The physician examines the patient on a routine basis for existing and potential medical problems. The patient is seen as needed when new symptoms or problems develop. The physician ensures that dialysis services are being provided as prescribed and makes adjustments to the dialysis prescription as needed. Laboratory data are reviewed. Medications and nutritional supplements are monitored, and changes are made as needed. The physician also establishes, monitors, and coordinates care, which may include social service interventions, nutritional support, kidney transplant planning, and services provided by other medical and/or surgical specialists.

90967-90969

90967   End-stage renal disease (ESRD) related services for dialysis less than a full month of service, per day; for patients younger than 2 years of age

90968   End-stage renal disease (ESRD) related services for dialysis less than a full month of service, per day; for patients 2-11 years of age

90969   End-stage renal disease (ESRD) related services for dialysis less than a full month of service, per day; for patients 12-19 years of age

End-stage renal disease (ESRD) services are provided per day in an outpatient setting when less than a full month of service is required. Outpatient ESRD services may be provided for only part of a month due to inpatient hospitalization or initiation of the services after the first of the month. The physician establishes the dialyzing cycle, performs outpatient evaluation and management services related to the dialysis services, and provides oversight and management of the patient during the dialysis as well as telephone follow-up as needed. The physician examines the patient on a routine basis for existing and potential medical problems. The patient is seen as needed when new symptoms or problems develop. The physician ensures that dialysis services are being provided as prescribed and makes adjustments to the dialysis prescription as needed. The physician monitors the patient's weight, makes recommendations regarding the patient's diet and fluid intake, and prescribes special renal supplement formula as needed. Laboratory data are reviewed. Medications and nutritional supplements are monitored and changes are made as needed. The physician initiates the necessary interventions for delays in growth or development, which may include injection of growth hormones. Social development is monitored and any behavioral or school problems are addressed by making referrals and intervening as needed. The physician counsels the parents and caregivers and responds to their questions and concerns. These ESRD services are age-specific and reported on a daily basis. Code 90967 is for patients younger than 2; code 90968 is for patients aged 2-11; and code 90969 is for patients 12-19 years of age.

90970

90970   End-stage renal disease (ESRD) related services for dialysis less than a full month of service, per day; for patients 20 years of age and older

End-stage renal disease (ESRD) services are provided per day in an outpatient setting when less than a full month of service is required. Outpatient ESRD services may be provided for only part of a month due to inpatient hospitalization or initiation of the services after the first of the month. The physician establishes the dialyzing cycle, performs outpatient evaluation and management services related to the home dialysis services, and provides oversight and management of the patient during the dialysis as well as telephone follow-up as needed. The physician examines the patient on a routine basis for existing and potential medical problems. The patient is seen as needed when new symptoms or problems develop. The physician ensures that dialysis services are being provided as prescribed and makes adjustments to the dialysis prescription as needed. Laboratory data is reviewed. Medications and nutritional supplements are monitored and changes are made as needed. The physician also establishes, monitors, and coordinates care, which may include social service interventions, nutritional support, kidney transplant planning, and services provided by other medical and/or surgical specialists. Code 90970 is reported on a per day basis for patients aged 20 or older.

90989-90993

90989   Dialysis training, patient, including helper where applicable, any mode, completed course

90993   Dialysis training, patient, including helper where applicable, any mode, course not completed, per training session

The physician performs administrative, routine professional services, and supervision or direction of a dialysis patient, including a helper where applicable, during self-dialysis training. During self-dialysis training the physician provides the following administrative services: training and supervision of staff, participation in staff conferences and management of the facility, advising staff on procurement of supplies, and medical direction of staff delivering the self training services to the patient. The physician's routine professional services may include such things as direction of and participation in training of dialysis patients; review of family, home status , and environment of the patient, counseling and training of family members; review of the training process; review of laboratory results, nurses' notes, and any other medical documentation; adjustment of patient's medication, diet, or the dialysis procedure; prescription of medical supplies; evaluation of patient's psychosocial status; evaluation of the appropriateness of

the treatment; pre-dialysis and post-dialysis patient examinations; and observation of a complete successful self-dialysis procedure by the patient. Code 90989 is used for a completed self-dialysis training course which typically includes at least 25 training sessions. Code 90993 is used when the course is not completed and is reported for each training session performed.

90997

90997   Hemoperfusion (eg, with activated charcoal or resin)

A hemoperfusion procedure is performed using activated charcoal or resin. Hemoperfusion is used to remove drugs, poisons, or other toxic substances from the blood that are harmful to the kidneys, to remove waste products from the blood in patients with kidney disease, or to provide supportive treatment to patients with liver failure before and after liver transplant. Hemoperfusion can clear toxins from a larger volume of blood than other filtration methods, such as hemodialysis, and can process over 300 ml of blood per minute. Two catheters are placed in the arm, one in an artery and one in a nearby vein, and connected to plastic tubing. The tubing from the arterial access site removes blood from the body and passes it through a hemoperfusion system. In the hemoperfusion system, the blood is passed over a column or cartridge containing the activated charcoal or resin, and the toxic molecules or particles are trapped within the column or cartridge. The cleansed blood flows out of the hemoperfusion system through the second tube and is returned to the body through the venous access site.

91010-91013

91010   Esophageal motility (manometric study of the esophagus and/or gastroesophageal junction) study with interpretation and report

91013   Esophageal motility (manometric study of the esophagus and/or gastroesophageal junction) study with interpretation and report; with stimulation or perfusion (eg, stimulant, acid or alkali perfusion) (List separately in addition to code for primary procedure)

These diagnostic procedures are performed to help determine the cause of swallowing difficulties and non-cardiac chest pain. Esophageal motility studies evaluate muscle contractions in the esophagus. Most commonly it is used to help diagnose esophageal achalasia which is characterized by failure of the lower esophageal sphincter to relax along with uncoordinated contractions of the thoracic esophagus, resulting in functional esophageal obstruction. One of the nostrils is numbed with lidocaine. A catheter containing a manometer is passed through the nostril and advanced through the pharynx into the esophagus. The patient is asked to swallow to help advance the catheter. In 91010, the catheter is advanced to the lower esophageal sphincter and contractility of the sphincter is measured. The catheter is retracted to the middle of the pharynx. The patient is given water to sip and muscle contractility of the mid-esophagus is measured and displayed on the manometry monitor as a 2-dimensional graph. The catheter is then withdrawn. The physician reviews the test results and provides a written evaluation of esophageal motility. In 91013, the motility study is performed as described above and then a stimulant such as mecholyl is administered, or an acid perfusion study is also performed. Mecholyl is a cholinergic agent that increases secretions and smooth muscle contractions. Patients with esophageal contractility dysfunction show increased smooth muscle contractions in response to mecholyl. Alternatively, a mild hydrochloric acid solution is instilled through the esophageal catheter in the esophagus. This is followed by salt water solution. The patient is asked to describe any discomfort or pain associated with the instillation of the hydrochloric acid. Enhanced 2D images of the esophageal contractions are displayed on a manometry monitor. The physician reviews the test results and provides a written evaluation of findings.

91020-91022

91020   Gastric motility (manometric) studies

91022   Duodenal motility (manometric) study

Manometric studies of the stomach or duodenum are used to evaluate gastric and small intestine motor function. Using separately reportable fluoroscopic guidance, a catheter containing perfusion ports and/or transducers is passed through the nose or mouth and into the stomach or duodenum. The catheter is attached to a pump that slowly pushes water into the stomach through the perfusion ports. The pump is connected to a computer. A manometer measures and records changes in intraluminal pressure in the stomach or duodenum. The patient may also be given a meal while the catheter is in place and pressure or contractions in the stomach or duodenum measured and recorded. The results are analyzed by the physician and a written report of findings provided. Use 91020 for gastric motility studies; use 91022 for duodenal motility studies.

91030

91030   Esophagus, acid perfusion (Bernstein) test for esophagitis

This diagnostic procedure is performed to help differentiate between chest pain caused by gastroesophageal reflux disease (GERD) and pain caused by a cardiac condition. One of the nostrils is numbed with lidocaine. A catheter is passed through the nostril and advanced through the pharynx into the esophagus. The patient is asked to swallow to help advance the catheter. A mild hydrochloric acid solution is instilled through the esophageal

Medicine

catheter in the esophagus. This is followed by saline solution. The patient is asked to describe any discomfort or pain associated with the instillation of the hydrochloric acid.

91034-91035

91034 **Esophagus, gastroesophageal reflux test; with nasal catheter pH electrode(s) placement, recording, analysis and interpretation**

91035 **Esophagus, gastroesophageal reflux test; with mucosal attached telemetry pH electrode placement, recording, analysis and interpretation**

An esophageal pH test is used for patients with symptoms of gastroesophgeal reflux disease (GERD) or in patients with known GERD who are not responding to treatment. In 91034, a nasal catheter containing a small probe is inserted through the nose and positioned near the lower esophagus. The catheter probe is plugged into a small external monitor that is secured with a belt around the waist or shoulder. The probe monitors pH levels in the esophagus over a 24-hour period. The pH levels change when acid from the stomach enters the esophagus. The patient can initiate recordings during occurrence of symptoms, before, during, and after meals, and when lying down by pressing a button on the monitor. The patient returns to the physician office the next day and the catheter probe is removed from the esophagus. The data stored in the monitor is then reviewed and interpreted by the physician and a written report is provided. In 91035, a catheter that contains a capsule with a pH probe, a battery, and a transmitter is introduced into the nose or mouth and advanced into the esophagus. The capsule is positioned in the esophagus and attached to the esophageal mucosa with a clip. The capsule is then detached and the catheter is removed. The patient wears an external recorder that communicates by telemetry with the transmitter in the capsule. The capsule captures pH data which is transmitted to the recorder for 24-48 hours. The patient can initiate recordings during occurrence of symptoms, before, during, and after meals, and when lying down by pressing a button on the recorder. The patient returns to the physician office and returns the recorder. The capsule is not removed as it will detach from the esophageal mucosa in 5-7 days and be passed in the stool. The physician analyzes data captured by the recorder and provides a written report.

91037-91038

91037 **Esophageal function test, gastroesophageal reflux test with nasal catheter intraluminal impedance electrode(s) placement, recording, analysis and interpretation**

91038 **Esophageal function test, gastroesophageal reflux test with nasal catheter intraluminal impedance electrode(s) placement, recording, analysis and interpretation; prolonged (greater than 1 hour, up to 24 hours)**

Gastroesophageal reflux impedance testing is performed to evaluate esophageal peristalsis and monitor acidic and non-acidic reflux over an extended period of time. A nasal catheter containing intraluminal impedance electrodes (sensors) is inserted into the nose and advanced into the esophagus. The distal impedance electrode is positioned approximately 5 cm above the distal esophageal sphincter. The patient is then given a saline solution and takes 10 swallows of the solution at 20-30 second intervals. As the saline bolus passes through the esophagus, the electrodes along the length of the catheter measure and record bolus transit times and esophageal function, including the dynamics of esophageal function and the effectiveness of the esophagus in moving the bolus into the stomach. The patient is then given a viscous material to swallow, taking 10 swallows at 20-30 second intervals. The electrodes again measure and record bolus transit times and esophageal function. Following completion of the study, the catheter is removed. The physician evaluates the esophageal function using recordings captured by the electrodes and provides a written report. Use 91037 for an esophageal function test of less than 1 hour. Use 91038 for a prolonged gastroesophageal function test lasting from 1-24 hours.

91040

91040 **Esophageal balloon distension study, diagnostic, with provocation when performed**

A diagnostic esophageal balloon distension study is performed to evaluate the cause of recurrent unexplained chest pain and/or pain when swallowing (dysphagia). A catheter with a deflated balloon is inserted through the nose into the esophagus. The balloon is positioned in the mid-esophagus and inflated with air or water in 2 cc increments until up to 30 cc of air or water has been instilled. The instillation is performed in such a way that the patient is unaware of the amount of air or water being instilled. The patient is queried throughout the procedure about symptoms of chest pain. If the symptoms are reproduced by the balloon distension, the volume of air or water that has been instilled is noted. The air or water is removed. The procedure may be repeated several times to provoke symptoms. The physician may also pretend to instill water or air without actually doing so to confirm that the balloon distension is actually causing the symptoms. Following completion of the test, the balloon is deflated and the catheter is removed. The physician interprets the results of the test and provides a written report.

91065

91065 **Breath hydrogen or methane test (eg, for detection of lactase deficiency, fructose intolerance, bacterial overgrowth, or oro-cecal gastrointestinal transit)**

Breath hydrogen or methane test is performed to evaluate gastrointestinal tract disorders, such as lactose intolerance (lactase deficiency), fructose intolerance, bacterial overgrowth of the small intestine, and motility disorders such as rapid or prolonged oro-cecal gastrointestinal transit. Sugars (e.g., lactose, fructose, glucose) are normally absorbed in the small bowel. However, some people do not have enough of the enzyme lactase to allow complete absorption of lactose or they have other conditions that do not allow complete absorption of other sugars in the small intestine. This causes unabsorbed sugars to pass into the large bowel (colon) where fermentation occurs and hydrogen and methane gases are produced. Another cause of excess production of hydrogen and methane gas in the bowel is bacterial overgrowth which occurs when gas producing bacteria normally present only in the colon are also present in the small bowel. Individuals with gastrointestinal motility disorders and delayed oro-cecal transit time often have bacterial overgrowth in the small bowel. Rapid oro-cecal transit causes sugars to pass through the small intestine before they can be completely digested. When there is an excessive amount of hydrogen or methane in the bowel, some of it enters the blood stream and is exhaled through the lungs, which is why a breath test is performed to evaluate hydrogen and methane levels. Prior to performing the breath test, the patient must fast for at least 12 hours. A baseline test is performed using a balloon that the patient blows into and fills with air. A sample of breath is removed from the balloon and the level of hydrogen or methane is evaluated. The patient then ingests small amounts of test sugar (e.g., lactose, fructose, sucrose, sorbitol, or lactulose). Additional breath samples are collected and analyzed at 15 minute intervals for a period of 3-5 hours. Normally, when hydrogen or methane is present in the breath samples taken after the test sugar is ingested, it is indicative of malabsorption of the test sugar.

91110-91111

91110 **Gastrointestinal tract imaging, intraluminal (eg, capsule endoscopy), esophagus through ileum, with interpretation and report**

91111 **Gastrointestinal tract imaging, intraluminal (eg, capsule endoscopy), esophagus with interpretation and report**

Intraluminal gastrointestinal (GI) tract imaging is done by a non-invasive method in which the patient swallows an endoscopic capsule after 10 hours of fasting. The patient wears a data recorder around the waist. Sensors in the recorder receive the data transmitted from the capsule as it moves through the GI tract while the patient goes about daily activity as normal. Color video images of the inside of the GI tract lumen are recorded and later viewed and interpreted. Use 91111 for imaging of the esophagus and 91110 for imaging of the esophagus through the ileum.

91112

91112 **Gastrointestinal transit and pressure measurement, stomach through colon, wireless capsule, with interpretation and report**

A procedure is performed to evaluate gastric emptying, gastrointestinal transit time, pH, and pressure in patients with suspected gastroparesis. The patient is fitted with an external receiver and recording device. A wireless capsule capable of transmitting radio signals to the receiver and recording device is ingested. The receiver and recording device continuously track the capsule as it passes through the stomach and the small and large intestine. The data is recorded. The capsule is passed in the stool usually within 2-5 days. The recorded data is then analyzed for gastric transit time, small intestine transit time, large intestine transit time, whole gut transit time, antral and duodenal pressures, and motility indices. The physician reviews the recorded data and software analysis, and provides a written report of findings.

91117

91117 **Colon motility (manometric) study, minimum 6 hours continuous recording (including provocation tests, eg, meal, intracolonic balloon distension, pharmacologic agents, if performed), with interpretation and report**

This diagnostic test is used to evaluate severe constipation and determine if the cause is due to colonic inertia. A manometric study is performed to record and measure muscle and nerve activity in the colon. A small thin manometry probe with multiple microsensors and a small balloon is inserted into the rectum and advanced into the colon. The probe is attached to a computerized device that records muscle and nerve activity as the probe is advanced along the colon. The contractions are graphed and displayed on a computer monitor. A series of provocation tests are performed and muscle and nerve activity is recorded to monitor any changes in colon contractions. The patient may be fed a 1000 calorie meal and muscle tone and sensory changes are recorded over an hour or more following the meal. Intracolonic balloon distension may be performed. This involves inflating and deflating the balloon with small amounts of air multiple times. The balloon distention procedure helps the doctor assess muscle responses. A pharmacologic agent may be administered to stimulate colon contraction and muscle and nerve activity are measured

Medicine

and recorded. At the completion of the test, the manometry probe with the attached sensors and balloon is removed. The physician reviews the recordings and measurements and provides a written interpretation of findings.

91120

91120   Rectal sensation, tone, and compliance test (ie, response to graded balloon distention)

This test measures compliance and sensory properties of the rectal wall using controlled balloon distension of the rectum in patients with constipation or fecal incontinence. A probe with a balloon is inserted into the rectum and secured with tape. The balloon is connected to a computerized distending device. The balloon is then distended in a stepwise fashion over a 30-minute period. Intra-operating pressure (IOP) and rectal tone are assessed. Next, intermittent balloon distensions are performed until the patient reports sensation, desire to defecate, and urgency. The maximum tolerable volume is determined. The patient is then asked to expel the balloon. Following a 15-minute rest period, the balloon is reinserted and inflated to the previously determined IOP. The patient is then fed a 1,000-calorie meal and rectal tone and sensory changes are recorded for 60 minutes. The balloon is deflated and then removed along with the probe.

91122

91122   Anorectal manometry

A small thin manometry probe with multiple microsensors and a small balloon is inserted into the rectum. The probe is attached to a computerized device that records muscle and nerve activity as the balloon is inflated with small amounts of air and deflated multiple times. This test helps the doctor assess anorectal muscle responses. At the completion of the test the manometry probe with the attached sensors and balloon is removed.

91132-91133

91132   Electrogastrography, diagnostic, transcutaneous
91133   Electrogastrography, diagnostic, transcutaneous; with provocative testing

Diagnostic transcutaneous electrogastrography (EGG) is performed. Transcutaneous EGG uses sensors placed on the skin of the abdomen to record electrical activity of the stomach. EGG is used in patients with complaints of persistent nausea, vomiting, early satiety, and epigastric discomfort to diagnose gastrointestinal motility disorders and gastric dysrhythmias. In 91132, recordings are made from several standardized positions on the abdominal wall. The one with the highest amplitude is selected for further analysis and additional recordings are made. Changes in EGG amplitude and frequency are evaluated. The physician interprets the EGG recording and provides a written interpretation of the result. In 91133, the EGG is performed with provocative testing. After determining optimal placement of sensors, a fasting EGG recording is obtained followed by a post-prandial recording. The patient is then given a provocative test by intravenous infusion of a drug such as edrophonium or by water loading with addtional recordings being made. The recordings from the fasting, post-prandial, and provocative tests are then compared and evaluated. The physician interprets the results and provides a written report of findings.

91200

91200   Liver elastography, mechanically induced shear wave (eg, vibration), without imaging, with interpretation and report

Liver elastography by mechanically induced shear wave is a non-invasive procedure used to assess liver stiffness. A transducer attached to an ultrasound probe sends a shear wave (vibration) into the liver and then measures the velocity as it passes through the liver. This sound wave is then converted into a measurement (kilopascals) that represents liver stiffness. This technique can be used to monitor liver disease caused by infection, portal hypertension, drug or alcohol use, or to assess the status of a transplanted liver. The ultrasound probe is placed at the intercostal space near the right lobe of the liver. The shear wave is delivered and the results are recorded by the ultrasound machine. Results are immediately available to the clinician to read and interpret. The results of shear wave elastography may not be reliable in obese patients, those with ascites, or a large amount of chest wall fat.

92002

92002   Ophthalmological services: medical examination and evaluation with initiation of diagnostic and treatment program; intermediate, new patient

An intermediate level of general ophthalmological services is provided to a new patient. A new patient is one who has not received any services from that physician or other physicians of the same specialty belonging to the same group practice for three years. For an intermediate level service, the ophthalmologist focuses on evaluating a new condition or an existing condition now complicated by a new diagnosis or management problem, which need not necessarily be related to the primary diagnosis. The intermediate evaluation includes a history and general medical observations; external ocular and adnexal exam; visual field or acuity testing and basic motor evaluation; the use of slit lamp; routine ophthalmoscopy; biomicroscopy and tonometry for conditions that do not require comprehensive care; keratometry; retinoscopy; and the use of mydriasis to facilitate routine ophthalmoscopy by dilating the pupils to help visualize the ocular media and fundus. Following diagnostic evaluation, the physician initiates a diagnostic treatment program which includes any necessary medication prescriptions and arranging for additional special services, consultations, laboratory tests, or radiology services.

92004

92004   Ophthalmological services: medical examination and evaluation with initiation of diagnostic and treatment program; comprehensive, new patient, 1 or more visits

A comprehensive level of general ophthalmological services is provided to a new patient within the course of 1 or more visits. The entire service reported with 92004 need not be performed in a single session. A comprehensive evaluation describes a general diagnostic evaluation of the complete visual system. It includes a history and general medical observations; external ocular and adnexal exam that includes lids, lashes, brows, eye alignment and motility, conjunctiva, cornea, and iris; the use of slit lamp; examination of the gross visual field or visual acuity of each eye; sensorimotor examination, routine ophthalmoscopy to examine the ocular media, retina, and optic nerve; tonometry; keratometry; retinoscopy; biomicroscopy for acute, complicated conditions; and the use of mydriasis or cycloplegia to facilitate the exam. A mydriatic agent may be used to dilate the pupils to help visualize the ocular media and fundus. A cycloplegic agent is used to temporarily paralyze the ciliary muscle and dilate the pupil for accommodation. Following diagnostic evaluation, the physician initiates a diagnostic treatment program which includes any necessary medication prescription and arranging for additional special services, consultations, laboratory tests, or radiology services.

92012

92012   Ophthalmological services: medical examination and evaluation, with initiation or continuation of diagnostic and treatment program; intermediate, established patient

An intermediate level of general ophthalmological services is provided to an established patient. For an intermediate level service, the ophthalmologist focuses on evaluating a new condition or an existing condition now complicated by a new diagnosis or management problem, which need not necessarily be related to the primary diagnosis. The intermediate evaluation includes a history or interval history and general medical observations; external ocular and adnexal exam; visual field or acuity testing and basic motor evaluation; the use of slit lamp; routine ophthalmoscopy; biomicroscopy and tonometry for conditions that do not require comprehensive care; keratometry; retinoscopy; and the use of mydriasis to facilitate routine ophthalmoscopy by dilating the pupils to help visualize the ocular media and fundus. Following diagnostic evaluation, the physician either initiates a new diagnostic treatment program or makes arrangements for continuation of an established program. This may include medication prescription, and arranging for additional special services, consultations, laboratory tests, or radiology services.

92014

92014   Ophthalmological services: medical examination and evaluation, with initiation or continuation of diagnostic and treatment program; comprehensive, established patient, 1 or more visits

A comprehensive level of general ophthalmological services is provided to an established patient within the course of 1 or more visits. The entire service reported with 92014 need not be performed in a single session. A comprehensive evaluation describes a general diagnostic evaluation of the complete visual system. It includes a history or interval history and general medical observations; external ocular and adnexal exam that includes lids, lashes, brows, eye alignment and motility, conjunctiva, cornea, and iris; the use of slit lamp; examination of the gross visual field or visual acuity of each eye; sensorimotor examination, routine ophthalmoscopy to examine the ocular media, retina, and optic nerve; tonometry in the established patient, such as for known cataract; keratometry; retinoscopy; biomicroscopy for acute, complicated conditions; and the use of mydriasis or cycloplegia to facilitate the exam. A mydriatic agent may be used to dilate the pupils to help visualize the ocular media and fundus. A cycloplegic agent is used to temporarily paralyze the ciliary muscle and dilate the pupil for accommodation. Following diagnostic evaluation, the physician either initiates a new diagnostic treatment program or makes arrangements for continuation of an established program. This may include medication prescription, and arranging for additional special services, consultations, laboratory tests, or radiology services.

92015

92015   Determination of refractive state

The provider examines the patient's eyes for refractive errors in conditions such as hyperopia, myopia, and astigmatism. Refraction is the ability of the eye to refract or deflect light that enters it from a straight path to focus an image on the retina. This refractive ability is what determines the patient's need for glasses or contact lenses and the appropriate prescription. Lens prescription includes the specification of lens type (monofocal, bifocal, other), lens power, axis, prism, absorptive power, impact resistance, and other factors. The patient sits in a chair behind a special device called a phoropter, or refractor, and looks through it while focusing on an eye chart. The provider moves lenses with different strengths into place and the patient determines when the chart appears more or less clear. For those with normal uncorrected vision, the refractive error is zero. Those with a refractive error achieve the best corrected visual acuity through the refractive test using different combinations of lenses. The examiner may also use a keratometer to measure the curvature of the surface of the cornea, or a retinoscope to shine light into the patient's eye and observe the reflex off the retina. The streak or spot of light is moved across the pupil as the examiner observes this reflex, then uses the phoroptor to move different lenses over the eye to neutralize the reflex.

92018-92019

92018   Ophthalmological examination and evaluation, under general anesthesia, with or without manipulation of globe for passive range of motion or other manipulation to facilitate diagnostic examination; complete

92019   Ophthalmological examination and evaluation, under general anesthesia, with or without manipulation of globe for passive range of motion or other manipulation to facilitate diagnostic examination; limited

Prior to administration of general anesthesia for an ophthalmological examination and evaluation, mydriatic eye drops are instilled to dilate the pupil and an intravenous line is placed. Once the pupils are adequately dilated, a general anesthetic is administered. Using an ocular microscope, the anterior portion of the eye is examined, including the cornea, iris, and lens. Eye pressure is measured and eye measurements are taken, including eye length and width and corneal thickness. Refraction is performed as needed to determine the correct eyeglass prescription. The posterior portion of the eye is examined including the retina, optic disc, and optic nerve. Photos are taken as needed. Any abnormalities are noted. Use 92018 for a complete examination under anesthesia and 92019 for a limited examination. Both 92018 and 92019 report bilateral procedures.

92020

92020   Gonioscopy (separate procedure)

Gonioscopy is an eye exam that is done to look at the anterior chamber of the eye between the cornea and the iris to check for glaucoma or birth defects that may cause glaucoma; view the iridocorneal angle to see if drainage is open, closed, or nearly closed; and identify any scarring or damage. Gonioscopy can help the doctor determine which kind of glaucoma is present and can also help treat glaucoma by aiming a laser light at the drainage angle through a special lens during gonioscopy to decrease pressure within the eye. The patient may lie down or sit in a chair with the chin and forehead supported while looking straight ahead. The eyes are numbed with drops. A lens is placed lightly onto the front of the eye and a slit lamp is used to look in the eye. A narrow beam of light is then directed into the eye and the doctor looks through the slit lamp to view the width of the iridocorneal drainage angle.

92025

92025   Computerized corneal topography, unilateral or bilateral, with interpretation and report

Computerized corneal topography is also known as computer assisted keratography or videokeratography. This is a method of measuring the curvature of the cornea. A special instrument projects rings of light onto the eye, which are reflected back to the device, which then creates a color-coded map of the cornea's surface with a cross-sectional profile. Defects such as scarring, astigmatism, and other abnormal curvatures of the eye can be detected using this method, which is commonly performed prior to corrective eye surgery, such as LASIK.

92060

92060   Sensorimotor examination with multiple measurements of ocular deviation (eg, restrictive or paretic muscle with diplopia) with interpretation and report (separate procedure)

An extended sensorimotor examination is performed to evaluate eye movement. The test is performed bilaterally. Motor function is tested by taking ocular alignment measurements as the eyes focus on different locations. More than one field of gaze is tested at distance and/or near. In adults and children who are old enough and able to respond, at least one sensory test, such as Titmus fly, Worth 4 dot, Maddox rod, or Bagolini lens test, is also performed. Any deviations in normal eye movements are documented. Test results are interpreted and a report of findings provided.

92065

92065   Orthoptic and/or pleoptic training, with continuing medical direction and evaluation

The physician provides individual orthoptic/pleoptic training sessions to the patient. Orthoptics are exercises designed for improving eye muscle function and pleoptics are exercises designed for improving impaired vision in the absence of organic eye disease. The physician prescribes specific eye movement and focusing exercises aimed at improving visual tracking and correcting ocular problems, such as uncoordinated eye movement

(amblyopia, strabismus), and defects in binocular vision (convergence insufficiency, convergence excess). Convergence insufficiency is a disorder in which the eyes' ability to turn inward towards each other when looking at near objects is impaired. The physician determines the appropriate eye exercises and trains the patient to do the therapy. A wide variety of techniques and equipment is employed and may include the use of prisms, pencil push-ups, special tinted lenses, color cards, penlights and mirrors, video games, and tracing pictures. Some visual therapy may be done mainly in the office, while other exercises may be assigned to continue at home. This code includes ongoing direction and evaluation and is reported for each session.

92071-92072

92071   Fitting of contact lens for treatment of ocular surface disease
92072   Fitting of contact lens for management of keratoconus, initial fitting

Contact lenses are fitted for the purpose of treating a disease. Fitting includes instruction for the wearer and training on use. Supply of the lenses and any incidental revision during the fitting and training are included. Lens fitting reported with these codes is not for vision correction. In 92071, the lens is fitted to help treat diseases of the ocular surface such as corneal abrasions, keratitis, corneal ulcers, bullous keratopathy, and recurrent corneal erosion. These conditions are treated with bandage soft contact lenses (BSCL) to help heal the cornea. These lenses can relieve pain, encourage epithelial growth and migration, deliver antibiotics, and allow for oxygen transmissibility. The type and extent of corneal wound is assessed along with pain level. The hydrogel or silicone hydrogel lens is then fitted for complete corneal coverage and centered with minimal movement. Additional topical antibiotics and oral analgesics may be utilized. In 92072, an initial fitting is performed for management of keratoconus which is a progressive eye condition affecting the cornea. The normally spherical shaped cornea thins and becomes cone-shaped and irregular. This causes blurred and distorted vision. There are several different types of lenses available for correction of keratoconus. The exact fitting technique depends on the type of lens selected. The stage of the disease is evaluated. The lens is then selected based on corneal topography studies and the practitioner's evaluation. A trial lens is selected and the fit is checked. This is repeated until the best fitting lens is identified. The patient may need to return to fine-tune the lens selection and fit.

92081

92081   Visual field examination, unilateral or bilateral, with interpretation and report; limited examination (eg, tangent screen, Autoplot, arc perimeter, or single stimulus level automated test, such as Octopus 3 or 7 equivalent)

A visual field examination tests the total area in which the patient can see objects within the peripheral vision while focusing on a central point. This is done for one or both eyes and tests for blind spots or loss of peripheral vision. One eye is tested with the other completely covered. A limited examination is reported for using a widefield screening protocol that evaluates the static field of vision and is essentially a screening test at a single stimulus level. This includes a tangent screen test in which the patient sits 3 feet away from a target painted on a screen, stares at the centered target, and tells the examiner when he/she sees objects that move into the side vision. Automated perimetry may be done in which the patient sits in front of a concave dome staring at an object in the center and presses a button whenever a small flash of light is seen in the peripheral vision. Interpretation of the results and a written report is included.

92082

92082   Visual field examination, unilateral or bilateral, with interpretation and report; intermediate examination (eg, at least 2 isopters on Goldmann perimeter, or semiquantitative, automated suprathreshold screening program, Humphrey suprathreshold automatic diagnostic test, Octopus program 33)

A visual field examination tests the total area in which the patient can see objects within the peripheral vision while focusing on a central point. This is done for one or both eyes to test for loss of peripheral vision and detect causative conditions, such as glaucomatous optic nerve damage and retinal disease. One eye is completely covered while the other is tested. An intermediate examination evaluates the full visual field using manual perimetry tests such as 2 isopters on Goldman perimeter or an equivalent test, automated suprathreshold Humphrey testing or semiquantitative screening program, and automated testing at 2 or 3 threshold related luminance levels such as Octopus program 33. The Octopus and the Humphrey-Zeiss field analyzer are popular devices that test static perimetry. These automated devices run a choice of programs by an onboard computer and employ stationary pinpoint light sources or dots projected within a large, white bowl. The patient focuses on a central point and pushes a button when he/she sees the light or movement in different locations. The computer stores the data and generates a vision field report. The traditional Goldman perimeter is a kinetic perimetry test process that utilizes moving light sources. A trained technician moves the light source and monitors that the patient maintains central focus fixation throughout the test and then produces a map of peripheral vision perception. Interpretation and report is included.

Medicine

92083

92083 **Visual field examination, unilateral or bilateral, with interpretation and report; extended examination (eg, Goldmann visual fields with at least 3 isopters plotted and static determination within the central 30°, or quantitative, automated threshold perimetry, Octopus program G-1, 32 or 42, Humphrey visual field analyzer full threshold programs 30-2, 24-2, or 30/60-2)**

A visual field examination tests the total area in which the patient can see objects within the peripheral vision while focusing on a central point. One or both eyes are tested for loss of peripheral vision and causative conditions, such as glaucomatous optic nerve damage and retinal disease. One eye is completely covered while the other is tested. An extended examination includes more comprehensive quantitative automated perimetry tests with multilevel threshold testing or manual perimetry tests with 3 isopters on Goldman visual field and static determination within central 30 degrees. The Octopus and the Humphrey-Zeiss field analyzer are popular automated devices that test static perimetry running a choice of programs (such as Octopus program G-1, 32, or 42 or Humphrey full threshold programs 30-2, 24-2, or 30/60-2) by an onboard computer. They employ stationary pinpoint light sources or dots projected within a large, white bowl. The patient focuses on a central point and pushes a button when he/she sees the light or movement in different locations or at different intensities. The computer stores the data and generates a vision field report. The traditional Goldman perimeter is a kinetic perimetry test process that utilizes moving light sources. A trained technician moves the light source and monitors that the patient maintains central focus fixation throughout the test. A map of peripheral vision perception intensity within specified degrees is then produced. Interpretation and report is included.

92100

92100 **Serial tonometry (separate procedure) with multiple measurements of intraocular pressure over an extended time period with interpretation and report, same day (eg, diurnal curve or medical treatment of acute elevation of intraocular pressure)**

Serial tonometry is used to determine the pressure of intraocular fluid in the diagnosis of certain conditions, such as glaucom). Serial tonometry includes a series of pressure checks over the course of a day to measure peaks and acute elevations in intraocular pressure (diurnal curve). There are a variety of methods used, such as Goldmann's, applanation, and Perkins. Goldmann's is the most widely accepted type of tonometry and uses a technique where an area is flattened and force is applied to measure intraocular pressure. In applanation, a topical anesthetic is introduced into the eye. A disinfected prism is then mounted on the tonometer and placed against the cornea. A cobalt blue filter is used to view the green semi-circles. The tonometer head is adjusted until the inner edges of the green semi-circles meet. A Perkins tonometer is a portable tonometer, used for children, patients unable to undergo a slit lamp examination and those in a supine position.

92132

92132 **Scanning computerized ophthalmic diagnostic imaging, anterior segment, with interpretation and report, unilateral or bilateral**

This procedure may also be referred to as optical coherence tomography which is a noninvasive, noncontact imaging technique that allows visualization of anterior segment structures using backscattering of light. The procedure is used to diagnose glaucoma and selected macular abnormalities. The procedure may be performed on one or both eyes. The patient is seated in front of the scanning device and is instructed to fixate on a target contained in the scanning system. The scanner is aligned and centered and the scan is obtained. The scanned images are reviewed and accepted. The physician then reviews the images, using the computerized scanning software to help analyze the images and assist in diagnosis and treatment planning. The physician identifies key landmarks and takes measurements required to formulate a diagnosis and assist with treatment planning. The physician interprets the results of the scan and provides a written report of findings.

92133-92134

92133 **Scanning computerized ophthalmic diagnostic imaging, posterior segment, with interpretation and report, unilateral or bilateral; optic nerve**

92134 **Scanning computerized ophthalmic diagnostic imaging, posterior segment, with interpretation and report, unilateral or bilateral; retina**

These tests may be performed on one or both eyes to evaluate diseases affecting the optic nerve or retina. Two different types of laser scanning devices are available, confocal laser scanning opthalmoscopy (topography) and scanning laser polarimetry. Confocal laser scanning topography uses stereoscopic videographic digitized images to calculate measurements of anterior or posterior eye structures. Scanning laser polarimetry measures the change in linear polarization of light. This device employs a polarimeter, an optical device, and a scanning laser ophthalmoscope. The patient is told to fixate on an internal target generated by the computer. Multiple radial scans of the posterior segment of the eye are obtained. Scans may be obtained of the optic nerve head (92133) or the retina (92134). Digitized images are displayed on a monitor. The computer calculates optic nerve

head measurements, retinal thickness, or other measurements. The digitized images and measurements are evaluated by the physician and then interpreted, with a written report provided.

92136

92136 **Ophthalmic biometry by partial coherence interferometry with intraocular lens power calculation**

Ophthalmic biometry by partial coherence interferometry is performed preoperatively to calculate the intraocular lens power needed to attain optimal refraction following cataract surgery. This procedure may also be referred to as optical or ocular coherence biometry (OCB) or laser Doppler interferometry. In order to calculate the correct intraocular lens power, three measurements are needed – axial eye length, the corneal radius, and the anterior chamber length. Partial coherence interferometry measures the axial length of the eye. The axial eye length is calculated by illuminating the eye using a laser Doppler. Light from the laser Doppler is passed through a beam splitting prism and is then reflected at both the cornea and the retinal pigment epithelium. Interference of the reflected light from the cornea and retinal pigment epithelium is detected by a photodetector and processed by the device computer which measures the path difference between the cornea and the retinal pigment epithelium. These measurements are then used to calculate the axial length, which is displayed graphically. The same device is used to measure the corneal radius using keratometry and the anterior chamber length using a slit lamp illumination.

92145

92145 **Corneal hysteresis determination, by air impulse stimulation, unilateral or bilateral, with interpretation and report**

Corneal hysteresis (CH) is a viscoelastic property which can be measured by sending an external shear force in the form of a puff of air toward the cornea causing it to flatten, called applanate, and then using an infrared beam to track the change in shape. The CH is calculated as the difference in air pressure between force in and force out applanation and is used to determine the stiffness or rigidity of the cornea and its resistance to intraocular pressure (IOP). CH can provide independent information that will aide in the diagnosis and management of glaucoma and may also help identify eyes at risk for keratoconus. CH may be used with topographic measurements to determine the geometric attributes of the eye, or to monitor the accuracy of tonometers and provide corneal compensated intraocular pressure (IOPcc) measurement.

92225-92226

92225 **Ophthalmoscopy, extended, with retinal drawing (eg, for retinal detachment, melanoma), with interpretation and report; initial**

92226 **Ophthalmoscopy, extended, with retinal drawing (eg, for retinal detachment, melanoma), with interpretation and report; subsequent**

Extended ophthalmoscopy is a detailed examination of the inside of the back of the eye (fundus) and other structures, including the retina, optic disc, choroid, and blood vessels, that goes beyond an intermediate or comprehensive general ophthalmological exam. This is done for severe posterior segment pathology. Eyedrops are given to dilate the pupil and numb the eye surface. An ophthalmoscope about the size of a flashlight is used that shines a beam of light through the pupil and has several different tiny lenses through which the doctor examines the eye. The microscope of a slit-lamp and a tiny lens may also be used. The physician exams the back of the eye and makes a drawing using standard colors and labeling that details the extent of retinal detachment, location of holes or tears, areas of traction, vitreous opacities, hemorrhaging, lesions, and any other appropriate documentation for specific conditions, such as glaucoma in which cupping, disc rim, pallor, slope, and any pathology around the optic nerve should be identified. An interpretation is also written that provides pertinent conclusions, impressions, and findings. Report 92225 for the initial evaluation of disease in each eye examined and 92226 for a repeat evaluation of an established problem that is worsening or complicated by other pathology.

92227-92228

92227 **Remote imaging for detection of retinal disease (eg, retinopathy in a patient with diabetes) with analysis and report under physician supervision, unilateral or bilateral**

92228 **Remote imaging for monitoring and management of active retinal disease (eg, diabetic retinopathy) with physician review, interpretation and report, unilateral or bilateral**

Remote retinal imaging is performed on one or both eyes to screen for retinopathy (92227) in at risk patients, such as those with diabetes, or to evaluate active retinal disease (92228). The images are obtained by a provider at one facility, often the primary care provider, and then transmitted electronically, to be reviewed and interpreted at another site by an ophthalmologist or other qualified health care professional under the direction of a retinal specialist. One or both pupils are dilated. Images are then obtained using a computerized retinal imaging system. Most systems automatically center on the pupil, illuminate the retina, focus, estimate visual acuity, and then obtain digital images of the retina. The digital images are electronically transmitted to the eye center. The images are reviewed and a written interpretation of findings is provided. In 92227, the images of a patient at risk for retinal disease may be reviewed and interpreted by a specially trained individual under physician supervision. In 92228, a physician reviews, interprets, and provides a written report of the images in a patient with active retinal disease.

92230

92230   Fluorescein angioscopy with interpretation and report

Fluorescein angioscopy is done using a modified microscope to study capillary vessels and assess or evaluate lesions in the eye and around the retinal periphery. A fluorescein dye is injected into a peripheral vein or fluorescence sodium salt can also be applied externally. An indirect ophthalmoscope is used to shine light into the eye. The fluorescent dye or sodium allows the vascular area that is being examined to light up and appear in relation to the color and be demarcated against surrounded areas and landmarks. One technique uses a cobalt blue filter that is carefully adjusted so only blue light illuminates the retina and partial fluorescence appears through the microscope, causing a blue image that identifies the location of retinal lesions. Other types of interference bandpass filters, such as a barrier filter, may be used to block out all light from the fluorescence, except at a specific wavelength. Acidic, yellowish green fluorescent sodium is used to identify corneal trauma and injury. Digital imaging is produced that can be stored, printed, and transferred. The physician provides a written interpretation and report of the findings.

92235

▲ 92235   Fluorescein angiography (includes multiframe imaging) with interpretation and report, unilateral or bilateral

In 92235, fluorescein angiography is used in the diagnosis and treatment of retinal disorders. Fluorescein is a fluorescent dye that is injected into the bloodstream and used to highlight the blood vessels of the retina. In 92240, indocyanine-green angiography is used in the evaluation of the retina and the choroid for diseases such as macular degeneration, abnormal vessel growth, macular edema, and retinal detachment. The test is performed using indocyanine green dye that fluoresces in the infrared spectrum and allows imaging through pigmentation, fluid, and collections of blood in the retina and choroid. To perform either test, the pupil is dilated using Mydriatic drops and fundal photographs are obtained prior to the infusion of fluorescein or indocyanine-green (ICG). A bolus of fluorescein or ICG is then injected into a peripheral vein, usually in the arm, and fundus photographs are obtained using a rapid sequence or video camera as the fluorescein flows through the blood vessels in the retina, or the ICG flows through the blood vessels in the retina and the choroid. The photographs or video images are then reviewed by the physician and any retinal abnormalities or retinal and choroid abnormalities are identified. A written interpretation of findings is provided which may be for one eye or both eyes. Report 92242 when both the fluorescein angiography and the indocyanine-green angiography test are performed during the same patient encounter.

92240

▲ 92240   Indocyanine-green angiography (includes multiframe imaging) with interpretation and report

Indocyanine-green (ICG) angiography is used in the evaluation of the retina and choroid for diseases such as macular degeneration, abnormal vessel growth, macular edema, and retinal detachment. The test is performed using indocyanine green dye that fluoresces in the infrared spectrum and allows imaging through pigmentation, fluid, and collections of blood in the retina and choroid. Mydriatric drops are instilled into the eyes to dilate the pupil and fundal photographs are obtained. A vein, usually in the arm, is punctured and dye is injected. Fundus photographs are obtained using a rapid sequence or video camera as the dye flows through the blood vessels in the retina and choroid. The photographs or video images are then reviewed by the physician and any retinal or choroidal abnormalities are identified. A written interpretation of findings is provided.

92250

92250   Fundus photography with interpretation and report

Fundus photography is the use of a retinal camera to take pictures of the inside of the back of the eye. Fundus photography may look at the optic nerve, macula, vitreous, the retina, and its vasculature. The highly specialized retinal camera is mounted on a microscope that contains high-powered, intricate lenses and mirrors. The lenses capture images of the back of the eye when light is focused through the cornea, the pupil, and the lens. The pupils are dilated with drops to prevent them from constricting at the bright light. The patient is instructed to stare at one fixation point to keep the eyes still. Pictures are then taken as a series of flashes of bright light are focused through the eye and camera lens. Fundus photography is done to evaluate abnormalities, follow the progress of a disease, assess therapeutic effects and surgical treatments, and plan for future treatment. Diseases that indicate a need for fundus photography include retinal neoplasms, macular degeneration, diabetic retinopathy, glaucoma, multiple sclerosis, and other central nervous system problems.

92260

92260   Ophthalmodynamometry

Ophthalmodynamometry (ODM) is a method for measuring blood pressure within the central retinal artery or vein. This noninvasive method involves an ophthalmoscopic examination of the central retinal artery/vein while intraocular pressure is induced and gradually increased. The eyes are dilated and numbing drops are instilled. An ophthalmodynamometer is then used to exert pressure on the globe towards the center of the eyeball. The patient holds the gaze fixed straight ahead with the other eye. The calibrated plunger transmits the extent of eye compression to a unit scale on the ophthalmodynamometer. The reading is noted when the central retinal artery ceases pulsation and becomes completely collapsed and blanched by the pressure applied to give the systolic measurement. The pressure applied is slowly lessened and the reading is noted again when the artery first begins to pulsate after collapse and complete interruption of blood flow. This number is the diastolic pressure measurement. The average diastolic value of retinal pressure is 47 mm/Hg and the systolic value is 78 mm/Hg. Measurements are used to detect retinal hypertension and to test for the presence of disease in the internal carotid artery as the two measurements are correlated. Blood pressure measured in the central retinal vein is used as a non-invasive method for screening cases of suspected elevated intracranial pressure (ICP). The pressure in the central retinal vein depends on ICP because the optic nerve is surrounded by cerebrospinal fluid and when the vein collapses or pulsates, the ICP is at least equal to or greater than the pressure within the optic nerve.

92265

92265   Needle oculoelectromyography, 1 or more extraocular muscles, 1 or both eyes, with interpretation and report

Needle oculoelectromyography is performed to evaluate nerve and muscle function of the eye muscles. This test is commonly performed in the diagnosis and evaluation of myasthenia gravis as well as other neuromuscular conditions effecting eye movement. This test is typically performed using single fiber electromyography (EMG) which uses a very fine needle to evaluate function in a single muscle fiber. The recording needle electrode is inserted into the targeted nerve-muscle communication point in the selected extraocular muscle. The electrode cable is attached to a recording device with a visual display. Electrical activity of the muscle is recorded. Action potential is tested by stimulating the muscle fiber. Action potential evaluates the ability of muscle fibers to respond to nerve stimulation. The EMG recording is displayed graphically as a wave form. The physician reviews the needle EMG recording and provides a written report of findings.

92270

92270   Electro-oculography with interpretation and report

Electro-oculography (EOG) is used to evaluate function of the retinal pigment epithelium (RPE) of the eye. The test records changes in electrical potential across the RPE as the eye adapts to periods of dark and light. The RPE is a pigmented cell layer lying just outside the retina that is located between the vascular layer of the choroid and the light sensitive outer segments of the photoreceptors. The RPE along with the photoreceptors play a critical role in the maintenance of visual function. To perform EOG, the pupils are dilated. Pairs of electrodes are placed on the skin usually medial and lateral to the eye. The patient is positioned in a head and chin rest within a full-field dome with two red fixation lights located to the left and right of center. Dark phase adaptation is tested first. The dome is programmed for complete darkness with maximal dimming of the fixation lights. The fixation lights are then alternately activated, prompting the patient to move the eyes from side to side to focus on the activated light. The dark phase lasts for 15 minutes, with the fixation lights alternating from side to side for 10 seconds a minute during which recordings are taken alternating with 50 seconds of complete darkness. The light phase is tested next and also lasts 15 minutes. The dome background lights are turned on and light phase testing is performed in the same manner with 10 seconds of alternating fixation lights followed by 50 seconds of light. Upon completion of the procedure, the EOG recording is evaluated for dark/light adaptation. Dark adaptation is identified as a decrease in resting potential which typically reaches a minimum called the dark trough after several minutes. Light adaptation is identified as an increase in resting potential called the light peak that drops off as the retina adapts to light. Specific parameters are calculated either manually or using computer algorithms which include the Arden (light/dark) ratio), the dark trough amplitude, the time from light phase initiation to light peak, the pupil size, and the type of adapting light source. A written report of findings is provided.

92275

92275   Electroretinography with interpretation and report

Electroretinography (ERG) is peformed to diagnose and evaluate conditions affecting the retina. Mydriatic drops are instilled to dilate the pupil. The patient is dark adapted for 30 minutes. ERG electrodes are then placed on the surface of the eye using dim red illumination. There are several types of electrodes that can be used including contact lens electrodes placed over the cornea, or gold Mylar tape containing electrodes placed between the lower lid and the sclera or cornea. The electrodes are connected to a recording device. The head is kept stationary using head and chin supports. The eye is

Medicine

then stimulated by flashes of light from a bright light source such as LEDs or a strobe lamp. Alternatively, a full-field dome with its own light source can be used. The flash of light causes an electrical response in the retina that is captured by the electrodes, recorded, and represented digitally as a waveform. The response to light flashes are first recorded in the dark and then with background lighting. Following completion of the test, two components are typically evaluated, the a-wave and b-wave. The a-wave represents the amplitude from the baseline to the lowest point (trough) and correlates to the health of the photoreceptors in the outer retina. The b-wave represents the amplitude from the trough of the a-wave to the peak of the b-wave and correlates to the health of the inner layers of the retina. A written interpretation of findings is provided.

92283

92283   Color vision examination, extended, eg, anomaloscope or equivalent

A test is performed to determine whether color vision is within the normal range. Individuals who do not see all colors in the spectrum in the usual way suffer from a vision deficit called color blindness. Color vision deficits are caused by color sensing pigment deficiencies in the cone cells of the eye. The most common type of color vision deficit is called protanomaly, which is the reduced ability to process red light. Two less common types are dueteranomaly, which is the reduced ability to process green light and tritanomaly, which is the reduced ability to process blue light. The severity of each of these types of color vision deficits can vary significantly. In very rare cases, an individual may see no color at all, only shades of gray. An anomaloscope uses two light sources that display light of different colors and different brightness side-by-side. The light on one side must be blended to match the color and brightness of the opposite side. The patient is familiarized with the controls on the anomaloscope. Lights in the red and green spectrums are displayed and the patient turns the dials until a color and brightness match is perceived. The patient may also indicate that no match can be made. An initial review of results is made and if a color vision deficit is noted, the anomaloscope is recalibrated to test for the severity of the specific color deficit detected. The test results are displayed graphically to show deviations from normal color and brightness perception and the severity of the color vision deficit. The test may be repeated with colors in the blue and yellow spectrums. The physician reviews the test results and provides a written test of findings.

92284

92284   Dark adaptation examination with interpretation and report

Dark adaptation tests the ability of the eyes to recover sensitivity in the dark following exposure to bright light. Light and dark vision is mediated by cone and rod cells in the retina. Cone cells mediate vision in well-lit conditions, while rod cells mediate vision in low-light conditions. During dark adaption, following exposure to bright light, the eye adapts by shifting from cone cells to rod cells to mediate vision. However, this does not happen instantaneously. Depending on the intensity of the light and the duration of exposure it can take the eye up to 50 minutes to make a complete shift from cone cells to rod cells. During this time, dark vision gradually improves as the eye adapts to the dark. To test for dark adaptation, the patient is first exposed to bright light for about 5 minutes. The light source is turned off and the time it takes for the eye to adapt to the dark and reach peak dark or low-light vision is determined. This is accomplished by exposing the eye to flashes of light of varying intensities in the newly darkened environment. The patient is cued when a flash of light occurs and must indicate whether or not the flash was seen. If the patient is not able to see the flash, a higher intensity flash is used until the patient indicates that the flash can be seen. The flashes of light continue but are reduced in intensity to determine the lowest level of intensity that can be seen during dark adaptation. The time it takes to reach the lowest level of light intensity that is able to be seen is the dark adaptation time. The results are displayed graphically and a written interpretation of findings is provided.

92285

92285   External ocular photography with interpretation and report for documentation of medical progress (eg, close-up photography, slit lamp photography, goniophotography, stereo-photography)

External ocular photography is performed to document and track conditions or injuries affecting the external structures of the eye, including the eyelids, lashes, sclerae, conjunctiva, and cornea. It may also be used for some structures of the anterior chamber, including the iris and filtration angle. Photography may be performed using a slit lamp, goniophotography, stereophotography, or close-up photography. Pictures may be stored as prints, slides, videotape, or digital media. The physician reviews the external ocular photographs and describes the findings, compares them to previously obtained photographs, and notes any resolution, progression, or late effects of the condition or injury.

92286-92287

92286   Anterior segment imaging with interpretation and report; with specular microscopy and endothelial cell analysis

92287   Anterior segment imaging with interpretation and report; with fluorescein angiography

Anterior segment imaging is performed to evaluate the integrity of the cornea, iris and other anterior segment structures. In 92286, anterior segment imaging is performed

with specular microscopy and endothelial cell analysis of the cornea. The cornea has several layers including epithelium, stroma, and a single-celled endothelial layer with the endothelium being the most posterior layer. The health of the endothelial layer is critical for maintaining visual acuity. The endothelial cells prevent aqueous humor from entering the cornea and pump fluid from the corneal stroma into the anterior chamber. Maintaining the cornea in a relatively dehydrated state is necessary for corneal clarity. However, because the corneal endothelial cells do not replicate, if they are destroyed by disease or surgery, the remaining cells must spread out to cover an increased surface area. As the total number of endothelial cells decrease, the endothelial layer can no longer maintain the dehydrated state and the cornea becomes cloudy resulting in loss of visual acuity. Specular microscopy provides a magnified view of a small area of corneal endothelial cells. Images obtained using specular microscopy are recorded on videotape or photographic film. Endothelial cell density and configuration are evaluated and cell counts are provided. The images are compared with any previous images and changes documented. In 92287, anterior segment imaging is performed with fluorescein angiography to evaluate the iris and other anterior segment structures. An intravenous injection of sodium fluorescein is administered. Serial images of the anterior segment are obtained beginning 8 to 10 seconds following fluorescein injection and continuing until 1 minute after injection. Additional images may be obtained 5 to 10 minutes after injection. The images are viewed and a written interpretation of findings is provided.

92310-92313

92310   Prescription of optical and physical characteristics of and fitting of contact lens, with medical supervision of adaptation; corneal lens, both eyes, except for aphakia

92311   Prescription of optical and physical characteristics of and fitting of contact lens, with medical supervision of adaptation; corneal lens for aphakia, 1 eye

92312   Prescription of optical and physical characteristics of and fitting of contact lens, with medical supervision of adaptation; corneal lens for aphakia, both eyes

92313   Prescription of optical and physical characteristics of and fitting of contact lens, with medical supervision of adaptation; corneoscleral lens

Based on the patient's vision needs, the medical provider selects the best contact lens options for the patient. The provider discusses the pros and cons of the different types of contact lenses available and assists the patient in selecting the type of lens that will best meet his/her needs. The provider specifies the optical and physical characteristics of the selected lenses, such as power, size, curvature, flexibility (hard/soft), and gas-permeability. The lenses are inserted by the provider and the fit of the selected lenses is checked. Adjustments are made as needed to achieve the best visual acuity and the most comfortable fit. The patient is then instructed on how to insert and remove the lenses and practices inserting and removing the lenses under the guidance of the provider. The patient may be given sample contact lenses by different manufacturers to try for a period of time so that the lenses that best meet the patient's needs can be determined. During the trial period, incidental revisions to the optical and physical characteristics of the lenses may be made to improve visual acuity or comfort. All services are performed by the medical provider. Use code 92310 for corneal lenses for both eyes to correct a condition other than aphakia. Use code 92311 for a lens prescribed to treat aphakia in one eye, or code 92312 when lenses are prescribed to treat bilateral aphakia. Use code 92313 for a corneoscleral lens.

92314-92317

92314   Prescription of optical and physical characteristics of contact lens, with medical supervision of adaptation and direction of fitting by independent technician; corneal lens, both eyes except for aphakia

92315   Prescription of optical and physical characteristics of contact lens, with medical supervision of adaptation and direction of fitting by independent technician; corneal lens for aphakia, 1 eye

92316   Prescription of optical and physical characteristics of contact lens, with medical supervision of adaptation and direction of fitting by independent technician; corneal lens for aphakia, both eyes

92317   Prescription of optical and physical characteristics of contact lens, with medical supervision of adaptation and direction of fitting by independent technician; corneoscleral lens

Based on the patient's vision needs, the medical provider selects the best contact lens options for the patient. The provider discusses the pros and cons of the different types of contact lenses available and assists the patient in selecting the type of lens that will best meet his/her needs. The provider specifies the optical and physical characteristics of the selected lenses, such as power, size, curvature, flexibility (hard/soft), and gas-permeability. The lenses are inserted by the provider and the fit of the selected lenses is checked. Adjustments are made as needed to achieve the best visual acuity and the most comfortable fit. An independent technician then works with the patient, providing instruction on how to insert and remove the lenses. The technician observes and assists the patient as needed while the patient practices inserting and removing the lenses. The patient may be given sample contact lenses by different manufacturers to try for a period of time so that the lenses that best meet the patient's needs can be determined. During the trial period, incidental revisions to the optical and physical characteristics of the lenses may be made to improve visual acuity or comfort. Use code 92314 for corneal lenses for both eyes to correct a condition other than aphakia. Use code 92315 for a lens prescribed to treat aphakia in one eye, or code 92316 when lenses are prescribed to treat bilateral aphakia. Use code 92317 for a corneoscleral lens.

92325

92325   Modification of contact lens (separate procedure), with medical supervision of adaptation

Modification of the contact lens is performed during a separate procedure to improve the function, fit, and/or comfort of the lens. The medical provider evaluates the current fit of the contact lens and queries the patient regarding visual acuity and the comfort of the lens. The provider determines what modifications should be made. Possible modifications include reducing the overall lens diameter; reducing the optical zone diameter; flattening the peripheral curves; blending the peripheral curves; polishing the edges, anterior, and posterior surfaces; or modifying the lens power. The provider makes the necessary lens modifications, checks the fit and comfort, and then checks visual acuity.

92326

92326   Replacement of contact lens

A contact lens is replaced due to damage or loss, or because of problems related to fit, comfort, or vision. If the contact lens has been damaged or lost, the provider verifies the optical and physical characteristics and provides a replacement prescription. If the contact lens needs to be replaced because of poor fit, discomfort, or vision problems, the provider determines what changes should be made, which may include a different brand or type of contact lens, and a new prescription is provided. The patient may be given a trial supply of the new brand or type of lens to see if the new lens eliminates the problems that the patient was experiencing with the previous lens.

92340-92342

92340   Fitting of spectacles, except for aphakia; monofocal
92341   Fitting of spectacles, except for aphakia; bifocal
92342   Fitting of spectacles, except for aphakia; multifocal, other than bifocal

Following a separately reportable eye examination of a patient needing corrective lenses for a condition other than aphakia, the patient meets with an eyeglass (spectacle) technician who evaluates anatomical facial characteristics and determines the correct frame size. The technician measures the anatomical facial characteristics, including the distance between the pupils, and submits the measurements to a laboratory for manufacture of the lenses and insertion into the selected frame. The lab returns the completed eyeglasses to the technician, and the patient then returns for fitting of the eyeglasses. The fit of the bridge and the nose pads are evaluated and modified as necessary. The fit of the temples and the temple arms that curve around the ear are inspected and adjusted as needed. The technician makes sure that the frame is level on the face and makes adjustments to the nose pads and/or temple arms as needed. Use code 92340 for fitting of monofocal lenses, code 92341 for bifocal lenses, and code 93242 for other multifocal lenses.

92352-92353

92352   Fitting of spectacle prosthesis for aphakia; monofocal
92353   Fitting of spectacle prosthesis for aphakia; multifocal

Following a separately reportable eye examination of a patient with aphakia (absence of the lens), the patient meets with a technician who evaluates anatomical facial characteristics and fits the spectacle prosthesis. The technician first determines the correct frame size by measuring the anatomical facial characteristics, including the distance between the pupils. The specifications are then submitted to a laboratory for manufacture of the prosthetic lenses and insertion into the selected frame. The lab returns the completed prosthetic spectacles to the technician, and the patient then returns for fitting. The fit of the bridge and the nose pads are evaluated and modified as necessary. The fit of the temples and the temple arms that curve around the ear are inspected and adjusted as needed. The technician makes sure that the frame is level on the face and makes adjustments to the nose pads and/or temple arms as needed. Use code 92352 for fitting of monofocal spectacle prosthetic lenses and code 93253 for multifocal spectacle prosthetic lenses.

92354-92355

92354   Fitting of spectacle mounted low vision aid; single element system
92355   Fitting of spectacle mounted low vision aid; telescopic or other compound lens system

A technician fits a spectacle mounted low vision aid to the patient's eyeglasses (spectacles). Spectacle mounted low vision aids protrude from the frame. They may be designed for use with one or both eyes. Low vision aids may magnify objects. They may be telescopes which aid distance vision or microscopes which aid close-up vision. The existing frame is evaluated for proper fit and comfort. The low vision aid is then attached to the

spectacles and the patient is instructed on proper use. The patient tests the low vision aid by using a reading card, holding it against the tip of the nose, and then pushing the card away until the words come in to focus. The distance needed to achieve the best focus is dependent on the size of the print or object the patient is reading or looking at. Use code 92354 for a single element low vision aid system, such as a magnifier. Use 92355 for a telescopic, microscopic, or other compound lens system.

92358

92358   Prosthesis service for aphakia, temporary (disposable or loan, including materials)

A patient, whose natural lens has been removed, is fitted for a temporary lens that attaches to the patient's spectacles. The fit of the patient's current spectacles is checked and adjustments are made as needed to ensure that the best fit is achieved. The temporary prosthetic lens is positioned over the lens in the patient's current spectacles and secured. The temporary lens is only capable of providing the patient with somewhat improved vision. It does not completely correct vision. The patient is instructed on the characteristics of the temporary lens and assured that the permanent prosthetic lens will provide better visual acuity.

92370-92371

92370   Repair and refitting spectacles; except for aphakia
92371   Repair and refitting spectacles; spectacle prosthesis for aphakia

The patient's existing spectacles that have been damaged or that do not fit properly are repaired and refitted. This may involve replacement of nose pads or hinges or repair of broken rims, bridges, temples, or temple arms. Once the repairs are made, the technician makes sure that the frame is level on the face and makes adjustments to the nose pads and/or temple arms as needed. Report 92370 when this is done for spectacles except for aphakia, and use code 92371 when this is done for spectacle prosthetic lenses for aphakia.

92502

92502   Otolaryngologic examination under general anesthesia

An otolaryngologic (ear, nose, and throat) examination is performed under general anesthesia. The external ear (pinna) is examined for size, shape, inflammation, and ulcers. The external auditory meatus is examined for patency, inflammation, ad discharge. Any wax is removed and any drainage is aspirated. The tympanic membrane is assessed for color, perforations, and mobility. If a perforation is present, the middle ear is examined through the perforation for any edema, discharge, or lesions. The external nose is assessed for deformity and shape. Any inflammation, cysts, or other lesions are evaluated. An anterior and posterior rhinoscopy is performed to examine the vestibule, nasal cavity, and nasopharynx for obstruction, drainage, bleeding, polyps, other lesions, and anomalies. The oral cavity is examined including the lips, teeth, gums, tongue, hard and soft palates, floor, and cheeks. The oropharynx is evaluated including the uvula, soft palate, anterior and posterior tonsillar pillars, tonsils, and posterior pharyngeal wall. The larynx and piriform fossa are examined. The neck is inspected and palpated and any abnormalities are noted.

92504

92504   Binocular microscopy (separate diagnostic procedure)

A binocular microscopy is performed as a separate diagnostic procedure. The ear, nose, mouth, and/or throat are examined using a microscope that has two oculars allowing both eyes to be used to examine these structures. Any disease or abnormalities are noted.

92507-92508

92507   Treatment of speech, language, voice, communication, and/or auditory processing disorder; individual
92508   Treatment of speech, language, voice, communication, and/or auditory processing disorder; group, 2 or more individuals

A speech-language pathologist treats a speech, language, voice, communication, and/or auditory processing disorder. Using the information obtained from a separately reportable screening and in-depth evaluation of a speech or language disorder, the clinician develops an individualized treatment plan for the patient. The clinician defines specific treatment goals and sets baseline measures with which to assess the patient's progress. These goals are continuously monitored and fine-tuned throughout the treatment period. Once the goals and baseline measures have been established the clinician uses a number of intervention activities to correct the specific speech or language disorder identified. These can include games, stories, rhymes, drills, and other tasks. If the patient has a speech disorder, the clinician may demonstrate the sounds and have the patient copy the way the clinician moves the lips, mouth, and tongue to make the right sound. A mirror may be used so that the patient can practice making the sound while observing himself or herself in the mirror. Treatment of a language disorder might include help with grammar. If the patient is having difficulty with auditory processing, a game like Simon Says might be used to help improve understanding of verbal instructions. Code 92507 is used for individual treatment of speech, language, voice, communication, and/or auditory processing disorder. Code 92508 is used when these services are provided to a group of two or more individuals.

92511

92511   Nasopharyngoscopy with endoscope (separate procedure)

A nasopharyngoscopy is performed with an endoscope as a separate procedure. Nasopharyngoscopy is performed to visualize the back of the nose, to evaluate velopharyngeal function, and to identify the cause of Eustachian tube dysfunction or other ear problems. An endoscope is inserted through the nose into the nasal cavity and advanced into the nasopharynx. The nasal structures and nasopharynx are visualized on a monitor as the endoscope is advanced and any abnormalities are noted. With the endoscope in the nasopharynx, the patient may be asked to perform several speech tasks so that nasopharyngeal function can be assessed.

92512

92512   Nasal function studies (eg, rhinomanometry)

Nasal function studies, such as rhinomanometry or acoustic rhinometry, are performed. Rhinomanometry measures air pressure and the rate of airflow in the nasal airway during respiration. Measurements are used to calculate nasal airway resistance. The calculations are used to assess and quantify nasal airway patency or the degree of nasal airway obstruction. Another type of nasal function study, acoustic rhinometry is used to assess the configuration of the nasal cavity and nasopharynx and evaluate nasal obstruction. Sound waves are reflected from the nasal cavities and analyzed.

92516

92516   Facial nerve function studies (eg, electroneuronography)

Facial nerve function studies, such as electroneuronography (ENoG), are performed to evaluate the integrity of the facial nerve. Stimulating electrodes are placed bilaterally near the earlobe with a cathode (negative) electrode placed posteriorly to each ear and an anode (positive) electrode placed anteriorly to each ear. Recording electrodes are placed bilaterally at or near the stylomastoid foramen and at or near the nasolabial fold. The facial nerve on the unaffected side is electrically stimulated and the muscle response is recorded. Next, the affected or abnormal side is electrically stimulated and the facial nerve muscle response is recorded. The two sides are compared and a written interpretation of the results is provided. Other facial nerve function studies that may be performed include the Hilger test, electromyography, acoustic reflex testing, evoked accelerometry, and antidromic nerve potentials.

92520

92520   Laryngeal function studies (ie, aerodynamic testing and acoustic testing)

Laryngeal function studies, such as aerodynamic testing or acoustic testing, are performed. An aerodynamic test, also referred to as an aerodynamic voice analysis, uses an air transducer to demonstrate how air from the lungs passes between and drives the vocal folds as the patient vocalizes. An acoustic test, also referred to as an acoustic analysis, uses computerized instruments to measure and analyze the acoustic properties of the voice. As the patient vocalizes, the instruments translate factors such as hoarseness, pitch, and loudness onto a visual screen display. Voice characteristics are then measured, analyzed, and displayed on a digital readout. A spectrograph may also be used to chart the patient's voice on paper. All of these voice measures are then analyzed and a written interpretation of results is provided.

92521

92521   Evaluation of speech fluency (eg, stuttering, cluttering)

Speech fluency is the natural flow of spoken words. Speech fluency disorders can include stuttering and cluttering. In stuttering, a disruption in the production of speech sounds occurs. Characteristics of stuttering can include repeating words or parts of words, prolongation of speech sounds, and complete blocks or stops when speaking. With cluttering, the speech pattern is very fast or slurred and the intelligibility of words may be decreased. An evaluation of speech fluency is usually performed by a speech-language pathologist (SLP). Evaluation includes self-report tests (questionnaires) and observational data collection.

92522

92522   Evaluation of speech sound production (eg, articulation, phonological process, apraxia, dysarthria)

Speech sound production disorders affect an individual's ability to communicate. There may be an organic cause for the problem (hearing impairment, cleft lip/palate, cerebral palsy, ankyloglossia) or it may be functional with no known cause. Articulation disorders are characterized by substitution, distortion, omission or addition of sounds and words. Phonological processing disorders are characterized by a set pattern of sound errors. Although small mistakes are common and normal in young children who are developing language skills, when articulation disorders persist past the age of 8 or phonological processing mistakes continue past the age of 5, an evaluation by a speech-language

pathologist (SLP) that includes an audiogram to assess hearing, formal and informal observation of speech and standardized testing with tools such as the Clinical Assessment of Articulation and Phonology (CAAP) is typically performed. Verbal apraxia is a condition in which an individual who does not have a diagnosed weakness or paralysis of the speech muscles has difficulty stating what he/she wants to communicate correctly and consistently. Acquired verbal apraxia can occur at any age and is due to changes in an area of the brain. Stroke, head injury, tumor or illness/infection can cause this type of change. Developmental verbal apraxia is present from birth. It can manifest as an overall language disorder or a neurologic disorder affecting signals to and movement of the muscles involved with speech. There may be a genetic link to developmental apraxia as it is often occurs in multiple family members. Dysarthria is a speech disturbance that may be caused by a brain injury or by paralysis, spasticity or lack of coordination of the speech muscles. Evaluation by a speech-language pathologist (SLP) typically includes an audiogram to assess hearing (reported separately), formal and informal observation of speech and assessment using standardized testing tools such as Screening Test for Developmental Apraxia of Speech.

92523

92523   Evaluation of speech sound production (eg, articulation, phonological process, apraxia, dysarthria); with evaluation of language comprehension and expression (eg, receptive and expressive language)

Disorders of speech sound production that relate to language comprehension and expression usually manifest before the age of 4 years. Mixed language disorder (receptive and expressive) may be due to brain injury, developmental problems such as autistic spectrum disorders, hearing loss and learning disorders. In receptive language disorders an individual will have problems understanding what has been said, following directions and organizing thoughts. Expressive language disorders can manifest with difficulty putting words together to form coherent sentences, word finding and the use of placeholder words such as "um", decreased vocabulary for age, leaving out words when speaking, improper use of tenses (past, present, future) and repetition (echoing) of phrases. Evaluation by a speech-language pathologist (SLP) should include an audiogram to assess hearing (reported separately), formal and informal observation and assessment using standardized testing tools such as Receptive-Expressive Emergent Language Test (REEL).

92524

92524   Behavioral and qualitative analysis of voice and resonance

Behavioral and qualitative analysis of voice and resonance can be accomplished using high speed digital imaging (HSDI) of the larynx and simultaneous acoustic recording of speech. The merging of these two testing modalities provides better characterization of the vibratory behavior of vocal folds and the quality of vocal sound. It may be used to monitor neurological or laryngeal diseases/disorders, such as stroke or muscle tension dysphoria, and to assess for improvement following voice therapy.

92526

92526   Treatment of swallowing dysfunction and/or oral function for feeding

Swallowing dysfunction and/or oral function are treated in an individual with difficulty passing food or liquid from the mouth or throat into the stomach. A swallowing or oral function disorder can occur in any age group or at any point in the swallowing process as food or liquid passes from the mouth, through the pharynx and esophagus, into the stomach. Swallowing disorders are common in individuals with degenerative neurological disorders such as cerebral palsy, amyotrophic lateral sclerosis (ALS), postpolio syndrome, myasthenia gravis, multiple sclerosis, and Parkinson's disease. A swallowing disorder may also result from neurological damage such as a stroke or head or spinal cord injury, or from a congenital or acquired deformity of the mouth, pharynx, esophagus, or stomach. Medical treatment is provided for a patient with a swallowing or oral function disorder. The diet is modified. Swallowing posture is assessed and modified as needed. Swallowing technique is modified to strengthen oropharyngeal muscle groups and improve the mechanics of swallowing so that food and liquid can pass into the esophagus and then into the stomach without aspiration into the lungs.

92531

92531   Spontaneous nystagmus, including gaze

A spontaneous nystagmus test with gaze evoked nystagmus (GEN) is performed. Nystagmus is a rapid, involuntary movement of the eye. Nystagmus tests are performed to identify the presence of a vestibular disorder characterized by vertigo (dizziness) and balance disturbance, including the inability to maintain balance, stand upright, or walk with a normal gait. The physician observes eye movement with the naked eye. The patient's eyes may be observed directly or the patient may wear Frenzel optical goggles to magnify the eye. If Frenzel optical goggles are used, eye movement is observed in both the light and dark. If the test is performed under direct vision, the physician performs the test with the patient's eyes opened and closed. Gaze testing is accomplished by having the patient look straight ahead for 30 seconds and then directing the gaze to the right for 10 seconds. The eyes are then returned to the center. This is repeated with the eyes directed to the left, up, and down. Any abnormal eye movement is noted. The physician analyzes and interprets the results of the tests.

92532

92532   Positional nystagmus test

A positional nystagmus test is performed. Nystagmus is a rapid, involuntary movement of the eye. Nystagmus tests are performed to identify the presence of a vestibular disorder characterized by vertigo (dizziness) and balance disturbance, including the inability to maintain balance, stand upright, or walk with a normal gait. Positional nystagmus tests are performed to identify vertigo and nystagmus associated with certain movements of the head or body. Positional nystagmus is associated with disfunction of the semicircular canals of the middle ear. The physician observes eye movement with the naked eye. The patient's eyes may be observed directly or the patient may wear Frenzel optical goggles to magnify the eye. Standard testing positions include head hanging forward, supine, supine with head turned to the right, supine with head turned to the left, lateral left, lateral right, or any other position that causes dizziness. Eye movement is observed and any abnormal eye movement is noted. The physician analyzes and interprets the results of the test.

92533

92533   Caloric vestibular test, each irrigation (binaural, bithermal stimulation constitutes 4 tests)

A caloric vestibular test is performed by water irrigation of the ears. Caloric stimulation of the vestibular system allows assessment of the lateral semicircular canal and provides a measurement of inner ear function in each labyrinth individually. The patient is placed in a reclining position and the head is tilted at a 30 degree angle to orient the lateral semicircular canals in the most vertical plane possible. Spontaneous nystagmus is evaluated before performing the water irrigation. Caloric stimulation is accomplished using alternating binaural bithermal or monothermal protocols. Alternating binaural bithermal water irrigation is done using a cool irrigation in each ear followed by a warm irrigation in each ear. Caloric irrigation produces a predictable response in patients with a responsive vestibular system. Cool irrigation causes fast phase nystagmus beats in the direction opposite the stimulated ear and warm irrigation causes nystagmus beats in the direction of the stimulated ear. Monothermal irrigation is performed in the same manner except that only warm water irrigation is used in both ears. Any abnormal eye movement is noted. The physician analyzes and interprets the results. Code 92533 is reported for each irrigation.

92534

92534   Optokinetic nystagmus test

An optokinetic nystagmus (OKN) test is performed. The patient is placed in front of a rotating drum of alternating black and white vertical strips and told not to focus on any one stripe. The physician observes the eyes and notes the response. The rotation is reversed and the process is repeated. The OKN test generates eye movements that resemble nystagmus. The physician observes the eye movement and evaluates the symmetry of the response. If the response is not symmetrical, it may be indicative of central nervous system pathology. The physician analyzes and interprets the results of the test.

92540

92540   Basic vestibular evaluation, includes spontaneous nystagmus test with eccentric gaze fixation nystagmus, with recording, positional nystagmus test, minimum of 4 positions, with recording, optokinetic nystagmus test, bidirectional foveal and peripheral stimulation, with recording, and oscillating tracking test, with recording

A vestibular evaluation is performed for nystagmus, which is a rapid, involuntary movement of the eye. Nystagmus tests are performed to identify the presence of a vestibular disorder characterized by vertigo (dizziness) and balance disturbance including the inability to maintain balance, to stand upright, or to walk with a normal gait. The physician first observes eye movement with the naked eye. The tests are performed with recording using electronystagmography (ENG). Horizontal electrodes are placed on the skin at the inner and outer aspect of each eye. A spontaneous nystagmus test with eccentric gaze and fixation is performed. For gaze testing, the patient first looks straight ahead for 30 seconds and then fixates on a target 30 degrees to the right for 10 seconds. The gaze is then returned to center. This is repeated with gaze directed to the left, up, and down. A positional nystagmus test is performed in a minimum of four positions to identify vertigo and nystagmus associated with certain movements of the head or body. Positional nystagmus is associated with disorders of function of the semicircular canals of the middle ear. Standard testing positions include head hanging forward, supine, supine with head turned to right, supine with head turned to left, lateral left, lateral right, or any other position that causes dizziness. Eye movement is recorded. A minimum of four positions are tested and any abnormal eye movement noted. An optokinetic nystagmus (OKN) test with bidirectional, foveal, or peripheral stimulation is performed. Eye movements are recorded and measured as the patient watches a series of targets moving simultaneously to the right and then to the left. The types of targets used include stripes on a rotating drum, a stream of lighted dots across a light bar, or a full-field array of moving stars or trees. The targets are moved at a rate of 300, 400, or 600 feet per second. This test generates eye movements that

resemble nystagmus. The physician evaluates the symmetry of the response. If the response is not symmetrical it may be indicative of central nervous system pathology. An oscillating tracking test is performed. The test evaluates the patient's ability to keep a moving visual target registered on the fovea. The patient tracks a pendulum, metronome, light, or computer generated stimulus as it moves back and forth along a smooth arc or path. Eye movement is recorded. A computer is used to calculate the gain, expressed as target velocity divided by eye velocity. This calculation is compared to age-matched norms. Upon completion of the vestibular evaluation, the recordings are reviewed and interpreted, and the physician provides a written report of findings.

92541

92541   Spontaneous nystagmus test, including gaze and fixation nystagmus, with recording

A spontaneous nystagmus test with gaze evoked nystagmus (GEN) and fixation nystagmus is performed with recording using electronystagmography (ENG). Nystagmus is a rapid, involuntary movement of the eye. Nystagmus tests are performed to identify the presence of a vestibular disorder characterized by vertigo (dizziness) and balance disturbance including the inability to maintain balance, stand upright, or walk with a normal gait. The physician first observes eye movement with the naked eye. Tests are then conducted using a recording device. Horizontal electrodes are placed on the skin at the inner and outer aspect of each eye. Each eye is tested separately. For gaze testing, the patient first looks straight ahead for 30 seconds and then fixates on a target 30 degrees to the right for 10 seconds. The gaze is then returned to center. This is repeated with gaze directed to the left, up, and down. The test is conducted using targets placed on the wall or ceiling or with computer generated targets. To test spontaneous nystagmus, it is important to eliminate any suppression of eye movement in order to note abnormal movements. The physician reviews the ENG, and analyzes and interprets the results of the tests.

92542

92542   Positional nystagmus test, minimum of 4 positions, with recording

A positional nystagmus test is performed in a minimum of four positions with recording using electronystagmography (ENG). Nystagmus is a rapid, involuntary movement of the eye. Nystagmus tests are performed to identify the presence of a vestibular disorder characterized by vertigo (dizziness) and balance disturbance, including the inability to maintain balance, stand upright, or walk with a normal gait. Positional nystagmus tests are performed to identify vertigo and nystagmus associated with certain movements of the head or body due to functional disorders of the semicircular canals of the middle ear. The physician first observes eye movement with the naked eye. Tests are then conducted using a recording device. Horizontal electrodes are placed on the skin at the inner and outer aspect of each eye. Standard testing positions include head hanging forward, supine, supine with head turned to the right, supine with head turned to the left, lateral left, lateral right, or any other position that causes dizziness. Eye movement is then recorded. A minimum of four positions are tested and any abnormal eye movement is noted. The physician reviews the ENG recording, and analyzes and interprets the results.

92544

92544   Optokinetic nystagmus test, bidirectional, foveal or peripheral stimulation, with recording

An optokinetic nystagmus (OKN) test with bidirectional, foveal, or peripheral stimulation is performed with recording using electronystagmography (ENG). Horizontal electrodes are placed on the skin at the inner and outer aspect of each eye. Eye movements are recorded and measured as the patient watches a series of targets moving simultaneously to the right. The types of targets used include stripes on a rotating drum, a stream of lighted dots across a light bar, or a full-field array of moving stars or trees. The targets are moved at a rate of 300, 400, or 600 feet per second. The movement is then reversed and the procedure is repeated as the targets move simultaneously to the left. Eye movements are generated that resemble nystagmus. The physician reviews the recording and evaluates the symmetry of the response. If the response is not symmetrical, it may be indicative of central nervous system pathology.

92545

92545   Oscillating tracking test, with recording

An oscillating tracking test is performed with recording using electronystagmography (ENG). Horizontal electrodes are placed on the skin at the inner and outer aspect of each eye. The test evaluates the patient's ability to keep a moving visual target registered on the fovea. The patient tracks a pendulum, metronome, light, or computer generated stimulus as it moves back and forth along a smooth pendular path. Eye movement is recorded. A computer is used to calculate the gain, expressed as target velocity, divided by eye velocity. This calculation is compared to age-matched norms. The physician reviews and interprets the results.

Medicine

92546

92546   Sinusoidal vertical axis rotational testing

A sinusoidal vertical axis rotational test is performed with recording using electronystagmography (ENG). The test evaluates the integrity of the vestibular-ocular system. The test reflects the relationship between natural head and eye movements involved in the balance mechanism. Horizontal electrodes are placed on the skin at the inner and outer aspect of each eye. The patient sits in a rotational chair. A slow, harmonic acceleration rotation lasting 30-40 minutes is typically performed under computer control and eye movement is recorded. The physician reviews the recording and analyzes and interprets the results.

92547

92547   Use of vertical electrodes (List separately in addition to code for primary procedure)

Nystagmus tests are performed using electronystagmography (ENG) with vertical electrodes (leads). Electrodes with a vertical channel are placed around each eye. Eye movement is recorded. The physician reviews the recording and analyzes and interprets the results. The use of vertical electrodes is reported in addition to the code for the horizontal ENG recording of the primary procedure.

92548

92548   Computerized dynamic posturography

A computerized dynamic posturography (CDP) test is performed. CDP is used to evaluate balance impairments and differentiate between sensory, motor, and central adaptive causes of impaired balance. The patient stands on a moveable support surface inside a moveable enclosure. A computer is used to move the support surface and the enclosure. A sensory organization test (SOT), motor control test (MCT), and adaptation test (ADT) are performed. Sensory organization tests the patient's vestibular balance control and the adaptive responses of the central nervous system to perceived changes in the support surface resulting from changes in the visual display. Sensory conflict is created by eliminating useful visual and support surface information. SOT is performed with eyes open and closed, on a fixed and sway referenced surface, using fixed and sway referenced visual inputs. Motor control tests the patient's ability to quickly and automatically recover from unexpected movement in the support surface. During MCT. the support surface is moved backwards and forwards and the patient's postural responses are assessed for timing, strength, and lateral symmetry of the response. Adaptation tests the patient's ability to modify posture and minimize sway as the support surface is tilted in toes up and toes down positions. Measures are controlled and calibrated based on the patient's height and weight. Results are displayed using standardized graphical summaries that are compared to age-based norms.

92550

92550   Tympanometry and reflex threshold measurements

Tympanometry and acoustic reflex threshold testing are used to evaluate middle ear function. Tympanometry measures the flexibility of the eardrum and is helpful in detecting fluid in the middle ear, negative middle ear pressure, perforation of the tympanic membrane, disruption of the ossicles, and otosclerosis. The physician examines the ear with an otoscope. The tympantometry device is placed into the ear canal and a small amount of pressure is applied that changes the air pressure in the ear canal. This causes the eardrum to move back and forth. The movement is recorded on a graph referred to as a tympanogram. Acoustic reflex threshold testing is used to measure the movement of the stapedius muscle and tensor tympani in response to loud sound. The tensing of these muscles causes the stapes to move. The acoustic reflex threshold is a measurement of the softest sound that can elicit a reflex contraction of the stapedius muscle. Acoustic reflex testing is performed using the same device used to perform tympanometry. A loud sound is emitted and the stapedius muscle contracts which changes middle ear immittance. The change in immitance is seen as a deflection in the recording. The physician reviews and interprets the results of the tympanometry and acoustic reflex threshold test.

92551

92551   Screening test, pure tone, air only

A basic screening test for hearing is performed by pure tone air conduction without the use of audiometry. The test determines the faintest tones that a person can hear at different low to high frequencies or pitches. The test is typically performed using earphones so that hearing can be tested separately in each ear. In response to hearing a tone, the patient may be asked to raise a finger or hand or respond verbally by answering yes. More sophisticated testing equipment may require that the patient press a button when a sound is heard and to indicate whether it was heard in the right or left ear. A written interpretation of the basic screening test is provided.

92552-92553

92552   Pure tone audiometry (threshold); air only
92553   Pure tone audiometry (threshold); air and bone

Hearing is tested and recorded on an audiogram using pure tone air conduction alone (92552) or air and bone conduction (92553). In pure tone air conduction audiometry studies, earphones are used to determine the faintest tones that a person can hear at different low to high frequencies, or pitches. The use of earphones allows each ear to be tested separately. Bone conduction studies use sound transmitted through a bone oscillator that is placed on the skull behind the ear. In response to hearing a tone either through the earphones or the bone oscillator, the patient presses a button when each sound is heard. The patient may also be asked to indicate whether the sound was heard in the right or left ear. Upon completion of the test, the results are presented graphically showing hearing acuity measured at the various frequencies for each ear. A written interpretation of findings is provided.

92555-92556

92555   Speech audiometry threshold
92556   Speech audiometry threshold; with speech recognition

Hearing tests are performed to determine speech audiometry threshold (92555) or speech audiometry threshold with speech recognition (92556). These tests are performed in a soundproof room using earphones so that each ear can be tested separately. Speech audiometry threshold, also called speech reception threshold, is performed by recording the faintest speech levels that can be heard half the time in each ear. The results are presented on an audiogram. In speech recognition, the audiologist speaks at a comfortable loudness level and tests the ability of the patient to repeat back the words accurately that the audiologist says. Additional speech testing may be performed with background noise to evaluate the patient's ability to hear in a noisy environment. The audiogram presents results for each ear graphically. Test results are reviewed and a written report of findings is provided.

92557

92557   Comprehensive audiometry threshold evaluation and speech recognition (92553 and 92556 combined)

Hearing is tested and recorded on an audiogram using pure tone air conduction, bone conduction, speech audiometry threshold, and speech recognition. Tests are typically performed in a sound proof room using earphones so that each ear can be tested separately. In pure tone air conduction studies, earphones are used to determine the faintest tones that a person can hear at different low to high frequencies, or pitches. Bone conduction studies use sound transmitted through a bone oscillator that is placed on the skull behind the ear. In response to hearing a tone, either through the earphones or the bone oscillator, the patient presses a button when each sound is heard and indicates whether the sound was heard in the right or left ear. Speech audiometry threshold, also called speech reception threshold, is performed in a soundproof room using earphones and records the faintest speech levels that can be heard half the time in each ear. In speech recognition, the audiologist speaks at a comfortable loudness level and tests the ability of the patient to repeat back the words accurately that the audiologist says. Additional speech testing may be performed with background noise to evaluate the patient's ability to hear in a noisy environment. Test results are presented graphically for each ear in an audiogram. Test results are reviewed and a written report of findings is provided.

92558

92558   Evoked otoacoustic emissions, screening (qualitative measurement of distortion product or transient evoked otoacoustic emissions), automated analysis

Otoacoustic emission (OAE) tests are performed to determine cochlear status related to hair cell function. This information can be used to screen for hearing loss and is particularly valuable for screening neonates, infants, or individuals with developmental disabilities because no behavioral response is required. In addition to receiving sound, the cochlea also produces low-intensity sounds called OAEs which are believed to be a result of cochlear outer hair cells expanding and contracting. An evoked OAE screening test is a qualitative measurement that is performed using either distortion product evoked otoacoustic emissions (DPEOAEs) or transient evoked otoacoustic emissions (TEOAEs). The test is performed using a stimulus and a low noise microphone to record the otoacoustic emissions. Screening using DPEOAEs involves recording OAE emitted in response to acoustic stimuli using 2 simultaneous tones of different frequencies. Screening using TEOAEs involves recording OAE emitted in response to acoustic stimuli of very short duration such as clicks or tone bursts. A microphone probe is put in the external ear canal on the side to be tested. The stimulus is applied and recordings are obtained which are analyzed by software in the testing device. The physician reviews the test results and determines whether additional testing is needed.

92559

92559   Audiometric testing of groups

Special testing equipment that is capable of performing hearing tests on multiple individuals at the same time is used to perform audiometry on a group of individuals. Hearing may be tested using pure tone air conduction, bone conduction, speech audiometry threshold, and/or speech recognition. In pure tone air conduction studies, earphones are used to determine the faintest tones that a person can hear at different low to high frequencies, or pitches. Bone conduction studies use sound transmitted through a bone oscillator placed on the skull behind the ear. In response to hearing a tone, either through the earphones or the bone oscillator, the patient presses a button when each sound is heard and indicates whether the sound was heard in the right or left ear. Speech audiometry threshold, also called speech reception threshold, is performed in a soundproof room using earphones and records the faintest speech levels that can be heard half the time in each ear. In speech recognition, the audiologist speaks at a comfortable loudness level and tests the ability of the patient to repeat back accurately the words that the audiologist says. Additional speech testing may be performed with background noise to evaluate the patients' ability to hear in a noisy environment. Test results are presented graphically for each ear in an audiogram. Test results for each individual are reviewed and a written report of findings is provided. The written report should include the specific audiometry tests performed.

92560-92561

92560   Bekesy audiometry; screening
92561   Bekesy audiometry; diagnostic

The Bekesy audiometry test is a pure tone air conduction hearing test that differs from other hearing tests in that the patient controls the intensity of the stimulus. The Bekesy test may be performed to help differentiate between hearing loss that is cochlear or neural in origin. Tests are typically performed in a soundproof room using earphones so that each ear can be tested separately. The pure tone air conduction stimulus slowly moves through the entire audible range. The patient is given a button to press that controls the sound frequency (pitch) and intensity. The patient is instructed to continue to press the button until the sound can no longer be heard, at which time the button is released. As long as the button is depressed the sound intensity continues to decrease. When the button is released, the intensity begins to increase. When the patient can again hear the sound, the patient again presses the button and the sound begins to decrease. This continues through all sound frequencies (pitches), low to high, that are in the audible range. The test is also performed using continuous and interrupted tones. As the test is performed it is traced (recorded), resulting in a zigzag tracing. The test results are interpreted and a written report of findings is provided. Use code 92560 when Bekesy audiometry is performed as a screening test. Use code 92561 when a diagnostic test is performed.

92562

92562   Loudness balance test, alternate binaural or monaural

Hearing balance testing is performed to evaluate whether loudness recruitment is present in a patient with unilateral or bilateral sensorineural (cochlear) hearing loss. Recruitment in unilateral sensorineural hearing loss is described as a phenomenon in which sounds are heard with equal intensities in both the normal ear and hearing impaired ear when sounds are presented at higher intensity (loudness) levels. Bilateral sensorineural hearing loss recruitment is described as a phenomenon where loudness balances are made in the ear but at different frequencies. There are two variations to the test, the alternate bilateral loudness balance (ABLB) and the monaural loudness balance test. When unilateral sensorineural hearing loss is present with normal hearing in the other ear, alternate bilateral loudness balance (ABLB) testing is performed. To perform ABLB testing, a tone is presented alternately between the two ears. The intensity of the tone remains constant in one ear, called the fixed ear, while it is varied in the other ear, called the variable ear. The patient is told to indicate when the sound is louder in the fixed ear, louder in the variable ear, and when it sounds equally loud in both ears. The point at which the loudness is equal in both ears is noted. When sensorineural hearing loss is present in both ears, alternate monaural hearing balance testing is performed. This test compares the loudness growth of a frequency (pitch) that would normally be heard in an individual with normal hearing to the loudness growth of a frequency in the patient with the sensorineural hearing impairment. The test evaluates each ear separately and compares each ear to the normal baseline. Hearing balance test results may be presented in a table or graphically. A written report of findings is provided.

92563

92563   Tone decay test

A tone decay test to evaluate for sensorineural hearing loss is performed. Earphones are used to deliver a continuous tone generated at the hearing threshold of the patient for up to one minute. If the patient indicates that he/she can no longer hear the tone prior to one minute elapsing, the tone is increased by 5 decibels and the test is repeated. This continues until the patient can continue to hear the tone for an entire minute. If the tone must be increased by more than 5 decibels above the initial hearing threshold for

continued perception, additional separately reportable tests for evaluation of sensorineural hearing loss may be needed. The test results and a written interpretation of the findings are provided.

92564

92564   Short increment sensitivity index (SISI)

The short increment sensitivity index (SISI) is performed using earphones. The test uses a pure tone that is presented to the patient at a sound intensity (loudness) of 20 decibels. A second transient tone with a small increase in intensity (1-5 decibels) is superimposed on the tone presented at 20 decibels. The patient is tested for the ability to detect the transient increases in intensity. The ability to detect small changes in intensity is indicative of sensorineural hearing pathology. The test results and a written interpretation of findings are provided.

92565

92565   Stenger test, pure tone

The Stenger test is performed using pure tone audiometry. Using earphones, each ear is tested separately and then together. The hearing threshold of each ear is determined. A tone at the patient's hearing threshold is delivered to each ear separately. The patient is asked to indicate whether the tone is heard in the right or left ear. In a patient with normal hearing or functional hearing loss, a tone delivered to the right ear at the hearing threshold will be heard in the right ear and a tone delivered to the left ear at the hearing threshold will be heard in the left ear. Tones delivered simultaneously to both ears at the hearing threshold will be perceived in the center of the head if the sensitivity levels of both ears are the same. If the sensitivity levels are different, the sound will be perceived in the ear with the higher sensitivity level until the intensity in the less sensitive ear is increased to the hearing threshold in that ear. In a patient with nonorganic hearing loss, which may be psychogenic or feigned, the test results will not show the expected pattern. Generally the Stenger test is integrated with other pure tone tests and the patient is not aware that a test is being performed to differentiate between functional hearing loss and nonorganic hearing loss. The test results are presented on an audiogram. A written interpretation of findings is provided.

92567

92567   Tympanometry (impedance testing)

Tympanometry is used to evaluate middle ear function. The test measures the flexibility of the eardrum and is helpful in detecting fluid in the middle ear, negative middle ear pressure, perforation of the tympanic membrane, disruption of the ossicles, and otosclerosis. The physician examines the ear with an otoscope. The tympantometry device is placed into the ear canal and a small amount of pressure is applied that changes the air pressure in the ear canal. This causes the eardrum to move back and forth. The movement is recorded on a graph referred to as a tympanogram. The physician reviews and interprets the tympanogram results.

92568

92568   Acoustic reflex testing, threshold

Acoustic reflex threshold testing is used to measure the movement of the stapedius muscle and tensor tympani in response to loud sound. The tensing of these muscles causes the stapes to move. A given sound threshold should cause the stapes to tighten in response to the loudness of the sound. The acoustic reflex threshold is a measurement of the softest sound that can elicit a reflex contraction of the stapedius muscle. Acoustic reflex testing is typically performed using the same device used to perform tympanometry. A loud sound is emitted and the stapedius muscle contracts which changes middle ear immittance. The change in immitance is seen as a deflection in the recording. The physician reviews and interprets the results.

92570

92570   Acoustic immittance testing, includes tympanometry (impedance testing), acoustic reflex threshold testing, and acoustic reflex decay testing

Acoustic immittance testing refers to a battery of tests used to evaluate middle ear function, cranial nerve (CN) VIII disorders, and hearing. Tympanometry measures the flexibility of the eardrum and is helpful in detecting fluid in the middle ear, negative middle ear pressure, perforation of the tympanic membrane, disruption of the ossicles, and otosclerosis. The physician examines the ear with an otoscope. The tympantometry device is placed into the ear canal and a small amount of pressure is applied that changes the air pressure in the ear canal. This causes the eardrum to move back and forth. The movement is recorded on a graph referred to as a tympanogram. Acoustic reflex threshold testing is used to measure the movement of the stapedius muscle and tensor tympani in response to loud sound. The tensing of these muscles causes the stapes to move. The acoustic reflex threshold is a measurement of the softest sound that can elicit a reflex contraction of the stapedius muscle. Acoustic reflex testing is performed using the same device used to perform tympanometry. A loud sound is emitted and the stapedius muscle contracts which changes middle ear immittance. The change in immitance is seen as

Medicine

a deflection in the recording. The acoustic reflex decay test is used to evaluate CN VIII. Following the determination of the acoustic reflex threshold, a continuous tone is presented in the contralateral ear for a period of 10 seconds at a stimulus level 10 decibels above the reflex threshold in the ear being tested. The response is recorded. If the amplitude of the deflection decreases by 50% or more within 10 seconds the test is considered positive which may indicate a retrocochlear lesion. The physician reviews and interprets the results of the tympanometry, acoustic reflex threshold and acoustic reflex decay tests.

92571

92571   Filtered speech test

There are a number of versions of the filtered speech test. The basic test uses a degraded or frequency-distorted speech sample. The words used in the test are common one syllable words that most children aged 10 or older and adults would recognize in a normal speech sample, such as hide, home, more, root. The words are passed through an electronic filter that degrades the sound or distorts the frequency of the words. Using earphones, these degraded or distorted words are then presented to the patient. The patient is asked to say the distorted word. An individual with normal auditory functioning can recognize the filtered words at least 70% of the time. However, an individual with an auditory processing disorder affecting the thalamo-cortical neural pathways and auditory cortex will typically not be able to recognize at least 70% of the words. Following the test, the test results are recorded and a written interpretation of findings is provided.

92572

92572   Staggered spondaic word test

The staggered spondaic word test is used to evaluate auditory processing function and to help diagnose certain types of auditory function impairments. The test uses two-syllable words that are pronounced with equal stress on each syllable (e.g., airplane, hotdog, padlock, baseball, railroad, mushroom). Using earphones, the first part of the first word and the last part of the second word are staggered between the two ears while the last part of the first word and first part of the second word are presented equally to both ears. The listener is asked to repeat the spondaic words. The test is scored and a written interpretation of findings is provided.

92575

92575   Sensorineural acuity level test

The sensorineural acuity level (SAL) test requires comparing data obtained from subjects with normal hearing to a patient with hearing loss. This test is performed to evaluate both sensorineural and conductive hearing loss. A baseline is determined with data collected from a group of individuals with normal hearing. Normative data required includes: air conduction thresholds in a quiet environment for each ear; air conduction thresholds with maximum masking presented using bone conduction in each ear; and the average normal shift in air conduction thresholds from quiet to maximum noise levels. This will usually be in the 55-60 decibel range. The test is performed using an audiometer with the capability of presenting narrow band noise signal using bone conduction. Insert-type earphones are placed in the patient's ears. A bone oscillator dedicated to (SAL) testing is placed on the forehead using an adjustable headband. The patient's air conduction thresholds in a quiet environment are determined for each ear followed by air conduction thresholds with maximum masking presented using bone conduction for each ear. The patient's shift from air conduction thresholds in quiet to bone conduction with noise is determined. The calculated shift in decibels is then subtracted from the air conduction thresholds obtained in quiet which provides the estimated bone conduction hearing threshold. The results are compared to the baseline to determine the type and extent of the patient's hearing loss. A report is generated and a written interpretation of findings is provided.

92576

92576   Synthetic sentence identification test

The synthetic sentence identification test is used to evaluate central auditory processing function. Earphones are used to present a nonsensical sentence in one ear while competing speech, such as a story, is heard in the opposite ear. The patient is asked to repeat the nonsensical sentence. An individual with normal central auditory function will be able to repeat the nonsensical sentence the majority of the time. However, an individual with an auditory processing disorder will typically not be able to repeat the sentence. Following the test, the test results are recorded and a written interpretation of findings is provided.

92577

92577   Stenger test, speech

The speech Stenger test is performed using spondee words. Spondee words are two syllable words that are pronounced with equal stress on each syllable (e.g., airplane, padlock, baseball). Using earphones, each ear is tested separately and then together. The hearing threshold of each ear is determined. A spondee word at the patient's hearing threshold is delivered to each ear separately. The patient is asked to repeat the word and indicate whether the word was heard in the right or left ear. In a patient with normal hearing or functional hearing loss, a word delivered to the right ear at the hearing threshold will be

heard in the right ear and a word delivered to the left ear at the hearing threshold will be heard in the left ear. Words delivered simultaneously to both ears at the hearing threshold will be perceived in the center of the head if the sensitivity levels of both ears are the same. If the sensitivity levels are different, the sound will be perceived in the ear with the higher sensitivity level until the intensity in the less sensitive ear is increased to the hearing threshold in that ear. In a patient with nonorganic hearing loss, which may be psychogenic or feigned, the test results will not show the expected pattern. Generally, the Stenger test is integrated with other hearing tests and the patient is not aware that a test is being performed to differentiate between functional hearing loss and nonorganic hearing loss. The test results are presented on an audiogram. A written interpretation of findings is provided.

92579

92579   Visual reinforcement audiometry (VRA)

Visual reinforcement audiometry (VRA) is a type of pure tone audiometry performed on infants and young children to evaluate hearing. The child is brought into a special testing room with toys. The toys are housed in boxes that are to the right and left of the child. When activated by the audiologist, the toy lights up and moves in the box. Typically, when an infant or young child hears a sound, he/she will look toward the sound to see what it is. Conditioning trials are performed. The trial begins with sounds of higher intensity and the visual reinforcement is presented at the same time as the sound. Reinforcement occurs as the child associates the sound with a light-up toy. Next, the sound is initiated. The toy is only lit-up if the child turns to look at the box with the toy. Once the child has demonstrated that conditioning has occurred, hearing is tested by lowering the intensity of the sound until the child can no longer hear it as demonstrated by the child no longer looking toward the toy. The test is repeated on the opposite side with a sound of a different pitch. The audiologist records the test results and provides a written report of findings.

92582

92582   Conditioning play audiometry

Conditioning play audiometry uses a play-oriented activity to test hearing on younger children. The child is first conditioned to perform an activity, such as move an object, in response to hearing a sound. Once the child can demonstrate the ability to respond to a sound stimulus by performing the play-oriented activity, testing is initiated. Earphones are used to deliver the sound stimulus so that each ear can be tested separately. The sound stimulus begins at a volume that the child can easily hear. Once the child has responded to the sound stimulus with the conditioned play activity, another sound stimulus is delivered at a decreased intensity and the child is allowed to respond to that stimulus. The audiologist records the responses for each ear and provides a written report of findings.

92583

92583   Select picture audiometry

Select picture audiometry is used to screen for hearing disorders in younger children. The test uses a picture board containing pictures of things that the child will recognize, such as an airplane, hotdog, cupcake, and sailboat. All the pictures also represent spondees which are two syllable words that are pronounced with equal stress on each syllable. The child wears earphones and receives instructions to touch or point to the objects beginning with a decibel level of 50 dB. Instructions are phrased as questions such as "Can you point to the airplane?" or "Where is the cupcake?" The decibel level is decreased in 5 dB increments until the child can no longer hear and follow the instructions. The clinician records the child's responses on a picture graph that represents the child's ability to hear and correctly identify the object at each decibel level. A written report of findings is provided.

92584

92584   Electrocochleography

Electrocochleography is performed to evaluate conditions of the inner ear such as Meniere's disease or endolymphatic hydrops that are characterized by fluid and pressure in the inner ear. An electrode attached to a recording device is placed on the forehead. Foil covered earphones are placed in the ear canals. The earphones deliver a sound that stimulates activity in the cochlea. The electrode on the forehead captures the electrical potentials generated by the sound stimulus which are recorded and displaced digitally as a waveform. The digital waveform is interpreted and a written report is provided.

92585-92586

92585   Auditory evoked potentials for evoked response audiometry and/or testing of the central nervous system; comprehensive

92586   Auditory evoked potentials for evoked response audiometry and/or testing of the central nervous system; limited

Auditory evoked potentials for evoked response audiometry and/or testing of the central nervous system is performed to evaluate hearing loss and help identify conditions such as acoustic neuroma or vestibular schwannoma. In 92585, a comprehensive auditory evoked response (AER) examination is performed, which includes brainstem response with middle latency and late cortical responses. AER tests brainstem response to auditory (click) stimuli. The click is transmitted from an acoustic transducer by an earphone or headphone.

Medicine

The elicited waveform response is measured by surface electrodes typically placed on the forehead (vertex of the scalp) and earlobes. Another electrode configuration is placement on the forehead, nape of the neck (inverting), and either the shoulder or cheek. The amplitude of the signal is averaged and charted against time, similar to an EEG recording. The recording is then interpreted and a written report of findings is provided. In 92586, a limited audiometry examination is performed which tests only brainstem response and may also be referred to as an auditory brainstem response (ABR).

92587-92588

92587 **Distortion product evoked otoacoustic emissions; limited evaluation (to confirm the presence or absence of hearing disorder, 3-6 frequencies) or transient evoked otoacoustic emissions, with interpretation and report**

92588 **Distortion product evoked otoacoustic emissions; comprehensive diagnostic evaluation (quantitative analysis of outer hair cell function by cochlear mapping, minimum of 12 frequencies), with interpretation and report**

Otoacoustic emission (OAE) tests are performed to determine cochlear status related to hair cell function. This information can be used to screen for hearing loss and is particularly valuable for screening neonates, infants, or individuals with developmental disabilities because no behavioral response is required. In addition to receiving sound, the cochlea also produces low-intensity sounds called OAEs which are believed to be a result of cochlear outer hair cells expanding and contracting. In 92587, a limited evaluation is performed using distortion product evoked otoacoustic emissions (DPEOAEs) or transient evoked otoacoustic emissions (TEOAEs) to confirm the presence or absence of a hearing disorder. The test is performed using a stimulus and a low noise microphone to record the otoacoustic emissions. A limited evaluation using DPEOAEs involves recording OAE emitted in response to acoustic stimuli using multiple tones, frequencies, and intensities. A limited evaluation requires the use of 3-6 frequencies. Alternatively, an evaluation can be performed using TEOAEs, which involves recording OAE emitted in response to acoustic stimuli of very short duration such as clicks or tone bursts. A microphone probe is put in the external ear canal on the side to be tested. The stimulus is applied at multiple frequencies and recordings are obtained. The test is repeated on the contralateral ear. The physician reviews the test results and provides a written report of findings. In 92588, a comprehensive diagnostic evaluation is performed using DPEOAEs with cochlear mapping to provide a quantitative analysis of outer hair cell function using a minimum of 12 frequencies. A microphone probe is put in the external ear canal and recordings are made that separate OAEs into different frequency bands. Different frequencies are picked up in different regions of the cochlea. Separating OAEs into different frequency bands allows mapping of the response in specific areas of the cochlea. The test is repeated on the contralateral ear. The recordings are interpreted by a physician and a written report of findings is provided.

92590-92591

92590 **Hearing aid examination and selection; monaural**
92591 **Hearing aid examination and selection; binaural**

Codes for hearing aid examination and selection do not have strict definitions as to what is included in the service. This is due in part to the lack of third party payer reimbursement for hearing aid examination and selection as well as to changes in technology that have resulted in changes to the services needed during the examination and selection of hearing aids. Generally, the patient is presented with a number of hearing aid options and the audiologist reviews the pros and cons of each type and discusses the differences in cost. The audiologist helps the patient weigh the pros and cons of the various types and then the patient selects the hearing aid that best meets their hearing and budget needs. If an internal hearing aid is selected, an ear mold is made so that a custom fitted hearing aid can be constructed. The hearing aid order is placed. When the hearing aid is received it has typically been preprogrammed for the patient's hearing prescription. The audiologist checks the programming to ensure that the parameters of the hearing aid have been accurately set. The patient returns for the initial fitting. Specialized ear measurements are taken to verify that the gain and output of the hearing aid are properly set to amplify speech for the patient's dynamic hearing range. This is validated with sound field testing that checks the ability of the patient to hear soft sounds and to recognize speech at normal levels in both a quiet and a noisy environment. The audiologist queries the patient on the quality of the sound and the comfort of the hearing aid. Additional adjustments are made to the hearing aid as needed. Codes 92590 and 92591 are reported only once for the selection and fitting of a new hearing aid. Use code 92590 for hearing aid selection and exam for one ear only, and code 92591 for both ears.

92592-92593

92592 **Hearing aid check; monaural**
92593 **Hearing aid check; binaural**

A hearing aid check is performed. Following dispensing and fitting a new hearing aid, the patient returns to have the function and fit of the hearing aid checked. The audiologist queries the patient about any problems with the hearing aid and the patient's assessment of the sound quality. Based on the patient's responses, the audiologist will make any

necessary adjustments. Use code 92592 for a monaural hearing aid check, and code 92593 for a hearing aid check for both ears.

92594-92595

92594 **Electroacoustic evaluation for hearing aid; monaural**
92595 **Electroacoustic evaluation for hearing aid; binaural**

During a follow-up visit, the information stored on the hearing aid is downloaded. The audiologist performs an electronic (computerized) analysis. The analysis provides the average number of hours that the hearing aid is being used per day, the noise environment of the patient (e.g., quieter or louder than average) as well as other factors based on the characteristics of the hearing aid. Based on this analysis, programming changes may be made. Use code 92594 for an electroacoustic evaluation of a hearing aid for one ear only, and code 92595 for a binaural electroacoustic evaluation.

92596

92596 **Ear protector attenuation measurements**

The adequacy of noise protection provided by an ear protector is evaluated. This procedure is rarely performed as most ear protectors are now rated for adequacy based on parameters set by the Environmental Protection Agency. Ear protectors are tested during the manufacturing process and have a Noise Reduction Rating (NRR) listed on the packaging. The NRR must be related to the actual noise environment of the individual to assess the adequacy of the attenuation of the ear protector. In the work environment, the employer is required to test the noise level of the work environment and to ensure that the NRR of the ear protectors used by employees is adequate to protect hearing.

92597

92597 **Evaluation for use and/or fitting of voice prosthetic device to supplement oral speech**

The provider evaluates the patient's needs related to a voice prosthetic device and selects the one with the features that best meet the patient's needs for supplementing his or her oral speech. Features of the prosthesis that must be evaluated include the diameter of the body, the thickness and diameter of the esophageal flange, and the length of the esophageal end. Measurements are obtained to determine the correct size of the prosthesis and it is ordered. When the prosthesis arrives, the patient returns for fitting. An esophageal retention collar in the correct diameter is selected and the prosthesis is inserted. The patient is instructed on use and care of the prosthetic device.

92601-92604

92601 **Diagnostic analysis of cochlear implant, patient younger than 7 years of age; with programming**
92602 **Diagnostic analysis of cochlear implant, patient younger than 7 years of age; subsequent reprogramming**
92603 **Diagnostic analysis of cochlear implant, age 7 years or older; with programming**
92604 **Diagnostic analysis of cochlear implant, age 7 years or older; subsequent reprogramming**

A cochlear implant is an electronic device that can restore useful hearing in patients with severe bilateral sensorineural hearing loss. Cochlear implants work by transforming speech and other sounds into electrical energy that stimulates auditory nerve fibers in the inner ear. The cochlear device has both an internal and external component. In codes 92601 and 92603, approximately 4 weeks following surgery to implant the internal processor, the external components are connected to the cochlear implant, analyzed, and programmed. The external components include a microphone, a speech processor that digitizes the sound into electrical signals, transmitting cables, and a transmitting coil that sends the electrical signals across the skin to the implanted receiver/stimulator. The implant is programmed for each individual based on his/her response to electrical stimuli. First, a map is created by setting threshold levels for the minimal amount of electrical stimulation needed for the perception of sound (T-level) and the upper limit of electrical stimulation perceived by the individual to be the most comfortable in intensity or loudness (M or C-levels). The external device is then programmed. In 92602 and 92604, periodic evaluation and reprogramming of the external device is performed in the same manner. Use codes 92601 and 92602 if the patient is younger than 7 years of age. Use 92603 and 92604 if the patient is age 7 years or older.

92605

92605 **Evaluation for prescription of non-speech-generating augmentative and alternative communication device, face-to-face with the patient; first hour**

Non-speech-generating augmentative and alternative communication (AAC) devices include any device that aids, supplements, or replaces speech and allows for expression of thoughts, needs, wants, and ideas without producing voice output. These types of devices include communication books, boards, or electronic devices with pictures, letters, words and/or phrases that allow communication without verbalization. The physician or speech language pathologist evaluates the patient in a face-to-face encounter to determine which

Medicine

AAC device is best suited to the patient's needs. This includes a thorough assessment of speech limitations and any other physical or learning disabilities. AAC devices that will best meet the patient's communication needs are reviewed with the patient, family, or caregiver. The various devices are demonstrated and the patient may practice using different devices to determine which device is best. Based on the evaluation, the physician or other professional may help the patient select the device that will best meet his/her communication needs. Use 92605 for the first hour of face-to-face evaluation. Use 92618 for each additional 30 minutes of face-to-face evaluation.

92606

92606   **Therapeutic service(s) for the use of non-speech-generating device, including programming and modification**

Non-speech-generating communication devices include any device that aids, supplements, or replaces speech and allows for expression of thoughts, needs, wants, and ideas without producing voice output. These types of devices include communication books, boards, or electronic devices with pictures, letters, words, and/or phrases that allow communication without verbalization. The speech language pathologist (SLP) evaluates a previously prescribed non-speech generating communication device to determine if the current programming is meeting the patient's needs. The SLP considers any changes in the patient's communication needs since acquiring the device, including changes in speech limitations and physical and/or learning disabilities. The device is reprogrammed or modified as needed to meet these needs.

92607-92608

92607   **Evaluation for prescription for speech-generating augmentative and alternative communication device, face-to-face with the patient; first hour**

92608   **Evaluation for prescription for speech-generating augmentative and alternative communication device, face-to-face with the patient; each additional 30 minutes (List separately in addition to code for primary procedure)**

Speech generating devices (SGD), also called voice-output communication aids (VOCA), are electronic devices that can produce synthetic or digital speech for an individual who has a communication impairment. A speech-language pathologist (SLP) performs a face-to-face evaluation of the cognitive and communication abilities of the patient. The evaluation identifies the type and severity of the communication impairment and includes an evaluation of current language skills and cognitive ability. Based on the evaluation, the SLP identifies the SGD that will best meet the patient's needs and identifies any accessories to the device that are required. Report 92607 for the first hour of the evaluation and 92608 for each additional 30 minutes.

92609

92609   **Therapeutic services for the use of speech-generating device, including programming and modification**

Speech generating devices (SGD), also called voice-output communication aids (VOCA), are electronic devices that can produce synthetic or digital speech for an individual who has a communication impairment. The speech language pathologist (SLP) evaluates a previously prescribed speech generating device to determine if the current programming is meeting the patient's needs. The provider considers any changes in the patient's communication needs since acquiring the device, including changes in speech limitations and physical and/or learning disabilities. The device is reprogrammed or modified as needed to meet these needs.

92610

92610   **Evaluation of oral and pharyngeal swallowing function**

An evaluation of the oral and pharyngeal phase of the swallowing function is performed in a patient who is suspected of having oropharyngeal dysphagia. The initial evaluation represented by code 92610 is typically performed by a dysphagia specialist, usually a speech-language pathologist. This evaluation is performed to determine whether more extensive studies are warranted. Swallowing function is divided into oral, pharyngeal, and esophageal phases. The oral and pharyngeal phases are made up of oral preparation for solid foods (not required for liquids or pureed foods), oral transfer, and initiation of the swallow. Both oral and pharyngeal movements are necessary in preparing, transferring, and swallowing food. The patient is given both solids and liquids to swallow. During oral preparation of solid food the ability of the tongue to move the food from side-to-side so that the solid can be chewed and prepared for swallowing is evaluated. Once the solid food is prepared and transferred to the back of the throat, the swallowing movements are evaluated. Propelling solids or liquids requires a complex set of movements including retraction of the base of the tongue, elevation of the hyolarynx, closure of the velopharyngeus, contraction of the pharynx, opening of the upper esophageal sphincter, and closure of the airway. The speech-language pathologist observes the patient to determine whether solids and liquids are being prepared, transferred, and propelled from the pharynx into the esophagus. A written report of findings is provided.

92611

92611   **Motion fluoroscopic evaluation of swallowing function by cine or video recording**

A dysphagia specialist working with a radiologist evaluates swallowing function by video (cine) fluoroscopic swallowing examination (VFSE). The dysphagia specialist observes the patient as he/she is given liquid barium and solids coated with barium to drink and eat. As the patient drinks and eats these substances, video fluoroscopy is used to capture the movement of the liquids and solids as they are swallowed. The radiologist reviews the fluoroscopic studies and provides a written report of findings.

92612-92613

▲ 92612   **Flexible endoscopic evaluation of swallowing by cine or video recording**

▲ 92613   **Flexible endoscopic evaluation of swallowing by cine or video recording; interpretation and report only**

Flexible endoscopic evaluation of swallowing function is performed using cine or video recording. The test is performed in a seated position. The nose and throat are numbed as needed using an analgesic spray. The endoscope is inserted through the nose or mouth and into the throat. Liquid and solid food is then ingested as cine or video images are recorded and displayed on a computer screen. The images are reviewed and a written report on the swallowing function is provided. Use 92612 for the complete procedure. Use 92613 when the provider performs only the interpretation with a written report of findings.

92614-92615

▲ 92614   **Flexible endoscopic evaluation, laryngeal sensory testing by cine or video recording**

▲ 92615   **Flexible endoscopic evaluation, laryngeal sensory testing by cine or video recording; interpretation and report only**

Flexible endoscopic evaluation of laryngeal sensory function is performed using cine or video recording. The test is performed in a seated position. The nose and throat are numbed as needed using an analgesic spray. The endoscope is inserted through the nose or mouth and into the throat. Puffs of air are then delivered through the endoscope into the throat to test sensory function. As the puffs of air are delivered, cine or video images are recorded. The images are reviewed and a written report on sensory function is provided. Use 92614 for the complete procedure. Use 92615 when the provider performs only the interpretation with a report of findings.

92616-92617

▲ 92616   **Flexible endoscopic evaluation of swallowing and laryngeal sensory testing by cine or video recording**

▲ 92617   **Flexible endoscopic evaluation of swallowing and laryngeal sensory testing by cine or video recording; interpretation and report only**

Flexible endoscopic evaluation of swallowing function and laryngeal sensory testing is performed using cine or video recording. The test is performed in a seated position. The nose and throat are numbed as needed using an analgesic spray. The endoscope is inserted through the nose or mouth and into the throat to the hypopharynx where both the laryngeal and pharyngeal structures are visible. To test swallowing function, liquid and solid food is ingested as cine or video images are recorded and displayed on a computer screen and all aspects of swallowing function are assessed. The ability to protect the airway and sustain airway protection for several seconds is determined. The ability to swallow promptly without spillage of liquid or food into the hypopharynx is evaluated. Timing of swallowing movements and the direction of the liquid or food bolus as it is propelled through the hypopharynx is noted, including whether the bolus has been completely cleared from the pharynx during the swallow or whether there is bolus pooling or residue in the pharynx following the swallow. To perform laryngeal sensory testing, puffs of air are delivered through the endoscope into the throat. As the puffs of air are delivered, cine or video images are recorded. Sensory function of the pharyngeal and laryngeal structures is evaluated and observed as the swallowing function test is performed. The images are reviewed and a written report of findings is provided. Use 92616 for the complete procedure. Use 92617 when the provider performs only the interpretation with a report of findings.

92618

92618   **Evaluation for prescription of non-speech-generating augmentative and alternative communication device, face-to-face with the patient; each additional 30 minutes (List separately in addition to code for primary procedure)**

Non-speech-generating augmentative and alternative communication (AAC) devices include any device that aids, supplements, or replaces speech and allows for expression of thoughts, needs, wants, ideas without producing voice output. These types of devices include communication books, boards, or electronic devices with pictures, letters, words and/or phrases that allow communication without verbalization. The physician or speech language pathologist evaluates the patient in a face-to-face encounter to determine which AAC device is best suited to the patient's needs. This includes a thorough assessment of speech limitations and any other physical or learning disabilities. AAC devices that will best meet the patient's communication needs are reviewed with the patient, family, or caregiver. The various devices are demonstrated and the patient may practice using different devices to determine which device is best. Based on the evaluation, the physician or other professional may help the patient select the device that will best meet his/her communication needs. Use 92605 for the first hour of face-to-face evaluation. Use 92618 for each additional 30 minutes of face-to-face evaluation.

92620-92621

92620 **Evaluation of central auditory function, with report; initial 60 minutes**
92621 **Evaluation of central auditory function, with report; each additional 15 minutes (List separately in addition to code for primary procedure)**

Central auditory function refers to the ability of the brain to process neural auditory impulses received from the peripheral nervous system. The audiologist obtains a medical, developmental, and family history related to auditory processing skills. Testing is then performed. Each test is standardized using a CD that is routed through a diagnostic audiometer, and is presented at standardized decibel levels. One type of test is word recognition. The audiologist describes the test that is going to be performed and provides instructions on what the patient is to do for each test. For word recognition, the patient repeats the word to the best of his/her ability. The audiologist records the responses and scores each test administered using raw and standard scores. The scores are then plotted on a graph. As each new test is administered the audiologist provides new instructions and monitors the patient throughout the test. After testing is complete, the audiologist compiles the results and interprets the results based on the patient's age. The audiologist identifies the types of stimuli and environments that adversely affect central auditory function. A report is prepared for the referring physician. If an interdisciplinary team is involved in evaluating central auditory function, the team is also provided with a report of findings. Use 92620 for the first 60 minutes of central auditory function evaluation. Use 92621 for each additional 15 minutes.

92625

92625 **Assessment of tinnitus (includes pitch, loudness matching, and masking)**

Tinnitus is any sound that emanates from the inner ear or head as opposed to the external environment. Typically tinnitus is audible only to the patient in which case it is referred to as subjective tinnitus. Rarely, in objective tinnitus, the provider can also hear the tinnitus. The patient may describe the sound as hissing, buzzing, ringing, squealing, whining, clicking, or popping in nature. Tinnitus may be continuous or intermittent. Assessment of tinnitus includes pitch (frequency) matching, loudness (intensity) matching, and minimum masking level (MML) of the tinnitus. Earphones are used to deliver auditory stimuli and an audiometer is used to display and record findings. Each ear is tested separately. To match pitch, auditory stimuli are delivered through the earphones and the patient is instructed to match the stimulus closest in pitch to the tinnitus. Loudness matching is performed in the same manner with stimuli of varying intensities delivered through the earphones. The patient must identify the loudness of the stimulus that matches the tinnitus. The masking evaluation uses a sound stimuli to mask the tinnitus and the patient must identify the lowest level of stimulus that makes the tinnitus inaudible. The test results are interpreted and a written report of findings is provided.

92626-92627

92626 **Evaluation of auditory rehabilitation status; first hour**
92627 **Evaluation of auditory rehabilitation status; each additional 15 minutes (List separately in addition to code for primary procedure)**

Evaluation of auditory rehabilitation status involves determining the best rehabilitation strategies given the hearing disability of the patient and the family's needs, periodically evaluating the effectiveness of the rehabilitation process, and making rehabilitation modifications as needed. For children, evaluation of auditory rehabilitation status focuses on assessing the effectiveness of auditory awareness training, the use of visual cues, speech improvement, language development, managing communication needs, and the use of hearing aids and other assistive listening devices. For adults, auditory rehabilitation typically focuses on strategies to improve participation of the hearing impaired patient in conversations which may include modifications or behavior changes to promote easier participation in conversation and modifications to deal with background noise. Both the patient and family members may participate in the auditory rehabilitation status evaluation. The patient and family are queried on how well the current techniques are working to help facilitate communication. When the hearing impaired individual is a child, the effectiveness of the rehabilitation plan in regard to the child's developmental needs is also addressed. The techniques being used to improve communication and develop skills are reviewed. Suggestions are made for changes that may further improve communication. A written report detailing the patient's current status, the effectiveness of current rehabilitation strategies, and changes to the rehabilitation plan is provided. Use code 92626 for the first hour of the evaluation service and 92627 for each additional 15 minutes.

92630-92633

92630 **Auditory rehabilitation; prelingual hearing loss**
92633 **Auditory rehabilitation; postlingual hearing loss**

Auditory rehabilitation is provided to help improve communication skills. In prelingual hearing loss, the focus is on language acquisition as well as developing alternative communication techniques such as sign language so that the child will be able to communicate effectively. Some rehabilitative techniques used include auditory awareness training, the use of visual cues, speech improvement, and language development exercises. Auditory awareness perception training uses activities to increase the prelingual child's awareness of sound and responses to sound using any remaining hearing. It also involves developing skill in using hearing aids and other assistive listening devices. The child is taught to use visual cues, such as focusing on the speaker's facial expression and body language. In order to improve speech, speaking exercises are performed to facilitate the production of speech and voice quality, and also to control the volume, rate, and rhythm of speech. Developing language includes rehabilitation techniques designed to teach both language understanding (reception) and language usage (expression). Rehabilitation may also include helping the child understand hearing loss and helping the child deal with communication difficulties by modifying behaviors and environmental factors that may make communication more difficult. In auditory rehabilitation for post-lingual hearing loss, the rehabilitation is much the same except that there is less intense focus on speech improvement and language development because those skills have already been at least partially developed. Use 92630 for auditory rehabilitation of a patient with prelingual hearing loss and code 92633 if the patient has postlingual hearing loss.

92640

92640 **Diagnostic analysis with programming of auditory brainstem implant, per hour**

Diagnostic analysis and programming of an auditory brainstem implant is done on a per hour basis. An auditory brainstem implant is used to treat hearing loss in patients who have damage to the nerve which conducts sound impulses from the inner ear to the brain. An external device must be worn by the patient to interface with the implant, and this device requires periodic calibration and programming to function properly.

92920-92921

92920 **Percutaneous transluminal coronary angioplasty; single major coronary artery or branch**
92921 **Percutaneous transluminal coronary angioplasty; each additional branch of a major coronary artery (List separately in addition to code for primary procedure)**

The physician performs a percutaneous transluminal coronary angioplasty (PTCA). The skin over the access artery, usually one of the femoral arteries, is prepped and the artery is punctured with a needle and a sheath is placed. A guidewire is inserted and advanced from the access artery through the aorta and into the blocked (occluded) coronary artery. A catheter with a balloon tip is advanced over the guidewire to the site of the occlusion. The balloon is inflated and the plaque compressed against the artery wall. The balloon may be inflated several times to achieve the desired result. The angioplasty catheter is withdrawn. Contrast is then injected and a completion angiography performed to ensure that the treated artery is patent. Use 92920 for PTCA of a single major coronary artery or branch and report code 92921 for each additional branch of a major coronary artery.

92924-92925

92924 **Percutaneous transluminal coronary atherectomy, with coronary angioplasty when performed; single major coronary artery or branch**
92925 **Percutaneous transluminal coronary atherectomy, with coronary angioplasty when performed; each additional branch of a major coronary artery (List separately in addition to code for primary procedure)**

The physician performs a percutaneous transluminal coronary atherectomy by mechanical or other method with or without angioplasty. The skin over the access artery, usually one of the femoral arteries, is prepped and the artery is punctured with a needle and a sheath placed. A guidewire is inserted and advanced from the access artery through the aorta and into the blocked (occluded) coronary artery. Atherectomy is performed using a specialized balloon catheter that has a window on one side through which a cutting piston is advanced. The cutting piston shaves plaque from the artery wall. As the plaque is shaved from the arterial wall, it is pushed into the nose of the atherectomy device and is removed upon completion of the procedure when the catheter is withdrawn. The physician may make several passes with the atherectomy device to achieve the desired result. The atherectomy device is then withdrawn. Following completion of the atherectomy procedure, a balloon tipped angioplasty catheter may be advanced to the site of the blockage and the balloon inflated to smooth out and compress any remaining plaque. The angioplasty catheter is then withdrawn. Contrast is injected and a completion angiography performed to ensure that the treated artery is patent. Use 92924 for treatment of a single major coronary artery or branch and report 92925 for treatment of each additional branch of a major coronary artery.

Medicine

92928-92929

92928   Percutaneous transcatheter placement of intracoronary stent(s), with coronary angioplasty when performed; single major coronary artery or branch

92929   Percutaneous transcatheter placement of intracoronary stent(s), with coronary angioplasty when performed; each additional branch of a major coronary artery (List separately in addition to code for primary procedure)

The physician performs a percutaneous transcatheter placement of an intracoronary stent with or without coronary angioplasty. A stent is a wire mesh tube used to open and support the artery walls in a narrowed or stenosed segment of the artery. The skin over the access artery, usually one of the femoral arteries, is prepped and the artery is punctured with a needle and sheath placed. A guidewire is inserted and advanced from the access artery through the aorta and into the blocked (occluded) coronary artery. Percutaneous transluminal coronary angioplasty (PTCA) is then performed using a catheter with a balloon tip that is advanced over the guidewire to the site of the occlusion. The balloon is inflated and the plaque compressed against the artery wall. The balloon may be inflated several times to achieve the desired result. The compressed stent is delivered using a balloon tip catheter. Once the stent is properly positioned, the balloon is inflated to expand and seat the stent. The stent forms a scaffold that holds the artery open. Contrast is injected and a completion angiography performed to ensure that the treated artery is patent. Use 92928 for stent placement in a single major coronary artery or branch and 92929 for each additional branch of a major coronary artery that is stented.

92933-92934

92933   Percutaneous transluminal coronary atherectomy, with intracoronary stent, with coronary angioplasty when performed; single major coronary artery or branch

92934   Percutaneous transluminal coronary atherectomy, with intracoronary stent, with coronary angioplasty when performed; each additional branch of a major coronary artery (List separately in addition to code for primary procedure)

The physician performs a percutaneous transluminal coronary atherectomy by mechanical or other method with placement of an intracoronary stent, with or without balloon angioplasty. The skin over the access artery, usually one of the femoral arteries, is prepped and the artery is punctured with a needle and a sheath placed. A guidewire is inserted and advanced from the access artery through the aorta and into the blocked (occluded) coronary artery. Atherectomy is performed using a specialized balloon catheter that has a window on one side through which a cutting piston is advanced. The cutting piston shaves plaque from the artery wall. As the plaque is shaved from the arterial wall, it is pushed into the nose of the atherectomy device and is removed upon completion of the procedure when the catheter is withdrawn. The physician may make several passes with the atherectomy device to achieve the desired result. The atherectomy device is then withdrawn. Following completion of the atherectomy procedure, a balloon tipped angioplasty catheter may be advanced to the site of the blockage and the balloon inflated to smooth out and compress any remaining plaque. The angioplasty catheter or atherectomy device is then withdrawn and a collapsed stent advanced to the site of the blockage. The compressed stent is delivered using the balloon tip catheter. Once the stent is properly positioned, the balloon is inflated to expand and seat the stent. The stent forms a scaffold that holds the artery open. Contrast is injected and a completion angiography performed to ensure that the treated artery is patent. Use 92933 for treatment of a single major coronary artery or branch and 92934 for treatment of each additional major coronary artery branch.

92937-92938

92937   Percutaneous transluminal revascularization of or through coronary artery bypass graft (internal mammary, free arterial, venous), any combination of intracoronary stent, atherectomy and angioplasty, including distal protection when performed; single vessel

92938   Percutaneous transluminal revascularization of or through coronary artery bypass graft (internal mammary, free arterial, venous), any combination of intracoronary stent, atherectomy and angioplasty, including distal protection when performed; each additional branch subtended by the bypass graft (List separately in addition to code for primary procedure)

The physician revascularizes an occluded or stenosed coronary artery bypass graft using angioplasty, atherectomy, and/or transluminal stent placement. The skin over the access artery, usually one of the femoral arteries, is prepped, the artery is punctured with a needle and a sheath is placed. Using radiological supervision as needed, a guidewire is inserted and advanced from the access artery into the occluded coronary artery bypass graft. A catheter is advanced over the guidewire and the bypass graft is evaluated. A distal embolic protection device is placed as needed. If angioplasty is performed, a catheter with a balloon tip is advanced over the guidewire to the site of the occlusion. The balloon is inflated and the plaque is compressed against the wall of the artery. The balloon may be inflated several times to achieve the desired result. Alternatively, an atherectomy may be performed with or without angioplasty. Atherectomy is performed using a specialized

balloon catheter that has a window on one side through which a cutting piston is advanced. The cutting piston shaves plaque from the arterial wall. As the plaque is shaved, it is pushed into the nose of the atherectomy device and removed upon completion of the procedure when the catheter is withdrawn. The physician may make several passes with the atherectomy device to achieve the desired result. If an intravascular stent is needed to maintain patency of the artery, the stent delivery catheter is advanced to the site, carefully positioned and deployed. The stent delivery catheter is removed. A balloon catheter may again be advanced and inflated to seat the stent. Contrast is injected and a completion angiography is performed to ensure that the artery is patent. All catheters are removed. Pressure is applied to the vascular access site and a pressure dressing is applied. Use 92937 when a single vessel is treated and 92938 for each additional branch subtended by the bypass graft.

92941

92941   Percutaneous transluminal revascularization of acute total/subtotal occlusion during acute myocardial infarction, coronary artery or coronary artery bypass graft, any combination of intracoronary stent, atherectomy and angioplasty, including aspiration thrombectomy when performed, single vessel

During acute myocardial infarction (MI) the physician revascularizes a partially or completely occluded coronary artery or coronary artery bypass graft using percutaneous transluminal coronary angioplasty, atherectomy and/or transluminal stent placement. The skin over the access artery, usually one of the femoral arteries, is prepped, the artery is punctured with a needle and a sheath is placed. Using radiological supervision as needed, a guidewire is inserted and advanced from the access artery into the occluded coronary artery bypass graft. A catheter is advanced over the guidewire and the coronary artery or bypass graft is evaluated. The site and size of the thrombus is noted. An aspiration catheter is advanced and the thrombus evacuated as needed. If angioplasty is performed, a catheter with a balloon tip is advanced over the guidewire to the site of the occlusion. The balloon is inflated and the plaque is compressed against the wall of the artery. The balloon may be inflated several times to achieve the desired result. Alternatively, an atherectomy may be performed with or without angioplasty. Atherectomy is performed using a specialized balloon catheter that has a window on one side through which a cutting piston is advanced. The cutting piston shaves plaque from the arterial wall. As the plaque is shaved, it is pushed into the nose of the atherectomy device and removed upon completion of the procedure when the catheter is withdrawn. The physician may make several passes with the atherectomy device to achieve the desired result. If an intravascular stent is needed to maintain patency of the artery, the stent delivery catheter is advanced to the site, carefully positioned and deployed. The stent delivery catheter is removed. A balloon catheter may again be advanced and inflated to seat the stent. Contrast is injected and a completion angiography is performed to ensure that the artery is patent. All catheters are removed. Pressure is applied to the vascular access site and a pressure dressing is applied.

92943-92944

92943   Percutaneous transluminal revascularization of chronic total occlusion, coronary artery, coronary artery branch, or coronary artery bypass graft, any combination of intracoronary stent, atherectomy and angioplasty; single vessel

92944   Percutaneous transluminal revascularization of chronic total occlusion, coronary artery, coronary artery branch, or coronary artery bypass graft, any combination of intracoronary stent, atherectomy and angioplasty; each additional coronary artery, coronary artery branch, or bypass graft (List separately in addition to code for primary procedure)

Percutaneous transluminal revascularization of a chronic total occlusion of a coronary artery, coronary artery branch, or coronary artery bypass graft is performed. Chronic total occlusion is defined as complete blockage (> 99 percent) of the native coronary artery or bypass graft for a duration of more than 3 months. The physician may use any combination of percutaneous procedures including angioplasty, atherectomy, and/or stenting to accomplish the revascularization. The skin over the access artery, usually one of the femoral arteries, is prepped, the artery is punctured with a needle and a sheath is placed. Using radiological supervision as needed, a guidewire is inserted and advanced from the access artery into the totally occluded native coronary artery or bypass graft. If angioplasty is performed, a catheter with a balloon tip is advanced over the guidewire to the site of the occlusion and the balloon is inflated and the plaque is compressed against the wall of the artery. Alternatively, an atherectomy may be performed with or without angioplasty using a specialized balloon catheter that has a window on one side through which a cutting piston is advanced. The cutting piston shaves plaque from the arterial wall and as the plaque is shaved, it is pushed into the atherectomy device and removed when the catheter is withdrawn. If an intravascular stent is needed to maintain patency of the artery, the stent delivery catheter is advanced to the site, carefully positioned and deployed. The stent delivery catheter is removed. A balloon catheter may again be advanced and inflated to seat the stent. Contrast is injected and a completion angiography is performed to ensure that the artery is patent. All catheters are removed. Pressure is applied to the vascular access site and a pressure dressing is applied. Use code 92943 to report percutaneous transluminal revascularization of chronic total occlusion of a single coronary

Medicine

artery, coronary artery branch, or coronary artery bypass graft. Report code 92944 for each additional coronary artery, coronary artery branch, or bypass graft treated.

92950

92950   Cardiopulmonary resuscitation (eg, in cardiac arrest)

Cardiopulmonary resuscitation (CPR) is a manual atttempt at restarting a patient's heart and lungs when cardiopulmonary arrest occurs. Typically led by a health care provided certified in CPR, the lungs are filled with air by holding the nose and breathing throught the mouth or performed with a ventilating bag. Chest compressions are also performed at intervals, alternating with the the air in the lungs. A defibrillator may be used to shock the heart into starting.

92953

92953   Temporary transcutaneous pacing

Temporary transcutaneous pacing is performed to regulate heart rhythm in patients with abnormally slow heart rates. Temporary pacing is performed until the cause of the patient's dysrhythmia can be determined and corrected either with medications or by placement of a permanent pacemaker. Three leads are placed to monitor the heart rhythm, one on the right side below the right clavicle, a second on the left side below the left clavicle, and a third lead on the left side over the heart. Two pacing pads are then placed, one on the chest to the left of the sternum and one on the back to the left of the spine. The pacing device is then set at the target rate, usually between 60-70 beats per minute, and the pacing device is turned on.

92960-92961

92960   Cardioversion, elective, electrical conversion of arrhythmia; external
92961   Cardioversion, elective, electrical conversion of arrhythmia; internal (separate procedure)

Elective external cardioversion (92960) is performed to restore normal cardiac rhythm in patients who are experiencing an abnormally rapid heart rate (arrhythmia). Sedation is administered. Two defibrillator pads or paddles are used. One pad/paddle is placed on the patient's chest near the sternum and the second is placed either in the lower left chest or on the back under the left scapula. Electrical impulses (shocks) are delivered that restore normal cardiac rhythm. The strength of the electrical impulse depends on the type of arrhythmia and the patient's response. If the first attempt to restore the heart to normal rhythm is unsuccessful, a higher electrical impulse may be used and the procedure repeated. Internal cardioversion (92961) involves placing the defibrillator pads directly on the heart during open chest surgery. Electrical impulses (shocks) are delivered directly to the heart muscle.

92971

92971   Cardioassist-method of circulatory assist; external

Internal cardioassist, in which the patient's circulation is assisted by a catheter with a balloon or other device is entered through the femoral artery and expanded in the aorta in order to widen the artery and promote blood flow. Code 92971 for an external procedure.

92973

92973   Percutaneous transluminal coronary thrombectomy mechanical (List separately in addition to code for primary procedure)

There are several types of thrombectomy devices, including an extraction device, an aspiration device, a saline jet device, a cutter device, and a laser device. Using the guidewire placed during the cardiac catheterization procedure, a thrombectomy device is passed over the guidewire and positioned in the coronary artery in proximity to the thrombus. For mechanical thrombectomy, the extraction device being used is passed to a point distal to the thrombus. The device is activated and pulled back across the thrombus and the thrombus is extracted. An aspiration device uses suction to remove the thrombus. A saline jet device uses a double lumen catheter to simultaneously disrupt the thrombus by flushing the thrombus with a high pressure saline wash and suctioning the debris. The mechanical cutter device uses a blade to break up the thrombus while simultaneously suctioning the debris into a vacuum bottle. The laser device also breaks up the thrombus which is then suctioned from the coronary artery. Once the thrombus has been removed, the physician performs separately reportable therapeutic interventions, such as angioplasty, atherectomy, or stenting to treat the coronary artery stenosis.

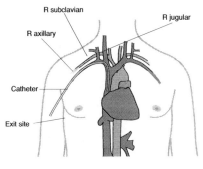

Percutaneous transluminal coronary thrombectomy

A blood clot is cleared by inserting a double-lumen catheter to the site, flushing the clot with a high-pressure saline wash and suctioning the debris

92974

92974   Transcatheter placement of radiation delivery device for subsequent coronary intravascular brachytherapy (List separately in addition to code for primary procedure)

The physician performs transcatheter placement of a radiation delivery device for subsequent delivery of intravascular brachytherapy during a separately reportable cardiac catheterization procedure. This procedure is performed to treat primary coronary stenosis or restenosis following coronary artery stenting. Using the guidewire placed during the cardiac catheterization procedure, a catheter containing the brachytherapy delivery device is passed over the guidewire and positioned in the stenotic lesion. The brachytherapy delivery device consists of a wire also called a seed train or ribbon that contains the radiation. Once the brachytherapy delivery device is properly positioned, a dose of radiation is delivered. The brachytherapy delivery device and catheter are removed. The physician then performs separately reportable therapeutic interventions, such as angioplasty, atherectomy, or stenting to treat the coronary artery stenosis or restenosis.

92975-92977

92975   Thrombolysis, coronary; by intracoronary infusion, including selective coronary angiography
92977   Thrombolysis, coronary; by intravenous infusion

Coronary thrombolysis is performed by intracoronary infusion of a thrombolytic agent (92975) or by intravenous infusion (92977). In 92975, a catheter is inserted from an access vessel, such as the femoral or brachial artery and advanced to the site of the intracoronary thrombus (blood clot). A thrombolytic agent, such as streptokinase, alteplase, or reteplase is then injected directly into the affected coronary artery to dissolve the blood clot. Contrast material is then injected and a selective coronary angiography performed to verify that the clot has been dissolved and that the artery is patent. In 92977, an intravenous infusion is performed. A vein in the arm is selected and a needle or intracatheter inserted. The thrombolytic agent is then injected into the vein to help dissolve the blood clot in the coronary artery.

92978-92979

▲ **92978   Endoluminal imaging of coronary vessel or graft using intravascular ultrasound (IVUS) or optical coherence tomography (OCT) during diagnostic evaluation and/or therapeutic intervention including imaging supervision, interpretation and report; initial vessel (List separately in addition to code for primary procedure)**
▲ **92979   Endoluminal imaging of coronary vessel or graft using intravascular ultrasound (IVUS) or optical coherence tomography (OCT) during diagnostic evaluation and/or therapeutic intervention including imaging supervision, interpretation and report; each additional vessel (List separately in addition to code for primary procedure)**

Intravascular ultrasound (IVUS) or optical coherence tomography (OCT) is performed on a native coronary artery or bypass graft during a separately reportable diagnostic and/or therapeutic intravascular cardiac procedure. IVUS allows visualization of the blood vessel from the inside with a cross sectional view of the vessel showing the circular layers which include the outer covering (adventitia), the vessel wall (media), the inner endothelial layer (intima), and the open channel through which blood flows (lumen). OCT is another type of noninvasive imaging that uses near/short wave infrared light to produce 3D cross-sectional images of the inside of the vessel with micrometer level resolution that can diagnose the presence of more severe coronary artery disease than IVUS. OCT has greater ability to detect much smaller dimensions in lumen areas and provide more detailed evaluation of the build-up of atherosclerotic plaques or tissue response to grafting than IVUS. During the separately reportable intravascular cardiac procedure, an IVUS catheter

Medicine

with a miniaturized transducer, or an OCT catheter with a single optical fiber that emits infrared light, is advanced over a guidewire to the site requiring endoluminal evaluation. The physician reviews the ultrasound or OCT images obtained and provides a written report of the findings. Use 92978 for the initial coronary artery or bypass graft imaged and 92979 for each additional artery or graft.

92986-92990

92986	Percutaneous balloon valvuloplasty; aortic valve
92987	Percutaneous balloon valvuloplasty; mitral valve
92990	Percutaneous balloon valvuloplasty; pulmonary valve

Percutaneous balloon valvuloplasty is performed on the aortic valve (92986), mitral valve (92987), or pulmonary valve (92990) to treat a stenosed (narrowed) heart valve. The skin over the access artery, usually one of the femoral arteries, is prepped and the artery is punctured with a needle and a sheath placed. Using continuous imaging guidance, a guidewire is inserted and advanced from the access artery through the aorta and into the heart to the opening of the stenosed heart valve. A catheter is advanced over the guidewire and positioned in the heart. The guidewire is withdrawn. Intracardiac and intra-arterial pressures are obtained by placing the catheter tip in the appropriate heart chambers and arteries. To measure pressures prior to aortic balloon valvuloplasty, the catheter is advanced to the pulmonary capillary wedge and measurement recorded at the right atrium, right ventricle and pulmonary artery. To measure pressures prior to mitral balloon valvuloplasty, the catheter is advanced into the left atrium and left ventricle and pressures obtained. To measure pressures prior to pulmonary balloon valvuloplasty, the catheter is placed in the right ventricle and the pulmonary artery and pressures are obtained. Contrast is injected and angiography performed. Still frames are reviewed and the valve annulus is measured. The first catheter is exchanged for a wire-positioning catheter. A guidewire is advanced through the wire positioning catheter and the guidewire tip advanced through the stenosed valve. The wire guiding catheter is removed and a balloon valvuloplasty catheter advanced over the guidewire and positioned in the center of the valve annulus. The valve is dilated by inflating the balloon. The balloon may be deflated and reinflated several times in order to achieve the desired amount of dilation. Upon completion of the dilation procedure, intracardiac and intra-arterial pressures are again measured and a completion angiogram performed to evaluate valve mobility and filling of cardiac chambers and great vessels.

92992-92993

| 92992 | Atrial septectomy or septostomy; transvenous method, balloon (eg, Rashkind type) (includes cardiac catheterization) |
| 92993 | Atrial septectomy or septostomy; blade method (Park septostomy) (includes cardiac catheterization) |

Atrial septectomy or septostomy is a palliative procedure performed to improve oxygen saturation in patients with complete transposition of the great arteries. A small incision is made in the groin and the femoral vein exposed. In 92992, a balloon septectomy or septostomy, also referred to as a Rashkind balloon septostomy, is performed. The femoral vein is punctured and a balloon tip catheter is threaded through the femoral vein to the right atrium. The balloon tip catheter is then passed through the foramen ovale into the left atrium. The balloon is inflated in the left atrium and forcefully pulled back across the atrial septum through the foramen ovale. The causes the atrial septum to tear enlarging the hole in the interatrial septum. In 92993, a blade septectomy or septostomy, also referred to as a Park septostomy is performed. A blade tipped catheter is threaded through the femoral vein to the right atrium. The blade tipped catheter is then passed through the foramen ovale into the left atrium. The blade is opened and pulled back through the foramen ovale incising the atrial septum. The blade may be passed several times between the left and right atrium until an optimal sized opening is created.

92997-92998

| 92997 | Percutaneous transluminal pulmonary artery balloon angioplasty; single vessel |
| 92998 | Percutaneous transluminal pulmonary artery balloon angioplasty; each additional vessel (List separately in addition to code for primary procedure) |

The physician performs a percutaneous transluminal pulmonary artery balloon angioplasty to treat pulmonary artery stenosis. The skin over the access artery, usually one of the femoral arteries, is prepped and the artery is punctured with a needle and a sheath placed. A guidewire is inserted and advanced from the access artery through the aorta and heart and into the stenosed (narrowed) pulmonary artery. A catheter is advanced over the guidewire, contrast is injected, and measurements of the narrowed area obtained. The first catheter is exchanged for a catheter with a balloon tip which is advanced to the site of the stenosis. The balloon is inflated and the narrowed segment of pulmonary artery dilated. The balloon may be deflated and reinflated several times to achieve the desired result. The first balloon tipped catheter is sometimes exchanged for a larger balloon-tipped catheter if the pulmonary artery requires additional dilation. Contrast is again injected, a completion angiography performed, and measurements obtained to ensure that the treated pulmonary artery is sufficiently dilated. Use 92997 for treatment of a single pulmonary artery and 92998 for each additional pulmonary artery treated.

93000-93010

93000	Electrocardiogram, routine ECG with at least 12 leads; with interpretation and report
93005	Electrocardiogram, routine ECG with at least 12 leads; tracing only, without interpretation and report
93010	Electrocardiogram, routine ECG with at least 12 leads; interpretation and report only

An ECG is used to evaluate the electrical activity of the heart. The test is performed with the patient lying prone on the exam table. Small plastic patches are attached at specific locations on the chest, abdomen, arms, and/or legs. Leads (wires) from the ECG tracing device are then attached to the patches. A tracing is obtained of the electrical signals from the heart. Electrical activity begins in the sinoatrial node which generates an electrical stimulus at regular intervals, usually 60 to 100 times per minute. This stimulus travels through the conduction pathways to the sinoatrial node causing the atria to contract. The stimulus then travels along the bundle of His which divides into right and left pathways providing electrical stimulation of the ventricles causing them to contract. Each contraction of the ventricles represents one heart beat. The ECG tracing includes the following elements: P wave, QRS complex, ST segment, and T wave. The P wave, a small upward notch in the tracing, indicates electrical stimulation of the atria. This is followed by the QRS complex which indicates the ventricles are electrically stimulated to contract. The short flat ST segment follows and indicates the time between the end of the ventricular contraction and the T wave. The T wave represents the recovery period of the ventricles. The physician reviews, interprets, and provides a written report of the ECG recording taking care to note any abnormalities. Use 93000 to report the complete procedure, including ECG tracing with physician review, interpretation, and report; use 93005 to report the tracing only; and use 93010 to report physician interpretation and written report only.

93015-93018

93015	Cardiovascular stress test using maximal or submaximal treadmill or bicycle exercise, continuous electrocardiographic monitoring, and/or pharmacological stress; with supervision, interpretation and report
93016	Cardiovascular stress test using maximal or submaximal treadmill or bicycle exercise, continuous electrocardiographic monitoring, and/or pharmacological stress; supervision only, without interpretation and report
93017	Cardiovascular stress test using maximal or submaximal treadmill or bicycle exercise, continuous electrocardiographic monitoring, and/or pharmacological stress; tracing only, without interpretation and report
93018	Cardiovascular stress test using maximal or submaximal treadmill or bicycle exercise, continuous electrocardiographic monitoring, and/or pharmacological stress; interpretation and report only

An ECG is used to evaluate the electrical activity of the heart using treadmill, bicycle exercise, and/or pharmacologically induced stress. Small plastic patches are attached at specific locations on the chest, abdomen, arms, and/or legs. Leads (wires) from the stress ECG device are then attached to the patches. A baseline ECG is obtained. The exercise portion of the study is then initiated. Heart rate and blood pressure are monitored. Staged stress protocol is used and the patient's response to stress is monitored as the stress ECG is recorded. Unless contraindicated, exercise or pharmacological stress continues until the patient is unable to continue or until the target heart rate is achieved. Upon completion of the study, the stress ECG is reviewed and a written interpretation of findings is provided. Use 93015 for the complete procedure. Code 93016 is reported for supervision only without interpretation and report. Code 93017 is reported for the tracing only without interpretation and report. Code 93018 is reported for the interpretation and report only.

93024

| 93024 | Ergonovine provocation test |

Ergonovine, also referred to as ergometrine or Methergin¬Æ, is used to evaluate chest pain in a patient who does not have evidence of atherosclerotic coronary artery disease or other coronary abnormalities on arteriography. The ergonovine provocation test helps to differentiate chest pain due to coronary artery spasm and chest pain associated with esophageal spasm. With the patient on continuous electrocardiographic (ECG) monitoring, ergonovine is administered intravenously in incremental doses of 0.1 mg starting with 0.1 mg every 5 minutes until pain occurs. If the patient experiences coronary artery spasm as evidenced by changes in the ECG, the chest pain is determined to be cardiac in origin and is due to spasm-induced angina. If no ECG changes are identified, the chest pain is due to esophageal spasm. At the onset of pain, the patient is immediately given a medication to stop the coronary artery or esophageal spasm.

93025

| 93025 | Microvolt T-wave alternans for assessment of ventricular arrhythmias |

Microvolt T-wave alternans testing is performed to assess patients who are at risk for sudden cardiac arrest due to previous heart attack, heart failure, left ventricular dysfunction, unexplained syncope, or family history of sudden cardiac arrest. A set of 14 electrodes are distributed on the torso and attached to the ECG machine. Seven are standard electrodes while the other seven are special microvolt T-wave alternans sensors. ECG recordings are obtained while the patient walks on a treadmill while slowly increasing treadmill speed to increase the heart rate gradually. Alternatively, heart rate may be increased pharmacologically or using a pacer. The special microvolt T-wave alternans sensors are able to detect extremely small changes in the T-wave portion of the ECG that are not visible to the naked eye on the ECG recording. The test continues until T-wave changes are detected or until the patient achieves the desired heart rate without evidence of T-wave changes. The physician reviews the ECG and provides an interpretation of findings with a written report.

93040-93042

93040   Rhythm ECG, 1-3 leads; with interpretation and report
93041   Rhythm ECG, 1-3 leads; tracing only without interpretation and report
93042   Rhythm ECG, 1-3 leads; interpretation and report only

Electrocardiography (ECG or EKG) is an interpretation of the electrical activity of the heart over time captured and externally recorded by skin electrodes placed in the thoracic area. It is a noninvasive recording produced by an electrocardiographic device that transmits information, displayed on a report which indicates the overall rhythm of the heart and weaknesses in different parts of the heart muscle. It measures and diagnoses abnormal rhythms of the heart. In 93040, 1-3 leads are used and a report is generated. In 93041, only the procedure is reported. In 93042, only a a physician report is generated without the procedure portion.

93224-93227

93224   External electrocardiographic recording up to 48 hours by continuous rhythm recording and storage; includes recording, scanning analysis with report, review and interpretation by a physician or other qualified health care professional
93225   External electrocardiographic recording up to 48 hours by continuous rhythm recording and storage; recording (includes connection, recording, and disconnection)
93226   External electrocardiographic recording up to 48 hours by continuous rhythm recording and storage; scanning analysis with report
93227   External electrocardiographic recording up to 48 hours by continuous rhythm recording and storage; review and interpretation by a physician or other qualified health care professional

Electrocardiographic (ECG) rhythm-derived data is gathered for up to 48 hours of monitoring as the patient goes about regular daily activity while wearing an external ECG recording device, also called a Holter monitor. Electrodes or leads are placed on the patient's chest, and the patient is instructed on the use of the monitor. The recording device makes continuous, original ECG wave recordings for a 12 to 48 hour period. The recordings are captured on magnetic tape or digitized medium to be reviewed later. At the end of the recording period, the patient returns to the office with the device. Stored data derived from the continuous recordings of the electrical activity of the heart include heart rhythm and rate, ST analysis, variability in heart rate and T-wave alternans. Visual superimposition scanning is done to give a 'page review' of the entire recording, identifying different ECG waveforms with selective samples of rhythm strips. A report is made after analysis of the scanning, and the physician or other qualified health care professional reviews and interprets the data for heart arrhythmias. Report 93224 for the complete procedure, including recording, scanning with report, review and interpretation. Report 93225 for the recording portion only, which includes connection, recording, and disconnection. Report 93226 for analysis of the scanning with report only. Report 93227 for the review and interpretation only.

93228-93229

93228   External mobile cardiovascular telemetry with electrocardiographic recording, concurrent computerized real time data analysis and greater than 24 hours of accessible ECG data storage (retrievable with query) with ECG triggered and patient selected events transmitted to a remote attended surveillance center for up to 30 days; review and interpretation with report by a physician or other qualified health care professional
93229   External mobile cardiovascular telemetry with electrocardiographic recording, concurrent computerized real time data analysis and greater than 24 hours of accessible ECG data storage (retrievable with query) with ECG triggered and patient selected events transmitted to a remote attended surveillance center for up to 30 days; technical support for connection and patient instructions for use, attended surveillance, analysis and transmission of daily and emergent data reports as prescribed by a physician or other qualified health care professional

The patient is fitted with a telemetry transmitter connected to an external cardiovascular monitoring system. The telemetry transmitter receives data from the external monitoring system and transmits the data via a wireless connection such as a radio frequency link to a telemetry receiver at a monitoring station. Clinical personnel at the monitoring station acquire and analyze the data transmissions and notify the physician or other qualified health care professional of cardiac events requiring immediate review. Monitoring software

may also be used to alert the clinician to these cardiac events. The transmitted ECG and other data is reviewed using either a printed readout or on a computer screen. The data may include periodic ECGs, stored cardiac episodes, paced and sensed events from heart chambers, and histograms. Device function, such as battery voltage and impedance, pacing and shocking lead impedance, and sensed ECG voltage amplitude are reviewed. Programmed parameters are also evaluated and changes are made as needed. The patient may be monitored for up to 30 days. Previously generated data and current data are compared and any changes noted. The data is interpreted and a report is provided that includes medical findings and recommended treatment. Use code 93228 for physician or other qualified health care professional review and interpretation with report. Use code 93229 for technical support including fitting and connection of the external system, patient instructions related to use, attended surveillance at the monitoring station, and analysis and acquisition of physician prescribed daily and emergent data reports.

93260

93260   Programming device evaluation (in person) with iterative adjustment of the implantable device to test the function of the device and select optimal permanent programmed values with analysis, review and report by a physician or other qualified health care professional; implantable subcutaneous lead defibrillator system

An in-person programming evaluation is performed on an implantable subcutaneous lead defibrillator system with iterative adjustment of the implantable device, testing its function and selecting optimal permanent programmed values, including physician or other qualified health care professional analysis and review with a written report. The patient is connected to the electrocardiogram (ECG) monitor. A connection is established between the defibrillator system and the programming device. Cardiac rhythm is assessed. Current stored data related to cardiac rhythm and tachyarrhythmia episodes is interrogated, reviewed, and compared with previous data acquisitions. Pacing capture threshold is assessed in each chamber. Pacing function is assessed, including the leads and battery, and any pacing or integrity issues are addressed. Sensing threshold data are obtained from each chamber. Cross-talk, as evidenced by stimulation of one chamber with sensing and activation of other chambers, is evaluated. Atrial and ventricular stimulation is performed to evaluate the presence or absence of phrenic nerve stimulation. In order to attain optimal settings, an iterative programming process is used for fixed or dynamic atrioventricular interval timing. Parameters are adjusted based on effects on ventricular pacing, hemodynamics, and heart response. Exercise and physiologic stress data are reviewed, and heart rate adaptations are noted. Programmed parameters are adjusted as needed. Any necessary reprogramming of the implantable subcutaneous lead defibrillator system is performed after careful evaluation of all parameters. The patient is given instructions regarding any required follow-up services or procedures.

93261

93261   Interrogation device evaluation (in person) with analysis, review and report by a physician or other qualified health care professional, includes connection, recording and disconnection per patient encounter; implantable subcutaneous lead defibrillator system

An in-person interrogation evaluation of an implantable subcutaneous lead defibrillator system with physician or other qualified health care professional analysis, review, and report is performed, including connection, recording, and disconnection. In-person interrogation device evaluation is performed when a patient presents with symptoms or complaints that might be due to device malfunction or a change in cardiac function. The patient is connected to the electrocardiogram (ECG) monitor. A connection is established between the defibrillator device and the interrogation device and the defibrillator is interrogated. The physician or other qualified health care professional reviews the data to assess function and current programmed parameters. Electrocardiogram recordings are reviewed for the presence of arrhythmia. Stored data are reviewed and compared with previous data acquisitions. The number and duration of events such as arrhythmias, ectopic beats, and mode switch episodes are reviewed. Exercise and physiologic stress data are reviewed and heart rate adaptations are noted. The implantable defibrillator system is evaluated for appropriate sensing and capture of cardiac rhythm. Function is assessed, including the leads and battery. Any alerts generated by the device are reviewed. The patient is informed of the findings and a written report is provided. This code is reported on a per encounter basis.

Medicine

93268-93272

93268 External patient and, when performed, auto activated electrocardiographic rhythm derived event recording with symptom-related memory loop with remote download capability up to 30 days, 24-hour attended monitoring; includes transmission, review and interpretation by a physician or other qualified health care professional

93270 External patient and, when performed, auto activated electrocardiographic rhythm derived event recording with symptom-related memory loop with remote download capability up to 30 days, 24-hour attended monitoring; recording (includes connection, recording, and disconnection)

93271 External patient and, when performed, auto activated electrocardiographic rhythm derived event recording with symptom-related memory loop with remote download capability up to 30 days, 24-hour attended monitoring; transmission and analysis

93272 External patient and, when performed, auto activated electrocardiographic rhythm derived event recording with symptom-related memory loop with remote download capability up to 30 days, 24-hour attended monitoring; review and interpretation by a physician or other qualified health care professional

Electrocardiographic (ECG) rhythm derived data is gathered with 24-hour attended monitoring as the patient goes about regular daily activity while wearing an external ECG recording device. Electrodes or leads are placed on the patient's chest and the patient is instructed in the use of the monitoring device. The monitor records in a continuous loop mechanism and is capable of storing a single channel of ECG data in refreshed memory. When symptoms occur, the patient activates the monitor. The ECG data is then permanently saved from the memory loop including the 60-90 seconds prior to the episode, the symptomatic period, and a period of time following cessation of the episode. This allows capture and recording of the onset of arrythmias or other transient event. The patient then transmits the data to a receiving station where a printout is generated and the physician or other qualified health care professional reviews and interprets the ECG data. Report 93268 for transmission and professional review and interpretation. Report 93270 for recording only, including connection and disconnection. Report 93271 for receipt of transmissions and analysis only. Report 93272 for physician or other qualified health care professional review and interpretation only. These codes are reported only once per 30-day time period.

93278

93278 Signal-averaged electrocardiography (SAECG), with or without ECG

Signal averaged ECG is performed with the patient at rest, lying on an exam table. Electrodes are placed on the chest, abdomen, and back. Lead wires connected to the ECG machine are then attached to the electrodes. Multiple ECG tracings are obtained over a 20 minute period which allows capture of several hundred cardiac cycles. The extended length of the ECG testing increases the probability of capturing subtle abnormalities that would not be seen on a standard ECG. A computer captures the electrical signals and averages them. This provides the physician with additional information about function of the cardiac conduction system. The physician reviews the signal averaged ECG recording and computer analysis and provides a written interpretation of findings.

93279-93281

93279 Programming device evaluation (in person) with iterative adjustment of the implantable device to test the function of the device and select optimal permanent programmed values with analysis, review and report by a physician or other qualified health care professional; single lead pacemaker system

93280 Programming device evaluation (in person) with iterative adjustment of the implantable device to test the function of the device and select optimal permanent programmed values with analysis, review and report by a physician or other qualified health care professional; dual lead pacemaker system

93281 Programming device evaluation (in person) with iterative adjustment of the implantable device to test the function of the device and select optimal permanent programmed values with analysis, review and report by a physician or other qualified health care professional; multiple lead pacemaker system

A programming evaluation is performed on a pacemaker device with iterative adjustment of the implantable device, testing its function and selecting optimal permanent programmed values, including physician or other qualified health care professional analysis and review with a written report. The patient is connected to the electrocardiogram (ECG) monitor. A connection is established between the pacemaker device and the programming device. Cardiac rhythm is assessed. Stored pacemaker data is interrogated, reviewed, and compared with previous data acquisitions. Pacemaker function is assessed, including the leads and battery. Summary data and recorded rhythm data are reviewed for evidence of arrhythmias. Rhythm alerts and parameters are noted; pacing capture threshold is measured; and voltage and pulse width parameters are reviewed. The sensing threshold is measured and adjusted as needed. Exercise and physiologic stress data is reviewed;

heart rate adaptations are noted; and programmed parameters are adjusted as needed. Any necessary reprogramming of the device is performed after careful evaluation of all parameters. The patient is given instructions regarding any required follow-up services or procedures. Use code 93279 for programming evaluation of a single lead pacemaker system, code 93280 for a dual lead system, or code 93281 for a multiple lead system.

93282-93284

93282 Programming device evaluation (in person) with iterative adjustment of the implantable device to test the function of the device and select optimal permanent programmed values with analysis, review and report by a physician or other qualified health care professional; single lead transvenous implantable defibrillator system

93283 Programming device evaluation (in person) with iterative adjustment of the implantable device to test the function of the device and select optimal permanent programmed values with analysis, review and report by a physician or other qualified health care professional; dual lead transvenous implantable defibrillator system

93284 Programming device evaluation (in person) with iterative adjustment of the implantable device to test the function of the device and select optimal permanent programmed values with analysis, review and report by a physician or other qualified health care professional; multiple lead transvenous implantable defibrillator system

An in-person programming evaluation is performed on a transvenous implantable defibrillator system with iterative adjustment of the implantable device, testing its function and selecting optimal permanent programmed values, including physician or other qualified health care professional analysis and review with a written report. The patient is connected to the electrocardiogram (ECG) monitor. A connection is established between the defibrillator system and the programming device. Cardiac rhythm is assessed. Current stored data related to cardiac rhythm and tachyarrhythmia episodes is interrogated, reviewed, and compared with previous data acquisitions. Pacing capture threshold is assessed in each chamber. Pacing function is assessed, including the leads and battery, and any pacing or integrity issues are addressed. Sensing threshold data are obtained from each chamber. Cross-talk, as evidenced by stimulation of one chamber with sensing and activation of other chambers, is evaluated. Atrial and ventricular stimulation is performed to evaluate the presence or absence of phrenic nerve stimulation. In order to attain optimal settings, an iterative programming process is used for fixed or dynamic atrioventricular interval timing. Parameters are adjusted based on effects on ventricular pacing, hemodynamics, and heart response. Exercise and physiologic stress data are reviewed, and heart rate adaptations are noted. Programmed parameters are adjusted as needed. Any necessary reprogramming of the defibrillator system is performed after careful evaluation of all parameters. The patient is given instructions regarding any required follow-up services or procedures. Use code 93282 for programming evaluation of a single lead transvenous implantable defibrillator system, code 93283 for a dual lead system, and code 93284 for a multiple lead system.

93285

93285 Programming device evaluation (in person) with iterative adjustment of the implantable device to test the function of the device and select optimal permanent programmed values with analysis, review and report by a physician or other qualified health care professional; implantable loop recorder system

A programming evaluation is performed on an implantable loop recorder system (ILR) with iterative adjustment of the implantable device and selection of optimal permanent programmed values, including physician or other qualified health care professional analysis and review with a written report. The patient is connected to the electrocardiogram (ECG) monitor. A connection is established between the ILR system and the programming device. Stored data from the ILR is retrieved. Alert conditions are identified and reviewed. Current data is compared with historical data. ILR function is assessed, including signal strength, battery voltage, and impedance. Sensing threshold is evaluated using a step-by-step process which includes recording the ILR signal and adjusting the sensing threshold until the optimal threshold has been attained. Sensing and gain parameters are revised and programmed as needed. Patient-activated and automatically recorded rhythm episodes are reviewed. The data is downloaded and reviewed for atrial fibrillation, premature atrial or ventricular contractions, supraventricular or ventricular tachycardia, and atrioventricular block. Rhythm alerts and recording parameters are reviewed, and programming is performed as needed to optimize capture of rhythm episodes. Total device memory capacity is checked, as is the recording capacity for the number of patient-activated and automatically detected episodes. The pre- and post-episode recordings are assessed and adjusted as needed. Any necessary reprogramming of the ILR system is performed after careful evaluation of all parameters. The patient is given instructions regarding any required follow-up services or procedures.

93286-93287

93286   Peri-procedural device evaluation (in person) and programming of device system parameters before or after a surgery, procedure, or test with analysis, review and report by a physician or other qualified health care professional; single, dual, or multiple lead pacemaker system

93287   Peri-procedural device evaluation (in person) and programming of device system parameters before or after a surgery, procedure, or test with analysis, review and report by a physician or other qualified health care professional; single, dual, or multiple lead implantable defibrillator system

A peri-procedural device evaluation is performed with programming of the device system parameters before or after surgery, a procedure, or other test including physician or other qualified health care professional analysis, review, and report. The patient is informed regarding the need to temporarily change the cardiac device parameters, the planned pre-procedure parameter changes and duration of the change, and the timing of the planned restoration of the pre-procedure baseline settings. A connection is established between the pacemaker or defibrillator system and the programming device. The necessary pre-procedure programming changes are made and the device is interrogated to verify the programming changes. The physician or other qualified health care professional evaluates the patient to ensure that the temporary changes are being tolerated and the patient's cardiac condition is stable. Following the procedure, the patient is evaluated and, if appropriate, the cardiac device parameters are returned to the pre-procedure settings. The patient is again evaluated and adjustments are made as needed to the settings. The patient is given instructions regarding any required follow-up services or procedures. Use code 93286 for a peri-procedural device evaluation and programming of a single, dual, or multiple lead pacemaker and code 93287 for a single, dual, or multiple lead implantable defibrillator system.

93288

93288   Interrogation device evaluation (in person) with analysis, review and report by a physician or other qualified health care professional, includes connection, recording and disconnection per patient encounter; single, dual, or multiple lead pacemaker system

An in-person interrogation evaluation of a pacemaker system (single, dual, or multiple lead) with physician or other qualified health care professional analysis, review, and report is performed, including connection, recording, and disconnection. In-person interrogation device evaluation is performed when a patient presents with symptoms or complaints that might be due to pacemaker malfunction or a change in cardiac function. The patient is connected to the electrocardiogram (ECG) monitor. A connection is established between the pacemaker device and the interrogation device. The pacemaker is interrogated. The physician or other professional reviews the interrogated data to assess pacemaker function and current programmed parameters. Electrocardiogram recordings are reviewed for the presence of arrhythmia. Stored pacemaker data are reviewed and compared with previous data acquisitions. The number and duration of events such as arrhythmias, ectopic beats, and mode switch episodes are reviewed. Exercise and physiologic stress data are reviewed and heart rate adaptations are noted. The pacemaker is evaluated for appropriate sensing and capture of cardiac rhythm. Pacemaker function is assessed, including the leads and battery. Any alerts generated by the pacemaker device are reviewed. The patient is informed of the findings and a written report is provided. This code is reported on a per encounter basis.

93289

93289   Interrogation device evaluation (in person) with analysis, review and report by a physician or other qualified health care professional, includes connection, recording and disconnection per patient encounter; single, dual, or multiple lead transvenous implantable defibrillator system, including analysis of heart rhythm derived data elements

An in-person interrogation evaluation of a transvenous implantable defibrillator system (single, dual, or multiple lead) with physician or other qualified health care professional analysis, review, and report is performed, including connection, recording, and disconnection. In-person interrogation device evaluation is performed when a patient presents with symptoms or complaints that might be due to device malfunction or a change in cardiac function. The patient is connected to the electrocardiogram (ECG) monitor. A connection is established between the defibrillator device and the interrogation device and the defibrillator is interrogated. The physician or other qualified health care professional reviews the data to assess function and current programmed parameters. Electrocardiogram recordings are reviewed for the presence of arrhythmia. Stored data are reviewed and compared with previous data acquisitions. The number and duration of events such as arrhythmias, ectopic beats, and mode switch episodes are reviewed. Exercise and physiologic stress data are reviewed and heart rate adaptations are noted. The implantable defibrillator is evaluated for appropriate sensing and capture of cardiac rhythm. Function is assessed, including the leads and battery. Any alerts generated by the device are reviewed. The patient is informed of the findings and a written report is provided. This code is reported on a per encounter basis.

93290

93290   Interrogation device evaluation (in person) with analysis, review and report by a physician or other qualified health care professional, includes connection, recording and disconnection per patient encounter; implantable cardiovascular monitor system, including analysis of 1 or more recorded physiologic cardiovascular data elements from all internal and external sensors

An in-person interrogation evaluation of an implantable cardiovascular monitor (ICM) system with analysis of one or more recorded physiologic cardiovascular data elements from all internal and external sensors is performed with physician or other qualified health care professional analysis, review, and report, including connection, recording, and disconnection. ICMs provide hemodynamic monitoring of intracardiac pressure, body temperature, physical activity, and heart rate in patients with cardiac conditions such as heart failure or unexplained syncope and collapse. In-person interrogation device evaluation is performed when a patient presents with symptoms or complaints that might be due to device malfunction or a change in cardiac function. The patient is connected to the electrocardiogram (ECG) monitor. A connection is established between the ICM device and the interrogation device and the ICM is interrogated. The physician or other qualified health care professional reviews interrogated data to assess ICM function and current programmed parameters. Electrocardiogram recordings are reviewed for the presence of arrhythmia. Stored data are reviewed and compared with previous data acquisitions. Data elements reviewed may include the following as well as other data elements: weight, systemic blood pressure, atrial and ventricular pressures, pulmonary artery pressure, and intra-thoracic impedance measurements. The ICM is evaluated for appropriate sensing and capture of data. ICM function is assessed, including the leads and battery. Any alerts generated by the device are reviewed. The patient is informed of the findings and a written report is provided. This code is reported on a per encounter basis.

93291

93291   Interrogation device evaluation (in person) with analysis, review and report by a physician or other qualified health care professional, includes connection, recording and disconnection per patient encounter; implantable loop recorder system, including heart rhythm derived data analysis

In-person interrogation device evaluation is performed when a patient presents with symptoms or complaints that might be due to implantable loop recorder (ILR) malfunction or to a change in cardiac function. A connection is established between the ILR device and the interrogation device. The ILR is interrogated. The physician or other qualified health care professional reviews interrogated data to assess ILR function and current programmed parameters. Stored ILR data including any stored events are reviewed and compared with previous data acquisitions. Patient-activated and automatically recorded rhythm episodes are reviewed. The data is downloaded and reviewed for atrial fibrillation, premature atrial or ventricular contractions, supraventricular or ventricular tachycardia, and atrioventricular block. Rhythm alerts and recording parameters are reviewed. The ILR is evaluated for appropriate sensing and capture of cardiac rhythm. Total device memory capacity is checked as is the recording capacity for the number of patient activated and automatically detected episodes. The pre- and post-episode recordings are assessed. ILR function is assessed including the leads and battery. Any alerts generated by the ILR device are reviewed. The patient is informed of the findings and a written report provided. This code is reported on a per encounter basis.

93292

93292   Interrogation device evaluation (in person) with analysis, review and report by a physician or other qualified health care professional, includes connection, recording and disconnection per patient encounter; wearable defibrillator system

An in-person interrogation evaluation of a wearable defibrillator system with physician or other qualified health care professional analysis, review, and report is performed, including connection, recording, and disconnection. In-person interrogation device evaluation is performed when a patient presents with symptoms or complaints that might be due to device malfunction or a change in cardiac function. The patient is connected to the electrocardiogram (ECG) monitor. A connection is established between the wearable defibrillator system and the interrogation device, and the defibrillator is interrogated. The physician or other qualified health care professional reviews interrogated data to assess defibrillator function and current programmed parameters. Electrocardiogram recordings are reviewed for the presence of arrhythmia. Stored data are reviewed and compared with previous data acquisitions. The number and duration of events such as arrhythmias, ectopic beats, and mode switch episodes are reviewed. Exercise and physiologic stress data are reviewed and heart rate adaptations are noted. The defibrillator is evaluated for appropriate sensing and capture of cardiac rhythm. Defibrillator function is assessed, including the leads and battery. Any alerts generated by the device are reviewed. The patient is informed of the findings and a written report is provided. This code is reported on a per encounter basis.

Medicine

93293

93293   Transtelephonic rhythm strip pacemaker evaluation(s) single, dual, or multiple lead pacemaker system, includes recording with and without magnet application with analysis, review and report(s) by a physician or other qualified health care professional, up to 90 days

One or more transtelephonic rhythm strip pacemaker (single, dual, multiple lead) evaluations, including recording with and without magnet application, with physician or other qualified health care professional analysis, review, and report for up to 90 days is performed. An initial transtelephonic rhythm strip is recorded for 30 seconds and evaluated for sensing and capture of heart rate and any arrhythmias. A second strip may then be recorded with a magnet placed over the pacemaker. This second strip is evaluated for sensing and capture of heart rate and any arrhythmias and for the magnet response, which includes a paced rate. A technician receives the rhythm strip data, which is reviewed. Any patient symptoms are noted. The technician reviews selected parameters and reports on any abnormalities. The technician documents findings into the database, verifies that leads and battery are functioning appropriately, and identifies arrhythmia events, noting both normal and abnormal events. Following review of the data, the technician provides a written report for the physician or other qualified health care professional who then reviews the report and the adequacy of the data, and communicates results as well as any required follow-up to the patient and the technician.

93294

93294   Interrogation device evaluation(s) (remote), up to 90 days; single, dual, or multiple lead pacemaker system with interim analysis, review(s) and report(s) by a physician or other qualified health care professional

One or more remote interrogation evaluations of a pacemaker system (single, dual, or multiple lead) with physician or other qualified health care professional analysis, review, and report is performed for up to 90 days. The pacemaker is interrogated by telemetric communication. The physician or other qualified health care professional reviews interrogated data to assess pacemaker function and current programmed parameters. Electrocardiogram recordings are reviewed for the presence of arrhythmia. Stored pacemaker data, including any stored events, are reviewed and compared with previous data acquisitions. The number and duration of events such as arrhythmias, ectopic beats, and mode switch episodes are reviewed. Exercise and physiologic stress data are reviewed and heart rate adaptations are noted. The pacemaker is evaluated for appropriate sensing and capture of cardiac rhythm. Pacemaker function is assessed, including the leads and battery. Any alerts generated by the pacemaker device are reviewed. The patient is informed of the findings and a written report is provided.

93295

93295   Interrogation device evaluation(s) (remote), up to 90 days; single, dual, or multiple lead implantable defibrillator system with interim analysis, review(s) and report(s) by a physician or other qualified health care professional

One or more remote interrogation evaluations of an implantable defibrillator system (single, dual, or multiple lead) with physician or other qualified health care professional analysis, review, and report is performed for up to 90 days. The defibrillator is interrogated by telemetric communication. The physician or other qualified health care professional reviews interrogated data to assess function and current programmed parameters. Electrocardiogram recordings are reviewed for the presence of arrhythmia. Stored data, including any stored events, are reviewed and compared with previous data acquisitions. The number and duration of events such as arrhythmias, ectopic beats, and mode switch episodes are reviewed. Exercise and physiologic stress data are reviewed and heart rate adaptations are noted. The defibrillator system is evaluated for appropriate sensing and capture of cardiac rhythm. Function is assessed, including the leads and battery. Any alerts generated by the device are reviewed. The patient is informed of the findings and a written report is provided.

93296

93296   Interrogation device evaluation(s) (remote), up to 90 days; single, dual, or multiple lead pacemaker system or implantable defibrillator system, remote data acquisition(s), receipt of transmissions and technician review, technical support and distribution of results

One or more remote interrogation evaluations of a pacemaker or an implantable defibrillator system (single, dual, or multiple lead), including remote data acquisitions, receipt of transmissions with technician review, and support and distribution of results, is performed for up to 90 days. The patient is registered for remote interrogation at a monitoring facility, which provides the patient with the necessary equipment and installation instructions, with additional phone support as needed to ensure that the patient has the equipment properly installed. An interrogation schedule is established based on the physician orders. Pacemaker or defibrillator interrogation is performed. The technician receives the data at the remote facility, reviews the data, and compares it to the parameters established by the physician. The technician also evaluates the device function, including leads and battery. The technician identifies any variations from the

parameters, along with any alerts, and communicates this information to the physician or other qualified professional along with any patient complaints or symptoms. The technician transfers all interrogated data and findings to the database and provides a comprehensive report of evaluated parameters for review.

93297

93297   Interrogation device evaluation(s), (remote) up to 30 days; implantable cardiovascular monitor system, including analysis of 1 or more recorded physiologic cardiovascular data elements from all internal and external sensors, analysis, review(s) and report(s) by a physician or other qualified health care professional

One or more remote interrogation evaluations of an implantable cardiovascular monitor (ICM) system with analysis of one or more recorded physiologic cardiovascular data elements from all internal and external sensors with physician or other qualified health care professional analysis, review, and report are performed for up to 30 days. ICMs provide hemodynamic monitoring of intracardiac pressure, body temperature, physical activity, and heart rate in patients with cardiac conditions such as heart failure or unexplained syncope and collapse. The ICM is interrogated by telemetric communication. The physician or other qualified health care professional reviews interrogated data to assess ICM function and current programmed parameters. Electrocardiogram recordings are reviewed for the presence of arrhythmia. Stored data, including any stored events, are reviewed and compared with previous data acquisitions. Data elements reviewed may include the following as well as alternatives: weight, systemic blood pressure, atrial and ventricular pressures, pulmonary artery pressure, and intra-thoracic impedance measurements. The ICM is evaluated for appropriate sensing and capture of data. ICM function is assessed, including the leads and battery. Any alerts generated by the device are reviewed. The patient is informed of the findings and a written report is provided.

93298

93298   Interrogation device evaluation(s), (remote) up to 30 days; implantable loop recorder system, including analysis of recorded heart rhythm data, analysis, review(s) and report(s) by a physician or other qualified health care professional

One or more remote interrogation evaluations of an implantable loop recorder (ILR) system with physician or other qualified health care professional analysis, review, and report are performed for up to 30 days. The ILR is interrogated. The physician or other qualified health care professional reviews interrogated data to assess ILR function and current programmed parameters. Stored ILR data, including any stored events, are reviewed and compared with previous data acquisitions. Patient-activated and automatically-recorded rhythm episodes are reviewed. The data is downloaded and reviewed for atrial fibrillation, premature atrial or ventricular contractions, supraventricular or ventricular tachycardia, and atrioventricular block. Rhythm alerts and recording parameters are also reviewed. The ILR is evaluated for appropriate sensing and capture of cardiac rhythm. Total device memory capacity is checked, as is the recording capacity for the number of patient-activated and automatically detected episodes. The pre- and post-episode recordings are assessed. ILR function is assessed, including the leads and battery. Any alerts generated by the ILR device are reviewed. The patient is informed of the findings and a written report is provided.

93299

93299   Interrogation device evaluation(s), (remote) up to 30 days; implantable cardiovascular monitor system or implantable loop recorder system, remote data acquisition(s), receipt of transmissions and technician review, technical support and distribution of results

One or more remote interrogation evaluations of an implantable cardiovascular monitor (ICM) system or implantable loop recorder (ILR) system, including remote data acquisitions, receipt of transmissions with technician review, technical support, and distribution of results are performed for up to 30 days. The patient is registered for remote interrogation at a monitoring facility. The facility provides the patient with the necessary equipment, installation instructions, and additional phone support as needed to ensure that the patient has the equipment properly installed. An interrogation schedule is established based on the physician orders. ICM or ILR interrogation is performed. The technician receives the data at the remote facility, reviews the data, and compares it to the parameters established by the physician. The technician also evaluates the device function, including leads and battery. Any variations from the parameters and device alerts are also identified and communicated to the physician, along with any patient complaints or symptoms. The technician transfers all of the interrogated data and findings to the physician's database and provides a comprehensive report of evaluated parameters for the physician to review.

Medicine

93303-93304

93303 Transthoracic echocardiography for congenital cardiac anomalies; complete
93304 Transthoracic echocardiography for congenital cardiac anomalies; follow-up or limited study

Transthoracic echocardiography uses ultrasonic sound waves to visualize the heart and great vessels. The sound waves are converted into electrical pulses displayed as a picture on a computer screen. In 93303, a complete transthoracic echocardiogram (TTE) is performed on a patient with a congenital cardiac anomaly. TTE uses real-time ultrasound scanning to display both the two-dimensional picture of the heart and movement as it occurs. Multiple views are obtained using ultrasound transducers on the chest to get a comprehensive functional and anatomic evaluation of the left and right chambers, the valves, the pericardium, and additional structures, such as the aorta, pulmonary vessels, and the vena cava. Selective M mode recording, also known as T-M mode, displays more specific time-motion information from a stationary beam, superimposed on the 2-D image. Depth is oriented along the vertical axis and time on the horizontal axis. M-mode is used primarily for cardiac measurements, such as septal wall thickness and valve timing. A complete TTE is reported when the examination includes at least the left and right atria, left and right ventricles, the aortic, mitral, and tricuspid valves, the pericardium, and adjacent portions of the aorta. A follow-up or limited TTE performed to evaluate a congenital cardiac anomaly (93304) is performed in the same manner; however, not all heart structures are evaluated. Typically a follow-up or limited study focuses on one area of clinical concern.

93306

93306 Echocardiography, transthoracic, real-time with image documentation (2D), includes M-mode recording, when performed, complete, with spectral Doppler echocardiography, and with color flow Doppler echocardiography

The physician performs complete transthoracic real-time echocardiography with image documentation (2-D) including M-mode recording, if performed, with spectral Doppler and color flow Doppler echocardiography. Cardiac structure and dynamics are evaluated using a series of real-time tomographic images with multiple views recorded digitally or on videotape. Time-motion (M-mode) recordings are made as needed to allow dimensional measurement. Blood flow and velocity patterns within the heart, across valves and within the great vessels are evaluated by color flow Doppler. Normal blood flow patterns through these regions have a characteristic pattern defined by direction, velocity, duration, and timing throughout the cardiac cycle. Spectral Doppler by pulsed or continuous wave technique is used to evaluate antegrade flow through inflow and outflow tracts and cardiac valves. Multiple transducer positions or orientations may be required. The physician reviews the echocardiography images and orders additional images as needed to allow evaluation of any abnormalities. Digital or videotaped images are then reviewed by the physician. Abnormalities of cardiac structure or dynamics are noted. The extent of the abnormalities is evaluated and quantified. Any previous cardiac studies are compared to the current study and any quantitative or qualitative changes are identified. The physician provides an interpretation of the echocardiography with a written report of findings.

93307-93308

93307 Echocardiography, transthoracic, real-time with image documentation (2D), includes M-mode recording, when performed, complete, without spectral or color flow Doppler echocardiography
93308 Echocardiography, transthoracic, real-time with image documentation (2D), includes M-mode recording, when performed, follow-up or limited study

A complete transthoracic echocardiogram obtains ultrasonic images of the heart and great vessels in real time with two-dimensional image documentation and selective M-mode recording, when done. Ultrasound visualizes the body internally using sound waves bounced off interior structures and reflected back to a receiving unit at varying speeds as the waves pass through different tissue densities. The waves are converted into electrical pulses displayed as a picture on screen. Real-time ultrasound scanning displays both the two-dimensional picture of the structure being viewed and movement as it occurs. Multiple views are obtained with ultrasound transducers on the chest to get a comprehensive functional and anatomic evaluation of the left and right chambers, the valves, the pericardium, and additional structures, such as the pulmonary valve or vessels, and the inferior vena cava. Selective M mode recording, also known as T-M mode, displays more specific time-motion information from a stationary beam, superimposed on the 2-D image. Depth is oriented along the vertical axis and time on the horizontal axis. M-mode is used primarily for cardiac measurements, such as septal wall thickness and valve timing. Report a follow-up or limited study (93308) when all the structures comprising a complete study are not evaluated, typically when one area of clinical concern is the focus.

93312-93314

93312 Echocardiography, transesophageal, real-time with image documentation (2D) (with or without M-mode recording); including probe placement, image acquisition, interpretation and report
93313 Echocardiography, transesophageal, real-time with image documentation (2D) (with or without M-mode recording); placement of transesophageal probe only
93314 Echocardiography, transesophageal, real-time with image documentation (2D) (with or without M-mode recording); image acquisition, interpretation and report only

Transesophageal echocardiography (TEE) is performed using a miniature high-frequency ultrasound transducer mounted on the tip of a flexible tube, or probe that is passed down through the mouth, advanced into the esophagus, and positioned behind the heart. The transducer directs ultrasound waves into the heart. The sound waves are then reflected back to the transducer and translated by a computer into an image of the heart that is displayed on a videoscreen. TEE uses real-time ultrasound scanning to display both the two-dimensional picture of the heart and movement as it occurs. Multiple views are obtained by manipulating the transducer within the esophagus to get a comprehensive functional and anatomic evaluation of the left and right chambers, the valves, the pericardium, and additional structures, such as the aorta, pulmonary vessels, and the vena cava. Selective M mode recording, also known as T-M mode, displays more specific time-motion information from a stationary beam, superimposed on the 2-D image. Depth is oriented along the vertical axis and time on the horizontal axis. M-mode is used primarily for cardiac measurements, such as septal wall thickness and valve timing. Use code 93312 when the physician performs probe placement, image acquisition, and a written report of findings. Use code 93313 when only the transesophageal probe placement is performed. Use 93314 when only the image acquisition and a written report of findings are performed.

93315-93317

93315 Transesophageal echocardiography for congenital cardiac anomalies; including probe placement, image acquisition, interpretation and report
93316 Transesophageal echocardiography for congenital cardiac anomalies; placement of transesophageal probe only
93317 Transesophageal echocardiography for congenital cardiac anomalies; image acquisition, interpretation and report only

Transesophageal echocardiography (TEE) is performed on a patient with a congenital cardiac anomaly using a miniature high-frequency ultrasound transducer mounted on the tip of a flexible tube, or probe that is passed down through the mouth, advanced into the esophagus, and positioned behind the heart. The transducer directs ultrasound waves into the heart. The sound waves are then reflected back to the transducer and translated by a computer into an image of the heart that is displayed on a videoscreen. TEE uses real-time ultrasound scanning to display both the two-dimensional picture of the heart and movement as it occurs. Multiple views are obtained by manipulating the transducer within the esophagus to get a comprehensive functional and anatomic evaluation of the left and right chambers, the valves, the pericardium, and additional structures, such as the aorta, pulmonary vessels, and the vena cava. Selective M mode recording, also known as T-M mode, displays more specific time-motion information from a stationary beam, superimposed on the 2-D image. Depth is oriented along the vertical axis and time on the horizontal axis. M-mode is used primarily for cardiac measurements, such as septal wall thickness and valve timing. Use code 93315 when the physician performs probe placement, image acquisition, and a written report of findings. Use code 93316 when only the transesophageal probe placement is performed. Use 93317 when only the image acquisition and a written report of findings are performed.

93318

93318 Echocardiography, transesophageal (TEE) for monitoring purposes, including probe placement, real time 2-dimensional image acquisition and interpretation leading to ongoing (continuous) assessment of (dynamically changing) cardiac pumping function and to therapeutic measures on an immediate time basis

Transesophageal echocardiography (TEE) is performed for monitoring purposes during surgery or other interventions that produce acute dynamic changes in cardiovascular function, such as procedures on the heart or aorta. The procedure includes probe placement, real time two-dimensional image acquisition, and interpretation with continuous assessment of cardiac pumping function and the effect of therapeutic measures as they are performed. A miniature high-frequency ultrasound transducer mounted on the tip of a tube is passed down through the mouth and advanced into the esophagus. The transducer directs ultrasound waves into the heart. The sound waves are then reflected back to the transducer and translated by a computer into an image of the heart that is displayed on a videoscreen. The images of the heart are continuously monitored as the surgical procedure or other intervention is performed. The monitoring physician reports changes to the physician performing the procedure or other intervention so that additional measures can be taken to minimize or counteract adverse changes in heart function.

Medicine

93320-93321

93320 Doppler echocardiography, pulsed wave and/or continuous wave with spectral display (List separately in addition to codes for echocardiographic imaging); complete

93321 Doppler echocardiography, pulsed wave and/or continuous wave with spectral display (List separately in addition to codes for echocardiographic imaging); follow-up or limited study (List separately in addition to codes for echocardiographic imaging)

Spectral Doppler is used to evaluate and measure the flow of blood through the heart chambers, valves, and arteries. A gel is placed on the chest and a handheld transducer that sends and receives sound waves is then moved over the chest. Spectral Doppler by pulsed or continuous wave technique is used to evaluate antegrade flow through inflow and outflow tracts and cardiac valves. Multiple transducer positions or orientations may be required. The physician reviews the initial echocardiography images and orders additional images as needed to allow evaluation of any abnormalities. Digital or videotaped images are then reviewed by the physician. Abnormalities of cardiac structure or dynamics are noted. The extent of the abnormalities is evaluated and quantified. Any previous cardiac studies are compared to the current study and any quantitative or qualitative changes identified. The physician provides an interpretation of the spectral Doppler echocardiography with a written report of findings. Use 93320 for an initial complete study or 93321 for a follow-up or repeat study.

93325

93325 Doppler echocardiography color flow velocity mapping (List separately in addition to codes for echocardiography)

Color flow Doppler provides two-dimensional images of the beating heart. Color is used to show the direction and speed of blood flow through the heart chambers, valves, and arteries. A gel is placed on the chest and a handheld transducer that sends and receives sound waves is then moved over the chest. The physician reviews the initial color flow Doppler echocardiography images and orders additional images as needed to allow evaluation of any abnormalities. Videotaped images are then reviewed by the physician and any abnormalities of blood flow are noted. The extent of the abnormalities is evaluated and quantified. Any previous cardiac studies are compared to the current study and any quantitative or qualitative changes identified. The physician provides an interpretation of the color flow Doppler echocardiography with a written report of findings.

93350-93352

93350 Echocardiography, transthoracic, real-time with image documentation (2D), includes M-mode recording, when performed, during rest and cardiovascular stress test using treadmill, bicycle exercise and/or pharmacologically induced stress, with interpretation and report

93351 Echocardiography, transthoracic, real-time with image documentation (2D), includes M-mode recording, when performed, during rest and cardiovascular stress test using treadmill, bicycle exercise and/or pharmacologically induced stress, with interpretation and report; including performance of continuous electrocardiographic monitoring, with supervision by a physician or other qualified health care professional

93352 Use of echocardiographic contrast agent during stress echocardiography (List separately in addition to code for primary procedure)

If an ECG is needed for gating, a three-lead ECG is hooked up. A baseline echocardiogram is obtained with the patient at rest. Cardiac structure and dynamics are evaluated using a series of real-time tomographic images with multiple views recorded digitally or on videotape. Time-motion (M-mode) recordings are made as needed to allow dimensional measurement. Ventricular function, chamber sizes, wall thickness and motion, aortic roots, and cardiac valves are assessed. Multiple transducer positions or orientations may be required to obtain images from multiple cardiac windows. The physician or other qualified health care professional reviews the resting ECG and orders additional images as needed to evaluate any abnormalities. The exercise portion of the study is then initiated. Heart rate and blood pressure are monitored. A continuous ECG may also be obtained and monitored. Staged stress protocol is used and the patient's response to stress is monitored. Unless contraindicated, exercise or pharmacological stress continues until the patient is unable to continue or until the target heart rate is achieved. Images of left ventricular wall motion are obtained immediately following completion of the stress component. The images are organized and submitted for review and interpretation. Abnormalities of cardiac structure or dynamics are noted, evaluated, and quantified. Any previous cardiac studies are compared to the current study, and any changes are identified. The physician or other qualified health care professional provides an interpretation of the ECG with a written report of findings. Use code 93350 for rest and stress echocardiography performed without continuous ECG or code 93351 when continuous ECG monitoring, with supervision by a physician or other qualified health care professional is required. Use add-on code 93352 when an echocardiographic contrast agent is used during the stress component. The prescribed dose of contrast is administered intravenously and titrated to achieve the necessary left ventricle opacification. Pre-stress images are obtained. Additional images are obtained at peak stress or immediately post-stress following administration of a second dose of

contrast. The patient is monitored until heart rate returns to normal. The intravenous catheter is removed. The physician or other qualified health care professional reviews and interprets the contrast-enhanced images and provides a written report of findings.

93355

93355 Echocardiography, transesophageal (TEE) for guidance of a transcatheter intracardiac or great vessel(s) structural intervention(s) (eg, TAVR, transcathether pulmonary valve replacement, mitral valve repair, paravalvular regurgitation repair, left atrial appendage occlusion/ closure, ventricular septal defect closure) (peri-and intra-procedural), real-time image acquisition and documentation, guidance with quantitative measurements, probe manipulation, interpretation, and report, including diagnostic transesophageal echocardiography and, when performed, administration of ultrasound contrast, Doppler, color flow, and 3D

Transesophageal echocardiography (TEE) uses high frequency sound waves to image the heart and great vessels through a flexible probe with transducer tip inserted orally into the esophagus. The esophagus is located directly behind the heart and the transducer picks up the sound waves and sends them back to a computer which displays in real time clear images of heart structures (aorta, pulmonary artery, valves, both atria, atrial septum, left atrial appendage, and coronary arteries) and measures heart function. TEE can image the size of the heart and thickness of the walls, show how well the heart pumps blood, aide in visualizing abnormal tissue around the heart valves indicating infection, tumor, regurgitation, or stenosis, and tears or dissection of the aorta. TEE may be performed preoperatively to evaluate and diagnose cardiac conditions and/or intra-procedurally when using a transcatheter approach to repair heart valves, vessels, and septal defects. TEE can be used with M-mode ultrasound to measure heart structure, size, and wall thickness, Doppler echocardiography to track the flow of blood through the heart chambers and valves, Color Doppler to help delineate the direction of blood flow, 2-dimensional echocardiography to visualize the actual structure and motion of the heart, and 3-dimensional echocardiography for real time image, greater depth of heart structure, and measurement of function while in motion.

93451

93451 Right heart catheterization including measurement(s) of oxygen saturation and cardiac output, when performed

The skin is cleansed over the catheter access site, usually the right femoral vein in the groin. A local anesthetic is injected. A small stab incision is made in the skin and a needle is inserted into the blood vessel followed by a sheath. A guidewire is threaded through the femoral vein, external iliac vein, inferior vena cava, and into the right atrium. The catheter is inserted into the access vein and threaded over the guidewire to the right atrium, then passed through the right atrium, right ventricle, and into the pulmonary arteries. As the catheter is passed through the right side of the heart and into the pulmonary arteries, the right heart chambers are inspected and pressures are obtained. Oxygen levels and cardiac output are measured as needed. The tricuspid and pulmonary valves are inspected. A separately reportable angiogram of the right heart and/or pulmonary arteries may be obtained. When the procedure is completed, the catheter is withdrawn, compression is applied to the venous access site, and a dressing is applied.

93452

93452 Left heart catheterization including intraprocedural injection(s) for left ventriculography, imaging supervision and interpretation, when performed

The skin over the selected artery, such as the brachial, axillary, or femoral artery is cleansed and a local anesthetic is administered. The artery is punctured with a needle and a sheath is placed. Using radiological supervision, a guidewire is inserted and threaded retrograde (against the flow of blood) through the artery, into the aorta, and into the left side of the heart (left ventricle and left atrium), followed by a catheter threaded over the guidewire. The guidewire is removed. The aortic valve, left ventricle, mitral valve, and left atrium are inspected. Left ventricular and atrial pressures are obtained and pressure gradients across the aortic and mitral valves are also obtained. Contrast media is injected and a left ventriculogram is obtained as needed. A separately reportable angiogram of the aorta may also be obtained. When the procedure is completed, the catheter is withdrawn, compression is applied over the arterial puncture site, and a compression dressing is applied. Results of the left heart catheterization and ventriculogram are reviewed and a written report of findings is provided.

93453

93453 Combined right and left heart catheterization including intraprocedural injection(s) for left ventriculography, imaging supervision and interpretation, when performed

For right heart catheterization, the access site is usually the right femoral vein in the groin. A small stab incision is made in the skin and a needle is inserted into the blood vessel followed by a sheath. A guidewire is threaded through the femoral vein, external iliac vein, inferior vena cava, and into the right atrium followed by a catheter threaded over the guidewire. Once the catheter is positioned, the guidewire is withdrawn. As the catheter is passed through the right side of the heart and into the pulmonary arteries, the right heart chambers are inspected and pressures are obtained. Oxygen levels are measured. The tricuspid and pulmonary valves are inspected and pressure gradients are obtained. A separately reportable angiogram of the right heart and/or pulmonary arteries may be obtained. The left heart catheterization is then performed. The skin over the brachial, axillary, or femoral artery is cleansed and a local anesthetic is administered. The artery is punctured with a needle and a sheath is placed. A guidewire is then inserted and threaded retrograde through the artery, into the aorta, and into the left side of the heart. A catheter is threaded over the guidewire and positioned in the left heart. The guidewire is removed. The aortic valve, left ventricle, mitral valve, and left atrium are inspected. Left ventricular and atrial pressures and pressure gradients across the aortic and mitral valves are obtained. Contrast is injected and a left ventriculogram is obtained as needed. Separately reportable angiograms of the aorta and/or right heart chambers may be obtained. When the procedure is completed, the catheters are withdrawn, pressure is applied over the venous and arterial puncture sites, and compression dressings are applied. Results of the right and left heart catheterization and ventriculogram are reviewed and a written report of findings is provided.

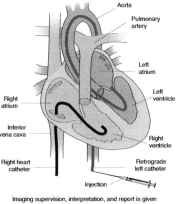

Combined left/right heart catheterization left ventriculography

Aorta

Pulmonary artery

Left atrium

Left ventricle

Right atrium

Inferior vena cava

Right ventricle

Right heart catheter

Retrograde left catheter

Injection

Imaging supervision, interpretation, and report is given

93454-93455

93454 Catheter placement in coronary artery(s) for coronary angiography, including intraprocedural injection(s) for coronary angiography, imaging supervision and interpretation

93455 Catheter placement in coronary artery(s) for coronary angiography, including intraprocedural injection(s) for coronary angiography, imaging supervision and interpretation; with catheter placement(s) in bypass graft(s) (internal mammary, free arterial, venous grafts) including intraprocedural injection(s) for bypass graft angiography

A catheter is placed in the coronary arteries, arterial and/or venous coronary bypass grafts for coronary angiography without concomitant right and/or left heart catheterization. The skin over the arterial access site is cleansed and a local anesthetic is administered. The artery is punctured with a needle and a sheath is placed. Using radiological supervision, a guidewire is then inserted. The guidewire is threaded through the artery, into the aorta, and positioned in the right or left coronary artery, and/or an arterial or venous coronary bypass graft. A catheter is threaded over the guidewire. The guidewire is removed. Contrast media is injected. The coronary arteries and bypass grafts are visualized and angiograms are obtained. When the angiogram procedure is completed, the catheter is withdrawn, pressure is applied to the puncture site, and a compression dressing is applied. The angiograms are reviewed and a written interpretation of findings is provided. Use 93454 when the catheterization, injection procedure, and angiography are performed on native coronary arteries only. Use 93455 when the procedure is performed on native coronary arteries and bypass grafts.

93456-93457

93456 Catheter placement in coronary artery(s) for coronary angiography, including intraprocedural injection(s) for coronary angiography, imaging supervision and interpretation; with right heart catheterization

93457 Catheter placement in coronary artery(s) for coronary angiography, including intraprocedural injection(s) for coronary angiography, imaging supervision and interpretation; with catheter placement(s) in bypass graft(s) (internal mammary, free arterial, venous grafts) including intraprocedural injection(s) for bypass graft angiography and right heart catheterization

The skin over the arterial access site is cleansed and a local anesthetic is administered. The artery is punctured with a needle and a sheath is placed. Using radiological supervision, a guidewire is inserted. The guidewire is threaded through the artery, into the

aorta, and positioned in the right or left coronary artery, or an arterial or venous coronary bypass graft, followed by a catheter threaded over the guidewire. The guidewire is removed. Contrast media is injected. The coronary arteries and bypass grafts are visualized and angiograms are obtained. When the angiogram procedure is completed, the catheter is withdrawn, pressure is applied to the puncture site, and a compression dressing is applied. The angiograms are reviewed and a written interpretation of findings is provided. Right heart catheterization is then also performed. A small stab incision is made in the skin and a needle is inserted into the femoral vein. A sheath is placed over the needle and the needle is withdrawn. A guidewire is threaded through the femoral vein, external iliac vein, inferior vena cava, and into the right atrium, followed by a catheter threaded over the guidewire. The guidewire is withdrawn. The catheter is passed into the right atrium, right ventricle, and into the pulmonary arteries. As the catheter is passed through the right side of the heart into the pulmonary arteries, the right heart chambers are inspected and pressures are obtained. Oxygen levels and cardiac output are measured as needed. The tricuspid and pulmonary valves are inspected. A separately reportable angiogram of the right heart and/or pulmonary arteries may be obtained. When the procedure is completed, the catheter is withdrawn, compression is applied to the venous access site, and a dressing is applied. A written report of findings is provided. Use 93456 for combined native coronary artery and right heart catheterization and evaluation. Use 93457 when coronary artery bypass grafts are also evaluated in conjunction with native coronary arteries and right heart structures.

93458-93459

93458 Catheter placement in coronary artery(s) for coronary angiography, including intraprocedural injection(s) for coronary angiography, imaging supervision and interpretation; with left heart catheterization including intraprocedural injection(s) for left ventriculography, when performed

93459 Catheter placement in coronary artery(s) for coronary angiography, including intraprocedural injection(s) for coronary angiography, imaging supervision and interpretation; with left heart catheterization including intraprocedural injection(s) for left ventriculography, when performed, catheter placement(s) in bypass graft(s) (internal mammary, free arterial, venous grafts) with bypass graft angiography

The skin over the arterial access site is cleansed and a local anesthetic is administered. The artery is punctured with a needle and a sheath is placed. Using radiological supervision, a guidewire is inserted. The guidewire is threaded through the artery, into the aorta, and positioned in the right or left coronary artery, or an arterial or venous coronary bypass graft, followed by a catheter threaded over the guidewire. The guidewire is removed. Contrast media is injected. The coronary arteries and bypass grafts are visualized and angiograms are obtained. A left cardiac catheterization is also performed. The catheter is advanced into the left ventricle. The aortic valve, left ventricle, mitral valve, and left atrium are inspected. Left ventricular and atrial pressures are obtained as well as pressure gradients across the aortic and mitral valves. Contrast media is injected and a left ventriculogram is obtained as needed. A separately reportable angiogram of the aorta may also be obtained. When the procedure is completed, the catheter is withdrawn, compression is applied over the arterial puncture site, and a compression dressing is applied. Results of the native coronary artery and coronary artery bypass graft studies, left heart catheterization, and left ventriculogram are reviewed and a written report of findings is provided. Use 93458 for combined native coronary artery and left heart catheterization and evaluation. Use 93459 when coronary artery bypass grafts are also evaluated in conjunction with native coronary arteries and left heart structures.

93460-93461

93460 Catheter placement in coronary artery(s) for coronary angiography, including intraprocedural injection(s) for coronary angiography, imaging supervision and interpretation; with right and left heart catheterization including intraprocedural injection(s) for left ventriculography, when performed

93461 Catheter placement in coronary artery(s) for coronary angiography, including intraprocedural injection(s) for coronary angiography, imaging supervision and interpretation; with right and left heart catheterization including intraprocedural injection(s) for left ventriculography, when performed, catheter placement(s) in bypass graft(s) (internal mammary, free arterial, venous grafts) with bypass graft angiography

The skin over the arterial access site is cleansed and a local anesthetic is administered. The artery is punctured with a needle and a sheath is placed. Using radiological supervision, a guidewire is inserted. The guidewire is threaded through the artery, into the aorta, and positioned in the right or left coronary artery, or an arterial or a venous coronary bypass graft, followed by a catheter threaded over the guidewire. The guidewire is removed. Contrast media is injected. The coronary arteries and bypass grafts are visualized and angiograms are obtained. Right and left heart catheterizations are also performed. For the right heart catheterization, the access site is usually the right femoral vein in the groin. A small stab incision is made in the skin and a needle is inserted into the blood vessel followed by a sheath. A guidewire is threaded through the femoral vein, external iliac vein, inferior vena cava, and into the right atrium, followed by a catheter threaded

Medicine

over the guidewire. Once the catheter is positioned, the guidewire is withdrawn. As the catheter is passed through the right side of the heart and into the pulmonary arteries, the right heart chambers are inspected and pressures are obtained. Oxygen levels are measured. The tricuspid and pulmonary valves are inspected and pressure gradients are obtained. A separately reportable angiogram of the right heart and/or pulmonary arteries may be obtained. The left heart catheterization is then performed. The left heart is typically accessed via the same vessel used to access the coronary arteries and/or bypass grafts. The catheter is advanced into the left ventricle. The aortic valve, left ventricle, mitral valve, and left atrium are inspected. Left ventricular and atrial pressures are obtained as well as pressure gradients across the aortic and mitral valves. Contrast is injected and a left ventriculogram is obtained as needed. A separately reportable angiogram of the aorta may be obtained. When the procedure is completed, the catheters are withdrawn, pressure is applied over the venous and arterial puncture sites, and compression dressings are applied. Results of the native coronary artery and coronary artery bypass graft studies, right and left heart catheterization and ventriculogram are reviewed and a written report of findings is provided. Use 93460 for combined native coronary artery and right and left heart catheterization and evaluation. Use 93461 when coronary artery bypass grafts are also evaluated in conjunction with the native coronary arteries and right and left heart structures.

93462

93462   Left heart catheterization by transseptal puncture through intact septum or by transapical puncture (List separately in addition to code for primary procedure)

During a separately reportable heart catheterization procedure, the heart catheter is passed into the left heart through the intact septum by transeptal puncture or by transapical puncture. To perform a transeptal puncture, the catheter is advanced into the right side of the heart. The intra-atrial septum is then punctured and the catheter is advanced into the left atrium. The catheter may remain in the left atrium or it may be passed into the left ventricle. If it remains in the left atrium, the left atrium and mitral valve are inspected and pressures are obtained. If it is passed into the left ventricle, the left ventricle and aortic valve are inspected and pressures are obtained. To perform transapical puncture, the left ventricle is approached percutaneously via a stab incision in the left chest. The catheter is advanced to the heart and a transapical stab incision is made in the left ventricle. The separately reportable evaluation of left heart structures can then be performed. This code for left heart catheterization via the puncturing of an intact heart structure must be used in addition to the main left heart catheterization procedure.

93463

93463   Pharmacologic agent administration (eg, inhaled nitric oxide, intravenous infusion of nitroprusside, dobutamine, milrinone, or other agent) including assessing hemodynamic measurements before, during, after and repeat pharmacologic agent administration, when performed (List separately in addition to code for primary procedure)

During a separately reportable heart catheterization procedure, a pharmacologic agent is administered and additional hemodynamic measures are obtained to evaluate the response to the agent. Hemodynamic measurements are obtained prior to administration of the pharmacologic agent. Measurements may include: cardiac index, cardiac output, central venous pressure, mean arterial pressure, preload, afterload, pulmonary artery pressure, pulmonary capillary wedge pressure, pulmonary vascular resistance, right ventricular pressure, stroke index, stroke volume, and systemic vascular resistance. The pharmacologic agent is then administered. Hemodynamic measurements are performed during the administration and again after the administration. An additional dose of the same agent or a different agent may be administered and hemodynamic measurements repeated. The measurements are compared and interpreted by the physician and a written report of findings is provided. This code may only be reported once in addition to the main heart catheterization procedure.

93464

93464   Physiologic exercise study (eg, bicycle or arm ergometry) including assessing hemodynamic measurements before and after (List separately in addition to code for primary procedure)

During a separately reportable heart catheterization procedure, a pharmacologic agent is administered and additional hemodynamic measures are obtained to evaluate the response to the agent. Hemodynamic measurements are obtained prior to administration of the pharmacologic agent. Measurements may include: cardiac index, cardiac output, central venous pressure, mean arterial pressure, preload, afterload, pulmonary artery pressure, pulmonary capillary wedge pressure, pulmonary vascular resistance, right ventricular pressure, stroke index, stroke volume, and systemic vascular resistance. The pharmacologic agent is then administered. Hemodynamic measurements are performed during the administration and again after the administration. An additional dose of the same agent or a different agent may be administered and hemodynamic measurements repeated. The measurements are compared and interpreted by the physician and a written

report of findings is provided. This code may only be reported once in addition to the main heart catheterization procedure.

93503

93503   Insertion and placement of flow directed catheter (eg, Swan-Ganz) for monitoring purposes

A flow directed catheter, also referred to as a pulmonary artery catheter (PAC), Swan-Ganz, or right heart catheter, is inserted and placed for monitoring purposes. The skin over the planned insertion site in the side of the neck, upper chest, or groin is cleansed and a local anesthetic is injected. A small incision is made in the skin overlying a major vein, most commonly the jugular, subclavian, or femoral vein. A small nick incision is made in the vein, and the flow directed catheter is threaded through the vein, into the right atrium, and advanced into the pulmonary artery. Separately reportable radiographs are obtained to ensure correct positioning of the catheter. The catheter is then connected to the monitoring equipment. The flow directed catheter monitors cardiac pressures, pulmonary artery pressure, and pulmonary capillary wedge pressure as well as cardiac output, mixed venous oxygen saturation, and oxygen saturations in the right heart chambers.

93505

93505   Endomyocardial biopsy

The physician performs an endomyocardial biopsy. The venous or arterial cannulation site is cleansed and a local anesthetic is injected. For right ventricular heart biopsy, the cannulation site is typically the right internal jugular vein and for left ventricular heart biopsy, it is usually the right or left femoral artery. A small incision is made in the skin over the access vein or artery and a needle is used to puncture the vessel. A guidewire is placed and a self sealing sheath is introduced over the guidewire. The sheath is advanced through the blood vessel and positioned in the right or left ventricle. The bioptome is introduced through the sheath, advanced into the right or left ventricle, and oriented toward the septum. The bioptome forceps are directed into the desired biopsy site and a tissue sample is obtained. The bioptome and sheath are removed and pressure is applied to the access site. The skin incision is closed and a pressure dressing is applied.

93530

93530   Right heart catheterization, for congenital cardiac anomalies

A right heart catheterization is performed on a patient with a congenital cardiac anomaly. The skin is cleansed over the catheter access site, usually the right femoral vein in the groin. A local anesthetic is injected. A small stab incision is made in the skin and a needle is inserted into the blood vessel followed by a sheath. A guidewire is threaded through the femoral vein, external iliac vein, inferior vena cava, and into the right atrium. The catheter is then inserted into the vein and threaded over the guidewire into the inferior vena cava. The catheter is then passed into the right atrium, right ventricle, and into the pulmonary arteries. As the catheter is passed through the right side of the heart and into the pulmonary arteries, the right heart chambers are inspected and the congenital cardiac anomaly is evaluated. Blood pressure in the right atrium and ventricle is obtained. Oxygen levels are measured. The tricuspid and pulmonary valves are inspected and evaluated for any anomalies. A separately reportable angiogram of the right heart and/or pulmonary arteries may be obtained. When the procedure is completed, the catheter is withdrawn, compression is applied to the venous access site, and a dressing is applied.

93531

93531   Combined right heart catheterization and retrograde left heart catheterization, for congenital cardiac anomalies

A combined right heart and retrograde left heart catheterization is performed on a patient with a congenital cardiac anomaly. The skin is cleansed over the catheter access sites. For right heart catheterization, the access site is usually the right femoral vein in the groin. A small stab incision is made and a needle is inserted into the vein followed by a sheath. A guidewire is threaded through the femoral vein, external iliac vein, inferior vena cava, and into the right atrium. The catheter is then inserted and threaded over the guidewire into the right atrium, right ventricle, and pulmonary arteries. Once the catheter is positioned, the guidewire is withdrawn. As the catheter is passed through the right side of the heart and into the pulmonary arteries, the right heart chambers are inspected and pressure and oxygen levels are measured. The tricuspid and pulmonary valves are inspected and pressure gradients are obtained. A separately reportable angiogram of the right heart and/or pulmonary arteries may be obtained. A retrograde left heart catheterization is also performed. The skin over the brachial, axillary, or femoral artery is prepped, the artery is punctured with a needle, and a sheath is placed. A guidewire is then inserted and threaded retrograde (against the flow of blood) through the artery, into the aorta, and into the left ventricle and left atrium. A catheter is then threaded over the guidewire and positioned in the left heart and the guidewire is removed. The aortic valve, left ventricle, mitral valve, and left atrium are inspected and any congenital cardiac anomalies of these structures are evaluated. Left ventricular and atrial pressures are obtained as are pressure gradients across the aortic and mitral valves. The catheter may also be positioned in the right and

Medicine

left coronary arteries and any anomalies of these vessels evaluated. When the procedure is completed, the catheters are withdrawn and compression dressings are applied.

93532

**93532	Combined right heart catheterization and transseptal left heart catheterization through intact septum with or without retrograde left heart catheterization, for congenital cardiac anomalies**

A combined right heart catheterization and transseptal left heart catheterization through an intact septum is performed with or without retrograde left heart catheterization for evaluation of a congenital cardiac anamoly. For right heart catheterization, the access site is usually the right femoral vein in the groin. A small stab incision is made and a needle is inserted into the vein followed by a sheath. A guidewire is threaded through the femoral vein, external iliac vein, inferior vena cava, and into the right atrium. The catheter is then inserted and threaded over the guidewire into the right atrium, right ventricle, and pulmonary arteries. Once the catheter is positioned, the guidewire is withdrawn. As the catheter is passed through the right side of the heart and into the pulmonary arteries, the right heart chambers are inspected and pressure and oxygen levels are measured. The tricuspid and pulmonary valves are inspected and pressure gradients are obtained. A separately reportable angiogram of the right heart and/or pulmonary arteries may be obtained. The intra-atrial septum is then punctured and the catheter is advanced into the left atrium. If the catheter remains there, the left atrium and mitral valve are inspected and congenital anomalies are evaluated. If the catheter is passed into the left ventricle, the left ventricle and aortic valve are inspected and any cardiac anomalies evaluated. Left ventricular and atrial pressures are obtained as are pressure gradients across the aortic and mitral valves. The right and left coronary arteries may be inspected. Separately reportable angiograms may be obtained. If a retrograde left heart catheterization is also performed, a second catheter is introduced through the brachial, axillary, or femoral artery and threaded over a guidewire that has been placed retrograde (against the flow of blood) through the artery, into the aorta, and into the left side of the heart. The left heart structures are inspected, cardiac anomalies are evaluated, and additional pressures are obtained.

93533

**93533	Combined right heart catheterization and transseptal left heart catheterization through existing septal opening, with or without retrograde left heart catheterization, for congenital cardiac anomalies**

A combined right heart and left heart transseptal catheterization through an existing septal opening is performed with or without retrograde left heart catheterization for evaluation of congenital cardiac anomalies. For right heart catheterization, the access site is usually the right femoral vein in the groin. A small stab incision is made and a needle is inserted into the vein followed by a sheath. A guidewire is threaded through the femoral vein, external iliac vein, inferior vena cava, and into the right atrium. The catheter is then inserted and threaded over the guidewire into the right atrium, right ventricle, and pulmonary arteries. Once the catheter is positioned, the guidewire is withdrawn. As the catheter is passed through the right side of the heart and into the pulmonary arteries, the right heart chambers are inspected and pressure and oxygen levels are measured. The tricuspid and pulmonary valves are inspected and pressure gradients are obtained. A separately reportable angiogram of the right heart and/or pulmonary arteries may be obtained. The catheter is then advanced through the existing septal opening into the left heart. The left atrium, mitral valve, left ventricle, and aortic valve are inspected and any congenital anomalies evaluated. Left ventricular and atrial pressures are obtained as are pressure gradients across the aortic and mitral valves. The right and left coronary arteries may be inspected and any anomalies evaluated. Separately reportable angiograms may be obtained. If a retrograde left heart catheterization is also performed, a second catheter is introduced through the brachial, axillary, or femoral artery and threaded over a guidewire that has been placed retrograde (against the flow of blood) through the artery, into the aorta, and into the left side of the heart. The left heart structures are inspected, cardiac anomalies are evaluated, and additional pressures obtained.

93561-93562

**93561	Indicator dilution studies such as dye or thermodilution, including arterial and/or venous catheterization; with cardiac output measurement (separate procedure)**

**93562	Indicator dilution studies such as dye or thermodilution, including arterial and/or venous catheterization; subsequent measurement of cardiac output**

Indicator dilution studies with cardiac output measurement are performed to evaluate intracardiac shunts and valvular regurgitation. Cardiac output is a measurement of the amount of blood pumped into the systemic circulation per minute. The procedure differs slightly depending on whether dye or a thermal dilution is used. For indicator dilution studies using a dye, venous and arterial catheters are inserted. A blood sample is obtained and the densitometer is calibrated using known concentrations of the dye mixed with the patient's blood sample. Dye is injected into the catheterized vein. The dye mixes with the blood, circulates through the heart, and is then pumped into the arteries. A blood sample is obtained from the catheterized artery. The densitometer is used to analyze and measure

the amount of dye present in the sample. The densitometer then calculates cardiac output. For indicator dilution studies using cold thermal dilution, a Swan Ganz catheter is inserted through the internal jugular or subclavian vein into the right atrium and ventricle and the tip is advanced into a branch of the pulmonary artery. Cold dextrose is injected via the port in the Swan Ganz catheter that lies in the right atrium. The cold dextrose mixes with the blood in the right atrium and ventricle and then passes into the pulmonary artery where the fall in temperature is sensed by a thermistor on the tip of the catheter lying in the pulmonary artery. Cardiac output is calculated using a temperature-time curve. For indicator dilution studies using warm thermal dilution, a Swan Ganz catheter with a heating coil is introduced into the right heart as described above. A series of heat pulses are administered and signal analysis is used to calculate cardiac output. Use 93561 for a single cardiac output measurement. Use 93562 for a subsequent cardiac output measurement.

93563

**93563	Injection procedure during cardiac catheterization including imaging supervision, interpretation, and report; for selective coronary angiography during congenital heart catheterization (List separately in addition to code for primary procedure)**

An injection procedure is performed for selective opacification of native coronary arteries during a separately reportable cardiac catheterization procedure on a patient with congenital cardiac anomalies. The catheter is positioned in the coronary artery. Contrast media is injected. The artery is visualized and the selective angiograms are obtained. If studies of additional coronary arteries are needed, the catheter is repositioned in the next coronary artery and the procedure is repeated until angiograms have been obtained for all coronary arteries requiring evaluation. The angiograms are reviewed by the physician and a written interpretation of findings is provided. Report this code in addition to the main anomalous heart catheterization procedure.

93564

**93564	Injection procedure during cardiac catheterization including imaging supervision, interpretation, and report; for selective opacification of aortocoronary venous or arterial bypass graft(s) (eg, aortocoronary saphenous vein, free radial artery, or free mammary artery graft) to one or more coronary arteries and in situ arterial conduits (eg, internal mammary), whether native or used for bypass to one or more coronary arteries during congenital heart catheterization, when performed (List separately in addition to code for primary procedure)**

An injection procedure is performed for selective opacification of aortocoronary venous or arterial bypass grafts during a separately reportable cardiac catheterization procedure on a patient with congenital cardiac anomalies. The catheter is positioned in the venous or arterial bypass graft. Contrast media is injected. The bypass graft is visualized and the selective angiograms are obtained. If studies of additional bypass grafts are needed, the catheter is repositioned in the next bypass graft and the procedure is repeated until angiograms have been obtained for all bypass grafts requiring evaluation. The angiograms are reviewed by the physician and a written interpretation of findings is provided. Report this code in addition to the main anomalous heart catheterization procedure.

93565-93566

**93565	Injection procedure during cardiac catheterization including imaging supervision, interpretation, and report; for selective left ventricular or left atrial angiography (List separately in addition to code for primary procedure)**

**93566	Injection procedure during cardiac catheterization including imaging supervision, interpretation, and report; for selective right ventricular or right atrial angiography (List separately in addition to code for primary procedure)**

An injection procedure is performed for selective left ventricular and/or atrial angiography (93565) or selective right ventricular and/or atrial angiography (93566) during a separately reportable cardiac catheterization procedure. In 93565, the catheter is positioned in the left heart. Contrast is injected. The left ventricle and/or atrium are visualized and angiograms are obtained. The angiograms are reviewed by the physician and a written interpretation of findings is provided. Use 93565 in addition to an anomalous heart catheterization procedure. In 93566, the catheter is positioned in the right heart during a separately reportable cardiac catheterization. Contrast media is injected. The right ventricle and/or atrium are visualized and the selective angiograms are obtained. The angiograms are reviewed by the physician and a written interpretation of findings is provided. Use 93566 in conjunction with the primary heart catheterization code.

Medicine

93567

93567   **Injection procedure during cardiac catheterization including imaging supervision, interpretation, and report; for supravalvular aortography (List separately in addition to code for primary procedure)**

An injection procedure is performed for supravalvular ascending aortography during a separately reportable cardiac catheterization procedure. Supravalvular aortography is used to evaluate conditions such as aortic regurgitation, aortic aneurysm or dissection, and congenital anomalies of the aorta. The catheter is positioned in the aorta at the time of the heart catheterization. Contrast media is injected. The aorta is visualized and the aortogram is obtained and processed, then reviewed by the physician. A written interpretation of findings is provided. Report this aortography in conjunction with the primary heart catheterization code.

93568

93568   **Injection procedure during cardiac catheterization including imaging supervision, interpretation, and report; for pulmonary angiography (List separately in addition to code for primary procedure)**

An injection procedure for pulmonary angiography is performed during a separately reportable right heart catheterization procedure. The catheter is positioned in the pulmonary artery. Contrast media is injected to visualize the pulmonary vessels and pulmonary angiography is performed. The resulting angiograms are processed, reviewed by the physician, and a written interpretation of findings is provided. Report this pulmonary angiography in conjunction with the primary right heart catheterization code.

93571-93572

93571   **Intravascular Doppler velocity and/or pressure derived coronary flow reserve measurement (coronary vessel or graft) during coronary angiography including pharmacologically induced stress; initial vessel (List separately in addition to code for primary procedure)**

93572   **Intravascular Doppler velocity and/or pressure derived coronary flow reserve measurement (coronary vessel or graft) during coronary angiography including pharmacologically induced stress; each additional vessel (List separately in addition to code for primary procedure)**

During a separately reportable coronary angiography procedure, a miniaturized Doppler or pressure transducer mounted on a guidewire is advanced through the existing catheter to a point just distal to the coronary vessel or graft being evaluated. Baseline blood flow velocity and/or pressure are obtained. Pharmacologically induced stress is accomplished using an injection of medication directly into the coronary artery to make the heart beat harder and faster. During the pharmacologically induced period of increased bloodflow (hyperemia), additional measurements of blood flow velocity and/or pressure are obtained. These measurements are compared and the difference between baseline blood flow velocity and/or pressure and hyperemic blood flow velocity and/or pressure is determined. These calculations are then used to determine the severity of the coronary artery or coronary graft stenosis or other lesion. Use code 93571 for the initial vessel evaluated and 93572 for each additional vessel studied during the same session.

93580

93580   **Percutaneous transcatheter closure of congenital interatrial communication (ie, Fontan fenestration, atrial septal defect) with implant**

The physician performs a percutaneous transcatheter closure of a congenital interatrial communication, such as an atrial septal defect, using an implant. This procedure may also be used for transcatheter closure of surgically created fenstrations, such as a Fontan fenestration, or for closure of leaks in surgically created baffles or patches. The skin over the access artery, usually one of the femoral arteries, is prepped and the artery is punctured with a needle and a sheath placed. A guidewire is inserted and advanced from the access artery through the aorta and into the heart. A catheter is advanced over the guidewire. A right heart catheterization with left heart catheterization through the existing septal opening is performed. Contrast is injected and angiography performed for visualization of the atrial septal defect. The catheter is passed from the right atrium across the atrial septal defect and into the left atrium. The catheter is advanced into the upper pulmonary vein. Following the diagnostic cardiac catheterization procedure, the first catheter is exchanged for a sizing balloon which is positioned across the defect and inflated to obtain the stretched diameter of the defect. Intracardiac pressures and oxygen saturation may be obtained while occluding the defect to ensure that closure of the defect will be tolerated by the patient. The sizing balloon is exchanged for a dilator that is advanced over a guidewire and positioned in the left atrium. The implant device is positioned in the defect and checked using separately reportable echocardiography. The implant is then deployed and the position checked again using echocardiography and/or angiography.

93581

93581   **Percutaneous transcatheter closure of a congenital ventricular septal defect with implant**

The physician performs a percutaneous transcatheter closure of a congenital ventricular septal defect (VSD) using an implant. The procedure requires percutaneous transcatheter placement through the femoral vein and artery. Depending on the exact nature of the defect an additional venous access may be required via the contralateral femoral vein and/or the jugular vein. The skin over the access vessels is prepped and the vessels are punctured with a needle and sheaths placed. Guidewires are inserted and advanced from the access vessels into the heart. Catheters are advanced over the guidewires. A right and left heart catheterization is performed. Closure of the VSD using an implant device requires crossing of the VSD, sizing of the defect, and delivery of the implant device. Crossing of the defect is dependent on the exact nature of the defect, but usually the VSD is crossed from left to right. Once the catheter is positioned in the left ventricle, a guidewire is advanced through the catheter across the defect and into the right ventricle and then into the pulmonary artery or right atrium. The guidewire is snared using one of the venous access vessels (femoral or jugular vein). An angiography catheter is advanced over the guidewire, contrast is injected, and angiography performed for visualization of the VSD. A sizing balloon catheter is positioned across the defect and inflated to obtain the stretched diameter of the defect. Intracardiac pressures and oxygen saturation may be obtained while occluding the defect to ensure that closure of the defect will be tolerated by the patient. The sizing balloon catheter is exchanged for the implant device. The implant device is positioned in the defect and checked using separately reportable echocardiography. The implant is then deployed and the position checked again using echocardiography and/or angiography.

93582

93582   **Percutaneous transcatheter closure of patent ductus arteriosus**

The ductus arteriosus is a normal structure of fetal circulation that connects the aorta and main pulmonary artery. It normally closes shortly after birth. However, in some newborns the ductus arteriosus fails to close and this is referred to as patent ductus arteriosus (PDA). Transcatheter closure using an occlusive device has largely replaced open surgical closure. With the patient under conscious sedation, the access blood vessel, usually one of the femoral veins, is punctured and a trocar is placed. A guide wire is advanced from the femoral vein through the vena cava, right atrium, right ventricle, and into the main pulmonary artery. The guide wire is then advanced through the PDA and into the descending aorta. The introducer is advanced over the guide wire and into the aorta. The catheter and sheath containing the occluding device are carefully positioned in the descending aorta to provide coverage of the PDA. Angiograms are obtained to confirm correct placement of the occlusion device. The sheath is removed and the occlusion device is deployed. Angiograms are again obtained to evaluate positioning of the device and to ensure that the PDA is closed. All catheters are removed and pressure is applied to the puncture site in the groin.

93583

93583   **Percutaneous transcatheter septal reduction therapy (eg, alcohol septal ablation) including temporary pacemaker insertion when performed**

Percutaneous transcatheter septal reduction therapy, also referred to as percutaneous transluminal septal myocardial ablation (PTSMA), is performed to treat dynamic left ventricular outflow tract (LVOT) obstruction which is a complication of hypertrophic obstructive cardiomyopathy (HOCM). Prior to the start of the septal reduction procedure, a temporary pacemaker is inserted if needed. An incision is made in the upper chest over the access vessel, usually the cephalic, subclavian, or jugular vein. A sheath is inserted into the selected vein and the pacemaker wire is advanced under radiological guidance into the selected heart chamber. The lead is positioned against the wall of the heart chamber. This is repeated if a temporary dual chamber pacemaker is placed. The lead is tested to ensure it is working properly and attached to an external generator that is taped to the skin. The PTSMA is then performed. The skin over the access site, usually the femoral artery, is cleansed and a local anesthetic is administered. The artery is punctured with a needle and a sheath is placed. Using radiological supervision, a guide wire is inserted. The guide wire is threaded through the access artery, into the aorta, and advanced from the aorta into the left anterior descending coronary artery. A catheter is advanced over the guide wire and angiograms are obtained to delineate the coronary artery vasculature. The angiogram catheter is removed and a balloon catheter is advanced over the guide wire. One of the small septal branches of the left anterior descending coronary artery is selected and an angioplasty balloon is positioned in the septal branch, inflated, and the artery is temporarily occluded. Alcohol is then instilled causing a localized myocardial infarction. The procedure may be repeated on a second septal branch. The myocardial infarction resulting from the instillation of alcohol causes necrosis of septal tissue. When the tissue heals, scarring causes thinning of the septum at the LVOT, reducing the obstruction and improving left ventricular function. Upon completion of the procedure, the balloon catheter and guide wire are removed and pressure is applied to the puncture site. The temporary pacemaker may remain in place while the septum heals.

93600-93603

93600 Bundle of His recording
93602 Intra-atrial recording
93603 Right ventricular recording

The physician obtains recordings from the bundle or His, the atria, or the right ventricle. One or more access veins are selected, such as the femoral or jugular veins. The skin over the access veins are prepped and the veins are punctured with a needle and sheaths placed. Using continuous fluoroscopic guidance, guidewires are inserted and advanced from the access veins into the heart. Catheters are advanced over the guidewire and positioned in the heart. The guidewires are removed. Recordings are then obtained using an electrode-mounted catheter. In 93600, a bundle of His recording is performed. The bundle of His, also referred to as the atrioventricular bundle, is a tract of conducting fibers that distribute an electrical impulse over the medial surfaces of the ventricles to the Purkinje fibers. The Purkinje fibers stimulate the ventricles to contract. This test measures electrical activity in the bundle of His. Interruption or blockage of electrical impulses in the bundle of His causes an irregular heartbeat. Recordings are obtained of electrical activity in the bundle of His. The physician reviews the recordings and provides a written report. In 93602, intra-atrial recording is performed. This test is performed to determine whether there is an atrial flutter or atrial fibrillation that cannot be detected by transthoracic electrocardiography (ECG). Intra-atrial electrical activity is recorded. The physician reviews the recordings and provides a written report. In 93603, right ventricular recording is performed. This test is performed to determine whether electrical impulses in the right ventricle are causing a dysynchronous contractions. The physician reviews the recordings and provides a written report.

93609

93609 Intraventricular and/or intra-atrial mapping of tachycardia site(s) with catheter manipulation to record from multiple sites to identify origin of tachycardia (List separately in addition to code for primary procedure)

Standard intraventricular and/or intra-atrial mapping of tachycardia sites is performed. Mapping is used to trace the origin of the tachycardia site and/or identify the electrical path of the tachycardia through the heart during a separately reportable arrhythmia induction procedure. Intra-cardiac catheters are placed in a separately reportable procedure. Standard mapping uses a sequential mapping technique. Electrode-mounted catheters are repositioned from one point to the next within the heart and sequential recordings taken from each site. A mapping of the tachycardia sites is then constructed from the sequential recordings. The physician reviews the recordings, mapping, and provides a written report.

93610-93612

93610 Intra-atrial pacing
93612 Intraventricular pacing

Intra-atrial or intraventricular pacing is performed. Pacing uses electrical impulses to change the heart rhythm. One or more access veins are selected, such as the femoral or jugular veins. The skin over the access veins are prepped and the veins are punctured with a needle and sheaths placed. Using continuous fluoroscopic guidance, guidewires are inserted and advanced from the access veins into the heart. Catheters are advanced over the guidewire and positioned in the atria or ventricles. The guidewires are removed. The physician then initiates the pacing procedure. Pacing is used to determine whether the patient needs an electrophysiological procedure, pacemaker, cardioverter, or other interventional procedure or device. The physician reviews the results of the pacing procedure and provides a written report. Use 93610 when intra-atrial pacing is performed and 93612 for intraventricular pacing.

93613

93613 Intracardiac electrophysiologic 3-dimensional mapping (List separately in addition to code for primary procedure)

The physician performs 3-dimensional (3D) mapping of tachycardia sites. Mapping is used to trace the origin of the tachycardia site and/or identify the electrical path of the tachycardia through the heart during a separately reportable arrhythmia induction procedure. Intra-cardiac catheters are placed in a separately reportable procedure. Using 3D mapping, simultaneous recordings from multiple electrodes on the same catheter are obtained. A computer reconstruction is then used to provide a 3D mapping of the tachycardia sequence. Additional recordings are obtained as needed to confirm the arrhythmia origin, to study additional arrhythmias and their sources, and at the conclusion of the mapping procedure. The physician reviews the recordings, mapping, and provides a written report.

93615-93616

93615 Esophageal recording of atrial electrogram with or without ventricular electrogram(s)
93616 Esophageal recording of atrial electrogram with or without ventricular electrogram(s); with pacing

Esophageal recording of atrial electrocardiogram (ECG) is performed with or without ventricular ECG with or without pacing. An esophageal probe with electrodes for monitoring heart rhythm is inserted through the mouth and advanced into the esophagus. The probe is positioned in the esophagus at a point just behind the heart. Atrial ECG recordings are obtained. Ventricular ECG recordings may also be obtained. The physician may then initiate the pacing procedure and obtain additional ECG recordings. Pacing is used to determine whether the patient needs an electrophysiological procedure, pacemaker, cardioverter, or other interventional procedure or device. The physician reviews the results of the esophageal ECG recordings and the pacing procedure and provides a written report. Use 93615 when esophageal ECG recordings are obtained without a pacing procedure and 93616 when a pacing procedure is performed in conjunction with the esophageal ECG recordings.

93618

93618 Induction of arrhythmia by electrical pacing

Electrical pacing is performed to induce an arrhythmia in a patient experiencing intermittent episodes of irregular heart rhythm. One or more access veins are selected, such as the femoral or jugular veins. The skin over the access veins are prepped and the veins are punctured with a needle and sheaths placed. Using continuous fluoroscopic guidance, guidewires are inserted and advanced from the access veins into the heart. Catheters are advanced over the guidewire and positioned in the atria or ventricles. The guidewires are removed. The physician then initiates the pacing procedure. Pacing is at different rates or programmed stimulation is performed using timed electrical impulses to induce an arrhythmia. Catheters may be repositioned during the arrhythmia induction and pacing or programmed stimulation performed at multiple sites in the heart. The physician reviews the results of the pacing procedure and the resulting arrhythmia and provides a written report.

93619

93619 Comprehensive electrophysiologic evaluation with right atrial pacing and recording, right ventricular pacing and recording, His bundle recording, including insertion and repositioning of multiple electrode catheters, without induction or attempted induction of arrhythmia

A comprehensive electrophysiologic study (EPS) of the right atrium and right ventricle is performed without induction or attempted induction of arrhythmia. A comprehensive study includes right atrial pacing and recording, right ventricular pacing and recording, His bundle recording, and insertion and repositioning of multiple electrode catheters. The skin is punctured or a small incision made over one or more blood vessels, usually in the groin. One or more catheters are inserted into the blood vessel(s). The catheters contain recording and stimulating electrodes. These catheters are threaded from the insertion site into the right atrium and right ventricle of the heart. Once inside the heart the recording electrode catheters measure and record electrical activity in the right side of the heart, and the stimulating electrode catheters pace the right side of the heart. Electrical activity in the bundle of His is recorded. The bundle of His is a group fibers that carry electrical impulses through the center of the heart. The bundle of His emerges from the atrioventricular (AV) node, lies along the upper intraventricular septum, and forms three branches, the right and left anterosuperior bundle branches and the left posteroinferior bundle branch. Interruption or blockage of these impulses in the bundle of His can cause irregular heart rhythm. When the procedure is completed, the catheter(s) are withdrawn and pressure applied to the puncture/incision sites.

93620-93622

93620 Comprehensive electrophysiologic evaluation including insertion and repositioning of multiple electrode catheters with induction or attempted induction of arrhythmia; with right atrial pacing and recording, right ventricular pacing and recording, His bundle recording
93621 Comprehensive electrophysiologic evaluation including insertion and repositioning of multiple electrode catheters with induction or attempted induction of arrhythmia; with left atrial pacing and recording from coronary sinus or left atrium (List separately in addition to code for primary procedure)
93622 Comprehensive electrophysiologic evaluation including insertion and repositioning of multiple electrode catheters with induction or attempted induction of arrhythmia; with left ventricular pacing and recording (List separately in addition to code for primary procedure)

A comprehensive electrophysiologic study (EPS) of the right atrium and right ventricle is performed with induction or attempted induction of arrhythmia. In 93620, a comprehensive study including right atrial pacing and recording, right ventricular pacing and recording, His bundle recording, and insertion and repositioning of multiple electrode catheters

© 2017 DecisionHealth   CPT © 2016 American Medical Association. All Rights Reserved.   ● New Code   ▲ Revised Code

Medicine

is performed. The skin is punctured or a small incision made over one or more blood vessels, usually in the groin. One or more catheters are inserted into the blood vessel(s). The catheters contain recording and stimulating electrodes. These catheters are threaded from the insertion site into the right atrium and right ventricle of the heart. Once inside the heart the recording electrode catheters measure and record electrical activity in the right side of the heart, and the stimulating electrode catheters pace the right side of the heart. Electrical activity in the bundle of His is recorded. The bundle of HIS is a group fibers that carry electrical impulses through the center of the heart. The bundle of HIS emerges from the atrioventricular (AV) node, lies along the upper intraventricular septum, and forms three branches, the right and left anterosuperior bundle branches and the left posteroinferior bundle branch. Interruption or blockage of these impulses in the bundle of His can cause irregular heart rhythm. Following the EPS study, pacing with induction or attempted induction of arrhythmia is performed. The arrhythmia is induced using pacing at different rates or programmed stimulation using timed electrical impulses. Catheters may be repositioned during the arrhythmia induction and pacing or programmed stimulation performed at multiple sites in the heart. When the procedure is completed, the catheter(s) are withdrawn and pressure applied to the puncture/incision sites. The physician interprets the results of the procedure and provides a written report. In 93621, the physician performs left atrial pacing and recording from the coronary sinus or left atrium at the time of the separately reportable comprehensive EPS. An electrode catheter is placed in the coronary sinus or left atrium. The catheter is manipulated to a position where optimum ECG recordings from the left atrium can be obtained. The physician may also perform pacing and attempt to induce the arrhythmia from this site. In 93622, the physician performs left ventricular pacing and recording at the time of the separately reportable comprehensive EPS. The catheter is manipulated to a position where optimum ECG recordings from the left ventricle can be obtained. The physician may also perform pacing and attempt to induce the arrhythmia from this site.

93623

93623 **Programmed stimulation and pacing after intravenous drug infusion (List separately in addition to code for primary procedure)**

The physician performs programmed stimulation and pacing following intravenous drug infusion performed during a separately reportable electrophysiologic study (EPS). An intravenous infusion of a drug, such as isoproterenol or procainamide, is performed to aid in the evaluation of an arrhythmia. The drug infused may help induce or suppress the arrhythmia. Following the drug infusion the physician performs additional stimulation and pacing procedures. The physician induces or attempts to induce the arrhythmia using pacing at different rates or programmed stimulation using timed electrical impulses. Catheters may be repositioned during the arrhythmia induction and pacing or programmed stimulation performed at multiple sites in the heart. The physician interprets the results of the procedure and provides a written report.

93624

93624 **Electrophysiologic follow-up study with pacing and recording to test effectiveness of therapy, including induction or attempted induction of arrhythmia**

A follow-up electrophysiologic study (EPS) to test the effectiveness of therapy is performed with pacing, recording, and induction or attempted induction of arrhythmia. Following a separately reportable therapy for treatment of a cardiac arrhythmia, an EPS follow-up study is performed. One or more catheters containing recording and stimulating electrodes are inserted into the access blood vessel(s), usually in the groin, and threaded through the vascular system into the right atrium and right ventricle. Once inside the heart, the recording electrode catheters measure and record electrical activity in the heart, and the stimulating electrode catheters pace the heart. Arrhythmia is induced or attempts are made to induce arrhythmia using pacing at different rates or programmed stimulation using timed electrical impulses. Catheters may be repositioned during the arrhythmia induction and pacing or programmed stimulation may be performed at multiple sites in the heart. These measurements and recordings, pacing procedures, and attempts to induce arrhythmia are evaluated and compared to EPS studies performed prior to therapy to determine the effectiveness of the arrhythmia treatment.

93631

93631 **Intra-operative epicardial and endocardial pacing and mapping to localize the site of tachycardia or zone of slow conduction for surgical correction**

The physician performs intra-operative epicardial and endocardial pacing and mapping to localize the site of a tachycardia or the zone of slow conduction so that it can be surgically corrected. During a separately reportable open heart surgery, electrodes are placed on the surface of the heart and within the heart chambers. The physician induces or attempts to induce the arrhythmia using pacing at different rates or programmed stimulation using timed electrical impulses. Catheters placed within the heart may be repositioned during the arrhythmia induction and pacing or programmed stimulation performed at multiple sites in the heart. Standard or 3-dimensional (3D) mapping of the arrhythmia sites is also performed. Mapping is used to trace the origin of the tachycardia site and/or identify the electrical path of the tachycardia through the heart. Standard mapping uses a sequential

mapping technique. Electrode-mounted catheters are repositioned from one point to the next within the heart and sequential recordings taken from each site. A mapping of the tachycardia sites is then constructed from the sequential recordings. Using 3D mapping, simultaneous recordings from multiple electrodes on the same catheter are obtained. A computer reconstruction is then used to provide a 3D mapping of the tachycardia sequence. Additional recordings are obtained as needed to confirm the arrhythmia origin, to study additional arrhythmias and their sources, and at the conclusion of the mapping procedure. The physician interprets the recordings, pacing, and mapping procedures and provides a written report.

93640-93641

93640 **Electrophysiologic evaluation of single or dual chamber pacing cardioverter-defibrillator leads including defibrillation threshold evaluation (induction of arrhythmia, evaluation of sensing and pacing for arrhythmia termination) at time of initial implantation or replacement**

93641 **Electrophysiologic evaluation of single or dual chamber pacing cardioverter-defibrillator leads including defibrillation threshold evaluation (induction of arrhythmia, evaluation of sensing and pacing for arrhythmia termination) at time of initial implantation or replacement; with testing of single or dual chamber pacing cardioverter-defibrillator pulse generator**

An electrophysiologic evaluation of single or dual chamber pacing cardioverter-defibrillator leads is performed at the time of initial implantation or replacement with an evaluation of the defibrillation threshold including induction of arrhythmia and evaluation of sensing and pacing for arrhythmia termination. The pacing cardioverter-defibrillator leads are checked to make sure that they are placed and functioning correctly. After placement of the transvenous leads, an arrhythmia is induced and the leads are checked to verify that they are optimally placed for sensing the arrhythmia. A threshold evaluation is performed to verify that the energy level of the shock delivered by the cardioverter-defibrillator is sufficient to terminate the arrhythmia. The leads are also checked to verify that the arrhythmia has been converted to a normal rate and rhythm. Use 93641 when the pulse generator is also tested.

93642

93642 **Electrophysiologic evaluation of single or dual chamber transvenous pacing cardioverter-defibrillator (includes defibrillation threshold evaluation, induction of arrhythmia, evaluation of sensing and pacing for arrhythmia termination, and programming or reprogramming of sensing or therapeutic parameters)**

A periodic electrophysiologic evaluation of single or dual chamber transvenous pacing cardioverter-defibrillator is performed with an evaluation of defibrillation threshold including induction of arrhythmia and evaluation of sensing and pacing for arrhythmia termination. This procedure includes any required programming or reprogramming of sensing or therapeutic parameters. Previously placed transvenous pacing cardioverter-defibrillators are evaluated periodically to verify that they are functioning properly and are able to sense the arrhythmia. A threshold evaluation is performed to verify that the energy level of the shock delivered by the cardioverter-defibrillator is sufficient to terminate the arrhythmia. The leads are also checked to verify that the arrhythmia has been converted to a normal rate and rhythm. Following evaluation of the transvenous leads, the pacing cardioverter-defibrillator sensing or therapeutic parameters may be changed to enhance the effectiveness of the device.

93644

93644 **Electrophysiologic evaluation of subcutaneous implantable defibrillator (includes defibrillation threshold evaluation, induction of arrhythmia, evaluation of sensing for arrhythmia termination, and programming or reprogramming of sensing or therapeutic parameters)**

The implanted subcutaneous defibrillator requires evaluation and interrogation every 1-6 months by a cardiologist and/or electrophysiologist. Additional evaluation and reprogramming may be required if the patient's medical condition changes or when the device fails to deliver appropriate treatment. Stored data is retrieved from the device by using an external magnet or sensor to download the information into a computer program. This information may include the number of ventricular tachycardia (VT) and/or ventricular fibrillation (VF) events appropriately detected and treated, and any inappropriate shocks that were delivered. Inappropriate treatment may occur with supraventricular tachycardia (SVT) when the heart rate satisfies the VT or VF rate threshold programmed into the device or when environmental noise such as exposure to an antitheft device in a store triggers a therapeutic shock. Interval testing of the device is also necessary to monitor battery life and voltage delivery during treatment. Following the retrieval of stored data, with the patient on a cardiac monitor, sedated as necessary and appropriate resuscitative equipment on standby, an arrhythmia is induced and the device is monitored for appropriate interpretation of the arrhythmia and response. The sensing and therapeutic parameters are reprogrammed as necessary for optimal device function.

93650

93650   Intracardiac catheter ablation of atrioventricular node function, atrioventricular conduction for creation of complete heart block, with or without temporary pacemaker placement

Intracardiac catheter ablation of atrioventricular node function and/or atrioventricular conduction for creation of complete heart block is performed to treat patients with atrial fibrillation. In another separately reportable procedure, the site of the arrhythmia is identified and mapped and the arrhythmia cycle is measured following the induction of arrhythmia. Ablation catheters are inserted and positioned at the atrioventricular (AV) junction using either a transaortic or transseptal approach. Radiofrequency or cryoablation is used to interrupt the conduction pathway of electrical impulses and create a complete right heart block. An attempt is made to induce arrhythmia. If arrhythmia occurs, the catheter is repositioned and the AV junction is again ablated. This is repeated until a complete AV block has been created as demonstrated by the inability to induce the arrhythmia. A temporary pacemaker may be placed to manage the resulting AV block.

93653-93655

93653   Comprehensive electrophysiologic evaluation including insertion and repositioning of multiple electrode catheters with induction or attempted induction of an arrhythmia with right atrial pacing and recording, right ventricular pacing and recording (when necessary), and His bundle recording (when necessary) with intracardiac catheter ablation of arrhythmogenic focus; with treatment of supraventricular tachycardia by ablation of fast or slow atrioventricular pathway, accessory atrioventricular connection, cavo-tricuspid isthmus or other single atrial focus or source of atrial re-entry

93654   Comprehensive electrophysiologic evaluation including insertion and repositioning of multiple electrode catheters with induction or attempted induction of an arrhythmia with right atrial pacing and recording, right ventricular pacing and recording (when necessary), and His bundle recording (when necessary) with intracardiac catheter ablation of arrhythmogenic focus; with treatment of ventricular tachycardia or focus of ventricular ectopy including intracardiac electrophysiologic 3D mapping, when performed, and left ventricular pacing and recording, when performed

93655   Intracardiac catheter ablation of a discrete mechanism of arrhythmia which is distinct from the primary ablated mechanism, including repeat diagnostic maneuvers, to treat a spontaneous or induced arrhythmia (List separately in addition to code for primary procedure)

A comprehensive electrophysiologic study (EPS) of the right atrium and right ventricle is performed including right atrial pacing and recording, and insertion and repositioning of multiple electrode catheters in conjunction with intracardiac catheter ablation. Right ventricular pacing and recording, and His bundle recording may also be performed when necessary. The skin is punctured or a small incision made over one or more blood vessels, usually in the groin. The catheters containing recording and stimulating electrodes are threaded from the insertion site into the right atrium and right ventricle of the heart. Once inside the heart, the recording electrode catheters measure and record electrical activity in the right side of the heart, and the stimulating electrode catheters pace the right side of the heart. Electrical activity in the bundle of His is recorded. Following the EPS study, pacing with induction or attempted induction of arrhythmia is performed. The arrhythmia is induced using pacing at different rates or programmed stimulation using timed electrical impulses. Catheters may be repositioned during the arrhythmia induction and pacing or programmed stimulation performed at multiple sites in the heart. The arrhythmogenic focus is identified and an ablation catheter tip advanced to the focus or pathway. Radiofrequency electrical energy, microwave energy, or cryoablation is applied to the cardiac tissue and the arrhythmogenic focus interrupted or destroyed. After the ablation procedure, testing is performed to ensure that tachycardia cannot be induced. Use code 93653 for treatment of supraventircular tachycardia by ablation of fast or slow atrioventricular pathways, accessory atrioventricular connections, or other atrial foci. Use 93654 when intracardiac catheter ablation of an arrhythmogenic focus is performed to treat life-threatening ventricular tachycardia or a focus of ventricular ectopy. Use add-on code 93655 when intracardiac catheter ablation is performed to treat a discrete mechanism of arrhythmia that is distinct from the primary site. Ablation catheters are inserted and positioned at the separate and distinct site. The site is ablated. Testing is again performed to ensure that the arrhythmia cannot be induced. This is repeated until the anomalous pathway has been obliterated as demonstrated by the inability to induce the arrhythmia. When the procedure is completed, the catheter(s) are withdrawn and pressure is applied to the puncture/incision sites. The physician interprets the results of the procedure and provides a written report.

93656-93657

93656   Comprehensive electrophysiologic evaluation including transseptal catheterizations, insertion and repositioning of multiple electrode catheters with induction or attempted induction of an arrhythmia including left or right atrial pacing/recording when necessary, right ventricular pacing/recording when necessary, and His bundle recording when necessary with intracardiac catheter ablation of atrial fibrillation by pulmonary vein isolation

93657   Additional linear or focal intracardiac catheter ablation of the left or right atrium for treatment of atrial fibrillation remaining after completion of pulmonary vein isolation (List separately in addition to code for primary procedure)

A comprehensive electrophysiologic study (EPS) is performed with induction or attempted induction of arrhythmia in conjunction with intracardiac catheter ablation. This procedure includes transseptal catheterizations and insertion and repositioning of multiple electrode catheters. The EPS study also includes as needed left or right atrial pacing and recording, right ventricular pacing and recording, and His bundle recording. All areas involved in triggering or maintaining atrial fibrillation are evaluated. The skin is punctured or a small incision is made over one or more blood vessels, usually in the groin. The catheters containing recording and stimulating electrodes are threaded from the insertion site into the right and/or left atrium and/or right ventricle of the heart. Once positioned, the recording electrode catheters measure electrical activity and the stimulating electrode catheters pace the left or right side of the heart. Electrical activity in the bundle of His is recorded. Following the EPS study, pacing with induction or attempted induction of arrhythmia is performed. The arrhythmia is induced using pacing at different rates or programmed stimulation using timed electrical impulses. Catheters may be repositioned during the arrhythmia induction and pacing or programmed stimulation performed at multiple sites in the heart. To treat atrial fibrillation by ablation by pulmonary vein isolation (93656), the intracardiac ablation catheter is applied to the targeted tissue around the connections of the pulmonary veins to the left atrium. When the procedure is completed, the catheter(s) are withdrawn and pressure applied to the puncture/incision sites. The physician interprets the results of the procedure and provides a written report. Report code 93657 for additional linear or focal intracardiac catheter ablation of the left or right atrium performed to treat atrial fibrillation remaining after completion of the initial pulmonary vein isolation.

93660

93660   Evaluation of cardiovascular function with tilt table evaluation, with continuous ECG monitoring and intermittent blood pressure monitoring, with or without pharmacological intervention

Cardiovascular function is evaluated using a tilt table with continuous ECG and intermittent blood pressure monitoring. Tilt table testing is used to diagnose the cause of syncope (fainting). Following placement of ECG electrodes and a blood pressure monitor, the patient is placed supine on a tilt table with restraints attached to keep the patient in position when the tilt table is raised and lowered. The table is then rapidly raised to a 60 degree angle and kept at that angle while heart rate and blood pressure are monitored and any resulting syncope is observed. If the test does not induce syncope, a pharmacological agent that causes venous pooling or increases adrenergic stimulation is administered intravenously and the test is repeated. Any hypotensive changes in blood pressure, heart rate slowing (bradycardia), or syncope is noted and monitored.

93662

93662   Intracardiac echocardiography during therapeutic/diagnostic intervention, including imaging supervision and interpretation (List separately in addition to code for primary procedure)

Intracardiac echocardiography (ICE) is performed during a therapeutic or diagnostic intervention including imaging supervision and interpretation. ICE provides images of the whole heart and surrounding structures throughout the entire duration of a separately reportable cardiac procedure. The femoral vein is punctured and the ICE catheter is advanced over a guidewire into the inferior vena cava and then into the right atrium. Alternatively, the ICE catheter may be inserted into the internal jugular or left subclavian vein, passed over a guidewire into the superior vena cava, and then into the right atrium. Ultrasound images are obtained using M-mode or B-mode with Doppler images which may include pulsed wave, continuous wave, and/or color wave imaging. Typically, 2D images are obtained with 3D reconstruction performed as needed. The real-time images of heart structures are used to identify normal and abnormal conduction pathways and facilitate placement of catheters within the heart, such as the tip of an ablation catheter. ICE is also used to monitor for complications, such as cardiac perforation, pericardial effusion, or cardiac tamponade. Upon completion of the diagnostic or therapeutic intervention, the ICE catheter is removed. The physician provides an interpretation of the ICE images with a written report of findings.

Medicine

93668

93668   Peripheral arterial disease (PAD) rehabilitation, per session

Peripheral artery disease (PAD) rehabilitation is performed. Patients with intermittent claudication, or recent peripheral vascular surgery such as angioplasty, stenting, or grafting may benefit from these rehabilitation services. Under the direction of a physician, a non-physician health care provider, such as an exercise physiologist or nurse, develops a rehabilitation program that uses exercise sessions on a motorized treadmill or track to determine the patient's symptom-limited exercise threshold. The supervising provider monitors and adjusts the workload based on the patient's response. When the symptom-limited threshold has been reached, the patient rests until symptoms diminish and then resumes exercise until a total of 30-45 minutes of total exercise time has been accrued. The supervising physician must be immediately available during the rehabilitation sessions, but does not need to be in the room. The physician provides ongoing supervision of the rehabilitation program including training and evaluation of personnel and development of safety standards. The physician is also available to intervene should patients develop angina, arrhythmia, or other complications. Typically, the patient receives 3 days of PAD rehabilitation per week for a period of at least 12 weeks. Services are provided in a group setting and are reported once per patient per session.

93701

93701   Bioimpedance-derived physiologic cardiovascular analysis

Bioimpedence is a noninvasive test used to evaluate cardiac physiology and may also be referred to as thoracic electrical bioimpeedance (TEB). Bioimpedance is a form of plethysmography that is used to measure cardiac output, respiration and other cardiovascular parameters. New bioimpedance technology allows measurement of cardiac index (CI) (blood flow per minute), stroke index (SI) (blood flow per beat), heart and respiratory rates, ventricular ejection time, pre-ejection period, ejection phase contractility index, inotropic state index, estimate of ejection fraction, and end-diastolic index. Bioimpedance-derived analysis of cardiac physiology uses eight electrodes (four on each side) placed over the lateral aspects of the neck and chest or upper abdomen. The electrodes are attached via a cable to the bioimpedance machine. A low magnitude current is passed though the thorax parallel to the spine between the electrodes in the neck and upper abdomen. As the current travels through the thorax, most of the current is deflected to through the thoracic aorta and inferior and superior vena cava. The electrical signals are recorded by the bioimpedance machine which can produce a printed readout of the various parameters recorded. The physician reviews and interprets the recordings and provides a written report of findings.

93702

93702   Bioimpedance spectroscopy (BIS), extracellular fluid analysis for lymphedema assessment(s)

Analysis of extracellular fluid using bioimpedance spectroscopy (BIS) may be used to identify individuals at risk for lymphedema following surgery or radiation and also to monitor the disease and response to treatment. Lymphedema is a chronic condition caused by impairment, disruption, or dysfunction of the lymphatic drainage system. Protein rich extracellular fluid accumulates in dependent tissue causing fibrotic changes and lipid accumulation that may lead to pain, paresthesias, and/or infection in the affected extremity. BIS is a minimally invasive technique used for detecting alterations in extracellular fluid volume by applying an alternating current though a set of cutaneous electrodes. The patient is positioned supine on a non-conducting surface, and the limbs are slightly abducted with upper extremities pronated. The skin is cleansed with alcohol and two measurement electrodes are placed at the wrist of the affected upper extremity and 2 drive electrodes placed about 5 cm below on the hand. When assessing lower extremities, the measurement electrode is placed at the ankle and the drive electrode on the foot. The low frequency current travels through the path of least resistance (extracellular fluid) with the higher frequency current passing through both extracellular and intracellular fluid creating a picture of total fluid volume. When assessing an individual with unilateral lymphedema, the non-affected limb may be tested using BIS to obtain (normal) control values.

93724

93724   Electronic analysis of antitachycardia pacemaker system (includes electrocardiographic recording, programming of device, induction and termination of tachycardia via implanted pacemaker, and interpretation of recordings)

A periodic evaluation of an antitachycardia pacemaker system is performed in an office or clinic setting. Heart rhythm is monitored using electrocardiography (ECG) as the antitachycardia pacemaker system is evaluated. The generator is interrogated using an external sensing device. The antitachycardia leads are checked to make sure they are functioning correctly. Tachycardia is induced using the implanted pacemaker. The leads are checked to verify that they have sensed the change in heart rate and rhythm. The feedback system of the leads and generator is evaluated to ensure that the increased heart rate and rhythm is sensed, and that the antitachycardia generator is promptly triggered to deliver

a shock that terminates the arrhythmia. The timing of the shock is evaluated to ensure the device has sensed and terminated the arrhythmia within the set time parameters. The energy level of the shock is also evaluated to ensure it is sufficient to terminate the arrhythmia. The leads are again checked to verify that they have sensed the return of the patient's heart rate and rhythm to normal. The physician may reprogram the device based on the evaluation. A written interpretation of the antitachycardia pacemaker evaluation and the ECG recordings is provided.

93740

93740   Temperature gradient studies

Temperature gradient studies are performed to evaluate the heart and circulatory system using contrasting temperatures of the blood vessels. An intravenous catheter is advanced into the blood vessels to be studied. Intravascular temperatures of the internal walls of the blood vessels are obtained. The temperatures are compared and a written interpretation of the variations in temperature of the blood vessel walls is provided.

93745

93745   Initial set-up and programming by a physician or other qualified health care professional of wearable cardioverter-defibrillator includes initial programming of system, establishing baseline electronic ECG, transmission of data to data repository, patient instruction in wearing system and patient reporting of problems or events

A wearable cardioverter defibrillator may be used temporarily by a patient following a myocardial infarction, coronary artery bypass surgery, or percutaneous coronary intervention such as angioplasty, atherectomy or stent placement. It may also temporarily in patients considered to have other risks for sudden cardiac arrest. During the initial set-up and programming, the patient is connected to the electrocardiogram (ECG) monitor. A connection is established between the wearable cardioverter-defibrillator system and the programming device. Cardiac rhythm is assessed and baseline programming is performed. The patient is instructed on use of the device including transmission of data to the physician or other qualified health care professional and the need to report any problems or cardiac events. Data is transmitted as needed and stored data related to cardiac rhythm and any tachyarrhythmia episodes is reviewed.

93750

93750   Interrogation of ventricular assist device (VAD), in person, with physician or other qualified health care professional analysis of device parameters (eg, drivelines, alarms, power surges), review of device function (eg, flow and volume status, septum status, recovery), with programming, if performed, and report

An in-person interrogation and evaluation of a ventricular assist device (VAD) with physician or other qualified health care professional analysis, review, programming, and report is performed. In-person interrogation and device evaluation may be performed on a routine basis or when the patient presents with symptoms or complaints that might be due to device malfunction or to a change in cardiac function. A connection is established between the VAD device and the interrogation device. The VAD is interrogated. The physician reviews interrogated data to assess VAD function and current programmed parameters. Parameters analyzed include drivelines, alarms, and power surges. Device function is evaluated for flow and volume status, septum, status and recovery. The physician may reprogram the device if needed. The patient is informed of the VAD interrogation findings. The physician provides a written report of findings.

93784-93790

93784   Ambulatory blood pressure monitoring, utilizing a system such as magnetic tape and/or computer disk, for 24 hours or longer; including recording, scanning analysis, interpretation and report
93786   Ambulatory blood pressure monitoring, utilizing a system such as magnetic tape and/or computer disk, for 24 hours or longer; recording only
93788   Ambulatory blood pressure monitoring, utilizing a system such as magnetic tape and/or computer disk, for 24 hours or longer; scanning analysis with report
93790   Ambulatory blood pressure monitoring, utilizing a system such as magnetic tape and/or computer disk, for 24 hours or longer; review with interpretation and report

Ambulatory blood pressure monitoring is performed to identify blood pressure fluctuations over a 24-hour or longer period. It may be performed to determine whether blood pressure is normal outside a clinic setting or whether blood pressure medications are working properly throughout the day. The blood pressure cuff and portable monitoring device are set up at the office or clinic. The device is programmed to take and record blood pressure readings at regular intervals throughout the day. At the end of the designated time period the device is returned and the readings are reviewed. Use code 93784 when recording and interpretation and report are performed; code 93786 for the recording only; code 93788 for a scanning analysis and report only; or code 93790 if only a review of the procedure with an interpretation and report is performed.

93797-93798

93797 Physician or other qualified health care professional services for outpatient cardiac rehabilitation; without continuous ECG monitoring (per session)

93798 Physician or other qualified health care professional services for outpatient cardiac rehabilitation; with continuous ECG monitoring (per session)

Cardiac rehabilitation is a professionally supervised program of exercise and education designed to help with recovery from a heart attack, open heart surgery or other coronary intervention procedures such as stenting or angioplasty. The physician or other qualified health care professional provides education and counseling services aimed at increasing physical fitness levels, reducing cardiac symptoms, improving overall health and reducing the risk of future heart problems, including heart attack. A medical evaluation is performed to determine the patient's needs and limitations and a rehabilitation program is then designed that includes supervised physical activity. Physical activity may include the use of a treadmill or exercise bike. Heart rate and blood pressure are monitored and continuous electrocardiography (ECG) is used as needed during the supervised physical activity. The patient is taught how to monitor heart rate and adjust the level of activity as needed. Counseling is provided on diet, smoking cessation, and stress reduction. Counseling may also address depression or anger issues. Use 93797 for outpatient cardiac rehabilitation without the use of continuous ECG monitoring and 93798 if continuous ECG monitoring is performed. Cardiac rehabilitation is reported per rehabilitation session.

93880-93882

93880 Duplex scan of extracranial arteries; complete bilateral study

93882 Duplex scan of extracranial arteries; unilateral or limited study

A vascular ultrasound study is performed to evaluate the extracranial arteries which include the common carotid and external carotid arteries. A duplex scan uses both B-mode and Doppler studies. A clear gel is placed on the skin over the arteries to be studied. A B-mode transducer is placed on the skin and real-time images of the artery are obtained. A Doppler probe within the B-mode transducer provides information on pattern and direction of blood flow in the artery. The B-mode transducer produces ultrasonic sound waves that move through the skin and bounce off the arteries when the probe is placed over the arteries at various locations and angles. The Doppler probe produces sound waves that bounce off blood cells moving within the artery. The reflected sound waves are sent to an amplifier that makes the sound waves audible. The pitch of the sound waves changes if there is reduced blood flow, or ceases altogether if a vessel is completely obstructed. A computer converts the sound waves to images that are overlaid with colors to produce video images showing the speed and direction of blood flow as well as any obstruction. Spectral Doppler analysis is performed to provide information on anatomy and hemodynamic function, including information on the presence of narrowing and plaque formation within the arteries. The physician reviews the duplex scan and provides a written interpretation of findings. Use code 93880 for a complete bilateral study of the common and external carotid arteries. Use code 93882 for a unilateral or limited study.

93886-93888

93886 Transcranial Doppler study of the intracranial arteries; complete study

93888 Transcranial Doppler study of the intracranial arteries; limited study

A transcranial vascular Doppler ultrasound study is performed to evaluate the intracranial arteries. The intracranial arteries are divided into three regions which include the right and left anterior circulation territories, and the posterior circulation territory. Doppler studies provide information on the pattern and direction of blood flow within the region being studied. For a complete transcranial Doppler study, clear gel is placed on the skin on the back of the neck, above each cheek bone, in front of both ears and over both eyelids. The Doppler probe is placed on the skin over each site. The probe produces sound waves that bounce off blood cells moving within the artery. The reflected sound waves are sent to an amplifier that makes the sound waves audible. The pitch of the sound waves changes if there is reduced blood flow, or ceases altogether if a vessel is completely obstructed. A computer converts the sound waves to images that are overlaid with colors to produce video images showing the speed and direction of blood flow as well as any obstruction. Spectral Doppler analysis is performed to provide information on anatomy and hemodynamic function, including information on the presence of narrowing and plaque formation within the intracranial arteries. The physician reviews the Doppler study and provides a written interpretation of findings. Use code 93886 for a complete study of all three regions. Use code 93888 for a limited study which includes two regions or less.

93890

93890 Transcranial Doppler study of the intracranial arteries; vasoreactivity study

A transcranial Doppler study is performed to evaluate cerebrovascular reactivity which provides information on the reserve capacity of the cerebrovascular system in a patient with known cerebrovascular disease of the carotid and/or vertebrobasilar arteries. The study may also be performed prior to surgery affecting blood flow to the brain to assess cerebrovascular reserve. Vasoreactivity studies measure the change in intracranial blood flow velocity resulting from a change in the level of carbon dioxide following inhalation of a gas mixture higher in carbon dioxide than normal room air and/or with breath holding or

hyperventilation. Alternatively, intracranial blood flow velocity can be evaluated following injection of acetazolamide or another drug that alters blood flow to the brain. Gel is applied to the skin. A hand-held Doppler probe is positioned on the skin and directed at the middle cerebral arteries (MCA) bilaterally. Continuous monitoring of the MCAs is performed during the rest phase and following the physiological challenge (breath holding, hyperventilation, and/or administration of CO_2 or medication) altering blood flow velocity to the brain. A computer program determines the blood flow reserve by calculating the change in blood flow from the baseline to following the physiological challenge. The physician reviews the images and the computer calculations and provides a written report detailing the findings, including whether there are adequate collateral blood flow channels that can maintain blood flow to the brain in the event of an interruption caused by stroke or a procedure that would temporarily alter blood flow to the brain.

93892-93893

93892 Transcranial Doppler study of the intracranial arteries; emboli detection without intravenous microbubble injection

93893 Transcranial Doppler study of the intracranial arteries; emboli detection with intravenous microbubble injection

A transcranial Doppler study is performed for emboli detection. Emboli are identified by short-duration, high-intensity signals on Doppler studies. The intensity of the signal is dependent on the density difference between the embolus and the blood cells with gaseous emboli showing the highest intensity signals and solid emboli (thrombotic, platelet, or atheromatous) showing slightly lower high intensity signals. Gel is applied to the skin. A hand-held Doppler probe is positioned on the skin and directed at the middle cerebral arteries (MCA) bilaterally. Continuous transcranial Doppler monitoring of the MCAs is performed through the temporal bone window. These are recorded on a designated computer system that provides both sound and visual images. A computer algorithm provides an analysis of the recording. Following completion of the recording, the physician reviews it for embolic signals, which are differentiated from artifacts. The physician then provides a written report detailing the findings. Use 93892 when emboli detection is performed without intravenous microbubble injection. Use 93893 when emboli detection is performed with an intravenous injection of agitated saline. Intravenous access is obtained and agitated saline is rapidly injected as a contrast agent. Monitoring begins immediately prior to the injection and is continued until after the agitated saline clears the MCAs. The physician reviews the contrast studies and provides a written report of findings.

93895

93895 Quantitative carotid intima media thickness and carotid atheroma evaluation, bilateral

Quantitative carotid intima media thickness (CIMT) and carotid atheroma evaluation is performed using ultrasound and a special software program to measure the mean and maximum CIMT. Carotid atheroma is an accumulation of degenerative material such as macrophage cells, lipids, calcium, and fibrous connective tissue that collects in the inner layers of the artery wall, called the intima media. The atheroma may cause swelling and narrowing of the vessel(s) and restrict blood flow to the brain. The information obtained by ultrasound examination of the carotid arteries can be used as a surrogate marker for atherosclerosis and a prognostic risk for cardiovascular disease. CIMT may also be used to monitor atherosclerosis disease progression and the regressive effects of treatment. A neck ultrasound is performed imaging both the right and left carotid arteries. Unlike traditional ultrasound studies that simply identify stenosis, this software program identifies the amount of soft plaque accumulation in segments of the vessels that do not exhibit overt atherosclerotic disease.

Medicine

93922-93923

93922   Limited bilateral noninvasive physiologic studies of upper or lower extremity arteries, (eg, for lower extremity: ankle/brachial indices at distal posterior tibial and anterior tibial/dorsalis pedis arteries plus bidirectional, Doppler waveform recording and analysis at 1-2 levels, or ankle/brachial indices at distal posterior tibial and anterior tibial/dorsalis pedis arteries plus volume plethysmography at 1-2 levels, or ankle/brachial indices at distal posterior tibial and anterior tibial/dorsalis pedis arteries with, transcutaneous oxygen tension measurement at 1-2 levels)

93923   Complete bilateral noninvasive physiologic studies of upper or lower extremity arteries, 3 or more levels (eg, for lower extremity: ankle/brachial indices at distal posterior tibial and anterior tibial/dorsalis pedis arteries plus segmental blood pressure measurements with bidirectional Doppler waveform recording and analysis, at 3 or more levels, or ankle/brachial indices at distal posterior tibial and anterior tibial/dorsalis pedis arteries plus segmental volume plethysmography at 3 or more levels, or ankle/brachial indices at distal posterior tibial and anterior tibial/dorsalis pedis arteries plus segmental transcutaneous oxygen tension measurements at 3 or more levels), or single level study with provocative functional maneuvers (eg, measurements with postural provocative tests, or measurements with reactive hyperemia)

Noninvasive physiologic studies of the upper or lower extremity arteries are performed to evaluate arterial disease and may include Doppler ultrasound waveform bidirectional studies, plethysmography, oxygen tension measurements, and/or provocative functional maneuvers. To perform Doppler ultrasound waveform bidirectional studies, a Doppler probe is placed on the skin over the vessel to be studied. The probe detects blood flow signals from the artery that are recorded and displayed on a computer monitor. The Doppler waveform system is also able to detect forward and reverse (bidirectional) blood flow during the various phases of the cardiac cycle. Plethysmography measures the amount of blood flow present or passing through a body region and is helpful in identifying deep vein thrombosis and arterial occlusive disease. There are two common types of plethysmography used to evaluate extremity arteries—electrical impedance plethysmography and segmental plethysmography. To perform segmental plethysmography, pneumatic cuffs are placed at several levels along the extremity. A measured volume of air is injected into the cuffs and pulsatile volume change is measured and recorded at each level. Oxygen tension measurements are taken transcutaneously using an oximetry device to measure oxygen saturation in capillaries at various levels along the extremity. Provocative functional maneuvers provoke changes in blood flow using postural changes or temporary occlusion of blood vessels using a tourniquet placed around the extremity at various levels. Changes in blood flow are measured before and after the provocative maneuver. Which studies are performed and at what levels is dependent upon the type, site, and extent of the arterial disease. Use 93922 for limited noninvasive studies generally defined as bilateral studies at 1-2 levels. Use 93923 for complete noninvasive physiologic studies generally defined as bilateral studies at 3 or more levels or provocative functional maneuvers at a single level. The studies are evaluated by a physician and a written report of findings is provided.

93924

93924   Noninvasive physiologic studies of lower extremity arteries, at rest and following treadmill stress testing, (ie, bidirectional Doppler waveform or volume plethysmography recording and analysis at rest with ankle/brachial indices immediately after and at timed intervals following performance of a standardized protocol on a motorized treadmill plus recording of time of onset of claudication or other symptoms, maximal walking time, and time to recovery) complete bilateral study

Noninvasive physiologic studies of the lower extremity arteries are performed to evaluate peripheral artery disease (PAD) and include Doppler ultrasound waveform bidirectional studies or plethysmography performed with ankle/brachial indices. PAD is a condition in which extremity arteries are narrowed or blocked. PAD of the legs can cause intermittent claudication which is a symptom of ischemia. Intermittent claudication refers to pain and numbness in the legs brought on by exercise, particularly walking. Testing for PAD involves performing a series of noninvasive physiologic studies both at rest and following treadmill stress testing, both immediately after the motorized treadmill protocol and at timed intervals that note the onset of symptoms and recovery time. To perform Doppler ultrasound waveform bidirectional studies, a Doppler probe is placed on the skin over the vessel to be studied. The probe detects blood flow signals from the artery that are recorded and displayed on a computer monitor. The Doppler waveform system is also able to detect forward and reverse (bidirectional) blood flow during the various phases of the cardiac cycle. Plethysmography measures the amount of blood flow present or passing through a body region and is helpful in identifying deep vein thrombosis and arterial occlusive disease. There are two common types of plethysmography used to evaluate extremity arteries—electrical impedance plethysmography and segmental plethysmography. To perform segmental plethysmography, pneumatic cuffs are placed at several levels along the extremity. A measured volume of air is injected into the cuffs and pulsatile volume change is measured and recorded at each level. The ankle/brachial index test compares blood pressure at the ankle with blood pressure in the arm. A low ankle/brachial index is an

indicator of PAD. The studies are evaluated by a physician and a written report of findings is provided.

93925-93926

93925   Duplex scan of lower extremity arteries or arterial bypass grafts; complete bilateral study

93926   Duplex scan of lower extremity arteries or arterial bypass grafts; unilateral or limited study

A vascular ultrasound study is performed to evaluate the lower extremity arteries or arterial bypass grafts. A duplex scan uses both B-mode and Doppler studies. A clear gel is placed on the skin of the lower extremity over the region to be studied. A B-mode transducer is placed on the skin and real-time images of the arteries or arterial bypass grafts are obtained. A Doppler probe within the B-mode transducer provides information on the pattern and direction of blood flow in the artery. The B-mode transducer produces ultrasonic sound waves that move through the skin and bounce off the arteries when the probe is moved over the region being studied. The Doppler probe produces sound waves that bounce off blood cells moving within the artery. The reflected sound waves are sent to an amplifier that makes the sound waves audible. The pitch of the sound waves changes if there is reduced blood flow, or ceases altogether if a vessel is completely obstructed. A computer converts the sound waves to images that are overlaid with colors to produce video images showing the speed and direction of blood flow as well as any obstruction. Spectral Doppler analysis is performed to provide information on anatomy and hemodynamic function, including information on the presence of narrowing and plaque formation within the arteries. The physician reviews the duplex scan and provides a written interpretation of findings. Use code 93925 for a complete bilateral study. Use code 93926 for a unilateral or limited study.

93930-93931

93930   Duplex scan of upper extremity arteries or arterial bypass grafts; complete bilateral study

93931   Duplex scan of upper extremity arteries or arterial bypass grafts; unilateral or limited study

A vascular ultrasound study is performed to evaluate the upper extremity arteries or arterial bypass grafts. A duplex scan uses both B-mode and Doppler studies. A clear gel is placed on the skin of the upper extremity over the region to be studied. A B-mode transducer is placed on the skin and real-time images of the arteries or arterial bypass grafts are obtained. A Doppler probe within the B-mode transducer provides information on the pattern and direction of blood flow in the artery. The B-mode transducer produces ultrasonic sound waves that move through the skin and bounce off the arteries when the probe is moved over the region being studied. The Doppler probe produces sound waves that bounce off blood cells moving within the artery. The reflected sound waves are sent to an amplifier that makes the sound waves audible. The pitch of the sound waves changes if there is reduced blood flow, or ceases altogether if a vessel is completely obstructed. A computer converts the sound waves to images that are overlaid with colors to produce video images showing the speed and direction of blood flow as well as any obstruction. Spectral Doppler analysis is performed to provide information on anatomy and hemodynamic function, including information on the presence of narrowing and plaque formation within the arteries. The physician reviews the duplex scan and provides a written interpretation of findings. Use code 93930 for a complete bilateral study. Use code 93931 for a unilateral or limited study.

93970-93971

93970   Duplex scan of extremity veins including responses to compression and other maneuvers; complete bilateral study

93971   Duplex scan of extremity veins including responses to compression and other maneuvers; unilateral or limited study

A vascular ultrasound study is performed to evaluate veins in the extremities. A duplex scan uses both B-mode and Doppler studies. A clear gel is placed on the skin of the extremity over the region to be studied. A B-mode transducer is placed on the skin and real-time images of the veins are obtained. A Doppler probe within the B-mode transducer provides information on the pattern and direction of blood flow in the veins. The B-mode transducer produces ultrasonic sound waves that move through the skin and bounce off the veins when the probe is moved over the region being studied. The Doppler probe produces sound waves that bounce off blood cells moving within the veins. The reflected sound waves are sent to an amplifier that makes the sound waves audible. The pitch of the sound waves changes if there is reduced blood flow, or ceases altogether if a vessel is completely obstructed. A computer converts the sound waves to images that are overlaid with colors to produce video images showing the speed and direction of blood flow as well as any obstruction. Spectral Doppler analysis is performed to provide information on anatomy and hemodynamic function. The duplex scan may include a baseline evaluation followed by additional scans obtained with compression or using other maneuvers that alter blood flow. The physician reviews the duplex scan and provides a written interpretation of findings. Use code 93970 for a complete bilateral study of the upper or lower extremity veins. Use code 93971 for a unilateral or limited study.

Medicine

93975-93976

93975 Duplex scan of arterial inflow and venous outflow of abdominal, pelvic, scrotal contents and/or retroperitoneal organs; complete study

93976 Duplex scan of arterial inflow and venous outflow of abdominal, pelvic, scrotal contents and/or retroperitoneal organs; limited study

A vascular ultrasound study is performed to evaluate the arterial inflow and venous outflow of abdominal, pelvic, and scrotal contents and/or retroperitoneal organs. A duplex scan uses both B-mode and Doppler studies. A clear gel is placed on the skin over the region to be studied. A B-mode transducer is placed on the skin and real-time images of the arteries and veins are obtained. A Doppler probe within the B-mode transducer provides information on the pattern and direction of blood flow in the arteries and veins. The B-mode transducer produces ultrasonic sound waves that move through the skin and bounce off the arteries and veins when the probe is moved over the region being studied. The Doppler probe produces sound waves that bounce off blood cells moving within the arteries and veins. The reflected sound waves are sent to an amplifier that makes the sound waves audible. The pitch of the sound waves changes if there is reduced blood flow, or ceases altogether if a vessel is completely obstructed. A computer converts the sound waves to images that are overlaid with colors to produce video images showing the speed and direction of blood flow as well as any obstruction. Spectral Doppler analysis is performed to provide information on anatomy and hemodynamic function, including information on the presence of narrowing and plaque formation within the blood vessels. The physician reviews the duplex scan and provides a written interpretation of findings. Use code 93975 for a complete study. Use code 93976 for a limited study.

93978-93979

93978 Duplex scan of aorta, inferior vena cava, iliac vasculature, or bypass grafts; complete study

93979 Duplex scan of aorta, inferior vena cava, iliac vasculature, or bypass grafts; unilateral or limited study

A vascular ultrasound study is performed to evaluate the aorta, the inferior vena cava, arterial inflow and venous outflow of the iliac vasculature, or bypass grafts. A duplex scan uses both B-mode and Doppler studies. A clear gel is placed on the skin over the region to be studied. A B-mode transducer is placed on the skin and real-time images of the arteries and veins are obtained. A Doppler probe within the B-mode transducer provides information on the pattern and direction of blood flow in the arteries and veins. The B-mode transducer produces ultrasonic sound waves that move through the skin and bounce off the arteries and veins when the probe is moved over the region being studied. The Doppler probe produces sound waves that bounce off blood cells moving within the blood vessels. The reflected sound waves are sent to an amplifier that makes the sound waves audible. The pitch of the sound waves changes if there is reduced blood flow, or ceases altogether if a vessel is completely obstructed. A computer converts the sound waves to images that are overlaid with colors to produce video images showing the speed and direction of blood flow as well as any obstruction. Spectral Doppler analysis is performed to provide information on anatomy and hemodynamic function, including information on the presence of narrowing and plaque formation within the blood vessels. The physician reviews the duplex scan and provides a written interpretation of findings. Use code 93978 for a complete study. Use code 93979 for a unilateral or limited study.

93980-93981

93980 Duplex scan of arterial inflow and venous outflow of penile vessels; complete study

93981 Duplex scan of arterial inflow and venous outflow of penile vessels; follow-up or limited study

A vascular ultrasound study is performed to evaluate the arterial inflow and venous outflow of the penile vessels. A duplex scan uses both B-mode and Doppler studies. A clear gel is placed on the skin. The B-mode transducer is then placed on the skin and real-time images of the arteries and veins are obtained. A Doppler probe within the B-mode transducer provides information on the pattern and direction of blood flow in the penile blood vessels. The B-mode transducer produces ultrasonic sound waves that move through the skin and bounce off the blood vessels when the probe is moved over the penis. The Doppler probe produces sound waves that bounce off blood cells moving within the penile vessels. The reflected sound waves are sent to an amplifier that makes the sound waves audible. The pitch of the sound waves changes if there is reduced blood flow, or ceases altogether if a vessel is completely obstructed. A computer converts the sound waves to images that are overlaid with colors to produce video images showing the speed and direction of blood flow as well as any obstruction. Spectral Doppler analysis is performed to provide information on anatomy and hemodynamic function, including information on the presence of narrowing and plaque formation within the blood vessels. The physician reviews the duplex scan and provides a written interpretation of findings. Use code 93980 for a complete study. Use code 93981 for a follow-up or limited study.

93982

93982 Noninvasive physiologic study of implanted wireless pressure sensor in aneurysmal sac following endovascular repair, complete study including recording, analysis of pressure and waveform tracings, interpretation and report

A noninvasive physiologic study is performed on a previously implanted wireless pressure sensor placed in an aneurysmal sac during endovascular repair of an abdominal aortic aneurysm (AAA). A complete study including recording, pressure analysis and waveform tracings is required at yearly or half-yearly intervals subsequent to the endovascular repair to ensure that there are no complications, such as repressurization or an endoleak. The highly specialized wireless sensor the size of a grain of rice measures pressure, flow, and temperature and allows for direct, noninvasive monitoring for the risk of rupture. The device uses acoustic waves, which transmit effectively through soft tissue, bone, and fluid without being absorbed, and requires very little energy for a high signal-to-noise ratio when accessing deep locations in the body. There is no battery, no antenna, and no connecting leads. The device has a special external unit that both powers the implant and receives the information directly from the implant. A technologist obtains the data from the sensor. The data is then reviewed by the physician, including waveform tracings of the activated sensor and aneurysm sac pressure measurements taken from different positions by the external unit. These are compared for pulsatility. The waveform tracings are compared with data obtained from prior studies including the presurgical study, the immediate post-operative study, and any other previously obtained post-discharge interval studies. Raw pressure measurements are normalized to the brachial systolic pressure, plotted, and then compared with previous pressure measurements. Any clinically significant change is noted. A report is dictated and the waveforms and pressure measurements to be submitted in the final report are identified.

93990

93990 Duplex scan of hemodialysis access (including arterial inflow, body of access and venous outflow)

A vascular ultrasound study is performed to evaluate a hemodialysis graft or fistula. Periodic evaluation of the hemodialysis access site is performed to identify abnormalities such as reduced flow and stenosis that may threaten the function of hemodialysis access if left untreated. A duplex scan uses both B-mode and Doppler studies. A clear gel is placed on the skin over the hemodialysis access site. A B-mode transducer is placed on the skin and real-time images of the arterial inflow and venous outflow are obtained. A Doppler probe within the B-mode transducer provides information on the pattern and direction of blood within the hemodialysis access. The B-mode transducer produces ultrasonic sound waves that move through the skin and bounce off the hemodialysis graft/fistula when the probe is moved over the site. The Doppler probe produces sound waves that bounce off blood cells moving within the graft/fistula. The reflected sound waves are sent to an amplifier that makes the sound waves audible. The pitch of the sound waves changes if there is reduced blood flow, or ceases altogether if the graft/fistula is completely obstructed. A computer converts the sound waves to images that are overlaid with colors to produce video images showing the speed and direction of blood flow as well as any obstruction. Spectral Doppler analysis is performed to provide information on anatomy and hemodynamic function including information on the presence of narrowing and plaque formation within the blood vessels. The physician reviews the duplex scan and provides a written interpretation of findings.

94002-94004

94002 Ventilation assist and management, initiation of pressure or volume preset ventilators for assisted or controlled breathing; hospital inpatient/observation, initial day

94003 Ventilation assist and management, initiation of pressure or volume preset ventilators for assisted or controlled breathing; hospital inpatient/observation, each subsequent day

94004 Ventilation assist and management, initiation of pressure or volume preset ventilators for assisted or controlled breathing; nursing facility, per day

Ventilation assist management is done for patients requiring breathing assistance. Ventilator use initiated by the therapist is either a pressure preset type (pressure support ventilator), or a volume preset type, (volume support ventilator). On a pressure preset ventilator, the therapist sets the inspiratory and expiratory positive airways pressure, the breath rate, and inspiratory time to match the patient's spontaneous respiratory effort, then sets the ventilator timing to allow the patient to trigger the breaths spontaneously and/or the machine to trigger breaths when apneic spells or slowed respiratory rate occur. Although a constant level of positive pressure is maintained with a pressure support ventilator, the tidal volume varies with the patient's effort and pulmonary mechanics, often resulting in ineffective respiratory efforts. The volume support machine uses the tidal volume as the feedback control. The therapist sets the tidal volume and respiratory frequency and the machine calculates a preset minute volume. The pressure support level is continuously adjusted to deliver the preset tidal volume, depending on the patient's respiratory efforts, breath by breath. Use 94002 for the initial day of ventilation assist and

Medicine

management for a hospital inpatient/observation stay, and 94003 for each subsequent day. Use 94004 for a nursing facility, per day.

94005

94005 **Home ventilator management care plan oversight of a patient (patient not present) in home, domiciliary or rest home (eg, assisted living) requiring review of status, review of laboratories and other studies and revision of orders and respiratory care plan (as appropriate), within a calendar month, 30 minutes or more**

A physician or other qualified health care professional provides ventilator management care oversight for a patient residing at home or a domiciliary, rest home, or assisted living center. An initial ventilator management care plan is developed or an existing plan is reviewed and revised as needed. The patient's current respiratory status is evaluated. Separately reportable laboratory studies are obtained and reviewed. Additional pulmonary function or other studies are obtained as needed and the results are reviewed. The ventilator management care plan is created or revised as needed. The new or revised care plan is provided in writing and integrated into the overall plan of care. The new or revised ventilator management care plan is discussed with other health care professionals assisting in the patient's care and communicated to family members or other caregivers. The physician or other health care professional must document the amount of time spent developing or revising the care plan and communicating with others involved in the care of the patient. Report code 94005 only once per calendar month for ventilator management care oversight of 30 minutes or more.

94010

94010 **Spirometry, including graphic record, total and timed vital capacity, expiratory flow rate measurement(s), with or without maximal voluntary ventilation**

Spirometry is a pulmonary function test that is used to help diagnose the cause of shortness of breath and to monitor existing pulmonary disease, such as chronic bronchitis, emphysema, pulmonary fibrosis, chronic obstructive pulmonary disease (COPD), and asthma. A spirometry device consisting of a mouthpiece and tubing connected to a machine that records and displays results is used to perform the test. The patient inhales deeply and then exhales through the mouthpiece. Inhalation and exhalation measurements are first taken with the patient breathing normally. The patient is then instructed to perform rapid, forceful inhalation and exhalation. The spirometer records the volume of air inhaled, exhaled, and the length of time each breath takes. The test results are displayed on a graph that the physician reviews and interprets in a written report.

94011-94012

94011 **Measurement of spirometric forced expiratory flows in an infant or child through 2 years of age**

94012 **Measurement of spirometric forced expiratory flows, before and after bronchodilator, in an infant or child through 2 years of age**

To perform spirometric forced expiratory flow (FEF) measurement, the infant or child is given a medication before the test to induce sleep. Once asleep, the infant or child is placed in a chest compression jacket. A spirometry device consisting of a mouthpiece and tubing connected to a machine that records and displays results is used to perform the test. Air is forced into the lungs which are expanded to maximum capacity. Forced maneuvers to express the air are then performed using automatic jacket inflation and chest compression. A spirometer is used to measure FEF as the air is expelled from the lungs. The test may be performed a second time after administration of a bronchodilator medication. The test results are displayed on a graph that the physician reviews and interprets in a written report. Use 94011 for FEF performed without use of a bronchodilator on an infant or child through age 2. Use 94012 when FEF is performed before and after administration of a bronchodilator on an infant or child through age 2.

94013

94013 **Measurement of lung volumes (ie, functional residual capacity [FRC], forced vital capacity [FVC], and expiratory reserve volume [ERV]) in an infant or child through 2 years of age**

Lung volumes are measured using a variety of pulmonary function tests for lung volume and capacity. In an infant or child through 2 years of age, lung volume tests require medications and additional testing equipment due to the inability of infants and young children to voluntarily perform the necessary breathing exercises. The infant or child is given a medication before the test to induce sleep. Once asleep, a spirometry device consisting of a mouthpiece and tubing connected to a machine that records and displays results is used to perform the test. Functional residual capacity measures the lung volume following a normal expiration when the respiratory muscles are completely relaxed. Not all air is exhaled during normal respiration and functional residual capacity measures the amount of remaining lung capacity following normal expiration. For other tests, the infant or child is placed in a chest compression jacket. Air is forced into the lungs which are expanded to maximum capacity. Forced maneuvers to express the air are then performed using automatic jacket inflation and chest compression. Forced vital capacity, the maximum

amount of air that can be forcibly exhaled, is measured. Residual volume measures the remaining volume of the lungs following a maximal expiration. Expiratory reserve volume is a calculation of the difference between functional residual capacity and residual volume. The physician may perform other lung volume tests as needed. The test results are displayed on a graph that the physician reviews and interprets in a written report.

94014-94016

94014 **Patient-initiated spirometric recording per 30-day period of time; includes reinforced education, transmission of spirometric tracing, data capture, analysis of transmitted data, periodic recalibration and review and interpretation by a physician or other qualified health care professional**

94015 **Patient-initiated spirometric recording per 30-day period of time; recording (includes hook-up, reinforced education, data transmission, data capture, trend analysis, and periodic recalibration)**

94016 **Patient-initiated spirometric recording per 30-day period of time; review and interpretation only by a physician or other qualified health care professional**

Patient initiated spirometric recordings are obtained over a 30 day period using a spirometer and recording device. The procedure is typically performed on patient's following lung transplant to evaluate for signs of organ rejection or respiratory complications such as infection or bronchiolitis obliterans. The patient is provided with the spirometry device which is tested and calibrated. The patient is instructed on how and when to perform spirometric recordings and how to transmit the data. The patient then performs daily spirometry at the designated time each day. The spirometry device records the data. Data is then transmitted electronically to the provider's office at scheduled intervals. The spirometry recordings are trended and analyzed to evaluate for lung transplant rejection or other respiratory complications. A written report of findings is provided by the physician or other qualified health care professional. The patient may return periodically to the provider's office for recalibration of the device. Report code 94014 when the complete procedure is performed by a single provider. Report code 94015 when only the technical component is performed which includes hook-up, education, data transmission, data capture, trend analysis and periodic recalibration. Report code 94016 when only the review and written interpretation is performed.

94060

94060 **Bronchodilation responsiveness, spirometry as in 94010, pre- and post-bronchodilator administration**

Spirometry with bronchodilation responsiveness is a pulmonary function test that is used to help diagnose the cause of shortness of breath and to monitor existing pulmonary disease, such as chronic bronchitis, emphysema, pulmonary fibrosis, chronic obstructive pulmonary disease (COPD), and asthma. The test is first performed without administration of a bronchodilator. A spirometry device consisting of a mouthpiece and tubing connected to a machine that records and displays results is used to perform the test. The patient inhales deeply and then exhales through the mouthpiece. Inhalation and exhalation measurements are first taken with the patient breathing normally. The patient is then instructed to perform rapid, forceful inhalation and exhalation. The spirometer records the volume of air inhaled, exhaled, and the length of time each breath takes. A bronchodilator medication is administered and the test is repeated. The test results are displayed on a graph that the physician reviews and interprets in a written report.

94070

94070 **Bronchospasm provocation evaluation, multiple spirometric determinations as in 94010, with administered agents (eg, antigen[s], cold air, methacholine)**

A bronchospasm provocation evaluation is performed using multiple spirometric determinations. The test is performed with the patient breathing normally followed by forced inhalation and exhalation and finally with administered agents such as antigens, cold air, or methacholine in an attempt to provoke bronchospasm. Spirometry is a pulmonary function test that is used to help diagnose the cause of shortness of breath and to monitor existing pulmonary disease, such as chronic bronchitis, emphysema, pulmonary fibrosis, chronic obstructive pulmonary disease (COPD), and asthma. A spirometry device consisting of a mouthpiece and tubing connected to a machine that records and displays results is used to perform the test. The patient inhales deeply and then exhales through the mouthpiece. Inhalation and exhalation measurements are first taken with the patient breathing normally. The patient is then instructed to perform rapid, forceful inhalation and exhalation. The spirometer records the volume of air inhaled, exhaled, and the length of time each breath takes. The spirometry tests are repeated with administration of one or more agents in an attempt to provoke bronchospasm. The test results are displayed on a graph that the physician reviews and interprets in a written report.

94150

94150 **Vital capacity, total (separate procedure)**

Vital capacity is determined using a spirometry device consisting of a mouthpiece and tubing connected to a machine that records and displays results. The patient inhales deeply and then forcibly exhales through the mouthpiece. The spirometer measures the maximum amount of air that the patient can expel from the lungs after maximum inhalation. The amount of air exhaled is combined with the patient's other physiological characteristics including height, weight, sex, age, and ethnicity to evaluate vital capacity and to determine if the patient has an underlying lung condition.

94200

94200   Maximum breathing capacity, maximal voluntary ventilation

The maximum breathing capacity, also called the maximal voluntary ventilation (MVV) represents the largest volume of air that can be breathed per minute. It provides an estimate for the peak ventilation available to meet physiologic demands of the body. Using a spirometer, a device consisting of a mouthpiece and tubing connected to a machine that records and displays results, the patient breathes as hard and fast as possible for 12-15 seconds. This measurement is then extrapolated to 1 minute and expressed as liters per minute.

94250

94250   Expired gas collection, quantitative, single procedure (separate procedure)

Expired gas collection uses a testing device with a breathing mouthpiece and tubing connected to an airtight collection container such as a Douglas bag. The tubing has a one way valve that allows the patient to inhale room air and then exhale gas contained in the lungs directly into the airtight collection container for a defined period of time. When the defined period of time has elapsed, the expired gas is sampled and the relative concentrations of O_2 and CO_2 are determined using an electronic gas analyzer. The values of O_2 and CO_2 in the room air is also determined and the results are compared to evaluate oxygen uptake (VO_2) and the rate of carbon dioxide elimination (VCO_2).

94400

94400   Breathing response to CO2 (CO2 response curve)

This pulmonary function test measures the patient's breathing response to the introduction of more carbon dioxide (CO_2), or a state of hypercapnia, in their air mixture. A mask is placed over the patient's mouth and nose. The test is performed using a gas mixture containing increasing levels of CO_2 (1%-7%). The patient breathes the gas mixture in through the mask and the exhaled gas mixture is then captured by gas analyzers that determine the values in the exhaled gases. As CO_2 levels in the air mixture being delivered through the mask are increased, the body's response to the increased CO_2 levels are recorded and a CO_2 hypercapnic response curve is generated by a computer. The physician reviews the changes in the values of the exhaled gases and the CO_2 response curve, and provides a written interpretation of findings.

94450

94450   Breathing response to hypoxia (hypoxia response curve)

This pulmonary function test measures the patient's breathing response to the reduction of oxygen, or a state of hypoxia, in their air mixture. A mask is placed over the patient's mouth and nose. The test is performed with a gas mixture containing decreasing amounts of oxygen (20%-12%). During the test, CO_2 is added to maintain alveolar PCO_2 at a normal level. The patient breathes the gas mixture in through the mask and the exhaled gas mixture is then captured by gas analyzers that determine the values in the exhaled gases. At the same time, peripheral artery oxygen (PaO_2) levels are measured either by pulse oximetry or by an indwelling arterial catheter. As oxygen levels in the air mixture being delivered through the mask are reduced, the body's response to the reduced oxygen levels are recorded and a hypoxic response curve is generated by a computer. The physician reviews the changes in exhaled gases and peripheral artery oxygen levels as well as the oxygen response curve, and provides a written interpretation of findings.

94452-94453

94452   High altitude simulation test (HAST), with interpretation and report by a physician or other qualified health care professional

94453   High altitude simulation test (HAST), with interpretation and report by a physician or other qualified health care professional; with supplemental oxygen titration

High altitude simulation test (HAST) is performed on a patient with a respiratory condition to evaluate whether supplemental oxygen is needed during plane travel or travel to a high-altitude location. HAST simulates conditions found at high altitude (8,000 feet) so that the patient can be screened for significant risk factors such as hypoxia or arrhythmias. A baseline blood pressure, heart rate and rhythm, SaO_2, and dyspnea rating is obtained. The patient is then placed on a hypoxic mixture of gases, approximately 15.1 percent oxygen, for 20-30 minutes or less, depending on symptoms. The patient is closely monitored during rest and mild exertion, and vital signs and dyspnea ratings are recorded. If significant symptoms occur, the test is repeated with supplemental oxygen to determine the amount of oxygen needed at higher altitude to ensure adequate treatment of symptoms. A written interpretation and report is provided. Use 94452 for HAST without a second test using

supplemental oxygen and 94453 when the test is performed without and then with supplemental oxygen.

94610

94610   Intrapulmonary surfactant administration by a physician or other qualified health care professional through endotracheal tube

The physician or other qualified health care professional administers intrapulmonary surfactant through an endotracheal tube. Surfactant reduces the surface tension of the pulmonary alveoli and prevents them from collapsing. This is most often given to premature neonates, whose underdeveloped lungs have a surfactant deficiency, to improve their survival and reduce chronic lung disease. The patient is intubated with an endotracheal tube and a bolus of surfactant (Curosurf) is administered with a dosage of approximately 100mg/kg.

94620-94621

94620   Pulmonary stress testing; simple (eg, 6-minute walk test, prolonged exercise test for bronchospasm with pre- and post-spirometry and oximetry)

94621   Pulmonary stress testing; complex (including measurements of CO2 production, O2 uptake, and electrocardiographic recordings)

Pulmonary stress testing is performed to evaluate how well the lungs, heart, and muscles function during exercise. For patient's experiencing respiratory symptoms such as shortness of breath, pulmonary stress testing is performed to help determine the cause of the symptoms. The test is typically performed using a treadmill or stationary bicycle, although for a simple test the patient may simply walk back and forth along a long hallway. Prior to the stress test, baseline spirometry and oximetry values are obtained. In the simple pulmonary stress test (94620), the patient exercises for a prescribed amount of time without being monitored. At the end of the exercise period, spirometry and oximetry values are again obtained and compared to the baseline values. In a complex pulmonary stress test (94621), a number of measurements are taken during the exercise phase for both lung function and heart function. An oximeter is placed on one of the fingers to monitor oxygen saturation. The patient breathes through a mouthpiece attached to a spirometer which is used to monitor CO_2 production and O_2 uptake. A nose clip is used to prevent breathing through the nose. Electrocardiography is also performed to monitor heart function. Upon completion of the exercise phase of the test, additional oximetry and spirometry readings are obtained. The physician reviews the results of the simple or complex pulmonary stress test and provides a written interpretation of findings.

94640

94640   Pressurized or nonpressurized inhalation treatment for acute airway obstruction for therapeutic purposes and/or for diagnostic purposes such as sputum induction with an aerosol generator, nebulizer, metered dose inhaler or intermittent positive pressure breathing (IPPB) device

The patient is placed on intermittent inhalation treatment for acute airway obstruction or to induce sputum production for therapeutic and/or diagnostic purposes. To treat acute airway obstruction, pressurized or nonpressurized bronchodilator medication is delivered for short intervals several times a day using an inhaler, nebulizer, aerosol generator, or an intermittent positive pressure breathing (IPPB) device. Bronchodilator medication is suspended as fine particles within a gaseous propellant and taken into the lungs as a fine spray. The medication acts to relax the smooth muscle of the bronchioles and lung tissue, which has constricted in conditions such as an asthma attack or hypersensitivity reaction, severely restricting air flow. The patient uses the prescribed pressurized or nonpressurized inhalation device as directed by the physician typically for 10-15 minutes several times during the day. To induce sputum production for diagnostic purposes, an isotonic or hypertonic solution is delivered using a nebulizer or other device. These solutions induct secretion of sputum in the lower airways. The patient must cough to expectorate the secretions which are collected in a sterile container and sent to the laboratory for separately reportable analysis.

94642

94642   Aerosol inhalation of pentamidine for pneumocystis carinii pneumonia treatment or prophylaxis

The medication pentamidine is used primarily to treat or prevent pneumonia caused by Pneumocystis jiroveci, also called Pneumocystis carinii. Pentamidine is suspended as fine particles within a gaseous propellant and taken into the lungs as a fine spray, or aerosol, using a nebulizer. A prepared dose of pentamidine is administered via a nebulizer following the administration instructions as provided in the medication prescription.

Medicine

94644-94645

94644 Continuous inhalation treatment with aerosol medication for acute airway obstruction; first hour

94645 Continuous inhalation treatment with aerosol medication for acute airway obstruction; each additional hour (List separately in addition to code for primary procedure)

The patient is placed on continuous inhalation treatment, also called continuous bronchodilator therapy (CBT), using the appropriate dose of a bronchodilator medication. The medication is suspended as fine particles within a gaseous propellant and is taken into the lungs as a fine spray when the aerosol pressure is released. The medication acts to relax the smooth muscle of the bronchioles and lung tissue, which have constricted in conditions such as an asthma attack or hypersensitivity reaction, severely restricting air flow. Periodic assessments are performed to monitor the response to treatment as the medication is administered. The dosage is changed as needed over the course of the inhalation treatment until the desired response to treatment is achieved. Once the symptoms of acute airway obstruction have resolved the inhalation treatment is discontinued. Use code 94644 for continuous inhalation treatment for up to one hour and code 94645 for each additional hour.

94660

94660 Continuous positive airway pressure ventilation (CPAP), initiation and management

Continuous positive airway pressure (CPAP) ventilation is used primarily to treat sleep apnea. It may also be prescribed to treat preterm infants whose lungs have not fully developed. CPAP uses a mask or other breathing device that fits over the nose and mouth which is connected via a tube to a CPAP device. The CPAP machine delivers an air mixture at a continuous low level of pressure. The continuous positive airway pressure keeps the airways open and prevents mechanical obstruction of the flow of air caused by relaxation and collapse of airway structures during sleep. This code is used for initial set-up and management. A durable medical device provider delivers the CPAP device and other required equipment to the home or a residential facility. The device is set up and programmed to the settings indicated by the written prescription obtained from the physician or other qualified health care professional. The patient or caregiver is instructed on correct use of the CPAP and then is asked to demonstrate understanding by placing the mask over the mouth and nose and turning on the machine.

94662

94662 Continuous negative pressure ventilation (CNP), initiation and management

Continuous negative pressure (CNP) ventilation uses a combination of subatmospheric pressure to which the surface of the thorax is exposed to cause thoracic expansion and inspiration. This is followed by an increase in pressure surrounding the thorax back to atmospheric pressure or greater than atmospheric pressure causing the recoil of the lung and chest wall resulting in expiration. CNP is used to treat conditions such as stable or slowly progressive respiratory failure due to neuromuscular diseases, chest wall deformity, or central hypoventilation syndromes. This code is used for initial set-up and management of the CNP ventilation device. A durable medical device provider delivers the CNP device and other required equipment to the home or a residential facility. The device is set up and programmed to the settings indicated by the written prescription obtained from the physician or other qualified health care professional. The patient or caregiver is instructed on correct use of the CNP and then is asked to demonstrate understanding on the use of the device.

94664

94664 Demonstration and/or evaluation of patient utilization of an aerosol generator, nebulizer, metered dose inhaler or IPPB device

A patient or caregiver receives a demonstration of and training in the use of an aerosol generator, nebulizer, metered dose inhaler, or IPPB device. The effectiveness of inhaled medications is in part dependent on the proficiency of the patient or a caregiver in using the prescribed device. The delivery device is selected based on the type of medication being administered and the ability of the patient or caregiver to master use of the device. The provider, usually a respiratory therapist, demonstrates use of the device and explains in detail why and how the medication and device must be used for maximum effectiveness. The patient or caregiver is then observed as he/she uses the device. The respiratory therapist offers help and clarification on the use of the device as needed. Correct use of the device may require more than one demonstration and training session. Code 94644 may be reported once each day for the demonstration and/or evaluation of correct use of the device by the patient or caregiver.

94667-94668

94667 Manipulation chest wall, such as cupping, percussing, and vibration to facilitate lung function; initial demonstration and/or evaluation

94668 Manipulation chest wall, such as cupping, percussing, and vibration to facilitate lung function; subsequent

Manual manipulation of the chest wall is performed to help break up secretions and facilitate improved lung function. Manipulation is accomplished using the hands or a hand-held oscillating device. The patient lies or sits in various positions so that percussion, vibration, and gravity can be used to help beak up secretions. Using cupped hands, the portion of the lung that is to be drained is percussed by a respiratory therapist or other qualified health care professional using a forceful study beat against the chest wall. Next the chest is vibrated by firmly placing flat hands over the area of the lung to be drained and then moving the chest musculature with the hands which vibrates the lungs. Following the percussion and vibration, the patient then deep breathes to get air as deep in the lungs as possible. Taking deep breaths followed by a forced exhalation is performed to stimulate the cough reflex in the patient. If coughing becomes too tiring, the patient can also huff by taking a breath and forcefully exhaling to clear the airways. This process is repeated with the patient in different positions until all portions of the lungs requiring percussion and vibration have been treated. Code 94667 is reported for the initial demonstration of the procedure and/or the initial evaluation of the caregiver performing the manual manipulation. Code 94668 is reported for evaluation and treatment on subsequent days.

94669

94669 Mechanical chest wall oscillation to facilitate lung function, per session

Mechanical chest wall oscillation is one type of chest physiotherapy used to mobilize and remove airway secretions in patients with chronic lung conditions. Mechanical chest wall oscillation uses a mechanical device such as a pneumatic vest connected to an air pulse generator to apply positive pressure air pulses to the chest wall. These air pulses vibrate (massage) the chest wall in a way that mimics the sheer forces caused by coughing thereby improving airflow, loosening mucus, and helping the patient expel sputum from the respiratory tract. The patient is placed upright in a sitting position. The pneumatic vest is put on the patient and attached to the air pulse generator. An aerosol bronchodilator is administered. Mechanical chest wall oscillation is initiated beginning with low pressures and frequency. The pressure and frequency is slowly increased to prescribed levels. Total treatment time per session is typically 30 minutes.

94680-94690

94680 Oxygen uptake, expired gas analysis; rest and exercise, direct, simple

94681 Oxygen uptake, expired gas analysis; including CO2 output, percentage oxygen extracted

94690 Oxygen uptake, expired gas analysis; rest, indirect (separate procedure)

Oxygen (O2) uptake is a pulmonary function test performed to determine how much oxygen is taken up by the lungs during respiration. In 94680, O2 uptake is determined using a direct method during rest and exercise. The procedure is performed first at rest. The patient breathes in room air through a one-way valve and exhales into an airtight container. The expired gases are collected and analyzed using an electronic gas analyzer. The concentrations of oxygen and carbon dioxide are determined. The procedure is repeated during exercise. The relative concentrations of O2 and CO2 at rest and during exercise are compared. The physician provides a written report of findings. In 94681, the procedure is performed in the same manner; however, in addition to oxygen uptake with expired gas analysis, CO2 output is determined and the percentage of oxygen extracted is calculated. In 94690, the procedure is performed in the same manner except that oxygen uptake at rest is determined indirectly by arterial puncture and analysis of blood gases as a separate procedure.

94726

94726 Plethysmography for determination of lung volumes and, when performed, airway resistance

Lung volume plethysmography is performed to determine the maximum volume of air that the lungs can hold. The test is performed in a small airtight room called a body box. Clips are placed on the nose to prevent air from entering the nostrils. The patient then breathes and/or pants into a mouthpiece that is in an open position. If airway resistance is measured, the patient then breathes and/or pants into a closed mouthpiece. As the chest moves during breathing or panting, the pressure and amount of air in the room and against the mouthpiece is measured. Changes in these variables allow the physician to measure lung volume with an open mouthpiece and airway resistance with a closed mouthpiece. The physician analyzes the test results and provides a written report of findings.

94727

94727 Gas dilution or washout for determination of lung volumes and, when performed, distribution of ventilation and closing volumes

Gas dilution is performed using helium and a spirometry device. Gas dilution measures mixing of helium and other gases in the lung. The test gas consists of air with added oxygen of 25-30 percent. Approximately 10 percent helium is then added. The lung volume is calculated using a known volume of inhaled gases containing a known fraction of helium. Clips are placed on the nose to prevent air from entering the nostrils. The patient then breathes into a mouthpiece. Initially the mouthpiece delivers room air. The test gas containing the helium is then delivered and the patient is instructed to take regular tidal breaths. Helium concentration is noted at 15 second intervals. When the change in helium concentration is less than 0.02 percent for 30 seconds, the patient is disconnected from the test gas and room air is delivered. Helium concentration and tidal volume are displayed graphically. The physician reviews the test results and provides a written report of findings. Gas washout measures the amount of expired nitrogen (N2) over a specific period of time which is used to calculate the maximum volume of air that the lungs can hold. An initial N2 alveolar concentration is obtained. Clips are placed on the nose to prevent air from entering the nostrils. The patient then breathes into a mouthpiece. Initially the mouthpiece delivers room air. Nitrogen (N2) washout is performed by having the patient breath 100 percent oxygen (O2). The expired N2 concentration is monitored throughout the test. When N2 concentration is less than 1.5 percent for three successive breaths, the washout is considered to be complete. The N2 wash out is displayed graphically. The physician reviews the test results and provides a written report of findings. During the test, the physician may also measure distribution of gases throughout the lung and closing volumes.

94728

94728   Airway resistance by impulse oscillometry

Impulse oscillometry is used to evaluate airway obstruction and to differentiate between central and peripheral airway obstruction. This test uses sound waves to detect airway changes in patients with asthma and other obstructive pulmonary diseases. An impulse oscillometry device is used. Clips are placed on the nose to prevent air from entering the nostrils. The patient then breathes normally into the mouthpiece of a pneumotachnograph while a sound wave generated by a loudspeaker is superimposed over the breathing. Airflow and sound wave response are transmitted to the impulse oscillometry device and various components of airway obstruction are recorded and measured. The physician reviews the test results and provides a written report of findings.

94729

94729   Diffusing capacity (eg, carbon monoxide, membrane) (List separately in addition to code for primary procedure)

The diffusing capacity of the lungs using carbon monoxide (CO) measures the ability of the lungs to transfer gas from inhaled air across the alveolar-capillary membrane to the red blood cells. This test is performed in conjunction with other separately reportable pulmonary function tests to determine whether lung restriction is due to parenchymal (intrapulmonary, interstitial) disease or to decreased cardiac output (extrapulmonary). The patient breathes all the way out. The patient then breathes in through the mouthpiece of the diffusion capacity testing device which delivers a gas mixture containing 0.3 percent CO, 10 percent Helium, 21 percent oxygen and 68.7 percent nitrogen. When total lung capacity is reached, the patient holds his/her breath for 10 seconds. The patient then breathes out, expelling the gas that has been in the dead space (mouth, trachea, and two main bronchi), which is discarded. The remainder of the gas is exhaled and collected. The amount of the various exhaled gases in the sample is then analyzed and diffusing capacity is evaluated. The physician reviews the test results and provides a written report of findings.

94750

94750   Pulmonary compliance study (eg, plethysmography, volume and pressure measurements)

Pulmonary compliance studies are performed to evaluate lung elasticity using plethysmography, volume and pressure measurements. Plethysmography measures changes in volume of a body part. Volume and pressure measurements are taken indirectly using a pressure sensing balloon in the esophagus. The patient swallows the deflated esophageal balloon which is attached to a pressure device and inflated. The pressure device records changes in pressure as the patient inhales and exhales. At the same time, lung volume is calculated by comparing the pressure changes on inhalation and exhalation. The physician reviews the volume and pressure measurements and provides a written report of findings.

94760-94762

94760   Noninvasive ear or pulse oximetry for oxygen saturation; single determination

94761   Noninvasive ear or pulse oximetry for oxygen saturation; multiple determinations (eg, during exercise)

94762   Noninvasive ear or pulse oximetry for oxygen saturation; by continuous overnight monitoring (separate procedure)

Ear or pulse oximetry measures the percentage of hemoglobin (Hb) that is satured with oxygen and is used to monitor oxygen saturation of blood and detect lower than normal levels of oxygen in the blood. Oximeters also record pulse rate and provide a graphical display of blood flow past the probe. A probe is attached to the patient's ear lobe or finger. The probe is connected to a computerized unit. A light source from the probe is emitted at two wavelengths. The light is partially absorbed by Hb in amounts that differ

based on whether the Hb is saturated or desatured with oxygen. The absorption of the two wavelengths is then computed by the oximeter processer and the percentage of oxygenated Hb is displayed. The oximeter can be programmed to sound an audible alarm when the oxygen saturation of blood falls below a certain level. Use code 94760 for a single oxygen saturation determination, 94761 for multiple determinations, such as that obtained during exercise, or 94762 for continuous overnight monitoring.

94770

94770   Carbon dioxide, expired gas determination by infrared analyzer

A carbon dioxide (CO2) expired gas determination is performed using an infrared analyzer. Because CO2 absorbs light in a specific infrared range, an infrared analyzer can be used to determine the amount of CO2 exhaled. The patient inhales room air and exhales into an infrared analyzer. The infrared analyzer then measures the amount of CO2 in the exhaled air. The physician reviews the results and provides a written report of findings.

94772

94772   Circadian respiratory pattern recording (pediatric pneumogram), 12-24 hour continuous recording, infant

A circadian respiratory pattern recording, more commonly called a pediatric pneumogram or pneumocardiogram (PCG), is performed continuously for 12-24 hours on an infant. A pediatric pneumogram records breathing effort, heart rate, oxygen level, and air flow from the lungs. Breathing and heart rate electrodes are placed on the chest. An oxygen sensor is placed on the infant's finger or toe. These are connected to the recording device and the recording is made for the prescribed period. The physician reviews the pneumogram recording and provides a written report of findings.

94774-94777

94774   Pediatric home apnea monitoring event recording including respiratory rate, pattern and heart rate per 30-day period of time; includes monitor attachment, download of data, review, interpretation, and preparation of a report by a physician or other qualified health care professional

94775   Pediatric home apnea monitoring event recording including respiratory rate, pattern and heart rate per 30-day period of time; monitor attachment only (includes hook-up, initiation of recording and disconnection)

94776   Pediatric home apnea monitoring event recording including respiratory rate, pattern and heart rate per 30-day period of time; monitoring, download of information, receipt of transmission(s) and analyses by computer only

94777   Pediatric home apnea monitoring event recording including respiratory rate, pattern and heart rate per 30-day period of time; review, interpretation and preparation of report only by a physician or other qualified health care professional

Pediatric home apnea monitoring is done on a child to screen for sleep apnea, bradycardia, and hypoventilation that may cause a life threatening event during sleep, or lead to sudden infant death syndrome. Event recording includes the respiratory rate and pattern as well as the heart rate per 30-day time period. The monitor is attached to the child with appropriate leads placed and the parameters set for apnea and low heart rate events that are physiologically significant for the child's age to avoid false alarms in pauses in respiration or variable heart rate. Typical data collected includes chest wall motion, EKG, or recording of airflow at the nose and mouth. The data is recorded and stored for transmission or download and further interpretation and analysis, whether by computer or physician review. The physician or other qualified health care professional must review raw tracings and separate the true abnormalities from normal variance and technical problems. Use code 94774 for monitor attachment, downloading data, physician review, interpretation, and preparation of a report. Code 94775 includes only monitor attachment with hook-up, initiation of recording, and disconnection. Use code 94776 for monitoring, downloading and receiving transmission(s) of data, and computer analyses. Code 94777 reports review, interpretation, and preparation of report.

94780-94781

94780   Car seat/bed testing for airway integrity, neonate, with continual nursing observation and continuous recording of pulse oximetry, heart rate and respiratory rate, with interpretation and report; 60 minutes

94781   Car seat/bed testing for airway integrity, neonate, with continual nursing observation and continuous recording of pulse oximetry, heart rate and respiratory rate, with interpretation and report; each additional full 30 minutes (List separately in addition to code for primary procedure)

The car seat test for airway integrity in neonates, also referred to as the car seat challenge test, is used primarily in preterm infants prior to hospital discharge to determine whether the neonate experiences episodes of apnea, bradycardia, or desaturation while in a car seat/bed. The neonate is placed in the car seat/bed with pulse oximetry, and heart and respiratory monitors in place. The nurse remains in constant attendance and monitors the neonate for any indication of compromised airway integrity which may include episodes of apnea, bradycardia, or low oxygen levels. The physician reviews the test and provides a

Medicine

written report of findings. Use 94780 for the first 60 minutes of testing. Use 94781 for each additional 30 minutes of testing.

95004

95004   Percutaneous tests (scratch, puncture, prick) with allergenic extracts, immediate type reaction, including test interpretation and report, specify number of tests

Percutaneous allergy tests are performed with allergenic extracts that provoke an immediate reaction. The skin is scratched, punctured, or pricked with one or more allergenic extracts and the test sites are then observed and evaluated by a physician or other qualified health care professional to identify any allergic reaction, such as redness and inflammation. The results are interpreted and a written report is provided that specifies the number of allergens tested, the specific allergenic extracts used, and the absence/presence/degree of allergic reaction to each allergen.

95012

95012   Nitric oxide expired gas determination

This test determines the amount of nitric oxide (NO) expelled from the lungs. Patients with asthma have elevated levels of expired nitric oxide compared with normal individuals. Expired nitric oxide is a marker of airway inflammation. Measuring expired NO is a noninvasive method of assessing the severity of an acute asthma exacerbation in the clinical setting. The patient exhales into an NO-impermeable Mylar balloon through a mouthpiece and the expirate is analyzed with a chemiluminescence device. Treatment with glucocorticoids has been shown to lower expired NO in asthmatics with acute exacerbation and in patients with stable asthma.

95017-95018

95017   Allergy testing, any combination of percutaneous (scratch, puncture, prick) and intracutaneous (intradermal), sequential and incremental, with venoms, immediate type reaction, including test interpretation and report, specify number of tests

95018   Allergy testing, any combination of percutaneous (scratch, puncture, prick) and intracutaneous (intradermal), sequential and incremental, with drugs or biologicals, immediate type reaction, including test interpretation and report, specify number of tests

Percutaneous and intracutaneous (intradermal) allergy tests are performed using drugs, biologicals, or venoms placed into the skin to provoke an immediate reaction. The physician scratches, punctures, or pricks the skin with a small amount of each test substance (percutaneous) or injects a small amount of each test substance into and under the skin (intracutaneous), and observes the test sites for allergic signs, such as swelling, redness, and itching sensation. The physician interprets the results and provides a written report that specifies the number of test sites, the specific allergenic extracts used, and the absence/presence/degree of allergic reaction to each allergen. Use code 95017 to report percutaneous and intracutaneous allergy tests performed using venoms and code 95018 to report tests performed using drugs or biological.

95024-95027

95024   Intracutaneous (intradermal) tests with allergenic extracts, immediate type reaction, including test interpretation and report, specify number of tests

95027   Intracutaneous (intradermal) tests, sequential and incremental, with allergenic extracts for airborne allergens, immediate type reaction, including test interpretation and report, specify number of tests

Intracutaneous (intradermal) tests are performed with allergenic extracts that provoke an immediate reaction. One or more allergenic extracts are injected just under the skin. The injection sites are then observed and evaluated by a physician or other qualified health care professional to identify any allergic reaction, such as redness and inflammation. The results are interpreted and a written report is provided that specifies the number of allergens tested, the specific allergenic extracts used, and the absence/presence/degree of allergic reaction to each allergen. Use 95027 for intracutaneous allergy tests performed to identify airborne allergens.

95028

95028   Intracutaneous (intradermal) tests with allergenic extracts, delayed type reaction, including reading, specify number of tests

Intracutaneous (intradermal) tests are performed with allergenic extracts that provoke a delayed reaction over a period of several days. One or more allergenic extracts are injected just under the skin. The specific allergens tested and the allergen extracts used are documented. The patient is instructed on what to expect from a delayed type reaction and is told when to return to have the results read. The patient returns to the office, usually 48 hours later, and the injection sites are then evaluated by a physician or other qualified health care professional to identify any allergic reaction, such as redness and inflammation. The results are interpreted and a written report is provided that specifies the absence/presence/degree of allergic reaction to each allergen tested.

95044

95044   Patch or application test(s) (specify number of tests)

Patch tests are typically performed to test for contact allergies that cause dermatitis. Patch tests expose the skin to multiple allergenic extracts, typically between 20 to 30 possible allergens. The patches are applied to the arm or back and are left in place for 48 hours. The patient is instructed not to bath or engage in physical activity that causes heavy perspiration. The patient returns to the office 48 hours later, the patches are removed, and the physician or other qualified health care professional identifies any allergic reaction, such as redness and inflammation. The results are interpreted and a written report is provided that specifies the absence/presence/degree of allergic reaction to each allergen applied to the skin on a patch.

95052

95052   Photo patch test(s) (specify number of tests)

Photo patch tests are performed in a process that combines patch testing and photo testing in order to diagnose photoallergic contact dermatitis and to identify the allergens responsible. Two patches are prepared with each allergen and the patches are applied symmetrically on each side of the back. The patches are left in place for 48 hours. During this time the patient is instructed not to bath or engage in activities that cause heavy perspiration. The patient returns to the office 48 hours later, the patches are removed, and the physician or other qualified health care professional identifies any allergic reaction, such as redness and inflammation. The initial results are interpreted and a written report is provided that specifies the absence/presence/degree of allergic reaction to each allergen tested. Next, one side of the back is shielded and the other side is exposed to an ultraviolet (UV) light source. An initial evaluation is performed of the side exposed to UV light approximately 30 minutes later and the results are documented. The patient returns again 48 to 76 hours later for a final evaluation of the side exposed to UV light. The physician provides a final evaluation that specifies the absence/presence/degree of photoallergic reaction for each allergen tested.

95056

95056   Photo tests

Photo tests are performed to identify an abnormal reaction to sun exposure. The test evaluates exposure to both short wave ultraviolet radiation (UVB) and long wave ultraviolet radiation (UVA). The abnormal reaction to sunlight is sometimes due to the use of specific medications which react to sunlight but may also be due to an allergic reaction to UVB and/or UVA radiation which can cause chronic photosensitivity dermatitis. The test involves the use of UVB and UVA light sources. An area of the lower back or buttocks is typically used. Small areas of skin are then exposed to different doses of UVB and UVA radiation. The type of radiation (UVA/UVB), the radiation dose, and the location of each exposure is documented. The patient returns 24 hours later to have the photo tests evaluated. The physician provides an evaluation that specifies the absence/presence/degree of photoallergic reaction for each type and dose of radiation (UVA/UVB) tested.

95060

95060   Ophthalmic mucous membrane tests

Ophthalmic mucous membrane tests, also called conjunctival challenge tests, are performed to identify allergens that affect the mucous membrane of the eye. An allergenic extract is placed into the conjunctival sac of the eye. The eye is then evaluated for redness, itchiness, tearing, or other symptoms indicative of an allergic response. More than one allergen may be tested. The physician evaluates any symptoms that occur in response to each allergen and provides a written report of findings.

95065

95065   Direct nasal mucous membrane test

Direct nasal mucous membrane test, also called nasal challenge or nasal challenge/provocation test, is performed for evaluation of allergic rhinitis. A suspected antigen is delivered to the nasal mucous membrane using an applicator. The response to the application of the allergen directly to the nasal mucous membrane is observed for symptoms and signs of an allergic response including redness, itching, and increased mucus production. The physician provides a written interpretation that identifies the specific allergen(s) tested and the patient's response.

95070-95071

95070   Inhalation bronchial challenge testing (not including necessary pulmonary function tests); with histamine, methacholine, or similar compounds

95071   Inhalation bronchial challenge testing (not including necessary pulmonary function tests); with antigens or gases, specify

An inhalation bronchial challenge test is used in the diagnosis and management of asthma. A nebulizer is used that disperses a mist containing a specific concentration of histamine, methacoline, or another testing compound. The patient inhales the mist for a prescribed period of time and then exhales forcefully into a spirometer. The spirometer records the volume of air inhaled and exhaled and the length of time each inhalation and exhalation takes. The test results are displayed on a graph. The concentration of the testing compound may be adjusted during the test in an effort to provoke a response. If the concentration is adjusted, the patient again inhales the mist for a period of time and then spirometric readings are obtained. The physician reviews and interprets the response to the bronchial challenge test and the spirometer recordings and provides a written report of findings. Report code 95071 when the bronchial challenge test is performed using antigens or specific gases dispersed within the mist (which must be identified), instead of histamine, methacholine, or similar compound.

95076-95079

95076 Ingestion challenge test (sequential and incremental ingestion of test items, eg, food, drug or other substance); initial 120 minutes of testing

95079 Ingestion challenge test (sequential and incremental ingestion of test items, eg, food, drug or other substance); each additional 60 minutes of testing (List separately in addition to code for primary procedure)

The physician observes reactions to determine specific allergies during an ingestion test in which the patient ingests certain foods and/or medications. To study the consequences of food ingestion, normal food consumption (i.e., amount and state) is replicated and the patient is observed after the ingestion for the usual amount of time between ingestion and onset of symptoms based on the patient's history. Use code 95076 to report the initial 120 minutes of testing. Code 95079 is reported for each additional 60 minutes of testing.

95115-95117

95115 Professional services for allergen immunotherapy not including provision of allergenic extracts; single injection

95117 Professional services for allergen immunotherapy not including provision of allergenic extracts; 2 or more injections

Allergen immunotherapy is performed to treat seasonal allergies, such as allergies to pollen from grasses, weeds, and trees or to treat indoor perennial allergies, such as allergies to dust mites, pet dander, and molds. Following separately reportable allergy testing to identify the specific allergen(s), an allergen immunotherapy schedule is developed consisting of two phases, the build-up phase and the maintenance phase. During the build-up phase, small but increasing doses of the allergen extract(s) are administered by injection, usually into the upper arm, one, two or three times a week. The build-up phase usually lasts for 3 to 6 months. During the maintenance phase, monthly injections are given for a period of 3 to 5 years. An allergist or outside supplier formulates and provides the allergenic extract for the patient and bills separately for the supply of the allergenic extract. Another physician or other qualified health care professional administers the allergenic extract and observes the patient for a period of time following each injection. Use code 95115 per encounter for a single injection and 95117 for a single encounter where two or more injections are given.

95120-95125

95120 Professional services for allergen immunotherapy in the office or institution of the prescribing physician or other qualified health care professional, including provision of allergenic extract; single injection

95125 Professional services for allergen immunotherapy in the office or institution of the prescribing physician or other qualified health care professional, including provision of allergenic extract; 2 or more injections

Allergen immunotherapy is performed to treat seasonal allergies, such as allergies to pollen from grasses, weeds and trees or to treat indoor allergies, such as allergies to dust mites, pet dander, and molds. Following separately reportable allergy testing to identify the specific allergen(s), an allergen immunotherapy schedule is developed consisting of two phases, the build-up phase and the maintenance phase. During the build-up phase small but increasing doses of the allergen extract(s) are administered by injection, usually into the upper arm, one, two or three times a week. The build-up phase usually lasts for 3 to 6 months. During the maintenance phase, monthly injections are given for a period of 3 to 5 years. The allergenic extract is prepared and provided by the physician or other qualified health care professional. Use code 95120 per encounter for a single injection and 95125 for a single encounter where two or more injections are given.

95130-95134

95130 Professional services for allergen immunotherapy in the office or institution of the prescribing physician or other qualified health care professional, including provision of allergenic extract; single stinging insect venom

95131 Professional services for allergen immunotherapy in the office or institution of the prescribing physician or other qualified health care professional, including provision of allergenic extract; 2 stinging insect venoms

95132 Professional services for allergen immunotherapy in the office or institution of the prescribing physician or other qualified health care professional, including provision of allergenic extract; 3 stinging insect venoms

95133 Professional services for allergen immunotherapy in the office or institution of the prescribing physician or other qualified health care professional, including provision of allergenic extract; 4 stinging insect venoms

95134 Professional services for allergen immunotherapy in the office or institution of the prescribing physician or other qualified health care professional, including provision of allergenic extract; 5 stinging insect venoms

Allergen immunotherapy is performed to treat allergies to stinging insects such as bees, wasps, hornets, or yellow jackets. Following separately reportable allergy testing to identify the specific stinging insect allergen(s), an allergen immunotherapy schedule is developed consisting of two phases, the build-up phase and the maintenance phase. During the build-up phase small but increasing doses of the allergen extract(s) are administered by injection, usually into the upper arm, one, two or three times a week. The build-up phase usually lasts for 3 to 6 months. During the maintenance phase, monthly injections are given for a period of 3 to 5 years. The allergenic extract is prepared and provided by the physician or other qualified health care professional. Use code 95130 per encounter for injection of a single stinging insect venom extract; 95131 for 2 stinging insect venoms; 95132 for 3 stinging insect venoms; 95133 for 4 stinging insect venoms; and 95134 for 5 stinging insect venoms.

95144

95144 Professional services for the supervision of preparation and provision of antigens for allergen immunotherapy, single dose vial(s) (specify number of vials)

An allergist or other supplier prepares or supervises the preparation of single dose vials of antigens for allergen immunotherapy. Using results obtained from separately reportable allergy testing services, the correct dose of the allergen is formulated and provided to the patient in single dose vials. A single dose vial provides the correct formulation for a single injection of the antigen. The total number of single dose vials that are needed for a course of immunotherapy are prepared and the physician reports code 95144 for each single dose vial supplied. The allergist typically administers the first dose which is reported separately and observes the patient for adverse effects. The patient then takes the single dose vials to another physician who administers the remaining doses.

95145-95149

95145 Professional services for the supervision of preparation and provision of antigens for allergen immunotherapy (specify number of doses); single stinging insect venom

95146 Professional services for the supervision of preparation and provision of antigens for allergen immunotherapy (specify number of doses); 2 single stinging insect venoms

95147 Professional services for the supervision of preparation and provision of antigens for allergen immunotherapy (specify number of doses); 3 single stinging insect venoms

95148 Professional services for the supervision of preparation and provision of antigens for allergen immunotherapy (specify number of doses); 4 single stinging insect venoms

95149 Professional services for the supervision of preparation and provision of antigens for allergen immunotherapy (specify number of doses); 5 single stinging insect venoms

An allergist or other supplier prepares or supervises the preparation of multiple dose vials of antigens for one or more stinging insects to be used for allergen immunotherapy. Using results obtained from separately reportable allergy testing services, the correct dose of one or more stinging insect allergens is formulated and provided to the patient in multiple dose vials. A multiple dose vial provides the correct formulation for a specific number of injections of the antigen. The total number of doses that are needed for a course of immunotherapy are prepared and the physician reports a single code for each multiple dose vial supplied. The allergist typically administers the first dose which is reported separately and observes the patient for adverse effects. The patient then takes the multiple dose vials and another physician administers the remaining doses. Use code 95145 when the allergist or other supplier prepares or supervises the preparation of a single stinging insect venom, code 95146 for 2 single stinging insect venoms, code 95147 for 3 single stinging insect venoms, 95148 for 4 single stinging insect venoms, and 95149 for 5 single stinging insect venoms.

Medicine

95165-95170

95165 **Professional services for the supervision of preparation and provision of antigens for allergen immunotherapy; single or multiple antigens (specify number of doses)**

95170 **Professional services for the supervision of preparation and provision of antigens for allergen immunotherapy; whole body extract of biting insect or other arthropod (specify number of doses)**

An allergist or other supplier prepares or supervises the preparation of multiple dose vials of antigens for allergen immunotherapy. Using results obtained from separately reportable allergy testing services, the correct dose of the allergen is formulated and provided to the patient in multiple dose vials. A multiple dose vial provides the correct formulation for a specific number of injections of the antigen. The multiple dose vials that are needed for a course of immunotherapy are prepared and the physician reports code 95165 for each multiple dose vial of a single or multiple antigens supplied or code 95170 for a whole body extract of a biting insect or other arthropod and specifies the number of doses in each vial. The allergist typically administers the first dose which is reported separately and observes the patient for adverse effects. The patient then takes the multiple dose vials to another physician who administers the remaining doses.

95180

95180 **Rapid desensitization procedure, each hour (eg, insulin, penicillin, equine serum)**

A patient who has experienced a hypersensitivity reaction to an essential or life-saving drug such as insulin, penicillin, other antibiotics, or equine or other serums undergoes a rapid desensitization procedure so that the required drug can be administered. Desensitization involves administration of the essential drug in a very small dose initially and then increasing the dose incrementally over several hours until the target dose is reached. The initial dose may be as little as one ten-thousandth of the target dose. As each subsequent dose is administered, the patient is carefully monitored for adverse effects. The physician provides a written report of the rapid desensitization procedure.

95250-95251

95250 **Ambulatory continuous glucose monitoring of interstitial tissue fluid via a subcutaneous sensor for a minimum of 72 hours; sensor placement, hook-up, calibration of monitor, patient training, removal of sensor, and printout of recording**

95251 **Ambulatory continuous glucose monitoring of interstitial tissue fluid via a subcutaneous sensor for a minimum of 72 hours; interpretation and report**

Continuous ambulatory glucose monitoring of interstitial fluid is done via a subcutaneous sensor for at least three days (72 hours). Interstitial fluid glucose measurement automatically monitors glucose values throughout the day to supply additional information on trends not available with isolated measurements from traditional self-monitoring. A temporary sensor is implanted in the subcutaneous tissues and attached to a small plastic disc taped to the skin to hold it in place. A thin wire connects the sensor to a monitor, where the information is stored. An electric signal is continuously relayed to the sensor, which takes interstitial glucose measurements and records the levels every five minutes. The sensor transmits values for a minimum of three days (72 hours), after which it is removed. The data captured in the monitor are downloaded and reviewed by the physician. Some models transmit readings in real time to a receiving unit that displays the current reading as well as trends. The devices are also designed to be used with an insulin pump. The monitor sends glucose readings every five minutes to the pump. Use code 95250 for sensor placement and hook-up, monitor calibration, patient instruction, sensor removal, and recording printout. Use code 95251 for interpretation and report.

95782-95783

95782 **Polysomnography; younger than 6 years, sleep staging with 4 or more additional parameters of sleep, attended by a technologist**

95783 **Polysomnography; younger than 6 years, sleep staging with 4 or more additional parameters of sleep, with initiation of continuous positive airway pressure therapy or bi-level ventilation, attended by a technologist**

Polysomnography is performed with sleep staging by a sleep technologist on a patient younger than 6 years old. Sleep studies are performed to evaluate and diagnose a variety of sleep disorders including sleep apnea, narcolepsy, insomnia, sleep walking, restless leg syndrome, and other periodic movements during sleep. Sleep staging is accomplished using electroencephalography (EEG), electro-oculogram (EOG), and electromyogram (EMG). EEG is performed using one to four electrodes attached to the scalp. Electrodes are attached around the eyes and an EOG performed to monitor eye movement. A submental EMG is performed by placing an electrode under the chin to record muscle tone. Four or more additional parameters of sleep are recorded and analyzed including: heart rate and rhythm; airflow; ventilation and respiratory effort; gas exchange by oximetry, transcutaneous monitoring, or end tidal gas analysis; extremity muscle activity or motor activity-movement; extended EEG monitoring; penile tumescence; gastroesophageal reflux; continuous blood pressure monitoring; snoring; and/or body position. Brain activity, eye and muscle movement are recorded. Other parameters of sleep are monitored and recorded as

needed. The physician analyzes the recorded data obtained during the polysomnography and provides a written interpretation of the test results. Use code 95782 when four or more additional parameters of sleep are measured. Use code 95873 when four or more additional parameters of sleep are measured and continuous positive airway pressure therapy or bilevel ventilation is performed. If CPAP is performed a nasal mask is applied to the nose to keep the airway open during inhalation. If bi-level ventilation is performed, a ventilator is used to augment respiration while still allowing spontaneous unassisted respiration.

95800-95801

95800 **Sleep study, unattended, simultaneous recording; heart rate, oxygen saturation, respiratory analysis (eg, by airflow or peripheral arterial tone), and sleep time**

95801 **Sleep study, unattended, simultaneous recording; minimum of heart rate, oxygen saturation, and respiratory analysis (eg, by airflow or peripheral arterial tone)**

Unattended sleep study is performed using a portable sleep study system in the patient's home or other ambulatory setting. Use of portable systems is growing due to the backlog at sleep study centers and the large number of patients who do not live in close proximity to sleep study centers. These codes report unattended sleep study systems that record fewer parameters than full-night polysomnography performed at a sleep center or comprehensive portable devices. Ambulatory sleep studies reported by these codes include recording of heart rate, oxygen saturation, and respiratory analysis performed by either airflow or peripheral arterial tone (PAT). There are two types of airflow devices, one type uses a heat (thermal) sensor placed on the upper lip and the other uses a mask placed over the nose or mouth to evaluate airflow. Airflow is combined with heart rate and pulse oximetry data to evaluate respiratory disturbance. PAT measures arterial pulsatile volume changes in the finger which is reflective of sympathetic nervous system activity. PAT indirectly detects apnea events by identifying surges of sympathetic activation associated with the end of an apnea event. PAT data is combined with heart rate and pulse oximetry data, which is then analyzed by the device and used to calculate the PAT respiratory disturbance index (RDI). The portable device is set up and programmed. If airflow is measured, a tight fitting mask is placed over the mouth and nose or a thermal device is placed on the upper lip. The heart rate monitor and oximetry device is attached to the finger. If PAT is measured, a finger device that includes a PAT device, heart rate and oximetry monitor is attached to the finger. The ambulatory system then records data as the patient sleeps. Use 95800 when sleep time is also measured and 95801 when sleep time is not measured.

95803

95803 **Actigraphy testing, recording, analysis, interpretation, and report (minimum of 72 hours to 14 consecutive days of recording)**

Actigraphy testing is performed for a minimum of 72 hours up to a maximum of 14 consecutive days. Actigraphy provides data on circadian rhythms and sleep patterns over a period of days or weeks that can be used to evaluate the adequacy of total sleep time and the time to waking after the onset of sleep. An actigraph is placed on the patient's wrist, which records digital data related to movement. Some actigraphs also collect data on light exposure and core body temperature. Data is recorded for the prescribed period of time and downloaded weekly. Weekly calibration and battery checks are also performed. The patient is instructed to keep a sleep diary to help correlate the recorded data. The diary lists bedtime, wake time, approximate number and duration of nocturnal awakenings, lights-off and lights-on times, estimated total sleep time, caffeine and alcohol consumption, the number and duration of naps during the day, and the level of daytime alertness. The patient also records personal information, such as level of stress, and any unusual occurrences that might have affected sleep. After the prescribed time period has elapsed, a technician reviews all downloaded data. Raw data is evaluated to ensure that the test results are valid. The raw data is edited using the information provided in the sleep diary. Objective data from the actigraph recording is correlated to subjective data in the sleep diary. A written interpretation and report of the objective and subjective data is provided. The physician reviews the results of the actigraphy with the patient.

95805

95805 **Multiple sleep latency or maintenance of wakefulness testing, recording, analysis and interpretation of physiological measurements of sleep during multiple trials to assess sleepiness**

A multiple sleep latency test (MSLT) or maintenance of wakefulness test is performed. The test is performed to evaluate the presence and severity of daytime sleepiness as well as detect sleep abnormalities associated with narcolepsy. The patient presents to the sleep study center in the morning approximately two hours after a normal nighttime sleep period has ended. Electrodes are attached to the scalp for electroencephalography (EEG). Electrocardiogram (ECG) electrodes are placed on the chest to monitor heart rate. Electrodes are also attached around the eyes, under the chin, and on the shoulders to monitor eye and muscle movement. An oxygen probe is attached to the finger to monitor oxygen saturation of the blood and air flow measurement devices are taped to the nose and mouth. MSLT consists of a series of timed naps taken at two hour intervals

● New Code   ▲ Revised Code   CPT © 2016 American Medical Association. All Rights Reserved.   © 2017 DecisionHealth

followed by periods of wakefulness. The room is darkened for the nap periods and a sleep technologist observes the patient using closed circuit television. Brain activity, eye and muscle movement, heart rate, oxygen saturation of the blood, and air flow through the nose and mouth are monitored and recorded. During the wakeful period the patient is allowed to read, watch television, have a visitor, or perform other activities to keep occupied. The patient's ability to maintain wakefulness is evaluated during the wakeful period. The physician analyzes the recorded data obtained during the MSLT and provides a written interpretation of the physiological measurements of sleep obtained during the testing period.

95806

95806   Sleep study, unattended, simultaneous recording of, heart rate, oxygen saturation, respiratory airflow, and respiratory effort (eg, thoracoabdominal movement)

Sleep studies are performed to evaluate and diagnose a variety of sleep disorders including sleep apnea, narcolepsy, insomnia, sleep walking, restless leg syndrome, and other periodic movements during sleep. An unattended sleep study may be performed as an outpatient procedure or at the patient's home. If a home sleep study is performed, the necessary sleep study equipment is delivered to the patient. A heart monitor is used to measure heart rate. A band is placed over the chest to monitor respiratory effort as indicated by thoracoabdominal movement. An oxygen probe is attached to the finger to monitor oxygen saturation of the blood. An airflow measurement device is placed over the nose and mouth to monitor respiratory airflow. The room is darkened and heart rate, ventilation, respiratory effort, oxygen saturation of the blood, and air flow through the nose and mouth are monitored and recorded. If the study has been performed at the patient's home, the testing equipment is picked up at the patient's home and the recorded data delivered to the physician. The physician analyzes the recorded data obtained during the sleep study and provides a written interpretation of the test results.

95807

95807   Sleep study, simultaneous recording of ventilation, respiratory effort, ECG or heart rate, and oxygen saturation, attended by a technologist

Sleep studies are performed to evaluate and diagnose a variety of sleep disorders including sleep apnea, narcolepsy, insomnia, sleep walking, restless leg syndrome, and other periodic movements during sleep. The patient presents to the sleep study center in the evening. Electrocardiogram (ECG) electrodes are placed on the chest to monitor heart rate. A band is placed over the chest to monitor respiration. An oxygen probe is attached to the finger to monitor oxygen saturation of the blood. A positive airway pressure device or other air flow measurement device is placed over the nose and mouth. The room is darkened and heart rate, ventilation, respiratory effort, oxygen saturation of the blood, and air flow through the nose and mouth are monitored and recorded. A sleep technologist observes the patient using closed circuit television during the sleep study. The physician analyzes the recorded data obtained during the sleep study and provides a written interpretation of the test results.

95808-95811

95808   Polysomnography; any age, sleep staging with 1-3 additional parameters of sleep, attended by a technologist

95810   Polysomnography; age 6 years or older, sleep staging with 4 or more additional parameters of sleep, attended by a technologist

95811   Polysomnography; age 6 years or older, sleep staging with 4 or more additional parameters of sleep, with initiation of continuous positive airway pressure therapy or bilevel ventilation, attended by a technologist

Polysomnography is performed with sleep staging by a sleep technologist. Sleep studies are performed to evaluate and diagnose a variety of sleep disorders including sleep apnea, narcolepsy, insomnia, sleep walking, restless leg syndrome, and other periodic movements during sleep. The patient presents to the sleep study center in the evening. Sleep staging is accomplished using electroencephalography (EEG), electro-oculogram (EOG), and electromyogram (EMG). EEG is performed using one to four electrodes attached to the scalp. Electrodes are attached around the eyes and an EOG performed to monitor eye movement. A submental EMG is performed by placing an electrode under the chin to record muscle tone. One or more additional parameters of sleep are recorded and analyzed including: heart rate and rhythm; airflow; ventilation and respiratory effort; gas exchange by oximetry, transcutaneous monitoring, or end tidal gas analysis; extremity muscle activity or motor activity-movement; extended EEG monitoring; penile tumescence; gastroesophageal reflux; continuous blood pressure monitoring; snoring; and/or body position. The room is darkened and brain activity, eye and muscle movement are recorded. Other parameters of sleep are monitored and recorded as needed. The physician analyzes the recorded data obtained during the polysomnography and provides a written interpretation of the test results. Use code 95808 when one to three additional parameters of sleep are measured on a patient of any age. Use code 95810 when four or more additional parameters of sleep are measured on a patient age 6 years or older. Use code 95811 when four or more additional parameters of sleep are measured and continuous positive airway pressure therapy or bilevel ventilation is performed on a patient age 6 years or older. If CPAP is

performed a nasal mask is applied to the nose to keep the airway open during inhalation. If bi-level ventilation is performed, a ventilator is used to augment respiration while still allowing spontaneous unassisted respiration.

95812-95813

95812   Electroencephalogram (EEG) extended monitoring; 41-60 minutes

95813   Electroencephalogram (EEG) extended monitoring; greater than 1 hour

An electroencephalogram (EEG) with extended monitoring is performed. An EEG may be performed to diagnose a seizure disorder, to determine the cause of confusion, to investigate periods of unconsciousness, to evaluate a head injury, or to identify other conditions affecting the brain such as a tumor, infection, degenerative disease, or metabolic disturbance. An EEG may also be used to evaluate a sleep disorder. An EEG technician applies sixteen or more electrodes in different positions on the scalp using a sticky paste. The electrodes are connected by wires to an amplifier and recording machine. The patient is instructed to lie still with the eyes closed. The machine is activated and the recording period begins. The machine converts electrical signals from the brain to wavy lines that are recorded on a moving piece of graph paper. During the recording the patient may be asked to hyperventilate or photic stimulation may be used in an attempt to trigger seizure activity. The physician reviews the EEG and provides a written interpretation of the test results. Use code 95812 for extended EEG monitoring lasting 41 to 60 minutes. Use code 95813 when the extended monitoring is for more than an hour.

95816-95822

95816   Electroencephalogram (EEG); including recording awake and drowsy

95819   Electroencephalogram (EEG); including recording awake and asleep

95822   Electroencephalogram (EEG); recording in coma or sleep only

An EEG may be performed to diagnose a seizure disorder, to determine the cause of confusion, to investigate periods of unconsciousness, to evaluate a head injury, or to identify other conditions affecting the brain such as a tumor, infection, degenerative disease, or metabolic disturbance. An EEG may also be used to evaluate a sleep disorder. An EEG technician applies sixteen or more electrodes to different positions on the scalp using a sticky paste. The electrodes are connected by wires to an amplifier and recording machine. The patient is instructed to lie still with the eyes closed. The machine is activated and the recording period begins. The machine converts electrical signals from the brain to wavy lines that are recorded on a moving piece of graph paper. During the awake portion of the recording the patient may be asked to hyperventilate or photic stimulation may be used in an attempt to trigger seizure activity. To identify some types of abnormal electrical activity of the brain, the patient must be drowsy or asleep. In order to accomplish the asleep or drowsy portion of the test, the patient should sleep less than normal the night before the EEG. The patient is tested while drowsy or asleep and brain activity recorded. An EEG may also be performed on a patient in a coma to evaluate the presence of brain activity. The physician reviews the EEG and provides a written interpretation of the test results. Use 95816 for EEG recording with the patient awake and drowsy. Use 95819 for EEG recording with the patient awake and asleep. Use 95822 for EEG recording for a patient who is in a coma or asleep.

95824

95824   Electroencephalogram (EEG); cerebral death evaluation only

An electroencephalogram (EEG) is performed to evaluate for suspected cerebral death in a comatose patient. An EEG technician applies sixteen to eighteen leads to different positions on the scalp using a sticky paste. The electrodes are connected by wires to an amplifier and recording machine. The machine is activated and the recording period begins. The machine converts electrical signals from the brain into wavy lines that are recorded on a moving piece of graph paper. Patients with suspected cerebral death are tested for a minimum of 30 minutes to determine whether any electrical brain activity is present. The physician reviews the EEG and provides a written interpretation of the test results.

95827

95827   Electroencephalogram (EEG); all night recording

An all night electroencephalogram (EEG) recording is performed. An EEG may be performed to diagnose a seizure disorder, determine the cause of confusion, investigate periods of unconsciousness, evaluate a head injury, or identify other conditions affecting the brain such as tumor, infection, degenerative disease, or metabolic disturbance. An EEG may also be used to evaluate a sleep disorder. To identify some types of abnormal electrical activity of the brain, the patient must be asleep. An all night EEG recording begins at the usual bedtime and ends at the time the patient normally awakes in the morning. An EEG technician applies sixteen or more electrodes to different positions on the scalp using a sticky paste. The electrodes are connected by wires to an amplifier and recording machine. The machine is activated at bedtime and the electrical activity of the brain is recorded for the entire night. The physician reviews the EEG and provides a written interpretation of the test results.

Medicine

95829

95829   Electrocorticogram at surgery (separate procedure)

Electrocorticogram (ECoG) is an electroencephalogram (EEG) that is performed directly on the exposed cerebral cortex during a surgical procedure. ECoG is typically performed to identify critical regions in the sensory cortex. ECoG allows the surgeon to identify the limits of a surgical resection in a patient with a neoplasm or brain injury or in a patient with epilepsy where the epileptogenic regions are to be resected. Following exposure of the brain in a separately reportable procedure, ECoG electrodes are placed on the brain, either on the outside of the dura (epidural) or under the dura (subdural). The electrodes may be configured in arrays, strips, or grids and are positioned based on the results of separately reportable preoperative EEGs and imaging procedures. Brain activity is continuously monitored as the surgical procedure is performed. A written report of the intraoperative ECoG is provided.

95830

95830   Insertion by physician or other qualified health care professional of sphenoidal electrodes for electroencephalographic (EEG) recording

Placement of sphenoidal electrodes is performed to capture an electroencephalogram (EEG) recording of the temporal lobe of the brain in a patient with a seizure disorder. The patient is placed on his/her back and the skin of one side of the face is cleaned with an antiseptic. A local anesthetic is injected into the deeper tissues of the face. Using X-ray guidance, a needle with an electrode is placed into the soft tissues at the base of the skull underneath the temporal lobe of the brain. The needle is removed and the electrode remains in place. The electrode is secured with tape and bandage. The same procedure is repeated on the opposite side. X-ray images are obtained to verify correct placement of the electrodes. A separately reportable EEG recording is obtained. Upon completion of the EEG, the sphenoidal electrodes are removed.

95831-95834

95831   Muscle testing, manual (separate procedure) with report; extremity (excluding hand) or trunk

95832   Muscle testing, manual (separate procedure) with report; hand, with or without comparison with normal side

95833   Muscle testing, manual (separate procedure) with report; total evaluation of body, excluding hands

95834   Muscle testing, manual (separate procedure) with report; total evaluation of body, including hands

Manual muscle testing is performed to evaluate function and strength of individual muscles and muscle groups. To perform manual muscle testing, a specific muscle or muscle group is isolated and then a movement such as flexion, extension, abduction, or adduction is performed while resistance is applied using either gravity or manual force. The patient is positioned for testing of the muscle or muscle group and stabilized as needed which may involve the use of a railing, bars, or external support belt. The patient is instructed on the movement, which may be demonstrated by the provider. Function is evaluated using passive range of motion as the provider moves the patient through the test movements, evaluating range of motion and any weakness or instability. The patient then performs the movements while resistance is applied to evaluate strength. The provider supplies a written report of findings and may quantify function and strength using a grading system such as the Medical Research Council's Manual Muscle Testing Grades. Use code 95831 for muscle testing of the trunk or an extremity excluding the hand. Use code 95832 for testing the hand with or without comparison to the hand on the normal side. Use code 95833 for a total evaluation of the body excluding the hands. Use code 95834 for total evaluation of the body including the hands.

95851-95852

95851   Range of motion measurements and report (separate procedure); each extremity (excluding hand) or each trunk section (spine)

95852   Range of motion measurements and report (separate procedure); hand, with or without comparison with normal side

Range of motion measurements are performed as a separate procedure to evaluate the function of specific joints and muscles or muscle groups. Passive range of motion is used. The provider moves the patient through the test movement while evaluating the patient's range of motion and noting any limitations to movement as well as any weakness or instability. Use code 95851 for range of motion testing of each extremity except the hand, or each section of the spine. Use code 95852 for range of motion testing of the hand with or without comparison to the hand on the normal side.

95857

95857   Cholinesterase inhibitor challenge test for myasthenia gravis

Myasthenia gravis is a relatively rare autoimmune disorder in which antibodies form against acetylcholine nicotinic post-synaptic receptors at the myoneural junction. This results in progressively impaired muscle strength with continued use of the muscle and recovery of muscle strength following a period of rest. Myasthenia gravis may be generalized or limited to bulbar muscles causing facial muscle weakness, ptosis, double or blurred vision, difficulty swallowing, and speech disturbances. A cholinesterase challenge test is performed to diagnose myasthenia gravis or to determine treatment requirements. A cholinesterase inhibitor, such as edrophonium (generic for Tensilon), is administered intravenously. The patient is evaluated for improved muscle strength. If muscle strength does not improve with the initial dose, progressively higher doses may be administered in an attempt to elicit a positive response. If muscle strength improves, the test is positive for myasthenia gravis.

95860-95864

95860   Needle electromyography; 1 extremity with or without related paraspinal areas

95861   Needle electromyography; 2 extremities with or without related paraspinal areas

95863   Needle electromyography; 3 extremities with or without related paraspinal areas

95864   Needle electromyography; 4 extremities with or without related paraspinal areas

Needle electromyography (EMG) is a diagnostic test used to evaluate pain, weakness, numbness, or tingling in the upper or lower extremities. The test records the electrical activity of the muscles. Abnormal electrical activity of muscles can be caused by a number of diseases or conditions including inflammation of the muscles, pinched nerves, intervertebral disc herniation, peripheral nerve damage, muscular dystrophy, amyotrophic lateral sclerosis (ALS), myasthenia gravis, as well as other conditions. One or more pin electrodes are inserted through the skin and into the muscle. The electrode cable is attached to a recording device with a visual display. Electrical activity of the muscle is recorded. The patient may be asked to move the extremity so that electrical recordings can be obtained with the muscle flexed and extended. The ability of muscle fibers to respond to nervous stimulation, called the action potential, is displayed graphically as a wave form. The test includes any EMG recordings of related paraspinal areas. The physician reviews the EMG recordings and provides a written report of findings. Use 95860 for needle EMG of one extremity; 95861 for two extremities; 95863 for three extremities; and 95864 for four extremities.

95865

95865   Needle electromyography; larynx

Needle electromyography (EMG) is performed on the larynx to diagnose and evaluate laryngeal nerve and muscle disorders. It may also be used when botox injections in the larynx are performed, or intraoperatively during procedures on the larynx. Small EMG needles are advanced through the skin and cricothyroid membrane and positioned in the muscles that move the vocal cords. The patient then performs a series of vocal exercises which cause movement of the vocal cords. Electrical responses are recorded. Upon completion of the test, the EMG needles are removed and pressure is applied at the puncture sites. The physician reviews the EMG recording and provides a written report of findings.

95866

95866   Needle electromyography; hemidiaphragm

Needle electromyography (EMG) is performed to evaluate muscle and nerve function of the right or left hemidiaphragm. It may also be used intraoperatively during procedures on the diaphragm. An EMG electrode is advanced through the skin, abdominal fascia, and abdominal wall muscles into the costal insertion of the diaphragm under the 8th, 9th, or 10th rib cartilage. Electrical responses are recorded with the patient breathing and holding the breath. The physician reviews the EMG recording and provides a written report of findings.

95867-95868

95867   Needle electromyography; cranial nerve supplied muscle(s), unilateral

95868   Needle electromyography; cranial nerve supplied muscles, bilateral

Needle electromyography (EMG) is performed to evaluate muscle and nerve function of cranial nerve supplied muscles. Cranial nerves and their branches that can be tested by EMG include: CN III Oculomotor, CN IV Trochlear, CN V Trigeminal, CN VI Abducens, CN VII Facial, CN IX Glossopharyngeal, CN X Vagus, CN XI Spinal, and CN XII Hypoglossal. An EMG electrode needle is advanced through the skin and into the targeted muscle supplied by the cranial nerve. Electrical responses are recorded. The physician reviews the EMG recording and provides a written report of findings. Use code 95867 when the EMG is performed on one of the paired cranial nerves on only one side of the body. Use code 95868 when both of the paired cranial nerves are tested.

95869

95869   Needle electromyography; thoracic paraspinal muscles (excluding T1 or T12)

Needle electromyography (EMG) is performed to evaluate muscle and nerve function of the thoracic paraspinal muscles, excluding those at levels T1 and T12. The paravertebral level where there is pain or other nerve or muscle symptoms is palpated. An EMG electrode needle is advanced through the skin and into the paravertebral gutter and positioned in the targeted thoracic paravertebral muscles. Electrical responses are recorded. The physician reviews the EMG recording and provides a written report of findings.

95870

95870   Needle electromyography; limited study of muscles in 1 extremity or non-limb (axial) muscles (unilateral or bilateral), other than thoracic paraspinal, cranial nerve supplied muscles, or sphincters

Needle electromyography (EMG) is a diagnostic test used to evaluate pain, weakness, numbness, or tingling in the muscles. In this procedure a limited study is performed on one extremity or the axial muscles excluding thoracic paraspinal muscles, cranial nerve supplied muscles or sphincters. The test records the electrical activity of the muscles. Abnormal electrical activity of muscles can be caused by a number of diseases or conditions including inflammation of the muscles, pinched nerves, intervertebral disc herniation, peripheral nerve damage, muscular dystrophy, amyotrophic lateral sclerosis (ALS), myasthenia gravis, as well as other conditions. One or more pin electrodes are inserted through the skin and into the muscle. The electrode cable is attached to a recording device with a visual display. Electrical activity of the muscle is recorded. The patient may be asked to move the extremity so that electrical recordings can be obtained with the muscle flexed and extended. The ability of muscle fibers to respond to nervous stimulation, called the action potential, is displayed graphically as a wave form. The physician reviews the EMG recordings and provides a written report of findings.

95872

95872   Needle electromyography using single fiber electrode, with quantitative measurement of jitter, blocking and/or fiber density, any/all sites of each muscle studied

Single-fiber electromyography (SFEMG) uses a specialized electrode with a 25 micrometer (¬µm) recording surface that is exposed at a port on the side of the electrode and a high pass filter of 500 hertz (Hz). The small recording surface allows the recording of action potentials from individual muscle fibers and also allows measurement of fiber density and evaluation of neuromuscular jitter and blocking. Neuromuscular jitter refers to abnormal transmission of nerve impulses and neuromuscular blocking refers to the failure of nerve transmission. One or more SFEMG electrode needles are positioned in the muscle fiber. The muscle is then activated by voluntary contraction by the patient or by electrical stimulation using a stimulating needle electrode. Recordings are then taken from 20 fibers of the same muscle. The recordings are then analyzed to identify jitter, blocking, and/or fiber density. The physician provides a written report of findings.

95873

95873   Electrical stimulation for guidance in conjunction with chemodenervation (List separately in addition to code for primary procedure)

Electrical stimulation is performed prior to chemodenervation to allow more precise localization of the chemodenervation injection site. A combination stimulation needle electrode and hypodermic containing the chemodenervation toxin is advanced through the skin and into the targeted injection site in the muscle. The stimulating device is activated and the stimulation needle is repositioned as needed until muscle contraction is observed or palpated by the physician. The position of the stimulation needle is manipulated until maximal contraction with a low level stimulus is achieved to ensure that the needle is in the most optimal position closest to the motor endplate of the nerve. The chemodenervation toxin is then injected in a separately reportable procedure. The stimulation and injection needle may be advanced along the muscle or may be withdrawn and reinserted at different sites in the muscle and the process repeated until the desired results are achieved.

95874

95874   Needle electromyography for guidance in conjunction with chemodenervation (List separately in addition to code for primary procedure)

Needle electromyography (EMG) is performed prior to chemodenervation to allow more precise localization of the chemodenervation injection site. A combination recording needle electrode and hypodermic containing the chemodenervation toxin is advanced through the skin and into the targeted injection site in the muscle. The recording device is activated to ensure that the needle is positioned in the spastic muscle and not in nearby blood vessels. The chemodenervation toxin is then injected in a separately reportable procedure. The recording and injection needle may be advanced along the muscle or may be withdrawn and reinserted at different sites in the muscle and additional injections performed until the desired results are achieved.

95875

95875   Ischemic limb exercise test with serial specimen(s) acquisition for muscle(s) metabolite(s)

An ischemic limb exercise test is performed to determine whether there is a metabolic cause of muscle weakness, fatigue, and/or cramps such as disorders of glycolysis and myoadenylate deaminase. A venous catheter is placed in the hand or forearm to be tested and an initial blood sample is obtained to establish baseline levels of lactate and ammonia. A blood pressure cuff is placed on the upper arm and inflated above the patient's systolic blood pressure level. The patient then uses a hand grip dynamometer to exercise the muscles of the hand and lower arm. The patient squeezes and releases the dynamometer at a set pace until muscle fatigue, pain, and cramping occurs usually for a minimum of 2 minutes. The blood pressure cuff is deflated and serial blood specimens are obtained at prescribed times to test lactate and ammonia levels.

95885-95886

95885   Needle electromyography, each extremity, with related paraspinal areas, when performed, done with nerve conduction, amplitude and latency/velocity study; limited (List separately in addition to code for primary procedure)

95886   Needle electromyography, each extremity, with related paraspinal areas, when performed, done with nerve conduction, amplitude and latency/velocity study; complete, five or more muscles studied, innervated by three or more nerves or four or more spinal levels (List separately in addition to code for primary procedure)

Needle electromyography (EMG) is a diagnostic test used to evaluate pain, weakness, numbness, or tingling in the extremities. EMG is often performed in conjunction with nerve conduction studies. Needle EMG records the electrical activity of the muscles. Abnormal electrical activity of muscles can be caused by a number of diseases or conditions including inflammation of the muscles, pinched nerves, intervertebral disc herniation, peripheral nerve damage, muscular dystrophy, amyotrophic lateral sclerosis (ALS), myasthenia gravis, and other conditions. Nerve conduction studies are performed to diagnose and evaluate damage to nerves, nerve disorders, and symptoms such as numbness, tingling, or other abnormal sensations. Needle EMG is performed using one or more pin electrodes inserted through the skin and into the muscle. The electrode cable is attached to a recording device with a visual display. Electrical activity of the muscle is recorded. The patient may be asked to move the extremity so that electrical recordings can be obtained with the muscle flexed and extended. The ability of muscle fibers to respond to nerve stimulation, called the action potential, is displayed graphically as a wave form. The test includes any EMG recordings of related paraspinal areas. Nerve conduction studies are performed using several flat metal disc electrodes that are attached to the skin with paste or tape. A shock-emitting electrode is placed over the nerve to be studied and a recording electrode is placed over the muscles innervated by that nerve. Electrical pulses are sent through the shock-emitting electrode. The conduction time, which is the time it takes for the muscle to contract in response to the shock, is recorded. The amplitude or strength of the response and the speed as reflected by latency or velocity of the response is also recorded. The physician reviews the needle EMG and nerve conduction recordings and provides a written report of findings. Use 95885 and 95886 when EMG and nerve conduction studies are performed with another separately reportable diagnostic neuromuscular procedure. Use 95885 for a limited study of each extremity. Use 95886 for a complete study of each extremity.

95887

95887   Needle electromyography, non-extremity (cranial nerve supplied or axial) muscle(s) done with nerve conduction, amplitude and latency/velocity study (List separately in addition to code for primary procedure)

Needle electromyography (EMG) is a diagnostic test used to evaluate pain, weakness, numbness, or tingling in the muscles. EMG is often performed in conjunction with nerve conduction studies. This test is performed on non-extremity muscles, such as cranial nerve supplied or axial muscles. Needle EMG records the electrical activity of the muscles. Nerve conduction studies are performed to diagnose and evaluate damage to nerves, nerve disorders, and symptoms such as numbness, tingling, or other abnormal sensations. Needle EMG is performed using one or more pin electrodes inserted through the skin and into the muscle. The electrode cable is attached to a recording device with a visual display. Electrical activity of the muscle is recorded. The ability of muscle fibers to respond to nerve stimulation, called the action potential, is displayed graphically as a wave form. Nerve conduction studies are performed using several flat metal disc electrodes that are attached to the skin with paste or tape. A shock-emitting electrode is placed over the nerve to be studied and a recording electrode is placed over the muscles innervated by the nerve. Electrical pulses are sent through the shock-emitting electrode. The conduction time, which is the time it takes for the muscle to contract in response to the shock, is recorded. The amplitude or strength of the response as well as the speed as reflected by latency or velocity of the response is also recorded. The physician reviews the needle EMG and nerve conduction recordings and provides a written report of findings. Use 95887 when EMG

Medicine

and nerve conduction studies are performed with another separately reportable diagnostic neuromuscular procedure.

95905

95905 **Motor and/or sensory nerve conduction, using preconfigured electrode array(s), amplitude and latency/velocity study, each limb, includes F-wave study when performed, with interpretation and report**

Nerve conduction studies are performed to diagnose and evaluate damage to nerves, nerve disorders such as carpal tunnel syndrome, and symptoms such as numbness, tingling, or other abnormal sensations. Automated systems are now available to perform tests on sensory and/or motor nerves. These automated systems are more commonly used on nerves of the wrist (median and ulnar nerves) and of the foot (peroneal, posterior tibia, and sural nerves). A preconfigured electrode array is attached to the skin of the limb being tested. Electrical pulses are sent through the array. The conduction time, which is the time it takes for the muscle to contract in response to the shock is recorded. The amplitude or strength of the response as well as the speed as reflected by latency or velocity of the response is also recorded. An F-wave study may also be performed. F-waves are small amplitude, long latency responses invoked by maximal stimulation of the motor nerve with the electrode directed away from the muscle being recorded. F-wave study provides information on the function of the proximal aspect of the nerve. Usually 10 or more F-wave recordings are made at each stimulus site. Recordings may be made on site or sent to a remote computer via a modem. The physician reviews the recordings and provides a written report of findings.

95907-95913

95907 **Nerve conduction studies; 1-2 studies**
95908 **Nerve conduction studies; 3-4 studies**
95909 **Nerve conduction studies; 5-6 studies**
95910 **Nerve conduction studies; 7-8 studies**
95911 **Nerve conduction studies; 9-10 studies**
95912 **Nerve conduction studies; 11-12 studies**
95913 **Nerve conduction studies; 13 or more studies**

Nerve conduction studies are performed to diagnose and evaluate damage to nerves, nerve disorders such as carpal tunnel syndrome, and symptoms such as numbness, tingling, or other abnormal sensations. Several flat metal disc electrodes are attached to the skin with paste or tape. A shock-emitting electrode is placed over the nerve to be studied and a recording electrode over the muscles innervated by the nerve. Electrical pulses are sent through the shock-emitting electrode. The conduction time, which is the time it takes for the muscle to contract in response to the shock, is recorded. The amplitude or strength of the response as well as the speed as reflected by latency or velocity of the response is also recorded. The physician reviews the recordings and provides a written report of findings. Use 95907 for 1-2 nerve conduction studies; 95908 for 3-4 nerve conduction studies; 95909 for 5-6 studies; 95910 for 7-8 studies; 95911 for 9-10 studies; 95912 for 11-12 studies; and 95913 for 13 studies or more.

95921-95922

95921 **Testing of autonomic nervous system function; cardiovagal innervation (parasympathetic function), including 2 or more of the following: heart rate response to deep breathing with recorded R-R interval, Valsalva ratio, and 30:15 ratio**
95922 **Testing of autonomic nervous system function; vasomotor adrenergic innervation (sympathetic adrenergic function), including beat-to-beat blood pressure and R-R interval changes during Valsalva maneuver and at least 5 minutes of passive tilt**

The autonomic nervous system (ANS) is divided into two parts, the sympathetic and parasympathetic nervous system. The sympathetic nervous system helps control blood pressure while the parasympathetic nervous system helps control heart rate. In 95921, cardiovagal innervation (parasympathetic function) is tested. An ECG rhythm strip is used to record heart rate, which varies in response to deep breathing, the Valsalva maneuver and moving from a lying to standing position if parasympathetic function is normal. The patient performs deep breathing and the recorded R-R interval on the ECG is evaluated. The Valsalva maneuver which involves attempting to forcibly exhale with the glottis closed so that no air escapes from the nose or mouth is also evaluated using the R-R interval on the ECG. The last test involves having the patient lie quietly on an exam table. The patient is then told to stand and the ratio of the longest R-R interval around 30th beat to the shortest R-R interval around the 15th beat is calculated (30:15 ratio). The physician reviews the tests and provides a written report of findings. In 95922, vasomotor adrenergic innervation (sympathetic adrenergic function) is tested. An ECG rhythm strip is used to record heart rate and R-R intervals and a blood pressure monitor is used to track changes in blood pressure. During the Valsalva maneuver beat-to-beat blood pressure and R-R intervals are recorded. The Valsalva maneuver increases intrathoracic pressure and reduces venous return which in turn should cause BP changes and reflex vasoconstriction if sympathetic adrenergic function is normal. A tilt test is also performed. The patient is placed on a tilt table in head down position for five minutes. The tilt table is then moved

to a head-up position which causes blood to shift from the head to the extremities. If sympathetic adrenergic function is normal reflex responses occur in blood pressure.

95923

95923 **Testing of autonomic nervous system function; sudomotor, including 1 or more of the following: quantitative sudomotor axon reflex test (QSART), silastic sweat imprint, thermoregulatory sweat test, and changes in sympathetic skin potential**

Sudomotor autonomic nervous system function is performed to evaluate small nerve fibers linked to sweat glands. There are a number of test methods available and the physician may use one or more of these methods. Quantitative sudomotor axon reflex test (QSART) begins by first measuring resting skin temperature and sweat output. Measurements are taken on the arms and/or legs. A plastic cup-shaped device is placed on the skin and the resting temperature and sweat output is measured. The patient is then given a chemical to stimulate sweat production which is delivered electrically through the skin to the sweat gland. Sweat production is measured. A computer is used to analyze the data to determine function of the portion of the autonomic nervous system that controls the sweat glands. Silastic sweat imprint uses silastic material placed on the skin a device that records the imprint of the sweat droplets on the silastic material. The thermoregulatory sweat test is performed by dusting the skin with an indicator powder. The patient is then placed in a heat cabinet to stimulate sweat production. The indicator powder changes color in response to sweat production. Changes in sympathetic peripheral autonomic skin potentials (PASP) are evoked using electrical stimulation of the skin. Electrical potential recordings are then made over the palms and soles of the feet to evaluate whether autonomic nerve fibers are functioning normally. The physician reviews the test results and provides a written report of findings.

95924

95924 **Testing of autonomic nervous system function; combined parasympathetic and sympathetic adrenergic function testing with at least 5 minutes of passive tilt**

The autonomic nervous system (ANS) is divided into two parts, the sympathetic and parasympathetic nervous system. The sympathetic nervous system helps control blood pressure while the parasympathetic nervous system helps control heart rate. Testing of the parasympathetic nervous system typically includes two or more of the following tests: heart rate response to deep breathing with R-R interval, Valsalva ratio, and 30:15 ratio. An ECG rhythm strip is used to record heart rate, which varies in response to deep breathing, the Valsalva maneuver and moving from a lying to standing position if parasympathetic function is normal. The patient performs deep breathing and the recorded R-R interval on the ECG is evaluated. The Valsalva maneuver which involves attempting to forcibly exhale with the glottis closed so that no air escapes from the nose or mouth is also evaluated using the R-R interval on the ECG. The last test involves having the patient lie quietly on an exam table. The patient is then told to stand and the ratio of the longest R-R interval around 30th beat to the shortest R-R interval around the 15th beat is calculated (30:15 ratio). Testing of the sympathetic nervous system typically includes: vasomotor adrenergic innervation with beat-to-beat blood pressure and R-R interval changes during Valsalva maneuver and at least 5 minutes of passive tilt. An ECG rhythm strip is used to record heart rate and R-R intervals and a blood pressure monitor is used to track changes in blood pressure. During the Valsalva maneuver beat-to-beat blood pressure and R-R intervals are recorded. The Valsalva maneuver increases intrathoracic pressure and reduces venous return which in turn should cause BP changes and reflex vasoconstriction if sympathetic adrenergic function is normal. A tilt test is also performed. The patient is placed on a tilt table in head down position for five minutes. The tilt table is then moved to a head-up position which causes blood to shift from the head to the extremities. If sympathetic adrenergic function is normal reflex responses occur in blood pressure.

95925-95927

95925 **Short-latency somatosensory evoked potential study, stimulation of any/all peripheral nerves or skin sites, recording from the central nervous system; in upper limbs**
95926 **Short-latency somatosensory evoked potential study, stimulation of any/all peripheral nerves or skin sites, recording from the central nervous system; in lower limbs**
95927 **Short-latency somatosensory evoked potential study, stimulation of any/all peripheral nerves or skin sites, recording from the central nervous system; in the trunk or head**

Somatosensory evoked potentials (SEPs) are electrical signals generated by afferent peripheral nerve fibers in response to sensory stimuli. SEPs are divided into three categories: short-latency, middle-latency, and long-latency. Short-latency SEPs refers to the portion of the SEP waveform that has the shortest delay (latency) time. The latency time varies depending on which nerve is being tested. Short-latency SEPs for the upper extremity nerves is the portion of the waveform occurring within 25 milliseconds of stimulation, while stimulation of the tibial nerve refers to the portion of the SEP waveform occurring within 50 milliseconds of stimulation. An abnormal SEP result indicates that

Medicine

there is dysfunction within the somatosensory pathways. Testing SEPs involves the use of electrical stimulation. Electrodes are placed on the skin over the selected peripheral nerve. A ground electrode is placed on the selected limb or other site to reduce stimulus artifact. Recording electrodes are placed over the scalp, spine, and peripheral nerves proximal to the stimulation site. Monophasic rectangular pulses are delivered using either constant voltage or a constant current stimulator. The stimulus causes the muscle to twitch and generates a SEP waveform. SEPs are recorded in a series of waves that reflect sequential activation of neural structures along the somatosensory pathways. The physician reviews the SEP recording and provides a written report of findings. Use 95925 for a short-latency SEP study of the upper limbs; use 95926 for the lower limbs; use 95927 for the trunk and head.

95928-95929

95928   Central motor evoked potential study (transcranial motor stimulation); upper limbs

95929   Central motor evoked potential study (transcranial motor stimulation); lower limbs

A central motor evoked potential (MEP) study uses electrical stimulation of the motor area of the cerebral cortex with recording from peripheral muscles in the extremities to evaluate motor pathway function. In 95928, motor pathway function in the upper extremities is evaluated. Prior to MEP recording, baseline nerve conduction studies of the upper extremities are performed. Electrodes are placed on the skin over the appropriate muscles, usually the biceps, triceps, abductor pollicis brevis, and abductor digiti minimi muscles. Impedances are checked and the electrodes are adjusted as needed. Beginning with the abductor digiti minimi muscles, and for each additional muscle tested, the optimal scalp location for electrical stimulation is identified. The MEP threshold is then determined. The motor area of the cerebral cortex is stimulated and MEPs are recorded. Transcranial MEP amplitude or strength of response as well as the speed of response as reflected by onset latency is measured and compared to the baseline nerve conduction study. Next, compound muscle action potential (CMAP) is tested. For the abductor digiti minimi CMAP, the ulnar nerve is stimulated. The relative abductor digiti minimi MEP strength of response reflected as a percentage of CMAP strength of response is measured. The central motor conduction time (CMCT) is calculated. Stimulator output is reduced in 5% increments so that the dissociation between MEP threshold and the cortical stimulation silent period (CSSP) can be measured. Stimulator output is reduced until stimulation no longer alters the appearance of the average EMG for the muscle being tested. Dissociation between excitory and inhibitory effects of transcranial stimulation is defined as EMG inhibition without a preceding MEP at 2 or more stimulus intensities. The data is replicated and the signals are stored. The procedure is repeated on 3-4 muscles on the ipsilateral upper extremity and then the contralateral upper extremity is tested in the same manner. The physician reviews the recordings and provides a written report of findings. In 95929, motor pathway function of the lower extremities is evaluated. The procedure is performed as described above except that electrodes are placed over selected muscles in the legs.

95930

95930   Visual evoked potential (VEP) testing central nervous system, checkerboard or flash

Visual evoked potential (VEP) tests, also called visually evoked response (VER) and visually evoked cortical potential (VECP), are performed to evaluate the function of the visual pathways. The visual pathways originate in the retina, travel along the optic nerves, and terminate in the visual cortex. VEPs use scalp electrodes to record electrical potentials that result from brief visual stimuli. The VEP waveforms are recorded and extracted from an electroencephalogram recording using signal averaging. The planned electrode sites on the scalp are cleansed and recording and grounding electrodes are placed. Either a flash or checkerboard stimulus is used to evoke a response from the visual cortex. Flash uses strobe light that rapidly flashes on and off. The most common stimulus uses the checkerboard reversal pattern. The patient looks at a black and white checkerboard stimulus where the black and white boxes reverse colors every half second. The patient focuses on the stimulus as the VEP waveforms are recorded. The waveforms are displayed on a computer screen and may be printed out on paper. The physician reviews the waveform and provides a written interpretation of the test results.

95933

95933   Orbicularis oculi (blink) reflex, by electrodiagnostic testing

Electrodiagnostic studies of the blink reflex, also called the orbicularis oculi reflex, are performed to help diagnose and localize pathology in the trigeminal cranial nerve (CN V), facial nerve (CN VII), or brainstem. The neural circuit of the blink reflex begins in the nerve endings in the cornea. From the cornea the nerve impulse travels along the trigeminal nerve and ganglion to the spinal trigeminal tract and nucleus to the interneurons in the reticular formation and then to the motor neurons in the facial nucleus and nerve, ending in the oribicularis oculi muscles. Electrodiagnostic studies of the blink reflex use a brief electrical shock, usually to the supraorbital nerve, to elicit a blink response. Electrodes are placed on the skin around the eyes. The supraorbital nerve is stimulated using an electrode placed above each eyebrow. The responses to the electrical stimuli applied to

the supraorbital nerves above each eye are recorded and displayed on a computer screen. The recordings are printed out and reviewed by the physician who provides a written interpretation of the test results.

95937

95937   Neuromuscular junction testing (repetitive stimulation, paired stimuli), each nerve, any 1 method

The neuromuscular junction is the site where neurotransmitters are released from the end of the nerve, cross the synapse, a small gap between the end of the nerve and the muscle surface, to the receptors in the muscle which then cause the muscle to contract. To test neuromuscular junction function, either repetitive or paired stimuli are used to stimulate muscle contraction. A shock-emitting electrode is placed over or inserted percutaneously near the motor nerve to be studied. Recording surface or percutaneous electrodes are placed in the muscle innervated by that nerve. Repetitive electrical pulses are then sent through the shock-emitting electrode. The corresponding surface electrode records the evoked muscle action potentials and the recording is displayed on a computer screen. The conduction time, which is the time it takes for the muscle to contract in response to the shock, is recorded. The amplitude or strength of the response, as well as the speed reflected by latency or velocity of the response, are recorded. The physician reviews the recordings and provides a written report of findings.

95938

95938   Short-latency somatosensory evoked potential study, stimulation of any/all peripheral nerves or skin sites, recording from the central nervous system; in upper and lower limbs

Somatosensory evoked potentials (SEPs) are electrical signals generated by afferent peripheral nerve fibers in response to sensory stimuli. SEPs are divided into three categories: short-latency, middle-latency, and long-latency. Short-latency SEPs refers to the portion of the SEP waveform that has the shortest delay (latency) time. The short-latency time varies depending on which nerve is being tested. Short-latency SEPs for the upper extremity nerves comprise the portion of the waveform occurring within 25 milliseconds of stimulation, while stimulation of the tibial nerve refers to the portion of the SEP waveform occurring within 50 milliseconds of stimulation. An abnormal SEP result indicates that there is dysfunction within the somatosensory pathways. Testing SEPs involves the use of electrical stimulation. Electrodes are placed on the skin over the selected peripheral nerve. A ground electrode is placed on the selected limb or other site to reduce stimulus artifacts. Recording electrodes are placed over the scalp, spine, and peripheral nerves proximal to the stimulation site. Monophasic rectangular pulses are delivered using either constant voltage or a constant current stimulator. The stimulus causes the muscle to twitch and generates a SEP waveform. SEPs are recorded in a series of waves that reflect sequential activation of neural structures along the somatosensory pathways. The physician reviews the recording and provides a written report of findings. Use 95938 for a short-latency SEP study of the upper limbs and lower limbs.

95939

95939   Central motor evoked potential study (transcranial motor stimulation); in upper and lower limbs

A central motor evoked potential (MEP) study uses electrical stimulation of the motor area of the cerebral cortex with recording from peripheral muscles in the extremities to evaluate motor pathway function. In 95939, motor pathway function in the upper and lower extremities is evaluated. Prior to MEP recording, baseline nerve conduction studies of the upper and lower extremities are performed. Electrodes are placed on the skin over the appropriate muscles. For the upper extremity, response is usually tested in the biceps, triceps, abductor pollicis brevis, and abductor digiti minimi muscles. Impedances are checked and the electrodes are adjusted as needed. Beginning with the abductor digiti minimi muscles, and for each additional muscle tested, the optimal scalp location for electrical stimulation is identified. The MEP threshold is then determined. The motor area of the cerebral cortex is stimulated and MEPs are recorded. Transcranial MEP amplitude or strength of response and the speed of response as reflected by onset latency is measured and compared to the baseline nerve conduction study. Next compound muscle action potential (CMAP) is tested. For the abductor digiti minimi CMAP, the ulnar nerve is stimulated. The relative abductor digiti minimi MEP strength of response reflected as a percentage of CMAP strength of response is measured. The central motor conduction time (CMCT) is calculated. Stimulator output is reduced in 5% increments so that the dissociation between MEP threshold and the cortical stimulation silent period (CSSP) can be measured. Stimulator output is reduced until stimulation no longer alters the appearance of the average EMG for the muscle being tested. Dissociation between excitory and inhibitory effects of transcranial stimulation is defined as EMG inhibition without a preceding MEP at 2 or more stimulus intensities. The data is replicated and the signals are stored. The procedure is repeated on 3-4 muscles on the ipsilateral upper extremity and then the contralateral upper extremity is tested in the same manner. Motor pathway function of the lower extremities is then evaluated. The procedure is performed as described above except that electrodes are placed over selected muscles in the legs. The

Medicine

physician reviews the recordings for the upper and lower extremities and provides a written report of findings.

95940-95941

95940 Continuous intraoperative neurophysiology monitoring in the operating room, one on one monitoring requiring personal attendance, each 15 minutes (List separately in addition to code for primary procedure)

95941 Continuous intraoperative neurophysiology monitoring, from outside the operating room (remote or nearby) or for monitoring of more than one case while in the operating room, per hour (List separately in addition to code for primary procedure)

Neurophysiology monitoring is performed during the course of a procedure which includes ongoing electrophysiological monitoring of sensory evoked potentials and EMG potentials performed intraoperatively to reduce permanent postoperative neurological deficits. Report code 95940 for each 15 minutes of one-on-one continuous intraoperative neurophysiology monitoring. Code 95941 is reported per hour of continuous intraoperative neurophysiology monitoring of more than one case in the operating room.

95943

95943 Simultaneous, independent, quantitative measures of both parasympathetic function and sympathetic function, based on time-frequency analysis of heart rate variability concurrent with time-frequency analysis of continuous respiratory activity, with mean heart rate and blood pressure measures, during rest, paced (deep) breathing, Valsalva maneuvers, and head-up postural change

The autonomic nervous system (ANS) is divided into two parts, the sympathetic and parasympathetic nervous system. The sympathetic nervous system helps control blood pressure while the parasympathetic nervous system helps control heart rate. Measurement of heart rate variability (HRV) obtained during deep breathing and Valsalva is a non-invasive technique that can be used to investigate the functioning of the autonomic nervous system. HRV combined with concurrent analysis of respiratory activity is performed to obtain quantitative, independent, simultaneous, noninvasive measures of both autonomic branches. This test is typically performed using automated equipment.

95950

95950 Monitoring for identification and lateralization of cerebral seizure focus, electroencephalographic (eg, 8 channel EEG) recording and interpretation, each 24 hours

The patient is admitted to an epilepsy unit of a hospital where long term monitoring is performed to identify seizure focus—the region of the brain where the seizure activity originates, and to determine whether the focus is on the left or right side of the brain. Multiple EEG electrodes are placed on the scalp. Electrodes may also be placed on other body sites. The electrodes transmit the electrical activity of the brain continuously to a recording and storage device either by a cable or by radio telemetry. The patient is continuously monitored by technicians under the supervision of a physician usually over a 1-3 day period. The physician periodically reviews and analyzes the EEG recordings both during and between seizures. Once sufficient EEG data has been captured, and the seizure focus has been identified and lateralized, the patient is discharged. The physician provides a written interpretation of the long term EEG recordings. Code 95950 is reported for each 24-hour monitoring period.

95951

95951 Monitoring for localization of cerebral seizure focus by cable or radio, 16 or more channel telemetry, combined electroencephalographic (EEG) and video recording and interpretation (eg, for presurgical localization), each 24 hours

The patient is admitted to an epilepsy unit of a hospital where long term monitoring is performed to localize the seizure focus—the region of the brain where the seizure activity originates. The site of the seizure focus must be determined prior to surgery to ensure that the origin of the seizure is in a region that can be treated with surgical excision or destruction of the seizure focus. Multiple EEG electrodes are placed on the scalp. Electrodes may also be placed on other body sites. The electrodes transmit the electrical activity of the brain continuously to a recording and storage device either by a cable or by radio telemetry. During the continuous EEG monitoring procedure, a video recording of the patient's behavior and activities is also captured. The EEG recording and video recording of the patient are time synchronized so that both the brain wave activity and the behavior and motor activity before, during, and after a seizure can be reviewed. The patient is continuously monitored by technicians under the supervision of a physician usually over 1-3 days. The physician periodically reviews and analyses the EEG and video recordings both during and between seizures. Once sufficient EEG and video data has been captured and the seizure focus has been localized, the patient is discharged. The physician provides a written interpretation of the long term EEG and video recordings. Code 95951 is reported for each 24-hour monitoring period.

95953

95953 Monitoring for localization of cerebral seizure focus by computerized portable 16 or more channel EEG, electroencephalographic (EEG) recording and interpretation, each 24 hours, unattended

An electroencephalogram (EEG) is performed to record electrical current potentials from nerve cells in the brain. Variations in the wave characteristics of the electrical current potentials are then used to localize cerebral seizure focus. This test uses a portable, ambulatory recording device for long-term EEG recordings performed on an outpatient basis. The EEG leads are strategically placed on the skin of the scalp. A miniature recording device attached to a belt or shoulder harness is then placed around the patient's waist or shoulder. The leads and recording device are tested to ensure that they are working properly. The recording device is activated and EEG recordings are obtained for the prescribed amount of time. The patient is allowed to leave the facility and perform normal daily activities while the EEG is obtained. Recordings may be taken for several days. When the prescribed amount of time has passed, the patient returns to the facility where the leads and recorder are removed. The physician downloads the EEG recordings onto a computer, evaluates the recordings, and provides a written report of findings. Report 95953 for each 24-hour period.

95954

95954 Pharmacological or physical activation requiring physician or other qualified health care professional attendance during EEG recording of activation phase (eg, thiopental activation test)

During a separately reportable EEG recording, seizure activity is stimulated using a drug such as thiopental or another form of physical activation. The physician or other qualified health care professional administers the medication or supervises other forms of physical activation and remains in attendance to monitor the patient during the activation phase of the EEG recording.

95955

95955 Electroencephalogram (EEG) during nonintracranial surgery (eg, carotid surgery)

An electroencephalogram is performed during a non-intracranial procedure, such as carotid endarterectomy, aneurysm repair requiring clamping of the carotid artery, or cardiac surgery requiring hypothermic cardiac arrest. Electrodes are secured to the scalp. Typically 10-20 electrodes are applied and an 8-32 channel EEG is used. Electrical activity of the brain is recorded and continuously monitored during the surgical procedure. Any changes indicating decreased blood flow to the brain are communicated to the surgical team so that necessary interventions can be initiated. The physician provides a written report of the EEG monitoring.

95956

95956 Monitoring for localization of cerebral seizure focus by cable or radio, 16 or more channel telemetry, electroencephalographic (EEG) recording and interpretation, each 24 hours, attended by a technologist or nurse

An electroencephalogram (EEG) is performed to record electrical current potentials from nerve cells in the brain. Variations in the wave characteristics of the electrical current potentials are then used to localize cerebral seizure focus. This test uses a cable or radio telemetry to transmit the electrical current captured by the EEG leads to a digitized receiver that records the EEG. The transmitted EEG recordings are monitored by a technologist or nurse. The EEG leads are strategically placed on the skin of the scalp. A cable or radio device is used to capture and transmit the digitized EEG waves to an offsite center where the digitized data is displayed on a computer screen. The leads and cable or radio device are tested to ensure that they are working properly. The cable or radio device is activated and EEG recordings are obtained and transmitted to the offsite center for the prescribed amount of time. When the prescribed amount of time has passed, the leads and cable or radio device are removed. The physician evaluates the recordings, and provides a written report of findings. Report 95956 for each 24-hour period.

95957

95957 Digital analysis of electroencephalogram (EEG) (eg, for epileptic spike analysis)

An electroencephalogram is analyzed digitally using tools that allow changes in filtering, horizontal and vertical display scales, and montage reformatting. The digital EEG is recorded using only minimally restrictive analog filtering and a single common reference for all electrodes. The technician uses a computer to reformat the EEG recording to the desired referential or bipolar montage. The EEG is also digitally filtered as needed. Segments of the EEG showing abnormalities may be reformatted multiple times using different montages and filters. Digital reformatting allows better display of abnormalities and helps the physician differentiate elliptiform brain wave patterns from nonelliptiform patterns. The physician reviews the original EEG and the digitally reformatted EEG and provides a written report of findings.

Medicine

95958

95958 Wada activation test for hemispheric function, including electroencephalographic (EEG) monitoring

The Wada test determines which hemisphere (right or left) of the brain controls language function and how important each side of the brain is with regard to memory. Typically, language is controlled by the left side of the brain and memory function is controlled by both sides but one side is dominant. However, there are variations between individuals so for patients who are considering surgical interventions for epilepsy or other conditions, the Wada activation test is performed prior to surgery. Electroencephalogram (EEG) monitoring is used during the procedure. Electrodes are placed on the scalp and connected to the recording device. The physician then injects an anesthetic into the right or left internal carotid artery to put one side of the brain to sleep. EEG recordings are analyzed to ensure that the brain on the side that was injected is asleep. The physician then tests the patient's ability to speak and also shows the patient cards with individual pictures and words. The side of the brain that is awake will try to speak and will try to recognize and remember the pictures and words. After the anesthetic wears off and the side of the brain that was anesthetized wakes up, the physician queries the patient about the cards to determine if the patient can remember the pictures and words that were displayed. The patient's responses are recorded. The opposite internal carotid artery is then injected with anesthetic and the test is repeated with the opposite side of the brain anesthetized. The results for each side of the brain are compared and the physician determines which side of the brain is dominant for language and memory and provides a written report of findings.

95961-95962

95961 Functional cortical and subcortical mapping by stimulation and/or recording of electrodes on brain surface, or of depth electrodes, to provoke seizures or identify vital brain structures; initial hour of attendance by a physician or other qualified health care professional

95962 Functional cortical and subcortical mapping by stimulation and/or recording of electrodes on brain surface, or of depth electrodes, to provoke seizures or identify vital brain structures; each additional hour of attendance by a physician or other qualified health care professional (List separately in addition to code for primary procedure)

Functional and cortical mapping of the brain is performed during a separately reportable neurosurgical procedure to identify regions of the brain cortex responsible for eloquent motor and sensory functions or to provoke seizures. The patient is sedated and a craniotomy is performed to expose the region of the brain were the surgical procedure will be performed. The patient is awakened. Electrodes are placed on the surface of the brain and or depth electrodes are placed in deeper brain tissue. Regions of the brain responsible for vital functions are stimulated and mapped. The separately reportable surgical procedure is then carried out using the mapping information to avoid as much as possible vital regions of the brain. Code 95961 is reported the first hour of attendance and mapping by a physician or other qualified health care professional and code 95962 reports each additional hour.

95965-95967

95965 Magnetoencephalography (MEG), recording and analysis; for spontaneous brain magnetic activity (eg, epileptic cerebral cortex localization)

95966 Magnetoencephalography (MEG), recording and analysis; for evoked magnetic fields, single modality (eg, sensory, motor, language, or visual cortex localization)

95967 Magnetoencephalography (MEG), recording and analysis; for evoked magnetic fields, each additional modality (eg, sensory, motor, language, or visual cortex localization) (List separately in addition to code for primary procedure)

Magnetoencephalography (MEG) is a noninvasive method used to diagnose and evaluate abnormal brain function typically used in conjunction with other separately reportable studies, such as electroencephalogram (EEG) and magnetic resonance imaging (MRI), for evaluating brain disorders. MEG is used to localize epileptic foci prior to surgery and to localize eloquent cortical areas in the brain prior to surgery for brain tumors, arteriovenous malformations, or epilepsy. A multichannel superconducting quantum interference device (SQUID) biomagnetometer system is used to observe and measure the magnetic field generated by brain activity. The MEG SQUID uses more than 100 sensors positioned on the scalp to record the magnetic fields in the brain associated with neuronal activity. The magnetic field recording is then mapped and the site of the epileptic foci or eloquent cortical region is located in the brain. The MEG mapping is then overlayed on separately reportable MRI studies of the brain to locate precisely the site of the epileptic foci or eloquent cortical regions of the brain. The physician reviews the MEG recording and mapping and provides a written interpretation of findings. Use code 95965 for MEG recording and analysis for spontaneous brain magnetic activity such as epileptic cerebral cortex localization. Use code 95966 for single modality evoked magnetic fields for localization of eloquent cortical areas of the brain (sensory, motor, language, or visual cortex localization). Use code 95967 in conjunction with 95966 for each additional modality for evoked magnetic fields (sensory, motor, language or visual cortex).

95970

95970 Electronic analysis of implanted neurostimulator pulse generator system (eg, rate, pulse amplitude, pulse duration, configuration of wave form, battery status, electrode selectability, output modulation, cycling, impedance and patient compliance measurements); simple or complex brain, spinal cord, or peripheral (ie, cranial nerve, peripheral nerve, sacral nerve, neuromuscular) neurostimulator pulse generator/transmitter, without reprogramming

An implanted neurostimulator pulse generator system consists of a generator that is placed in a subcutaneous pocket and electrical leads that are tunneled from the nerve being stimulated to the generator. Electrical impulses are sent from the generator to the brain, spinal cord, peripheral nerve (cranial, sacral, or other peripheral nerve) or to a neuromuscular region to treat a variety of conditions such as pain, epilepsy, and depression. A simple neurostimulator system is defined as one that affects three or fewer of the following: pulse amplitude, pulse duration, pulse frequency, eight or more electrode contacts, cycling, stimulation train duration, train spacing, number of programs, number of channels, alternating electrode polarities, dose time, treatment of more than one clinical feature (rigidity, dyskinesia, tremor). A complex neurostimulatory system affects more than three of the parameters listed above. Neurostimulator pulse generator systems require periodic evaluation to verify that the device is working properly, that the desired results for the condition being treated are being achieved, that the programmed parameters have not changed, and that the battery does not need to be replaced. All device parameters are checked during the evaluation, which may include: rate, pulse amplitude and duration, configuration of waveform, battery status, electrode selectability, output modulation, cycling, impedance, and patient compliance. Use 95970 for electronic analysis of a previously implanted, simple or complex neurostimulator pulse generator system that does not require reprogramming.

95971

95971 Electronic analysis of implanted neurostimulator pulse generator system (eg, rate, pulse amplitude, pulse duration, configuration of wave form, battery status, electrode selectability, output modulation, cycling, impedance and patient compliance measurements); simple spinal cord, or peripheral (ie, peripheral nerve, sacral nerve, neuromuscular) neurostimulator pulse generator/transmitter, with intraoperative or subsequent programming

An implanted neurostimulator pulse generator system consists of a generator that is placed in a subcutaneous pocket and electrical leads that are tunneled from the nerve being stimulated to the generator. Electrical impulses are sent from the generator to the brain, spinal cord, peripheral nerve (cranial, sacral, or other peripheral nerve) or to a neuromuscular region to treat a variety of conditions such as pain, epilepsy, and depression. A simple neurostimulator system is defined as one that affects three or fewer of the following: pulse amplitude, pulse duration, pulse frequency, eight or more electrode contacts, cycling, stimulation train duration, train spacing, number of programs, number of channels, alternating electrode polarities, dose time, treatment of more than one clinical feature (rigidity, dyskinesia, tremor). Neurostimulator pulse generator systems require periodic evaluation to verify that the device is working properly, that the desired results for the condition being treated are being achieved, that the programmed parameters have not changed, and that the battery does not need to be replaced. All device parameters are checked during the evaluation, which may include: rate, pulse amplitude and duration, configuration of waveform, battery status, electrode selectability, output modulation, cycling, impedance, and patient compliance. In 95971, a previously implanted simple spinal or peripheral neurostimulator pulse generator system is subsequently analyzed and programmed or evaluated intraoperatively and programmed.

95972

95972 Electronic analysis of implanted neurostimulator pulse generator system (eg, rate, pulse amplitude, pulse duration, configuration of wave form, battery status, electrode selectability, output modulation, cycling, impedance and patient compliance measurements); complex spinal cord, or peripheral (ie, peripheral nerve, sacral nerve, neuromuscular) (except cranial nerve) neurostimulator pulse generator/transmitter, with intraoperative or subsequent programming

A complex spinal cord or peripheral neurostimulator pulse generator system is electronically evaluated and programmed. An implanted neurostimulator pulse generator system consists of a generator/transmitter placed in a subcutaneous pocket and electrical leads tunneled from the nerve being stimulated to the generator. Electrical impulses are sent from the generator to the spinal cord, a peripheral or sacral nerve (except cranial nerves), or neuromuscular region to treat a variety of conditions such as pain, epilepsy, and depression. A complex neurostimulator system is defined as one that affects more than three of the following: pulse amplitude, pulse duration, pulse frequency, eight or more electrode contacts, cycling, stimulation train duration, train spacing, number of programs and channels, alternating electrode polarities, dose time, and treatment of more than one clinical feature such as rigidity, dyskinesia, and tremor. Neurostimulator pulse generator

Medicine

systems require periodic evaluation to verify that the device is working properly, that the desired results for the condition under treatment are being achieved, that the programmed parameters have not changed, and that the battery does not need to be replaced. All device parameters are checked during the evaluation, which may include: rate, pulse amplitude and duration, configuration of waveform, battery status, electrode selectability, output modulation, cycling, impedance, and patient compliance. The device is then programmed. The analysis and programming may be performed intraoperatively at the time the device is implanted or revised, or programming may be performed during a subsequent evaluation of the implanted device.

95974-95975

95974 Electronic analysis of implanted neurostimulator pulse generator system (eg, rate, pulse amplitude, pulse duration, configuration of wave form, battery status, electrode selectability, output modulation, cycling, impedance and patient compliance measurements); complex cranial nerve neurostimulator pulse generator/transmitter, with intraoperative or subsequent programming, with or without nerve interface testing, first hour

95975 Electronic analysis of implanted neurostimulator pulse generator system (eg, rate, pulse amplitude, pulse duration, configuration of wave form, battery status, electrode selectability, output modulation, cycling, impedance and patient compliance measurements); complex cranial nerve neurostimulator pulse generator/transmitter, with intraoperative or subsequent programming, each additional 30 minutes after first hour (List separately in addition to code for primary procedure)

A complex cranial nerve neurostimulator generator/transmitter is evaluated and programmed. An implanted neurostimulator pulse generator system consists of a generator that is placed in a subcutaneous pocket and electrical leads that are tunneled from the nerve being stimulated to the generator. Electrical impulses are sent from the generator to the cranial nerves to treat a variety of conditions such as pain, epilepsy, and depression. A complex neurostimulator system is defined as one that affects more than three of the following: pulse amplitude, pulse duration, pulse frequency, eight or more electrode contacts, cycling, stimulation train duration, train spacing, number of programs, number of channels, alternating electrode polarities, dose time, treatment of more than one clinical feature (rigidity, dyskinesia, tremor). Neurostimulator pulse generator systems require periodic evaluation to verify that the device is working properly, that the desired results for the condition being treated are being achieved, that the programmed parameters have not changed, and that the battery does not need to be replaced. All device parameters are checked during the evaluation, which may include: rate, pulse amplitude and duration, configuration of waveform, battery status, electrode selectability, output modulation, cycling, impedance, and patient compliance. The device is then programmed. The evaluation and programming may be performed intraoperatively at the time the device is implanted or revised, or programming may be performed during a subsequent evaluation of the device. Use 95974 for the initial hour of evaluation and programming. Use 95975 for each additional 30 minutes.

95978-95979

95978 Electronic analysis of implanted neurostimulator pulse generator system (eg, rate, pulse amplitude and duration, battery status, electrode selectability and polarity, impedance and patient compliance measurements), complex deep brain neurostimulator pulse generator/transmitter, with initial or subsequent programming; first hour

95979 Electronic analysis of implanted neurostimulator pulse generator system (eg, rate, pulse amplitude and duration, battery status, electrode selectability and polarity, impedance and patient compliance measurements), complex deep brain neurostimulator pulse generator/transmitter, with initial or subsequent programming; each additional 30 minutes after first hour (List separately in addition to code for primary procedure)

Deep brain stimulation is used to treat conditions such as Parkinson's disease, essential tremor, and dystonia. It is accomplished by placing stimulating electrodes in various regions of the brain. The electrodes are connected to a pulse generator that is usually implanted in a subcutaneous pocket in the supraclavicular region. The generator is programmed by a physician to reduce symptoms of the neurological condition being treated. Because these neurological conditions may evolve over time, the generators must be reprogrammed periodically for optimal benefits. During initial programming or a subsequent reprogramming of the device, the physician first checks the general functioning of the system. Once proper function is verified, the physician interrogates the device to obtain information on the use of the device if this is a reprogramming service. The physician queries the patient as to his/her experience with the device since the last reprogramming to address any problems or concerns. Any medications that are being used in conjunction with the device are also evaluated to determine if any adjustments to medication are required. Using this information, the physician then sets the parameters for the initial programming or reviews all of the current parameters of the deep brain neurostimulator system for reprogramming including rate, amplitude and duration, battery status, electrode selectability and polarity, and impedance. The physician then programs or reprograms the

device. Use code 95978 for first hour of initial programming or subsequent reprogramming. Use code 95979 for each additional 30 minutes of initial programming or subsequent reprogramming.

95980-95982

95980 Electronic analysis of implanted neurostimulator pulse generator system (eg, rate, pulse amplitude and duration, configuration of wave form, battery status, electrode selectability, output modulation, cycling, impedance and patient measurements) gastric neurostimulator pulse generator/transmitter; intraoperative, with programming

95981 Electronic analysis of implanted neurostimulator pulse generator system (eg, rate, pulse amplitude and duration, configuration of wave form, battery status, electrode selectability, output modulation, cycling, impedance and patient measurements) gastric neurostimulator pulse generator/transmitter; subsequent, without reprogramming

95982 Electronic analysis of implanted neurostimulator pulse generator system (eg, rate, pulse amplitude and duration, configuration of wave form, battery status, electrode selectability, output modulation, cycling, impedance and patient measurements) gastric neurostimulator pulse generator/transmitter; subsequent, with reprogramming

An intraoperative electronic analysis of an implanted gastric neurostimulator pulse generator and transmitter system is performed. Gastric electrical stimulation (GES) is used to treat gastroparesis, a digestive disorder characterized by delayed emptying of the stomach. GES uses an electrical gastric pacemaker device to provide mild stimulation to the lower stomach nerves, which encourages the stomach to contract and move food through the digestive tract. The gastric neurostimulator system is checked during separately reportable placement or replacement. The neurostimulator device and memory card are programmed with patient specific criteria prior to insertion of the electrodes in the stomach. Following placement of the electrode wires, an interrogation procedure is performed. The interrogating head is attached and placed in a plastic bag. The stimulating wires are placed in the neurostimulator and impedance between the wires is checked. If impedance is out of range, the interrogation procedure is repeated while switching the polarity of the electrodes, removing and reinserting the wires into the stimulator, and/or removing and replacing the wires in the stomach until the impedance is within range. Following the interrogation, the surgeon completes the separately reportable implantation procedure. Upon completion of implantation, the interrogation procedure and impedance analysis is repeated and steps taken to bring impedance within range, including switching polarity of the electrodes, and cleansing and reattaching wires in the stimulator, or, removing and replacing the wires in the stomach. Once impedance is in range, incisions are closed and the interrogation procedure is repeated. When the correct impedance range has been attained, the stimulation settings are programmed and reviewed. The stimulation rate, pulse width, cycling times, stimulating electrode settings, and battery status are checked and recorded. When proper functioning of all components has been verified, the device is turned on and the interrogating head is removed. Use 98981 to report subsequent electronic analysis of an implanted neurostimulator device without programming. Subsequent analysis is typically performed at six month intervals to verify that the GES system is functioning properly. The interrogation head is placed over the subcutaneous stimulator in the abdomen. Impedance, voltage, and current are measured along with stimulation rate, pulse width, cycling times, stimulating electrode selections, and battery status. These are compared with previous settings, but no adjustments are necessary. Use 98982 when subsequent electronic analysis is performed with reprogramming, when an adjustment of one of the parameters is required. The physician performs the required reprogramming and verifies the results using the interrogator.

95990-95991

95990 Refilling and maintenance of implantable pump or reservoir for drug delivery, spinal (intrathecal, epidural) or brain (intraventricular), includes electronic analysis of pump, when performed

95991 Refilling and maintenance of implantable pump or reservoir for drug delivery, spinal (intrathecal, epidural) or brain (intraventricular), includes electronic analysis of pump, when performed; requiring skill of a physician or other qualified health care professional

An implantable spinal or brain infusion pump provides long-term continuous or intermittent drug infusion. Because drugs are infused over an extended period of time, the pump or reservoir must be periodically refilled. When the pump is refilled, any pump or reservoir maintenance is performed and an electronic analysis may also be done. The drug is received from the pharmacy and the prescription and patient information are verified. An external needle is used to inject the drug into the pump or reservoir through a self-septum in the implantable infusion pump. Electronic analysis is performed as needed using an interrogation device. A connection is established between the programmable pump and the interrogation device, which provides information on reservoir status, alarm status, and drug flow rates, which are evaluated to ensure that they are all within normal parameters. Use 95991 when refilling and maintenance requires the skill of a physician or other qualified health care professional.

Medicine

95992

95992   Canalith repositioning procedure(s) (eg, Epley maneuver, Semont maneuver), per day

One or more canalith repositioning procedures, such as the Epley or Semont maneuver, are performed to alleviate vertigo (dizziness) caused by calcium crystal debris in the semicircular canal. This type of vertigo is referred to as benign paroxysmal positional vertigo (BPPV). The repositioning procedure redeposits the debris into a neutral area where it no longer causes vertigo. The Epley maneuver is performed by placing the patient in a series of positions that change the orientation of the head. The patient is placed upright in a sitting position. The patient then quickly lies on the back with the head turned to the symptomatic side at a 45 degree angle. The head is also slightly hyperextended. This position is held for 30 to 60 seconds. The patient's eyes are observed for nystagmus, which indicates that the patient is experiencing vertigo. When the vertigo subsides, the head is turned and placed at a 45 degree angle on the opposite side. This position is maintained for another 30 to 60 seconds and the eyes again observed for nystagmus. The patient's body is then turned in the same direction as the head and the patient lies on the side with the head maintained at the 45 degree angle from the body for 30 seconds. The patient may experience another episode of dizziness. The patient is then returned to a sitting position with the head tilted slightly forward. The patient may be very dizzy at this point and may need support to maintain the sitting position. The maneuver is repeated one or more times as needed to alleviate the dizziness. The Semont maneuver is not as popular in the United States. The maneuver begins in a sitting position as described for the Epley maneuver. The patient then lies down on the affected side and is rapidly moved to the opposite side and then returned to sitting position. The maneuver is repeated one or more times. Canalith repositioning may require several treatment sessions over several days and is reported on a per day basis.

96000-96004

96000   Comprehensive computer-based motion analysis by video-taping and 3D kinematics

96001   Comprehensive computer-based motion analysis by video-taping and 3D kinematics; with dynamic plantar pressure measurements during walking

96002   Dynamic surface electromyography, during walking or other functional activities, 1-12 muscles

96003   Dynamic fine wire electromyography, during walking or other functional activities, 1 muscle

96004   Review and interpretation by physician or other qualified health care professional of comprehensive computer-based motion analysis, dynamic plantar pressure measurements, dynamic surface electromyography during walking or other functional activities, and dynamic fine wire electromyography, with written report

Comprehensive computer based motion analysis studies are performed to assist in determining the best therapeutic services or procedures for a patient with a complex movement problem such as that associated with cerebral palsy, spina bifida, traumatic brain injury, amputation, stroke or any other condition that affects movement. These studies may be performed to help determine the need for and the best type of brace or prosthetic and to determine the best surgical intervention. The studies are performed in a dedicated motion analysis laboratory with the capability of performing videotaping from the front, back and both sides; computerized 3-D kinematics; 3-D kinetics and dynamic electromyography. In 96000, markers are placed on specific boney landmarks on the pelvis and lower extremities. The patient then walks in a designated area while cameras track the markers. As the patient walks over force plates, information is collected on joint movement and power. Stride characteristics are also measured by electronic sensors placed on the feet or by the tracking markers. In 96001, dynamic plantar pressure measurements are taken. This involves placement of electronic sensors on the feet. As the patient walks, the sensors record and measure weight bearing pressures on the bottom of the foot. In 96002, surface electrodes are placed bilaterally on the muscles of the lower extremities including the adductors, rectus femoris, quadriceps, hamstrings, and calf muscles. As the patient walks or performs other functional activities, the activity of each individual muscle is recorded including timing and magnitude of muscle response. In 96004, the physician or other qualified health care professional reviews and analyses the results of the computer based motion analysis studies performed and provides a written report of findings. Code 96004 is reported only once regardless of the types or number of motion studies performed.

96020

96020   Neurofunctional testing selection and administration during noninvasive imaging functional brain mapping, with test administered entirely by a physician or other qualified health care professional (ie, psychologist), with review of test results and report

During functional brain imaging, the brain structures are observed while participating in specific mental operations. Images are taken at rest or during a lack of stimulation for a baseline reference and then a series of images are acquired while undergoing certain mental task(s), such as specific body movement, speech function, or processing hearing, visual, or tactile stimulation. The type of neurological function tested and the manner in which the test is applied to the patient during functional brain imaging is determined and administered by a physician or or other qualified health care professional (i.e., psychologist) and includes review of test results and report.

96040

96040   Medical genetics and genetic counseling services, each 30 minutes face-to-face with patient/family

A trained genetic counselor provides a medical genetics evaluation and genetic counseling services to a patient, couple, or family. Genetic counseling is provided to assist the patient and family members in understanding a diagnosed genetic disorder or predisposition for a genetic disorder. The counselor first obtains a family genetic history and may construct a family pedigree chart to illustrate the incidence of the genetic disorder within the family. The specific risk of the patient or the patient's offspring carrying or inheriting the genetic disorder is also assessed. The genetic counselor then helps the patient and family to understand the medical implications of the disorder by explaining the specific disorder, the probable course of the genetic condition, and what medical interventions are available to manage the genetic condition. The genetic counselor explains the hereditary features of the disorder and the risk of occurrence for the patient and the patient's offspring. Options are presented for dealing with a known fetal genetic disorder or the possibility that future offspring may inherit the disorder. The genetic counselor assists the patient and family in choosing a course of action based on their risk tolerance, family considerations, and ethical and religious beliefs. When a child or other family member is affected by a disorder, the genetic counselor also helps the patient and family members adjust to the needs of the affected individual and understand his or her reactions, fears, and concerns related to the diagnosis. Report code 96040 for each 30 minutes of face-to-face counseling with the patient and/or family.

96101

96101   Psychological testing (includes psychodiagnostic assessment of emotionality, intellectual abilities, personality and psychopathology, eg, MMPI, Rorschach, WAIS), per hour of the psychologist's or physician's time, both face-to-face time administering tests to the patient and time interpreting these test results and preparing the report

Psychological testing that may include psychodiagnostic assessment of emotionality, intellectual abilities, personality, and psychopathology using standardized tests such as MMPI, Rorschach, and WAIS. This code reports a time-based testing service and is reported per hour of face-to-face psychologist or physician time spent administering the test(s). The code also includes time spent interpreting the test results and preparing the report by a qualified professional. The appropriate test(s) to be administered are selected and in a face-to-face encounter, the test(s) is administered. Following the testing, raw and standardized scores are derived and analyzed. Additional test data acquired from computer or technician testing is reviewed and integrated and a written report is prepared.

96102-96103

96102   Psychological testing (includes psychodiagnostic assessment of emotionality, intellectual abilities, personality and psychopathology, eg, MMPI and WAIS), with qualified health care professional interpretation and report, administered by technician, per hour of technician time, face-to-face

96103   Psychological testing (includes psychodiagnostic assessment of emotionality, intellectual abilities, personality and psychopathology, eg, MMPI), administered by a computer, with qualified health care professional interpretation and report

Psychological testing that may include psychodiagnostic assessment of emotionality, intellectual abilities, personality, and psychopathology using standardized tests such as MMPI, Rorschach, and WAIS. This code reports a time-based testing service and is reported per hour of face-to-face technician time spent administering the test(s). The code includes time spent interpreting the test results and preparing the report by a qualified professional. The appropriate test(s) to be administered are selected and in a face-to-face encounter, the test(s) is administered. Following the testing, raw and standardized scores are derived and analyzed. Additional test data acquired from computer or technician testing is reviewed and integrated and a written report is prepared. Use 96102 when the psychological testing is administered by a technician and the test(s) is returned to the qualified health care professional for interpretation of the data and written report. Use 96103 when the psychological testing is administered by computer and the patient completes the computerized test. The qualified health care professional reviews the computer test results, interprets the data, and prepares a written report.

Medicine

96105

96105 **Assessment of aphasia (includes assessment of expressive and receptive speech and language function, language comprehension, speech production ability, reading, spelling, writing, eg, by Boston Diagnostic Aphasia Examination) with interpretation and report, per hour**

Aphasia is defined as a disturbance in the comprehension or production of speech caused by a neurological condition or brain injury, such as atherosclerotic disease leading to a cerebral infarction or a skull fracture with intracranial bleeding due to a blow to the head. Assessment of aphasia involves an evaluation of spontaneous speech; word, phrase, and sentence repetition; speech comprehension; recognition and naming of objects; reading; and writing. Assessment involves both the use of an aphasia assessment tool such as the Boston Diagnostic Aphasia Examination and the training, knowledge, and skill of the medical professional performing the assessment. The medical professional administers the test using appropriate testing protocols. The medical professional then reviews the test results and provides a written interpretation of the results. The interpretation will generally identify the specific type of aphasia, such as expressive aphasia or receptive aphasia and will further describe the patient's specific speech and language deficits, such as receptive aphasia with the inability to recognize spoken words (pure word deafness) and the inability to comprehend the meaning of words (transcortical sensory aphasia) or expressive aphasia with the inability to translate thoughts into spoken language. Code 96105 is reported per hour for the assessment, interpretation, and written report.

96110

96110 **Developmental screening (eg, developmental milestone survey, speech and language delay screen), with scoring and documentation, per standardized instrument**

Developmental screening is performed to identify or rule-out developmental delays in children using an age-appropriate standardized screening tool. The screening typically uses a combination of performance-based assessment and parent reporting. Areas of development evaluated include fine motor, gross motor, visual motor/adaptive, speech and language, and personal and social skills. The individual administering the screening selects items based on the age of the patient for each functional area screened, and scores and documents whether performance in each functional area meets developmental milestones or is outside the normal expected range. The number of items in which performance is below the normal expected range determines whether development is classified as within the normal range, suspect, or delayed. Children in the suspect range are monitored by more frequent screening. Children with delayed development are referred for additional developmental testing.

96111

96111 **Developmental testing, (includes assessment of motor, language, social, adaptive, and/or cognitive functioning by standardized developmental instruments) with interpretation and report**

Developmental testing using standardized developmental instruments is performed on a child identified as having one or more developmental delays in motor skills, language, social, adaptive, or cognitive functioning. The individual administering the developmental test selects items based on the age of the patient for each functional area tested. Testing is used to identify the type and severity of the developmental delays more specifically so that appropriate interventions can be initiated and an individual education program (IEP) can be developed for the child. Upon completion of the developmental tests, the individual administering the test interprets the results and provides a written report of findings.

96116

96116 **Neurobehavioral status exam (clinical assessment of thinking, reasoning and judgment, eg, acquired knowledge, attention, language, memory, planning and problem solving, and visual spatial abilities), per hour of the psychologist's or physician's time, both face-to-face time with the patient and time interpreting test results and preparing the report**

A neurobehavioral status exam is performed by a psychologist or physician to assess brain dysfunction. The causes of brain dysfunction and resulting neurobehavioral changes are diverse and include conditions such as vascular disorders, metabolic disorders, head injuries, infections, toxins, brain tumors, developmental disorders (e.g. autism spectrum disorders), and degeneration of the nervous system. Neurobehavioral status exams often involve lengthy observation and evaluation of the patient's development and behavior without the use of direct testing tools. The neurobehavioral status exam can be used as an initial assessment tool to help diagnose and characterize the brain dysfunction, or following diagnosis to assess the progression of brain dysfunction and to evaluate changes in symptoms over time. The psychologist or physician evaluates thinking, reasoning, and judgment. Examples of areas assessed include acquired knowledge, attention, language, memory, the ability to plan and problem solve, and visual spatial abilities. Following the exam the psychologist or physician interprets the test results and provides a written report. Code 96116 is reported per hour for the exam, interpretation, and written report.

96118-96120

96118 **Neuropsychological testing (eg, Halstead-Reitan Neuropsychological Battery, Wechsler Memory Scales and Wisconsin Card Sorting Test), per hour of the psychologist's or physician's time, both face-to-face time administering tests to the patient and time interpreting these test results and preparing the report**

96119 **Neuropsychological testing (eg, Halstead-Reitan Neuropsychological Battery, Wechsler Memory Scales and Wisconsin Card Sorting Test), with qualified health care professional interpretation and report, administered by technician, per hour of technician time, face-to-face**

96120 **Neuropsychological testing (eg, Wisconsin Card Sorting Test), administered by a computer, with qualified health care professional interpretation and report**

A psychologist or physician performs neuropsychological testing in 96118 to evaluate brain function and impairment using standardized tests such as Halstead-Reitan Neuropsychological Battery, Wechsler Memory Scales and Wisconsin Card Sorting Test. This code reports a time-based testing service and is reported per hour of face-to-face time spent administering the test(s), interpreting the results, integrating acquired data, and preparing the report. The psychologist, neuropsychologist, neurologist, or other physician identifies and selects the appropriate test(s) to be administered. In a face-to-face encounter, the test(s) is administered. Raw and standardized scores are derived and analyzed. Additional test data from computer or technician testing is also reviewed and integrated and a written report is prepared. Use 96119 when the neuropsychological testing is administered by a technician and the test data is returned to a qualified health care professional for interpretation and written report. Code 96119 is reported per hour of face-to-face technician time. Use 96120 when the testing is administered by computer and the qualified health care professional reviews the results, interprets the data, and prepares a written report.

96125

96125 **Standardized cognitive performance testing (eg, Ross Information Processing Assessment) per hour of a qualified health care professional's time, both face-to-face time administering tests to the patient and time interpreting these test results and preparing the report**

Standardized cognitive performance testing, such as Ross Information Processing Assessment, is performed by a qualified health care professional such as a speech-language pathologist or occupational therapist. This code reports a time-based testing service and is reported per hour of face-to-face time spent administering the testing, interpreting the results, and preparing the report are included in the total time reported. The qualified health care professional identifies and selects the appropriate test(s) to be administered. Following face-to-face testing, raw and standardized scores are derived and analyzed. A written report is prepared and sent to the requesting physician.

96127

96127 **Brief emotional/behavioral assessment (eg, depression inventory, attention-deficit/hyperactivity disorder [ADHD] scale), with scoring and documentation, per standardized instrument**

Emotional/behavioral assessments may be performed by medical and mental health professionals in the clinical setting and also by trained professionals in the educational setting. These assessments gather information regarding feelings and emotions and problem behaviors through direct observation of the individual and/or questionnaires completed by the individual, caregivers, teachers, and others. Areas assessed can include activities of daily living (ADL), relationships, attitude, adaptability, aggression, anxiety, attention, atypicality, conduct problems, depression, functional communication, hyperactivity, social skills, somatization, withdrawal, and self-esteem. Assessment tools may include the Behavior Assessment System for Children-Second Edition (BASC-2), Behavior Rating Profile-Second Edition (BRP-2), Child Behavior Checklist (CBCL), Conners' Rating Scale, Pervasive Developmental Disorder Behavior Inventory (PDDBI), Brief Infant Toddler Social Emotional Assessment (BITSEA) and the Patient Health Questionnaire for Depression and Anxiety (PHQ-4, PHQ-9). The individual tests can take from 10-45 minutes to complete with additional time allocated for the results to be compiled and scored. Code 96127 can be applied for each standardized test that is administered, scored, and reported.

96150-96151

96150 **Health and behavior assessment (eg, health-focused clinical interview, behavioral observations, psychophysiological monitoring, health-oriented questionnaires), each 15 minutes face-to-face with the patient; initial assessment**

96151 **Health and behavior assessment (eg, health-focused clinical interview, behavioral observations, psychophysiological monitoring, health-oriented questionnaires), each 15 minutes face-to-face with the patient; re-assessment**

A health and behavior assessment or reassessment may be performed by any health care professional with specialized training in health and behavior assessment including physicians, psychologists, advanced practice nurses, or clinical social workers. Health and behavioral assessment procedures are performed to identify biopsychosocial factors that may impact physical health problems and treatments in patients that have acute or chronic illnesses or disabilities. The patient is interviewed regarding medical, emotional, and social history. The patient's ability to manage problems related to the acute or chronic illness is assessed. Standardized questionnaires that evaluate anxiety, pain, coping strategies, and other contributing factors are used to obtain additional information. A treatment plan is developed that includes health and behavioral interventions including a plan for modifying any social factors that may be impacting the patient's health. Use 96150 for the initial face-to-face assessment and report once for each 15-minute time increment. Use 96151 for subsequent face-to-face reassessments and report once for each 15-minute time increment.

96152-96155

96152 Health and behavior intervention, each 15 minutes, face-to-face; individual
96153 Health and behavior intervention, each 15 minutes, face-to-face; group (2 or more patients)
96154 Health and behavior intervention, each 15 minutes, face-to-face; family (with the patient present)
96155 Health and behavior intervention, each 15 minutes, face-to-face; family (without the patient present)

Health and behavior intervention services are performed that may include cognitive, behavioral, social, psychophysiological, or other procedures designed to improve health and treatment outcomes, reduce frequency and severity of disease-related problems, and improve overall well-being. The intervention services may be provided by any health care professional with specialized training in health and behavior interventions including physicians, psychologists, advanced practice nurses, or clinical social workers. Intervention services are specifically designed for the individual patient based on a separately reportable assessment. Techniques used might include education related to biopsychosocial factors influencing health, stress reduction techniques including relaxation and guided imagery, social support such as group discussions, social skills training. The family may be included in the intervention services if family dynamics are exacerbating the health issues of the patient. The provider may help improve communication, conflict resolution, and problem solving skills within the family by providing instruction during the encounter and interpersonal communication exercises to be performed at home. Family members may also be instructed on how to manage biopsychosocial factors related to the care of children or terminally ill patients. For parents of young children, this may include behavior modification techniques such as praise and reward or distraction techniques to reduce fear and anxiety. In terminally ill patients, the caregiver may receive instruction and support related to improving communication, pain monitoring, and issues related to death and dying. Report the appropriate intervention code for each 15 minute time increment. Use 96152 for individual face-to-face encounters with the patient. Use 96153 for group face-to-face encounters. Use 96154 for family face-to-face encounters with the patient present and 96155 for family encounters without the patient present.

96360-96361

96360 Intravenous infusion, hydration; initial, 31 minutes to 1 hour
96361 Intravenous infusion, hydration; each additional hour (List separately in addition to code for primary procedure)

An intravenous infusion is administered for hydration. An intravenous line is placed into a vein, usually in the arm, and fluid is administered to provide additional fluid levels and electrolytes to counteract the effects of dehydration or supplement deficient oral fluid intake. The physician provides direct supervision of the fluid administration and is immediately available to intervene should complications arise. The physician provides periodic assessments of the patient and documentation of the patient's response to treatment. Use 96360 for the initial 31 minutes to one hour of hydration. Use 96361 for each additional hour.

96365-96368

96365 Intravenous infusion, for therapy, prophylaxis, or diagnosis (specify substance or drug); initial, up to 1 hour
96366 Intravenous infusion, for therapy, prophylaxis, or diagnosis (specify substance or drug); each additional hour (List separately in addition to code for primary procedure)
96367 Intravenous infusion, for therapy, prophylaxis, or diagnosis (specify substance or drug); additional sequential infusion of a new drug/substance, up to 1 hour (List separately in addition to code for primary procedure)
96368 Intravenous infusion, for therapy, prophylaxis, or diagnosis (specify substance or drug); concurrent infusion (List separately in addition to code for primary procedure)

An intravenous infusion of a specified substance or drug is administered for therapy, prophylaxis, or diagnosis. An intravenous line is placed into a vein, usually in the arm, and the specified substance or drug is administered. The physician provides direct supervision

of the administration and is immediately available to intervene should complications arise. The physician provides periodic assessments of the patient and documentation of the patient's response to treatment. Use code 96365 for an intravenous infusion up to one hour. Use add-on code 96366 for each additional hour of the same infusion. Use add-on code 96367 for another, sequential infusion of a different substance or drug for up to one hour. Use add-on code 96368 when a different substance or drug is administered at the same time as another drug in a concurrent infusion.

96369-96371

96369 Subcutaneous infusion for therapy or prophylaxis (specify substance or drug); initial, up to 1 hour, including pump set-up and establishment of subcutaneous infusion site(s)
96370 Subcutaneous infusion for therapy or prophylaxis (specify substance or drug); each additional hour (List separately in addition to code for primary procedure)
96371 Subcutaneous infusion for therapy or prophylaxis (specify substance or drug); additional pump set-up with establishment of new subcutaneous infusion site(s) (List separately in addition to code for primary procedure)

A subcutaneous infusion for therapy or prophylaxis of up to one hour is performed (96369), including pump set-up and establishment of infusion site(s). Using aseptic technique, a sterile syringe and needle are used to withdraw the prescribed amount of the substance or drug to be infused. The pump reservoir is filled and the pump and tubing are prepared. The number and location of infusion sites are selected based on the total dosage of the prescribed medication. Common infusion sites include the abdomen, upper buttocks, lateral thigh or hip, and/or upper arm. The infusion sites are prepped with antiseptic solution and a needle is placed in the subcutaneous tissue at each site and tested to verify that it has not been placed in a blood vessel by pulling back on the syringe and checking for blood flow. As each needle is inserted and verified to be placed in subcutaneous tissue, it is secured with tape. When all sites are secured, the drug or medication is administered. Use 96370 for each additional hour of subcutaneous therapeutic or prophylactic infusion beyond the initial hour. Use 96371 for each additional pump set-up beyond the first with establishment of new subcutaneous infusion site(s).

96372

96372 Therapeutic, prophylactic, or diagnostic injection (specify substance or drug); subcutaneous or intramuscular

A subcutaneous or intramuscular injection of a therapeutic, prophylactic, or diagnostic substance or drug is given. A subcutaneous injection is administered just under the skin in the fatty tissue of the abdomen, upper arm, upper leg, or buttocks. The skin is cleansed. A two-inch fold of skin is pinched between the thumb and forefinger. The needle is inserted completely under the skin at a 45 to 90 degree angle using a quick, sharp thrust. The plunger is retracted to check for blood. If blood is present, a new site is selected. If no blood is present, the medication is injected slowly into the tissue. The needle is withdrawn and mild pressure is applied. An intramuscular injection is administered in a similar fashion deep into muscle tissue, differing only in the sites of administration and the angle of needle insertion. Common sites include the gluteal muscles of the buttocks, the vastus lateralis muscle of the thigh, or the deltoid muscle of the upper arm. The angle of insertion is 90 degrees. Intramuscular administration provides rapid systemic absorption and can be used for administration of relatively large doses of medication.

96373

96373 Therapeutic, prophylactic, or diagnostic injection (specify substance or drug); intra-arterial

An intra-arterial injection of a therapeutic, prophylactic, or diagnostic substance or drug is given. Intra-arterial injection delivers medication directly to an artery or organ. Very few medications are delivered into an artery. The arterial site is identified and the skin is cleansed. The artery is punctured and the specified substance or drug is injected.

96374-96376

96374 Therapeutic, prophylactic, or diagnostic injection (specify substance or drug); intravenous push, single or initial substance/drug
96375 Therapeutic, prophylactic, or diagnostic injection (specify substance or drug); each additional sequential intravenous push of a new substance/drug (List separately in addition to code for primary procedure)
96376 Therapeutic, prophylactic, or diagnostic injection (specify substance or drug); each additional sequential intravenous push of the same substance/drug provided in a facility (List separately in addition to code for primary procedure)

A therapeutic, prophylactic, or diagnostic injection is administered by intravenous push (IVP) technique. The specified substance or drug is injected using a syringe directly into an injection site of an existing intravenous line or intermittent infusion set (saline lock). The injection is given over a short period of time, usually less than 15 minutes. Use 96374 for a single or initial substance or drug. Use 96375 as an add-on code for each additional sequential push of a new substance or drug provided through the same venous access site.

Medicine

Use 96376 for the facility component for each additional sequential intravenous push of the same substance/drug when the interval between each administration is 30 minutes or more.

96401-96402

96402 **Chemotherapy administration, subcutaneous or intramuscular; hormonal anti-neoplastic**

96401 **Chemotherapy administration, subcutaneous or intramuscular; non-hormonal anti-neoplastic**

A subcutaneous injection is administered just under the skin in the fatty tissue of the abdomen, upper arm, upper leg, or buttocks. The skin is cleansed. A two-inch fold of skin is pinched between the thumb and forefinger. The needle is inserted completely under the skin at a 45 to 90 degree angle using a quick sharp thrust. The plunger is retracted to check for blood. If blood is present, a new site is selected. If no blood is present, the medication is injected slowly into the tissue. The needle is withdrawn and mild pressure is applied at the injection site. An intramuscular injection is administered in a similar fashion deep into muscle tissue. Common intramuscular sites include the gluteal muscles of the buttocks, the vastus lateralis muscle of the thigh, or the deltoid muscle of the upper arm. The angle of insertion is a 90 -degree angle. Intramuscular administration provides rapid systemic absorption and can be used for administration of relatively large doses of chemotherapy substances or drugs. Use 96401 for a non-hormonal anti-neoplastic agent and 96402 for a hormonal anti-neoplastic.

96405-96406

96405 **Chemotherapy administration; intralesional, up to and including 7 lesions**
96406 **Chemotherapy administration; intralesional, more than 7 lesions**

One or more malignant lesions in the skin or subcutaneous tissues are injected with an antineoplastic agent to eradicate or reduce the size of the lesion. The skin is cleansed around the planned injection site. The physician then injects the antineoplastic agent in and around the lesion. If more than one lesion is to be treated, the process is repeated until all lesions have been injected. Use code 96405 for injection of up to 7 lesions. Use 96406 for injection of more than 7 lesions. Report these codes based on the number of lesions, not on the number of injections as a single lesion may be injected at multiple sites.

96409-96411

96409 **Chemotherapy administration; intravenous, push technique, single or initial substance/drug**

96411 **Chemotherapy administration; intravenous, push technique, each additional substance/drug (List separately in addition to code for primary procedure)**

A chemotherapy substance or drug is administered by intravenous push (IVP) technique for treatment of a malignant neoplasm. The specified chemotherapy substance or drug is injected using a syringe directly into the vein via an existing intravenous line or an intermittent infusion set (saline lock). The injection is given over a short period of time, usually less than 15 minutes. Use 96409 for IVP of a single or initial chemotherapy substance or drug. Use 96411 as an add-on code for each additional sequential push of a new chemotherapy substance or drug provided through the same venous access site.

96413-96417

96413 **Chemotherapy administration, intravenous infusion technique; up to 1 hour, single or initial substance/drug**

96415 **Chemotherapy administration, intravenous infusion technique; each additional hour (List separately in addition to code for primary procedure)**

96416 **Chemotherapy administration, intravenous infusion technique; initiation of prolonged chemotherapy infusion (more than 8 hours), requiring use of a portable or implantable pump**

96417 **Chemotherapy administration, intravenous infusion technique; each additional sequential infusion (different substance/drug), up to 1 hour (List separately in addition to code for primary procedure)**

An intravenous infusion of a chemotherapy substance or drug is administered for treatment of a malignant neoplasm. An intravenous line is placed into a vein, usually in the arm, and the specified chemotherapy agent is administered. The physician provides direct supervision of the administration of the chemotherapy agent and is immediately available to intervene should complications arise. The physician provides periodic assessments of the patient and documentation of the patient's response to treatment. Use code 96413 for an intravenous infusion up to one hour of a single or initial chemotherapy substance or drug. Use add-on code 96415 for each additional hour of the chemotherapy substance or drug. Use 96416 for prolonged chemotherapy intravenous infusion of more than eight hours requiring the use of a portable or implantable pump. Use add-on code 96417 for an additional sequential infusion of a different substance or drug for up to one hour.

96420

96420 **Chemotherapy administration, intra-arterial; push technique**

A chemotherapy substance or drug is administered by intra-arterial push technique for treatment of a malignant neoplasm. This technique may also be referred to as regional or isolation chemotherapy perfusion. An intra-arterial injection delivers medication directly to an artery or organ. Separately reportable arterial catheterization under radiologic supervision is performed so that the chemotherapy substance or drug can be delivered directly to the site of the neoplasm. The chemotherapy substance or drug is injected directly into the artery supplying blood to the organ or site over a short period of time, usually less than 15 minutes.

96422-96425

96422 **Chemotherapy administration, intra-arterial; infusion technique, up to 1 hour**

96423 **Chemotherapy administration, intra-arterial; infusion technique, each additional hour (List separately in addition to code for primary procedure)**

96425 **Chemotherapy administration, intra-arterial; infusion technique, initiation of prolonged infusion (more than 8 hours), requiring the use of a portable or implantable pump**

A chemotherapy substance or drug is administered by intra-arterial infusion technique for treatment of a malignant neoplasm. This technique may also be referred to as regional or isolation chemotherapy perfusion. An intra-arterial injection delivers medication directly to an artery or organ. Separately reportable arterial catheterization under radiologic supervision is performed so that the chemotherapy substance or drug can be delivered directly to the site of the neoplasm. The chemotherapy substance or drug is injected directly into the artery supplying blood to the organ or site. Use code 96422 for an intra-arterial infusion up to one hour and add-on code 96423 for each additional hour. Use 96425 for prolonged chemotherapy by intra-arterial infusion for more than eight hours using a portable or implantable pump.

96440

96440 **Chemotherapy administration into pleural cavity, requiring and including thoracentesis**

One or a combination of antineoplastic drugs is injected directly into the pleural cavity. The physician inserts a chest tube into the pleural space. The skin is cleansed and a local anesthetic is administered. A small incision is made between the ribs on the side or the front of the chest and a trocar is used to puncture into the pleural cavity. A small track is then made through the chest wall and a tube is inserted into the pleural cavity and fluid is drained. The antineoplastic drugs are then infused through the chest tube, which is repositioned as needed and the process is repeated. The antineoplastic drugs are left in the pleural cavity for a prescribed period of time and then the pleural cavity is drained by connecting the chest tube to a thoracic drainage and collection system. The chest tube remains in place until drainage is complete.

96446

96446 **Chemotherapy administration into the peritoneal cavity via indwelling port or catheter**

Intraperitoneal chemotherapy is used to treat both primary and secondary malignancies of the peritoneum, a serous membrane composed of mesothelial cells with a rich vascular and lymphatic capillary network. Peritoneal neoplasms may originate in the peritoneal tissues or metastasize from adjacent or remote sites. An indwelling port or intraperitoneal catheter is placed during a separately reportable procedure. A chemotherapeutic or other anti-neoplastic agent is administered via the existing port or catheter. This allows the agent to come into direct contact with malignant tissue resulting in higher exposure to the chemotherapeutic or other anti-neoplastic agent. The patient is placed supine with the head of the bed slightly elevated. The chemotherapeutic or other anti-neoplastic agent is then infused via the port or catheter. Upon completion of the infusion, the patient is repositioned from side-to-side every 15 minutes for a total of one hour to promote dispersal of the agent throughout the peritoneal cavity.

● New Code   ▲ Revised Code   CPT © 2016 American Medical Association. All Rights Reserved.   © 2017 DecisionHealth

Medicine

Chemotherapy administration, peritoneal cavity

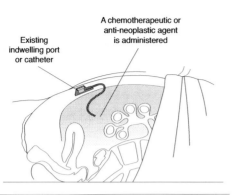

A chemotherapeutic or anti-neoplastic agent is administered

Existing indwelling port or catheter

96450

96450   Chemotherapy administration, into CNS (eg, intrathecal), requiring and including spinal puncture

One or a combination of antineoplastic drugs is injected into the central nervous system. This procedure is also referred to as intrathecal chemotherapy. The skin over the lumbar spine is disinfected and a local anesthetic is administered. A lumbar puncture needle is then inserted into the spinal canal. CSF specimens are collected as needed. A spinal catheter is advanced through the lumbar puncture needle. The antineoplastic drugs are then injected into the spinal fluid in the spinal canal. The spinal fluid containing the antineoplastic drugs then circulates around the spinal canal and brain delivering the drugs to the central nervous system. Upon completion of the procedure, the spinal catheter is removed and pressure is applied at the puncture site as needed.

96521-96522

96521   Refilling and maintenance of portable pump
96522   Refilling and maintenance of implantable pump or reservoir for drug delivery, systemic (eg, intravenous, intra-arterial)

External and implantable pumps or reservoirs are used for prolonged infusion of chemotherapy drugs, monoclonal antibody agents, other biologic response modifiers, and other antineoplastic substances. Prolonged infusion is defined as infusion over more than eight hours. The pump is filled with the prescribed amount of the chemotherapy drug or other highly complex drug or biologic agent. The pump is programmed to continuously deliver the prescribed amount of the drug over a prolonged period of time. The pump is checked to ensure that the pump is working properly and the drug is being delivered as prescribed. Use 96521 for an external portable pump. Use 92522 for an implantable pump or reservoir.

96523

96523   Irrigation of implanted venous access device for drug delivery systems

Implanted venous access devices require periodic irrigation to keep blood clots from forming and obstructing the device. The site of the venous access device is cleansed with alcohol and/or betadine and then allowed to air dry. A needle connected to a syringe is inserted into the device and the heparin in the tubing aspirated. When blood return is achieved, a syringe that is preloaded with the appropriate amount of saline is used to flush the venous access device. Another syringe with a preloaded amount of heparin is then injected into the venous access device to prevent blood clots from forming in the device. Use 96523 for periodic irrigation services that are not provided in conjunction with an injection or infusion service.

96542

96542   Chemotherapy injection, subarachnoid or intraventricular via subcutaneous reservoir, single or multiple agents

One or a combination of antineoplastic drugs is injected into the subarachnoid or intraventricular spaces of the central nervous system via a previously placed subcutaneous reservoir. A subcutaneous reservoir is used for injection of chemotherapy drugs, monoclonal antibody agents, other biologic response modifiers, and other antineoplastic substances. The skin is prepped over the reservoir site. A special needle is used to puncture the skin and the needle is then advanced into the reservoir. The reservoir is filled with the prescribed amount of the chemotherapy drug or other highly complex drug or biologic agent. The reservoir may then be manually compressed to deliver the drug to the subarachnoid space or ventricles or a pump may be used to deliver the drug. The drug circulates with the cerebrospinal fluid and is delivered to the site of the neoplasm.

96567

96567   Photodynamic therapy by external application of light to destroy premalignant and/or malignant lesions of the skin and adjacent mucosa (eg, lip) by activation of photosensitive drug(s), each phototherapy exposure session

Photodynamic therapy (PDT) uses photosensitive (photoreactive) chemicals and light to destroy premalignant and malignant lesions of the skin and adjacent mucosa. Photoreactive chemicals may be administered intravenously or applied topically to the lesion. If the chemicals are applied topically, the lesion may be prepared by removing overlying crust and scale. The lesion is then irradiated with light of the appropriate wavelength which activates the photoreactive chemical resulting in destruction of the lesion. More than one lesion may be treated per PDT session. Code 96567 is reported once per PDT session.

96570-96571

96570   Photodynamic therapy by endoscopic application of light to ablate abnormal tissue via activation of photosensitive drug(s); first 30 minutes (List separately in addition to code for endoscopy or bronchoscopy procedures of lung and gastrointestinal tract)
96571   Photodynamic therapy by endoscopic application of light to ablate abnormal tissue via activation of photosensitive drug(s); each additional 15 minutes (List separately in addition to code for endoscopy or bronchoscopy procedures of lung and gastrointestinal tract)

Photodynamic therapy (PDT) involves administration of a light-activated drug followed by application of light from a laser to destroy abnormal tissue in the lungs or gastrointestinal tract. Approximately 48 hours prior to the planned PDT procedure, an intravenous injection is given of the light-activated drug (Photofrin). The drug is absorbed by body tissue including cancerous or abnormal tissue. During a separately reportable gastrointestinal endoscopy or bronchoscopy procedure, a low-intensity laser is directed at the cancerous or abnormal tissue. The drug reacts to the light and which causes destruction of the cancerous or abnormal tissue. Use code 96570 for the first 30 minutes of PDT and code 96571 for each additional 15 minutes.

96900

96900   Actinotherapy (ultraviolet light)

Actinotherapy, also referred to as phototherapy, involves the use of ultraviolet light (UVA or UVB) to treat skin conditions. The site of the skin condition is exposed. The appropriate wave-length of UVA or UVB light is selected and the site of the skin condition is exposed to the light for the prescribed period of time.

96902

96902   Microscopic examination of hairs plucked or clipped by the examiner (excluding hair collected by the patient) to determine telogen and anagen counts, or structural hair shaft abnormality

Hair that is plucked or clipped is examined microscopically to determine the phase of growth and help diagnose disorders of hair growth and/or disorders of the hair shaft. If hair is plucked, about 50 individual hairs are grasped and sharply pulled out by the roots. The hair roots are examined microscopically and the hair growth phase of each hair is determined. Hair growth is divided into three phases—anagen (hair with sheaths attached to roots), telogen (hair with bulbs but not sheaths at the roots), and catagen (short transition phase between the anagen and telogen phase). In the anagen phase, hair is actively growing; in the catagen phase, hair growth has ceased; and in the telogen phase, hair is resting prior to falling out. Typically at any point in time, 85-90% of individual hairs are in the anagen phase, 10-15% are in the telogen phase, and less than 1% are in the catagen phase. Hair shaft disorders may be diagnosed by clipping the hair and looking for abnormalities in the hair such as bubble hair, beaded hair, or bamboo hair. All of these hair shaft disorders result in fragility and breakage of hair which can be diagnosed by examining the hair microscopically. A written report of the microscopic findings is provided.

96904

96904   Whole body integumentary photography, for monitoring of high risk patients with dysplastic nevus syndrome or a history of dysplastic nevi, or patients with a personal or familial history of melanoma

Whole body integumentary photography is done to monitor high risk patients with current dysplastic nevus syndrome, those with a history of dysplastic nevi, or a personal or familial history of melanoma. This procedure involves taking extensive photographs of the patient's skin to detect abnormal moles, which can be a sign or precursor of skin cancer. Dysplastic nevus syndrome is a condition in which the patient experiences the sudden appearance of multiple abnormal moles, typically at a young age.

Medicine

96910-96912

96910 Photochemotherapy; tar and ultraviolet B (Goeckerman treatment) or petrolatum and ultraviolet B

96912 Photochemotherapy; psoralens and ultraviolet A (PUVA)

Photochemotherapy, such as Goeckerman, petrolatum and UVB, or psoralen plus ultraviolet A light therapy (PUVA), is used to treat severe photoresponsive dermatoses, such as psoriasis, eczema, vitiligo, and mycosis fungoides. Using PUVA therapy, psoralen, a medication that increases sensitivity to UVA light, is administered orally approximately 2 hours before exposure to the light. Goeckerman therapy uses a combination of coal tar applied to the affected areas of the skin and UVB light therapy. Alternatively, petrolatum and UVB light may be used. Following administration of the psoralen or application of the coal tar or petrolatum, the patient is placed in a UVA or UVB light booth for a specified period of time. The length of exposure to the UVA or UVB light will depend on the nature of the dermatosis being treated. Following treatment, any topical medications are removed from the skin, the skin is inspected, and dressings are applied as needed. Use code 96910 for Goeckerman or petrolatum photochemotherapy using UVB light exposure. Use code 96912 for PUVA therapy.

96913

96913 Photochemotherapy (Goeckerman and/or PUVA) for severe photoresponsive dermatoses requiring at least 4-8 hours of care under direct supervision of the physician (includes application of medication and dressings)

Photochemotherapy, such as Goeckerman or psoralen plus ultraviolet A light therapy (PUVA), is used to treat severe photoresponsive dermatoses, such as psoriasis, eczema, vitiligo, and mycosis fungoides. Using PUVA therapy, psoralen, a medication that increases sensitivity UVA light, is administered orally approximately 2 hours before exposure to the light. Goeckerman therapy uses a combination of coal tar applied to the affected areas of the skin and UVA light therapy. The patient is then placed in a UVA light booth for a specified period of time depending on the nature of the dermatosis being treated. The patient remains under direct physician supervision for a period of 4-8 hours which includes the time following administration of the medication or application of coal tar and the time during which the light therapy is administered. Following treatment the physician may apply dressings as needed to affected areas of the skin.

96920-96922

96920 Laser treatment for inflammatory skin disease (psoriasis); total area less than 250 sq cm

96921 Laser treatment for inflammatory skin disease (psoriasis); 250 sq cm to 500 sq cm

96922 Laser treatment for inflammatory skin disease (psoriasis); over 500 sq cm

Laser treatment for inflammatory skin disease such as psoriasis is performed. A clarifying agent such as mineral oil is applied to the affected area. The site to be treated is inspected and the lesions are evaluated for redness and erythema. If there is any blistering or pain due to a previous laser treatment or other treatment modality that is also evaluated. Laser dosage is determined and the area is treated. The physician monitors the skin surface and the patient's pain level throughout the procedure. Use 96920 for a total area of less than 250 sq cm, 96921 if total area is between 250 sq cm and 500 sq cm, and 96922 if total area is greater than 500 sq cm.

97010

97010 Application of a modality to 1 or more areas; hot or cold packs

Hot or cold packs are applied to one or more sites. Cold packs are applied to reduce blood flow, inflammation, and pain. Cold packs are typically used as an initial treatment for an acute soft tissue injury. The physical therapist applies the cold pack to the site of the injury. Hot packs are used to increase blood flow, promote muscle relaxation, promote healing, and to prepare muscles for stretching or other exercise. Typically moist hot packs are used. The physical therapist places the moist hot pack on or around the site to the treated. Hot and cold packs are a supervised physical medicine modality that does not require direct (one-on-one) patient contact.

97012

97012 Application of a modality to 1 or more areas; traction, mechanical

Mechanical traction involves the use of a pulling force to the head/neck, pelvis, or extremities. The pulling force is used to stretch and distract muscles, ligaments, and tendons to relieve pain and increase connective tissue flexibility. The patient is fitted with halters or straps to which weights are applied to provide the pulling force. Alternatively, body weight may be used to provide the pulling force for distraction of the cervical spine. Mechanical traction is used to treat conditions such as extremity pain or tingling, spinal nerve root impingement, and loss of mobility in the spine. Mechanical traction is a supervised physical medicine modality that does not require direct (one-on-one) patient contact.

97014

97014 Application of a modality to 1 or more areas; electrical stimulation (unattended)

Electrical stimulation involves the use of a transcutaneous electrical nerve stimulation device (TENS), functional electrical stimulation device (FES), or a neuromuscular electrical stimulation device (NMES). The physical therapist or other physical therapy aid places the electrodes of the selected device over the region to be stimulated. The electrical impulse is set to the desired strength and the control unit is turned on. Electrical impulses are transmitted to the skin. The electrical stimulation device causes the muscles to contract. The muscle contraction stimulates both muscle and nerve tissues to relieve pain and promote healing. Electrical stimulation may be provided as a supervised modality that does not require direct (one-on-one) patient contact or it may be provided under constant attendance with direct (one-on-one) patient contact. Code 97014 reports an unattended, supervised physical medicine modality that does not require direct (one-on-one) patient contact.

97032

97032 Application of a modality to 1 or more areas; electrical stimulation (manual), each 15 minutes

Electrical stimulation involves the use of a transcutaneous electrical nerve stimulation device (TENS), functional electrical stimulation device (FES), or a neuromuscular electrical stimulation device (NMES). The physical therapist or other physical therapy aid places the electrodes of the selected device over the region to be stimulated. The electrical impulse is set to the desired strength and the control unit is turned on. Electrical impulses are transmitted to the skin. The electrical stimulation device causes the muscles to contract. The muscle contraction stimulates both muscle and nerve tissues to relieve pain and promote healing. Electrical stimulation may be provided as a supervised modality that does not require direct (one-on-one) patient contact or it may be provided under constant attendance with direct (one-on-one) patient contact. Code 97032 reports electrical stimulation with constant attendance and direct (one-on-one) patient contact per 15 minutes.

97033

97033 Application of a modality to 1 or more areas; iontophoresis, each 15 minutes

Iontophoresis uses electric current to treat hyperhidrosis (excessive sweating). It may also be used to relieve pain and inflammation of tendons, bursae, and muscles, which involves the use of a drug applied topically, such as lidocaine or dexamethasone, and the use of electrodes to help the drug penetrate the skin so that it can be absorbed by deeper tissues. Iontophoresis uses mild electrical currents that are generated and regulated using a control unit and electrodes that are placed on the site to be treated. A drug may be applied topically or a drug patch may be placed on the skin prior to placing the electrodes. The iontophoresis machine is then activated for the prescribed period of time. Alternatively for treatment of hyperhidrosis of the hands and feet, a tray filled with water to which the electrodes are attached may be used. Iontophoresis is a physical therapy modality that requires constant attendance with direct (one-on-one) patient contact. Iontophoresis is a time-based service reported in 15-minute increments.

97035

97035 Application of a modality to 1 or more areas; ultrasound, each 15 minutes

Ultrasound uses high frequency sound waves applied to produce heat and/or vibration to promote the circulation, reduce inflammation, and improve the flexibility of connective tissue. A water-soluble gel is applied to the site to be treated. A hand-held device is used to deliver the sound waves. The device is moved over the site using a circular motion. Ultrasound is helpful in treating acute soft tissue injures. Ultrasound is a physical therapy modality that requires constant attendance with direct (one-on-one) patient contact. Ultrasound is a time-based service reported in 15-minute increments.

97530

97530 Therapeutic activities, direct (one-on-one) patient contact (use of dynamic activities to improve functional performance), each 15 minutes

In a one-on-one physical therapy session, the provider instructs and assists the patient in therapeutic activities designed to address specific functional limitations. The therapeutic activities are specifically developed and modified for the patient. Dynamic/movement activities, also called kinetic activities, that are designed to improve functional performance such as lifting, bending, pushing, pulling, jumping and reaching are included in this service. For example, the patient may be given therapeutic activities to perform to improve the ability to sit, stand, and get out of bed after an injury without straining or risking reinjury. This code is reported for each 15 minutes of one-on-one therapeutic activity provided.

● New Code   ▲ Revised Code   CPT © 2016 American Medical Association. All Rights Reserved.   © 2017 DecisionHealth

Medicine

97532

97532   **Development of cognitive skills to improve attention, memory, problem solving (includes compensatory training), direct (one-on-one) patient contact, each 15 minutes**

Direct, one-on-one cognitive skill training is provided by an occupational therapist to improve attention, memory, and problem solving skills. This type of training may be used for patients with psychiatric disorders, traumatic brain injuries, or cerebral vascular accidents. Cognitive skill training includes activities designed to improve short and long term memory, apply logic, develop the ability to remember, and perform a sequence of activities, such as dressing or taking medications. The occupational therapist first evaluates the patient's home environment and daily routine. The therapist then develops a program that will help the patient develop the necessary skills to live independently, return to work, and function safely in their home and/or work environment. Once the training program has been defined and therapy goals are established, the therapist then works with the patient on a one-to-one basis until the goals have been met. Cognitive skill training is reported per 15 min interval.

97533

97533   **Sensory integrative techniques to enhance sensory processing and promote adaptive responses to environmental demands, direct (one-on-one) patient contact, each 15 minutes**

Direct, one-on-one sensory integrative techniques are used to enhance sensory processing and promote adaptive responses to environmental demands. Sensory integration services may be used in the treatment of autism, developmental disorders, attention deficit disorders, cerebral palsy, or motor ataxia. Sensory integration refers to the ability of the brain to properly integrate and adapt to information coming through the senses. Patients with sensory integration dysfunction have difficulty adapting and functioning because they are unable to filter and appropriately respond to sensory stimuli. These patients may then respond with sensory defensiveness, over-reaction to stimuli, behavioral problems, or attention deficits. The occupational therapist first evaluates the patient to determine which sensory systems are affected and may include one or more of the following: vestibular, proprioceptive, tactile, visual, or auditory. Once the affected sensory systems are identified, the therapist designs activities to help the patient regulate behavioral responses to stimuli that they find disturbing or painful. The therapist also establishes treatment goals. For example, an individual who is oversensitive to touch might begin with exercises designed to improve response to light touch. Then as behavioral responses improve, activities that involve progressively heavier touch or touch involving different textures are introduced. Sensory integrated services are reported per 15 minute interval.

97535

97535   **Self-care/home management training (eg, activities of daily living (ADL) and compensatory training, meal preparation, safety procedures, and instructions in use of assistive technology devices/adaptive equipment) direct one-on-one contact, each 15 minutes**

Self-care/home manageme The patient receives one-on-one training to improve the ability to care for himself/herself and maintain independence. This may include training in activities of daily living (ADL), such as bed mobility, transfers, dressing, grooming, eating, bathing and toileting. The patient is given instruction on compensatory measures that can be taken to overcome any physical, mental or emotional disabilities. The patient receives training in how to adapt meal preparation to his/her specific needs and how to perform activities safely. The patient may also receive instruction in the use of assistive technology devices and adaptive equipment which includes any item used to improve the functional capability of the patient in the home and with ADL. This code is reported for each 15 minutes of one-on-one self-care/home management training designed to meet the specific needs of the patient.nt training, which includes instructions in the use of any assisting equipment.

97537

97537   **Community/work reintegration training (eg, shopping, transportation, money management, avocational activities and/or work environment/ modification analysis, work task analysis, use of assistive technology device/adaptive equipment), direct one-on-one contact, each 15 minutes**

The patient receives one-on-one training designed to facilitate community and/or work reintegration and to live as independently as possible. This may include taking the patient out into the community to use public transportation or shop, helping the patient set up a budget and develop a system for managing money, and assessing and modifying the work environment so that the patient can perform job related tasks. The patient may also receive instruction in the use of assistive technology devices and adaptive equipment which includes any item used to improve the functional capability of the patient in the community or at work. This code is reported for each 15 minutes of one-on-one communication/work reintegration training.

97597-97598

97597   **Debridement (eg, high pressure waterjet with/without suction, sharp selective debridement with scissors, scalpel and forceps), open wound, (eg, fibrin, devitalized epidermis and/or dermis, exudate, debris, biofilm), including topical application(s), wound assessment, use of a whirlpool, when performed and instruction(s) for ongoing care, per session, total wound(s) surface area; first 20 sq cm or less**

97598   **Debridement (eg, high pressure waterjet with/without suction, sharp selective debridement with scissors, scalpel and forceps), open wound, (eg, fibrin, devitalized epidermis and/or dermis, exudate, debris, biofilm), including topical application(s), wound assessment, use of a whirlpool, when performed and instruction(s) for ongoing care, per session, total wound(s) surface area; each additional 20 sq cm, or part thereof (List separately in addition to code for primary procedure)**

An open wound is evaluated for size, depth, and evidence of inflammation, ulceration, or necrosis. Whirlpool is used as needed prior to the debridement procedure. The involved tissue, including fibrin, devitalized epidermis and/or dermis, exudate, debris, or biofilm, is selectively debrided using a high pressure waterjet or sharp debridement. A high pressure waterjet system consists of a power console, foot pedal, disposable hand held waterjet/ aspirator, sterile water, tubing, and evacuation receptacle. The target tissue is identified. A high-pressure stream of water is projected at the target tissue which is simultaneously "cut" and aspirated into an evacuation receptacle. Sharp debridement involves using scissors, scalpel, and/or forceps to selectively remove devitalized tissue and debris. Topical agents to promote healing and dressings are applied as needed following the debridement. The patient or caregiver is instructed on dressing changes and wound evaluation. Use 97597 for debridement of the first 20 sq cm of wound surface area. Use 97598 for each additional 20 sq cm debrided or portion thereof.

97602

97602   **Removal of devitalized tissue from wound(s), non-selective debridement, without anesthesia (eg, wet-to-moist dressings, enzymatic, abrasion), including topical application(s), wound assessment, and instruction(s) for ongoing care, per session**

Non-selective debridement is performed without anesthesia to remove devitalized tissue from wounds including topical applications, wound assessment, and instructions for ongoing care. Non-selective debriement includes debridement performed by wet, wet-to-dry, and wet-to-moist dressings; the use of enzymes; or by autolysis or abrasion. Previously placed dressings are removed. The wound is lightly cleansed. The wound is evaluated for size, depth, and evidence of inflammation, ulceration, or necrosis. Involved tissue is prepared using pulsatile lavage, irrigation, or hydrotherapy to soften and loosen the tissue. The tissue is then removed using one of the above techniques. Ointments, cleansers, sealants, and dressings are applied as needed to the wound. Non-selective debridement is reported per treatment session.

97605-97606

97605   **Negative pressure wound therapy (eg, vacuum assisted drainage collection), utilizing durable medical equipment (DME), including topical application(s), wound assessment, and instruction(s) for ongoing care, per session; total wound(s) surface area less than or equal to 50 square centimeters**

97606   **Negative pressure wound therapy (eg, vacuum assisted drainage collection), utilizing durable medical equipment (DME), including topical application(s), wound assessment, and instruction(s) for ongoing care, per session; total wound(s) surface area greater than 50 square centimeters**

Negative pressure wound therapy (NPWT) may be used to promote healing of acute or chronic wounds and enhance healing of first and second degree burns. NPWT is the controlled application of sub-atmospheric, intermittent or continuous pressure to a local wound area which has been sealed with a bio-occlusive dressing and connected to a vacuum pump. This technique allows the wound to remain moist but protected, and removes excess fluid, reduces edema, and increases blood circulation. The dressing consists of cell foam or gauze filler material fitted to the wound contours which is then sealed with a transparent bio-occlusive film. The drainage tube is inserted into the wound through a small slit in the film and connected to the vacuum pump. The dressing is changed 2-3 times per week, disposing of old dressing material and drainage tubing in biohazard bags. The wound is then assessed for healing and infection. The wound may be irrigated and cleaned and topical medications may be applied. The wound is then redressed and the patient/caregiver is given instructions for ongoing care. Code 97605 is used when the wound(s) surface area is less than or equal to 50 square centimeters. Code 97606 is used when the total wound(s) surface area is greater than 50 square centimeters.

Medicine

97607-97608

97607 Negative pressure wound therapy, (eg, vacuum assisted drainage collection), utilizing disposable, non-durable medical equipment including provision of exudate management collection system, topical application(s), wound assessment, and instructions for ongoing care, per session; total wound(s) surface area less than or equal to 50 square centimeters

97608 Negative pressure wound therapy, (eg, vacuum assisted drainage collection), utilizing disposable, non-durable medical equipment including provision of exudate management collection system, topical application(s), wound assessment, and instructions for ongoing care, per session; total wound(s) surface area greater than 50 square centimeters

Negative pressure wound therapy (NPWT) may be used to promote healing of acute or chronic wounds and enhance healing of first and second degree burns. NPWT is the controlled application of sub-atmospheric, intermittent or continuous pressure to a local wound area which has been sealed with a bio-occlusive dressing and connected to a vacuum pump. This technique allows the wound to remain moist but protected, and removes excess fluid, reduces edema, and increases blood circulation. The dressing consists of cell foam or gauze filler material fitted to the wound contours which is then sealed with a transparent bio-occlusive film. The drainage tube is inserted into the wound through a small slit in the film and connected to the vacuum pump. The dressing is changed 2-3 times per week, disposing of old dressing material and drainage tubing in biohazard bags. The wound is then assessed for healing and infection. The wound may be irrigated and cleaned and topical medications may be applied. The wound is then redressed and the patient/caregiver is given instructions for ongoing care. Code 97607 is used when the wound(s) surface area is less than or equal to 50 square centimeters. Code 97608 is used when the total wound(s) surface area is greater than 50 square centimeters. Nondurable equipment used in NPWT may consist of a single use, disposable, and ultra small, portable vacuum assist device that delivers wound therapy for a prescribed number of days, allowing the patient to remain mobile.

97610

97610 Low frequency, non-contact, non-thermal ultrasound, including topical application(s), when performed, wound assessment, and instruction(s) for ongoing care, per day

Low frequency, non-contact, non-thermal ultrasound is applied to promote wound healing. This procedure is reported on a per day basis and includes topical applications when performed, wound assessment, and instructions for ongoing care. Low frequency, non-contact, non-thermal ultrasound is a new modality for treating chronic wounds such as pressure ulcers, diabetic foot ulcers, vascular ulcers, and surgical wound dehiscence. The ultrasound system consists of an ultrasonic generator and disposable sterile applicator. The ultrasound device uses continuous low-frequency acoustic and sound energy to atomize saline delivered as a continuous mist to the wound bed through low frequency ultrasound. The treatment results in cavitation and acoustic mainstreaming that promote wound healing by stimulating tissue granulation and cell repair. The wound is assessed and measured. Photographs are taken. The wound and surrounding tissue are cleansed. The disposable applicator is attached to the transducer and treatment parameters are selected. The saline source is inserted into the applicator and the wound is treated with low frequency, non-contact, non-thermal ultrasound for the prescribed time period by moving the applicator in a serpentine fashion over the entire wound bed at a distance of 5-10 mm above the wound surface. Following completion of the procedure, the applicator and saline source are discarded and other device components are disinfected. The wound bed is wiped with sterile gauze and a dressing is applied.

97755

97755 Assistive technology assessment (eg, to restore, augment or compensate for existing function, optimize functional tasks and/or maximize environmental accessibility), direct one-on-one contact, with written report, each 15 minutes

An assistive technology assessment is performed to evaluate the patient's needs and to identify the most appropriate assistive technology devices and adaptive equipment for the patient based on the patient's current functional capacity. Assistive technology may be used to improve, augment, or restore the patient to the highest level of function and to maximize the patient's ability to maintain independence both at home and in the community or at work. The provider assesses the patient's current function and provides a variety of devices and types of equipment for the patient to test. The provider helps the patient select the appropriate devices and types of equipment and identifies any modifications or customization that may need to be made to devices or equipment. The provider also assesses the patient's home, work and transportation needs to ensure that the prescribed devices and equipment will work in these environments. The assessment is reported in 15 minute time increments.

97802

97802 Medical nutrition therapy; initial assessment and intervention, individual, face-to-face with the patient, each 15 minutes

A registered dietician (RD) provides medical nutrition therapy (MNT) to an individual. In 97802, initial assessment and intervention is provided to an individual in a face-to-face encounter. During the initial assessment, the RD determines the need for therapy, develops a plan, and determines how the therapy will be provided. A detailed medical history is obtained of all acute and chronic illnesses and other conditions. A psychosocial assessment is also performed including economic status, ethnic and cultural background, education level, occupation, and mental status. The RD determines whether the patient has access to the foods required to maintain health. Handicaps are noted, specifically those affecting the ability to obtain and/or prepare food. A list of current medications, including all vitamin, mineral, and herbal supplements, is obtained and reviewed for interactions between food and medications, particularly adverse reactions related to nutrient absorption and excretion. Vitamin and mineral supplements are also evaluated to determine whether they are adequate or if toxic levels of supplements are being used. A diet history is obtained including number of meals per day and what the patient eats in a typical 24 hour period. Food preparation techniques may also be evaluated to determine the amount of sodium or fat consumed each day. The patient may be asked to rate appetite from poor to good. Any taste alterations, food allergies, or religious restrictions are noted as are chewing or swallowing difficulties and bowel habits. A physical examination is performed including height, weight, body mass index, and arm or wrist circumference. Any recent weight changes are noted. The appearance of hair, skin, and nails is also evaluated for evidence of nutritional deficiencies. The RD then develops a nutrition therapy plan that addresses the patient's needs. Initial MNT is reported per 15 min interval.

97803-97804

97803 Medical nutrition therapy; re-assessment and intervention, individual, face-to-face with the patient, each 15 minutes

97804 Medical nutrition therapy; group (2 or more individual(s)), each 30 minutes

In 97803, a registered dietician (RD) provides medical nutrition therapy (MNT) re-assessment and intervention to an individual in a face-to-face encounter. The RD evaluates the effectiveness of the previously developed nutrition therapy plan. The patient is weighed. If the patient has been keeping a daily food diary, it is reviewed. Changes to the diet are suggested. The RD may provide food and recipe suggestions to help the patient meet nutritional needs. Re-assessment is reported per 15 min interval. In 97804, MNT is provided in a group setting of two or more individuals, usually for patients with similar health problems, such as diabetes or renal disease. Nutrition and lifestyle of each individual is evaluated. On-going nutrition counseling is provided along with counseling related to managing lifestyle factors affecting diet and exercise. The patient's progress in managing specific dietary needs is monitored. Group MNT is reported per patient per 30 min interval.

980834-90836

90836 Psychotherapy, 45 minutes with patient and/or family member when performed with an evaluation and management service (List separately in addition to the code for primary procedure)

Forty-five minutes of individual psychotherapy is provided to a patient and/or family member utilizing reeducation, support and reassurance, insight discussions, and occasionally medication to affect behavior-modification through self-understanding or to evaluate and improve family dynamics as they relate to the patient's condition. If psychotherapy is provided alone, report 90834. If medical evaluation and management services are also provided, report code 90836.

98960-98962

98960 Education and training for patient self-management by a qualified, nonphysician health care professional using a standardized curriculum, face-to-face with the patient (could include caregiver/family) each 30 minutes; individual patient

98961 Education and training for patient self-management by a qualified, nonphysician health care professional using a standardized curriculum, face-to-face with the patient (could include caregiver/family) each 30 minutes; 2-4 patients

98962 Education and training for patient self-management by a qualified, nonphysician health care professional using a standardized curriculum, face-to-face with the patient (could include caregiver/family) each 30 minutes; 5-8 patients

A physician or other health care professional provides education and training to a patient on how to manage a disease, injury, or other health problem. Family members of the patient or other caregivers may also be present. The instruction is based on a standard curriculum, though it may be modified slightly as circumstances dictate. Code 98961 if the education session is given to 2-4 patients at the same time, and 98962 if 5-8 patients are present.

● New Code   ▲ Revised Code

98966-98968

98966 Telephone assessment and management service provided by a qualified nonphysician health care professional to an established patient, parent, or guardian not originating from a related assessment and management service provided within the previous 7 days nor leading to an assessment and management service or procedure within the next 24 hours or soonest available appointment; 5-10 minutes of medical discussion

98967 Telephone assessment and management service provided by a qualified nonphysician health care professional to an established patient, parent, or guardian not originating from a related assessment and management service provided within the previous 7 days nor leading to an assessment and management service or procedure within the next 24 hours or soonest available appointment; 11-20 minutes of medical discussion

98968 Telephone assessment and management service provided by a qualified nonphysician health care professional to an established patient, parent, or guardian not originating from a related assessment and management service provided within the previous 7 days nor leading to an assessment and management service or procedure within the next 24 hours or soonest available appointment; 21-30 minutes of medical discussion

An established patient, parent, or guardian initiates a telephone conversation that results in a telephone assessment and management service provided by a qualified nonphysician health care professional, such as a registered dietician, physical therapist, occupational therapist, or speech-language pathologist. The phone call is not related to any previous face-to-face assessment and management service within the last seven days prior to the telephone service nor does it lead to a subsequent face-to-face assessment and management service within the following 24 hours or the soonest available urgent care appointment. The telephone assessment and management service is also not performed during the post-operative period of a related surgical procedure. During the telephone conversation, the qualified nonphysician health care professional listens to the patient's complaints and concerns, answers questions, requests additional related information, provides counseling and instruction as needed, and modifies the treatment plan, if necessary. The conversation is documented in the medical record and the amount of time spent conversing with the patient is noted. Use 98966 for a medical discussion lasting 5-10 minutes, 98967 for 11-20 minutes, and 98968 for 21-30 minutes.

98969

98969 Online assessment and management service provided by a qualified nonphysician health care professional to an established patient or guardian, not originating from a related assessment and management service provided within the previous 7 days, using the Internet or similar electronic communications network

An established patient, parent, or guardian initiates an online (e-mail), or similar electronic communication encounter that results in an online assessment and management service provided by a qualified nonphysician health care professional. Examples of qualified nonphysician health care professionals include registered dietician, physical therapist, occupational therapist, and speech-language pathologist. The online encounter is not related to any previous assessment and management service within the last seven days. The online assessment and management service is also not performed during the post-operative period of a related surgical procedure. During the online service the qualified nonphysician health care professional reviews complaints and concerns, answers questions, requests additional related information, provides counseling and instruction as needed, and modifies the treatment plan, if necessary. The online service is documented in the medical record.

99000-99001

99000 Handling and/or conveyance of specimen for transfer from the office to a laboratory

99001 Handling and/or conveyance of specimen for transfer from the patient in other than an office to a laboratory (distance may be indicated)

A specimen is transported from the office (99000) or from another setting (99001) where it was obtained to the laboratory where the requested laboratory study will be performed. Prior to transport the specimen is stored in the office or other location where it was obtained following the specific protocol for handling of the specimen. The specimen is transported as required by the laboratory protocol designed for the specific specimen which may include keeping the specimen at a specific temperature (frozen or refrigerated). All safety precautions are adhered to when handling and transporting the specimen.

99002

99002 Handling, conveyance, and/or any other service in connection with the implementation of an order involving devices (eg, designing, fitting, packaging, handling, delivery or mailing) when devices such as orthotics, protectives, prosthetics are fabricated by an outside laboratory or shop but which items have been designed, and are to be fitted and adjusted by the attending physician or other qualified health care professional

Services performed by an outside laboratory or shop in connection with the provision of a device including designing, fitting, packaging, handling, mailing or delivery are provided. The orthotic, prosthetic, protective or other device is designed in the provider office but is then fabricated by the laboratory or shop and must be delivered to the office of the physician or other qualified health care provider for final fitting and adjustment.

99026-99027

99026 Hospital mandated on call service; in-hospital, each hour

99027 Hospital mandated on call service; out-of-hospital, each hour

Code 99026 is reported for each hour the physician spends in the hospital on call. Code 99027 reports on-call time a physician spends when not located in the hospital. Both codes do not include physician time spent on other reportable services and/or procedures.

99078

99078 Physician or other qualified health care professional qualified by education, training, licensure/regulation (when applicable) educational services rendered to patients in a group setting (eg, prenatal, obesity, or diabetic instructions)

Educational services are provided in a group setting by a physician or other qualified health care professional. Qualified health care professionals include those with the necessary education and training and/or those with the necessary licensure or other credentials as required by federal or state statute. The group educational services may relate to prenatal health, obesity, diabetes, or other health care topics. Topics might include diet, exercise, or medication administration. It should be noted that educational services reported with code 99078 may be considered a bundled service and may not be allowed by all payers.

99091

99091 Collection and interpretation of physiologic data (eg, ECG, blood pressure, glucose monitoring) digitally stored and/or transmitted by the patient and/or caregiver to the physician or other qualified health care professional, qualified by education, training, licensure/regulation (when applicable) requiring a minimum of 30 minutes of time

Physiologic data such as ECG, blood pressure, glucose monitoring that has been digitally stored by the patient or caregiver and then transmitted to the physician or other qualified health care professional is collected and interpreted. Qualified health care professionals include those with the necessary education and training and/or those with the necessary licensure or other credentials as required by federal or state statute. The physiologic data is collected, reviewed and a written interpretation of the data is provided. Code 99091 may only be reported if the work involved requires 30 minutes or more of dedicated time.

99170

99170 Anogenital examination, magnified, in childhood for suspected trauma, including image recording when performed

A pediatric anogenital examination is performed for suspected trauma resulting from suspected sexual abuse. This exam is performed with a colposcope. A colposcope is an instrument that looks like a pair of binoculars mounted on a pedestal with a light attached. The colposcope lenses magnify the tissue of the anogenital region (vagina, anus, and perineum), allowing better visualization of any trauma. The colposcope is placed at the vaginal or anal opening. A speculum is then placed into the vagina or anus to separate the vaginal or anal wall. The vaginal or anal wall is inspected in its entirety by rotating the speculum so that the entire circumference can be examined. Tissues are examined under two or three different magnifications. A videocolposcope may be used to record images of vaginal and anal tissue and to document any trauma to these sites. Pediatric anogenital examination with magnified images using an endoscope designed specifically for the vagina and cervix, or the anus, done in cases of suspected sexual abuse, including any image recordings.

99172

99172 Visual function screening, automated or semi-automated bilateral quantitative determination of visual acuity, ocular alignment, color vision by pseudoisochromatic plates, and field of vision (may include all or some screening of the determination[s] for contrast sensitivity, vision under glare)

A vision function screening test is performed including automated or semi-automated bilateral quantitative determination of visual acuity, ocular alignment, color vision by

Medicine

pseudoisochromatic plates, and field of vision. The test may also include screening for determination of contrast sensitivity and vision under glare. This type of vision test is performed primarily on individuals whose occupations require that specific vision parameters be met for safety purposes. Typically, the specific vision requirements for the job are stated in the screening request so that the most appropriate evaluation of vision function is performed. Visual acuity is checked using a method that allows a quantitative determination, such as a Snellen chart. Both near and far vision may be evaluated, i.e., from 14 in to 20 ft. Ocular alignment tests extraocular muscle balance for both vertical and lateral phorias. Testing for phorias evaluates the relative directions assumed by the eyes during binocular fixation in the absence of a fusion stimulus. Color vision is evaluated using pseudoisochromic plates to determine any color deficiencies. One type commonly used is the Ishihara color test. Pseudoisochromic plates are composed of differently shaded dots that contain a number within the dot pattern. In a color vision deficient person, the number will not be visible on one or more of the plates. Field of vision testing is done to determine if peripheral vision is normal. This may be accomplished using an apparatus onto which lights are projected. The patient fixates on a central spot and then indicates when he/she sees a small spot of light off to the side. Another method is to use a screen on which a white spot is moved horizontally and the patient indicates when the spot disappears. If needed, contrast sensitivity is tested to determine how well the patient sees low contrast images under conditions of low visibility. There are a number of tests available for contrast sensitivity including Pelli-Robson test, Bailey-Lovie chart, and Vision Contrast Test System (VCTS). Individuals with poor contrast sensitivity may fail to see edges, borders, or variations in brightness. Testing vision under glare may be performed using a Brightness Acuity Tester, which simulates three bright light conditions, including bright overhead sunlight, partly cloudy day, and bright overhead artificial light. If vision is diminished under these conditions, a glare disability may be present. The physician or technician performing the visual function screening interprets the results and provides a written report of findings.

99173

99173   Screening test of visual acuity, quantitative, bilateral

A bilateral quantitative visual acuity screening test is performed, primarily on children, and used to test visual acuity only. Visual acuity is checked using a method that allows quantitative determination, such as a Snellen chart, which determines the smallest letters that the patient can read 14 to 20 ft away. Each eye is checked individually. Near vision may also be checked using a card held 14 inches away. In younger children, symbols, numbers, or gratings may be used instead of letters. Gratings are used to test vision in infants and consist of one gray and one black and white striped stimulus. The gray stimulus is placed over the striped stimulus. As the gray stimulus is slowly moved to expose the striped stimulus, an infant with normal vision will follow the striped stimulus. The physician or technician performing the visual acuity screening interprets the results and provides a written report of findings.

99174-99177

99174   Instrument-based ocular screening (eg, photoscreening, automated-refraction), bilateral; with remote analysis and report

99177   Instrument-based ocular screening (eg, photoscreening, automated-refraction), bilateral; with on-site analysis

Instrument based ocular screening such as photoscreening or automated refraction is performed on both eyes. Ocular photoscreening with interpretation and report is performed on an infant or child to screen for amblyogenic factors that reduce, dim, or blur vision, such as esotropia, exotropia, anisometropia, cataracts, ptosis, hyperopia, and myopia. Ocular photoscreening uses a specialized camera to detect and record eye reflexes in response to stimuli. The ocular photoscreening system is set up and the patient is positioned so that images can be obtained. Depending on the specific ocular photoscreening system used, the images may be reviewed by the physician, transmitted to a screening laboratory to be read analyzed remotely, and a report of findings submitted back to the physician (99174), or an automated analysis may be performed on site (99177) and the data provided to the physician. Automated refraction is performed with an automated refraction system which is used to obtain an auto-refractor reading which is then analyzed by the software. A reading is also taken from the patient's glasses. Patient information is entered into the software. An automated perocter is then used to obtain subjective refractions of both eyes. The results are compared with the automated refraction and the patient is again tested using the automated and subjective test results to ensure that the subjective testing results are those that the patient feels provide the best correction.

99183

99183   Physician or other qualified health care professional attendance and supervision of hyperbaric oxygen therapy, per session

Hyperbaric oxygen therapy is performed to treat decompression sickness, also referred to as "the bends" which is caused by surfacing too quickly when scuba diving. It may also be performed for air embolism or to treat serious infections, severe anemia, and wounds that won't heal, such as those seen in diabetics or in patients with radiation injuries. The patient is placed in a special chamber or room where the air pressure is raised to a level up to 3 times higher than normal air pressure. The increased air pressure causes the lungs to take

in more oxygen than is possible under normal air pressure. The increased levels of oxygen in the lungs then enter the blood increasing oxygen levels and restoring normal blood gases. Adequate oxygen levels in the blood are essential for normal tissue function and also for healing of injured tissues. The patient may remain in the hyperbaric oxygen chamber or room for up to 2 hours. During the treatment period the patient is observed and the response to treatment monitored by a physician or other qualified health care professional.

99184

99184   Initiation of selective head or total body hypothermia in the critically ill neonate, includes appropriate patient selection by review of clinical, imaging and laboratory data, confirmation of esophageal temperature probe location, evaluation of amplitude EEG, supervision of controlled hypothermia, and assessment of patient tolerance of cooling

Head or total body hypothermia may be initiated in term or near term neonates (gestational age >36 weeks) who have suffered birth related oxygen deprivation (hypoxic ischemic encephalopathy, perinatal asphyxia) and have signs of brain injury. The brain cells remain normal for a brief time following the initial hypoxic episode. However, a second delayed brain injury can often occur hours later. Mild hypothermia lowers the cerebral metabolic rate for glucose and oxygen and reduces the delayed onset of cerebral lactic alkalosis. Hypothermic therapy can decrease the incidence of hypoxic ischemic encephalopathy (HIE) and may increase the infant's chances for normal survival. Criteria for initiation of hypothermia includes documented metabolic acidosis (cord blood pH of 7.0 or less), base deficit of at least 12 mmol/L, and multisystem organ dysfunction with exclusion of other possible causes. Brain activity is monitored by amplitude integrated electroencephalography (aEEG) and an MRI may be performed. The infant is intubated and placed on mechanical ventilation for respiratory support. An esophageal temperature probe is inserted and placement is checked with x-ray. The umbilical artery and vein are catheterized to facilitate blood draws and administer fluids. A urinary catheter is inserted to monitor urine output and kidney function. Baseline laboratory values are obtained including serum electrolytes, blood gases, clotting time, and CBC/hemoglobin. Hypothermia is induced by placing the infant on a cooling blanket or applying a cooling cap to the head. The core body temperature is lowered to between 33.5 and 35 degrees Centigrade. The infant is closely monitored for the duration of the therapy averaging 72 hours, and during re-warming.

99188

99188   Application of topical fluoride varnish by a physician or other qualified health care professional

Topical fluoride varnish contains highly concentrated fluoride in a fast drying resin base. When painted onto flat tooth surfaces and the pits/fissures of molars, fluoride varnish forms a sticky residue that hardens when it comes in contact with saliva. Fluoride varnish may be used as a desensitizing agent and to prevent and/or reverse dental caries. The compound can be applied by a dentist, dental hygienist, or other trained health care professional such as a physician, nurse, or medical/dental assistant. Before application, the patient should have an oral examination and a risk based assessment. Fluoride varnish should only be used on patients at medium to high risk for dental caries. The teeth are cleaned and dried and the varnish is painted on tooth surfaces using a small brush or applicator. The patient should refrain from eating or drinking for 30 minutes, and from brushing for 12 hours following application of the varnish.

99190-99192

99190   Assembly and operation of pump with oxygenator or heat exchanger (with or without ECG and/or pressure monitoring); each hour

99191   Assembly and operation of pump with oxygenator or heat exchanger (with or without ECG and/or pressure monitoring); 45 minutes

99192   Assembly and operation of pump with oxygenator or heat exchanger (with or without ECG and/or pressure monitoring); 30 minutes

Assembly and operation of a pump with an oxygenator or heat exchanger by the physician. This code may or may not include a pump with ECG and/or pressure detection. Code this code for each hour of assembly. Code 99191 for treatment lasting three-quarters of an hour, and 99192 for treatment lasting half an hour.

99195

99195   Phlebotomy, therapeutic (separate procedure)

Drawing blood as a therapeutic procedure is done to correct dangerously imbalanced blood chemistry.

99500

99500   Home visit for prenatal monitoring and assessment to include fetal heart rate, non-stress test, uterine monitoring, and gestational diabetes monitoring

A home visit by a physician or other health care provider for prenatal monitoring and assessment, including the fetal heart rate and uterine condition. May include drawing blood to check for gestational diabetes.

99501

99501   Home visit for postnatal assessment and follow-up care

A home visit by a physician or other health care provider for postnatal follow-up and assessment. This may also include parental education and planning, setting dates for immunizations, and directing parents to other resources, etc.

99502

99502   Home visit for newborn care and assessment

Home visit for newborn (36-72 hours after delivery) to help the family make the transition from the hospital. This visit is not a replacement for a complete medical assessment, but may diagnose early problems.

99503

99503   Home visit for respiratory therapy care (eg, bronchodilator, oxygen therapy, respiratory assessment, apnea evaluation)

Home visit for respiratory therapy care, which may include patient and/or family education, inspection of equipment, follow-up examination, etc.

99504

99504   Home visit for mechanical ventilation care

Home visit for patients receiving mechanical ventilation care, which may include patient and/or family education, inspection of equipment, follow-up examination, etc.

99505

99505   Home visit for stoma care and maintenance including colostomy and cystostomy

A health care professional provides colostomy (an artificial connection between two body cavities, or between a body cavity and the surface of the skin, e.g. a colostomy) and/or cystostomy care to a patient at home, which may include patient and/or family education, inspection of equipment and/or surgical site, follow-up examination and taking of samples, etc.

99506

99506   Home visit for intramuscular injections

A health care professional provides an injection(s) to a patient at home, which may include patient and/or family education, inspection injeciton site, follow-up examination and taking of samples, etc.

99507

99507   Home visit for care and maintenance of catheter(s) (eg, urinary, drainage, and enteral)

A health care professional provides catheter (e.g. a urinary catheter, or one placed for feeding, etc.) care to a patient at home, which may include patient and/or family education, inspection of equipment and/or surgical site, follow-up examination and taking samples, etc. It may also include wound and dressing inspection.

99509

99509   Home visit for assistance with activities of daily living and personal care

Home visit for assistance with two or more activities of daily living and personal care, such as eating, using the bathroom, bathing, dressing, moving about the living area, etc.

99510

99510   Home visit for individual, family, or marriage counseling

Home visit for individual, family, or marriage counseling.

99511

99511   Home visit for fecal impaction management and enema administration

Home visit for bowel impaction (blockage) management, including administration of an enema. May include dietary instruction and/or prescription of medication to prevent future impaction.

99512

99512   Home visit for hemodialysis

Home visit for hemodialysis for kidney failure patients, commonly done three times per week, with each treatment lasting 1-2 hours.

99601-99602

99601   Home infusion/specialty drug administration, per visit (up to 2 hours)
99602   Home infusion/specialty drug administration, per visit (up to 2 hours); each additional hour (List separately in addition to code for primary procedure)

Home infusion of a specialty drug (e.g. intravenously). Code this code for the first two hours. Add 99602 for each additional hour.

99605-99607

99605   Medication therapy management service(s) provided by a pharmacist, individual, face-to-face with patient, with assessment and intervention if provided; initial 15 minutes, new patient
99606   Medication therapy management service(s) provided by a pharmacist, individual, face-to-face with patient, with assessment and intervention if provided; initial 15 minutes, established patient
99607   Medication therapy management service(s) provided by a pharmacist, individual, face-to-face with patient, with assessment and intervention if provided; each additional 15 minutes (List separately in addition to code for primary service)

A pharmacist provides individual, face-to-face medication therapy management services to a patient, including assessment and intervention as needed. The pharmacist reviews the patient's pertinent history and medication profile, including both prescription and nonprescription medications, and identifies possible interactions and problems. The pharmacist then fine tunes the drug therapy for the best results, makes recommendations to improve health outcomes, and encourages compliance with the drug treatment regimen. Use 99605 for an initial new patient service of 15 minutes, 99606 for an established patient service of 15 minutes, and 99607 for each additional 15 minutes during the initial or established patient encounter.

Medicine

0042T

0042T Cerebral perfusion analysis using computed tomography with contrast administration, including post-processing of parametric maps with determination of cerebral blood flow, cerebral blood volume, and mean transit time

Cerebral perfusion is the injection of fluid (contrast) into a blood vessel in order to measure the blood flow through the cerebral microvascular system, aided by computer tomography. Code 0042T includes post-processing of parametric maps, with determination of cerebral blood flow, cerebral blood volume (CBV), and mean transit time.

0051T-0053T

0051T Implantation of a total replacement heart system (artificial heart) with recipient cardiectomy

0052T Replacement or repair of thoracic unit of a total replacement heart system (artificial heart)

0053T Replacement or repair of implantable component or components of total replacement heart system (artificial heart), excluding thoracic unit

A heart system is implanted into a patient until a donor heart can be found. The heart is exposed by median sternotomy. Cardiopulmonary bypass is established. The patient's diseased heart is removed (cardiectomy) The artificial heart is inserted into the chest and the coronary arteries are connected to the appropriate outlets. The patient is weaned off cardiopulmonary bypass; chest tubes are placed; and chest incisions are closed. In 0052T, the pump of the artificial heart is replaced; in 0053T, a component, such as an oxygenator is replaced.

0054T-0055T

0054T Computer-assisted musculoskeletal surgical navigational orthopedic procedure, with image-guidance based on fluoroscopic images (List separately in addition to code for primary procedure)

0055T Computer-assisted musculoskeletal surgical navigational orthopedic procedure, with image-guidance based on CT/MRI images (List separately in addition to code for primary procedure)

A computer-assisted musculoskeletal surgical navigation orthopedic procedure is performed with image guidance based on fluoroscopic images (0054T) or CT/MRI images (0055T). Computer-assisted surgical navigational procedures allow surgeons to perform complex procedures, such as joint replacement (arthroplasty) or fixation of a femoral or pelvic fracture, through small incisions. Use of navigation systems provide greater surgical accuracy, reduce surgery time and blood loss, and shorten the postoperative rehabilitation period. The computer-assisted surgical navigation procedure is a three-step process involving data acquisition, registration, and tracking. A separately reportable complex orthopedic procedure is performed. Tracker pins are placed at selected sites and fluoroscopic, CT or MRI images are obtained. Registration techniques are then used to relate the anatomic surface data to the bony anatomy in the surgical field. A computer-generated model is prepared from the radiographic images and matched to the surface data points. The radiographic images are used in conjunction with a computer-assisted navigational system to track position and orientation of surgical tools and/or internal fixation devices as the complex orthopedic procedure is performed.

0058T-0059T

0058T Cryopreservation; reproductive tissue, ovarian

During a separately reportable procedure, ovarian reproductive tissue or oocytes are harvested for cryopreservation and use in a subsequent assisted reproduction procedure. The harvested ovarian reproductive tissue or oocytes are assessed and a series of cryoprotectant solutions specifically formulated for ovarian reproductive tissue or oocytes is prepared. In 0058T, the ovarian reproductive tissue is minced and moved through the prepared solutions that contain progressively more cryprotectant. The tissue may be frozen by direct contact and then placed in straws or vials or it may be placed in straws or vials and then frozen. The straws or vials are labeled with identifying information, including patient name, number, and contents. The reproductive tissue is gradually cooled to -270 degrees centigrade in a controlled rate freezing chamber and stored in vapor phase or submerged under liquid nitrogen until needed for use. In 0059T, cryopreservation of individual oocytes is performed. Two techniques are available for oocyte freezing, the traditional slow freezing method described above or a rapid freezing process referred to as vitrification. Vitrification uses a high concentration of cryoprotectant that results in a solid glass-like frozen oocyte free of ice crystals. Following freezing by either method, the oocyte(s) are stored as described above until they are needed for use in an assisted reproduction procedure.

0071T-0072T

0071T Focused ultrasound ablation of uterine leiomyomata, including MR guidance; total leiomyomata volume less than 200 cc of tissue

0072T Focused ultrasound ablation of uterine leiomyomata, including MR guidance; total leiomyomata volume greater or equal to 200 cc of tissue

Focused ultrasound ablation of uterine leiomyomata is performed including magnetic resonance (MR) guidance. Focused ultrasound ablation is a noninvasive technique that uses a thermal ablation device to precisely target and destroy soft tissue within the body. The ablation system is fully integrated with the MR imaging system which provides guidance and monitoring throughout the procedure. Prior to performing the ablation procedure, a three plane localizer MR scan is performed to ensure that the patient is properly positioned on the treatment table. The target fibroid is identified. Treatment software is used to determine the appropriate treatment routes and ablation dose delivery settings. 3D renderings are created on the computer and dose simulations are reviewed. The treatment plan and beam path simulations are also reviewed in 3D on the computer. This procedure is performed using conscious sedation so that the patient remains awake and able to communicate sensations to the assistant and physician during the procedure. The patient, assistant, and treating physician all have access to an emergency shut off button to terminate the procedure if needed. Using continuous MR imaging, the leiomyoma is destroyed using focused sonification. If multiple leiomyomata are treated, the process is repeated, including targeting, imaging, analysis, and destruction at each site until all leiomyomata are destroyed. Use 0071T if total leiomyomata volume is less than 200 cc of tissue or 0072T if total volume is 200 cc or greater.

0075T-0076T

0075T Transcatheter placement of extracranial vertebral artery stent(s), including radiologic supervision and interpretation, open or percutaneous; initial vessel

0076T Transcatheter placement of extracranial vertebral artery stent(s), including radiologic supervision and interpretation, open or percutaneous; each additional vessel (List separately in addition to code for primary procedure)

A stent is placed in an extracranial vertebral or intrathoracic carotid artery through a catheter. A needle is used to insert the catheter and the stent is threaded through a partially-blocked blood vessel. This allows the artery to remain open for good blood flow. Report 0075T for the initial blood vessel stented. Code 0076T for any additional blood vessels stented.

0095T-0098T

0095T Removal of total disc arthroplasty (artificial disc), anterior approach, each additional interspace, cervical (List separately in addition to code for primary procedure)

0098T Revision including replacement of total disc arthroplasty (artificial disc), anterior approach, each additional interspace, cervical (List separately in addition to code for primary procedure)

The physician revises an additional cervical total-disc arthroplasty, which may include replacement of the artificial disc using an anterior approach. An incision is made in the front of the neck just off the midline of the spine. The esophagus is retracted. Nerves and arteries are identified and protected as the soft tissues of the neck are dissected and the spine is exposed. The intervertebral muscles are retracted, and the previously placed artificial disc is exposed. In 0098T, following separately reportable revision of the first artificial disc, an additional one is revised. The existing artificial disc is revised, which may include removal and replacement with a new one. Revision may be required due to pain, degenerative changes, or improper alignment of the spine at the treated or adjacent disc spaces. The existing artificial disc is dissected off the end plates and removed. The amount of bone loss and damage to the vertebral bodies is evaluated. If a new disc can be placed, the intervertebral space is prepared for a new artificial disc. The end plates above and below the space are milled and shaped to accommodate the new artificial disc. Tension is applied to the vertebral bodies above and below the disc space to open it and allow placement of the artificial disc. The new artificial disc is inserted, and the two metal plates that surround the polyurethane core and saline cushion are pressed into the prepared bony end plates, taking care to ensure that normal cervical lordotic curvature is maintained. Tension is released from the vertebral bodies above and below the artificial disc, which compresses it and holds it in place. Report 0098T for each additional revision of an artificial disc. Use 0095T to report each additional existing artificial disc being removed as described above, without replacement, following separately reportable removal of the first disc.

● New Code ▲ Revised Code

Category III Codes

0100T

0100T   Placement of a subconjunctival retinal prosthesis receiver and pulse generator, and implantation of intra-ocular retinal electrode array, with vitrectomy

The physician replaces the patient's eye with an artifical retina, which consists of a small video camera affixed to a pair of eyeglasses which transmits information to an implant in the back of the eye which interfaces with the optic nerve.

0106T-0110T

0106T   Quantitative sensory testing (QST), testing and interpretation per extremity; using touch pressure stimuli to assess large diameter sensation

0107T   Quantitative sensory testing (QST), testing and interpretation per extremity; using vibration stimuli to assess large diameter fiber sensation

0108T   Quantitative sensory testing (QST), testing and interpretation per extremity; using cooling stimuli to assess small nerve fiber sensation and hyperalgesia

0109T   Quantitative sensory testing (QST), testing and interpretation per extremity; using heat-pain stimuli to assess small nerve fiber sensation and hyperalgesia

0110T   Quantitative sensory testing (QST), testing and interpretation per extremity; using other stimuli to assess sensation

A device is used that provides specific sensory stimulation to test the sensory response of one of the patient's limbs. If the physician tests pressure stimulation, use 0106T. If vibration sensation is tested, use 0107T. If the patient's sensory response to cool temperatures is tested, use 0108T. For the testing of heat and/or pain stimuli, use 0109T. If other stimuli not found in codes 0106T-0109T are used to test sensation, use 0110T.

0111T

0111T   Long-chain (C20-22) omega-3 fatty acids in red blood cell (RBC) membranes

A blood sample is tested to determine the levels of long-chain omega-3 fatty acids in the bloodstream. These essential fatty acids may prevent some heart disease, and research has shown it to be an effective treatment for migraine headaches and borderline personality disorder.

0126T

0126T   Common carotid intima-media thickness (IMT) study for evaluation of atherosclerotic burden or coronary heart disease risk factor assessment

An ultrasound is used to measure the thickness of the carotid artery. Excessive thickness of the carotid artery is an early indicator of atherosclerosis, which can lead to cardiocascular disease and disorders of the heart.

0159T

0159T   Computer-aided detection, including computer algorithm analysis of MRI image data for lesion detection/characterization, pharmacokinetic analysis, with further physician review for interpretation, breast MRI (List separately in addition to code for primary procedure)

This code reports computer-aided lesion detection or characterization by algorithm analysis of MRI breast image data, including additional physician interpretive review. This is an add-on code to be used in conjunction with the primary procedure. MRI images of the breast are run through computer analysis, using a methodical, step-by-step pattern of analyzing the data on video display to identify or characterize any unusual or suspicious areas in the breast, which the physician reviews.

0163T

0163T   Total disc arthroplasty (artificial disc), anterior approach, including discectomy to prepare interspace (other than for decompression), each additional interspace, lumbar (List separately in addition to code for primary procedure)

Total disc arthroplasty is done for complete, artificial replacement of an extremely damaged or diseased intervertebral disc. This code reports an anterior approach through an abdominal incision to reach a lumbar vertebra for each additional interspace treated beyond the first. When the spinal column is reached, the intervertebral muscles are retracted and the target disc is identified using x-ray for confirmation. The pathogenic cartilaginous disc matter is cleaned out with a rongeur to prepare the intervertebral disc space for the artificial implant. There are different designs or types of artificial disc implants, but a common one used has two metal endplates with a convex, weight-bearing polyethylene insert. The metal endplates are inserted into the prepared disc space in a collapsed state; seated into the vertebrae above and below; then opened with distraction. The polyethylene, weight bearing disc material insert is then placed in the space and seated into the endplates by a snap-lock mechanism. When the total disc replacement is assembled, the wounds are closed and a drain is left in place.

0164T

0164T   Removal of total disc arthroplasty, (artificial disc), anterior approach, each additional interspace, lumbar (List separately in addition to code for primary procedure)

A previously placed, artificial total disc arthroplasty is removed by anterior approach from each additional lumbar interspace beyond the first removed. An incision is made in the abdomen and muscle and tissue are retracted to reach the spinal column. The artificial disc implant is located. Adhesions and fibrous tissue are freed and distraction is applied to open the intervertebral space. The implant is unseated from its position between the vertebrae above and below and is removed. The space is explored and debrided. Muscle and tissue are closed in position for wound repair.

0165T

0165T   Revision including replacement of total disc arthroplasty (artificial disc), anterior approach, each additional interspace, lumbar (List separately in addition to code for primary procedure)

Revision of each additional lumbar artificial total disc arthroplasty, beyond the first interspace, including replacement, is done by anterior approach through an incision in the abdomen. When the spinal column is reached, the intervertebral muscles are retracted and the artificial disc is identified. Adhesions and fibrous tissue are freed and the area is explored. Distraction is applied to open the intervertebral space. The implant may be unseated from an improper position in the vertebrae above and below and may then be reseated, or implant components may be replaced or adjusted for proper functioning. When replacement is to be done, the failed implant or component is removed and the interspace is explored and prepared for insertion of another prosthesis or component, which is seated into position. The fascia and muscle tissue are repaired and the wound is closed with a drain left in place.

0174T-0175T

0174T   Computer-aided detection (CAD) (computer algorithm analysis of digital image data for lesion detection) with further physician review for interpretation and report, with or without digitization of film radiographic images, chest radiograph(s), performed concurrent with primary interpretation (List separately in addition to code for primary procedure)

0175T   Computer-aided detection (CAD) (computer algorithm analysis of digital image data for lesion detection) with further physician review for interpretation and report, with or without digitization of film radiographic images, chest radiograph(s), performed remote from primary interpretation

Computer-aided detection (CAD) using computer algorithm analysis of digital image data for detecting a lesion, such as a pulmonary nodule, is performed in conjunction with separately reportable routine chest radiographs. This may be done with or without digitization of the radiographic film. CAD is performed concurrently with primary interpretation of the routine radiographs in 0174T and at a site remote from where the primary radiographs are obtained and interpreted in 0175T. CAD is then supplemented with further physician review, interpretation, and a written report. Interpreting standard two-dimensional images of three-dimensional structures is difficult. Determining true depth, location, and feature characterization of abnormalities is complicated by the fact that lesions are embedded in tissue, making detection, discrimination, and integration of distinct lesion features difficult. CAD image processing technology aids in detecting and classifying lesions. It enhances standard radiographs using computer software that analyzes and marks regions of interest. The marks do not necessarily represent a malignancy, but areas that require additional scrutiny. An experienced radiologist uses his/her expertise to determine whether the marked regions of interest represent potential malignancies. The CAD scanner is used to scan and digitize the radiograph. If the original was captured digitally, this step is not necessary. The computer software analyzes the digitized radiograph and marks regions of interest and the enhanced radiograph is displayed on the monitor. The radiologist reviews the original routine radiographs and identifies abnormalities and then reviews the CAD analysis and the marked regions of interest. The two sets of radiographs, before and after CAD are compared. The physician interprets the findings and provides a written report.

0178T-0180T

0178T   Electrocardiogram, 64 leads or greater, with graphic presentation and analysis; with interpretation and report

0179T   Electrocardiogram, 64 leads or greater, with graphic presentation and analysis; tracing and graphics only, without interpretation and report

0180T   Electrocardiogram, 64 leads or greater, with graphic presentation and analysis; interpretation and report only

The standard placement for a 12-lead ECG provides optimal location for recording ventricular activity. The addition of more leads with optimal placement allows for better graphic representation of cardiac electrical activity and better diagnostic information. Conditions that can be diagnosed and localized with more confidence include myocardial infarction, ventricular tachycardia, and/or ventricular fibrillation with an increased risk of sudden cardiac death, and atrial arrhythmias. Placement of the additional leads is dependent on the suspected condition. The physician reviews a separately reportable 12-lead ECG to determine if a 64-lead or greater ECG is required for a more definitive diagnosis. Additional leads totaling 64 or greater are placed on both the back and the chest, uniformly distributed or concentrated in specific areas, such as over the heart. A 64-lead ECG produces both an ECG tracing and a graphic presentation. The ECG signals over intervals lasting several minutes are stored for later processing to provide the graphic presentation in the form of a torso body map, localizing the site of concern. Using the map in conjunction with the ECG tracing, the physician is able to identify the lead(s) that has captured the definitive data. The ECG tracing from this lead(s) is carefully inspected and any abnormalities are noted and characterized. The information from the separately reportable 12-lead ECG, the 64-or greater lead ECG, the graphic image (body torso map), and the data stored on the computer disc, is compiled and interpreted. A written report is provided. Use 0178T to report the complete study, with analysis and interpretation and report. Use 0179T for the tracing and graphic presentation only (without an interpretation and report), and 0180T for the interpretation and report portion only.

0184T

0184T   Excision of rectal tumor, transanal endoscopic microsurgical approach (ie, TEMS), including muscularis propria (ie, full thickness)

The TEMs approach requires specially designed equipment consisting of a TEMs set that includes components for attachment to the operating table and an armrest and other components that provide insufflation, irrigation, light, and magnification. Proctoscopy is performed to verify the location and extent of the tumor. The anal sphincter is dilated using a 40 mm resectoscope with a stereoscopic binocular viewing eyepiece. The dilation is maintained by a constant flow of carbon dioxide. A vasoconstrictor is injected beneath the tumor to prevent excessive bleeding. The rectal mucosa around the lesion is scored. The incision is carried through the full thickness of the rectal wall and the lesion is excised. Adjacent mesorectum is also excised. The lesion and mesorectum are sent for separately reportable pathology examination. The rectal wall is repaired.

0188T-0189T

0188T   Remote real-time interactive video-conferenced critical care, evaluation and management of the critically ill or critically injured patient; first 30-74 minutes

0189T   Remote real-time interactive video-conferenced critical care, evaluation and management of the critically ill or critically injured patient; each additional 30 minutes (List separately in addition to code for primary service)

The physician provides off-site critical care evaluation and management services to a critically ill or critically injured patient using remote real-time interactive video-conferencing. This service is provided to supplement on-site critical care services when the required critical care is not available or the on-site services require the expertise of a more specialized physician located at a remote site. The off-site physician reviews pertinent information with the on-site physician and they develop a plan of care. The off-site physician then monitors the patient, interacting with the on-site physician, nursing staff, and other ancillary personnel as needed to provide the required critical care. The off-site physician may be responsible for monitoring specific conditions and/or complications that arise and for ordering and following up on the necessary medical interventions. The remote physician visually monitors the patient via a video screen; assesses the patient's condition; and may order tests as well as review and interpret the results. The off-site physician initiates changes to the treatment plan and orders interventions as needed. Use code 0188T for the first 30-74 minutes of remote critical care on a given date and code 0189T for each additional 30 minutes provided on the same calendar day.

0190T

0190T   Placement of intraocular radiation source applicator (List separately in addition to primary procedure)

An intraocular radiation source applicator is placed in a procedure performed to treat choroidal neovascularization caused by age-related macular degeneration. Choroidal neovascularization is a disorder characterized by the growth of new blood vessels at the site of a break in the Bruch membrane. The new blood vessels grow into the subretinal pigment epithelium or subretinal space causing loss of vision. A separately reportable vitrectomy is performed to gain access to the vitreous cavity. An applicator containing a radiation source enclosed in a protected storage compartment is inserted into the vitreous cavity and positioned over the choroidal neovascular lesion. The radiation source is advanced out of the storage compartment of the applicator and into the closed-chamber cannula tip. The radiation source is placed in contact with the retina at the site of the neovascular lesion for a prescribed amount of time. When the time has elapsed (usually not more than five minutes), the radiation source is retracted back into the protected storage compartment of the applicator, which is removed from the eye.

0191T

0191T   Insertion of anterior segment aqueous drainage device, without extraocular reservoir, internal approach, into the trabecular meshwork; initial insertion

An anterior segment aqueous drainage device without an extraocular reservoir is inserted via an internal approach to treat chronic or progressive open angle glaucoma. A small, self-sealing incision is made in the cornea and the incision is deepened to access the anterior chamber. A magnification lens such as a gonioscope is used to place and position the drainage device (shunt) at the angle of the anterior chamber. The terminal end of the drainage device is positioned in the trabecular meshwork. It is not necessary to close the small corneal incision as it is so small that it will self-seal.

0195T-0196T

0195T   Arthrodesis, pre-sacral interbody technique, disc space preparation, discectomy, without instrumentation, with image guidance, includes bone graft when performed; L5-S1 interspace

0196T   Arthrodesis, pre-sacral interbody technique, disc space preparation, discectomy, without instrumentation, with image guidance, includes bone graft when performed; L4-L5 interspace (List separately in addition to code for primary procedure)

Lumbar arthrodesis is performed using a pre-sacral interbody technique with imaging and discectomy to prepare the interspace. The pre-sacral interbody technique, also referred to as transsacral or paracoccygeal, uses a minimally invasive percutaneous approach to the anterior portion of the disc space. The patient is placed in a prone position and a small incision is made at the level of the coccyx slightly lateral to the midline. A trocar is advanced anterior to the sacrum under fluoroscopic guidance. A small presacral channel is created in the disc space. The two adjacent vertebral bodies are distracted, and the disc interspace is prepared by removing the intervertebral disc material and the cartilage from the end plates of the adjacent vertebrae. Separately reportable bone allografts (donor) or autografts are obtained. Spinal fusion (arthrodesis) is accomplished by packing the bone graft material into the disc space. Use code 0195T for arthrodesis of L5-S1 interspace. Code 0196T is reported additionally when arthrodesis of the L4-5 interspace is performed during the same surgical session.

0198T

0198T   Measurement of ocular blood flow by repetitive intraocular pressure sampling, with interpretation and report

This test is performed using a miniaturized sensor embedded in a tonometer tip. The concave tonometer tip is designed in such a way that the cornea will take on the shape of the tonometer tip when positioned on the cornea. The tonometer tip is placed on the cornea and when a portion of the central cornea has conformed to the shape of the tip, the pressure sensor begins to take intraocular pressure (IOP) readings. The sensor can take up to 100 IOP readings per second. Measurement of ocular blood flow is obtained as the device generates a pulse wave that reflects heart rate and the mean difference between diastolic and systolic IOP. This measurement is called ocular pulse amplitude (OPA) and is a good indicator of the quality of ocular blood flow. This test is helpful in diagnosing normal tension glaucoma.

0200T-0201T

0200T   Percutaneous sacral augmentation (sacroplasty), unilateral injection(s), including the use of a balloon or mechanical device, when used, 1 or more needles, includes imaging guidance and bone biopsy, when performed

0201T   Percutaneous sacral augmentation (sacroplasty), bilateral injections, including the use of a balloon or mechanical device, when used, 2 or more needles, includes imaging guidance and bone biopsy, when performed

Percutaneous sacroplasty is performed to treat sacral insufficiency fractures most commonly seen in postmenopausal women with osteoporosis. Other risk factors include: rheumatoid arthritis, steroid therapy, previous hip replacement, and radiation therapy to the pelvis. While these fractures will heal with bed rest and pain management, the fractures are often associated with severe debilitating pain. Using fluoroscopic guidance, one or more trocar needles are placed into the sacrum on the right or left side. The needle is advanced into the marrow cavity of the sacrum. If a single needle is used it is positioned midway between the sacroiliac joint and sacral foramen. Polymethylmethacrylate (PMMA) is mixed with sterile barium and injected into the marrow space through the indwelling needle(s). The PMMA solution is visualized as it fills the marrow space to ensure proper placement. The procedure is repeated on the opposite side as needed. Use 0200T for a unilateral injection and 0201T for a bilateral injection.

Category III Codes

0202T

0202T Posterior vertebral joint(s) arthroplasty (eg, facet joint[s] replacement), including facetectomy, laminectomy, foraminotomy, and vertebral column fixation, injection of bone cement, when performed, including fluoroscopy, single level, lumbar spine

Paired posterior vertebral joints, also known as the facet joints, are located between the vertebrae of each vertebral segment. The facet joints have a flat articular surface and provide the posterior articulation between adjacent vertebrae. They also provide stability to the vertebral joint when the intervertebral disc has been damaged. The facet joints can become damaged resulting in nerve compression and back pain. Facet joint repair which may include replacement of the facets is performed. The back is incised over the affected lumbar segment. Fluoroscopy is used to aid in visualization of the joint. The intervertebral ligament is divided and the lamina exposed. Part or all of the lamina is excised and the involved nerve root is exposed. The facet joints are explored. The facet joint is excised. Typically only the lower facet is excised but the upper facet may also be excised depending on the extent of the damage. The vertebral foramen is enlarged using a rongeur or a foraminotomy punch. The spine is then stabilized using a facet joint prosthesis or a vertebral column fixator device. Bone cement is injected as needed. Upon completion of the procedure, bleeding is controlled by coagulation, the wound is irrigated and incisions closed.This code reports surgery on a single level of the lumbar spine.

0205T

0205T Intravascular catheter-based coronary vessel or graft spectroscopy (eg, infrared) during diagnostic evaluation and/or therapeutic intervention including imaging supervision, interpretation, and report, each vessel (List separately in addition to code for primary procedure)

During a separately reportable diagnostic cardiac catheterization or therapeutic percutaneous coronary angioplasty, atherectomy, or stent procedure the coronary vessel or bypass graft is visualized using spectroscopy to evaluate the chemical composition of the intraluminal plaque. Use of infrared or other spectroscopic technology allows analysis of the plaque without temporary displacement of blood. Using infrared or near infrared technology, the vessel is exposed to a light beam that contains a broad spectrum of wavelengths. Some of the wavelengths are absorbed by the plaque and blood vessel tissues. The remaining wavelengths traverse the tissue. The wavelengths that have been absorbed are evaluated to determine the chemical composition of the plaque. Another type of spectroscopy called Raman spectroscopy uses a single wavelength light beam. Shifts in the wavelength caused by interaction of photons with vessel tissue and plaque are monitored and evaluated to determine the substances with which the photons have interacted. The physician provides imaging supervision and interprets the resulting images. A written report is provided. This code is reported for each vessel evaluated.

0206T

0206T Computerized database analysis of multiple cycles of digitized cardiac electrical data from two or more ECG leads, including transmission to a remote center, application of multiple nonlinear mathematical transformations, with coronary artery obstruction severity assessment

Computerized resting electrocardiogram (ECG) analysis is performed using 2 or more ECG leads to evaluate the severity of coronary artery disease (CAD). An ECG tracing is obtained. Using computerized hardware and software, the analog tracing is then amplified and digitized. The digitized information is transmitted to a central server where multiple nonlinear mathematical transformations are applied. Following these transformations, the patterns found in the ECG tracing are compared to a large reference database and a severity score is generated that indicates the likelihood of clinically significant CAD. This results are then transmitted to the physician or other qualified health care provider.

0207T

0207T Evacuation of meibomian glands, automated, using heat and intermittent pressure, unilateral

The meibomian glands are located in the eyelids and secret the lipid layer of tear film that prevents rapid evaporation of tears. Dysfunction of meibomian glands is caused by blockage or thickening of the meibum. This can cause dry eye symptoms even in individuals who appear to produce adequate tearing. Using an automated device heat and intermittent pressure are applied unilaterally to the eyelid to relieve obstruction of the meibomian glands. The device consists of a compress and a sealed container that contains a heat source. Heat is released by an exothermic reaction. The compress remains on the eye and heat is applied for a predetermined length of time to help melt and liquefy the lipid secretions. Once the secretions have been liquefied, the device applies intermittent pressure to the eyelids to help express the lipid secretions.

0208T-0209T

0209T Pure tone audiometry (threshold), automated; air and bone
0208T Pure tone audiometry (threshold), automated; air only

Automated pure tone audiometry uses a computerized system to evaluate hearing. Ambient noise microphones are placed near the patient's ears. Ear inserts are placed in the ear. These inserts are attached to transducers and a bone oscillator outside the ear. The ear inserts do not completely occlude the ear canal. The automated otography device is then programmed and the desired tests are performed. In 0208T, automated pure tone air audiometry testing is performed. This test measures hearing sensitivity. Pure tone thresholds identify the softest sound audible to the patient at least 50 percent of the time. The computer displays a graphic representation of hearing sensitivity. In 0209T, both air and bone pure tone audiometry is performed. Air pure tone audiometry is performed as described above. A second hearing test is then performed using a signal transmitted through the bones of the skull to the cochlea and then through auditory pathways in the brain. The computer displays graphic representations of both the air and bone hearing thresholds.

0210T-0211T

0211T Speech audiometry threshold, automated; with speech recognition
0210T Speech audiometry threshold, automated

Automated hearing tests are performed using a computerized system. Ambient noise microphones are placed near the patient's ears. Ear inserts are placed in the ear. These inserts are attached to the speakers. The ear inserts do not completely occlude the ear canal. The automated testing device is then programmed and the desired tests are performed. In 0210T, automated speech audiometry testing is performed. This test measures the lowest intensity speech stimulus audible to the patient at least 50 percent of the time. The computer scores the speech audiometry threshold. In 0211T, speech recognition is performed in conjunction with speech audiometry threshold. Speech recognition, also referred to as speech discrimination or word recognition, tests the patient's ability to repeat correctly a set of words delivered by the computerized program. The computer scores the number of words repeated correctly as a percentage of all words delivered.

0212T

0212T Comprehensive audiometry threshold evaluation and speech recognition (0209T, 0211T combined), automated

Automated hearing tests are performed using a computerized system. Ambient noise microphones are placed near the patient's ears. Ear inserts are placed in the ear. These inserts are attached to the transducers and a bone oscillator outside the ear for the air and bone pure tone audiometry portion of the test and to speakers for the speech recognition portion of the test. The ear inserts do not completely occlude the ear canal. The automated testing device is then programmed and the desired tests are performed. Automated pure tone air audiometry measures hearing sensitivity. Pure tone thresholds identify the softest sound audible to the patient at least 50 percent of the time. The computer displays a graphic representation of the hearing sensitivity. Pure tone bone audiometry is performed using a signal transmitted through the bones of the skull to the cochlea and then through auditory pathways in the brain. The computer displays graphic representations of the bone conduction thresholds. Automated speech audiometry measures the lowest intensity speech stimulus audible to the patient at least 50 percent of the time. The computer scores the speech audiometry threshold. Speech recognition, also referred to as speech discrimination or word recognition, tests the patient's ability to repeat correctly a set of words delivered by the computerized program. The computer scores the number of words repeated correctly as a percentage of all words delivered.

0213T-0215T

0215T Injection(s), diagnostic or therapeutic agent, paravertebral facet (zygapophyseal) joint (or nerves innervating that joint) with ultrasound guidance, cervical or thoracic; third and any additional level(s) (List separately in addition to code for primary procedure)
0214T Injection(s), diagnostic or therapeutic agent, paravertebral facet (zygapophyseal) joint (or nerves innervating that joint) with ultrasound guidance, cervical or thoracic; second level (List separately in addition to code for primary procedure)
0213T Injection(s), diagnostic or therapeutic agent, paravertebral facet (zygapophyseal) joint (or nerves innervating that joint) with ultrasound guidance, cervical or thoracic; single level

Paravertebral facet joints, also called zygapophyseal joints, are located on the back (posterior) of the spine on each side of the vertebra at the point where one vertebra overlaps the next. Facet joint pain may be associated with post-laminectomy syndrome or other spinal surgery with destabilization of the spinal joints, scar tissue formation, or recurrent disc herniation. Other causes include spondylosis, spondylolisthesis, and arthritis. Using ultrasound guidance, a diagnostic or therapeutic facet joint injection or injection of nerves innervating the joint is performed. The skin overlying the facet joint is prepped and a local anesthetic is injected. A spinal needle is directed into the facet joint space until bone or cartilage is encountered. A small amount of contrast material is injected to verify that the needle is correctly positioned. This is followed by injection of a local anesthetic and/or steroid. Diagnostic facet joint injection uses a local anesthetic to identify the specific area generating the pain. If the patient experiences pain relief for a significant period of time following a diagnostic injection, the physician will perform a therapeutic injection on a subsequent date of service using a long acting local anesthetic in conjunction with a steroid. Use 0213T for a single cervical or thoracic facet joint injection; use 0214T for the second level; use 0215T for the third and any additional cervical or thoracic levels injected.

0216T-0218T

0218T Injection(s), diagnostic or therapeutic agent, paravertebral facet (zygapophyseal) joint (or nerves innervating that joint) with ultrasound guidance, lumbar or sacral; third and any additional level(s) (List separately in addition to code for primary procedure)

0217T Injection(s), diagnostic or therapeutic agent, paravertebral facet (zygapophyseal) joint (or nerves innervating that joint) with ultrasound guidance, lumbar or sacral; second level (List separately in addition to code for primary procedure)

0216T Injection(s), diagnostic or therapeutic agent, paravertebral facet (zygapophyseal) joint (or nerves innervating that joint) with ultrasound guidance, lumbar or sacral; single level

Paravertebral facet joints, also called zygapophyseal joints, are located on the back (posterior) of the spine on each side of the vertebra at the point where one vertebra overlaps the next. Facet joint pain may be associated with post laminectomy syndrome or other spinal surgery with destabilization of the spinal joints, scar tissue formation, or recurrent disc herniation. Other causes include spondylosis, spondylolisthesis, and arthritis. Using ultrasound guidance, a diagnostic or therapeutic facet joint injection or injection of nerves innervating the joint is performed. The skin overlying the facet joint is prepped and a local anesthetic is injected. A spinal needle is directed into the facet joint space until bone or cartilage is encountered. A small amount of contrast material is injected to verify that the needle is correctly positioned. This is followed by injection of a local anesthetic and/or steroid. Diagnostic facet joint injection uses a local anesthetic to identify the specific area generating the pain. If the patient experiences pain relief for a significant period of time following a diagnostic injection, the physician will perform a therapeutic injection on a subsequent date of service using a long acting local anesthetic in conjunction with a steroid. Use 0216T for a single lumbar or sacral facet joint injection; use 0217T for the second level; use 0218T for the third and any additional lumbar or sacral levels injected.

0219T-0222T

0222T Placement of a posterior intrafacet implant(s), unilateral or bilateral, including imaging and placement of bone graft(s) or synthetic device(s), single level; each additional vertebral segment (List separately in addition to code for primary procedure)

0221T Placement of a posterior intrafacet implant(s), unilateral or bilateral, including imaging and placement of bone graft(s) or synthetic device(s), single level; lumbar

0220T Placement of a posterior intrafacet implant(s), unilateral or bilateral, including imaging and placement of bone graft(s) or synthetic device(s), single level; thoracic

0219T Placement of a posterior intrafacet implant(s), unilateral or bilateral, including imaging and placement of bone graft(s) or synthetic device(s), single level; cervical

Paired posterior vertebral joints, also known as the facet joints, are located between the vertebrae of each vertebral segment. The facet joints have a flat articular surface and provide the posterior articulation between adjacent vertebrae. They also provide stability to the vertebral joint when the intervertebral disc has been damaged. The facet joints can become damaged resulting in nerve compression and back pain. Placement of a posterior intrafacet implant is performed. The back is incised over the affected vertebral segment. Imaging guidance is used as needed to aid in visualization of the joint. The intervertebral ligament is divided and the lamina is exposed. Part or all of the lamina is excised and the involved nerve root is exposed. The facet joints are explored. The spine is then stabilized using a posterior intrafacet implant, such as a facet screw system, locking screw and nut device, or other device placed between the facets in the intervertebral space. If a bone graft is needed, it is harvested locally or from the iliac crest or other site. The bone graft is prepared and placed between the facets. Bone cement is injected as needed. The procedure may be performed on one side only or bilaterally on both of the paired facet joints. Upon completion of the procedure, bleeding is controlled by coagulation, the wound is irrigated, and incisions are closed. Use 0219T when the procedure is performed on a single level in the cervical spine; use 0220T for a single level in the thoracic spine; use 0221T for a single level in the lumbar spine; and use 0222T for each additional vertebral segment in the cervical, thoracic or lumbar spine.

0228T-0229T

0229T Injection(s), anesthetic agent and/or steroid, transforaminal epidural, with ultrasound guidance, cervical or thoracic; each additional level (List separately in addition to code for primary procedure)

0228T Injection(s), anesthetic agent and/or steroid, transforaminal epidural, with ultrasound guidance, cervical or thoracic; single level

A transforaminal epidural injection is performed to treat foraminal stenosis and large or lateral disc herniations. The patient is positioned prone on the treatment table. Using fluoroscopic guidance, a needle is advanced through the skin and nerve root foramen of the affected vertebra and into the epidural space. Contrast is injected to ensure proper placement of the needle within the epidural space. An anesthetic agent and/or steroid is then injected. Use 0228T for the first injection of a cervical or thoracic vertebral level. Use 0229T for each additional cervical or thoracic level injected.

0230T-0231T

0231T Injection(s), anesthetic agent and/or steroid, transforaminal epidural, with ultrasound guidance, lumbar or sacral; each additional level (List separately in addition to code for primary procedure)

0230T Injection(s), anesthetic agent and/or steroid, transforaminal epidural, with ultrasound guidance, lumbar or sacral; single level

A transforaminal epidural injection is performed to treat foraminal stenosis and large or lateral disc herniations. The patient is positioned prone on the treatment table. Using fluoroscopic guidance, a needle is advanced through the skin and nerve root foramen of the affected vertebra and into the epidural space. Contrast is injected to ensure proper placement of the needle within the epidural space. An anesthetic agent and/or steroid is then injected. Use 0230T for the first injection of a lumbar or sacral vertebral level. Use 0231T for each additional lumbar or sacral level injected.

0232T

0232T Injection(s), platelet rich plasma, any site, including image guidance, harvesting and preparation when performed

Platelet rich plasma is used to treat non-healing injuries. Platelet rich plasma contains concentrated platelets that release growth factors including platelet derived growth factor and transforming growth factor, as well as other types. When injected into a non-healing injury, platelet rich plasma causes a chain reaction beginning with the release of growth factors that in turn act on fibroblasts, causing them to increase in number, which then accelerates repair of injured tissues. The procedure begins with collection of blood from the patient. The blood is centrifuged to separate the plasma from other blood constituents and concentrate the platelets. The platelet rich plasma is then placed in a syringe. A local anesthetic is administered as needed. The platelet rich plasma is injected into the injured tissue. Depending on the site of the injury, imaging guidance may be used to ensure proper placement of the needle into the injured tissue.

0234T-0235T

0234T Transluminal peripheral atherectomy, open or percutaneous, including radiological supervision and interpretation; renal artery

0235T Transluminal peripheral atherectomy, open or percutaneous, including radiological supervision and interpretation; visceral artery (except renal), each vessel

The physician performs an open or peripheral transluminal atherectomy of a renal (0234T) or other visceral artery (0235T). If an open approach is used, the skin over the access artery is prepped and incised, and the artery is exposed. The artery is nicked and a sheath is placed. If a percutaneous approach is used, the skin over the access artery, usually one of the femoral arteries, is prepped and the artery is punctured with a needle. A sheath is placed. Using radiological supervision, a guidewire is inserted and advanced from the access artery to the occluded renal or visceral artery. The atherectomy catheter is advanced over the guidewire and the guidewire is withdrawn. Atherectomy is performed using a specialized balloon catheter that has a window on one side through which a cutting piston is advanced. The cutting piston shaves plaque from the arterial wall. As the plaque is shaved, it is pushed into the nose of the atherectomy device and removed upon completion of the procedure when the catheter is withdrawn. The physician may make several passes with the atherectomy device to achieve the desired result. The atherectomy device is exchanged for a guidewire. An angiography catheter is advanced over the guidewire and the guidewire is withdrawn. Contrast is injected and a completion angiography is performed to ensure that the renal or visceral artery or aorta is patent. The angiography catheter is withdrawn. Upon completion of the procedure, if an open approach has been used, the access artery is repaired and the skin incision is closed. If a percutaneous approach has been used, pressure is applied over the puncture site to control bleeding and a pressure dressing is applied. Report 0234T for a renal artery treated by open or percutaneous atherectomy and 0235T for each visceral artery other than renal treated by atherectomy.

Category III Codes

0236T

0236T   **Transluminal peripheral atherectomy, open or percutaneous, including radiological supervision and interpretation; abdominal aorta**

The physician performs an open or percutaneous transluminal atherectomy of the abdominal aorta. If an open approach is used, the skin over the access artery is prepped and incised, and the artery is exposed. The artery is nicked and a sheath is placed. If a percutaneous approach is used, the skin over the access artery, usually one of the femoral arteries, is prepped and the artery is punctured with a needle. A sheath is placed. Using radiological supervision, a guidewire is inserted and advanced from the access artery into the occluded portion of the abdominal aorta. The atherectomy catheter is advanced over the guidewire and the guidewire is withdrawn. Atherectomy is performed using a specialized balloon catheter that has a window on one side through which a cutting piston is advanced. The cutting piston shaves plaque from the arterial wall. As the plaque is shaved, it is pushed into the nose of the atherectomy device and removed upon completion of the procedure when the catheter is withdrawn. The physician may make several passes with the atherectomy device to achieve the desired result. The atherectomy device is exchanged for a guidewire. An angiography catheter is advanced over the guidewire and the guidewire is withdrawn. Contrast is injected and a completion angiography is performed to ensure that the artery is patent. The angiography catheter is withdrawn. Upon completion of the procedure, if an open approach has been used, the access artery is repaired and the skin incision is closed. If a percutaneous approach has been used, pressure is applied over the puncture site to control bleeding and a pressure dressing is applied.

0237T

0237T   **Transluminal peripheral atherectomy, open or percutaneous, including radiological supervision and interpretation; brachiocephalic trunk and branches, each vessel**

The physician performs an open or percutaneous transluminal atherectomy of the brachiocephalic trunk and branches. If an open approach is used, the skin over the access artery is prepped and incised, and the artery is exposed. The artery is nicked and a sheath is placed. If a percutaneous approach is used, the skin over the access artery, usually one of the femoral arteries, is prepped and the artery is punctured with a needle. A sheath is placed. Using radiological supervision, a guidewire is inserted and advanced from the access artery into the occluded brachiocephalic trunk or branch. The atherectomy catheter is advanced over the guidewire and the guidewire is withdrawn. Atherectomy is performed using a specialized balloon catheter that has a window on one side through which a cutting piston is advanced. The cutting piston shaves plaque from the arterial wall. As the plaque is shaved, it is pushed into the nose of the atherectomy device and removed upon completion of the procedure when the catheter is withdrawn. The physician may make several passes with the atherectomy device to achieve the desired result. The atherectomy device is exchanged for a guidewire. An angiography catheter is advanced over the guidewire and the guidewire is withdrawn. Contrast is injected and a completion angiography is performed to ensure that the artery is patent. The angiography catheter is withdrawn. Upon completion of the procedure, if an open approach has been used, the access artery is repaired and the skin incision is closed. If a percutaneous approach has been used, pressure is applied over the puncture site to control bleeding and a pressure dressing is applied. Report 0237T for each brachiocephalic vessel treated by atherectomy.

0238T

0238T   **Transluminal peripheral atherectomy, open or percutaneous, including radiological supervision and interpretation; iliac artery, each vessel**

The physician performs an open or percutaneous transluminal atherectomy of iliac artery. If an open approach is used, the skin over the access artery is prepped and incised, and the artery is exposed. The artery is nicked and a sheath is placed. If a percutaneous approach is used, the skin over the access artery, usually one of the femoral arteries, is prepped and the artery is punctured with a needle. A sheath is placed. Using radiological supervision, a guidewire is inserted and advanced from the access artery into the occluded iliac artery. The atherectomy catheter is advanced over the guidewire and the guidewire is withdrawn. Atherectomy is performed using a specialized balloon catheter that has a window on one side through which a cutting piston is advanced. The cutting piston shaves plaque from the arterial wall. As the plaque is shaved, it is pushed into the nose of the atherectomy device and removed upon completion of the procedure when the catheter is withdrawn. The physician may make several passes with the atherectomy device to achieve the desired result. The atherectomy device is exchanged for a guidewire. An angiography catheter is advanced over the guidewire and the guidewire is withdrawn. Contrast is injected and a completion angiography is performed to ensure that the artery is patent. The angiography catheter is withdrawn. Upon completion of the procedure, if an open approach has been used, the access artery is repaired and the skin incision is closed. If a percutaneous approach has been used, pressure is applied over the puncture site to control bleeding and a pressure dressing is applied. Report 0238T for each iliac vessel treated by atherectomy.

0249T

0249T   **Ligation, hemorrhoidal vascular bundle(s), including ultrasound guidance**

Submucosal vascular beds composed of connective tissue, smooth muscle, and blood vessels surround the anal canal. When the vascular beds become enlarged and protrude into the anal canal, they are called hemorrhoids. This procedure involves ligation of the entire vascular bundle. Using ultrasound guidance, the involved vascular bundle is located and grasped with forceps. The entire vascular bundle is then suture ligated to cut off the blood supply and tissue distal to the ligature is excised.

0253T

0253T   **Insertion of anterior segment aqueous drainage device, without extraocular reservoir, internal approach, into the suprachoroidal space**

An anterior segment aqueous drainage device without an extraocular reservoir is inserted to treat chronic or progressive open angle glaucoma. The anterior chamber is accessed via a small, self-sealing incision in the cornea. The suprachoroidal space is accessed using a deep posterior scleral flap. A magnification lens such as a gonioscope is used to place and position the drainage device (shunt) at the angle of the anterior chamber. The drainage device traverses the sclera with the terminal end positioned in the suprachoroidal space.

0254T-0255T

0255T   **Endovascular repair of iliac artery bifurcation (eg, aneurysm, pseudoaneurysm, arteriovenous malformation, trauma) using bifurcated endoprosthesis from the common iliac artery into both the external and internal iliac artery, unilateral; radiological supervision and interpretation**

0254T   **Endovascular repair of iliac artery bifurcation (eg, aneurysm, pseudoaneurysm, arteriovenous malformation, trauma) using bifurcated endoprosthesis from the common iliac artery into both the external and internal iliac artery, unilateral**

Endovascular graft placement is performed to repair an iliac artery aneurysm, false aneurysm, arteriovenous malformation, or traumatic injury spanning both the external and internal iliac arteries. Both femoral arteries are exposed. The ipsilateral (same side) femoral artery is incised. A guidewire is introduced and advanced to a point just above the external iliac artery defect. An introducer sheath containing the endovascular bifurcated graft is advanced over the guidewire and positioned over the external iliac artery defect using fluoroscopic guidance. The contralateral (opposite side) femoral artery is incised and a guidewire is advanced into the contralateral iliac artery, aorta, and then into the ipsilateral external iliac artery. An angled guidewire is used to access the internal iliac artery. Correct positioning of the endograft in the external iliac artery is verified fluoroscopically and the guidewire is removed. The sheath is then removed and the external iliac portion of the endograft is deployed. The limb is manipulated into the internal iliac artery and the position is verified fluoroscopically. The internal iliac limb is deployed. A balloon catheter is used as needed to seat the endograft. The balloon catheter is removed and a pigtail or sidehole catheter is introduced over the guidewire. Angiography is performed to evaluate the endograft position and to ensure that there are no endoleaks. Catheters and guidewires are removed and the groin incision is closed. Use 0254T for placement of the endograft. Use 0255T for the radiological supervision and interpretation portion of the endograft placement.

0263T-0265T

0263T   **Intramuscular autologous bone marrow cell therapy, with preparation of harvested cells, multiple injections, one leg, including ultrasound guidance, if performed; complete procedure including unilateral or bilateral bone marrow harvest**

0264T   **Intramuscular autologous bone marrow cell therapy, with preparation of harvested cells, multiple injections, one leg, including ultrasound guidance, if performed; complete procedure excluding bone marrow harvest**

0265T   **Intramuscular autologous bone marrow cell therapy, with preparation of harvested cells, multiple injections, one leg, including ultrasound guidance, if performed; unilateral or bilateral bone marrow harvest only for intramuscular autologous bone marrow cell therapy**

Bone marrow cell therapy is performed on a patient with peripheral artery [occlusive] disease (PAD), complicated by severe limb ischemia with amputation the only other viable treatment option. If possible, three months prior to bone marrow harvest, separately reportable Doppler-guided arterial segment pressures of the dorsal pedis and tibial arteries are documented. Immediately before the autologous bone marrow harvest, a separately reportable routine angiography is performed to identify the location of the stenosis and/or occlusion in the limb. An anterior incision is made over the anterior superior iliac spine. A bone marrow needle with a syringe is used to enter the medullary canal and the bone marrow is aspirated. The bone marrow is then placed in a centrifuge to concentrate the bone marrow cells. The bone marrow cells are immediately re-injected intramuscularly into the stenotic and/or occlusive sites in the leg using ultrasound guidance as needed. Ankle-brachial index (ABI) measurements, rest pain, and ischemic ulceration status are obtained before and after the bone marrow cell therapy. In 0263T, a complete procedure is performed, including unilateral or bilateral bone marrow harvest. In 0264T, the bone marrow cell therapy is performed without the bone marrow harvest. In 0265T, only a unilateral or bilateral bone marrow harvest is performed without the intramuscular injection(s).

0266T-0268T

0266T   **Implantation or replacement of carotid sinus baroreflex activation device; total system (includes generator placement, unilateral or bilateral lead placement, intra-operative interrogation, programming, and repositioning, when performed)**

0267T   **Implantation or replacement of carotid sinus baroreflex activation device; lead only, unilateral (includes intra-operative interrogation, programming, and repositioning, when performed)**

0268T   **Implantation or replacement of carotid sinus baroreflex activation device; pulse generator only (includes intra-operative interrogation, programming, and repositioning, when performed)**

A carotid sinus baroreflex activation device is implanted in a patient with refractory hypertension. The carotid sinus baroreflex helps to regulate arterial blood pressure and heart rate by sending electrical impulses to the brainstem. In patients with refractory hypertension, the ability of the carotid sinus baroreflex to modulate blood pressure and heart rate is impaired. Implantation of a baroreflex activation device increases electrical activity in the carotid baroreceptor afferent nerves which is interpreted by the brainstem as elevated arterial blood pressure. The central nervous system responds by modulating the sympathetic and vagus nerve outflows which results in a lowering of blood pressure and heart rate. The implantable device activates the carotid baroreflex using electrodes that are implanted on the exterior surface of the carotid sinus wall. An incision is made over the carotid bifurcation on one side. The common carotid artery is exposed. The vagus nerve is identified and protected. The carotid artery bifurcation is mobilized circumferentially without disturbing the neurovascular bundle contained within the bifurcation. The first electrode is positioned on the bifurcation in the area of the carotid sinus. The electrode is attached to the battery powered impulse generator (IPG), tested, and hemodynamic response is evaluated. The electrode is repositioned as needed until optimal hemodynamic response is attained. The electrode is sutured in place. The procedure is repeated on the contralateral side. The leads are then tunneled to the infraclavicular region where the subcutaneous pocket for the IPG is developed. An incision is made in the skin and a subcutaneous pocket is fashioned. The leads are connected to the IPG and the impulse generator is tested. The optimal frequency and intensity of impulses is determined and the generator is programmed. Once it has been determined that the leads and IPG are working properly and that the desired reduction in blood pressure and heart rate has been attained, the IPG is placed into the pocket, sutured to underlying tissue, and the pocket is closed. Use 0266T for implantation or replacement of the entire system including unilateral or bilateral leads and pulse generator. Use 0267T for implantation or replacement of the lead only (unilateral). Use 0268T for implantation or replacement of the pulse generator only.

0269T-0271T

0269T   **Revision or removal of carotid sinus baroreflex activation device; total system (includes generator placement, unilateral or bilateral lead placement, intra-operative interrogation, programming, and repositioning, when performed)**

0270T   **Revision or removal of carotid sinus baroreflex activation device; lead only, unilateral (includes intra-operative interrogation, programming, and repositioning, when performed)**

0271T   **Revision or removal of carotid sinus baroreflex activation device; pulse generator only (includes intra-operative interrogation, programming, and repositioning, when performed)**

A carotid sinus baroreflex activation device is revised or removed due to mechanical malfunction, pain, infection, extravascular tissue stimulation, bradycardia, or failure to respond to the therapy. The carotid sinus baroreflex helps to regulate arterial blood pressure and heart rate by sending electrical impulses to the brainstem. In patients with refractory hypertension, the ability of the carotid sinus baroreflex to modulate blood pressure and heart rate is impaired. The baroreflex activation device increases electrical activity in the carotid baroreceptor afferent nerves which is interpreted by the brainstem as elevated arterial blood pressure. The central nervous system responds by modulating the sympathetic and vagus nerve outflows which results in a lowering of blood pressure and heart rate. The implantable device activates the carotid baroreflex using electrodes that are implanted on the exterior surface of the carotid sinus wall. For revision of the generator and/or leads, the old incision over the subcutaneous pocket is opened. The generator and distal aspect of the leads are exposed. The connections between the leads and the impulse generator are checked and repositioned or revised as needed. Once it has been determined that the generator is functioning properly, attention is turned to the leads. If it is determined that one or both leads are not delivering impulses to the carotid sinuses, the lead insertion site(s) at the carotid artery bifurcation is(are) exposed. One or both leads are repositioned or revised as needed. Once the leads and generator are functioning properly, the optimal frequency and intensity of impulses is determined and the generator is programmed. Programming and placement of the leads is adjusted until the

desired reduction in blood pressure and heart rate has been attained. The IPG is placed into the pocket, sutured to underlying tissue, and the pocket is closed. For removal of the entire system, the pulse generator is exposed, detached from the leads, and removed. The insertion sites of the leads at the carotid bifurcations are exposed. The leads are dissected from surrounding tissues and removed. Incisions are closed. Use 0269T for revision or removal of the entire system including unilateral or bilateral leads and pulse generator. Use 0270T for revision or removal of the lead only (unilateral). Use 0271T for revision or removal of the pulse generator only.

0272T-0273T

0272T   **Interrogation device evaluation (in person), carotid sinus baroreflex activation system, including telemetric iterative communication with the implantable device to monitor device diagnostics and programmed therapy values, with interpretation and report (eg, battery status, lead impedance, pulse amplitude, pulse width, therapy frequency, pathway mode, burst mode, therapy start/stop times each day)**

0273T   **Interrogation device evaluation (in person), carotid sinus baroreflex activation system, including telemetric iterative communication with the implantable device to monitor device diagnostics and programmed therapy values, with interpretation and report (eg, battery status, lead impedance, pulse amplitude, pulse width, therapy frequency, pathway mode, burst mode, therapy start/stop times each day); with programming**

An in-person interrogation evaluation of a carotid sinus baroreflex activation device system is performed. In patients with refractory hypertension, the ability of the carotid sinus baroreflex to modulate blood pressure and heart rate is impaired. An implanted baroreflex activation device system increases electrical activity in the carotid baroreceptor afferent nerves which is interpreted by the brainstem as elevated arterial blood pressure. The central nervous system responds by modulating the sympathetic and vagus nerve outflows which results in a lowering of blood pressure and heart rate. In 0272T, in-person interrogation device evaluation is performed as a routine evaluation or when a patient presents with symptoms or complaints that might be due to device malfunction or a change in cardiac function. The patient is connected to an electrocardiogram (ECG) monitor. A connection is established between the carotid sinus baroreflex activation device and the interrogation device. The interrogation is performed. The physician reviews the interrogated data to assess device function and current programmed parameters. Stored device data are reviewed and compared with previous data acquisitions. The number and duration of events as evidenced by changes in blood pressure and heart rate are evaluated. Exercise and physiologic stress data are reviewed and blood pressure and heart rate adaptations are noted. The device is evaluated for appropriate sensing and capture of blood pressure and heart rate. Mechanical function is assessed, including the integrity of the leads and battery. No programming of the device is performed. The patient is informed of the findings and a written report is provided. In 0273T, the device interrogation is performed as described above and the device is programmed. This may include changes in pulse amplitude, pulse width, therapy frequency, pathway mode, burst mode, and daily therapy start/stop times. These codes are reported on a per encounter basis.

0274T-0275T

▲ **0274T**   **Percutaneous laminotomy/laminectomy (interlaminar approach) for decompression of neural elements, (with or without ligamentous resection, discectomy, facetectomy and/or foraminotomy), any method, under indirect image guidance (eg, fluoroscopic, CT), single or multiple levels, unilateral or bilateral; cervical or thoracic**

▲ **0275T**   **Percutaneous laminotomy/laminectomy (interlaminar approach) for decompression of neural elements, (with or without ligamentous resection, discectomy, facetectomy and/or foraminotomy), any method, under indirect image guidance (eg, fluoroscopic, CT), single or multiple levels, unilateral or bilateral; lumbar**

A percutaneous laminotomy or laminectomy is performed for neural decompression. Separately reportable preoperative MRI, CT, or myelography is performed to identify the target entry site over the spine. CT or C-arm fluoroscopy is used intraoperatively to visualize the spine. Percutaneous devices are designed to access the interlaminar space using a posterior approach. Contrast is injected as needed into the epidural space to facilitate better visualization of surrounding structures and to evaluate the degree of decompression achieved. A guiding portal and inner trocar are inserted percutaneously inferior to the vertebral segment being decompressed and lateral to the spinous process margin. The guiding portal and inner trocar are advanced to the inferior vertebral segment lamina toward the border of the interlaminar space using imaging guidance. The inner trocar is removed leaving the hollow access portal in the interlaminar space. The portal is secured against the skin surface using plate and guide devices which are used to ensure proper placement of the surgical instruments. A bone sculptor is advanced through the portal to the free edge of the lamina. Small pieces of bone are removed from the superior and inferior lamina (laminotomy/laminectomy). Once the interlaminal space has been enlarged, the bone sculptor is removed and a tissue sculptor is advanced through the portal. The ligamentum flavum is resected as needed. The openings under the facet joints where the nerve runs through are checked and a portion of the bone around the opening may be

Category III Codes

removed for additional pressure relief, if necessary (foraminotomy). Ruptured disc fragments or bulging nucleus pulposus is also removed to decompress the nerve(s). Decompression is then visually confirmed by changes in the epidurogram and flow of contrast. The procedure may be performed as a unilateral or bilateral procedure at each vertebral level and it may be performed at one or more levels. Use 0274T for percutaneous decompression of neural elements in the cervical or thoracic spine, unilateral or bilateral, single or multiple levels. Use 0275T for percutaneous decompression of neural elements in the lumbar spine, unilateral or bilateral, single or multiple levels.

0278T

0278T   Transcutaneous electrical modulation pain reprocessing (eg, scrambler therapy), each treatment session (includes placement of electrodes)

Transcutaneous electrical modulation pain reprocessing (TEMPR), also referred to as scrambler therapy, is used to treat intense, chronic pain, such as oncologic/cancer pain, pain due to failed back surgery, low back pain and sciatica, post-herpetic pain, trigeminal neuralgia, post-surgical nerve lesion neuropathy, pudendal neuropathy, brachial plexus neuropathy and other types of neuropathic pain. It works by interfering with pain signal transmission using transmission of non-pain impulses via surface electrodes that are picked up by the same nerve fibers transmitting the pain impulses. This mixes or scrambles the pain signal, modifying or overriding the pain signal received by the brain. Surface electrodes are applied to the skin at the sites of the pain. The electrodes are attached to a multiprocessor apparatus that stimulates the nerves with non-pain impulses during a treatment session which typically consists of 1-5 applications, each lasting approximately 30 minutes. Pain response is evaluated before and after each application. Patients may receive multiple treatment sessions over the course of several days or weeks. Report 0278T for each treatment session which may consist of 1 or more 30-minute applications.

0293T-0294T

0293T   Insertion of left atrial hemodynamic monitor; complete system, includes implanted communication module and pressure sensor lead in left atrium including transseptal access, radiological supervision and interpretation, and associated injection procedures, when performed

0294T   Insertion of left atrial hemodynamic monitor; pressure sensor lead at time of insertion of pacing cardioverter-defibrillator pulse generator including radiological supervision and interpretation and associated injection procedures, when performed (List separately in addition to code for primary procedure)

An implantable left atrial hemodynamic (LAH) monitor device is used to monitor left atrial pressure (LAP) in patients with heart failure. Precise measurement of cardiac hemodynamics is used to manage fluid status in acutely decompensated heart failure. The monitoring system can be used as a stand-alone device or in combination with implantable cardioverter defibrillator (ICD) or cardiac resynchronization therapy defibrillator (CRT-D). The LAH monitor device consists of an implantable sensor lead coupled with a subcutaneous antenna coil and a sealed sensor module with a pressure sensing membrane and circuitry for measuring and communicating LAP, temperature, and intracardiac electrogram. Using a Seldinger technique, sheaths are placed in the right femoral vein and transseptal puncture is performed. After closed femoral transseptal puncture, heparin 5000 IU is administered and a delivery sheath is placed in the left atrium. The sensor system is implanted under fluoroscopic guidance by advancing the sensor lead until the distal anchor unfolds and contacts the left side of the atrial septum. The antenna coil is then connected to the proximal end of the sensor lead and placed in a subcutaneous pocket. Use code 0293T for implantation of a stand-alone system. Use code 0294T to report insertion of a pressure sensor lead at the time of insertion of a cardioverter-defibrillator pulse generator.

0295T-0298T

0295T   External electrocardiographic recording for more than 48 hours up to 21 days by continuous rhythm recording and storage; includes recording, scanning analysis with report, review and interpretation

0296T   External electrocardiographic recording for more than 48 hours up to 21 days by continuous rhythm recording and storage; recording (includes connection and initial recording)

0297T   External electrocardiographic recording for more than 48 hours up to 21 days by continuous rhythm recording and storage; scanning analysis with report

0298T   External electrocardiographic recording for more than 48 hours up to 21 days by continuous rhythm recording and storage; review and interpretation

Long-term, continuous, unmonitored electrocardiographic (ECG) rhythm recording is obtained as the patient goes about regular daily activity while wearing an external ECG recording device. These new devices typically include both the electrodes and the recording device in a single, compact, lightweight unit that is waterproof and can be worn continuously for up to 21 days. The device is placed on the upper aspect of the left chest and tested, then an initial recording is obtained. The patient is instructed in the use and care of the recording device. The device is activated and ECG rhythm is recorded and stored continuously for a period of more than 48 hours up to 21 days. After the prescribed

period of time has elapsed, the patient returns the device to the office or clinic. The data is downloaded, a computerized analysis is performed, and a report is generated. A physician or other qualified health care professional reviews the ECG data and scanning analysis and provides a written interpretation of findings. Report code 0295T for the complete procedure including rhythm recording, scanning analysis with report, and review and interpretation by the physician or other qualified health care professional. Report code 0296T for recording only, including connection and initial recording. Report code 0297T for scanning analysis and report only. Report code 0298T for physician or other qualified health care professional review and interpretation only.

0299T-0300T

0299T   Extracorporeal shock wave for integumentary wound healing, high energy, including topical application and dressing care; initial wound

0300T   Extracorporeal shock wave for integumentary wound healing, high energy, including topical application and dressing care; each additional wound (List separately in addition to code for primary procedure)

High energy extracorporeal shock wave therapy (HE-ESWT) is a non-invasive treatment with few adverse side effects. High-pressure shock (sound) waves are generated through a fluid medium (water or a coupling gel) to a focused area of tissue. This therapy may be used to treat burns, acute traumatic injuries, chronic skin ulcerations and skin flaps. The therapeutic effect of HE-ESWT is increased blood flow and reduction of inflammation at the targeted area which leads to tissue regeneration and healing. HE-ESWT is usually performed in an outpatient setting by a physician trained in the technique. The wound is examined and targeted area for therapy marked. A mild sedative or local anesthetic may be administered. HE-ESWT may be performed using a number of different modalities including electrohydrolic shock wave, electromagnetic shock wave and piezoelectric shock wave. Following the procedure the wound is covered with an appropriate dressing. Use 0299T for the initial wound and 0300T for each additional wound treated.

0301T

0301T   Destruction/reduction of malignant breast tumor with externally applied focused microwave, including interstitial placement of disposable catheter with combined temperature monitoring probe and microwave focusing sensocatheter under ultrasound thermotherapy guidance

Focused microwave therapy (FMT) is a non-invasive or minimally invasive technique that can be used to destroy malignant breast tumors and/or make them more sensitive to radiation therapy and chemotherapeutic drugs. Malignant breast tumor cells have higher water content than the surrounding healthy breast tissue making them more sensitive to high temperatures. FMT may be an effective primary or adjunctive treatment option for patients who decline or are poor candidates for traditional surgery (lumpectomy, mastectomy). A local anesthetic is injected followed by insertion of a multiprobe catheter directly into the tumor using ultrasound for guidance. The patient is then positioned on the treatment table (modified stereotactic breast needle biopsy table) and the breast is compressed between two plates. A probe in placed into the catheter and secured to the skin. Microwave applicators are positioned at opposing angles. The microwaves are focused on the target area of the isolated breast and a skin cooling device is applied. The target area of the isolated breast is then exposed to high temperature microwave currents for a prescribed period of time. The FMT treatment typically lasts 20-30 minutes. Following treatment the probes and catheter are removed and a sterile dressing is placed over the small puncture sites in the skin.

0302T-0304T

0302T   Insertion or removal and replacement of intracardiac ischemia monitoring system including imaging supervision and interpretation when performed and intra-operative interrogation and programming when performed; complete system (includes device and electrode)

0303T   Insertion or removal and replacement of intracardiac ischemia monitoring system including imaging supervision and interpretation when performed and intra-operative interrogation and programming when performed; electrode only

0304T   Insertion or removal and replacement of intracardiac ischemia monitoring system including imaging supervision and interpretation when performed and intra-operative interrogation and programming when performed; device only

An intracardiac ischemia monitoring system measures electrocardiogram (specifically ST) changes in real time and alerts the patient to seek medical care when a cardiac ischemic event occurs. In some individuals, warning signs such as chest pain, shortness of breath, nausea or diaphoresis (sweating) do not occur or are ignored. The monitoring device has the potential to decrease the elapsed time from the ischemic event to presentation in the emergency room (ER). The monitoring system is comprised of a programmable implantable monitoring device (IMD), right ventricular lead wire, lead wire adapter, external alarm device (EXD) and a programming unit. Insertion of the device usually takes place in the cardiac catheterization lab under monitored anesthesia care (MAC) or sedation. The physician injects a local anesthetic in the area of the upper left chest and makes a skin incision 2-3 inches long. Using fluoroscopy the lead wire is advanced through a (chest) vein to the apex of the right ventricle. The lead wire is attached to the IMD and the IMD programmed. The IMD is then inserted into the chest incision, tested, and the skin is closed with sutures. When a real time ten second electrocardiogram is determined by the device to be outside of the programmed baseline, the EXD will alarm using vibration, flashing lights and/or audible beeps indicating to the patient they should seek emergent medical care. Information from the device can be retrieved via computer and analyzed by the treating physician. The device is recommended for use in patients with previous acute coronary events, diabetes, or renal insufficiency who are considered high-risk for ischemic cardiac events. Use 0302T for insertion or removal and replacement of the complete system (device and electrode); Use code 0303T for insertion or removal and replacement of the electrode only. Use 0304T for insertion or removal and replacement of the device only.

0305T-0306T

0305T **Programming device evaluation (in person) of intracardiac ischemia monitoring system with iterative adjustment of programmed values, with analysis, review, and report**

0306T **Interrogation device evaluation (in person) of intracardiac ischemia monitoring system with analysis, review, and report**

An intracardiac ischemia monitoring system measures ST changes in real time and alerts the patient to seek medical care when a cardiac ischemic event occurs. In some individuals, warning signs such as chest pain, shortness of breath, nausea or diaphoresis (sweating) do not occur or are ignored. The monitoring device has the potential to decrease the elapsed time from the ischemic event to presentation in the ER. The monitoring system is comprised of a programmable implantable monitoring device (IMD), right ventricular lead wire, lead wire adapter, external alarm device (EXD) and a programming unit. The IMD is capable of storing event information that is downloadable via computer for interpretation by the treating physician. Regular monitoring of the device is necessary to ensure that it is programmed correctly and capturing data. Use code 0305T for in person programming device evaluation including any adjustment to the programmed values. Adjustments can be made using the external programming device. An analysis, review and written report is provided as part of the evaluation service. Use code 0306T for in person interrogation device evaluation. Data is downloaded, reviewed and a written report provided as part of the interrogation service.

0307T

0307T **Removal of intracardiac ischemia monitoring device**

The intracardiac ischemia monitoring device is removed in the operating room (OR) or cardiac catheterization lab under monitored anesthesia care (MAC) or general anesthesia. A local anesthetic is infiltrated into the skin over the implanted device. The device is turned off using the external programmer. The previous incision is reopened and the implanted programmable monitoring device (IMD) is freed from scar tissue and carefully removed. The lead wire is separated from the IMD and a sheath is passed over the wire. Using fluoroscopy and/or ultrasound the sheath is then threaded down the wire toward the heart. The sheath may have a laser or electrocautery heating device to vaporize scar tissue encountered along the length of the lead wire. Once the lead wire is completely freed from scar tissue it is removed along with the sheath. An alternate method of removal is to pass a snare wire alongside the lead wire to the apex of the right ventricle. The snare is used to free the tip of the lead wire and using tension the lead wire is pulled back through the vein. The incision is closed with sutures.

0308T

0308T **Insertion of ocular telescope prosthesis including removal of crystalline lens or intraocular lens prosthesis**

An ocular telescopic prosthesis is used to improve visual acuity in patients with end stage age-related macular degeneration (AMD). The wide angle micro optic telescope works in combination with optics of the cornea to create a telephoto system that can magnify objects 2.2-2.7 times their actual size. AMD typically causes a loss of vision in the central portion of the eye. When the telescopic lens is implanted into the cornea, incoming images are reflected onto the undamaged periphery of the retina. The procedure begins with a fairly large incision (12 mm) in the cornea or sclera and is followed by removal of most of the crystalline lens which is located behind the iris. The posterior capsule (elastic lens capsule) is left in place to help support the weight of the telescopic lens. The lens is secured to the posterior capsule with sutures brought through haptic loops on the lens. The patient will usually notice improved vision in the immediate post-operative period and will have the ability to focus on near and far objects using natural eye movements.

0309T

0309T **Arthrodesis, pre-sacral interbody technique, including disc space preparation, discectomy, with posterior instrumentation, with image guidance, includes bone graft, when performed, lumbar, L4-L5 interspace (List separately in addition to code for primary procedure)**

Arthrodesis is the artificial ossification or fusion of a joint which results from surgical intervention. The pre-sacral interbody technique is minimally invasive and requires

fluoroscopy (x-ray imagining). This technique is recommended only for pseudoarthritis, unsuccessful previous disc fusion, spinal stenosis, spondylolisthesis (Grade I) and degenerative disc disease documented by history and x-rays. A small (15-20 mm) incision is made lateral to the coccyx. Under fluoroscopy, a blunt guide introducer is inserted through the incision and advanced along the midline, anterior surface of the sacrum. Guide pins are then inserted and tapped into the sacrum followed by graduated dilators that create a working channel for the surgical instruments. The nucleus pulposus is debulked and bone graft material is injected to fill the disc space. A bone autograft from the patient's own body or allograft of donor bone may be used. A threaded rod is then inserted to maintain the disc and neural foramen height. The instruments are withdrawn and the incision is closed with sutures.

0310T

0310T **Motor function mapping using non-invasive navigated transcranial magnetic stimulation (nTMS) for therapeutic treatment planning, upper and lower extremity**

Navigated transcranial magnetic stimulation (nTMS) is a non-invasive technique that maps motor function in the upper and lower extremities prior to therapeutic treatment or surgical procedures. TMS is used to induce cortical (brain) activity which leads to peripheral nerve response. When TMS is enhanced with magnetic resonance imaging (MRI) it allows continuous visualization (navigation) of the induced electric field in 3-dimension. Mapping motor function using nTMS provides a framework for the surgeon and minimizes the risk of paralysis or impaired function when performing a procedure near the motor cortex. This allows for more complete resection of tumors or an epileptic trigger area while preserving motor function.

0312T

0312T **Vagus nerve blocking therapy (morbid obesity); laparoscopic implantation of neurostimulator electrode array, anterior and posterior vagal trunks adjacent to esophagogastric junction (EGJ), with implantation of pulse generator, includes programming**

Vagus nerve blocking (VBLOC) therapy is used to treat for morbid obesity. The vagus nerve (pneumogastric nerve, cranial nerve X) arises from the brainstem and is comprised of two branches that travel along the esophagus, bronchi and great vessels, through the diaphragm and terminate in the upper portion of the stomach. Impulses travel back and forth along the nerve sending signals of hunger or satiety. In VBLOC therapy, an intermittent, high frequency, low energy electrical stimulus is used to block nerve impulses between the stomach/pancreas and the brain. A small portal incision is made in the upper abdomen and a trocar is placed. A pneumoperitoneum is established by insufflation of carbon dioxide. Two to three additional small incisions are made in the upper abdomen for introduction of surgical instruments. Another small incision is made just above the umbilicus and the laparoscope is introduced through a port. The liver is retracted and the esophagogastric junction is exposed. The electrode arrays are introduced under laparoscopic visualization and are secured around the anterior and posterior trunks of the vagus nerve at the distal aspect of the esophagus. The leads are attached to the neuroregulator and tested. A subcutaneous pocket is created for the pulse generator. A skin incision is made in the side of the body usually over the lower ribs and carried down to the subcutaneous tissue. A pocket is fashioned and the neuroregulator is placed in the pocket. The leads are tunneled to the neuroregulator, connected and again tested. The leads are secured in the subcutaneous tissue and the skin is closed over the neuroregulator. The neuroregulator is activated and programmed using a transmit coil and external mobile charging unit.

0313T-0316T

0313T **Vagus nerve blocking therapy (morbid obesity); laparoscopic revision or replacement of vagal trunk neurostimulator electrode array, including connection to existing pulse generator**

0314T **Vagus nerve blocking therapy (morbid obesity); laparoscopic removal of vagal trunk neurostimulator electrode array and pulse generator**

0315T **Vagus nerve blocking therapy (morbid obesity); removal of pulse generator**

0316T **Vagus nerve blocking therapy (morbid obesity); replacement of pulse generator**

Vagus nerve blocking (VBLOC) therapy is used to treat for morbid obesity. The vagus nerve (pneumogastric nerve, cranial nerve X) arises from the brainstem and is comprised of two branches that travel along the esophagus, bronchi and great vessels, through the diaphragm and terminate in the upper portion of the stomach. Impulses travel back and forth along the nerve sending signals of hunger or satiety. In VBLOC therapy an intermittent, high frequency, low energy electrical stimulus is used to block nerve impulses between the stomach/pancreas and the brain. Before replacing the leads and/or neuroregulator, the device is programmed off. A small portal incision is made in the upper abdomen and a trocar is placed. A pneumoperitoneum is established by insufflation of carbon dioxide. Two to three additional small incisions are made for introduction of surgical instruments. Another small incision is made just above the umbilicus, and the laparoscope is introduced through a port. The liver is retracted and the previously implanted electrode arrays at the anterior and posterior esophagogastric junction are exposed. If the procedure involves relocation of the existing electrode array(s), one or both arrays are located and repositioned around the vagus nerve trunks as needed. If one or both arrays require replacement, a skin incision is made over the neuroregulator, old lead(s) are disconnected and removed and new lead (s) are placed. If the neuroregulator also requires replacement, it is removed and new device implanted. The repositioned or new leads are connected to the neuroregulator and tested. If new leads have been placed they are tunneled to the neuroregulator, connected and again tested. The neuroregulator is returned to the subcutaneous pocket which is closed with sutures. The neuroregulator is activated and programmed using a transmit coil and external mobile charging unit. Use code 0313T for revision or replacement of one or both electrode arrays with connection to the existing neuroregulator. Use code 0314T for removal of the neurostimulator electrode array and pulse generator. Use code 0315T for removal of the neuroregulator only and code 0316T for replacement of the neuroregulator.

0317T

0317T   Vagus nerve blocking therapy (morbid obesity); neurostimulator pulse generator electronic analysis, includes reprogramming when performed

The vagus nerve blocking (VBLOC) therapy system is used to treat morbid obesity. The system includes a neuroblocking pulse generator (neurogenerator) implanted in subcutaneous tissue near the ribs, and leads (electrodes, electrode arrays) placed along the vagus nerve at the esophagogastric junction (EGJ) that are connected to the neurogenerator. The neurogenerator sends out intermittent, high frequency, low energy electrical pulses during waking hours. A mobile charger is worn externally for short periods. The mobile charger connects to a transmit coil placed on the skin over the neurogenerator and delivers radiofrequency battery charging and programming information. Using a clinician programming unit connected to the mobile charger, the physician or other qualified health care professional retrieves reports stored by the system components including patient use and system performance. These reports are reviewed and the therapy settings are reprogrammed as needed to optimize the effects of treatment.

0329T

0329T   Monitoring of intraocular pressure for 24 hours or longer, unilateral or bilateral, with interpretation and report

A soft, hydrophilic, single use contact lens with an embedded pressure sensor is used to monitor intraocular pressure for a period of 24 hours or longer. The lens is inserted and the device activated during an outpatient visit with a physician/eye care professional. The pressure sensor in the contact lens detects circumferential changes (fluctuations in diameter) of the corneoscleral junction which correlates to intraocular pressure (IOP). The readings are sent wirelessly to an antenna located in a circular adhesive worn around the eye. The antenna is connected to a portable recording unit where the data is saved and later downloaded to a computer program by the physician/eye care professional. The physician/eye care professional interprets the data collected, reports the results, and formulates an optimal treatment plan for the patient.

0330T

0330T   Tear film imaging, unilateral or bilateral, with interpretation and report

Ocular tear film is comprised of three layers, a lipid outer layer that helps retard tear evaporation, an aqueous middle layer and a mucus inner layer that anchors the tear film to the corneal epithelium. Tear film imaging is used to quantify the tear film by measuring the height of the tear meniscus, assess for instability of the tear film and identify dry spots. Tear film imaging can be accomplished using optical coherence tomography (OCT) or ellipsometry. OCT uses light waves to outline the anterior segment of the eye and the tear boundaries in a non-invasive, high resolution imaging technique. Ellipsometry measures the polarization states of light determined by the thickness and refractive index of the tear film lipid layer. Ellipsometry and OCT are often used together for multimodal tear film evaluation. These measurements aid in obtaining accurate refraction for fitting of corrective lenses and in successful outcome of cataract and refractive surgeries.

0331T-0332T

0331T   Myocardial sympathetic innervation imaging, planar qualitative and quantitative assessment

0332T   Myocardial sympathetic innervation imaging, planar qualitative and quantitative assessment; with tomographic SPECT

The heart is densely populated with nerves of the sympathetic nervous system (SNS). Myocardial sympathetic innervation imaging uses radiolabeled metaiodobenzylguenidine (I-mIBG) to map the distribution of cardiac nerves and measure heart to mediastinum (H/M) ratio of norepinephrine (NE) reuptake. The ratio of uptake and changes in sympathetic nerve activity can identify disease processes and mortality risks. With the patient at rest, I-mIBG is administered intravenously. In 0331T, radiologic (x-ray) planar (anterior) views of the chest are obtained 10-30 minutes following administration of I-mIBG and again at 3-4 hours. In 0332T, both planar and single-proton emissions computed tomography (tomographic SPECT) are used to evaluate heart function.

Qualitative assessment of uptake and distribution of mIBG by the heart muscle is performed by visual assessment of the planar and/or tomographic SPECT images. A quantitative or semi-quantitative assessment is then performed by identifying regions of interest in the heart and mediastinum and quantitating mIBG uptake by calculating the heart to mediastinum ratio to determine the retention of norepinephrine by sympathetic neurons. The physician reviews the images, calculates the mIBG uptake heart to mediastinum ratio, and provides a written report of findings.

0333T

0333T   Visual evoked potential, screening of visual acuity, automated

Visual evoked potential (VEP) measures the functional integrity of the visual pathway (retina and optic nerve) to the visual cortex of the brain. Screening of visual acuity using an automated device is accomplished by placing the patient in front of a monitor, applying electrodes to the head/scalp, stimulating the visual field, and recording the brain's response. Automated visual stimuli can be in the form of strobe flash, flashing light-emitting diodes (LEDs), transient and steady state pattern reversal and pattern onset/offset (checkerboard). The test is useful for diagnosing amblyopia, refractive errors such as myopia (near-sightedness) and hyperopia (far-sightedness), astigmatism and strabismus in very young and/or non-verbal patients.

0335T

0335T   Extra-osseous subtalar joint implant for talotarsal stabilization

An extra-osseous subtalar joint implant is inserted to prevent excessive motion of the joint and/or correct flat foot deformity. Excessive motion of the subtalar joint is evidenced by failure of the talar and tarsal facets to maintain normal contact causing excessive motion along the talotarsal axis. This leads to hyperpronation of the joint which causes misalignment of other foot structures. Under monitored anesthesia care (MAC) and local anesthetic, the anterior foot is prepped and draped. A small skin incision is made and a percutaneous guide wire is inserted into the sinus tarsi (joint space) transecting the soft tissue. The stent device is then inserted and oriented into the sinus from an anterior-lateral-distal position to a posterior-medial-proximal location. The guide wire is removed and the incision closed.

0337T

0337T   Endothelial function assessment, using peripheral vascular response to reactive hyperemia, non-invasive (eg, brachial artery ultrasound, peripheral artery tonometry), unilateral or bilateral

The endothelial membrane lines the inside of the heart and blood vessels. The membrane releases a substance that controls vascular relaxation and contraction and enzymes that control blood clotting, immune function and platelet adhesion. Function/dysfunction of the endothelial membrane can be correlated to cardiovascular risk factors and coronary artery disease. There are two methods of non-invasive assessment that are used to monitor peripheral response to reactive hyperemia, which is a temporary increase in organ blood flow following a brief period of ischemia. These methods are high resolution ultrasound of the brachial artery which measures changes in vascular dimension and peripheral artery tonometry which measures finger arterial pulse wave amplitude. Endothelial function assessment using brachial artery ultrasound uses longitudinal ultrasound images of the brachial artery to establish a baseline. A blood pressure cuff is placed above the ultrasound transducer and inflated to supra-systolic pressure for 5 minutes to induce inschemia. The percent flow-mediated dilation of the brachial artery is assessed and calculated after 60 seconds of reactive hyperemia. To assess function using peripheral artery tonometry, pneumatic probes are placed on the index fingers of each hand and a baseline of pulse wave amplitude is established. A blood pressure cuff is applied to one arm and inflated to supra-systolic pressure to induce ischemia. The pulse wave amplitude is measured and compared to baseline in the hyperemic finger and contralateral, non-ischemic finger. This procedure may be performed on one or both sides.

0338T-0339T

0338T   Transcatheter renal sympathetic denervation, percutaneous approach including arterial puncture, selective catheter placement(s) renal artery(ies), fluoroscopy, contrast injection(s), intraprocedural roadmapping and radiological supervision and interpretation, including pressure gradient measurements, flush aortogram and diagnostic renal angiography when performed; unilateral

0339T   Transcatheter renal sympathetic denervation, percutaneous approach including arterial puncture, selective catheter placement(s) renal artery(ies), fluoroscopy, contrast injection(s), intraprocedural roadmapping and radiological supervision and interpretation, including pressure gradient measurements, flush aortogram and diagnostic renal angiography when performed; bilateral

Renal sympathetic denervation is used to treat hypertension, heart failure and renal dysfunction, improve glucose control and control sleep apnea when lifestyle changes and pharmacologic interventions are not effective. Elevated sympathetic nervous system activity emanating from the renal plexus is one of the major causes of hypertension. Disruption of nerve impulses from the renal plexus is effective in reducing sympathetic nervous system activity which reduces hypertension. This procedure can now be performed using a transcatheter endovascular technique. Renal sympathetic denervation is accomplished using low-level radiofrequency energy that is delivered through the wall of the renal artery to the sympathetic nerves of the kidney. The skin over the access artery, usually one of the femoral arteries, is prepped and the artery is punctured with a needle and a sheath is placed. Heparin administered via bolus. A guide wire is inserted and advanced from the access artery into the aorta and positioned at or below the renal arteries for flush aortogram or diagnostic renal angiography. A flush catheter is advanced over the guide wire and the guide wire is withdrawn. Contrast is injected and refluxed into the renal arteries with a flush of contrast into the infrarenal aorta. Images are obtained of renal vasculature and of the infrarenal aorta. The guide wire is reinserted to the level of the renal artery and the flush catheter removed. Using fluoroscopic guidance, a renal double curved (RDC) or left internal mammary artery (LIMA) renal guiding catheter and a soft tip straight delivery catheter with radiofrequency (RF) energy electrode tip is delivered over the guidewire and into the right or left renal artery. The guidewire is removed. Radiofrequency (RF) energy is delivered at 4-6 carefully selected treatment points along the vessel to interrupt nerve impulses from the renal plexus. The same procedure is repeated on the contralateral renal artery as needed. Intraprocedural roadmapping and pressure gradient measurements are obtained during the procedure as needed. Following completion of the procedure, the catheters are removed and pressure is applied to the vascular access site. Use 0338T for treatment of one renal artery (right or left) and 0339T when both renal arteries (right and left) are treated.

0387T-0388T

0387T   **Transcatheter insertion or replacement of permanent leadless pacemaker, ventricular**

0388T   **Transcatheter removal of permanent leadless pacemaker, ventricular**

A procedure is performed to insert, replace, or remove a permanent leadless pacemaker into or out of the right ventricle using a transcatheter approach. A leadless pacemaker consists of a pulse generator with a built-in battery and electrode. The device is indicated for single chamber ventricular pacing in patients with arrhythmias including atrial fibrillation and atrioventricular heart block. Using fluoroscopic guidance, the femoral vein is accessed by percutaneous or cut down approach and upsized to accommodate a large diameter sheath. The sheath is advanced through the femoral vein to the apex of the right ventricle. Using a steerable catheter inserted through the sheath, the pacemaker is delivered across the tricuspid valve through the delivery catheter and anchored to the ventricular endocardium via a screw helix or prongs. Once the catheter is properly positioned, the delivery catheter is withdrawn, the sheath is removed, and the incision is closed. To retrieve or remove a pacemaker, the femoral vein is accessed identically as for insertion; however, a catheter-based snare system is delivered through the sheath into the right ventricle. The pacemaker is grasped with the snare and the device is withdrawn via the sheath. The sheath is then removed and the incision is closed. Code 0387T includes transcatheter insertion or replacement of a permanent ventricular leadless pacemaker. Code 0388T includes removal of a permanent ventricular leadless pacemaker.

0389T

0389T   **Programming device evaluation (in person) with iterative adjustment of the implantable device to test the function of the device and select optimal permanent programmed values with analysis, review and report, leadless pacemaker system**

The patient with a leadless pacemaker system is evaluated at designated intervals to review stored and measured information including parameter settings and battery life, capture and sensing function, and heart rhythms. The programming evaluation may also include sensor and rate response, upper and lower heart rate, AV interval, pacing voltage, and pulse duration. Electrocardiogram electrodes are placed on the patient's chest and extremities. The electrodes are connected to a computer with a software program that downloads information from the pacemaker onto a display screen or printout. The clinician reviews the current functioning of the device, makes any adjustments, analyzes the programmed parameters and selects the optimal permanent settings, and provides a written report of the leadless pacemaker system.

0390T

0390T   **Peri-procedural device evaluation (in person) and programming of device system parameters before or after a surgery, procedure or test with analysis, review and report, leadless pacemaker system**

The patient with a leadless pacemaker system may require adjustments to the device prior to and/or after undergoing surgery, medical tests, or procedures. Electrocardiogram electrodes are placed on the patient's chest and extremities. The electrodes are connected to a computer with a software program that downloads information from the pacemaker onto a display screen or printout. The clinician reviews and analyzes the data, makes adjustments to the programmed parameters of the device, and provides a written report of the leadless pacemaker system.

0391T

0391T   **Interrogation device evaluation (in person) with analysis, review and report, includes connection, recording and disconnection per patient encounter, leadless pacemaker system**

The patient with a leadless pacemaker system is evaluated at designated intervals to review stored and measured information including parameter settings and battery life, capture and sensing function, and heart rhythms. Electrocardiogram electrodes are placed on the patient's chest and extremities. The electrodes are connected to a computer with a software program that downloads information from the pacemaker onto a display screen or printout. The clinician reviews and analyzes the data from the recording after the connection, and provides a written report of the leadless pacemaker system.

0395T

0395T   **High dose rate electronic brachytherapy, interstitial or intracavitary treatment, per fraction, includes basic dosimetry, when performed**

High dose rate (HDR) electronic brachytherapy uses an x-ray tube that delivers electronically generated photons as the radiation source, eliminating the need for radioactive isotopes. Currently, the primary use of HDR electronic brachytherapy is for treatment of breast cancer following lumpectomy. During a separately reportable implantation procedure, the brachytherapy applicator device is inserted into the body at the site of the malignant neoplasm or the tumor bed site of the lumpectomy. The application device may be inserted into tissue (interstitial) or into a body cavity (intracavitary). The radiation oncologist verifies the target volume to be treated and the prescribed dose of radiation. Any necessary refinements in the treatment plan are made using computerized brachytherapy dosimetry. The x-ray generator is attached to the application device. A shielding device is applied to protect normal tissue. External shielding may also be applied as needed. The prescribed dose is set on the control panel and a check run of the x-ray generator is first performed. The control panel is then set to deliver the prescribed dose of radiation; the x-ray generator is activated; and the high dose electronic brachytherapy is delivered to the tumor or tumor bed for the prescribed period, which may range from 10 to 40 minutes. If a multichannel applicator is used, the process is repeated as needed. Treatments are broken down into fractions with a typical treatment following lumpectomy being 10 fractions, with two fractions delivered per day for five days. Each fraction is reported separately. The brachytherapy applicator is left in place until the entire treatment course is complete.

0396T

0396T   **Intra-operative use of kinetic balance sensor for implant stability during knee replacement arthroplasty (List separately in addition to code for primary procedure)**

A procedure is performed during total knee arthroplasty (TKA) to measure alignment and rotational congruency between the prosthetic tibial and femoral contact points, and quantify pressure across the weight bearing surfaces. Standard cuts are made to the distal femur and proximal tibia and a trial spacer embedded with microelectronic sensors is inserted. Once the spacer is in place and the sensors are activated, the patella is cut and patellar button is applied. A pin is placed to stabilize the joint which is then taken into extension and the tibial baseplate is rotated until medial and lateral femoral contact points are parallel with the graphic user interface (GUI). A second pin is placed to prevent malrotation and the knee is assessed in full extension, mid flexion, and 90 degree flexion. Load measurements taken from the GUI are transmitted wirelessly to a computer software program. The computer provides feedback to the surgeon as the prosthesis is manipulated in the joint space. Soft tissue release of the ligaments is performed by making multiple small punctures using a needle or blade and progressively stretching the ligaments until the intercompartmental pressures are optimal. The soft tissue pocket (muscle, tendon, ligaments) is fashioned, and the final load measurements are calculated and recorded prior to cementing the prosthesis in place. Standard closure of the incision is then performed. Report code 0396T separately as an adjunct code to the primary total knee arthroplasty procedure.

0397T

0397T   **Endoscopic retrograde cholangiopancreatography (ERCP), with optical endomicroscopy (List separately in addition to code for primary procedure)**

Endoscopic retrograde cholangiopancreatography (ERCP) is performed with optical endomicroscopy. An endoscope is passed through the esophagus, stomach, and into the duodenum to the point where the pancreatic duct and the common bile duct meet, (the Ampulla of Vater), at the major duodenal papilla. A smaller catheter is placed through the scope, the Ampulla of Vater is cannulated, and contrast dye is injected into the ducts. The common bile duct, biliary tract, gallbladder, and pancreas are visualized on x-rays, taken as soon as the dye is injected. Optical endomicroscopy provides in vivo visualization and characterization of the mucosal tissue in the biliary and/or pancreatic ducts and the pathophysiological processes occurring there at the microscopic level. This allows the physician to see histological details during the ERCP. With the contrast

● New Code   ▲ Revised Code

Category III Codes

agent administered, endomicroscopy is performed with a miniaturized endomicroscope integrated into or inserted through the endoscope with a blue laser light that scans the biliary ductal mucosa from the surface to the deepest mucosal layer. Endomicroscopy allows the physician to obtain separately reportable targeted biopsies when needed from areas with microscopic changes rather than taking random tissue samples and also provides instant histological information for immediate treatment.

0399T

0399T Myocardial strain imaging (quantitative assessment of myocardial mechanics using image-based analysis of local myocardial dynamics) (List separately in addition to code for primary procedure)

A procedure is performed to assess myocardial function using echocardiography and two dimensional (2D) speckle tracking. Strain imaging is a non-invasive technique that measures longitudinal, radial, and circumferential deformation of the left ventricle (LV) during systole and diastole. It can be used to quantify myocardial dysfunction, assess myocardial viability, detect acute allograft rejection and early allograft vasculopathy following heart transplant, and may also be helpful in detecting sub-clinical cardiac manifestations in patients with diabetes, systemic sclerosis, myocardial ischemia, arterial hypertension, mitral or aortic regurgitation, non-ischemic cardiomyopathies, as well as for predicting the outcome of patients with acute heart failure. Ultrasound images are obtained with ECG gating in apical 4 chamber, 3 chamber, and 2 chamber views and short axis view at the basal, mid, and apical levels with a minimum of 3 cardiac cycles for each loop. The patient should hold the breath for all images. Special software is then applied to the images to analyze cardiac motion by tracking speckles (natural acoustic markers) in the 2D ultrasound. The markers are tracked frame by frame to determine velocity and strain rate is then calculated from those measurements. Report code 0399T separately as an adjunct code to a primary echocardiography procedure.

0402T

0402T Collagen cross-linking of cornea (including removal of the corneal epithelium and intraoperative pachymetry when performed)

A procedure is performed using riboflavin (Vitamin B2) and ultraviolet-A (UV-A) light to strengthen collagen bonds in the cornea. Collagen cross linking increases the number of fiber anchors that bond collagen together and is a first line treatment for keratoconus, pellucid marginal degeneration, and ectasia caused by LASIK. Collagen cross linking may also be used to treat corneal ulcers and infection, and to bond Intacts, tiny plastic discs, following surgical implantation within the cornea. With the patient reclining, a lid speculum is placed and anesthetic eye drops are instilled. Ultrasound pachymetry may be performed to measure the pre-treatment thickness of the cornea. A thin layer of epithelium may be removed for more rapid absorption of riboflavin, or the treatment may proceed with the epithelium in place as a transepithelial procedure. Riboflavin eye drops are instilled at measured intervals or until the riboflavin is detected in the anterior chamber of the eye using a blue filter on a slit lamp. The UV-A light is then applied to the corneal apex for a prescribed period of time. Ultrasound pachymetry may be performed to measure the post-treatment thickness of the cornea as well. Antibiotic eye drops are instilled and a bandage contact lens is applied following the treatment.

0404T

0404T Transcervical uterine fibroid(s) ablation with ultrasound guidance, radiofrequency

A procedure is performed to ablate uterine fibroid(s) using a transvaginal approach with ultrasound (US) guidance and radiofrequency. A uterine fibroid, or leiomyoma, is a benign solid tumor that forms in the smooth muscle tissue (myometrium) of the uterus. Symptoms include abnormal uterine bleeding, pelvic pressure and pain, and the presence of fibroid(s) may cause suboptimal fertility conditions. US guided radiofrequency is a minimally invasive procedure that destroys the fibroid(s) by thermal fixation and coagulation necrosis while preserving the architecture of the uterus. The cervix is dilated to permit insertion of a probe containing the ultrasound transducer and radiofrequency electrode. Ultrasound is used to confirm the location and size of the fibroid(s) and a graphic map of the treatment area is created. The radiofrequencies and safety parameters are calculated based on the size and location of the fibroid(s). Once the treatment settings have been determined, the radiofrequency electrode is introduced into the fibroid, and thermal energy is deployed under continuous US visualization until the fibroid is reduced in size. The procedure is repeated if multiple fibroids are present and the transducer is removed.

0405T

0405T Oversight of the care of an extracorporeal liver assist system patient requiring review of status, review of laboratories and other studies, and revision of orders and liver assist care plan (as appropriate), within a calendar month, 30 minutes or more of non-face-to-face time

The medical professional provides clinical oversight of the patient with liver failure receiving support from an extracorporeal liver assist system. This system may be employed as a bridge to liver transplant or to support the liver until it can recover. Liver failure

and elevated levels of toxins in the body can lead to coagulopathy, hemodynamic dysregulation such as vasodilation or low mean arterial pressure, and multisystem organ failure from poor perfusion and oxygenation. Extracorporeal liver assistance utilizes a hemodialysis machine that removes blood from the patient and processes it through filters to remove water soluble and albumin-bound toxins including small fatty acids, metabolites of aromatic amino acids, and tryptophan, bilirubin, nitric oxide, and vasoactive substances. The patient in liver failure will be monitored for cognitive changes, renal function, glucose, electrolytes, acid-base balance, and anticoagulation (activated clotting time, partial thromboplastin time). Hemodialysis access points such as an A-V fistula or central venous catheter must also be monitored and maintained. Code 0405T includes 30 minutes or more of non-face-to-face time to review a patient's clinical status, laboratory and other tests, and make revisions to orders and the patient's liver assist care plan as required during a calendar month.

0421T

● 0421T Transurethral waterjet ablation of prostate, including control of post-operative bleeding, including ultrasound guidance, complete (vasectomy, meatotomy, cystourethroscopy, urethral calibration and/or dilation, and internal urethrotomy are included when performed)

A procedure is performed using water-jet hydrodissection (aqua ablation) to treat benign prostatic hypertrophy (BPH) with lower urinary tract symptoms (LUTS) of bladder outlet obstruction. Transrectal ultrasound imaging is used to map the target area and the surgeon programs a robotic system with precise tissue contours/depth. Using electromechanical control and real time ultrasound guidance, a high velocity stream of saline is delivered to the prostate via the urethra, which may require meatotomy, internal urethrotomy, and urethral calibration or dilation for access and successful ablation. The water jet selectively ablates the glandular tissue, which is simultaneously collected for post procedural laboratory analysis. A laser beam captured by a low pressure water jet may be employed to obtain surface coagulation and hemostasis. Ultrasound guidance and control of post procedural bleeding is included as well as vasectomy and cystourethroscopy, when performed.

0438T

● 0438T Transperineal placement of biodegradable material, peri-prostatic (via needle), single or multiple, includes image guidance

A procedure is performed to place a hydrogel spacer between the prostate gland and the anterior rectum prior to radiation therapy for prostate cancer. When in place, the anatomical spacer material pushes the rectum away from the prostate, protecting rectal tissue from radiation toxicity and damage during external beam radiotherapy or brachytherapy. Transrectal ultrasound is performed in both longitudinal and transverse planes to identify the area of perirectal fat between Denonvilliers' fascia and the anterior rectal wall. An 18 gauge needle is inserted through the perineum and into the targeted area and a small amount of saline is injected to confirm placement and allow hydrodissection of the space. Syringes containing the biodegradable material are then connected to the needle and injected under real time ultrasound guidance. Once satisfactory placement has been confirmed, the needle is removed. The injected material solidifies into a soft, firm hydrogel within seconds of injection and remains effective for about 3 months. The hydrogel will biodegrade and liquefy, and is absorbed by the body and excreted in the urine.

0443T

● 0443T Real-time spectral analysis of prostate tissue by fluorescence spectroscopy, including imaging guidance (List separately in addition to code for primary procedure)

A procedure is performed to identify malignant prostate tissue using real-time spectral analysis during separately reportable needle or punch prostate biopsy. Fluorescence spectroscopy (FS) analyzes naturally fluorescing endogenous proteins and enzymes in body tissue that scatter signals after undergoing photon-electron stimulation. Since the amount of endogenous fluorophores in prostate tissue differs with disease states, FS is used to help quantify the variation and identify malignant lesions. The FS signals are read by a custom fluorometer interfaced with software to differentiate benign from malignant tissue and provide a histopathological grade to suspected malignant tumors. An optical biopsy needle containing a built-in light sensitive optical probe/sensor with fibers for tissue excitation and collection of the spectral data is advanced into the prostate under FS guidance. The custom fluorometer has light-emitting diodes and spectrometer and reads the acquired spectral data acquired for real time in vivo prostate cancer diagnosis or recognition of suspicious target areas within the prostate gland, thereby increasing the yield of diagnostic information attained with the biopsy sample.

Evaluation and Management Services

Correct code selection with supporting documentation has proven difficult for many providers to consistently produce. For the most common categories of Evaluation and Management (E/M) service, there are five levels of service, yet many providers cluster their code selection towards the middle, and thus continually generate bell-shaped productivity curves that may not capture the actual levels of work being performed. Physicians and NPPS have long selected codes based on combinations of uncertainty, a vague notion of time spent or even what the charge for a given level might be. It often seems that codes are rarely selected based on the criteria set forth on the AMA's CPT* book and CMS documentation guidelines for E/M services.

Regardless of the reason for code selection and the method of documentation, federal audit and regulatory activity consistently turn up high levels of either over-coding or under-documentation, depending on how it is reviewed. If federal and commercial payer reviews included the larger spectrum of claims submitted rather than just the higher levels, it is likely that significant amounts of under-coding of services would also be detected.

Medicare, Medicaid and commercial payers audit claims based on the definitions for E/M category and service levels found in either or both the CPT book and CMS documentation guidelines. When auditing a provider or practice, payers typically ask for a patient's medical record and compare the recorded progress note or chart entry with the requirements for the level of service reported on the claim. Should the information in the medical chart not support the level of service reported, the payer may demand that the provider pay the difference between the amounts received and the amount that would have been paid for the level of service as documented in the chart.

Federal programs expenditures were close to $30 billion for E/M services in fiscal 2007, and E/M codes have recently accounted for over $4 billion in overpayments based on audit findings. With the proliferation of electronic health records new concerns of replicating and an excessive volume of documentation have begun to equal historic concerns of missing or inadequate documentation. The concept of medical necessity is playing a larger role in audit activity such that the savvy practice will take care to provide clear documentation of the important parts of the chart, not just computer generated data.

Classification of Evaluation and Management Services

The E/M section is divided into broad categories such as office visits, hospital visits, and consultations. Most of the categories are further divided into two or more subcategories of E/M services. For example, there are two subcategories of office visits (new patient and established patient) and there are two subcategories of hospital visits (initial and subsequent). The subcategories of E/M services are further classified into levels of E/M services that are identified by specific codes. This classification is important because the nature of work varies by type of service, place of service, and the patient's status.

The basic format of the levels of E/M services is the same for most categories. First, a unique code number is listed. Second, the place

and/or type of service is specified, eg, office consultation. Third, the content of the service is defined, eg, comprehensive history and comprehensive examination. Fourth, the nature of the presenting problem(s) usually associated with a given level is described. Fifth, the time typically required to provide the service is specified.

Definitions of Commonly Used Terms

Certain key words and phrases are used throughout the E/M section. The following definitions are intended to reduce the potential for differing interpretations and to increase the consistency of reporting by physicians in differing specialties. E/M services may also be reported by other qualified health care professionals who are authorized to perform such services within the scope of their practice.

New and Established Patient

Solely for the purposes of distinguishing between new and established patients, professional services are those face-to-face services rendered by a physician and other qualified health care professionals who may report evaluation and management services reported by a specific CPT code(s). A new patient is one who has not received any professional services from the physician/qualified health care professional or another physician/qualified health care professional of the exact same specialty and subspecialty who belongs to the same group practice, within the past three years.

An established patient is one who has received professional services from the physician/qualified health care professional or another physician/qualified health care professional of the exact same specialty and subspecialty who belongs to the same group practice, within the past three years.

In the instance where a physician/qualified health care professional is on call for or covering for another physician/qualified health care professional, the patient's encounter will be classified as it would have been by the physician/qualified health care professional who is not available. When advanced practice nurses and physician assistants are working with physicians, they are considered as working in the exact same specialty and exact same subspecialties as the physician.

No distinction is made between new and established patients in the emergency department. E/M services in the emergency department category may be reported for any new or established patient who presents for treatment in the emergency department.

Chief Complaint

A chief complaint is a concise statement describing the symptom, problem, condition, diagnosis, or other factor that is the reason for the encounter, usually stated in the patient's words.

Concurrent Care and Transfer of Care

Concurrent care is the provision of similar services (eg, hospital visits) to the same patient by more than one physician or other qualified health care professional on the same day. When concurrent care is provided, no special reporting is required.

Transfer of care is the process whereby a physician or other qualified health care professional who is providing management for some or all of a patient's problems relinquishes this responsibility to another physician who explicitly agrees to accept this responsibility and who, from the initial encounter, is not providing consultative services. The physician or other qualified health care professional transferring care is then no longer providing care for these problems though he or she may continue providing care for other conditions when appropriate. Consultation codes should not be reported by the physician or other qualified health care professional who has agreed to accept transfer of care before an initial evaluation but are appropriate to report if the decision to accept transfer of care cannot be made until after the initial consultation evaluation, regardless of site of service.

Counseling

Counseling is a discussion with a patient and/or family concerning one or more of the following areas:

- Diagnostic results, impressions, and/or recommended diagnostic studies
- Prognosis
- Risks and benefits of management (treatment) options
- Instructions for management (treatment) and/or follow-up
- Importance of compliance with chosen management (treatment) options
- Risk factor reduction
- Patient and family education (For psychotherapy, see 90832-90834, 90836-90840)

Family History

A review of medical events in the patient's family that includes significant information about:

- The health status or cause of death of parents, siblings, and children
- Specific diseases related to problems identified in the Chief Complaint or History of the Present Illness, and/or System Review
- Diseases of family members that may be hereditary or place the patient at risk

History of Present Illness

A chronological description of the development of the patient's present illness from the first sign and/or symptom to the present. This includes a description of location, quality, severity, timing, context, modifying factors, and associated signs and symptoms significantly related to the presenting problem(s).

Levels of E/M Services

Within each category or subcategory of E/M service, there are three to five levels of E/M services available for reporting purposes. Levels of E/M services are not interchangeable among the different categories or subcategories of service. For example, the first level of E/M services in the subcategory of office visit, new patient, does not have the same definition as the first level of E/M services in the subcategory of office visit, established patient.

The levels of E/M services include examinations, evaluations, treatments, conferences with or concerning patients, preventive pediatric and adult health supervision, and similar medical services, such as the determination of the need and/or location for appropriate care. Medical screening includes the history, examination,and medical decision-making required to determine the need and/or location for appropriate care and treatment of the patient (eg, office and other outpatient setting, emergency department, nursing facility).

The levels of E/M services encompass the wide variations in skill, effort, time, responsibility, and medical knowledge required for the prevention or diagnosis and treatment of illness or injury and the promotion of optimal health. Each level of E/M services may be used by all physicians or other qualified health care professionals.

The descriptors for the levels of E/M services recognize seven components that are used in defining levels of E/M services. These components are:

- History
- Examination
- Medical decision making
- Counseling
- Coordination of care
- Nature of presenting problem
- Time

The first three of these components, history, examination, and medical decision making, are the key components in selecting the level of E/M services. (See section "Determine the Extent of History Obtained".)

The next three components (counseling, coordination of care, and the nature of the presenting problem) are considered contributory factors in the majority of encounters. Although the first two of these contributory factors are important E/M services, it is not required that these services be provided at every patient encounter.

Coordination of care with other physicians, or other qualified health care professionals, or agencies without a patient encounter on that day is reported using the case management codes. The final component, time, is discussed in detail in the section "Time."

Any specifically identifiable procedure (ie, identified with a specific CPT code) performed on or subsequent to the date of initial or subsequent E/M services should be reported separately.

The actual performance and/or interpretation of diagnostic tests/studies ordered during a patient encounter are not included in the levels of E/M services. Physician performance of diagnostic tests/studies for which specific CPT codes are available may be reported separately, in addition to the appropriate E/M code. The physician's interpretation of the results of diagnostic tests/studies (ie, professional component) with preparation of a separate distinctly identifiable signed written report may also be reported separately, using the appropriate CPT code with modifier 26 appended.

The physician or other qualified health care professional may need to indicate that on the day a procedure or service identified by a CPT code was performed, the patient's condition required a significant separately identifiable E/M service above and beyond other services provided or beyond the usual preservice and postservice care associated with the procedure that was performed. The E/M service may be caused or prompted by the symptoms or condition for which the procedure and/or service was provided. This circumstance may be reported by adding modifier 25 to the appropriate level of E/M service. As such, different diagnoses are not required for reporting of the procedure and the E/M services on the same date.

Nature of Presenting Problem

A presenting problem is a disease, condition, illness,injury, symptom, sign, finding, complaint, or other reason for encounter, with or without a diagnosis being established at the time of the encounter. The E/M codes recognize five types of presenting problems that are defined as follows:

Minimal: A problem that may not require the presence of the physician or other qualified health care professional, but service is provided under the physician's or other qualified health care professional's supervision.

Self-limited or minor: A problem that runs a definite and prescribed course, is transient in nature, and is not likely to permanently alter health status OR has a good prognosis with management/compliance.

Low severity: A problem where the risk of morbidity without treatment is low; there is little to no risk of mortality without treatment; full recovery without functional impairment is expected.

Moderate severity: A problem where the risk of morbidity without treatment is moderate; there is moderate risk of mortality without treatment; uncertain prognosis OR increased probability of prolonged functional impairment.

High severity: A problem where the risk of morbidity without treatment is high to extreme; there is a moderate to high risk of mortality without treatment OR high probability of severe, prolonged functional impairment.

Past History

A review of the patient's past experiences with illnesses, injuries, and treatments that includes significant information about:

- Prior major illnesses and injuries
- Prior operations
- Prior hospitalizations
- Current medications
- Allergies (eg, drug, food)
- Age appropriate immunization status
- Age appropriate feeding/dietary status

Social History

An age appropriate review of past and current activities that includes significant information about:

- Marital status and/or living arrangements
- Current employment
- Occupational history
- Use of drugs, alcohol, and tobacco
- Level of education
- Sexual history
- Other relevant social factors

System Review (Review of Systems)

An inventory of body systems obtained through a series of questions seeking to identify signs and/or symptoms that the patient may be experiencing or has experienced. For the purposes of the CPT codebook the following elements of a system review have been identified:

- Constitutional symptoms (for example, fever, weight loss)
- Eyes
- Ears, Nose, Mouth, Throat
- Cardiovascular
- Respiratory
- Gastrointestinal
- Genitourinary
- Musculoskeletal
- Integumentary (skin and/or breast)

- Neurological
- Psychiatric
- Endocrine
- Hematologic/Lymphatic
- Allergic/Immunologic

The review of systems helps define the problem, clarify the differential diagnosis, identify needed testing, or serves as baseline data on other systems that might be affected by any possible management options.

Time

The inclusion of time in the definitions of levels of E/M services has been implicit in prior editions of the CPT codebook. The inclusion of time as an explicit factor beginning in *CPT 1992* is done to assist physicians in selecting the most appropriate level of E/M services. It should be recognized that the specific times expressed in the visit code descriptors are averages and, therefore, represent a range of times that may be higher or lower depending on actual clinical circumstances.

Time is not a descriptive component for the emergency department levels of E/M services because emergency department services are typically provided on a variable intensity basis, often involving multiple encounters with several patients over an extended period of time. Therefore, it is often difficult for physicians to provide accurate estimates of the time spent face-to-face with the patient.

Studies to establish levels of E/M services employed surveys of practicing physicians to obtain data on the amount of time and work associated with typical E/M services. Since "work" is not easily quantifiable, the codes must rely on other objective, verifiable measures that correlate with physicians' estimates of their "work." It has been demonstrated that physicians' estimations of intraservice time (as explained on the next page), both within and across specialties, is a variable that is predictive of the "work" of E/M services. This same research has shown there is a strong relationship between intraservice time and total time for E/M services. Intraservice time, rather than total time, was chosen for inclusion with the codes because of its relative ease of measurement and because of its direct correlation with measurements of the total amount of time and work associated with typical E/M services.

Intraservice times are defined as face-to-face time for office and other outpatient visits and as unit/floor time for hospital and other inpatient visits. This distinction is necessary because most of the work of typical office visits takes place during the face-to-face time with the patient, while most of the work of typical hospital visits takes place during the time spent on the patient's floor or unit. When prolonged time occurs in either the office or the inpatient areas, the appropriate add-on code should be reported.

Face-to-face time (office and other outpatient visits and office consultations): For coding purposes, face-to-face time for these services is defined as only that time that the physician spends face-to-face with the patient and/or family. This includes the time spent performing such tasks as obtaining a history, performing an examination, and counseling the patient.

Time is also spent doing work before or after the face-to-face time with the patient, performing such tasks as reviewing records and tests, arranging for further services, and communicating further with other professionals and the patient through written reports and telephone contact.

This non-face-to-face time for office services—also called pre- and postencounter time—is not included in the time component described in the E/M codes. However, the pre- and post-non-face-to-face work associated with an encounter was included in calculating the total work of typical services in physician surveys.

Thus, the face-to-face time associated with the services described by any E/M code is a valid proxy for the total work done before, during, and after the visit.

Unit/floor time (hospital observation services, inpatient hospital care, initial inpatient hospital consultations, nursing facility): For reporting purposes, intraservice time for these services is defined as unit/floor time, which includes the time present on the patient's hospital unit and at the bedside rendering services for that patient. This includes the time to establishe and/or review the patient's chart, examine the patient, write notes, and communicate with other professionals and the patient's family.

In the hospital, pre- and post-time includes time spent off the patient's floor performing such tasks as reviewing pathology and radiology findings in another part of the hospital. This pre- and postvisit time is not included in the time component described in these codes. However, the pre- and postwork performed during the time spent off the floor or unit was included in calculating the total work of typical services in physician surveys. Thus, the unit/floor time associated with the services described by any code is a valid proxy for the total work done before, during, and after the visit.

Unlisted Service

An E/M service may be provided that is not listed in this section of the CPT codebook. When reporting such a service, the appropriate unlisted code may be used to indicate the service, identifying it by "Special Report," as discussed in the following paragraph. The "Unlisted Services" and accompanying codes for the E/M section are as follows:

99429   Unlisted preventive medicine service

99499   Unlisted evaluation and management service

Special Report

An unlisted service or one that is unusual, variable, or new may require a special report demonstrating the medical appropriateness of the service. Pertinent information should include an adequate definition or description of the nature, extent, and need for the procedure and the time, effort, and equipment necessary to provide the service. Additional items that may be included are complexity of symptoms, final diagnosis, pertinent physical findings, diagnostic and therapeutic procedures, concurrent problems, and follow-up care.

Clinical Examples

Clinical examples of the codes for E/M services are provided to assist in understanding the meaning of the descriptors and selecting the correct code. Each example was developed by physicians in the specialties shown.

The same problem, when seen by different specialties, may involve different amounts of work. Therefore, the appropriate level of encounter should be reported using the descriptors rather than the examples.

Medical Decision-Making

Medical decision-making is the third component of the component-based codes. This component is most often the equivalent of the Assessment and Plan portion of the standard provider's note. The cognitive work here reflects the amount of experience, training and knowledge a provider uses to address a problem or problems in addition to the quantifiable indicators below. The CPT has defined three sub-components of decision-making and CMS has provided further guidance on decision-making indicators.

Per the CPT book, medical decision-making refers to the complexity of establishing a diagnosis and/or selecting a management option as measured by:

- The number of possible diagnoses and/or the number of management options that must be considered

- The amount and/or complexity of medical records, diagnostic tests, and/or other information that must be obtained, reviewed, and analyzed

- The risk of significant complications, morbidity, and/or mortality, as well as comorbidities, associated with the patient's presenting problem(s), the diagnostic procedure(s), and/or the possible management options

Four types of medical decision-making are recognized: straight-forward; low complexity; moderate complexity; and high complexity. To qualify for a given type of decision-making, two of the three elements in the following table should be met or exceeded.

Comorbidities/underlying diseases, in and of themselves, are not considered in selecting a level of E/M services unless their presence significantly increases the complexity of the medical decision-making.

Number of diagnoses or management options	Amount and/or complexity of data to be reviewed	Risk of complications and/or morbidity or mortality	Type of Decision Making
Minimal	Minimal or None	Minimal	Straightforward
Limited	Limited	Low	Low Complexity
Multiple	Moderate	Moderate	Moderate Complexity
Extensive	Extensive	High	High Complexity

Number of Diagnoses/Management Options

This element is based on the number and type of problems addressed during the encounter, the complexity of establishing a diagnosis, and the management decisions that must be made. The number and type of diagnostic tests may be an indicator of the number of possible diagnoses. Problems that are improving or resolving are less complex than those that are worsening are. The need to seek advice from others is another indicator of complexity of diagnostic or management problems.

DG: For each encounter, an assessment, clinical impression, or diagnosis should be documented. It may be explicitly stated or implied in documented decisions regarding management plans and/or further evaluation.

- For a presenting problem with an established diagnosis, the record should reflect whether the problem is (a) improved, well controlled, resolving, or resolved; or (b) inadequately controlled, worsening, or failing to change as expected.

- For a presenting problem without an established diagnosis, the assessment or clinical impression may be stated in the form of a differential diagnosis or as "possible," "probable," or "rule out (R/O)" diagnoses.

DG: Initiation of, or changes in, treatment should be documented. Treatment may involve a wide range of management options, including patient instructions, nursing instructions, therapies, and medications.

DG: If referrals are made or consultations requested, the record should indicate to whom or where the referral or consultation is made

CMS does not really define what a self-limited problem is, and what determines if other entries are established or new problems. Self-limited measures degree or significance while established and new pertains to time or chronicity. There is also uncertainty about what 'additional work-up' means.

Amount and/or Complexity of Data to be Reviewed

This element is based on the types of testing ordered or reviewed. A decision to obtain and review old medical records and/or obtain history from sources other than the patient increases the amount/complexity of data.

Discussion of unexpected test results with the physician who performed or interpreted the test, or if the physician who ordered a test personally reviews the image, tracing, or specimen to supplement information from the physician who prepared the report or interpretation are indicators of the complexity of the data being reviewed.

DG: If a diagnostic service is ordered, planned, scheduled, or performed at the time of the E/M encounter, the type of service should be documented.

DG: The review of tests should be documented. An entry such as "WBC elevated" or "chest x-ray unremarkable" is acceptable. Or, the review may be documented by initialing and dating the report containing the test results.

DG: A decision to obtain old records or to obtain additional history from the family, caretaker, or other source to supplement that obtained from the patient should be documented.

DG: Relevant findings from the review of old records or additional history should be documented. If there is no relevant information beyond that already obtained, that fact should be documented. A notation of "old records reviewed" or additional history obtained from family "without elaboration" is insufficient.

DG: The results of discussion of laboratory, radiology, or other tests with the physician who performed or interpreted the study should be documented.

DG: The direct visualization and independent interpretation of an image, tracing or specimen previously or subsequently interpreted by another physician should be documented.

Risk of Significant Complications/Morbidity/Mortality

This element is based on the risks associated with the presenting problem(s), the diagnostic procedure(s), and the possible management options.

DG: Comorbidities/underlying diseases or other factors that increase the complexity of medical decision-making by increasing the risk of complications, morbidity, and/or mortality should be documented.

DG: If a surgical or invasive diagnostic procedure is ordered, planned, or scheduled at the time of the E/M encounter, the type of procedure should be documented.

DG: If a surgical or invasive diagnostic procedure is performed at the time of the E/M encounter, the type of procedure should be documented.

DG: The referral or decision to perform a surgical or invasive diagnostic procedure on an urgent basis should be documented or implied.

The Table of Risk

The Table of Risk may be used to help determine the risk level. Because this determination is complex and not readily quantifiable, the table includes common clinical examples rather than absolute measures of risk. The highest level of risk in any one category (presenting problem(s), diagnostic procedure(s), or management option(s) determines the overall risk.

Level of Risk	Presenting problem(s)	Diagnostic procedure(s) ordered	Management options selected
Minimal	• One self-limited or minor problem, e.g. cold, insect bite, tinea corporis	• Laboratory test requiring venipuncture • Chest x-rays • Urinalysis • KOH Prep • EKG/EEG • Ultrasound, e.g. echo	• Rest • Gargles • Elastic bandages • Superficial dressing
Low	• Two or more self-limited or minor problems • One stable chronic illness, e.g. well controlled hypertension of non-insulin dependent diabetes, cataract, BPH • Acute uncomplicated illness or injury, e.g. cystitis, allergic rhinitis, simple sprain	• Physiologic tests not under stress, e.g. pulmonary function tests • Non-cardiovascular imaging studies w/ contrast, e.g. barium enema • Superficial needle biopsies • Clinical lab tests requiring arterial puncture • Skin biopsies	• Over-the-counter drugs • Minor surgery with no identified risk factors • Physical therapy • Occupational therapy • IV fluids without additives
Moderate	• One or more chronic illnesses w/ mild exacerbation, progression, or side effects of treatment • Two or more stable chronic illnesses • Undiagnosed new problem w/ uncertain prognosis, e.g. lump in breast • Acute illness w/ systemic symptoms, e.g. pyelonephritis, pneumonitis, colitis • Acute complicated injury, e.g. head injury with brief loss of consciousness	• Physiologic tests not under stress, e.g. cardiac stress tests, fetal contraction stress test • Diagnostic endoscopies w/ no identified risks • Deep needle or incisional biopsies • Cardiovascular imaging w/ contrast and no identified risk factors, e.g. arteriogram cardiac cath • Obtain fluid from body cavity, e.g. lumbar puncture, thoracentesis, culdocentesis	• Minor surgery with identified risk factors • Elective major surgery (open, percutaneous or endoscopic) with no identified risk factors • Prescription drug management • Therapeutic nuclear medicine • IV fluids with additives • Closed treatment of fracture or dislocation without manipulation
High	• One or more chronic illnesses w/ severe exacerbation, progression or side effects of treatment • Acute or chronic illnesses or injuries that may pose a threat to life or bodily function, e.g. multiple trauma, acute MI, pulmonary embolus, severe respiratory distress, progressive severe rheumatoid arthritis, psychiatric illness with potential threat to self or others, peritonitis, acute renal failure • An abrupt change in neurologic status, seizure, TIA, weakness or sensory loss	• Cardiovascular imaging studies w/ contrast w/ identified risk factors • Cardiac electrophysiological tests • Diagnostic endoscopies w/ identified risk factors • Discography	• Elective major surgery (open, percutaneous, or endoscopic with identified risk factors • Emergency major surgery (open, percutaneous, or endoscopic) • Parenteral controlled substances • Drug therapy requiring intensive monitoring for toxicity • Decision not resuscitate or to de-escalate care because of poor prognosis

Although the table above is the one that most often appears in federal and commercial payer audit worksheets, it was first published over 12 years ago and has some elements that can be used somewhat mechanically to artificially boost service levels beyond current understanding of medical necessity. The inclusion of the 'prescription drug management' element associated with moderate level complexity, when combined with the 'new problem' option, can have the effect of nudging codes higher than practical sense may indicate.

Although the instructions indicate that the highest level of risk in any given category determines the overall risk, it may be better stated that the level or indicator of risk that best characterizes the patient's condition may be a better indicator of overall risk. For example, an acute uncomplicated problem such as otitis media may be treated with an antibiotic, but it is better characterized as that acute uncomplicated illness or injury than as an example of prescription drug management. Many commercial payers are beginning to clarify that they don't consider antibiotics and other lower level prescriptions to be prescription drug management. Check in with each carrier for guidance.